NANDA-ACCEPTED DIAGNOSES

Activity intolerance
Activity intolerance, potential
Adjustment, impaired
Airway clearance, ineffective
Anxiety
Aspiration, potential for
Body image disturbance
Body temperature, altered, potential
Breastfeeding, effective
Breastfeeding, ineffective
Breathing pattern, ineffective
Cardiac output, decreased
Communication, impaired verbal
Constipation
Constipation, colonic
Constipation, perceived
Coping, defensive
Coping, family: potential for growth
Coping, ineffective family: compromised
Coping, ineffective family: disabling
Coping, ineffective individual
Decisional conflict (specify)
Denial, ineffective
Diarrhea
Disuse syndrome, potential for
Diversional activity deficit
Dysreflexia
Family processes, altered
Fatigue
Fear
Fluid volume deficit (1)
Fluid volume deficit (2)
Fluid volume deficit, potential
Fluid volume excess
Gas exchange, impaired
Grieving, anticipatory
Grieving, dysfunctional
Growth and development, altered
Health maintenance, altered
Health seeking behaviors (specify)
Home maintenance management, impaired
Hopelessness
Hyperthermia
Hypothermia
Incontinence, bowel
Incontinence, functional
Incontinence, reflex
Incontinence, stress
Incontinence, total
Incontinence, urge
Infection, potential for
Injury, potential for
Knowledge deficit (specify)
Mobility, impaired physical
Noncompliance (specify)
Nutrition, altered: less than body requirements
Nutrition, altered: more than body requirements
Nutrition, altered: potential for more than body requirements
Oral mucous membrane, altered
Pain
Pain, chronic
Parental role conflict
Parenting, altered
Parenting, altered, potential
Personal identity disturbance
Poisoning, potential for
Post-trauma response
Powerlessness
Protection, altered
Rape-trauma syndrome
Rape-trauma syndrome; compound reaction
Rape-trauma syndrome; silent reaction
Role performance, altered
Self care deficit, bathing/hygiene
Self care deficit, dressing/grooming
Self care deficit, feeding
Self care deficit, toileting
Self-esteem disturbance
Self-esteem, chronic low
Self-esteem, situational low
Sensory/perceptual alterations (specify) (visual, auditory, kinesthetic, gustatory, tactile, olfactory)
Sexual dysfunction
Sexuality patterns, altered
Skin integrity, impaired
Skin integrity, impaired, potential
Sleep pattern disturbance
Social interaction, impaired
Social isolation
Spiritual distress (distress of the human spirit)
Suffocation, potential for
Swallowing, impaired
Thermoregulation, ineffective
Thought processes, altered
Tissue integrity, impaired
Tissue perfusion, altered (specify type) (renal, cerebral, cardiopulmonary, gastrointestinal, peripheral)
Trauma, potential for
Unilateral neglect
Urinary elimination, altered patterns
Urinary retention
Violence, potential for: self-directed or directed at others

From the Proceedings of the Ninth National Conference of the North American Nursing Diagnosis Association, 1990.

FOUNDATIONS OF NURSING

FOUNDATIONS OF NURSING

Edited by

BARBARA LAURITSEN CHRISTENSEN, RN, MS
Nurse Educator
Mid-Plains Community College
North Platte, Nebraska

ELAINE ODEN KOCKROW, RN, MS
Nurse Educator
Mid-Plains Community College
North Platte, Nebraska

With 808 *illustrations*

Mosby Year Book

St. Louis Baltimore Boston Chicago London Philadelphia Sydney Toronto

Mosby
Year Book
Dedicated to Publishing Excellence

Editor: Linda L. Duncan
Project Manager: Patricia Tannian
Production Editor: Betty Hazelwood
Book Design: Gail Morey Hudson
Cover Design: Susan Lane

A Mosby imprint of Mosby–Year Book, Inc.

Printed in the United States of America

Mosby–Year Book, Inc.
11830 Westline Industrial Drive, St. Louis, Missouri 63146

Library of Congress Cataloging in Publication Data

Foundations of nursing/edited by Barbara Christensen, Elaine Kockrow.
p. cm.
Includes bibliographical references.
Includes index.
ISBN 0-8016-0168-1
1. Practical nursing. I. Christensen, Barbara. II. Kockrow, Elaine.
[DNLM: 1. Nursing. WY 100 F771]
RT62.F68 1991
610.73—dc20
DNLM/DLC
for Library of Congress 90-13594
CIP

GW/CD/VH 9 8 7 6 5 4 3 2 1

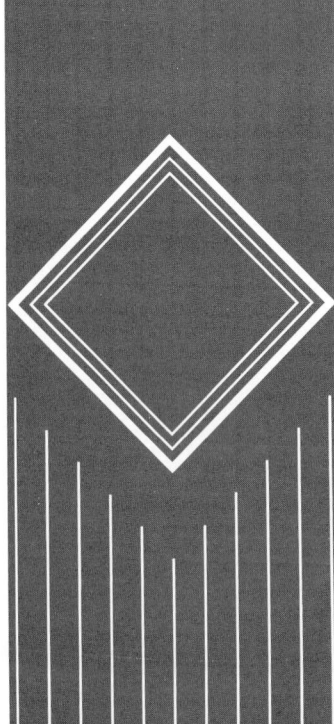

Contributors

M. LYNNE ACHESON, RN, BSN
Staff Education Coordinator
Great Plains Regional Medical Center
North Platte, Nebraska

PERSEPHONE C. AGRAFIOTIS, RN, PhD
Management Consultant
Manchester, New Hampshire

JENANN ALLEN, RN, BS
Vocational Nursing Instructor
Grayson County College
Denison, Texas

LORA JEAN ALLEY, RN
Medical Assistant Instructor
Draughons Junior College
Bristol, Tennessee;
LPN Instructor, Jacksboro Vocational Technical School
Jacksboro, Tennessee

DONNA M. BABAO, RN, MA, MSN
Nursing Instructor, Yuba College
Marysville, California

SYLVIA LONG BALDWIN, RN, BSN
Instructor, Howard College Vocational Nursing Program
San Angelo Campus, San Angelo, Texas

SALLY L. PERSONS BECK, RN, MS, CPC
Rehabilitation Nurse Counselor
Centennial Rehabilitation Associates, Inc.
Lincoln, Nebraska

BOBBIE BLOCH, RN, MSN
Doctoral Student
Department of Educational Technology
University of Toledo, Toledo, Ohio

GLORIA DePOLE COSCHIGANO, RN, MSN
Assistant Professor of Nursing
Iona College, Elizabeth Seton School
Yonkers, New York

LINDA CUTCHEN-CLARK, RN, MSN
Chair, Nursing Department
Butte College, Oroville, California

CYNTHIA M. DAVIS, MEd
Associate Professor of Nursing
Bainbridge College
Bainbridge, Georgia

CAROLYN DEAN, RN, BSN
Coordinator, Practical Nursing Program
North Central Missouri College
Trenton, Missouri

CAROLYN S. EDWARDS, RN, MEd
Coordinator, Wood County Vocational School of Practical Nursing
Parkersburg, West Virginia

JOSEPHINE M. ESTRADA, RN, BSN
Patient Care Coordinator for Home Health/Hospice
Great Plains Regional Medical Center
North Platte, Nebraska

JEANETTE M. JEFFERS, RN, C, PhD
Assistant Professor, Department of Nursing, The Wichita State University
Wichita, Kansas

FRANCES JEAN KELLEY, RN, PhD
Instructor, The University of Texas Health Science Center
Houston, Texas

SANDRA KLOCKE, RN, MS
Administrator
Statewide Home Health Program and Horizon Home Health Care Subunit
Nebraska State Health Department
Division of Community Health Nursing, North Platte, Nebraska

GRETCHEN H. LeGAULT, RN, MSN
Instructor, Fundamentals of Nursing, Psychiatric, Mental Health Nursing
Pima Community College, Tucson

KRISTEN KARTCHNER MAUGHAN, BS, RD

Nutrition Instructor, Mid-Plains Community College
North Platte, Nebraska

MARY MILLER-WERLINGER, RN, MSN, ANP

Staff Development Coordinator
Goodall-Witcher Hospital Foundation
Clifton, Texas

IVA L. MUELLER, RN, BSN

Assistant Director, Home Health Aides
Visiting Nurses' Association of Omaha; Graduate Student, Creighton University—Pastoral Ministry, Omaha, Nebraska

RUTH BECKMANN MURRAY, RN, EdD

Professor and Coordinator
Psychiatric/Mental Health Nursing Graduate Major
St. Louis University School of Nursing, St. Louis, Missouri

JOYCE ELIZABETH MYERS, RN, MSN

Nursing Professor, Florida Community College at Jacksonville
Jacksonville, Florida

CHRISTINE NEFF, RN, BSN

Nursing Instructor, Mid-East Ohio Vocational School
Zanesville, Ohio

LINDA NORTH, RN, MSN

LPN Coordinator and Instructor
Reid State Technical College, Evergreen, Alabama

PATRICIA HELMER OLES, RN, MSN

Assistant Professor of Nursing
Pasco-Hernando Community College
New Port Richey, Florida

KAREN H. RICHARDSON, RN, MA

Assistant Professor of Nursing
Pasco-Hernando Community College
New Port Richey, Florida

LINDA RICKEL, RNP, MSN

University of Arkansas at Pine Bluff;
John L. McClellan Veterans Hospital
Little Rock, Arkansas

ELIZABETH SCHENK, RN, MSN

Vice President of Nursing, Heather Hill, Inc.
Chardon, Ohio;
Clinical Faculty Member
Frances Payne Bolton School of Nursing
Case Western Reserve University, Cleveland, Ohio

GLADYS M. SCIPIEN, RN, MS

Assistant Professor, University of Massachusetts Boston, Harbor Campus
Boston, Massachusetts

ALITA SELLERS, RN, MDEd, PhD

Course Coordinator and Instructor
Western Pennsylvania Hospital, School of Nursing
Pittsburgh, Pennsylvania

ANNABELLE SITLER, RN, BSN

Instructor, Hannah E. Mullins School of Practical Nursing
Salem, Ohio

GEORGEANNA TEMRES SMITH, RN, MEd

Nursing Program Director
Northern Nevada Community College, Elko, Nevada

MARTHA E. SPRAY, RN, BSN

Adult Practical Nursing Instructor
Mid-East Ohio Vocational School District
Zanesville, Ohio

AUDREY WADMAN SZCZESIUL, RN, MS

Instructor, Practical Nurse Education Program
A.I. Prince Regional Vocational School
Hartford, Connecticut

PHYLLIS J. TURNER, RN, MS

Coordinator of Health Occupations Education
Jefferson Technical Institute
Metairie, Louisiana

HAZEL WALKER, RN, MNEd

Formerly Administrative Director, Division of Nursing
St. Francis Regional Medical Center
Wichita, Kansas

CONNIE M. WALLACE, RN, MSN

Nurse Educator, Jennie Edmundson Memorial Hospital
School of Nursing
Council Bluffs, Iowa

LOIS WHITE, RN, PhD

Director, Vocational Nursing
Del Mar College, Corpus Christi, Texas

GLORIA E. WOLD, RN, MS

Instructor, Laboratory Manager
Milwaukee Area Technical College
Milwaukee, Wisconsin

Consultants

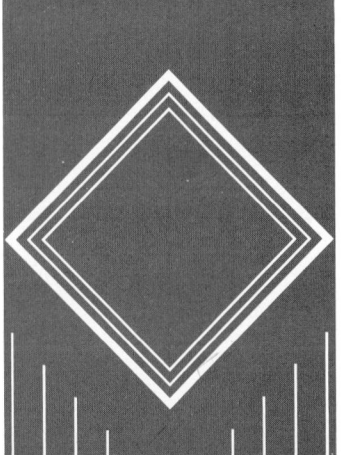

PAMELA ANDERSON, BSN

Cliffview Medical Group, P.C.;
Independence, Missouri

BETTY GLORE BECKER, RN, BS

Our Lady of Victories
St. Louis, Missouri

LINDA L. BLAND, RN, MSN

Trinity Valley Community College
Vocational Nursing Program
Palestine, Texas

SUSAN BODTKE, RN, CNM, MSN

Oklahoma State University
Oklahoma City, Oklahoma

JUDY BREWER, BSN

Crockett Hospital
Lawrenceburg, Tennessee

JUDITH BRYANT, RN, MS

Niagara County Community College
Sanborn, New York

CATHERINE FRAHER BURKE, RN, MS

Kankakee Community College
Kankakee, Illinois

VIRGINIA E. CLEVENGER, RN, MA

Mercer County Vocational School
Trenton, New Jersey

BETTY R. COFFMAN, RN, MEd

Coosa Valley Technical Institute
Rome, Georgia

ZELMA L. COLEMAN, RN, BGS, MEd

Hocking College
Nelsonville, Ohio

MARY ANN COSGAREA, BA, BSN

W. Howard Nicol School of Practical Nursing
Greensburg, Ohio

PRUDENCE D'ANGELO, RN, BSN

Springfield Hospital Center School of Practical Nursing
Sykesville, Maryland

BARBARA DISBENNETT, BSN

Valley Baptist Medical Center
Harlingen, Texas

ROBYN HUMPHREY D'ORIA, RN, MA

Medical Center at Princeton
Princeton, New Jersey

Sr. KAREN DUFAULT, RN, PhD

St. Elizabeth Medical Center
Yakima, Washington

BETTY DUNCAN, RN, BSOE, MEd

Director of Vocational Nursing
Vernon Regional Junior College
Wichita Falls, Texas

RUTH S. DZIK, RN, MEd

Riveredge Hospice of St. Francis Medical Center
Breckenridge, Minnesota

ELIZABETH S. FAYRAM, MSN

Edgewood College, Madison, Wisconsin

ALICE GLOOR, RN, MEd

Salem Community College
Carney's Point, New Jersey

CATHERINE HALL, RN, MS

Kingsport School of Practical Nursing
Kingsport, Tennessee

JANET R. HAMILTON, RN, MSN, OCN

Lamar University at Orange
Orange, Texas

PERSIS MARY HAMILTON, RN, EdD

Formerly of Napa Valley College
Associate Degree Nursing
Napa, California

CAROLYN L. HICHS, RN, BSN
Butte College, Oroville, California

SALLY R. HOLLAND, RN, BSEd
James L. Walker Vocational-Technical Center
Naples, Florida

CATHLEEN HOYEM, RN, BSN
Idaho State Veterans' Home, Boise, Idaho

GARNET LAURITSEN JOHNSTON, RN
Mercy Hospital, Cincinnati, Ohio

RELDA KELLY, RN, MSN
Kankakee Community College, Kankakee, Illinois

NORMA R. LOWDEN, RN, BSN
Kokomo School of Practical Nursing, Kokomo, Indiana

MARY McCARTHY, RN, MEd
Department of Health and Hospitals, Boston, Massachusetts

SANDRA R. MILLER, RNC
Hotel Pawnee—Assisted Living Program
North Platte, Nebraska

MARY MILLER-WERLINGER, RN, MSN, ANP
Goodall-Witcher Hospital Foundation, Clifton, Texas

MARY JANE LARSON NELSON, RN, BSN
Nebraska Home Health Care, Ogallala, Nebraska

MARILYN POWELL, RN, MSN
Assistant Professor of Nursing
Pasco-Hernando Community College
New Port Richey, Florida

LINDA N. SAMUELS, BS, MA
New Rochelle Board of Education, New Rochelle, New York

JOANNA CLIFFONE SCALABRINI, RNC, MN
Westchester Community College, Valhalla, New York

SANDRA SCHULER, RN, MSN
Montgomery College, Takoma, Maryland

ELAINE L. SMITH, RN, MA
Pinellas Technical Education Center—St. Petersburg
St. Petersburg, Florida

JACQUELINE SMITH, BSN
Midlands Technical College, Columbia, South Carolina

WANDA SPRATT, MSN
College of the Redwoods, Eureka, California

ELINOR SWANSON, RN, MA
Knox County Career Center, Mt. Vernon, Ohio

JULIE THELEN, RN
Great Plains Regional Medical Center, North Platte, Nebraska

MARILYN FUQUA THOMPSON, RN, MS
Lake Land College, Mattoon, Illinois

DONNA MAZZA WAGNER, RN, MSEd
Woodland Hills School District, Pittsburgh, Pennsylvania

SALLY R. WALKER, RN, BSN
Walker Vocational Technical Center, Naples, Florida

BEVERLY WANKO, RN, BSN
Anson Community College, Ansonville, North Carolina

NANCY WARSCHAW, RN, BSN
Casaloma College, Lakeview Terrace, California

COSETTE WHITMORE, RN, MS
Erwin Technical Center, Tampa, Florida

JOANN PREISENDORF WIELAND, RN, MS
Central Community College, Hasting, Nebraska

PATRICIA ANN WINBERG, RN, BSN
Kansas City Missouri Board of Education Program of Practical Nursing, Kansas City, Missouri

GLORIA E. WOLD, MS
Milwaukee Area Technical College, Milwaukee, Wisconsin

KATHRYN A. WOOD, MS Community Health Nursing
Erie Community College, North Williamsville, New York

LAURA J. WRIGHT, RN, MSN
Health Care Specialists, Inc., Greeley, Colorado

BEVERLY POST YESHION, RN, BSN, ACCE
Southwest Florida Blood Bank, Tampa, Florida

LULA M. ZLOMKE, RN, MS
Mid-Plains Community College, North Platte, Nebraska

To my parents
Nels and **Mable Lauritsen,**
who gave me the gift of compassion.
To my beloved children
Jennifer Holly, Jessica Heather, and **Jason Heath,**
whose presence in my life gives meaning to all things.
BARBARA LAURITSEN CHRISTENSEN

To my husband
Don *and children* **Ann, Philip, Amy,** and **Brad,**
whose pride in my accomplishments brings me fulfillment.
ELAINE ODEN KOCKROW

Preface

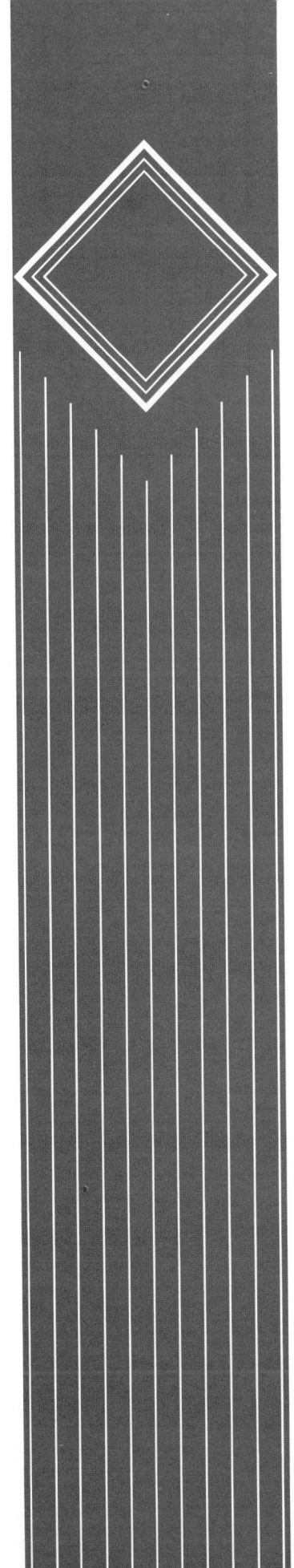

Foundations of Nursing has been developed as a comprehensive nursing textbook with the goal of providing practical and vocational nursing students (RNA Students in Canada) with the knowledge necessary to provide competent nursing interventions to a variety of patients in numerous settings. This textbook is ideally suited for the nursing programs involved in the ladder concept of nursing education. This textbook is distinctive in that it covers all areas of the practical/vocational nursing curriculum without presenting the material too briefly. It includes coverage of anatomy and physiology, mathematics review, basic nursing skills, medical-surgical, pediatrics, geriatrics, maternity, mental health, nutrition, and medications. The text may stand alone or be used in conjunction with a few supplement titles, thereby reducing the need to purchase a book for every core area. Sensitive to reading level, we have also strived to present content in a concise and well-organized manner that is conducive to student learning.

ORGANIZATION

The text contains 57 chapters organized into 17 units. Unit I presents foundation for the practical/vocational nursing curriculum, including important chapters on the evolution of nursing, legal aspects, and ethical concerns. Unit II emphasizes the importance of communication, the nursing process, and documentation. The nursing process is introduced in Chapter 5 and is integrated throughout all appropriate chapters. Unit III incorporates growth and development throughout the life span, as well as sociocultural and family influences. Unit IV focuses on signs, symptoms, physical assessment, and vital signs. Unit V includes seven chapters on basic nursing skills needed by the practical/vocational nursing student to function knowledgeably at the bedside. Skills in these chapters are presented in two formats: standard step-by-step and step-by-step within a nursing process framework. Unit VI covers basic nutrition principles and therapeutic diets. Unit VII presents a valuable mathematics review, followed by principles and practice of medication administration. Unit VIII focuses on the surgical patient and addresses all aspects of preoperative and postoperative nursing interventions within the realm of the practical/vocational nurse. Unit IX focuses on therapeutic management of adult health disorders in ten body systems chapters, each including an anatomy and physiology overview preceding the medical-surgical presentation. Also featured in this unit are chapters on immune disorders, cancer and AIDS. Unit X presents maternal/newborn nursing and a separate chapter on complications and high-risk maternity nursing. Unit XI contains 2 chapters devoted to pediatric nursing, covering both normal and abnormal conditions. Remaining units and chapters focus on such specialty areas as geriatrics, mental health, home health, rehabilitation, emergency nursing, dying and death, and hospice care. The final chapter gives the graduating student nurse helpful information on methods of job seeking, leadership and management styles, and professional development.

FEATURES

- We have presented clear and measurable learning objectives to allow students to more easily comprehend the significance of chapter content and measure their success in mastering difficult concepts.
- A list of key terms is presented at the beginning of each chapter; the terms are then bold-faced where they are defined or discussed in the text.
- A glossary at the end of the text allows students quick access to important nursing and medical terminology.
- Major disorders within Unit IX have been presented in a consistent format, focusing on etiology/pathophysiology, clinical manifestations, assessment, presentation of collection of subjective and objective data, diagnostic tests, medical management, and nursing diagnosis and nursing interventions with patient teaching. We have endeavored to present the art of nursing, as well as the science of nursing. The nursing model with a holistic approach is emphasized throughout the textbook.
- 9th conference NANDA-approved nursing diagnoses help students participate in the development of nursing care plans. Nursing interventions are correlated with the appropriate diagnosis.
- Sample nursing care plans for a variety of common disorders provide students with guidelines for participating in the development of care plans for their own patients
- Numerous documentation examples stress the importance of timely and accurate charting.
- In addition to the basic skills presented in Unit V, many skills have been integrated throughout the medical-surgical unit, presented in step-by-step fashion with rationales where appropriate.
- Therapeutic dialogues give students examples of effective nurse-patient interactions and emphasize the importance of good communication skills.
- Chapter Challenge at the end of each chapter includes key points, covering important concepts in the chapter, and multiple-choice study questions (answer key at end of book).
- Each unit begins with an essay written by a student on what it means to be a practical/vocational nurse.
- The attractive two-color design provides visual appeal and enhances student learning.
- Numerous illustrations throughout the text enhance student understanding of difficult concepts.
- Where possible, illustrations of anatomy and physiology are presented in full color, allowing students to better view the intricacies of the human body.
- References and suggested readings highlight up-to-date research and point students to further areas of study.
- The inside front and back covers feature a quick reference guide to information within the text, including a brief table of contents, a list of current NANDA diagnoses, a list of commonly used abbreviations, and a list of skills and care plans included in the text.

TEACHING-LEARNING PACKAGE

We recognize that educators have limited time in which to prepare classrooms and clinical activities. We have therefore provided an instructor's resource manual, which provides suggested activities, as well as a test bank of approximately 600 questions.

To help students make better use of their study time, we have provided a comprehensive study guide (prepared by Brenda Goodner). This guide includes learning objectives, prerequisite and suggested readings, chapter summaries, key points, and a variety of questions for classroom discussion or independent study. Clinical simulations and a test at the end of each chapter promote decision-making skills in the clinical setting.

EDITORS, CONTRIBUTORS, AND REVIEWERS

Practical and vocational nursing have undergone dramatic changes in the past decade, and keeping abreast of these changes could not have been possible without the selection of a team of expert editors, contributors, and reviewers from all walks of education and practice and from diverse geographical areas. They have been involved in the 3-year research and development of this project, as well as the numerous drafts of manuscript. These professionals have contributed not only their knowledge of their particular subject areas, but their love of nursing and its continued success, and for this we are indebted.

Barbara Christensen
Elaine Kockrow

Acknowledgment

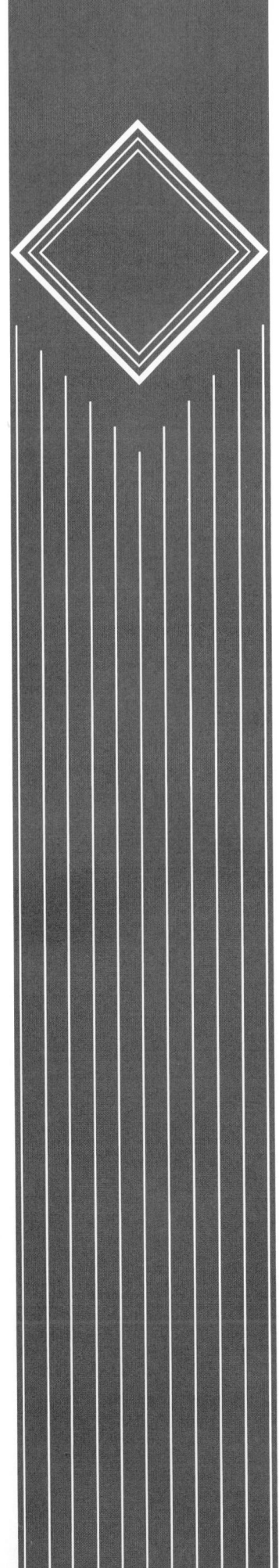

This textbook culminates a lifelong love for the art and science of nursing. To produce a text of this magnitude requires the creativity, intellect, steadfastness of purpose, and energy of numerous persons.

We would like first to acknowledge the editorial staff of Mosby–Year Book: Linda Duncan, Senior Editor, for her belief in our ability to coedit this textbook, for her organizational skills, and for her keen awareness of the needs of student nurses; Joanna May, Developmental Editor, for her patience, creativity, quiet, good humor, and faith in our expertise in the nursing field; Teri Merchant, Developmental Editor, for her commitment to detail and her insight into what is necessary for a superior text; Betty Hazelwood, Senior Production Editor, for her perfectionism, energy, time management, and superior command of the English language; Becky Sweeney, editorial Assistant, for her courtesy and willingness to contribute to the many details necessary to complete this textbook; and Gail Hudson, Book Designer, for her diligence and expertise in preparing the presentation of this book.

We thank Lydia Kibiuk, medical illustrator, for her meticulous detail in illustrating and all of the Mosby–Year Book authors for the use of their artwork in our textbook.

We are indebted to the knowledge, dedication, and perseverance of our talented contributors and reviewers. Their special skills span the nation.

We extend our special acknowledgment to Christine Neff for her forthright authoring of all the anatomy and physiology sections of (Chapters 27-37); to Gloria Wold for her boundless energy and talent for task completion in preparing the instructors' manual; to Brenda Goodner for her resourceful contribution in authoring the study guide; and to Joan Browning for her conscientious endeavor to present an accurate glossary.

We are grateful to Great Plains Regional Medical Center for the use of various documents that were made available to us. Our special thanks to Cindy Bradley, Nancy Hudson, and John Gonzales.

We are indebted to our mentors, who gave us the tools to practice the art of nursing, and to our patients, who have allowed us to practice this art. We acknowledge our students, who bring their enthusiasm to nursing and challenge us to continue to strive for perfection.

We extend our thanks to Mid-Plains Community College for the support, confidence, and encouragement throughout this laborious task. We appreciate the efforts of Pauline Shahan, Director of Health Occupations; it was with her encouragement that we began to coedit this textbook. We also appreciate the support of Dr. William Hasemeyer, College President, and Jim Doyle, retired Dean of Vocational Instruction. In addition, we thank our typists, Ginger Snodgrass and Debbie Beebout. To Doris Israelson we give our special thanks for her friendship and ceaseless support for this project.

This book could not have been completed without the love, patience, sacrifices, and forbearance of our families. Their willingness to give us the gift of time allowed us to coedit a textbook that we believe to be unique.

Finally, we wish to acknowledge a unique 16-year friendship, which has allowed us to contribute our knowledge and skills to the formation of this textbook. We share a bond of respect, trust, and devotion that encompasses our philosophy of nursing, pursuit of education, and love of family.

Contents

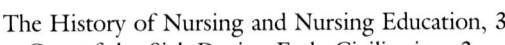

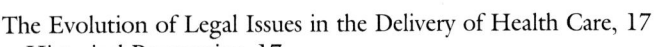

UNIT I
INTRODUCTION TO NURSING

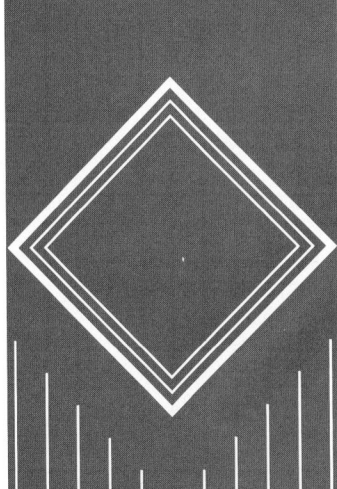

UNIT VI
NUTRITION

I

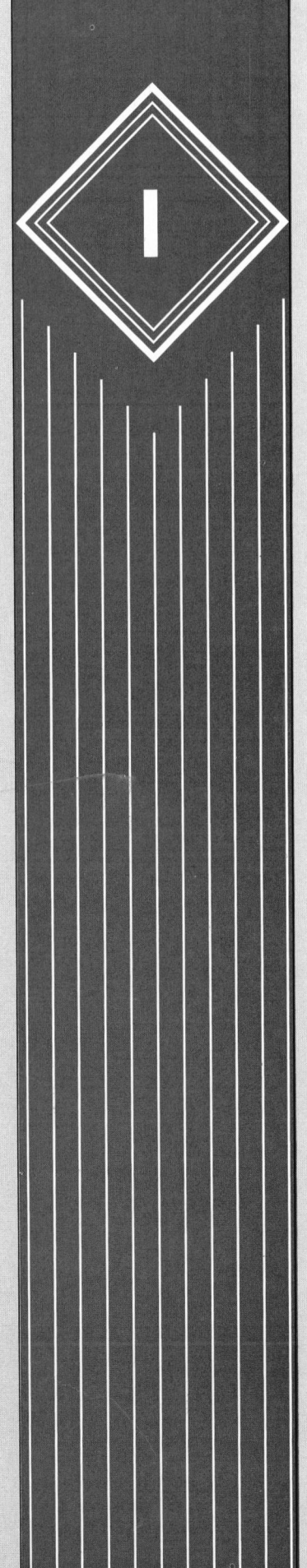

Introduction to Nursing

Nursing—the profession of treating human responses to actual or potential health problems. The definition doesn't seem to give nursing justice. Nursing to me is a feeling: one of compassion, love, understanding, and always being there when a patient needs you. I really feel deep in my heart that being a nurse is what I've always wanted to be. The feeling I get when I go into a patient's room, knowing that I'm really needed and trusted, is one of the most wonderful feelings I know and I will carry it with me for a lifetime.

SUSAN HAND
Student Nurse

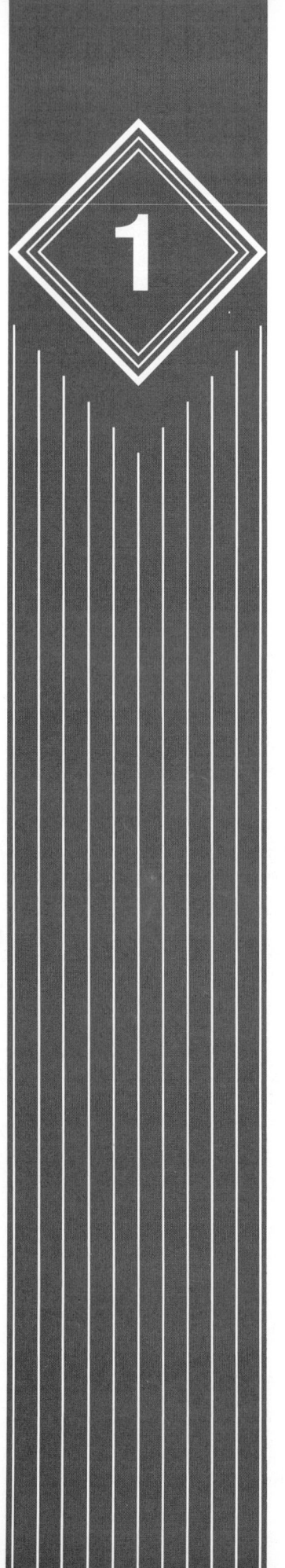

1

The Evolution of Nursing

PERSEPHONE C. AGRAFIOTIS

LEARNING OBJECTIVES

After reading this chapter, the student should be able to do the following:

- Define the key terms.
- Describe the evolution of nursing and nursing education from early civilization to the twentieth century.
- List the major developments of practical/vocational nursing.
- Identify the components of the health care system.
- Identify the participants of the health care system.
- Describe the complex factors involved in the delivery of patient care.
- Define practical/vocational nursing.
- Describe the purpose, role, and responsibilities of the practical/vocational nurse.

RELATED TOPICS OF INTEREST

- Legal aspects of nursing (Chapter 2)
- Ethical aspects of nursing (Chapter 3)
- Communication (Chapter 4)
- The nursing process (Chapter 5)
- Documentation (Chapter 6)

KEY TERMS

Define the following:

- accreditation
- approved
- health
- health care system
- holistic health care
- illness
- licensure
- medicine
- nursing
- patient
- wellness

THE HISTORY OF NURSING AND NURSING EDUCATION

Nursing has evolved over many years, influenced by the means by which the sick were cared for. Changes in the way people live, the interrelationship of people with their environment, the search for knowledge and truth through education, and technological advances have made nursing and nursing education what it is and what it will be.

Care of the Sick During Early Civilization

In 5000 BC there was little reference to nursing, per se. **Illness** was considered to be directly related to disfavor with God. Primitive people believed that a person became sick when an evil spirit entered the body and that the presence of a good spirit kept disease away.

Medicine men performed witchcraft on the affected part of the body to induce the bad spirits to leave the body. Some of the techniques involved the use of frightening masks, noises, incantations, vile odors, charms, spells, and even sacrifices.

Men assisted the medicine men in treating illnesses. They used purgatives, emetics, application of hot and cold substances, cauterization, cupping, blistering, and massage. Few women assisted the medicine men. They assisted mostly women in childbirth.

The Babylonians were intellectually, socially, and scientifically well developed. Many wars brought misery, suffering, illness, and injury to their people. There is evidence that some form of medical service existed and that lay persons provided this service. It is believed that these caregivers were usually men. If they were women, they were probably of low status because the actions of Babylonian women were dominated by men.

The ancient Hebrews, according to the Talmud and the Old Testament, attributed their misfortunes and illnesses to God's wrath. They depended on Him to restore them to **health** when they were sick. They combined their religious beliefs with the hygienic practices that they acquired from Babylonia, where they had been in captivity. These practices included the inspection of all meats and the careful selection and preparation of all foods. They prevented the spread of communicable disease by burning infected garments and scrubbing the homes of those infected with the disease. Nurses were mentioned occasionally in the Talmud as persons caring for the sick in their homes. This appears to have been a demonstration of the first public health/home care movement.

Ancient records of early Egyptian civilization described nursing procedures, such as feeding a **patient** with tetanus and dressing wounds.

Records of pre-Christian India reported the establishment of hospitals where the sick were cared for. The reports described a body of attendants, probably male, who were of good behavior, who were distinguished for purity and cleanliness of habits, and who were clever, skillful, and endowed with kindness. They bathed patients, made beds, and were always willing to do whatever they could to assist the sick.

By 500 BC the Hellenic civilization showed keen intellect, independent thinking, democratic action, and a thirst for knowledge and truth. **Medicine** progressed from the belief that demons and spirits caused human ills to the founding of temples suitable for rest and restoration of health. These temples, often referred to as hospitals, resembled our health centers of today: they had spas, mineral springs, baths, gymnasiums, and treatment and consultation rooms. The religious influence was still present in the form of prayer, thanks offerings, and rituals. Priestesses served as attendants and cared for the sick. Pregnant women and people with incurable diseases were not admitted.

Hippocrates, born in 460 BC on the island of Cos in the Mediterranean, was a brilliant, progressive physician and teacher. He rejected the belief in the supernatural origin of disease and adopted a system of physical assessment, observation, and record keeping as an integral part of patient care. As his patient-centered care approach and medical ethics were adopted, Hippocrates was named the "Father of Medicine" and was credited for the Hippocratic Oath, still taken by physicians today. The work of Hippocrates is the basis for the holistic approach to patient care.

The Greek influence on the care of the sick changed the belief from mysticism to public health and safety. The religious influence was still prevalent, but with an emphasis on the poor, the sick, the widowed, and the children. Deacons and deaconesses were designated by the Roman bishops to assist the church by providing services, such as visiting the sick women in their homes, visiting and tending to the needs of prisoners, and watching over the sick in the hospitals. One of the first deaconesses, Phoebe, performed nursing functions about AD 60. She was known as a visiting nurse, attending the sick and poor in their homes. Another Roman woman, Fabiola, spent her wealth and time nursing the sick and poor. She is credited with providing the first free hospital in Rome in AD 390.

Monastic and military orders were charged with caring for the sick over the next period, but the rise and fall of feudalism in Central Europe hindered the progress made in Greece and Rome. Famine, disease, war, and the emphasis on survival resulted in an increased need to care for the sick and poor, but the ongoing battles between the church and state hindered the development of any one approach to patient care. Care of the sick was performed by both men and women. Female religious orders were concerned with the care of the sick and needy, but the concern for religious problems took priority. Male military personnel served the medical needs of soldiers on the battlefield.

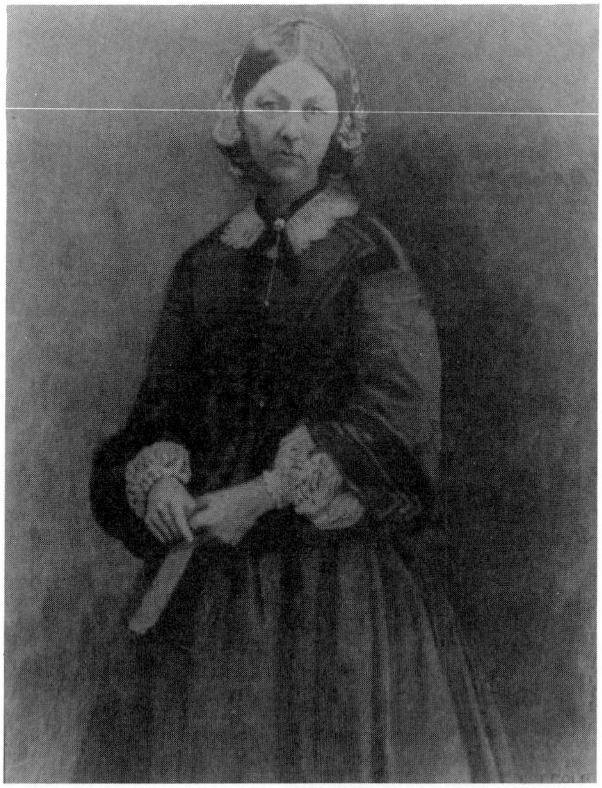

FIG. 1-1 Florence Nightingale. (From Cole T: Florence Nightingale, Wood engraving, National Library of Medicine, Bethesda, Md.)

Organized Nursing Education in the Nineteenth Century

In the early nineteenth century, hospitals were overcrowded, and there was a lack of trained and qualified people who were interested in caring for the sick and the infirm. Hospitals were a place to contract diseases rather than be cured of them, because of patients with open wounds and unchecked infection and the dirty physical conditions of the plant itself. Women of "proper upbringing" did not work outside of the home during this time. As a result, nursing attracted inferior and undesirable lower-class women who drank heavily and engaged in prostitution. The best sources of nurses were the religious nursing orders, but these orders could not begin to meet the ever-increasing need for nursing services.

The Lutheran Order of Deaconesses established the first real school of nursing under the guidance of Theodor Fliedner, a German pastor in Kaiserswerth, Germany. The reputation of the school spread throughout Europe. It reached a young woman in England whose interest in nursing overshadowed the opposition of her family, her friends, and the social class to which she belonged. Florence Nightingale (Fig. 1-1), a strong-minded, intelligent, and determined young woman, joined the Kaiserswerth program in 1851 at the age of 31.

Armed with the education and training she received at Kaiserswerth and with her administrative and organizational skills, Florence Nightingale became the superintendent of a charity hospital for ill governesses in 1853. The governing board of the hospital was not always pleased with the changes and innovations she made and the guidance she gave her uneducated nurses, even though the quality of patient care improved.

In the following year, when she was preparing to become Superintendent of King's College Hospital in London, news of the atrocious conditions befalling the wounded soldiers in the Crimean War reached England. People were greatly concerned over the number of casualties and deaths that were reported. The Secretary of War, a long-standing friend of Miss Nightingale, asked her to lead a group of nurses to Scutari, Turkey, to care for the wounded. Ironically she had sent him a letter offering her services at about the same time. Within a week of receiving the Secretary's letter, she and 38 nurses left England for Turkey.

Once again Florence Nightingale applied the principles of nursing she had learned at Kaiserswerth. These concepts, coupled with her dedication and leadership, turned the tide. The hospital units were cleaned, clothes were washed regularly, and sanitary conditions, which were nonexistent before her coming, were established. The mortality among the casualties dropped significantly. Not only had the physical environment of the hospital been changed by Florence Nightingale's actions, but through her patience, dedication, and empathetic treatment of the soldiers, a psychological change took place as well. The soldiers grew to respect her and looked forward to her presence on the wards. They looked for her smile and took strength from her self-fulfilled personality. When she made her rounds through the wards late at night, she carried a lamp to light her way through the rows of beds of the injured and sick. This practice became a ritual, and soon she was known as "The Lady With the Lamp." The small lamp that she carried became her trademark and continues to be the symbol of the nursing profession around the world.

The standards of nursing care established by Florence Nightingale gained the respect of the medical community and led to improved care for the sick and a much improved image of nursing in general. The need for educated and trained nurses became painfully evident, and the time was right for a shift in the approach to nursing education.

In 1860 Florence Nightingale began the reformation of nursing from occupation to profession by establishing the nursing school at Saint Thomas Hospital in London. She chose this hospital for the location of the school because of its reputation as a progressive medical facility and thereby the ideal place to promote the new standards of nursing she so strongly believed in.

The nursing program operated separately from the hospital and was financially independent to ensure that the major emphasis of its activity was directed exclusively toward educating nursing students. A nurses' residence was provided for the students who passed the strict admission procedures. The length of nurses' training was 1 year and included both formal instruction and practical experience. Complete records were kept on each student's progress while at the school. This practice became known as the "Nightingale Plan," which was to become the model for nursing education in the twentieth century. After the students graduated, records were also kept on where they were employed. This eventually became a "register," which was the beginning of a movement to exercise control over the nursing graduate and to establish a standard for the practicing nurse.

Students admitted into the nursing program at Saint Thomas had to provide excellent character references, show a strong commitment to a career in nursing, and demonstrate that they were intellectually capable of passing the course of study before them. The resultant demand for "Nightingale Nurses" was overwhelming. The improved patient care provided by this new breed of nurse included such measures as good hygiene, sanitation, patient observation, accurate record keeping, nutritional improvements, and the introduction and use of certain new medical equipment.

During the time that Florence Nightingale was active in Europe, the same kinds of patient care problems were occurring in America. Both the American Revolution and the Civil War produced severe casualties, disease, infected wounds, and archaic medical care. As in the Crimean War, nurses were scarce and those who were available were poorly trained to handle the horrors of war. Women such as Dorothy Dix, Superintendent of Female Nurses of the Union Army in 1861, and Clara Barton, the founder of the Red Cross, tried to meet the needs of both the battlefield casualties and civilian casualties.

By the end of the nineteenth century, three schools of nursing had been established in the United States. All three of these schools were modeled after the Nightingale Plan. In May of 1873 the Bellevue Hospital School of Nursing in New York established itself as the foremost proponent of the Nightingale Plan in America. In October of that same year the Connecticut Training School was opened in New Haven. In November the Boston Training School at the Massachusetts General Hospital began operating.

In the interest of establishing standards for the new nursing schools, dedicated women such as Isabelle Hampton Robb and Lavinia Dock organized The American Society of Superintendents of Training Schools of Nursing in 1894. The major goal of this organization was to set educational standards for nurses. The structure of the organization was modeled after the American Medical Association. A code of ethics for nurses was adopted by the Society, and this code, known as the Nightingale Pledge, is subscribed to by the nursing profession of today.

Changes in Nursing Practice and Education in the Twentieth Century

While the superintendents of the nurses' training schools organized at the national level, the graduates of those training schools organized in their own fashion at the local levels. They established the Alumnae Association in an attempt to establish standards for the actual practice of nursing.

However, change in nursing education and practice could not come about in a vacuum. Any change had to be affected by the social issues of the times. This resulted in the need for rigid standards and laws, which were bound to affect the supply of well-trained nurses. In 1903 the first nursing **licensure** laws to protect the public were passed in North Carolina, New Jersey, New York, and Virginia. As a result, the nursing organizations recognized the need to amend their purpose and redirect their focus. As part of the reorganization that followed, The American Society of Superintendents of Training Schools became the Education Committee of the National League For Nursing Education in 1903. The Alumnae Association became the American Nurses Association in 1911.

Concurrent with these changes, Isabelle Hampton Robb and Mary Adelaide Nutting developed a program at Columbia University to train and develop teachers of nursing. They were convinced that nurses needed not only a college education and clinical practice, but also specific training in theoretical knowledge. The belief that nurses needed such a balance of liberal arts education and nursing practice skills brought a new, balanced perspective to the profession of nursing.

World War I brought about an increased demand for nurses. The newly formed Army and Navy Nurse Corps sought nurses whom school superintendents certified as having "good moral character and professional qualifications." The available supply of nurses could not meet the demand, so once again untrained women volunteered their services to their country. Nursing leaders, concerned that these untrained personnel would be caring directly for wounded and ailing soldiers without adequate training, quickly established the Army School of Nursing.

After the war the women who served as military nurses returned to their homes and their previous jobs and careers. They had no desire to remain in nursing as civilians. The image attached to professional nurses still posed a problem for most women. Furthermore, they were disenchanted because nurses' training still focused heavily on "service to the patient" rather than on a comprehensive professional education. This was far removed from what the Nightingale Plan had proposed for aspiring nurses.

Twenty-five years later, the demand for trained nurses was once again escalated almost overnight because of World War II. Although medicine had advanced, so had the art of war, and the casualties were high and severe. Early in the war, the Cadet Nurse Corps was established to provide nursing education and training. The Corps provided an abbreviated training program designed to meet the needs of the war effort. Additionally, federally subsidized programs in nursing were developed and implemented to offer to women and, for the first time, to men an education and career in nursing while serving their country in the war. After the war, many of the nurses trained by these programs remained in military service. Prestige, pay, and the opportunity for advancement were much greater in the military service when compared with the same benefits, or lack of benefits, for civilian nurses. Civilian nurses received low pay and worked long shifts under atrocious conditions in the major hospitals, particularly in urban areas. These conditions in no way could attract those who became nurses as a result of the war and who, ironically, enjoyed a certain life-style that war invariably provides. As a result, the shortage of nurses in the United States and other countries continued to grow.

The effects of World War I, the Great Depression, and World War II strongly influenced this deficit. Pressure was exerted on the state boards of nursing, which had licensure responsibility, to mandate requirements for nurses. State-administered licensing examinations were no longer considered adequate for the country's needs. The parochial state examinations were in no way standardized and allowed a wide spectrum of competence to enter nursing. National norms of competence were needed and quickly established.

The characteristics of health care changed rapidly as health care became an industry. Growth and diversity became the major emphasis as the industry of health care became increasingly lucrative. The need for nurses, particularly well-educated nurses, increased at a rate much greater than could be provided.

The nursing organizations continued to deliberate on the future of nursing as a profession. In 1965 the American Nurses Association (ANA) took the position that nursing education should take place in institutions of learning within the general system of education, much as Robb and Nutting had proposed in 1903. Their position paper further delineated that the minimum preparation for the beginning professional nurse should be a baccalaureate degree in nursing and the minimum education for technical nursing practice should be an associate degree in nursing. Assistants to nurses, they said, should have preservice programs in vocational education rather than just on-the-job training. This position has had a profound effect. Since 1965 many hospital-based nursing programs have been disbanded and an increasing number of baccalaureate and associate degree nursing programs have been established in the colleges and universities. The intent is obviously to change the trend from "training" nurses to "educating" nurses.

Development of Practical/Vocational Nursing in the United States

Practical/vocational nursing in the United States is not as clearly defined as registered nursing in the history of nursing. The first school for training the practical nurse started in Brooklyn, New York, in 1892 and was conducted under the auspices of the Young Women's Christian Association (YWCA). The Ballard School, as it was known, was approximately 3 months in duration and trained its students to care for the chronically ill, the invalid, children, and the elderly. The main emphasis was on home care and included cooking, cleaning, nutrition, basic science, and simple nursing procedures. Graduates of this program were referred to as *attendant nurses*.

Two other programs were started, and they were patterned after the Ballard School. In 1907 the Thompson Practical Nursing School opened in Brattleboro, Vermont, and in 1918 the Household Nursing Association School of Attendant Nursing (later changed to the Shepard-Gill School of Practical Nursing) opened in Boston. The focus of these programs continued to be on home nursing care, cooking, laundry, and other light housekeeping duties. Hospital experience was not a part of the training in the early programs. The Ballard School closed in 1949 because of the reorganization of the YWCA. The Shepard-Gill School closed in 1984. The Thompson School is still in operation and continues to be accredited by the National League for Nursing (NLN).

Practical nursing programs developed slowly during the first half of the twentieth century. Robb, Nutting, and others active in the two nursing organizations emphasized professionalizing nursing rather than promoting the vocational/technical aspects. A total of 36 schools opened during this period.

The increased demand for nursing services brought on by World War II and the postwar years resulted in the opening of 260 practical/vocational nursing programs between 1948 and 1954. These programs varied in administrative design. Some were affiliated with hospitals or chronic care institutions, whereas others aligned themselves with private agencies or private schools. Their general commitment was meeting the needs of the sick and the infirm. Students in these programs once again provided nursing services while they were obtaining their education and training. This on-the-job, or apprentice, training again emphasized vocational/technical education. The allocation of federal funds for training practical/vocational nurses helped recruit men and women.

The rapid growth of practical nursing programs and the diverse administrative controls of such programs were a concern to nursing leaders of the country. The need to establish standards again became a major issue. The Association of Practical Nurse Schools was founded in 1942 and was dedicated exclusively to practical nursing. Its membership was multidisciplinary and included licensed practical nurses, registered nurses, physicians, hospital and nursing home administrators, students, and public figures. Together they planned the first standard curriculum for practical nursing. By 1945 they saw the need to change the name to the National Association of Practical Nurse Education and Service (NAPNES). They broadened their focus to include education and practice and established an accrediting service for schools of practical/vocational nursing.

Accreditation of a program differs from program approval. An **approved** program is one that meets minimum standards set by the respective state responsible to oversee educational programs. The state seeks to ensure that a given program, for example, meets the needs of the student, has adequate course content and qualified faculty, is of sufficient length, has adequate facilities, and provides clinical experience. All of these elements are needed for licensure. The state also ensures that the welfare of the public is protected by maintaining minimum standards. Approval is required for the program to operate. **Accreditation,** on the other hand, involves the administration of a program voluntarily seeking a review by a given organization to determine if the program meets the preestablished criteria of that organization. Many times the standards that are established by professional organizations that accredit are far higher than those established by the state. Although graduates of nonaccredited programs can take the **licensure** examination required in most states, accreditation is extremely important when programs seek federal funding.

In 1961 the NLN broadened its scope of service because of the growth of practical/vocational nursing programs. It established a Department of Practical Nursing Programs and developed an accreditation service for these programs.

For 20 years both the NLN and NAPNES provided accreditation services. Nursing programs had the option of selecting either organization from which to seek accreditation. In recent years, however, the NAPNES board of directors has discontinued this service.

Practical/vocational nursing programs continued to proliferate, and by 1987-1988 there were 1095 practical/vocational nursing programs in the United States, which produced 26,912 graduates in that year. Nursing programs are still offered by various organizations, such as high schools, trade or technical schools, hospitals, junior and community colleges, colleges and universities, and private education agencies. However, they must all meet minimum state standards. The length of the programs is usually 12 months, with a focus on nursing skills and theory that is correlated with clinical practice. On completing the program, the graduate is eligible to take the National Council Licensing Examination for Practical Nursing (NCLEX-PN).

Creative educational programs in nursing today offer various approaches to educating student practical/vocational nurses. The combination of practical/vocational nurse education with associate degree programs in 2-year colleges is available. At the successful completion of the first academic year, the student can either exit and take the licensure examination for practical/vocational nursing or continue for another year and earn an associate degree in nursing, becoming eligible to take the licensure examination for registered nursing. Many other programs offering other combinations of education and degree-granting are available throughout the United States.

Events That Changed Practical/Vocational Nursing (Box 1-1)

The history of practical nursing in the United States before 1940 is vague. Early sources make reference to "assistants to priests" and "assistants to physicians." Before 1860 nursing care in the United States was provided generally by persons who were self-taught and who gained what experience they could as they practiced their nursing skills. Registration, licensing, and title differentiation were not clear or were nonexistent. Clearly defined duties and responsibilities were absent. The term *nurse* was used only in the broadest sense as "a person who takes care of the sick." It is difficult to determine where, in the ambiguously defined group of persons called nurses, the practical/vocational nurse of today fits.

The early creation and development of practical nursing in the United States was not planned, but rather evolved from the need for a caregiver who could be trained and ready for service in a short time. The cost of the services provided by these caregivers was expected to be low and easily affordable by the common person. There was also the need at that time to provide a vocation for the many unskilled women who were migrating to the larger cities to seek better lives. This need prompted the YWCA in New York City to start the first practical nursing program in the late 1800s. During this time women generally were not skilled or trained for jobs other than manual labor. Practical/vocational nursing education enabled women to secure a vocation, and at the same time it expanded the availability of health care nursing.

World War I escalated the need for trained nurses abroad, while in the United States, the Spanish influenza epidemic strained the resources of the nursing community. The Smith-Hughes Act was passed in 1917 to provide vocational and public education. Federal funding then provided the means for vocational-based practical/vocational nursing programs throughout the country. Even with these resources, the demand for nurses caused by the war and the epidemic could not be met.

By 1940 thousands of self-taught "practical nurses"

BOX 1-1 IMPORTANT DATES OF MAJOR EVENTS

1892 The Ballard School at the YWCA in Brooklyn, New York, established the first school to train practical nurses.

1907 The Thompson Practical Nursing School in Brattleboro, Vermont, was the second practical nursing school to be established.

1914 The Mississippi State Legislature was the first political body to pass license laws controlling practical nurses.

1917 The Smith-Hughes Act was passed. It provided federal funding for vocationally oriented practical nursing programs.

1918 The Household Nursing Association School of Attendant Nursing in Boston, Massachusetts, later called the Shepard-Gill School of Practical Nursing, was the third practical nursing school established.

1942 The Association of Practical Nursing Schools was founded. It set standards for practical nursing education.

1944 The U.S. Department of Vocational Education commissioned an intensive study to differentiate tasks of the practical nurse.

1945 The Association of Practical Nursing Schools became the National Association of Practical Nurse Education and Service (NAPNES).

1945 New York became the only state to have mandatory licensure laws for practical nurses.

1949 The Ballard School in Brooklyn, New York, closed.

1955 All of the states passed licensure laws affecting practical/vocational nursing.

1961 The National League for Nursing established a Department of Practical Nursing.

1965 The American Nurses Association published a position paper defining two levels of nursing, which did not include practical/vocational nursing.

1985 The Shepard-Gill School of Practical Nursing closed.

were working to meet the needs of the country. However, they lacked the education and experience that can be obtained only under supervision in an established program. They could not really be called practical/vocational nurses nor could they be licensed by the states. In fact, few states had even established minimum standards for the practice of practical/vocational nursing. Only 19 states and one territory had considered or passed legislation dealing with practical/vocational nursing. Licensure of the practical/vocational nurse was mandatory in only one state by the end of 1945. Many job descriptions and titles were used in referring to the work done by the practical/vocational nurse. There was no agreement on the duties, the role, or the responsibilities of these people. These facts and the absence of standards and licensing practices created difficulties.

Even before the United States entered World War II, the Depression caused a great demand for nurses. The Cadet Navy Corps and the American Red Cross provided expedient training in nursing. Practical nursing programs flourished throughout the United States. The need for skilled medical care personnel, although important, was upstaged by the need to prepare people for nursing in the shortest time. A 1-year program provided the minimum amount of training for practical/vocational nursing. As the shortage of nurses in the hospitals and other health care facilities became critical, the practical/vocational nurse, practicing in the home environment, was hired to work in those institutions. Furthermore, because of the shortage of registered nurses, the responsibilities given to the practical/vocational nurses in the hospitals often far exceeded their scope of training.

In 1944 the United States Department of Vocational Education commissioned an intensive study of practical/vocational nursing tasks. The outcome of this study differentiated the tasks performed by the practical/vocational nurse in relation to those tasks performed by the registered nurse. As a result of this study, individual state boards of nursing began to specify the duties and responsibilities that could be accomplished by both groups of nurses. These new practices of defining and differentiating the roles of the registered nurse and the practical/vocational nurse with respect to what tasks each could or could not perform again reflected the desire of nursing leaders to separate the registered nurse (the professional) from the practical nurse (the technician).

Another event that influenced change in attitude about practical/vocational nursing was the position paper of the American Nurses Association published in 1965. This position paper clearly defined two levels of nursing practice: that of the registered nurse and that of the technical nurse. The term *practical nurse* was not included in the paper as if to nullify their existence and their contribution to health care. This debate continues.

Licensure for Practical/Vocational Nursing

Licensing laws have been passed throughout the states to protect the public from unqualified persons practicing in almost any field or profession. Every state and the District of Columbia, American Samoa, the Northern Mariana Islands, and the Virgin Islands have licensing laws that apply to the practical/vocational nurse. These laws are promulgated through various state agencies, usually the state boards of nursing and the Nurse Practice Acts of the respective states.

Licensing for practical nurses in the United States began in 1914 when the state legislature in Mississippi passed the first laws pertaining to that group. This followed the passage of laws on licensing registered nurses by 11 years. The passage of such laws governing practical/vocational nursing in other states was slow in coming. Only six states passed such laws between 1920 and 1940. This may have been because there were not many practical nurses' training programs initiated during that period. After the outbreak of World War II and the opening of a large number of practical/vocational nurses' training programs, all of the states were forced to pass legislation concerning the licensing of practical/vocational nurses. By 1955 all states had passed laws in this area in consonance with the standards set by NAPNES. The State Board Test Pool of the NLN Education Committee established a testing mechanism for all states and administered the examination several times a year throughout the United States. Graduates of a state-approved practical/vocational nursing education program were eligible to take the examination and, if they passed, became licensed practical nurses (LPNs) or licensed vocational nurses (LVNs), as they are called in Texas and California. Each state established its own required passing score on the examination.

Currently graduates of a state-approved LPN/LVN education program are eligible to take the NCLEX-PN. On completing the examination with a "pass" score (numerical scores are no longer given), the graduate is issued a license to practice as an LPN or an LVN.

Licensing laws for nursing are now established in all states. It is the individual's responsibility to be informed regarding licensure in the state in which she resides or intends to practice. Interstate endorsement (reciprocity between states) exists, and licensing for practice in other states can be obtained without repeating the NCLEX-PN if resident state requirements are met.

HEALTH CARE DELIVERY SYSTEMS

LPNs/LVNs will be practicing within the established health care delivery system. For them to practice to their fullest, they must recognize the complexity of this system and particularly how they fit into it.

Identification of the Health Care System

The **health care system** in the United States is an open system that depends on a variety of health care professionals who interact with their external environment. This environment includes the patient, the patient's family, the community in which the system is operating, the current technology, governmental agencies, the medical profession in the community, third-party participants, such as insurance companies, and many other forces that affect the patient's care. The major goal of the system is to achieve optimal levels of health care for a defined population through adequate and appropriate health care services. The LPN/LVN is an integral member of the team of health care professionals within the overall system who will provide her services within the scope of practice as defined by the state's Nurse Practice Act.

Wellness/illness continuum. Health care services provided by the LPN/LVN depend on the wellness/illness continuum of the consumer, as well as the environment where the services are provided.

The wellness/illness continuum is defined as the range of a person's total health. This continuum is ever changing and is influenced by the individual's physical condition, mental condition, and social well-being. **Wellness,** at one end of the spectrum, represents the highest level of optimum health. **Illness,** at the opposite end of the spectrum, represents a diminished or impaired state of health (Fig. 1-2).

Wellness- - - - - - - - - - - - - - - - - Illness

Highest level of optimum health — Diminished or impaired state of health

FIG. 1-2 Wellness/illness continuum.

Maintaining one's health requires constant effort to achieve a balance of all aspects of life. To achieve this equilibrium, a number of interrelated factors must be considered when providing health care to the consumer. Such factors include age, sex, family relationships, cultural influences, and economic status. This comprehensive approach to health care is known as **holistic health care.**

Health promotion and illness prevention. From the earliest recorded civilizations to the twentieth century, the primary focus on health care has been on the care of the sick. As time passed, the focus broadened to include the determination of the cause of illness and the prevention of its spread.

Hospitals, which were historically dirty, unsanitary, and ill-kept institutions where unsuspecting patients acquired diseases, slowly became clean, sterile, well-kept places where patients were fairly well assured that their disease or illness would be attended and, it was hoped, cured, without risking the added exposure to additional medical problems. The phenomenal death rates in the hospitals during the Crimean War decreased dramatically when the hospital units were cleaned and strict sanitary requirements were imposed.

As more and more standards were established and adhered to, health statistics gathered by the U.S. Department of Public Health began to identify what types of diseases were most prevalent, which age groups seemed to be affected by certain illnesses, and which illnesses were predominant in various parts of the country. These statistics identified problem areas for researchers and health care providers, whose efforts were then directed at developing treatment for the illness, establishing methods to decrease its spread, and isolating its cause. Childbirth without prenatal care increased the mortality of infant and mother; lack of milk in an infant's diet affected bone development and contributed to crippling deformities; coal miners' constant exposure to coal dust and contaminated air in the mines deteriorated their lungs.

Once causes for these and other problems were found, the focus shifted from curing the problem to preventing it. With the focus on decreasing the risk factors for a given illness or disease and thereby preventing it, the quality of life and life expectancy in general were enhanced in the United States. General medical research and specific research for the cause and cure of cancer, cystic fibrosis, heart disease, and many other life-threatening conditions continue to be integral parts of the health care system in this country.

Continuity of care. The patient is the most important person in the health care system. However, he is not the only factor in the total scheme of the holistic health care system that has evolved. The number of health care providers and health care agencies involved in the care and treatment of a single patient is extensive. Increased specialization by the health care providers and health care institutions, reimbursement procedures by third-party payers (such as insurance companies), cumbersome federal regulatory organizations, and state health care regulatory agencies all affect the consumer (the patient) and the type and quality of care provided.

Maintaining one's autonomy and ensuring that continuity of care is received within the maze of the present health care delivery system is an ongoing challenge for the medical care consumer. Understanding what procedures are done, why, and by whom is a frustrating and often impossible task for patients already bewildered and frightened by medical conditions that threaten their well-being. The right to choose which method of care will be provided or who will provide that care becomes a terrifying dilemma, which many times cannot be resolved by the patient.

Delivery of Patient Care

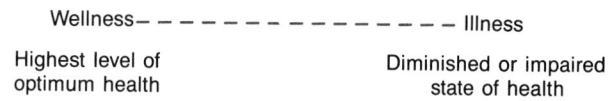

The delivery of patient care is an extremely humanistic activity. It is the delivery of services by human beings to human beings. It involves not only the treatment of disease and injury but the prevention of disease, the restoration of optimum wellness through rehabilitation, the maintenance of a desirable level of wellness through such procedures as kidney dialysis, the care of the chronically ill, the provision of assistance to the patient in the arduous process of self-care, and patient education.

The development of an individualized care plan is needed to identify individual needs of the patient and to plan a systematic approach to meet those needs. The nursing process (discussed in Chapter 5) provides the means by which a patient's individual needs are identified, and a plan of health care is developed to meet those expressed needs. The care plan involves both professional and paraprofessional health care providers who, through a coordinated and cooperative effort, work toward meeting the patient's total needs in a holistic, caring manner.

Participants in the health care system. The **patient,** the consumer of health care services, is the central focus of those activities performed by more than 200 types of health providers identified in the health care system in the United States. Physicians, dentists, osteopathic physicians, surgeons, psychiatrists, and other professional health care specialists must pass examinations in their specialty to become *board certified* and be permitted to practice in their area of specialization. In many cases physicians employ persons who have specialized training to function in cooperation with the physician. These people may be physician assistants or nurse practitioners.

The registered nurse (RN), a direct health care giver, has completed one of three types of nursing education programs: a 4-year baccalaureate degree program; a 2-year associate degree program; or a 3-year diploma program. On satisfactory completion of one of these programs, the graduate nurse is eligible to take the National Council Licensing Examination for Registered Nurses (NCLEX-RN). The registered nurse practices in a variety of settings, performing skills within the parameters of the education received and the scope of nursing practice as outlined in the state's Nurse Practice Act.

The LPN/LVN functions under the supervision of the registered nurse. Working together, they are the direct patient caregivers in most institutions. The activity of the LPN/LVN is based on the scope of practice outlined in a given state's Nurse Practice Act.

Other caregivers are required to be registered and to have specialized education and training that are dictated by their professional organizations. For example, the social worker is trained to counsel patients who may have social, emotional, or environmental problems. The patient may be referred to other agencies or professionals for specific care and treatment. The physical therapist, on the other hand, uses precise methods of massage, exercise, and hydrotherapy that may help restore physical muscular functioning of the body. The dietician is trained to provide the intake of foods that will meet the nutritional requirements of the patient. The respiratory therapist assists the patient by administering oxygen, monitoring and maintaining ventilators, drawing blood for blood gas analysis, and performing other pulmonary function tests.

Technologists and medical technicians are among the group of laboratory, radiology, and other diagnostic personnel who are prepared to assist the medical professional staff in their attempt to diagnose and treat disease and injury. The term *technologist* refers to those who have a baccalaureate degree, whereas the term *technician* refers to those who have an associate degree or less. Paraprofessionals are those persons educated to assist the professional in providing care for the patient. The nursing assistant is educated in basic nursing techniques and performs under the supervision of the registered nurse. The ward clerk is mainly a secretary, preparing and maintaining patients' records, ordering supplies, scheduling diagnostic tests, performing receptionist duties, and directing the flow of traffic in the patient care unit. These are only a sampling of the health care participants in the health care system.

Environmental factors affecting health and illness. Social and physical environmental factors do not necessarily cause illness, but they do influence the development or progression of an illness. Personal financial hardship, life-style, social pressures, and major societal issues, such as AIDS, abortion, and drug abuse, are some of the more obvious social factors. Stress, conflict, smoking, excessive weight, alcoholism, and the impact of today's high technology are among the physical factors.

Reactions to these factors vary from patient to patient. Fear of illness and dehumanization, loss of identity, and loss of control can affect one's mental state, whereas an imbalance in body functions can affect one's physical condition. Although we tend to separate social factors from physical factors, it must be emphasized that one group affects the other and vice versa.

Early recognition of the effect of environmental factors on a patient and prompt intervention by family, health care providers, or the patient himself can decrease or minimize any negative impact.

Expectations of the patient and health care team. Each patient is unique, possessing a personality, different background, different life-style, and various levels of education. His needs, expectations, and response to health care are influenced by all of these factors.

The belief held by most people in the United States is that everyone has a right to health care, regardless of race, color, creed, or economic status. This health care includes the treatment of disease, as well as preventive medicine. The acute awareness of preventive medicine today has resulted in an emphasis on the wellness continuum through education about issues such as smoking, heart disease, drug and alcohol abuse, weight control, stress syndrome, and social diseases.

Ironically, there is less emphasis on the treatment of illness than on its prevention in the mind of most people. They believe that once they become ill, they are no longer in control of their health. Subsequently, when a person does become ill and seeks medical attention, there is an expectation that it will be provided in a knowledgeable, safe, expeditious manner that will lead to a cure. It is expected that the health care providers will work in a cooperative manner for the benefit of the patient and that the cost of the care will be reasonable and, most important, paid for by somebody else (an insurance company or the government). It is presumed that the service will be highly satisfactory, and it is hoped that a cure will follow.

There is one more expectation that is not as obvious as those stated above and most often overlooked by health care workers. Patients expect to be treated like human beings and to have their rights respected. In 1972 the

BOX 1-2 THE PATIENT'S BILL OF RIGHTS Very important!

- The patient has the right to considerate and respectful care.
- The patient has the right to obtain from his physician complete current information concerning his diagnosis, treatment, and prognosis in terms the patient can be reasonably expected to understand. When it is not medically advisable to give such information to the patient, the information should be made available to an appropriate person in his behalf. He has the right to know by name, the physician responsible for coordinating his care.
- The patient has the right to receive from his physician information necessary to give informed consent prior to the start of any procedure and/or treatment. Except in emergencies, such information for informed consent, should include, but not necessarily be limited to, the specific procedure and/or treatment, the medically significant risks involved, and the probable duration of incapacity. Where medically significant, alternatives for care or treatment exist, or when the patient requests information concerning medical alternatives, the patient has the right to such information. The patient also has the right to know the name of the person responsible for the procedures and/or treatment.
- The patient has the right to refuse treatment to the extent permitted by law, and to be informed of the medical consequences of his action.
- The patient has the right to every consideration of his privacy concerning his own medical care program. Case discussion, consultation, examination, and treatment are confidential and should be conducted discreetly. Those not directly involved in his care must have permission of the patient to be present.
- The patient has the right to expect that all communications and records pertaining to his care should be treated as confidential.
- The patient has the right to expect that within its capacity a hospital must make reasonable response to the request of a patient for services. The hospital must provide evaluation, service, and/or referral indicated by the urgency of the case. When medically permissible the patient may be transferred to another facility only after he has received complete information and explanation concerning the needs for and alternatives to such a transfer. The institution to which the patient is to be transferred must first have accepted the patient for transfer.
- The patient has the right to obtain information as to any relationship of his hospital to other health care and educational institutions insofar as his care is concerned. The patient has the right to obtain information as to the existence of any professional relationships among individuals, by name, who are treating him.
- The patient has the right to be advised if the hospital proposes to engage in or perform human experimentation affecting his care or treatment. The patient has the right to refuse to participate in such research projects.
- The patient has the right to expect reasonable continuity of care. He has the right to know in advance what appointment times and physicians are available and where. The patient has the right to expect that the hospital will provide a mechanism whereby he is informed by his physician or a delegate of the physician of the patient's continuing health care requirements following discharge.
- The patient has the right to examine and receive an explanation of his bill regardless of source of payment.
- The patient has the right to know what hospital rules and regulations apply to his conduct as a patient.

American Hospital Association issued a "Patient's Bill of Rights" (Box 1-2) in an effort to ensure that this expectation be realized. This document assured patients that they have the right to high-quality care, the right to respect and dignity, the right of access to information about the illness and/or treatment, the right to be involved in decisions about the care being provided, the right of informed consent, the right to express concerns about the care being provided, and the right to refuse care.

The delivery of health care needs to be a process of mutual exchange between patients and health care givers. Whereas patients expect the "rights" as outlined, health care workers expect something as well. Health care professionals expect that patients will actively participate in their care as much as possible by taking an active role in the planning process, by having an understanding of the care and the treatment given, by asking questions, by following the treatment plan prescribed, by acting responsibly with respect to their own conditions, and by giving health care workers the same respect that patients are entitled to.

Interdisciplinary approach to health care. The primary goal of the health care team is the optimal physical, mental, and social well-being of the patient. This goal is achieved by promoting and restoring health within the wellness/illness continuum. It is imperative that health care personnel, when working to meet the needs of the patient, work together as a health care team. Each member of the team must coordinate his or her activity with every other member of the team by developing a comprehensive care plan, by effectively communicating, and by keeping accurate records. A care plan is a document that outlines the individual needs of the patient and the approach to meeting these needs. It further identifies who will assist in treating the patient. The document guides and directs the activities surrounding the patient's care and ensures that continuity and consistency of care will be provided.

Good communication is essential for the exchange of information among the members of the health care team. This communication ensures that either the care plan is meeting the needs of the patient or if it is not, there is opportunity to make appropriate changes. (See Chapter 4 for a further discussion of communication.)

Documentation in any form is the permanent record of the patient's progress and treatment. It constitutes the formal and legal record of care received by the patient and the patient's response to that care. The information recorded during the entire course of treatment serves many purposes. It provides a progress record of treatment so that all of the involved health care members are aware of what treatment the patient is receiving. It also provides a history of events, which may be valuable in the future treatment of the same condition. (See Chapter 6 for a further discussion of documentation.)

Following this interdisciplinary approach to treatment prevents the fragmentation of patient care. Just as the plan of care for patients is developed in a holistic manner, so is the actual delivery of health care. Health care providers must never forget that the central focus of all of their activity is the patient.

PRACTICAL/VOCATIONAL NURSING

The role of the practical/vocational nurse is not new within the health care delivery system. The role and responsibilities have expanded from bathing patients, cooking, and light housekeeping to performing skilled tasks needed to provide health care to people within the wellness/illness continuum.

The role of the LPN/LVN continues to evolve in the midst of a nursing shortage and the controversy of the future of nursing as a profession. This evolution is influenced by the various states' Nurse Practice Acts, individual changes within the health care agencies that use the LPN/LVN, the availability of health care workers, and the needs of patients.

The blend of nursing history and today's health care delivery system sets the foundation for the career of an LPN/LVN.

Definition of Practical/Vocational Nursing

Practical/vocational nursing is defined as the activity of providing specific services to patients under the direct supervision of a licensed physician or dentist and/or registered nurse. The services are provided in a structured setting surrounding the caring for the sick, the rehabilitation of the sick and injured, and the prevention of sickness and injury. This definition is adapted from the NAPNES and several states' Nurse Practice Acts.

Objectives, Components, and Characteristics of Practice

The stated objectives for practical/vocational nursing practice are the following:

- To acquire specialized knowledge and skill that is needed to meet the health care needs of patients in a variety of settings
- To be a graduate of a state-approved practical/vocational nursing program
- To take and pass the NCLEX-PN examination
- To acquire a state license to practice

To accomplish these objectives, the students must assume the responsibility for their own education, intensive study, and dedication to duty. Organizing one's time effectively helps accomplish these objectives and ultimately assures the patient safe and competent care.

Distinguishing characteristics for practice by the LPN/LVN are shown in Box 1-3.

BOX 1-3

CHARACTERISTICS, ROLE, AND RESPONSIBILITIES OF THE PRACTICAL/VOCATIONAL NURSE

- Being a responsible and accountable member of the health care team
- Maintaining a current license
- Practicing within the scope of the Nurse Practice Act
- Performing within the limits of one's educational preparation
- Participating in continuing education activities
- Recognizing one's limitation and seeking assistance
- Being an effective member of the health care team
- Using the nursing process in meeting patient's needs
- Promoting and maintaining health, preventing disease, and encouraging and assisting in rehabilitation
- Maintaining a professional appearance
- Subscribing to recognized ethical practices
- Performing within legal parameters
- Participating in activities of professional organizations
- Assisting in developing the role of the licensed practical/vocational nurse of tomorrow

Roles and Responsibilities of the Practical/Vocational Nurse

In 1981 NAPNES issued the following statement of responsibilities required for practice as a practical/vocational nurse:

- Recognizes the LPN/LVN's role in the health care delivery system and articulates that role with those of other health care team members
- Maintains accountability for one's own nursing practice within the ethical and legal framework
- Serves as a patient advocate
- Accepts their role in maintaining developing standards of practice in providing health care
- Seeks further growth through educational opportunities

Practical/vocational nursing is an exciting, challenging career that provides an opportunity to care for others while receiving personal satisfaction. The focus is on bedside/personal care of patients in a variety of settings that requires knowledge, skill, and expertise to perform in a responsible, accountable manner.

REFERENCES AND SUGGESTED READINGS

1. Alfano GJ: A rose is a rose . . . . licensed nurse, Geriatr Nurs 9(2):87, 1988.
2. Becker BG and Fendler DJ: Vocational and personal adjustments in practical nursing, ed 6, St Louis, 1990, The CV Mosby Co.
3. Carlson R and Newman B: Issues and trends in health care, St Louis, 1987, The CV Mosby Co.
4. Cress L and others: LP/VNs: the modern Nightingale, vocal, vigilant, valuable, Pract Nurs 37(2):28, 1987.
5. Donahue MP: Nursing: the finest art—an illustrated history, St Louis, 1986, The CV Mosby Co.
6. Ellis JR and Hartley CL: Nursing in today's world: challenges, issues, and trends, ed 3, Philadelphia, 1988, JB Lippincott Co.
7. Forfa L and others: Building a better place to practice for the LP/VN, J Pract Nurs 37(2):33, 1987.
8. Glanze WD and others: Mosby's medical and nursing dictionary, ed 3, St Louis, 1990, The CV Mosby Co.
9. Harkness-Hood G and Dincher JR: Total patient care: foundations and practice, ed 7, St Louis, 1988, The CV Mosby Co.
10. Kalish PA and Kalish BJ: The advance of American nursing, ed 2, Boston, 1985, Little, Brown & Co, Inc.
11. Kelly LY: Dimensions of professional nursing, ed 5, New York, 1985, Macmillan Publishing Co.
12. Kelly LY: The nursing experience: trends, challenges, and transitions, New York, 1987, Macmillan Publishing Co.
13. Kenney E: An LPN looks at the developing LPN role, Issues 7(2):6, 1986.
14. Levey S and Loomba NP: Health care administration, ed 2, Philadelphia, 1984, JB Lippincott Co.
15. McCloskey JC and Grace HK: Current issues in nursing, ed 3, St Louis, 1990, The CV Mosby Co.
16. Nightingale F: Notes on nursing: what it is and what it is not, London, 1859, Harrison & Sons.
17. Nivens B: Careers without a degree, Essence Magazine, p 124, Sept 1, 1988.
18. O'Brien P: All a woman's life can bring, Nurs Res 36(1):12, 1987.
19. Reverby S: A caring dilemma: womanhood and nursing in historical perspective, Nurs Res 36(1):5, 1987.
20. Southmayd N and others: A clinical ladder for the LPN, Pract Nurs 35(3):20, 1985.
21. Strickland P and others: Characteristics of nursing staff in long-term care facilities: their training, experience, and perceived proficiency levels, Nursing Home 36(1):22, 1987.
22. Walters S: Why I want to be an LPN, J Pract Nurs 39(1):42, 1989.
23. Walters S: And why I choose to remain an LPN, J Pract Nurs 39(1):44, 1989.

CHAPTER CHALLENGE

KEY POINTS

- The evolution of nursing was greatly influenced by the way the sick and injured were cared for.
- The influence of Florence Nightingale on nursing practice and nursing education was highly significant in the nineteenth century.
- Nursing practice and education in the United States were significantly influenced by activities of Florence Nightingale.
- Practical/vocational nursing rapidly developed to meet the increasing demand for nursing services facing the health care consumer.
- Mandatory licensure laws were established for practical/vocational nursing education and practice.
- The wellness/illness continuum is the range of a person's total health situation.
- Prevention of illness and injury and continuity of patient care is an integral component of holistic health care.
- The practical/vocational nurse is one of many of the large groups of health care workers who provide health care services.
- The role and responsibilities of the practical/vocational nursing community function in accordance with the several states' Nurse Practice Acts.

STUDY QUESTIONS

Like "Adjustments" Test

1. Factor(s) that influence a change in nursing and nursing education is/are:
   a. The interrelationship of man with his environment
   b. The search for knowledge and truth through education
   c. Technological advances
   d. All of the above
2. Medicine men performed witchcraft on the affected part of the body to induce evil spirits to leave the body by using:
   a. Frightening masks, vile odors, and sacrifices
   b. Proven therapeutic techniques
   c. Advanced medical practices
   d. Prayers to the gods
3. Florence Nightingale was a strong-minded, intelligent young woman whose interest in nursing was a result of all but one of the following:
   a. Strong desire to excel in nursing
   b. Dominance over the opposition of her family and friends
   c. Influence by Theodor Fliedner
   d. Strong desire to help others
4. A deviation from standards of nursing education and practice during the early twentieth century became commonplace because of:
   a. The effects of World War I, the Depression, and World War II
   b. National norms of competence established by states' licensure laws
   c. Characteristics of the health care industry that remained unchanging
   d. None of the above
5. The focus of practical/vocational nursing programs has historically been on:
   a. The care of patients in a hospital setting
   b. Home nursing care, cooking, laundry, and light housekeeping duties
   c. Complex nursing procedures
   d. All of the above
6. The components of the health care system today include:
   a. Professional and paraprofessional health care providers
   b. Consumers who are the recipients of health care services
   c. Health care agencies, such as hospitals and nursing homes
   d. All of the above
7. Licensed practical/vocational nursing is:
   a. Total, independent nursing practice
   b. The practice of specific services under the supervision of a registered nurse or a licensed physician
   c. Institutional licensure only
   d. Achieved through on-the-job training only

2

Legal Aspects of Nursing

PERSEPHONE C. AGRAFIOTIS

LEARNING OBJECTIVES

After reading this chapter, the student should be able to do the following:

- Define the key terms.
- Outline the development of the legal influence on health care.
- Describe the parts of the legal process.
- Define the legal relationship between the patient and the practical/vocational nurse.
- Describe the legal protection system and controls available for both the patient and practical/vocational nurse.

RELATED TOPICS OF INTEREST

- The evolution of nursing (Chapter 1)
- Ethical aspects of nursing (Chapter 3)
- Communication (Chapter 4)
- Documentation (Chapter 6)
- Principles and practice of medication administration (Chapter 25)
- The world of the graduate (Chapter 57)

KEY TERMS

Define the following:

- answer
- appeal
- complaint
- damages
- defendant
- deposition
- discovery
- interrogatories
- judgment
- law
- liability
- litigate
- malpractice
- mandatory
- negligence
- plaintiff
- statute
- summons
- tort

situational ethics

THE EVOLUTION OF LEGAL ISSUES IN THE DELIVERY OF HEALTH CARE

No system operates in a vacuum, and the health care delivery system is no exception. As the health care providers within the system deliver numerous services to the consumer, they must practice within the limits established by federal and state legislation. Court-rendered definitions of health care and court decisions that establish precedents have operational implications that affect how, when, where, and to whom health care will be provided.

The law requires that a minimum standard should be met. Ethical standards may require a higher standard and are set by the requirements and/or needs of a particular situation.

Historical Perspective

In early times laws were developed by a monarch, the church, the ruling class, or other persons whom the people accepted as having the "right" to make decisions for them. Either these persons were given the right to make these decisions because of their knowledge, expertise, and position or they assumed the right based on power they were able to exert over the people.

Laws were developed from **judgments** that came forth when those having the right or the power to make decisions did so on a case-by-case basis. Future laws and rules continued to be developed on such decisions and contributed to the establishment of a system of rules by which the people lived. This form of case law established by a given society's rulers, and later by judges, became known as "common law" or "judge-made law".

With the advent of societal development, governing rules for the people became more formal and legislative bodies were added to the common law approach. The formation of the legislative bodies followed the creation of parliament in England and congress in the United States.

Law became known as the reference to a rule, principle, or regulation established and made known by a government to protect or to restrict the people affected.

As we have seen from the historical perspective of nursing, clearly defined laws for health care were nonexistent well into the nineteenth century. Until then, laws that were passed emphasized human freedom, personal liberty, and property rights.

In the health care field, the fundamental principles that governed behavior came from people such as Hippocrates, Florence Nightingale, Dorothea Dix, and Clara Barton. Their efforts to assist the poor, the sick, and the infirm brought about significant changes in the delivery of health care that became the foundation for the standards of practice and eventually the passage of laws for the protection of the consumer.

THE LEGAL PROCESS

The legal process enables a person to look at societal issues and to respond to problems with a broad background of experience that is based on laws established by the people and for the people that they ultimately affect. The laws provide fundamental rights and establish relationships between governmental bodies and the citizenry. The validity of the legislation passed and the regulations established is measured against either federal or state constitutional standards, or both, depending on the issue in question.

The Legal System in the United States and Its Influence on the Health Care System

Law refers to man-made rules and regulations that derive their authority from various sources. In the United States there are three levels of government involved with establishing law: the federal, the state, and the local levels. These bodies produce statutory law. These laws are passed by the legislative bodies created by the United States Congress, state legislative bodies, and city councils. **Statutes** are officially acted on or voted on by the legislative bodies and are compiled into codes, collections of statutes, or city ordinances.

To enact these laws, administrative agencies are established with the power to implement the rules and regulations that enforce statutory law. These rules and regulations are known as administrative laws.

Judicial or decision laws are those made by courts of law and that interpret legal issues that are being disputed. The interpretation of statutes and regulations decides which of two conflicting approaches applies to a given situation. Once decided, a precedent is established for future interpretation of the law in question.

Legal health care issues began to surface in the courts as early as 1852 when a case before the North Carolina Supreme Court asked that court to define the health care status of a slave suffering with myopia (near-sightedness). The court noted that healthy meant "free from disease or bodily ailments." The court extended the definition by adding the word "sound," which in their opinion meant "whole, right, nothing the matter, and free from any defect." The court's interpretation and subsequent decision supported the claim that the slave was unfit to work because of his condition.

Five years later the North Carolina Supreme Court was again asked to determine the level of health of a slave who had a contracted finger. In a lengthy opinion, the court interpreted health, healthy, and soundness with regard to the contracted finger. It decided that the condition was somewhat less than healthy but not totally unhealthy and therefore the slave could perform the work required of him.

Such questions surrounding health care continue to be debated in the courts today. However, the complexity of the cases and the adequacy of the treatment or care of the patient have increased dramatically as evidenced by some of the malpractice suit judgments and awards made by the courts. The outcome of these court debates, from the seemingly insignificant to the more serious, continue to influence the health care delivery system and the individual behavior of everyone working in that system, including the practical/vocational nurse. An example of a court case is presented as follows:

Rodriquez V. Columbus Hospital, 326 N.Y.S.2d. 438 (New York 1971). A 49-year-old died of anaphylactic shock following an injection of penicillin. The allegation made by the family of the deceased was that the licensed practical nurse injected the drug into the patient's bloodstream instead of muscle tissue. The jury awarded $100,000.

Components and Characteristics of the Legal Process

Judicial or decision law involving the health care delivery system is increasing because of issues being litigated between the consumer and the health care provider.

Litigation (a lawsuit) begins when a complaining party (the **plaintiff**) files a document known as a **complaint** with the court. This document states the basis for the complaint and outlines the **damages** (compensation) sought by the plaintiff. The person at whom the complaint is directed is known as the **defendant.** The filing of a complaint is followed by the issue of a **summons,** which is a court order advising the defendant that a lawsuit against him is pending. It further notifies the defendant what he must do with respect to the lawsuit and the time constraints involved.

If the defendant, once served, chooses to do nothing in response to the summons, such as hire an attorney or file a countercomplaint, the court may enter a default judgment against the defendant, which is based on the uncontested testimony of the plaintiff.

A defendant presented with a summons normally retains an attorney, who then files a document called an appearance, which prevents the court from entering a default judgment. The defendant, through his attorney, then files a response **(answer)** to the allegations made in the complaint. This response either admits or denies the allegations made. If the response by the defendant includes significant information not referred to in the original complaint, the plaintiff, through his attorney, has the option to file a reply.

When all of the allegations by both parties have been addressed, the case is ready to move forward and the parties are said to be "at issue." **Discovery** procedures are then initiated, whereby relevant information is gathered by both sides. **Depositions** (testimony taken under oath) and **interrogatories** (written questions) of witnesses are taken from witnesses before the scheduled trial. During this pretrial period, efforts may be made by either side to influence the outcome of the lawsuit. Such efforts include, but are not limited to, motions to dismiss the complaint, requests to change the trial date, and offers of a settlement out of court.

If motions to dismiss the lawsuit are denied and all other motions have been resolved by the court, the case then goes to trial. The court hears the evidence, comes to certain conclusions, and decides on a verdict. Once the judge or jury reaches a decision and a verdict is declared, either party may **appeal** that verdict to an appellate court. If an appeal is granted, the testimony and the procedures of the trial are reviewed by the appellate court. That court may choose to uphold or reverse the decision of the lower court. The right to an appeal is a constitutional right and serves as part of the system of checks and balances on the court system of the United States.

The time period for the process of litigation and the outcome of that litigation varies, depending on many factors that are peculiar to each case. Predominant factors are (1) the severity of the complaint, (2) whether an injury or a death is involved, and (3) the backlog of cases pending before the court.

The Legal Relationship of the Patient and the Practical/Vocational Nurse

The role of the practical/vocational nurse is changing rapidly in the dynamic world of health care today. This ever-changing environment contributes to the uncertainty that exists while performing the duties and accepting the responsibilities of a practical/vocational nurse. These changes require a keen awareness of the state laws that control and regulate the activities of both the nurses and the institutions employing them.

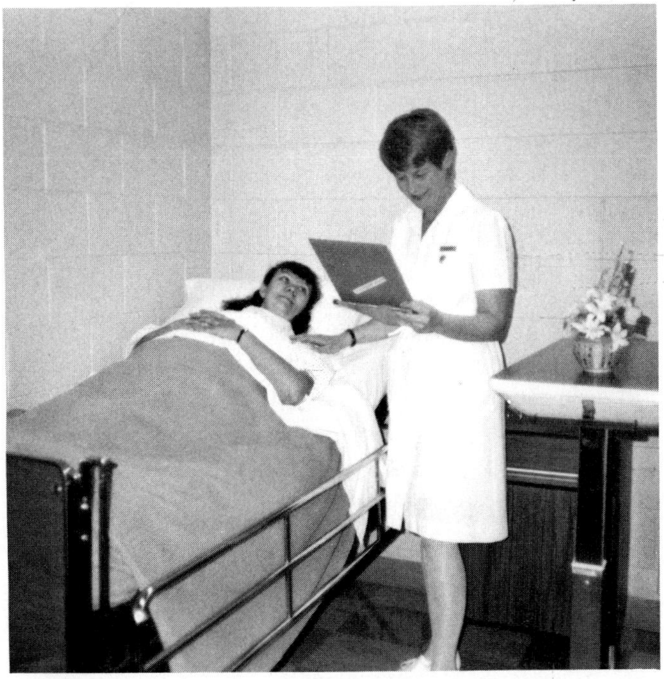

Knowledge of the law, rules and regulations, and even existing institutional policy is essential to (1) make informed decisions concerning the care given to patients; (2) become a responsive and responsible employee in the health care system; and (3) achieve personal and professional satisfaction.

LEGAL ISSUES

Legal precedents that have been made over the years have well established the right of both patient and nurse to be protected when involved in receiving or giving health care services.

The patient has the right to expect that the practical/vocational nurse will act in the patient's best interest by providing proper care based on existing standards, the Patient's Bill of Rights, and the principle of informed consent. See Box 2-1 for a list of common legal terms.

Nurses, on the other hand, must rely on the rights granted in their respective states' Nurse Practice Acts. These rights vary from state to state but generally are intended to provide basic legal protection for nurses provided they are operating professionally, prudently, and within the scope of their authority.

Controls for the Protection of the Patient

Devotion to duty by the health care professional is an expectation that every patient depends on when suffering from an illness or injury and under medical care. However, the legal system requires more stringent and tangible controls that can be recorded, observed, and measured against a standard. It is these standards that provide the key control for patient protection.

Standards of care. Standards of care are determined in a variety of ways. They are devised by professional organizations, the Nurse Practice Acts of each state, guidelines established by accrediting bodies for hospitals, nursing homes, educational programs, and other health care agencies, and finally by the people who are charged with providing that care.

These standards define those acts that are permitted to be performed or prohibited from being performed by a prudent person working within the parameters of his or her training, license, and experience and the conditions existing at the time. These standards are the ruler against which the practical/vocational nurse's performance is measured with respect to providing patient care.

Patients' rights. Today's consumers of health care services are more knowledgeable than ever about their own medical and health care needs. They are also extremely knowledgeable about what they can and cannot expect in health care services.

Over the years, a number of documents regarding patients' rights have been published. The National League

BOX 2-1 COMMON LEGAL TERMS

abandonment To desert, surrender, or give up rights
affidavit Written or printed statement of facts
assault Any willful attempt to injure another person
battery Unlawful application of force to another person
breach Breaking a law by either commission or omission
burden of proof Proving a fact or facts in a dispute
commission The authority or instructions given to a person to conduct business
competent Duly qualified
complaint The original pleading by which an action begins under Rules of Civil Procedure
crime Any act done in violation of performing a duty
defamation The act of using ridicule and contempt as a means of negatively affecting one's reputation
due process of law Law in its regular course of administration through the courts of justice
felony A crime graver than or more serious than a misdemeanor
fraud False representation of a present or past fact
liable Accountable by law
libel A malicious written document or oral pronouncement intended to blacken a person's reputation
malpractice Misconduct or failure to render the degree of skill and learning common to a professional service
maltreatment Improper or unskilled treatment
misdemeanor Offense lower than a felony and generally punishable by fines
negligence Omission to do something that a reasonable or prudent person would do
omission Neglect or failure to perform a duty
prudent The use of good judgment and reason
slander Speaking words intended to defame or prejudice another in reputation
statute An act of the legislature declaring, commanding, or prohibiting something
suit Any proceeding against another in a court of law
testimony Evidence given by a competent witness under oath
tort Private or civil wrong or injury
victim A person who is the object of a crime

Adapted from Black HC: Black's law dictionary, ed 5, St Paul, Minn, 1979, West Publishing Co.

for Nursing (NLN) in 1959 published a document titled "What People Can Expect of Modern Nursing Practice." In 1972 the American Hospital Association (AHA) issued the "Statement on a Patient's Bill of Rights" (see Box 1-2, p. 12). In that same year the Pennsylvania Insurance Department issued a document called the "Citizen's Bill of Hospital Rights."

In 1973 Minnesota became the first state to incorporate patients' rights into a law and the Congress of the United States passed the Rehabilitation Act, which granted services to handicapped persons. In 1980 the Mental Health Patient's Bill of Rights and the Pregnant Patient's Bill of Rights came into law.

The Joint Commission on Accreditation of Healthcare Organizations (JCAHO) includes an entire section on the "Rights and Responsibilities of Patients" in its accreditation manual. Among the rights that hospitals must provide to patients to be accredited are access to health care, the right to respect and dignity, the right to privacy and confidentiality, the right to personal safety, the right to their identity, the right to information about their treatment and hospital rules and regulations, the right to communication with the health care staff, the right to give or not give consent, the right to consultation, the right to refuse treatment, the right to know what the charges for their treatment or care will be, and the right to transfer and continuity of care.

On the other hand, patients also have responsibilities, such as providing information about themselves and their condition, complying with instructions given them in conjunction with their care and treatment, and behaving within the rules and regulations of the institution.

Informed consent. One important aspect of the Patient's Bill of Rights is the matter of informed consent (Fig. 2-1). Before any invasive treatments or procedures can be performed on patients, they must consent to treatment. Not only must they give their consent, they must also be allowed to make an informed choice as to whether an alternate method of treatment and/or care will be provided or whether the proposed treatment is, in fact, necessary.

Procedures must be followed that provide in nontechnical terms an explanation to patients of the preferred treatment, the risks involved, alternative courses of treatment, and who will be perfoming the treatment or procedure. Included in these procedures should be a method to ensure that patients understand what they are told.

Following such procedures not only helps to avoid unnecessary lawsuits but establishes a relationship of trust between the patient and the health care providers.

Controls for the Protection of the Practical/Vocational Nurse

Standards of care not only assure patients that practical/vocational nurses will perform their duties based on the criteria established by the profession, they also protect the nurses.

INFORMED CONSENT FOR AMNIOCENTESIS

I. I hereby request and authorize Doctor ______________________ to perform a diagnostic amniocentesis (pass a needle through the abdominal wall and withdraw some of the amniotic fluid). I further request that an attempt be made to perform the following test(s) on my unborn child:

A. Chromosome analysis __________ (Initial)

B. Alpha-fetoprotein __________ (Initial)

C. Acetylcholinesterase (If indicated) __________ (Initial)

D. __________________ __________ (Initial)

II. I consent to the performance of an ultrasound examination for the purpose of dating the pregnancy, locating the placenta and selecting a site for placement of the needle.

III. I understand that:

A. the procedure of amniocentesis involves a small risk to both mother and fetus and that these risks include; discomfort at the site where the needle was inserted, cramping, bloody spotting, leakage of amniotic fluid, intrauterine infection and miscarriage.

B. there is a possibility that growing the fetal cells may not be successful and that repeat amniocentesis would then be required.

C. although the liklihood of an error is considered to be extremely small, a complete and correct diagnosis of the condition of the fetus based on the test(s) performed cannot be guaranteed.

D. the results provided of normal chromosomes or normal biochemical status of the fetus does not eliminate the possibility that the child may have birth defects and/or mental retardation because of other disorders.

E. in the case of twins, the results may apply to only one of the pair.

F. in some Rh negative mothers Rh sensitization has occurred following amniocentesis.

IV. I have had my questions answered and understand and accept the risks and limitations of this test.

Signed: ______________________________ (Patient)

______________________________ (Spouse)

______________________________ (Witness)

Date: ______________________________

FIG. 2-1 Sample consent form for a special procedure. A signed informed consent is **mandatory** for invasive procedures for the protection of the patient, physician, and facility. (Courtesy The Children's Mercy Hospital, Kansas City, Mo.)

The standards of care that a reasonable person would use in a particular circumstance are made known through the Nurse Practice Acts of each state, the rules and regulations established by administrative law, standing operating procedures of the various health care agencies, and employee policies of the health care institutions.

Deviations from the standards of care provide grounds for charges of **negligence** or **malpractice.** The nurse has a responsibility to behave in a reasonable and prudent manner within the parameters of the accepted standards of care. The best protection that nurses have against potential lawsuits is that they act within the scope of the standards of care that are expected in a given circumstance.

Nurse Practice Acts. The Nurse Practice Act of each state contains a legal definition of nursing practice and delineates the area of practice that the law seeks to regulate.

Included in the acts are the duties and functions that the various levels of nurses can perform and under what circumstances they can be performed. The acts provide definitions for nursing practice, registered nursing, practical/vocational nursing, and advanced practice for nurses.

Rules and regulations. Administrative rules and regulations are written within the scope of the authority granted by the legislative body of the respective state.

Administrative agencies, such as the board of nursing in each state, develop the rules and regulations that ensure that the Nurse Practice Act can be effectively implemented. These rules and regulations detail how the act will be implemented and describe procedures that are measurable and enforceable.

Standard operating procedures. Each health care agency has established standard operating procedures that have been approved by its administrative body.

Standard operating procedures are written documents that contain rules, policies, procedures, regulations, and orders for the conduct of patient care in various stipulated circumstances that are unique to the agency making them known. In such procedures, conditions are usually specified under which a prescribed action is to be taken. Health care providers are guided as they provide care in their institution or agency. The standard operating procedures of an organization are the means of establishing and maintaining the standards for the organization.

Employee policies. Employee policies, often described in a handbook that is distributed to all newly hired employees, should provide personnel with key information about the operation of the organization. These policy statements should include such information as the organization's philosophy, goals, rules, regulations, procedures, and behavioral expectations. It is important for all employees to understand the operation and responsibility of the organization as it relates to their positions in that organization.

BOX 2-2 DO'S AND DO NOT'S

Do document all unusual incidences.
Do report all unusual incidences.
Do follow policies and procedures as established by your employing agency.
Do keep current your license to practice.
Do perform procedures that you have been taught and that are within the standard scope of your practice.
Do protect patients from injuring themselves.

Do not remove side rails on patients' beds unless there is an order or hospital policy to do so.
Do not allow patients to leave the hospital or nursing home unless there is an order or signed release.
Do not accept money or gifts from patients.
Do not give advice that is contrary to doctor's orders or the nursing care plan.
Do not give medical advice to friends and neighbors.
Do not witness a patient's will.
Do not take medications that belong to patients.
Do not work as a licensed practical/vocational nurse in a state in which you are not licensed.

Good Samaritan Acts. Good Samaritan Acts provide rules that govern how a citizen within a state can, by law, act in lending assistance to another citizen. It is especially written to encourage health care providers to render assistance to people in distress or at the scene of an accident.

These acts protect health care providers from civil liability while rendering help to people in need. Because of these acts, health care providers are immune from any liability from suit that might be brought against them.

Liability protection. The ever-changing environment of health care and the complexity of the legal system contribute to a higher incidence of medical malpractice lawsuits in the United States than ever before. Whereas in the past, the physician and the health care institution were usually the targets of lawsuits, health care providers at every level are now equally vulnerable.

Health care agencies and institutions usually provide an adequate level of malpractice insurance to cover their employees under normally adverse situations. However, this coverage does not always provide the full range of protection that is sometimes needed under unusual or unforeseen circumstances. This kind of protective insurance can be found only in a personal, professional **liability** insurance policy. Carrying malpractice insurance, once the burden only of a physician, now is a consideration for the nurse as well. Malpractice insurance provides personal protection by paying damages, when warranted, against the nurse. It also pays for legal fees, bonds, and lost wages under certain circumstances.

Although this is neither an endorsement of malpractice insurance for the nurse nor an indictment of society's view of the medical and health care profession's behavior, it is a fact that every nurse must accept. Box 2–2 contains *do's* and *do not's* for the practical/vocational nurse as guidelines for safe practice.

REFERENCES AND SUGGESTED READINGS

1. Cowdrey ML: Basic law for the allied health professional, Monterey, Calif, 1984, Wadsworth Health Sciences.
2. Creighton H: Law every nurse should know, ed 5, Philadelphia, 1986, WB Saunders Co.
3. Cushing M: Nursing jurisprudence, Norwalk, Conn, 1988, Appleton & Lange.
4. Fiesta J: The law and liability: a guide for nurses, ed 2, New York, 1988, John Wiley & Sons, Inc.
5. Guido GW: Legal issues in nursing: a source book for practice, Norwalk, Conn, 1988, Appleton & Lange.
6. Intentional and unintentional acts: malpractice, Regan Rep Nurs Law 28:4, 1988.
7. Luguire R: Six common causes for nursing liability, Nurs 88 18(11):61, 1988.
8. Northrup CE and Kelly ME: Legal issues in nursing, St Louis, 1987, The CV Mosby Co.
9. Rocerto LR and Maleski CM: Following orders . . . and other obligations: 8 legal questions, NursingLife 4:6, 1984.
10. Sandroft R: Why you really ought to have your own malpractice policy, RN 46:28, 1983.
11. Willis-Long SL: Off duty emergency care: do you know your legal rights? NursingLife 8:31, 1988.

CHAPTER CHALLENGE

KEY POINTS

- Laws were developed on a case-by-case basis and were known as common law.
- The interpretation of statutes and regulations decides which of two conflicting approaches applies to a given situation, thus establishing precedent.
- Laws control the practice of the practical/vocational nurse.
- The patient has the right to expect care that is based on an established standard of care.
- The legal process is becoming more and more prevalent in today's health care delivery system.
- The Nurse Practice Act of each state contains a legal definition of nursing practice and delineates the area of practice that the law seeks to regulate.
- The Patient's Bill of Rights outlines what the patient can expect from the health care delivery system.
- Liability protection for the practical/vocational nurse provides personal protection in a society where increased malpractice lawsuits are filed.

STUDY QUESTIONS

1. During early times, persons who made laws, rules, and regulations were given the right to make them based on:
   a. Their knowledge and expertise
   b. Their demand that people follow their rules
   c. A and b
   d. Neither a nor b
2. A litigation includes:
   a. A plaintiff and a defendant
   b. A summons
   c. Depositions and interrogatories
   d. All of the above
3. Controls and protection for patients receiving health care include:
   a. Informed consent
   b. Standards of care
   c. A Patient's Bill of Rights
   d. All of the above
4. The Nurse Practice Act in each state includes:
   a. The legal definition of nursing
   b. Liability protection for nurses
   c. Outlines of the duties and functions of the nurse
   d. All of the above
   e. A and c
5. Administrative law is written within the scope of the authority granted by:
   a. The hospital
   b. The legislative body
   c. The nursing home
   d. None of the above

3

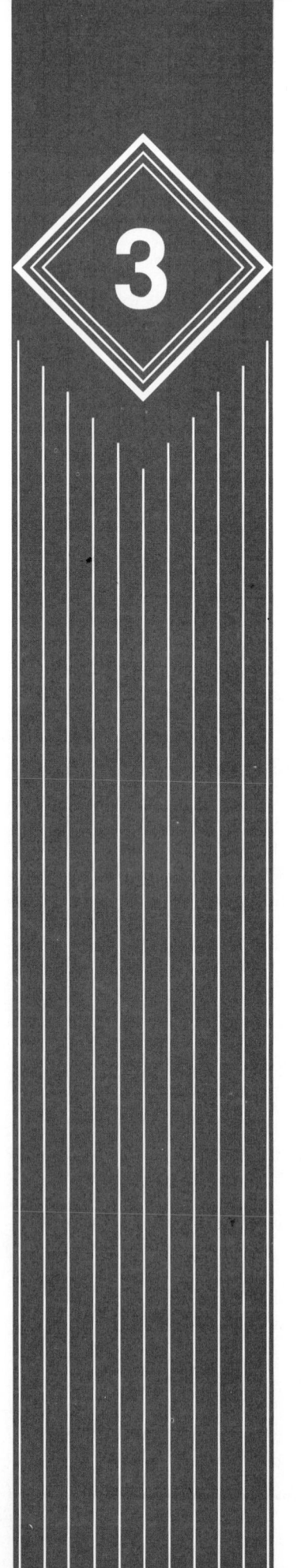

Ethical Aspects of Nursing

PERSEPHONE C. AGRAFIOTIS

LEARNING OBJECTIVES

After reading this chapter, the student should be able to do the following:

- Define the key terms.
- Describe the evolution of ethical codes involved in the delivery of health care.
- Identify the importance of value clarification in the delivery of patient care.
- Outline the ethical issues of health care.
- List ethical dilemmas faced in practicing as a practical/vocational nurse.

RELATED TOPICS OF INTEREST

- The evolution of nursing (Chapter 1)
- Legal aspects of nursing (Chapter 2)
- Care of the patient with AIDS (Chapter 40)
- Care of the patient with cancer (Chapter 41)
- Care of the mother and newborn at risk (Chapter 45)
- Hospice care (Chapter 56)

KEY TERMS

Define the following:

- autonomy
- customs
- dilemma
- ethics
- morals
- mores
- value system

THE EVOLUTION OF ETHICAL CODES AND CONSIDERATIONS

Shifting of today's attitudes and values is an obvious consequence of the tremendous change in society as a whole. Advances in medical knowledge and technology, combined with these societal changes, have greatly influenced ethical considerations of the health care delivery system. These ethical considerations are placing stress on the interpersonal and intrapersonal relationships of members of the health care community.

The role of the practical/vocational nurse has also changed significantly since the first school of practical/vocational nursing was started in 1892. This new role is one where the nurse must meet the demands of a dynamic and pluralistic society by providing effective, responsible, and ethical health care.

Practical/vocational nurses should explore, assess, and determine their own personal values and should recognize their own priorities in the decision-making process. This process must consider the patient's value system and needs.

Daily contact with patients over extended periods requires that the practical/vocational nurse respect patients as human beings and make every effort to meet their needs.

This respect is essential if meaningful, individual, and holistic patient care is to be provided.

Historical Perspective

Early history defines man as a member of a well-defined group known as the family. This family group was organized to provide solidarity and a means of survival against the hardships and adversities of the environment.

The primary means of perpetuating the family, or tribe as it was called early on, was to hand down the customs and mores that represented the way all members of the family were expected to behave. These **customs** and **mores** became the law of the land, and strict enforcement by the family leaders strongly influenced family members to obey them. Noncompliance with these customs and mores meant banishment from the group or even death.

The health care needs of the family were provided by the members themselves, usually the women. As the need for care of the sick and infirm increased and became more complex, the need evolved for a designated "expert" to provide health care. This person was the family or tribal "medicine man." The medicine man learned how to care for the sick and to keep people well. The primary method used was to ward off evil spirits, which were believed to be the cause of all illness.

The medicine man was the primary caregiver until approximately 525

BC, when the Egyptians established the position of priest physician. The priest physician was responsible for performing both the religious and medical tasks required in Egyptian society. These combined practices assured the people that not only would they be cared for while they were alive, their status in life would be preserved after death.

Hippocrates did not accept this combination of medical and religious practice. He sought to dispel the mystical approach to a healthy body. His approach saw man as having three faculties; the mind, the body, and the spirit. These faculties, he believed, existed in unison, and for an individual to attain the ideal virtuous state, these faculties must be in perfect balance. He further proposed that physician and patient share a common set of values that would allow them to agree on what is considered beneficial or harmful to one's health. This was the basis for the Hippocratic Oath.

Over the years, the affiliation between the physician and the nurse was not always equitable. The ethical standards and practices of the physician did not include the nurse. As a result, the nursing profession sought to establish its own code of ethics as the ethical issues involved with medicine and health care increased.

The work of Florence Nightingale, Lavinia Dock, and Isabel Hampton Robb persuaded the members of the American Society of Superintendents of Training Schools of Nursing to include the development of a code of ethics as one of the objectives of that organization. In 1893 Lystra E. Gretter, of the Farrand School of Nursing in Detroit, Michigan, developed an oath resembling the Hippocratic Oath, called the Nightingale Pledge. It was not until 1961 that the Code for Licensed Practical/Vocational Nurses was adopted by the National Federation of Licensed Practical Nurses.

Ethics has always been an integral part of nursing. Throughout history one can find codes of ethics, statements of **moral** principles, treatises on maintaining high ideals, and recorded discussions of moral and ethical issues. Caring for and comforting the sick and protecting the suffering are human activities of nurses. These human activities and how society views them directly affect the mores, customs, and beliefs of humankind.

Values Associated with Health Care

A person's value system is the accepted mode of conduct and set of norms, goals, and values that the person has developed over many years, beginning in childhood. This system serves as a guide for the individual to determine what is right and what is wrong, what is good and what is bad, and what is desirable and what is undesirable. A person uses his **value system** in making decisions and achieving a meaningful life.

A person holds many values simultaneously and without conflict until faced with a severe state of stress or serious illness. When these situations occur, some values become more prominent and take precedence over all others. Most evident are the values of self-determination, well-being, and equity.

The principle of self-determination recognizes that people define their values and assume responsibility for particular life-styles and certain health practices. They are entitled to accept or reject health care interventions on the basis of these values and their personal goals.

The principle of well-being preserves and improves one's state of health by avoiding harm and seeking good physical and mental health care practices. The person's own best interest becomes the first priority and allows the choice of many options in health care.

The principle of equity causes the person to expect fair and equal treatment by sharing in the health care decision-making process as it relates to him or her. Common areas where shared decision making is needed include: the question of when life begins; abortion; contraception; sterilization; surrogate mother; organ transplant; AIDS; and drug testing.

In all cases, the right of free choice is an important value and must be respected by all who work in the health care delivery system.

Patient Advocacy

An advocate is a person who works on behalf of another person who is in a vulnerable or underprivileged position. Patients often are vulnerable when in the high-technology environment of a health care facility. Such an environment tends to threaten their **autonomy** (independent functioning) because they do not always have the knowledge or the control to make meaningful decisions about their care. When this occurs, the patient advocate, acting on the patients' behalf, provides information to patients about their situation, assists in helping patients understand their situation, assists health care providers in understanding patients and patients' perceptions of what is happening, and helps patients negotiate therapeutic relationships as these relationships pertain to their care and well-being.

The patient advocate provides relief and remedies against wrongdoing by members of the health care system. The advocates' activities, if accomplished within the scope of their charter, safeguard patients against possible abuse and violation of their basic rights.

BOX 3-1 **THE NIGHTINGALE PLEDGE**

I solemnly pledge myself before God and in the presence of this assembly:
To pass my life in purity and to practice my profession faithfully;
I will abstain from whatever is deleterious and mischievous and will not take or knowingly administer any harmful drug;
I will do all in my power to maintain and elevate the standard of my profession, and will hold in confidence all personal matters committed to my keeping and all family affairs coming to my knowledge in the practice of my calling;
With loyalty will I endeavor to aid the physician in his work, and devote myself to the welfare of those committed to my care.

BOX 3-2 **THE PRACTICAL NURSE'S PLEDGE**

Before God and those assembled here, I solemnly pledge:
To adhere to the code of ethics of the nursing profession;
To cooperate faithfully with the other members of the nursing team and to carry out faithfully and to the best of my ability the instructions of the physician or the nurse who may be assigned to supervise my work;
I will not do anything evil or malicious and I will not knowingly give any harmful drug or assist in malpractice;
I will not reveal any confidential information that may come to my knowledge in the course of my work;
And I pledge myself to do all in my power to raise the standards and the prestige of practical nursing.
May my life be devoted to service, and to the high ideals of the nursing profession.

BOX 3-3 **1973 CODE OF ETHICS OF INTERNATIONAL COUNCIL OF NURSES**

The fundamental responsibility of the nurse is fourfold: to promote health, to prevent illness, to restore health, and to alleviate suffering.
The need for nursing is universal. Inherent in nursing is respect for life, dignity, and rights of man. It is unrestricted by considerations of nationality, race, creed, colour, age, sex, politics, or social status.
Nurses render health services to the individual, the family, and the community and coordinate their services with those of related groups.

NURSES AND PEOPLE

The nurse's primary responsibility is to those people who require nursing care.
The nurse, in providing care, respects the beliefs, values, and customs of the individual.
The nurse holds in confidence personal information and uses judgment in sharing this information.

NURSES AND PRACTICE

The nurse carries personal responsibility for nursing practice and for maintaining competence by continual learning.
The nurse maintains the highest standards of nursing care possible within the reality of a specific situation.
The nurse uses judgment in relation to individual competence when accepting and delegating responsibilities.
The nurse when acting in a professional capacity should at all times maintain standards of personal conduct that would reflect credit upon the profession.

NURSES AND SOCIETY

The nurse shares with other citizens the responsibility for initiating and supporting action to meet the health and social needs of the public.

NURSES AND CO-WORKERS

The nurse sustains a cooperative relationship with coworkers in nursing and other fields.
The nurse takes appropriate action to safeguard the individual when his care is endangered by a co-worker or any other person.

NURSES AND THE PROFESSION

The nurse plays the major role in determining and implementing desirable standards of nursing practice and nursing education.
The nurse is active in developing a core of professional knowledge.
The nurse, acting through the professional organization, participates in establishing and maintaining equitable social and economic working conditions in nursing.

From The International Council of Nurses, 3, rue de l'Ancien-Port, CH-1201, Geneva, Switzerland, Telephone (022) 31 29 60.

Code of Ethics

Within any given profession, a code of ethics serves as a means of self-regulation and a source of guidelines for individual behavior and responsibility. Ideally, codes of ethics are a response to a society's needs for trustworthy, competent, and accountable practitioners. Professional codes of ethics are a system of rules and principles by which that profession is expected to regulate its members and demonstrate its responsibility to society. They provide an enforceable standard of minimal conduct and indicate the ethical considerations of professional conduct.

A code of ethics provides a standard of behavior that serves as a guide for (1) education and practice of nurses, (2) legislation affecting nurses, (3) licensing of nurses, and (4) public participation of nurses.

The Nightingale Pledge (Box 3-1), prepared by Gretter, included the basic principles governing ethical practices.

The pledge that was prepared for the practical nurses addressed similar aspects of the Nightingale Pledge (Box 3-2).

As ethical decision making became prevalent with the advancement of medical technology, the need for a code of ethics became apparent. In 1965 the International Council of Nurses, which met in Geneva, Switzerland, decided that these pledges may not meet the needs of nurses in some countries, so they adopted an International Code of Ethics. In 1973 it was revised to reflect the changes of the health care delivery system (Box 3-3).

VALUE CLARIFICATION

Value clarification is the expression of a person's preferences, likes, and dislikes about those things affecting life and living that are important to him or her.

Issues such as life and death, belief in God or disbelief in God, what is good and what is bad, the concept of truth, and the concept of love are only a few of the values that must be considered when the health care provider must make a health care decision.

Patient's Values

Each patient's character is defined by the value choices he or she makes and then incorporates into his or her value system. These values are statements (nonverbal) that a patient makes through behavior, expression of need, or actions. They define what is important to the patient at a time when health care decisions must be made.

These value choices (1) contribute to the development of health care goals, attitudes, and feelings experienced when people are patients and (2) grow from their experiences to become a permanent part of their value systems.

Choices made by patients, then, are based on what is perceived as important to them at the time they are confronted with a traumatic situation.

Practical/Vocational Nurse's Practice Values

The practical/vocational nurse is active in decision making involved in caring for a patient. This is accomplished in an ever-changing environment of new developments in health care technology. Such developments include human experimentation, euthanasia, right to life, abortion, living wills, informed consent, Do Not Resuscitate orders, drug and alcohol abuse and testing, sterilization, use of blood, care of the elderly, and organ transplant.

The ultimate goals in health care are to achieve maximum health potential, to maintain good health, to prevent disease, and to provide rehabilitative care.

The practical/vocational nurse is responsible for assisting the patient to achieve these goals by adhering to the standards of ethical practice and conduct set forth in the Code for Licensed Practical/Vocational Nurses adopted by the National Federation of Licensed Practical/Vocational Nurses (NFLPN) last revised in 1979 (Box 3-4).

BOX 3-4 **CODE FOR LICENSED PRACTICAL/VOCATIONAL NURSES**

1. Know the scope of maximum utilization of the LP/VN and function within this scope.
2. Recognize and respect cultural backgrounds, spiritual needs, and religious beliefs of individual patients.
3. Safeguard the confidential information acquired from any source about the patient.
4. Refuse to give endorsements to the sale and promotion of commercial products or services.
5. Uphold the highest standards in personal appearance, language, dress, and demeanor.
6. Accept responsibility for membership in the NFLPN and participate in its efforts to maintain the established standards of nursing practice and employment policies conducive to quality patient care.

From the National Federation of Licensed Practical Nurses, Inc, 250 West 57th Street, New York, NY 10019.

ETHICAL ISSUES

Nursing has a commitment to keep the well-being of a patient the primary focus in the delivery of health care. Ethical codes of practice emphasize the obligation to fulfill this commitment.

Ethical decisions, as seen, are not made in a vacuum. Many factors influence the process as one searches for the right decision. It is important to understand all of the factors involved in the decision-making process and to appreciate that these factors are not independent or mutually exclusive, but act and react with one another.

Right to Know

In response to patient's demands and as an outcome of court decisions regarding the methods in which health care is delivered, the "right to know movement" has had a significant effect on the health care system. This movement prompted the American Hospital Association to issue its "Patient's Bill of Rights" in 1973.

Patients who receive health care in the context of organized institutions, such as hospitals, nursing homes, and ambulatory care centers, depend on health care providers for all aspects of care. Patients should not be treated as persons incapable of learning, and they should not be manipulated and coerced into making decisions about their care that suit the health care provider. Rather, the health care provider should assist the patient in making intelligent decisions based on adequate information regarding his or her condition and within the scope of the patient's values.

BOX 3-5 ETHICAL DILEMMAS: WHAT WOULD YOU DO IF . . .

You had just received confirmation that you are 10 weeks pregnant. Your obstetrician cautioned you to avoid exposure to infectious diseases because of the effects it may have on the fetus. You were assigned to take care of a newly admitted patient with AIDS. What would you do?

You were assigned to the operating room as an assistant scrub nurse. You were scheduled to assist with an abortion. Abortion is contrary to your religious belief. What would you do?

You attended a party with a nurse with whom you work. She was drinking heavily and began to brag that she was addicted to drugs such as morphine, Librium, Valium, and codeine. She showed you a handful of the drugs that she was taking. The next day you were assigned to work on the same unit with her. At the end of the shift, the narcotic count was incorrect. What would you do?

You were assigned to care for a 75-year-old female patient who had a cerebral vascular accident, had brain damage, and was on a respirator. You overheard family members arguing about whether they should give approval for a "Do Not Resuscitate" order to be written by their physician. The respirator alarm has just gone off. What would you do?

Confidentiality

The development of a trusting relationship contributes positively to the total environment of patient care. The practical/vocational nurse has an obligation to preserve patients' privacy by holding information regarding their care in strict confidence.

All information about a patient and his or her care belongs to that patient. Maintaining patient confidentiality is a valuable tool because by creating an atmosphere of trust, the health care provider makes it possible for patients to feel comfortable about telling the truth about their condition. Furthermore, there may be serious legal ramifications when the privacy of a patient is invaded, misused, or otherwise compromised.

Policies have been adopted within health care agencies that provide specific guidelines about what information must be revealed according to existing freedom-of-information laws. In most cases this information does not violate patient confidentiality.

Accountability and Responsibility

Practical/vocational nurses are held accountable for the quality of their practice and the actions taken during the course of that practice. These actions must be performed within the scope of the standards of practice established by the profession, the Nurse Practice Acts, and the policies, rules, and regulations of the health care agency.

Accepting responsibility for one's actions in the total context of a patient's care and treatment cannot be overemphasized. This is a shared responsibility because seldom is one person totally responsible for a patient's well-being.

ETHICAL DILEMMAS

A **dilemma** is defined as a situation requiring a choice between two equally desirable or undesirable alternatives. In an ethical dilemma, each alternative course of action can be justified by the way in which a person views the course of action based on his or her value system.

Issues in health care delivery practices present different alternatives based on whether the issue or course of action is viewed by the patient, the health care agency, the legal system, or the practical/vocational nurse.

The dilemma occurs when opposing views are seen for the solution of an issue and a decision must be made. There are no set procedures or easy answers for how an ethical dilemma should be resolved. A list of challenging ethical dilemmas is presented in Box 3-5.

ETHICS COMMITTEES

The patient's rights movement, in conjunction with the complexity and rising costs of health care, has accelerated the consumer movement in today's society. Consumers are demanding greater participation in the decision-making process as it affects them in the delivery of health care.

Ethics committees, which at one time were attended only by physicians, now include administrators, relevant health care professionals, public policymakers, and consumers. These committees are the formal mechanism by which ethical decision making is shared on such issues as the behavior of health care providers, appropriateness of certain procedures and treatments, and other ethical dilemmas as they occur.

REFERENCES AND SUGGESTED READINGS

1. Bandman EL and Bandman B: Nursing ethics in the life span, Norwalk, Conn, 1985, Appleton-Century-Crofts.
2. Becker BG and Fendlerd T: Vocational and personal adjustments in practical nursing, ed 6, St Louis, 1990, The CV Mosby Co.
3. Benjamin M and Curtis J: Ethics in nursing, ed 2, New York, 1986, Oxford University Press, Inc.
4. Cody M: Witholding treatment: is it ethical? J Gerontol Nurs 12:24, 1986.
5. Gaze H: Ethics: a question of morality, Nurs Times 83:44, 1987.
6. Jameton A: Nursing practice, Englewood Cliffs, NJ, 1984, Prentice Hall, Inc.
7. Melia K: Everyday ethics for nurses, Nurs Times 83:28, 1987.
8. Reisman EC: Ethical issues confronting nurses, Nurs Clin North Am 23(4):789, 1988.
9. Saylor DC: The LP/VN's role in bioethical decision-making, J Pract Nurs Clin North Am 23(4):789, 1988.
10. Viens DC: A history of nursing's code of ethics, Nurs Outlook 37(1):45, 1989.

CHAPTER CHALLENGE

KEY POINTS

- Early civilization contributed to the development of humans' value systems as they exist in today's pluralistic society.
- A person's value system influences the ethical decisions made regarding health care.
- Codes of ethics are systems of rules and principles that guide the members of a profession in meeting the ethical standards of that profession.
- Value clarification is the process whereby personal values of the practical/vocational nurse and the patient are both considered when providing holistic health care.
- Early ethical principles for nurses were outlined in the Nightingale Pledge.
- The quality of a practical/vocational nurse's practice is performed within the scope of the standards of practice established by the profession, the Nurse Practice Acts, and the policies, rules, and regulations of the health care agency.

STUDY QUESTIONS

1. The primary means of perpetuating the family or the tribe were:
   a. The customs and mores that influenced behavior
   b. The right and proper manner in which each person was expected to behave
   c. The law of the land, because violation meant punishment or death
   d. All of the above
2. When faced with illness or stress, the person's values that become dominant and take precedence over all others include all but one of the principles listed below:
   a. Self-determination
   b. Inequity
   c. Equity
   d. Well-being
3. The Code of Ethics for the licensed practical/vocational nurse was adopted:
   a. At the same time as the Hippocratic Oath
   b. By the National Federation of Licensed Practical Nurses last revised in 1979
   c. By Florence Nightingale and commonly known as the "Nightingale Pledge"
   d. By the American Hospital Association in 1973
4. Ethical dilemmas occur when opposing views are seen for the solution of an issue and involve:
   a. The patient
   b. The health care provider
   c. The legal system
   d. All of the above
5. Ethics committees are established as the formal mechanism whereby ethical decision making is discussed. The membership of these committees includes:
   a. Physicians only
   b. Administrators only
   c. A combination of physicians, administrators, health care providers, and consumers
   d. Consumers only
   e. Health care providers only

II

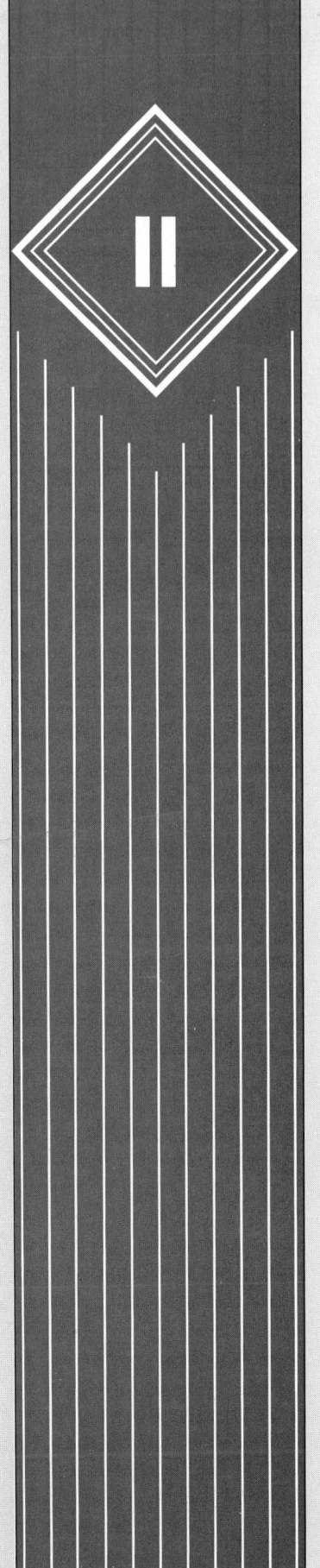

Communicating Health Care

I am a forty-year-old woman who is fulfilling a lifelong dream. When I was a little girl, people would ask, “What do you want to be when you grow up?” I would always say, “I want to be a nurse!” I feel nursing is a very honorable and gratifying profession. I love nursing because it is a fulfilling and rewarding job. It gives me the greatest pleasure and feeling of satisfaction to know I have perhaps eased someone’s pain and suffering or discomfort, listened to a concern or question and been able to help in some small way, and maybe, just a little, brightened the day with a smile or a touch to say I care and understand. I have great empathy for someone who is ill and suffering and less fortunate than me. There have been times when I have cried when a patient has passed away and times I have been elated when someone recovers and goes home.

PATRICIA PIKE
Student Nurse

4

Communication

GRETCHEN H. LeGAULT

LEARNING OBJECTIVES

After reading this chapter, the student should be able to do the following:

- Define the key terms.
- Identify six major reasons why communication skills are important.
- Describe the process of communication.
- Discuss the components of the communication process.
- Identify the three phases of an interview, and explain the significance of each phase.
- Differentiate between therapeutic and nontherapeutic communication.
- Identify significant components of nonverbal communication.
- Discuss blocks and barriers to effective communication.
- Describe means to facilitate communication.
- Relate techniques used to enhance therapeutic interactions.
- Discuss factors considered when communicating with a child or an elderly person.

RELATED TOPICS OF INTEREST

- The nursing process (Chapter 5)
- Documentation (Chapter 6)
- Cultural aspects of nursing care (Chapter 12)

KEY TERMS

Define the following:

- affective
- cognitive
- communication
- congruent
- context
- feedback
- perception
- therapeutic communication
- values

Communication is a process in which a message is transferred from one person to another. Communication may be verbal or nonverbal. It may be direct, such as face to face interchange or observation of an expression or gesture, or it may be indirect, such as written, printed, or recorded. Communication is basic to nursing, and therefore communication skills are some of the most important skills the nurse will learn.

Good communication skills can be learned by integrating observation and learned principles of communication into daily life and then adapting those skills to nursing practice.

We often hesitate to try to learn a new skill for fear of appearing foolish. A beginning skier would not expect to start skiing on the expert slopes. He would start on the easy slopes and then with much practice would progress to the more difficult slopes. So it is with communication. The nurse starts at a beginning level and through practice of techniques acquires this important skill. Why are communication skills so important? Six major reasons are as follow:

1. Communication is the vehicle the nurse uses to provide assistance to a patient.
2. Communication allows a person to establish, maintain, and improve contacts with others.
3. Communication enables the nurse to establish a working relationship with patients and eventually help them meet their health care needs.
4. Communication creates ways to effect change.
5. Communication establishes relationships among the health care team and promotes continuity of care.
6. Everything one uses or does has communicative value:
   a. Use of the senses—hearing, sight, taste, smell, touch
   b. Sending verbal, nonverbal, written, or recorded messages

The quality of communication influences the quantity of communication.

PROCESS OF COMMUNICATION

To understand communication, it is necessary to understand the process of communication. Although it may seem simple, communication is complex because of the number of variables. Communication is an ongoing, dynamic, ever-changing series of events, each of which affects all others.

The communicator, or sender, is the individual who initiates or delivers the message. The communicator has a thought, idea, or message he wishes to share with another person or persons. The communicator must consider the best way to send the message so that the receiver attains an accurate perception of the message sent (Fig. 4-1).

The channel of communication must be appropriate for the abilities and knowledge of the receiver. Often the message is sent through several channels.

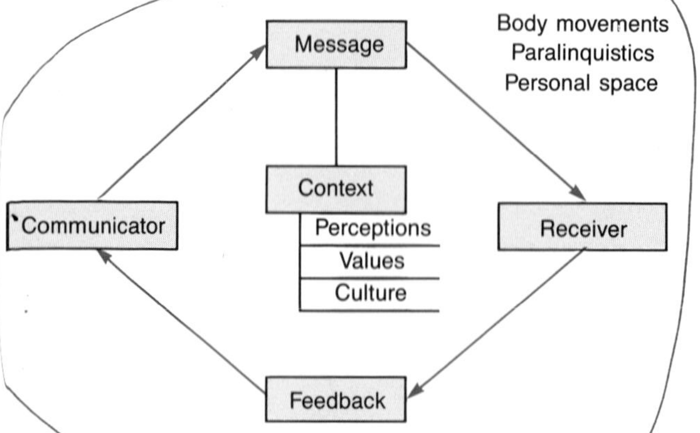

FIG. 4-1 The process of communication.

Verbal and nonverbal messages are perceived through hearing and sight. Touch may also be used, affecting the tactile senses. When possible, it is best to use more than one channel of communication. For example, verbal instructions should be followed by written instructions to ensure accurate compliance.

The message is the actual idea, thought, or feeling that is conveyed to the other party. It is important that the message be organized in a clear, simple format to be perceived accurately. The message is affected by body movements, paralinguistics, and personal space.

Body movements include the use of gestures, facial expressions, eyes, posture, and body physique, that is, height, weight, and general appearance. Paralinguistics includes how the voice is used, that is, voice level, pitch, rate, and rhythm. Many people are sensitive to their personal space. Personal space is an area with invisible boundaries surrounding the person's body. It includes four distinct zones, primarily in front of the person: (1) intimate zone, as far as 18 inches; (2) personal zone, 18 inches to 4 feet; (3) social zone, 4 feet to 12 feet; (4) public zone, 12 feet and beyond. Nurses often "invade" a patient's intimate or personal zone. When a patient moves away or attempts to pull back from the nurse, it is a cue to invasion of personal space.

The receiver receives the message through one of the senses. The receiver must actively listen to receive all of the verbal and nonverbal messages. The receiver then interprets the message within the context.

No communication is complete without feedback. **Feedback** is the receiver's response to the communicator's message. Feedback may be positive or negative; it may be verbal or nonverbal. For example, the nurse enters the room with a big smile and says, "Good morning, isn't this a beautiful day?" The patient bursts into tears and says, "I'm so afraid; am I going to die?" All communication falls within the context of both the communicator and the receiver. The **context** is affected by the perceptions, values, and culture of both the communicator and the receiver.

Perception is the conscious recognition and interpretation of sensory stimuli, which serves as a basis for understanding. It is a personal internal reaction to present stimuli or could be based on other experiences. No two people perceive the world or an event in the same way; therefore human communication is initially affected by the participants' perception of one another. It is important to know oneself and how one's experiences affect one's perceptions.

A **value** is a guideline for determining what is right or wrong, good or bad, that serves as a frame of reference for the individual to reach decisions. A value identifies what is of worth to a person. An individual's values continually change as he or she matures and gains knowledge and experience. Age, role, and financial circumstances may have a significant impact on values.

Culture is the development of intellectual and moral beliefs, usually attained through the ethnic group to which one belongs. Culture determines the unique style of communication when interacting with others. Cultural beliefs are learned early in life, and because they are often unrecognized as beliefs, they can lead to false conclusions. (See Chapter 12, Cultural Aspects of Nursing Care.)

The content of the message is determined by what the *sender* thinks, feels, and perceives and how the sender wants to be perceived. The *receiver's* perception of the message is structured by the following:

1. The perceiver's perception of the world
2. The perceiver's perception of self within the context of the message received

PHASES OF AN INTERVIEW

When using the nursing process, the nurse often interviews the patient. Every patient interview has three phases: a beginning, a middle, and an end. The purpose of the interview determines how much emphasis is placed on each phase.

Introduction Phase

The beginning of the interview, or introduction phase, is usually short and concise. It is important for the nurse to greet the patient by name, introduce herself, and define her role. The tone and the guidelines for the interview are set. Expectations may be clarified and mutual goals discussed. Appropriate nonverbal behavior, such as smiling and maintaining eye contact, should accompany the verbal greeting. "Good morning, Mrs. Bailey. My name is Jean Baker. I am a student practical nurse from Douglas

Community College. I will be caring for you for the next three mornings. If you have any questions about your care, please feel free to ask me."

Working Phase

The middle phase of the interview, or the working phase, is the major portion of the interview. The middle phase is used to accomplish identified goals or objectives. A health history may be taken to obtain information about the patient's health problems. Giving instructions might be one of the goals. A patient's knowledge about his health problem should not be overestimated. It is wise to find out how much the patient knows and build from this. It is better to repeat areas of knowledge than to assume the patient already knows. Many patients do not know what questions to ask or are embarrassed to say they do not know. Feedback to determine understanding of instructions should always be requested. The nurse should also realize the patient may have an emotional reaction to the information given and should encourage the patient to verbalize his feelings.

The working phase has two important factors. The *functional* factor indicates direct action. For example, the patient has a poor appetite. The nursing goal is to increase food intake. The action taken is to encourage small, frequent meals. The *expressive* factor is the patient's emotional state, sentiments, or feelings. Both factors are present and must be in harmony to reach a goal. If the patient with the poor appetite is a patient with anorexia nervosa, the two factors would be in disharmony, with the patient and the nurse working toward different goals. Whenever possible, goals should be mutual between patient and nurse.

Termination Phase

The final phase of the interview is termination. Some nurses have difficulty ending an interview. However, it is important to end the interview smoothly, because most nurses are under a fairly rigid time schedule. The nurse should give the patient verbal cues, such as, "I have another 2 minutes to discuss this with you. Do you have any questions you would like to ask?" If the patient has questions that cannot be answered in the time frame, the nurse should tell the patient that she will return. If the nurse cannot answer or does not know the answer to a patient's question, she should tell him the truth. A short summary of what was discussed and follow-up instructions, followed by an exit cue (i.e., "Good-bye" and turn to door) helps to end the interview. It is important that the patient does not feel rejected when the interview is terminated.

THERAPEUTIC VERSUS NONTHERAPEUTIC COMMUNICATION

What is therapeutic communication? **Therapeutic communication** is the act of an educated nurse. Elianor Hein said, "Any nursing procedure, any act of reassurance, or any measure of comfort or relief, regardless of how small or seemingly incidental, is preceded by communication." Every communicative act initiated in the presence of a patient has an impact on him. The use of communication skills should demonstrate to the patient that his welfare is the primary concern of the nurse. The primary purpose of a therapeutic relationship with a patient is the optimal well-being of the patient. The nurse's knowledge, skill, and expertise are critical. The nurse must be able to establish and maintain a relationship, and the patient must feel free to reveal facts about himself and his life. Outcomes depend on the nurse's communication skills. In understanding and using therapeutic communication skills for the patient's best interest, the nurse needs to practice the following:

1. Be aware of self-interests and prejudices
2. Respect the patient as a person
3. Keep dependence within bounds
4. Encourage patient participation and cooperation in his own care

Therapeutic interaction differs from social interaction in several ways (Table 4-1). Nurses have many time limitations placed on them. Often nurses have only a few minutes to talk to a patient. Therefore the nurse must use those few minutes in a meaningful way. Most interviews with a patient are not only purposeful but very structured and goal directed. Although social interactions may be purposeful, usually they are not structured, because there is no particular goal. Time constraints are important. If the goal is not reached in the given time period, the nurse will schedule another interview. A social interview is more task oriented. The participants continue until they complete their task or agree the task cannot be

Table 4-1 Differences Between Therapeutic and Social Interaction

Therapeutic	Social
1. Goal directed	1. No set goal
2. Patient centered	2. Mutually beneficial to all participants
3. Time limited	3. Task limited
4. Content specific to patient needs	4. Superficial content
5. Deliberative, planned, purposeful	5. Casual, intuitive, unplanned
6. Structured	6. No structure

concluded in a satisfactory manner. A social interaction usually benefits all the participants. A therapeutic interaction is directed primarily at the needs of the patient. Although the nurse gains satisfaction in helping the patient, the patient is the primary concern. In a social interaction, responses are casual, intuitive, and unplanned.

The content of a therapeutic interaction is specific and structured and responses are directed toward meeting the patient's needs. The degree of skill and sensitivity a nurse brings to a therapeutic interaction often determines the amount of relief and comfort the patient attains.

TYPES OF COMMUNICATION

Messages are communicated in a number of ways: verbal, nonverbal, written, or recorded. For the purpose of this chapter we will address only verbal and nonverbal communication.

Nonverbal Communication

Nonverbal communication includes the use of body movements, paralinguistics, and personal space. Nonverlanguage delivers a powerful message. It is usually motivated by subconscious feelings and is therefore a more reliable indication of true feelings than the spoken word. Observation of nonverbal cues is an important skill. The patient might voice a thought, but the nonverbal cues are not **congruent.** For example, a patient is going to have surgery. He states he is not nervous, but he jokes with the nurses and talks very rapidly, and his fingers twist and roll a corner of the sheet. The diversion of focus to jokes, rapid speech, and finger movements indicates anxiety. The nurse must also be aware of the nonverbal cues *she* is emitting: the patient may be astute at picking up the nurse's nonverbal cues. The nurse should be able to project a feeling of warmth and caring toward the patient.

Body motion may add significant meaning to a verbal statement or total communication. Total body movement or posture may indicate strong emotions. Squirming, rocking back and forth, or extreme rigidity may indicate worry, tension, or anxiety. Slouching or sitting at an angle may show unwillingness to interact. Facing the other person directly and leaning forward in a relaxed manner usually indicate openness.

Eyes have been called a window to a person's soul. Eyes are expressive. They can show joy, sadness, dislike, and many other emotions. Eye contact indicates willingness to interact. Lack of eye contact or looking away may indicate embarrassment, dislike, withdrawal, or possibly an attempt to remember or process what is being said. Different cultures have different interpretations of eye contact or lack of contact. In some cultures, direct eye contact shows lack of respect, for instance in native American and Japanese cultures. Facial expressions are sometimes difficult to interpret. Usually the face shows a mixture of feelings, as shown in the eyes and the mouth. Decreased tension and an open mouth may show surprise or disbelief. A smile may indicate joy or happiness, whereas tight lips may indicate anger. Movement of the head up and down may indicate agreement. Shaking the head from side to side indicates disagreement or disbelief. Bowing the head indicates sadness or concern.

The arms or hands may indicate a person's emotional state. Relaxed hands and arms indicate openness. Arms that are rigid with hands clenched indicate anger, tension, or explosiveness. Hands that are busy in a meaningless fashion, such as finger tapping, indicate anxiety. Feet and legs that appear relaxed and comfortable with both feet flat on the floor indicate openness. Shuffling feet, toe tapping, and crossing and uncrossing legs usually indicate anxiety or impatience. The nurse or patient who leans back in the chair with his or her arms and legs crossed indicates a closed attitude toward the interaction procedure, a "show me" attitude, or that the person is more interested in comfort than in the person with whom he or she is interacting.

Body language is used to emphasize paralinguistic cues and the spoken word. Paralinguistics relates to how a message is delivered. Voice level refers to the volume of speech, whereas pitch refers to intonation. A soft voice can be used to control, forcing a person to be quiet to hear. The soft voice may also indicate embarrassment at discussing a sensitive topic, or it may show lack of self-esteem. A loud voice may indicate anger, force, or power. Variable pitch is normal and often relays a change in the content of the message. Rate and rhythm of speech reflect changes in the content. Increased rate may indicate anxiety. Slow, methodical speech may show lack of decisiveness.

Mirror imaging is an intervention used to alter pitch, rate, and rhythm. For example, if the patient is speaking loudly and rapidly, the nurse will do the opposite. If the nurse speaks slowly and softly, the effect will usually slow and quiet the patient. Language patterns affect understanding and being understood. A common language and understanding regional dialects is important.

Personal space. Most people feel comfortable talking at a distance of 3 to 5 feet. Nursing procedures often require less distance. Nurses must realize this is invading the patients' personal space and might make them uncomfortable.

Touch is a powerful expression of communication. It is a meaningful personal mode of communication, and its meaning is different to different people. Touch can convey warmth and interest: "I am here, I understand." Because touch is more spontaneous, it often seems more genuine. However, there are many social guidelines that govern the use of touch. Health status and culture both have implications for the use of touch. Some nurses or patients are uncomfortable touching or being touched. The nurse must recognize her feelings and be sensitive to the patient's feelings.

Verbal Communication

Verbal communication includes the spoken or written word. It is either speaking to others or writing to or about others. To be effective, a message should be short, clear, relevant, and timed appropriately. Many people tend to overcommunicate. They give wordy explanations or ask several questions at once. Thus the patient wonders, "What did the nurse say?" or "Which question should I answer?" Another area of confusion is the use of abbreviations or initials, such as saying "q day" or "bid" instead of "every day" or "twice a day." Time is wasted in explanations, or the patient may be embarrassed to admit he does not understand and therefore does not ask for an explanation. The choice of words used by the nurse is dictated by the patient's level of understanding. For example, the nurse would address a child differently from a well-educated adult. The nurse should be cautious when using complex medical terms, because they are often misunderstood. Communication is enhanced by keeping the message short and simple, speaking slowly, enunciating clearly, and using words the patient understands. Timing and relevancy are also important to enhance understanding of a message. A patient will not be interested in learning how to plan a diabetic menu when he is nauseated. The patient must be free from distraction and open to listening for effective communication to take place.

Blocks and Barriers

Blocks are verbal techniques and attitudes that jeopardize communication. An example of blocking communication is to ask "why?" When the nurse does not understand a patient's actions or behavior, the most frequent response is "why?" or "why did you do that?" The "why" question places the patient on the defensive. This causes insecurity and resentment. There are better ways to gain information. Rather than asking, "Why did you stop taking your medication?" it is better to say, "You appear to have a problem with your medications; let's talk about what has happened."

Changing the subject inappropriately might be harmful. For example, the patient asks, "Am I going to die?" The nurse replies, "You have a lovely bouquet of flowers. Did you just receive it today?" The patient will feel as though no one is listening or cares about what is happening to him.

The use of *excessive questioning* places too much pressure on the patient and is upsetting, particularly when more than one question is asked at a time. It becomes an interrogation rather than an interaction.

Making judgments labels a patient as good or bad and does not accept him as an individual. A patient needs to be encouraged to make independent decisions.

False reassurance is nonfactual information that makes the nurse feel good but may harm the patient. It is patronizing and actually devalues a patient's feelings. For example, the nurse says to a patient who is apprehensive about moving to a nursing home, "You can't go back to your trailer alone, you know. I'm sure you will enjoy your new home." It would be better to say, "You seem apprehensive about moving to the nursing home. Let's talk about how you see the move changing your life."

Highly emotional words, such as "angry," "crazy," "hostile," and "guilty," should be avoided because many patients will not admit to having these strong feelings.

Giving advice is inappropriate. This takes decision making away from the patient. The patient therefore no longer has an investment in the outcome. He should be encouraged to develop a solution to the problems.

Focusing on self is one way some nurses maintain distance from a patient. They listen just long enough to relate the conversation to something that happened to them. For example, "Oh, you're having a hysterectomy tomorrow. Don't worry. I had one 2 years ago and got along fine. I was in the hospital only. . . ." This type of response shows patients that their feelings are unimportant and the nurse is preoccupied with herself and does not really care about the patients.

In *listening* the nurse needs to listen not only to the patient, but to self. People are often unaware of what they are saying. They talk just to be talking. They will often respond, "Did I say that?" or "I did not say that." Nurses must think before speaking and listen to what they say. *Listening* is the most effective technique to facilitate communication. If the nurse inadvertently blocks communication, the mistakes should be acknowledged and corrected. Removing blocks to communication requires sensitivity and ingenuity on the part of the nurse. Physical barriers, such as language differences and muteness, hinder communications.

Speaking a different language may occur at several levels. The language difference may be cultural, such as English, Spanish, German; it may be ethnic, such as minority groups; or it may be regional, such as idioms specific to a region in the country (e.g., the "deep south").

BOX 4-1 BLOCKS AND BARRIERS TO COMMUNICATION

BLOCKS (Verbal)	BARRIERS (Physical)
1. Asking why	1. Language difference
2. Inappropriately changing subject	2. Deafness
3. Excessive questioning	3. Stuttering
4. Making judgments	4. Muteness
5. Giving false reassurance	5. Blindness
6. Using highly emotional words	
7. Giving advice	
8. Focusing on self	

Physical barriers, such as deafness, stuttering, muteness, or blindness, demand some specific strategies for effective communication. These blocks and barriers are summarized in Box 4-1.

COMMUNICATION ENHANCERS

Just as there are blocks and barriers to communication, there are ways to facilitate communication (Box 4-2). *Active listening* is listening with all senses and requires energy and concentration. It is trying to understand the complete message. Active listening is not selective listening, but focusing solely on the needs of the patient. The nurse can convey an attitude of active listening by the following:

1. Facing the patient squarely, with both feet on the floor and staying relaxed
2. Maintaining good eye contact without staring
3. Leaning forward, showing interest, maintaining a nondefensive position
4. Positioning self on the same level as the patient (not towering over the patient)
5. Providing privacy where appropriate, for example, if subject is embarrassing or personal or may invoke loss of control

There are several ways to use *silence*. It may be used to help patients organize their thoughts or gain control of their emotions. It may be combined with touch to show concern or support. It may be used to place some of the responsibility of the interaction on the patient. When silence is used for reflection or reminiscence, caution must be used so that the patient can keep his thoughts in perspective.

An *accepting attitude* is important on the part of the nurse. Anyone who has been a patient can probably think

BOX 4-2 FACILITATORS OF COMMUNICATION

1. Active listening
2. Silence
3. Accepting attitudes
   Empathy
   Respect
   Trust
   Competence
4. Identifying affective cues
5. Presenting self honestly

of a nurse who did not portray a compassionate attitude. A patient may think, "What an indifferent person" or "That nurse certainly doesn't seem to have a high regard for the patient."

Empathy and *respect* are the two most important attitudes. Empathy is the ability to put oneself in other persons' shoes and feel what they are feeling; this is critical in a therapeutic relationship. Empathy is not only an attitude, it is a skill used to gain rapport and obtain information from a patient. If empathy turns to sympathy, the nurse will lose objectivity in the approach to the patient.

Every person deserves respect and to be considered a person of worth and dignity. It is important for the nurse to view the person as an individual in need rather than to judge the person on his deeds. Respect is often shown not only by accepting without judging the person as he is, but also by conveying warmth in caring for him. Nurses often convey warmth and caring by actions rather than words, that is, facial expression, eye contact, and gentleness of hands-on procedures. It is critical that the patient trust the nurse. Usually that trust is implicit unless the nurse's actions suggest that she is not trustworthy. The best way the nurse can maintain the trusting relationship is by showing *competence* in doing the job. Competence, or the ability do the job well, indicates the nurse puts a high value on caring for the patient.

When the nurse responds to a patient, she must be able to identify both the **cognitive** (thought content) and the **affective** (feeling) cues. It is particularly important to be able to respond to affective cues to understand what this experience means to the patient and how he is feeling. Cormier and others present a list of commonly used affect words in categories of four negative feelings and one positive feeling (Table 4-2).

When identifying or reflecting a feeling, it is important to consider the intensity of the feeling the patient portrays. It takes skill for the nurse to select appropriate interchangeable words to show she is listening to the

Table 4-2 List of Commonly Used Affect Words

Positive	Negative			
Happiness	**Sadness**	**Fear**	**Uncertainty**	**Anger**
happy	discouraged	anxious	puzzled	upset
pleased	disappointed	tense	confused	frustrated
satisfied	miserable	nervous	uncertain	annoyed
content	unhappy	uptight	undecided	irritated
cheerful	hopeless	uneasy	insecure	hassled
excited	lonely	worried	bothered	offended

From Cormier SL and Cormier WH: Interviewing and helping skills for health professionals, Boston, 1983, Jones & Bartlett Publishers, Inc.

patient. While a patient is using energy to deal with feelings, he cannot use that energy to get well.

Nurses should present themselves and their abilities honestly. If they do not know answers to patients' questions, they should say so and assure the patients that they will find the answers if possible or if appropriate. When telling a patient that a question will be followed up, the nurse must do so. If this is not done, not only the nurse but nursing as a profession loses credibility.

THERAPEUTIC TECHNIQUES

Every person communicates in his or her own way. The nurse will learn a number of techniques to become proficient in therapeutic communication. No one technique is sufficient. The nurse should adapt the following techniques to his or her style and to the patient's individuality and circumstance.

Focusing is used to keep the communications specific and concrete. Some patients have difficulty staying with the subject matter. Focusing is used to keep the patient's responses relevant to the issue. The following is an example:

Mr. Jones states he does not want to move to a nursing home. "People do not get good care there. My grandmother lived at home until she died." He then talks further about his grandmother—when she came to this country, her life, etc. It will be necessary to bring Mr. Jones back to the issue. "Mr. Jones, your grandmother's life is interesting, but we need to discuss what specifically we can do for you when you move to a nursing home."

Acceptance and understanding are often conveyed through active listening. The nurse can use nonverbal expressions. "Yes" or "uh-huh" and nodding appropriately indicate approval. The nurse contributes to the accepting atmosphere by not interrupting or arguing when in disagreement. It is often helpful to identify themes in recognizing a patient's feelings or concerns. By recognizing patterns of thought, the nurse may also identify thoughts the patient repeatedly avoids. Often further exploration can help the patient talk about the concern or feeling.

Reflection is demonstrated when the nurse restates the cognitive part of the message, the affective part of the message, or both. Reflection is used to indicate the nurse hears what is being said and encourages the patient to continue. The following is an example:

MRS. ELLIOT: I'm really nervous about my surgery tomorrow. My sister had similar surgery a couple years ago and had a terrible time. She had a lot of pain and had an infection after she got home. I'm very frightened, and I don't know if I can handle it.

NURSE: You are anxious (*affective*) about your surgery (*cognitive*). You're afraid (*affective*) of pain and possible complications (*cognitive*) and your ability to handle them (*cognitive*).

Paraphrasing is similar to reflection, except the patient's message is rephrased in the nurse's own words. For example:

NURSE: You are afraid you might have complications from your surgery tomorrow.

Clarification is asking the patient to rephrase or add to a message to correct a misunderstanding. When the nurse is unclear about the message a patient is conveying, it is appropriate to ask for clarification. Usually clarification is requested in the form of a question. For example:

PATIENT: I don't know why I gain weight. With the way my appetite is, I eat hardly anything.

NURSE: I'm not sure I understand. You say you don't have an appetite, yet you gain weight. Would you tell me what you ate yesterday?

Broad openings help determine the focus of the interview and encourage the patient to express problems and concerns. They are helpful at the beginning of an interview. For example:

NURSE: Mrs. Miller, I wonder if you would like to talk about your new job. It seems your health problems have increased since you took your new position.

Giving information is a method of supplying the patient with information, often used in conjunction with the other techniques for health teaching. For example:

NURSE: Mrs. Jones, this is your prescription to take home. You will need to have the prescription filled at your pharmacy. Take one pill three times a day until they are all gone. Here is an instruction sheet with the directions written on it.

Summarization is several brief statements reviewing the content of the interview or series of interviews. Summary can be used to identify key issues to be discussed during the next interview, or it can be used to show progress toward a goal. For example:

MR. JORGENSEN: We have been discussing the importance of your being able to give your own insulin injections. You have practiced giving injections. Tomorrow we will review what you went over today, and you will demonstrate giving a self-injection of insulin.

QUESTIONING

Questioning is an acceptable method of obtaining information. Several types of questions are used to obtain patient information. Most helpful is the open-ended question.

The *open-ended question* requests information but does not specify the exact content. An open-ended question requires an explanation and is not easily answered with a one-word or "yes" or "no" answer. Open-ended questions encourage or give the patient permission to express thoughts, feelings, and concerns. For example:

NURSE: How do you see your new living arrangements differing from your past ones?

The *closed question* asks for specific information and can be answered with a one-word or "yes" or "no" answer. This type of question is included in most hospital health history forms. Most closed questions elicit more complete information if asked in the open-question form. For example:

Closed: NURSE: Have you ever had any problems with your heart?

Open: NURSE: Describe any heart problems you have had in the past.

The *related question* asks for more complete information within a topic. It is usually an open-ended question. For example:

NURSE: Tell me more about your most recent heart attack.

The *laundry list* is used when the patient has a problem speaking, such as one who has had a cerebral vascular accident (CVA) or one who has a problem understanding (e.g., a child or patient with a knowledge deficit). The nurse gives a list of adjectives from which the patient can choose. When using this method, the nurse must be careful not to indicate the "right" answer. Many patients will tell the nurse what they think she wants to hear. For example:

Mr. Jepson is unable to talk but is diaphoretic (perspiring profusely) and holding his abdomen.

NURSE: Mr. Jepson, you appear to be having pain. I know you can't describe your pain to me, but I will give you a list of words. Please nod if one describes the pain you are having. Is the pain dull, medium, sharp? (*Give patient time to react to each word.*) Is the pain constant (all the time) or intermittent (once in a while)?

The terms the nurse uses would depend on the patient's level of understanding. When asking the question, the nurse should phrase the question in a short, clear manner and should ask only one question at a time.

CONFRONTATION

Confrontation is used when a discrepancy or incongruency has been identified. Confrontation should be used carefully and never used to place blame or guilt on a patient. A confrontation will almost always elicit a response from a patient. Therefore it should be used only when there is enough time for the patient to discuss a response. The nurse should try to make the confrontation tentative. Patients may respond with acceptance, false acceptance, or anger, or actually not understand what is being discussed. For example:

NURSE: Mr. Shelby, when you left the hospital, we discussed the medications you were to take at home. This is your third checkup with the doctor, and I notice you are no longer taking your medications.

MR. SHELBY: Oh, I wasn't having those dizzy spells or pain any more, so I just stopped taking them.

Mr. Shelby obviously needs more education about his medications.

COMMUNICATION WITH SPECIAL GROUPS

Children

Communication with children takes special consideration. Some people talk down to children. Children are very quick to recognize this and often resent it. It is

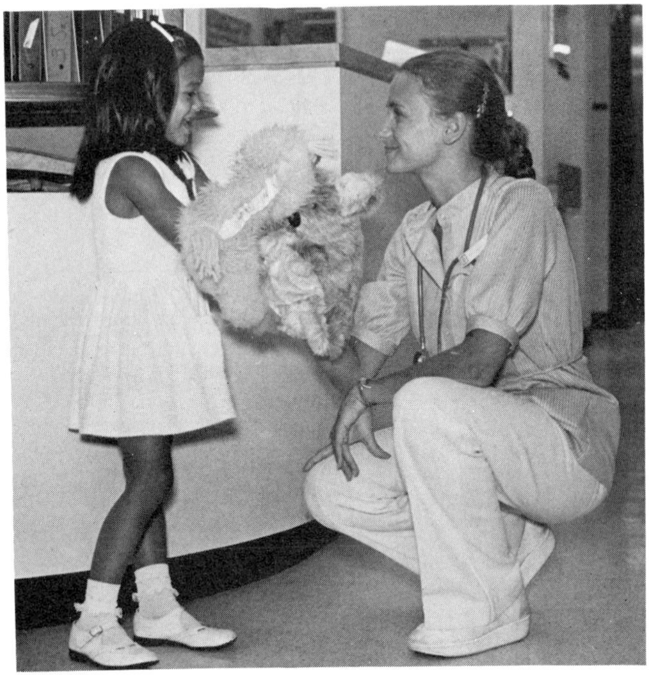

FIG. 4-2 A nurse talks to a child, using puppets and assuming a position at the child's level.

important to consider the age and stage of development of the child and to assess the degree of understanding. It is also important always to be honest and use simple, direct language. It often helps to use play therapy in communicating with children (Fig. 4-2). Children should be given the opportunity to act out what is happening to them. Painting or drawing also helps them relate their feelings in a nonthreatening way. It helps if the nurse can be at eye level with the child, and often exaggerated gestures and fake formality help put the child at ease (e.g., "GOOD MORNING, Mr. Brian," and shake hands). The child often feels vulnerable in the hospital environment. The child's family or significant person must be included in the therapy.

The Elderly

Good communication skills are particularly important when interacting with the elderly. Several factors must be carefully considered: (1) environment, (2) physiological barriers, (3) psychological tone, and (4) communication techniques.

The setting of the interview is important. The environment should be comfortable—free of drafts and probably a little warmer than for a younger person. Proper lighting and a minimum of distracting noises are important. A firm but comfortable chair, preferably with armrests, should be provided. There should be adequate space to maneuver if the older person uses a walker or wheelchair. Water, tea, coffee, or other beverage should be provided for the following reasons:

1. It is a social custom to provide beverages during conversation. It shows caring. Also, as people talk their throats often become dry. They will stop talking, not realizing that it is from lack of fluids.
2. Many older people do not have adequate fluid intake. Having fluids available may increase fluid intake.

It is important to assess any physiological barriers. Three major barriers are blindness, deafness, and confusion. If the patient is blind, it is important for the nurse to speak to him, introduce herself when she enters the room, and state her reason for being there: "Mr. Elliot, I am Nurse Black, and I have some medication for you." The nurse should always speak to a blind patient before touching him to forewarn him of her presence. If the patient is deaf, the nurse should determine which ear he hears better from, and then speak close to that ear. If the patient wears a hearing aid, it should have batteries and be turned to the proper volume. The nurse should face the patient directly, so he can read her lips. Many elderly people function well with minimal hearing not only by listening but also by lip reading. Because most elderly people lose the ability to hear high tones first, the nurse should speak slowly and in a low, clear voice, accenting key words. She should not shout because the patient might perceive this as threatening.

Communicating with the older, confused patient takes special skill and patience. This skill requires much practice to develop. The key concepts are the use of eye contact and key words, listening for themes, and showing kindness and respect.

The patient's self-esteem may be enhanced by the nurse setting the psychological tone. The nurse should introduce herself by the title she prefers to be called. It is helpful if the nurse wears a name tag that is easily read. It is proper to call an older person by his last name preceded by the appropriate title (Mr., Mrs., Ms., or Miss). If the name is difficult to pronounce, the nurse should ask the patient for the proper pronunciation. The nurse may ask the patient what he would like to be called; however, it is never correct for health care personnel to address an older patient in the familiar terms of "Pops," "Gramps," "Granny," and "Sweetie."

It is helpful for the nurse to give complete explanations of why a question is asked, how it pertains to the patient's care, and how the information will be used. The elderly are usually more cooperative when someone cares enough to explain. The nurse must also be aware of what her body language is saying to the patient, both positive and negative, and what the patient's body language is saying to the nurse. Is the body language congruent with what is being said?

Common methods beyond general communication techniques will assist the nurse to gain information. The first rule is for the nurse to go slowly. Older people need more time to process what is said. The nurse should speak slowly, enunciate clearly, and give the patient time to process the message and respond. Younger people tend to get impatient and do not give the older person adequate time to respond.

Reminiscence is often used to gain valuable information from an older person. For many older people, recalling the past is clearer than considering current happenings. By recognizing common themes, much can be ascertained about a person's life-style, feelings, and relationships. It helps to emphasize the positive areas of the interaction and downplay or ignore, where possible, the negative aspects. Much can be gained from observations of nonverbal behavior.

Although closed questions are acceptable to obtain some information, such as "Where do you buy your medications?" elderly patients will respond more freely to open-ended questions. This reveals something about their skills and style in communication.

REFERENCES AND SUGGESTED READINGS

1. Bernstein L and Bernstein RS: Interviewing: a guide for health professionals, ed 4, East Norwalk, Conn, 1985, Appleton & Lange.
2. Burggraf V and Stanley M: Nursing the elderly: a care plan approach, Philadelphia, 1989, JB Lippincott Co.
3. Burnside I: Nursing and the aged: a self-care approach, ed 3, St Louis, 1988, The CV Mosby Co.
4. Cormier SL and others: Interviewing and helping skills for health professionals, Boston, 1984, Jones & Bartlett Publishers, Inc.
5. Eliopoulas C: Gerontology nursing, Philadelphia, 1987, JB Lippincott Co.
6. Ellis JR and Nowlis EA: Nursing: a human needs approach, ed 3, Boston, 1985, Houghton Mifflin Co.
7. Hollinger L: Communicating with the elderly, J Gerontol Nurs 12(3):8, 1981.
8. Lumin L and Rysticken N: Aids to bridge the communication barrier, Geriatr Nurs 6(6):348, 1985.
9. Potter P and Perry A: Fundamentals of nursing: concepts, process, and practice, ed 2, St Louis, 1989, The CV Mosby Co.

CHAPTER CHALLENGE

KEY POINTS

- Communication is one of the most important skills a student nurse will learn.
- It is necessary to understand how the components of communication affect the quality and quantity of communication.
- An interview has three phases: the beginning (introduction), the middle (working), and the end (termination).
- Nonverbal communication is usually a more accurate reflection of the patient's thoughts than verbal communication.
- There are verbal blocks and physical barriers to communication.
- There are techniques that facilitate therapeutic communication.
- Children and the elderly require some special considerations in communication.

STUDY QUESTIONS

1. The process of communication has five major components and six subcomponents. The five major components are:
   a. Context, perception, values, culture, proxemics
   b. Kinesics, receiver, values, sender, message
   c. Communicator, message, receiver, feedback, context
   d. Communicator, message, culture, receiver, feedback
2. The tone and guidelines are set during which phase of the interview:
   a. Introductory phase
   b. Working phase
   c. Termination phase
3. Therapeutic communication differs from social communication in that therapeutic communication is:
   a. Time limited
   b. Mutually beneficial to all participants
   c. Goal directed
   d. Patient centered
   e. Little structure
   f. a, b, c, e
   g. a, c, d, e
   h. a, c, d
   i. All of the above

Identify the technique used in the following questions (an answer may be used only once):

a. Open-ended question
b. Closed question
c. Reflection
d. Confrontation
e. Clarification

4. _____ PATIENT: I don't know why I have to have these tests. It is such a waste of time.
   NURSE: You're upset about the time it takes to have these tests.
5. _____ PATIENT: I don't know why I have to go to a nursing home. I can get along just fine at home.
   NURSE: What do you mean when you say "fine" at home?
6. _____ PATIENT: I have been having terrible headaches the last 3 months. Nothing seems to help. My husband finally made me come in.
   NURSE: Tell me what has changed in your life in the last 3 months.
7. _____ PATIENT: I have been having terrible headaches the last 3 months. Nothing seems to help. My husband finally made me come in.
   NURSE: Have you ever had a problem with headaches before?
8. _____ PATIENT: I don't know why I keep coming in to see the doctor. I try everything, and I still don't lose weight.
   NURSE: You say you want to lose weight and you have tried everything, yet I see by your food charts you haven't kept to your diet.

5

The Nursing Process

GRETCHEN H. LeGAULT

LEARNING OBJECTIVES

After reading this chapter, the student should be able to do the following:

- Define the key terms.
- List the five phases of the nursing process.
- Discuss how the five phases of the nursing process are used in nursing practice.
- Explain the essential components of each phase of the nursing process.
- Describe methods of collecting data.
- Discuss the steps in forming a nursing diagnosis.
- Describe the process of developing nursing goals and outcome criteria.
- Describe the process of developing nursing orders.
- Develop a nursing care plan using the nursing process.
- Discuss assignment of patient care.
- Explain the use of evaluation in patient care and quality assurance.

RELATED TOPICS OF INTEREST

- Communication (Chapter 4)
- Documentation (Chapter 6)

KEY TERMS

Define the following:

- ANA Standards of Nursing Practice
- assessment
- cues
- data base
- etiology
- evaluation
- goal
- health history
- implementation
- medical diagnosis
- NANDA
- nursing diagnosis
- nursing process
- objective data
- planning
- problem
- PSRO
- quality assurance
- signs and symptoms
- subjective data

Historically nurses focused on treating specific diseases and implementing physicians' orders. Little planning was done to individualize nursing care for a specific patient. The nursing process has evolved from the earlier trial and error method of administering nursing care. The **nursing process** is a systematic problem-solving approach to nursing care, based on broad theoretical knowledge combined with technical and communication skills. Today nursing is diversified, and nurses at all levels of practice use the nursing process in a variety of settings. Therefore it is very important that the nursing process be dynamic, flexible, and goal directed. Use of the nursing process has allowed increased individualization and continuity of care and has resulted in a higher quality of patient care.

The term **process** means a series of events, one event leading to another toward a goal. The five steps of the nursing process are interrelated, dynamic, and goal directed. Each phase builds on the preceding phase; therefore each phase builds on the accuracy of the prior phase. The five steps of the nursing process are assessment, nursing diagnosis, planning, implementation, and evaluation (Box 5-1).

BOX 5-1 NURSING PROCESS STEPS AND RELATED ACTIONS

ASSESSMENT

Collect data
- Observe (physical assessment)
- Interview (health history)
- Explore secondary sources

Validate data

NURSING DIAGNOSIS

Interpret data
Form nursing diagnosis

PLANNING

Set priorities
Form realistic goals
Identify outcomes
Write nursing actions
Develop nursing care plan

IMPLEMENTATION

Delegate care
Carry out nursing actions

EVALUATION

Reassess patient
Compare patient progress with identified outcomes
Modify care plan

ASSESSMENT

Assessment is an organized system for collecting data to determine a patient's health status. The first phase of assessment is to determine and establish a data base. Assessment will be continuous throughout the other phases of the nursing process as new data are compared with the data base to determine the patient's progress or lack of progress. To collect data the nurse employs observation and interviewing skills to obtain a health history, the technical skills of a physical assesment, and secondary sources of information such as significant others, medical records, and laboratory/diagnostic tests.

Types of Data

Five types of data are collected by the nurse during the assessment: historical, current, potential, subjective, and objective. Historical data involve events that have taken place before the patient's current illness. These might include childhood diseases, previous hospitalizations, or previous illnesses. Current data include what is happening to the patient now. The nurse must be aware that some patients talk about past and current problems together; therefore it is important for the nurse to put data in chronological order. Potential problems are identified by an analysis of the data that indicate the patient is at risk. For example, a 38-year-old man who is obese, smokes three packs of cigarettes a day, has a highly stressful job, and whose father and uncle died of myocardial infarction at ages 40 and 41, respectively, would be potentially at high risk for myocardial infarction. **Subjective data** are the patients' perceptions and feelings about themselves and what is happening to them. Only the patient can give subjective data. The nurse can observe relevant physiological objective data. A patient may describe a continuous, sharp pain in the right lower quadrant of the abdomen (subjective data); the nurse observes that the patient is holding his abdomen, is grimacing, is diaphoretic, and has an elevated pulse rate (objective data). **Objective data** are observable and measurable. Vital signs and diagnostic reports are examples of objective data.

Sources of Data

The sources of data are primary and secondary. The patient will always be the primary source of data, except in instances in which the patient is too young, too ill, too confused, or unwilling or unable to communicate. Secondary sources are all other sources of data. Significant others, such as family members, and members of the health care team often supply data. They provide their perceptions of stressors and events preceding the current illness; they may also give additional information and/or validate patient information.

Methods of Data Collection

The primary methods of data collection are observation, interviewing, obtaining a health history, physical assessment, and gathering diagnostic data and medical records. Observation is the gathering of data by systematically using the five senses (sight, hearing, touch, smell, and taste). Observation begins with the first contact with the patient and is ongoing. Observation requires a broad knowledge base, recognition of "normal" health states, and practice to recognize abnormal findings. Nurses should automatically do a rapid, systematic observation every time they see a patient; expression, posture, and gait can give many cues about how the patient is feeling. If any observation should reveal a deviation from normal, it warrants further investigation.

Health Interview

Interviewing is a goal-directed method of communication. Many hospitals have a specific format to be used. The interview should be more than a question-and-answer session: questions should be open ended to allow the patient to freely express thoughts and feelings. Closed questions are restrictive and generally elicit a yes or no or similar one-word answer. Unless the nurse asks the right question, valuable information may not be elicited. Open-ended questions broaden the range of discussion and encourage the expression of feelings. (See Chapter 4, Communication, on communication skills and conducting an interview.)

Observing and interviewing are the primary skills used in obtaining a health history. The **health history** provides a systematic format to gather facts from which an assessment is made regarding past, current, and potential health problems. If a standardized health history form is not available, the content presented in Box 5-2 should be used.

Physical Assessment

The physical assessment is done to obtain data about the patient's physical status. (See Chapter 13, Physical Assessment, for a discussion of assessment skills.)

Diagnostic Data

Diagnostic tests are ordered to provide a data base and to confirm or negate findings from the health history and physical assessment. The results of the diagnostic tests are compared with established norms. Some diagnostic tests are routine for all patients; others are ordered according to the patient's symptoms. Some diagnostic tests that may be ordered are radiographic examinations, ECG, computerized tomography (CT) scans, ultrasound studies, barium enema, and laboratory tests, such as blood chemistry profile, complete blood count, and blood, urine, or wound culture and sensitivity.

BOX 5-2 HEALTH HISTORY CONTENT

Statistical data
Record name, address, phone number, age, sex, marital status, educational level, occupation, employment status, and income/insurance

Chief complaint
Record patient's statement about seeking medical assistance

History and development of the complaint

Medical history

Family medical history

Medication history
Include all medications patient is currently taking, including over-the-counter medications and vitamins; include allergies to medication

Tobacco, alcohol, and drug history
Determine amount per day, age started, type, and frequency of use

Social history
Identify strengths and weaknesses, need for referrals, and living arrangements

Activities of daily living
Identify patterns of sleep, activity, nutrition, and elimination

Medical Records

Medical records may be a valuable source of a patient's past health and illness patterns. It is important to check the dates of the records to determine their relevancy.

NURSING DIAGNOSIS

Validating Data

To *validate* or *verify* means to confirm, substantiate, or establish the truth. By validating the data received it is possible to identify discrepancies, errors, or possible gaps where additional information may be needed. Not all data need validation, such as vital signs. Data that are incomplete, unclear, or show discrepancies must be verified. If inaccurate data are used, the entire plan of care will be inaccurate. Data may be confirmed through the primary source, the patient. Data may also be confirmed through secondary sources, e.g., family, significant others, physician, health care team, diagnostic data, medical records, and nursing home histories.

Grouping and Analyzing Data

During the assessment phase of data collection the nurse collects an enormous amount of information. These data must be organized to be used effectively. The first step is to sort out the data that are relevant to the patient's current health problem; the relevant data are then organized into categories that are related to each other. The **cues** within the categories are compared with normal standards and are assessed for patterns or trends. The categories are used to make *inferences.* An inference, or the interpretation of categories, is based on identified **cues.** For example:

CUES	INFERENCE
Loose-fitting dentures Unable to feed self Has lost 15 pounds in 2 months	Altered nutrition: less than body requirements

For many nurses the patient's areas of need or weakness are easily identified, e.g., persistent cough, pain, and anxiety. However, areas of strength are often overlooked. Some strengths might include a strong support system, strong self-concept or self-image, no history of smoking or the patient's having quit smoking, and financial security. Strengths aid a person's ability to cope and hasten the recovery time.

To relate and categorize data the nurse should consider areas of need. Maslow has identified basic human needs in hierarchical order (see p. 51); this structure not only aids the nurse in setting priorities, but also assists in developing the diagnostic statement.

Errors in Data Interpretation

Several factors may interfere with accurate interpretation of the data base:

1. Inadequate clinical knowledge or lack of clinical experience will seriously impede the nurse's ability to knowledgeably group cues or make inferences from cues. Extra emphasis may be placed on areas within the nurse's experience, while important cues outside the nurses experience may be overlooked.
2. Inaccurate information will lead to errors. This emphasizes the importance of validation.
3. Identification of the nurse's needs rather than the patient's needs indicates the nurse must be aware of how her values and beliefs affect her ability to interpret cues correctly.
4. Inappropriate interpretation of cues may lead to error. Cues must be compared with identified standards of both medical knowledge and of the individual patient. Cues should be grouped according to identified patient needs or problems. Use of a single cue on which to base a nursing diagnosis is usually insufficient.

A nursing diagnosis should not be formulated until all similar cues have been grouped.

Identifying the Problem or Need

When a patient's health status is altered or he is unable to meet his own needs, a problem results. Correct identification of the problem is necessary before the nursing diagnosis can be made. When cues and inferences have been compared with normal standards and problems are identified, the problems are classified as actual, potential, or possible problems. Actual problems are those currently affecting the health status of the patient. For a patient who is dehydrated, the diagnosis might be actual fluid volume deficit related to inability to reach fluids for self. Potential problems indicate that the patient is at risk as a result of predictable responses to disease complications or health history. For example, a recently widowed patient might receive a diagnosis of potential altered nutrition: less than body requirements related to loneliness (recent loss of spouse). Possible problems indicate that there may be a problem but more data are needed. For example, for a patient in a nursing home who stays in her room and becomes very agitated when unfamiliar people enter her room, the nurse might write a nursing diagnosis such as possible social isolation related to unknown factors.

Once the problems are accurately identified, the nurse refers to the list of NANDA-approved nursing diagnoses to assist in writing the diagnostic statement.

Formulating the Nursing Diagnosis

Making the **nursing diagnosis** statement is the second phase of the nursing process. The diagnostic statement is based on accurate data and identification of the patient's actual or potential health problems. The statement is related to one patient problem that lies within the scope of independent nursing practice. Only those problems treatable within the scope of nursing practice are included in the nursing care plan. The PES form is used when writing the nursing diagnosis statement:

P = Problem
E = Etiology
S = Signs and symptoms

The **problem** (*P*) is a description of the patient's actual or potential health problem. To promote quality of nursing care only the nursing diagnoses approved by the North American Nursing Diagnosis Association **(NANDA)** are used. Because of continual change in health care delivery, the list of nursing diagnoses is continually being revised. NANDA meets every 2 years to consider additions to the NANDA list of approved nursing diagnoses (see inside front cover for Ninth NANDA-approved nursing diagnoses).

Etiology (*E*) reflects the factors believed to be related to or contributing to the identified problem, e.g., environmental (excessive noise), sociological (inability to speak English), spiritual (conflict between beliefs and prescribed medical practice), psychological (fear of loss of control), and physiological (incisional pain).

The problem and the etiology are connected by "related to" (R/T), which shows a relationship, not "cause and effect." To use the term "due to" or "caused by" would indicate cause, which then invades the realm of the physician. Etiology can be stated in two parts, e.g., self-care deficit, bathing/hygiene, related to inability to wash body parts secondary to (2°) obesity. At times the etiology will be unknown, e.g., pain related to unknown etiology. **Medical diagnosis** is never used as part of the nursing diagnosis.

Signs and symptoms (*S*) are the objective and subjective cues that give evidence that a problem exists. Signs and symptoms are connected to the etiology by "as shown by" or "manifested by" (M/B), e.g., anticipatory grieving related to potential loss of spouse (M/B) (1) changes in eating and sleeping patterns, and (2) expression of distress of potential loss.

It is not always necessary to show signs and symptoms; however, both the etiology and the signs and symptoms assist in determining the nursing interventions. A well-written diagnostic statement prepares the nurse for phase three of the nursing process (Box 5-3).

PLANNING

Planning, phase three of the nursing process, consists of four major tasks:

1. Setting priorities
2. Developing realistic goals and outcome criteria
3. Writing nursing orders
4. Developing the nursing care plan

BOX 5-3 GUIDELINES FOR NURSING DIAGNOSES

1. The medical diagnosis should not be included in the diagnostic statement.
2. The diagnostic statement must be written within the scope of independent nursing functions.
3. The nursing diagnosis should not be influenced by personal bias.
4. The problem and etiology should be linked by "related to" (R/T), not "due to" or "caused by."
5. Etiology and signs and symptoms are connected by "as shown by" or "manifested by" (M/B).
6. Use only NANDA-approved diagnoses for the problem.
7. Always write the problem first and related etiology second.
8. Use legally advisable terms.
9. State in terms of a problem, not a need.
10. The elements of the diagnostic statement should not say the same thing.
11. The diagnostic statement should give direction for nursing interventions.

BOX 5-4 MASLOW'S BASIC HUMAN NEEDS

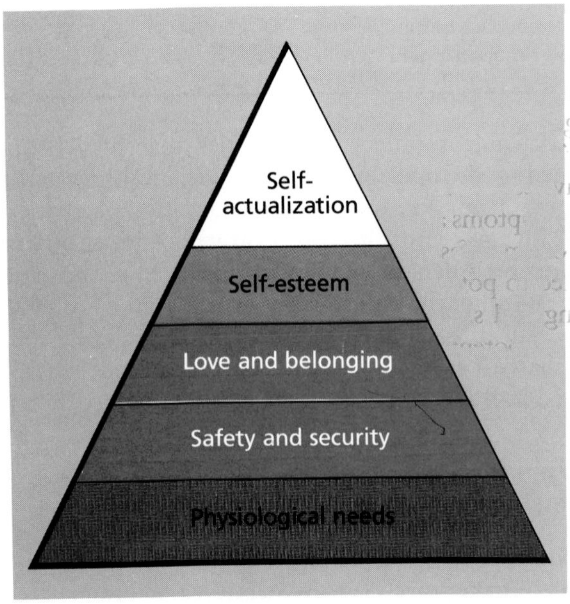

I. Physical needs
  A. Physiological needs
    1. Personal hygiene
    2. Activity
    3. Sexuality
  B. Homeostatic
    1. Eating and drinking
    2. Vital functions (oxygenation)
    3. Sleep and rest
    4. Elimination

II. Safety and security
  A. Safety and accident prevention
  B. Religion and philosophy
  C. Feeling of well-being

III. Love and belonging
  A. Communication
  B. Affection
  C. Identity
  D. Modesty
  E. Companionship
  F. Dependence

IV. Self-esteem
  A. Recognition

V. Self-actualization
  A. A desire for self-fulfillment

Setting Priorities

Most patients have more than one nursing diagnosis; thus it is necessary to set priorities to establish a preferential order for nursing interventions. Setting priorities is facilitated by using a framework such as Maslow's hierarchy of needs (Box 5-4). Emphasis in nursing is placed on the first four levels. Maslow's physiological needs of oxygen, fluid, nutrition, and elimination are basic to life and therefore would receive a higher priority than activity or love and belonging. Life-threatening problems must have immediate attention and thus receive the highest priority. Priorities change as the patient's health problems change. When possible it is important for the patient to have input into setting priorities. Priorities must also be congruent with treatment by other medical personnel.

According to Maslow's theory, human needs at the lower levels must be met before higher needs, in a hierarchy of five levels. The basic or first level is physiological: oxygen, water, and food. The second level consists of safety and security needs, which are divided into psychological and physiological safety. The third level is the need for love and belonging; everyone needs social relationships. On the fourth level is self-esteem, which includes thinking well of yourself and feeling that others think well of you. The fifth level is self-actualization, the state of having reached one's full potential and being able to cope with problems.

Establishing Realistic Goals and Outcome Criteria

A nursing **goal** is the desired change in the patient's health status after nursing intervention. When possible, goals are made jointly by the patient and nurse (Box 5-5). Realistic goals give direction to the formation of nursing interventions and provide the basis for evaluation. Goals may be short term or long term. The short-term goal is used most frequently. When the long-term goal is used, it builds on the short-term goal. For example, on a patient's second postoperative day, a short-term goal might be that the patient will walk from the bed to chair with assistance twice a day for 2 days. A long-term goal would be that the patient will walk the length of the hall independently three times a day until discharge. The nurse must write patient goals in clear, concise, measur-

BOX 5-5 GUIDELINES FOR GOALS

1. Must be written in terms of patient behavior
2. Must be observable and measurable
3. Must be realistic
4. Must be time oriented
5. Must be clear and concise

able terms. Evaluation of nursing interventions is possible only if this criterion is met. The goal is written with (1) a statement of patient intent (the patient will), (2) an action verb (eat), (3) a behavior (80% of three meals served), and (4) a time factor (every day for 4 days).

Outcome criteria must be identified so the nurse can determine whether the goal was met. Outcome criteria may be included as part of the goal statement (No. 3, behavior), or in some institutions they are stated as actual behavior at the end of the evaluation period: "The patient ate 75% of breakfast meals, 80% of dinner meals, and 100% of supper meals for 4 days."

Selecting Nursing Interventions

Nursing interventions are actions designed to achieve the identified nursing goals or meet the outcome criteria. Two to four nursing interventions are usually adequate for each identified nursing problem. For each nursing intervention the nurse must consider the consequences as well as the merits. Alternative actions should also be considered; then the best intervention for the individual patient should be chosen.

Writing Nursing Orders

Nursing interventions are written as nursing orders. Nursing orders are clear, concise statements of action the nurse will take to achieve nursing goals. Nursing orders are not statements of routine hospital procedures (e.g., "vital signs AM and PM") or of medical orders (e.g., "pain medication prn"). Nursing orders are written so that all nurses caring for that patient will have clear instructions for expected nursing interventions. Nursing orders must be specific, clear, concise, and action oriented. Nursing orders may be dependent, interdependent, or independent.

A dependent order indicates how a medical order will be carried out. For example, if the physician's order states "up in chair bid," the nursing orders might read:

8/15:
Up in chair for 30 minutes at 10 AM and 8 PM.
Needs two-person assist.
Elevate (R) leg on pillow.

Interdependent orders are activities the nurse carries out with other health care workers. For example, for a patient who speaks only Spanish and tends to isolate himself from other patients and staff, the social worker and nurse might write the following orders:

3/18:
A Spanish-speaking staff member will interact with patient for 30 minutes q shift q day.
Patient will make his needs known by interacting with Spanish-speaking staff person q day.

BOX 5-6 GUIDELINES FOR WRITING NURSING ORDERS

1. Date: date order was written
2. Action verb
3. Subject: who is to carry out the order
4. Descriptive phrase: what, where, when, how much, and how long
5. Signature: who wrote order

Independent orders are activities that may be performed by the nurse without a physician's order and are within the nurse's experience and education. Activities of daily living are usually covered in independent orders.

Nursing orders should be individualized to the patient and be consistent with the prescribed plan of care. It is important that all nursing orders be theoretically sound and based on scientific rationales. The guidelines presented in Box 5-6 will assist the nurse in writing nursing orders.

Developing the Nursing Care Plan

The final stage of the planning phase is development of the nursing care plan. A well-developed nursing care plan facilitates communication to other health care personnel, continuity of care for the patient, and the evaluation process. The professional nurse is responsible for writing the nursing care plan; however, both the patient and other nursing personnel should be involved in the development of the plan of care (see sample, p. 53).

IMPLEMENTATION

Implementation is the fourth phase of the nursing process. Implementation is putting the interventions in the care plan into action. Actions, like nursing orders, may be dependent, interdependent, or independent. A nurse may carry out the interventions alone or may assign patient care to other nursing personnel. When a nurse assigns patient care to other nursing personnel, she must assess three areas: (1) the degree to which the patient can help himself, (2) the needs and acuity of the patient, and (3) the educational level, licensure, and expertise of the caregiver. When the assignment is based on complexity, the caregiver with the higher level of education and expertise is assigned to give the most complex care. Less prepared or less experienced caregivers are assigned to the patients with less complex needs. As the nurse implements nursing orders, she must continue to collect pertinent data and assess patient response to the interventions. The care plan must be flexible and reflect changes in the patient's health care. Knowledge based on critical thinking and expertise aids the nurse in decision

NURSING CARE PLAN: SAMPLE

64-year-old Hispanic male admitted posttrauma—car accident.

Patient received fracture of left humerus, fracture of second cervical vertebra, fracture of 4th rib; has halo brace; is obese; osteoarthritis consistent with age. Discharge date: 1 week. Primary caregiver for wife, who is unable to care for herself.

GOAL: Patient will be independent in all ADLs before going home.

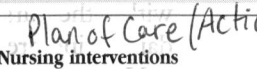

Nursing diagnoses/supporting data	Nursing interventions	Rationale	Expected outcome/actual outcome
Self-care deficit, related to disruption of ability to perform activities of daily living as a result of multiple fractures as shown by need for assistance with bathing, dressing, grooming, and toileting	Discuss ADLs with patient to determine areas where assistance will be necessary at home; determine wife's ability to assist. Teach other family members how to assist in areas where she is unable. Contact social worker with discharge data and advise of home needs; arrange meeting with patient.	An important objective in treating fractures is to help patients return to their normal activities as soon as possible. Evaluate patient's ability to care for self at home. Ensure patient's ability to manage fracture at home. Lack of knowledge and poor preparation of self-care at home contribute to anxiety and nonadherence to therapeutic regimen.	Patient will verbalize areas of self-care that require assistance in the home. Patient will plan with nurse and social worker for the necessary assistance from family member or health care professional at home before discharge fom hospital.
Impaired skin integrity, related to application of halo brace (secondary to spinal fracture) M/B erythema, drainage, tenderness, vesicles, or pain under the halo vest.	Clean pin sites with half-strength hydrogen peroxide; then apply Neosporin ointment q shift. Check for erythema or vesicles under halo vest. Ask patient if halo vest is causing any discomfort q shift.	Nursing care is directed toward promoting comfort, wound healing, and reducing hazards of immobility. Interruption in skin continuity may lead to infection. Therefore special care must be taken to keep pin sites clean.	Patient will not complain of pain at pin sites or under halo vest. Patient will remain free of erythema, drainage, or tenderness (or loosening) at pin sites q shift. Patient will remain free of erythema, tenderness, or vesicle formation under halo vest q shift.

making when changes must be made as a result of reassessment. Interventions and their results should be recorded in the patient's chart for evaluation and legal purposes.

EVALUATION

Evaluation is the fifth phase of the nursing process. To evaluate is to determine what progress has been made toward meeting the patient's goals. The outcomes of care are compared with the established outcome criteria. Evaluation must be carried out within the time line stated in the outcome criteria.

As in all other phases of the nursing process, data obtained in reassessing the patient will show the degree of progress or lack of progress the patient has made toward the stated goals. Progress is judged in the following ways: (1) the goal was met, (2) the goal was partially met, (3) the goal was not met. If the goal was partially met or not met, the nurse needs to reexamine all phases of the nursing process and modify the nursing care plan where necessary.

The **ANA Standards of Nursing Practice** (Box 5-7), which give specific direction to the use of the nursing process, are reexamined to assist in meeting identified standards of practice. **Quality assurance** has become in-

BOX 5-7 ANA STANDARDS OF NURSING PRACTICE

I. The collection of data about the health status of a client/patient is systematic and continuous. The data are accessible, communicated, and recorded.
II. Nursing diagnoses are derived from health status data.
III. The plan of nursing care includes goals derived from the nursing diagnoses.
IV. The plan of nursing care includes priorities and the prescribed nursing approaches or measures to achieve the goals derived from the nursing diagnoses.
V. Nursing actions provide for participation in health promotion, maintenance, and restoration.
VI. Nursing actions assist the client/patient to maximize his health capabilities.
VII. The client's/patient's progress or lack of progress toward goal achievement is determined by the client/patient and the nurse.
VIII. The client's/patient's progress or lack of progress toward total achievement directs reassessment, reordering of priorities, new goal setting, and revision of the plan of nursing care.

creasingly important in determining the quality of care provided in health care settings. Areas evaluated are the standards of nursing care used, the quality and effectiveness of nursing care, and the organization of the patient care system. Since 1972 the Joint Commission on Accreditation of Hospitals (JCAH)* has required a systematic evaluation of the quality of care given to all patients in hospitals. A nursing audit is a review of patients' charts to evaluate nursing performance. An audit may be retrospective (evaluation of the patient's chart after the patient is discharged) or concurrent (a review of current practices). The Professional Standards Review Organization **(PSRO)** has developed peer review as a method of evaluation. In peer review a person reviews documented nursing interventions in a patient's chart to determine if the nursing actions meet accepted nursing standards. The reviewer is a peer who is equal in education and other qualifications to the nurses who are charting.

There are three types of nursing audits:

1. A structural audit focuses on how care is structured. It includes policies and procedures, staffing, equipment, management, physical facilities, and safety of the environment.
2. A process audit focuses on the activities of the nurse within the nursing process. The nurse is evaluated on her competency in all five phases of the nursing process.
3. An outcomes audit focuses on the end result of nursing interventions. As a result of quality assurance, specific problems are being carefully monitored and corrected and preventive actions are being taken.

*Now referred to as Joint Commission on Accreditation of Healthcare Organizations (JCAHO).

REFERENCES AND SUGGESTED READINGS

1. Alfaro R: Application of nursing process, ed 3, Philadelphia, 1986, JB Lippincott Co.
2. Arnold E and Boggs K: Interpersonal relationships, Philadelphia, 1989, WB Saunders Co.
3. Carpenito LJ: Nursing diagnosis: applications to clinical practice, Philadelphia, 1989, JB Lippincott Co.
4. Crosby FS and others: Teaching nursing diagnosis to school nurses: a standardized measure of cognitive effect, J Contin Educ Nurs 19(5):211, 1988.
5. Douglass LM: The effective nurse: leader and manager, ed 3, St Louis, 1988, The CV Mosby Co.
6. Ellis JR and Nowles EA: Nursing: a human needs approach, ed 3, Boston, 1985, Bartin-Houghton-Mifflin.
7. Frisch N and others: Nursing diagnosis: a curricular model based on the NANDA list, Nurs Educ 13(5):14, 1988.
8. Gordon M: Manual of nursing diagnosis, New York, 1986, McGraw-Hill Book Co.
9. Gordon M: The concept of nursing diagnosis, Nurs Clin North Am 14:487, 1979.
10. Iyer PW, Taptich BJ, and Losey DB: Nursing process and nursing diagnosis, Philadelphia, WB Saunders Co.
11. Krenz M: Linking nursing diagnosis, quality assurance, and nursing standards, J Adv Med Surg Nurs 1(3):53, 1989.
12. Potter PA and Perry AG: Fundamentals of nursing, ed 2, St Louis, 1989, The CV Mosby Co.
13. Scheffer B and others: LEAD: learning efficient and accurate diagnosing. Nurs Diagn Proc Eighth Conf, 1989, p 246.
14. Taylor CM and Cress SS: Nursing diagnosis cards, Springhouse, Pa, 1987, Springhouse Corp.
15. Tucker SM and others: Patient care standards: nursing process, diagnosis and outcome, ed 4, St Louis, 1988. The CV Mosby Co.

CHAPTER CHALLENGE

KEY POINTS

- The nursing process is a systematic problem-solving approach that is dynamic, flexible, and goal directed.
- The five phases of the nursing process are assessment, nursing diagnosis, planning, implementation, and evaluation.
- The patient is the primary source of data, except in instances in which the patient is too young, too ill, too confused, or unwilling or unable to communicate.
- All of the senses are used when observing and assessing a patient.
- An understanding of "normal" is essential when making or assisting with a head-to-toe assessment of a patient.
- Nursing diagnoses are based on accurate data and identification of patient needs.
- The nursing diagnosis is formulated according to the PES format, using the current NANDA list of approved diagnoses.
- A nursing goal indicates a desired change in a patient's status after nursing intervention.
- Nursing orders are clear, concise statements of actions that the nurse will take to achieve the goals.
- Implementation, like nursing orders, may be dependent, interdependent, or independent.
- A nurse may carry out the orders or assign patient care to other nursing personnel.
- The outcome of care is evaluated according to outcome criteria.
- The ANA Standards of Nursing Practice is used to identify standards of practice.

STUDY QUESTIONS

1. The nursing process consists of the following five sequential, interrelated phases:
   a. Observation, interaction, validation, implementation, and evaluation
   b. Assessment, nursing diagnosis, planning, implementation, and evaluation
   c. Define the problem, collect data, analyze data, devise solution, and evaluate
   d. Analyze, make inferences, validate, reassess, and implement
2. Maslow's hierarchy of needs is useful in assisting the nurse in:
   a. Identifying cultural and ethnic needs
   b. Identifying developmental factors of care
   c. Setting priorities of care
   d. Documenting care
3. The nursing diagnosis statement is written according to the PES format. PES means all of the following except:
   a. Medical diagnosis
   b. Description of the problem
   c. Etiology
   d. Signs and symptoms
4. The nursing process is a deliberate problem-solving approach directed at meeting the needs of the patient:
   True ______ False ______
5. Consistent problem identification is assisted by using the NANDA list of accepted nursing diagnoses:
   True ______ False ______
6. The goal should clearly state what the nursing action will be:
   True ______ False ______
7. Quality assurance is a planned, systematic evaluation of patient care:
   True ______ False ______

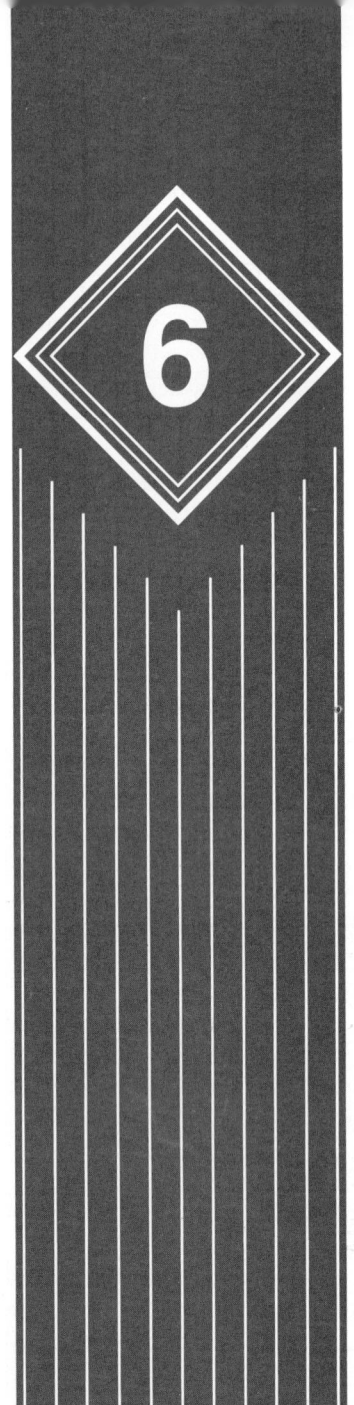

6

Documentation

DONNA M. BABAO

LEARNING OBJECTIVES

After reading this chapter, the student should be able to do the following:

- Define the key terms.
- List the five purposes for written patient records.
- Describe the differences between traditional and problem-oriented medical records.
- State important legal aspects of chart ownership, access, confidentiality, and patient care documentation.
- Describe the purpose of and relationship between the Kardex and the nursing care plan.
- Explain the relationship of the nursing care plan to care documentation and patient care reimbursement.
- Describe the basic guidelines for and mechanics of charting.
- Describe the differences in documenting care using activity of daily living and physical assessment forms, narrative, SOAPE, and focus formats.
- Discuss the use of computers for record keeping and documentation in health care facilities.

RELATED TOPICS OF INTEREST

- Legal aspects of nursing (Chapter 2)
- Communication (Chapter 4)
- The nursing process (Chapter 5)
- Principles and practice of medication administration (Chapter 25)

KEY TERMS

Define the following:

- auditors
- chart (health care record)
- charting
- charting by exception
- computer terminal
- confidentiality
- defensive charting
- diagnosis related groups (DRGs)
- documenting
- focus charting
- Kardex
- narrative charting
- nursing care plan
- nursing notes
- peer review
- physician's orders
- problem list
- problem-oriented medical record (POMR)
- progress notes
- quality assurance
- Rand recording
- SOAPE
- SOAPIER
- traditional or block chart

A medical record should furnish all health care providers with a concise, accurate, written picture of a patient's medical and nursing problems, care planned and given, and the patient's response to treatments. The **chart,** or **health care record,** has never been more important in the health care system than it is today; it is a legal record that is used to meet the many demands of the health, accreditation, medical insurance, and legal systems.

A nurse must understand how to use these records effectively and efficiently. This chapter will cover the purposes for written records, common types of records, basic guidelines and rules for documentation, and legal concerns. The knowledge and ability to chart completely, accurately, and legibly is a requirement for licensure and employment as a nurse.

The process of adding written information to the chart is called **charting, recording,** or **documenting.** Although there are many details to remember when documenting in the chart, the process is not difficult but can be time consuming. Documentation is part of the implementation phase of the nursing process (see Chapter 5) and is necessary for the evaluation of patient care as well as for care cost reimbursement.

PURPOSES OF PATIENT RECORDS

There are five basic purposes for written patient records: (1) written communication, (2) permanent record for accountability, (3) legal record of care, (4) teaching, and (5) research and data collection.

The patient's chart provides a permanent written record of past and current medical and nursing problems, plans for care, care given, and the patient's responses to various treatments. The record facilitates accurate communication and continuity of care among all members of the health care team. Written information is not as easily lost or accidentally altered as is the spoken word.

This permanent written record may also be used by various government and other agencies to evaluate the institution's patient care and to prove that care was given for cost reimbursement. Current regulations require chart audits (review of specific chart components for completion and appropriateness) by officially appointed **auditors.** Institutions have medical and **peer review** systems plus specific procedures to provide for **quality assurance** audits. Accurate and legible records are the only means institutions have to prove that they are providing care to meet the patient's needs and established standards.

Cost reimbursement rates by the government plans (Medicare, Medicaid) are based on **diagnosis related groups (DRGs).** Many private insurance companies now use similar illness categories when setting hospital payment rates. The **nursing notes** are carefully reviewed when deciding whether the necessary and ordered care is being or was given. Institutions are reimbursed by insurance companies or government programs only for the patient care documented.

The patient chart or health record is a legal document and can be called into court. While the physician or institution owns the original record, lawyers and courts can gain access to it. That is why it is important to chart in a very detailed, defensive manner. Most states now also grant patient access through channels established by the individual facility. The patient usually does not have immediate access to his full record (see Chapter 2).

Patient health records are also used for teaching. Students in the health care professions can learn more quickly and easily if examples of good charting are shared. Individuals can also learn from their mistakes and the mistakes of others.

Individuals involved in research and data collection in the health field have many uses for patient records. For example, the government periodically publishes data on certain diseases and the effectiveness of new treatments. The usual length of hospitalization and the cost of treatment for specific illnesses or surgeries have become very important to the government and other health insurance providers because of the pressure to contain or limit health care costs.

COMMON MEDICAL ABBREVIATIONS AND TERMINOLOGY

A nurse cannot effectively and efficiently use a health record until some understanding and knowledge of common abbreviations and medical terms have been developed. This information is also required for concise and accurate documentation of care. Most facilities have a published list of generally accepted medical abbreviations and terms approved for use in charting. The use of ambiguous abbreviations and terms should be avoided, because their use may lead to misinterpretations and errors. (Consult the inside front cover of this text.)

TYPES OF PATIENT RECORDS

There are basically two types or forms for patient health records: the traditional or block chart and the problem-oriented medical record (POMR). Both formats, while different in style, contain the same information.

Traditional Chart

The **traditional** or **block chart** is divided into specific sections or blocks. Emphasis is placed on specific sheets of information. Typical blocks are admission sheet, **physician's orders, progress notes,** history and physical examination data, nurse's admission information, care plan, and nursing notes, graphics, and laboratory and x-ray reports. The order, content, and number of the sections vary among institutions. Nurses use flow sheets, graphics, and **narrative notes** to chart observations, care, and responses (Fig. 6-1).

Problem-Oriented Medical Record

The organization of the **problem-oriented medical record (POMR)** is based on the scientific problem-solving system or method. The principal sections are data base, **problem list,** initial plan, and progress notes. The accumulated data or data base from the history, physical examination, and diagnostic tests are used to identify and prioritize the health problems on the master medical and other problem list.

This problem list of active, inactive, potential, and resolved problems serves as the index for chart documentation. All health care providers—physicians, nurses, social workers, and therapists—chart on the same progress notes. This is done to facilitate and enhance communication between care providers. The charting format used is called **SOAPE,** or the more specific **SOAPIER.**

SOAPIER is an acronym for seven different aspects of charting. For notes on specific patient problems, only the necessary parts needed for completeness are used.

- **S** *Subjective* information is what the patient states or feels; *only* the patient can provide subjective information.
- **O** *Objective* information is what the nurse can measure or factually describe.
- **A** *Assessment* refers to an analysis or potential diagnosis of the cause of the patient's problem or need.
- **P** *Plan* is the general statement of the plan of care to be given or action to be taken.
- **I** *Implementation* is the specific care given or action taken.
- **E** *Evaluation* is an appraisal of the response and effectiveness of the plan.
- **R** *Revision* includes the changes that may be made to the original plan of care.

SOAPE (Box 6-1) is the briefer adaptation of the charting format for the problem-oriented record. In this more compact form, the care given or action taken *(I)* is in-

BOX 6-1 SOAPE CHARTING FORMAT

Subjective
Objective
Assessment
Plan
Evaluation

000 – 123
Spaur, Phyllis Room 348 A
female – 60
Dr. Pearson – Bennett

ADDRESSOGRAPH

NURSE'S RECORD

Great Plains Regional Medical Center
NORTH PLATTE, NEBRASKA

Code: ✓ = Yes 0 = No ⓧ = Refer to Nurse's Notes

DATE: 12/7/90 1

CODE for 23:00 to 7:00 A = Awake S = Sleeping C = Comatose

23:00	24:00	1:00	2:00	3:00	4:00	5:00	6:00
A	S	S	S	A	S	S	A

DIET	Cl Liq	APPETITE
B	Cl Liq	100%
D		
S		

G = Good F = Fair P = Poor

	OBSERVATIONS:	23-7	7-15	15-23
SYSTEMS	CardioVascular, Regular.	✓	✓	
	G.I.,soft	✓	✓	
	G.U., voiding	✓	ⓧ	
	Neuro., no deficit	✓	✓	
	Resp., Regular	✓	✓	
ROUTINE	Bath	✓	BB	
	Oral Care	✓	✓	
	Side Rails up	✓	✓	
	Call Light in reach	✓	✓	
	Back Care	✓	✓	
	Bed in Lo Position	✓	✓	
OTHER	IV – D5W c̄ 30 mEq KCl @ 125 ml/hr	✓	✓	
	dressing chg		✓	
	INITIALS:	FE	DP	

NURSE'S NOTES: 0600 awake and alert. Skin pink, warm and dry. T-tube draining dark green liquid. IV infusing in lt. antecubital area @ 20 gtts/minute. No evidence of erythema or edema. Sleeping well for 2 hour intervals. Has obtained relief from pain since 11 p.m. medication. Ambulated to bathroom, voided 100 ml. of dark amber urine. C/o slight vertigo and assisted to bed. Dressings dry and intact. ~~~~~ F Ellefson RN.
0700–1100 0700 alert and oriented x3. Skin pink, warm c̄ dry. 99⁸–88–22. Denies incisional discomfort. Coughs well c̄ splinting of incision. Cough nonproductive, lungs clear, bowel sounds hypoactive. Abdominal dressing dry and intact. T-tube draining dark green liquid, 30 ml drainage in bag. IV infusing @ 20 gtts/minute in lt. antecubital space, no erythema or edema @ site D. Phillips LPN
0900 ambulated to bathroom with 1 assist. C/o burning on urination. Voided 100 ml of dark, amber, cloudy urine. T. 101² (0), c/o feeling hot and flushed. Dr. Pearson-Bennett notified. Fluids encouraged. #16 Fr. catheter inserted s̄ difficulty. 300 ml of dark, amber, cloudy urine obtained. Specimen to laboratory for C c̄ S. IV antibiotic started after catheterization by G Johnston RN
Oral fluids taken well. Abd. dressings changed – incision approximated. Staples intact – no erythema noted. T-tube in place. T. 100 (0). Resting comfortably. ~~~~~ D. Phillips LPN.

Continue on reverse side if necessary

SIGNATURES: G. J. Garnet Johnston RN F.E. Francis Ellefson RN
DP Dorothy Phillips LPN.

Form N-55 (1-87) 2647

FIG. 6-1 Narrative notes.

Great Plains Regional Medical Center
North Platte, Nebraska 69101

PROGRESS NOTES

Last Name	First Name	Attending Physician	Room No.	Hosp. No.
Spaur	Phyllis	Dr. Pearson-Bennett	348 A	000-123

Date	Notes Should Be Signed by Physician
12/7	0930 Problem #3 elevated temperature
	(Nursing diagnosis: alteration in body temperature: fever.)
	S: Feels hot & flushed. Has burning on urination and
	heavy feeling over bladder area. c/o some discomfort in lt. flank
	O: Temperature 101² (o) elevated from 99⁸ @ 7³⁰ A.M. Skin
	warm, flushed, dry. Urinating in 100-200 ml am'ts. Urine dark,
	amber and cloudy. Foley cath. dc'd 12/6 @ 10 P.M. Lungs clear.
	A: Possible bladder infection secondary to foley catheter.
	P: Notify Dr. Pearson-Bennett of temperature elevation,
	dysuria and back discomfort. Assess for other signs of
	infection. To x-ray for chest evaluation. Begin oral
	antibiotics after catheterization and urine specimen to
	laboratory for C & S per Dr. Pearson-Bennett orders.
	Encourage increase oral fluids.
	E: Urine to laboratory, x-ray of chest ordered, chest and
	breath sounds clear. Nonproductive cough. Taking fluids
	well. 10:30 urine less concentrated.
	11 A.M. problem #2 pain
	(Nursing diagnosis: pain)
	S: Uncomfortable from incisional pain when ambulating -
	splinting helps alleviate some discomfort.
	O: Dressings dry and intact. Incision and sutures intact,
	no drainage or erythema on first dressing change. Temp 100° (o)
	A: Minimal postoperative pain.
	P: Medicate for pain PRN as ordered.
	E: States pain is less severe, able to ambulate more
	easily. ~~~~ G. Johnston LVN

N-8 2640 PROGRESS NOTES

FIG. 6-2 SOAPE charting progress notes.

GREAT PLAINS
REGIONAL MEDICAL CENTER

Page 1 of 2 PATIENT CARE PLAN

Admitting Diagnosis: Cholelithiasis/Cholecystitis Operation: Cholecystectomy Surgery Date: 12/5/90

Additional Diagnosis: Surgeon: Dr. Pearson-Bennett Adm. Date: 12/4 Dism. Date:

Nursing Diagnosis with outcome	Start Date	Nursing Interventions	Date D/Cd	Init	Reassessment	Date D/Cd	Init
#1 Knowledge deficit preoperative and postoperative care R/T Scheduled surgery Goal: will verbalize routines and demonstrate postop. deep breathing, coughing and leg exercises	12/5	Explain preoperative routine NPO laboratory blood work. Demonstrate postoperative deep breathing, coughing and leg exercises. Explain about I.V., tubes, vital signs, pain control c̄ medication.	12/6	DP	Has learned to cough, deep breath and do leg exercises		DP
#2 Pain R/T incision and muscle spasms M/B verbalization of pain, guarded movements. Goal: Relate that she feels more comfortable, moves more easily, rests and sleeps well @ intervals	12/6	Review incisional splinting. Assist c̄ splinting by using pillow or bath blanket. Encourage requesting medication for pain before complaints are too severe. Teach relaxation exercises. Administer analgesics PRN. Assess response to medication within 1/2 hour.	12/7	DP	Is moving more easily, resting well for several hours. Is splinting incision well and able to cough and deep breath.		DP

INITIALS AND SIGNATURE: DP D. Phillips, RN

GREAT PLAINS
REGIONAL MEDICAL CENTER

Page 2 of 2 PATIENT CARE PLAN

Admitting Diagnosis: Cholelithiasis Operation: Cholecystectomy Surgery Date: 12/5/90

Additional Diagnosis: UTI Surgeon: Dr. Pearson-Bennett Adm. Date: 12/4/90 Dism. Date:

Nursing Diagnosis: with outcome	Start Date	Nursing Interventions	Date D/Cd	Init	Reassessment	Date D/Cd	Init
#3 Alteration in body temperature R/T UTI M/B temperature >101°(O) feeling flushed and c/o dysuria Goal: maintain normal body temperature and dysuria will subside.	12/7	Vital signs q̄ 4 and PRN Encourage fluids as tolerated I & O, provide high calorie in between meal snacks. Assess comfort. Medicate for temperature >102° (O) q̄ 4 PRN		DP			

INITIALS AND SIGNATURE: DP D. Phillips, RN

FIG. 6-3 Patient care plan with nursing diagnosis.

MASTER PROBLEM LIST

Date	Problem	Resolved	Reviewed	Reactivate
12/5/90	#1 Knowledge deficit R/T Preoperative and postoperative procedures.	12/6/90		
12/6/90	#2 Pain R/T incision.	12/7		
12/7/90	#3 Temperature elevation 2° to bladder infection.			

Addressograph

FIG. 6-4 Master problem list.

DATE	12/7	
TIME	**FOCUS**	**NURSES NOTES**
2 p.m.	post-op pain	Ambulating in hall c̄ moderate assist. I.V. infusing @ 20 gtts/min. Still feels warm, main concern is incisional pain, splinting is helpful. Positioned in bed c̄ pillows for support. Medicated for pain. Practiced relaxation breathing exercises. D Phillips LPN.
2:30 p.m.	pain / fever	Feels more comfortable. Appears relaxed. Skin warm and dry. T. 99^6 (o). C/o some burning on urination, less than in a.m. Taking fluids well. Urine light yellow and less cloudy. D Phillips LPN

FIG. 6-5 Focus charting nurses' notes.

BOX 6-2 FOCUS CHARTING FORMAT

Data
Action
Response

cluded in the plan notations. The needed plan revisions *(R)* are noted after the evaluation of the response to treatment in the evaluation section. The commonly used charting forms in the progress notes in medical records are shown in Figs. 6-2 through 6-4.

Focus Charting Format

One other charting form used in some institution has similarities to the problem list for the POMR. This **focus charting format** (Box 6-2), developed by nurses, could be used with both traditional and POMR charting. In focus charting, instead of problem lists, a modified list of nursing diagnoses is used as an index for nursing documentation. This form of charting uses the nursing process and the more positive concept of the patient's needs rather than medical diagnoses and problems.

The focus can be a current patient concern or behavior, significant change in patient status or behavior, or significant event in the patient's therapy. A focus is not a medical diagnosis.

Data *(D)* is equivalent to the assessment step of the nursing process. Action *(A)* is a combination of planning and implementation. Response *(R)* is the same as evaluation. Not all the DAR steps need to be used each time notes are made on a particular focus (Fig. 6-5).

BASIC GUIDELINES FOR DOCUMENTATION

The quality and accuracy of the nurse's notes are very important. The words used can clearly and concisely convey the intended message or can cause confusion and errors in communication and patient care. Correct spelling, grammar, and punctuation, as well as penmanship and other writing skills, are important in documentation.

The information recorded in the chart should be clear, concise, complete, and accurate. The forms used to make these notes vary, but each institution's policy should be followed. Each facility uses a combination of graphics, care flow sheets, and narrative or SOAPE notes to document observations, care, and responses. The nurse's notes should always correlate with the medical orders, Kardex information, and nursing care plan.

The registered nurse has primary responsibility for each patient's initial admission nursing history, physical assessment, and development of the care plan based on the nursing diagnoses identified. Contributions by all team members during this initial process and during later updating sessions are very important.

Some facilities want a minimum of three entries per shift made on the narrative notes, as well as all care given or not given charted on a flow sheet. This is a policy that fulfills the charting concept that care was not given if it was not charted. While all care should be charted, this is a time-consuming and detailed manner of **defensive charting.**

Many hospitals now have a policy called **charting by exception.** Complete physical assessments, observations, vital signs, IV site and rate, and other pertinent data are charted at the beginning of each shift. During the shift only additional treatments done or withheld, changes in patient condition, and new concerns are charted. All active nursing diagnoses on the nursing care plan should have notations reflecting progress or revisions. More detailed flow sheets, which cut down on the time needed to chart, are used with this method of documentation.

Auditors will check to see whether all ordered care was charted as given and whether responses to specific care plan items and treatments were noted. Accuracy and completeness of documentation are important for communication, continuity of patient care, legal matters, accreditation and quality assurance audits, and cost reimbursement purposes. Charting should cover all areas of patient needs and concerns: physical, emotional, psychological, social, and spiritual.

NARRATIVE NOTES

The idea of writing narrative notes is often intimidating to students. This form of nurse's notes is easier to complete if the writer remembers that the steps of the nursing process are followed and that the notes should include the same information as a SOAPE note. The narrative note should include the basic patient need or problem data (subjective and/or objective), whether someone was contacted, care and treatments provided (implementation), and the patient's response to treatment (evaluation). The type of note is written in an abbreviated story form instead of in the outline style of the POMR note format (see Fig. 6-1).

CHARTING RULES

Generally accepted charting rules were developed to provide consistency in documentation between health care providers and facilities (Box 6-3). These rules also meet the standards expected by the individuals and agencies using the charts.

BOX 6-3 BASIC RULES FOR CHARTING

- All sheets should have the correct patient name, date, and time if appropriate.
- Use only approved abbreviations and medical terms.
- Be timely, specific, accurate, and complete.
- Write legibly (print if handwriting is not legible).
- Follow rules of grammar and punctuation.
- Fill all spaces; leave no empty lines.
- Chart after care, not before.
- Chart as soon and as often as possible.
- Chart only your own care, observations, and teaching; *never* chart for anyone else.
- Use direct quotes when appropriate.
- Describe each item as you see it—"white metal ring with clear stone."
- Be objective in charting—only what you hear, see, feel, smell.
- Chart facts; avoid judgmental terms and placing blame.
- Sign each block of charting or entry with full legal name and title.
- When a patient leaves a unit (e.g., to go to x-ray, lab, or office) chart the time and method of transportation on departure and return.
- Chart all ordered care as given or explain the deviation (NPO for lab, off unit, refused, etc.).
- Note patient response to treatments and response to analgesics or other special medications.
- Use only hard-pointed, permanent ink pens; no erasures or correcting fluids are allowed on charts.
- If a charting error is made, draw one line through the faulty information, mark error, initial if required, and make the correct entry (~~simple~~ error sample).
- When making a late entry note it as a late entry, and then proceed with your notation: for example, Late entry __ __ __ __ __ .
- Follow each institution's policies and procedures for charting.

OTHER DOCUMENTATION FORMS AND EXAMPLES

The nursing **Kardex** or **Rand** is a card system used to consolidate patient orders and care needs in a centralized, concise way. The cumulative card file or Rand is kept at the nursing station for quick reference. Card forms vary between institutions based on information required for care (Fig. 6-6).

The **nursing care plan** is developed to meet the nursing care needs of a patient. A standard care plan for a certain condition or surgery may be used and special needs added for individualized care. This plan is based on nursing assessment and nursing diagnosis; it is developed by nurses for nurses. Nursing care plans include the pertinent nursing diagnoses, goals, and plans of care, and specific actions for care implementation and evaluation (Fig. 6-3).

SPECIAL ISSUES IN DOCUMENTATION

Record Ownership and Access

As mentioned earlier, the original health care record or chart is the property of the institution or physician. On admission to the health care facility the patient is usually asked to sign a form granting permission for appropriate persons to have access to the record as necessary.

Patients have gained access rights to their records in most states, but only if they follow the established policy of each facility. Usually a written request for chart access must be submitted, and institutions state an allowed period of time for the physician and the facility to review the record and give a response. The institution may require that a staff member or physician be present while the individual looks through the chart to answer questions and to protect the integrity of the record.

A lawyer can gain access to a chart with the patient's written permission. Courts can legally obtain records for their review and use.

Confidentiality

Health care personnel must respect the **confidentiality** of the patient's record. The Patient's Bill of Rights and the law guarantee that the patient's medical information will be kept private, except if the information is needed in providing care or the patient gives permission for others to see it. The nurse should not read a record unless there is a good reason and should never gossip about patients. Trust is necessary for good nurse-patient relationships, and breaking confidences is a way to lose patient trust. If laws concerning record confidentiality are broken, a nurse can also face a lawsuit.

The Use of Computers by Nurses for Documentation Purposes

Many institutions are installing mainframe computers for data processing tasks. Most billing information is now stored and processed on this type of computer. Individuals enter data through desktop **computer terminals** that include a screen, keyboard, and printer. It is a very efficient means of retrieving individual records to change or add information.

Some progressive hospitals have installed computer systems that can handle physician orders, pharmacy, laboratory, and x-ray orders, central supply requests, care planning, documentation, and billing. All departments are interconnected in the system. Information is relayed

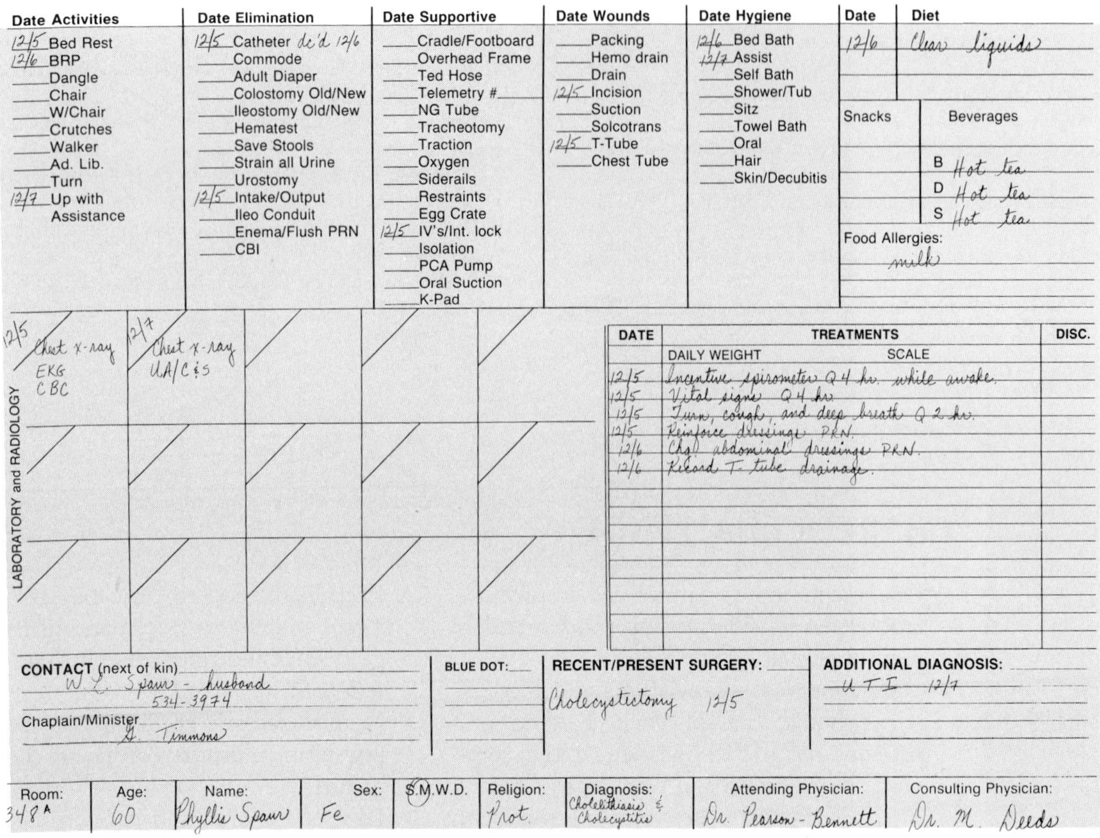

Date Activities	Date Elimination	Date Supportive	Date Wounds	Date Hygiene
12/5 Bed Rest	12/5 Catheter dc'd 12/6	Cradle/Footboard	Packing	12/6 Bed Bath
12/6 BRP	Commode	Overhead Frame	Hemo drain	12/7 Assist
Dangle	Adult Diaper	Ted Hose	Drain	Self Bath
Chair	Colostomy Old/New	Telemetry #	12/5 Incision	Shower/Tub
W/Chair	Ileostomy Old/New	NG Tube	Suction	Sitz
Crutches	Hematest	Tracheotomy	Solcotrans	Towel Bath
Walker	Save Stools	Traction	12/5 T-Tube	Oral
Ad. Lib.	Strain all Urine	Oxygen	Chest Tube	Hair
Turn	Urostomy	Siderails		Skin/Decubitis
12/7 Up with Assistance	12/5 Intake/Output	Restraints		
	Ileo Conduit	Egg Crate		
	Enema/Flush PRN	12/5 IV's/Int. lock		
	CBI	Isolation		
		PCA Pump		
		Oral Suction		
		K-Pad		

Date: 12/6 Diet: Clear liquids

Snacks / Beverages: B Hot tea; D Hot tea; S Hot tea

Food Allergies: milk

LABORATORY and RADIOLOGY: 12/5 Chest x-ray, EKG, CBC; 12/7 Chest x-ray, UA/C&S

DATE	TREATMENTS	DISC.
	DAILY WEIGHT SCALE	
12/5	Incentive spirometer Q 4 hr. while awake.	
12/5	Vital signs Q 4 hr.	
12/5	Turn, cough, and deep breath Q 2 hr.	
12/5	Reinforce dressings PRN.	
12/6	Chg. abdominal dressings PRN.	
12/6	Record T-tube drainage.	

CONTACT (next of kin): W. E. Spaur - husband 534-3974

Chaplain/Minister: G. Timmons

BLUE DOT:

RECENT/PRESENT SURGERY: Cholecystectomy 12/5

ADDITIONAL DIAGNOSIS: U T I 12/7

Room:	Age:	Name:	Sex:	S.M.W.D.	Religion:	Diagnosis:	Attending Physician:	Consulting Physician:
348A	60	Phyllis Spaur	Fe	(M)	Prot.	Cholelithiasis & Cholecystitis	Dr. Pearson-Bennett	Dr. M. Deeds

FIG. 6-6 Nursing Kardex or Rand card.

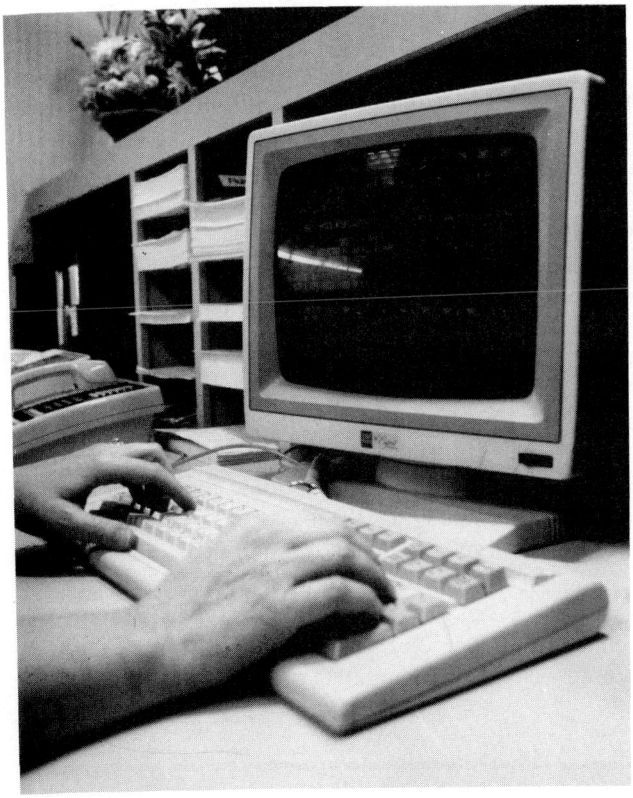

quickly and efficiently, and use of the computer avoids duplication of efforts. Time is not wasted recording data in several places and relying on runners or a tube system to deliver messages.

A computerized system is very expensive to install, and nurses must be willing to attend classes to learn how to use it. Computers are becoming easier to understand and use; they are an effective tool to save nurses documentation time and energy so that they can spend that time caring for patients.

REFERENCES AND SUGGESTED READINGS

1. Bergerson S: More about charting with a jury in mind, Nurs 88 18:51, April 1988.
2. Eggland, E: Charting: how and why to document your care daily—and fully, Nurs 88 18:76, Nov 1988.
3. Fitzpatrick J: How can we enhance nursing knowledge and practice? Nurs Health Care 9(9):517, 1988.
4. Heller B and Romano C: Nursing informatics: the pathway to knowledge, Nurs Health Care 9(9):483, 1988.
5. Hood G and Dincher J: Total patient care: foundations and practice, ed 7, St Louis, 1988, The CV Mosby Co.
6. Kim M, McFarland G, and McLane A: Pocket guide to nursing diagnosis, ed 3, St Louis, 1989, The CV Mosby Co.
7. Lampe S: Focus charting: streamlining documentation, Nurs Manage 16(7):43, 1985.
8. Lewis L and Timby B: Fundamental skills and concepts in patient care, ed 4, Philadelphia, 1988, JB Lippincott Co.

9. Long B and Phipps W: Essentials of medical-surgical nursing: a nursing process approach, ed 2, St Louis, 1989, The CV Mosby Co.
10. Luquire R: 6 common causes of nursing liability, Nurs 88 18:61, Nov 1988.
11. McPhee A: Teaching students how to chart, Nurse Educ 12(4):33, 1987.
12. Mosby's medical and nursing dictionary, ed 3, St Louis, 1990, The CV Mosby Co.
13. Philpott M: 20 rules for good charting, Nurs 86 16(8):63, Aug 1986.
14. Potter P and Perry A: Basic nursing: theory and practice, ed 2, St Louis, 1991, Mosby-Year Book, Inc.
15. Rich P: Make the most of your charting time, Nurs 87 17:68, May 1987.
16. Rutkowski B: How D.R.G.'s are changing your charting, Nurs 85 15:49, Oct 1985.
17. Sullivan G: The right way to fill out an incident report, RN 53, Dec 1988.
18. Thornton L: We teach nurses to chart defensively, RN 57, April 1986.
19. Tribulski J: Nursing diagnosis: waste of time or valued tool? RN 30, Dec 1988.
20. Walker B: Charting chuckles, Nurs 86 16:25, Oct 1986.

CHAPTER CHALLENGE

KEY POINTS

- Documentation is part of the implementation phase of the nursing process and is used in evaluation.
- Only approved abbreviations and medical terms should be used when charting in a patient's record. Knowledge of the common abbreviations and terms is required.
- There are five purposes for written patient records. Records are (a) a means of written communication to facilitate continuity of care, (b) a permanent record for accountability (audits, accreditation, and cost reimbursement), (c) a legal record, (d) used in teaching, and (e) used for research and data collection.
- Two common types of medical records or charts are the traditional or block chart and the problem-oriented medical record (POMR).
- The POMR uses a master patient problem list as an index to the chart. These listed problems are usually medical diagnoses.
- SOAPIER is one format for charting in the POMR. The letters stand for subjective *(S)*, objective *(O)*, assessment *(A)*, plan *(P)*, implementation *(I)*, evaluation *(E)*, and revision *(R)*.
- Two other common formats for charting nurse's notes are narrative and focus. Focus charting has a data *(D)*, action *(A)*, and response *(R)* format.
- Charting needs to be legible, clear, concise, accurate, and complete. These guidelines serve as a national standard for licensed nurses.
- Each institution or unit may have specific forms and charting format, but the general guidelines and rules for charting should be followed.
- Medical records are legal documents. The physician or institution owns the original record.
- Lawyers, courts, and patients can gain access to the record but must follow specified access procedures.
- The contents of a health record are confidential information protected by the law and the Patient's Bill of Rights.
- The nursing Kardex or Rand is a card-filing system used by nurses to condense all the orders and other care information needed quickly for each patient. It is kept at the nursing station for quick reference and is updated frequently.
- The nursing care plan is a plan of care for a patient and a part of the health record. The nurse uses the assessment data to make nursing diagnoses of the patient's responses to illness and problems. This plan includes the nursing diagnosis, treatment goals, specific directions for care implementation, and evaluation guidelines. The care plan should serve as a guide for individualized nursing care delivery and recording.
- Nursing access to computer terminals and care documentation systems has the potential to save time and energy needed for patient care services. These systems are expensive but are a great benefit to the nurses able to use them.

STUDY QUESTIONS

1. Charting rules include all of the following except:
   a. Permanent, nonerasable ink is used
   b. Each charting block or entry is signed with the person's name and title
   c. Errors can be erased or correcting fluid used
   d. Notes should be timely, concise, and accurate
   e. Chart is done after, not before, giving care
2. The purposes for written care records are:
   a. To improve communication and continuity of care
   b. To provide information for cost of care reimbursement
   c. To have a written record of the care given for legal purposes
   d. To provide information for teaching and research
   e. All of the above
3. The nursing care plan is:
   a. Based on a problem list of medical diagnoses
   b. Based on nursing assessment data and developed by nurses
   c. A work sheet for nurses and not a part of the record
   d. Not useful for planning nursing care and charting
   e. Part of the assessment step of the nursing process
4. The nursing care plan includes:
   a. Nursing diagnosis of a patient's actual or potential health problems
   b. Plans or goals of treatment
   c. Specific actions for care implementation
   d. Evaluation guidelines
   e. All of the above
5. The nursing Kardex is:
   a. A card-filing system used as a quick reference
   b. A formal part of the patient record
   c. A guide for charting patient care
   d. Never changed
6. Which form is used to quickly chart physical assessment data and basic care and treatments:
   a. Graphics sheet
   b. Flow sheets
   c. Narrative nurse's notes
   d. Progress notes
7. When charting patient care a nurse should:
   a. Wait until the end of the shift to chart all at one time
   b. Leave empty lines so another nurse can add a note
   c. Chart in whatever type and color of pen is available
   d. Chart after care is given and as often as possible
8. Documenting is part of which step of the nursing process:
   a. Assessment
   b. Diagnosis
   c. Planning
   d. Implementation
   e. Evaluation
9. Which are accepted forms of charting for nurses:
   a. Narrative
   b. Graphics, ADL, and flow sheets
   c. SOAPE
   d. DAR
   e. All of the above
10. Patient health records are:
    a. Owned by the patient
    b. Confidential records protected by law
    c. Not admissible in court
    d. Not mentioned in the Patient's Bill of Rights
11. Means used to assess the standard of care given by institutions or individuals are:
    a. Peer review
    b. Quality assurance audits
    c. Accreditation audits
    d. All of the above
12. Computers are:
    a. Not a useful tool for nurses
    b. Inexpensive and used in many hospitals by nurses
    c. A potentially useful and time-saving charting tool
    d. Not used in the health care system

III

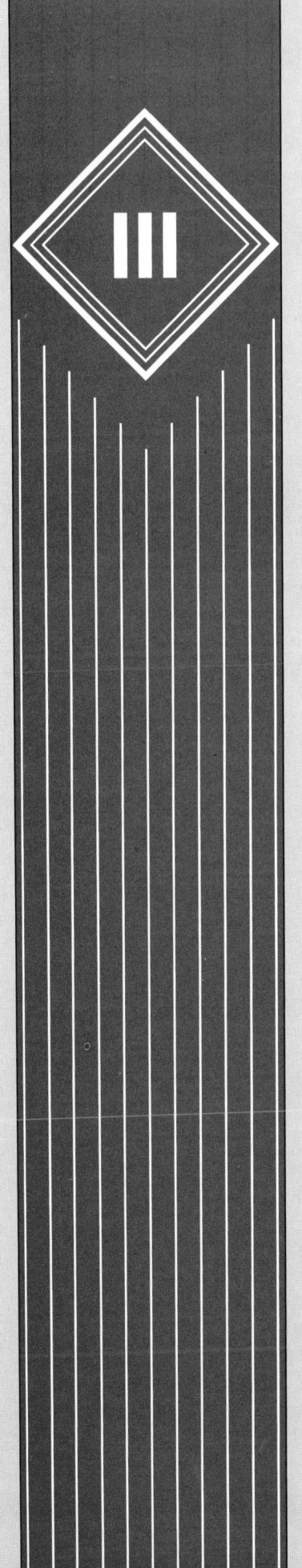

Developmental, Sociocultural, and Family Influences

Nursing means caring and understanding toward all people, whether it be patients, family, or staff. It is the feeling of joy I get inside from being able to help others. Sometimes the nurse is the only person that the patient has. Your caring and understanding can help the healing as much as anything. I enjoy a challenge, and every day there is a new challenge to meet in the nursing field. I love people and care just as much for them as I do myself. Their feelings come first. When they are happy and feel good, I feel wonderful. If they are upset or angry, I feel it also. Nursing comes from the heart of a special person. My heart is wide open to nursing and all that comes with it.

SHELLY MCNULTY

Student Nurse

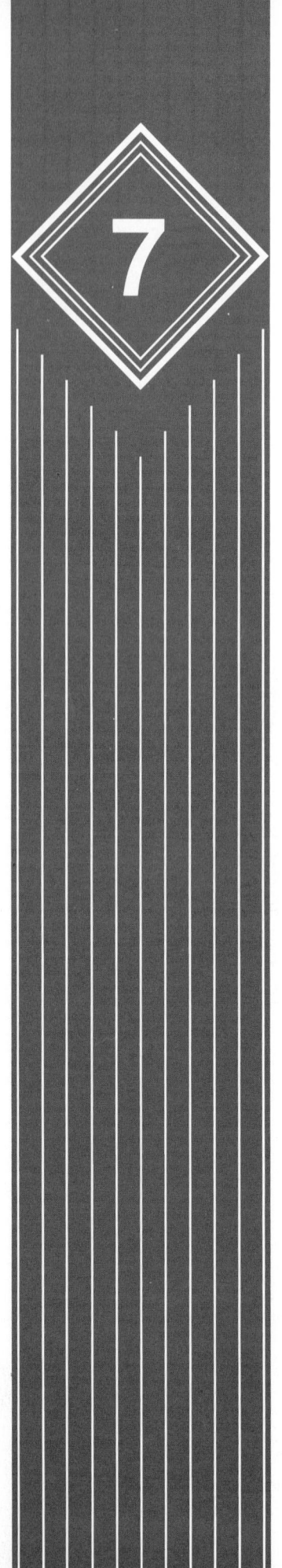

7

The Family

RUTH BECKMANN MURRAY

LEARNING OBJECTIVES

After reading this chapter, the student should be able to do the following:

- Define the key terms.
- Discuss the various forms of family structure commonly seen in health care settings.
- Describe developmental tasks for the establishment, expectancy, parenthood, and disengagement stages.
- Relate the impact of feelings about the self and childhood experiences on later family interaction patterns.
- Discuss factors that affect the relationship between parent and child.
- Describe characteristics of the abused woman and the abused child.
- Describe factors that contribute to abuse of family members.

RELATED TOPICS OF INTEREST

- The infant and young child (Chapter 8)
- The school-age child (Chapter 9)
- The adolescent (Chapter 10)
- The adult (Chapter 11)
- Cultural aspects of nursing care (Chapter 12)
- Basic nutrition (Chapter 22)

KEY TERMS

Define the following:

- adoptive family
- battered woman syndrome
- child abuse
  - emotional
  - physical
  - sexual
- cohabitation
- couvade syndrome
- disengagement stage
- engagement
- establishment stage
- expectant stage
- extended family
- family
- family interaction
- matrifocal/matriarchal family
- neglect
- nuclear family
- parenthood stage
- patrifocal/patriarchal family
- reconstituted/blended family
- single parent family

INTRODUCTION TO THE FAMILY

The **family** is a primary reference group. The family unit is characterized by face-to-face contact; bonds of affection; sense of loyalty and concern for each other; a continuity of past, present, and future; and shared goals, identity, values, and behaviors common only to the specific unit. The family is responsible for various roles, communication patterns, socialization, and physical and emotional care of the members in each developmental stage.[9,16,29]

Healthy families are characterized by the following[16,18,28]:

1. A sense of togetherness that promotes capacity for change
2. A balance between mutual and independent action on the part of family members
3. Nurturance and resources for growth and sustenance
4. Stability and integrity of structure
5. Mastery of developmental tasks leading to interdependence and ability to meet demands for survival and development

Families have difficulty in maintaining these characteristics. Assisting the family during illness helps them to maintain togetherness.

The family may take one of several forms: **nuclear** (mother, father, children), **extended** (nuclear plus other relatives), **patrifocal** or **patriarchal** (father is authority), **matrifocal** or **matriarchal** (mother is authority), and reconstituted/blended. Or the family may be made up of siblings (especially in middle or late life), homosexuals, or a man and woman living together without being married **(cohabitation)**. The dead or missing family member may remain clearly in the other members' memory and affect behavior of the family.

Family Developmental Tasks

The family is considered responsible for the child's growth and development and behavioral outcomes and for the welfare of its members. The family is strongly influenced by its environment, as is the child himself, and should not bear full responsibility for what the child is or becomes. Few parents deliberately set out to rear a disturbed or delinquent offspring, although such failures occur.[16]

The family is expected to perform tasks shown in Box 7-1, which continue to be met in various ways, including during illness of one of its members.

The family's ability to complete its tasks depends on the maturity of the adult members and support given by the social system—nursing and other health care workers and educational, work, religious, social, welfare, and governmental institutions. The family that is most successful as a unit has a working philosophy and value system that is understood and lived, uses healthy adaptive patterns most of the time, uses available community services, and develops linkages with nonfamily units and organizations.[9]

Signs of Strained or Unhealthy Family Relationships

During assessment, various behaviors indicate that the family is not relating in a constructive or harmonious way. The behaviors in Box 7-2 should be reported to a nurse manager.

BOX 7-1 FAMILY DEVELOPMENTAL TASKS

- Provide for physical safety, daily routines, and economic needs of its members and obtain enough resources to survive
- Create a sense of family loyalty and security and a mentally healthy environment for the family's well-being
- Reproduce and socialize the child(ren), teaching values and appropriate behavior
- Teach members to effectively communicate their needs, ideas, feelings, and respect for each other
- Provide social togetherness simultaneously with division of labor, patterning of sexual roles, and performance of family roles with flexibility and cooperation
- Help members to develop physically, emotionally, intellectually, and spiritually and to develop a personal and family identity while adjusting to the demands of family life
- Release family members into the larger society—school, church, organizations, employment, and eventually another family unit[6,16]

BOX 7-2 SIGNS OF STRAINED OR UNHEALTHY FAMILY RELATIONSHIPS

- Lack of communication between spouses or other family members
- Disregard shown by family members to each other, alternating with harassment through arguments or harshness with each other
- Lack of decision making or inability to cooperate with caregivers
- Over-possessiveness of children, mate, or other family members; extreme behavior or incest
- Derogatory remarks by children to parents or vice versa
- Blame placed among family members for difficulties
- High level of anxiety, tension, or insecurity present in the interactions between family members
- Pattern of immature or regressive behavior in family members[9,16,27]

STAGES OF FAMILY DEVELOPMENT

The natural history of the family is a continuum: marriage or cohabitation; choosing whether to have children; rearing biological or adoptive offspring, if any; and releasing children into society to establish homes of their own. In later life the aging parents or grandparents are a couple once again, unless divorce occurs or until death occurs. The nurturing of spouse or children goes on simultaneously with a multitude of other activities: employment, managing a household, participation in community groups, pursuit of leisure and hobbies, and maintaining friendships and family ties. Or the person may decide to remain single and live alone or live with another person. The tasks and stages of family life must also be worked out, even during illness. The nurse must observe how illness, hospitalization, and recovery are influencing the patient and family members in relation to family tasks and stages.

Engagement and Establishment Stages

Courtship and **engagement** precede establishment of the family unit. During this time the couple prepare for marriage and they become free of parental domination. The **establishment stage** begins with marriage. The couple's main emotional tie is no longer with the parents. The couple commit themselves to living together. They must work out the developmental tasks previously listed.[6,27]

The establishment stage ends when the woman becomes pregnant or when the couple work out their living pattern and philosophy of life that may include a decision not to have children.

Expectant Stage

During the **expectant stage** (pregnancy) many domestic and social adjustments must be made. The couple (or the single mother and her significant others) are learning new roles and gaining new status in the community. Attitudes toward pregnancy and the physical and emotional status of the mother and father, as well as of significant others, will affect future parenting abilities. Now the couple think in terms of family instead of a pair. They explore beliefs about childrearing and plan for the new member in terms of space, budget, and necessary supplies.[6]

The woman may initially dislike being pregnant because it interferes with her personal plans, or she may feel proud and fulfilled. Usually she is more preoccupied with herself, her new feelings, and changing body image, and she experiences fantasies and fears regarding the baby and the childbirth experiences.

The man experiences a variety of feelings when he learns of the woman's pregnancy. The feelings change during the pregnancy. The reality of the pregnancy to the man increases with time. The man may feel happy or scared, proud of his virility, or guilty about the woman's physical symptoms. Concerns identified by fathers are (1) ability to care for the infant, (2) adequacy as a father, (3) financial security, and (4) the effect of the baby on the couple's relationship.[12,14,17]

Both the woman and the man may experience similar physical and emotional symptoms, such as nausea, indigestion, backache, distention, and depression. Symptoms in the woman may result from hormonal changes or feelings about the pregnancy. In the man they are part of the **couvade syndrome,** which may be a reaction based on identification with or sympathy for the woman, uncertainty about the pregnancy, or envy of the woman's childbearing ability.[4,20,21]

Major decisions for the couple are whether to attend childbirth preparation classes and whether the man should be present in the labor and delivery rooms. The woman may feel eager to have the man with her, or she may feel that he will think of her as sexually unattractive or be repulsed. The man may be curious about what is happening and want to attend his child's birth, or he may feel guilty about not wanting to when he feels others expect him to be there. He may be embarrassed about his wife's behavior and appearance during labor and delivery. Or he may feel he cannot cope with the childbirth event if he is present. Some men and women do not want to participate in childbirth preparation classes and should not be made to feel guilty about their decision. Childbirth preparation classes improve the woman's self-image and physical condition for labor. The nurse must assess the couple's preparation for and preferences about childbirth.

The woman needs extra "mothering" from the partner (or others) during pregnancy. The man also needs extra attention and nurturing, or he may be unable to continue to support the mother-to-be emotionally.[12] The nurse should listen to the woman's and man's concerns and help them understand that what they are experiencing is normal. Various teaching aids that explain pregnancy and what to expect during the birth experience are useful. Care should be family centered and directed toward both parents-to-be.

Parenthood Stage

With the **parenthood stage** the couple assume a status that they will never lose as long as each has memory and life—that of parent.

During the time after birth parents feel excited about the new baby but also uncertain about parenthood. A parent/child attachment is being formed. Difficult adjustments must be made. New roles and behaviors are learned by the parents with each stage of the child's development. They are concerned with carrying out the tasks of the family and, for the welfare of the child and family, must suppress their own desires.[6,16]

Disengagement Stage of Parenthood

Sometimes the final or **disengagement stage** does not last too long for various reasons. The young adult who is unemployed, a college dropout, or divorced may return home to live. The aged parents or other relatives may be unable to continue to live independently and then are included in the household of middle-aged offspring. Or one of the spouses may die. In these situations or if the couple live alone, the tasks and relationships of the family must be reworked. Space and other resources must be redivided. Time schedules for daily activities may be reworked. Privacy, communication, and respectful use of possessions must be ensured.[6,16] The nurse may be of assistance.

FAMILY RELATIONSHIPS

Interaction of the husband and wife and other members living in the same house is basic to the mental and sometimes physical health of the adults, as well as to the eventual health of the children. While caring for a patient, the nurse may learn of difficulties in the following areas and may help the patient or refer him to other resources.

Importance of Self-Esteem

To feel a sense of self-esteem, to love, and to have a positive self-image evolves through interaction with parents from birth and in turn affects how the person interacts in later life with others, including spouse and offspring.[16] The adult in the family who lacks self-acceptance and self-respect is not likely to be a loving spouse or parent. The person may react in ways designed to defend self from the rejection that he or she thinks will be received. The person may criticize, get angry, brag, demand perfection from others, or withdraw. In turn, others are not likely to respond to the person's basic needs for love, acceptance, and respect. To remain open and giving in such situations is difficult, but that may be the only way to elevate the person's self-esteem.

Family Interaction

Long before the child learns to speak, sensory, emotional, and intellectual exchanges are made between the child and other family members. Through such exchanges, and later with words, the child learns how to live. The games and toys purchased for and played with by the child, the books selected and read, and the television programs allowed can provide key learning experiences. **Family interaction** for the child and adult is affected by the stage of family development and gender of the child. Presence of an only child, of multiple births (such as twins), or of an adoptive child or stepchild also influences interaction.

Parents tend to identify with their children and to treat

them according to how they were treated as children. A parent can identify best with the child who matches his or her own gender and sibling position. A man from a family of boys may not know how to interact with a daughter. In the process of identifying with the parent, the child adopts many of the parent's characteristics, especially if the child is the oldest or only child.[16]

Family Size

One child. The only child may feel more loneliness but develops more rapidly and may seem older and more serious than peers who have siblings. He or she lacks the opportunities siblings could provide. He or she may not share feelings and experiences with someone close, unless there is a close friend. The only child learns less about compromising with peers and sharing adult attention. He or she is often brought into the parents' conflicts and is likely to help maintain harmony and preserve equilibrium in the household.[6,26] The only child may be forced prematurely to assume adult roles.

Certainly the only child can develop into a wholesome, well-adjusted person. The qualities of being more serious, assertive, responsible, independent, curious, and able to entertain self and find satisfaction in personal pursuits frequently develop because of parental and home demands and are useful adult characteristics. The adult contact develops the only child's creativity, language skills, planning abilities, and intellectual potential. The child has a high need to achieve and prefers the novel or complex.

Multiple births. There are fewer families with three or more children now than in the past. The last born may be less wanted than the first or middle born, although parents feel more skilled and confident in rearing the younger children. Large families have advantages. Of necessity, the children learn thrift and reuse of material goods and to share time, space, and possessions. The children learn responsibility. In a loving home, they have not only their parents', but also siblings', love, listening ear, and help. If the parent does not have time to read to the 4-year-old, the older sibling does. Each child learns cooperation, compromise, tolerance, and how to handle peer pressure. For parents, the effort, work, expense, and self-denial of having a large family can be offset by the rewards of watching children grow and develop and by a sense of contribution to the generations to come.[16,24,26]

Twins may each receive less parental affection and communication, because parents have less time to devote to each child. Thus twins are often slower to talk, and many have a slower intellectual growth unless parents work to prevent it. Multiple-birth children are likely to be closer to one another than other siblings (Fig. 7-1). Their experiences are different from those of having siblings of other ages. Twins or other multiple births have considerable impact on family interaction. The needs and tasks of these parents will differ from the parents who have a single birth. Because multiple births are often premature, the first 4 or 5 months is demanding on the parents in terms of the amount of energy and time spent in child care. This means that the parents have less energy and time for each other or other children. Financial worries and concern about space and material needs may intrude on normal husband/wife relationships. Twins meet the world as a pair. It takes longer to separate in childhood and adolescence (they may not, emotionally or physically). Twins learn about the extra attention resulting from their birth status and may take advantage of the situation. Interaction between them is often complementary; one twin may be dominant and the other submissive.[15,16,26]

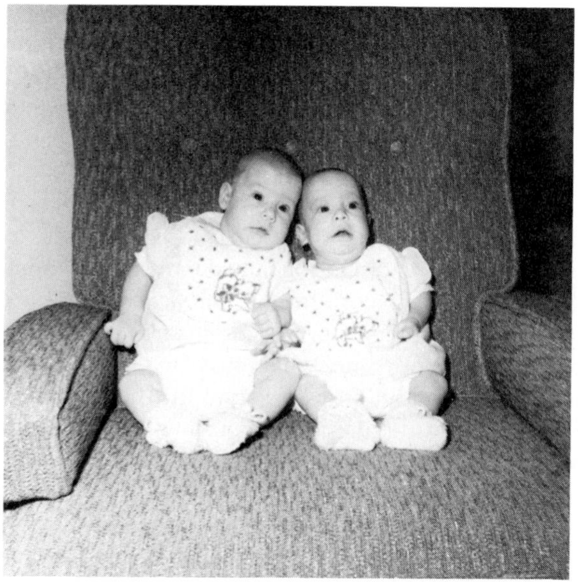

FIG. 7-1 Twins pose a unique challenge to parents.

Ordinal position of the child. Birth order is important to development. Siblings have an important influence on each other. The first born, who is an only child until the second one is born, may enjoy some advantages in achievement of intellectual superiority, perspective about life, and responsibility. He or she has more contact with adults and is the sole recipient of attention for a time. He or she becomes dominant over younger siblings. Younger children benefit from the parents' experience with child raising and from having older siblings to imitate. Last borns are also more sociable, possibly to ensure acceptance by older siblings or to gain parental attention. The last born may be more dependent. The middle child is likely to become caught between the jealousy of the older child and the envy of the younger. He or she learns double or triple roles and is prepared for more kinds of relationships in adulthood.[16,26]

Gender of the child. Gender of the child influences development within the family.[1] In most cultures a higher value is placed on boys than on girls. In some cultures only a boy's birth is welcomed or celebrated. If a boy arrives in a family that hopes for a girl, he may receive pressure to be feminine. If the boy arrives after a family has two or three girls, he will receive much attention but also the jealousy of his sisters. Developing a masculine identity may be more difficult for him, especially if there is no male nearby with whom to relate. In spite of being pampered, he will be expected by his family to be manly. The boy may feel envious of his sisters' position and their freedom from such great expectations. The girl who arrives in a family with a number of boys may also receive considerable attention, but she may have to become tomboyish to compete with her brothers and receive their esteem. Feminine identity may be difficult for her.[16,26] Such feelings and interactions begin before birth and are seen while the mother and baby are in the obstetrical unit.

Family Structure

The adoptive family. In the **adoptive family** the adopted child may suffer some problems of the only child. In addition, the adopted child has to work through feelings about rejection and abandonment by the biological parents versus being wanted and loved by the adoptive parents. Usually by the preschool years he or she can be told about adopting and of being a wanted child. The adopted child may ask questions, which can be answered by the nurse or referred to another staff member.

Adopted children bring their own genes, birth experiences, and life history to the family. The adoptive family is not the same as a biological family. Both adoptive parents and adopted children tend to feel they have less control over their situation. It is not unusual for the adoptive child to seek the biological parents in late adolescence or adulthood, even when the adoptive parents are considered the true parents. The adoptive parents' personal qualifications, marital harmony, love and acceptance of the child, and the child's friendships are major determinants of the child's adjustment and development.[3,13,16]

The reconstituted/blended family. The **reconstituted, blended family** is also common. The remarriage of a divorced or widowed parent with children from one or both partners may form a composite family unit known as the reconstituted, complex, blended, or stepparent family. These families may be formed in a variety of ways. All members of this new family bring a history of values, life experiences, relationships, and expectations to the stepfamily. Conflict often occurs when the values and rules of individuals or the former single-parent family differ from those of the second or blended family. Conflicts about how to care for ill family members can be the most explosive issue with which the nurse becomes involved.

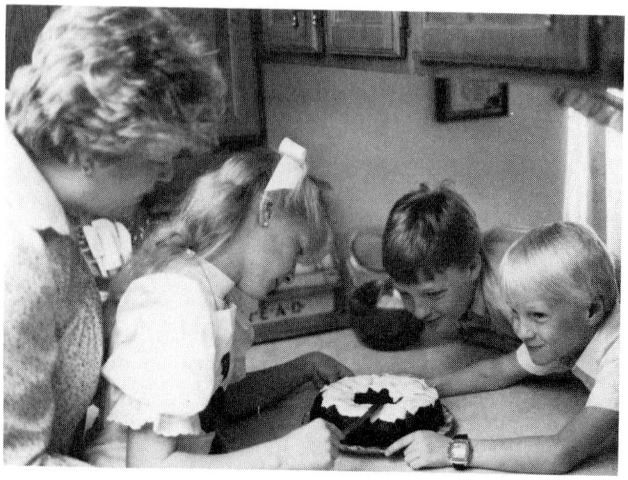

FIG. 7-2 Single parents take every opportunity to engage in activities with their children.

The single-parent family. Death and illegitimacy may cause the family to have only one parent; however, divorce of the natural parents is the more common reason. In most cases these families have undergone a major change in life-style or disruption before the family breakup. In a **single-parent family** the children may experience grief for the absent parent, guilt for their real or imagined part in the loss, shame for the change in their family structure, and fear about what changes the future may bring. Each person may need to assume additional responsibilities and tasks (Fig. 7-2). An adolescent may serve as a parent substitute to younger siblings. Other children assume new household tasks. Health care may be neglected. The nurse can refer to appropriate community agencies.

Abuse in the Family

Battering is a social and emotional health problem of all socioeconomic levels. The man may be abused, but female and child abuse—physically, emotionally, and sexually—is a greater problem. Woman and child are the man's property in some cultures, and beating is accepted behavior. Traditionally, the woman has been too ashamed or too hopeless to admit the problem or seek help. Frequently no help existed. Perhaps acknowledgment of and efforts to overcome child abuse and the women's liberation movement together helped to initiate change. The nurse may listen carefully, assess the problem, and report to the nursing manager for other assistance.

Battered or abused women. A woman of any age who suffers adult abuse often reveals the following typical signs or characteristics of the **battered woman syndrome** that can be assessed by the nurse[10,11,16,22]:

1. She is isolated socially or physically from neighbors, relatives, and friends.
2. She feels increasingly helpless, guilty, and isolated,

and has low self-esteem; she feels trapped and dependent on the man.
3. Her educational and occupational status is higher than the man's.
4. Beating or other abuse began early in marriage and increased in frequency and intensity over the decades.
5. Violence occurs more typically in the evening, on weekends, and in the kitchen, and is not witnessed by nonfamily members.
6. Frequently she is unable to leave the home because of lack of money, transportation, a place to go, support people, or support agencies in the community; further, she has learned helpless behavior patterns and feels unable to try to escape.
7. Injuries from abuse may not be visible, but she usually talks about the problem freely when asked directly if abuse is occurring.
8. Increasing incidence of abuse and the physical and emotional consequences of abuse causes more passivity, less flexibility, less ability to think logically, more depression, and possibly suicide attempts.
9. Eventually the frustration, stress, and anger may be externalized into physical behavior that is more than protective of the self or the child(ren); she may in turn become violent to the point of killing the battering partner.

Sexual abuse. Another form of battering that may affect either the male or female, but more commonly affects the female, is incest or other sexual abuse. Symptoms and problems in adulthood may result from childhood sexual abuse and incest. When the nurse cares for anyone with the following conditions, a health history may reveal relationship of these conditions to abuse[10,16,25]:

1. Chronic depression, hopelessness related to shame and guilt
2. Drug and alcohol abuse
3. Various physical complaints, including symptoms of panic attacks, headaches, hysterical seizures
4. Problems with trusting or intimate relationships with the opposite gender
5. Character disorders, such as borderline or narcissistic states
6. Multiple personality disorders
7. Sexual dysfunction, gynecological problems

Many communities now have shelters or homes for abused women and children. These homes (1) provide emergency shelter, peer discussion, and support, (2) assist in working through feelings in a positive way, and (3) provide information on how to cope with the situation and how to find an alternative life-style. Some communities have organizations that also work with the abusing man in an effort to help him recognize anger and frustration feelings in self, realize it is not acceptable to vent feelings through violent behavior to the spouse, and learn alternate coping and behavior patterns. The nurse can refer people to these agencies.

Child abuse. In **child abuse,** the following three factors must be present for physical neglect or abuse, emotional neglect or abuse, verbal abuse, or sexual abuse:

1. The parents must have the potential for neglectful, abusive behavior because of their own background.
2. The child is perceived as different or deserving of the neglect or abuse.
3. The family is undergoing severe or numerous stresses.

Parents who abuse their children are from every race, color, creed, ethnic origin, and economic level.[3] Abused children range in age from neonate through adolescence. Abuse should be considered when the nurse assesses any injured or ill child/adolescent. Physical abuse or nonaccidental physical injury includes multiple bruises or fractures from severe beatings, poisonings, overmedication, burns from immersion in hot water or from lighted cigarettes, excessive use of laxatives or enemas, and human bites. The trauma to the child may be great enough to cause permanent blindness, scars on the skin, neurological damage, subdural hematoma, permanent brain damage, or death. **Sexual abuse** includes rape, incest, exhibitionism to the child, or fondling of the child's/adolescent's genitals. **Emotional abuse** includes excessively aggressive or unreasonable parental behavior to the child; placing unreasonable demands on the child; constantly verbally attacking, belittling, or teasing the child; or withdrawing love, support, or guidance. **Neglect** involves inadequate mothering, or inadequate emotional, moral, and social care.[1,10,16] The parents' lack of concern is usually obvious. Abandonment may occur. In all forms of abuse, the child frequently acts fearful of the parents, or adults in general. The child is usually too fearful to tell how he or she was injured.[16]

REFERENCES AND SUGGESTED READINGS

1. Bettelheim B: A good enough parent: a book on child rearing, New York, 1987, Alfred A Knopf, Inc.
2. Bowlby J: The making and breaking of affectional bonds, Br J Psychiatry 130:201, 1977.
3. Brockhaus JP: Foster care, adoption, and the grief process, J Psychiatr Nurs Mental Health Serv 20(9):9, 1982.
4. Clinton J: Expectant fathers at risk for couvade, Nurs Res 35(5):290, 1986.
5. Drake VK: Battered women: a health care problem in disguise, Image 14(2):40, 1982.
6. Duvall E and Miller B: Marriage and family development, ed 6, New York, 1984, Harper & Row Publishers, Inc.
7. Edwards MP and Boyd FE: Adoption for adolescents, Child Welfare 54(4):298, 1975.
8. Erikson E: Childhood and society, ed 2, New York, 1963, WW Norton & Company, Inc.
9. Friedman M: Family nursing: theory and assessment, ed 3, Norwalk, Conn, 1985, Appleton-Century-Crofts.
10. Garbarino J, Guttman E, and Seeley J: The psychologically battered child: strategies for identification, assessment, and intervention, San Francisco, 1987, Jossey-Bass, Inc, Publishers.
11. Helton A and others: Battered and pregnant: a prevalence study, Am J Public Health 77(10):1337, 1987.
12. Hott J: The crisis of expectant fatherhood, AJN 76(9):1436, 1976.
13. Krementz J: How it feels to be adopted, New York, 1982, Alfred A Knopf, Inc.
14. Lamb M: The fathers' role, New York, 1986, John Wiley & Sons, Inc.
15. Moshman D, Glover J, and Bruning R: Developmental psychology, Boston, 1987, Little, Brown & Co, Inc.
16. Murray R and Zentner J: Nursing assessment and health promotion through the life span, ed 4, Norwalk, Conn, 1988, Appleton & Lange.
17. Obrzut L: Expectant father's perceptions of fathering, AJN 76(9):1440, 1976.
18. Roberts C and Feetham S: Assessing family functioning across three areas of relationships, Nurs Res 31(4):231, 1982.
19. Rosenthal K and Keshet H: Fathers without partners, Totowa, NJ, 1981, Rowman & Littlefield, Publishers.
20. Rubin R: Attainment of the maternal role, Part I: processes, Nurs Res 16(3):237, 1967.
21. Rubin R: Attainment of the maternal role, Part II: models and referrants, Nurs Res 16(4):342, 1967.
22. Schechter S: Women and male violence: the visions and struggles of the battered women's movement, Boston, 1982, South End Press.
23. Schuster CS and Ashburn SS: The process of human development: a holistic life-span approach, ed 2, Boston, 1986, Little, Brown & Co, Inc.
24. Smith S: Big families can be happy, too, Newsweek, p 12, Jan 14, 1985.
25. Sonkin D, Martin D, and Walker L: The male batterer: a treatment approach, New York, 1985, Springer Publishing Co, Inc.
26. Toman W: Family constellation, ed 3, New York, 1976, Springer Publishing Co.
27. Wachtel E and Wachtel P: Family dynamics in individual psychotherapy: a guide to clinical strategies, New York, 1986, The Guilford Press.
28. Williams D: Black problems become white, Newsweek, p 7, Aug 18, 1986.
29. Wright L and Leahey M: Nurses and families: a guide to family assessment and intervention, Philadelphia, 1984, FA Davis Co.

CHAPTER CHALLENGE

KEY POINTS

- The family has a major role in shaping the person in development, health, or illness.
- The family is considered responsible for the child's growth and development and behavioral outcomes and for the welfare of its members.
- During assessment, various behaviors indicate that the family is not relating in a constructive or harmonious way.
- The tasks and stages of family life must be worked out, even during illness.
- The nurse must assess the couple's preparation for and preferences about childbirth.
- Family interaction for the child and adult is affected by the stage of family development and gender of the child.
- Birth order is important to development.
- Conflicts about how to care for family members can be the most explosive issue with which the nurse becomes involved.
- Battering is a social and emotional health problem of all socioeconomic levels.
- A woman of any age who suffers abuse often reveals typical signs or characteristics that can be assessed by the nurse.
- Parents who abuse their children are from every race, color, creed, ethnic origin, and economic level.
- Abuse should be considered when the nurse assesses any injured or ill child/adolescent.

STUDY QUESTIONS

1. Healthy families are characterized by all of the following *except*:
   a. Sense of togetherness that promotes capacity for change
   b. Nurturance and resources for growth and sustenance
   c. Instability and lack of harmony
   d. Balance between mutual and independent action on the part of family members
2. The family form in which there is a mother, father, and child(ren) in a family unit is called:
   a. Nuclear family
   b. Extended family
   c. Blended family
3. Choose the behavior that indicates the family is not relating in a constructive or harmonious way:
   a. Pattern of immature or regressive behavior in a family member
   b. Communication between spouses or other family members
   c. Decision making and ability to cooperate with caregivers
   d. Children's favorable remarks to parents or vice versa
4. During pregnancy, both the woman and the man may experience similar physical and emotional symptoms, such as nausea, backache, distention, and depression. In the man this syndrome is called:
   a. Patrifocal
   b. Couvade
   c. Disengagement
5. A time in family life when the child(ren) leave home, leaving the couple or individual living alone, is called:
   a. Disengagement
   b. Reconstituted
   c. Matrifocal
6. A parent can identify best with the child who:
   a. Is opposite gender and matches his or her sibling position
   b. Matches his or her gender and sibling position
7. An only child is more prone to which of the following characteristics:
   a. More serious, assertive, responsible, independent, curious, intellectually superior
   b. Tolerant of others, thrifty, slower to talk, slower in intellectual growth
8. Characteristics of the last-born child in the family are often seen as:
   a. Dominant over others
   b. Having the ability to learn double or triple roles
   c. Being more sociable and a dependent person
9. The remarriage of a divorced or widowed parent with children may form a composite family unit known as the:
   a. Reconstituted, blended family
   b. Nuclear family
   c. Extended family
10. An abused woman often reveals the following typical signs or characteristics:
    a. Sociable with neighbors, relatives, friends
    b. Educational and occupational status inferior to the male
    c. Helpless behavior patterns
11. When the nurse cares for anyone with the conditions of chronic depression, drug and alcohol abuse, panic attacks, or hysterical seizures, a health history often reveals:
    a. Incest and other sexual abuse
    b. Genetic pathology
    c. Congenital anomalies

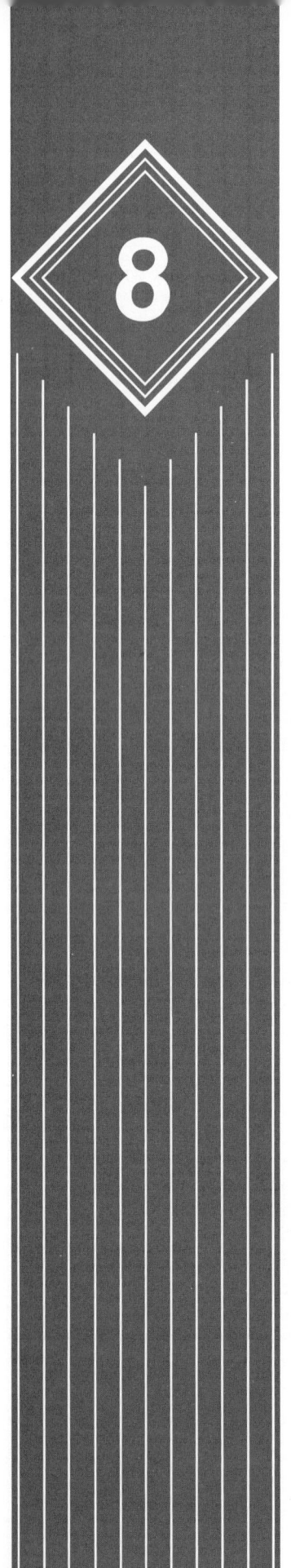

8

The Infant and Young Child

RUTH BECKMANN MURRAY

LEARNING OBJECTIVES

After reading this chapter, the student should be able to do the following:

- Define the key terms.
- Give examples of basic developmental principles pertinent to the young child.
- Describe the crisis of birth for the family.
- Compare parental behaviors that indicate attachment behavior and difficulty with parenting.
- Discuss developmental tasks for the family in relation to infants, toddlers, and preschoolers.
- Describe discipline to be used with the young child.
- Describe the neonate's physical characteristics and the manner in which psychosocial needs begin to be filled.
- Contrast major physiological, motor, cognitive, and emotional characteristics of the infant, toddler, and preschooler.
- Discuss the nutritional, sleep, and play needs of the infant, toddler, and preschooler.
- Explain the immunization schedule for the young child.
- Discuss the developmental tasks for the infant, toddler, and preschooler.

RELATED TOPICS OF INTEREST

- The family (Chapter 7)
- Basic nutrition (Chapter 22)
- Care of the mother and newborn (Chapter 44)
- Basic pediatric nursing care (Chapter 46)
- Care of children with physical and emotional problems (Chapter 47)

KEY TERMS

Define the following:

- anterior fontanel
- Apgar score
- attachment
- autonomy
- bonding
- cognitive development
- colostrum
- crisis
- denial
- despair
- egocentric
- engrossment
- guilt
- immunization
- infant
- initiative
- meconium
- mistrust
- neonate
- parallel play
- posterior fontanel
- preoperational stage
- preschooler
- protest
- rapid eye movement (REM)
- reflex
- sensorimotor stage
- separation anxiety
- shame and doubt
- sibling
- toddler
- trust
- umbilical cord
- weaning

FAMILY DEVELOPMENT AND RELATIONSHIPS

Parenting

The coming of the child is a **crisis,** felt by the woman first as she recognizes body changes and new emotional responses. The crisis may also relate to determining how long she can work in a career or profession and whether she can balance working and childrearing. The crisis may involve making spatial changes in the home or moving to a new home to accommodate the baby and balancing the budget to meet additional expenses.

If pregnancy and parenting create a crisis for a couple who want a baby, they create even more upheaval for the adolescent or for the woman who heads the single-parent family—either unmarried or if married, left by the husband or father to face pregnancy, birth, and childrearing alone. This mother needs the support of and help from at least one other person during this period. A parent, relative, friend, or nurse can be a resource.

After a baby joins the family, a number of problems must be resolved. The realities of child care and managing a household may be a disillusionment after exposure to the American ideals promoted by the media and advertising. Partners must allow time to be together without interruption by the child and must maintain a mutually effective communication and a mutually satisfying sexual relationship. Joy and involvement increase as the parent/child **attachment** is developed. Establishing attachment is crucial to the long-term nurturing of the child and parental interest in the child.

Child/Parent Attachment

Table 8-1 outlines behaviors of the infant, mother, and father that occur in establishing **bonding, engrossment,** and **attachment**.* The extent to which these behaviors are shown will depend on how much contact is permitted between parents and baby by the nursing staff. Some mothers and fathers may at first be hesitant in relating to the child. The infant's behavior also affects interactional behavior, affection, and comfort toward the infant and later, the child.

Factors that interfere with mothering behaviors include the following:

1. The mother's immaturity or lack of mothering
2. Stressful situations
3. Financial worries
4. Lack of a supportive partner
5. The gender and appearance of the child

Separating mother and infant the first few days of life, depersonalized care by the nurses or doctors, rigid hospital routines, and premature discharge

---

*References 4, 5, 15, 17, 21, 25, 36.

Table 8-1 Infant/Parent Attachment Behaviors

Infant	Mother	Father
Reflexly looks into mother's face, establishes eye-to-eye contact or "face tie"; molds body to mother's body when held.	Reaches for baby; holds baby high against breast-chest-shoulder area; handles baby.	Has great interest in baby's face and notes eyes.
Vocalizes and stretches out arms in response to mother's voice.	Talks softly and in high-pitched voice; intense interest in baby; puts baby face-to-face with hers (en face position); eye contact gives baby sense of identity to mother; mother feels identity of baby.	Desires to touch and hold baby; cradles baby; shows more fingertip touching and smiling to male baby; has more eye contact with infant delivered by forceps or cesarean section.
Roots, licks, then sucks mother's nipple if in contact with mother's breasts. Cries; smiles.	Touches baby's extremities, examines, strokes, and kisses baby shortly after delivery; puts baby to breast if permitted.	Looks for distinct features; thinks newborn resembles self; perceives baby as beautiful.
Reflexly embraces, clings, using hands, feet, head, and mouth to maintain body contact.	Calls baby by name; notes desirable traits; expresses pleasure toward baby; attentive to reflex actions.	Feels proud after birth; has desire to protect and care for child.

Modified from Murray R and Zentner J: Nursing assessment and health promotion strategies through the lifespan, ed 4, East Norwalk, Conn, 1989, Appleton & Lange.
NOTE: Similar behaviors are seen with a premature baby, but the timing will vary.

from the hospital without adequate help also interfere with establishing attachment and maternal behaviors.[21,25,34-36] The nurse's nurturing behavior to the mother and assistance to her to find additional help may offset the negative impact of these factors.

Box 8-1 presents patterns of relating to and holding the infant that indicate the mother's or father's difficulty in establishing attachment. All of these behaviors may not be observed, but a combination of several indicates actual or potential difficulty with being a parent and should be reported to the nurse manager and physician.

Development of attachment between parent and baby continues through childhood. The nurse can teach about the importance of emotional, cognitive, and socialization processes: loving through cuddling, touching, stroking, kissing, talking to, laughing, playing with, and reinforcing and teaching the child. Such contact should be *consistent* and *done during physical care* and play with the child. The touching, talking, and laughing can also be focused on the child while the parent is preparing a meal, doing a household task, or waiting in a grocery line. The parent's voice across the room can also soothe and contributes to attachment.

Response to Separation in Hospitalization

The nurse will encounter **separation anxiety** at 7 or 8 months and at about 18 and 24 months in the hospitalized child. The child who is more accustomed to strangers will suffer less from a brief separation. When separated, the child experiences feelings of anger, fear, grief, and revenge. An apathetic, resigned reaction in the young child is a sign of abnormal development. The child who is separated from the parent for a time, as with hospitalization, goes through three phases of grief or mourning as a result of separation anxiety: protest, despair, and denial.[5,25]

During **protest,** the need for mother is conscious, persistent, and grief laden. The child cries continuously, tries to find her, is terrified, fears he has been deserted, feels helpless and angry that mother left him, and clings to her on her return. If the child is also ill, additional uncomfortable bodily sensations assault him. The child needs mother at this time.[5,25]

Despair is characterized by less activity. The child does not cry continuously, but is in deep mourning. He does not understand why mother isn't present. The child neither makes demands on the environment nor responds to overtures from others, including, at times, the mother. Yet the child clings to her if permitted. Mother may feel guilty and want to leave to relieve her distress, since she may feel her visits are disturbing to the child, especially when the child does not respond to her.[5,25]

Denial defends against anxiety by repressing the image of and feelings for mother and may be misinterpreted as recovery. The child begins to take more interest in the environment, eats, plays, and accepts other adults. Anger and disappointment at mother are so deep that the child acts as if he does not need her, shows revenge by rejecting

BOX 8-1

INDICATIONS OF DIFFICULTY WITH PARENT/CHILD ATTACHMENT

- Maintains little or no eye contact with the child
- Does not readily touch child, or holds child at times to meet personal needs
- Does not support baby's head or take safety precautions with the child
- Holds child at a distance, at arm's length, loosely, or not at all
- Appears disinterested in child or preoccupied with something else when child is present, and has a fixed facial expression or unconvincing smile in response to other's enthusiasm about child
- Perceives child as unattractive or looking like someone who is disliked
- Talks or coos to child little or not at all
- Has passive response to child; allows child to be placed in the arms rather than reaching out to child
- Calls child "it" rather than saying "my baby" or calling child by name
- Notes defects or undesirable traits in child even if child is normal, or is convinced the child is abnormal
- Avoids talking about child even when someone else initiates the topic
- Expresses dissatisfaction with or revulsion about care of child
- Ignores child's communications or cries, grunts, sneezes, and yawns
- Gets upset when child's secretions, feces, or urine touch the body or clothes; perceives care of child as revolting
- Readily gives child to someone else
- Handles the child roughly, even after the child has eaten or vomited
- Gives inappropriate responses to child's needs, such as overfeeding or underfeeding, overhandling or underhandling
- Thinks child does not love him/her
- Complains of being too tired to take care of child
- Expresses fears that child might die of a minor illness[7,8,17,25,35]

her, and sometimes even rejects gifts she brings. To prevent further estrangement, mother should understand that the child's need for her is more intense than ever.[5,25]

The mother should be told that immediate aftereffects of separation include changes in the child's behavior, such as regression, clinging, and seeking extra attention and reassurance. If extra affection is given to the child, trust is gradually restored. When separation is prolonged, the child's behavior can be changed and disturbed for months after return to the parents. The child's expressions of hostility should be accepted and demands met. Harsh discipline of or withdrawal from the child will cause further loss in trust and regression.

Influence of the Child on the Parents

Some children have a high activity level and from birth respond easily to the parent. Some are quiet and withdrawn and have a low activity level. Various other mixtures of activity level and temperament exist. The child's dominant reaction pattern to new situations manifests an innate temperament, and the temperament affects the reactions of parents. They in turn will mold the child's reaction pattern. It is easy to love a lovable baby and child, but parents have to work harder with children who are not highly responsive. Reactions between baby, and then the child, and parents affect the style of child care that will develop. A highly active mother who expects an intense reaction may have a hard time mothering a low-activity, quiet baby and child, because she may misinterpret the behavior, feel rejected, and in turn reject the child. The child will be denied the stimulation necessary for development. If mother is withdrawn, quiet, unexpressive, and has a high-activity child, she may punish normal energetic or assertive behavior and ignore the bids for affection and stimulation. Extreme parental rejection or lack of reaction causes emotional illness and autistic behavior. An assertive child may become controlling with an indecisive mother and not learn that others also have needs and rights. If the child is controlled by mother, he cannot develop trust, independence, or ability to cope with persons on equal terms.[2] The nurse should assess for and teach the parents about how the child can affect parental behavior.

The family unit, regardless of the specific form, is important to the young child. The close relationship of baby to mother and father gradually expands to include other significant adults living in the home, siblings, and other relatives. Through these relationships the child learns how to interact with men and women and how to act like a boy or girl. Gender identity is also reinforced through name, clothing, color of clothing and room, and behavior toward and expectations of the child. The ongoing contacts between the child and significant adults contribute to gender or sexual identification and should occur in early childhood.

Teaching sexuality to the child enables him or her to acquire gender identity and positive feelings about self. The basis for sex education begins prenatally with the parents' attitudes toward the coming child. Parents and other caregivers continue daily thereafter to form attitudes in the child and impart factual knowledge in response to questions. Parents may need help in acquiring information to answer the child's questions. If parent/child communication has been open—if the child feels free to ask questions about sex and other topics and if the parent gives satisfactory and correct answers without embarrassment—the basis for a healthy sexual attitude exists.

Although *sex education* must be tailored to the individual child's needs and interests, as well as to the cultural, religious, and family values, the following suggestions may be given by the nurse to parents of young children[25]:

1. Education about the self as a sexual person is best given by example through parents' showing respect and love for the self, mate, and the child.
2. The child who learns to trust others and to give, as well as receive, love has begun preparation for satisfactory adulthood, marriage, and parenthood.
3. The child's questions should be answered by giving information honestly, in a relaxed, accepting manner, and on the child's level of understanding. Isolated facts, myths, or animal analogies should be avoided. Religious beliefs can be worked into the explanation while acknowledging human realities.
4. The child should be taught anatomical names rather than other words for body parts and processes.
5. Grabbing the genitals and some masturbation are normal. Children explore their bodies, especially body parts that are not easily seen and that give pleasurable sensations when touched. The child should be taught that this is not normal behavior in public.
6. Playing doctor or examining each other's body parts is normal for preschool children. Parents should not overreact. If children seem to be using each other in a sexual way, they should be told that this is not acceptable.
7. The child's changing self motivates the same or different questions again and again. Explanation about reproduction may begin with a simple explanation of sperm and egg. Later the child can be given more detail.

Relationships with Siblings

The discussion in Chapter 7 on the effect of the child's gender and ordinal position on family interaction is significant for understanding and interacting with the young child, and for teaching parents.

Often the young child experiences the arrival of a **sibling.** The preschooler is no longer the center of attention but is expected to delight in the baby. It is important for parents to prepare the young child for a new arrival (Fig. 8-1). The nurse can assist parents with this task. Accepting the family's affection toward the baby is difficult, and jealousy is likely to occur if too much attention is focused on the baby. As a result, the preschooler may regress or act like a baby. He may ask for the bottle, soil self, lie in the baby's crib, or demand extra attention. He may appear to love the baby more than is normal but then harm the baby through play or rough handling. The child may show hostility toward the mother by direct physical or verbal attacks or by ignoring or rejecting her.

The older sibling who is given attention for accomplishments may cause feelings of envy and frustration in the preschooler. To get attention, the preschooler may try to engage in activity beyond his ability. If the younger child can identify with the older sibling and take pride in the accomplishments while simultaneously getting recognition, the child will feel positive about self. If the younger child feels defeated and is not given realistic recognition for his abilities, he may stop imitating the older sibling. In turn, the older sibling can be helpful to the younger child if he does not feel emotionally deprived or is not reprimanded excessively because of the preschooler's behavior.

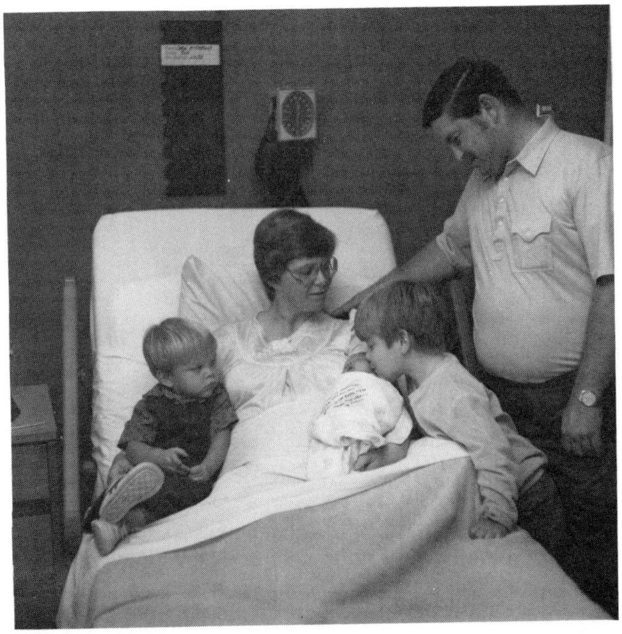

FIG. 8-1 Sibling visitation shortly after birth can be significant in the attachment process.

The nurse can assist the parents and young child in understanding effects of sibling rivalry, during both the parent's and child's hospitalization.

THE NEONATE

Physical Development

The **neonatal** period, the first 30 days of life, includes the critical transition from fetal existence to general physiological independence. Transition begins at birth with the first cry. Air is sucked in to inflate the lungs. Complex chemical changes are initiated in the cardiorespiratory system so that the baby's heart and lungs can assume the burden of oxygenating the body. The foramen ovale closes during the first 24 hours; the ductus arteriosus closes after several days. For the first time, baby experiences light, gravity, cold, and firm touch.[30,39]

Apgar scoring system. The physical status of the newborn is determined with the **Apgar score** 1 minute after birth and then 5 minutes later. A maximum score of 2 is given to each sign, so that the score could range from 0 to 10, as indicated by Table 8-2. A score under 7 means that the newborn is having difficulty adapting, needs even closer observation than usual, and may need life-saving intervention.[39]

Table 8-2 Apgar Scoring System in the Newborn

Sign	0	1	2
1. Heart rate	Absent	Below 100 per min	Above 100 per min
2. Respirations	Absent	Slow, irregular	Cry; regular rate
3. Muscle tone	Flaccid	Some flexion of extremities	Active movements
4. Reflex irritability	None	Grimace	Cry
5. Color	Body cyanotic or pale	Body pink, extremities cyanotic	Body completely pink

Appearance. The nurse can help parents adjust to the newborn's appearance. The head is misshapen. The nose is flat, and the eyelids are edematous. Often undistinguished is eye color. Discolored skin, large tongue, undersized lower jaw, short neck, small, sloping shoulders, short limbs, large abdomen, protruding umbilical stump (which remains to 3 weeks), and bowed, skinny legs are normal. The head, which accounts for one fourth of the total body size, appears large in relation to the body.

The **anterior fontanel** and the **posterior fontanel** are often called soft spots. These areas and the suture lines of the skull bones are not calcified and allow the bones to overlap during delivery and also allow for expansion of the brain as they gradually fill in with bone cells. The posterior fontanel closes by 2 or 3 months; the anterior fontanel closes between 6 and 18 months. These soft spots may add to the parents' impression that the newborn is too fragile to handle.[30,39] The head and fontanels can be gently touched without harm, but should be protected against strong pressure or direct injury.

The baby's characteristic position during this period closely imitates the fetal position: fists tightly closed and arms and legs drawn up against the body. Baby is aware of disturbances in equilibrium and will change position, reacting with the Moro reflex (see Chapter 44).

General measurements

Weight and length. In newborns, weight and length provide an index to normal development, and measurements should be accurate. The average birth weight of Caucasian males in the United States is 7½ pounds (3400 g) and of females is 7 pounds (3180 g). African-American, Indian, and Oriental newborns are smaller, on the average, at birth.[19,38] Maternal age, parity, and the woman's previous state of nutrition influence birth weight. Shortly after birth, the newborn loses weight, as much as 10% of birth weight, because of water loss, and parents should be told that this is normal before a steady weight gain, which begins in 1 or 2 weeks.[30]

The average length of American infants at birth is just under 20 inches (50.8 cm). Boys range from 19 to 21 inches (48.2 to 53.3 cm); girls average slightly less. The bones are soft, consisting chiefly of cartilage. The back is straight and curves with sitting. The muscles feel hard and are slightly resistant to pressure.[45] Ethnic differences for weight, length, head circumference, and other measurements have been noted.[19]

Head circumference. Measurement of head circumference throughout infancy is important to determine if any abnormalities are present. The measurement is taken over the brow just above the eyes and across the posterior occipital protuberance. Head size averages about 14 inches, or 35 cm, at birth; variations of one-half inch are common. Chest circumference is usually about an inch less than head size.[39]

Vital signs. In the newborn, vital signs are not stable. Respirations range from 50 to 80 per minute during the first hour after birth and then decrease to 30 to 60 per minute. Respirations are irregular, quiet, and shallow and may be followed by a 5- to 10-second pause intermittently. Causes of respiratory initiations may include physical stimulation of the birth process, the sudden change in baby's environment at birth, exposure to firm touch, and cool air. If mother was medicated during labor or if the baby is premature, the respiratory center of the brain is less operative and baby will have more difficulty breathing.[39]

Body temperature ranges from 97° to 100° Fahrenheit (F) (36.1° to 37.7° Celsius [C], because (1) the heat-regulating mechanism in the hypothalamus is not fully developed; (2) shivering to produce heat does not occur; (3) there is less subcutaneous fat; and (4) heat is lost to the environment. At birth, amniotic fluid increases temperature loss by evaporation; thus diligent efforts to dry the skin are necessary. The wet newborn can lose up to 200 calories of heat per kilogram per minute (90 calories per minute is the maximum the adult can lose). If the room is cool and baby is placed in contact with cold objects, heat loss occurs by convection, radiation, and conduction.[39]

Baby should be placed next to mother's abdominal skin or breasts initially and then wrapped well in blankets before placed in a warm crib. Several mechanisms occur to help the newborn conserve heat: (1) vasoconstriction—constricted blood vessels maintain heat in the inner body; (2) flexion of the body to reduce total amount of exposed skin (the premature baby does not assume a flexion of the extremities onto the body); (3) increased metabolic rate and heat production; and (4) metabolism of adipose tissue that has been stored during the eighth month of gestation. Thus fat between the scapulae around the neck, behind the sternum, and around the kidneys and adrenal glands accounts for 2% to 6% of the neonate's body weight and is metabolized quickly.[39,45]

Body temperature of the baby normally drops 1° to 2° F immediately after birth, but in a warm environment it begins to rise slowly after 8 hours. Prevention of heat loss, especially during the first 15 minutes, is crucial to extrauterine life.

Heart rate ranges at birth from 100 to 160 beats per minute because of the immature cardiac regulatory mechanism in the medulla. The heart rate may increase to 170 to 180 beats per minute when the newborn cries and drop to 90 during sleep. The pulse rate gradually decreases during the first and subsequent years.[39]

Blood pressure may range from 40 to 50 millimeters of mercury (mm Hg) systolic. By the end of the first month, blood pressure averages 80/40.[45]

Development of body systems

Integument. The neonate's skin is thin, delicate, usually mottled, varies from pink to red, and becomes very ruddy when the baby cries. Characteristics of the skin are given in Box 8-2.[39]

The epidermal layers in the baby are permeable, causing greater fluid loss from the body. Dry, intact skin is the greatest deterrent to bacterial invasion. The inability of the skin to contract and shiver in response to cold or perspire in response to heat causes ineffective thermal regulation.[30,39,40]

Umbilical cord. The **umbilical cord** is cut 1½ to 3 inches from baby's abdominal wall. Because of the high water content, the stump of the cord dries and shrinks rapidly. By the second day, it is a very hard, yellow or black (blood) tab on the skin. Slight oozing where the cord joins the abdominal wall is common.

Gastrointestinal. The baby urinates at birth. Fecal material, **meconium,** is sticky, odorless, and tarry and is passed from 8 to 24 hours after birth. Transitional stools for a week are loose, contain mucus, are greenish yellow and pasty, and have a sour odor. There will be 2 to 4 stools daily. If the baby is fed formula, the stools will become yellow, harder, and average 1 to 2 daily.

Neuromuscular. **Reflexes** indicate neurological function. Individual differences in the newborn's response are apparent at birth. Some respond vigorously to the slightest stimulation; others respond slowly. The nervous system of the newborn is both anatomically and physiologically immature, and **reflexes** should be observed for their presence and symmetry. These reflexes are described in Table 8-3.[25,30,38,39,45]

Sensory. The newborn has more highly developed sensory abilities than was once supposed. A moderately enriched environment without too much or too little stimulation is best suited for sensory motor development. Premature babies placed in a stimulus-rich environment until discharged from the hospital learn more quickly and are healthier at 4 months than premature babies who lived in the traditional environment.[18,45]

Twenty minutes of extra handling a day will result in earlier exploring and grasping behavior by the infant. The baby is very sensitive to touch, rocking, and being held upright, which are necessary for development of the nervous system, skin sensitivity, and emotional health.[18,24,25,38] Extra touch and movement each day results in a baby who is quieter, gains weight faster, and shows improved socioemotional function and ability to cope with stress.

Sensitivity to pain, pressure, and temperature extremes is present at birth; pain is shown by a distinct cry.[23] The baby is especially sensitive to touch around the mouth and on the palms and soles. Girls are more responsive to touch and pain than boys.[40] Visceral sensations of discomfort, such as hunger, overdistention of the stomach, passage of gas and stool, and extremes of temperature, apparently account for much of the newborn's crying. In a few weeks, baby acquires subtle modifications in the cry that provide clues to the attentive parent and nurse about the nature of the discomfort.[30]

The visual abilities of the newborn are apparent as he visually follows large moving objects beginning a day after birth. The eyes are as sensitive to changes in light intensity as adult eyes. Because eye movements are not yet fully coordinated and the neonate's eyeball is shorter than that of the adult, the newborn cannot focus on objects unless they are held about 8 to 20 inches from his face. Pupils respond sluggishly to light.[28]

Hearing is blurred the first few days of life because fluid is retained in the middle ear, but hearing loss can

BOX 8-2 CHARACTERISTICS OF NEONATAL SKIN

Vernix caseosa Cheesy covering that rubs off in a few days

Lanugo Downy hair remaining from fetal life that is replaced by other hair growth in several months

Acrocyanosis Bluish discoloration of hands and feet, which lasts only several days after birth

Milia Tiny white spots of sebaceous secretion collection on nose, chin, and forehead

Hemangiomas Pink spots on various regions of the face, neck, or back that may or may not be permanent

Mongolian spots Slate-colored areas in buttocks or lower back in African-American, Oriental, or Mediterranean babies that fade gradually

Physiological jaundice Yellow discoloration that appears about the third or fourth day as a result of hemolysis of excess number of red blood cells

Table 8-3 Assessment of Infant Reflexes

Reflex	Description	Appearance/ Disappearance
Rooting	Touching baby's cheek causes head to turn toward the side touched	Present in utero at 24 wk; disappears 3 to 4 mo; may persist in sleep 9 to 12 mo
Sucking	Touching lips or placing something in baby's mouth causes baby to draw liquid into mouth by creating vacuum with lips, cheeks, and tongue	Present in utero at 28 wk; persists through early childhood, especially during sleep
Pupillary response	Flashing light across baby's eyes or face causes constriction of pupils	Present at 32 wk of gestation; persists throughout life
Blink	Baby closes both eyes	Remains throughout life
Moro or startle	Making a loud noise or changing baby's position causes baby to extend both arms outward with fingers spread, then bring them together in a tense, quivery embrace	Present at 28 wk of gestation; disappears 4 to 7 mo
Palmar grasp	Placing object or finger in baby's palm causes his fingers to close tightly around object	Present at 32 wk of gestation; disappears 3 to 4 mo; replaced by voluntary grasp at 4 to 5 mo
Plantar grasp	Placing object or finger beneath toes causes curling of toes around object	Present at 32 wk of gestation; disappears 9 to 12 mo
Tonic neck reflex (TNR) or fencing	Postural reflex seen when infant lies on back with head turned to one side; arm and leg on the side toward which he is looking are extended while opposite limbs are flexed	Present at birth; disappears about 4 mo
Orienting	Turning head and eyes toward stimulus of noise, accompanied by cessation of other activity, heartbeat change, and vascular constriction	Present at birth; comes under voluntary control later; persists throughout life
Attending	Fixing eyes on a stimulus that changes brightness, movement, or shape	Present shortly after birth; comes under voluntary control later; persists throughout life
Trunk incurvation	Stroking one side of spinal column while baby is on his abdomen causes crawling motions with legs, lifting head from surface, and incurvature of trunk on the side stroked	Present in utero; then seen about third or fourth day; persists 2 to 3 mo
Babinski	Stroking bottom of foot causes big toe to raise while other toes fan out and curl downward	Present at birth; disappears about 9 to 10 months; presence of reflex later may indicate disease
Biceps	Tap on tendon of biceps causes biceps to contract quickly	Brisk in first few days, then slightly diminished; permanent
Knee jerk	Tap on tendon below patella or on patella causes leg to extend quickly	More pronounced first 2 days; permanent

Modified from Murray R and Zentner J: Nursing assessment and health promotion strategies through the life span, ed 4, East Norwalk, Conn, 1989, Appleton & Lange.

be tested as early as the first day. The neonate responds to voice pitch changes. A low pitch quiets; a high pitch increases alertness. Baby responds to sound direction—left or right—but responds best to mother's voice and to sounds directly in front of the face.[30,40] Baby often sleeps better with background songs or a tape recording of mother's heartbeat.[37]

Other characteristics. Several other characteristics are also normal and resolve shortly after birth: swollen breasts, which contain liquid in boys and girls; swollen genitalia with undescended testicles in the boy; and vaginal secretions in the girl, caused by maternal hormones. Genitalia size varies for boys and girls. Urine is present in the bladder, and the baby voids at birth.

THE INFANT

Physical Development

Appearance. During the first year of life, the growing **infant** changes in appearance as he changes size and proportion. The face grows rapidly; trunk and limbs lengthen; back and limb muscles develop; and coordination improves. Physical growth and emotional, social, and neuromuscular learning are interrelated and rapid in the first year. The first year of life is one of two periods of rapid physical growth after birth. (The other period is prepuberty and at puberty.) Birth weight normally doubles by 5 to 6 months and triples by 12 months; many babies gain more weight in the first year. The baby grows about 12 inches in the first year.[30,38,39]

Physical and motor abilities are heavily influenced by genetic, biological, and environmental factors; nutrition, maturation of the central nervous system, skeletal formation, and overall physical health status; stimulation; and consistent loving care. African-American infants mature ahead of Caucasian infants in motor skills, bone ossification, and walking. This is apparently because of genetic factors and has evolutionary adaptive value.[19,45]

Table 8-4 divides developmental sequence into 3-month periods for specific assessment,[14,25,30,39,45] but it is only a guide. Great individual differences occur among infants. Girls usually develop more rapidly than boys, although the activity level is generally higher for boys. Overall behavior patterns rather than isolated characteristics are the key to understanding development and nursing assessment.

Table 8-4 Physical Characteristics of the Infant

1 to 3 Months	3 to 6 Months	6 to 9 Months	9 to 12 Months
Many characteristics of newborn, but more stable physiologically	Most neonatal reflexes gone Temperature stabilizes at 99.4° F (37.5° C)		Temperature averages 99.7° F (37.7° C)
Heartbeat about 120 to 130 beats per min		Pulse about 115 per min	Pulse about 100 to 110 per min
Blood pressure about 80/40; gradually increases		Blood pressure about 90/60	Blood pressure about 96/66
Respirations more regular at 30 to 40 per min; prone to respiratory infection			Respirations 20 to 40 per min; respiratory tract lining more mature
Weight gain of 5 to 7 oz (141.75 to 198.45 g) per wk	Weight gain of 3 to 5 oz (85.05 to 141.75 g) per wk		Weight gain of 3 to 5 oz (85.05 to 141.75 g) per wk
Weight at 8 to 13 lb (3629 to 5897 g)	Weight at 15 to 16 lb by 6 mo (6.8 to 7.3 kg)	Birth weight doubled by 6 mo	Birth weight tripled; average 22 lb (10 kg)
Head circumference increases 1 inch for a total circumference of up to 16 inches (40 cm)	Head size increases 1 inch (2.54 cm)	Head size 17.8 inches (43.21 cm)	Head size about two thirds of adult size (18.3 inches or 45 to 46 cm)
Chest circumference 16 inches (40 cm)	Chest size increases over 1 inch (17.3 inches or 43 to 44 cm)	Chest circumference increases ½ inch (17.8 inches or 44 to 45 cm)	Chest circumference increases about ½ inch (18.3 inches or 45 to 46 cm)

Modified from Murray R and Zentner J: Nursing assessment and health promotion strategies through the life span, ed 4, East Norwalk, Conn, 1989, Appleton & Lange.

Table 8-4 Physical Characteristics of the Infant—cont'd

1 to 3 Months	3 to 6 Months	6 to 9 Months	9 to 12 Months
Growth of 1 inch (2.54 cm) monthly	Growth of ½ inch (1.27 cm) monthly	Growth of ½ inch (1.27 cm) monthly	Growth of ½ inch monthly; height 29 to 30 inches (72.5 to 75 cm), increased by 50% since birth
Limbs used simultaneously, but not separately	Movements more symmetrical		
Clenched fists giving way to open hands that bat at objects			
Reaches for objects	Reaches for objects with flexed fingers; objects transferred from one hand to another by 6 mo; bangs with objects held in one hand; scoops objects with hands; begins to use fingers separately	Palmar grasp developed; picks up objects with both hands; bottle held with hands; preference for the use of one hand; probes with index finger; thumb opposition to finger (prehension)	Brings hands and thumb and index finger together at will to pick up small objects; releases objects at will
Can follow moving objects with eyes when supine; begins to use both eyes together about age 2 months	Binocular depth perception by about 5 mo	Explores, feels, pulls, tastes, objects	Makes mark on paper
	Looks for objects when they are dropped		
	Improving eye/hand coordination	Hand/mouth coordination	
		Feeds self cracker and other finger foods	Eats with fingers; holds cup, spoon
Stomach emptying time from 2½ to 4 hours; 2 bowel movements daily, or more if breast-fed	Stomach capacity about 150 ml; bowel movements of breast-fed baby lighter colored than those of bottle-fed baby		
	Eruption of one or two lower incisors	Begins weaning process; peristaltic waves slower; needs iron replacement	Has six teeth: central and lateral incisors; eruption of first molars about 12 mo
Attends to voices	Turns head to sound		
Raises chin while lying on stomach at 1 mo			
Raises chest while lying on stomach at 2 mo			
Holds head erect in prone position at 3 mo			
	Rolls over completely by 6 mo		Rolls easily from back to stomach

Continued.

Table 8-4 Physical Characteristics of the Infant—cont'd

1 to 3 Months	3 to 6 Months	6 to 9 Months	9 to 12 Months
Sits if supported	Sits with support at 4 mo		
	Holds head steady while sitting		
	Pulls self to sitting position		
	Begins to sit alone for short periods	Sits erect unsupported by 7 mo	Sits alone steadily
	Plays with feet		Puts feet in mouth
	Begins to scoot backward while sitting	Creeps or crawls by 9 mo	Hitches with backward locomotion while sitting
	Bears portion of own weight when held in standing position	Pulls self to feet by holding onto support	Sits from standing position without help
	Pushes feet against hard surface by 3 or 4 mo	Cruises (walking sideways while holding onto object with both hands) by 10 mo	Stands alone briefly
			Walks when led by 11 mo
		Begins to walk with help	Walks with help by 12 to 14 mo
			Lumbar and dorsal curves developed while learning to walk
			Turning of feet and bowing of legs
			Beginning to show regular bladder and bowel patterns; has one or two stools per day; interval of dry diaper does not exceed 1 to 2 hr
			Not ready for toilet training
Smiles reflexly	Smiles deliberately during interaction	Experiences separation anxiety about 7 to 9 mo	
			Begins to cooperate in dressing; puts arm through sleeve; takes off socks
			Improves previously acquired skills throughout this period

Emotional Development

According to Erikson,[11] the infant should learn to **trust.** Basic trust involves optimism, acceptance of and reliance on self and others, and a sense of hope. A sense of trust forms the basis for later identity formation, social responsiveness to others, and ability to care about and love others. Presence of trust may be demonstrated in the infant by the ease of feeding, the depth of sleep, and the overall appearance of contentment. If trust is not developed, mistrust develops. **Mistrust** is a sense of feeling dissatisfied emotionally or physically, an inability to believe in or rely on others or self. It is characterized by lethargy, lack of weight gain, poor eating, excessive colic, lack of sleep, and failure to thrive. Later, predominant feelings and behaviors are pessimism, suspicion, bitterness toward others, and antagonism. The person may be dependent or withdrawn, or he may bully others to gain control.[25]

Security and trust are fostered by the prompt, loving, and consistent response of parents or other caregivers, including the nurse, to the infant's distress and needs, as well as by the positive response to happy, contented behavior. The infant who is in a nurturing, loving environment and who has developed trust is a happy baby most of the time. He is sociable and responsive to others.[1,2,25]

Cognitive/Intellectual Development

Psychosocial, physical, and motor development greatly influence each other. A level of physiological maturation of the nervous system must be present before environmental stimulation and learning opportunities can be effective in promoting emotional and cognitive development. In turn, without love and tactile, kinesthetic, verbal, and other environmental stimuli, some nervous system structures do not develop. **Cognitive development** or learning depends on innate capacity, maturation, nutrition, gross and fine motor stimulation, touch, stimulation of all senses through various activities, language imitation, and social interaction.[25,43,44]

The infant is in the **sensorimotor stage** of cognitive development, according to Piaget. During the neonatal period, behavior is entirely reflexive. Yet all stimuli to each of the senses are being assimilated into beginning mental images.[28,29] From 1 to 4 months, life is a series of random events, but hand/month and ear/eye coordination are developing. The infant's eyes follow moving objects; eyes and ears follow sounds and novel stimuli. Responses to different objects vary. Baby smiles at familiar faces and anticipates a routine, such as diapering. From 4 to 8 months, baby learns to initiate and recognize new experiences and repeat pleasurable ones. Reaching, grasping, listening, and laughing become better coordinated. Baby anticipates familiar events or a moving object's position. From 8 to 12 months, baby's behavior is showing clear acts of beginning intelligence and experimentation. Baby uses certain actions to attain goals. He realizes for the first time that someone other than self can cause activity. He searches for and retrieves a toy that disappeared from view. Shapes and sizes of familiar objects are recognized. Because of the baby's increased sense of separateness, he experiences separation or eighth month anxiety when the mothering figure leaves. Sitting, creeping, standing, or walking gives baby a new perception of the environment.*

Communication and Language

Communication between people involves facial expressions, body movements, other nonverbal behavior, vocalizations, speech, and use of language. A newborn is ready to communicate if parents and caretakers know how to read the messages. The first communications are through eye contact, crying, and body movements.[23,32] Later, vocalizations are self-reinforcing; that is, the baby finds pleasure in making and hearing his own sounds, and responses from others provide further reinforcement. Reinforcement from caregivers, including the nurse, when desired sounds are made is necessary for the infant to progress to language development. The child must also hear others speak, to further reinforce using the sounds and language of the culture.[25,43,45] Between 9 and 12 months, baby learns to recognize his name and the names of several familiar objects, responds to "no," and may occasionally obey the parents' command.[26]

Promoting Optimum Health

Nutrition. Feeding time is a crucial time for the baby and mother: a time to strengthen attachment so that the child feels love and security, and a time for the child to learn about the environment.

Breast-feeding. The American Academy of Pediatrics recommends breast-feeding for the first year of life. However, the bottle-fed baby can thrive equally well.[46] Human milk is sterile, digestible, available, inexpensive, and contains the necessary nutrients except vitamins C and D and iron. In undernourished women, the composition of breast milk is adequate, although vitamin content depends on the mother's diet.[20,31] Breast milk is all that baby needs the first 6 months of life. Immunoglobulins (antibodies) to many types of microorganisms and enzymes that destroy bacteria are also obtained from human milk. Breast-fed babies are also less prone to allergies.[31,46] The baby may be put to breast immediately after delivery and fed within 8 hours after birth to reduce hypoglycemia and hyperbilirubinemia.[30,39]

The nurse can assist the mother with breast-feeding, which should be a comfortable, uninterrupted time.

---

* References 14, 25, 28, 29, 32, 44.

Mother needs (1) an encouraging partner or family member, (2) supportive nursing personnel to assist, (3) acquaintance with other successful nursing mothers, and (4) after delivery, hospital routines that allow access to the baby when the baby is hungry and her breasts are full. The mother should not automatically receive medication to stop lactation; baby should not be fed in the nursery between breast feedings. Mother should be encouraged to increase her fluid intake and meet the increased recommended dietary allowances (RDA) for lactating women.[31,46]

The first nourishment the baby receives from breastfeeding is **colostrum,** a thin secretion. Colostrum is rich in carbohydrates, which the newborn needs. It serves as a laxative to clean out the gastrointestinal tract. Colostrum fed immediately after birth triggers antibody production.[31,46] True milk comes in the first few days after delivery.

Baby may nurse every 1 or 2 hours at first, perhaps 15 to 30 minutes each time, and then every 3 to 4 hours. A large or active infant may need supplemental feeding. Usually extra formula or baby food is not necessary before the fourth month. Food in addition to breast milk (or formula) should be introduced by the end of the sixth month. If mother received ample amounts of iron during pregnancy, her baby's iron stores should last 4 to 12 months.[31,46]

Commercial formulas. Commercial formulas are similar to each other and to human milk, but they are not exactly the same. Special formulas have been developed to meet the needs of infants who cannot take regular formula. Formula-fed infants vary in the amount they drink and their demand for food. Table 8-5 lists average formula and feeding patterns during infancy.[31,39,45,46]

Solid foods. What and when solid food is offered seems to be a matter of preference of the pediatrician and mother. The infant's needs and developmental achievements, such as eye/hand/mouth coordination and fine pincer grasp, should be considered when introducing solids.

Introducing baby to solid foods should be a pleasant experience. The foods offered should be smooth and well diluted with milk or formula. The infant should not be hurried, coaxed, or allowed to linger more than 30 minutes. New foods should be offered one at a time and early in the feeding while baby is still hungry. Developmentally, a child of 6 or 7 months is ready to chew solids rather than ingest only thickened feedings.[31]

When baby is first fed pureed foods with a spoon, he expects and wants to suck. Protrusion of the tongue, which is needed in sucking, makes it appear as if baby is pushing food out of the mouth. This is not a dislike for the food, but is really the result of immature muscle coordination and possibly surprise at the taste and feel of the new items in the diet. This reflex gradually disappears

Table 8-5 Infant Feeding Patterns

Age	Amount	Frequency
1-7 days	60-90 ml	Every 3-4 hours
8-30 days	90-120 ml	Every 4 hours
2-3 months	120-180 ml milk; accepts cereal	Every 3-4 hours; 5 feedings; sleeps through night
4-5 months	150-210 ml milk; other strained foods added gradually (vegetables, meat, fruit, egg yolk)	Every 3-4 hours; 5 feedings during day
6-7 months	210-240 ml milk; enjoys finger foods, especially when teething	Every 4 hours; 4-5 feedings during day
8-10 months	240 ml milk; regular food	Eats 3 meals; drinks extra fluid

by 7 to 8 months. The baby should not be punished for spitting out food.

Food is a learning experience. Baby gains motor control and coordination in self-feeding. He learns to recognize color, shape, and texture. Use of mouth muscles stimulates speech movements, and trust develops with the consistent, loving atmosphere of mealtime.[46]

Weaning. **Weaning** is usually started at 6 months and completed by the end of the first year as baby shows signs of readiness. Muscle coordination increases; teeth erupt; and he resists being held close while feeding. Mother's consistency in meeting the new feeding schedule is important to development of a sense of trust. The most difficult feeding to give up is usually the bedtime feeding, because baby is tired. During times of stress, baby is then more likely to want the "old method." After the maxillary central incisory teeth erupt, a night bottle should contain no carbohydrate, to reduce decay in the deciduous teeth. Baby is also learning to wait longer for food and may object vigorously to this new condition.

Water intake. Baby needs about 100 to 150 ml of water per kilogram of body weight daily to offset normal fluid losses. Some of this is obtained in the milk. Hot weather, fever, diarrhea, or vomiting quickly leads to dehydration, because babies have a smaller total fluid volume in the body relative to body size.[31,46]

Nutrient intake. Baby needs daily an average of 2.2 g of protein and 117 calories per kilogram (or 36 per pound) of body weight to grow and gain weight satisfactorily. Some fats are necessary, because they contain essential fat-soluble vitamins and furnish more energy per unit than carbohydrates and protein. Adequate vitamins and minerals are essential. If the water supply is not fluorinated, supplementation should be given until 12 years of age to prevent dental caries.[46]

Sleep, rest, and exercise. The nurse is in a key position to teach parents about the child's sleep patterns and to promote sleep in the child. Every infant has a unique sleep pattern. The following are some generalizations that can serve as a guide for the baby's first months[40]:

1. During regular or quiet sleep, eyes are closed, breathing is regular, and the only movements are sudden; baby makes little sound and cannot be awakened with mild stimuli.
2. During irregular, active **rapid eye movement** (REM) sleep, baby's eyes are closed, breathing is irregular, muscles twitch slightly from time to time, and there are smiles or pouts in response to sounds or lights.
3. During quiet wakefulness, eyes are open, body is more active, breathing is irregular, and there is varying spontaneous response to external stimuli.
4. During active wakefulness, eyes are open and follow interesting sights and sounds.

As the infant's nervous system develops, periods of sleep and wakefulness gradually become longer and more regular. By 6 to 8 weeks, baby's biological rhythms usually coincide with day and night hours. Babies sleep an average of 16 to 20 hours a day for the first week. By 12 to 16 weeks, these hours will be reduced to 14 or 15 hours a day. By 7 or 8 months, baby may sleep through the night without awakening. By the end of the first year, the baby may sleep 12 to 14 hours at night and nap 1 to 4 hours during the day.[30,39] The baby goes through the stage of separation anxiety about 7 or 8 months of age; bedtime becomes more difficult because he does not want to leave mother. The parent should be firm, but not harsh, about getting the child ready for bed. Prolonging bedtime adds to fatigue and separation fears. Caressing or singing softly while holding baby in a sleeping position in bed is calming. If the mother is available when the baby first awakes, baby anticipates this pleasure and sleep is associated with return of mother. If the baby awakes and cries during the night, the parent should wait briefly. The crying will usually subside with the baby's development. Persistent crying indicates unmet needs and should be attended.[25]

A baby can sleep comfortably in an infant crib or bassinet during the first few weeks, but as soon as active arms and legs begin to hit the sides, he should be moved to a full-size crib. The crib slats should be no more than 2½ inches apart. No pillows should be used. The crib should have a crib border placed at the bottom of the slats to prevent the head getting caught between the bars. It should be fitted with a firm, waterproofed, easy-to-clean mattress and with warm, light covers loosely tucked in. The sides of the crib should fit closely to the mattress so that the infant will not get caught if he rolls to the edge. Thin plastic sheeting should never be used on or around the baby's crib; it can cause suffocation.[25]

Immunization. Immunizations in the infant are as follows[1,9,12,41,42]:

AGE	VACCINE IMMUNIZATION
2 months	DTP (diphtheria, tetanus, pertussis)
	OPV (live oral polio virus)
4 months	DTP
	OPV
6 months	DTP
	OPV (optional)
15 months	MMR (rubeola or long measles, mumps, rubella)

At 12 months the child should be given a tine test to detect possible tuberculosis.

Injury prevention. Safety promotion and injury control are based on the understanding of behavior of the infant and young child. The nurse is responsible for giving safe care and can teach parents and others about safety measures for the child.

Contrary to common belief, baby is not immobile. Baby rolls, crawls, creeps, walks, reaches, and explores. And because he is helpless in water, baby should never be left alone or with an irresponsible person while in water. The home and car have many often unnoticed hazards; baby should never be left alone in either and should never roam freely in the car while it is in motion.[25] Parents should use an approved car infant seat or harness.[33]

Falls can be avoided if the parents or nurses do the following[25,30,45]:

- Keep crib rails up
- Maintain a firm grasp of baby while carrying or caring for him, and support the head during the first few months
- Use a sturdy high chair and car infant seat or harness with fasteners in place
- Have a gate at the top of the stairs or in front of windows or doors that are above the first story

Suffocation at home and in the health care setting can be avoided by the following[23,30,45]:

- Removing small objects that could be inhaled or ingested (safety pins, small beads, coins, toys, nuts, raisins, popcorn, balloons)
- Keeping plastic bags, venetian blind cords, or other cords out of reach
- Avoiding pillows in the crib or excessively tight clothing or bedcovers

Burns can be avoided by the following[25,30,45]:

- Placing the crib away from radiators or fireplaces
- Using warm-air vaporizers with caution
- Covering electrical outlets
- Avoiding tablecloths that hang over the table's edge
- Turning pot handles inward on the stove
- Avoiding excessive sun exposure
- Avoiding smoking around the baby

Developmental tasks. The following developmental tasks are to be accomplished in infancy[10]:

- Achieve overall physiological equilibrium of organ systems
- Perceive self as a dependent person but a separate being from others
- Become aware of the alive versus inanimate, and familiar versus unfamiliar
- Develop a feeling of and desire for affection and response from others
- Begin to manage the changing body and learn new motor skills, begin eye/hand coordination, and establish rest/activity rhythm
- Begin to understand the immediate environment through exploration
- Develop a beginning language system
- Direct emotional expressions to indicate needs and wishes

Table 8-7 Muscular Development of the Toddler

Age	Muscular Skill
12-15 months	Walks alone; reaches for objects without superfluous movement
17 months	Walks backward and sideways
20 months	Climbs stairs with help
24 months	Climbs up or down stairs without help, holding rail; places both feet on a step before climbing to next step; vision is 20/10 (farsighted)
28 months	Jumps off floor with both feet
30 months	Throws ball overhand; balances on one foot; walks on tiptoes
32 months	Jumps from chair; pedals tricycle
36 months	Climbs up stairs with alternate feet; jumps 10-12 inches

THE TODDLER

Physical Development

Appearance. The chubby look of infancy is gone by 12 to 15 months. Limbs are growing faster than torso, giving a different proportion to the body. By 12 to 15 months, chest circumference is larger than head circumference. The child increasingly looks like a family member as the face contours with the presence of deciduous teeth. By age 2, there are 16 teeth. Muscle tone becomes firmer as the fat-storing mechanisms change.

Rate of growth. During the **toddler** period, age 12 to 15 months up to 36 months, growth is slower than in infancy, but it is even. Bone growth continues with the development of about 25 new ossification centers during the second year. Height and weight progression is shown in Table 8-6. By 2 years, the girl has grown to 50% of final adult height; by 2½ years, the boy to 50% of adult height.[39]

Neuromuscular development. Increasing gross motor coordination is shown by leg and hand/arm movements. Spontaneous scribbles are followed by circular motions and then vertical and horizontal lines. The child enjoys handling a spoon and glass and feeding self, but he frequently spills fluid from a glass or tips food from a container. Table 8-7 shows major muscular abilities of the toddler.[30,39,40,45]

Table 8-6 Toddler Height and Weight Norms

Age	Height	Weight
12-24 months	Increase 4-5 inches (10-12 cm)	Increase 5 pounds (2.27 kg)
24-36 months	Increase 2½-3½ inches (6-8 cm)	Birth weight quadrupled by 24 months

Vital signs. The pulse averages 105 beats per minute. Blood pressure averages 80 to 100 systolic and 64 diastolic. The capillary bed has increased ability to respond to environmental temperatures, thus aiding thermoregulation. Body temperature averages 99° F (39.2° C). Respirations average 20 to 30 per minute. Lung volume increases, and susceptibility to respiratory infections decreases as respiratory tract structures increase in size.[39,40,45]

Other characteristics. The skin becomes more protective against outer invasion from microorganisms. It becomes tougher, with more resilient epithelium and less water content; less fluid is lost through the skin as a result. The skin remains dry, because sebum secretion is limited. At this age, eczema improves and the frequency of rashes declines.[40]

Toilet Training

This is a major developmental accomplishment and relates directly to development of the neuromuscular system and to development of autonomy.[11] The toddler gradually learns to control bowel and bladder. Neuromuscular maturity, which occurs from 18 months to 3 years, with bowel before bladder control, is necessary for regular, self-controlled evacuation.[30,39,40]

Bowel training is a less complex task than bladder training and should be attempted first. The toddler shows readiness for bowel training when he defecates regularly and shows some signs of being aware of defecation, such as grunting, straining, or tugging at the diaper. It also helps if the child can speak, understand directions, and manipulate the clothing somewhat.

Some toddlers cry after defecation and indicate distress until their diaper or training pants are changed. Others play with and smear feces. Play with feces must be restricted because it is unsanitary and nonaesthetic. Changing diapers immediately after defecation, keeping the diaper on snugly, having well-fitted training pants, and showing disapproval are ways to prevent such play. Opportunities for play and smearing with clay, sand, mud, paste, and finger paints help the child divert instinctual urges into socially accepted behavior.

Parents should approach toilet training in a matter-of-fact and relaxed way, expect some resistance, and not push the child or reflect anxiety. Every child by age 3 is able to carry on this task with some help. Encourage the parents to have the child use a potty chair (Fig. 8-2), since it is mechanically easier than the family toilet. Recommend that the child wear training pants and that training take place when disruptions in regular routine are at a minimum. The toddler should be praised for success. Toilet training should not be started in difficult or insecure periods, such as hospitalization, homecoming of a new baby, absence of the main caretaker from home, or a family crisis.

Bladder training is more complex, because neurological maturation comes later. Bladder control demands more self-awareness and self-discipline from the toddler and is usually achieved between the ages of 2½ and 3½ years when physiological development has progressed enough that the bladder can retain urine for about 2 hours.

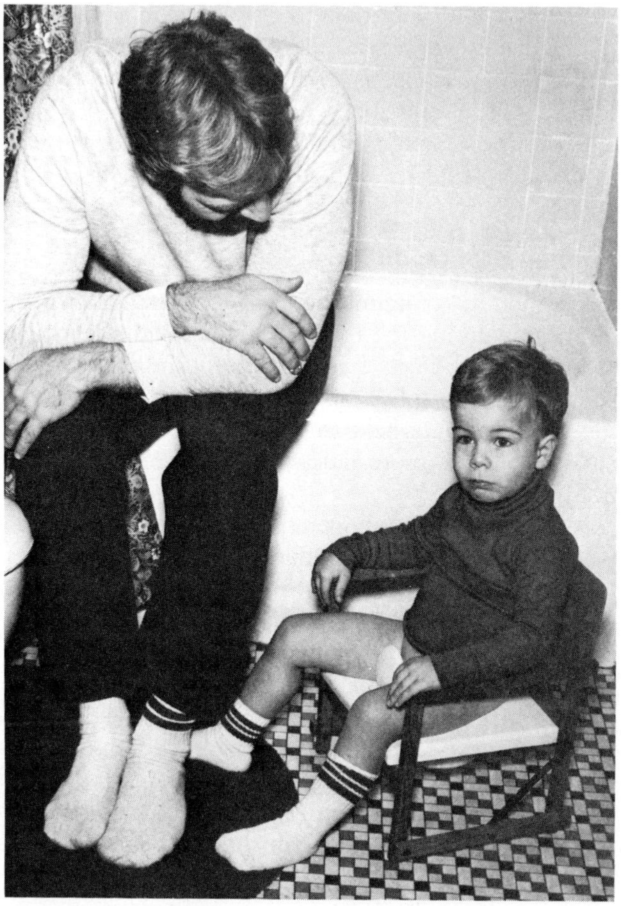

FIG. 8-2 Toddler on freestanding potty chair.

Emotional Development

The toddler is an uninhibited, energetic little person, always seeking attention, approval, and personal goals. Sometimes the toddler is cuddly and loving. At other times, he bites, hits, or pinches. The toddler only slowly realizes that he cannot have everything desired and that some behavior annoys others. He tries to be independent, yet becomes easily frightened and runs to the parent for protection, security, reassurance, and approval. The toddler laughs frequently, especially at surprise sounds and startling incongruities, and laughs with others who are laughing at his antics.[25,45]

The toddler should develop autonomy instead of shame and doubt.[11] **Autonomy** is shown in the ability to gain self-control; to feel able to cope adequately with problems or get the necessary help; to give generously or to hold on; to distinguish between himself, his possessions or wishes, and others and their possessions; and to have a feeling of goodwill and pride. Autonomy is characterized by the often-heard statement, "Me do it." Displaying temper, dawdling, and rituals; exploring even when parents object; developing language skills; saying "no" although he may do as asked; and increasing control over his body or situations are some apparent ways the toddler is demonstrating developing autonomy and maintaining a sense of security and control. Ritualistic behavior is normal and at a peak at 2½ years, especially at bedtime and during illness.[25]

Shame and doubt are felt if autonomy and a positive self-concept are not achieved.[11] Shame is the feeling of being fooled, embarrassed, exposed, or small. Doubt is fear, uncertainty, and feeling that nothing done is any good and that one is controlled by others rather than being in control of self. There is a limit to how exposed, dirty, mean, and vulnerable one can feel. If the child is pushed past the limit, disciplined, or toilet trained too harshly, the child cannot know what he should be and can do. If everything is planned and done for and to the child, he cannot develop autonomy. The child may become defiant, excessively negativistic, stubborn, physically overactive, or impulsive, and develop behaviors opposite to expectations. A low frustration tolerance and difficulty with eating, digestion, elimination, and sleep may be seen.[25]

Temper tantrums result in the toddler because he does not want to feel helpless. Once the feelings are discharged, the child regains composure quickly and without revenge. If temper tantrums (a form of negativism) occur, the best advice is to ignore the outburst if the child is not harming self or another being. It will soon disappear.

BOX 8-3 RULES FOR DISCIPLINING THE YOUNG CHILD

1. Provide an environment in which the child feels respected.
2. Decide what is important and what is not worth a battle of wills; avoid negativism and an angry scene.
3. Changing the mind, pursuing an alternate activity, or letting the child have his way is not giving in, losing face, being a poor parent, or letting the child be manipulative. When limits are consistent, changing a direction of behavior can be a positive learning experience for the child. The child is becoming aware of being a separate person, able to assert self and influence others.
4. Avoid having to repeatedly say "no," by removing or avoiding temptations, such as breakable objects within reach or candy that should not be eaten.
5. Try not to ask open-ended questions for the child to decide about an activity when the decision is not really one the child can make.
6. Consider limits as more than restrictions but also as a distraction from one prohibited activity to another in which the child can freely participate. Distraction with alternatives or a substitute is effective with the toddler, because attention span is short.
7. Reinforce appropriate behavior through approval and attention. The child will continue behavior that gains attention, even if the attention is punitive, because negative attention is better than none to the child.
8. Set limits consistently so that the child can rely on the adult's judgment rather than testing the adult's endurance in each situation.
9. Set limits only when necessary. Some rules promote a sense of security, but too many confuse the child.
10. Provide a safe area where the child is free to do whatever he wants to do.
11. Do not overprotect the child; he should learn that some things have a price, such as a bruise or a scratch.
12. Do not terminate the child's activity too quickly: tell him that the activity is ending.

Cognitive/Intellectual Development

According to Piaget, the toddler from 12 to 24 months is in the last phases of the sensorimotor stage. The toddler from 24 months to 3 years and the preschooler are in the **preoperational stage,** which extends from age 2 to 7 years.[28,29]

The toddlers attention span lengthens, but he does not fully understand simple explanations. He can name pictures on repeated exposure. The child is aware that objects continue to exist even though they cannot be seen. The toddler manipulates objects in new and various ways to learn what they will do. Activities are now linked to memories, ideas, and feelings about past events.

From 18 to 24 months, the child does less trial-and-error thinking, but uses memory and imitation to act as if he arrived at an answer. The toddler begins to solve problems, to foresee maneuvers that will succeed or fail, and to remember an object that is absent and search for it until it is found. The toddler can understand simple ideas, but thinking is basically related to observable events. He knows only one word for any object and cannot understand how the one word can refer to many objects. If the flower is called flower and plant, the child will not understand that more than one word can refer to the same object. Concept of time is now. Concept of distance is whatever can be seen.

From 2 to 4 years of age, the child gathers facts as they are encountered but cannot separate reality from fantasy or classify or define events in a logical manner. He is capable of perceiving gross outward appearances but sees only one aspect of an object or situation at a time. The child remains **egocentric** or self-centered, perceives ideas and situations from his own perspective only, but has gradually increasing ability to develop concepts. He defines one property at a time. The child goes from general to specific in explanation and understanding.*

Communication and Language Development

Learning to communicate in an understandable manner begins during the toddler era. Through speech the toddler will gradually learn to control unacceptable behavior, exchange physical activity for words, and share the view of reality held by society. Speech enables the child to become more independent and to better make needs known.

As the child and parents respond verbally and nonverbally to each other, the child learns attitudes and values, as well as behaviors and ideas. The normal child will begin to speak by 14 months, although some children may make little effort to speak until after 2 years. By age 3, he may still mispronounce more than half the sounds.[3,25]

The toddler speaks in the present tense. Single words represent entire sentences. By 18 to 20 months, he uses two- to four-word expressions that contain a noun and verb and maintain word order, such as "go play" and "go night-night." The toddler frequently says "no," perhaps

*References 14, 25, 28, 29, 32, 44.

in imitation of the parents and their discipline techniques, but may often do what is asked even while saying "no." Stuttering is common, because ideas come faster than the ability to speak.[14,25]

Effective ways of talking with the young child include the following[2,25,45]:

1. Try to maintain mutual respect as you talk with the child.
2. Do not discourage talking, questions, or the make-believe in the child's language: verbal explorations are essential to learn the language.
3. Tell the truth to the best of your ability and on the child's level of understanding; admit if the answer is unknown, and seek the answer with the child.
4. Do not make a promise unless you can keep it.
5. Talk about the child's feelings instead of only the event or only agreeing or disagreeing with what he says. Help the child understand what he feels rather than why he feels it.
6. Precede statements of advice and instruction with a statement of understanding the child's feelings; when the child is upset emotionally, he cannot listen to instructions.
7. Do not give undue attention to slang or curse words, and do not punish the child for using them. Attention or punishment emphasizes the importance of the words. Remain relaxed and give the child a more difficult or different word to say. Ask him not to say the word again, since it may hurt others; or use distraction.
8. Sit down if possible when talking with children.
9. Through attentive listening and interested facial expression, convey a tell-me-more-about-it attitude to encourage the child to communicate.
10. Regard some speech difficulties as normal; ignore stuttering that does not persist; often the child thinks faster than he can articulate.

Promoting Optimum Health

Immunizations. The child at 18 months should receive DTP and OPV boosters. From 18 to 24 months, *Haemophilus influenzae* type B immunization should be given.

Nutrition. The nurse is in a key position to teach parents about nutrition and feeding of the child. The daily diet of a toddler should include one serving of meat or fish, an egg or cheese, two or more servings of green and yellow vegetables, at least two servings of fruit, cereal, and bread to meet caloric needs, butter or margarine, and a maximum of 1 quart of milk, preferably low fat, to lower caloric and fat intake. Too much milk without adequate amounts of other foods is undesirable, because omission of meats and vegetable could lead to iron-deficiency anemia.[36,46] Average serving size for the child of 2 to 3 years is the following[31,46]:

Milk	6 oz (¾ glass)
Juice	3 to 4 oz (⅓ to ½ cup)
Meat	⅙ lb
Egg	1 medium size
Cereal	3 tbs cooked, ½ cup ready-to-eat
Bread	½ slice
Fruits and vegetables	½ cup of raw fruit, 1 to 2 tbs cooked

Food intake or its refusal is one way for the toddler to show increasing independence. Decreased food intake may result from (1) slower growth rate; (2) short attention span and distraction by other stimuli; and (3) increased interest in the surroundings. How well the toddler eats is determined to a great extent by how parents manage mealtime and parental behavior toward food. The well or ill toddler eats best when the following conditions are met: (1) food is served in small portions; (2) finger foods are served, or food is cut so that it can be eaten with the fingers; (3) toddler is allowed to choose—it is not necessary for the toddler to sample every food served; and (4) high-carbohydrate foods, such as soda, candy, cake, or similar snack foods, are not served.[25]

Sleep, rest, and exercise. Sleep and rest are essential. Rest periods should follow periods of exploration and exertion. The toddler needs an average of 10 to 12 hours of sleep nightly plus a daytime nap.

Play. The infant engages in play with self: with the hands or feet and by rolling, getting into various positions, and making sounds. Playful activity from the parent(s) and caretakers or the nurse is needed to stimulate development in all spheres. The toddler engages in solitary and later **parallel play,** playing alongside other children.[13,35] The toddler often cannot share toys with other children.

Purposes of play. The natural mode of expression for the child is play. Purposes of play include the following[14,25,30,43,45]:

- Develop and improve muscular strength, coordination, and balance
- Develop spatial and sensory perception
- Work off excess physical energy
- Communicate with others, establish friendships, and develop concern for others
- Learn cooperation and sharing
- Express imagination, creativity, and initiative
- Translate feelings, drives, and fantasies into action
- Imitate and learn about social activity and adult roles
- Test and deal with reality
- Explore, investigate, and manipulate features of the adult world
- Build self-esteem
- Feel a sense of power, make things happen, explore and experiment

- Provide for intellectual, sensory, and language development and deal with concrete experiences in symbolic terms
- Assemble novel aspects of the environment
- Learn about self and how others see him
- Practice leader and follower roles
- Have fun, express joy, and feel the pleasure of mastery
- Work through a painful physical or emotional state by repetition in play so that it is more bearable and assimilated into the child's self-concept

Injury prevention. Situations in the yard or the street have greater hazard because there is more contact with them. Normal developmental characteristics of the toddler increase the chance of accidents. The child moves quickly and is impulsive. The inquisitive, assertive behavior helps him enjoy learning by touch, taste, and sight, but the curiosity can lead to hazards. The toddler enjoys playing with small objects, which can be hazardous. He likes to attract attention, has a short attention span and unreliable memory, lacks judgment, has incomplete self-awareness, and imitates the actions of others.[1,14,25]

The toddler and preschooler need clear-cut safety rules, explained simply, repeatedly, and consistently. As the child learns to protect self, he should be allowed to take added responsibility for personal safety and should be given appropriate verbal recognition and praise that reinforces safe behavior.

The following safety suggestions are necessary for the young child[6,25,30,33,45]:

- When a behavior must be forbidden, use simple command words in a firm voice without anger to convey that the child is expected to obey; for example, "stop," "no."
- Never leave the child alone at home, in public, or in a car.
- Never allow play in or near a busy driveway or garage; forbid street play. Teach children to look carefully for and to get away from cars.
- Keep matches in containers and out of reach.
- Dispose of or store out of reach and in a locked cabinet as many poisons as possible: rat and roach killer, insecticides, weed killer, kerosene, cleaning agents, medicines. Bright-colored pills can be mistaken for candy.
- Observe the child closely while he plays near water; cover wells and cisterns; fence ponds or swimming pools.
- Keep stairways and nighttime play areas well lit.
- Equip upstairs windows with sturdy screens and guards; have hand rails for stairways.
- Store knives, saws, and other sharp objects or power tools out of reach.
- Remove doors from abandoned appliances or cars, and campaign for legislation for appropriate disposal of these, as well as mandatory door removal.
- Discourage playing with or in the area of appliances or power tools while they are in operation: a washing machine with a wringer, a lawn mower, a saw, or a clothes dryer.
- Use safety glass in glass doors or shower stalls; place decals on sliding doors at child's eye level (and adult's eye level, too) to prevent walking or running through them.
- Use adhesive strips in the bathtub.
- Avoid scatter rugs, debris, or toys cluttered on the floor in the areas of traffic or slippery, waxed floors.
- In the car use seatbelts that are appropriate for the weight of the child.
- Begin safety teaching early; teaching done in the toddler years, for example, pays off later.
  - —Phrase safety rules and their reasons in positive rather than negative terms when possible.
  - —Teach the child his full name, address (including zip code), and telephone number, and teach the child how to use the police or adults in service roles for help.
  - —Teach the child not to give information over the phone about self or family.
  - —Teach the child to share any "secrets," and emphasize that he should not be afraid to say anything to the family.
  - —Teach the child not to leave home alone or with a stranger; he should use a "buddy" system when going somewhere.
  - —Teach the child escape techniques, for example, how to unlock home doors or car doors.
  - —Teach the child how to safely cross the street.
  - —Teach the child to refuse gifts or rides from strangers, to avoid walking or playing alone on a deserted street, road, or similar area, and to be aware of the possibility of child molesters or abductors.

Developmental tasks. By the end of the toddler period, the child should have achieved the following developmental tasks[10]:

1. Settled into a daily routine
2. Mastered eating habits
3. Mastered the basics of toilet training
4. Developed physical skills appropriate to the stage of motor development
5. Achieved feeling like a family member
6. Learned to communicate more effectively

THE PRESCHOOLER

Physical Development

General measurements. Growth during the **preschool** years is stable and relatively slow, but changes occur that transform the chubby toddler into a sturdy child who appears taller and thinner. Trunk and limb growth is apparent. Although development does not proceed at a uniform rate in all areas or for all children, development follows a logical, precise pattern or sequence.[13,30] The preschool child grows about 2 to 2½ inches (5 to 6 cm) and gains less than 5 pounds (2.2 kg) per year. The child appears tall and thin because he grows proportionately more in height than in weight. The average height of the 3-year-old is 37 inches (94 cm). The 4-year-old is 41 inches (104 cm), or double the birth length. The 5-year-old is 43 to 52 inches (110 to 130 cm). At age 3, the child weighs about 33 pounds (15 kg); at 4 years, 38 pounds (17 kg); and at 5 years, about 40 to 50 pounds (18 to 23 kg).[14,25,30]

Vital signs. Temperature is 98° to 99° F (36.7° to

Table 8-8 Physical Characteristics and Muscle Control

Three Years	Four Years	Five Years
Occasional accident in toileting when busy at play; responds to routine times; tells when going to bathroom; needs help with back buttons and drying self; night control of bowel and bladder most of time	Independent toilet habits; manages clothes without difficulty; insists on having door shut for self but wants to be in bathroom with others; asks many questions about elimination	Takes complete charge of self; self-conscious about exposing self; voids 4 to 6 times during waking hours; occasional nighttime accident
Runs more smoothly; turns sharp corners; suddenly stops	Runs with coordination; skips clumsily; hops on one leg; legs, trunk, shoulder, arms move in unison; aggressive physical activity	Runs with skill, speed, and agility and plays games simultaneously; increases strength and coordination in limbs
Walks backward; climbs stairs with alternate feet; jumps from low step	Heel-toe walk; walks a plank; climbs stairs without holding onto rail; climbs and jumps without difficulty	May still be knock-kneed; jumps from 3 or 4 steps
Tries to dance but inadequate balance	Enjoys motor stunts and gross gesturing	Balances self on toes; dances with some rhythm; balances on one foot about 10 seconds
Pedals tricycle; swings	Enjoys new activities rather than repeating same ones	Jumps rope; roller skates; hops and skips on alternate feet; enjoys jungle-bar gym
Undresses self; helps dress self; undoes buttons on side or front of clothing; washes hands; feeds self; may brush own teeth	Dresses and undresses self except tying bows, closing zipper, putting on boots and snow suit; does buttons; distinguishes front; brushes teeth alone	Dresses self without assistance; ties shoelaces; requires less supervision of personal duties; washes self without wetting clothes
Catches ball with arms fully extended 1 of 2 or 3 times; increasing coordination in vertical direction; pours fluid from pitcher, occasional spills; hits large pegs on board with hammer	Greater flexion of elbow; catches ball thrown at 5 feet 2 of 3 times; throws ball overhand; judges where a ball will land; helps dust objects; likes water play	Uses hands more than arms in catching ball; pours fluid from one container to another with few spills; uses hammer to hit nail on head; interest and competence in dusting; likes water play
Builds tower of 9 or 10 blocks; builds 3-block gate from model; imitates a bridge	Builds complicated structure extending vertically and laterally; builds 5-block gate from model; notices missing parts or broken objects; requests parents to fix	Builds things out of large boxes; builds complicated 3-dimensional structure and may build several separate units; able to disassemble and reassemble small object
Copies circle or cross; begins to use scissors; strings large beads; shows hand preference	Copies a square; uses scissors without difficulty; enjoys finer manipulation of play materials	Copies triangle or diamond from model; folds paper diagonally; definite hand preference
Trial-and-error method with puzzle	Surveys puzzle before placing pieces; matches simple geometric forms	Does simple puzzles quickly and smoothly
Scribbles; tries to draw a picture and name it	Less scribbling; form and meaning in drawing apparent to adults	Prints some letters correctly; prints first name; draws clearly recognized lifelike representatives; differentiates parts of drawing

Modified from Murray R and Zentner J: Nursing assessment and health promotion strategies through the life span, ed 4, East Norwalk, Conn, 1989, Appleton & Lange.

37.2° C). Pulse rate is normally 80 to 110. Respiratory rate averages 30 per minute. Blood pressure is about 90/60 mm Hg, systolic and diastolic.[39]

Other characteristics. Vision in the preschooler is farsighted; the 5-year-old has 20/40 to 20/30 vision. By the end of the preschool period, the child is beginning to lose deciduous teeth.[30,44]

Physical characteristics for the 3-, 4-, and 5-year-old are listed in Table 8-8.* Each child is unique; the normative listings indicate only where most children of a given age are in their development.

Emotional Development

The preschooler displays beginning motor self-control, high energy level, greater use of language, some ability to delay immediate gratification, ability to tolerate separation from mother, curiosity, strong imagination, and a desire to move. The child likes to plan, start tasks, learn, direct behavior with some thought, and appear self-confident and relaxed. Tolerance of frustration is still limited, but flares of temper and frustrations pass quickly. The child is learning to handle independence and dependence, so he is increasing mastery of self and others, learning to get along with more people—children and adults. The preschooler attempts to behave like an adult in realistic activity and play and is developing a conscience and beginning to learn rules and social roles, moral responsibility, and cooperation, although he still grabs, hits, and quarrels for short bursts of time.[25] The preschool child should learn a sense of **initiative** rather than guilt, and all the aforementioned behaviors are part of achieving initiative.[11] Initiative is enjoyment of energy displayed in action, assertiveness, learning, increasing dependability, and ability to plan.

If the child does not achieve initiative, there is an overriding sense of **guilt** from the tension between the demands of the superego, or others' expectations, and actual performance.[15] Guilt is a sense of defeatism, anger, feeling responsible for things for which he is not really responsible, feeling easily frightened from what he wants to do, and feeling bad, shameful, and deserving of punishment. A sense of guilt can develop from sibling rivalry, lack of opportunity to try things, restriction on or lack of guidance in response to fantasy, or interference by parents with the child's activity. Parents stifle initiative by doing for the child or by frequently asking, "Why didn't you do it better?" If the guilt feelings are too strong, the child is anxious and easily frightened, he cannot organize activity and cannot do what he is neuromuscularly, mentally, and socially ready to do. At the same time, he feels resentment and bitterness toward the restrictive adult. Excessive guilt and lack of initiative development may be shown in a variety of behaviors: poor motor coordination; stammering speech; fears; nightmares; eating and elimination problems; irritability; regressed behavior; inability to separate from mother without panic; fear of strangers; temper tantrums; or lack of interest in peers or childhood activities.[2,25]

Cognitive/Intellectual Development

Table 8-9 summarizes cognitive development in the preschool child.*

Promoting Optimum Health

Immunizations. A tine test should be taken at 3 years of age. At age 4, the child should receive a DTP booster and an OPV.

Nutrition. The preschooler needs the same four basic food groups as the adult daily, but in smaller quantities. The slower growth rate and heightened interest in exploring the environment may lessen interest in eating. The preschool child needs 1 to 1½ pints (2 to 3 glasses) of milk servings per day, 4 or more servings of vegetables and fruits, 2 servings of 1½ or 2 ounces of meat or meat substitutes, and 4 servings of bread and cereals. A rule of thumb for the size of servings is 1 tablespoon for each year of age: 3 tablespoons of fruit or vegetables for a 3-year-old; as much as 5 tablespoons for a 5-year-old.[33,41]

Midmorning, midafternoon, and evening snacks are necessary because of the child's high activity level, but should be wisely chosen: milk, juice, fruit wedges, vegetable strips, cereal without sugar, cheese cubes, peanut butter with crackers or bread, or plain cookies. Sweets (candy, raisins, sodas) should be offered only occasionally, not as a reward for behavior and not before a meal.[25]

There may be periods of overeating or not wanting to eat certain foods, but these do not persist. The sense of taste is keen; color, flavor, form, and texture are important. Foods should be attractively served and preferably lukewarm rather than too hot or too cold, including drinks. The preschooler likes to eat one thing at a time. Vegetables and fruits should be cut into bite-sized pieces. Meats should be easily chewed and cut into bite-sized pieces. New foods can be gradually introduced; if a food is refused once, offer it again after several days.[14,31]

Sleep and rest. The 3-year-old needs 10 to 12 hours of sleep at night; at naptime he may sleep or rest and play quietly for 1 or 2 hours. The 4-year-old resists naps but needs a quiet period. The 5-year-old is unlikely to nap if he gets adequate sleep (9 to 11 hours) at night.[14,30]

The preschooler may take a favorite toy to bed. He

*References 13, 14, 25, 30, 40, 45.

*References 14, 25, 28, 29, 32, 44.

Table 8-9 Mental Development in the Preschool Child

Three Years	Four Years	Five Years
Knows he is a person separate from another; knows own sex and some sex differences	Senses self one among many	Aware of differences between people and the two sexes; can tell full name and address; remains calm if lost away from home
Resists commands but distractible and responsive to suggestions; can ask for help; desire to please; friendly; sense of humor	States alibis because more aware of attitude and opinions of others; self-critical; does not like to admit inabilities; praises self; bosses or criticizes others; likes recognition for achievement, heeds others' thoughts and feelings; expresses own	Dependable; increasing independence; can direct own behavior, but fatigue, excessive demands, fantasy, and guilt interfere with assuming self-responsibility; admits when needs help; moves from direct to internalized action; uses clues
Uses language rather than physical activity to communicate	Active use of language; likes to make rhymes, to hear stories with exaggeration and humor, and dramatic songs; knows nursery rhymes; tells action implied in picture books	Improves use of symbol system, concept formation; repeats long sentences accurately; carries plot in story; defines objects in terms of use; states relationship between two events
Imaginative; egocentric; better able to organize thoughts; can be bargained with; sacrifices immediate pleasure for promise of future gain	Highly imaginative yet literal, concrete thinking; fantasy age; increasing reasoning power and critical thinking capacity; makes crude comparisons	More realistic; asks details; can be reasoned with logically; more accurate, relevant, practical, sensible than 4-year-old; asks to have words defined
Understands simple directions	Concept of 1, 2, 3; counts to 5; generalizes ideas	Begins to understand money; can determine which of two weights heavier; idea in head precedes drawing on paper or physical activity; interested in meaning of relatives/family
Knows age; meager comprehension of past and future; knows mostly today	Conception of time; knows when next birthday is; birthday and holidays significant because aware of units of time; loves parties related to holiday; knows day of week	Understands week as a unit of time; knows day of week; knows month and year; sense of time and duration increasing; knows how old will be on next birthday; memory surprisingly accurate
Has attention span of 10 to 15 minutes	Has attention span of 20 minutes	Has attention span of 30 minutes

Modified from Murray R and Zentner J: Nursing assessment and health promotion strategies through the life span, ed 4, East Norwalk, Conn, 1989, Appleton & Lange.

likes to postpone bedtime in an effort to remain with others and activities, and is ritualistic about bedtime routines. Dreams and nightmares may awaken the 3- or 4-year-old, causing fear and a move into bed with parents or older siblings. The 5-year-old sleeps quietly through the night without getting up to urinate, and has fewer nightmares.[35]

Exercise and play. The preschool child is capable of cooperative play with other children. Purposes of play are described on pp. 97 and 98.

Injury prevention. Safety rules described on p. 98 apply to the preschooler.

Guidance and discipline. Guidance and discipline help the child learn to understand and care for self and to get along with others. It is not just punishing, correcting, or controlling behavior.[2] In moving away from complete dependency, the child demonstrates energy and drive and requires sufficient restrictions to ensure physical and psychological protection and, at the same time, enough freedom to permit exploration and autonomy. Because mother must now set limits, a new dimension is added to the relationship established between mother or the nurse or other caregivers, and the young child. Before, mother met basic needs immediately. Now with the child's increasing ability, freedom, and demands, the parent sometimes makes him wait or denies a wish if it will cause him harm. The transition should be made in a loving and consistent, yet flexible, manner so that the child maintains trust and moves in the quest for independence. Excessive limitations might cause an overly rebellious or passive child. Complete lack of limitations can cause accidents, poor health, and insecurity. Through guidance and the parent's reaction, the child is being socialized, learning what is right and wrong. The child cannot adequately reason and must depend on and trust the parents as a guide for all activities. The child can obey simple commands, learn rules, and become self-disciplined as a result of having been patiently disciplined.[2,25] Some rules of discipline are listed in Box 8-3.[2,25,30,40,45]

The communication techniques for guidance and limit setting that are useful in caring for young children are listed below[2,25,30,40,45]:

- Convey authority without anger or threat to avoid feelings of resentment, fear, or guilt.
- Be positive, clear, and consistent; let the child know what is acceptable behavior.
- Recognize the child's wish, and put it into words: "You wish you could have that, but . . ."; point out ways the wish can be partially fulfilled when possible.
- Help the child express some resentment likely to arise when restrictions are imposed: "I realize you don't like the rules, but . . . ."
- State limits clearly, concisely, simply, positively, and in a calm voice. For example, if the child cannot touch a certain object, say, "Look with your hands behind your back" or "Look with your eyes, not your hands," rather than, "Don't touch."
- Positive suggestions rather than commands and "don'ts" help the child to learn how to get what is wanted and also form happy relationships with others.
- If the child has no choice about a situation, give direction that conveys what he must do, for example, "It is time now to . . . ."
- Convey that adults are present to help the child solve problems that cannot be solved alone.
- Control the situation if the child has temporarily lost self-control: remove him from the stimulating event; stay with the child; talk quietly; use distraction if necessary; encourage thinking through the problem and finding a fair solution after he becomes calm; convey that you feel the child can regain self-control.

Developmental tasks. Development tasks for the toddler and preschooler may be summarized as follows[10]:

- Settle into a healthful daily routine of adequate food, exercise, and rest.
- Master basic physical skills of large- and small-muscle coordination and movement.
- Become a participating member in the family; identify with the same-sex parent.
- Conform to others' expectations; develop a conscience.
- Express emotions healthfully and for a wide variety of experiences.
- Learn to communicate effectively with an increasing number of peers and adults.
- Learn to use initiative tempered by a conscience and realistic guilt.
- Develop ability to handle potentially dangerous situations.
- Develop basic concepts for increasing depth of understanding about the meaning of life, self, the world, and ethical, religious, and philosophical ideas.

REFERENCES AND SUGGESTED READINGS

1. Allen DW: Health maintenance procedures in family practice: a critical appraisal, Fam Med Rev 1(3):50, 53, 1982.
2. Bettelheim B: A good enough parent: a book on child-rearing, New York, 1987, Alfred A Knopf, Inc.
3. Bishop B: A guide to assessing parenting capabilities, Am J Nurs 76(11):1784, 1976.
4. Bowen S and Miller B: Paternal Attachment behavior as related to presence at delivery and preparenthood classes: a pilot study, Nurs Res 29(5):307, 1980.
5. Bowlby J: Attachment and loss, vol I, Attachment, New York, 1969, Basic Books, Inc, Publishers.
6. Budnick L and Ross D: Bathtub drownings in the United States, 1979-81, Am J Public Health 75(6):630, 1985.
7. Carruth B: Modifying behavior through social learning, Am J Nurs 76(11):1804, 1976.
8. Clark AL: Recognizing discord between mother and child and changing it to harmony, Matern Child Nurs J 1(2):100, 1976.
9. Doster S and others: Measles and rubella: our remaining responsibilities, Am J Nurs 83(5):490, 1983.
10. Duvall E and Miller B: Marriage and family development, ed 6, New York, 1984, Harper & Row, Publishers, Inc.
11. Erikson E: Childhood and society, ed 2, New York, 1963, WW Norton & Co, Inc.
12. General recommendations on immunizations, Morbidity and Mortality Weekly Report, 32, no 1, Atlanta, 1983, US Department of Health and Human Services, Public Health Service Center for Disease Control.
13. Gesell A and Ilg F: The child from five to ten, New York, 1946, Harper & Brothers.
14. Gesell A and others: The first five years of life, New York, 1940, Harper & Brothers.
15. Greenburg M and Morris N: Engrossment: the newborn's impact upon the father, Am J Orthopsychiatry 44:520, 1974.
16. Hartwick N: Infant formula: a threat to third-world babies, Graduate Woman 75(6):26, 1981.
17. Klaus M and Kennell J: Parent-infant bonding, ed 2, St Louis, 1982, The CV Mosby Co.
18. Kramer M and others: Extra tactile stimulation of the premature infant, Nurs Res 24(5):324, 1975.
19. Krantz L: Comparison of body proportions of one-year-old Mexican American and Anglo children, Am J Public Health 71(3):280, 1981.
20. Lactation and composition of milk in undernourished women, Nutr Rev 33(2):42, 1975.
21. Lamb M: The father's role, New York, 1986, John Wiley & Sons, Inc.
22. Ludington-Hoe S: What can newborns really see? Am J Nurs 83(9):1286, 1983.
23. McDonald B: Heeding the baby's cry, Washington University School of Medicine Outlook 24(1):17, 1987.
24. Montagu A: Touching: the human significance of the skin, New York, 1971, Columbia University Press.
25. Murray R and Zentner J: Nursing assessment and health promotion strategies through the life span, ed 4, East Norwalk, Conn, 1989, Appleton & Lange.
26. Out of the mouths of babes, Newsweek, p 84, Dec 15, 1986.
27. Owens M: A crying need, Am J Nurs 86(1):73, 1986.
28. Piaget J: The origins of intelligence in children, New York, 1952, International Universities Press, Inc.
29. Piaget J: The construction of reality in the child, New York, 1954, Basic Books, Inc, Publishers (Translated by M Cook).
30. Pillitteri A: Child health nursing: care of the growing family, ed 4, Boston, 1982, Little, Brown, & Co, Inc.
31. Pipes P: Nutrition in infancy and childhood, ed 4, St. Louis, 1989, The CV Mosby Co.
32. Pontious S: Practical Piaget: helping children understand, Am J Nurs 82(1):114, 1982.
33. Richi F and Krzy R: The child in the car: what every nurse should know about safety, Am J Nurs 83(10):1421, 1983.
34. Rubin R: Attainment of the maternal role. I. Nurs Res 16(3):237, 1967.
35. Rubin R: Attainment of the maternal role. II. Nurs Res 16(4):342, 1967.
36. Rubin R: Binding-in in the postpartum period, Matern Child Nurs J 6:67, 1977.
37. Salk L: The role of the hearbeat in the relations between mother and infant, Sci Am 228:24, 1973.
38. Schuster CS and Ashburn SS: The process of human development: a holistic life-span approach, ed 2, Boston, 1986, Little, Brown & Co.
39. Scipien GM and others: Comprehensive pediatric nursing, ed 3, New York, 1986, McGraw-Hill, Inc.
40. Turner J and Helms D: Lifespan development, ed 3, New York, 1987, Holt, Rinehart & Winston, Inc.
41. US Department of Health and Human Services: New recommended schedule for active immunization of normal infants and children, Morbidity and Mortality Weekly Report 35(37):577, 1986.
42. Vaccinating children against *H. influenzae,* Am J Nurs 85(6):642, 1985.
43. Verzemnieks I: Developmental stimulation for infants and toddlers, Am J Nurs 84(6):749, 1984.
44. Wadsworth B: Piaget's theory of cognitive and affective development, ed 4, New York, 1989, Longman, Inc.
45. Whaley L and Wong D: Nursing care of infants and children, ed 4, St Louis, 1991, The CV Mosby Co.
46. Williams S: Nutritional and diet therapy, ed 6, St Louis, 1989, The CV Mosby Co.

CHAPTER CHALLENGE

KEY POINTS

- Establishing attachment is crucial to the long-term nurturing of the child and parental interest in the child.
- The child who is separated from the parent for a time goes through three phases of grief and mourning: protest, despair, and denial.
- The child's dominant reaction pattern to new situations manifests an innate temperament, and the temperament affects the reactions of the parents, just as the parents' responses affect the child.
- Teaching sexuality to the child is a part of the acquisition of gender identity and positive feelings about self.
- It is important for parents to prepare the young child for arrival of a baby sibling.
- The nurse can assist the parent and young child in understanding effects of sibling rivalry.
- The neonatal period includes the critical transition from fetal existence to basic physiological independence.
- Physical and motor abilities are heavily influenced by genetic, biological, and environmental factors.
- Emotional, cognitive, physical, and motor development greatly influence each other.
- According to Erikson, the infant should develop a sense of trust instead of mistrust.
- The nurse is responsible for giving safe care and can teach parents and others about safety measures for the child.
- According to Erikson, the toddler should develop autonomy and a positive self-concept instead of shame and doubt.
- The preschooler attempts to behave like an adult in realistic activity and play.
- The natural mode of expression for the child is play.
- Toddler and preschooler need clear-cut safety rules, explained simply, repeatedly, and consistently.
- According to Erikson, the preschooler should develop a sense of initiative rather than overwhelming or unrealistic guilt.

STUDY QUESTIONS

1. Factors that interfere with mothering behaviors include all of the following except:
   a. The mother's immaturity or lack of mothering
   b. Personalized care of mother and infant by nurses and physicians
   c. Financial worries
   d. Lack of a supportive partner
   e. The gender and appearance of the child
2. The nurse will encounter separation anxiety at what ages in the hospitalized child:
   a. 7 to 8 months, 18 to 24 months
   b. 3 to 6 months, 12 to 16 months
   c. Birth to 3 months, 6 to 12 months
   d. 2½ to 3 years, 3 to 5 years
3. The child who is separated from the parent for a time, as with hospitalization, goes through three phases of grief and mourning; these are:
   a. Anger, grief, revenge
   b. Regression, hostility, rejection
   c. Protest, despair, and denial
4. The basis for a healthy sexual attitude exists if all of the following occur *except:*
   a. Parent/child communication has been open
   b. The child feels free to ask questions about sex
   c. The parent gives satisfactory and correct answers without embarrassment
   d. The parent redirects the child's questions to a more knowledgeable resource
5. The evaulation of an infant's physical condition, usually performed at 1 minute and again 5 minutes after birth, based on heart rate, respirations, muscle tone, reflex irritability, and colors, is called:
   a. Enterobacteriaceae
   b. Apgar score
   c. Apex cardiogram
   d. Enisyl score

STUDY QUESTIONS (cont'd)

6. The average birth weight of Caucasian male infants in the United States is:
   a. 7½ pounds
   b. 7 pounds
   c. 6½ pounds
   d. 8 pounds
7. Heart rate ranges at birth from:
   a. 80 to 90 beats per minute
   b. 70 to 96 beats per minute
   c. 100 to 160 beats per minute
   d. 100 to 110 beats per minute
8. A yellow discoloration that appears about the third or fourth day of life as a result of hemolysis of an excessive number of red blood cells is called:
   a. Physiological jaundice
   b. Direct bilirubin elevation
   c. Mongolian spots
   d. Acrocyanosis
9. According to Erikson, the infant should develop:
   a. Initiative
   b. Industry
   c. Autonomy
   d. Basic trust
10. The first nourishment from breast-feeding the baby receives after delivery is:
    a. True milk
    b. Colostrum
11. Immunization in the infant at age 2 months should include:
    a. Haemophilic influenza type B and OPV (live polio virus)
    b. MMR (rubeola or long measles, mumps, rubella)
    c. DTP, OPV
    d. OPV
12. The child should be able to walk alone at what age:
    a. 17 to 20 months
    b. 20 to 24 months
    c. 12 to 15 months
    d. 16 to 24 months
13. According to Erikson, the toddler should develop:
    a. Autonomy
    b. Basic trust
    c. Initiative
    d. Industry
14. Decreased food intake for the toddler may result from:
    a. Slower growth rate
    b. Longer attention span and distractibility by other stimuli
    c. Decreased interest in surroundings
    d. Rapid growth rate
15. Which is a less complex task and should be attempted first with the toddler:
    a. Bowel training
    b. Bladder training
16. Growth during the preschool years is relatively:
    a. Fast
    b. Slow
17. According to Erikson, the preschooler should develop:
    a. Basic trust
    b. Initiative
    c. Autonomy
    d. Industry
18. For the most effective means of guidance and discipline for a young child, it is best to have:
    a. Excessive limitations to protect from injury
    b. A loving, consistent, yet flexible, manner
    c. Complete dependency until school age

9

The School-Age Child

RUTH BECKMANN MURRAY

LEARNING OBJECTIVES

After reading this chapter, the student should be able to do the following:

- Define the key terms.
- Describe major aspects of the family relationships of the school-age child.
- List family developmental tasks.
- Compare the physical changes, including nutrition, rest, exercise, safety, and health protection, for the school-age child at different ages.
- Compare cognitive, communication, play, emotional, and sexuality development in children during the school years and preadolescence.
- Discuss school entry and ways children adapt to the experience of formal education.
- Discuss the significance of peers and the chum relationship to the psychosocial development of the child.
- Explore guidance of the child to foster health development in all spheres of personality.
- Analyze the influences of media on behavior.
- State the developmental tasks of the school-age child.

RELATED TOPICS OF INTEREST

- The family (Chapter 7)
- Basic nutrition (Chapter 22)
- Basic pediatric nursing care (Chapter 46)
- Care of children with physical and emotional problems (Chapter 47)

KEY TERMS

Define the following:

- animistic
- chum
- classification
- cognitive
- concrete operations
- conservation
- decentering
- gang
- industry
- inferiority
- menarche
- nesting
- preadolescence (prepubescence)
- reversibility
- school age
- seriation
- sex eduation
- sexuality education
- syntaxic mode of experience (consensual validation)
- transformation

FAMILY DEVELOPMENT AND RELATIONSHIPS

Relationships with Parents

Parents continue to be a vital part of the **school-age** child's life. The child channels energy into intellectual pursuits, widens social horizons, and becomes familiar with the adult world. He or she has identified with the parent of the same sex, and through imitation continues to learn a social role.[18]

Parental support is needed: school-age children pull away from overt signs of parental or adult affection—yet during illness, they turn to parents for affection and protection. Parents get frustrated with behavioral changes, antics, and infractions of household rules.[18]

The child needs to be given time—physically, emotionally, mentally, and socially—to be a child, and to learn about the community and world at an individual pace. Too often parents want to hurry the child into adulthood. Television, films, advertisements, peers, and neighbors all exert pressure to be adultlike, to have fewer limits and less guidance. Parents sometimes feel their child must be the early maturer. The pressures and hurry, especially in middle and upper class suburban families, are contributing to a growing number of troubled children who are emotionally distressed or antisocial in behavior.[8,14,16,18]

Relationships with Siblings

Although parental influence is of primary importance, the child's relationship with siblings affects personality formation.

School-age children need privacy and personal space. Quarrels and conflicts erupt when this need is violated. The older child may be jealous of the attention given to younger siblings and may resent having to help with their care. The younger school-age child may feel jealous of the freedom given to older siblings. School-age children may feel the need to compete for parental attention and academic excellence. Yet siblings feel protection and affection for each other.[18,30,34]

Family Developmental Tasks

Family activities with the school-age child revolve around expanding the child's world. Family development tasks include the following[7]:

1. Continue parenting roles.
2. Adjust the marital system and the life-style to allow physical, emotional, and social care of the child(ren).
3. Keep lines of communication open among family members.
4. Work together to achieve common goals.

5. Plan a life-style within economic means.
6. Find creative ways to continue a mutually satisfactory married life, or satisfactory single parenthood.
7. Maintain close ties with relatives.
8. Expand family life into the community through various activities.
9. Validate the family philosophy of life when the child brings home new ideas and talks about different life-styles.

Relationships Outside the Family

With entry into school, the child's position within the family is altered. The child's social environment widens. The influence of the family and the time spent with the family decrease. Although parents continue to be role models, teachers and other adults such as nurses also begin to function as adult models and to influence the child.[44] The child learns new ideas, attitudes, perspectives, and modes of behavior that may conflict with those of the family. Parents may feel a loss of control and may actually experience ambivalent feelings toward teachers as well as toward their child's peers. The child may demonstrate less love and respect for parents and may resent limits imposed by the family. Through contacts with the peer group, children learn that parents can make mistakes, and they acquire a basis for judging parents and other adults as individuals.[27,28,44] Box 9-1 gives guidelines for parental support during the school years.

BOX 9-1 WAYS IN WHICH PARENTS CAN HELP CHILDREN IN SCHOOL

GENERAL GUIDELINES

Be supportive—through companionship share ideas and thoughts

Be positive—every child should experience some success each day

Share an interest in reading—use the library, discuss books they are reading

Support and encourage activity rather than passivity

Encourage originality—help children make their own projects from discarded articles or other available materials

Foster the development of hobbies and collections

Encourage children to wonder and reflect during free time

Encourage family experiences and trips to places of interest

Encourage questions—help children discover sources for information or places in which to explore and investigate

Stimulate creative thinking and problem solving—help children try out new solutions to problems without fear of making mistakes

Use rewards rather than punishment

SPECIFIC GUIDELINES

Meet the teacher at the beginning of school and plan to visit the school to see what is taught and expected

Send the child to school every day—teachers are concerned when parents make other plans for their children; it conveys the impression that school is unimportant

Demonstrate an interest in what the child is learning

Demonstrate an interest in content and growth more than in grades

Set goals that the child can achieve

Take advantage of situations that support and reinforce school learning

Share information with teachers that will help them understand the child better

Communicate with the teacher if there appears to be a problem—avoid waiting for a scheduled conference

Provide a quiet, well-lighted area for study that is safe from interruption; do not allow television, radio

Enforce regular study time—some children can do their work at a single session; others do best in 20- to 30-minute sessions with breaks between study times

Support the child in home study; offer guidance for finding answers but do not give the answers; before providing explanations, determine what the child understands about the problem, read the material aloud, and discuss it briefly with the child

Teach the child to break large tasks (such as a report) into smaller manageable tasks spread over the allotted time rather than attempt the entire project the night before it is to be completed

PHYSICAL DEVELOPMENT

General measurements. Children between 6 and 12 years old exhibit considerable change in physical appearance. The growth rate is usually slow and steady, characterized by periods of somewhat faster growth in the spring and fall and by rapid growth during preadolescence.[18,24,34,39]

Weight, height, and girth. Measurements vary among children and depend on genetic, environmental, and cultural influences. For example, African-American children and Caucasian children from lower socioeconomic groups tend to be smaller in weight and height at this age.[6,29] There is a large proportion of relatively short but heavy children among Mexican-Americans.[15]

The average school-age child grows 2 to 2½ inches (5 to 6 cm) per year to gain 1 to 2 feet (30 to 60 cm) in height by age 12. A weight gain of 4 to 7 pounds (2 to 3.5 kg) occurs per year. The average weight for a 6-year-old boy is 48 pounds (21.5 kg); the average height is 46 inches (117 cm). By age 12 the average child weighs approximately 88 pounds (40 kg) and is over 59 inches tall (150 cm). In early school age, girls and boys may differ little in size. Their bodies are usually lean, with narrow hips and shoulders. There is a gradual decrease in the amount of baby fat, with an increase in muscle mass and strength. Males usually have more muscle cells, whereas females have more adipose tissue. The muscles are changing in composition and becoming more firmly attached to the bones. Muscles may be immature in regard to function, causing the child to be prone to injury stemming from overuse, awkwardness, and inefficient movement. As the skeletal bones lengthen, they become harder. Formation of bone continues at a steady pace. The schoolchild loses the pot-bellied, sway-back appearance of early childhood; abdominal muscles become stronger; the pelvis tips backward; posture becomes straighter.[18,30,33,39]

Head. The growth of the head is nearly complete; head size measures about 21 inches (53 cm) in circumference by age 12. Children lose the childish look as their faces take on features that will characterize them as an adult. Girls lose teeth earlier than boys; deciduous or baby teeth are lost and replaced at the rate of four teeth per year until about the age of 11 or 12. Evaluation for braces should not be complete until all four 6-year molars have appeared. The second permanent molars erupt by age 14. The third molars (wisdom teeth) come in as late as age 30, or may never erupt.[18,24,30,34]

Vital signs. Temperature, pulse, and respiration gradually approach adult norms. The average temperature is 98° to 98.6° F (36.7° to 37° C). Pulse rate is 70 to 80 per minute; resting pulse rate is 60 to 76 per minute. Respiratory rate is 18 to 21 per minute. The average systolic blood pressure is 94 to 112, and average diastolic blood pressure is 56 to 60 millimeters of mercury. The ribs shift from a horizontal to a more oblique position; the chest broadens and flattens to allow for increased lung size and capacity.[18,30,34]

Development of Body Systems

Cardiovascular. The heart grows slowly during this age period; the left ventricle of the heart enlarges. After 7 years of age, the apex of the heart lies at the interspace of the fifth rib at the midclavicle line. Before this age, the apex can be palpated at the fourth interspace just to the left of the midclavicle line. Because the heart is smaller proportionately to body size, the child may tire easily. The school-age child should not be pushed to run, jog, or engage in excessively vigorous sports such as football, hockey, or racquetball.[18,24,30,34]

Sensory. The normal farsightedness of the preschool child is converted to 20/20 vision by age 8. Binocular and peripheral vision is well developed in most children by 6 years of age. Girls tend to have poorer visual acuity than boys, but their color discrimination is superior. Large print is recommended for reading matter.[18,34]

Neuromuscular. By age 7 the child's brain has reached 90% of adult size. By age 12 the brain has virtually reached adult size. Myelinization is complete. Memory improves. The child can more astutely listen and make associations. Neuromuscular coordination is sufficient to permit the schoolchild to learn most skills he or she wishes.[34] The transformation of the clumsy 6-year-old into the coordinated 12-year-old results in part from maturation of the central nervous system. Table 9-1 summarizes neuromuscular development.[10,11,17,34,39]

Other systems. Lymphoid tissues reach the peak of development by age 7, exceeding the amount found in adults. Enlargement of adenoidal and tonsillar lymphoid tissue is normal. Sore throats, upper respiratory infections, and ear infections are caused by the excessive tissue growth and increased vulnerability of the mucous membranes to congestion and inflammation. Frontal sinuses are developed by about age 6; thereafter, all sinuses are potential sites for infection.[18,24,34] Secretion, digestion, absorption, and excretion of the digestive system and urinary function become more efficient and similar to the adult. Maturity of the gastrointestinal system is reflected in fewer stomach upsets, better maintenance of blood sugar levels, and an increased stomach capacity.[18,34]

Prepubertal Sexual Development

During the **preadolescent** or **prepuberty** period, both males and females begin development of sexual maturity. This period is characterized by a physical growth spurt, changes in body proportion, the beginning of secondary sex characteristics, and increased self-consciousness and

Table 9-1 Neuromuscular Development of the School-Age Child

Age (Years)	Motor Skill
6	Hops, runs, rollerskates, walks chalk mark with balance; hammers nail, fastens clothing, ties shoes; awkward grasp of pencil or crayon. Makes large letters or figures. Movement is constant.
7	Lower activity level. Enjoys active and quiet games. Sees small print without difficulty; reverses letters less frequently. Able to print.
8	Energetic but graceful and balanced. Increased myelination improves reaction time and coordination; better small muscle coordination. Longer arms permit more skillful throwing.
9	Less restless. Refined eye-hand coordination; uses both hands independently. Works to perfect physical skills, coordination, strength, and endurance.
10-12	Energetic, active; movements are restless. Skillful manipulative movements nearly equal to those of adults. Physical changes of prepuberty appear. Girls undergo growth spurt: average of 3 inches (7.5 cm) yearly until **menarche.**

modesty. There is an increase in fat deposition approximately 1 year before the height spurt. These fat deposits last approximately 2 years or until skeletal growth and muscle mass increase. Females have more subcutaneous fat deposits; fat is lost at a slower rate, accounting for the fuller appearance of the female figure. For both males and females, the growth spurt begins in the hands and feet and progresses to the calves, forearms, hips, chest, and shoulders; the trunk is the last to grow appreciably.[24,30,34,39] The nurse may be asked questions about these physical changes and the associated emotional and social effects.

As sebaceous glands of the face, back, and chest become active, acne (pimples) may develop. These blemishes are caused by collected sebaceous material being trapped under the skin in small pores. This condition usually disappears when physical growth is completed. However, the child should be taught to thoroughly cleanse the skin to reduce blemishes. Vasomotor instability with rapid vasolidation causes excessive and uncontrollable blushing.

Physical or secondary sex changes that occur in the female, in sequence, during prepuberty or preadolescence are as follows[18,24,34,39]:

1. Increase in transverse diameter of the pelvis
2. Broadening of hips
3. Tenderness in developing breast tissue and enlargement of areola diameter
4. Axillary perspiring
5. Change in vaginal secretions from alkaline to acid pH
6. Change in vaginal layer to thick, gray, mucoid lining
7. Change in vaginal flora from mixed to Doederlein's lactic acid—producing bacilli
8. Appearance of pubic hair from 8 to 14 years; hair first appears on labia and then spreads to mons; adult triangular distribution does not occur for approximately 2 years after initial appearance of pubic hair

Physical or secondary sex changes that occur in the male, in sequence, during the same period are as follows:

1. Growth spurt at 12 to 16 years old (14 years average); average of 4 inches (10 cm) for 2½ years
2. Axillary perspiring
3. Increased testicular sensitivity to pressure
4. Increase in testes size
5. Changes in scrotum color
6. Temporary enlargement of breasts
7. Increase in height and shoulder breadth
8. Appearance of lightly pigmented hair at base of penis
9. Increase in length and width of penis

EMOTIONAL DEVELOPMENT

School-age children develop a sense of industry, according to Erikson.[19] They like to learn and solve problems (Fig. 9-1) and have greater body competence and apply themselves to skills and tasks. School-age children get tired of play, want to participate in the real world, and seek attention and recognition for efforts and concentration on a task. Pride comes from succeeding in either a physical or cognitive task. A sense of **industry** involves self-confidence, perseverance, diligence, self-control, cooperation, and compromise rather than just competition. Parents, teachers, and nurses may see this industry at times as restlessness, irritability, rebellion toward authority, and lack of obedience.[9,18]

The danger of this period is that children may develop a sense of **inferiority.**[9] Children—and later adults—who feel inferior will not like to work or try new tasks. They will be moody, anxious, oversensitive to and isolated from others, excessively meek, and lacking in perseverance. Regressive or withdrawn behavior, excess fear of bodily injury or illness, speech disorders, or psychosomatic disorders may be observed. Children may try to prove themselves by various acting-out behaviors, such as lying or stealing or other destructive acts. Sometimes opposite behavior may occur as they try to cope with feelings of inferiority or inadequacy. Instead, children might immerse themselves in tasks to prove personal worth and gain attention, become aggressive, bossy, and excessively competitive, and want their own way regularly. There is no time for play.[28]

A 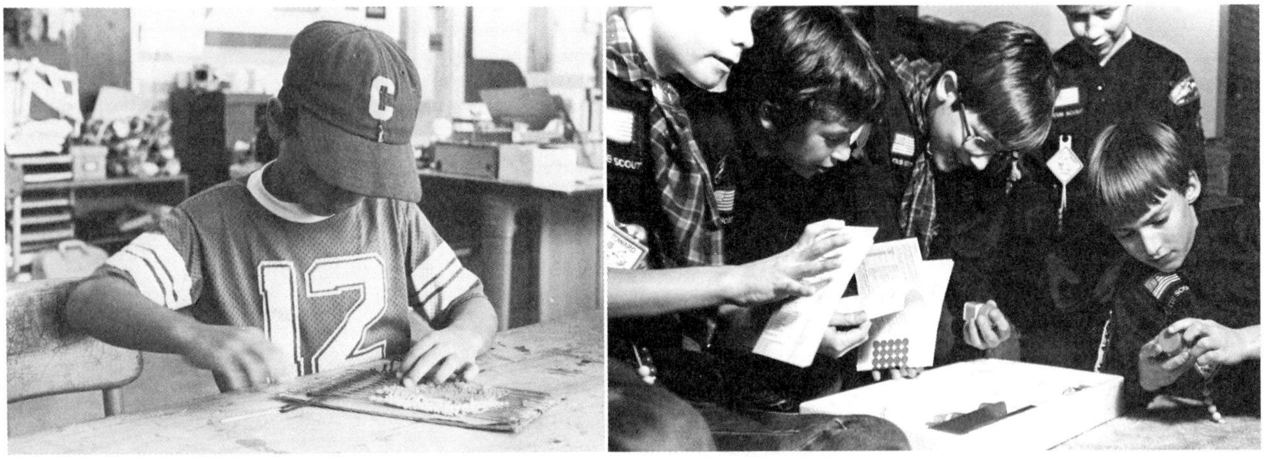 B

FIG. 9-1 School-age children are motivated to complete tasks. **A,** Working alone. **B,** Working with others.

Self-Concept

Until the child goes to school, self-perception is derived primarily from the parents' attitudes and reactions toward him or her. The child who is loved learns to love and accept himself and others. A positive self-concept is necessary for happiness, personality unity, and developing a sense of industry. The child with a positive self-concept enjoys life, believes he or she can be successful and can solve problems, and has a realistic self-estimate.

If parental reactions have been rejecting, if the child has been made to feel ugly, ashamed, or guilty, he or she enters school feeling bad, inadequate, or inferior. A negative self-image causes the child to feel defensive and hinders adjustment to school and academic progress.[17,18,33,34]

Sex education, begun earlier, should continue. By 7 or 8, children usually know that both sexes are required for childbirth to occur, but they are not sure how. Parents, teachers, or the nurse may use the following guidelines for sex and **sexuality education**[18]:

1. Know the facts and explain them on the child's level.
2. Do not lecture or preach.
3. Do not skip anything because the youngster says, "I already know." Chances are the child has some misinformation.
4. Answer all questions as honestly as possible.
5. Do not force too much at one sitting.
6. Aim the information at the child's immediate interest.
7. Do not pry into the child's feelings and fantasies.
8. Try to make the conversation as relaxed as possible.

COGNITIVE-INTELLECTUAL DEVELOPMENT

According to Piaget, the school-age child is in the concrete operations stage. Operations characteristic of this stage include **classification, seriation, nesting,** multiplication, **reversibility, transformation, conservation,** and **decentering.**[10,11,20,21,37]

These operations increase in complexity as the child matures. The child can look at a situation, analyze it, and come up with an answer without purposefully going through each step. Table 9-2 summarizes **cognitive** development in the school-age child.[10,11,17,34,37]

Entering School

The school experience has considerable influence on children, because they are in formative years and spend much time in school. School should help children learn to do the following:

1. Think critically
2. Make judgments based on reason
3. Accept criticism
4. Develop social skills
5. Cooperate with others
6. Accept other adult authority
7. Be leaders and followers

Every child should have a sense of successful accomplishment in some area. In addition to school, the home, and other groups, peer or organized clubs are important for intellectual and social development and for promoting a sense of achievement and industry.[18,34] Illness may interfere with the child's school experience.

Communication Patterns

Many factors influence the child's communication pattern, vocabulary, and diction, including the following[17,18,34]:

1. Speech and verbal and nonverbal communication patterns of parents, siblings, other adults, such as teacher or nurse, and peers

Table 9-2 Cognitive Characteristics of the School-Age Child

Age (Years)	Cognitive Ability
6	Preoperational stage: thinking is concrete and **animistic.** Beginning to understand semiabstract concepts; defines objects in relation to their use and effect on self. Ability depends on prior opportunity. May not be able to consider parts and wholes in words at the same time. Likes to hear about his past. Future important in relation to holidays.
7	Entering stage of **concrete operations.** Learns best from interaction with actual materials or visible props. Becoming less egocentric, less animistic. Better able to do cause-effect and logical thinking. More reflective; deeper understanding of meanings and feelings. Interested in conclusions and logical endings. Attention span lengthened, may work several hours on activity of interest. More aware of environment and people in it; also interested in magic and fantasy. Understands length, area, or mass. Sense of time practical, detailed, present; plans the day. Knows months, seasons, years.
8	More aware of people and impersonal forces of nature. Improvises simple activities. Likes to learn about history, geography, science, and social science. Tolerant and accepting of others. Understands logical reasoning and implications. Learns from own experience. Extremely punctual. Can read a compass.
9	Realistic in self-appraisal and tasks, reasonable, self-motivated, curious. Needs minimal direction. Likes to be involved with activities and complex tasks, plan in advance, make lists and collections. Believes in laws. Enjoys history. Tells time without difficulty. Likes to know length of time for task.
10	Matter-of-fact. Likes to participate in discussions about social problems. Likes a challenge. Likes to memorize, identify facts, locate sites on a map, make lists. Easily distracted; many interests and concentrates on each for the moment. Greater interest in present than past.
11	Curious but not reflective; concrete, specific thinking. Likes action or experimentation in learning. Concentrates well when competing with one group against another. Prefers routine. Better at rote memorization than generalization. Defines time as distance from one event to another.
12	Likes to consider all sides of a situation. Enters self-chosen task with initiative. Likes group work but more inner motivated than competitive. Able to classify and generalize. Likes to discuss and debate. Beginning formal operation, or abstract thinking. Verbal formal reasoning is possible. Defines time as duration, a measurement. Plans ahead so feels life is under own control. Interested in present and future. Understands abstractness of space.

2. Attitudes of others toward the child's efforts to speak and communicate
3. General environmental stimulation
4. Opportunity to communicate with a variety of people in a variety of situations, thus building vocabulary skills
5. Intellectual development
6. Ability to hear and articulate speech
7. Contact with television, movies, or other media

The 6-year-old has command of nearly every form of sentence structure. The child experiments less with language, using it more as a tool and less for the mere pleasure of talking than during the preschool period. He or she also swears and uses slang to test others' reactions.[10,17,21]

At 7, the child can print several sentences, and at 8, write instead of print. By 9, the child participates in family and health care discussions. Common objects are described in detail. Writing skill has improved; he or she usually writes with small, even letters. By 10, the child can write for a relatively long time with speed. The preadolescent may seem less talkative, withdrawing when frustrated instead of voicing anger. Sharing feelings with a best friend is a healthy outlet.[10,11,17,34]

As the child shares ideas and feelings, he or she learns how someone else thinks and feels about similar matters. The child expresses self in a way that has meaning to others, at first to a chum and then to others; thus he or she is checking vocabulary, ideas, and feelings. The child learns that a friend's family has similar life patterns, demands of the child, and frustrations. The child learns about himself or herself in the process of learning more about another. He or she recalls what has happened in the past, realizes how this has affected the present, and considers what effect present acts will have on future events. This is called using a **syntaxic mode of experience** or **consensual validation** in communication.[18,33] The nurse is in a key position to foster effective communication skills in the school-age child and to encourage the child to ask questions about health care.

Effect of TV on Child

Television and movies have a powerful influence on a child's communication and behavior patterns.[17,25,31,32,38] If watching television is controlled by responsible adults, learning can be enhanced. Geographical, sports, science, historical, humorous, dramatic, and religious presentations are useful.

Understanding television can involve active mental

work for the young child, but often the child does not understand content, motives, or feelings, integrate the events shown, or infer conditions not shown.[31,32] Those mental processes are stimulated by adult and peer interactions and reading literature. Television can stifle family and peer interaction. Stereotypical, simplistic, and romanticized views of family life and physical appearance shown by most programs are unrealistic. False expectations about events and people are raised. Science fiction may convey that life in the future may be scary and difficult at best or may fire a child's imagination to become a scientist, writer, researcher, or explorer, and may influence the child's present and future values system.[17,35] Some television programming is frankly pornographic.

The violence in television programming is graphic, explicit, too realistic, and intensely involving. Portrayals of violence suggest that violence is normal and justified. Realistic or punitive consequences of violent behavior are not shown. Continual viewing of violence desensitizes the person to violence in general; it is no longer a noteworthy act in the home or society.* The nurse may need to monitor television viewing of the ill child and can educate parents about negative effects of television viewing.

Children who have grown up in stable families, who feel secure and loved, and who have a variety of interests and relationships will not be adversely affected by the aggression, violence, and sex seen on televison. They can separate fantasy from fact.

SOCIAL DEVELOPMENT

Friendship Patterns

Peer groups, including the gang and the close chum, provide companionship with a widening circle of persons outside the home. Peers teach the child new roles and use of rules, more independence, and the abilities to compete, compromise, and cooperate.

In preadolescence the **gang** becomes important. Gang rules take precedence over almost everything.[3,18,30,34,39] In the gang, children discharge hostility and aggression against peers rather than adults and begin to work out their own social patterns without adult interference. On a hospital division, a group of preadolescents may form a gang and may turn their hostility toward the nurses. Working with the gang can also be an effective way to encourage healthy behavior.

The chum stage. The **chum** stage occurs at about 9 or 10 years of age, and sometimes later, when affection moves from the peer group and gang to a special friend. The friend becomes an extension of the child's own self. As children share ideas and feelings, they learn a great deal about themselves as well as about their chums. The child learns self-acceptance, which increases acceptance of others, so that the child of this age is very sociable, generous, and sympathetic, enjoys differences in people, and is liberal in ideas about the welfare of others. Also, through the chum relationship the child learns the syntaxic mode of communication.[33] Loyalty to the chum at this age may be greater than loyalty to the family.[18]

Cooperation and compromise are gradually learned from peers as well as teachers and family. The child becomes less rigid in behavior and begins to understand the social implications of acts.[33]

*References 5, 19, 31, 32, 35, 36.

PROMOTING OPTIMUM HEALTH

Nutrition

Although caloric requirements per unit of body weight continue to decrease for the school-age child, nutritional requirements remain relatively greater than the adult's. By age 10 there is a decrease in the calories per kilogram for both boys (45 calories per kg) and girls (38 calories per kg). An individual child may require more or less calories than the Recommended Dietary Allowances, depending on size, activity, and growth rate.[30,40] Daily caloric needs can be approximated for the school-age child by using the following formula[18,40]: 1000 calories for the 6-year-old plus 100 calories for each additional year in this age period. Water intake may be overlooked; the school-age child needs 1.5 to 3 quarts daily, depending on his or her size. The nurse can refer the child to the nutritionist for instruction.

Nutritional needs for the school-age child include daily servings of the following foods[18,30,40]:

Meats and eggs, or dry beans, dry peas, and lentils	2 or more 2- or 3-ounce servings
Milk (whole, skim, or powdered)	2-6 cups (1-1½ quarts)
Fruits and vegetables, including a dark-green or deep-yellow vegetable for vitamin A and a fruit or vegetable that contains high vitamin C	4 or more servings
Breads and cereals	4 or more servings to meet caloric needs
Fats and carbohydrates	Based upon need for added calories

Sleep and Rest

Hours of sleep needed depends on age, health status, and the day's activities. Schoolchildren usually do not need a nap. A 6-year-old usually requires about 11 hours of sleep nightly; an 11-year-old may need only 9 hours.[18,39] The school-age child may need firm discipline from the parent or nurse to go to bed at the prescribed hour. Sleep may be disturbed with dreams and nightmares, especially if he or she has considerable emotional stimulation before bedtime.

BOX 9-2 INJURY PREVENTION DURING SCHOOL-AGE YEARS

MOTOR VEHICLES

Educate regarding proper use of seat belts while a passenger in a vehicle

Maintain discipline while a passenger in a vehicle, for example, keep arms inside, do not lean against doors or interfere with driver

Emphasize safe pedestrian behavior

Teach safety and maintenance of two-wheeled vehicles, such as bicycles

Insist on wearing of safety apparel (e.g., helmet) where applicable, such as riding a motorcycle

DROWNING

Teach to swim

Teach basic water safety, especially swimming with a buddy

BURNS

Instruct in behavior in the areas involving contact with potential burn hazards, for example, gasoline, matches, bonfires or barbecues, firecrackers, lighters, cooking utensils, chemistry sets; avoid climbing around high-tension wires

Instruct in proper behavior in the event of fire (e.g., fire drills at home or school)

Teach proper behavior if clothing becomes ignited

Advise regarding excessive exposure to sunlight (ultraviolet burn)

POISONING

Educate regarding hazards of taking nonprescription drugs and chemicals, including aspirin and alcohol

Keep potentially dangerous products in properly labeled receptacles—preferably out of reach

FALLS

Instruct in proper use of playground equipment

Instruct in proper use and care of sports equipment, especially the more hazardous devices (e.g., skateboards, skis)

Emphasize use of protective equipment when engaged in individual activities such as skateboarding and cycling and team sports such as soccer or hockey

BODILY DAMAGE

Help provide facilities for supervised activities

Encourage playing in safe places

Keep firearms safely locked up except during adult supervision

Teach proper care of, use of, and respect for devices with potential danger (e.g., power tools, firecrackers)

Stress eye protection when using potentially hazardous objects or devices or when engaged in potentially hazardous sports

Teach safety regarding use of corrective devices (glasses); if child wears contact lenses, monitor duration of wear to prevent corneal damage

Stress careful selection and maintenance of sport and recreation equipment

Emphasize proper conditioning for sports or other recreational activities

Caution against engaging in hazardous sports, such as those involving trampolines

Have identification on child, such as plastic "shoe pocket" attached to shoe laces

Exercise and Play

Exercise is essential for increasing muscular development, coordination, balance, strength, and enhancing other body functions such as circulation, aeration, and waste elimination. School-age children should have a safe place to play and simple pieces of equipment. When children cannot play outside, they should have opportunities to exercise indoors.

Parents and other adults should play actively with their children and encourage them in exercise. Children benefit from adults' knowledge of various activities and are encouraged by the attention.[18]

Both sexes enjoy some active and quiet activities, such as painting, music, crafts, reading, simple table games, television, video and computer games, digging, riding a bicycle, running games, skating, and swimming. The parent can sometimes enjoy these activities with the child. The child imitates the roles of his or her own sex and becomes increasingly realistic in play. By age 8, collections are a favorite pastime, and loosely formed, short-lived clubs with changing rules develop.[3,10,14] By age 10, sex differences in play are more apparent.

Immunization

Booster doses of DTP should be given by 6 years of age. Pertussis vaccine is not necessary for children over this age. Girls should receive rubella vaccine before they enter puberty to prevent congenital defects in the newborn should they be exposed to rubella during pregnancy. Boys should be immunized against mumps before the age of 12; mumps contracted during or after puberty can cause sterility. The need for tuberculin tests depends on the prevalence of tuberculosis and the risk of exposure.* The influenza virus vaccine, pneumococcal vaccine, and hepatitis B vaccine are recommended for children in certain high-risk groups.[1,4,34,39]

Injury Prevention

Although school-age children have developed more refined muscular coordination and control, their use of bicycles, skateboards, and roller skates and participation in sports increases their risk for injury. Incidence of injury is significantly higher in school-age boys than girls. Some of the injuries sustained during sporting activities may cause permanent disability.[30,39] Guidelines for injury prevention during school-age years are presented in Box 9-2.

Guidance and Discipline

In guidance, parents or other adults and the nurse should invite confidence of the child. The atmosphere should be open and inviting for the child to talk with the parents or adults, but the child's privacy should not be invaded. Parents should see the child realistically, not as an idealized extension of themselves.[18]

The school-age child has a rather strict conscience and also uses various rituals to maintain self-control. He or she prefers to initiate self-control rather than be given commands or overt discipline. The child needs some alternatives from which to choose to learn different ways of behaving and coping. If development has been normal during the preschool years, the child is now well on the way to absorbing and accepting the standards, codes, and attitudes of society. Ongoing guidance rather than an emphasis on disciplinary measures is needed.[18]

DEVELOPMENTAL TASKS

While the school-age child continues working on past developmental tasks, he or she is confronted with a series of new ones[7]:

1. Decreasing dependence on family and gaining some satisfaction from peers and other adults
2. Increasing neuromuscular skills so that he or she can participate in games and work with others
3. Learning basic adult concepts and knowledge to be able to reason and engage in tasks of everyday living
4. Learning ways to communicate with others realistically
5. Becoming a more active and cooperative family participant
6. Giving and receiving affection among family and friends without immediately seeking something in return
7. Learning socially acceptable ways of getting money and saving it for later satisfactions
8. Learning how to handle strong feelings and impulses appropriately
9. Adjusting the changing body image and self-concept to come to terms with the masculine or feminine social role
10. Discovering healthy ways of becoming acceptable as a person
11. Developing a positive attitude toward his or her own and other social, racial, economic, and religious groups

The accomplishment of these tasks gives the school-age child a foundation for entering adolescence, an era filled with dramatic growth and changing attitudes. The nurse can assist the child in achieving these developmental tasks through assessment, planning care with the child, and teaching the child and parents as indicated.

*References 4, 12, 18, 24, 27, 30.

REFERENCES AND SUGGESTED READINGS

1. American Academy of Pediatrics, Committee on Infectious Diseases: Prevention of hepatitis B virus infections, Pediatrics 75(2):364, 1985.
2. American Academy of Pediatrics, Committee on Infectious Diseases: Recommendations for using pneumococcal vaccine in children, Pediatrics 75(6):1153, 1985b.
3. Bettelheim B: A good enough parent: a book on child-rearing, New York, 1987, Alfred A Knopf.
4. Carlstrom JA and Nelson S: Measles and rubella: old problems in a new generation, J Commun Health Nurs 4(2):69, 1987.
5. Comer J: Television, sex, and violence, Parents 160, July 1986.
6. Diseker R and others: A comparison of height, weight, and triceps skinfold thickness of children ages 5-12 in Michigan (1978), Forsyth County, North Carolina (1978), and Hanes, Texas, Part I (1971-1974), Am J Publ Health 72(7):730, 1982.
7. Duvall E and Miller B: Marriage and family development, 6, New York, 1984, Harper & Row Publishers.
8. Elkind D: Why children need time, Parade 14, Jan 10, 1982.
9. Erikson E: Childhood and society, ed 2, New York, 1963, WW Norton.
10. Gesell A and Ilg F: The child from five to ten, New York, 1946, Harper & Brothers.
11. Gesell A, Ilg F, and Ames L: Youth: the years from ten to sixteen, New York, 1956, Harper & Brothers.
12. Immunizations still important for children, Health Scene 11, Fall 1987.
13. Katz L: Telling children about divorce, Parents 152, July 1986.
14. Kids need more time to be kids, Newsweek 56, Feb 2, 1987.
15. Malina R, Zuvaleta A, and Little B: Body size, fatness, and leanness of Mexican-American children in Brownsville, Texas: changes between 1972 and 1983, Am J Publ Health 77(5):573, 1987.
16. Manning M: Disappearing childhood: 6 going on 16, Kappa Delta Pi Record 14, Fall 1985.
17. Mosham D, Glover J, and Bruning R: Developmental psychology, Boston, 1987, Little, Brown & Co.
18. Murray R and Zentner J: Nursing assessment and health promotion strategies through the lifespan, ed 4, East Norwalk, Conn, 1989, Appleton-Century-Crofts.
19. Parke R and Slaby R: The development of aggression. In Hetherton E and Mussen P, editors: Handbook of child psychology, vol 4, Socialization, personality, and social development, New York, 1983, John Wiley & Sons.
20. Piaget J: Judgment and reasoning in the child, New York, 1928, Humanities Press.
21. Piaget J: The growth of logical thinking from childhood to adolescence, New York, 1958, Basic Books.
22. Piaget J: The origins of intelligence in children, New York, 1963, WW Norton.
23. Piaget J: The child's conception of numbers, New York, 1965, WW Norton.
24. Pillitteri A: Child health nursing: care of the growing family, ed 3, Boston, 1987, Little, Brown & Co.
25. Porter C: Grade school children's perceptions of their internal body parts, Nurs Res 23(5):384, 1974.
26. R ratings: most violent programming shown as children watch, St Louis Post Dispatch, Sept 11, 1986, Sec C, pp 17-18.
27. Robbins K, Brandling-Bennett D, and Hinman A: Low measles incidence: association with enforcement of school immunization laws, Am J Publ Health 71(3):270, 1981.
28. Rubenstein E: Television and behavior: research conclusions of the 1982 NIMH report and their policy implications, Am Psychol 38:820, 1983.
29. Scholl T and others: Ethnic differences in growth and nutritional status: a study of poor schoolchildren in southern New Jersey, Publ Health Reports 102(3):278, 1987.
30. Scipien GM and others: Comprehensive pediatric nursing, ed 3, New York, 1986, McGraw-Hill Book Co.
31. Singer DC: A time to re-examine the role of television in our lives, Am Psychol 38:815, 1983.
32. Singer JL and Singer DE: Implications of childhood television viewing for cognition, imagination, and emotion. In Bryant J and Anderson D, editors: Children's understanding of television: research on attention and comprehension, New York, 1983, Academic Press.
33. Sullivan HS: The interpersonal theory of psychiatry, New York, 1953, WW Norton.
34. Turner J and Helms D: Lifespan development 3, New York, 1987, Holt, Rinehart & Winston.
35. US Department of Health and Human Services: Television and behavior: Ten years of scientific progress and implications for the eighties, Washington, DC, 1982, US Government Printing Office.
36. US Department of Health and Human Services: New recommended schedule for active immunization of normal infants and children, Morbidity and Mortality Weekly Report 35(37)577, Sept 19, 1986.
37. Wadsworth B: Piaget's theory of cognitive and affective development, ed 4, New York, 1989, Longman.
38. Warning from Washington: violence in television is harmful to children, Time, 77, May 17, 1982.
39. Whaley L and Wong D: Nursing care of infants and children, ed 4, St Louis, 1991, The CV Mosby Co.
40. Williams S: Nutrition and diet therapy, ed 6, St Louis, 1989, Times Mirror/Mosby College Publishing.

CHAPTER CHALLENGE

KEY POINTS

- The school-age child channels energy into intellectual pursuits, widens social horizons, and becomes familiar with the adult world.
- Although parental influence is of primary importance, the school-age child's relationship with siblings affects personality formation.
- The child's growth rate is usually slow and steady.
- The preadolescent at puberty is characterized by a spurt of physical growth and changes in body proportion.
- The school-age child develops a sense of industry, according to Erikson.
- In addition to school, the home and other groups and peer or organized clubs are important for the school-age child.
- Although caloric requirements per unit of body weight continue to decrease for the school-age child, nutritional requirements remain relatively greater than for the adult.
- A systematic schedule of immunization should be followed for the school-age child.
- Exercise and play are essential for increasing the school-age child's muscular development, coordination, balance, and strength.

STUDY QUESTIONS

1. African-American children and Caucasian children from lower socioeconomic groups tend to be:
   a. Smaller in weight and height
   b. Short in height, overweight
   c. Tall in height, underweight
   d. None of the above
2. The following vital signs are within the normal range for the school-age child:
   a. Temperature 98°-99°, pulse rate 100-110 per minute, respiratory rate 30-34 per minute, blood pressure 84/50
   b. Temperature 97°-97.4°, pulse rate 60-65 per minute, respiratory rate 12-16 per minute, blood pressure 120/70
   c. Temperature 98°-98.6°, pulse rate 70-80 per minute, respiratory rate 18-21 per minute, blood pressure 100/60
3. According to Erikson, the school-age child develops:
   a. Initiative, expanding sense of mastery, and responsibility
   b. Industry, a stage of systematic instruction, movement from play to a sense of work, problem solving skills
   c. Autonomy, begins to exert control over self and some of the surrounding world
   d. Generativity, general concern for guiding and supporting the next generation
4. According to Piaget, the school-age child is in the concrete operations stage. Operations characteristic of this stage include:
   a. Classification
   b. Prehension
   c. Locomotion
   d. Trapping
5. At what age do most children begin to write instead of just print:
   a. 7 years
   b. 8 years
   c. 9 years
6. The school-age child needs approximately how much water per day:
   a. 1.5 to 3 quarts
   b. 1 to 2 pints
   c. 0.5 to 1 quart
7. Pertussis vaccine is not necessary for children after what age:
   a. 3 years
   b. 6 years
   c. 10 years
8. Syntaxic mode of experience or consensual validation means:
   a. Ability to mentally shift from one state to another
   b. Mentally ordering objects according to height, weight, or strength
   c. Communication in which two people can understand the meaning of their dialogue, speaking cause-effect relationships
9. During the school-age years, the heart is:
   a. Larger proportionate to body size
   b. Smaller proportionate to body size
   c. The same size as an adult heart
10. For both males and females, the school-age growth spurt begins:
    a. In the trunk, then the arms and legs
    b. In the chest, then the forearms
    c. In the hands and feet and progresses to the calves

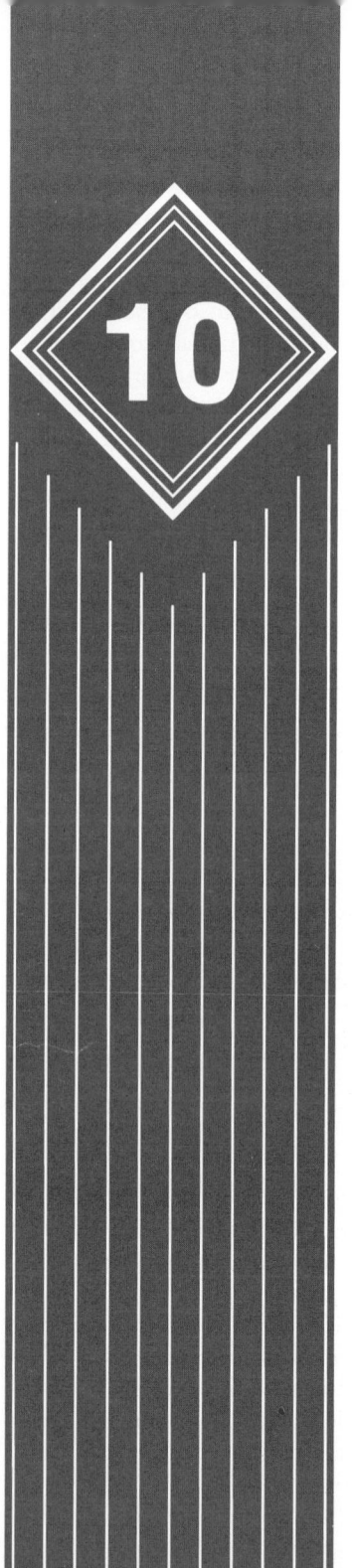

10

The Adolescent

RUTH BECKMANN MURRAY

LEARNING OBJECTIVES

After reading this chapter, the student should be able to do the following:

- Define the key terms.
- Compare characteristics of the adolescent in early, middle, and late adolescence.
- Discuss the impact of adolescence on family life.
- List family developmental tasks.
- Describe physiological changes and needs, including nutrition, exercise, and rest.
- Describe health promotion measures of immunizations.
- Discuss cognitive and social development of the adolescent.
- Describe emotional development of the adolescent.
- Explore identity formation and its significance for ongoing maturity.
- Discuss the developmental tasks of adolescence.

RELATED TOPICS OF INTEREST

- The family (Chapter 7)
- Basic nutrition (Chapter 22)
- Basic pediatric nursing care (Chapter 46)
- Care of children with physical and emotional problems (Chapter 47)

KEY TERMS

Define the following:

- adolescence
- androgens
- estrogens
- formal operations
- identity diffusion
- identity formation
- menarche
- menstruation
- nocturnal emissions
- ovulation
- progesterone
- puberty
- sex hormones
- spermatogenesis
- testosterone

The practical/vocational nurse may care for the adolescent in a variety of settings, or the adolescent may be a family member of the patient. Understanding and helping the family to understand the adolescent's behavior is an important aspect of nursing care.

Early **adolescence** begins with **puberty** and lasts for several years (11 or 12 to 13 or 14 for females and 12 or 14 to 16 for males). The growth spurt focuses attention on self and becoming comfortable with body changes. The teenager tries to separate from parents; the dependency-independency struggle is shown by less involvement in family activities (and chores, if possible), being critical of the parents, and rebellion against parental and other adult discipline and authority. Peer friendships are gaining in importance. Although the peer group usually consists of friends of the same sex, the adolescent has an increased interest in the opposite sex. Group activities with peers are popular, and conformity to peer behavior is important.[1,14,18]

Middle adolescence begins when physical growth is nearly completed and usually extends from age 13 to 16 for females and 14 to 18 for males. The major tasks are achievement of ego **identity,** attainment of greater independence, interest in the future, career planning, and establishment of heterosexual relationships. Peer group allegiance, at a peak in 15- to 16-year-olds, is manifested by choices of clothing, food, and other fads, preferred music, and common jargon. Experimentation with adultlike behavior and risk taking is common to prove oneself to peers. Sexual experimentation often begins now (or earlier) as a result of social exploration and physical maturation. The person moves to more abstract thinking, returning to more concrete operations during times of stress.[1,14,18,23] Some teenagers are expected to take on the tasks of young adulthood at this point. While they may be employed or independent in other ways, developmentally they are still emotionally immature.

Late adolescence may continue until about 20 to 25 years of age. The person has finished adolescent rebellion, has established a stable sense of self, and is more realistically aware of strengths and limits in self and others. The youth is selecting an occupation and questions existing social, vocational, and emotional roles and life-styles. He or she may be a student or an apprentice.[11] The value system is being clarified; issues of philosophy, religion, life and death, and ethical decisions are being analyzed. The peer group has lost its primary importance. The youth may establish independence from parents by moving away from home; a more adult form of friendship begins between late adolescents and their parents. The person establishes a deeper, more lasting emotionally intimate relationship with a member of the opposite sex. At that point, the person is developmentally a young adult, having made the transition from adolescence.[1,14,18]

FAMILY DEVELOPMENT AND RELATIONSHIPS

Family Relationships

During early adolescence, the teenager remains involved in family activities and functions. Gradually family relationships change; the adolescent develops more social ties and close relationships outside the family during the teen years. The family's beliefs, life-style, values, and patterns of interaction influence development of these relationships.[19]

During middle and late adolescence, the most severe changes occur in the parent-child relationship. The relationship must evolve from a dependency status to mutual affection, equality, and autonomy. Achieving independence usually creates family turmoil, conflict, and ambivalence as parents and the adolescent learn new roles. Parents should gradually increase the teenager's responsibilities and allow privileges formerly denied. The adolescent wants to make independent decisions and to have increased freedom of movement, yet have basic needs being met in the family. Parents must resist granting instant adult status when the child reaches the teen years. The adolescent needs to be independent yet dependent; the adolescent feels more self-confident in exploring the environment if reasonable restraints are imposed. The adolescent's viewpoints may offer hints about the readiness for more independence and freedom.[14,19,27] Most ambivalence and negative behavior in the adolescent stem from perceived external restrictions. Teenagers may fight for grown-up privileges that they never use; the battle is more important than the actual privilege.[23,27]

In addition to other conflicts, youths must also work through feelings for the parent of the opposite sex and ambivalence toward the parent of the same sex. The adolescent reworks some of the gender identity and family triangle problems that remain from the preschool era. In an attempt to resolve this ambivalence, the adolescent may strive to be as different as possible from the parent of the same sex. Frequently affection is turned to an adult outside the family. Idolizing another adult person causes the adolescent to want to please that person; therefore the adolescent's actions and language may change when the idolized person is present. Frequently the adolescent identifies so completely with this person that some of the person's adult characteristics are taken into the personality. These relationships are not harmful to the adolescent unless the person who is chronologically an adult still feels confused and rebellious toward society and fosters immaturity.[14]

Parental and adolescent responses to the ambivalence and conflicts of this period vary. Parents may adhere to rules and the status quo to bolster their own security rather than change for the offspring's benefit, and they may overprotect. Others may be reluctant to admit that their child is establishing independence; they may dread facing the empty-nest stage.[23] If adolescents have come from a family who have provided past opportunities to learn responsibility, self-reliance skills, and self-respect, they will make a smoother transition from childhood dependency to adulthood independence. If parents have been too liberal, overly permissive, or uninterested, the adolescent will have more difficulty adjusting because the past lacked structure and a system of standards or values—the youth will have no point of reference to determine whether the behavior is suitable and decisions are appropriate.[13]

The practical/vocational nurse can encourage parents to relate to the adolescent in a way to promote maturity.

Family Developmental Tasks

The overall family goal at this time is to allow the adolescent increasing freedom and responsibility for preparation for young adulthood. The family unit as a whole has the following developmental tasks[4]:

1. Provide opportunities and facilities for individual differences and needs of family members.
2. Work out a system of financial responsibility with the family.
3. Establish a sharing of responsibilities between family members.
4. Continue a mutually satisfying marriage relationship.
5. Strengthen communication within the family.
6. Rework relationships with relatives, friends, and associates.
7. Broaden horizons of the adolescent and parents.
8. Formulate a workable philosophy of life as a family.

Generally speaking, developmental tasks for a family at this time involve maintaining a grasp on the facets of life that continue to have meaning while striving for a deeper awareness and understanding of the present situation.

PHYSICAL DEVELOPMENT

The practical/vocational nurse may be asked about physical changes and should be prepared to explain the processes that are part of puberty. Knowledge of physical development is basic for assessment.

General Measurements

Weight and height. Adolescence is the second major period of accelerated growth (infancy was the first). The adolescent growth spurt occurs about 2 years earlier in females than in males. During the years of the growth spurt, females grow 2½ to 5 inches (6 to 12.5 cm) and

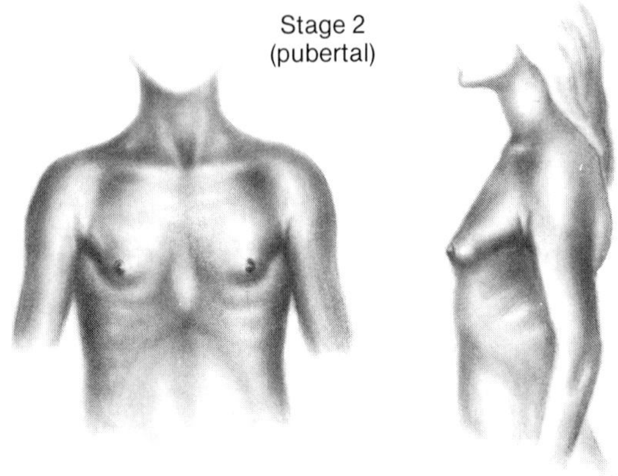

Breast bud stage—small area of elevation around papilla; enlargement of areolar diameter

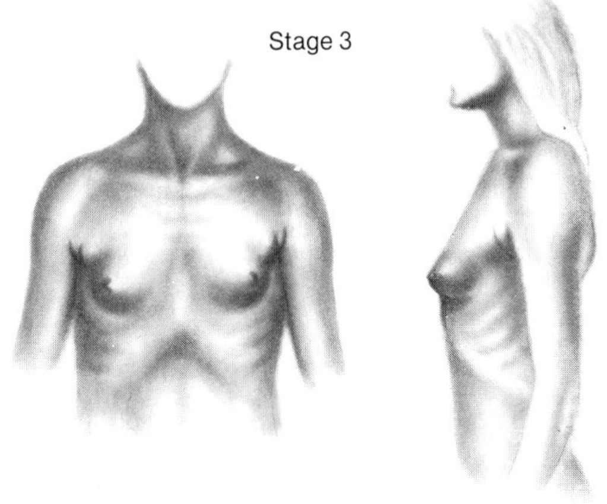

Further enlargement of breast and areola with no separation of their contours

gain 8 to 10 pounds (3.5 to 4.5 kg). Males grow an average of 3 to 6 inches (7.5 to 15 cm) and gain 12 to 14 pounds (5.5 to 6.5 kg). In the initial phase of the growth spurt, the increase in height results from lengthening of the legs; later, most of the increase is in the trunk length. The total process takes about 3 years in females and 4 years in males.[13,14,23] Every system of the body is growing rapidly, but physiological changes do not occur evenly or at one time within the person.

Sexual Development

Four physical characteristics that define puberty for most adolescents, as they observe themselves and each other, are as follows[12,14,18,23,27]:

FEMALES	MALES
Height spurt: ages 8 to 17 years; peak age 12	Height spurt: 10 to 20 years; peak age 14
Menarche: 10 to 16 years; average age 12.5	Penis development: 10 to 16 years
Breast development: 8 to 18 years	Testes development: 9 to 17 years
Pubic hair: 11 to 14 years	Pubic hair: 12 to 16 years

Menarche is the indicator of puberty and sexual maturity in the female. Ovulation usually first occurs 12 to 24 months after menarche. The onset of menarche varies among population groups and is influenced by heredity, nutrition, health care, and other environmental factors. In the United States, the average age of onset is 12.6 to 12.9 years.[19,23]

Secondary sex characteristics in the female begin to develop in prepuberty (see Chapter 9) and may take 2 to 8 years for completion (Figs. 10-1 and 10-2). Breast enlargement and elevation occur; areola and papillae project to form a secondary mound. Axillary and pubic hair grows thicker and becomes darker, and pubic hair spreads over the pubic area.[18]

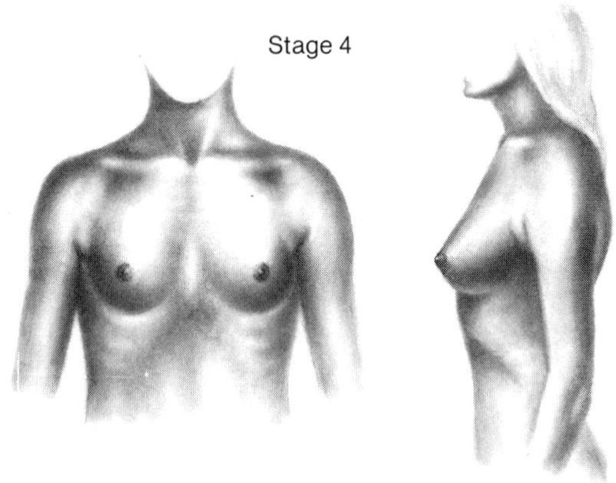

Projection of areola and papilla to form a secondary mound (may not occur in all girls)

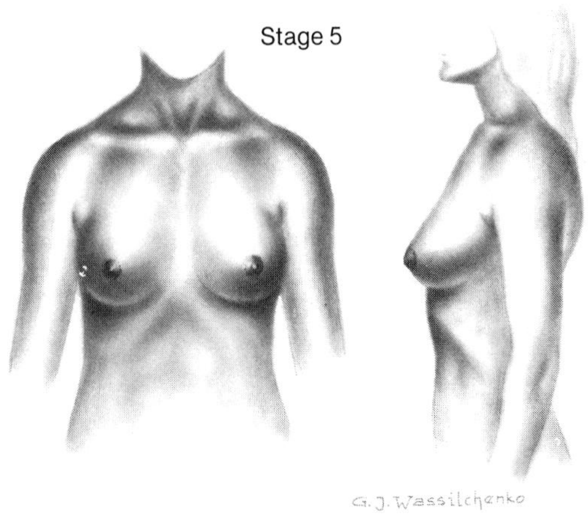

Mature configuration; projection of papilla only caused by recession of areola into general contour

FIG. 10-1 Development of the breast in girls—average age span: 11 to 13 years. Stage 1 (prepubertal: elevation of papilla only) is not shown. (Adapted from Marshall WA and Tanner JM, Arch Dis Child 44:291, 1969; and Daniel WA and Paulshock BZ, Patient Care, May 13, 1979, p.122.

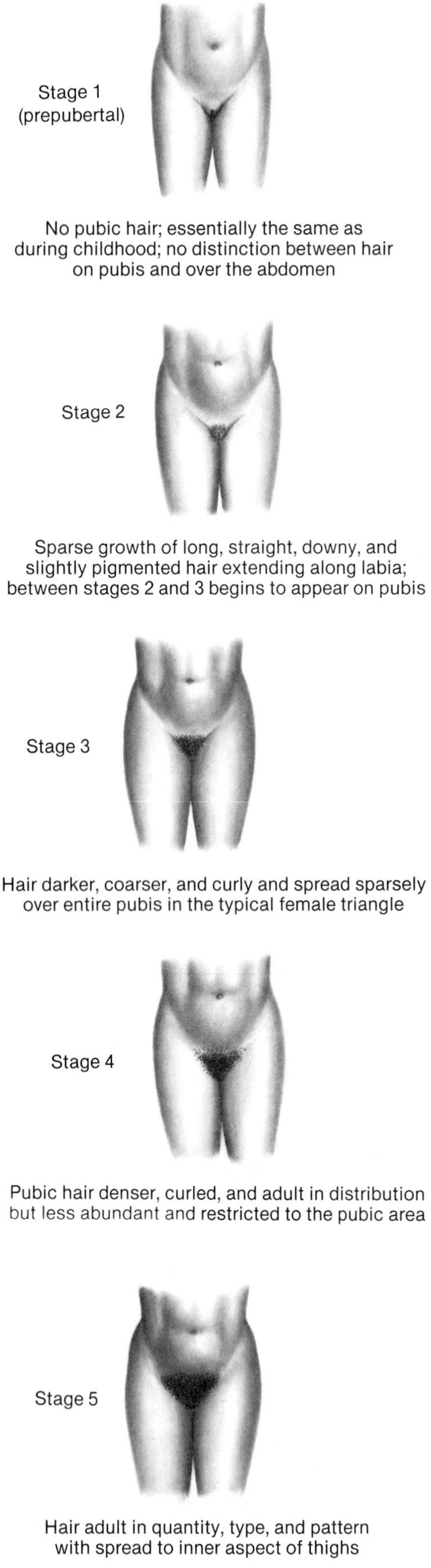
Stage 1
(prepubertal)
No pubic hair; essentially the same as during childhood; no distinction between hair on pubis and over the abdomen
Stage 2
Sparse growth of long, straight, downy, and slightly pigmented hair extending along labia; between stages 2 and 3 begins to appear on pubis
Stage 3
Hair darker, coarser, and curly and spread sparsely over entire pubis in the typical female triangle
Stage 4
Pubic hair denser, curled, and adult in distribution but less abundant and restricted to the pubic area
Stage 5
Hair adult in quantity, type, and pattern with spread to inner aspect of thighs

FIG. 10-2 Growth in pubic hair in girls—average age span for stages 2 through 5: 11 to 14 years. (Adapted from Marshall WA and Tanner JM, Arch Dis Child 44:291, 1969; and Daniel WA and Paulshock BZ, Patient Care, May 13, 1979, p. 122.

Spermatogenesis and seminal emissions mark puberty and sexual maturity in the male. The first ejaculate of seminal fluid occurs about 1 year after the penis has begun its adolescent growth. **Nocturnal emissions** occur at about age 14.[18]

The development of secondary sex characteristics in the male also begins in the prepubertal period (see Chapter 9) and may take 2 to 5 years for completion (Fig. 10-3). Body shape changes, growth of body hair, and muscle development may continue until 19 or 20 years of age, or even until the early twenties. North American males complete growth in stature by 18 or 19 years, with an additional ½ to 1 inch (1 to 2 cm) in height occurring during the twenties because of continued vertebral column growth.[18] The penis, scrotum, and testes enlarge; the scrotum reddens and scrotal skin changes texture. Hair grows at the axilla and base of the penis and spreads over the pubis. Body hair generally increases, especially facial hair. The voice deepens.[19]

Menstrual cycle. The 28-day menstrual or reproductive cycle is controlled by an intricate feedback system involving (1) the hypothalamus, which audits the level of hormones in the bloodstream, (2) the anterior lobe of the pituitary and its hormones, follicle-stimulating hormone (FSH) and luteinizing hormone (LH), (3) the ovaries and their hormones, **estrogen** and **progesterone,** and (4) the interplay between ovarian hormones and FSH and LH.[13]

At the onset of the menstrual cycle, when the estrogen level is lowest, the shedding of the endometrium (lining of the uterus) occurs. The hypothalamus, because of the low estrogen level, stimulates the pituitary gland to release FSH, which causes the maturation of one of the ova-containing ovarian or graafian follicles as well as increased production of estrogen. This is the time of highest estrogen levels in the bloodstream. In response to estrogen, the endometrium begins to thicken to prepare the uterus to receive the zygote if fertilization occurs.[13,18]

In response to the high level of estrogen, the anterior pituitary releases LH. The sudden increase of LH triggers **ovulation** from the follicle, which happens about 14 days after the onset of the cycle. The LH moves to the ruptured follicle, which causes the development of the glandular corpus luteum. This produces both estrogen and progesterone, which, when acting together, cause the glands of the endometrium to prepare further for the nourishment of a possible zygote.

If fertilization of the ovum by a sperm cell does not occur, the ovum deteriorates. The pituitary stops pro-

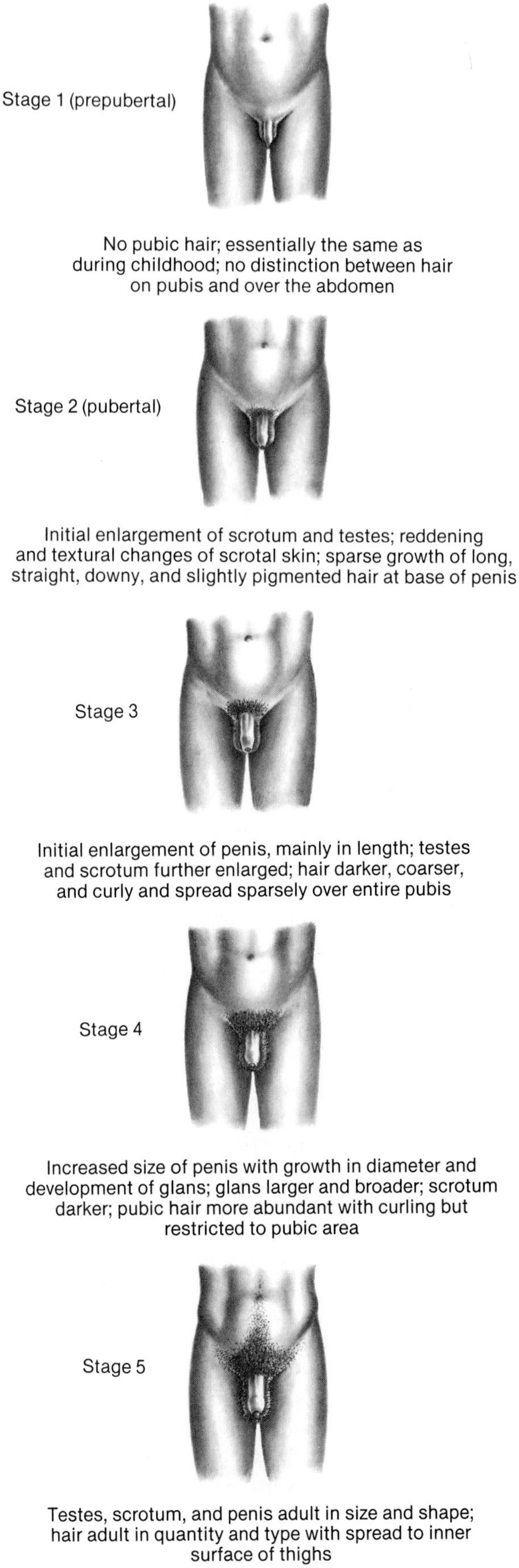
Stage 1 (prepubertal)
No pubic hair; essentially the same as during childhood; no distinction between hair on pubis and over the abdomen
Stage 2 (pubertal)
Initial enlargement of scrotum and testes; reddening and textural changes of scrotal skin; sparse growth of long, straight, downy, and slightly pigmented hair at base of penis
Stage 3
Initial enlargement of penis, mainly in length; testes and scrotum further enlarged; hair darker, coarser, and curly and spread sparsely over entire pubis
Stage 4
Increased size of penis with growth in diameter and development of glans; glans larger and broader; scrotum darker; pubic hair more abundant with curling but restricted to pubic area
Stage 5
Testes, scrotum, and penis adult in size and shape; hair adult in quantity and type with spread to inner surface of thighs

FIG. 10-3 Developmental stages of secondary sex characteristics and genital development in boys—average age span: 12 to 16 years. (Adapted from Marshall WA and Tanner JM, Arch Dis Child 45:13,1970; and Daniel WA and Paulshock BZ, Patient Care, May 13, 1979, p. 122.

duction of both FSH and LH, and the corpus luteum becomes dormant and atrophies. The resulting drop in estrogen and progesterone levels stimulates the shedding of the endometrial lining. This consists of blood, mucus, and tissues—the menstrual discharge. **Menstruation** lasts 3 to 5 days. The cycle then begins anew.[18] Menstrual cramps may be the result of these hormonal changes but do not occur in all females.

Hormonal changes in the male. In the male, the hormonal system for reproductive behavior is much simpler because there is no cyclical pattern. The male gonads, the testes, produce sperm continuously and secrete **androgens.** The major androgen is **testosterone.** Just as FSH promotes the development of the ovum in females, FSH promotes the development of sperm in males. A continuous level of sperm production takes place in the seminiferous tubules inside the testes. The secretion of LH (also called interstitial cell–stimulating hormone or ICSH) stimulates the Leydig cells lying between these tubules to secrete the androgen.[18]

Influences on Physical Growth

The precise physiological cause for onset of the physical changes characteristic of this period is unknown, and cultural and possibly hereditary differences in size and onset of changes exist. The hypothalamus initiates puberty through secretion of substances that stimulate the anterior pituitary gland to release gonadotropic hormones, somatotropic hormone (STH), or growth hormone (GH), thyroid-stimulating hormone (TSH), and adrenocorticotropic hormone (ACTH).[18,27]

Both male and female hormones are produced in varying amounts in each sex throughout life. During prepubescent years, the adrenal cortex secretes a small amount of **sex hormones.** However, it is sex hormone production that accompanies maturation of ovaries and testes that is responsible for the physiological changes observed in puberty. Both forms of gonadal hormones stimulate epiphyseal fusion by repression of the pituitary growth hormone, thus slowing physical growth at the end of puberty.[14,27]

Development of Body Systems

Musculoskeletal. Structural changes—growth in skeletal size, muscle mass, adipose tissue, and skin—are significant in adolescence. The skeletal system grows faster than the supporting muscles. Hands and feet grow out of proportion to the body. Large muscles develop faster than small muscles; poor posture and decreased coordination result. Males and females differ in skeletal growth patterns: males have greater length in arms and legs relative to trunk size, in part because of a prolonged prepubertal growth period in boys. (Males are also more clumsy than females.) Males also have a greater shoulder width, a difference which begins in prepuberty. Ossification of the skeletal system occurs later for boys than girls. In girls, estrogen influences bone ossification and early unity of the epiphyses with shafts of the long bones, resulting in shorter stature.[19,27] Muscle growth continues in males during late adolescence because of androgen production. Muscle growth in females is proportionate to growth of other tissue. Adipose tissue distribution over thighs, buttocks, and breasts occurs predominantly in females and is related to estrogen production.[18]

Integumentary. Skin texture changes. Sebaceous glands become active and increase in size, and thus acne may develop. Sweat glands are fully developed, are more responsive to emotional stimuli, and are more active in males.

Cardiovascular. The heart grows slowly at first, compared with the rest of the body, resulting in inadequate oxygenation and fatigue. The heart continues to enlarge until age 17 or 18.[13,18] The heart should be found at the fifth left intercostal space, as in the adult, and most functional murmurs should be outgrown. Systolic blood pressure and pulse pressure increase; blood pressure averages 100 to 120/50 to 70. Pulse rate averages 60 to 68 beats per minute. Females have a slightly higher pulse rate, basal body temperature, and lower systolic pressure than males.[27]

Respiratory. The respiratory system also grows slowly relative to the rest of the body, contributing to inadequate oxygenation. Respiratory rate averages 16 to 20 per minute. Males' greater shoulder width and chest size result in greater respiratory volume, greater vital capacity, and increased respiration; however, lung capacity in males matures later than in females, in whom lung capacity matures at about 17 or 18 years.[27]

Hematological. Red blood cell mass and hemoglobin concentration increase in both sexes because of increased hormone production. Hematocrit levels are high in males. Platelet count and sedimentation rate are higher in females. White blood cell count is lower in both sexes than it was earlier.[27]

Gastrointestinal. This system matures rapidly from 10 to 20 years. By age 21 all 32 teeth have usually appeared. Stomach capacity increases to about 1 quart (more than 900 cubic centimeters), which correlates with increased appetite, as the stomach becomes longer and less tubular. Increased gastric acidity occurs to facilitate digestion of the increased food intake. Intestines grow in length and circumference. Muscles in the stomach and intestinal wall become thicker and stronger. The liver attains adult size, location, and function.[18,19]

Changes in fluid and electrolyte balance reflect changes in body composition in terms of bones, muscle, and adipose tissue. The percentage of body water decreases, reaching adult levels. About 60% of the male's total body weight is fluid, compared with 50% in the female; the difference is the greater percentage of muscle mass in the male. Because of their greater muscle mass, males have a 15% higher potassium concentration.[19]

Renal. Urinary bladder capacity increases; the adolescent voids up to 1½ quarts (1500 cubic centimeters) daily. Renal function is like that of the adult.[19,27]

Special senses. The eyeball lengthens, increasing the incidence of myopia in early adolescence. Auditory acuity peaks at age 13, and from that age on, hearing acuity gradually decreases. Sensitivity to odors develops at puberty; the female's increased sensitivity to musklike fragrances may be related to estrogen levels.[19,27]

COGNITIVE DEVELOPMENT

Formal Operations Stage

Tests of mental ability indicate that adolescence is the time when the mind has great ability to acquire and use knowledge.

According to Piaget, the **formal operations** period differs from concrete operations in that a much larger range of symbolic processes and logic is used.[15,25] Adolescents use available information to look for further facts, consider alternate solutions to problems, project thinking into the future, and try to categorize thoughts into usable forms. They are capable of highly imaginative thinking. The adolescent's ideas may be oversimplified and lack originality, but the structure is set for adult thinking patterns. The adolescent can solve hypothetical, mental, and verbal problems; use scientific reasoning; deal with the past, present, and future; and understand causality.[14]

Keniston[10] describes cognitive development of late adolescence as proceeding from a simple understanding of right and wrong and either-or of an issue, to an awareness of multiplicity, a realization of less-well-defined areas in life, and a more existential sense of truth. Now the person thinks about thinking, achieves a new level of consciousness, and manifests a higher level of creativity. This stage involves being very aware of inner processes, focusing on states of consciousness as something to be controlled and altered, and thinking about the ideal self and society.[10,11]

If the adolescent does not stay in school, his intellectual potential will not be developed. Dropping out of school occurs for a variety of reasons and has unfortunate consequences. The LPN/LVN can encourage the adolescent to complete formal education.

SOCIAL DEVELOPMENT

Peer Group Influences

The peer group influences the adolescent to a greater extent than parents, teachers, popular heroes, religious leaders, or other adults do[13] (Fig. 10-4). Because peer groups are so important, the adolescent has intense loyalty to them. Social relationships take precedence over family and counteract feelings of emptiness, isolation, and loneliness. Significance is attached to activities deemed important by peers. Peers serve as models or instructors for skills yet to be acquired. Explanations by peers may be more readily understood than adult explanations.[26] The practical/vocational nurse may need to include peers in the teaching plan if it is to be successful. Peer groups provide a sense of acceptance, prestige, belonging, approval, and opportunities for learning how to behave now and in later adult roles. The peer group helps the adolescent define personal identity and adapt to a changing body image and heightened sexual feelings. The peer group has well-defined types of behavior for masculinity and femininity. As the adolescent tries a variety of acceptable behaviors within the safety of the group, he or she incorporates new ideas and develops more mature relationships. The adolescent who is rejected by peers may not learn the social skills and ability to form relationships necessary for the adult culture.[14]

Peer group relations are beneficial, but they can also direct the adolescent into antisocial behavior through pressure to conform and the need to gain approval. Adolescents may participate in drug and alcohol abuse, sexual intercourse, or various delinquent acts not entirely because they want to or enjoy them, but rather to prove themselves, vent aggression, or gain superiority over younger or fringe members of the group. They may even gain pleasure from sadistic activities toward others.[14,18] Parents have reason to be concerned about their adolescent's peers and to guide their child into wholesome activities and groups that will reinforce the values they have taught.[19] The practical/vocational nurse can support parents in their efforts.

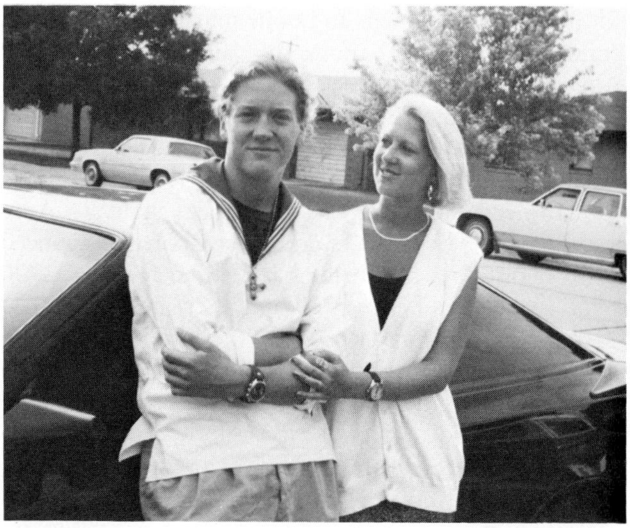

FIG. 10-4 Peer interaction is essential to healthy adolescent development.

EMOTIONAL DEVELOPMENT

Emotional Characteristics

Emotional characteristics of the personality cannot be separated from family, physical, intellectual, and social development. Emotionally the adolescent is characterized by mood swings and extremes of behavior. Table 10-1 lists typical contradictions.[9,14,18] Emotional development requires an interweaving and organization of opposing tendencies into a sense of unity and continuity. This process occurs during adolescence in a complex and truly impressive way to move the person toward psychological maturity.[9] The practical/vocational nurse needs to be understanding and flexible with the adolescent's changing moods.

Development of Identity

The psychosexual crisis of adolescence, according to Erikson, is **identity formation** versus identity diffusion: "Who am I?" "How do I feel?" "Where am I going?"

Table 10-1 Contrasting Emotional Responses of Adolescents

Independent Behaviors	Dependent Behaviors
Happy, easy-going, loving, self-confident, sense of humor	Sad, irritable, withdrawn, fearful, worried
Energetic, self-assertive	Apathetic, passive
Questioning, critical of others	Strong allegiance to others
Exhibitionistic or at ease with self	Excessively modest or self-conscious
Interested in intellectual pursuits	Daydreaming, fantasizing
Cooperative, seeking responsibility	Rebellious, evading work, ritualistic behavior, dropping out from society
Suggestible to outside influences	Unaccepting of new ideas
Desirous of adult privileges	Apprehensive about adult responsibilities

"What meaning is there in life?" Identity formation results through synthesis of biopsychosocial characteristics from a number of sources, for example, earlier gender identity, parental and friend relationships, and social class, ethnic, religious, and occupational group influences.[5-7,14] Identity formation implies emerging from this era with a sense of wholeness, knowing the self as a unique person, feeling responsibility, loyalty, and commitment as a unique person—and feeling responsibility, loyalty, and commitment to a value system.

Identity diffusion results if the adolescent fails to achieve a sense of identity. With identity diffusion, he or she feels impotent, insecure, and disillusioned. The adolescent feels that he or she is losing grip with reality; is impatient but unable to initiate action or decision making; cannot delay gratification and appears brazen or arrogant; and is apprehensive about and avoids adult behavior, fearing loss of uniqueness by entering adulthood. The real danger of identity diffusion looms when a youth finds a negative solution to the quest for identity. He or she gives up, feels defeated, and pursues antisocial behavior, since "it's better to be bad than nobody at all." Identity diffusion is more likely to occur if the teenager has close contact with an adult who is still confused about personal identity and who is rebellious against society.[5-7,14] The practical/vocational nurse can foster identity formation by reinforcement of positive behavior, listening, providing support during trying times, and being a role model of maturity.

Self-Concept and Body Image Development

Development of self-concept and body image is closely akin to cognitive organization of experiences and identity formation. Earlier experiences that were helpful enabled the adolescent to feel good about the body and self. If the youngster enters adolescence feeling negative about self or the body, this will be a difficult period.[14]

Other factors influence the adolescent's self-concept, including (1) age of maturation, (2) degree of attractiveness, (3) name or nickname, (4) size and physique appropriate to gender, (5) degree of identification with the same-sex parent, (6) level of aspiration and ability to reach ideals, and (7) peer relationships.

The rapid growth of the adolescent period is an important factor in body image revision. Growth changes cannot be denied; to function, adolescents are forced to alter their mental picture of themselves. More important than the growth changes is the meaning attached to the changes. The adult who says, "That's all right, John, we all have our clumsy moments," is providing the understanding that a comment such as, "Can't you ever walk through the room without knocking something down?" denies. The adolescent needs this understanding because of fear of rejection and oversensitivity to others' opinions.[14] If the teen does not seem to care about appearance, he or she may have already decided, "I'm so ugly, what's the use?" Adolescents may overemphasize a defect and underevaluate themselves as persons. If adolescents do not get much acceptance for themselves and their bodies, they may try to compensate for real or imagined defects through sports, vocational or academic success, a religious commitment, or a date or group of friends that enhances prestige, which can promote healthy development and improve self-esteem.[19]

By late adolescence overall self-image development is complete. Self-esteem should be high, and self-concept should have stabilized. Adolescents feel autonomous but no longer believe they are so unique that no one has ever experienced what they are currently experiencing. Late adolescents no longer believe everyone is watching or being critical of their physical or personality characteristics. Egocentricity has declined. Interactions with the opposite sex are more comfortable, although awareness of gender is keen.[14]

PROMOTING OPTIMUM HEALTH

Nutrition

During this time of accelerated physical and emotional development the body's metabolic rate increases and nutritional needs increase. The peak requirements occur in the year of maximum growth; calorie and protein requirements during this year are higher than at almost any other time of life. The adolescent female's requirements are equaled or surpassed only during pregnancy and lactation. Even after the obvious period of accelerated growth has ended, nutritional intake must be adequate for muscle development and bone mineralization, which continues. Table 10-2 shows the daily requirements for adolescents.[14,28]

Both males and females have an increased appetite. A fast-growing boy's stomach capacity may be too small to accommodate the amount of food he requires to meet growth needs unless he eats at frequent intervals. Adolescent females between 11 and 14 years of age may need 2200 calories per day; males of the same age need 2700 calories. Females between 15 and 18 years of age need 2100 calories and males need 2800 calories.[28] However, the stage of sexual maturation, rate of physical growth, and amount of physical and social activity should be considered before determining exact caloric needs. In addition, the nutritional needs differ for pregnant and nonpregnant adolescents.

Protein must be increased to maintain a positive nitrogen balance within the body during the metabolic pro-

Table 10-2 Recommended Minimum Daily Serving of Basic Four Food Groups

Food Group	Nonpregnant Teenager	Pregnant Teenager
Dairy products	4 servings	4 servings
Meat and meat alternatives	2 servings	3 servings
Fruit, vegetables, or juices	4 servings	5 servings
Breads and cereals	4 servings	4 servings

NOTE: the following amounts equal one serving[14]:
Dairy products: 1 C milk, 1 oz cheese, 1¼ C cottage cheese, ⅓ C dry milk, 1¾ C ice cream.
Meat and meat alternatives: 2 eggs, 2 oz lean meat, 1 C beans or split peas, 4 Tbsp peanut butter, 2 oz cheddar cheese, ½ C cottage cheese.
Fruits, vegetables, or juices: ½ C or a medium fresh fruit or vegetable.
Breads and cereals: 1 slice bread, ½ C cooked cereal, ¾ C ready-to-eat cereal, ½ to ¾ C cooked macaroni, spaghetti, rice, or grits.

cess.[28] More iron is needed because of the increased muscle, soft tissue, and red cell growth. Girls may be especially susceptible to iron deficiency at menarche.[28] Calcium (1200 mg daily) is needed for bone growth and continued teeth formation. If the adolescent drinks 1 quart of milk daily, this dietary requirement can be met. The practical/vocational nurse can teach about and encourage good nutrition.

Exercise, Rest, and Sleep

The teenager is expending large amounts of energy and functioning with an inadequate oxygen supply; both these contribute to fatigue and need for additional rest. In addition, protein synthesis and growth hormone production occur more readily during sleep.[27]

Limit setting may be necessary to ensure adequate opportunities for rest, especially for the ill adolescent. Rest is not necessarily sleep. A period of time spent with some quiet activity is also beneficial for the well adolescent. Every afternoon should not be filled with extracurricular activities or home responsibilites. When there is school the next morning, the adolescent should be in bed at a reasonable hour.[14]

Leisure

Sports, dancing, hobbies, reading, listening to the radio or stereo, talking on the telephone, daydreaming, experimenting with hairstyles, cosmetics, or new clothes, or just loafing have been teenagers' favorite activities for decades. Motorcycle riding, sports, driving and working on cars, watching television, working with a computer, and playing video games are also popular. Political activism draws some youths; various causes rise and then fade in interest as the youth matures. "Everybody's doing it" is a strong influence on the adolescent's interests and activities.[14]

Many parents consider a party in the home for a group of teenagers a safe use of leisure time. This is undoubtedly true if parents and other adults are on the premises and can give guidance as needed, and if the parents are not themselves supplying the teens with alcohol and drugs. In spite of protests to the contrary, teenagers may also feel more secure when their parents are actively interested in knowing about the youths' activities. Parental limits can reduce feelings of conflict and give an excuse to avoid an activity he or she does not want to engage in.[19] The practical/vocational nurse can encourage parents to give the necessary guidance and limits.

For some teenagers, there is little leisure time. They may have considerable home responsibility or may work to earn money for their own needs or to help support the family. Other youths are active in volunteer work. Ideally, the adolescent has some free time for personal pursuits, to stand around with friends, and to sit and daydream.

Immunizations

Immunizations are a part of health protection to the adolescent, although they may be overlooked by that time of life. The practical/vocational nurse should teach adolescents and parents directly or through informational flyers that if the immunizations discussed in relation to other age groups have not been received, they should be given as indicated. If the adolescent has been routinely immunized, combined tetanus and diphtheria toxoids (adult-type Td) should be given about 14 to 16 years of age and every 10 years thereafter. Pertussis vaccine should not be given to anyone over 6 years of age. The oral form of polio virus (OPV) immunization is recommended for all children younger than 18 years of age unless contraindicated. Influenza virus vaccine, pneumococcal polysaccharide vaccine, and hepatitis B vaccine should be given to adolescents in selected high-risk groups. For clean wounds, no tetanus booster is needed by a fully immunized person unless more than 10 years has elapsed since the last inoculation. For dirty or contaminated wounds, a booster dose can be given if more than 5 years has elapsed since the last inoculation. Periodic testing for tuberculosis should be included in all adolescent immunization programs.[14,20,24]

Injury Prevention and Safety Education

Safety courses should be required for every adolescent, including driver education, knowledge of safety programs in the community, water safety, routine safety practices, and emergency care measures. Many accidents and deaths could be avoided if the adolescent were better equipped to handle their new freedom.* Parents and youths should be informed of the dangers, as well as exercise and prestige value, involved with certain sports and privileges. The practical/vocational nurse should include teaching safety measures along with other teaching of the parent and adolescent.

Developmental Tasks

The following developmental tasks should be met by the end of adolescence.[4,14]:

1. Accept one's changing body size, shape, and function and understand the meaning of physical maturity.
2. Learn to handle one's body in a variety of physical skills and to maintain good health.
3. Achieve a satisfying and socially acceptable feminine or masculine role, recognizing how these roles have similarities and distinctions.
4. Become a member of one or more peer groups and develop skills in relating to a variety of people, including those of the opposite sex.
5. Achieve independence from parents and other adults while maintaining an affectionate relationship with them.
6. Select an occupation in line with interests and abilities (although the choice of occupation may later change) and prepare for economic independence.
7. Prepare to settle down, frequently for marriage and family life, or for a close relationship with another, by developing a responsible attitude, acquiring needed knowledge, making appropriate decisions, and forming a relationship based on love rather than infatuation.
8. Develop the intellectual and work skills and social sensitivities of a competent citizen.
9. Desire and achieve socially responsible behavior in the cultural setting.
10. Develop a workable philosophy, a maturing set of values, and worthy ideals, and assume standards of social morality.

Until these tasks are accomplished, the person remains immature—an adolescent regardless of chronological age.

* A teenage safety checklist can be obtained from the National Society for Crippled Children and Adults, 2023 W Ogden Avenue, Chicago, IL, 60612, to help the adolescent be aware of how to improve safety behavior.

REFERENCES AND SUGGESTED READINGS

1. Adams B: Adolescent health care: needs, priorities, and services, Nurs Clin North Am 18(2):237-248, 1983.
2. Advance Report of Final Mortality Statistics, 1983, National Center of Health Statistics, DHHS P#85-1120, Monthly Vital Statistics Report, 34, no 6 (Sept 26, 1985), 18-20.
3. Cangelosi A, Gressard C, and Mines R: The effects of a rational thinking group on self-concept in the adolescent, School Counselor 27(5):357, 1980.
4. Duvall E and Miller B: Marriage and family development, ed 6, New York, 1984, Harper & Row Publishers.
5. Erikson EH: Childhood and society, ed 2, New York, 1963, WW Norton.
6. Erikson EH: Identity: you and crisis, New York, 1968, WW Norton.
7. Erikson EH: Memorandum on youth. In Sze W, editor: Human life cycle, New York, 1975, Jason Aronson.
8. Freeman E and others: Adolescent contraceptive use: comparisons of male and female attitudes and information, Am J Publ Health 70(8):790, 1980.
9. Gesell A, Ilg F, and Ames L: Youth: the years from ten to sixteen, New York, 1956, Harper & Brothers.
10. Keniston K: Youth: a new stage of life, Am Scholar 39:631, 1970.
11. Keniston K: Youth as a stage of life. In Sze W, editor: Human life cycle, New York, 1975, Jason Aronson.
12. Manning M: Disappearing childhood: 6 Going on 16, Kappa Delta Pi Record 14, Fall 1985.
13. Moshman D, Glover J, and Bruning R: Developmental psychology, Boston, 1987, Little, Brown & Co.
14. Murray R and Zentner J: Nursing assessment and health promotion strategies through the lifespan, ed 4, East Norwalk, Conn, 1989, Appleton-Century-Crofts.
15. Piaget J: The growth of logical thinking from childhood to adolescence, New York, 1961, Basic Books.
16. Poll: most adults favor sex education in school, Health Link 45, March 1987.
17. Scales P: Promoting adolescent health: the need to model positive skills and challenge assumptions, Health Education 17(1):27, 1986.
18. Schuster CS and Smith-Ashburn S: The process of human development: a holistic life-span approach, ed 2, Boston, 1986, Little, Brown & Co.
19. Scipien GM and others: Comprehensive pediatric nursing, ed 4, St Louis, 1990, The CV Mosby Co.
20. Selekman J: Immunization: what's it all about? Am J Nurs 80(8):1440, 1980.
21. Smith D: Meeting the psychosocial needs of teenage mothers and fathers, Nurs Clin North Am 19(2):369, 1984.
22. Turner J and Helms D: Lifespan development, ed 3, New York, 1987, Holt, Rinehart & Winston.
23. US Department of Health and Human Services: New recommended schedule for active immunization of normal infants and children, Morbidity and Mortality Weekly Report, 35, no 37 (September 19, 1986), 577-579.
24. Wadsworth B: Piaget's theory of cognitive and affective development, ed 3, New York, 1984, David McKay Co. Inc.
25. Webb P: Piaget: implications for teaching, Theory Into Practice 19(2):93, 1980.
26. Whaley L and Wong D: Nursing care of infants and children, ed 4, St Louis, 1991, The CV Mosby Co.
27. Williams SR: Nutrition and diet therapy, ed 6, St Louis, 1989, Times Mirror/Mosby College Publishing.

CHAPTER CHALLENGE

KEY POINTS

- Behavioral differences exist in early, middle, and late adolescence.
- During middle and late adolescence, most severe changes occur in the parent/child relationship.
- Developmental tasks for a family with adolescents involve maintaining a grasp on the facets of life that continue to have meaning while striving for a deeper awareness and understanding of the present situation.
- Adolescence is the second major period of accelerated growth (infancy was the first). Every system is growing rapidly, but physiological changes do not occur evenly.
- Nutritional needs are increased because of rapid growth and higher metabolism.
- The adolescent can solve hypothetical, mental and verbal problems; use scientific reasoning; deal with the past, present, and future; and understand causality.
- The peer group influences the adolescent to a greater extent than do parents, teachers, popular heroes, religious leaders, and other adults.
- The psychosexual crisis of adolescence, according to Erikson, is identity formation versus identity diffusion. Identity formation occurs with successful emotional development.
- Developmental self-concept and body image are closely akin to cognitive organization of experience and identity formation.
- Adolescents need additional rest because they are expending large amounts of energy and functioning with an inadequate oxygen supply.
- Peer group relationships and leisure activities affect mental, emotional, and social development and relationships.
- Immunization and safety education must be continued with the adolescent.
- Successful accomplishment of developmental tasks is essential for a person to mature into young adulthood.

STUDY QUESTIONS

1. In early adolescence, the dependency-independency struggle is demonstrated by:
   a. Less involvement in family activities
   b. Peer friendships decreasing in importance
   c. Peer group nonallegiance
   d. Compliance with parental and other adult discipline
2. Late adolescence may still be present by:
   a. 14 to 16 years of age
   b. 16 to 18 years of age
   c. 20 to 25 years of age
3. Most ambivalence and negative behavior in the adolescent stems from:
   a. Actual external restrictions imposed
   b. Perceived external restrictions
4. In the initial phase of the growth spurt, the adolescent's increase in height results from:
   a. Increase in trunk length
   b. Lengthening of the legs
   c. Increase in the chest length
5. Nocturnal emissions of seminal fluid first occur at about what age:
   a. 14 years
   b. 16 years
   c. 18 years
6. North American males complete growth in stature at approximately what age:
   a. 14 to 15 years
   b. 14 to 16 years
   c. 15 to 17 years
   d. 18 to 19 years
7. In the male, the hormonal system for reproductive behavior is:
   a. Not a cyclical pattern
   b. A cyclical pattern
8. In the female adolescent, what influences bone ossification and early unity of epiphyses with the shaft of the long bones:
   a. Progesterone
   b. Estrogen
   c. Luteinizing hormone
9. The formal operations period differs from concrete operations in that:
   a. The individual uses nonscientific reasoning
   b. An unawareness of multiplicity is noted
   c. A much longer range of symbolic processes and logic is used
10. The following are independent behaviors of the adolescent *except:*
    a. Self-assertion
    b. Questioning
    c. Excessive modesty
    d. Desire for adult privileges
11. The psychosexual crisis of adolescence, according to Erikson, is:
    a. Trust versus nontrust
    b. Identity formation versus identity diffusion
    c. Autonomy versus shame
    d. Ego integrity versus despair
12. Development of self-concept and body image is closely akin to:
    a. Cognitive organization of experiences and identity formation
    b. Degree of identity diffusion
13. Adolescent males between 15 and 18 years of age need at least how many calories per 24 hours:
    a. 2200 calories
    b. 2000 calories
    c. 2800 calories
    d. 4800 calories
14. An adolescent requires how much milk to meet nutritional requirements of calcium:
    a. 1 quart
    b. 1 pint
    c. 1½ quarts
15. If the adolescent has been routinely immunized during infancy and early childhood, what vaccines should be given at 14 to 16 years of age:
    a. Tetanus and diphtheria toxoid (adult-type Td)
    b. Pertussis vaccine
    c. Pneumococcal polysaccharide vaccine

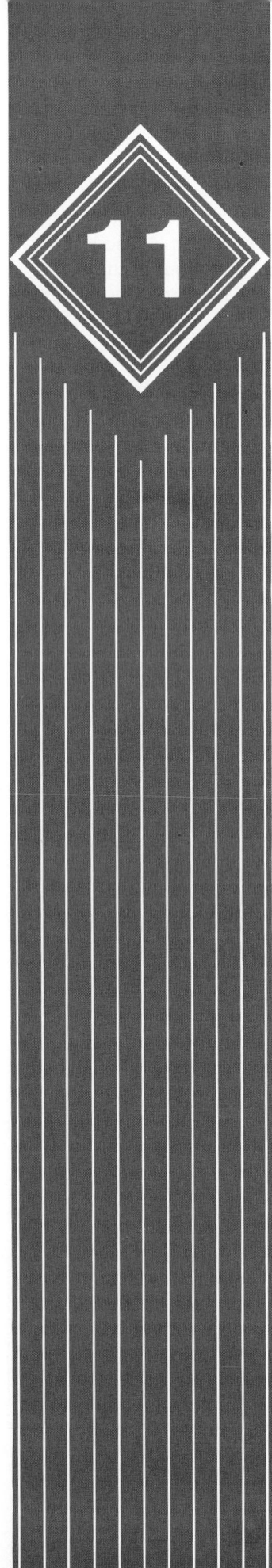

11

The Adult

RUTH BECKMANN MURRAY

LEARNING OBJECTIVES

After reading this chapter, the student should be able to do the following:

- Define the key terms.
- Contrast family relationships in young, middle, and older adulthood.
- List the developmental tasks of the young, middle-aged, and older adult's family.
- Contrast the physical characteristics of the young, middle-aged, and older adult.
- Describe nutritional requirements for the adult.
- Compare the stages of the sleep cycle.
- Discuss the adult's need for rest, sleep, exercise, and leisure.
- Discuss health promotion measures in adulthood.
- Contrast cognitive characteristics of the young, middle-aged, and older adult.
- Describe emotional characteristics during adulthood.
- Describe developmental tasks for the young, middle-aged, and older adult.

RELATED TOPICS OF INTEREST

- The family (Chapter 7)
- Care of the patient with a reproductive disorder (Chapter 36)
- Care of the aging (Chapter 48)

KEY TERMS

Define the following:

- ageism
- aging
- atrophy
- caregiver role
- chronological age
- climacteric
- dysmenorrhea
- ego integrity
- generation gap
- generativity
- intimacy
- isolation
- leisure
- lentigo senilis
- menopause
- middle age
- midlife crisis
- premenstrual syndrome
- presbycusis
- presbyopia
- psychological age
- self-despair
- stagnation or self-absorption
- turgor
- widow(er)hood
- young adulthood

THE YOUNG ADULT

The practical/vocational nurse will care for adults in many health care settings. Many patients will be middle-aged or elderly. Information in this chapter will assist in assessment and planning for intervention. The chapter describes changes through the adult years as a basis for nursing care.

Childhood and adolescence are the periods for growing up; adulthood is the time for settling down. The changes in **young adulthood** relate more to sociocultural forces and expectations and to value and cognitive changes than to physical development.

The young adult in the 20s is expected to enter new roles of finding an occupation, establishing a family, and demonstrating responsibility at work, at home, and in society and to develop values, attitudes, and interests in keeping with these roles. Young adults may have difficulty through their 30s and 40s if they work at primarily one of these roles at a time and neglect the others, which can create problems for persons in any of these areas.

Family Development and Relationships

The young adult's offspring and parents. The major family goal is the reorganization of the family into a continuing unity while releasing maturing young people into lives of their own. Most families actively prepare their children to leave home.

In the United States the young adult is expected to be independent from the parents' home and care. Sometimes the young adult does not leave the parents' home as quickly as parents would like, or returns because of prolonged education, divorce, unemployment, and increasing apartment rent. Parents may resent the intrusion. If young adults do live at home, they should expect and be expected to assume a share of the home responsibilities and to adjust life-style to that of the parents. Sometimes the adult offspring can be a help. Some parents delay their adult children's independence because of their own needs. As young adult offspring establish families, parents should take the complementary roles of letting go and standing by with encouragement, reassurance, and appreciation. The practical/vocational nurse may be in the role of assisting the adult sort through these issues.

Family developmental tasks. The following family developmental tasks must be accomplished by the family of the young adult. Listening, teaching, and referral to other sources of help are ways the practical/vocational nurse can assist the parents of adult offspring with these tasks[9]:

1. Rearrange the home physically, and reallocate resources (space, material, objects) to meet the needs of remaining members.
2. Meet the expenses of releasing the offspring, and redistribute the budget.
3. Redistribute the responsibilities among grown and growing children and finally between the husband and wife or among the adult members living in the household on the basis of interests, ability, and availability.
4. Maintain communication within the family to contribute to harmony and happiness while remaining available to young adult and other offspring.
5. Enjoy companionship and sexual intimacy as a husband/wife team while incorporating changes.
6. Widen the family circle to include the close friends or spouses of the offspring, as well as the entire family of in-laws.
7. Reconcile conflicting loyalties and philosophies of life.

Physical Development

Although body and mind changes continue through life, physical structures are completed when the person reaches young adulthood. Changes that occur during adult life are different from those in childhood; they are slower and smaller in increment. The practical/vocational nurse will assess the body systems during patient care and teach about physical characteristics described in the following material.

General measurements

Weight and height. An average adult person is described only in physiology texts or insurance tables. Normal values cover a wide range in healthy individuals. Height and weight depend on many factors: heredity, sex, socioeconomic class, geographical area, food habits and preferences, level of activity, and emotional and physical environment.

Development of body systems

Musculoskeletal. Skeletal growth for the young adult is completed by age 25, when the epiphyseal line calcifies and fuses with the main shaft of the long bones. By the 40s, the bones may have lost some mass and density. The process may begin earlier in women. With increasing age, the cartilage in all joints has a more limited ability to regenerate itself. Normally, posture is erect.[26,33]

Body systems are functioning at their peak efficiency. Peak muscle strength is attained between the ages of 19 and 30. There is a 10% loss of strength between the ages of 30 and 60; this loss usually occurs in the back and leg muscles. However, a person can maintain peak performance throughout the 30s and much of the 40s with regular exercise and dietary moderation.[26]

Integumentary. The skin of the young adult is smooth, and skin **turgor** is taut. The skin of the African-American manifests some conditions that are not typically seen in Caucasians. Refer to the article by Sykes, Kelly, and Kennedy on African-American skin problems for a pictorial and descriptive summary.[52] In late young adulthood, the skin begins to dry and wrinkle.

Cardiovascular. Heart and circulatory changes occur gradually with age, depending on exercise and diet patterns. Maximum cardiac output is achieved and peaks between 20 and 30 years of age. Heart rate averages 72 beats per minute. Blood pressure averages 120/80 to 100/60.

Respiratory. Respirations average 12 to 20 breaths per minute. Chest muscles are strong; lung tissue is elastic. The maximum breathing capacity decreases between ages 20 and 40. Breathing rates and capacity will differ according to the size and condition of the individual.[26]

Gastrointestinal. The digestive organs function smoothly. Digestive juices gradually decrease after age 30. The last four molars (wisdom teeth) may erupt in the 20s.

Neurological. The brain continues to grow into young adulthood and reaches maximum weight during adulthood. Visual and auditory sensory perception should be at peak. Women in this age group can detect high auditory tones better than men.

Endocrine. Adrenal secretion of cortisol (hydrocortisone) decreases about 30% over the entire adult life span. Because plasma cortisol levels remain constant, the young adult maintains good response to stress.[33]

Reproductive

Sexual maturity. Sexual maturity for men is usually reached in the late teens, but their sexual drive remains high through young adulthood. In healthy women, menstruation is well established and regular by the late teens. Female organs are fully matured. Optimal period for reproduction is between 20 and 30 years of age.

Premenstrual syndrome. **Premenstrual syndrome** (PMS) and **dysmenorrhea** occur in about 10% of women. Box 11-1 shows physiological symptoms and signs and emotional reactions that are reported by some women.

Not all of these signs and symptoms appear together; they are variable in degree, and they decrease after menses begins.[26,36]

The following measures can offset or prevent symptoms.[26] The practical/vocational nurse should teach these practices to the woman who has PMS:

1. Consume less caffeine, sugar, alcohol, and salt, especially during the premenstrual period.
2. Eat four to six small meals a day rather than two or three meals, to minimize the risk of hypoglycemia that accompanies PMS.

BOX 11-1 PREMENSTRUAL SYMPTOMS, SIGNS, AND REACTIONS

PHYSIOLOGICAL SYMPTOMS AND SIGNS	EMOTIONAL REACTIONS
Appetite change, craving salty or sweet foods	Apprehension/anxiety
Acne/hives	Confusion
Abdominal distention	Sadness/depression
Breast tenderness	Forgetfulness
Clumsiness	Frequent crying
Constipation or diarrhea	Indecisiveness
Dizziness	Irritability
Edema around eyes, in fingers, feet, legs, thighs, hips, breasts, abdomen	Restlessness
	Suspiciousness
Fatigue; need for sleep increases	Tension
Headache/backache	Withdrawal
Menstrual cramps	
Nausea	
Sex drive change	
Weight gain	

3. Snack on complex carbohydrates, such as fresh fruits, vegetable sticks, and whole wheat crackers, which provide energy without excessive sugar.
4. Drink 6 to 8 glasses of water; it will help prevent fluid retention by flushing excess salt from the body.
5. Limit fat intake, especially in red meat, which builds hormones that cause breast tenderness and fluid retention; choose low-fat dairy products.
6. Eat more whole grains, nuts, and raw greens, which are high in vitamin B, magnesium, and potassium, and add vitamin B_6 and calcium, nutrients that reduce symptoms.
7. Develop a variety of activities, including exercise, rest, relaxation techniques, massage, and creative activity, so that focus is not on symptoms.
8. Discuss feelings with family and friends so that they can be more understanding of behavior.

Ovulation. Ovulation normally occurs in every menstrual cycle, but not necessarily midcycle. The ovum is capable of being fertilized for 24 to 48 hours postovulation.

The mucous cycle by which to predict ovulation is as follows; the nurse may give information to the young adult about the cycle[16]:

1. The cycle begins with menstruation.
2. The period is usually followed by a few "dry days," when no mucus is seen or felt.
3. As the ovum begins to ripen, some mucus is felt at the vaginal opening and can be seen if the woman wipes the vaginal area with toilet tissue; this mucus is generally yellow or white, but definitely opaque and tenacious.
4. When the blood estrogen level (derived from the ripening ovum) reaches a critical point, the glands of the cervix respond with a different mucus; this fertile mucus starts out cloudy, is not tenacious, and becomes very clear, like raw egg white.
5. After ovulation, progesterone causes the abrupt cessation of the clear, slippery, fertile mucus and causes production of mucus that is tenacious and sometimes not present at the vagina.
6. Progesterone prepares the uterine lining for the reception of the egg if the egg has been fertilized.
7. Usually the egg is ovulated within 24 hours of the peak wetness, but this interval may be as long as 48 hours.

If this method is used to avoid pregnancy, there should be abstinence from intercourse from the beginning of the slippery, fertile mucus until the height of wetness ("peak day," when there may be so much wetness that mucus is not only seen, but moisture is noted on the underclothing), plus a full 72 hours to ensure that the ovum will not be impregnated.[26]

Human sexual response. The human sexual response cycle involves physiological reactions, psychological components, and psychosocial influences on behavior. The nurse may teach the adult about the physiological reactions of the cycle.

The four phases of the cycle are excitement, plateau, orgasm, and resolution; the phases vary with each person and from time to time[22]:

1. The excitement phase develops from any source of bodily or psychic stimuli; this phase may be interrupted, prolonged, or ended by distracting stimuli.
2. The plateau phase follows excitement, during which sexual tension intensifies.
3. Orgasm is the climax of sexual tension increase, which lasts for a few seconds, during which vasocongestion and myotonia occur as a result of forceful muscle contractions.
4. The resolution phase returns the body to the preexcitement physiology; the woman may begin another cycle immediately if stimulated, but the man is unable to be restimulated for about 30 minutes.

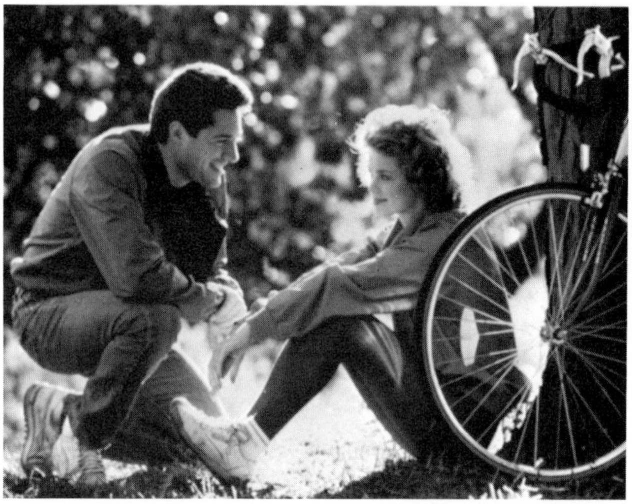

FIG. 11-1 Young adulthood—interacting and gaining a greater respect for others.

Emotional Development

The nurse may contribute to emotional development by the care that is given. Understanding emotional development assists in modifying the approach during care.

Young adulthood is a time when there is increased clarity and consistency of personality and identity, established interests and activities, increased coping ability, less defensiveness, a responsibility for self and others, and more appreciation of surroundings.

Developmental crisis. According to Erikson, the psychosexual crisis is intimacy versus self-isolation. **Intimacy** involves mutual love and trust, sharing of feelings, and responsibility to and cooperation with each other. Intimacy includes intercourse, but it means more than physical or genital contact. The person is involved with people, work, hobbies, and community issues (Fig. 11-1). Intimacy is when two people (in marriage or in a close relationship) accept all aspects of the other and adjust their behavior to each other's behavior and needs for mutual satisfaction.[26]

Isolation involves becoming withdrawn, lonely, and conceited and behaving in a stereotyped manner.[21] The isolated person often experiences a long succession of unsuccessful relationships, overextends self without any real interest or feeling, and then cannot sustain close friendships. No real exchange of fellowship occurs.

Cognitive Development

Erikson believed that the basis for adult cognitive performance is established during the school years when the child accomplishes the task of industry, learns how to learn and win recognition by producing and achieving, and learns to enjoy learning. Children learn an attitude that lasts into adulthood: how much effort a task takes and how long and hard they should work for what is desired or expected. The sense of industry is necessary in adult life, as a worker, family member, and citizen.

Promoting Optimum Health

Nutrition. Table 11-1 lists the recommended daily number of servings for each food group and the recommended daily caloric intake for young adults and pregnant and lactating women.[26,42]

Caloric intake should be based on occupation, amount of physical activity or mental effort, emotional state, age, body size, climate, individual metabolism, and presence of disease. Women have a 5% to 10% lower metabolism than men of comparable height and weight; thus healthy,

Table 11-1 Recommended Daily Average Calories and Number of Servings from Each Food Group

Food Group/Calories	Young Adult	Pregnant Woman	Lactating Woman
Milk and milk products	2 or more cups	3 or 4 cups	4 or more cups
Meat, fish, or protein equivalent	2 (2 to 3 oz) servings	3 (2 to 3 oz) servings	3 to 4 (2 to 3 oz) servings
Fruits and vegetables (including a high vitamin C source)	4 (½ cup) servings	4 to 5 (½ cup) servings	4 to 5 (½ cup) servings
Grain, bread, and cereals	4 servings	4 or more servings	4 or more servings
Recommended daily calories			
Man	2700		
Woman	2000	2300	2500

nonpregnant women need fewer calories. The obese person requires fewer calories for size, because adipose tissue consumes less oxygen than muscles.[26,42]

Rest and sleep. Rest and sleep patterns vary with the individual. However, 7 or 8 hours of sleep daily is the normal requirement.

Exercise, work, and leisure. The adult often focuses on work but must also engage in exercise and leisure activities for both physical and mental health.

Immunizations. The practical/vocational nurse can teach adults the importance of immunizations. Young adults may need immunizations, depending on their history. In young adults, 5% to 20% remain susceptible to both types of measles and should be vaccinated.

Developmental Tasks

For the young adult in general, the following tasks must be achieved, regardless of the station in life[9,26]:

1. Accepting self and stabilizing self-concept and body image
2. Establishing independence from parental home and financial aid
3. Working in a vocation or profession that provides personal satisfaction, economic independence, and a feeling of contributing to society
4. Learning to appraise and express love responsibly through more than sexual contact
5. Establishing an intimate bond with another, either through marriage or with a close friend
6. Establishing and maintaining a home and managing a time schedule and life stresses
7. Finding a congenial social and friendship group
8. Deciding whether to have a family and carry out the tasks of parenting and family development (Fig. 11-2)
9. Formulating a meaningful philosophy of life and reassessing priorities and values
10. Becoming involved in the community as a citizen

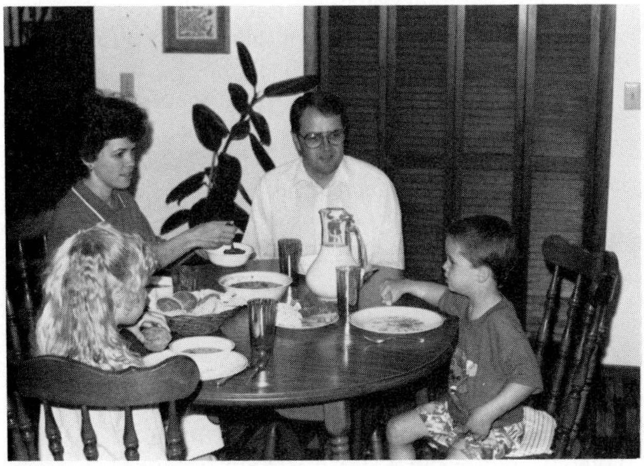

FIG. 11-2 Middle adulthood—the development of a family.

MIDDLE AGE

Chronological age of 45 to 65 years is only one definition of middle age. The person will also consider the physiological age condition of the body and **psychological age:** how old he or she acts and feels.

In the past 20 years, middle age has become a distinct life period. Middle age is attributed to improved nutrition, control of communicable disease, discovery and control of familial disease, and other medical advances. Life has been lengthened in the middle because people stay younger longer. What was old age is now middle age. **Middle age** is a time of relatively good health, new personal freedom, maximum command of self, and influence over the social environment.

Many patients are middle aged. Nurse can listen to and teach middle-aged persons concerning problems related to offspring, spouse, or aging parents or relatives.

Family Development and Relationships

Middle-agers and their offspring. The experience, values, and expectations of middle-aged persons differ from those of their offspring, creating a **generation gap.** Yet the younger and older generations can successfully combine efforts to work for legislation, policy changes, or social justice.[5,17]

The effect of divorced children on middle-aged parents cannot be overlooked. The parents may feel that their effort and help in getting the child "out of the nest" through marriage or their assistance to the couple to set up a home was to no avail. This feeling may be especially strong if the divorced family member decides to live at home again.[26] The sense of responsibility and loss of independence is heightened if the young adult offspring brings grandchildren. Having extra children and grandchildren in the home interferes with the relationship with the spouse and may also serve to prevent the middle-aged woman from attempting to pursue new career goals.

The marital couple. Equally important as relationship with the children and grandchildren is the middle-ager's relationship with the spouse. A happy marriage has security and stability, although there are also struggles. The couple know each other well. Each depends on the other. There is increased shared activity. Because the middle-ager probably has roots firmly implanted, he or she can cultivate warm friendships with members of the generation, as well as with family members. Marriage can be secure economically. Economic influence begins to wane as retirement nears, but the middle-aged working wife helps to offset this. Nationally, many working women are older than 45.[24] The literature discusses menopause and the "empty nest." Such feelings may not exist. Menopause and middle age may bring both men and women an enriched sense of self and enhanced capacity to cope with life. Not all marriages are happy and stable. Negative, critical feelings can gradually erode what was apparently a happy relationship. The wife and husband may have drifted apart instead of growing closer together with the years. Their relationship is changing because they are changing. Marital crisis may result from feelings of disappointment with self, feeling depleted emotionally because of lack of communication with the spouse, seeking rebirth or changing directions, or seeking escape from reality and superego pressures.[26] The result may be for one to reach outside the marriage to prove youthfulness, masculinity, or femininity, overlooking that they still love each other.

Widow(er)hood. Loss of spouse from death is a crisis in any life era, but it is more likely to first occur in middle age.

The loss of a spouse may mean many things: loss of a sexual partner and lover, companion, caretaker, audience for unguarded, spontaneous conversation, accountant, or plumber, depending on the roles performed by the mate. Secondary losses may involve reduced income, change in life-style and social involvements, return to the work force, and giving up some of what was previously taken for granted.[32] **Widow(er)hood** is a threat to self-concept and sense of wholeness; now the person is seen as "only one." Often the woman's identity is so tied to that of her husband that she feels completely lost, alone, and depressed after his death. The widow(er) misses having someone with whom he or she can share happy occasions, as well as sad news and problems. The emotional burden is increased if the woman still has children in the home to raise by herself. She has difficulty helping them work through their grief when she is in mourning. Friendship patterns and relationships with in-laws often change as well.

Although the widower is more accepted socially, he too will have painful gaps in his life. If the wife concentrated on keeping an orderly house, cooking meals, and keeping his wardrobe in order, he may suddenly realize that what he had taken for granted is gone. Even more significant is the loss if his wife was a "sounding board" or confidante in business matters and if she was actively involved in raising children still in the home.[26]

The bereavement of widow(er)hood affects physical health; somatic complaints related to anxiety are not unusual. The widow(er) may experience symptoms similar to those of the deceased spouse. The practical/vocational nurse should learn about widow(er)hood in assessment; that may be the reason for illness.

Relationship with aging parents and relatives. The middle-ager is in the middle in many ways, including in the middle of two demanding generations. They may still be considerably involved with offspring at the same time that they are caregivers for aging parents, aunts, uncles, or grandparents. Many families have four or five generations. Sometimes the middle-ager realizes the elderly person's dependence and need for help before the elderly person is ready to admit the need, which can become a source of frustration. The middle-aged woman who is the older daughter is often the caregiver; sometimes the aged parent or relative is brought to the middle-ager's home. Older relatives become more demanding just when the middle-ager feels he or she deserves time for self. Older relatives may complain and want their needs met immediately, which creates guilt in the middle-agers. The nurse can assist the middle-ager by listening to concerns about the **caregiver role** and by supporting decision making.

Certainly the older adult and middle-aged generations can give a great deal to each other. The older generation(s) can share insights and wisdom about life. Sometimes they can give assistance financially or with various tasks. The older generation(s) can be a source of joy, pride, and inspiration.[26]

A critical time for the adult is death of the parent(s), whether the relationship between parent(s) and offspring was harmonious or conflictual. The first parental death signals finiteness and mortality of the self, as well as of the other parent and other loved ones. Mourning may be done not only for the parent but for previously lost loved ones. Some mourning is an anticipation of future losses of the other parent, other beloved relatives, friends, and self. The middle-ager may be a patient while mourning the death of parents and may need referral to a spiritual advisor or counselor to resolve grief.

Family developmental tasks. The following developmental tasks must be accomplished for the middle-aged and older family to survive and achieve happiness, harmony, and maturity; acceptance, reinforcement, listening, teaching, and referral to other agencies are ways the practical/vocational nurse can help accomplish these tasks[9]:

1. Maintain a pleasant and comfortable home.
2. Assure security for later years, financially and emotionally.
3. Share household and other responsibilities, based on changing roles, interests, and abilities.
4. Maintain emotional and sexual intimacy as a couple, or regain emotional stability if death or divorce occurs.
5. Maintain contact with grown children and their families.
6. Adapt to departure of the child(ren).
7. Meet the needs of elderly parent(s), spouse, or other relatives in such a way as to make life satisfactory for each generation.
8. Participate in community life beyond the family, and maintain satisfactory social relations.
9. Use competencies built in earlier stages to expand or deepen interests and social or community involvement.

Physical Development

Physical appearance. Body parts age at different rates. One day the person may suddenly become aware of being "older" or middle-aged. Not all people decline alike. How quickly they decline depends partly on the stresses and strains they have undergone. Gray, thinning hair, wrinkles, coarsening features, decreased muscular tone, weight gain, varicosities, and capillary breakage may be the first signs of middle age. The listening and support of the practical/vocational nurse may help the middle-aged patient adjust to physical changes.

Hormonal changes in the female. Hormonal changes occur in the period known as the **menopause** for the woman or the **climacteric** for either sex. Basic to the changing physiology of the middle years is declining hormonal production. Contrary to myth, depression or other symptoms are neither inevitable nor clearly related to the perimenopausal or climacteric years. The nurse can teach others to overcome the myths about the menopause and climacteric.

The average age for menopause onset is 50; the usual range is between 45 and 55 years, although it may occur as early as age 35. Aging causes changed secretion of the follicle-stimulating hormone (FSH), which causes changes in the ovaries, leading to the menopause. Ovulation ceases, since all ova either are degenerated or have ovulated. Thus the cyclical production of progesterone fails to occur, and estrogen levels rapidly fall below the amount necessary to induce endometrial bleeding. The menstrual cycle becomes irregular. For 1 to 2 years, periods of heavy bleeding may alternate with no menses and then eventually stop altogether.[26]

For about 5 years before menopause, some discomforts may occur in a small percentage of women. Hormonal changes cause hot flashes associated with chilly sensations, dizziness, headaches, perspiration, palpitations, water retention, nausea, muscle cramps, fatigue, insomnia, and paresthesia of fingers and toes. Many symptoms, including irritability, depression, emotional lability, and palpitations, are frequently attributed to menopause, but only perspiring and hot flashes are found to be consistently related to menopause. Difficulties experienced during menopause may be associated with life changes or recent loss or stress.[20] The cause of symptoms appears to be more complex than simple estrogen deficit. Psychological factors, such as anger, anxiety, and excitement, are considered important.[26]

Hormonal changes in the male. This comes in the 50s or early 60s, although the symptoms may not be as pronounced as in the female climacteric. A few men may even complain of hot flashes, sweating, chills, dizziness, headaches, and heart palpitations. Unlike women, however, men do not lose their reproductive abilities, although these abilities decrease with age as output of sex hormones is reduced. The testes become less firm and smaller; sperm production decreases. Because of decreased testosterone production, the man may need a longer time to achieve erection and may experience premature or less forceful ejaculation. Testosterone level is likely to be lower in the middle-aged man who has high stress, lowered self-esteem, and depression. Testosterone therapy should be administered with caution because it may increase prostatic hypertrophy and risk of cancer.[22]

In about 20% of men, hypertrophy of the prostate begins naturally late in middle age, so that gradually the enlarging prostate around the uretha causes the embarrassment of frequent urination, dribbling, and nocturia. In addition, urine stasis may predispose to urinary infections.[26]

Related changes. Hormonal decline brings additional changes. The skin, subcutaneous tissue, and mucous membranes become dry and begin to **atrophy**. The loss of skin turgor and muscle tone results in wrinkles, pouches under the eyes, sagging chin, and loss of muscle tone, including of the pelvic floor. The loss of tone of the bladder mucosa and sphincter, urethral tissue, and supporting structures may cause embarrassing symptoms, such as frequent, urgent urination and stress incontinence, which may limit social activities. The uterus, ovaries, external genitalia, and breast tissue begin to atrophy. Atrophy, loss of elasticity of the vaginal mucosa, and less vaginal lubrication during sexual arousal may interfere with the pleasure of the sexual experience and cause painful urination. Regular sexual intercourse helps to maintain an adequate vaginal outlet and to prevent shrinkage of the vaginal mucosa.[22] If the couple experiences difficulty with sexual response and if the sexual problems result from changes in lubrication, use of estrogen vaginal cream can be effective in maintaining lubrication and distensibility.

Some of the changes in the woman result because the level of androgen in the body remains constant while the estrogen is decreasing. A small amount of hair growth may occur on chin or upper lip. There may be a loss of weight in the face and limbs at a time when diminishing muscle tone and additional adipose deposits make the woman look and feel larger at the waist. The coarseness of skin and sharpness of contours are the result of loss of some subcutaneous tissue.[26]

Metabolic changes. Metabolic changes include gradual decalcification of the bones, producing decreased bone density and a gradual osteoporosis. With the bone porosity and gradually shortening intervertebral disks, the woman will eventually be 1 to 2 inches shorter and the "dowager's hump" will form in the cervical and upper thoracic area. By age 55, a woman runs 10 times the risk of bone fractures as the 55-year-old man. Most vulnerable to fractures are forearms, hips, and spinal vertebrae.[26]

Presbyopia occurs at some point in middle age. The pupil takes in half as much light at 50 years as at 20 years. Pupils react more slowly in late middle age. Some degree of hearing is also gradually lost, especially for high-pitched sounds. Auditory reaction time slows; sound discrimination decreases. Other sensory acuity remains intact.[26,33]

Tooth decay is not caused by aging but chiefly by circulatory changes, poor dietary habits, poor mouth hygiene, or poor dental care over the years. Hence the middle-ager may have dentures or a partial plate or be in need of dental care for either dental caries or periodontal disease.[26]

Emotional changes related to physical changes. Depression, irritability, a change in sexual desire, or fear of loss of sexual identity may occur in response to physical changes and their meaning. Severe symptoms occur in fewer than 10% of women, so these symptoms may be minor and little noticed. Earlier personality patterns and attitudes are more responsible for the symptoms than the cessation of glandular activity.[26,27] Women who previously had low self-esteem and life satisfaction are more likely to have difficulties with menopause. Some women minimize the significance of the menopause. Some feel health is improved after menopause. Most couples feel there is no effect on sex life.

Cognitive Development

Piaget stated that the adult remains in formal operations, described in Chapter 9. The adult at any age is creative in thought but also engages in concrete operations of necessity, discussed in Chapter 8. The person begins at the abstract level and compares the idea mentally or verbally with previous memories, knowledge, or experience. The person combines or integrates a number of steps of a task mentally instead of thinking about or doing each step as a separate unit. Synthesizing and integrating ideas or information into the memory, beliefs, or solutions result in a unique product. Adult thought is different from adolescent thought. The adult can differentiate among many perspectives. The adult is objective, realistic, and less egocentric. Thinking and learning are problem centered, not just subject centered. The person can imagine and reason about events that are not occurring in reality but that are possible. Verbal ability and general knowledge increase until old age. Reaction time or speed of performance is individual and generally stays the same or diminishes during late middle age. Memory is maintained through young and middle adulthood; no major age differences are evident.

The older adult performs certain cognitive tasks more slowly for several reasons:

1. Decreased visual and auditory acuity
2. Slower motor response to sensory stimulation
3. Loss of recent memory
4. Changed motivation; less interest in competition

Reaction time is slower because of brain wave changes and when the person suffers significant environmental or social losses, is unable to engage in social contact, and is unable to plan daily routines. Persons who are ill often endure environmental and social losses by virtue of being in the patient role. Thus they may be slower responding to questions or requests.[26]

Emotional Development

In middle age (and beyond), the person perceives life as time left to live rather than time since birth. Death is a possibility. Middle-agers clock themselves by changes in body, family, and career, rather than primarily by chronological age. Time is measured in two ways: how much time to finish what the person wants to do and how much meaning and pleasure can be obtained in the time that is left. The person evaluates how achievements measure against goals and the entire value system.

Developmental crisis. The psychosexual crisis of middle age is **generativity** versus self-absorption/stagnation. The generative person has a sense of parenthood and creativity; of being vital in establishing and guiding the next generation, the arts, or a profession; and of feeling needed and being important to the welfare of humankind. A biological parent does not necessarily get to the psychosocial stage of generativity, and the unmarried person or the person without children can be very generative.[26] The middle-ager who is generative takes on the major work of providing for others, directly or indirectly. There is a sense of productivity, mastery, charity, altruism, and perseverance. These concepts motivate action. In church work, social work, community fund drives, cultural or artistic efforts, the profession, or political work, the person is active and often the leader. The person's goal is to leave the world a better place in which to live. For some, the middle years are the best years of life.[26]

If generativity is not achieved, **stagnation** or **self-absorption** results. The person hates the aging process and feels neither secure nor adept at handling self physically or interpersonally. The person is withdrawn, resigned, isolated, and introspective. The person becomes like a child, indulging self. Fear of old age may cause regression to inappropriate youthfulness in behavior or dress, or unfaithfulness in marriage. Or the opposite can occur: the middle-aged person can become resigned to old age too soon, seeing each physical change to an exaggerated degree. The chronic defeatism and depression that result from feeling too old also isolate the person in self-pity and egocentrism. Inability to emotionally adjust to physical and life change can result in **midlife crisis,** when the person's behavior becomes more immature.

Promoting Optimum Health

Nutrition. The basic food groups remain the same, but because of reduced basal energy requirements, caloric intake should be reduced. The exact level of calcium needed by the postmenopausal woman is still unknown. However, adequate calcium intake (100 mg per day) is necessary. Calcium intake may reduce the amount of estrogen the woman needs to prevent bone loss.

Sleep and rest. Throughout the adult years, factors such as emotional and physical status, occupation, and amount of physical activity determine the need for rest and sleep. Workers such as nurses, who alternate between day and night shifts, frequently feel exhausted and may need more sleep than people whose work schedules do not change. Surgery, illness, pregnancy, and the postpartum state all require that the individual receive more sleep. Mothers of infants, toddlers, and preschoolers may need daytime naps. The tradition that adults should have 7 to 8 hours of sleep seems valid, although some get along fine with less.[33]

Immunizations. Adults at risk for hepatitis should receive hepatitis B vaccination. Individuals who garden and participate in other outdoor activities should receive tetanus immunization as indicated.

Injury prevention. Safety promotion is important for all adults, and the practical/vocational nurse can emphasize safety measures while giving care. Accidents can be prevented in the home or while maintaining a yard through the following ways:

1. Handrails for stairways
2. Handgrip at the bathtub
3. Conveniently located electrical outlets
4. Indirect, nonglare, and thorough lighting
5. Tools, equipment, and home or yard machines kept in proper working condition.

Developmental Tasks

The following developmental tasks should be accomplished by middle-aged people:

1. Maintain or establish healthful life patterns.
2. Discover and develop new satisfactions as a mate, give support to mate, enjoy mutual activities, develop a deeper sense of unity and intimacy, and take pride in accomplishments of self and spouse.
3. Help growing and grown children become happy and responsible adults, take pride in their accomplishments, stand by to assist as needed, and accept their friends and mates.
4. Create a pleasant, comfortable home, appropriate to values, interests, time, energy, and resources; give, receive, and exchange hospitality.
5. Find pleasure in generativity and recognition in work if employed; gain knowledge, proficiency, and wisdom; be able to lead or follow.
6. Balance work with other roles.
7. Reverse roles with aging parents and parents-in-law; assist them as needed without dominating; prepare emotionally for the eventual death of parents unless they are already deceased.
8. Maintain a standard of living related to values, needs, and financial resources.
9. Achieve mature social and civic responsibility; be informed as a citizen; give time, energy, and resources to causes beyond self and home.
10. Develop or maintain an active organizational membership, deriving from it pleasure and a sense of belonging; refuse conflicting or too burdensome invitations with poise; work through intraorganizational tensions.
11. Accept and adjust to the physical changes of middle age; maintain healthful ways of living; enjoy maturing.
12. Make an art of friendship; cherish old friends and choose new; enjoy an active social life with friends.
13. Use **leisure** creatively and with satisfaction without yielding too much to social pressures and styles; learn to do some things well enough to become known for them among family, friends, and associates; share some leisure activities with a mate or others; balance active and passive leisure activities.
14. Continue to formulate a philosophy of life and religious or philosophical affiliation, discovering new depths and meanings in God or a creator, that include but also go beyond a particular religious denomination; gain satisfaction from altruistic activities.
15. Prepare for retirement with financial arrangements and development of hobbies and leisure activities, and rework philosophy and values.
16. Recognize the finiteness of life, and prepare for eventual personal death.

THE ELDERLY

The beginning age for the elderly actually depends on many factors. Historically, it was the decision to have age 65 as the beginning age for receiving Social Security benefits. Now Social Security benefits may be received at age 62 or 70, and retirement age is not a valid marker for old age. Studies consistently show that many people 65 years and older do not consider themselves old. However, members of ethnic minorities and lower socioeconomic levels may view onset of old age as taking place earlier.[44]

Many of the negative myths and stereotypes associated with **aging (ageism)** are culturally determined. The older adult in the United States lives in a culture oriented to youth, productivity, and rapid pace. Thus older Americans may feel that they are not respected, valued, or needed. Cultures and ethnic groups influence the role of the older adult in family relationships and determine health practices. For example, the older African-American family members are held in esteem. In Asian culture, the older adults have an important role, and the young are expected to respect and care for them.[26]

The practical/vocational nurse can listen to the older person and give information or support related to family concerns and issues.

Family Development and Relationships

Relations with spouse. In later life, responsibilities of parenthood and employment diminish, with few formal responsibilities to take their place. Declining health, limited income, and fewer daily responsibilities may create greater needs for social support. Thus having a spouse provides increased possibility for companionship. Sometimes marriages have not been filled with mutual emotional or social support in earlier years, so there is no foundation for increasing mutual emotional support. Women are often the sole support for men; older women tend to feel the husband is not supportive emotionally or helpful in health care. Women tend to rely more on family and friends for support.[8]

For the woman, continually having the spouse with her, wanting to share in her activities, can be distressing, even though it has been positively anticipated. The loss of privacy and solitude, doing tasks her own way and at her own pace, loss of independence, and loss of contact with friends may all be issues. However, the increased accommodation to meeting the husband's needs is offset by increased opportunities for nurturing and being nurtured and for sharing mutual interests.[26]

The spouse is the primary caregiver to the impaired husband or wife. In turn, the spouse may become at risk physically or emotionally because of the stresses of caregiving. Widowhood has even greater implications in old age for the remaining spouse.

Grandparenthood. Grandparents are often happy with their role; they enjoy the young person in a playful, informal, companion, confidante relationship. The grandchild is seen as a source of leisure activity. Grandparents typically do not want to get into an authoritarian or disciplinarian role, but have the experience to do so if necessary.[26]

Great-grandparents may wish to remain active in that role, but advanced age and sometimes distance may limit their participation. Also, this generation feels removed from the very young, whereas the grandparent generation often feels a special tie with the very young.

Social relationships. Family, friends, and neighbors provide assistance and support, especially during stressful events, and promote coping and self-esteem. These significant people may be the ones called on by the nurse to assist the elderly when ill, after discharge, or with rehabilitation in the home.

About 5% of elderly are single—never married. They may have living family members. They may or may not live alone. Having lived independently during adult life, the person may have developed effective adaptive mechanisms and a friendship network. Or the nurse may become the most significant person during the elder's illness, especially with decisions facing the ill or dying person.

Family developmental tasks. (See Family Developmental Tasks for middle age, p. 138).

Physical Development

General appearance. The general appearance of the older adult is determined in part by the changes that occur in the skin, face, hair, and posture. All physical changes are pertinent to the practical/vocational nurse's assessment, intervention, and teaching, and the elderly need help in accepting appearance and other changes.

Skin. The skin develops creases and furrows and begins to sag. **Lentigo senilis** appears, especially on the dorsum of hands, arms, and face. Some capillaries and small arteries on exposed portions of the skin surface enlarge and become more visible. Fair-skinned older adults lose the pink flesh tone. Berliner's two articles are excellent references and picture various conditions.[1]

Changes in the skin cells and cellular elements cause decrease in the skin turgor. The outer epidermal layer becomes thinner as cells are depleted. Skin cells are replaced more slowly in the older adult. Because the sebaceous glands, which normally lubricate the skin with oil, decrease activity, the skin becomes dryer and rougher. The inability of the aging skin to retain fluids also contributes to dryness and less turgor. A reduction in the number of sweat glands interferes with the body's ability to sweat freely, which interferes with heat regulation. Loss of subcutaneous fat, which functions as insulation for the body, can make the older adult susceptible to the cold. The loss of subcutaneous fat also accounts for the sagging tissues and thinner look of old age.[26,41]

Melanin production in the hair follicle diminishes. The hair gradually grays; the exact shade of gray depends on the original hair color. Loss of hair occurs on the scalp, in the pubic and axillary areas, and on the extremities. In most older adults, there is also increased growth of facial hair because of the change in androgen/estrogen ratio.[33,41]

Posture. The posture of the older adult is one of general flexion. The head is tilted forward; hips and knees are slightly flexed. Muscles in the torso are held rigidly. The older adult stands with the feet apart to provide a wide base of support. Shorter steps produce a shuffling gait.[33] A shift in the center of gravity occurs as well, which affects movement and balance.

Development of body systems

Neurological. The sensory response changes are as follows: (1) nerve transmission is slower; (2) nerve conduction velocity decreases; (3) electrical activity declines; (4) sensory threshold increases; and (5) integration of sensory and motor function declines. By age 70, slower voluntary movement, slower decision making, and slowed startle response are seen. Higher sensory threshold affects pain and tactile perception, so more intense stimuli are needed to examine or stimulate the person.[26,33]

Cardiovascular. The cardiovascular system is still able to maintain the daily cardiac and circulatory functions of the older adult. The cardiovascular system may not be able to meet the needs of the body when a disease process is present or when excess demands caused by stress or exercise occur.

Structural changes occur. The cardiac muscle has an increased amount of collagen and fat. Valves become more rigid. The left ventricle wall thickens. Atherosclerosis is present, and its effect on the aorta, coronary arteries, and carotid arteries is especially apparent. Large arteries have decreased elasticity. Varicose veins are common. The left ventricle is unable to pump large volumes of blood; thus the total cardiac output per minute is lower. Because the cardiac output is lower, less blood is sent to the brain and coronary arteries. Muscles and viscera may receive inadequate blood supplies when there is an increased demand for blood flow. Consistent exercise throughout life is the best way to maintain adequate cardiac output in later maturity.[26,41]

Respiratory. The rib cage becomes less mobile, and elasticity of the lung tissue decreases. Decline in structure and function of the respiratory muscles decreases strength of the muscles used in breathing. Decreased muscle tone and sensitivity to stimuli impair ability to cough. Less oxygen is delivered. There is a decrease in the vital capacity. Calcification of vertebral cartilages and kyphosis cause more shallow respirations.

Musculoskeletal. A gradual decrease in height occurs as the vertebrae shrink from loss of calcium and normal aging. Height is also affected by curvature of the thoracic spine, which frequently occurs in older adults. The older adult may experience a significant weight loss around 70 years of age. This is probably the result of the decreased number of body cells, the changes in cell composition, and the decrease in the amount of body tissues.[26,41]

There is a gradual loss of muscular strength and endurance. Muscle cells atrophy. Lean muscle mass is lost. As the elastic fibers in the muscle tissues decrease, the muscles become less flexible and stiffness is noted more frequently. Continued physical activity and proper nu trition can slow muscle atrophy and stiffness. Progressive loss of bone strength occurs because of loss of bone mineral content. Active exercise and proper nutrition decrease the rapidity of bone density loss.[41]

Genitourinary. There is a loss of nephron units in the kidneys. By age 70 or 80, the glomerular filtration rate is approximately one-half the rate of a 30-year-old. Impaired filtration rate causes slower excretion of urea nitrogen, creatinine, uric acid, and even drugs. Tubule cells change reabsorption, causing a loss of water and electrolytes. Kidneys also need more time to correct alkalosis, acidosis, and/or electrolyte disturbances. When both renal and respiratory functions are impaired, protection against shifts in blood pH is decreased.[26,41]

Some muscle tone loss occurs in the ureters and bladder. This may cause incomplete emptying of the bladder and increase the risk of retention and bladder infection in the older adult. The bladder capacity gradually decreases, and the older adult experiences frequent urination and nocturia. Older women may develop incontinence when relaxation of the pelvic muscles occurs.[26]

Gastrointestinal. Difficulty with chewing is the result of tooth decay, loss of teeth, degeneration of the jaw bone, progressive gum recession, and increased reabsorption of the dental arch. Saliva becomes more alkaline as the salivary glands secrete less ptyalin and amylase. These changes alter the digestive process at the onset.[26]

In the gastrointestinal tract, peristalsis slows, causing delayed emptying of the esophagus and stomach. There is reduction in digestive enzymes. Bile tends to be thicker, and the gallbladder empties more slowly. These changes result in a decreased digestion and decreased absorption of nutrients and drugs by the gastrointestinal tract.

Elimination of waste products is of equal importance to gastrointestinal function in the aged. Elimination depends on fluid intake, muscle tone, regularity of habits, exercise, state of health, and adequate nutrition. The changes in the cell, and therefore in tissue structure, and the loss of muscle tone may decrease intestinal mobility, resulting in constipation.

Endocrine. There is some general decrease in progesterone and estrogen secretion. There is a lack of response to some hormones, especially those of the adrenal and thyroid glands. Thus ability to respond to stress in old age is reduced.

Immune. The older adult has a delayed immune response to infection and a delayed or inadequate response to the stress of an infection. Both of these factors alter the normal inflammatory response, causing altered signs and symptoms of infection. The white blood count does not become as elevated in response to an infection as it does in the middle-aged individual.[26]

Reproductive

Changes that influence sexual function. Concentration of testosterone diminishes with aging, producing a gradual decline in sexual vigor, muscle strength, and active sperm. As a sexual partner, the older man experiences reduction in (1) the frequency of intercourse, (2) the intensity of sensation, (3) the speed of attaining erection, and (4) the force of ejaculation.

The older woman encounters little sexual difficulty if she is in good health, has an open and positive attitude toward sexual relations, and has an available and effective sexual partner. Effective sexual capacity and performance among women remains until late 70s or even older.[22,26] Neural and hormonal changes may combine to make the sex act less satisfying.

When one is old, the yearning for intimacy, security, and belonging becomes intensified as other privations are felt keenly: loss of friends, job status, active participation in parenting or career, and decision making. Too often the elderly consider themselves members of a third sex, nonpersons whom the functional world passes by.

Sensory

Vision. Changes in vision occur. The lens thickens and yellows; objects take on a yellow hue. The size of the pupil decreases; it is less responsive to light. Increased lens opacity causes light to scatter, causing sensitivity to glare and difficulty in adjusting when moving from a lighted to a darker room. Presbyopia, if not present before, occurs now. Lacrimal glands produce fewer tears, causing the cornea to become dry and irritated.[26,33]

Color vision is altered. Colors such as green, blue, and violet are more difficult to see than red, orange, and yellow. Pastels fade so that they are indistinguishable from each other. Monotones, whites, and dark colors are also difficult to see. Brighter colors compensate for decline in color discrimination and yellowing and opacity of the lens.

Hearing. Hearing changes of middle age continue through later life. Of all those over 65, 13% suffer severe **presbycusis**. The consonants *s*, *sh*, and *f* are examples of sounds that are difficult to hear. The ability to locate the direction from which sound is coming diminishes. Older people have difficulty hearing individuals who speak rapidly or in high tones. Hearing loss may be caused by changes in the nervous system or ear drum.

Taste and smell. These senses also are affected by aging. The number of taste buds decreases with age. The older adult experiences a decrease in taste sensation and an increased preference for more spices, highly seasoned foods, and more sugar and salt. The sense of smell decreases, which combined with the decline in taste sensation may account for a loss of appetite. The inability to smell presents hazards for the individual, since he or she cannot quickly detect leaking gas, spoiled food, smoke, or burning food.[13,26]

Cognitive Development

Habits, judgment, creativity, and problem-solving wisdom are maintained even into old age if there is no deterioration caused by extensive physical or neurological changes. The mental abilities of the adult, especially the aged, should be recognized during assessment and intervention. The attitude of the practical/vocational nurse when teaching the adult is to believe in the capacity of the elderly to learn, relearn, and problem solve. Many adults, especially the elderly, are apprehensive about new learning, particularly in competitive situations, and ask for more details and more specific directions because they anticipate difficulty in learning new tasks.[26] The nurse should be patient and proceed at the individual's pace.

Emotional Development

No specific personality changes occur as a result of **aging**. Values, life orientation, and personality traits remain consistent from at least middle age onward. The older person continues to develop emotionally and in personality, adding on characteristics instead of making drastic changes. If he or she were physically active, had a flexible personality, and participated in social activities in the young years, these characteristics will be apparent in later physical status and life situation. If the person were not compatible when younger, he or she will be harder to live with in old age. Stereotypes describe the older person as rigid, conservative, opinionated, self-centered, and disagreeable. Such characteristics are not likely to be new, but rather are an exaggeration of lifelong traits.

Developmental crisis. The psychosexual crisis in old age is ego integrity versus self-despair. **Ego integrity** is the coming together of all previous phases of the life cycle. Having accomplished the earlier tasks, the person accepts life as it has been. The person demonstrates the characteristics of maturity, achieving both wisdom and an enriched perspective about life and people.

Without a sense of ego integrity, the person feels a sense of **self-despair** and self-disgust. The person wants another chance to redo life's events. Death is feared. The person becomes hypercritical of others, and projects personal self-disgust, inadequacy, and anger onto others. Instead of the aged person feeling a sense of importance, there is a feeling of being a burden, too slow, and worthless.

Promoting Optimum Health

Nutrition. The Basic 4 food groups remain a foundation for nutrition. Although caloric requirements may be lower than in earlier life, the elderly require more of some of the vitamins and trace elements. Ensuring adequate nutrition is difficult because of aging changes that affect taste, digestion, and metabolism; emotional changes; living alone; income changes; and availability of shopping and cooking facilities. At least six or seven glasses (8 ounces) of water should be ingested daily to (1) soften stools; (2) maintain kidney function; (3) aid expectoration; (4) moisturize dry skin; and (5) aid absorption of medications, bulk laxatives, and high-fiber foods.[26,42]

Rest and sleep. The older person may sleep less soundly and awaken more frequently during the night, as well as nap during the day.

Exercise, work, and leisure. The middle-ager and older adult grew up under the hardships of the Depression and with the Protestant ethic, emphasizing the economic and moral importance of work. Thus work is respected and sought.

Retirement can be either anticipated or dreaded in late middle age or as the person approaches 62, 65, or 70 years of age. As corporations reduce their work force numbers, the older worker is most likely to be released, because of salary and pension costs. Yet the older worker may be less costly, because of retraining costs for newly hired employees and lower absenteeism of older workers.

Retirement affects all the other positions the person has held, relationships with others, and income. Inability to keep up with the former activities of an organization or group may result, and a change in status may require a changing social life.

Current information on Social Security benefits and Medicare coverage should be obtained. Government publications are available at little or no cost from the Superintendent of Documents of the Government Printing Office in Washington, D.C. Current lists of material pertinent to health and social programs may be obtained directly from the National Clearing House on Aging, U.S. Department of Health and Human Services, 330 Independence Avenue, S.W., Washington, D.C. 20201.

The middle-ager and older adult, because of their work ethic, may have difficulty with use of leisure time. Older adults value most the leisure activity that involves interaction with others, promotes development, and maintains contact with the broader community. Use of leisure time by serving as a volunteer may be rewarding (Fig. 11-3). Leisure time can also be spent playing with a pet.

Immunizations. Older adults are more susceptible to acute illnesses. Immunization for influenza and pneumococcal pneumonia is usually recommended for older adults, especially those with chronic respiratory and cardiovascular diseases.[38]

Injury prevention. Older people have a disproportionate share of accidents that cause bodily injury or death, especially in the home. Many of these accidents are directly related to physiological changes that result from normal aging discussed earlier. Changes in visual acuity and problems with color interpretation, light intensity, and depth perception produce numerous hazards for the older adult. Accidents from distorted vision can be prevented in the following ways[26]:

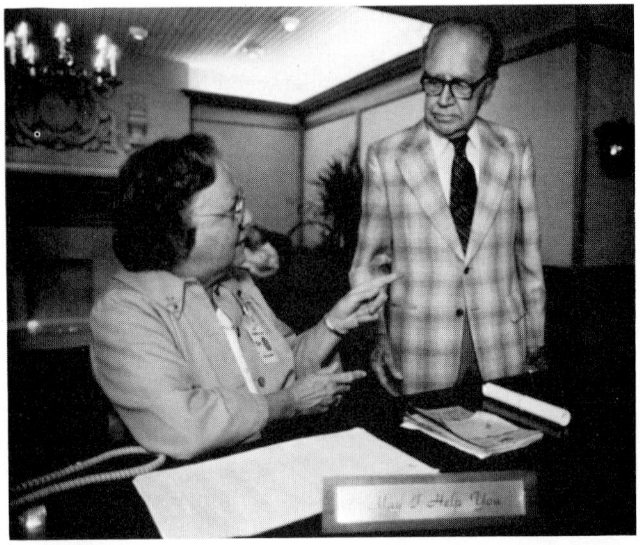

FIG. 11-3 Later adulthood—volunteer work enhances self-worth.

1. Use higher light intensity.
2. Avoid direct lights, exposed light bulbs, white surfaces, waxed floors, and glossy furniture, which produce glare.
3. Arrange lights so that they are not directed down from the ceiling, creating pools of light that may distort vision.
4. Use sharply contrasting colors for door facings and walls, brightly colored doors, stripes of contrasting color along the bottom of a wall and a yellow or red strip at the edge of each step to assist color and depth perception.
5. To prevent falls, avoid objects on the floor, furniture with sharp edges, and scatter rugs.
6. Prepare signs with dark backgrounds and light lettering; blues and greens should be avoided, because these colors are not seen clearly by the elderly.
7. Printed numbers on doors, elevators, and telephones should be large enough for the older adult to see.
8. Light fixtures should be at the entrance of a room, because vision of the older person takes longer to adjust when moving from a light to a dark area.

Other changes also cause hazards. Changes in hearing acuity may predispose the person to accident risks. Changes in temperature regulation and the inability to feel pain also produce safety problems. The elderly usually feel cold more easily and require more covering when in bed. A room temperature somewhat higher than usual may be desirable. Most hospitals and nursing homes do not have thermometers that register body temperature below 94° F (35° C). Therefore statistics are not available on how many elderly persons suffer and die from hypothermia. A nighttime room temperature of 66° F (18.3° C) is too low for an aged person. The victim may not be aware of the extreme loss of body heat, especially when supine and relatively inactive. Measures to prevent hypothermia in cold weather are as follows:

1. Stay indoors as much as possible, especially on windy, wet, and cold days.
2. Wear layered clothing, and cover the head when outdoors.
3. Eat high-energy foods, such as some fats, easily digested carbohydrates, and protein, daily.
4. Keep at least one room warm.
5. Use extra blankets, caps, socks, and layered clothing in bed.
6. Have contact with someone daily.

Dulling of tactile sensation occurs because of a decrease in the number of areas of the body responding to all stimuli and in the number and sensitivity of sensory receptors. Use caution when applying hot packs or other hot or cold applications. The elderly person may be burned or suffer frostbite before realizing any discomfort. Complaints of pain, such as abdominal discomfort or chest pain, may be more serious than the older person's perception might indicate. There may be clumsiness or difficulty in identifying objects by touch. Fewer tactile cues are received from the soles of the feet, so the older person may get confused about location and position, and stumble more easily.[21,26]

Developmental Tasks

The following developmental tasks are to be achieved by the aging couple as a family, as well as by the aging person living alone[9,26,31]:

1. Recognize the aging process and resulting limitations.
2. Adjust to decreasing physical strength and health changes.
3. Continue a supportive, close, warm relationship with the spouse or significant other, including a satisfying sexual relationship.
4. Find a satisfactory home or living arrangement, and establish a safe, comfortable household routine to fit health and economic status.
5. Adjust living standards to retirement income; supplement retirement income if possible with remunerative activity.
6. Maintain maximum level of health; care for self physically and emotionally by getting health examinations and needed medical or dental care, eating an adequate diet, and maintaining personal hygiene.
7. Maintain contact with children, grandchildren, and other living relatives, finding emotional satisfaction with them.
8. Establish and maintain affiliation with members of own age group.
9. Maintain interest in people outside the family and in social, civic, and political responsibility.
10. Pursue alternate sources of need satisfaction and new interests, and maintain former activities to gain status, recognition, and a feeling of being needed.
11. Find meaning in life after retirement and in facing inevitable illness and death of oneself and spouse, as well as other loved ones.

Through careful, ongoing assessment, listening and teaching during periods of physical caregiving, and referring to nursing supervisors or other team members, the practical/vocational nurse can assist the young, middle-aged, and older adult to meet developmental tasks.

REFERENCES AND SUGGESTED READINGS

1. Berliner H: Aging skin, Am J Nurs 86(10):1138, 1986.
2. Brody E: Parent care as a normative family stress, Gerontologist 25(1):19, 1985.
3. Brookes J: A study of the premenstrual syndrome, Health Visit 56:416, 1983.
4. Brown M: Primary dysmenorrhea, Nurs Clin North Am 17(1):145, 1982.
5. Carlson E: The phony war, Modern Maturity, p 34, Feb/Mar, 1987.
6. CDC, others call for an increased effort for hepatitis B vaccination, The Nation's Health, pp 1, 9, Jan, 1985.
7. Crocker K, Gerber F, and Sheerer J: Metabolism of carbohydrate, protein, and fat, Nurs Clin North Am 18(1):3, 1983.
8. Depner C and Ingersoll-Dayton B: Conjugal social support: patterns in later life, J Gerontol 40(6):761, 1985.
9. Duvall E and Miller B: Marriage and family development, ed 6, New York, 1984, Harper & Row Publishers, Inc.
10. Engel N: Menopausal stage, current life change, attitude toward women's roles, and perceived health status, Nurs Res 36(6):353, 1987.
11. Forrester D: Myths of masculinity: impact upon men's health, Nurs Clin North Am 21(1):15, 1986.
12. Harker J and Riegi W: Aging and delay effects on recognition of words and designs, J Gerontol 40(5):601, 1985.
13. Hayter J: Modifying the environment to help older persons, Nurs Health Care 4(5):265, 1983.
14. Henley EC and Bohl S: Nutrition across the woman's life cycle, Nurs Clin North Am 12(1):99, 1982.
15. Hoole AJ, Greenberg RA, and Pickard CG: Patient care guidelines for nurse practitioners, ed 3, Boston, 1988, Little, Brown & Co, Inc.
16. Irwin T: Male menopause: crisis in the middle years, New York, 1982, Public Affairs Pamphlets.
17. Kaplan S: The new generation gap, Common Cause Magazine p 13, March-April, 1987.
18. King L: The dual-career couple faces corporate relocation, St. Louis Post-Dispatch, pp 12-13, 33, Aug 1986.
19. Kohen J: Old but not alone: informal social supports among the elderly by mental status and sex, Gerontologist 23(1): 57, 1983.
20. Lindeman E: Symptomology and management of acute grief, Am J Psychiatry 101:141, 1944.
21. Loevinger J: Ego development, San Francisco, 1976, Jossey-Bass, Inc, Publishers.
22. Masters W and Johnson V: Human sexual response, Boston, 1966, Little, Brown & Co, Inc.
23. May RR: Mood shifts and the menstrual cycle, J Psychosom Res 20:125, 1985.
24. Moshman D, Glover J, and Bruning R: Developmental psychology, Boston, 1987, Little, Brown & Co, Inc.
25. Muhlenkamp A, Waller M, and Bourne A: Attitudes toward women in menopause: a vignette approach, Nurs Res 32(1):20, 1983.
26. Murray R and Zentner J: Nursing assessment and health promotion through the lifespan, ed 4, East Norwalk, Conn, 1989, Appleton & Lange.
27. Neugarten B: The awareness of middle age. In Owen R, editor: Middle age, London, 1967, British Broadcasting Corporation.
28. Notham M: Adult life cycles: changing roles and changing hormones. In Parsons J: The psychology of sex differences and sex roles, Washington, DC, 1980, Hemisphere Publishing Corp.
29. Older workers are bearing brunt of most down-sizing programs, AARP News Bulletin 28(11):1, 4, 1987.
30. Osteoporosis: estrogen connection clearer, Am J Nurs 88(1):13, 1988.
31. Peck RC: Psychological developments in the second half of life. In Neugarten B, editor: Middle age and aging, Chicago, 1968, University of Chicago Press.
32. Prock V: The midstage woman, Am J Nurs 75(6):1019, 1975.
33. Schuster C and Ashburn S: The process of human development, ed 2, Boston, 1986, Little, Brown & Co, Inc.
34. Some hypothermia deaths tied to lack of thermometers, The AARP News Bulletin 23(4):1982.
35. Spencer G: Commentary: dramatic growth of centenarian population, Statistical Bulletin 68(1):8, 1987.
36. Sykes JA, Kelly P, and Kennedy JA Jr: Black skin problems, Am J Nurs 79(6):1092, 1979.
37. Toth S and Toth A: Empathic intervention with the widow, Am J Nurs 80(9):652, 1980.
38. Vaccines for adult diseases, Newsweek, p 92, Oct 12, 1987.
39. Wadsworth B: Piaget's theory of cognitive and affective development, ed 3, New York, 1984, David McKay Co, Inc.
40. Walsleben J: Sleep disorders, Am J Nurs 82(6):936, 1982.
41. Whitbourne SK: The aging body: physiological changes and psychological consequences, New York, 1985, Springer-Verlag New York, Inc.
42. Williams SR: Nutrition and diet therapy, ed 6, St. Louis, 1989, The CV Mosby Co.
43. Windom R: Adult immunization should be routine, too, Public Health Rep 102(3):245, 1987.
44. Women and athletic endurance, Graduate Woman 79(4):5, 1985.

CHAPTER CHALLENGE

KEY POINTS

- The major family goal with young adults is the reorganization of the family into a continuing unit while releasing maturing young people into lives of their own.
- Developmental tasks must be achieved by the young adult, middle-aged adult, and older adult for a successful family developmental structure to continue.
- Physiological changes that occur during young adult life are different from those in childhood; they are slower and smaller in increment; body systems are functioning at peak efficiency.
- The human sexual response cycle involves physiological reactions, psychological components, and psychosocial influences on behavior.
- According to Erikson, in young adults, the psychosexual crisis is intimacy versus isolation.
- The basis for adult cognitive performance is laid during the school years when the child accomplishes the task of industry.
- Middle-aged adults experience family development and relationships with their children, and as a marital couple, widowerhood may occur and the caregiver role with aging parents and relatives begins.
- The first parental death signals finiteness and mortality of the self, as well as of the other parent and other loved ones.
- Basic to the changing physiology of the middle years is the declining hormonal production and gradually decreased basal metabolism rate.
- The middle-aged adult remains in formal operations stage of cognitive development, as well as the concrete operations stage.
- The psychosexual crisis of middle age is generativity versus self-absorption/stagnation.
- In the elderly adult, all body systems decrease in their peak efficiency. Many variables affect the physiology of the elderly.
- Cultures and ethnic groups influence the role of the older adult in family relationships and determine health practices.
- The psychosexual crisis of old age is ego integrity versus self-despair.
- Habits, judgment, creativity, and problem-solving wisdom are maintained into old age if there is no deterioration caused by extensive physical or neurological changes.

STUDY QUESTIONS

1. Peak muscle strength is attained at what age:
   a. 17 to 22 years
   b. 19 to 30 years
   c. 30 to 40 years
2. Maximum cardiac output is achieved and peaks at what age:
   a. 17 to 20 years
   b. 30 to 35 years
   c. 20 to 30 years
3. According to Erikson, the psychosexual crisis that occurs during the young adult years is:
   a. Intimacy versus self-isolation
   b. Ego integrity versus despair
   c. Generativity versus self-absorption/stagnation
4. Erikson believed that the basis of adult performance is laid during which years:
   a. Preschool-age years
   b. School-age years
   c. Adolescent years
5. A critical time for the adult is death of parent(s). The first parental death usually signals all of the following *except*:
   a. Finiteness and mortality of the self
   b. Anticipated loss of other parent
   c. Stagnation/self-absorption
6. Menopausal symptoms, such as hair growth on chin and upper lip, loss of weight in face and extremities, and coarseness of skin occur because:
   a. Level of androgen in the body remains constant while estrogen is decreasing
   b. Level of progesterone in the body remains constant while estrogen is decreasing
   c. Level of estrogen in the body remains constant while progesterone is decreasing
7. The older adult performs certain cognitive tasks more slowly for all of the following reasons *except*:
   a. Decreased visual and auditory acuity
   b. Quicker motor response to sensory stimulation
   c. Loss of recent memory
   d. Changed motivation; less interest in competition
8. The psychosexual crisis of middle age is:
   a. Intimacy versus isolation
   b. Ego integrity versus self-despair
   c. Generativity versus self-absorption/stagnation
9. The older adult in the United States lives in a culture:
   a. Oriented to youth, productivity, and rapid pace
   b. In which the elder is held in high esteem
   c. Where the older adults have an important role and the young are expected to respect and care for them
10. In most older women, there is an increase in growth of facial hair because of:
    a. Change in adrenal secretion of cortisol
    b. Change in thyroid-stimulating hormone secretions
    c. Change in androgen/estrogen ratio
11. Immunization for what disease usually is recommended for the older adult:
    a. Measles, mumps, polio
    b. Influenza and pneumococcal pneumonia
    c. Hepatitis B
12. The elderly usually need the room temperature higher or lower because of their metabolism:
    a. Higher
    b. Lower
13. According to Erikson, the psychosexual crisis in the older adult is:
    a. Intimacy versus isolation
    b. Generativity versus self-absorption
    c. Ego integrity versus self-despair

12

Cultural Aspects of Nursing Care

BOBBIE BLOCH

LEARNING OBJECTIVES

After reading this chapter, the student should be able to do the following:

- Define the key terms.
- Describe ways in which culture influences an individual.
- Explain how ethnocentrism can cause cultural conflicts in the nurse/patient relationship.
- Discuss how cultural variables may influence health behavior.
- Use cultural data to bring about change in health behavior of a patient.
- Evaluate the effects of nurses' values, beliefs, and practices on the patient related to their ethnicity.

RELATED TOPICS OF INTEREST

- The family (Chapter 7)
- The infant and young child (Chapter 8)
- The school-age child (Chapter 9)
- The adolescent (Chapter 10)
- The adult (Chapter 11)

KEY TERMS

Define the following:

- cultural healing beliefs
- culture
- dominant group
- ethnic stereotype
- ethnicity
- ethnocentrism
- minority group
- racism
- subculture
- values

The 1980 census shows that more than 20% of the United States population is of racial and ethnic groups: 11.5%, African-Americans; 6.4%, Hispanics; and the remaining 2.4%, Asians and American Indians. By the year 2020, African-Americans and Hispanics will make up between 25% and 30% of the United States population.[3] In the past 20 years, these American ethnic minority groups have increased their awareness about racial and cultural identity.

Recently new immigrants, such as Vietnamese, Cubans, and Haitians, have come to the United States. Like ethnic minority groups of the past, new immigrants tend to keep familiar cultural beliefs and practices as they adjust to their new environment. Often these new immigrants have difficulty adapting to the changes required by their new environment. For example, a Vietnamese peasant may experience confusion and stress because of (1) difficulty speaking English and (2) lack of skills to obtain a job.

In response to issues raised by both new and older ethnic minority groups, the following questions arise:

- What influence does a patient's or nurse's culture have on providing effective nursing care?
- What knowledge and nursing skills would be needed in providing the care of persons from different racial and cultural backgrounds?

To answer these important questions, it is necessary to understand the concept of culture and its influence on the patient's ability to adapt to health and illness. This chapter will give some examples of cultural characteristics of several ethnic minority groups, but it is beyond the scope of this discussion to present in greater detail every group known.

CULTURE

Definition of Culture

Culture may be defined as "the learned ways of acting and thinking which are transmitted by group members and which provide for each individual ready-made and tested solutions for vital problems."[5,16] Culture includes such areas as diet, language and communication process, religion, art and history, family life processes, social groups' interactive patterns, value orientations, and healing beliefs and practices. How persons resolve problems related to basic human needs is strongly influenced by these cultural elements. Because culture is devised by people to solve human problems, it is universal.

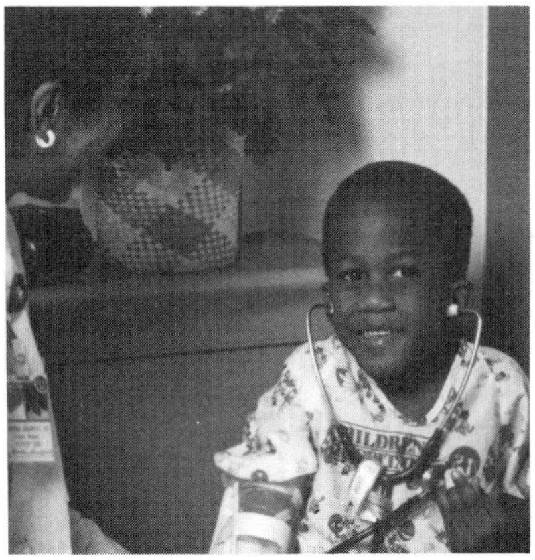

Characteristics of Culture

Murray and Zentner[9] have identified three major characteristics of culture as follows:

1. Culture is learned.
   A person learns behaviors, values, attitudes, and beliefs within his cultural family system. This learning is influenced mainly by the person's social status within a society and adaptation to his environment.
2. Culture is capable of change but remains stable.
   Language, traditions, and norms or customs may act as stabilizers for a culture.
3. Components or patterns are present in every culture.
   These include communication systems, means of economic and physical survival, transportation systems, family systems, social customs and mores, and religious systems.

Influences of Culture

Nurses providing care should consider all patients as individuals, because each person is unique. How a person is influenced, as well as the extent of the influence, depends on the individual. How a person is influenced by his culture depends on the unique life experiences of the individual (e.g., family factors, "critical events," age, and socioeconomic level). Culture influences behavior patterns, communications process, and health and illness beliefs and practices. The nurse and the patient each have their own cultural life-styles. It is not that a nurse should change her beliefs, values, and practices related to health and illness to fit those of her patients, but she needs to gain an understanding of her patient's characteristics to provide effective care. If a nurse is not aware of a patient's cultural background, she may (1) misjudge the culture's effect on health care, (2) make culturally incorrect and improper nursing care judgments, and (3) provide poor and even unsafe interventions.[11]

To provide individualized nursing care, it will be important for nurses to develop a positive approach in interacting with patients who are culturally and racially different. We all have a cultural background, and each person will decide which cultural characteristics are important. Even if a person considers himself to be mainstream American, he will also have a cultural life-style. Trends or similarities that exist among persons belonging to a distinct cultural or racial group can be seen in their behavior and communication in the clinical or community setting.

The cultural variables described in this chapter are group characteristics of ethnic minorities. Again, these characteristics may not be shown by every member of a cultural group. A person never acquires a culture as a complete and absolute pattern; instead, he merely learns the main components of a **subculture**. Variations within a cultural group usually occur because of individual differences.[10] Examples of these differences are displayed in Box 12-1.

Because culture influences different individuals' values, attitudes, and behaviors in various ways, the nurse must not stereotype members of any cultural group. Porter[13] defined stereotype as "attitudinal sets in which we assign characteristics to another person solely on the basis of the class or category to which that person belongs." An **ethnic stereotype** is a fixed concept of how all members of an ethnic group act or think. Stereotypes may or may not bear any relationship to reality. For example, stereotypes based on racism are unrelated to reality.[10] An example of a stereotype is the belief that all patients of Japanese ancestry are uncomplaining and cooperative.[11]

BOX 12-1 **FACTORS RELATED TO CULTURAL VARIATIONS AMONG ETHNIC/MINORITY GROUPS**

- Age
- Religion
- Dialect/language spoken
- Gender identity and roles
- Socioeconomic background
- Geographical location in country of origin or current residence
- Amount and type of interaction between younger and older generations
- Degree of adoption of values in current country

ETHNOCENTRISM AND CULTURAL CONFLICTS

Definition of Ethnocentrism

Ethnocentrism is the tendency to view members of other cultural or ethnic groups in terms of the standards of behavior and values of a person's own group.[13] Ethnocentrism restricts a person from accepting another culture favorably. For instance, an ethnocentric nurse might immediately view all non-Western healing methods as primitive and unscientific. Both ethnocentrism and stereotyping can affect the quality of patient care.

When ethnocentrism increases, cultural racism can result. **Racism** is any ethnocentric activity—cultural, individual, or institutional, deliberate or not, that is based on the belief of the superiority of one racial group over other racial groups to maintain the oppression and control of these groups.[10]

Racial/Cultural Conflicts

Cultural conflict between health professionals and their patients occurs when health care is perceived as unequal. For example, if a minority group has been stereotyped as dirty, a patient from the minority group may perceive a nurse's emphasis on cleanliness and bathing as prejudice.

Aggression occurs when **minority group** members strike out against their subordinate status by engaging in hostile acts against members of the **dominant group.** The patient from a minority group may react to prejudice and discrimination with overt (direct) or covert (indirect) aggression. One form in which hostility may find expression is in humor—the joke. For example, a Puerto Rican patient says to a nurse: "Hey, Mr. Jones changed his room. Is he afraid of catching something from me? He acted like I was a strange thing from outerspace or something (laughing)." The "joke" illustrates the patient's underlying feeling or belief that his roommate left because of his racial or ethnic minority status. It is safer to express it using humor versus anger or hostility. It is in reality not meant to be funny, but to mask the patient's true feelings in a clinical environment. The astute nurse can often pick up significant clues concerning the patient's real sentiments and attitudes from their jokes. In contrast, sullenness or stubbornness and verbal hostility might be used by patients of a minority group to express more direct forms of frustration. Nurses should interact by showing sympathy and understanding to break down the wall of resistance.[11]

Sometimes it is impossible to change a patient's ideas, but if a nurse has dealt with her own feelings of racial prejudice, this is a step in the right direction and offers an example for others. Piero said, "Think through beliefs about people of other races. Most of us harbor prejudices. To be fair with ourselves, fellow workers, and patients, we must find them and overcome them."[12] Nurses also need to expand their knowledge of culture and analyze nurse/patient interactions in an attempt to resolve cultural conflicts.

CULTURAL VARIABLES

Cultural variables (differences) are those characteristics generally identified with a particular cultural group. These variables may or may not be exhibited by every person from a cultural group. An understanding of the underlying development of the cultural variables is essential for carrying out an appropriate and effective cultural assessment. Box 12-2 highlights those variables that form the basis for cultural assessment.

Ethnic and Racial Identity

Werner[17] defines **ethnicity** as a group's "affiliation as a result of shared linguistic, racial, religious, and/or cultural background." For example, Africans and Puerto Ricans are members of ethnic groups, whereas the terms *Black* and *Oriental* describe membership in racial groups.

Value Orientations

Values are intrinsic beliefs about the worth of an entity or concept.[4] They provide the basis for attitudes and behaviors, and they help a person establish a hierarchy of needs and goals. For example, different cultures place different values on privacy, courtesy, respect for elders, and the work ethic. Value orientations are defined as principles that assist in the solution of common human problems.[6]

Language and Communication Process

The most difficult area for nurses and ethnic/cultural patients is in the communication process, since so much of the nursing process depends on communication. One example of communication variations is in the Filipino communication process. The patient who is Filipino is

BOX 12-2 CULTURAL VARIABLES

1. Ethnic and racial identity
2. Value orientations
3. Language and communication process
4. Family system
5. Healing beliefs and practices
6. Religious beliefs and practices
7. Nutritional behavior and cultural influences

likely to view the nurse as an authority figure who should be treated with formality; thus a patient who is Filipino may appear aloof and reserved, even in an anxiety-provoking clinical situation. Another example is the different traditional communications patterns of Caucasians and African-Americans: the White tradition relies on a relatively rigid pattern of expression characterized by heavy dependence on the written word, whereas the African-American tradition is more memory-oriented and favors oral communication.[15] Thus the nurse might find that visual aids are better received by African-American patients, whereas written pamphlets are more helpful with Caucasian patients.

BOX 12-3 **FACTORS TO CONSIDER IN ASSESSING FAMILY SYSTEM**

1. Consider the family as a unit when planning a patient's care.
2. Consider how the family structure influences the patient's response to health/illness.
3. Consider the family's participation in the patient's care.
4. Consider the family's role in health promotion or illness causation.

Family System

The extended family, including relatives beyond the basic family unit, is highly valued among many ethnic minority groups. Usually the entire family is involved when a person becomes ill. The elderly play a significant role in family functions in ethnic families. For example, the "issei" (first generation) Japanese expect their children, the "nisei" (second generation), to practice "oya koko," meaning caring for parents in old age.[11] McGoldrick, Pearce, and Giordano[7] state that "individual behavior cannot be understood in isolation from the family context and that family behavior makes sense only in the larger framework of culture." Known characteristics of groups may assist in formulating initial thoughts and concerns about health and illness behavior of ethnic families.[2]

For example, strong kinship bonds are highly prevalent among African-Americans as a means of survival, regardless of social class. If a family member cannot take care of a young child, often the child is informally adopted by another family member.[1] La Fargue[7] states that nurses are often not aware of this survival strategy among African-Americans "to immerse themselves in a domestic circle of kinfolk who will help them."

Four points to remember when assessing the ethnic/cultural importance of a patient's family system are described in Box 12-3.

Healing Beliefs and Practices

Cultural healing beliefs reflect a specific cultural group's orientation to health and illness. Alternative healing beliefs and practices may be the most difficult factors for the nurse to assess, because they differ greatly from the traditional scientific medical theories about health and illness with which nurses are familiar. Much research has been done to show these beliefs and practices are prevalent among ethnic/cultural groups.[14]

For example, the Hmong from Southeast Asia believe in the idea of a "bad fate" person. "Any child or adult who is disfigured or disabled is viewed as having become this way because the ancestor spirits and other spirits in nature have produced the malady."[18]

Healing practices among ethnic minority groups commonly involve using herbs, potions, oils, powders, tokens, rituals, ceremonies, candles, and incense. The nurse on occasion may ask patients who are from an ethnic minority group if they are using cultural healing practices or employing cultural healers (spiritualist, voodoo priests, curandero, or Asian herbalist) that may impact on Western orthodox medicine. Nurses must understand that these beliefs often have great psychological impact on whether the patient gets well.

Religious Beliefs and Practices

Religious beliefs and practices often overlap with the cultural beliefs about the cause of illness and methods of cure. For example, pledges, prayers, and the wearing of clothing identified with saints are still practiced by some Hispanics during illnesses. Many Hispanics also believe that wellness or illness is the will of God.[11] Religion is a major psychological support system for many ethnic minority patients. Patients should be encouraged to use this support system, and they should be allowed to keep or use talismans, tokens, or religious ceremonies that may help them combat the anxiety and stress associated with their illness and/or its treatment.

Nutritional Behavior and Cultural Influences

The nurse should assess food preferences and restrictions, meaning of foods, style of food preparation and consumption, frequency of eating, time of eating, and eating utensils that are culturally determined. Chinese believe that conditions such as dry mouth, constipation, or poor digestion are caused by eating too many hot foods (fried/spicy) and they must be balanced with cold foods (leafy vegetables). Finally, some American Indians use corn in many religious ceremonies, because corn is thought to possess medicinal qualities and may be sprinkled around an ill person to protect him.[11]

Understanding the cultural basis of a patient's behavior will help the nurse appreciate differences in custom or practice that might otherwise be viewed as harmful to the patient's health. To provide effective care to patients from diverse cultural backgrounds, nurses must develop an understanding of ethnic/cultural data for those populations in their communities.

REFERENCES AND SUGGESTED READINGS

1. Bloch B: The Black family: rules and modes of communication. In Wang F, Nath CL, and Simoni PS, editors: Living with change and choice in health, Morgantown, W Va, 1986, Sigma Theta Tau, Alpha Rho Chapter.
2. Capers CF: Cultural stereotypes of ethnic families, Cultural Connections 8(2):1, 4, 1988.
3. Crawford LA and Olinger BH: Recruitment and retention of nursing students from diverse cultural backgrounds, J Nurs Educ 27(8):379, 1988.
4. Frances GM and Munjas BD: Manual of social-psychologic assessment, New York, 1976, Appleton-Century-Crofts.
5. Haviland WA: Cultura. anthropology, ed 3, New York, 1981, Holt, Rinehart & Winston, Inc.
6. Kluckholn FR and Strodtbeck FL: Variations in value orientations, Elmsford, NY, 1961, Row, Peterson, & Co.
7. La Fargue JP: A survival strategy: kinship networks, Am J Nurs 80:1636, 1980.
8. McGoldrick M, Pearce JK, and Giordano J, editors: Ethnicity and family therapy, New York, 1982, The Guilford Press.
9. Murray RB and Zentner JP: Nursing concepts for health promotion, ed 2, Englewood Cliffs, NJ, 1979, Prentice-Hall, Inc.
10. Orque MS and Bloch B: Cultural factors in health. In Potter PA and Perry AG, editors: Basic nursing: theory and practice, St Louis, 1987, The CV Mosby Co.
11. Orque MS, Bloch B, and Monrroy LAS: Ethnic nursing care: a multicultural approach, St Louis, 1983, The CV Mosby Co.
12. Piero P: Black-White crisis, Am J Nurs 74:281, 1974.
13. Porter RE: An overview of intercultural communication. In Samovar LA and Porter RE, editors: Intercultural communication: a reader, Belmont, Calif, 1972, Wadsworth, Inc.
14. Roberson MHB: Home remedies: a cultural study, Home HealthC Nurse 5(1):35, 1987.
15. Smitherman G: Talkin' and testifyin': the language of Black America, Boston, 1977, Houghton Mifflin Co.
16. Walter PA: Race and culture relations, New York, 1952, McGraw-Hill, Inc.
17. Werner EE: Cross-cultural child development: a view from the planet earth, Monterey, Calif, 1979, Brooks/Cole Publishing Co.
18. Westermeyer J: Cultural beliefs and surgical procedures, JAMA 255(23):3301, 1986.

CHAPTER CHALLENGE

KEY POINTS

- Cultural background affects a person's health in all dimensions, and therefore the nurse should consider the patient's cultural background when planning care.
- The impact of culture on behaviors, attitudes, and values depends on individual factors and varies among members of a specific cultural group.
- How a person seeks to meet basic human needs is influenced by culture.
- Ethnocentrism can impede the delivery of care to ethnic minority patients and when pervasive can become cultural racism.
- Stereotyping ethnic group members can lead to mistaken assumptions about an individual ethnic minority patient.
- Cultural groups vary widely in value orientations, use of language, family systems, healing beliefs and practices, religious beliefs and practices, and food and eating habits.

STUDY QUESTIONS

1. Describe several ways in which nurses might obtain first-hand information from ethnic minority communities in their local area.
2. How can the nurse intervene if patient's cultural beliefs about physical symptoms are different from nursing beliefs about physical illness?
3. How can the nurse intervene if cultural healing practices conflict with traditional scientific methods of curing?
4. A sacred talisman was removed from Mr. Grayhorse, an American Indian, before surgery; this patient and family members became highly upset; what would be an appropriate intervention by the nurse in this situation?

IV

Vital Signs and Physical Assessment

I love nursing because every day brings new and different challenges for which I may use the skills I have been taught. I love nursing because it is very exciting and challenging to work in a field in which medical advancements are taking place seemingly every day. I love working with the whole medical team and realizing that their main concern, like mine, is to see the rapid recovery of the ill, as well as the new life that is being brought into the world. Yes, I love nursing because it is rewarding, challenging, and exciting, but most of all I love nursing because I love people.

MICHAEL A. PETERSON

Student Nurse

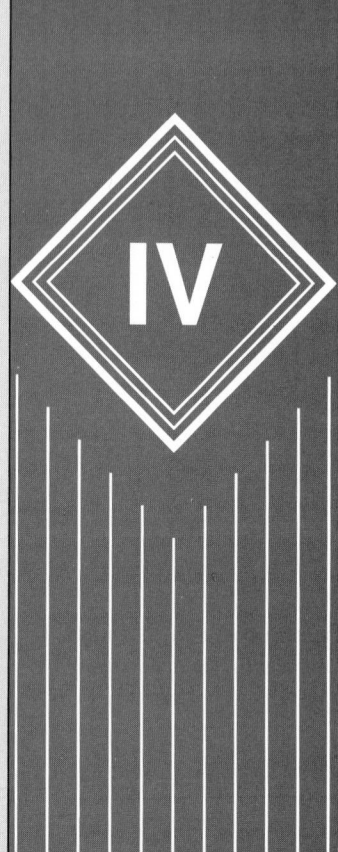

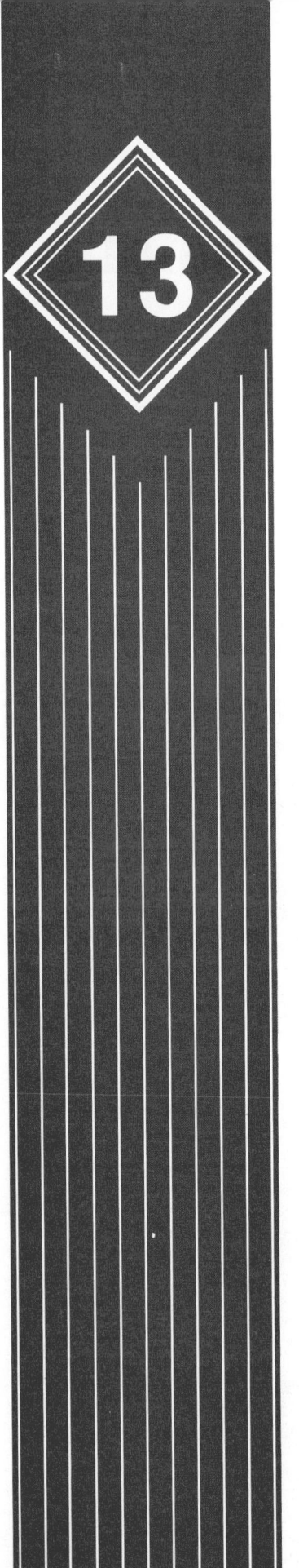

13

Signs, Symptoms, and Physical Assessment

AUDREY WADMAN SZCZESIUL

LEARNING OBJECTIVES

After reading this chapter, the student should be able to do the following:

- Define the key terms.
- Differentiate between a sign and a symptom.
- List the origins of disease.
- Discuss the four major risk categories for development of disease.
- Identify terms used to describe disease.
- List the universal signs of inflammation/infection.
- Identify frequently noted signs and symptoms in disease conditions.
- List methods to enhance the patient interview.
- Interview a patient.
- List the nursing responsibilities when assisting a physician with a physical examination.
- Describe the information obtained in a review of systems.
- Describe the sequence of steps when performing a physical assessment.
- List the equipment necessary to perform a physical assessment.
- Describe the positions assumed by the patient during a physical assessment.
- Describe methods of assessment.
- Describe normal assessment findings.

RELATED TOPICS OF INTEREST

- Communication (Chapter 4)
- Documentation (Chapter 6)
- Vital signs (Chapter 14)
- Care of the patient with cancer (Chapter 41)

KEY TERMS

Define the following:

- acute
- ADL
- adventitious
- anomalies
- assessment
- auscultation
- bruits
- chronic
- crepitus
- CVA
- data base
- edema
- etiology
- erythema
- Hemoccult
- inspection
- JVD
- leukoplakia
- leukorrhea
- LOC
- neoplastic
- objective data
- ophthalmoscope
- palpation
- percussion
- periorbital edema
- PERRLA
- PQRST
- ptosis
- pupillary reflex
- purulent
- reflecting
- review of systems
- ROM
- signs
- subjective data
- symptoms
- thrill
- TMJ
- turgor

SIGNS AND SYMPTOMS

Signs are **objective data,** as perceived by the examiner, in this case the nurse. Examples of signs are rashes, altered vital signs, and visible drainage. The nurse uses the senses of sight, hearing, touch, and smell to gather these objective data or signs.

Symptoms are subjective indications of illness that are perceived by the patient. Examples of symptoms are pain, nausea, and anxiety. The nurse is unaware of symptoms unless the patient describes the sensation. Symptoms are referred to as **subjective data.**

Disease and Diagnosis

A disease is a specific illness characterized by a recognizable set of signs and symptoms. These signs and symptoms are clustered into a group that allows the physician to make a medical diagnosis. The nurse also relies on assessment of signs and symptoms to formulate a nursing diagnosis. Unlike a medical diagnosis, which deals with pathophysiological factors and the cure of a disease, the nursing diagnosis recognizes holistic needs of the patient that can be treated with independent and dependent nursing interventions. These needs are patient problems, either real or potential.

Origins of disease. Disease or illness originates from many causes, including hereditary, congenital, infectious, metabolic, deficiency, neoplastic, traumatic conditions, and environmental factors. There are other diseases for which no apparent cause is known. These illnesses have an unknown **etiology** (cause).

Hereditary diseases are transmitted genetically from parent to offspring. An example of a genetically transmitted disease is cystic fibrosis. The offspring has a 25% chance of acquiring cystic fibrosis if both the parents have the recessive trait. The child with cystic fibrosis develops lifelong respiratory and digestive difficulties.

Congenital diseases are present at birth. The disease results from a condition during the pregnancy that interferes with the normal development of the fetus, such as the mother's having rubella (german measles) during early gestation (pregnancy). Congenital conditions include **anomalies** (structural defects) and defects in the functioning of a body organ. An example of an anomaly is clubfoot. Defects in the body's functioning include Down's syndrome or cretinism, both of which result in physical and mental retardation.

Infectious diseases result from the invasion of bacteria or viruses into the body. Examples of infectious diseases include acquired immunodeficiency syndrome (AIDS), tuberculosis, and measles.

Deficiency diseases result from the lack of a specific nutrient. Nutrients are minerals, vitamins, proteins, fats, and carbohydrate. Scurvy is a deficiency disease resulting from a lack of vitamin C. Kwashiorkor results from a severe deficiency of protein in the diet.

Metabolic disease is caused by a dysfunction that results in a loss of metabolic control of homeostasis in the body. The dysfunction usually involves endocrine glands, which secrete hormones to regulate body processes. Diabetes mellitus results from the dysfunction of the pancreas. Other examples of metabolic disease are hypothyroidism and acromegaly, which involve the thyroid and pituitary glands.

Neoplastic disease is described as an abnormal growth of new tissue. The new growth may be benign or malignant (cancerous). Malignant neoplasms are a serious threat to health, because the rapid growth of the cells robs nutrients from the body's normal cells.

Traumatic conditions result from both physical and emotional trauma. Physical trauma, such as a motor vehicle accident, can result in traumatic brain injury (TBI). TBI may leave the individual mentally and physically impaired. Emotional trauma, such as the loss of a loved one, can result in the individual being unable to function in activities of daily living **(ADLs)** as they did before the trauma.

Environmental diseases are a group of conditions that develop from exposure to a harmful substance in the environment. The "tight building syndrome" is an example of an environmental illness. The individual complains of headache, dizziness, and respiratory infections. These signs and symptoms result from the fact that the well-built buildings of today do not allow circulation of fresh air and instead recycle air containing fumes and microorganisms. Radon gas and asbestos are also substances in the environment that can lead to disease.

Although many disease conditions have an unknown cause, many conditions are now thought to result from autoimmune responses. In an autoimmune response, the body develops immunoglobulins (antibodies) against its own tissues or body substances. Rheumatoid arthritis and ulcerative colitis are being researched as possible autoimmune diseases.

Risk factors for development of disease. Risk factors are situations, habits, environmental conditions, physiological conditions, or other variables that increase the vulnerability of an individual or group to illness. Risk factors do not necessarily mean that a person will develop a disease condition but that the chances of disease are increased. For example, risk factors for the development of heart disease include cigarette smoking, high blood levels of cholesterol, and stressful work conditions. The nurse assesses the patients's risk factors, because nursing diagnoses are made for potential as well as actual patient problems.

Risk factors are placed into four major categories: genetic and physiological, age, environment, and life-style (Box 13-1).

BOX 13-1 RISK FACTORS FOR DISEASE

RISK CATEGORY	EXAMPLE
Genetic, physiological	A family history of cancer increases the risk of an individual's developing cancer (genetic). Malnourishment predisposes an individual to illness (physiological).
Age	Thinning skin in the elderly makes this group more susceptible to skin trauma.
Environment	Radon gas seeping from the earth into a basement can increase the risk of cancer development.
Life-style	Smoking increases the risk of lung cancer.

Terms used to describe disease. Diseases are described in terms of duration. **Chronic** disease develops slowly and persists over a long period, often for a person's lifetime. Diabetes mellitus (inability of the body to use glucose) is an example of a chronic disease. Chronic disease can be further described as early, late, or terminal. Chronic disease can also be described as being in remission. Remission means there has been a partial or complete disappearance of clinical and subjective characteristics of the disease. Remission may be spontaneous or a result of therapy.

In comparison, a disease described as **acute** begins abruptly with marked intensity of severe symptoms and then often subsides after a period of treatment. An episode of appendicitis would be considered acute.

Disease can also be described as functional or organic. Organic disease results from changes in an organ that interfere with its functioning. Cerebrovascular accident (CVA, stroke) is an organic disease of the brain. A functional disease may be manifested as an organic disease, but careful examination fails to reveal evidence of structural or physiological abnormalities. A headache can be an organic or a functional disorder.

Common signs and symptoms of disease (Box 13-2)

Signs and symptoms: inflammation/infection. Inflammation differs from infection. Infection is caused by invasion of a microorganism, such as a bacteria or a parasite. Inflammation does have similar signs and symptoms of infection but is not necessarily the result of an invading organism. The universal signs of inflammation/infection are pain, erythema (redness), **edema** (swelling), heat, purulent drainage (pus), and loss of function. The purulent drainage may also have a foul (fetid) odor.

BOX 13-2 FREQUENTLY NOTED SIGNS AND SYMPTOMS OF DISEASE

Jaundice	Yellow tinge to the skin and may indicate obstruction in the flow of bile from the liver.
Cyanosis	Bluish discoloration of the skin and mucous membranes caused by an excess of deoxygenated hemoglobin in the blood.
Pallor	An unnatural paleness or absence of color in the skin: It may result from a decrease in hemoglobin and erythrocytes (red blood cells).
Erythema	Redness or inflammation of the skin or mucous membranes that is the result of dilation and congestion of superficial capillaries; erythema is seen in a mild sunburn.
Edema	An abnormal accumulation of fluid in interstitial spaces. It may be caused by overhydration, excess sodium intake, or a loss of serum albumin (a protein), which causes fluid to leave the vessels and collect in the interstitial space. Skin that is edematous will be taut and shiny. Pitting may occur when the skin is pressed; a small indentation will remain after the finger is removed.
Pruritus	A symptom of itching and an uncomfortable sensation leading to an urge to scratch. Some causes are allergy, infection, jaundice, and skin irritation.
Nausea	A sensation often leading to the urge to vomit. Common causes include intense pain, gall bladder disease, inflammation of the stomach, and food poisoning.
Vomiting	To expel the contents of the stomach through the esophagus and out of the mouth. The quality of the vomitus can give a clue to the underlying cause. "Coffee ground" vomitus indicates bleeding in the stomach. The blood takes on a coffee ground appearance because of the effect of the digestive juices. Vomiting of bright red blood could be a sign of gastric hemorrhage.
Anorexia	Lack of appetite resulting in the inability to eat. This symptom can occur in many disease conditions.
Diarrhea	Frequent passage of loose liquid stools; generally results from increased motility in the colon. This is usually a sign of an underlying disorder. The characteristics of the diarrhea give evidence as to the source. Dark black tarry stools can mean there is bleeding in the intestines. Bright red blood in the feces indicates active bleeding from the lower portion of the intestinal tract.
Constipation	Difficulty in passing stools or an incomplete or infrequent passage of hard stools. There are many causes, both organic and functional.
Coughing	A sudden audible expulsion of air from the lungs. Coughing is an essential protective response that serves to clear the lungs, bronchi, or trachea of irritants and secretions or to prevent aspiration of foreign material into the lungs. It is a common sign of diseases of the chest and larynx.
Dyspnea	A shortness of breath or difficulty in breathing that may be caused by certain heart and lung conditions, strenuous exercise, or anxiety.
Orthopnea	An abnormal condition in which a person must sit or stand to breathe deeply or comfortably. Occurs in many disorders of the respiratory and cardiac system.
Tachypnea	an abnormally rapid rate of breathing seen in many diseased conditions.
Tachycardia	An abnormal condition in which the heart contracts regularly but at a rate greater than 100 beats per minute. The heart rate accelerates in response to fever, exercise, or nervous excitement.
Pain	An unpleasant sensation caused by noxious (extremely destructive or harmful) stimulation of the sensory nerve endings. It is a cardinal symptom of inflammation and is valuable in the diagnosis of many disorders and conditions. Pain may be mild or severe, chronic, acute, burning, dull, or sharp, precisely or poorly localized, or referred.
Fever Pyrexia Febrile	An abnormal elevation of the temperature of the body above 98.6° F (37° C) because of disease. It results from an imbalance between the elimination and production of heat. Infection and many different diseases may lead to elevated temperature.

The inflammatory process is actually a body defense against the causative agent. The erythema and edema are the result of increased blood flow to the area. Pain occurs because of increased pressure on pain sensors in the area. Heat occurs as blood flow and metabolism in the area are increased. Loss of function is the body's method of resting the injured part. Purulent drainage is the accumulation of the white blood cells, dead cells, bacteria, and other debris from the inflammatory process. The heat felt when fever is present during an illness is a body defense, since many bacteria will be destroyed by the higher temperature.

BOX 13-3 MAINTAINING EFFECTIVE COMMUNICATION

PROMOTING EFFECTIVE COMMUNICATION

Maintaining silence. Silence can help the nurse and patient to organize their thoughts. It also enables the nurse to observe the patient more closely.

Listening attentively. Attentive listening allows one to understand an entire message conveyed, verbally and nonverbally. It also facilitates trust.

Conveying acceptance. Acceptance means that one is nonjudgmental. Acceptance is not synonymous with agreement; rather, it is a willingness to hear the person's message. One conveys acceptance through positive feedback and making sure verbal and nonverbal cues match.

Asking related questions. Questioning is a direct method of communicating. Asking related questions allows the patient to give information logically. Open-ended questions are useful for eliciting more information from the patient about a subject.

Paraphrasing. Paraphrasing sends feedback to the patient that information has been accurately received.

Clarifying. Clarifying helps retain important information. Using examples can clarify abstract ideas. All clarification should be specific.

Focusing. When a discussion becomes vague or ill defined, focusing directs conversation to a specific topic or issue. It limits the area of discussion to which the patient can respond. The nurse seeks meaning in the patient's message.

Stating observations. Describing a patient's observed behavior can provide feedback as to whether an intended message was received. It can clarify conflicts between verbal and nonverbal cues.

Offering information. Offering information provides a patient with relevant data and prevents one-sided conversations. It is useful for health teaching and helps in decision making.

Summarizing. Summarizing is a concise review of main ideas from a discussion. It sets the tone for further interactions. By reviewing a conversation the participants can focus on key issues and any relevant information previously deleted.

INHIBITING EFFECTIVE COMMUNICATION

Giving an opinion. Giving an opinion takes decision making away from the patient. It inhibits spontaneity, stalls problem solving, and creates doubt. If offering suggestions, the nurse should stress that they are only options.

Offering false reassurance. Offering false reassurance can do more harm than good. False reassurance may allow the nurse to promise something that will not occur or is unrealistic.

Being defensive. Defensiveness in the face of criticism implies that the patient has no right to an opinion. The patient's concerns often become ignored. Attentive listening helps the patient open up but does not imply agreement.

Showing approval or disapproval. Showing approval or disapproval is judgmental and may halt a conversation. It inhibits the patient's ability to share ideas and make decisions independently. Disapproval can indicate rejection.

Asking why. Asking why may imply an accusation. It can cause resentment, insecurity, and mistrust. If additional information is needed, the nurse can phrase a question to avoid use of "why."

Changing the subject inappropriately. Changing the subject inappropriately is rude and shows a lack of empathy. It stalls communication. The patient may then give incomplete or inadequate information.

Forming communication barriers. Forming communication barriers by saying something inadvertently that blocks a patient's communication can break down communication. By acknowledging the mistake, the nurse can start the communication process anew.

Assessment

Nursing **assessment** is the identification by a nurse of the needs, preferences, and abilities of a patient. Assessment follows an interview with and observation of a patient by the nurse and considers the signs and symptoms of the condition, the patient's verbal and nonverbal communication, medical and social history, and any other information available. Assessment is extremely important, because it provides the scientific basis for a nursing diagnosis and a complete nursing care plan.

The patient interview. The physical assessment begins with the patient interview. The nurse conducts the interview in a relaxed, unhurried manner in a quiet, private, well-lighted setting. To conduct an effective and informative interview, the nurse must develop interviewing skills, gain the patient's trust, and convey feelings of compassion while remaining objective. The patient must feel that the information being given is important to the nurse; the nurse must demonstrate an interest in the patient's state of wellness.

The nurse initially establishes trust by introducing himself or herself and asking what name the patient wishes to be called by and then using that name during the interview. An accepting posture, in which the nurse is sitting in a relaxed manner at eye level with the patient, will foster trust. A pleasant facial expression will help, and eye contact makes the patient feel he has the nurse's full attention.

The nurse can enhance communication by using nonjudgmental language. Statements by the nurse such as "Yes, I see," or "What happened next?" can encourage the patient to explain without feeling threatened. **Reflecting** what the patient has said in his own words clarifies statements, as does summarizing and restating what the patient has said. The nurse's approving nods and gestures facilitate the exchange of information (Box 13-3).

After the nurse briefly explains the purpose of the interview, the questioning should proceed in a structured fashion, beginning with biographical data and proceeding to chief complaint, past history, psychosocial status, and a review of systems. In most facilities the biographical data are obtained in the admitting department, and the nurse may refer to this information to begin the interview. To elicit the chief complaint, the nurse simply asks, "What is the reason for your admission?" This allows the patient not only to describe the reason for admission but also to make his expectations known to the nurse. To get the most information from the patient about his health concerns, the nurse can use the **PQRST** method of questioning (Box 13-4).

The interview should proceed with questions about past illnesses, hospitalizations, psychosocial data including family relationships and support systems, and living situations. A psychosocial history should include questions about the use of alcohol and drugs. This may be an uncomfortable area for both the interviewer and the interviewee, but a more accurate response is obtained if the question is asked, "How much do you drink?" rather than asking the patient if he drinks. The patient's ability to perform ADLs should be questioned. Medications that the patient is taking or has taken should be recorded, and conditions for which the medications are taken are clarified.

The next portion of the interview is a **review of systems** (Box 13-5). When determining the status of each body system, the patient is asked specific questions relating to the functioning of the organ. For example, assessment of the respiratory system might begin with the question, "Do you have any trouble breathing?" If the reply is affirmative, then the questioning can continue with "Please explain," or a more specific question, such

BOX 13-4 HISTORY OF PRESENT ILLNESS

When discussing the history of present illness with your patient, make sure he describes his problems fully. To do this, ask him the following questions about each complaint:

Time of onset. When was the first date (the problem) happened? What time did it begin?

Type of onset. How did (the problem) start: suddenly? gradually?

Original source. What were you doing when you first experienced or noticed (the problem)? What seems to trigger it: stress? position? certain activities? arguments? If describing a discharge: thick? runny? clear? colored? If describing a psychological problem: Do the voices drown out other sounds? Whose voice does it sound like?

Severity. How bad is (the problem) when it's at its worst? Does it interfere with your normal activities? Does it force you to lie down, sit down, slow down?

Radiation. In the case of pain, does it travel down your back or arms, up your neck, or down your legs?

Time relationship. How often do you experience (the problem): hourly? daily? weekly? monthly? When do you usually experience it: daytime? at night? in the early morning? Are you ever awakened by it? Does it ever occur before, during, or after meals? Does it occur seasonally?

Duration. How long does an episode of (the problem) last?

Course. Does (the problem) seem to be getting better, to be getting worse, or does it remain the same?

Associations. Does (the problem) lead to anything else? Is it accompanied by other signs and symptoms?

Source of relief. What relieves (the problem): changing diet? changing position? taking medications? being active?

Source of aggravation. What makes (the problem) worse?

You can remember all these questions using the letters *PQRST:*

P Provocative/palliative
What causes it? What makes it better?
What makes it worse?

Q Quality/quantity
How does it feel, look, or sound, and how much of it is there?

R Region/radiation
Where is it? Does it spread?

S Severity scale
Does it interfere with activities?
How does it rate on a severity scale of 1 to 10?

T Timing
When did it begin? How often does it occur? Is it sudden or gradual?

BOX 13-5 **REVIEW OF SYSTEMS**

It is probable that all of the questions in each system will not be included every time you take a history. Nevertheless, some questions regarding each system should be included in every history. These essential areas are listed in bold type in the outline that follows. More comprehensive and detailed areas for questions relating to each system are listed afterward and should be included whenever the patient gives positive responses to the first group of questions for that system. Keep in mind that these lists do not represent an exhaustive enumeration of questions that might be appropriate within an organ system. Even more detailed questions may be required, depending on the patient's problem.

A. **General constitutional symptoms:** fever, chills, malaise, fatigability, night sweats; weight (average, preferred, present, change, appetite)
B. **Skin:** rash or eruption, pruritus, pigmentation or texture change; excessive sweating, abnormal nail or hair growth
C. **Skeletal:** joint stiffness, pain, restriction of motion, edema, erythema, heat, bony deformity
D. **Head**
   1. General: frequent or unusual headaches, dizziness, syncope, severe head injuries
   2. Eyes: visual acuity, blurring, diplopia (double vision), photophobia (abnormal sensitivity to light), pain, recent change in appearance or vision; glaucoma, use of eye drops or other eye medications; history of trauma or familial eye disease
   3. Ears: hearing loss, pain, discharge, tinnitus, vertigo
   4. Nose: sense of smell, frequency of colds, obstruction, epistaxis, postnasal discharge, sinus pain
   5. Throat and mouth: hoarseness or change in voice; frequent sore throats, bleeding or edema of gums; recent tooth abscesses or extractions; soreness of tongue or buccal mucosa, ulcers; disturbance of taste
E. **Endocrine:** thyroid enlargement or tenderness, heat or cold intolerance, unexplained weight change, diabetes, polydipsia (excessive thirst), polyuria, changes in facial or body hair, increased hat and glove size, skin striae
   1. Males: onset of puberty, erections, emissions, testicular pain, libido, infertility
   2. Females:
      a. Menses: onset, regularity, duration of flow, dysmenorrhea, last period, intermenstrual discharge or bleeding, pruritus, date of last Pap smear, age at menopause, libido, frequency of intercourse, sexual difficulties
      b. Pregnancies: number, miscarriages, abortions, duration of pregnancy in each and any complication during any pregnancy or postpartum period; use of oral or other contraceptives
      c. Breasts: pain, tenderness, discharge, lumps, mammograms
F. **Respiratory:** pain relating to respiration, dyspnea, cyanosis, wheezing, cough, sputum (character and quantity), hemoptysis (expectorating blood from respiratory tract), night sweats, exposure to TB; date and result of last chest x-ray examination
G. **Cardiac:** chest pain or distress, precipitating causes, timing and duration, relieving factors, palpitations, dyspnea, orthopnea (number of pillows needed), edema, claudication (weakness of legs accompanied by cramplike pain), hypertension, previous myocardial infarction, estimate of excerise tolerance, past ECG or other cardiac tests
H. **Hematological:** anemia, tendency to bruise or bleed easily, thromboses, thrombophlebitis, any known abnormality of blood cells, transfusions
I. **Lymph nodes:** enlargement, tenderness, suppuration (to produce purulent [pus] material)
J. **Gastrointestinal:** appetite, digestion, intolerance for any class of foods, dysphagia, heartburn, nausea, vomiting, hematemesis, regularity of bowels, constipation, diarrhea, change in stool color or contents (clay-colored, tarry, fresh blood, mucus, undigested food), flatulence, hemorrhoids, hepatitis, jaundice, dark urine; history of ulcer, gallstones, polyps, tumor; previous x-ray examinations (where, when, findings)
K. **Genitourinary:** dysuria, flank or suprapubic pain, urgency, frequency, nocturia, hematuria, polyuria, hesitancy, dribbling, loss in force of stream, passage of stone; edema of face, stress incontinence, hernias, sexually transmitted disease (inquire what kind and symptoms, and list results of serological test for syphilis [STS], if known)
L. **Neurological:** syncope (brief lapse in consciousness caused by transient cerebral hypoxia), seizures, weakness or paralysis, abnormalities of sensation or coordination, tremors, loss of memory; unusual frequency, distribution, or severity of headaches, serious head injury in past
M. **Psychiatric:** depression, mood changes, difficulty concentrating, nervousness, tension, suicidal thoughts, irritability, sleep disturbances

THERAPEUTIC DIALOGUE

■ Mr. Jones is admitted to the hospital with a diagnosis of possible peptic ulcer.

NURSE: Mr. Jones, can you tell me about your pain? What brings it on?
MR. JONES: I get the pain several times a day after I eat. *(provocative) (timing)*
NURSE: What does it feel like?
MR. JONES: It feels like burning. *(quality)*
NURSE: Where does the pain occur?
MR. JONES: In my stomach. *(region)*
NURSE: How does the pain rate on a scale of 1 to 10?
MR. JONES: About an 8. *(severity)*
NURSE: How long have you had this pain?
MR. JONES: It began about 6 months ago. *(timing)*

as "Do you have shortness of breath?" A review of systems guide can be used to guarantee a complete interview.

The patient interview at the beginning of the physical assessment gives the nurse much more information about the patient than what is actually spoken. The therapeutic dialogue above is an example of an interview using the PQRST technique. The nurse observes patient mobility and gains insight about the patient's intellect, level of orientation, and emotional and psychological state.

The nurse should assess the appropriateness of the patient's answers. By asking questions such as "Who are you?" "Why are you here?" and "Where are you?" the nurse determines the level of consciousness **(LOC)** and orientation of the individual is made.

Once the interview has been completed, the nurse can proceed to the physical assessment. When assessing the patient, the nurse should pay special attention to areas about which the patient has expressed concern.

THE NURSING PHYSICAL ASSESSMENT

The purpose of the nursing physical assessment is to determine the patient's state of health or illness. The physician performs a physical assessment to determine the medical diagnosis.

When the physical examination is performed by the physician, the nurse has specific responsibilities when assisting the physician. These responsibilities include psychological support for the patient, physical preparation of the patient and environment before the procedure, assisting with positioning of the patient during the examination (Table 13-1), and assisting the physician by handing needed equipment and labeling specimens.

Psychological support is provided by explaining what is going to happen during the examination and answering any questions the patient may have. During the examination, holding the patient's hand or relaying comforting words or gestures can help the patient feel at ease.

Physical preparation of the patient includes having the patient empty the bladder before the examination. A urine specimen may be obtained at this time if required. The patient should be wearing a hospital gown for the examination. The nurse assists the patient to assume the position most suitable for the assessment of each body area. The nurse drapes the patient appropriately with a sheet or blanket to maintain privacy.

Preparation of the environment includes providing privacy by closing curtains or doors, making sure the room temperature is warm enough, and decreasing extraneous noises as much as possible. All necessary equipment needed during the examination is anticipated and provided by the nurse so the examination can proceed uninterrupted.

When the examination is concluded, the nurse assists the patient with hygiene as necessary, perhaps removing lubricant used during the rectal or vaginal examination. The nurse assists the patient to dress if appropriate and leaves the patient comfortable.

The nurse can also perform an assessment to determine the actual or potential patient problems that will require nursing intervention for the safety and well-being of the patient. For example, if during the assessment the nurse observes that the patient has a need for oxygen (a basic human need), positioning, deep breathing, and coughing can be instituted to meet this need.

The nurse's ability to correctly assess the patient is also valuable, because the nurse is the person in constant contact with the patient and can evaluate the medical treatment. The nurse can also monitor the patient to discover developing complications.

When to Perform a Physical Assessment

The best time to assess the patient is as soon after admission as possible. In some facilities, policy dictates that the assessment be done within 24 hours of admission. The initial physical assessment is performed by a registered nurse; however, the ongoing assessment is the responsibility of both the registered nurse and the licensed practical/vocational nurse.

The formal head-to-toe assessment (which will be described in detail) is initially done when the patient is admitted; however, portions of the assessment can be performed when the nurse observes a change in the patient's condition. The nurse can make a modified physical assessment part of daily nursing care. A complete physical assessment performed initially on the patient will help establish a **data base** from which a nursing care plan can be developed.

Table 13-1 Positions for Examination

Position	Areas Assessed	Rationale	Limitations
Sitting 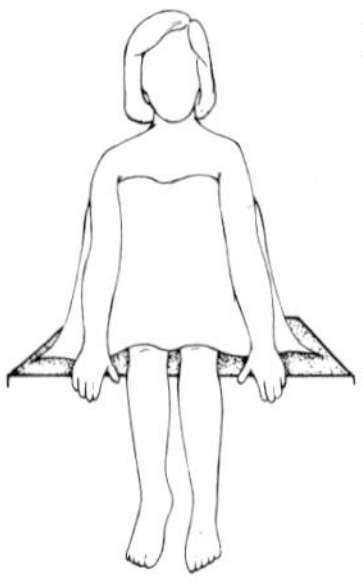	Head and neck, back, posterior thorax and lungs, anterior thorax and lungs, breasts, axillae, heart, vital signs, and upper extremities	Sitting upright provides full expansion of lungs and provides better visualization of symmetry of upper body parts.	A physically weakened patient may be unable to sit. Use supine position with head of bed elevated instead.
Supine 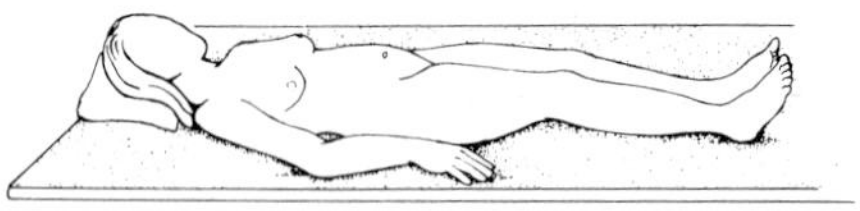	Head and neck, anterior thorax and lungs, breasts, axillae, heart, abdomen, extremities, pulses	This is the most normally relaxed position. It prevents contracture of abdominal muscles and provides easy access to pulse sites.	If patient becomes short of breath easily, examiner may need to raise head of bed.
Dorsal recumbent 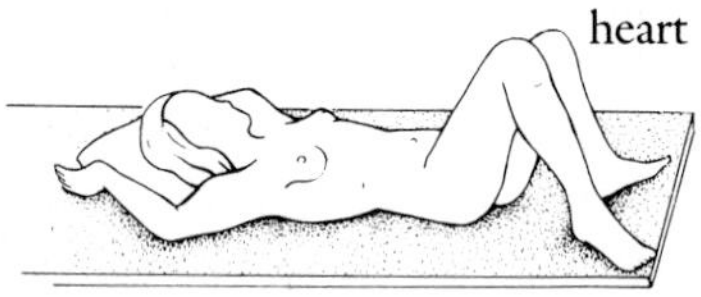	Head and neck, anterior thorax and lungs, breasts, axillae, heart	Certain patients with painful disorders are more comfortable with knees flexed.	Position is not used for abdominal assessment, because it promotes contracture of abdominal muscles.
Lithotomy 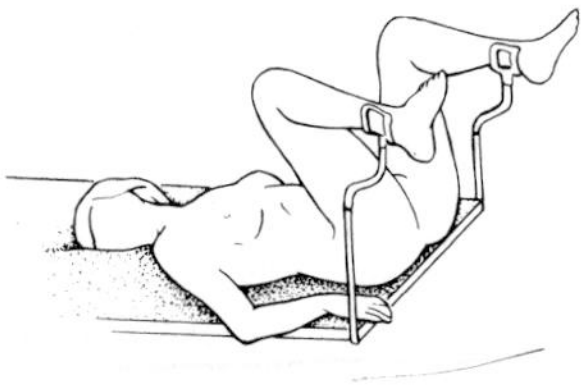	Female genitalia and genital tract	This position provides maximal exposure of genitalia and facilitates insertion of vaginal speculum.	This is an embarrassing and uncomfortable position, so minimize time the patient spends in this position. Keep patient well draped. A patient with severe arthritis or other joint deformity may be unable to assume this position.
Sims' 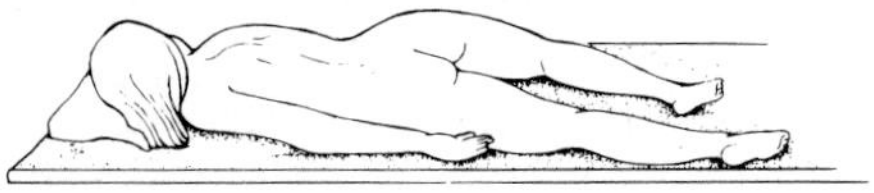	Rectum	Flexion of hip and knee improves exposure of rectal area.	Joint deformities may hinder the patient's ability to bend hip and knee.
Prone 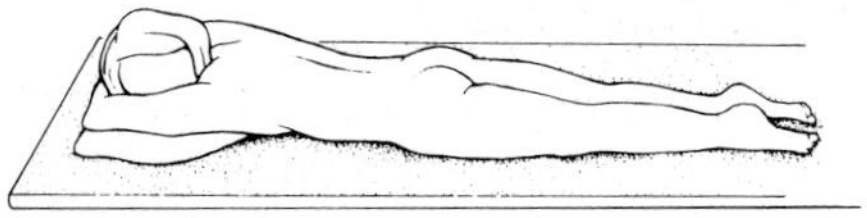	Musculoskeletal	This position is used only to assess extension of the hip joint.	This position is intolerable for a patient with respiratory difficulties.

Where to Perform a Physical Assessment

Regardless of the type of nursing care performed, whether it be home care, hospital care, or nursing in an extended care facility (ECF), the area in which the nursing assessment is performed should be comfortable for the patient, with a table or bed to allow for the positioning of the patient. It should provide for the patient's privacy and be free of distracting sights and sounds. In most cases the patient's own room works very well and is convenient for both patient and nurse.

Methods of Physical Assessment

The assessment may be organized as head-to-toe or system-by-system. In either case, the nurse must proceed systematically. If special concerns are expressed by the patient or noted by the nurse, it may be best to perform assessment of the system involved. For example, if the patient complains of abdominal pain, the nurse can then concentrate on assessment of the abdomen, employing percussion, palpation, and auscultation.

The head-to-toe method of assessment is best when performing a complete examination. The nurse begins with the head and neck, including the eyes, ears, nose, and mouth. The chest, back, arms, abdomen, perineal area, legs, and feet are examined in that order.

Nursing Skills for Assessment

To assess most accurately, the nurse must develop the skills of inspection, palpation, percussion, and auscultation.

Inspection. Inspection is purposeful observation of the patient. Observation begins the moment the nurse makes contact with the patient. Although during the actual physical assessment each part of the body is specifically inspected, casual observation is constantly being performed. If during inspection a physical abnormality is noted, it can then be further assessed by palpation, percussion, or possibly auscultation.

Palpation. Palpation involves using the fingers and hands to touch a body part. Hands are very sensitive to texture, temperature, and moisture and thus help to determine the quality of an area. Palpation is frequently used to assess the condition of lymph nodes and breasts and the abdomen for masses or distention. Palpation is used to clarify and verify an observation.

When using palpation, the nurse should warm the hands before touching the patient. Explanations to the patient as to what is being palpated and why will help relax him. Social conversation during palpation is appropriate at times to distract the patient and help him relax. Pads of the fingers should be used and placed flat against skin with slight pressure and gentle rotation of the area under examination. The thumb and forefinger can be used to palpate muscle mass on arms or legs. Pulses are palpated with the pads of the fingers.

Palpation can be light or deep, depending on the amount of downward pressure exerted. Light palpation depresses the skin to a depth of ½ inch. Deep palpation, used to locate internal organs, can be to a depth of 2 inches (Fig. 13-1).

During palpation the nurse should note the patient's facial expression; a grimace may indicate pain, which the patient can be asked to describe.

Auscultation. Auscultation is listening to the sounds produced by the body. This is usually accomplished with the aid of a stethoscope. The stethoscope should be in good working order and should have both a bell and a diaphragm. The areas to be assessed by auscultation are the heart, lungs, intestines, and blood vessels.

Mastering auscultation technique requires practice; when auscultating, the nurse realizes that the body produces many sounds that are normal and must be able to ignore these normal noises and concentrate on abnormal sounds. **Adventitious** (abnormal) breath sounds may be superimposed over normal sounds. The environment must be quiet for accurate assessment. Television, sounds from nasogastric suction, movement of bed linen, and patient conversation can all interfere with accurate auscultation. Auscultation should not be rushed; time is taken to locate each area to be assessed. The nurse listens critically to decide exactly what is being heard.

The stethoscope's diaphragm is placed gently over the patient's skin. If the area is hairy, the area can be dampened to decrease the sound made by the diaphragm on the hair. It is helpful to take the time to listen to one's own body sounds; audiotapes are available to help the nurse hear and recognize lung and heart sounds.

Percussion. Percussion is tapping on an area of the body to determine the density of the tissue beneath. Different organs of the body elicit different sounds (Table 13-2).

Percussion is used to determine consolidation in the lungs and also the contents of the intestines. To perform percussion, the flats of the fingertips of the nondominant hand are placed on the area to be percussed. The dominant hand then lightly taps the middle finger. Using the dominant hand allows control of pressure. Percussion should not be painful for the patient, but if it does cause discomfort, it should be discontinued and the result charted. Each area should be tapped two or three times. Experience can be gained by percussing the different areas of one's own body.

Performing the Physical Assessment

Items essential to the nurse's assessment are a penlight or flashlight, stethoscope, blood pressure cuff, thermometer, gloves, and a tongue blade. The nurse also makes

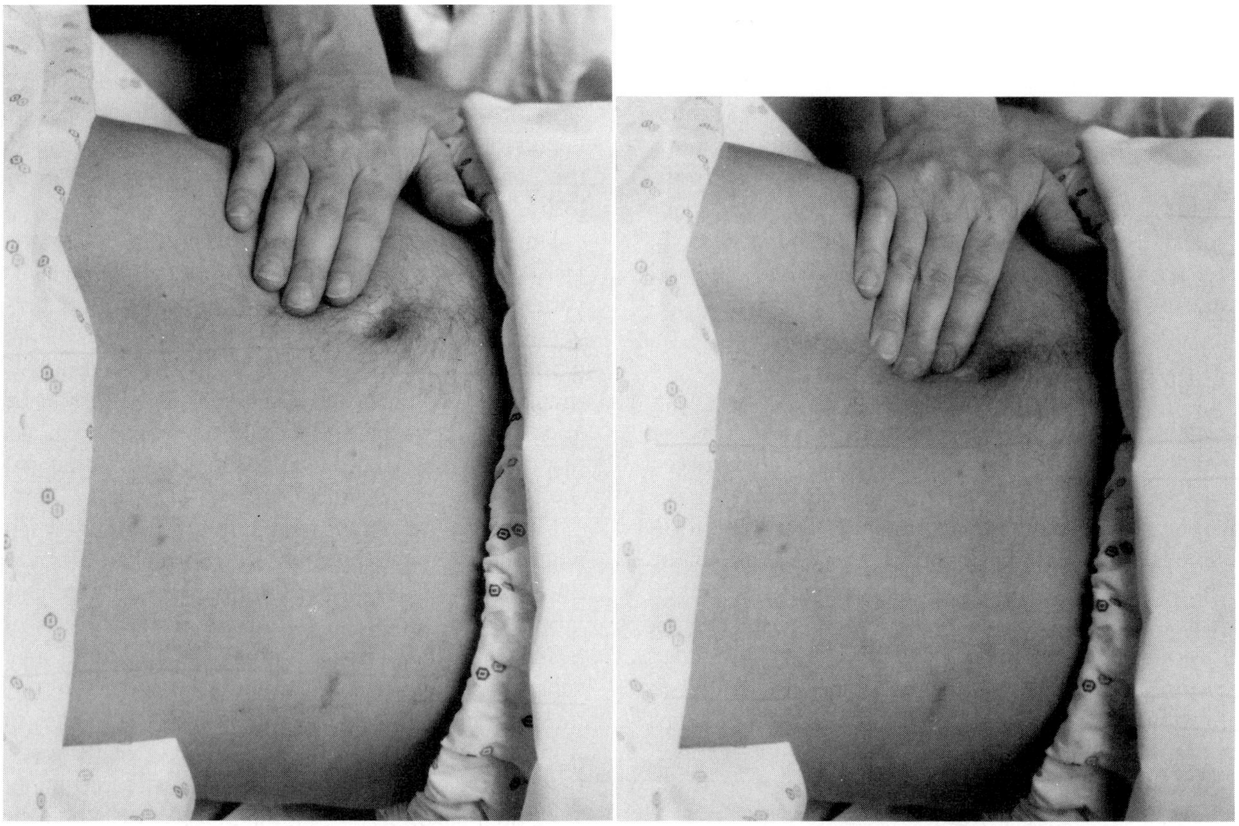

A B

FIG. 13-1 **A,** To perform light palpation, the examiner presses gently on the patient's skin, indenting approximately ½ to 1 inches. The hand is moved in a circular motion. **B,** To perform deep palpation, fingertip pressure is increased, indenting about 2 inches.

use of the senses of touch, smell, sight, and hearing. The nurse should always wash the hands before beginning the physical assessment.

The patient should be provided the opportunity to empty the bladder before the examination. This makes the patient more comfortable and allows easier assessment of the bladder.

The patient's vital signs are obtained, including temperature, pulse, respirations, and blood pressure. Height and weight can also be measured at the outset of the exam. Height and weight should be measured by the nurse for accuracy rather than taking the patient's stated height and weight. Vital sign data gathered at the beginning of the assessment may give the nurse a clue as to areas that will warrant more critical evaluation.

Head-to-toe assessment

Head and neck. Assessment of the head includes the eyes, ears, nose, and mouth. The neck involves assessment of arteries, veins, lymph nodes, and the thyroid gland.

Table 13-2 Sounds Produced by Percussion

Percussion Sound	Intensity	Pitch	Duration	Quality	Anatomical Location Where Examiner Hears Sounds
Tympany	Loud	High	Moderate	Drumlike	Enclosed air-containing space: gastric/ intestine
Resonance	Moderate to loud	Low	Long	Hollow	Normal lung
Hyperresonance	Very loud	Very low	Longer than resonance	Booming	Emphysematous lung
Dullness	Soft to moderate	High	Moderate	Thudlike	Liver
Flatness	Soft	High	Short	Flat	Muscle

Examination of the face begins with the assessment of the skin, including the hair.

The nurse should note the symmetry of the face; facial movements should also be symmetrical and appropriate. The facial expression can give clues to the emotional state of the patient. The hair should be of smooth texture and not oily or dry. The scalp should be free of dandruff, lesions, or parasites. The nurse may wish to wear gloves for the inspection of the hair and scalp. The skin's color, texture, temperature, and moisture can be noted. Normal skin tones vary with race, heredity, and exposure to the sun. Normally, the skin should be dry and smooth, with good **turgor** (resilience). The nurse should note whether the patient has a normal pattern of hair growth.

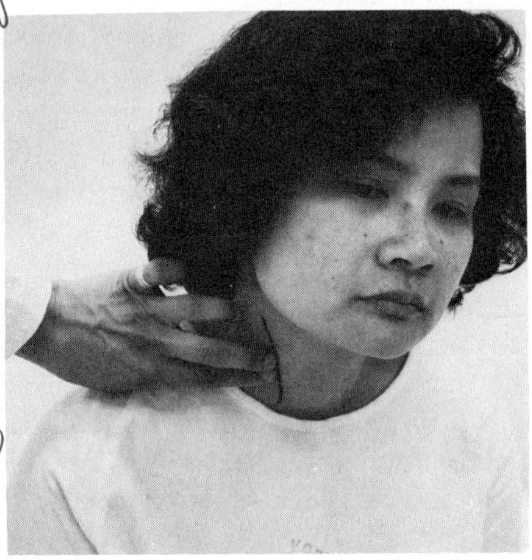

FIG. 13-2 Palpation of carotid artery.

Gross assessment of range of motion **(ROM)** can be done by having the patient move his head from side to side and in a nodding motion. The patient is asked to touch his chin to his chest; he should be able to move his head comfortably through these motions. The temporomandibular joint **(TMJ)** is palpated and the patient is directed to open and close his jaw. There should be no clicking or **crepitus** felt, crepitus being a "crackly" sensation beneath the skin. Using the pads of the fingers, the nurse palpates beneath the jaw and down each side of the neck to feel for enlarged lymph nodes. Although it is not abnormal for a person to have an enlarged node, it should not be tender. The nurse palpates the carotid pulses gently and one at a time (Fig. 13-2). The pulses should be even and palpable without a **thrill** (vibrating sensation).

The nurse next inspects for jugular vein distention **(JVD).** Normally, the veins will not be observable.

The thyroid gland can be palpated for enlargement. This is best done standing behind the patient. The pads of the fingers are placed on either side of the trachea below the Adam's apple, and the patient is asked to tilt his head back slightly and swallow. The nurse should be able to feel the gland sliding up beneath the fingers. The gland should not be noticeably enlarged, nor should it be tender or uneven. Palpation of the thyroid gland takes practice (Fig. 13-3).

Auscultation of the carotid artery can be performed at this point. The artery should be heard just below the mandible (lower jaw) with the bell of the stethoscope. There should be no bruits heard. **Bruits** are abnormal "swishing" sounds heard over organs, glands, and arteries.

Mouth and throat. Inspection of the lips and mucous

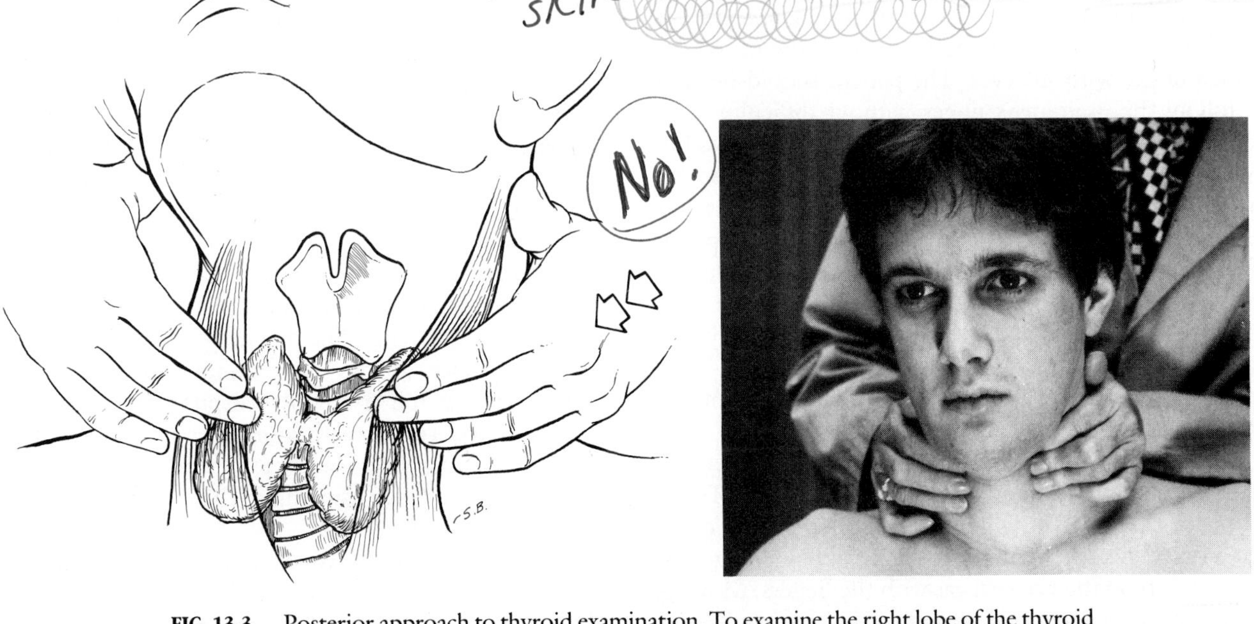

FIG. 13-3 Posterior approach to thyroid examination. To examine the right lobe of the thyroid gland, the examiner displaces the trachea slightly to the right with the fingers of the left hand and palpates for the right thyroid lobe with the fingers of the right hand.

membranes of the mouth is done with a tongue blade and penlight to assess all surfaces of the oral cavity. The mucous membrane should be pink and free of lesions. The lips should be smooth, moist, and free of cracking. The teeth and gums can be inspected for periodontal disease and dental caries. Assessment of the teeth can give the nurse insight into the health habits of the patient. To examine the throat, the patient is asked to say "ah." The movement of the tongue is noted, and the light is directed to the back surface of the throat to inspect the tonsils and throat for **erythema** (redness), **leukoplakia** (thickened white patches), **edema** (swelling), or **purulent discharge** (pus). Tonsils may be enlarged, but this is considered normal if other findings are negative. Breath odors can indicate disease; the breath should not be foul, fruity, or musty.

Eyes. The nurse should first note whether the eyes are symmetrical. There should be no drainage from the eyes, and the lids should be open. The sclera of the eye should be white and the conjunctiva pink. There should be no signs of icterus (yellowing of the sclera) or **ptosis,** which is drooping of the eyelid. The conjunctiva is observed by gently depressing the lower lid. **Periorbital edema** (edema around the eyes) is abnormal.

Both eyes should be assessed individually. The nurse also observes the eyes for **pupillary reflex.** This is done easily by darkening the room, using the penlight to shine the light into the pupil. The light should come from the side of the eye with the patient looking straight ahead at a focal point. The normal eye will show the pupil constricting when the light is applied. The rate and size of constriction should be equal. This finding can be recalled by using the acronym **PERRLA,** which stands for pupils equal, round, and reactive to light and accommodation.

Eye movement can be assessed by having the patient hold his head still and having him follow the tip of the nurse's finger with his eyes. The patient should be able to follow the examiner's finger without difficulty. The hand is moved in a star pattern to check all possible movements. The patient should have no extraocular movements. Visual acuity (clearness of perception) can be simply assessed by having the patient read newsprint. If the patient uses glasses or contact lenses, he should wear them. Examination with the **ophthalmoscope** is an advanced procedure, and the ophthalmoscope may not be available to the nurse in a particular setting. The screening mentioned above can give adequate information for the nurse to make a nursing diagnosis.

Ears. The nurse first notes that the ears are symmetrical and the level at which they are attached to the head. There should not be any discharge from the ears. The ear canal can be examined by using the penlight and pulling gently back and up on the external ear with the fingers. Moving the ear in this manner will straighten the canal and allow the nurse to look further into it. With a child under the age of 3, the ear is pulled back and down. There should not be any pain associated with this movement. The ear canal should be free of excess cerumen (earwax), blood, or any purulent discharge (pus).

During this assessment, the nurse should note whether the patient is appropriately following commands, indicating ability to hear. A simple hearing test can be conducted by standing behind the patient and having him repeat whispered words; another test involves rubbing the patient's hair between the fingers near the ear and asking the patient if he can hear the sound.

Nose. The nose should be symmetrical, although variations in size are considered normal. To test for patency (openness), the nurse presses against one nostril and asks the patient to breathe. Air should flow through the nose. Both nostrils are assessed, observing for bleeding or drainage. The nurse palpates on either side of the nose beneath the eyes with the fingertips to assess for sinus tenderness. Sinuses should not be tender. The functioning of the first cranial nerve is checked by having the patient smell and name a common odor. The first cranial nerve is the olfactory nerve for the sense of smell. An alcohol wipe or lemon glycerine swab can be used.

Chest, heart, and lungs. Assessment of the chest, heart, and lungs is performed with the patient in a sitting position. The nurse inspects the chest for bilateral chest expansion, which should be symmetrical. The respiratory rate and depth of respirations are noted. Audible congestion is noted and can later be auscultated to determine the quality. The normal respiratory rate for an adult is 12 to 20 breaths per minute. Breathing should be quiet. Posture can indicate pulmonary status: the patient who is unable to lie supine or who must lean forward to breathe may have respiratory difficulty. A large, rounded "barrel chest" may be a sign of increased respiratory effort such as in emphysema.

Lung sounds. Auscultation of breath sounds is a major method of assessing the lungs' status. When beginning to assess breath sounds, it is sufficient for the nurse to recognize the sound of normal respirations; this later allows recognition of abnormal sounds. Both the bell and diaphragm of the stethoscope should be used. Labeling the sounds as rales or wheezes will come with practice. Lung sounds are best heard by placing the stethoscope on the patient's back. The diaphragm of the stethoscope is used to pick up the lung sounds. The nurse should listen for one full inspiratory/expiratory cycle at each point. Adventitious breath sounds are superimposed over normal sounds. The nurse's eyes should be closed and the breath held when listening so that one can concentrate on the sounds (Fig. 13-4).

Breath sounds are classified as either rales (crackles) or wheezes (rhonchi). Rales can be fine, medium, or coarse. Fine rales sound like hair being rubbed between the fingers and are heard at the end of the inspiratory phase.

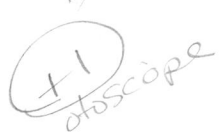

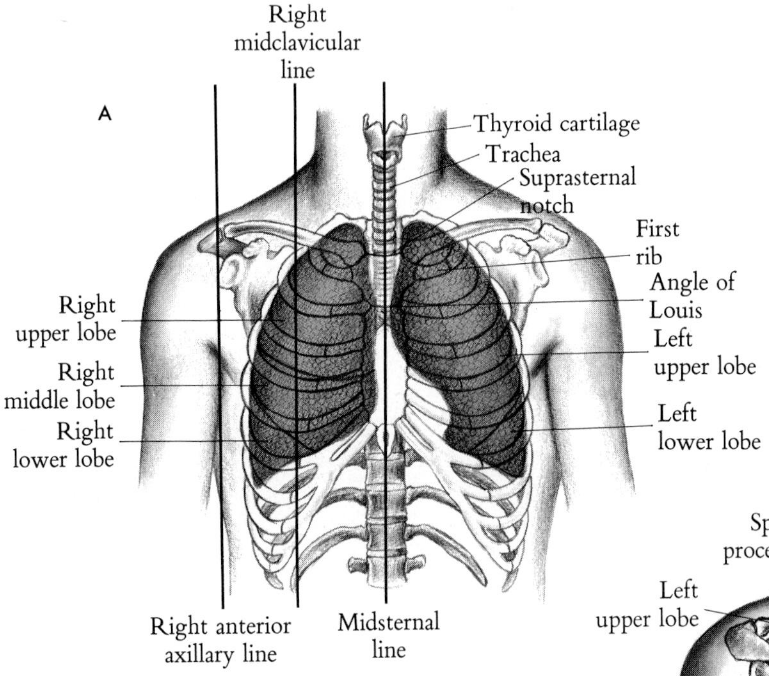

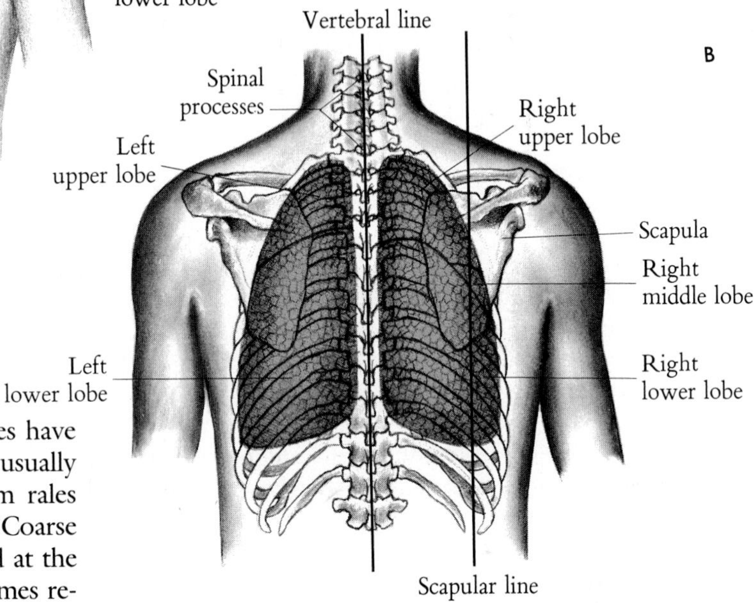

FIG. 13-4 Thoracic landmarks. **A,** Anterior thorax. **B,** Posterior thorax.

They are high pitched and discrete. Medium rales have a deeper tone and a more moist sound and are usually heard in the middle of the inspiration. Medium rales sound like the "fizzing" of a carbonated beverage. Coarse rales make a loud, bubbling sound and are heard at the beginning of inspiration. Coarse rales are sometimes referred to as the "death rattle." Wheezes or rhonchi are classified as sibilant or sonorous. Sibilant rhonchi may be heard on both inspiration and expiration and sound like high-pitched crowing. Sonorous rhonchi are lower-pitched sounds. Rhonchi characteristically clear when the patient coughs, whereas rales do not. As a rule, rales indicate congestion in the smaller alveoli and wheezes (rhonchi) indicate narrowing or congestion in the larger airways of the bronchial tree and trachea (Fig. 13-5). Pleural friction rubs can also be heard and sounds like "pieces of leather being rubbed together." This sound indicates inflammation of the pleura.

Spine. With the patient in a sitting position, the curvature of the spine is noted. The nurse should also assess the posture when the patient is standing. The nurse can run the fingers down the patient's spine. The spine should be straight. There should be a normal lumbosacral curve. The skin of the back should be of normal color, temperature, and moisture.

Heart sounds. Heart sounds are auscultated with the stethoscope. The nurse places the stethoscope at four points on the patient's chest and listens for several cardiac cycles at each point. The normal "lub-dub" sound of the heart occurs because of the contraction of the atria and ventricles respectively; these are designated S_1, S_2. When listening, the nurse uses both the bell and the diaphragm of the stethoscope to hear low- and high-pitched sounds (Fig. 13-6).

Breast. The nurse assesses a female patient's breast by inspection and palpation. Both breasts should be symmetrical, although it is normal for one breast to be slightly larger than the other.

The skin color on the breast should match the rest of the thorax. Examination of the breasts should begin with the patient in a sitting position. The patient is asked to raise her arms and place her hands behind her head. The nurse looks for any dimpling or noticeable nodules. With the patient then in a lying position, the nurse can begin the systematic palpation of the breast tissue. When the nipple is palpated, it is gently squeezed to note any drain-

Fine rales: high-pitched, discrete, noncontinuous crackling sounds heard during the end of inspiration

Medium rales: lower, more moist sound heard during the midstage of inspiration; not cleared by a cough

Coarse rales: loud, bubbly noise heard during inspiration; not cleared by a cough

Rhonchi: loud, low, coarse sounds like a snore heard at any point of inspiration or expiration; coughing may clear sound (usually means mucus accumulation in trachea or large bronchi)

Wheeze: musical noise sounding like a squeak; may be heard during inspiration or expiration; usually louder during expiration

Pleural friction rub: dry, rubbing, or grating sound, usually caused by inflammation of pleural surfaces; heard during inspiration or expiration; loudest over lower lateral anterior surface

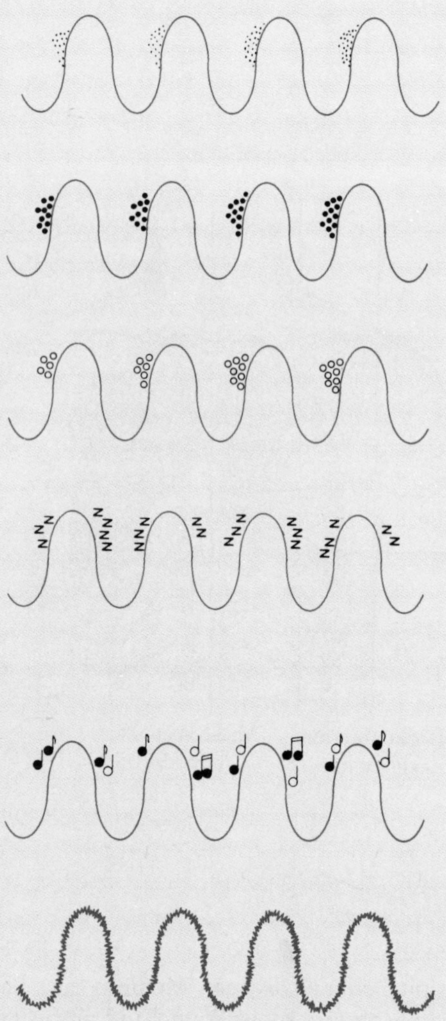

Modified from Thompson et al., 1986.

FIG. 13-5 Adventitious breath sounds.

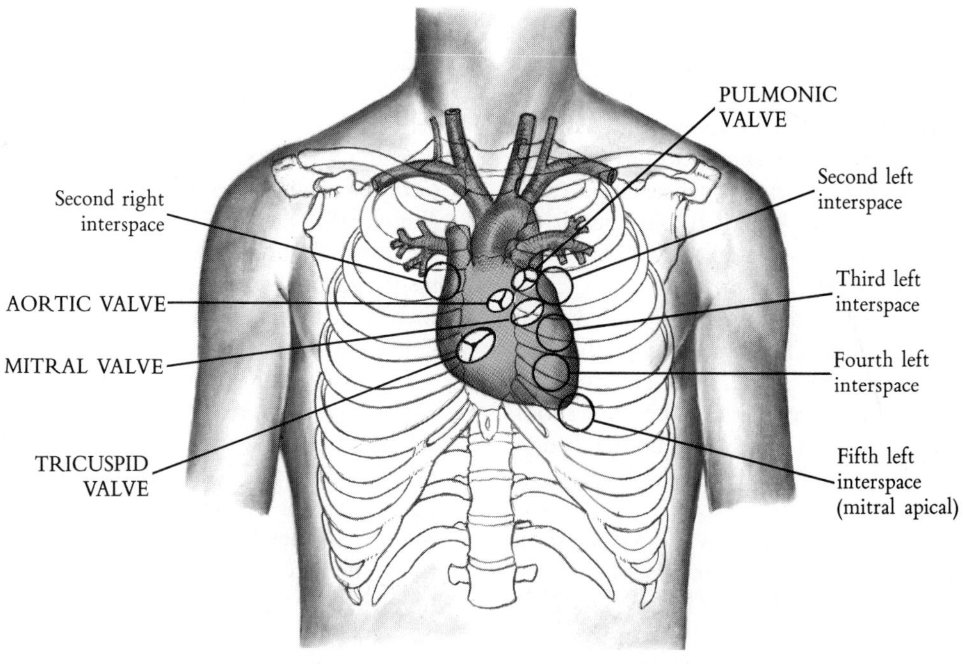

FIG. 13-6 Areas for auscultation of the heart.

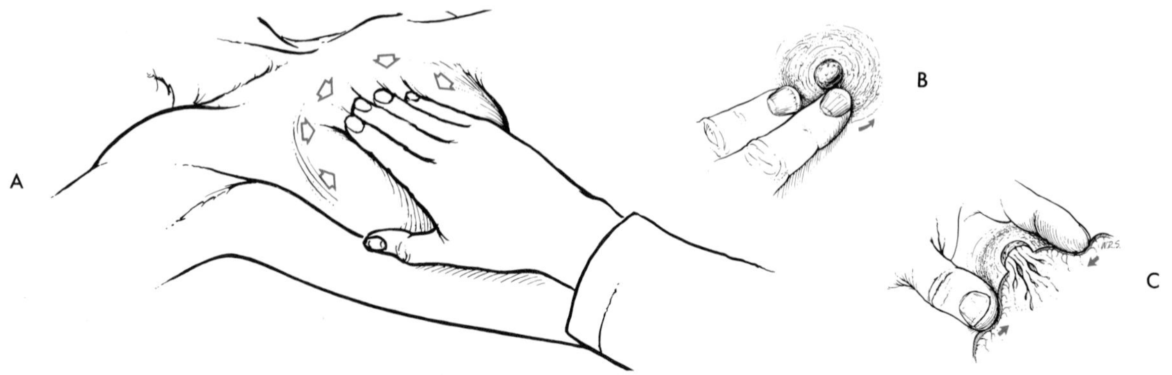

FIG. 13-7 Palpation of the breasts. **A,** Glandular area. **B,** Areololar area. **C,** Compression of the nipple.

age (Fig. 13-7). Included in the palpation is the area of breast tissue that extends into the axilla (tail of Spence), an area where a large percentage of breast cancers develop (Fig. 13-8). The nurse's fingers apply gentle pressure and use a rotating motion to feel for underlying lumps. Once the axillary nodes have been palpated, the nurse can begin the breast examination following a rotating pattern beginning from the outer edge of the breast and working inward (Fig. 13-9).

The breast should be soft and nontender, and there should be no drainage from the nipple. During the breast examination is a good time to instruct the patient on the importance of breast self-examination (BSE). This assessment should be performed once a month, usually the fifth to seventh day after the onset of the monthly menses. In postmenopausal women, the BSE should be performed the same day of each month. See Chapter 41 for discussion of care of the patient with cancer.

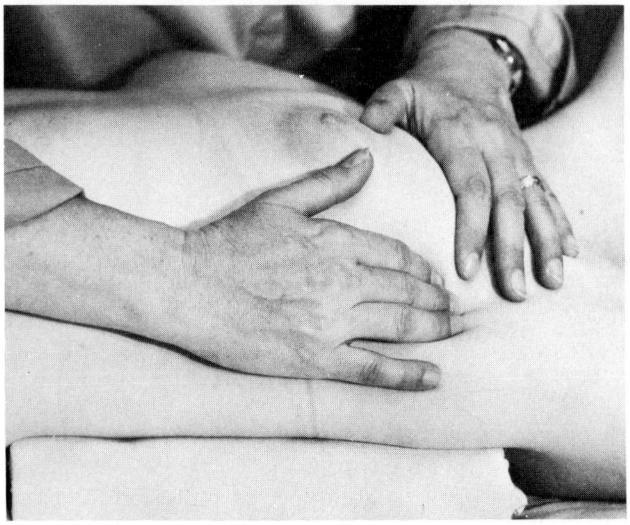

FIG. 13-8 Palpation of the axillary tail of spence.

Abdomen. During the remaining portion of the examination the patient can remain in the supine position. The nurse then examines the abdomen. During this portion of the assessment, the patient should be properly draped to decrease exposure of the pubic area. The nurse first inspects the abdomen for shape, contour, lesions, scars, lumps, or rashes. The abdomen's contour should be even, and skin color should be the same as that of the thorax. Before palpating, the nurse auscultates for bowel sounds by placing the diaphragm of the stethoscope over the divisions of the abdomen and listening for the peristaltic sounds produced by the intestines (Fig. 13-10). Because peristalsis (wavelike movements of the intestines) is continuous, sound should be present in all four quadrants. Bowel sounds occur every 15 to 60 seconds and are classified as being hyperactive, hypoactive, or absent. If the patient has nasogastric suction, the machine is turned off during auscultation. The nurse listens to bowel sounds for 1 full minute in all four quadrants. However, if the patient does not have any specific abdominal complaints, it is not necesary to listen to each quadrant for 1 full minute. The normal rate of bowel sounds is 4 to 32 per minute.

After auscultating for bowel sounds, the nurse can then palpate the underlying structures. Both light and deep palpation is used. Beginning with light palpation, the

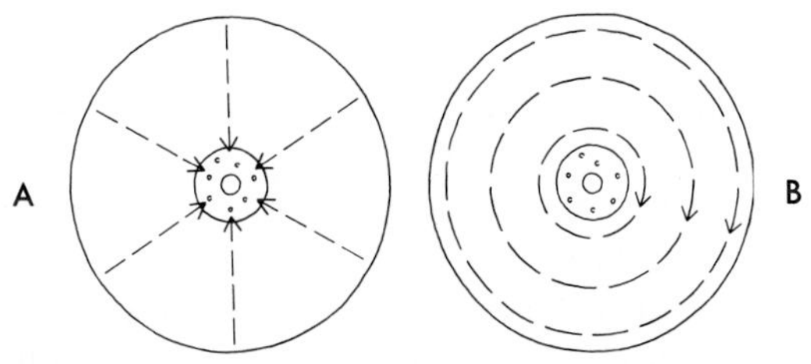

FIG. 13-9 Two methods of systematic breast palpation. **A,** Palpation in wedge sections from breast periphery to center. **B,** Palpation along concentric circles from periphery to center.

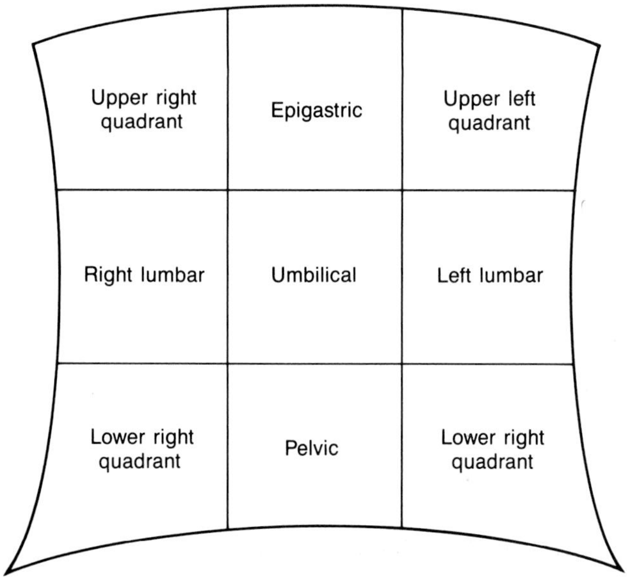

FIG. 13-10 Abdominal quadrants and descriptive areas.

nurse notes the texture, temperature, and moisture of the skin in all four quadrants. To ensure that the patient is relaxed during the palpation, the hands should be warmed, and conversation can be used to distract the patient. Light palpation can detect superficial lesions just below the skin. The skin of the abdomen should be smooth, dry, and warm. Deep palpation is used to detect tenderness or masses of the abdomen. In the upper right quadrant just below the rib cage, the liver may be palpated. If the liver can be felt, this may mean that it is enlarged. The liver should be smooth and nontender. The abdomen itself should be free of masses, and palpation should not be uncomfortable for the patient (Fig. 13-11). The nurse notes the patient's face when palpating and looks for grimacing. The patient may also guard a tender area, which means he will tighten up abdominal muscles when the area is touched.

Percussion is used on the abdomen to note the density of underlying tissue. It is also used to locate the margins of internal organs. The abdomen has a tympanic (drumlike) sound, with dullness noted over the liver. A hollow sound heard over the stomach or intestines indicates flatus.

Genitourinary system. Nurses do not perform the vaginal examination with a speculum unless they have had advanced training. Assessment of the urinary system is performed using observation and palpation. It is most convenient for the nurse to perform this inspection during the perineal care of the patient. Gloves should be worn when inspecting the labia for lesions. The pubic hair is inspected for lice, and any vaginal drainage is noted. Normal labia are pink, moist, and free of lesions.

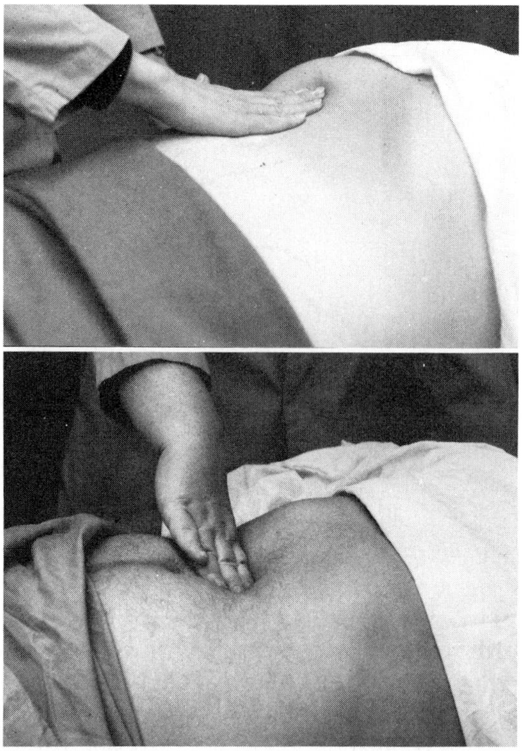

FIG. 13-11 Palpation of the abdomen to assess organs such as the liver and spleen.

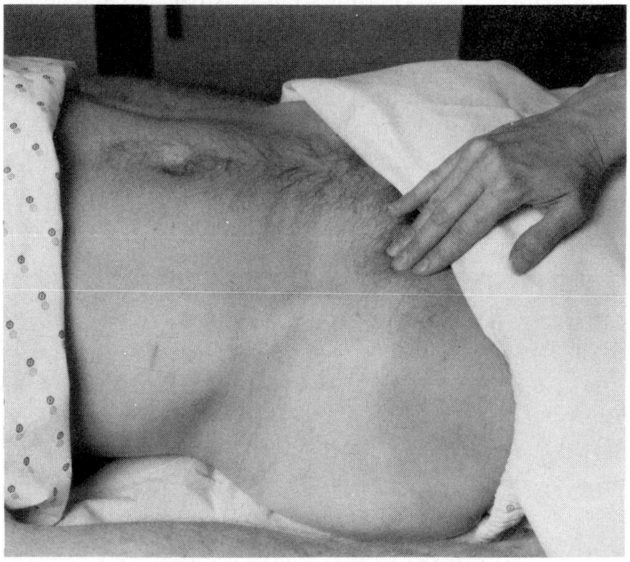

FIG. 13-12 Palpation of the femoral artery.

A normal white vaginal drainage known as **leukorrhea** can be present in the female.

The male genitalia are inspected for lesions and lice; the nurse looks for drainage from the penis. The scrotum is palpated for lumps or hernias. If the male is uncircumcised, the foreskin should be retracted to inspect for lesions on the glans penis.

While inspecting the genitalia on both the male and female, the nurse can palpate the femoral artery in that area (Fig. 13-12). Palpation of the suprapubic area can also be performed to determine bladder distention. Tenderness at the costovertebral angle **(CVA)** could indicate kidney disease.

Rectum. The rectal area is best examined with the patient in a Sims' position. The buttocks can be spread to look for hemorrhoids or lesions. Normal skin around the anus is darker than surrounding skin. To further assess the intestinal system, the nurse can explain the procedure for obtaining a stool specimen to the patient and leave a Hemoccult slide with the patient. The results of the test may indicate whether gastrointestinal bleeding is present.

Legs and feet. The legs and feet are the final area of assessment. Femoral, popliteal, posterior tibial, and pedal pulses should be palpated (Fig. 13-13). The legs and feet should be observed and palpated for edema. The nurse directs the patient to flex knees and ankles to test for ROM, although a better assessment of this is made by observing the patient's gait. Skin color on the legs should be similar to the rest of the body. Varicosities (enlarged veins) should not be present.

Check the CMS (color, motion, and sensation) of both feet. The nurse can test for sensation by touching the toes and asking the patient whether he feels it. The patient's feet should be equally warm. Pedal pulses should be present. Corns or bunions may interfere with the patient's mobility.

Neurological assessment. The neurological assessment can be integrated with the head-to-toe assessment. For instance, after taking a radial pulse the nurse can have the patient grasp the nurse's hands to test for equal grip. Gross motor and coordination skills can be assessed by having the patient touch the tip of his nose with his finger and then touch the tip of the nurse's finger as it is moved to different positions. The patient should be able to follow the movement of the nurse's finger.

Recording the Interview

Most institutions have a form to follow when conducting the patient interview and review of systems. The nurse should state the patient complaints in the patient's own words. It is acceptable to record information as it is obtained; therefore a pad and pencil are helpful during the assessment.

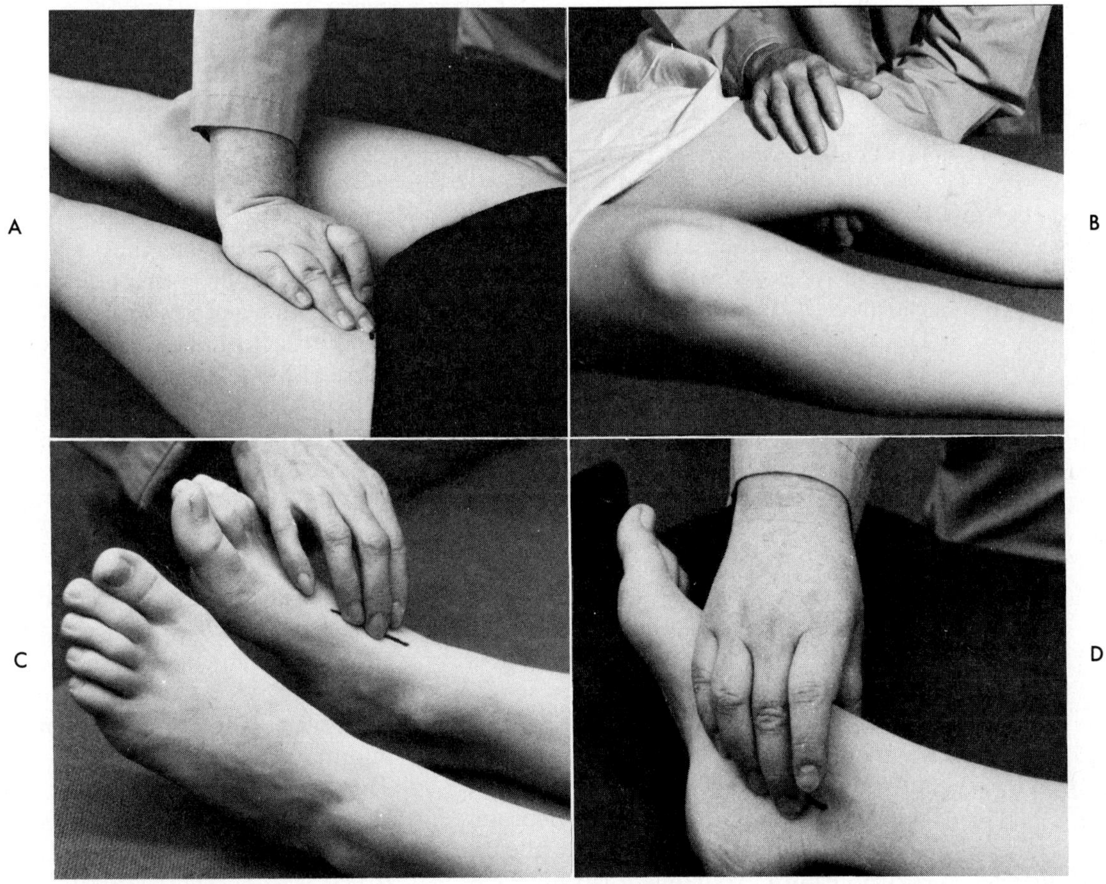

FIG. 13-13 Palpation of **A**, femoral, **B**, popliteal, **C**, pedal, and **D**, posterior tibial pulses.

Abnormalities are described by location, size, color, temperature, and tenderness. Absence of inspected pulses or sounds is also recorded. The nurse should not attempt to diagnose a medical condition but should describe what is seen, heard, felt, or smelled.

Concluding the Assessment

At the conclusion of the examination, the patient is asked what questions he has. The nurse assists the patient to a comfortable position and shares with him any significant findings.

The complete nursing assessment is reserved for gathering initial patient data. For patients who are hospitalized for long periods, the nurse can focus assessment on areas of patient concern. For example, with the patient who is admitted with a diagnosis of asthma, the nurse should perform a thorough assessment of the lungs.

REFERENCES AND SUGGESTED READINGS

1. Anthony ML and others: Nursing interventions: independent or not? Nurs Manage 19(12):14, 1988.
2. Billings DM and Stokes LG: Medical-surgical nursing, ed 2, St Louis, 1987, The CV Mosby Co.
3. Campbell J and others: A theoretical approach to nursing assessment, J Adv Nurs 10(2):111, 1985.
4. Erickson B: Detecting abnormal heart sounds, Nurs 86 16(1):58, 1986.
5. Flynn J and Heffron P: Nursing from concept to practice, Norwich, Conn, 1988, Appleton & Lange.
6. Ford R: Health assessment handbook, Springhouse, Pa, 1987, Springhouse Publishing Co.
7. Frank A and Murray S: A no-guess guide for urinary color assessment, RN 51(6):46, 1988.
8. Hood GH and Dincher JR: Total patient care, ed 7, St Louis, 1988, The CV Mosby Co.
9. Koph R: Handbook of nursing physical assessment, Rockville, Md, 1988, Aspen Publishers, Inc.
10. Malasanos L and others: Health assessment, ed 4, St. Louis, 1990, The CV Mosby Co.
11. Merry J: Take your assessment all the way down to the toes, RN 51(1):60, 1988.
12. Miracle V: Get in tune with cardiac assessment (part 2), Nurs 88 18(4):41, 1988.
13. Mosby's medical and nursing dictionary, ed 3, St Louis, 1990, The CV Mosby Co.
14. Popkess-Vawterm S and Pinnell N: Should we diagnose strengths? Am J Nurs 87(9):1211, 1987.
15. Potter P and Perry A: Basic nursing: theory and practice, ed 2, St Louis, 1991, The CV Mosby Co.
16. Rifas E: How to listen to breath sounds, RN 47(3):30, 1984.
17. Seidel HM and others: Mosby's guide to physical examination, St Louis, 1987, The CV Mosby Co.
18. Smith C: Assessing chest pain quickly and accurately, Nurs 88 18(5):52, 1988.
19. Stevens S and Becker K: Get in touch and in tune with cardiac assessment (part 1), Nurs 88 18(3):51, 1988.
20. Stevens S and Becker K: How to perform a picture-perfect respiratory assessment, Nurs 88 18(1):57, 1988.
21. Stevens S and Becker K: Performing in-depth abdominal assessment, Nurs 88 18(6):59, 1988.

CHAPTER CHALLENGE

KEY POINTS

- A sign is perceived by the nurse using the senses of sight, touch, smell, and hearing.
- A symptom is a sensation felt only by the patient, such as pain or dizziness.
- Diseases originate from several different causes, and may be hereditary, congenital, traumatic, neoplastic, infectious, deficiency, or environmental in nature.
- Risk factors for acquiring a disease include age, genetics, environment, and life-style variables.
- The universal signs of infection are erythema, edema, pain, heat, loss of function, and purulent malodorous drainage.
- A complete nursing physical assessment should be performed as soon after admission as possible.
- Continuous nursing assessment can be performed as part of the daily nursing care.
- Some frequently noted signs and symptoms of disease are cyanosis, pallor, erythema, edema, nausea, vomiting, diarrhea, dyspnea, tachycardia, and fever.
- The nursing physical assessment begins with the patient interview.
- Interviewing the patient first determines signs and symptoms and areas of patient concern that can be clarified by the examination.
- Vital signs and height and weight should be measured at the beginning of the physical assessment.
- The physical assessment should proceed in an orderly fashion: head-to-toe or system-by-system.
- Assessment should be performed in the specific order of observation, palpation, percussion, and auscultation.
- Results of laboratory evaluation of specimens such as urine and stool can add to the information about the patient.
- The practical/vocational nurse should be familiar with normal assessments and thus be able to identify abnormalities.

=objective

STUDY QUESTIONS

1. An example of a sign noted in a patient would be:
   a. Fatigue
   b. Nausea
   c. Pain
   d. Fever

   subjective

2. Disease may originate from all the following causes except:
   a. Exercise
   b. Trauma
   c. Infection
   d. Environmental
3. Categories of risk for development of disease include all except:
   a. Political preference
   b. Life-style
   c. Age
   d. Environment
4. A sign of infection is:
   a. Decreased turgor
   b. Coolness
   c. Increased function
   d. Erythema
5. A redness of the skin noted on a patient with an inflammation of the hand is called:
   a. Edema
   b. Pallor
   c. Erythema
   d. Jaundice
6. The patient stated he had a poor appetite; this symptom is called:
   a. Nausea
   b. Tachypnea
   c. Pruritus
   d. Anorexia
7. The condition in which a patient must sit or stand to breathe deeply is called:
   a. Orthopnea
   b. Tachycardia
   c. Cyanosis
   d. Bradycardia

Mr. Jones is admitted to the hospital with a diagnosis of gastrointestinal bleeding. The physician orders insertion of a nasogastric tube for suction. The patient complains of abdominal tenderness.

8. The physician plans to perform a physical examination of Mr. Jones. What action would the nurse perform initially:
   a. Remove the patient's clothing
   b. Explain the procedure
   c. Collect equipment
   d. Collect a stool specimen
9. When the physician assesses the abdomen, which position would the nurse help Mr. Jones assume:
   a. Sims'
   b. Supine
   c. Prone
   d. Fowler's
10. Which factor might interfere with auscultation of bowel sounds:
    a. The fact that the patient is NPO
    b. The nasogastric suction
    c. The patient's diarrhea
    d. The gastrointestinal bleeding
11. During the interview with Mr. Jones, communication was enhanced by all except:
    a. Questions requiring a "yes" or "no" answer
    b. Sitting down at Mr. Jones's bedside
    c. Maintaining eye contact
    d. Reflecting Mr. Jones's statements
12. During morning care to Mr. Jones, he complains of abdominal pain. To locate the site of the pain the nurse would use:
    a. Palpation
    b. Inspection
    c. Percussion
    d. Auscultation
13. Normal respiration sounds are:
    a. Crackly
    b. High-pitched
    c. Silent
    d. Fizzy

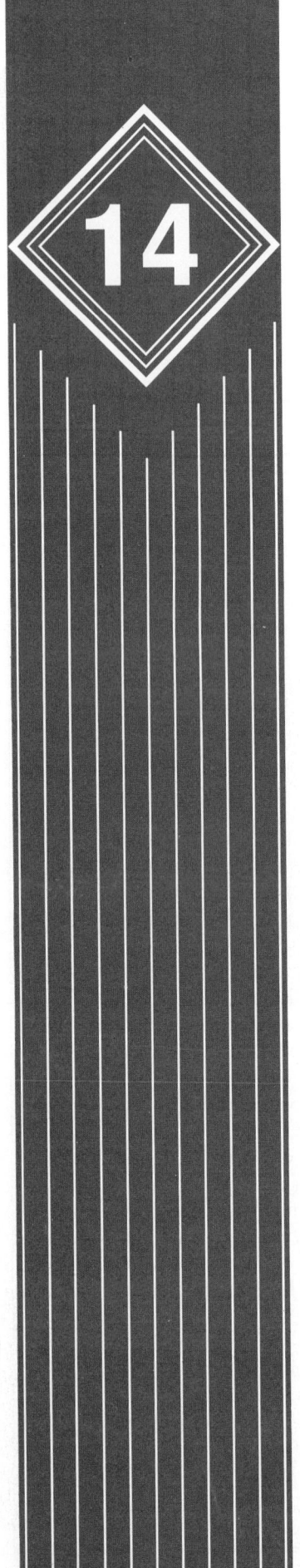

14

Vital Signs

AUDREY WADMAN SZCZESIUL

LEARNING OBJECTIVES

After reading this chapter, the student should be able to do the following:

- Define the key terms.
- Discuss the steps in obtaining an oral, rectal, and axillary temperature using glass and electronic thermometers.
- Describe the procedure for obtaining an apical rate and radial pulse.
- Describe the procedure for determining a respiratory rate.
- List the steps in obtaining a blood pressure.
- State the normal limits of vital signs.
- List the factors that affect vital sign readings.
- Describe the procedure for obtaining an accurate height and weight.
- Discuss methods by which the nurse can ensure accurate measurement of vital signs.

RELATED TOPICS OF INTEREST

- Signs, symptoms, and physical assessment (Chapter 13)
- Medical asepsis (Chapter 16)
- Care of the patient with a cardiovascular disorder (Chapter 32)
- Care of the patient with a respiratory disorder (Chapter 34)

KEY TERMS

Define the following:

- alveoli
- apical
- apnea
- auscultate
- axillary
- bradycardia
- bradypnea
- cardiac output
- Cheyne-Stokes respirations
- diaphragm
- diastolic
- dyspnea
- dysrhythmia
- expiration
- febrile
- hypertension
- hyperthermic
- hypotensive
- hypothermic
- inspiration
- Korotkoff sounds
- oxidation
- orthostatic
- pulse deficit
- pulse pressure
- pyrexic
- radial pulse
- retractions
- sphygmomanometer
- stethoscope
- syncope
- systolic
- tachycardia
- tachypnea
- vertigo
- vital signs

Vital signs include temperature, pulse, respirations, and blood pressure. It is necessary for the nurse to be able to obtain accurate measurements of these. Because vital signs are an indication of basic body functioning, it is appropriate to begin the physical assessment by obtaining this data.

TEMPERATURE

The body strives to maintain a temperature of 98.6° F (Box 14-1), which is considered normal. However, variations of from 97° F to 99.6° F are considered to be within normal range. Many factors can cause body temperature variances, including the environment, the time of day, the patient's state of health, activity levels, and stage of monthly menstrual cycle (Box 14-2).

Body temperature is regulated by the hypothalamus, which is located in the brain, forming the floor and part of the lateral wall of the third ventricle. The hypothalamus helps maintain a balance between heat lost and heat produced by the body.

The body produces heat by metabolism. The amount of heat produced can be increased by increasing metabolism, as with exercise and digestion. Constriction of peripheral vessels helps conserve heat by preventing loss of heat through the skin surface.

Temperature measurements are obtained by several methods. Glass and electronic thermometers are used to obtain oral, rectal, **axillary,** and groin temperatures. Groin temperature is measured mainly in pediatric patients. Heat-sensitive patches are used also. The patches are placed on an area of skin, such as the forehead. Color changes on the patch indicate temperature readings. Tympanic temperature measurement is quick and accurate. A small probe aimed at the eardrum uses infrared beam to determine body temperature. The temperature reading is displayed digitally (Fig. 14-1).

Glass thermometers have been widely replaced by the electronic thermometer, since the electronic method is fast and accurate (see Fig. 14-7). Determining body core temperature rectally is most accurate, since the thermometer is placed in a closed cavity. There are two basic styles of glass thermometers for oral and rectal temperature measure. They are usually color coded: red tipped for rectal, and blue or clear tipped for oral. The mercury bulb of the rectal thermometer is short and rounded; of the oral thermometer, long and narrow (Fig. 14-2, *A-C*). Because glass thermometers contain mercury (a hazardous material), the nurse should not clean up a broken thermometer without a mercury spill kit. This is a kit that includes a bulb syringe and sealed container. The mercury is aspirated with the syringe and transferred into a labeled container for safe disposal by the facility.

Temperature readings are documented in either *Celsius* degrees (C) or Fahrenheit degrees (F) (Fig. 14-2). Glass thermometers are calibrated in either F or C scales. The type of scale used is determined by facility policy.

BOX 14-1 NORMAL BODY TEMPERATURES ACCORDING TO SITES

	Oral	Rectal	Axillary	Tympanic
Fahrenheit (F)	98.6°	99.5°	97.6°	98.6°
Centigrade (C)	37.0°	37.5°	36.4°	37.0°

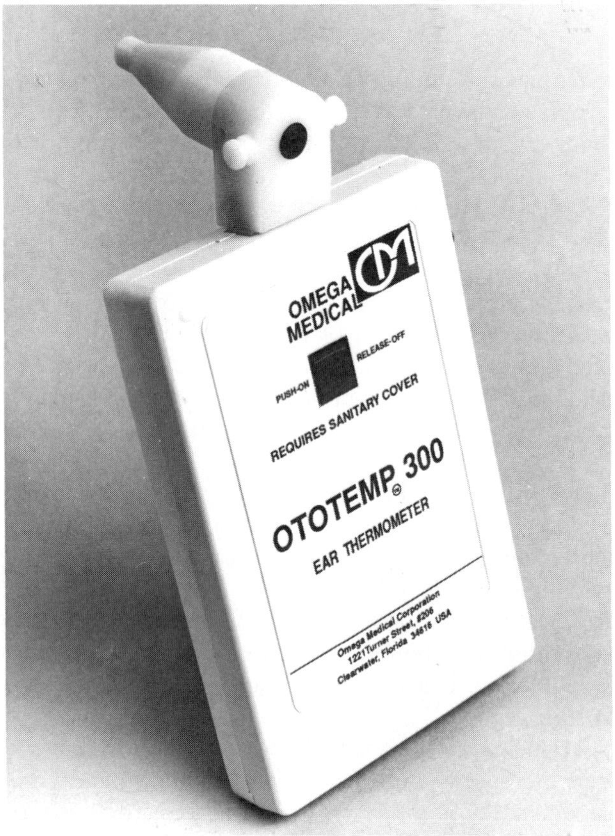

FIG. 14-1 Ototemp used for tympanic temperature measurement. The setting can be changed so the nurse can ascertain oral, rectal, or surface readings. (Courtesy Omega Medical Corporation, Clearwater, Fl.)

BOX 14-2 FACTORS AFFECTING BODY TEMPERATURE

Age. The neonate's temperature normally ranges from 35.5° to 37.5° C (96° to 99.5° F). Temperature regulation is labile during infancy because of immature physiological mechanisms. This can continue until puberty. With old age the normal range commonly lowers, with 35° C (95° F) not being unusual for some elderly patients in cold weather. With aging, sensitivity to temperature extremes develops because of deteriorating control mechanisms.

Exercise. Any form of exercise can increase body temperature. Prolonged strenuous exercise can temporarily raise body temperatures to as high as 41° C (105° F).

Hormonal influences. Women generally have greater variations in body temperature than men. Hormone changes during ovulation and menstruation cause body temperature fluctuations.

Diurnal variations. Body temperatures normally change throughout the day, with the lowest reading occurring between 1 AM and 4 AM (36.5° C [97.7° F] on average). The temperature usually peaks around 4 PM to 6 PM.

Stress. Physical or emotional stress, such as anxiety, may raise body temperature.

Environment. Environmental temperature extremes can raise or lower the body temperature. The changes depend on the extent of exposure, air humidity, and the presence of convection currents.

Ingestion of hot/cold liquids. Drinking hot or cold liquids can cause slight variations in actual oral temperature readings (−0.2° F to −1.6° F after drinking iced water) (Woodman et al., 1967).

Smoking. Smoking cigarettes or cigars may alter body temperature measurement (−0.2° F to 0.2° F) (Woodman et al., 1967).

Because glass thermometers are not disposable, several policies have been adopted by health facilities to prevent cross-contamination among patients. In some cases, each patient is issued his own thermometer, which is kept at the bedside. Also, disposable plastic sheaths are used to cover both glass and electronic thermometers when these thermometers are used for more than one patient. The nurse may be responsible for cleaning and disinfecting glass thermometers. A common method of cleaning/disinfecting is to first wipe the thermometer from fingers to bulb after patient use. The thermometer is then washed with detergent and rinsed with cool water to avoid breakage. The next step is to soak glass thermometers in a disinfectant, for example, alcohol, for a length of time specified by policy. The last step is to rinse thermometers in tepid water, dry, and store in a dry place.

Temperature elevations may be the first sign of illness. When body temperature is above normal, the patient is said to be **pyrexic, febrile,** or **hyperthermic.** Fever is actually a body defense. Elevated body temperature will destroy invading bacteria. Unfortunately, if temperature exceeds 105° F, normal body cells can be damaged.

Fevers are classified as constant, intermittent, and remittent. Constant fevers remain elevated with less than 1 degree variation during a 24-hour period. Intermittent

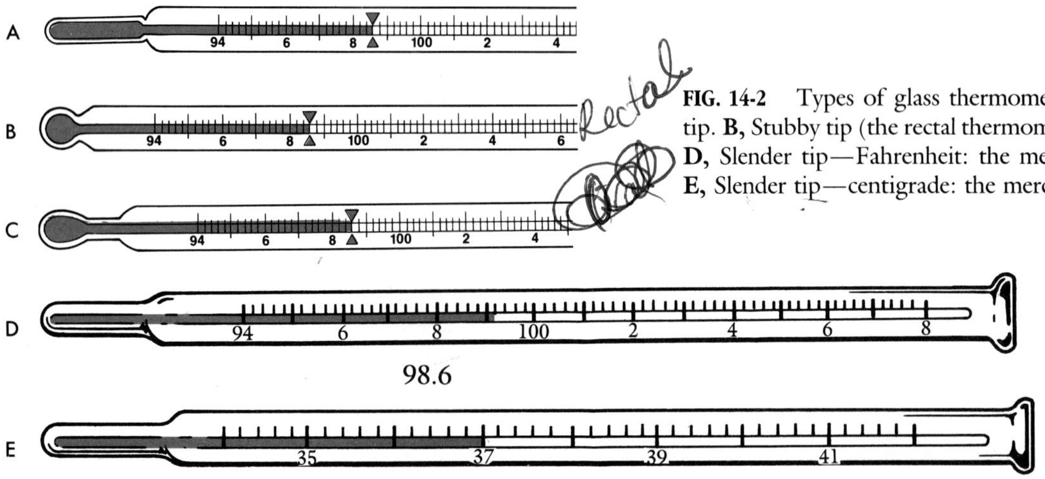

FIG. 14-2 Types of glass thermometers. **A,** Long or slender tip. **B,** Stubby tip (the rectal thermometer). **C,** Pear-shaped tip. **D,** Slender tip—Fahrenheit: the mercury level is at 99.2° F. **E,** Slender tip—centigrade: the mercury level is at 37° C.

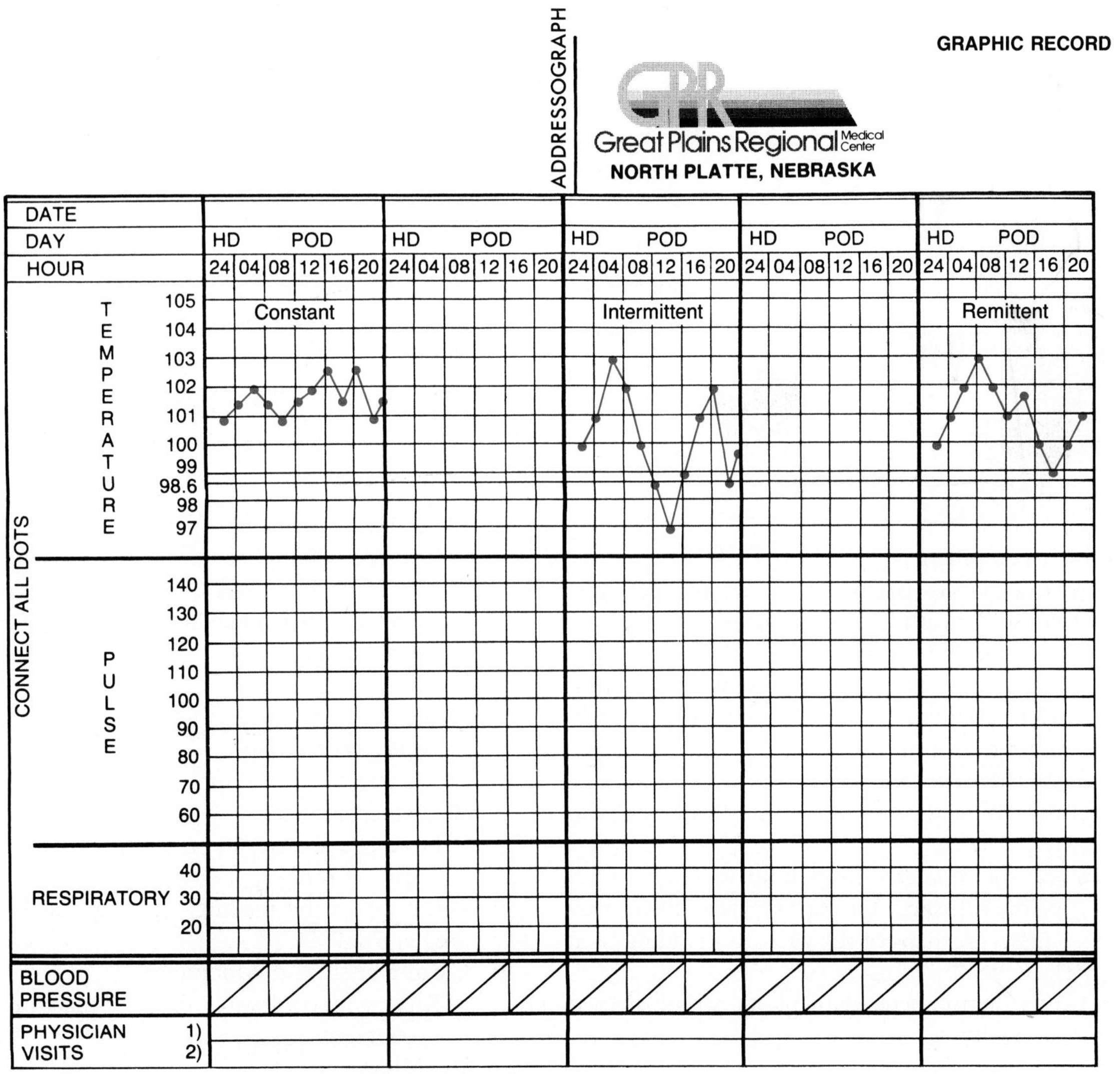

FIG. 14-3 Form for recording vital signs. Note temperature graphic showing types of fevers.

Table 14-1 Selection of Sites for Temperature Measurement

Site	Advantages	Disadvantages
Oral	Most accessible site; more comfortable for patient	Should not be used for patients who could be injured by thermometer, who are unable to hold thermometer properly, or who might bite down on thermometer; infants or small children, confused or unconscious patients, patients who have had oral surgery, patients with trauma to face or mouth, patients experiencing oral pain, patients who breathe only with mouth open, paitents with history of convulsions, patients experiencing a shaking chill
Rectal	Thought to provide most reliable measurement	Should not be used for patients after rectal surgery, patients who have a rectal disorder, such as tumor or hemorrhoids, or patients who cannot be positioned for proper thermometer placement, such as those in traction
Axilla	Safest method because noninvasive	Least accurate

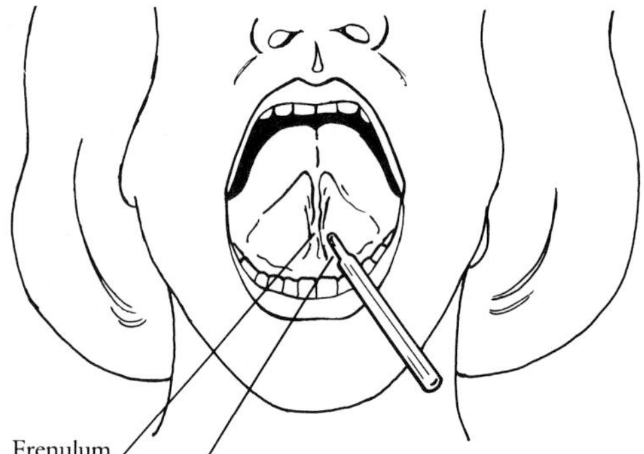

FIG. 14-4

SKILL 14-1 OBTAINING AN ORAL TEMPERATURE READING

1. Wash hands.
2. Gather equipment.
   An oral glass thermometer, alcohol pledgets, disposable sheath if used in facility.
3. Explain procedure to patient.
   If patient has eaten, drunk, or smoked in the past 15 to 30 minutes, wait 15 minutes before taking temperature.
4. Prepare thermometer.
   Rinse off disinfectant if necessary with cool water.
   Wipe thermometer from bulb to fingers with pledget. Inspect for cracks. Shake down mercury with snaps of the wrist to a reading of at least 96° F.
   Cover thermometer with plastic sheath if used at facility.
5. Place thermometer into patient's mouth.
   Place in sublingual pocket to the side of the tongue (Fig. 14-4). Have patient close lips around thermometer, and instruct patient not to talk.
6. Wait 5 minutes.
7. Remove thermometer, and wipe with pledget from fingers to bulb.
   If using a cover, remove and discard sheath.
8. Read thermometer.
   Hold at eye level, and rotate until mercury line can be read.
9. Write down the reading, for charting later: example, 98.6° F.
10. Clean and store thermometer.
    Rinse with cool water, dry, and place in storage container.
11. Wash hands.

SKILL 14-2 OBTAINING A RECTAL TEMPERATURE READING

1. Wash hands.
2. Gather equipment.
   A rectal safety thermometer with a short, blunt bulb (glass), alcohol pledgets, water-soluble lubricant, and disposable sheath if used in facility.
3. Explain the procedure to the patient.
4. Provide for privacy.
   Pull the curtains or close door. Have drape available for patient if necessary.
5. Don gloves.
6. Prepare thermometer.
   Rinse thermometer, and wipe from bulb to fingers with pledget. Shake down mercury with snaps of the wrist to a reading of at least 96° F.
   Cover thermometer with sheath if used. Lubricate tip of thermometer 1½ inches.
7. Position patient.
   Place in a Sims' position if possible.
8. Insert thermometer.
   Spread buttocks, and gently insert the thermometer 1½ inches (Fig. 14-5). Hold thermometer in place throughout procedure.
9. Wait 2 minutes.
10. Remove thermometer.
    Wipe from fingers to bulb with pledget, or remove and discard sheath.
11. Provide for patient comfort.
    Remove excess lubricant from rectal area, and assist to replace clothing if necessary. Repositon for comfort.
12. Read thermometer.
    Hold thermometer at eye level, and rotate until line of mercury is seen.
13. Write down the reading, for charting later: example, 99.6° F Ⓡ.
14. Clean and store thermometer.
    Rinse with cool water, dry, and replace in storage container.
15. Wash hands.

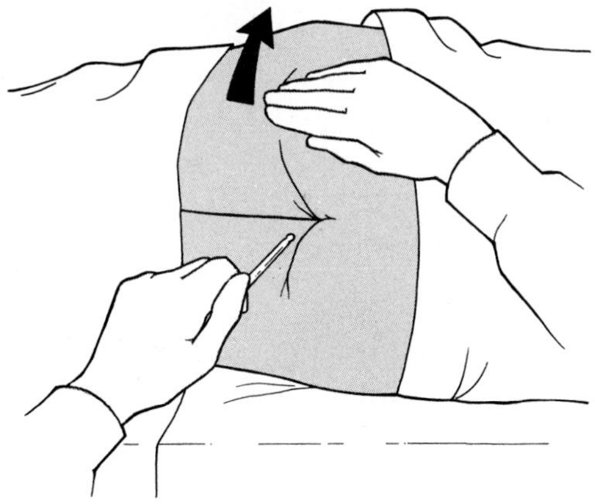

FIG. 14-5

fevers rise and fall, for example, normal in the morning and "spiking" in the afternoon. Remittent fevers are similar to intermittent fevers except the temperature never returns to normal until the patient becomes well (Fig. 14-3).

The patient with an abnormally low temperature is referred to as being **hypothermic.** Death can occur if the body temperature falls below 93.2° F. There have been documented cases of persons surviving with much lower temperatures. The patient may intentionally be placed in hypothermia for a surgical procedure. Certain conditions, such as hypothyroidism, produce a subnormal temperature.

The method to measure the temperature is determined by the nurse's assessment of the patient (Table 14-1). Oral temperature is not obtained in the comatose or confused patient or small infants, since this method requires patient cooperation (See Skill 14-1). Rectal temperatures are contraindicated for patients with recent rectal surgery or certain conditions of the perineum (See Skill 14-2). Axillary temperature is considered the least accurate method but in some cases is the only alternative (See Skill 14-3). The nurse should be aware that rectal readings are normally 1 degree higher than oral, and axillary readings 1 degree lower than oral. See Skill 14-4 for obtaining temperature reading with an electronic thermometer.

SKILL 14-3 OBTAINING AN AXILLARY TEMPERATURE READING

1. Wash hands.
2. Gather equipment.
   An oral thermometer, alcohol pledgets, disposable sheath if used in facility.
3. Explain procedure to patient.
   This decreases anxiety and elicits cooperation.
4. Provide privacy.
   Pull curtains; expose axillary area.
5. Prepare thermometer.
   Rinse thermometer in cool water, and wipe from bulb to fingers with pledget. Shake down mercury with snaps of the wrist to a reading of at least 96° F. Apply a sheath if used.
6. Place thermometer bulb against skin axilla.
   If the skin is wet, dry first for an accurate reading.
   Have the patient hold his upper arm snugly along side and his lower arm across chest (Fig. 14-6).
7. Wait 5-10 minutes.
8. Remove thermometer.
   Wipe from fingers to bulb with pledget. Remove and discard sheath if used.
9. Provide for patient comfort.
   Assist with replacing clothing. Position for comfort.
10. Read thermometer.
    Hold thermometer at eye level, and rotate until line of mercury is seen.
11. Write down the reading, for charting later: example, 97.6° F (A).
12. Clean and store thermometer.
    Rinse with cool water, dry, and replace in storage container.
13. Wash hands.

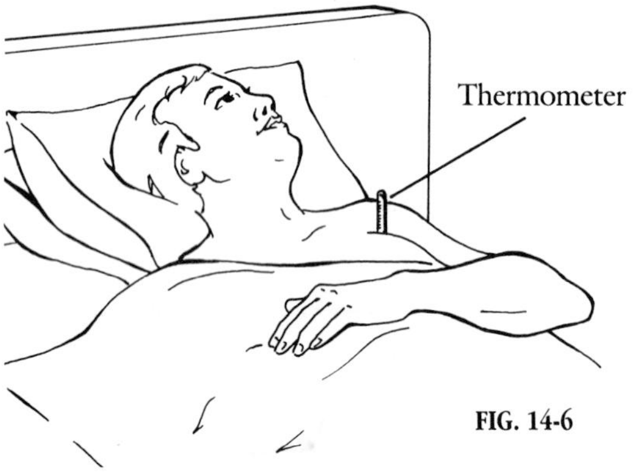

FIG. 14-6

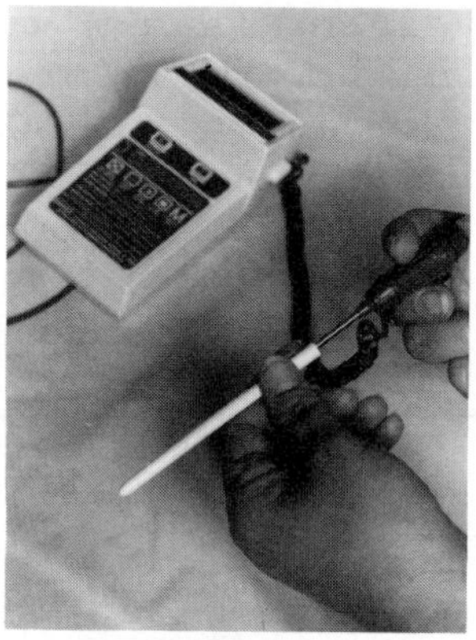

FIG. 14-7

SKILL 14-4 OBTAINING TEMPERATURE READINGS WITH AN ELECTRONIC THERMOMETER

1. Wash hands.
2. Gather equipment.
   Electronic thermometer with rectal or oral probe, probe covers, lubricant for rectal temperature.
3. Explain procedure to patient.
4. Remove probe from socket, and insert snugly into probe cover (Fig. 14-7).
   Use red-tipped probe for rectal*; blue-tipped probe for oral.
5. Place probe against body surface.
   Oral in sublingual pocket, axillary in axillary space, and rectal lubricated tip 1½ inches into rectum.
6. Wait for audible signal, which indicates temperature reading is complete.
7. Remove probe.
8. Remove and dispose of probe cover by pressing ejection button on top of probe.
9. Read temperature before reinserting probe into socket.
10. Write down the reading, for charting later.
11. Replace probe in socket, and return unit to battery charger.
12. Wash hands.

*If a rectal temperature is taken, don gloves.

PULSE

Pulse is a rhythmic beating or vibrating movement. It is the regular, recurrent expansion and contraction of an artery produced by waves of pressure caused by the ejection of blood from the left ventricle of the heart as it contracts. It corresponds to each beat of the heart. When taking the pulse, the nurse notes the rate, rhythm, and volume of the pulse. The adult pulse rate is normally between 60 to 80 beats per minute, but there are many factors that can influence the rate.

The patient's age, sex, emotional state, size, temperature, condition of the heart, and amount of physical activity can influence the pulse rate. If the pulse is faster than 100 beats per minute, the patient has **tachycardia;** if it is slower than 60, the patient has **bradycardia.** Tachycardia can result from shock, hemorrhage leading to hypovolemia, exercise, fever, and acute pain. Drugs such as adrenalin can also increase the rate. Bradycardia can result from unrelieved, severe pain, because it stimulates the parasympathetic nervous system, which slows the heart rate. Drugs such as digitalis may lower the heart rate. Resting in a supine position may decrease the heart rate, as will the cardiac condition *heart block* (Box 14-3). If the amount of time between beats varies, there will be an irregular pulse or **dysrhythmia.** The normal pulse reflects an equal amount of time between beats. The *volume* of the pulse refers to the amount of blood pushing against the artery wall with each beat. A *weak* pulse is difficult to palpate; a *bounding* pulse is easily felt with light palpation. A pulse that cannot be felt at all is *imperceptible* (Table 14-2).

The pulse rate is usually obtained at the radial artery, which is located on the thumb side of the inner wrist. When assessing the patient, the nurse should palpate all major pulses and should **auscultate** the apical rate. For example, a pulse palpated at the dorsalis pedis indicates blood flow to the foot. Major pulses include the temporal, facial, carotid, brachial, radial, femoral, popliteal, and posterior tibial and dorsalis pedis (Fig. 14-8).

Pulses are palpated using the pads of the index and middle finger. Only slight pressure is applied over the artery to avoid obliterating the pulse (by occluding blood flow). See Skill 14-5 for obtaining a radial pulse rate.

The **apical** rate is auscultated when the radial pulse is irregular or is difficult to palpate. The apical rate represents the actual beating of the heart. When auscultating the apical rate, the "lub dub" heard by the nurse represents one cardiac cycle, or heart beat. See Skill 14-6 for obtaining apical pulse rate.

The nurse may note a difference in the rates between the radial and apical rates. This is called a **pulse deficit.** To confirm a pulse deficit, the nurse listens to the apical rate, and a second nurse palpates the radial pulse at the same time, using the same watch. A deficit results when the radial rate is less than the apical rate. A pulse deficit signifies that the pumping action of the heart is faulty.

BOX 14-3 FACTORS INFLUENCING PULSE RATES

Exercise. Short-term exercise increases pulse rate. Long-term exercise strengthens heart muscle, resulting in lower than normal rate at rest and a quicker return to resting rate after exercise.

Fever, heat. Both increases the pulse rate because of increased metabolic rate.

Acute pain, anxiety. These increase the pulse rate because of sympathetic stimulation.

Unrelieved severe pain. This decreases the pulse rate because of parasympathetic stimulation.

Drugs. Various drugs alter pulse rate. For example, digitalis decreases the pulse rate; atropine increases the pulse rate.

Hemorrhage. Loss of blood increases the pulse rate because of the sympathetic stimulation.

Postural changes. Lying down decreases the pulse rate. Standing or sitting increases the pulse rate.

Table 14-2 Pulse Volume Variations

Type	Description
Absent pulse	None felt.
Thready pulse	Difficult to feel; not palpable when only slight pressure applied.
Weak pulse	Somewhat stronger than a thready pulse but not palpable when light pressure applied.
Normal pulse	Easily felt but not palpable when moderate pressure applied.
Bounding pulse	Feels full and spring like even under moderate pressure.

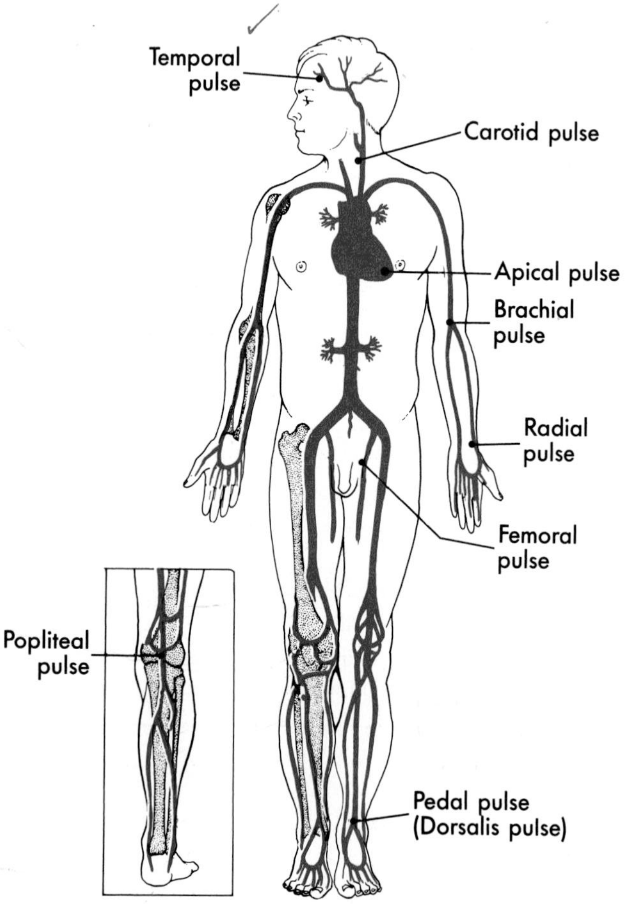

FIG. 14-8 The pulse sites.

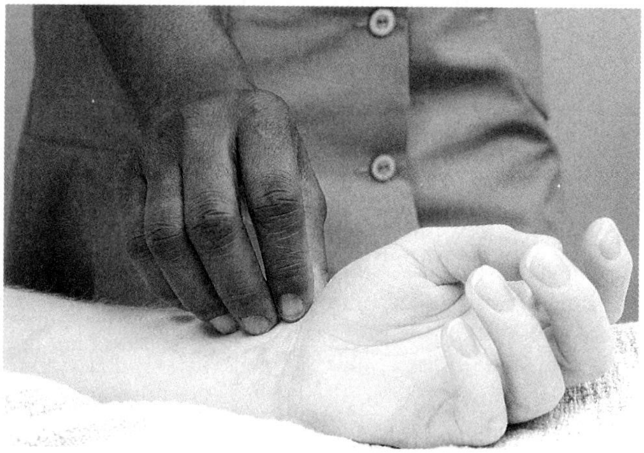

FIG. 14-9

SKILL 14-5 OBTAINING A RADIAL PULSE RATE

1. Wash hands.
2. Explain procedure to patient.
3. Palpate radial pulse.
   Use the pads of the index and middle finger. Gentle pressure is used so the pulse is not obliterated. Place fingers on the thumb side of the patient's wrist (Fig. 14-9).
4. Count pulse for 60 seconds.
5. Write down the pulse rate, for charting later: example, P—60, regular.
6. Wash hands.

SKILL 14-6

OBTAINING AN APICAL PULSE RATE

1. Wash hands.
2. Gather equipment.
   A stethoscope in good working condition.
3. Explain procedure to patient.
4. Provide privacy.
   Close curtains, expose patient's chest.
5. Place stethoscope against chest wall.
   Place diaphragm at apex of heart, which is located halfway between left nipple and sternum (Fig. 14-10).
6. Count rate for 60 seconds.
7. Write down apical rate, for charting later: example, P—64 (ap), regular.
8. Provide for patient comfort. Assist to redress if necessary.
9. Wash hands.

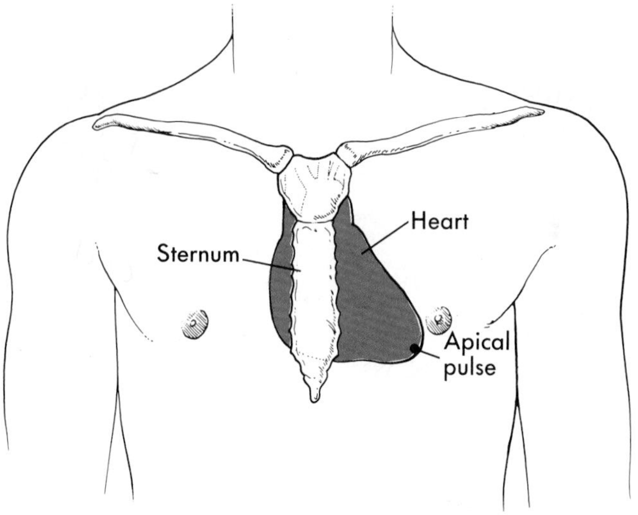

FIG. 14-10

RESPIRATIONS

Respirations can be internal or external. Internal respiration refers to the exchange of gas at the alveolar level. There is a molecule exchange of oxygen and carbon dioxide with the body's tissues, from the lungs to cellular **oxidation** processes. The breathing movements of the patient that can be observed by the nurse are called external respirations. External respirations have two parts in the cycle: inspiration and expiration. **Inspiration** is inhaling air into the lungs, and **expiration** is exhaling air. The rate of respiration is controlled by the medulla oblongata of the brain.

Any activity that increases metabolism will increase the need for oxygen by the body and will increase respiratory rate. In assessing respirations, the nurse notes the rate, depth, rhythm, and quality. The normal rate for an adult is between 12 to 20 respirations per minute (Box 14-4).

BOX 14-4 **FACTORS INFLUENCING RESPIRATION**

Disease or illness. Chronic lung disease (e.g., emphysema or bronchitis) alters the normal stimulus for ventilation. Lung tissue disease, reduced red blood cells, and chest pain alter the rate and depth of respiration.

Stress. An anxious or fearful patient will likely have increases in the rate and depth of respiration, and as a result, hyperventilation occurs.

Age. With growth from infancy to adulthood, the lungs' capacity increases and respiratory rate gradually declines. With old age, lung elasticity and depth of respiration decrease, and respiratory rate increases.

Sex. Men have a greater lung capacity than women.

Body position. In slumped or stooped position, ventilation is often impaired, with a reduced depth of respiration.

Drugs. Narcotics depress the patient's ability to increase the volume of air inspired and the rate of respiration is decreased. Other drugs may increase or decrease the rate and depth of respiration and may affect the rhythm.

Exercise. Exercise increases the rate and depth of respirations.

The patient with a rapid respiratory rate has **tachypnea.** Exercise and fever increase respiratory rate. A slow respiratory rate, below 12, is known as **bradypnea.**

The depth of respiration is determined by the amount of air taken in with inhalation. Normally 500 ml of air is inspired. Movement by the **diaphragm** and intercostal muscles allows the nurse to judge the depth of respirations. Shallow respirations make ventilation difficult to

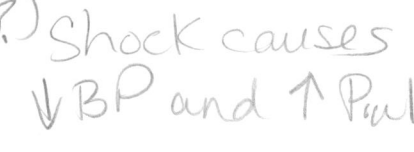

SKILL 14-7 OBTAINING A RESPIRATORY RATE

1. Wash hands.
2. Explain procedure to patient.
   Because the respiratory rate can be altered unconsciously by the patient if he knows he is being observed, it is best to assess the respiratory rate at the same time a pulse is counted.
3. Place fingertips as if to obtain a radial pulse.
4. Observe respiratory rate.
   One inhalation/exhalation = one respiration. Count each time the chest rises for inhalation. Count for 60 seconds.
5. Write down the count, for charting later: example R—20, regular.
6. Wash hands.

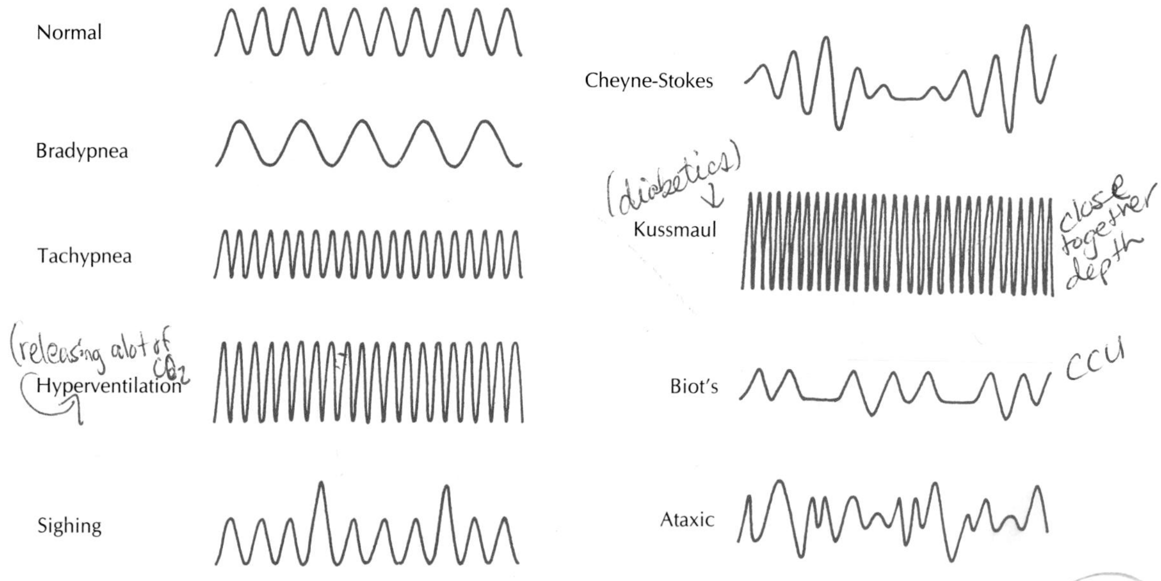

FIG. 14-11 Patterns of respiration.

observe and only a small amount of air is exchanged in the lungs. The rhythm of respiration should be regular and uninterrupted. Occasional sighing is normal and allows all **alveoli** to be aerated. Respirations should not be audible except with the aid of a **stethoscope** (See Skill 14-7).

Patterns of breathing should be assessed (Fig. 14-11). **Dyspnea** is breathing with difficulty. The patient may be laboring to get enough oxygen, with pursed lips, flared nostrils, and clavicular and costal **retractions. Apnea** is a lack of spontaneous respirations. **Cheyne-Stokes respirations** are an abnormal pattern of respiration characterized by alternating periods of apnea and deep, rapid breathing. The periods of apnea increase as time goes on. Cheyne-Stokes respirations are noted in the critically ill or terminal patient.

The best time to assess respirations is when counting a radial or apical pulse. The patient is unaware and unable to alter respirations.

BLOOD PRESSURE

The blood pressure is the pressure exerted by the circulating volume of blood on the arterial walls, veins, and chambers of the heart. Blood pressure is measured in millimeters of mercury (mm Hg). There are actually two pressures that make up blood pressure. The **systolic** pressure is the higher number and represents the ventricles contracting, forcing blood into the aorta and pulmonary arteries. This occurrence of systole is indicated by the first sound heard on ausculation. The second number is the **diastolic** pressure and represents the pressure within the artery between beats. It is the period between contractions of the atria or the ventricles during which blood enters the relaxed chambers from the systemic circulation and the lungs. Diastole represents the initial absence of sound. The difference between the two readings is called the **pulse pressure.**

Blood pressure reflects **cardiac output,** the quality of the arteries, the blood volume, and blood viscosity.

Whenever the blood is pumped by the heart into the arteries, the pressure within the arteries rises. Therefore the greater the amount of blood pumped by the heart, the greater the pressure. Likewise, if the blood volume is increased, the pressure within the artery will increase.

When the arteries' lumens, the channels within the arteries, narrow and become less flexible, blood pressure will rise because there is less space for the blood to enter.

Increased viscosity (thickness) of the blood causes a slower flow of blood in the capillaries, which causes back-up pressure in the larger vessels (Box 14-5).

Normal blood pressure in the adult is 120/80. **Hypertension** occurs when the sustained elevated pressure is above 140/90. Primary or essential hypertension is the most common form. The cause is unknown, but it is believed to be related to aging. Heredity, smoking, and high cholesterol, caffeine, and alcohol ingestion have been linked with hypertension.

The patient with a blood pressure below normal is **hypotensive.** It is considered healthy to have a low blood pressure providing there are no ill effects, such as **vertigo** or **syncope. Orthostatic** hypotension occurs when a person rises too quickly from a supine position. The patient may feel light-headed and unstable. This patient should be advised to rise slowly from lying to sitting to standing, thus preventing blood volume from shifting suddenly. Hypotension resulting from shock or massive hemorrhage is very serious and requires immediate medical intervention (Table 14-3).

The patient is assessed for hypertension and hypotension. The diagnosis of hypertension is not made with only one random elevated reading but by the average of elevated readings over 140/90 taken on several occasions.

Blood pressure readings are taken with a sphygmomanometer and a stethoscope. A **sphygmomanometer** consists of an inflatable cuff and a gauge. The gauge can be aneroid or mercury (Fig. 14-12). The cuff is inflated around the patient's arm to compress the artery, which will occlude blood flow; then it is slowly deflated, which will allow blood flow to resume. While performing this, the nurse listens to the brachial artery with the stethoscope and hears pulsating sounds. These are called **Korotkoff sounds.** The sounds go through five phases (Fig. 14-13). When the first sound is heard, the nurse

BOX 14-5 FACTORS INFLUENCING BLOOD PRESSURE

Age. Variables influence normal blood pressure:

AGE	ARTERIAL PRESSURE (mm Hg)
Newborn (3000 g [6.6 lb])	Systolic 50-52 Diastolic 25-30 Mean 35-40
4 years	85/60
6 years	95/62
10 years	100/65
12 years	108/67
16 years	118/75
Middle adult	120/80
Elderly	140-160/90-100

Anxiety, fear, pain, and emotional stress. May increase blood pressure because of increased heart rate and increased peripheral vascular resistance.

Drugs. Can either lower or increase blood pressure depending on their pharmacological action.

Hormones. Variations in blood pressure may be manifested as a person ages, because of hormonal alterations. Pregnancy may cause mild to severe elevations in blood pressure.

Diurnal. Variations may include a lower blood pressure in the morning, rising throughout the day, peaking in late afternoon or evening, and lowering at night; individual variations are significant.

Table 14-3 Conditions Causing Alterations in Blood Pressure

Conditions	Effect	Cause
Hemorrhage	Lowers pressure	Decreased blood volume
Increased intracranial pressure	Raises pressure	Disturbance of cardiovascular control mechanisms in brainstem resulting from pressure exerted on the medulla oblongata
Acute pain	Raises pressure	Increased vasomotor tone and peripheral vascular resistance as a result of sympathetic stimulation
Chronic renal failure	Raises pressure	Increased blood volume resulting from increased retention of sodium and water; release of renin, a vasopressor that increases peripheral vascular resistance
Essential hypertension	Raises pressure	Increased peripheral vascular resistance resulting from progressive thickening of arterial walls
General anesthesia	Lowers pressure	Decreased vasomotor tone resulting from depression of vasomotor center in brainstem

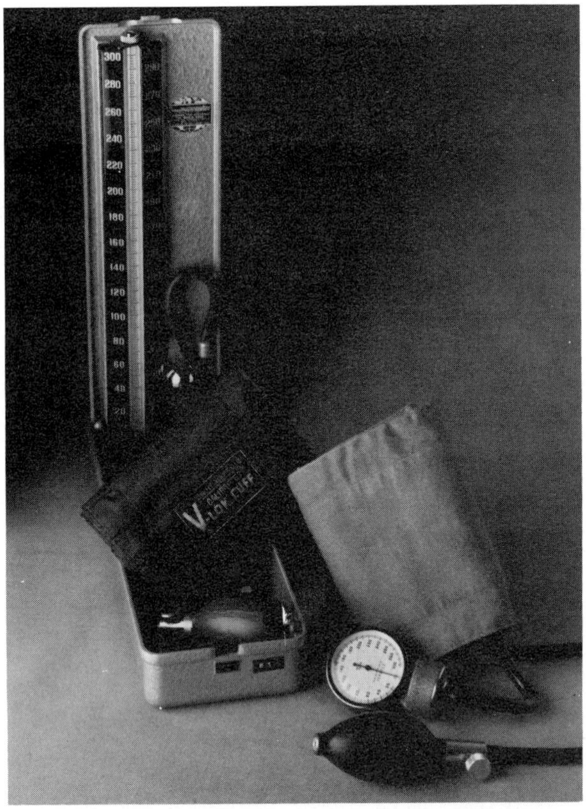

FIG. 14-12 Sphygmomanometer is composed of pressure manometer, cloth cuff with rubber bladder, and pressure bulb. Mercury manometer is at left; aneroid manometer at right.

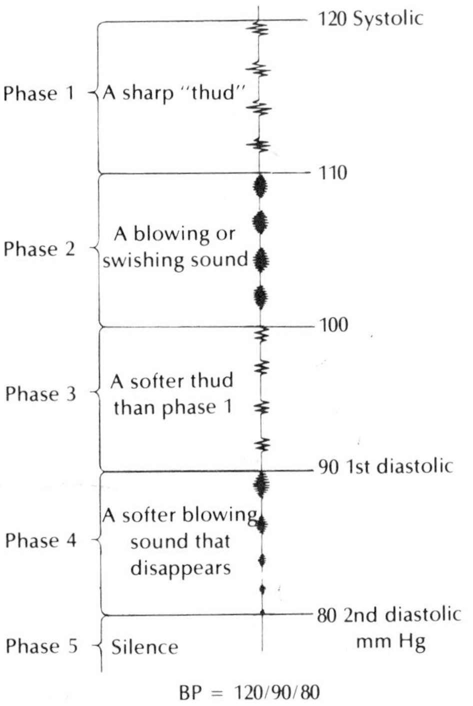

FIG. 14-13 Phases of the Korotkoff sounds.

makes a mental note of that point on the sphygmomanometer gauge and again notes when the sound disappears. The point when the first sound is heard is the systolic pressure. The point at which the last sound is heard is the diastolic pressure. At times the sounds are heard to zero. In this case the nurse must listen for a subtle change in the quality of the sound as it approaches the diastolic reading. This then is the diastolic pressure, and the blood pressure is written using the three readings, for example, 120/80/0.

Blood pressure measurements can also be obtained by the palpatory method. The nurse applies the blood pressure cuff as in the auscultatory method. The radial pulse is then palpated on that arm. The cuff is inflated until the pulse is obliterated. As the cuff is slowly deflated, the nurse notes the point at which the pulse is again felt. This corresponds to the systolic pressure.

To assure an accurate blood pressure reading, the environment must be quiet. The equipment must be in good working order, and the cuff should fit correctly. The gauge should be read at eye level (See Skill 14-8).

HEIGHT AND WEIGHT

With the initial measurement of vital signs, the nurse measures the patient's height and weight. Height and weight determination is important because it helps to assess normal growth and development, aids in proper drug dosage calculation, and may be used to assess the effectiveness of drug therapy, such as diuretics. A significant loss of weight may be a sign of an underlying disease.

Daily weights should be taken in the same manner each time; it is best to weigh the patient at the same time of day and in the same amount of patient clothing.

The nurse weighs malnourished patients, patients who are undergoing diuretic therapy, and patients who have diseases that increase fluid retention, such as heart, liver, and kidney disease (See Skill 14-9).

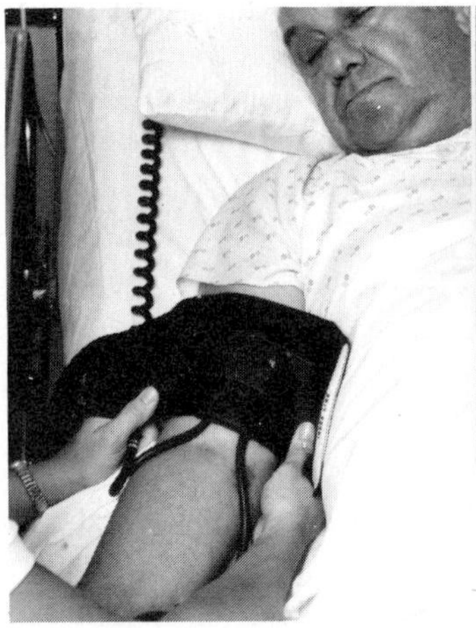

FIG. 14-14

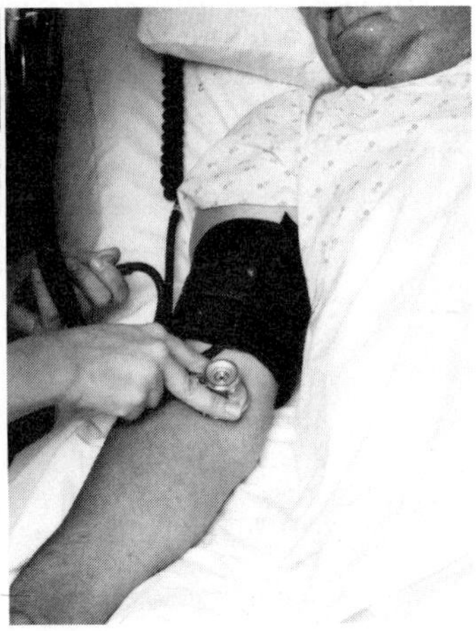

FIG. 14-15

SKILL 14-8

OBTAINING A BLOOD PRESSURE READING USING PALPATORY—AUSCULTATORY METHOD

1. Wash hands.
2. Gather equipment.
   A sphygmomanometer and stethoscope are needed.
   Use the correct cuff size. The improper size will give an inaccurate reading. The length of the cuff should be 80% of the upper arm circumference and be two-thirds the width of the upper arm.
   Ensure all connections are tight, the cuff inflates, and the stethoscope is functional.
3. Explain procedure to patient.
4. Apply the cuff to the arm.
   The arm should be bare. The cuff is applied 1 to 2 inches above the elbow (Fig. 14-14). The cuff should be centered over the brachial artery. The upper arm is held at the level of the heart, and the lower arm should rest comfortably on a firm surface.
5. Palpate the radial artery.
   The artery is located on the patient's thumb side of the wrist. Use index and middle finger to palpate.
6. Inflate the cuff.
   Note the point on the cuff gauge when the radial pulse is obliterated. This is the approximate systolic pressure.
7. Deflate the cuff.
   Allow the arm to rest for 30 seconds before reinflating to take the blood pressure reading. This allows the congestion to leave the arm and thus prevent a false high systolic reading.
8. Palpate the brachial artery and place stethoscope diaphragm/bell over it (Fig. 14-15).
   The artery is located on the inner aspect of the antecubital space. Hold the diaphragm down with thumb and place fingers behind the patient's elbow so that secure contact is made. Keep the stethoscope free so interfering noise will be minimal.
9. Reinflate the cuff.
   Inflate to 20 to 30 mm Hg above the point where the radial pulse disappeared.
10. Slowly deflate cuff.
    Cuff is deflated at a rate of 2 mm per second.
    Note the point at which the first pulse beat is heard. This is the systolic. Note the point at which the pulse beat disappears. This is the diastolic. If the blood pressure was not heard, wait 30 seconds with cuff deflated before repeating procedure.
11. Remove cuff.
12. Write down the reading, for charting later: example, BP—120/80.
13. Assist patient to replace clothing if necessary.
14. Return equipment to storage.
15. Wash hands.

SKILL 14-9

MEASURING HEIGHT AND WEIGHT

1. Wash hands
2. Gather equipment.
   A scale with measuring line.
3. Explain procedure to patient.
4. Balance scale to zero.
5. Have patient step onto scale.
   Have patient weighed in same amount of clothing each time—preferably gown and slippers.
6. Measure height.
7. Measure weight.
   Support patient gently if unstable, or use chair scale or bed scale.
8. Assist patient off scale.
   Have patient step to side instead of backwards, and assist to bed if necessary.
9. Write down the measurements for charting later: example, Ht/Wt—64 in/136 lb.
10. Store scale appropriately.
11. Wash hands.

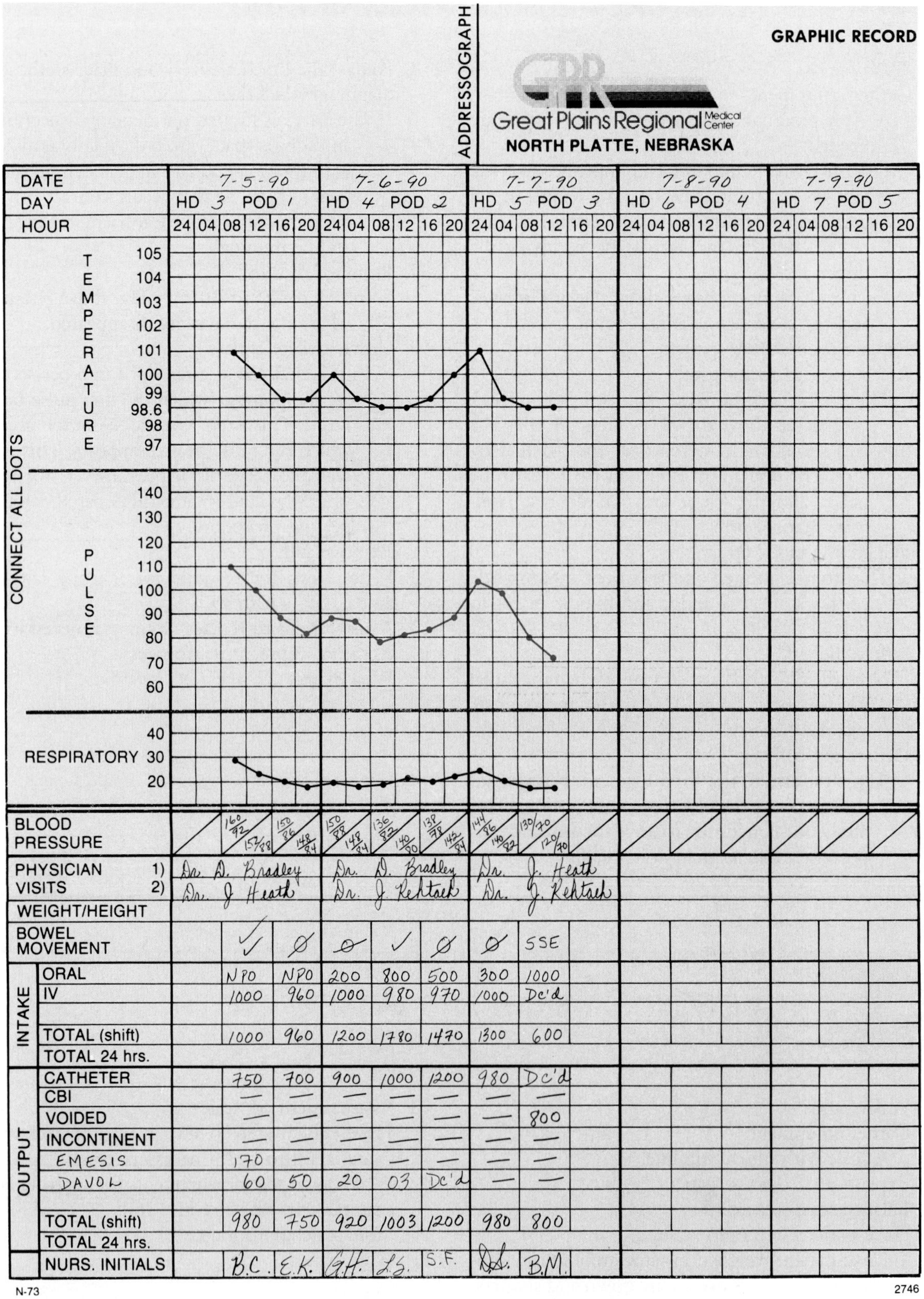

FIG. 14-16 Sample of a graphic flow sheet.

Table 14-4 Age-Related Vital Signs

Age Group	Heart Rate (per minute)	Respiratory Rate (per minute)	Blood Pressure (mm Hg)	
Neonate	130-150	36-60	Systolic	20-60
Infant	125-135	40-46	Systolic	70-80
Toddler	65-105	20-24		
School-age (6-10)	65-105	20-24	Systolic	90-100
			Diastolic	60-64
Adolescent (10-18)	65-100	16-22	Systolic	100-120
			Diastolic	70-80
Adult	60-100	12-20	Systolic	100-120
			Diastolic	70-89
Older adult	60-100	12-18	Systolic	130-140
			Diastolic	90-95

WHEN VITAL SIGNS ARE ASSESSED

Although temperature, pulse, respiration, and blood pressure are presented as separate procedures, all of them are usually assessed at the same time at set intervals. A set of vital signs is taken when a patient is admitted to a facility, and then as prescribed by the physician or as policy dictates, for example, every 4 hours, once a shift, or even weekly in some extended-care facilities. The more ill the patient, the more frequently vital signs are taken. The nurse uses her judgment in cases where the patient's condition worsens, at which times vital signs should always be obtained. Vital sign readings are interrelated. A rise in temperature of 1 degree will cause an increase in pulse rate of 4 beats per minute. Respiratory rate and blood pressure readings will likewise increase with a rise in temperature; however, when blood pressure falls because of hemorrhage, the pulse will increase. It is also important to recognize the age-related differences in vital signs (Table 14-4).

If there is a possibility of contact with body secretions, the nurse should wear gloves while obtaining vital signs.

Before measurement of vital signs, the patient should be given an explanation of the procedure to elicit cooperation and decrease anxiety, which may alter measurements.

RECORDING VITAL SIGNS

Most facilities have graphic flow sheets for charting vital signs. In some cases a rectal temperature would be indicated with a small circled Ⓡ, and axillary with a small circled Ⓐ next to the reading. Blood pressures are always written with the systolic first and the diastolic beneath: 120/80. When charting the pulse on a graphic sheet, note that the pulse was an apical measurement by writing "ap" next to the number: 78 ap. An example of graphic flow sheet is shown in Fig. 14-16.

REFERENCES AND SUGGESTED READINGS

1. American Heart Association: Technique for blood pressure measurement—palpatory and auscultatory method, 1988.
2. Billings D and Stokes L: Medical-surgical nursing: common health problems of adults and children across the life span, ed 2, St Louis, 1987, The CV Mosby Co.
3. Boylan A and Brown P: Student observations: more than "doing the obs" . . . the significance of pulse and blood pressure measurement, Nurs Times 81:24, 1985.
4. Boylan A and Brown P: Student observations: temperature, Nurs Times 81:36, 1985.
5. DiVito A and Kleven M: Dyspnea, RN 50(6):40, 1987.
6. Doyle JT: You swallowed your what! . . . the missing thermometer, RN 48:40, 1985.
7. Gurevich I: Fever: when to worry about it, RN 48(12):14, 1985.
8. The latest words for high blood pressure, Am J Nurs 89(5):504, 1989.
9. Malasanos L and others: Health assessment, ed 4, St Louis, 1990, The CV Mosby Co.
10. Mosby's medical and nursing dictionary, ed 3, St Louis, 1990, The CV Mosby Co.
11. Potter P and Perry A: Basic nursing, ed 2, St Louis, 1991, The CV Mosby Co.
12. Preparing to take a patient's blood pressure, Nurs '89, p 65, June 1989.
13. Rudy S: Take a reading on your blood pressure techniques, Nurs '86 16(8):46, 1986.
14. Samples JF, VanCott ML, and Long C: Circadian rhythms: basis for screening for fever . . . routine temperature assessments in hospitals, Nurs Res 34:377, 1985.
15. Seidel H and others: Mosby's guide to physical examination, ed 2, St Louis, 1991, The CV Mosby Co.
16. Stone S: A new concept in routine vital signs measurement, Nurs Manage 17:28, 1986.
17. Taking accurate blood pressure readings, Nurs '88, pp 32J-32N, April 1988.

CHAPTER CHALLENGE

KEY POINTS

- Vital signs are an indication of a person's overall health status.
- Vital signs should be obtained initially to establish a baseline.
- Vital signs should be obtained whenever the patient's condition changes adversely.
- The nurse is aware of factors that could influence vital sign readings.
- The nurse controls factors that may alter vital sign readings.
- The nurse knows the normal limits of vital sign readings.
- Pulses are an indication of blood flow to a body part.
- Temperatures can be obtained by oral, rectal, axillary, groin, and tympanic routes; the rectal temperature reflects core body temperature most accurately.
- When assessing blood pressure, proper equipment is as important as correct technique.
- Temperature, pulse, respirations, and blood pressure are interrelated; a change in one may alter another.
- Height and weight is a ratio. Knowing the weight or height alone usually does not supply useful information.

STUDY QUESTIONS

Mrs. Jones, 45, is admitted with a fever of unknown origin. She has a history of heart disease.

1. When assessing Mrs. Jones' temperature, the most accurate reading would be:
   a. Rectal
   b. Oral
   c. Axillary
   d. Tympanic
2. Mrs. Jones' oral temperature is 100.6° F. What rectal reading would you expect:
   a. 101.6° F
   b. 100.6° F
   c. 99.6° F
   d. 97.6° F
3. Mrs. Jones' temperature is elevated in the evening but returns to normal in the morning; this fever is classified as:
   a. Constant
   b. Intermittent
   c. Remittent
   d. Normal
4. With a history of heart disease, the most accurate pulse rate to assess would be:
   a. Carotid
   b. Brachial
   c. Apical
   d. Radial
5. Mrs. Jones' pulse rate is 110; she is said to have:
   a. Bradycardia
   b. Bradypnea
   c. Tachypnea
   d. Tachycardia
6. Which would be a normal respiratory rate for Mrs. Jones:
   a. 30-60
   b. 12-20
   c. 8-12
   d. 24-30
7. Mrs. Jones displays signs of dyspnea; signs would include *all except*:
   a. Cyanosis
   b. Nasal flaring
   c. Restlessness
   d. Pallor
8. When taking Mrs. Jones' blood pressure you palpate the radial pulse while inflating the cuff; the pulse disappears at 100 mm Hg; after waiting 30 seconds, you reinflate the cuff to ____mm Hg to obtain the blood pressure reading:
   a. 130
   b. 200
   c. 180
   d. 70
9. To be classified as hypertensive, Mrs. Jones would have a sustained elevated blood pressure of over:
   a. 160/100
   b. 140/90
   c. 130/70
   d. 120/80
10. The difference in rates between the radial and apical pulse is called:
    a. Pulse pressure
    b. Dysrhythmia
    c. Pulse deficit
    d. Systole

irregular

V

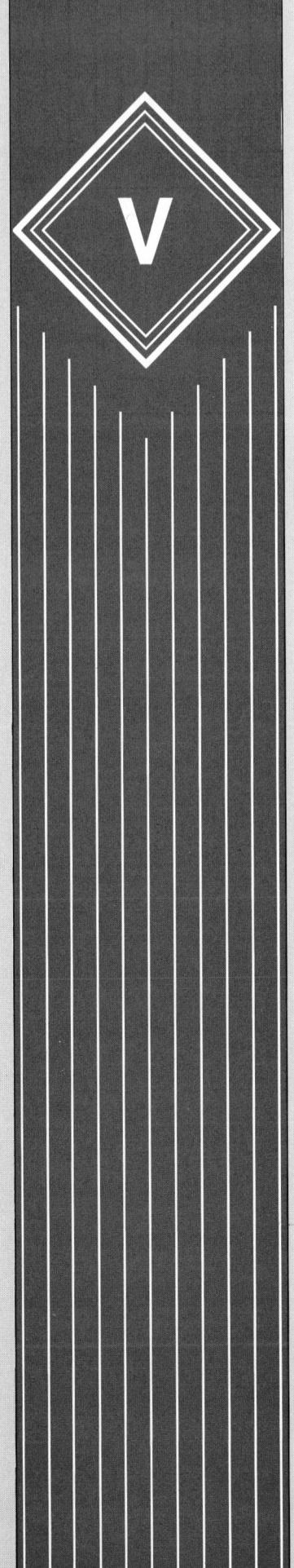

Basic Nursing Skills

Do I really want to empty a bed pan? Do I really want to take care of the contrary old man or woman? Do I really want to see the miracle of a baby born into the world? The answer lies within eyes filled with pain and a weak, frail hand grasping mine in a silent thank you. For within me lies a nurturing soul. Just to see the joy of life begin and end, knowing I did all I could, and maybe saving the life of someone's loved one.

JOYCE L. JESSE
Student Nurse

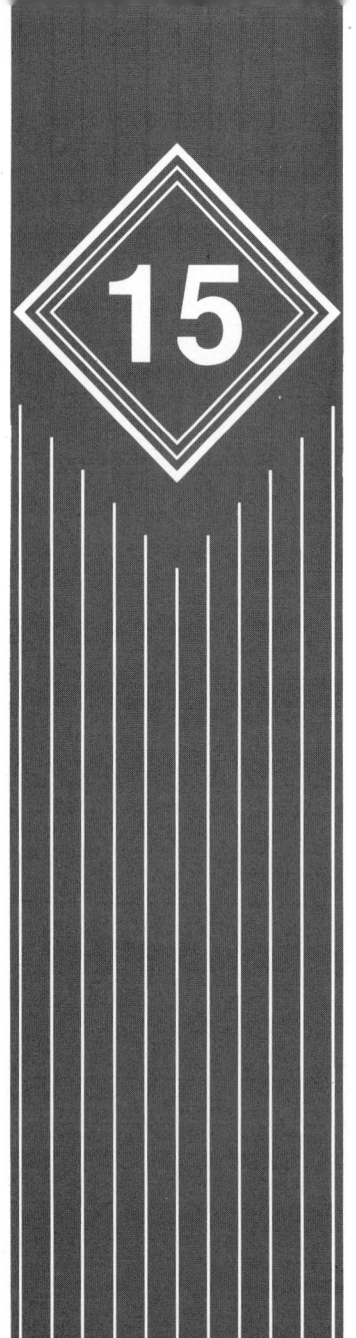

15

Admission, Transfer, and Discharge

LOIS WHITE

LEARNING OBJECTIVES

After reading this chapter, the student should be able to do the following:

- Define the key terms.
- Identify guidelines for admission, transfer, and discharge of a patient.
- Describe common patient reactions to hospitalization.
- Identify ways that the nurse can respond to these reactions.
- Identify the nurse's responsibilities in performing admission, transfer, and discharge.
- Describe how to prepare a room for patient admission.
- Describe how the nurse prepares a patient for transfer to another unit or facility.
- Describe how the nurse prepares a patient for discharge.
- Identify the nurse's role when a patient chooses to leave a hospital against medical advice.

SKILLS

15-1 Admitting a patient
15-2 Transferring a patient
15-3 Discharging a patient

KEY TERMS

Define the following:

- admission
- against medical advice (AMA)
- consumer
- continuity of care
- discharge
- disorientation
- empathy
- health care facility
- home health agency
- interagency
- intraagency
- orientation
- separation anxiety
- third-party payors
- transfer

COMMON PATIENT REACTIONS TO HOSPITALIZATION

Admission to a hospital or other **health care facility** is an anxious time for patients and their families. The patient is usually very concerned about health problems, or potential health problems, and the potential outcome of treatment. Often the patient is having pain or some other discomfort. The first contact with nurses and other health care workers is important; anxiety and fears can be lessened and a positive attitude regarding the care to be received can be initiated.

The environment of a health care facility differs from a patient's home and has new sights, sounds, and smells that may interfere with the patient's comfort. It is the nurse's responsibility to assist the patient in maintaining dignity and a sense of control and to become comfortable in this new environment.

Each person's reaction to hospitalization is unique; however, there are some common reactions the nurse can anticipate, such as fear of the unknown, loss of identity, **disorientation, separation anxiety,** and loneliness. These reactions are related to some of the needs described by Maslow.[6]

Fear of the unknown, which causes insecurity, may be the most common reaction. This relates to the need Maslow calls safety. Such questions as these can cause anxiety and insecurity if unanswered: How do I work the bed? how do I call the nurse? how or when do I get some food? when can my family visit? and what are they going to do to me next? A caring nurse can relieve some of the anxiety by orienting the patient and family to the room and explaining how the equipment works. Explanations about hospital policies, information about medical orders and procedures, and simple direct answers to questions the patient or family may ask help the person feel more comfortable and in control.

During the admission process to a health care facility, a patient may feel a loss of identity that reflects a need for esteem, including recognition, as described by Maslow.[6] When an identification band is put on the patient's wrist, the patient may feel recognized only as the number and name on the identification band rather than as a person. Thus it is important to explain that this is a necessary procedure to provide a positive means of identification, because medications, anesthesia, discomfort, and emotional reactions may cause the patient to be confused or unresponsive.

The nurse must learn new patients' names quickly and use Mr., Mrs., Ms., or Miss with the last name. First names are used only at the patient's request. Using "honey, dear, gramps, or grandma" is *never* appropriate.

The reactions of separation anxiety and loneliness reflect a need for belongingness and love that Maslow identified. **Separation anxiety** is widely recognized in young children, but adults and the elderly often have this reaction as well. It generally is expressed in children by crying; adults may be either very quiet or very talkative; the elderly may exhibit disorientation, depression, or confusion.

Liberal visiting hours in health care facilities encourage family and friends to visit. Many hospitals now allow small children to visit relatives, especially their mother with a new baby. Parents are encouraged to stay with their hospitalized child to prevent the anxiety of separation from the parents. This also gives the child a feeling of security. In some facilities pets are allowed to visit; pets may even live in some nursing homes.[1]

The nurse may help reduce the severity of these common reactions to hospitalization with a warm, caring attitude and with courtesy and **empathy.** Treating each patient with respect, maintaining his dignity, involving him in the plan of care, and, whenever possible, adjusting hospital routine to meet his desires will help the patient adapt.

SKILL 15-1: ADMITTING A PATIENT

Guidelines

The **admission** procedure generally begins in the admitting department. Here admissions staff gather information to start the patient's record. This information usually includes name, address, telephone number, age, birth date, Social Security number, next of kin, insurance company and policy number, place of employment, physician's name, and reason for this admission and previous admissions. This information is primarily used in the business office for billing purposes. The identification band is prepared with the patient's name, age, ID number, physician's name, and the room number. The admitting clerk usually puts the band on the patient's wrist. The unit where the patient is assigned for care is notified, and the patient is escorted to the room.

Some hospitals have telephone admitting. The day before a planned admission, a clerk from the admitting office calls the patient at home and gathers all the information needed to begin the records. Instructions are given regarding time to arrive at the hospital, items to bring to the hospital, and things that should not be brought to the hospital (e.g., jewelry and large sums of money). When the patient arrives the next day, the records and identification band need only the room number put on them.

Persons brought to the emergency room may be admitted directly to a patient care room or a special care unit such as an intensive care unit (ICU), coronary care unit (CCU), or burn unit. In these situations a family member, usually the next of kin, goes to the admitting office to provide the necessary information.

When the unit staff are notified that a new patient is being escorted to a room, the room should be made ready. A room that is neat and clean, with lighting and temperature appropriate, and personal care items in place, makes the patient feel expected and welcome. A room that is not prepared may make the patient feel unexpected or that arrival is inconvenient to the nurse. This makes a bad first impression on which to build a nurse-patient relationship.

If special equipment will be required by the new patient, such as oxygen or traction, it should be in place and ready when the patient arrives. A patient arriving on a stretcher will need the bed in the high position; the low bed position is best for a patient arriving by wheelchair or walking.

Greeting the patient by name and making him feel welcome is one of the most important aspects of the admission procedure. The nurse should introduce herself by name and title (e.g., Miss Doe, SPN [or SVN], or Mr. Smith, LPN [or LVN]). A person who is warmly welcomed will be more at ease in this new environment.

The new patient should be given an **orientation** to the unit and the room. The orientation should include the following:

1. The relationship of the room to the nurses' station
2. The location of lounge areas
3. The location of shower and bathroom facilities
4. How to call the nurse from the bed and the bathroom
5. How to use the intercom system
6. How to adjust the bed and lights
7. How to operate the television
8. How to operate the telephone and the radio
9. Explanation of policies that are applicable to the patient

The hospital routine should also be explained. Knowing when meals are served, when family and friends may visit, when laboratory tests or x-ray evaluations are scheduled, when the physician usually sees patients, and the policy on side rails at bedtime will give the patient a sense of security and lessen anxiety. Many hospitals have booklets for the patient explaining these routine activities; these serve as reminders of what the nurse explained. Some booklets include information about the availability of various social services, religious services, and facilities such as cafeteria, library, and gift shop.

The admitting procedure on the patient care unit is much more extensive than that in the admitting department. The nurse should check the identification band and verify the information with the patient. Assessment of immediate needs such as pain, shortness of breath, or severe anxiety should be made and reported. If there is another patient in the room, the roommate should be introduced.

Jewelry, money, and medication should be given to the family to take home. If no family member is present, the valuables may be put in the hospital safe. The nurse must carefully follow the hospital policy for patient valuables.

Losing a patient's valuables can have serious legal implications for both the hospital and the nurse. Disposition of valuables must be documented on the medical record.

The patient is usually asked to put on pajamas or a hospital gown. Sometimes the nurse must help the patient change clothes. If this help is not needed, give the patient a few minutes of privacy to change. Clothing should be inventoried along with other personal items the patient uses, such as glasses, contacts, dentures, prostheses, crutches, hearing aids, wigs, or Bible. Jewelry and money kept in the patient's room must also be recorded. Fig. 15-1. is a sample clothing and valuable inventory check.

Once the patient is settled, the nurse should take the health history and do the initial nursing assessment. The health history generally includes the reason for admission, signs and symptoms the patient is experiencing, past illnesses or hospitalizations, medications (both prescription and nonprescription), allergies (food, medications,

SPOHN HOSPITAL

VALUABLES FORM

VAUABLES BROUGHT WITH PATIENT TO HOSPITAL DATE ________

Clocks ________ Hearing Aids ________

Dentures: no. of plates ________ Jewelry ________

Bridgework: no. of pieces ________ Money (billfold) ________

Eyeglasses ________ Money (purse) ________

Contact lens ________ Radio ________

Watches ________ T.V. ________

Electric toothbrush ________ Electric razor ________

Prosthesis (any type) ________ Others ________

I take entire responsibility for retaining in my possesion the articles listed above. I am holding nothing in my possession which I have not declared here. I understand and agree that Spohn Hospital is not liable or responsible for any of patient's property left in the care, custody and control of the Hospital at patient's or patient representative's request if items are not secured in the Valuables Storage Envelope or in the Hospital safe.

SIGNATURE OF PATIENT ________

I have fully explained to this patient that Spohn Hospital takes no responsibility for articles retained by the patient.

SIGNATURE OF EMPLOYEE RECORDING ARTICLES ________

VALUABLES STORAGE ENVELOPE

When Valuables Storage Envelope is used, record the following information:

Envelope Number ________

Date property received ________

Employee taking envelope to Cashier ________

T 278 902830 Revised 7-88

FIG. 15-1 Clothing and valuables inventory check form. (Courtesy Spohn Hospital, Corpus Christi, TX.)

other), eating habits, elimination habits, sleep habits, and activity/exercise. Other information to be included in a history is the language spoken and understood, family members, home situation, and occupation.

The initial assessment should include level of consciousness, vital signs, height, weight, breath sounds, bowel sounds, range of motion, and condition of skin, vision, and hearing. Fig. 15-2 is an example of a record used to collect this information. The health history and initial nursing assessment may be performed by the RN in some hospitals. In others, either an RN or LPN/LVN may collect this information.

The physician is notified when the patient has been admitted. If no orders have been previously received, the physician will give the nurse orders at this time.

Skill 15-1 identifies the general steps to follow in admitting a patient. Specific hospital policies and the patient's condition may alter these steps.

Purposes

The nurse performs the accepted procedure for admitting a patient for the following reasons:

- to assist the patient to become comfortable in the hospital environment
- to obtain information about the patient that will serve as a basis for care
- to begin to establish a nurse/patient relationship

Related Knowledge and Skills

Before admitting a patient, the nurse should understand the following:

- principles of communication (see Chapter 4)
- accurate documentation (see Chapter 6)
- growth and development (see Chapters 7-11)
- physical assessment (see Chapter 13)
- vital sign assessment (see Chapter 14)

SKILL 15-1 ADMITTING A PATIENT

Nursing action	Rationale
1. Wash hands thoroughly.	Prevents spread of microoganisms.
2. Prepare the room before the patient arrives: care items in place; bed at proper height and open; light on.	Makes the patient feel expected and welcome.
3. Greet the patient and family. Introduce yourself. Introduce roommate(s) if any.	Gives recognition. Patient and family are more at ease when they know the people around them.
4. Check the identification band and verify accuracy.	Ensures identification before tests or surgery is performed or medication is given.
5. Assess immediate needs.	Establishes trust if needs are recognized and met.
6. Orient the patient to the unit, lounge, and nurses' station.	Provides security.
7. Orient the patient to the room. Explain the use of equipment, call system, bed, telephone, and television.	Allows the patient some control over the environment and prevents accidents.
8. Explain hospital routines, such as visiting hours, meal times, and morning wake-up.	Decreases fear of unknown and gives a feeling of security.
9. Provide privacy if the patient desires. Family may be asked to leave the room. Assist the patient to undress if needed.	Helps maintain dignity and shows respect for the patient. Helping the patient undress prevents fatigue and falling. Range of motion and the skin may be assessed.
10. Follow hospital policy for care of valuables, clothing, and medications.	Avoids loss of valuables, clothing, or medications which is upsetting to the patient and family and could result in legal problems.
11. Obtain the patient's health history, and do the initial nursing assessment.	Provides a basis for individualized care.

SKILL 15-1 ADMITTING A PATIENT—cont'd

Nursing action	Rationale
12. Provide for safety: bed low, side rails up.	Helps prevent accidents.
13. Begin care as ordered by the physician.	Patient and family develop a positive attitude about the institution when care is started immediately.
14. Invite the family back into the room if they left earlier.	Decreases family anxiety when they see the patient settled.
15. Wash hands thoroughly.	Prevents spread of microorganisms.
16. Record the information on the patient's chart according to hospital policy.	Provides information that can also be used by other health professionals. It is the beginning of the permanent record.

Sample charting

Date	Time	Notes
1/15/91	1445	17-year-old white male admitted per wheelchair accompanied by parents. T—96^6, P—78, R—18, BP 128/74. C/O pain in R knee. Limps when walking. Edema noted in R knee. To have right knee surgery in AM. Wallet given to mother. No known allergies. Health history taken and initial assessment completed.

(nurse's signature)

SPECIAL CONCERNS

When a patient is admitted in critical condition, only the most pertinent information need be collected immediately. The remaining information may be obtained at a later time.

Children. Admission of an infant or small child requires emotional support for both child and parents. Parents are generally encouraged to stay with their child to prevent separation anxiety for both the child and parents. The most reliable source of admission information is the parents.

Young children are very curious about what is happening to them and around them. Letting the child use equipment on dolls helps reduce anxieties. Children should be encouraged to express how they feel. It is generally best to perform invasive procedures (e.g., obtaining blood specimens, starting intravenous lines) in a treatment room so the child can make the association that his room is a safe area.

Older children and adolescents are often self-conscious about the changes in their bodies. Be aware of their modesty and provide them with privacy. Trust can be established by asking them the health questions instead of the parents.

Elderly. Elderly patients should be spoken to slowly and clearly, because hearing may be less acute with age. The nurse should face the patient to make lip-reading possible. Elderly patients should not be rushed; the nurse should wait for the patient to answer rather than letting family members answer. The change in environment and daily routine may cause confusion, loss of appetite, or reversal of sleeping-waking patterns. Anxiety about hospitalization may interfere with memory.

HOME HEALTH VARIATIONS

A patient requiring care at home may be referred to a **home health agency.** The services may include skilled nursing care or simply assistance with activities of daily living. There must be a physician's order for these services to be reimbursable from insurance or Medicare/Medicaid. A health history and initial assessment are performed, just as in the hospital (see Chapter 51).

NURSING HOME VARIATIONS

Admission to a nursing home may be a transfer from the hospital (see Skill 15-2) or a direct admission. A health history and initial nursing assessment are done to determine the patient's condition. The patient is encouraged to bring clothes and other personal items such as pictures; even personal furniture may be brought to place in the room to give a feeling of familiarity.

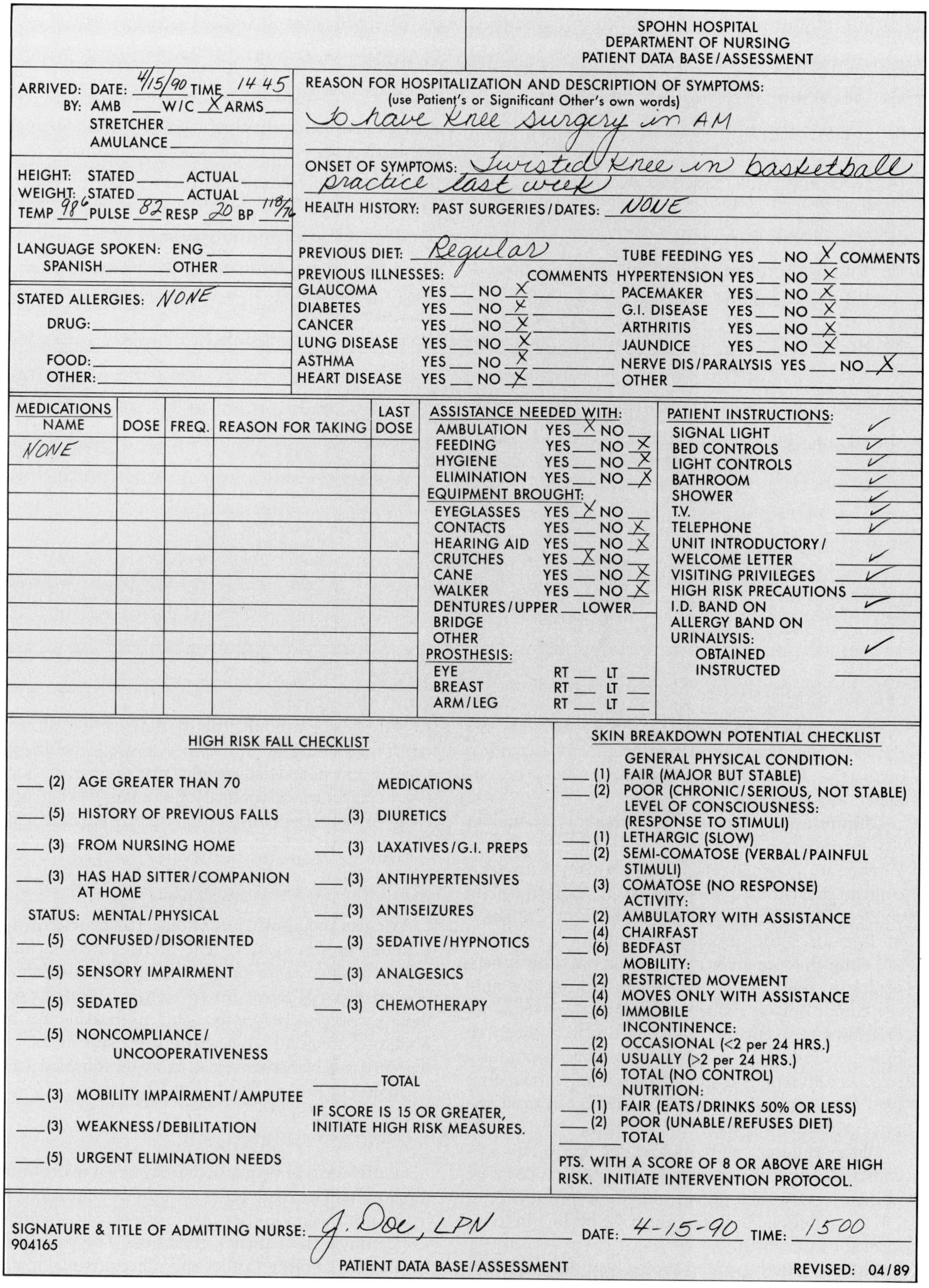

SPOHN HOSPITAL
DEPARTMENT OF NURSING
PATIENT DATA BASE/ASSESSMENT

ARRIVED: DATE: 4/15/90 TIME 1445
BY: AMB ___ W/C X ARMS ___
STRETCHER ___
AMULANCE ___

REASON FOR HOSPITALIZATION AND DESCRIPTION OF SYMPTOMS:
(use Patient's or Significant Other's own words)
To have knee surgery in AM

HEIGHT: STATED ___ ACTUAL ___
WEIGHT: STATED ___ ACTUAL ___
TEMP 98[6] PULSE 82 RESP 20 BP 118/76

ONSET OF SYMPTOMS: Twisted knee in basketball practice last week

HEALTH HISTORY: PAST SURGERIES/DATES: NONE

LANGUAGE SPOKEN: ENG ___
SPANISH ___ OTHER ___

PREVIOUS DIET: Regular TUBE FEEDING YES ___ NO X COMMENTS

STATED ALLERGIES: NONE
DRUG: ___
FOOD: ___
OTHER: ___

PREVIOUS ILLNESSES:			COMMENTS				
GLAUCOMA	YES ___	NO X		HYPERTENSION	YES ___	NO X	
DIABETES	YES ___	NO X		PACEMAKER	YES ___	NO X	
CANCER	YES ___	NO X		G.I. DISEASE	YES ___	NO X	
LUNG DISEASE	YES ___	NO X		ARTHRITIS	YES ___	NO X	
ASTHMA	YES ___	NO X		JAUNDICE	YES ___	NO X	
HEART DISEASE	YES ___	NO X		NERVE DIS/PARALYSIS	YES ___	NO X	
				OTHER			

MEDICATIONS NAME	DOSE	FREQ.	REASON FOR TAKING	LAST DOSE
NONE				

ASSISTANCE NEEDED WITH:
AMBULATION YES X NO ___
FEEDING YES ___ NO X
HYGIENE YES ___ NO X
ELIMINATION YES ___ NO X

EQUIPMENT BROUGHT:
EYEGLASSES YES X NO ___
CONTACTS YES ___ NO X
HEARING AID YES ___ NO X
CRUTCHES YES X NO ___
CANE YES ___ NO X
WALKER YES ___ NO X
DENTURES/UPPER ___ LOWER ___
BRIDGE
OTHER

PROSTHESIS:
EYE RT ___ LT ___
BREAST RT ___ LT ___
ARM/LEG RT ___ LT ___

PATIENT INSTRUCTIONS:
SIGNAL LIGHT ✓
BED CONTROLS ✓
LIGHT CONTROLS ✓
BATHROOM ✓
SHOWER ✓
T.V. ✓
TELEPHONE ✓
UNIT INTRODUCTORY/ WELCOME LETTER ✓
VISITING PRIVILEGES ✓
HIGH RISK PRECAUTIONS ___
I.D. BAND ON ✓
ALLERGY BAND ON ___
URINALYSIS:
OBTAINED ✓
INSTRUCTED ___

HIGH RISK FALL CHECKLIST

___ (2) AGE GREATER THAN 70
___ (5) HISTORY OF PREVIOUS FALLS
___ (3) FROM NURSING HOME
___ (3) HAS HAD SITTER/COMPANION AT HOME

STATUS: MENTAL/PHYSICAL
___ (5) CONFUSED/DISORIENTED
___ (5) SENSORY IMPAIRMENT
___ (5) SEDATED
___ (5) NONCOMPLIANCE/ UNCOOPERATIVENESS
___ (3) MOBILITY IMPAIRMENT/AMPUTEE
___ (3) WEAKNESS/DEBILITATION
___ (5) URGENT ELIMINATION NEEDS

MEDICATIONS
___ (3) DIURETICS
___ (3) LAXATIVES/G.I. PREPS
___ (3) ANTIHYPERTENSIVES
___ (3) ANTISEIZURES
___ (3) SEDATIVE/HYPNOTICS
___ (3) ANALGESICS
___ (3) CHEMOTHERAPY

___ TOTAL

IF SCORE IS 15 OR GREATER, INITIATE HIGH RISK MEASURES.

SKIN BREAKDOWN POTENTIAL CHECKLIST

GENERAL PHYSICAL CONDITION:
___ (1) FAIR (MAJOR BUT STABLE)
___ (2) POOR (CHRONIC/SERIOUS, NOT STABLE)
LEVEL OF CONSCIOUSNESS: (RESPONSE TO STIMULI)
___ (1) LETHARGIC (SLOW)
___ (2) SEMI-COMATOSE (VERBAL/PAINFUL STIMULI)
___ (3) COMATOSE (NO RESPONSE)
ACTIVITY:
___ (2) AMBULATORY WITH ASSISTANCE
___ (4) CHAIRFAST
___ (6) BEDFAST
MOBILITY:
___ (2) RESTRICTED MOVEMENT
___ (4) MOVES ONLY WITH ASSISTANCE
___ (6) IMMOBILE
INCONTINENCE:
___ (2) OCCASIONAL (<2 per 24 HRS.)
___ (4) USUALLY (>2 per 24 HRS.)
___ (6) TOTAL (NO CONTROL)
NUTRITION:
___ (1) FAIR (EATS/DRINKS 50% OR LESS)
___ (2) POOR (UNABLE/REFUSES DIET)
___ TOTAL

PTS. WITH A SCORE OF 8 OR ABOVE ARE HIGH RISK. INITIATE INTERVENTION PROTOCOL.

SIGNATURE & TITLE OF ADMITTING NURSE: J. Doe, LPN DATE: 4-15-90 TIME: 1500
904165
PATIENT DATA BASE/ASSESSMENT REVISED: 04/89

FIG. 15-2 Patient data base assessment form. (Courtesy Spohn Hospital, Corpus Christi, TX.)

SPOHN HOSPITAL
DEPARTMENT OF NURSING
PATIENT DATA BASE/ASSESSMENT

DISCHARGE PLANNING ADMISSION SCREEN

	YES	NO
Do you live in a nursing home?		X
Do you have a visiting nurse?		X
Do you have help at home with your daily care or needs?	X	
Do you have a dependent person at home with no one to care for him/her?		X

A yes answer to any of the above questions requires a referral to Social Services

ADDITIONAL COMMENTS: ______

SYSTEMS	YES	NO	COMMENTS
CNS			
L.O.C.			
- alert	✓		
- drowsy		✓	
- comatose		✓	
- disoriented		✓	
EYES			
- PEARL			
- vision normal	✓		
- prosthesis		✓	
EARS			
- responds to normal voice tone	✓		
- drainage		✓	
SPEECH			
- clear	✓		
- slurred			
- hoarse/raspy			
- aphasic			
INTEGUMENTARY			
SKIN - color normal	✓		
- warm, dry	✓		
- turgor good	✓		
- bruises, abrasions, lacerations		✓	
- rash, lesions		✓	
- scars		✓	
- decubitus		✓	
- dressing		✓	

SYSTEMS	YES	NO	COMMENTS
CARDIOVASCULAR			
PULSES			
- radial			82
- carotid		✓	
- pedal			80
APICAL RATE ____		✓	
CHEST PAIN			
RESPIRATORY			
RESPIRATIONS			
- rapid		✓	
- slow		✓	
- deep		✓	
- shallow		✓	
- labored		✓	
BREATH SOUNDS			
- clear	✓		
- wheezes		✓	
- rales		✓	
COUGH			
- present		✓	
- productive		✓	
GASTROINTESTINAL			
ABDOMEN			
- soft	✓		
- distended		✓	
- tenderness		✓	
ELIMINATION			
- bowel sounds	✓		
- diarrhea		✓	
- constipation		✓	
- incontinence		✓	
- ostomy		✓	
LAST B.M. this AM			

SYSTEMS	YES	NO	COMMENTS
MUSCLE/SKELETAL			
EXTREMITIES			
- moves all on command	✓		
- WEAKNESS (SPECIFY)			pain from injury
RA ____ LA ____			
RA ____ LA ____	✓		
- edema		✓	
- normal ambulation			c̄ crutches
- prosthesis (SPECIFY)			
GENITOURINARY			
VOIDING			
- normal	✓		
- frequency		✓	
- burning		✓	
- incontinence		✓	
- catheter		✓	
CATHETER INSERTION DATE ____			
DATE OF LAST MENSTRUAL PERIOD:			
PSYCHO-SOCIAL			
- cooperative	✓		
- agitated		✓	
- depressed		✓	
- frightened			anxious about surgery
- combative		✓	
HABITS			
- smoking		✓	
- alcohol		✓	
- drugs		✓	

After assessing this patient's physical condition, psycho-social needs, the Data Base and the Discharge Planning Admission screen, is Discharge Planning indicated at this time? ____ YES ____ NO

Referred to Social Services ____ YES X NO

Reviewed for Discharge Planning: High Risk ____ YES X NO

______ Signature of Registered Nurse ______ Date ______ Signature of Social Worker ______ Date

904165 PATIENT DATA BASE/ASSESSMENT REVISED: 04/89

FIG. 15-2, cont'd For legend see facing page.

SKILL 15-2: TRANSFERRING A PATIENT

Guidelines

The changing condition of a patient, whether improved or more critical, may require **transfer** either to another unit in the hospital or to another health care institution, such as a nursing home or rehabilitation hospital. A patient whose condition becomes critical may be moved to special care areas, such as the ICU or CCU. A patient whose condition improves may be moved from a special care area to a general care area. Other patients may be transferred to a nursing home for continued care at a lower cost. Transfers may also be done at the patient's request; for example, a patient may wish to have a private room or a room where smoking is allowed.

Transfer combines admission and discharge. The patient is discharged from one unit and received on the new unit, much like an admission. A physician's order is generally needed to begin the transfer process. The patient's family should be notified of the transfer. Skill 15-2 gives general steps to follow when transferring a patient.

Purposes

The nurse performs the accepted procedure for transferring a patient for the following reasons:

- to match the type and intensity of nursing care to the patient's needs
- to locate the patient in the facility best able to provide the care needed
- to accommodate the patient's request for a specific type of room

Related Knowledge and Skills

Before transferring a patient, the nurse should understand the following:

- principles of communication (see Chapter 4)
- accurate documentation (see Chapter 6)

SKILL 15-3: DISCHARGING A PATIENT

Guidelines

When a patient is ready to be released from a health care facility, the physician writes a **discharge** order. Planning for discharge should begin at the time of admission; this allows time for patient and family teaching and for adjustments to be made at home for the patient's return. Planning for discharge must be individualized to the patient's specific needs.

Throughout the hospital stay, the patient should be taught about medications, diet, activity, treatments, and any signs or symptoms to be reported to the physician. General health teaching must also be performed.

Daily teaching allows the patient time to think about the information and to ask questions and gives the nurse a chance to verify the patient's understanding of the information. All teaching and the level of the patient's understanding must be recorded on the chart. Having family members involved in this teaching ensures **continuity of care** at home.

At the time of discharge, a review of the medications, diet, activity, and treatments to be continued at home should be conducted with the patient and family. If the patient or family cannot manage this care, arrangements should be made for home health care or nursing home care.

Many hospitals have a form with written instructions and teaching documentation for the patient to sign acknowledging understanding of the instructions. These instructions serve as a guide for the patient to use at home (Fig. 15-3). The primary nurse may make a follow-up telephone call a day or two after discharge to discuss progress and/or problems.

Sometimes a patient will insist on leaving the hospital without the physician's consent, that is, **against medical advice (AMA).** A special form must be signed by the patient in which the patient acknowledges leaving without the physician's discharge order and that the physician, hospital, and hospital personnel will not be responsible for any problems that might occur because of this action.

A rational adult patient who will not sign the form cannot be forcibly detained. Only if a court order was issued for the admission, as in some cases of mental illness, can a patient be detained forcibly. A lawsuit for false imprisonment could be filed against the hospital and/or personnel for keeping patients against personal wishes. Documentation of the refusal to sign the form and the information given about the risks of leaving should be made in the patient's chart.

Skill 15-3 outlines the steps for discharging a patient.

SKILL 15-2 TRANSFERRING A PATIENT

Nursing action	Rationale
1. Wash hands thoroughly.	Prevents spread of microorganisms.
2. Check physician's order for transfer.	Verifies if and when a patient is to be transferred.
3. Inform the patient and family of the transfer.	Reduces the fear of the unknown and strengthens the nurse/patient relationship.
4. Notify the receiving unit that the patient is being transferred and when to be expected.	Allows time to prepare to welcome the new patient and begin care in an unhurried manner.
5. Gather *all* the patient's belongings and necessary care items to accompany the patient.	Builds trust and prevents loss of items.
6. Assist in transferring the patient, usually by stretcher or wheelchair.	Ensures patient safety. Condition will determine mode of transportation.
7. Introduce patient and family to nurses on new unit and to roommate.	Establishes the beginning of new nurse/patient relationships and gives a sense of belonging.
8. Provide a brief summary of medical diagnosis, treatment care plan, and medications. Review medical orders with nurse assuming care. If transfer is to another facility, complete an interagency transfer form.	Gives personnel on the receiving unit pertinent information for continuing care. Reviewing records together prevents errors.
9. Explain equipment, policies, and procedures that are different on the new unit.	Gives the patient some control and reduces anxiety.
10. Wash hands thoroughly.	Prevents spread of microorganisms.
11. Record condition of patient and means of transfer. The nurse on the new unit should also record an assessment of the patient's condition on arrival.	The chart should reflect all care given and the patient's response to that care while in the hospital.
12. Notify other hospital departments, such as x-ray, laboratory, switchboard, dietary, and business offices, of the transfer.	Keeps records current and avoids errors.

Sample charting

Date	Time	Notes
1/15/91	1230	Transferred by private car with personal belongings to *(name)* nursing home. Accompanied by son and daughter-in-law. Alert and smiling. Physician's orders and nursing care plan sent.

(nurse's signature)

SPECIAL CONCERNS

An **interagency** transfer may be made by ambulance or private car. The patient must be dressed or covered appropriately for the weather. If oxygen is required, a small transport tank may be used. A nurse generally accompanies a critically ill patient being transferred.

Children. Infants are generally transported in an Isolette that is returned to the sending health care facility. Parents usually accompany their child during transfer unless the transfer is by aircraft. Then parents would follow in family transportation.

HOME HEALTH AND NURSING HOME VARIATIONS

Following agency policies and requirements of **third-party payers** is important so that benefits will not be lost. Home care patients may be either transferred for a few hours to a clinic or outpatient services for tests or treatments, or transferred for admission to the hospital or nursing home.

Purposes

The nurse performs the accepted procedure for discharging a patient for the following reasons:

- to assist the patient in making the change from the hospital environment to the home environment
- to provide for continuity of care at home so that the patient can return to the best state of wellness possible

Related Knowledge and Skills

Before discharging a patient, the nurse should understand the following:

- principles of communication (see Chapter 4)
- accurate documentation (see Chapter 6)
- growth and development (see Chapters 7-11)

SPOHN HOSPITAL
DEPARTMENT OF NURSING

DISCHARGE INFORMATION RECORD

PATIENT/FAMILY TEACHING AND INSTRUCTIONS

Diet: __X__ Regular ______ Bland
______ Diabetic ______ (Specify)
______ Other ______ (Specify)
______ Diet list given to patient
Comments: ______

Activity: ______ Restricted __X__ Unrestricted
______ Ambulatory ______ With Assistance
Comments: ______

Treatments/Self-Care: __X__ Not Applicable
Specify: ______

MEDICATIONS	DOSAGE	FREQUENCY
Tylenol #3	1 tab	Every 4 hr. if needed for pain

OTHER: ______ ______ Not Applicable

Follow-up: To be seen in Dr. Smith's (Dr. Name) office in 1 week 8-26-90 (Period of time/date).
______ Transferred to Nursing Home ______ (Specify).
______ Transferred to another hospital ______ (Specify).
______ Home Health/Hospice Services ______ (Specify)
______ Other ______ (Specify)

[X] Preprinted Instructions From Physician's Office Given to Patient/Family.

I understand the above information: ______ (Patient/Family Signature)

Admission Date 4-15-90 Discharge Date 8-18-90 Via: Wheelchair Escorted by: J. Doe LPN
Time: 1 AM/PM Destination: Home

PATIENT DISCHARGE STATUS

Nursing Assessment of patient's condition at time of discharge: ______

Own meds from home returned to patient/family. ______ Yes ______ No __X__ N/A
Prescription(s) given to patient/family. __X__ Yes ______ No ______ N/A
Valuables returned to patient/family. ______ Yes ______ No __X__ N/A

Signature/Title Discharge Nurse: J. Doe, LPN

904008 DISCHARGE INFORMATION RECORD NEW: 7-84

FIG. 15-3 Patient discharge information record. (Courtesy Spohn Hospital, Corpus Christi, TX.)

SKILL 15-3

DISCHARGING A PATIENT

Nursing action	Rationale
1. Wash hands thoroughly.	Prevents spread of microoganisms.
2. Make certain there is a written discharge order.	Verifies physician's decision regarding time for the patient to be discharged.
3. If no discharge order has been written, have AMA form signed by patient.	Generally patients cannot be held against their wishes. The patient's signature acknowledges full responsibility for what happens after leaving.
4. Notify the family or person who will be transporting the patient home.	Avoids delay in discharge.
5. Verify that the patient and family understand the instructions for care: medications, special diet, exercise.	Helps ensure appropriate home care.
6. Gather equipment, supplies, and prescriptions that the patient is to take home.	Provides service patient is unable to do.
7. Check to see that business office has given a release.	Prevents undue waiting for the patient when leaving.
8. Assist the patient to dress and pack items to go home.	Conserves patient's strength.
9. Check clothing and valuables list made on admission according to policy.	Avoids patient leaving personal items at facility.
10. Transfer the patient and belongings via wheelchair to the vehicle. Assist patient into the vehicle if needed.	Provides patient safety and complies with policy of most hospitals.
11. Wash hands thoroughly.	Prevents spread of microorganisms.
12. Chart entire discharge procedure.	Documentation of teaching, patient's condition, and method of discharge completes the record. Legally this is important and may prevent problems in the future.

Sample charting

Date	Time	Notes
1/15/91	1300	Diet and activity instructions reviewed. Copy of instructions and prescription for Tylenol #3 given to mother. Mother can state name, dosage, frequency to give, desired and unexpected effects of Tylenol #3. Given appointment card to see Dr. Smith. Cleared through business office. Dismissed by wheelchair to parent's car.

____
(nurse's signature)

Continued.

SKILL 15-3 DISCHARGING A PATIENT—cont'd

SPECIAL CONCERNS

- **Children.** The parents must be included in all aspects of teaching and the entire discharge procedure for children. Some hospitals have a special form to be signed by the person legally responsible for taking the child away from the facility.
- **AMA.** If the patient is leaving without a physician's discharge order, the appropriate forms must be signed and the physician notified.

HOME HEALTH VARIATIONS

Discharge from a home health agency involves the same kind of teaching as from the hospital. The nurse must be sure the patient or family can provide any care still needed. Since the patient is already home, it is the nurse who must gather any equipment and supplies to be returned to the agency.

NURSING HOME VARIATIONS

Discharge from a nursing home is essentially the same as from a hospital. There will be more personal belongings to gather and pack.

REFERENCES AND SUGGESTED READINGS

1. Arkow P, editor: The loving bond: companion animals in the helping professions, Saratoga, Calif, 1987, R&E Publishers, Inc.
2. Cave L: Follow-up phone calls after discharge, Am J Nurs 89:942, 1989.
3. Feuer L: Discharge planning: home caregivers need your support too, Nurs Manag 18:58, 1987.
4. Hood GH and Dincher JR: Total patient care, ed 7, St Louis, 1988, The CV Mosby Co.
5. Lewis LW and Timby BK: Fundamental skills and concepts in patient care, ed 4, Philadelphia, 1988, JB Lippincott Co.
6. Maslow AH: Motivation and personality, New York, 1954, Harper & Row, Publishers.
7. Omdahl D: Home care strictly by the rules, Am J Nurs 89:511, 1989.
8. Perry A and Potter P: Clinical nursing skills, ed 2, St Louis, 1990, The CV Mosby Co.
9. Porter A and others: Patient needs on admission, Am J Nurs 77:112, 1977.
10. Potter P and Perry A: Fundamentals of nursing, ed 2, St Louis, 1989, The CV Mosby Co.
11. Vaughn B and Taylor K: Homeward bound, Nurs Times 84(15):28, 1988.
12. Weinberger B: Discharge planning, the sooner, the better, Nurs 89 2:75, 1989.

CHAPTER CHALLENGE

KEY POINTS

- The patient is a human being who deserves to be treated with dignity, courtesy, and respect.
- The nurse's attitude often influences the patient's feelings about the care received.
- Common reactions to hospitalization are fear of the unknown, loss of identity, disorientation, separation anxiety, and loneliness.
- An adult patient should always be addressed as Miss, Ms., Mrs., or Mr. (Jones) unless the patient requests otherwise.
- Plans for discharge should be started at the time of admission.
- Generally, a person may not be kept in a health care facility against his will.
- Coordination is the key to the efficient and safe transfer of a patient.

STUDY QUESTIONS

1. Plans for discharge should be started:
   a. On the day of admission
   b. No special plans need be made
   c. When the patient feels like it
   d. The day before the patient is scheduled for discharge
2. Admission to a health care facility may cause a person to feel a loss of identity. This reflects which of Maslow's needs:
   a. Safety
   b. Esteem
   c. Self-actualization
   d. Belongingness and love
3. The first thing the nurse should do when admitting a new patient is:
   a. Measure vital signs
   b. Notify the physician
   c. Introduce self and any roommates
   d. Help the patient undress and get into bed
4. Calling an elderly male patient "gramps" is:
   a. Never appropriate
   b. Just fine if he has grandchildren
   c. Acceptable if you cannot remember his name
   d. Acceptable if you feel comfortable calling him "gramps"
5. Transferring a patient from the assigned room in a hospital to the ICU is called a (an):
   a. Interagency transfer
   b. Intraagency transfer
   c. Business office transfer
   d. Patient-initiated transfer
6. An important principle to remember when admitting, transferring, or discharging a patient is:
   a. The nurse knows best and should tell the patient what to do
   b. The patient is a human being deserving dignity, courtesy, and respect
   c. The patient is ill and unable to make decisions or give accurate information
   d. Families get in the way and should be encouraged not to get involved in the patient's care
7. When a patient chooses to leave a health care facility without a physician's written order, the nurse should:
   a. Call the family so they can expect the patient at home
   b. Allow the patient to leave, because no one can be held against his will
   c. Call security, because there must be a physician's order before a patient may leave
   d. Explain the risks of leaving and have the patient sign a paper accepting responsibility for problems that may occur
8. The nurse's best response to a patient experiencing the common reaction of fear of the unknown is:
   a. "Let me explain the hospital policies, and answer any questions."
   b. "Don't worry, we know what to do. Just let us take care of you."
   c. "Your physician has ordered many tests to find out what is really wrong."
   d. "Your family may stay so they can tell what was done if you cannot remember."
9. When preparing a room for a new patient, the nurse should:
   a. Ask all visitors to leave the area
   b. Call housekeeping to dust and mop the floor
   c. Spray disinfectant and deodorant around the room
   d. Turn on lights, open the bed, and adjust it to the proper height

16

Medical Asepsis

ANNABELLE SITLER

LEARNING OBJECTIVES

After reading this chapter the student should be able to do the following:

- Define the key terms.
- Describe the characteristics of the six elements of the infection process.
- List five major classifications of pathogens.
- Differentiate between *Staphylococcus aureus* and *Staphylococcus epidermidis* as to virulence.
- Describe nursing interventions used to interrupt the sequence in the infection process.
- Describe situations where nosocomial infections most often occur (e.g., the environment and susceptible patients).
- Demonstrate the appropriate procedure for 2-minute handwashing.
- State the rationale for universal precautions.
- List the situations when specific isolation techniques should be used.
- Demonstrate appropriate gowning and gloving technique for protective asepsis.
- Demonstrate the appropriate method for double bagging contaminated articles.
- Demonstrate the accepted techniques of preparation for disinfection and sterilization.

SKILLS

16-1 Performing a 2-minute handwashing
16-2 Donning gloves
16-3 Gowning for isolation
16-4 Donning a mask
16-5 Double bagging
16-6 Providing protective asepsis
16-7 Preparing for disinfection and sterilization

KEY TERMS

Define the following:

- antibody
- antigen
- asepsis
- Centers for Disease Control (CDC)
- contaminated
- disinfection
- endogenous infection
- exogenous infection
- fomite
- host
- immune response
- immunoglobulin
- infection process cycle
- inflammation
- inhibit
- isolation
- lymphocyte
- medical asepsis
- microorganism infection
- portal of entry
- sterilization
- surgical asepsis
- universal precautions
- vehicle
- virulence

GUIDELINES

With research and the discovery that microorganisms cause infection came the realization that somehow their growth and reproduction must be inhibited or stopped to prevent infection. Although many scientists, researchers, and doctors contributed to the progress made in aseptic technique, Joseph Lister (1827-1912) is known as the father of aseptic technique.

Lister's method of aseptic technique helped reduce morbidity and mortality from surgery and wound care. These methods are still used in asepsis today.

ASEPSIS

There is a great societal concern regarding the increase of transmissible infections not only in health care institutions but also in the home. Microorganisms are naturally present on and in the human body, as well as in the environment. Many of these microorganisms are harmless (nonpathogenic) and do not produce disease in most individuals; some are even helpful. However, if an individual is highly susceptible to infection, the nonpathogenic microorganisms could be dangerous also. There are also known microorganisms (pathogens) that do cause specific diseases or infections.

Infection control is routine in whatever action a nurse performs. Any patient entering a health care facility because of lowered resistance or the need for an invasive procedure is at a greater risk of developing an infection. In many situations nurses are exposed to pathogenic microorganisms and should use both specialized and routine practices of cleanliness and disinfection to prevent the spread of infection. These techniques aid in accomplishing **asepsis**, or freedom from pathogenic microorganisms. Asepsis is divided into two categories:

1. **Medical asepsis** is a technique that inhibits the growth and spread of pathogenic microorganisms. This is also known as *clean technique* and is used in many daily activities, such as handwashing.
2. **Surgical asepsis** destroys all microorganisms and their spores. This is known as *sterile technique* and is used in specialized areas or skills, such as care of surgical wounds, urinary catheter insertion, invasive procedures, and surgery.

INFECTION PROCESS

For a microorganism to be transported and be effective in continuing contamination, it follows a definite cycle and must have the following six elements (Fig. 16-1):

1. The infectious agent—a pathogen
2. Reservoir—where the pathogen can grow

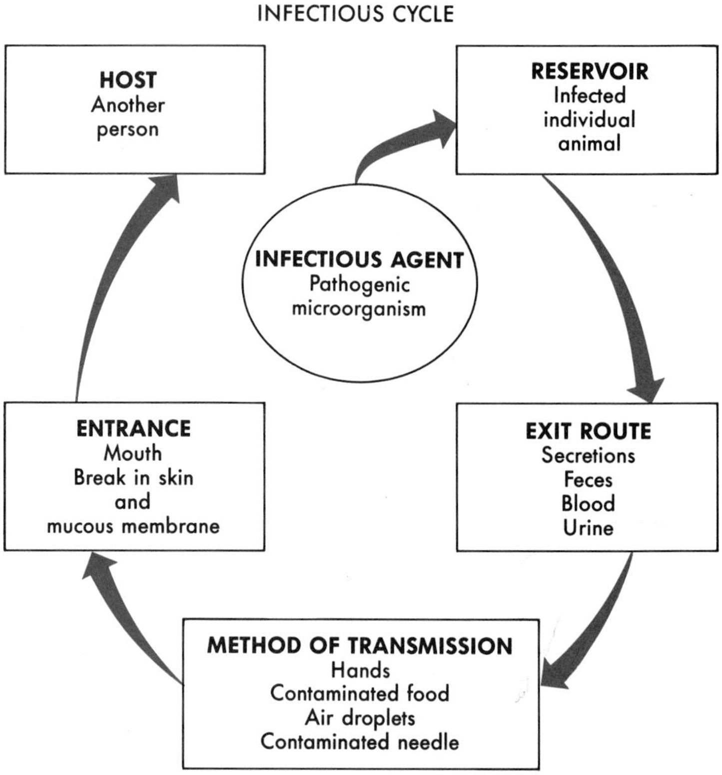

FIG. 16-1 The infectious cycle.

3. Exit from reservoir
4. Method of transportation, such as exudate, feces, and needles
5. Entrance through skin, mucous lining, or mouth
6. Host—another person or animal

To prevent the spread of a microorganism, the cycle must be interrupted. This is accomplished through daily practices of medical asepsis. These practices help to inhibit the growth and reduce the number of microorganisms, especially pathogens.

Infectious Agent

Bacteria. The study of bacteria has shown that they have many different characteristics. In addition to the three basic shapes—round, oblong, and spiral—there are many variations of these shapes. Some may be elongated or have pointed ends, or they may be flattened on one side. Some are shaped like a comma, and others may appear square. Spirilla may be tightly coiled like a corkscrew. During cell division some remain together to form pairs, whereas others may form long chains. All these modifications are important in identifying specific kinds of bacteria.

Bacteria may also have different chemical compositions, require different nutrients, and form different waste products. Aerobic bacteria grow only in the presence of oxygen, whereas anaerobic bacteria grow only in the absence of oxygen. Some bacteria are capable of movement. Their motility is possible because of fine, hairlike projections—flagella— that arise from the bacterial cell. These projections cause a wavelike motion that moves the cell. A bacterium may have only one flagellum attached to one end of the cell, or there may be many flagella surrounding the cell. Locomotion of the spirochete is achieved by a wiggling motion involving the entire cell body.

Some bacteria form a specialized structure called a spore. Spore formation appears to occur when conditions are unfavorable for growth of the bacterium. The spore is a round body that is formed by the bacterium in the presence or absence of oxygen. The spore enlarges until it is as large as the bacterial cell and is surrounded by a capsule. Eventually the portion of the cell surrounding the spore disintegrates. The spore remains dormant until environmental conditions become favorable for growth. At that time the spore will germinate and begin reproducing in a normal manner. Characteristically, spores have a high degree of resistance to heat and disinfectants. They cannot be stained by the usual laboratory methods but require special staining techniques.

Some bacteria have the ability to form capsules about the cell wall. These mucilaginous envelopes seem to form when the bacterial environment is unfavorable; it is also believed that the formation may be defensive to protect the bacteria. The composition of the capsules varies with the species of bacteria. However, they may be composed of protein or fat substances, and some may contain nitrogen and phosphorus. As with spores, staining in the laboratory may require special procedures. When capsules are present, antibiotic therapy may be ineffective because the capsule may prevent the drug from reaching the bacteria within the capsule.

Many diseases cannot be diagnosed and properly treated until the specific microorganism causing the illness has been identified. Identification of microorganisms is made by specially trained laboratory personnel. Most bacteria cannot be seen until a special staining process has been done. In some instances examination may be done before staining, but this is usually less satisfactory. Staining is accomplished by the use of a dye applied to a specially prepared glass slide containing a small amount of the material to be examined. Most bacteria can be identified by this simple process; however, other bacteria require additional staining. Depending on whether a color can be removed by a solvent or is retained after the use of the solvent, the organism is identified as being Gram positive or Gram negative. This identification is important in the treatment of the patient. This is a simple laboratory test that will assist in the selection of effective antibiotics. Different antibiotics may be required for their destruction. Some bacterias are known as acid-fast bacteria, depending on the staining process. Special staining is required for bacteria having flagella, spores, or capsules.

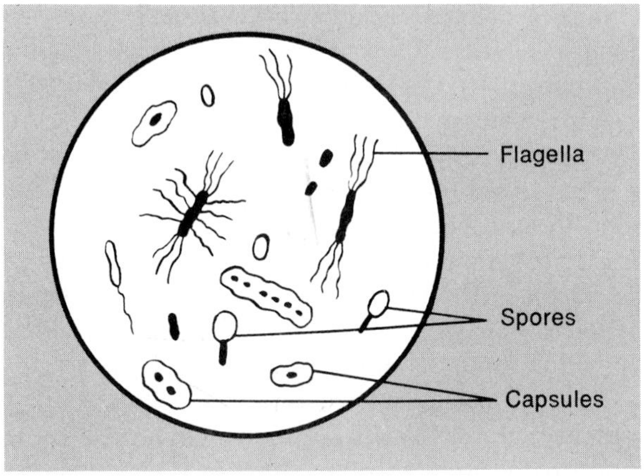

Flagella, spores, and capsules.

Body fluids and secretions suspected of containing pathogenic organisms can be collected in sterile containers and sent to the laboratory for culture and sensitivity tests. In the laboratory the collected specimens are transferred to a special culture medium that promotes growth. The culture is then studied, and the pathogens are identified. Sensitivity tests are carried out to determine which antibiotics will effectively inhibit the pathogens' growth. Appropriate antibiotics are ordered on the basis of these tests.

Bacterial infections are transmitted from person to person by direct contact, by inhaling droplet nuclei, and by indirect contact with articles contaminated with the pathogen. Some are also transmitted through the ingestion of contaminated food and drink.

Bacteria have been divided into three major groups: (1) cocci, (2) bacilli, and (3) spirilla. In addition, the rickettsiae are now classified as bacteria.

Streptococci, staphylococci, and diplococci. The streptococcus bacterium is responsible for more diseases than is any other organism. Some strains produce serious or even fatal diseases; other strains produce disease only under special conditions; and other strains are nonpathogenic. Disease-producing strains include beta-hemolytic streptococci and the viridans groups, also called alpha-hemolytic streptococci.

The beta-hemolytic group of streptococci is responsible for about 90% of streptococcal infections. Some of the diseases caused by this group are extremely serious and may be fatal. They include osteomyelitis, septicemia, scarlet fever, rheumatic fever, and pneumonia, as well as relatively common diseases like tonsillitis and impetigo. The organisms may also invade surgical wounds or malignant lesions. Wound infection may occur as the result of improper handwashing before changing dressings. The organisms live in the upper respiratory tract and may be spread from one person to another by direct or indirect contact.

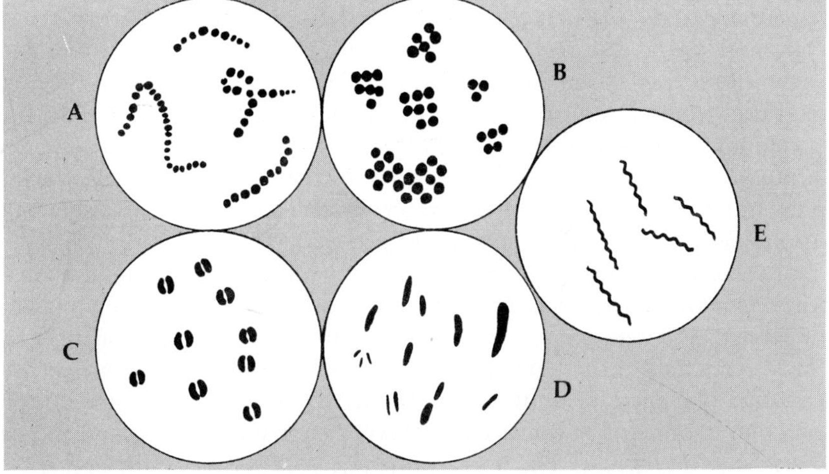

Some common disease-producing bacteria. **A,** Streptococci. **B,** Staphylococci. **C,** Diplococci. **D,** Bacilli. **E,** Spirilla.

Viridans streptococci may cause subacute bacterial endocarditis, in which the valves of the heart may be affected. Viridans streptococci may also be found in the nose and throat of well persons.

There are two primary species of staphylococcus bacteria: *Staphylococcus aureus* and *Staphylococcus epidermidis. Staphylococcus aureus* belongs to the pyogenic (pus-producing) group. Staphylococci may be found on the skin at all times and cause boils, abscesses, and carbuncles. Sometimes they get into the bloodstream and cause serious complications. (See Chapter 29.)

Staphylococcus epidermidis is a nonpathogenic species of the staphylococcus organism that inhabits the human skin. Although this species may cause minor infections, the incidence of such infections is low.

There are several kinds of diplococcus bacteria. One type causes pneumonia and was previously called the *pneumococcus;* it is now called *Streptococcus pneumoniae.* One characteristic of this organism is that it is encased in a capsule, or gelatinous envelope. Two other forms of diplococci cause gonorrhea (gonococcus) and meningitis (meningococcus).

Bacilli. The name *bacilli* means "little rod"; however, its rodlike shape is extremely variable. Certain forms of the bacillus produce spores. These forms are present in the intestinal tract of humans and animals and are discharged onto the soil. These spore-forming bacilli produce tetanus, gas gangrene, and anthrax. Numerous other diseases are caused by these organisms, including tuberculosis, diphtheria, pertussis, typhoid fever, and bacillary dysentery.

Spirilla. Spirilla organisms are spiral shaped, like a corkscrew. Some forms of spirilla are rigid, whereas others are flexible. One form, which resembles a comma, is the cause of Asiatic cholera. Most of the diseases caused by the spirilla bacteria are uncommon. The spirochetes that cause syphilis are spiral shaped, but they have been separated and classed in a different order of bacteria.

Rickettsiae. Rickettsiae are microorganisms now classified as bacteria. They are parasites that flourish only within living suspectible cells. The cells provide a suitable environment and the nutrients needed for their growth. The most serious diseases caused by rickettsiae are typhus fever and Rocky Mountain spotted fever. Typhus fever is spread from person to person through bites from infected body lice or fleas from rats. Epidemic typhus is an acute, severe disease associated with overcrowding, famine, and filth. It has caused devastating epidemics, responsible for the deaths of millions of persons over the past centuries. Although it is rare, cases can be found in the southern United States bordering Mexico.

Rocky Mountain spotted fever has been found in almost every area of the United States, and its prevalence seems to be increasing. It is transmitted to humans through the bite of an infected tick. Several varieties of ticks carry the disease. The ticks live on many different kinds of animals found in rural and wooded areas. They may also live on common house pets, such as cats and dogs. Persons working in areas where ticks are known to be abundant are more likely to become infected. The tick attaches itself to the skin, and the longer it remains attached to the skin, the more likely the person is to become infected. In removing the tick from the skin, great care should be taken not to crush or squeeze it.

Symptoms of Rocky Mountain spotted fever and typhus fever are similar; in both diseases patients are usually extremely ill. Preventive vaccines are available for both diseases, and persons going into areas where the diseases are known to exist should avail themselves of the preventive vaccines.

Viruses. Viruses are the smallest known agents that cause disease. They are not complete cells, but consist of a protein coat around a nucleic acid core and depend on the metabolic processes of the cell they enter. Before 1900, scientists discovered that certain agents, unlike bacteria, would pass through a laboratory filter. In addition, they were unable to observe these tiny bodies with the ordinary microscope. In 1898 Martinus W. Beijerinck called these small bodies *viruses,* and they became known as filterable viruses.

For years scientists knew little about viruses, even though they were able to observe their effect on humans and animals. In 1941 the electron microscope became available, and a whole new era in the study of human disease was opened. With this advancement the science of virology was born. In addition to the electron microscope, the use of certain dyes that become luminous when exposed to ultraviolet light (fluorescent microscopy), tissue culture methods, ultracentrifuge, cytochemistry, and the development of other technical laboratory aids has resulted in rapid advances in the study of viruses.

The virus may gain entrance to the body through the respiratory tract, the gastrointestinal tract, or the broken skin resulting from an animal bite, or it may be injected by a mosquito or hypodermic needle. Viruses are selective in the type of body cells they attack, but once they have found cells showing affinity, they enter the cell and reproduce rapidly. As they multiply, they interrupt the cell activities and use the cell material to produce new virus material.

Viral infections are usually self-limiting. They run a given course, and recovery occurs. One exception is rabies, which is almost always fatal. Another exception is AIDS (acquired immunodeficiency syndrome), which is the most severe disease state observed to date of a continuum of illnesses related to infection by the human immunodeficiency virus (HIV). See Chapter 40. Other viral diseases may be fatal if complications occur or if they attack extremely weak, elderly, or debilitated persons. The common cold is caused by a virus, and the aching feeling, fever, and chilling sensations may be relieved by staying in bed and taking certain medicines. No medicine will cure the cold, only relieve the discomfort that it causes. In nearly all viral diseases, antibiotics and sulfonamide agents do not alter the course of the disease.

Viruses are classified in various ways. They can be classified according to the human diseases they cause or by the characteristics of a specific group. In the latter classification system, each subgroup may have many types or strains.

Fungi. The fungal (mycotic) infections are among the most common diseases found in humans. Fungi belong to the plant kingdom, and although many of them are harmless, some are responsible for infections. Types of fungi that are familiar to everyone include the fuzzy, black, green, or white growth on stale bread, decayed fruit, or damp clothing. Fungi are among the most plentiful forms of life. Mycotic infections are diseases caused by yeasts and molds. They may be superficial, involving the skin and mucous membranes. The most frequently involved areas include the external layers of the skin, hair, and nails. These infections are commonly referred to as ringworm (dermatomycosis). The most frequent site in children is the scalp. The condition is considered infectious, and the child may not be permitted to attend school until the infection has been cured. Other sites include men's beard (barber's itch) and the feet (athlete's feet). The infection may also occur on other parts of the body, frequently about the nails. Domestic pets may also have ringworm infection and are frequently the source of infection for humans.

Fungi also invade the deeper tissues of the body. Most of these infections produce no symptoms; however, some become serious and may be fatal. Those most common in the United States are coccidioidomycosis (valley fever) and histoplasmosis.

1. *Coccidioidomycosis* was discovered in southern California, although the disease is found in other areas of the Southwest where the climate is hot and dry. The disease affects the lungs and is believed to be contracted by inhaling the spores present in soil, which are blown about in the wind.
2. *Histoplasmosis* also affects the lungs. This disease is widespread throughout the world; in some areas 80% of the population may be infected. The disease occurs as the result of inhaling spores present in the soil, and there is also a possibility that ingestion of the spores may cause the disease. Histoplasmosis has often been associated with various kinds of birds; however, it is now believed that the only relationship is that bird droppings enrich the soil, providing fertile media in which the fungi may proliferate.
3. *Candida albicans* may cause superficial or systemic infections. This fungus is a normal inhabitant of the gastrointestinal tract, the mouth, and the vagina. An infection develops when something, such as change in pH, interferes with the balance of the normal flora, allowing the organism to grow. This change in balance can occur as a result of antibiotic therapy.

Protozoa. The protozoa are single-celled animals existing everywhere in nature in some form. Some of the parasitic forms of protozoa are found in the intestinal tract, genitourinary tract, respiratory tract, and circulatory system of humans and animals. The disease-producing protozoa are responsible for malaria, amebic dysentery, and African sleeping sickness. In 1981 pneumonia caused by *Pneumocystis carinii,* which is a protozoan, was the first opportunistic infection reported in AIDS. It remains a serious life threatening infection in AIDS.[5] Another form of protozoa causes vaginal trichomoniasis in women, often as a complication of pregnancy. It may also live in the male urethra and may be acquired or transmitted through coitus. Of the diseases caused by protozoa, the three of importance in the United States are *Pneumocystis carinii* pneumonia, malaria, and amebic dysentery. The last is more prevalent where sanitation is poor and personal hygiene neglected. The source of infection can be the excreta of convalescent patients or carriers, and the disease is transmitted by food handlers, contaminated food, or contaminated water supplies. The common housefly may be an intermediary vector by transmitting the organism to food.

The malaria protozoan is transmitted to humans through the bite of the female *Anopheles* mosquito. Malaria is a worldwide health problem and is one of the most serious handicaps to the development of many countries.[6]

Pathogenic microorganisms are infectious agents. These pathogens could be bacteria, viruses, yeasts, fungi, or protozoa. All of these microorganisms require food for growth and the proper environment in which to live. Areas such as unwashed hands, wound dressings, soiled linen, or oral cavities are ideal for pathogenic growth. The strength of the microorganism, the number of microorganisms present, the effectiveness of a person's immune system, and the length of exposure to the microorganisms determine a pathogen's ability to produce disease. It is important for the nurse to provide a safe environment for a patient. This can be accomplished by handwashing, donning gloves, use of disinfectants, and sterilization techniques.

Reservoir

Any natural habitat of a microorganism that promotes growth and reproduction is a reservoir. There are different microorganisms found in many areas of the body, but the presence of these microorganisms does not always cause illnesss.

Examples of a reservoir are soiled or wet dressings, hospital equipment, such as a bedside stand, overbed table, suction equipment, and urinary drainage bags, and a carrier, or one who has pathogens present but shows no symptoms of the illness.

The role of the nurse is to prevent known carriers from coming into contact with the patient, appropriately change wet or soiled dressings, clean hospital equipment, change suction bottles routinely, and use medical asepsis when handling urinary drainage bags.

Exit Route

A microorganism cannot cause disease in another host unless it finds a point of escape from the reservoir. Human exit routes are gastrointestinal, respiratory, genitourinary, tissue, and blood.

By handwashing, the nurse can prevent the spread of microorganisms or cross-contamination. The nurse can also teach the patient to cover the nose when coughing or sneezing.

Method of Transmission

Once the microorganism has exited a reservoir there are many vehicles on or by which it can travel to the next host. These vehicles are then considered **contaminated.** If the vehicle is an inanimate (nonliving) object, it is called a **fomite,** which might be a stethoscope, thermometer, bandage scissors, tissue, drinking glass, needles, or one of many other objects. This is know as the *indirect* method of transmission.

The microorganism can be transmitted through *direct* contact, such as when the nurse turns or bathes a patient or uses inappropriate handwashing technique.

Air currents can carry microorganisms easily. Therefore when beds are made, the linens should not be shaken. A dampened or treated cloth should be used when dusting to prevent circulation of dust particles.

The floor is the dirtiest area in any building. Anything dropped, such as soiled linens and other supplies, should be discarded. Feet and furniture are the only items that belong on the floor.

Entrance of Microorganisms

Once the microorganism has exited one host and been transmitted, it must find a way to enter the susceptible host. Often the route or method of entrance is the same as the method of exit. When the host's defense mechanisms are reduced, the microorganism has a greater chance to enter. If the patient's skin is punctured with a contaminated needle, microorganisms may enter and be absorbed into the bloodstream. Incorrect handling of a wound dressing allows microorganisms to enter the open wound and cause an infection.

The methods used to prevent entrance of microorganisms are similar to the ones used in controlling the exit of microorganisms. The skin is the first line of defense and should be kept intact, lubricated, and clean. Areas of possible skin impairment should be closely observed, and

BOX 16-1 FACTORS AFFECTING IMMUNOLOGICAL DEFENSE MECHANISMS

1. Increasing age and the very young
2. Stress
3. Poor nutrition
4. Inherited conditions
5. Type of disease process
6. The environment

Accidental needle sticks are a hazard for all health personnel and should be reported immediately so that prophylactic measures can be started. There should be appropriate waste containers for safe disposal of sharp instruments. Needles should never be recapped.

Inappropriate care of Foley catheter or other drainage apparatus can provide an entrance for microorganisms and allow the infectious process to continue. Tubes should remain connected and intact. Care should be taken when turning, positioning, or transferring a patient to prevent tubes from becoming tangled or pulling apart.

Appropriate cleansing of wounds will prevent the entrance of microorganisms. This is accomplished by cleaning away from the wound, wearing sterile gloves, and using an antiseptic agent. Gloves should be worn when handling soiled dresssings, and the dressings should be placed in a container for infectious waste.

Host

How susceptible a person is to an infection is determined by the amount of resistance shown to the pathogen. Microorganisms are constantly in contact with people, but an infection will not develop unless a person is susceptible to the strength and numbers of the microorganism. As the pathogen's strength and number increase, the person becomes more susceptible. Factors that affect a person's immunological defense mechanisms are described in Box 16-1.

The microorganism must accept the host for it to continue to exist.

Immunizations have proven effective in providing additional protection against infectious disease. These may be given before a person has been exposed to a disease (to provide protection before contact) or after exposure (if the person's history indicates possible contact with an infectious microorganism).

NOSOCOMIAL INFECTIONS

The term *nosocomial* is taken from the Greek word *nosocomium* meaning health care facility. A *nosocomial infec-*

tion is one that is acquired while in a hospital or other health agency. This is a far-reaching and serious problem. More than 40 million people are admitted to hospitals each year, and, while there, as many as 10% of these people acquire infections. A hospital harbors microorganisms that may be highly virulent, making it a more likely place to acquire an infection. The patient's immune system may already be weakened from disease or therapy, which makes the patient more susceptible to pathogens. Nosocomial infections not only extend hospital care for the patient but increase cost for both patient and hospital.

An **exogenous infection** is a nosocomial infection caused by microorganisms from another person. An **endogenous infection** is an infection caused by the patient's own normal microorganisms becoming altered and overgrowing or being transferred from one body site to another (e.g., microorganisms found in fecal material can be transferred to skin by hands and infect a wound).

Nosocomial infections are most commonly transmitted by direct contact between health personnel and patients or from patient to patient. For this reason heavy emphasis is placed on sanitary procedures, such as handwashing.

To decrease the occurrence or continuation of nosocomial infections, many agencies have an infection control department, which investigates and establishes policies to develop sanitary procedures. These procedures include clean technique, which is used in all areas, and sterile technique, which is used in specialized areas.

The nurse is responsible for providing the patient with a clean and safe environment. The conscientiousness and accuracy of the nurse in performing clean and aseptic procedures increase the effectiveness of infection control.

UNIVERSAL PRECAUTIONS

With the increased awareness of contamination from blood-borne pathogens—for example, the hepatitis B virus (HBV) and the human immunodeficiency virus (HIV) that causes acquired immunodeficiency syndrome (AIDS)—came the realization that definite precautions should be taken to prevent infections. The **Centers for Disease Control (CDC)** is conducting studies on health care workers with documented skin or mucous membrane exposures to blood or body fluids of infected patients. The results have not been documented, but preliminary figures show infection when health care workers did not use protective measures.

It is difficult to accurately identify all patients infected with blood-borne pathogens. The CDC recommends that "universal blood and body fluid precautions" or **"universal precautions"** be used by health care workers when caring for all patients. These recommendations include the following precautions:

1. Gloves should be worn during any procedure that could result in contact with blood or body fluid, open skin lesions, or mucous membranes. Goggles, masks, or face shields should be worn if there is risk of droplets spraying. Aprons or gowns should be worn to protect uniforms.
2. Handwashing procedure should be performed immediately after removal of gloves and if known contamination with blood or body fluid has occurred.
3. The health care worker should prevent injury from needles, scalpels, and other sharp instruments. Disposable sharp instruments should be placed immediately in a puncture-resistant container for disposal.
4. Protective devices should be available for use when resuscitation is necessary.
5. Health care workers with draining lesions should not have patient contact or contact with patient equipment until the problem is corrected.

SKILL 16-1: PERFORMING A 2-MINUTE HANDWASHING

Guidelines

Handwashing is the most important preventive technique for interrupting the infectious process. Box 16-2 indicates when it is essential to initiate handwashing.

A 2-minute handwashing will provide appropriate protection before the nurse cares for a patient. A 30-second handwashing before caring for another patient should be sufficient to ensure minimal transmission of microorganisms between patients. If a nurse has handled organic material or a contaminated article, a 1-minute handwashing would be appropriate.

Teaching patients and visitors about appropriate times for handwashing is an important role for the nurse. This enables the patient and family to inhibit the spread of microorganisms when health care is continued at home. The importance of handwashing before and after handling food, after handling contaminated articles, and before and after elimination should be stressed in the teaching process.

In addition to handwashing, other actions can be taken

BOX 16-2 HANDWASHING IS ESSENTIAL

1. Before and after caring for a patient
2. After contact with organic material, such as feces, wound drainage, and mucus
3. In preparation for an invasive procedure, such as suctioning, catheterization, or injections
4. Before changing a dressing or contact with open wounds
5. Before preparing and administering medications
6. After removing disposable gloves or handling contaminated equipment

to reduce the chance of transmitting microorganisms. A patient should receive his own set of personal care articles, such as a bedpan, urinal, bath basin, thermometer, water pitcher, and drinking glass, to prevent cross-contamination.

Microorganisms are transmitted by indirect contact with contaminated equipment and soiled linen. These articles should be placed in special waste containers or laundry bags and kept away from the nurse's uniform.

By following these recommendations the health care worker will be protected from infection and will prevent the patient acquiring a nosocomial infection.

Purposes

The nurse performs routine handwashing for the following reasons:

- to prevent nosocomial infection
- to maintain a safe, clean environment for the patient
- to provide safety for the nurse and prevent cross-contamination of patients or the spread of microorganisms

SUPPLIES/EQUIPMENT

warm running water	orange stick
paper towels	hand lotion
liquid soap	

SKILL 16-1 PERFORMING A 2-MINUTE HANDWASHING

Nursing action	Rationale
1. Inspect hands, observing for visible soiling, breaks, or cuts in the skin and cuticles.	Poor personal hygiene and an open area of the skin provide areas in which microorganisms can grow.
2. Determine contaminant of hands.	Helps determine the need for a 2-minute handwash.
3. Assess areas around the sink that are contaminated or clean.	Prevents contamination of hands during and after handwashing procedure.
4. Explain to the patient the importance of handwashing.	Helps the patient understand that handwashing slows down the spread of infection.
5. Remove jewelry (except plain wedding band), and push watch and long sleeves above wrist.	Microorganisms can collect in jewelry and watch bands. Also, removing jewelry makes it easier to wash all areas of hands and wrist.
6. Adjust the water to appropriate temperature and force.	Water that is too hot can chap skin, and too much force will cause splashing and spread microorganisms to other areas.
7. Wet hands and wrists under the running water, always keeping hands lower than elbows.	Because hands are the most contaminated part of the arm, water should flow from the wrists (least contaminated area), over the hands, and then down the drain.

STEP 7

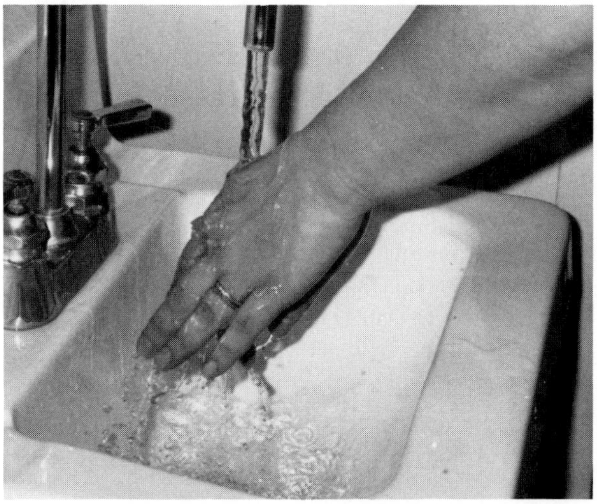

SKILL 16-1

PERFORMING A 2-MINUTE HANDWASHING—cont'd

Nursing action	Rationale
8. Lather hands with liquid soap (about 1 teaspoon).	Soap lather emulsifies fat and aids in cleansing.
9. Wash hands thoroughly using a firm, circular motion and friction on back of hands, palms, and wrists. Wash each finger individually, paying special attention to areas between fingers and knuckles by interlacing fingers and thumbs and moving hands back and forth.	Friction helps to loosen dirt and microorganisms—both resident (normally present) and transient (acquired from contamination).
10. Wash 1 minute, rinse thoroughly, relather, and wash another minute, using a continuous amount of friction.	Rinsing removes the loosened microorganisms, and relathering ensures more thorough cleaning. The greater the contamination, the more need for longer washing.
11. Rinse wrists and hands completely, keeping hands lower than elbows.	Water should run from cleaner area (the wrists) over the hands, and then down the drain, rinsing the dirt and microorganisms away.
12. Clean fingernails carefully under running water using fingernails of other hand or blunt end of an orange stick.	Reduces chance of microorganisms remaining under nails.
13. Dry hands thoroughly with paper towels. Start by patting at fingertips, hands, and then wrists and forearms.	Drying hands prevents chapping. The cleanest areas are now the fingers and hands, so drying should progress from clean to less clean.

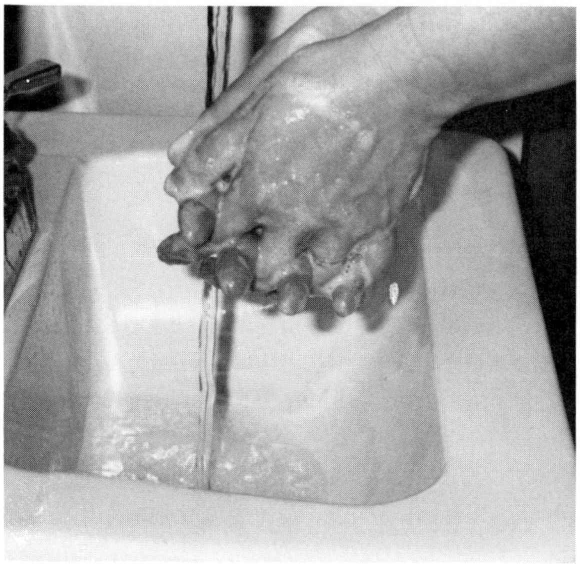

STEP 9

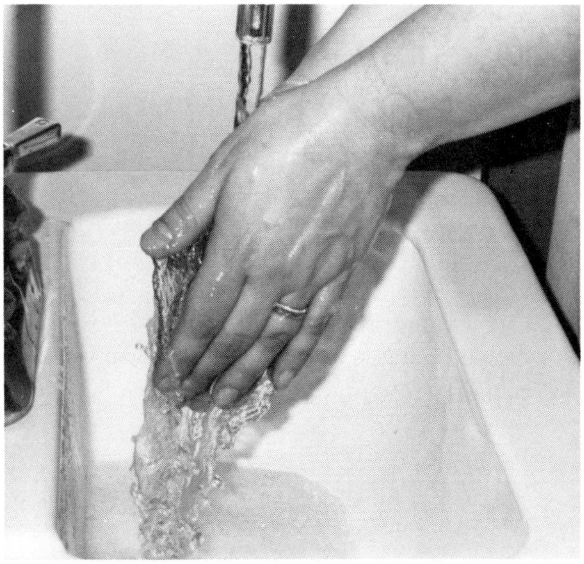

STEP 11

Continued.

SKILL 16-1

PERFORMING A 2-MINUTE HANDWASHING—cont'd

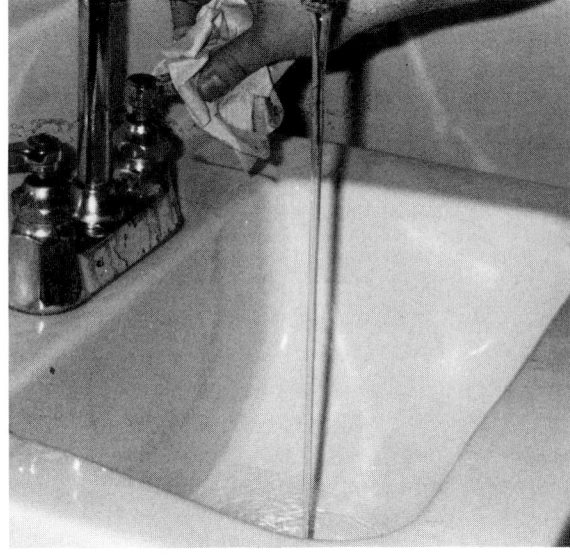

STEP 14

Nursing action	Rationale
14. Turn off faucets with a dry paper towel.	Clean hands prevents touching contaminated handles.
15. Use hand lotion if desired.	Keeps skin soft and lubricated so skin will not crack easily.
16. Inspect hands and nails for cleanliness.	Ensures cleanliness of hands and nails.

DOCUMENTATION

1. Record procedure.

Provides documentation of performance of 2-minute handwashing before administering patient care.

Sample charting

DATE	TIME	NOTES
1/12/91	0745	Two-minute handwashing procedure performed by the nurse.

____
(nurse's signature)

FOLLOW-UP

1. Two-minute handwashing should be performed each morning before beginning patient care.

Initial handwashing aids in removing surface soil from outside influences encountered on the way to work.

2. Perform handwashing between care of patients.

Additional handwashing prevents cross-contamination.

SPECIAL CONCERNS

- Avoid using water that is too hot or too cold when washing hands because breaks in the skin may occur and cause the hands to become contaminated when performing patient care.
- The very young and the elderly are highly susceptible to infection.

PATIENT TEACHING

- Demonstrate handwashing in view of the patient whenever possible to emphasize the importance of effective handwashing technique.
- Ask the patient questions or answer patient's questions regarding medical asepsis when necessary.

SKILL 16-2: DONNING GLOVES

Guidelines

Nurses or health care personnel don gloves if there is any possibility of contact with infectious material. Updated advice from CDC (1987) on wearing gloves includes the following:

1. Gloves are worn only once and then placed into infectious-waste containers for safe disposal.
2. If the nurse has not completed the patient's care but has come into contact with infectious material, the gloves should be changed before continuing patient's care.
3. There is a chance that gloves could be perforated during use, so hands should be washed after gloves are removed.

Family members should understand the importance of appropriate use of gloves. It is necessary for the nurse to explain that gloves will become contaminated if they have touched infected material or a contaminated object.

Purposes

The nurse wears gloves for all types of patient care for the following reasons:

- to protect the nurse and the nurse's family from disease
- to protect the patient from the nurse, who may be considered a contaminator to the patient
- to comply with 1987 CDC recommended use in order to (1) protect personnel from contact with infectious microorganisms, (2) reduce the possibility of patient contact with the health care worker's endogenous flora or normal bacteria, and (3) lessen the chance of personnel becoming infected with pathogenic microorganisms, which then could be carried to other patients

SUPPLIES/EQUIPMENT

pair of gloves

Related Knowledge and Skills

Before donning gloves the nurse should understand the following:

- patient teaching (see Chapter 4)
- assessment of the skin (see Chapters 13 and 29)

SKILL 16-3: GOWNING FOR ISOLATION

Guidelines

The use of gowns in isolation is important primarily to protect clothing from getting soiled while administering patient care. The gown also prevents contact with infectious microorganisms that could have exited from the patient. It is recommended that gowns not be reused but be discarded when leaving the patient's room. This aids in preventing the spread of pathogens to other patients or personnel. This procedure also applies to visitors. Reuse of an isolation gown might be acceptable in nurseries and special isolation units.

Another rationale for use is protection of a patient whose immune system is inadequate. In this case the gown is worn to prevent the transfer of pathogens from health care personnel and visitors to the patient.

There are many types of isolation, and some require wearing a gown, whereas others do not.

Donning an isolation gown is indicated when caring for patients with diseases characterized by heavy drainage, infectious and acute diarrhea, other gastrointestinal disorders, respiratory disorders, skin wounds or burns, and urinary disorders.

Isolation gowns open at the back with ties at the neck and the waist. This keeps the gown securely closed, protecting the back of the uniform, as well as the front. The gown should be long enough to cover the uniform and have long sleeves with cuffs for added protection.

To don gowns correctly, follow the procedures listed in Skill 16-3.

Purposes

The nurse gowns for isolation for the following reasons:

- to protect the nurse from contracting an infection from the patient
- to prevent medical personnel from contaminating the patient who has a disease affecting the immune system

SUPPLIES/EQUIPMENT

isolation gown

Related Knowledge and Skills

Before gowning the nurse should understand the following:

- patient teaching (see Chapter 4)
- assessment of the skin (see Chapters 13 and 29)

SKILL 16-2

DONNING GLOVES

Nursing action	Rationale
1. Remove gloves from dispenser.	Keeps gloves readily available for use.
2. Don gloves when ready to begin patient care.	Provides protection for the patient and nurse.
3. Inspect gloves for possibility of perforation.	Perforated gloves can allow entry of pathogenic microorganisms.
4. Change gloves after direct handling of infectious drainage.	Prevents contamination of patient.

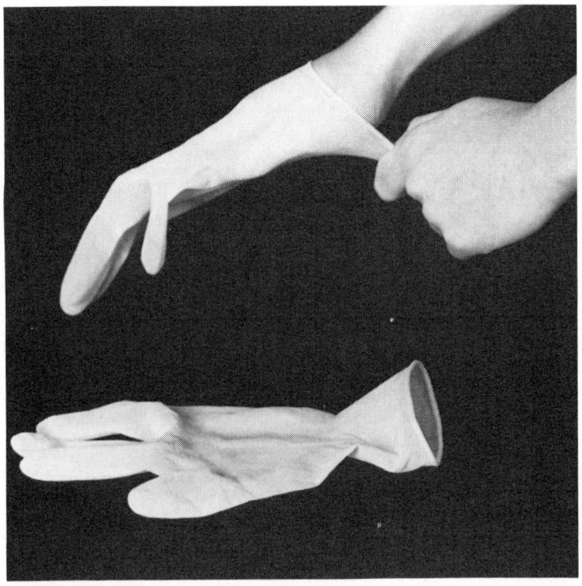

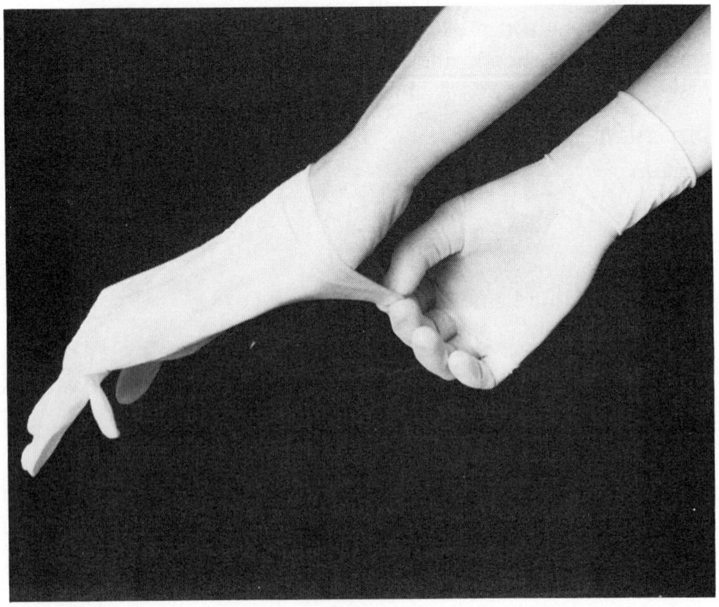

STEP 3

SKILL 16-2

DONNING GLOVES—cont'd

Nursing action	Rationale
5. Remove gloves by grasping at cuff edge and turning gloves inside out and drop into waste container.	Prevents nurse from touching outside area of gloves, which is considered contaminated.
6. Wash hands thoroughly.	Removes microorganisms that could be on nurse's hands.

STEP 5

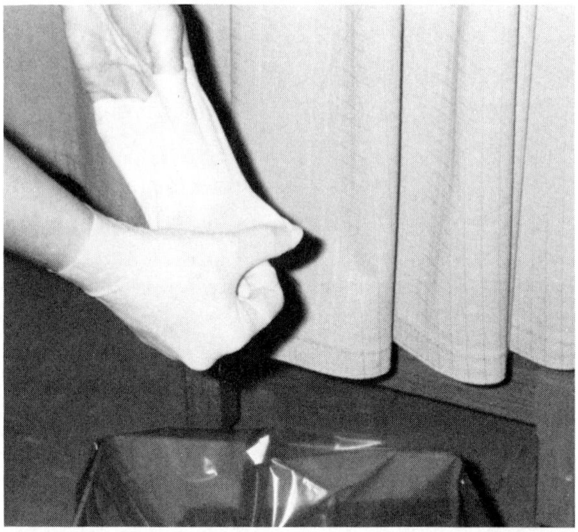

DOCUMENTATION

1. Record use of gloves during patient care.

Provides documentation of wearing gloves for protection of patient and nurse.

Sample charting

DATE	TIME	NOTES
1/12/91	0800	Gloves worn by nurse during administration of bed bath and AM care. Patient asked why gloves were worn. Explained reason for use of gloves. Patient seemed satisfied with explanation.

____
(nurse's signature)

FOLLOW-UP

1. Make certain patient knows nurse is not afraid of the patient.

Assists in patient's well-being and does not offend patient.

SPECIAL CONCERNS

- contamination of patient continues, nurse must ve technique reassessed.

PATIENT TEACHING

- Patient may need special assistance in understanding the universal precautions.
- The nurse should demonstrate donning gloves to patient.
- The nurse should allow a question and answer session for the patient.

SKILL 16-3

GOWNING FOR ISOLATION

Nursing action	Rationale
1. Remove watch and push up long sleeves.	Ensures that uniform sleeve is under gown sleeve for protection.
2. Place watch on a paper towel before taking vital signs.	Prevents cross-contamination of the watch.
3. Wash hands.	Inhibits spread of microorganisms.
4. Don gown by securely tying gown at neck and waist.	Provides protective covering of the entire uniform.
5. Remove gown.	Protects nurse.
6. Wash hands.	Prevents spread of microorganisms.

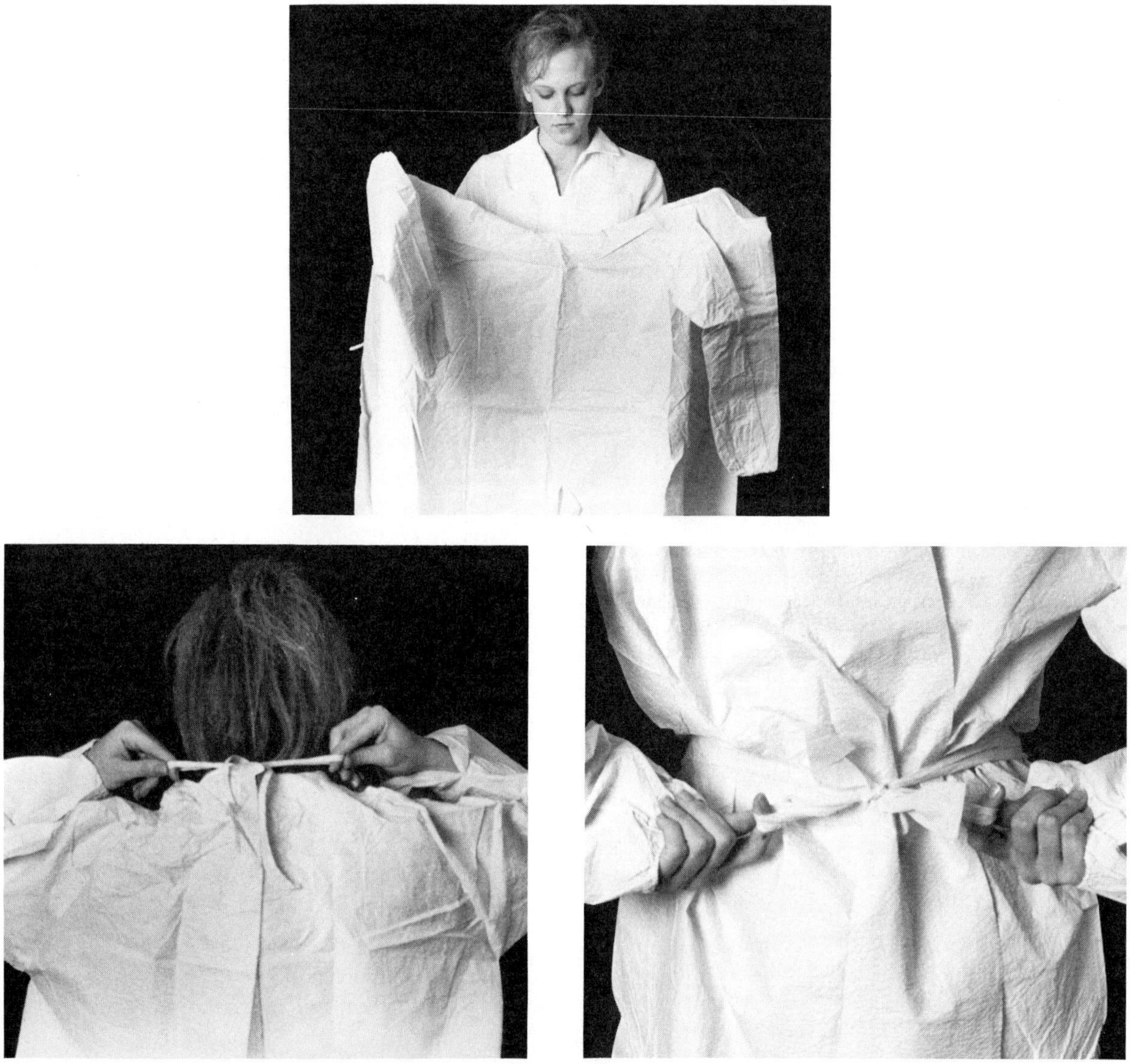

STEP 4

SKILL 16-3

GOWNING FOR ISOLATION—cont'd

DOCUMENTATION

1. Record use of gown in isolation procedure.	Provides proof that appropriate procedure was followed.

Sample charting

DATE	TIME	NOTES
1/23/91	0930	Followed strict isolation procedure for heavy drainage from wound. Explained purpose for carrying out isolation technique.

(nurse's signature)

FOLLOW-UP

1. Discard soiled gown appropriately.	Prevents contamination.

SPECIAL CONCERNS

- Gown must be disposed of appropriately.
- Patient should feel comfortable and accepted.

PATIENT TEACHING

- Teach universal precautions.
- Explain risks of inappropriate isolation technique.

SKILL 16-4: DONNING A MASK

Guidelines

When a mask is appropriately applied, it will fit snugly over the nose and the mouth and the top edge will fit below eyeglasses, if worn. (This prevents fogging of the glasses.) A mask should be changed at least every 20 to 30 minutes or if it becomes moist. Masks should not be reused or dangled around the neck and then reused. The patient and family members should be instructed on appropriate use of the mask.

Purposes

A mask should be worn for the following reasons:

- to protect the wearer from inhaling microorganisms that travel on airborne droplets for short distances or that remain suspended in the air for longer periods
- to prevent inhaling pathogens if resistance is reduced or if being transported to another area (patient use)
- to discourage the wearer from touching the mouth, nose, or eyes and from transmitting infectious material

SUPPLIES/EQUIPMENT

isolation mask

Related Knowledge and Skills

Before donning a mask, the nurse should understand the following:

- patient teaching (see Chapter 4)
- assessment of the skin (see Chapters 13 and 29)

SKILL 16-4

DONNING A MASK

Nursing action	Rationale
1. Remove mask from container.	Keeps mask readily available for use.
2. Don mask when ready to begin patient care by covering the nose and mouth with the mask. Secure mask in place with elastic band or by tying the strings behind the head.	Provides protection from microorganisms.
3. Wear mask until it becomes moist but no longer than 20 to 30 minutes.	Moisture renders a mask ineffective.
4. Remove mask by untying the strings or moving the elastic. Make certain not to touch contaminated area.	Protects nurse from coming into contact with contaminated mask.
5. Dispose of soiled mask.	Protects other health care workers.
6. Wash hands thoroughly.	Removes microorganisms

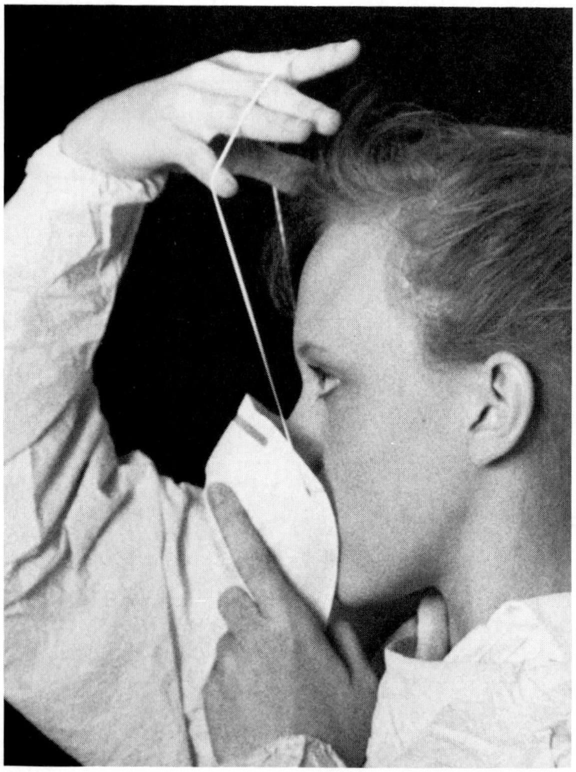

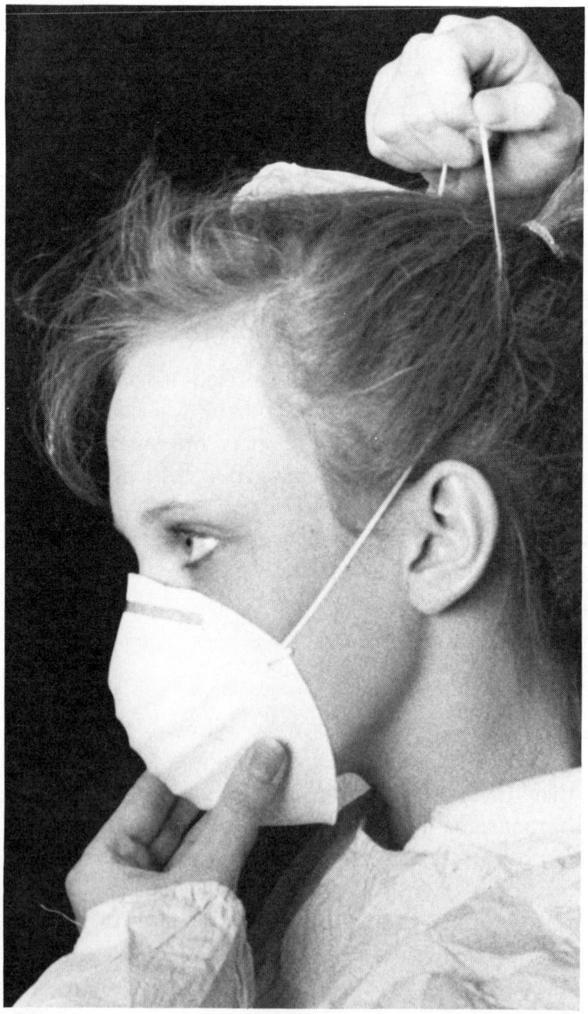

STEP 2

SKILL 16-4

DONNING A MASK—cont'd

DOCUMENTATION

1. Record use of mask during patient care.	Provides proof of wearing mask for protection of patient and nurse.

Sample charting

DATE	TIME	NOTES
1/30/91	0800	Mask worn by nurse during patient care.

____
(nurse's signature)

FOLLOW-UP

1. Make certain patient knows nurse is not afraid of the patient.	Assists in patient's well-being and prevents patient's being offended.

SPECIAL CONCERNS

- If contamination of patient continues, technique must be reassessed.

PATIENT TEACHING

- Patient may need special assistance in understanding the universal precautions.
- Allow a question and answer session for the patient.

SKILL 16-5: DOUBLE BAGGING

Guidelines

A single bag is adequate if the contaminated articles can be placed in the bag without contamination of the outside of the bag. Double bagging is recommended by the CDC when it is impossible to keep the outer surface of a single bag free from contamination. The second bag should be labeled or color-coded to alert nursing personnel and to prevent contamination of housekeeping personnel when handling contaminated material. Double bagging can be used for safe removal of any article from the room.

Purposes

The nurse uses special bagging technique to remove contaminated articles from the patient's environment for the following reasons:

- to prevent the spread of microorganisms to the surrounding environment
- to prevent potential accidental exposure of personnel to contaminated articles

SUPPLIES/EQUIPMENT

single isolation bag
special color-coded double bag
holder for isolation bag
isolation gown
isolation mask
clean gloves
holder for laundry bag

Related Knowledge and Skills

Before performing double bagging, the nurse should understand the following:

- communication (see Chapter 4)
- documentation (see Chapter 6)
- patient teaching (see Chapter 4)
- physical assessment (see Chapter 13)

SKILL 16-5 DOUBLE BAGGING

Nursing action	Rationale
1. Don gown, mask, and gloves before entering patient's room.	Prevents contact with contaminated articles.
2. Collect all contaminated disposable articles in isolation bag.	Prepares for double bagging.
3. Summon second health care worker to remain outside patient area.	Prevents risk of contamination of personnel.
4. Second person holds double bag with the top edge of bag covering hands.	Prevents risk of contamination of personnel.
5. First person drops contaminated bag in double bag without touching edges of bag.	Outside of double bag remains clean.
6. Bags are sealed or tied and labeled.	Prevents spread of infectious microorganisms.
7. First person places new bags in holders.	Keeps articles ready for use.
8. Remove gloves, gown, and mask without contamination.	Prevents spread of pathogens.
9. Wash hands thoroughly.	Prevents contamination of nurse and others.

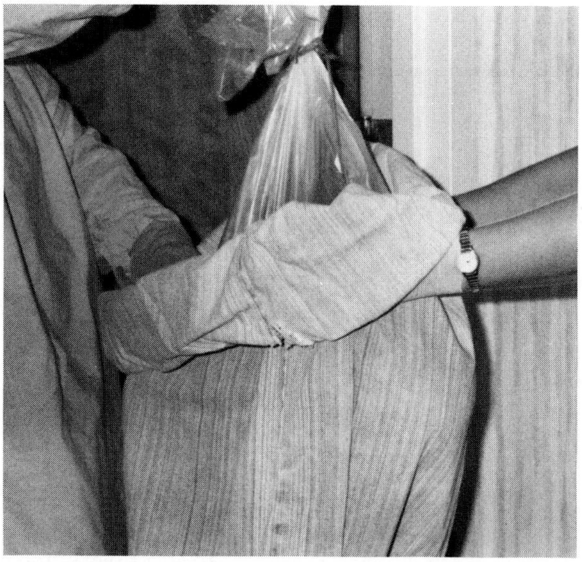

STEP 4

DOCUMENTATION

1. Record double bagging procedure.	Provides proof of use of appropriate technique.
2. Document patient's response to isolation.	Could indicate need for patient teaching.

SKILL 16-5

DOUBLE BAGGING—cont'd

Sample charting

DATE	TIME	NOTES
1/31/91	0940	All disposable, contaminated articles double bagged and placed outside room for pickup. Patient understands and cooperates with isolation procedures.
		____________ *(nurse's signature)*

FOLLOW-UP

1. Ensure positive feelings of patient toward being in isolation. — Prevents patient from feeling rejected.

SPECIAL CONCERNS

- If contamination of patient continues, the technique must be reassessed.

PATIENT TEACHING

- Patient may need special assistance in understanding universal precautions.
- Allow a question and answer session for the patient.

SKILL 16-6: PROTECTIVE ASEPSIS

Guidelines

The type of isolation technique followed will depend on how transmissible the pathogen. The use of environmental barriers will keep pathogens in a confined area. Examples of such barriers are a private room, isolation room, closed door, protective gown, mask, and gloves, and shoe covers.

There are specific guidlines issued by the CDC for protective asepsis in a controlled environment. There are two systems for implementing these guidelines: the disease-specific system, where certain procedures are performed for each type of infectious disease, and the category-specific system. The category-specific system recognizes eight ways a microorganism is transmitted (Box 16-3). In this category similar isolation precautions are used for different diseases because the microorganism is transmitted in the same manner. Although the disease-specific system has proven to be less time consuming and less costly because some diseases need only minimum precautions, the category-specific system is most commonly used in health care agencies.

There are some basic principles to be followed no matter what protective system is used. They are as follows:

1. Thorough handwashing should be performed before entering and after leaving a patient's room when using protective asepsis.
2. An understanding of the disease process and method of transmission of the infectious microorganism helps determine the use of protective barriers.
3. Contaminated equipment and articles are to be disposed of in a safe and effective manner to prevent transmission of pathogens to other individuals.
4. If the patient is to be transported to other areas in the agency (away from the isolation room), necessary measures should be taken to protect those who may be exposed. This is accomplished by having the patient wear a gown and mask.

The patient with an infectious disease should be placed in a private or isolation room equipped with the appropriate handwashing and toilet facilities. The routine care of a patient in isolation is the same hygienic care given to all patients. The health care worker should remember that all articles that come into contact with the patient are contaminated and should be handled in the correct manner to maintain protective asepsis. Equipment for assessing vital signs remains in the room if possible.

BOX 16-3 CATEGORY-SPECIFIC ISOLATION PRECAUTIONS

1. Strict isolation—Diseases transmitted by air or contact require full-isolation technique. Disease example: diphtheria.
2. Direct contact precautions—The nurse should wear gown, mask, and gloves only when coming into contact with the infectious substance. Disease examples: impetigo, herpes simplex, and acute respiratory infections in infants and small children.
3. Respiratory isolation—Health care personnel must wear a mask whenever in the room with the patient, because the pathogen is transmitted by airborne droplets over short distances. Disease examples: pneumonia, measles, or bacterial meningitis.
4. Enteric precautions—Disease spread through fecal material. The nurse should wear gown and gloves for protection against feces. Disease examples: viral hepatitis or infectious diarrhea.
5. Tuberculosis isolation—Pathogen transmitted by air droplet and sputum. The nurse may need to wear gown and a mask if the patient is coughing without covering the mouth, but gloves are not indicated.
6. Drainage/secretion precautions—The pathogen is transmitted by direct or indirect contact with drainage from an infected body site. The nurse should wear gown and gloves to prevent contact with the infectious material. A mask is not needed. Disease example: infected burns or wounds.
7. Blood/body fluid precautions—Direct or indirect contact with infected body fluids or blood requires the use of gown and/or gloves. Caring for a patient with acquired immunodeficiency syndrome (AIDS) requires blood/body fluid precautions.
8. Care of immunosuppressed patient—This was previously known as reverse isolation. Health care personnel caring for an immunosuppressed patient should wear a gown, mask, and gloves to prevent transmission of pathogens by contact or air droplet. Disease examples: leukemia, burns, or patients with organ transplants.

Otherwise, the equipment must be disinfected safely when removed from the room. The nurse's watch may be placed on a clean paper towel or sealed in a plastic bag and placed on the bedside unit stand before touching any article in the room.

It is important in the care of this patient to consider the psychological implications created by isolation. The patient is forced into solitude and deprived of normal social contacts. The patient should feel wanted and cared for like all other patients. Extra time should be spent with the patient, the room should be kept clean and pleasant, and the patient should be taught the rationale for use of this technique. The emotional state of the patient can interfere with recovery unless the nurse minimizes the feeling of psychological and physical isolation. The patient and family should have an understanding of the patient's disease and know the importance of following protective asepsis. Family and visitors should be taught how to wear isolation apparel, and the nurse should ensure that the procedure is followed.

Purpose

The nurse follows isolation procedure for the following reason:

- to prevent the transmission of infectious microorganisms by preventing pathogens from leaving the room of the infected patient or from entering the room of a highly susceptible patient

SUPPLIES/EQUIPMENT

Outside Patient's Room or in Anteroom:
isolation gowns
isolation masks
isolation gloves
clean linens
single isolation bags
double isolation bags
paper towels
running water
soap with dispenser

Inside the Patient's Room or in Anteroom:
holder for isolation bag
holder for laundry bag

Related Knowledge and Skills

Before performing isolation technique, the nurse should understand the following:

- communication and patient teaching (see Chapter 4)
- documentation (see Chapter 6)
- physical assessment (see Chapter 13)

SKILL 16-6

ISOLATION TECHNIQUE

Nursing action	Rationale
1. Determine causative microorganism or effectiveness of patient's immune system.	Helps nurse know virulence of causative pathogen.
2. Recognize mode of transmission and how microorganism exits the body.	Determines category or type of isolation to use.
3. Follow agency policy for specific type of isolation used.	Increases awareness of isolation categories available in the agency.
4. Provide an environment with adequate equipment and supplies:	
a. Private room or isolation with anteroom.	Reduces possibility of transmission of pathogens.
b. Sign stating isolation category.	Alerts personnel, patient, family, and visitors about special precautions to be followed.
c. Adequate handwashing facilities.	Handwashing can easily be performed on entering and leaving the area.
d. Special containers for trash, soiled linen, and sharp instruments, such as needles.	Ensures safe disposal of contaminated articles.
5. Plan time to explain isolation technique to patient, family, and visitors.	Relieves apprehension and promotes cooperation of those involved.
6. Post card on door of patient's room or wall outside room stating the protective measures in use for patient care.	Informs those entering room of precautions to be followed and encourages cooperation.
7. Supply the room with designated lined containers for soiled linens and for trash.	Prevents transmission of pathogens from seepage through container.

DOCUMENTATION

1. Report changes in patient's health status, whether positive or negative.	Ensures continued care and helps determine progress of patient.
2. Record assessments and performance of protective asepsis.	Provides proof of appropriate patient care.

Sample charting

DATE	TIME	NOTES
2/1/91	0745	Isolation procedure carried out. Patient answered questions clearly and showed understanding of procedures performed.

____

(nurse's signature)

Continued.

SKILL 16-6 ISOLATION TECHNIQUE—cont'd

FOLLOW-UP

1. Determine patient's understanding of activities in room.	Increases patient's comfort and feeling of well-being.

SPECIAL CONCERNS

- Make certain that patient does not feel alone and isolated from loved ones.
- Ensure patient safety.

PATIENT TEACHING

- Teach patient how to carry out handwashing precautions.

BOX 16-4 PRINCIPLES OF STERILIZATION OR DISINFECTION

PHYSICAL METHOD

1. **STEAM UNDER PRESSURE,** or moist heat, is the most practical and dependable method for destruction of all microorganisms. This technique is called *sterilization*. Examples of sterilization equipment are the autoclave, which is used in hospitals and other agencies, and the pressure cooker, which is used in a home environment.
2. **BOILING WATER** is the best method for home use and is the least expensive. However, this technique will not destroy bacterial spores and some viruses. The article should be boiled for a minimum of 20 minutes for disinfection.
3. **RADIATION** sterilizes pharmaceutical goods, foods, and heat-sensitive items. It is extremely effective on articles that are difficult to sterilize.
4. **DRY HEAT** is a method used for disinfecting articles that are destroyed by moisture. Health agencies seldom use this method, but in the home an article can be disinfected by placing it in the oven for 2 hours at 320° F or for 45 minutes at 350° F.

CHEMICAL PROCESS

1. **GAS** (ethylene oxide) is used for sterilization. It destroys spores formed by bacteria.
2. **CHEMICAL SOLUTIONS** are often used to disinfect instruments because they are effective in destroying microorganisms. Clinical thermometers can be stored in a chemical solution, and some articles are soaked in a solution to prepare them for another method of disinfection or sterilization.

SKILL 16-7: PREPARING FOR DISINFECTION AND STERILIZATION

Guidelines

Pathogenic microorganisms are believed to be present on most articles in the home and public areas, including health agencies. Disinfection and sterilization are two processes used to prevent spread of pathogens and disease.

Most health agencies have a central supply department, which sterilizes some supplies and disinfects reusable equipment and supplies. Although most supplies used today for patient care are disposable, there are situations that still require the use of sterilization and disinfection techniques. The patient and family can also be taught cleansing and disinfecting principles for the home environment.

There are two accepted methods of sterilization and disinfection (Box 16-4). One is a physical process that uses heat or radiation; the second process uses chemicals. Both methods destroy microorganisms. The method used depends on the following factors: (1) the type of microorganism present, since spore-forming bacteria are resistant to destruction; (2) how many microorganisms are present, since it takes longer to kill a large number; and (3) the type of article in need of cleansing, since some materials are so sensitive that heat or certain chemicals can destroy the article. Other determinants of the sterilization method used are (1) the intended use for the article (e.g., surgery requires all organisms be destroyed, whereas medical asepsis only requires removal of pathogens) and (2) the methods of sterilization available.

Effective chemicals used in disinfection and sterilization are iodine, alcohol, and chlorine compounds. Chlorine is useful for household disinfecting and in disinfection of water but should never be mixed with ammonia because of the resulting emission of toxic fumes. Chlorine has a tendency to corrode some metals. Iodine is a good bactericidal agent (i.e., it kills the bacteria but not spores). Iodine stains articles and is not used as widely as it once was.

Purpose

The nurse follows basic clean or aseptic technique for the following reason:

- to interrupt the infection process in order to prevent and control the spread of infection

SUPPLIES/EQUIPMENT

Disinfection
gloves
running water
scrub brush

Sterilization
cloth wrappers

Related Knowledge and Skills

Before preparing for disinfection and sterilization the nurse should understand the following:

- commonly accepted disinfectants
- methods for sterilization
- medical asepsis

SKILL 16-7 PREPARING FOR DISINFECTION AND STERILIZATION

Nursing action	Rationale
1. Prepare equipment and supplies.	Ensures organization of task.
a. Disinfectant to use for cleansing.	Aids in appropriate care of equipment and reusable supplies.
b. Method of sterilization.	Ensures that appropriate method is used.
c. Gloves.	Protects nurse from contamination.
d. Running water.	Aids in cleansing and rinsing of articles.
e. Scrub brush.	Aids in cleansing grooves.
f. Cloth wrappers.	Provides means for wrapping articles requiring sterilization.
2. Don gloves.	Protects nurse from contamination.
3. Rinse article under cool running water.	Emulsifies or softens dirt for removal.
4. Wash article with detergent.	Emulsifies or softens dirt for easy removal.
5. Use scrub brush to remove material in grooves.	Friction loosens material in corners and grooves.
6. Dry article thoroughly.	Prevents growth of microorganisms.
7. Prepare article for sterilization by wrapping it in cloth wrappers.	Ensures appropriate sterilization of the article.

RELATED ACTIVITIES

1. Clean work area and put in order.	Prevents growth of microorganisms.

SPECIAL CONCERNS

- In the home an oven or a pressure cooker may be used for sterilization.
- Exposure to sunlight is helpful.
- Boiling of contaminated articles destroys microorganisms.

PATIENT TEACHING

- Teach patient to recognize possible sources of infection to perform the necessary protective measures.
- Set a personal example of cleanliness.
- Teach patient and family members to understand the steps performed in protective asepsis to help prevent transmission of pathogens.
- Teach and assist patient and family to control infection in the home by improvising or using available materials to maintain hygienic techniques.
- Inform patient about nature of infections and techniques to control and prevent the spread of disease. Topics that can be discussed in teaching sessions are presented in Box 16-5.

BOX 16-5 **TOPICS FOR TEACHING INFECTION CONTROL**

1. The nurse should teach the patient about the infection process, especially how an infection is transmitted, and stress the importance of interrupting the process. A simple diagram can be used to illustrate this. The nurse should use an example for each step that is familiar to the patient.
2. Although handwashing is a basic aseptic technique, the nurse should stress when and how the procedure should be performed to be effective in preventing infection.
3. The nurse should emphasize the importance of adequate exercise, a well-balanced diet, and current immunizations. This is good preventive health care for patients to follow.
4. The nurse should discuss the susceptibility of the patient to infection.
5. The patient should be taught correct and safe methods of storing and preparing food.
6. The patient should practice good methods of hygiene to minimize microorganism growth and spread. The nurse may suggest a list of disinfectants that could be used in daily cleaning.
7. The patient should be aware of family members who are susceptible to infections.

REFERENCES AND SUGGESTED READINGS

1. Brunner L and Suddareh D: Textbook of medical–surgical nursing, ed 6, Philadelphia, 1988, JB Lippincott Co.
2. CDC: Recommendations for prevention of HIV transmission in health-care settings, MMWR 36(25): 1987.
3. DeCrosta T: Nosocomial infections, Nurs Life 6(5): 1986.
4. Department of Labor and Department of Health and Human Services: Joint advisory notice: protection against occupational exposure to hepatitis B virus (HBV) and human immunodeficiency virus (HIV), 1987.
5. Gayling G and Morgan T: AIDS: concepts in nursing practice, Baltimore, 1988, Williams & Wilkins.
6. Hood G and Dincher J: Total patient care, ed 7, St Louis, 1988, The CV Mosby Co.
7. Mosby's medical, nursing & allied health dictionary, ed 3, St Louis, 1990, The CV Mosby Co.
8. Potter PA and Perry AG: Fundamentals of nursing, ed 2, St Louis, 1989, The CV Mosby Co.

CHAPTER CHALLENGE

STUDY QUESTIONS

1. One purpose of protective asepsis is to:
   a. Prevent transmission of infectious microorganisms
   b. Control the environment of the patient and family
   c. Prevent the patient from continuously coughing
   d. Prevent caring for psychological needs of the patient
2. The most important method used in preventing the spread of microorganisms is:
   a. Wearing gown
   b. Placing patient in isolation
   c. Handwashing
   d. Wearing gloves
3. When setting up a protective asepsis, the main goal is to:
   a. Prevent transmission of microorganisms from patients' rooms to other areas
   b. Keep all articles sterile
   c. Prevent *only* visitors from coming into contact with microorganisms
   d. Protect *only* the patient from an invading microorganism
4. For appropriate isolation technique a mask is:
   a. Stored inside the isolation room
   b. Changed at least every 20 to 30 minutes or sooner if it becomes moist
   c. Saved and worn again if not soiled
   d. Worn from patient to patient if the wearer is careful
5. A private room is desired for a patient with an infectious disease because:
   a. It is easier to prevent the spread of the disease
   b. A "No Visitors" rule can be better controlled
   c. There is more room to use special equipment
   d. The patient will be kept isolated from others
6. Enteric precautions include the following:
   a. Mask only
   b. Gloves and mask if in contact with secretions
   c. Gowns only
   d. Gown and gloves if in contact with secretions
7. Precautions for respiratory isolation are:
   a. Gloves
   b. Gloves and masks
   c. Masks, gowns, and gloves
   d. Gowns and gloves
8. If the patient's immune system is inadequate, the nurse should protect the patient by wearing:
   a. Gown, gloves, mask
   b. Mask only
   c. Gloves and gown
   d. Gloves and mask
9. All contaminated articles used by a patient with an infectious disease should be:
   a. Placed with other soiled linens
   b. Double bagged and appropriately discarded
   c. Single bagged and placed at nurse's desk
   d. Left in the patient's room
10. When performing isolation technique, which of the following situations *require* gloves to be worn:
    a. Direct contact with blood or body fluids
    b. When infection is highly contagious
    c. When doing oral care
    d. All of the above

STUDY QUESTIONS

11. Nosocomial infections occur when:
    a. A doctor prescribes the wrong medicine
    b. A patient refuses treatment
    c. Protective asepsis is not followed correctly
    d. A laboratory report is positive for infection
12. The two general types of isolation practices the CDC has recommended are:
    a. Protective and reverse
    b. Category-specific and disease-specific
    c. Specific disease and reverse
    d. Category and protective
13. Universal precautions are practiced by health care personnel to protect:
    a. The nurse
    b. The patient
    c. The family
    d. All of the above
14. If the nurse's watch is needed in isolation to check a patient's vital signs, the most practical way to keep it clean is:
    a. Wear it outside cuff or gown
    b. Clean with disinfectant after use
    c. Place in clean plastic bag and lay on bedside stand when entering room
    d. Have a second person hold the watch while the nurse takes vital signs
15. An important goal for the nurse to have when teaching the patient medical asepsis is:
    a. To ensure the patient understands the need for basic methods of cleanliness
    b. To ensure the patient does *all* procedures correctly
    c. To ensure the patient *completely* understands the diagnosed infectious disease
    d. To ensure the patient has no questions regarding aseptic procedure
16. Which organism is responsible for more diseases than any other pathogen:
    a. Streptococcus
    b. Virus
    c. Fungus
    d. Protozoan
    e. Staphylococcus
17. Which organism is usually self-limiting and antibiotics do not alter the course of the disease:
    a. Diplococcus
    b. Fungus
    c. Virus
    d. Protozoan

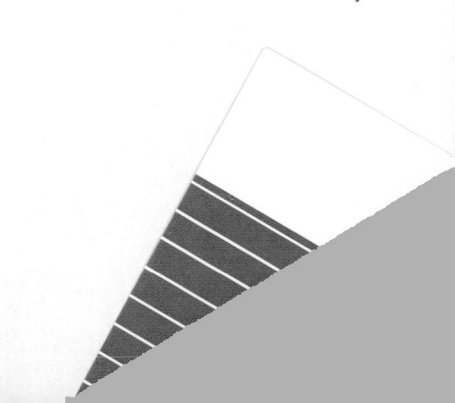

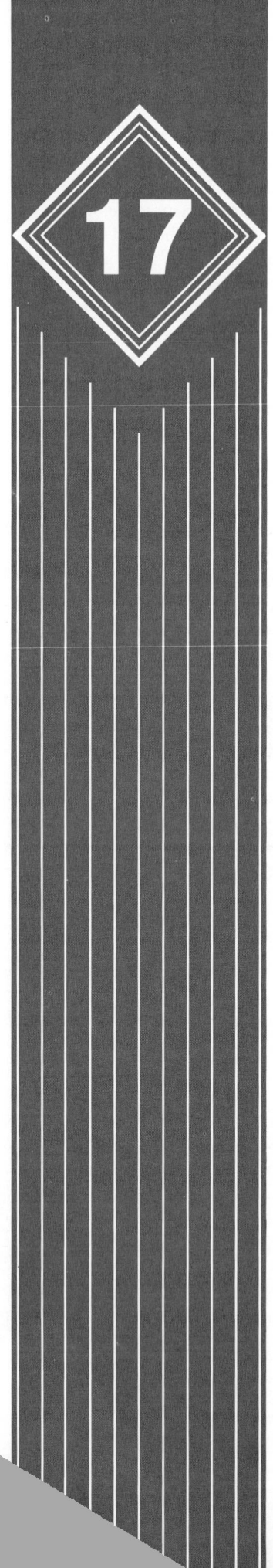

17

Safety

FRANCES JEAN KELLEY

LEARNING OBJECTIVES

After reading this chapter, the student should be able to do the following:

- Define the key terms.
- Summarize safety precautions that can be implemented to reduce falls.
- Discuss specific risks to safety as they pertain to the infant and young child.
- Discuss specific risks to safety as they pertain to the older adult.
- Discuss specific risks to safety as they pertain to the hospitalized patient.
- Discuss specific risks to safety as they pertain to the health care worker.
- List four reasons for applying restraints.
- Discuss applying restraints appropriately and safely.
- Describe nursing interventions that are specific to the patient requiring restraints.
- List the steps to be followed in the event of a fire.
- Discuss the role of the nurse in disaster planning.
- Describe nursing interventions in the event of accidental poisoning.

SKILLS

17-1 Applying restraints
17-2 Ensuring fire safety
17-3 Disaster planning
17-4 Accidental poisoning

KEY TERMS

Define the following

- CDC
- code
- disaster-preparedness plan
- Hazard Communication Act
- OSHA
- poisoning
- RACE
- restraint

GUIDELINES

The need for a safe environment is ever present and ranges from concerns about the immediate environment of a patient to local and national concerns about the environment in which one lives and works. Such issues as water and air pollution, disposal of waste and toxic materials, safety on the highways, protection of endangered species, and the preservation of forests illustrate general environmental concerns about safety. The hospital environment in terms of overall safety for the patient has traditionally been a primary concern of nursing. Today the focus on a safe hospital environment has expanded with the recognition and identification of potential hazards and threats faced by hospital personnel.

A safe environment implies freedom from injury with focus on helping to prevent falls, electrical injuries, fires, burns, and poisoning. The nurse must be aware of potential safety problems and must be knowledgeable about how to report and respond when safety is threatened.

The responsibility for providing and maintaining a safe environment involves the patient, visitors, and members of the health care team. Both protection and education are primary nursing responsibilities, with nurses directly and actively involved in ensuring a safe health care environment. Checking to see that the call light or signal system being used is working and accessible is an example of how the nurse helps maintain a safe environment.

Falls are a common problem, and nurses should be aware of patients who may fall. Not only the very young and the older adult, but also individuals who become ill or are injured, especially those requiring anesthesia or narcotics, are at risk. Various safety precautions can be taken to prevent falls (Box 17-1).

Ensuring the safety of the immediate environment of the infant and young child requires protection of the infant and child and education of the parents. Anticipating what injuries are likely to occur can assist nurses to individualize their care and teaching. Growth and the acquisition of new motor skills place the infant and child at great risk for injury.

For example, children younger than 6 years cannot read labels on cleaning materials or medication containers. All household cleaning items are potentially poisonous when ingested and should be kept out of the reach of children. Young infants in the oral stage of development put almost anything into their mouths, and as infants learn to crawl, electric sockets and cords become a danger. Toddlers and young children should be protected from burns: handles of pots on a stove should be turned away from the child's reach, and bath water temperature should be carefully monitored. No infant, toddler, or preschool child should be left unattended in a bathtub or pool of water, not even for a moment. Infants and toddlers should be protected from falling out of bed. Side rails must be up at all times. The nurse should always place

BOX 17-1 **SAFETY PRECAUTIONS TO PREVENT FALLS**

1. Bedside tables and overbed tables should be placed within the patient's reach.
2. Patients who have had surgery, who have received narcotics for analgesia, or who have been in bed for an extended period should be assisted when they get out of bed.
3. The environment should be kept free of litter, because such items as books, magazines, and shoes can cause the patient to trip and fall.
4. Facility policies should be followed regarding the use of side rails.
5. Adjustable beds should be in the low position except when care is given.
6. When ambulating, patients should be encouraged to wear slippers or shoes with low heels. Terry cloth slippers with rubber, skid-resistant soles are recommended; loose, poor-fitting soft shoes should be avoided.
7. Spilled liquids should be wiped up or mopped promptly. Personnel and patients should be alert to signs warning of wet or slippery floors.
8. The use of handrails in the bathrooms and halls should be encouraged.
9. The proper use of emergency call buttons or cords should be demonstrated.

her hand on the infant or toddler if she must turn to obtain supplies, for example.

Changes associated with aging significantly affect the ability of older adults to protect themselves from injury. For example, unsteadiness in gait causes falls. Age-related eye changes may affect the individual's ability to see the height of stairs. Vertigo (dizziness) is often related to a side effect of some medications and to chronic disease conditions (see Chapter 48). Eyeglasses, hearing aids, and assistive devices, such as canes, should be used bypatients with deficits. The nurse should be certain the frail or confused elderly patients are assisted when drinking hot liquids, such as soups, coffee, or tea. These persons are vulnerable to burns from spilled hot liquids. Long, loose clothing, which might cause tripping, should not be worn.

By using the nursing process, nurses can help reduce the risk of injury in the patient's immediate environment. Specific interventions can help ensure a safe environment by removing potential threats to safety. Should safety be threatened, appropriate guidelines should be followed to resolve the situation.

The hospital environment itself is a source of potential safety hazards to health care workers. Various biological, chemical, and physical hazards have been identified. Hazards range from smoke inhalation associated with laser use in the operating room to exposure to blood and body fluids, contaminated needles, and radiation.

The Occupational Safety and Health Administration's **(OSHA) Hazard Communication Act** requires hospitals to inform employees about the presence of or potential for harmful exposures and how to reduce the risk of exposure. The Centers for Disease Control **(CDC)** also provides guidelines for working with infected patients. The nurse should request information and follow recommended guidelines for reducing exposure to hazards in the hospital environment.

SKILL 17-1: APPLYING RESTRAINTS

Guidelines

A **restraint** is defined as any one of numerous devices used to immobilize a patient. The most common type of restraint is the soft restraint. This is often referred to as a *Posey* restraint after the company that manufactures this type of restraint.

Restraints are used for various reasons. Patient safety is the primary consideration. Restraints are employed to maintain treatment (e.g., wrist restraints to prevent patients removing intravenous lines and drainage tubes). Restraints also prevent the confused patient from wandering and prevent or reduce the risk of the patient falling from a bed, chair, or wheelchair. Movement of an aggressive patient may also be restricted to protect other patients and staff from harm.

The use of restraints is widespread in North America: 7% to 10% of the hospital population is restrained. Certain patient populations, such as the elderly and the confused, are more likely to be restrained. Today both ethical and legal issues surround the use of restraints. There is a focus on using other means to protect patients.

The use of restraints can also result in increased restlessness, anxiety, and a feeling of powerlessness. Restraint use contributes to immobility and the problems associated with immobility. Patients who are restrained often pull against the restraints, causing skin and circulation problems.

Documentation about the need for restraints, the type of restraints used, and patient response is crucial. A comprehensive assessment focusing on the patient's behavior, activity, and skin condition is necessary. All nursing interventions, including patient and family teaching about the restraints, must be noted.

Most health care facilities have specific policies and procedures related to the use of restraints. Most facilities require a specific order from a physician. The nurse should be familiar with the policies regarding the application of restraints. Restraints should be used judiciously and with kindness. The nurse should explain to the patient the need for the restraint even if the patient does not seem to understand the explanation. If the nurse has any questions, the supervisor should be consulted.

Purposes

The nurse, usually in response to a physician's order or facility unit policy, may apply restraints for the following reasons:

- to promote safety when the patient is in bed or up in a chair or wheelchair
- to prevent injury to the patient and/or others caring for the patient
- to prevent injury or an interruption of therapeutic interventions (e.g., dislodging tubes, pulling out an IV needle or catheter, or inadvertently removing a dressing)

Related Knowledge and Skills

Before applying restraints, the nurse should know the health care facility's policy concerning restraint use and documentation and should understand the following:

- assisting with the collection of subjective and objective data with a focus on an assessment of the skin (see Chapters 13 and 29)

SKILL 17-1 APPLYING RESTRAINTS

Nursing action	Rationale
Assessment	
1. Assess patient's potential for injury, including the patient and/or others.	Identifies need for protective devices, such as a restraint.
2. Identify reasons for the behavior or contributing medical conditions or treatments.	Identifies patients at risk for injury and determines ability to cooperate and understand.
3. Assess patient's level of consciousness and orientation.	
4. Assess skin status in the restrained extremities.	Determines adequacy of circulation and overall skin condition.
5. Assess possibility of using other nursing interventions for coping with the situation (e.g., moving patient nearer the nurses' station). Assess effectiveness of reality orientation. Also consider the availability of staff or family members to stay with the patient.	Permits interventions other than restraints.
6. Assess type of restraint needed.	Nursing assessment helps determine type needed.
7. Obtain or verify physician's order or follow health care facility policy.	Protects nurse from liability.
Nursing diagnoses	
1. Potential for injury, related to altered mental status (e.g., confusion or disorientation).	Patient is at risk for injury because of changes in mental status.
2. Potential impaired skin integrity, related to the presence of restraints.	Patient is at risk for impairment or alteration in the skin surface as a result of pulling against a restraint (shearing effect).

Continued.

SKILL 17-1

APPLYING RESTRAINTS—cont'd

Nursing action	Rationale
Planning	
1. Explain to both patient and family (1) why using a restraint is necessary, (2) the type of restraint to be used, and (3) approximately how long restraint use will be needed.	Restraint use is often misunderstood by both patient and family. Restraint use may also further agitate the patient. Explanations often reduce some of these feelings and may increase cooperation.
2. Obtain proper restraint and padding for use with wrist and ankle restraints. Never restrain all four extremities unless absolutely necessary.	Padding protects circulation to distal portion of extremity.
Implementation	
1. Follow physician order and/or facility restraint policy.	Directions are provided.
2. Wash hands.	Prevents the spread of microorganisms.
3. Apply appropriate type of restraint:	
a. **Wrist or ankle** (extremity restraint)	Designed to immobilize one or more extremities.
1) If using Kerlix gauze, make a clove hitch by forming a figure eight and then picking up the loops.	The clove hitch does not tighten when pulled.

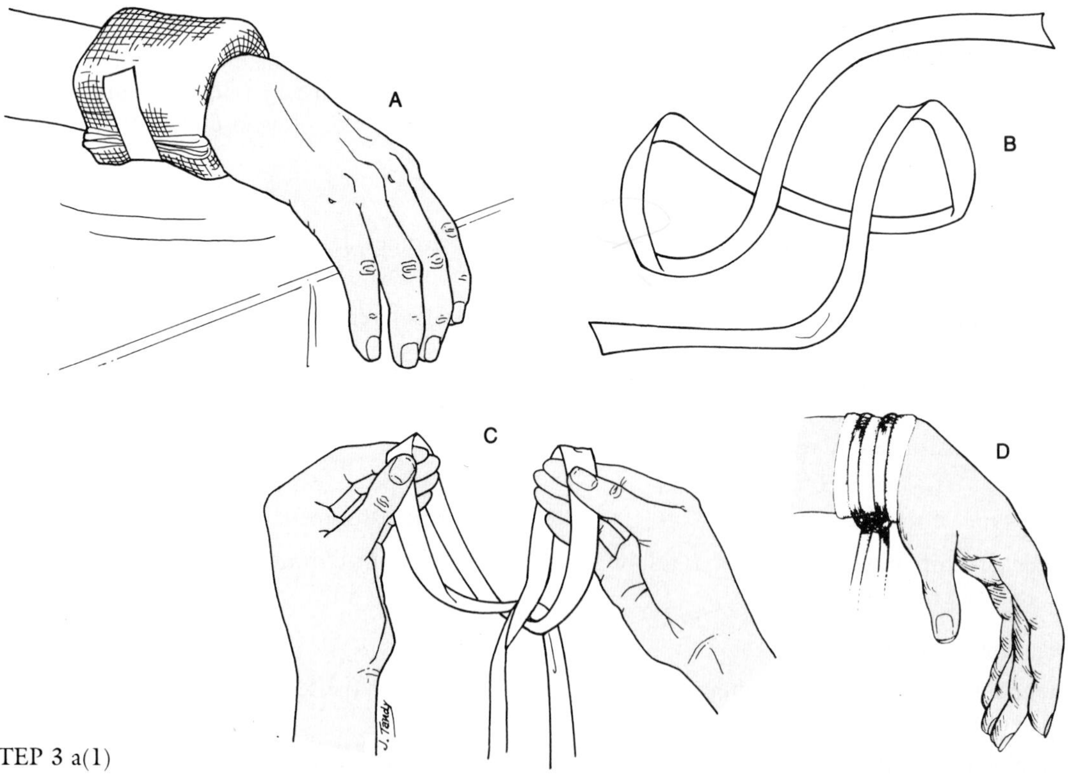

STEP 3 a(1)

SKILL 17-1 APPLYING RESTRAINTS—cont'd

Nursing action	Rationale
Implementation—cont'd	
2) Place gauze or padding around the extremity.	The use of padding decreases injury to underlying skin.
3) Slip the wrist(s) or ankle(s) through loops directly over the padding—if using a commercially made restraint, wrap the padded portion of the restraint around affected extremity, thread tie through slit in restraint, and fasten to second tie with a secure knot.	
4) Secure ends of ties to bed frame, NOT SIDE RAILS.	If side rails are lowered with the restraint attached, injury could result.

STEP 3 a(4)

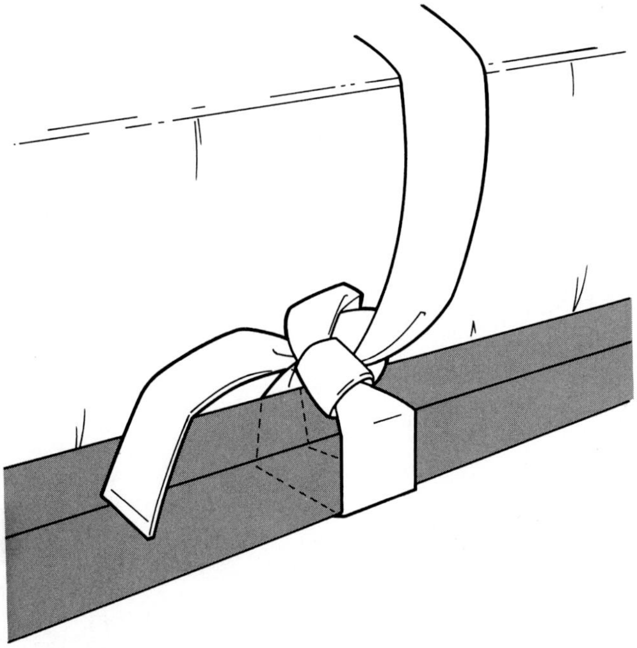

5) Leave as much slack as possible (1 to 2 inches).	Provides for movement.
6) Palpate pulses below the restraint.	Ensures that restraint is not too tight, thus occluding circulation.
7) Monitor for skin impairment.	Excessive pressure may lead to loss of skin integrity.
8) Assess extremity distal to restraint at least every 2 hours.	Identifies any problems or need to remove or adjust restraint.
9) Remove restraint on one extremity at a time at least every 2 hours for 5 minutes.	Allows supervised movement of extremity, enhances circulation, and reduces apprehension.

Continued.

SKILL 17-1 APPLYING RESTRAINTS—cont'd

Nursing action	Rationale
Implementation—cont'd	
b. **Elbow restraint**	Often used with children to prevent elbow flexion so they cannot disturb tubes, catheters, and dressings.
1) Place restraint (a piece of fabric with slots for the insertion of tongue blades to keep the elbow straight) over the elbow or elbows.	

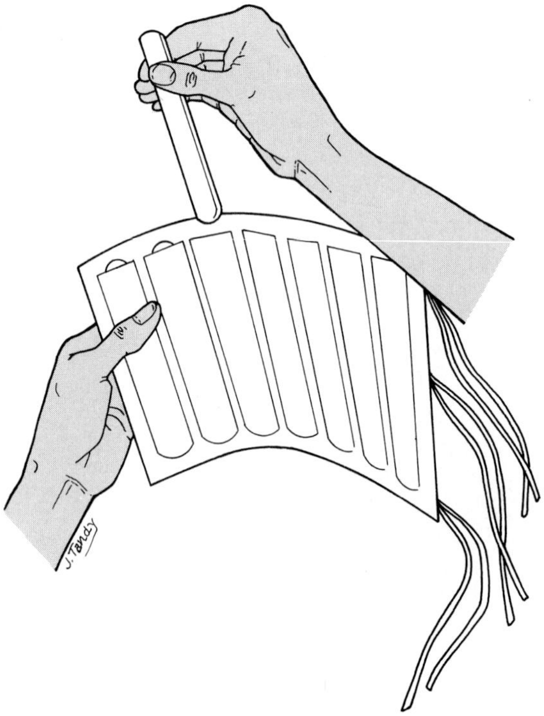

STEP 3 b

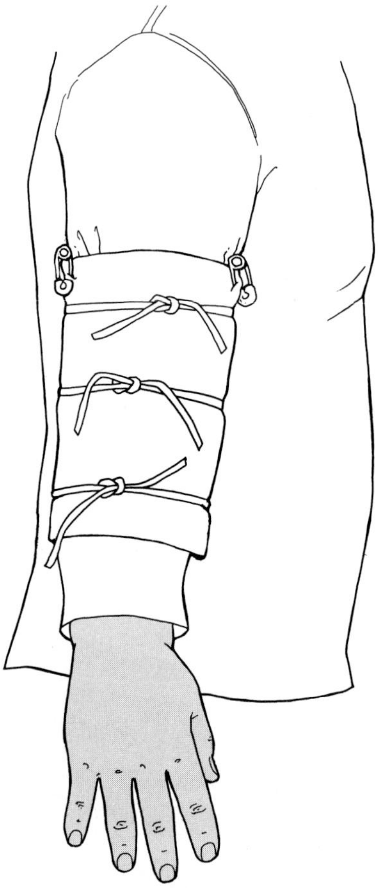
STEP 3 b(2)

Nursing action	Rationale
2) Wrap restraint snugly, tying the restraint at the top.	For small infants, tie or pin restraints to their shirts.
3) Monitor position of restraint, circulation, and skin condition frequently.	
c. **Vest** (may be referred to as the wrap jacket or chest restraint)	
1) Apply restraint over the patient's gown.	Protects the skin.
2) Put vest on patient with V-shaped opening in the front.	If vest is on backwards and patient becomes restless, choking could result.
3) Pull tie at end of vest flap across the chest and slip tie through slit on opposite side of vest.	

SKILL 17-1

APPLYING RESTRAINTS—cont'd

Nursing action	Rationale
Implementation—cont'd	
4) Wrap the other end of the flap across patient and tie the straps to frame of bed or behind wheelchair.	Helps secure vest restraint to the patient.

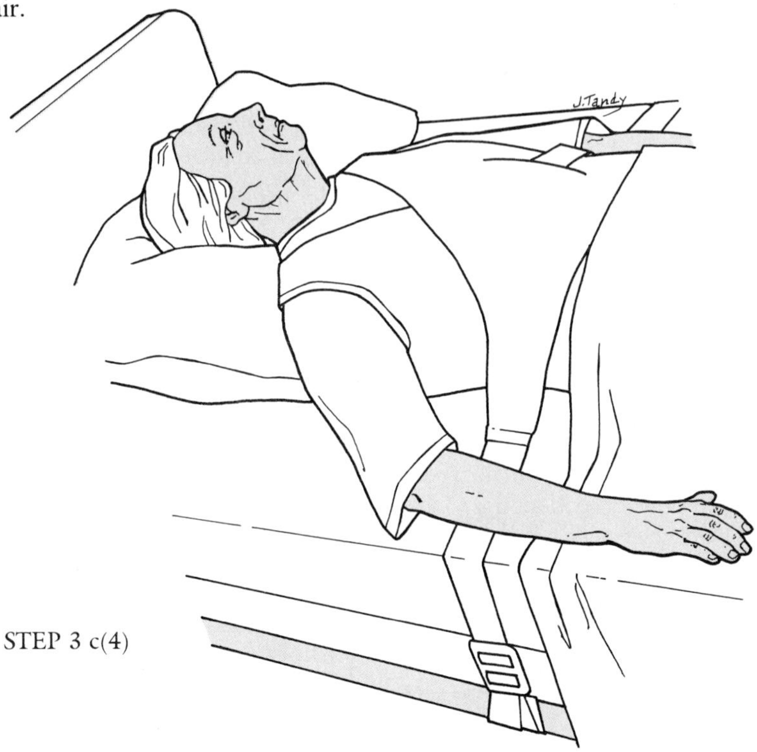

STEP 3 c(4)

Nursing action	Rationale
5) There should be room for a fist in the space between the vest and the patient.	Determines the vest is not too tight.
6) Monitor respiratory status.	Respiratory distress may occur if there is restriction from the vest.
4. A square knot rather than a regular knot should be used to secure the restraint to bed frame.	A square knot can be released quickly in an emergency.

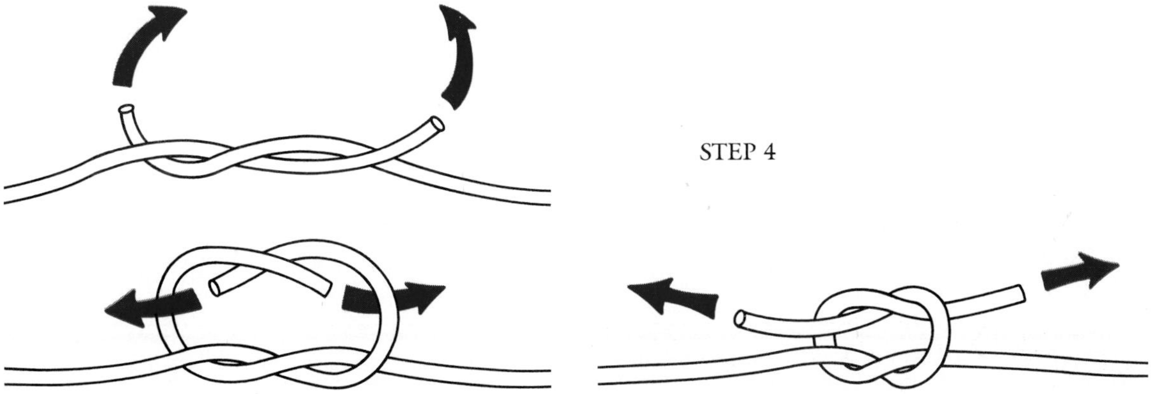

STEP 4

Continued.

SKILL 17-1

APPLYING RESTRAINTS—cont'd

Nursing action	Rationale
Implementation—cont'd	
5. Restraints should be removed at least every 4 hours; patient should NOT be left unattended during this time.	Patient's position can be changed and skin inspected.
6. Massage skin beneath restraint—lotion or powder may be applied if indicated.	Increases circulation.
7. Check frequently for tangled ties or pressure points from knots; adjust restraint as needed.	Excessive pressure leads to loss of skin integrity and impaired circulation.
8. Restraints should be secured so that the patient cannot untie them.	Injury may result.
9. Monitor physical and mental status, circulation, and need for restraints.	Restraints should be removed when they are no longer required.
10. Apply restraints with gentleness and compassion.	
Evaluation	
1. The restraint is adequate for the individual patient's condition: prevents interruption of treatment or therapy and/or prevents patient from falling from bed, chair, or wheelchair.	The correct application of the appropriate restraints promotes safety and comfort while restraints are indicated.
2. Restraints are correctly applied.	Correct application prevents injury to patient.
3. Assess for any related problems, i.e., to the skin or to the musculoskeletal system.	Complications can be prevented with timely intervention.

Sample charting

DATE	TIME	NOTES
12/4/90	22:30	Restless. Thrashing about in bed. Attempting to get out of bed. Explained to patient danger of falling. Attempts to quiet patient unsuccessful.
	22:45	Dr. D. Bradley notified. Orders to restrain patient with wrap jacket noted.
	22:55	Wrap jacket applied. Fastened to underside of bed frame. Patient offered no resistance.
	23:15	Quiet. Color pink. Pulse, 82. Fluids offered.
	23:45	Remains quiet. Respirations even and unlabored.

(*nurse's signature*)

SKILL 17-1 APPLYING RESTRAINTS—cont'd

SPECIAL CONCERNS

- A physician's order is usually required before restraints are applied.
- Some facilities may have specific requirements for restraint use in certain situations (e.g., the presence of an endotracheal tube).
- Older adults' skin is frequently very thin and fragile. Skin impairment can result also because of a decreased sensitivity to pressure. The older adult should be restrained loosely with soft restraints. The skin should be assessed more frequently, at least every 2 hours.
- A comprehensive nursing assessment of the patient's potential for injury and/or treatment-related need for restraints is critical before restraints are supplied.
- The use of restraints increases the need for observation and ongoing assessment.
- While restraints are in use, the patient will need assistance with activities of daily living.
- Restraining a patient without a physician's order or without a reasonable cause could result in being charged with false imprisonment.

PATIENT TEACHING

- Explain to the patient and members of the family why restraints are necessary.
- Provide information about the type of restraint to be used and approximate time frame for use.
- Inform patient and family that patient will still receive comfort measures such as repositioning and limb exercises.

NURSING HOME VARIATIONS

Recent legislation has greatly affected the use of restraints in the long-term facility. Under the Omnibus Budget Reconciliation Act (OBRA) of 1987, resident rights are specifically addressed in terms of restraint use. Restraints may be used only to ensure the physical safety of the resident or other residents. There must be a written order by the physician detailing the duration and circumstances under which the restraints are to be used.

SKILL 17-2: ENSURING FIRE SAFETY

Guidelines

Both the home and the health care facility are at risk for fires. Fires in the health care facility are often related to smoking in bed or faulty electrical equipment. Approximately 8100 hospital fires and 4300 nursing home fires are reported each year.

An established fire safety program is mandatory for all health care facilities. Most facilities have a safety committee that is actively involved in establishing and monitoring prevention and fire education programs. Fire prevention includes good housekeeping, maintenance, and employee discipline.

The housekeeping responsibilities include the elimination of all unnecessary combustible material, whereas maintenance responsibilities include ensuring the proper functioning of fire protection devices, such as alarms, extinguishers, and sprinklers. All mechanical and electrical equipment also must be regularly inspected and maintained to minimize fire hazards.

All employees should know the telephone number and procedure for reporting a fire, as well as the location of the nearest alarms and firefighting equipment. Additionally, health care workers must know their roles in the overall hospital evacuation plan. Checking for fire hazards should be ongoing.

An important element in any fire safety program is knowing what type of fire extinguisher to use on different types of fires.

Paper, wood, and cloth fires require a type **A** fire extinguisher.

Flammable liquid fires, such as those caused by grease and anesthetics, require a type **B** fire extinguisher.

Electrical fires require a type **C** fire extinguisher.

Fire extinguishers marked **ABC** can be used on any type of fire. Knowing which type of extinguisher is on the unit *before* a fire occurs is vital. Most fire safety programs afford health care workers the opportunity to handle the different types of fire extinguishers.

In the event of fire, patients in immediate danger should be rescued and then the facility's procedure should be followed for activating the fire alarm and reporting the location and extent of the fire. Measures should then be taken to contain or extinguish the fire until firemen arrive.

Measures to contain or extinguish the fire include closing doors and windows, turning off oxygen and electrical equipment, and using the appropriate fire extinguisher. By remembering the formula **RACE** (**R**escue patients, sound the **A**larm, **C**onfine the fire, and **E**xtinguish or **E**vacuate), nurses can be prepared when safety is threatened by fire.

Enforcing the facility's smoking policy and monitoring for potential electrical hazards help *prevent* fires. For example, frayed or broken electrical cords or a faulty piece of equipment should not be used. The maintenance department should be notified of any defects in the equipment. Any shocks felt while using equipment must be reported. *No Smoking* rules must be monitored carefully with patients receiving oxygen. The safety of both the patient and the staff depends on the staff's knowledge of fire prevention guidelines and fire procedures.

Purposes

The nurse is knowledgeable of fire safety practices and fire procedures for the following reasons:

- to prevent or decrease the likelihood of fires
- to provide safety and protection for patients, visitors, and health care workers
- to be prepared to respond to a simulated (fire drill) or actual fire

Related Knowledge and Skills

To be prepared to function effectively in preventing fires and in a fire emergency, the nurse should fulfill the following responsibilities:

- periodically review the facility's overall and unit fire emergency procedures, including patient evacuation procedures
- know where emergency exits are
- know where fire alarms and fire extinguishers are and how to appropriately use them
- participate, when possible, in fire drills to become familiar with the protocols

SKILL 17-3 DISASTER PLANNING

Guidelines

Disaster planning or emergency preparedness enables rescuers to respond effectively and efficiently when confronted with a disaster situation. A disaster situation is an uncontrollable, unexpected, psychologically shocking event. The disaster situation is unique and directly affects health care facilities. Examples of natural threats to safety are earthquakes, hurricanes, floods, and tornados. Bombings, arson, riots, and hostage taking represent acts of violence carried out by people.

Factors that affect disaster response include the time of the day, the scope and duration of the triggering event, readiness of the health care facility, personnel, equipment, and procedures, and the extent to which the various community agencies and institutions collaborate with each other. Health care facilities are expected to receive victims and survivors and to assist rescuers.

Disasters are also referred to as *external* or *internal*. The external disaster originates outside the health care facility and results in an influx of casualties brought to the facility. The emergency department is the main focus of activity. There is no immediate safety threat to staff, patients, or hospital property.

The internal disaster represents an extraordinary situation that is brought about by events within the health care facility. The organization's ability to function normally is threatened. The internal disaster often threatens the safety of patients, visitors, staff, and facility property.

Disaster planning represents the means by which health care facilities and personnel meet the responsibilities associated with managing the disaster. The conduction of disaster drills on a routine basis helps ensure that health care personnel respond effectively. Personnel should be familiar with the location and contents of the facility's disaster manual. Generally, disaster manuals specify departmental responsibilities, chain of command, callback procedures, assignment procedure, patient evacuation procedure and routes, procedures for the receipt and management of casualties, and policies related to the overall management of supplies and equipment.

Purposes

The nurse is knowledgeable of the health care facility's overall disaster plan for the following reasons:

- to recognize the various codes used by the health care facility to alert physicians and hospital personnel to the various emergencies affecting the facility
- to be prepared to respond to a simulated (drill) or actual disaster emergency

Related Knowledge and Skills

To function effectively in the event of a disaster, the nurse should do the following:

- periodically review the established facility's protocols related to disaster-preparedness
- participate, when possible, in disaster drills to become familiar with the protocols

SKILL 17-2 FIRE SAFETY

Nursing action	Rationale
Assessment	
1. Identify patient's age, sensory impairments, level of mobility, ability to comprehend instructions, and overall need for protection.	Protects and assists patient in interpreting environmental stimuli relevant to safety.
2. In case of fire, identify type of fire extinguisher needed.	The appropriate fire extinguisher must be used for each type of fire.
3. If indicated, assess patients for type of evacuation assistance needed.	Individuals at risk for injury must be moved to a safer area.
Nursing diagnosis	
1. Potential for injury, related to fire hazards in the environment (e.g., smoking in bed, faulty electric wires, and oxygen in use).	Patient is at risk for injury because of fire hazards in the evironment.
Planning	
1. Reduce the potential for fire-related injuries by: a. Knowing the location of fire alarm boxes and fire extinguishers. b. Knowing where the fire exits are. c. Being familiar with the hospital fire safety program and protocols for evacuation. d. Keeping hallways free of unnecessary supplies, furniture, and other obstacles. e. Checking to see that electrical equipment is operating safely.	Saves valuable time and improves overall performance.
2. Participate, when possible, in disaster drills.	Drills are helpful in evaluating the overall fire safety program and are required by accrediting agencies.
Implementation	
1. Follow facility fire plan in the event of a fire.	Plan outlines procedures to follow.
2. Provide clear explanations to patients and visitors in a calm manner.	Anxiety hinders understanding of situation and ability to follow instructions.
3. Assist with evacuations if needed: a. Usually patients are moved horizontally, i.e., out of rooms, across halls, and through next set of fire doors.	The fire and its potential for spreading may necessitate movement to a safer area.
b. If smoke or fire prevents the nurse from moving patients across the floor, proceed vertically down to a lower level.	Never use elevators to escape.
4. If a patient cannot walk or be moved by bed, stretcher, or wheelchair from the fire area, the patient may need to be carried.	Use the carrying method that is safe for both the nurse and the patient; fire department personnel can help with the evacuation.
Evaluation	
1. The immediate environment of the patient is safe from potential fire hazards.	Fire safety practices can help *prevent* fires.
2. In the event of a fire, established protocols are followed.	The emergency can be handled rapidly and appropriately.

Continued.

SKILL 17-2

FIRE SAFETY—cont'd

SPECIAL CONCERNS

- Certain areas of the health care facility require additional fire safety programs and precautions. For example, fires and smoke inhalation are potential problems associated with the use of lasers in surgery and with oxygen therapy.
- In the event of a fire, patients on life support systems may need manual respiratory support with an Ambu bag.
- Fire safety education programs are necessary to meet the requirements of accrediting agencies, such as the Joint Commission on Accreditation of Healthcare Organizations.
- Learning experiences are provided through participation in fire drills and formal critiques of the activity.
- Many facilities are adopting a *No Smoking* policy to promote a smoke-free environment for patients and employees.

PATIENT TEACHING

- The nurse should use the fire drill procedure as an opportunity to talk about fire safety.

HOME HEALTH VARIATIONS

Today, as more patients are discharged with follow-up care in the home, the nurse has an excellent opportunity to evaluate fire safety practices in the home environment. Patients who are elderly or patients with mobility limitations may require the assistance of the nurse to help achieve an environment that is free of potential fire hazards. Instructions should be given about the proper use of monitoring or therapy equipment used. Several electrical circuits should be used to prevent overloading. Electrical appliances and equipment should not be used near sinks, bathtubs, or showers.

Smoking practices should be reviewed with instructions to not smoke in bed or when sleepy. Smoking by either the patient, family, or visitors should not be permitted in areas where oxygen is used. The installation of fire alarms and detectors should be encouraged, as well as the purchase of a portable fire extinguisher.

SKILL 17-3 DISASTER PLANNING

Nursing action	Rationale
Assessment	
1. Identify the type of disaster emergency by recognizing the code that is used to announce the specified disaster.	Unfamiliarity with the codes could result in loss of valuable time and cause injury to patients and/or personnel.
2. Identify patient's age, sensory impairments, level of mobility, ability to comprehend instructions, and overall need for protection.	Provides protection and assists patient in interpreting environmental stimuli relevant to safety.
3. If indicated, assess patients for possible discharge and/or transfer.	Space may be needed for disaster victims.
Nursing diagnosis	
1. Potential for injury, related to environmental hazards.	Patient is at risk for injury because of hazards in the environment.
Planning	
1. Review facility disaster plan frequently to update knowledge.	Information helps health care workers anticipate role in the event of a disaster.
2. Know own particular responsibilities in a disaster emergency.	Valuable time is saved and overall performance improved.
3. Participate, when possible, in disaster drills.	Drills help evaluate the overall plan and are required by accrediting agencies.
Implementation	
1. Follow facility disaster plan for particular type of disaster.	The plan works best when personnel respond appropriately.
2. If an actual disaster occurs when off duty, health care personnel should report to the facility.	Additional personnel, e.g., student nurses and clinical faculty, could assist with inpatient care to free staff for more critical disaster victims.
3. Provide clear explanations to patients and visitors in a calm manner.	Anxiety limits understanding of situation and instructions.
4. Assist with "early" discharges and transfers as indicated.	Space may be needed for disaster victims.
5. If an internal disaster occurs, assist with planned evacuations if indicated.	The disaster may necessitate movement to a safer area.
Evaluation	
1. Compare actual outcomes and performances with disaster-preparedness plan (usually a critique session is held).	Allows facility to examine whether plan accomplished goals and objectives; necessary changes can be made.

Continued.

SKILL 17-3

DISASTER PLANNING—cont'd

FOLLOW-UP ACTIVITIES

A disaster can and does change lives. Disasters, because they are sudden and their scope is impossible to predict, cause unexpected emotional changes. Health care personnel are also at risk. Disaster planners should recognize that any personnel directly involved in the facility response will experience some level of emotional or somatic stress symptoms. Mental health services are valuable resources that should be included in the overall planned response to disaster. After a disaster, crisis support teams have also been formed to assist families and victims of disasters.

SPECIAL CONCERNS

- Protection of inpatients, as well as casualties from a disaster, is a top priority.
- The development of the **disaster-preparedness plan** is an evolving and ongoing process.
- The disaster-preparedness plan must prepare the facility and health care workers for both external and internal disasters.
- Learning experiences are provided through disaster drills and formal critiques of the responses.
- Community agencies and resources are incorporated into the overall plan.

PATIENT TEACHING

The amount of information the patient and family has about the situation (drill, disaster event) will affect their ability to cooperate and participate in any planned or unplanned activity.

NURSING HOME VARIATIONS

Nursing home residents may also require evacuation and relocation because of an internal disaster situation. The successful nursing home disaster-preparedness plan, like those for hospitals, outlines the sequence of events to be followed. Residents will require some type of identification card. At the designated triage site, nurses will decide where residents will go. Residents may require admission to a hospital or other building, such as a school or church, for temporary shelter and care. The disaster plan must include instructions and guidelines for what is to be done after the relocation is completed. Families and physicians must be notified. A log is usually kept to document events and transfers as they occur.

SKILL 17-4: ACCIDENTAL POISONING

Guidelines

Childhood **poisoning** is one of the major causes of death in children under 5 years of age. Whaley and Wong[14] note that there are more than 500 toxic substances in the average home. Although legislation that was passed in the early 1970s required the use of child safety packaging for certain substances, a significant number of accidental poisonings continue to occur. Specific antidotes and treatments are not available for all types of poisons.

The older adult is also at risk. Changes associated with aging interfere with the individual's ability to absorb or excrete drugs. Older adults may "share" drugs with friends or limit their medications because of the expense. Changes in eyesight may lead to an accidental ingestion. If there is any memory impairment, elderly patients may forget when they last took either prescribed or over-the-counter medication.

Hospitalized patients can be at risk for accidental poisoning because there are many poisonous substances in the environment (e.g., cleaning solutions). Drugs, of course, are potentially hazardous if prepared or administered inappropriately. Human carelessness can cause errors. Drug administration procedures should always be followed (see Chapter 25). Staff-development inservice programs that present new drugs or provide updated information on frequently used drugs should be attended when scheduled.

To prevent poisoning, toxic agents should be removed from areas where accidental poisoning could occur. Toxic or poisonous substances should not be removed from their original containers because substances may be incorrectly identified. Poisonous substances should be labeled conspicuously and after use should immediately be stored appropriately.

Poison control centers are valuable sources of information when poisoning is suspected or does occur. Information received from the center can aid in both treatment and referral if needed. Most health care facilities also have posted instructions about how to handle poisoning cases. The nurse should know where these are located. (See Chapter 54.)

Purposes

The nurse is aware of substances and practices that may contribute to accidental poisoning and is knowledgeable of procedures to be followed for the following reasons:

- to prevent or decrease the likelihood of accidental poisoning
- to take appropriate measures in the event of a poisoning

Related Knowledge and Skills

In the event of a poisoning, the nurse should know the following:

- the location of the emergency instructions for handling victims of poisonings

SKILL 17-4 ACCIDENTAL POISONING

Nursing action	Rationale
Assessment	
1. Obtain an accurate history: a. Identify the route (e.g., injected, ingested, inhaled), type, and amount of poisonous substances(s) received. b. Determine how long ago it happened. c. Obtain a history of allergies, prescribed medications, medical problems, and general state of physical and mental health.	To identify possible antidote(s) and method of treatment needed.
2. Assess for changes in mental status and the presence of motor and sensory deficits.	Incomplete data may result in incorrect identification of patient's health care needs.
Nursing diagnosis	
1. Potential for poisoning, related to the ingestion, injection, inhalation, or exposure to a poisonous substance.	The individual is at high risk for accidental poisoning (e.g., treatment related, maturational, or environmental factors).
Planning	
1. Reduce the potential for accidental poisoning by (1) being aware of potentially poisonous substances (e.g., drugs, plants, and cleaning solutions); (2) informing patients and families about how to handle a poisoning emergency; and (3) ensuring that poisonous substances are labeled, locked, and out of the reach of children.	The risk of accidental poisoning can be greatly reduced. Quick and appropriate action can decrease the effects of the poisoning.
2. Know where emergency instructions are located.	The procedure and guidelines for handling the emergency are outlined.
3. Know the number of the poison control center and be prepared to provide information about the poison.	The poison control center will provide information needed to treat the patient or offer referral assistance.
Implementation	
1. Notify the poison control center and/or follow facility protocols.	Treatment guidelines will be furnished.
2. If instructed to use ipecac syrup to induce vomiting, follow dose instructions (see Chapter 54). a. Make sure gag reflex is intact.	Ipecac syrup is considered the safest and most effective way to induce emesis.
b. Ipecac syrup should be administered with adequate amounts of fluids.	Home remedy methods, such as drinking salt water, are often unsafe and ineffective.
c. If instructed, save emesis; note the presence or absence of such material as pill particles.	For toxicological analysis.
d. Place individual with head turned to side.	Reduces risk of aspiration.

SKILL 17-4

ACCIDENTAL POISONING—cont'd

Nursing action	Rationale
Implementation—cont'd	
3. Do not induce vomiting if poisoning is related to the following substances: household cleaners, lye, furniture polish, grease, or petroleum products.	Vomiting can increase risk of internal burns.
4. Do not induce vomiting in an unconscious individual.	Vomiting increases danger of aspiration.
5. Continue to monitor vital signs and response to treatment.	Ongoing assessment is a part of the treatment.
Evaluation	
1. The immediate environment is safe from potential poisoning hazards (e.g., poisonous substances are labeled, locked, and properly stored).	Safety practices can reduce the risk of accidental poisoning.
2. In the event of an accidental poisoning, established protocols are followed.	The emergency is handled rapidly and appropriately.

SPECIAL CONCERNS

- Drug administration policies and procedures should always be followed. Nurses should have their dosage calculations checked, especially if a mixed or prepared drug is to be infused.
- Nurses should keep informed of new medications and recommended dosages.
- Cleaning solutions and disinfectants should be properly labeled and stored.
- Substances from unmarked containers should never be used.

PATIENT TEACHING

- Inform patients and parents about potential sources of poisoning found in the home and appropriate safety precautions.
- Inform patients and parents about poison control centers.
- Teach basic interventions to follow in the case of a poisoning.
- Inform that safety items, such as ipecac syrup or stickers with poison center information, should be available for use.
- Teach that to decrease problems associated with taking medication, label medications in print large enough to be seen, write instructions in a clear manner, or use a color-coded calendar or chart and pill holders to assist in proper administration of medications. Instruct to not give medications to others or take medication from others.
- Instruct to keep all medications, both prescribed and over-the-counter, out of the reach of children, to discard medications that do not have labels or medications no longer taken, and to check expiration dates.

REFERENCES AND SUGGESTED READINGS

1. Collins HL: Who'd survive a fire on your unit? RN 51(7):32, 1988.
2. Costa L: Residents' rights and the use of restraints under OBRA, Contemp Long Term Care 12(10):48, 1989.
3. Davis NM and Cohen MR: Today's poisons, Nurs '89 19(1):49, 1989.
4. Farrell J: Nursing care of the older person, Philadelphia, 1990, JB Lippincott Co.
5. Hayes G, Goodwin T, and Miars B: After disaster, Am J Nurs 90(2):61, 1990.
6. Jacobson E: New hospital hazards, Am J Nurs 90(2):36, 1990.
7. Luckman J and Sorensen KC: Medical-surgical nursing, ed 3, Philadelphia, 1987, WB Saunders Co.
8. McHutchion E and Morse JM: Releasing restraints, J Gerontol Nurs 15(2):16, 1989.
9. Needham JF: Planning for disaster, Nurs Homes 36(1):28, 1987.
10. Seliger JS and Simoneau JK: Emergency preparedness, Rockville, Md, 1986, Aspen Publishers, Inc.
11. Steele P and Spyker DA: Poisonings, Pediatr Clin North Am 32(1):77, 1985.
12. Turner JT: Handbook of hospital security and safety, Rockville, Md, 1988, Aspen Publishers, Inc.
13. Using restraints, Nurs '88 18(4):15, 1988.
14. Whaley LF and Wong DL: Nursing care of infants and children, ed 4, St Louis, 1991, Mosby–Year Book, Inc.

CHAPTER CHALLENGE

STUDY QUESTIONS

1. Restraints are frequently used in the hospital setting to prevent patient injury. Which of the following statements is correct:
   a. Restraints often decrease anxiety as the patient feels safer.
   b. All elderly patients should have some type of restraint at night.
   c. As much freedom of movement as possible should be allowed when the restraints are applied.
   d. When used to prevent injury from falling out of bed, the soft restraint should be tied to the side rail.
2. The initial step taken to protect the patient in the event of a fire is to:
   a. Notify the fire department
   b. Disconnect the oxygen supply
   c. Use any extinguisher on the fire
   d. Remove the patient from the area
3. You are working the 7 AM to 3 PM on the adult surgical unit and hear the code announced for an external disaster emergency. Which event best represents this type of situation:
   a. A school bus accident
   b. A bomb threat in the mail room
   c. A hostage-taking event in the emergency room
   d. An electrical fire in the maintenance department
4. Which factor MOST places a child at risk for specific types of injuries:
   a. Sex of the child
   b. Overall health
   c. Educational level
   d. Developmental level
5. An appropriate nursing intervention when caring for a patient requiring the use of restraints is to:
   a. Monitor the skin for signs of impairment
   b. Remove the restraints once every 24 hours
   c. Secure the ends of the ties to the side rails
   d. Ensure that the restraints are in place at all times
6. Your assessment of the patient who requires the use of an extremity restraint reveals an edematous extremity. The MOST appropriate nursing action is to:
   a. Elevate the involved extremity
   b. Increase the padding around the extremity
   c. Notify the physician for a different type of restraint
   d. Remove the restraint and watch the patient more closely
7. Type **C** fire extinguishers are required for the following type of fire:
   a. Paper
   b. Cloth
   c. Grease
   d. Electrical
8. Which action indicates the need for further fire safety instruction:
   a. Fire exits and corridors are kept clear
   b. A *No Smoking* sign is posted when oxygen is in use
   c. A heating pad cord is taped when a frayed area is noted
   d. Facility smoking policies are a part of the admission procedure
9. Vomiting would MOST likely be induced if poisoning is related to the ingestion of the following substance(s):
   a. Lye
   b. Petroleum products
   c. Household cleaners
   d. Salicylates, such as aspirin
10. A patient is brought to the emergency department for treatment of an accidental poisoning. The first step in the treatment is:
    a. To induce vomiting
    b. To assess the patient
    c. To place the patient in an upright position
    d. To notify the poison control center

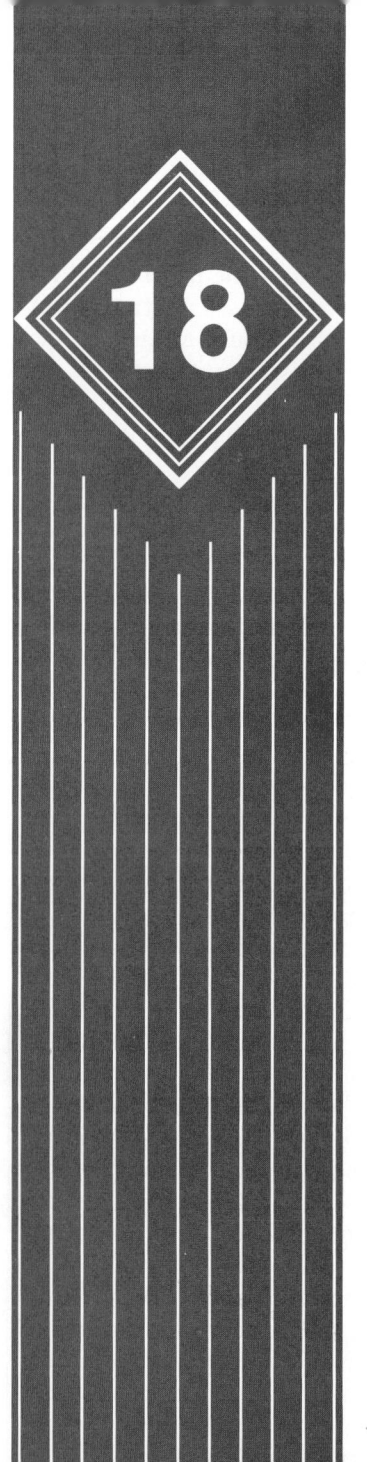

18

Body Mechanics

LORA JEAN ALLEY

LEARNING OBJECTIVES

After reading this chapter, the student should be able to do the following:

- Define the key terms.
- State the principles of body mechanics.
- Demonstrate using appropriate body mechanics.
- Describe the purposes for properly positioning the patient.
- Demonstrate positioning in Fowler's, supine (dorsal), Sims', side-lying, prone, dorsal recumbent, lithotomy.
- Explain range-of-motion exercises.
- Identify complications caused by inactivity.
- Explain appropriate technique for turning, moving, lifting, and carrying the patient.

SKILLS

18-1 Using appropriate body mechanics

18-2 Positioning the patient
- dorsal
- dorsal recumbent
- Fowler's
- knee-chest
- lithotomy
- orthopneic
- prone
- semi-Fowler's
- Sims'
- Trendelenburg

18-3 Performing range-of-motion exercises

18-4 Moving the patient
- lifting and moving the patient
- turning the patient
- dangling the patient
- logrolling the patient
- transferring the patient

18-5 Using the lift for moving the patient

KEY TERMS

Define the following:

- abduct
- adduct
- alignment
- base of support
- body mechanics
- contracture
- dorsal (supine)
- dorsiflexion
- extension
- hyperextension
- joint
- lithotomy
- orthopneic
- pronate
- prone
- recumbent
- ROM
- semi-Fowler's
- Sims'
- supinate
- Trendelenburg

SKILL 18-1: USING APPROPRIATE BODY MECHANICS

Using appropriate body mechanics or movements protects the nurse's large muscle groups from injury and provides safety for the patient when ambulating. Also the patient must be taught appropriate positioning for home care, and a family member must learn to assist the patient at home.

The nurse uses body mechanics daily in making beds, assisting the patient to walk, carrying supplies and equipment, lifting, providing patient care, and carrying out other procedures.

Understanding **body mechanics** includes understanding how certain muscle groups are used. The musculoskeletal system must be protected to prevent injury to the patient and nurse. The nurse must learn self-protection, as well as teach the patient to protect himself.

Guidelines

The nurse must maintain a wide **base of support** when standing. Keeping the feet slightly apart helps provide better stability (Fig. 18-1). This stability prevents becoming overbalanced while carrying out an activity such as assisting the patient in and out of bed or ambulating in the room.

Equilibrium, or balance, is maintained by skeletal muscles and the nervous system and aids appropriate body alignment when lifting, bending, moving, and other activities. The back can be well protected when the nurse bends the knees before attempting these activities.

If the base of support is widened in the direction of movement, less effort is required to carry out an activity. Standing in front of the object helps avoid twisting of the spine.

When stooping, the nurse flexes or bends the hips and knees and maintains appropriate body alignment. The nurse should avoid bending from the waist, since this will, in time, strain the lower back (Fig. 18-2).

Using large muscle groups helps in performing a greater work load more safely. The more muscle groups used, the more evenly the work load is distributed. The nurse's back is vulnerable to stress and to potential injury because of the physical work required in nursing.

Adjusting the working level to one of comfort and ease for the nurse helps prevent undue stress and strain of the back muscles. This can be accomplished by adjusting the height of the bed appropriate to the height of the nurse.

Carrying objects close to the midline of the body (Fig. 18-3), avoiding reaching too far, avoiding lifting when other means of movement are available, and alternating periods of rest and activity are ways in which both the patient and nurse can be protected from injury.

The appropriate use of body mechanics should be practiced daily and used in personal life. Maintaining appropriate body alignment is the key

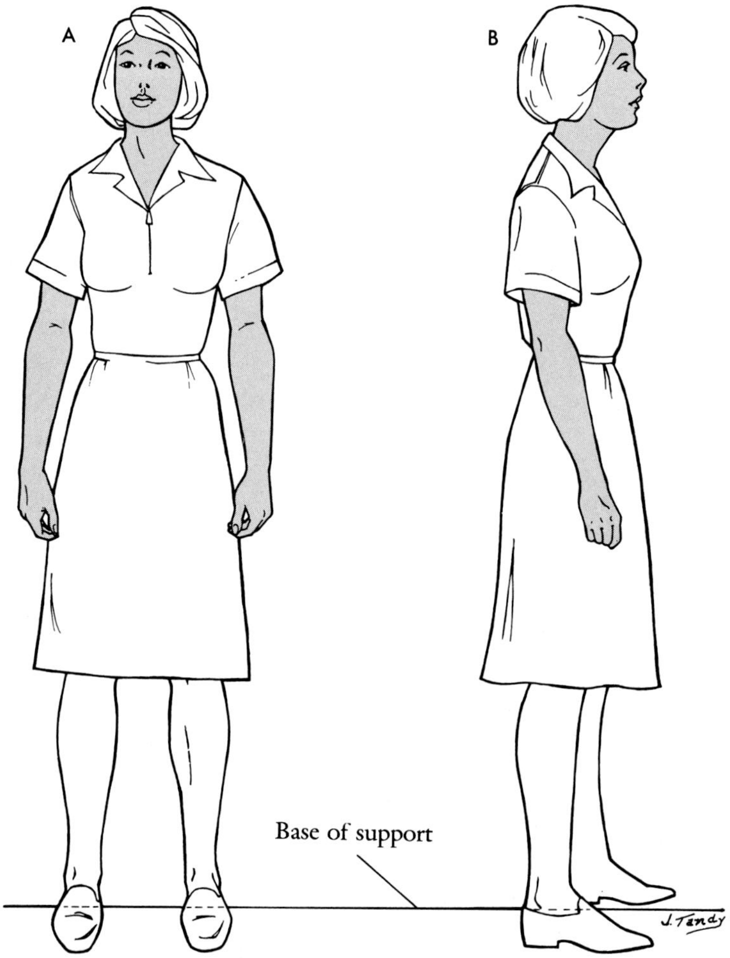

FIG. 18-1 **A,** Anterior view of adult in good body alignment with feet apart for a wide base of support. **B,** Lateral view of adult with good posture and alignment.

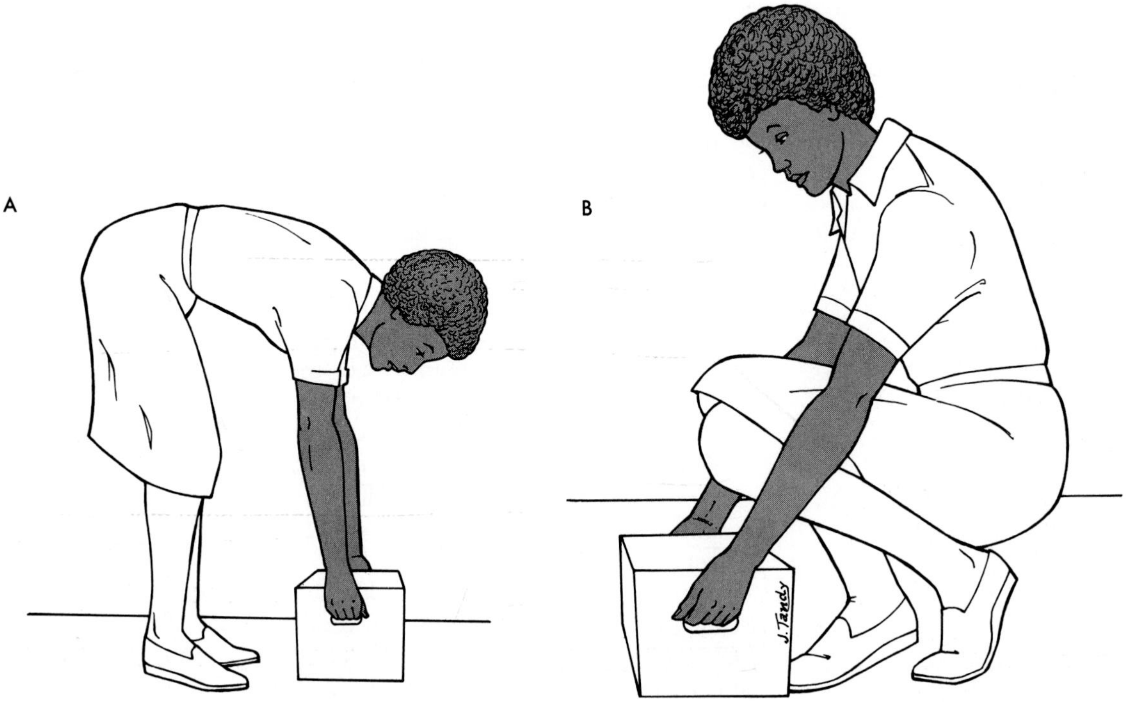

FIG. 18-2 **A,** Picking up a box with poor body mechanics. **B,** Picking up a box with good body mechanics.

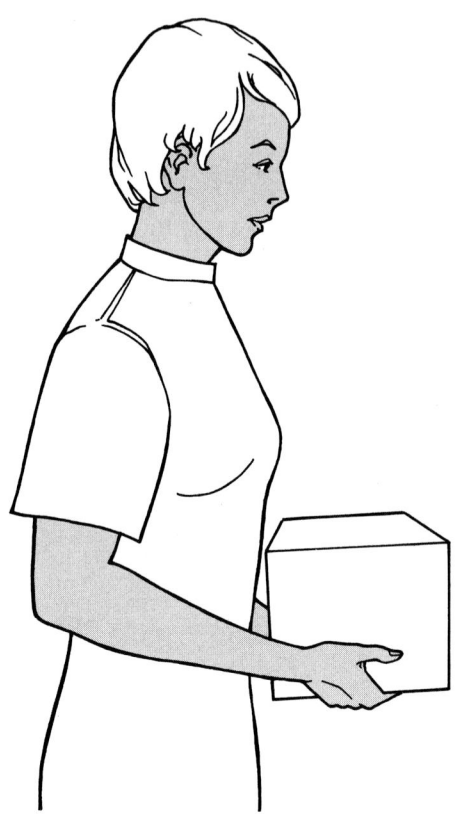

FIG. 18-3 Box carried close to the body and base of support.

factor in proper body mechanics. The term **alignment** refers to the relationship of various body parts to each other. Alignment helps balance and helps coordinate movements smoothly and effectively.

Purposes

The nurse uses appropriate body mechanics for the following reasons:

- to prevent strain and injury to the patient
- to prevent strain and injury to the nurse
- to use appropriate technique when moving the patient
- to provide safety for the patient

SUPPLIES/EQUIPMENT

chair

Related Knowledge and Skills

Before performing body mechanics, the nurse should understand the following:

- communication (see Chapter 4)
- documentation (see Chapter 6)
- vital signs (see Chapter 14)
- medical asepsis (see Chapter 16)
- safety measures (see Chapter 17)

SKILL 18-1

USING APPROPRIATE BODY MECHANICS

Nursing action	Rationale
1. Position feet 6 to 8 inches apart.	Provides adequate base of support.
2. Align and balance weight on both feet.	Distributes weight evenly.
3. Flex knees slightly.	Prevents **hyperextension** (extreme or abnormal stretching).
4. Tilt pelvis forward by pulling buttocks inward.	Helps straighten lumbar curve of spine.
5. Hold abdomen in and up.	Provides support and reduces muscle strain.
6. Hold chest up.	Allows better lung expansion.
7. Keep head erect.	Helps maintain appropriate alignment of spine.
8. Use appropriate body mechanics in all activities:	
a. standing	Demonstrates appropriate body movement.
b. sitting	Demonstrates appropriate body movement.
c. bending	Demonstrates appropriate body movement.
d. lifting	Demonstrates appropriate body movement.

SKILL 18-2: POSITIONING THE PATIENT

Guidelines

Positioning patients is performed daily by the nurse. There are many positions a nurse must learn to prevent the patient from developing complications. Permanent disability can occur from inappropriate positioning.

Purposes

The nurse positions the patient for the following reasons:
- to provide movement for the patient
- to prepare a patient for a procedure
- to provide patient comfort

SUPPLIES/EQUIPMENT

chair
hospital bed
pillow

Related Knowledge and Skills

Before positioning the patient, the nurse should understand the following:
- communication (see Chapter 4)
- documentation (see Chapter 6)
- vital signs (see Chapter 14)
- medical asepsis (see Chapter 16)
- safety measures (see Chapter 17)

Text continued on p. 270

SKILL 18-2

POSITIONING THE PATIENT

Nursing action	Rationale
Assessment	
1. Assess need for positioning patient.	Determines patient's need for movement.
2. Choose appropriate position.	Rotating positions prevents pressure areas.
Nursing diagnosis	
1. Cluster assessment data to reveal actual or potential nursing diagnoses:	
a. Potential impaired skin integrity.	Occurs from lack of change of position.
b. Impaired physical mobility.	Occurs from lack of movement.
Planning	
1. Read physician's order.	Provides basis of care.
2. Wash hands.	Helps prevent cross-contamination.
3. Obtain supplies.	Organizes procedure.
4. Develop individualized patient goals based on nursing diagnoses, including:	
a. Patient's skin integrity will be maintained.	Prevents impaired skin integrity.
b. Mobility will be maintained.	Helps prevent contractures.
Implementation	
1. Introduce self.	Decreases anxiety level.
2. Identify patient by identification band.	Identifies correct patient for procedure.
3. Explain procedure.	Seeks cooperation and decreases anxiety.
4. Wash hands.	

SKILL 18-2

POSITIONING THE PATIENT—cont'd

Nursing action	Rationale
Implementation—cont'd	
5. Position patient:	
a. **Dorsal (supine)**	
1) Slide patient and mattress to head of bed, and remove pillow.	Helps ensure appropriate body alignment.
2) Lower head of bed unless contraindicated.	Provides patient safety.
3) Turn patient onto back.	Positions patient.
4) Replace pillow.	Provides patient comfort.
5) Wash hands.	Helps prevent cross-contamination.
6) Document.	Documents procedure and patient's response.
b. Dorsal **recumbent**	
1) Slide patient and mattress to head of bed, and remove pillow.	Helps ensure appropriate body alignment.
2) Lower head of bed unless contraindicated.	Provides patient safety.
3) Turn patient onto back.	Positions patient.
4) Assist patient to raise legs, bend knees, and allow legs to relax.	Positions patient.
5) Replace pillow.	Provides patient comfort.
6) Wash hands.	Helps prevent cross-contamination.
7) Document.	Records procedures and patient's response.
c. Fowler's	
1) Slide patient and mattress to head of bed, and remove pillow.	Helps ensure appropriate body alignment.
2) Raise head of bed to 45 to 60 degrees.	Positions appropriately.
3) Replace pillow.	Provides patient comfort.
4) Raise foot of bed.	Helps prevent patient from slipping down in bed.
5) Wash hands.	Helps prevent cross-contamination.
6) Document.	Records procedure and patient's response.

STEP 5 a

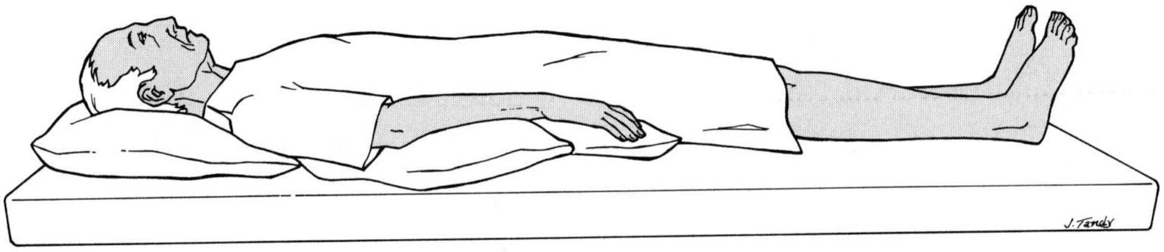

STEP 5 b

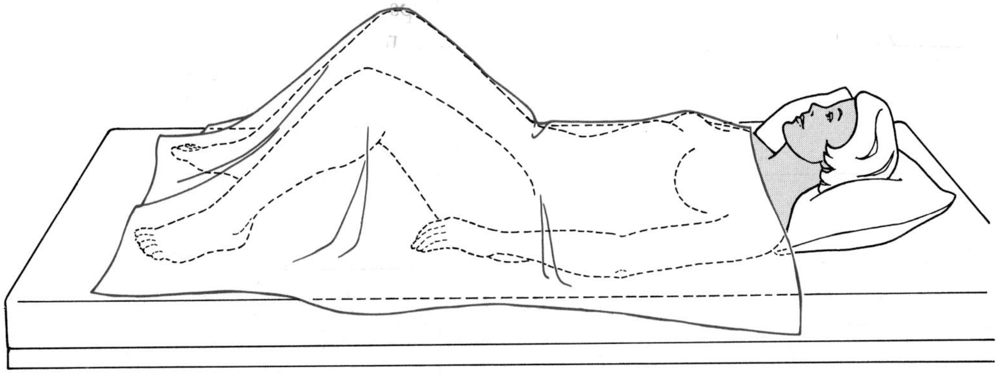

Continued.

SKILL 18-2 POSITIONING THE PATIENT—cont'd

Nursing action	Rationale
Implementation—cont'd	
d. Knee-chest	
1) Turn patient onto abdomen.	Facilitates positioning.
2) Assist patient to kneeling position; arms and head should rest on pillow while upper chest rests on bed.	Completes positioning.
3) Wash hands.	Helps prevent cross-contamination.
4) Document.	Records procedure and patient's response.
e. **Lithotomy**	
1) Request patient to slide buttocks to edge of examinating table.	Facilitates positioning.
2) Lift both legs, have patient bend knees, and place feet in stirrups.	Positions patient.
3) Drape patient.	Provides privacy and prevents exposure.
4) Wash hands.	Helps prevent cross-contamination.
5) Document	Records procedure and patient's response.

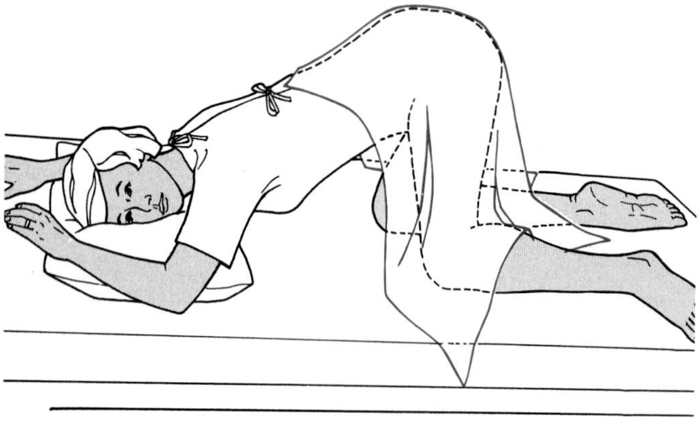

STEP 5 d

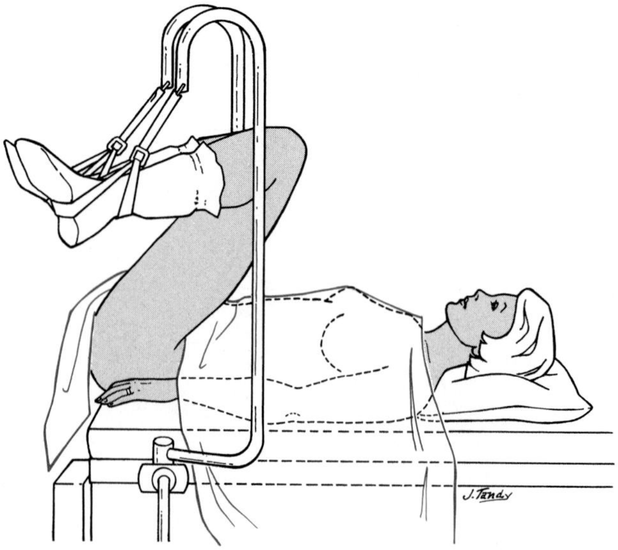

STEP 5 e

SKILL 18-2	POSITIONING THE PATIENT—cont'd

Nursing action	Rationale
Implementation—cont'd	
f. **Orthopneic**	
1) Elevate head of bed to 90 degrees.	Facilitates positioning.
2) Place pillow between patient's back and mattress.	Provides back support.
3) Place pillow on over-bed table, and assist patient to lean over, placing head on pillow.	Facilitates more ease of breathing.
4) Wash hands.	Helps prevent cross-contamination.
5) Document.	Records procedure and patient's response.
g. Prone	
1) Assist patient onto abdomen with face to one side.	Positions patient.
2) Flex arms toward the head.	Provides appropriate body alignment.
3) Wash hands.	Helps prevent cross-contamination.
4) Document.	Records procedure and patient's response.
h. **Semi-Fowler's**	
1) Slide patient and mattress to head of bed, and remove pillow.	Helps ensure appropriate body alignment.
2) Raise head of bed to about 30 degrees.	Positions appropriately.
3) Replace pillow.	Provides patient comfort.
4) Slightly raise foot of bed.	Helps prevent patient from slipping in bed.
5) Wash hands.	Helps prevent cross-contamination.
6) Document.	Records procedure and patient's response.

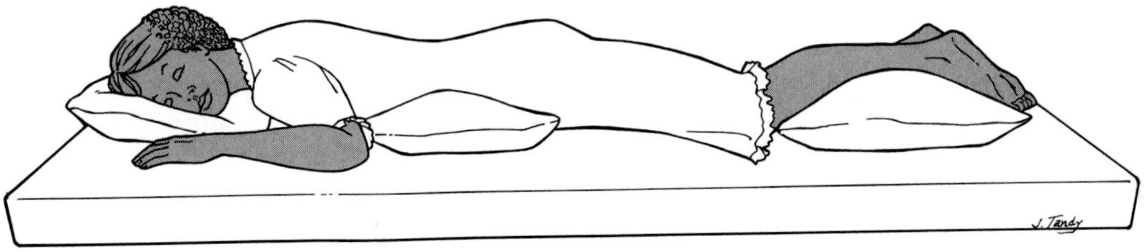

STEP 5 g

STEP 5 h

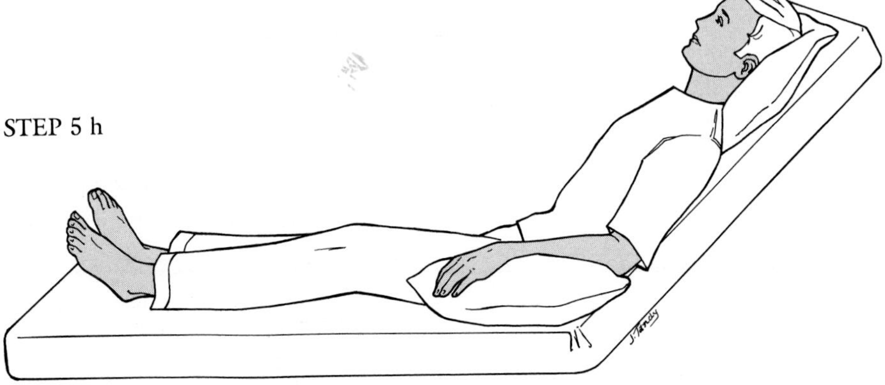

Continued.

SKILL 18-2 POSITIONING THE PATIENT—cont'd

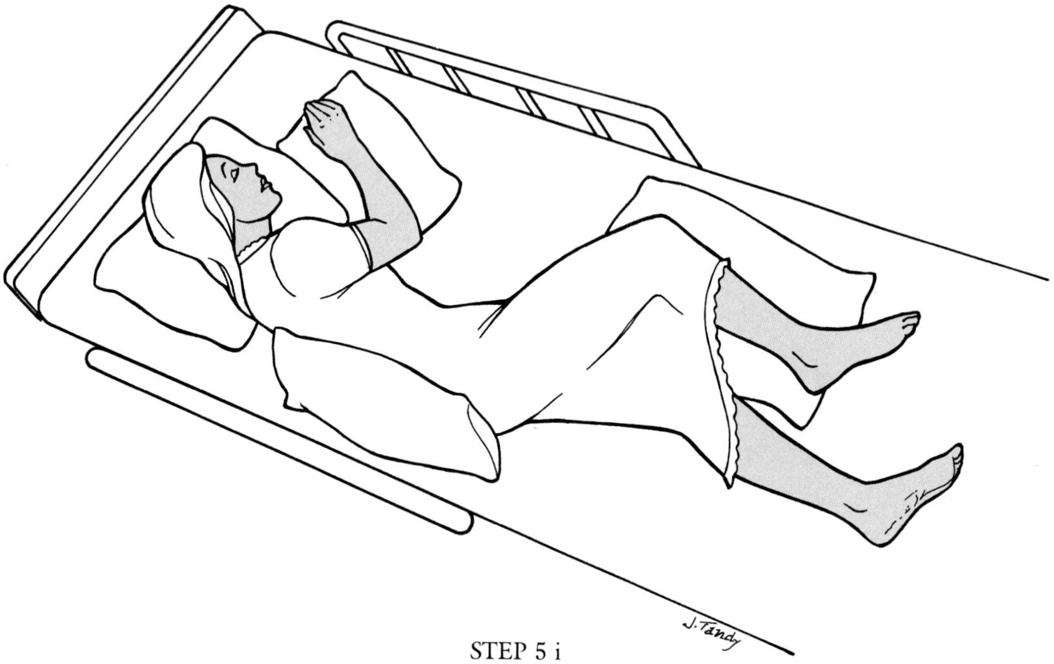

STEP 5 i

Nursing action	Rationale
Implementation—cont'd	
i. **Sims'**	
1) Turn patient to left side.	Initiates position placement.
2) Draw right knee and thigh up near abdomen.	Provides appropriate position for administering an enema.
3) Place patient's right arm along the back.	Provides appropriate body alignment.
4) Allow patient to lean forward to rest on chest.	Provides comfort.
5) Wash hands.	Helps prevent cross-contamination.
6) Document.	Records procedure and patient's response.
j. **Trendelenburg**	
1) Place patient's head lower than the body with body and legs elevated and on an incline (bed may be elevated on blocks).	Used in performing abdominal surgery (not used if patient has a head injury). Trendelenburg position is not usually used to treat shock because of the pressure it causes on the diaphragm by the organs in the abdomen.
2) Wash hands.	Helps prevent cross-contamination.
3) Document.	Records procedure and patient's response.

SKILL 18-2

POSITIONING THE PATIENT—cont'd

DOCUMENTATION

1. Record appropriate alignment and position of patient.

Provides documentation of patient's safety and welfare.

Sample charting

DATE	TIME	NOTES
12/30/90	0900	Positioned in semi-Fowler's position in appropriate body alignment. States feels comfortable.

____

(nurse's signature)

FOLLOW-UP

1. Make certain patient remains as appropriately positioned.

Provides appropriate patient care.

EVALUATION

1. Assess for appropriate body alignment and positioning of patient.

Determines safety and welfare of patient.

SPECIAL CONCERNS

- Performing a back massage after turning from one position to another helps prevent impaired skin integrity.
- Appropriate body alignment should be assessed after every change of position.
- Skin of the elderly is often thin and nonelastic and needs special care to prevent tearing and further impaired skin integrity.
- Small children must often be propped with pillows to help them maintain a position.

HOME HEALTH VARIATIONS

- Teach family members how to position and maintain body alignment.

PATIENT TEACHING

- Explain importance of maintaining skin integrity.
- Explain importance of appropriate body alignment.

SKILL 18-3: PERFORMING RANGE-OF-MOTION EXERCISES

Guidelines

Range-of-motion **(ROM)** exercises may be performed by the physical therapy department or by the nurse. The exercises are ordered for patients confined to bed for long periods. Range of motion may be performed passively by the nurse or actively by the patient. Designated body **joints** are moved to the point of resistance, using care to avoid injury. The nurse or therapist gradually increases the range of motion with subsequent exercises as tolerated.

Purposes

The nurse performs ROM exercises for the following reasons:

- to increase circulation
- to prevent **contractures**
- to provide joint motion and flexibility

Related Knowledge and Skills

Before performing ROM exercises, the nurse should understand the following:

- communication (see Chapter 4)
- documentation (see Chapter 6)
- physical assessment (see Chapter 13)
- patient safety (see Chapter 17)

SKILL 18-3 PERFORMING RANGE-OF-MOTION EXERCISES

Nursing action	Rationale
Assessment	
1. Assess need for ROM exercises.	Determines patient's impaired ability.
2. Assess joint movement.	Provides a baseline for performing the exercises.
Nursing diagnosis	
1. Cluster assessment data to reveal actual or potential nursing diagnoses:	
a. Impaired physical mobility.	Occurs from stiffened joints.
b. Potential for disuse syndrome.	Patient assumes a position of comfort to alleviate pain.
c. Potential for injury: joint.	Damaged joints become edematous and can be further injured.
Planning	
1. Read physician's order.	Provides basis for care.
2. Wash hands.	Helps prevent cross-contamination.
3. Obtain supplies.	Organizes procedure.
4. Develop individualized patient goals based on nursing diagnoses, including:	
a. ROM exercises will be effective.	Helps prevent permanent joint stiffness.
b. Flexibility of joints will be maintained.	Prevents **contractures.**
c. Patient will perform some active exercises.	Ensures joint mobility.
Implementation	
1. Introduce self.	Decreases anxiety level.
2. Identify patient by identification band.	Identifies correct patient for procedure.
3. Explain procedure to patient.	Seeks cooperation and decreases anxiety.
4. Wash hands.	Helps prevent cross-contamination.
5. Assist patient in putting each joint through full ROM (Table 18-1 and Figs. 18-11 to 18-22).	Provides baseline for impaired joint mobility and for appropriate information to report.
6. Adjust bed linen.	Provides privacy and comfort.
7. Wash hands.	Helps prevent cross-contamination.
8. Document.	Records procedure and patient's response.

Continued on p. 274.

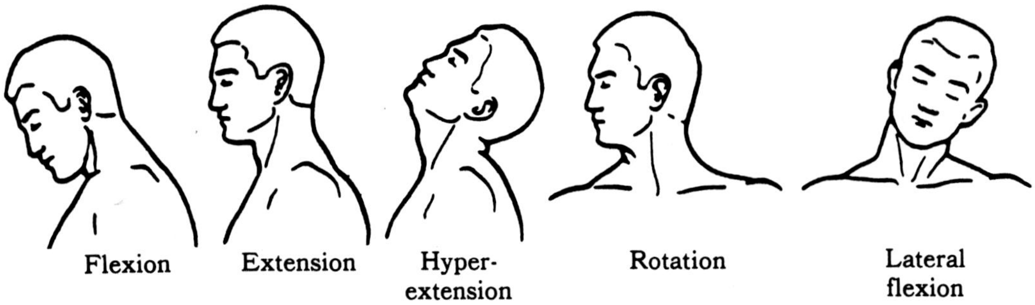

FIG. 18-11 Range-of-motion exercises for the neck.

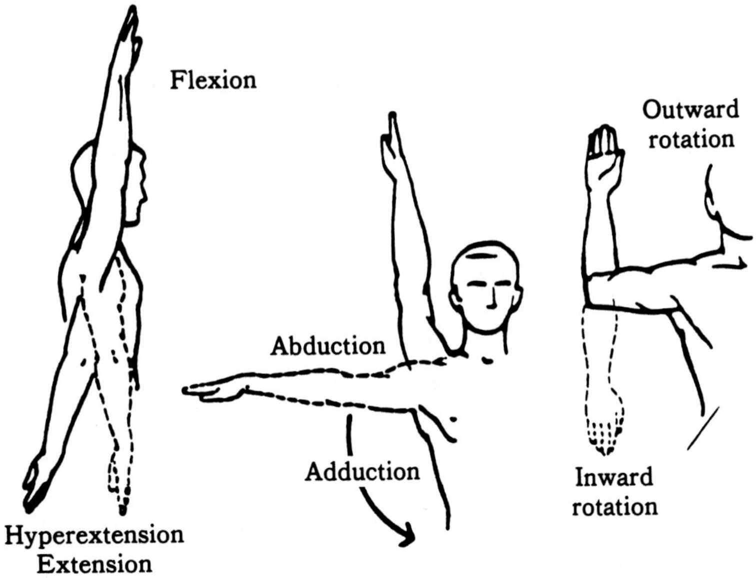

FIG. 18-12 Range-of-motion exercises for the shoulder.

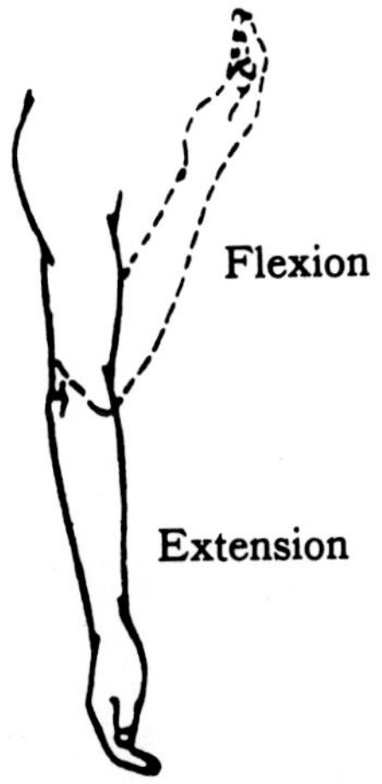

FIG. 18-13 Range-of-motion exercises for the elbow.

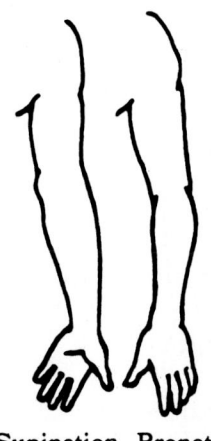

FIG. 18-14 Range-of-motion exercises for the forearm.

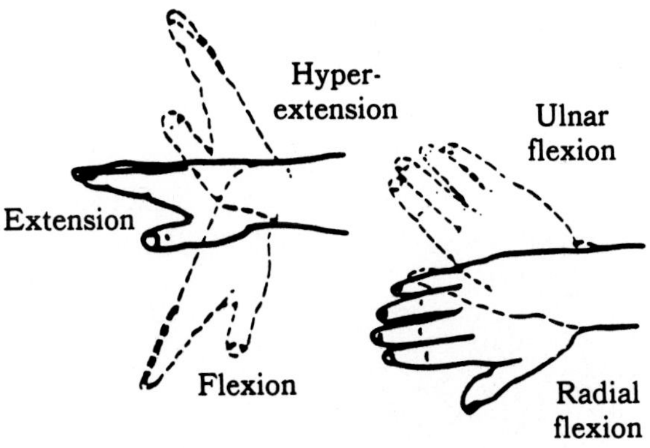

FIG. 18-15 Range-of-motion exercises for the wrist.

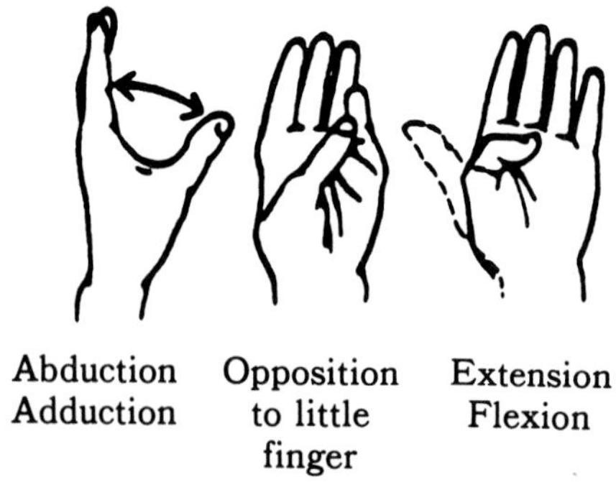

FIG. 18-16 Range-of-motion exercises for the thumb.

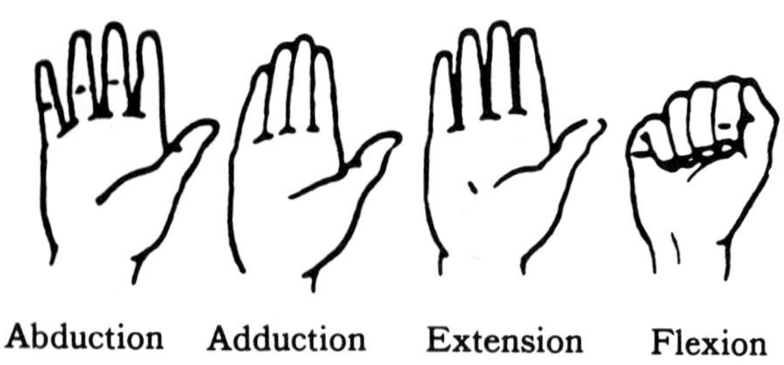

FIG. 18-17 Range-of-motion exercises for the fingers.

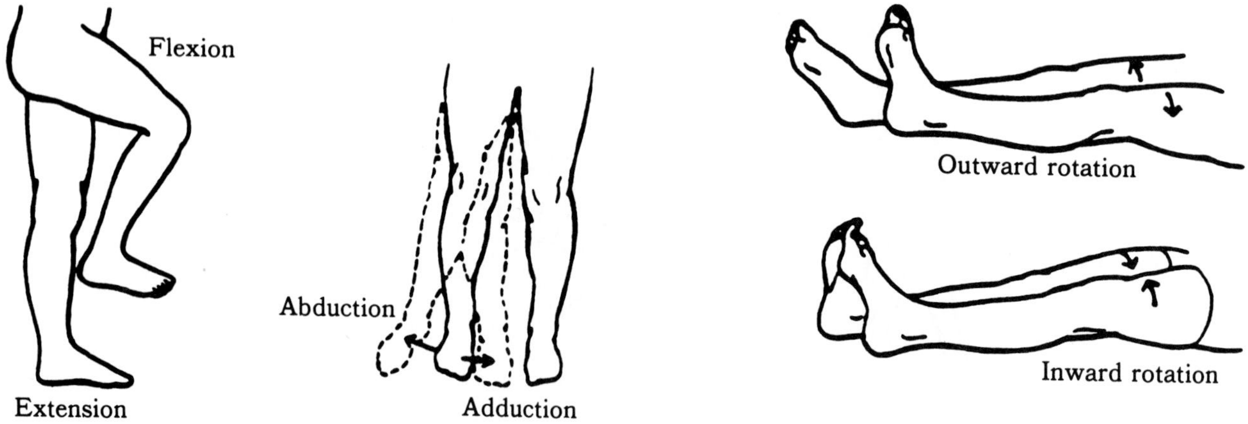

FIG. 18-18 Range-of-motion exercises for the hip.

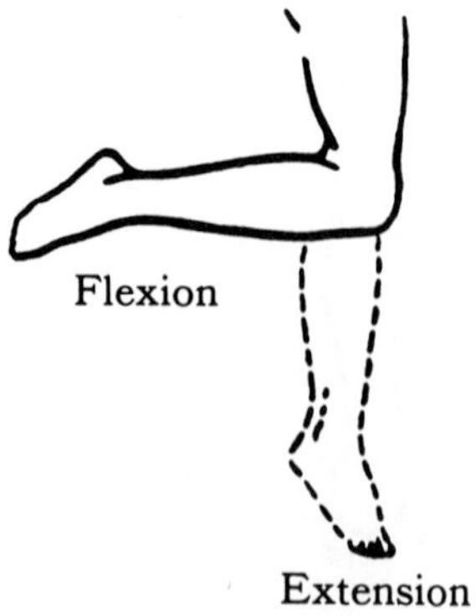

FIG. 18-19 Range-of-motion exercises for the knee.

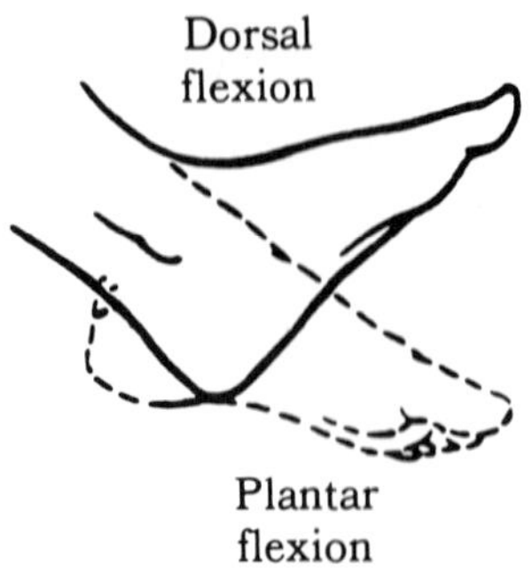

FIG. 18-20 Range-of-motion exercises for the ankle.

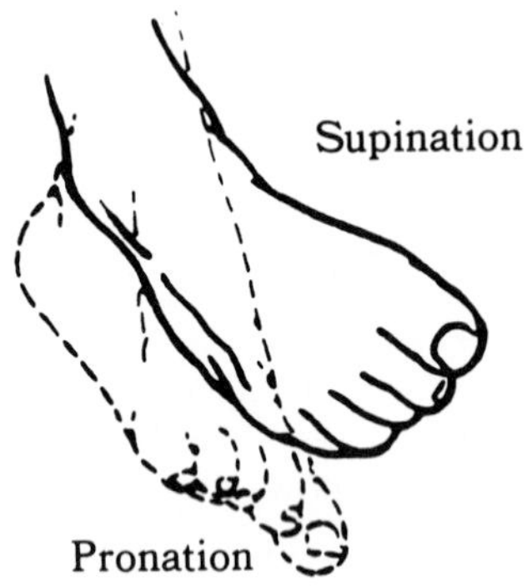

FIG. 18-21 Range-of-motion exercises for the foot.

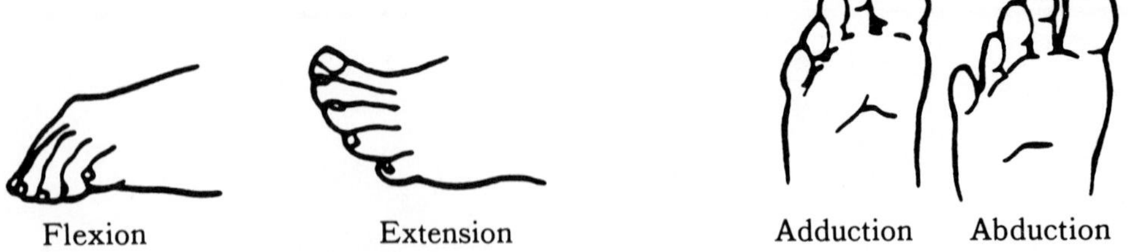

FIG. 18-22 Range-of-motion exercises for the toes.

SKILL 18-3

PERFORMING RANGE-OF-MOTION EXERCISES—cont

DOCUMENTATION

1. Report and record any abnormal findings. — Provides information for patient care.
2. Report and record normal findings. — Provides information of normal patient assessment.

Sample charting

DATE	TIME	NOTES
11/27/90	0800	Carried out full ROM to all joints. Stated felt pain in wrist joint left hand (patient is left-handed). Reported joint pain to M. McHarness, RN.

____

(nurse's signature)

FOLLOW-UP

1. Turn patient. — Prevents acquired deformities.
2. Maintain appropriate body alignment. — Prevents joint immobility.

EVALUATION

1. Compare information found with normal joint assessment. — Determines abnormal findings.

SPECIAL CONCERNS

- To prevent contractures, the nurse should not allow patients with joint pain to remain continuously in position of comfort; joints must be exercised routinely.
- The nurse should provide back massage periodically for patient comfort.

HOME HEALTH VARIATIONS

- Nurse must teach patient and family member ROM exercises.
- Full ROM exercises must be carried out on geriatric bedfast patients to prevent further complications of immobility.
- Avoid injury to joints in children because of more rapid metabolism.

PATIENT TEACHING

- Emphasize importance of patient performing active ROM exercises where possible.

Table 18-1 Normal Range of Motion

Body Part	Motion	Measurement
Jaw	Open and close jaw	Able to insert three fingers
	Move jaw side to side	Bottom side teeth overlapping top side teeth
	Move jaw forward	Top teeth behind lower teeth
Neck	Touch chin to sternum	Flexion 70°-90°
	Extend neck with chin pointing toward ceiling	Hyperextension 55°
	Bend neck laterally, ear toward shoulder	Lateral bending 35°
	Rotate neck with ear toward chest	Rotation 70° to left and right
Spine	Bend forward at the waist	Flexion 75°
	Bend backward	Extension 30°
	Bend to each side	Lateral bending 35°
Shoulder	**Abduct** arm straight up	Abduction 180°
	Adduct arm toward midline of trunk	Adduction 45°
	Abduct arm straight horizontally to floor; bring arm backward toward spine and forward across chest	Horizontal extension 45° Horizontal flexion 130°
	Flex or elevate forward with arm straight	Flexion 180°
	Extend backward with arm straight	Extension 60°
Elbow	Extend lower arm to normal extreme	**Extension** 150°
	Flex lower arm toward biceps	Flexion 150°
	Hyperextend arm beyond normal resting point	Hyperextension up to 10°
	Supinate lower arm (the palm of the hand turned up)	Supination 90°
	Pronate lower arm (the rotation of the forearm so that the palm of the hand faces downward and backward)	Pronation 90°
Wrist	Flex wrist toward lower arm	Flexion 80°-90°
	Extend wrist backward	Extension 70°
	Deviate wrist laterally toward radius	Radial deviation 20°
	Deviate wrist laterally toward ulna	Ulnar deviation 30°-50°
Fingers	Flex fingers into fist, and then extend them flat	Flexion 80°-100° (varies with joint) Extension up to 45°
	Spread fingers apart	Abduction 20° between fingers
	Cross fingers together	Adduction (fingers will touch)
	Oppose fingers: touch each fingertip with thumb	Includes abduction and flexion
Hip	Raise leg with knee straight	Flexion 90°
	Raise leg with knee flexed	Flexion 110°-120°
	Lying prone, extend leg straight back	Extension 30°
	Abduct partially flexed leg outward	Abduction 45°-50°
	Adduct partially flexed leg inward	Adduction 20°-30°
	Flex knee, and swing foot away from midline	Internal rotation 35°-40°
	Flex knee, and swing foot toward midline	External rotation 45°
Knee	Flex knee with calf touching thigh	Flexion 130°
	Extend knee beyond normal point of extension	Hyperextension 15°
	Rotate knee and lower leg toward midline	Internal rotation 10°
Ankle	Dorsiflex foot with toes pointing toward head	**Dorsiflexion** 20°
	Plantar flex foot with toes pointing down	Plantar flexion 45°
	Turn foot away from midline	Eversion 20°
	Turn foot toward midline	Inversion 30°
Toes	Curl toes under foot	Flexion 35°-60° (varies with joints)
	Raise toes to point upward	Extension up to 90° (varies with joints)
	Spread toes apart	Varies

SKILL 18-4: MOVING THE PATIENT

Guidelines

The nurse often will be required to assist in moving the patient. Moving includes lifting the patient up in bed, turning, dangling, and assisting the patient in and out of bed for ambulation. Other techniques include using mechanical equipment for lifting the patient, such as the hydraulic lift, roller board, and gurney lift.

Purposes

The nurse moves the patient for the following reasons:
- to move patient up toward head of bed
- to move patient for appropriate positioning
- to assist patient into bed
- to assist patient out of bed
- to turn patient

SUPPLIES/EQUIPMENT

hospital bed
chair
siderails
patient slippers
cotton blanket
pillows
extra personnel

Related Knowledge and Skills

Before moving the patient, the nurse should understand the following:
- communication (see Chapter 4)
- documentation (see Chapter 6)
- physical assessment (see Chapter 13)
- vital signs (see Chapter 14)
- safety measures (see Chapter 17)

SKILL 18-4 MOVING THE PATIENT

Nursing action	Rationale
Assessment	
1. Assess patient mobility.	Provides baseline for assistance required for safe movement.
2. Assess need for patient teaching related to patient safety.	Determines how much assistance will be needed to move patient.
Nursing diagnosis	
1. Cluster assessment data to reveal actual or potential nursing diagnoses:	
a. Impaired physical mobility.	Requires assistance for ambulation.
b. Activity intolerance.	Movement causes pain.
Planning	
1. Read physician's order.	Provides basis for care.
2. Wash hands.	Helps prevent cross-contamination.
3. Obtain supplies.	Organizes procedure.
4. Develop individualized patient goals based on nursing diagnoses, including:	
a. Appropriate mobility will be maintained.	Prevents contractures.
b. Patient safety will be maintained.	Prevents patient injury.
c. Patient will have minimal to no pain on movement.	Mechanics used for movement will help prevent pain.

SKILL 18-4 MOVING THE PATIENT—cont'd

Nursing action	Rationale
Implementation	
1. Introduce self.	Decreases anxiety level.
2. Identify patient by identification band.	Identifies correct patient for procedure.
3. Explain procedure to patient.	Seeks cooperation and decreases anxiety.
4. Wash hands.	Helps prevent cross-contamination.
5. Lifting and moving patient up in bed:	Takes one or more nurses.
a. Place patient supine with head flat.	Provides less resistance if on flat surface.
b. Face side of bed, and provide base of support.	Protects nurse's back.
c. Place one arm under axilla and opposite arm under shoulder and neck.	Supports patient.
d. Ask patient to flex knees and push up with feet on count of three while assisting or:	Protects nurse's back, and promotes patient mobility.
e. Nurse on each side of patient supports patient's back with one arm and the second arm under shoulder and neck.	Protects nurses, and provides patient safety.
f. On count of three, each nurse pulls patient up to head of bed.	Moves patient in unison.
6. Turning the patient:	
a. Stand with feet slightly apart, and flex knees.	Provides base of support for nurse.
b. Place one arm under patient's neck and shoulders and other arm under waist.	Provides patient safety.
c. Pull patient toward nurse.	Reduces strain on nurse.
d. Turn patient on side facing raised siderail.	Prevents falling out of bed.
e. Flex one leg over the other.	Reduces pressure on legs.
f. Align shoulders.	Ensures appropriate body alignment.
g. Support back with pillows if necessary.	Helps keep patient in position.
h. Assess appropriate body alignment.	Provides patient safety.

STEP 6 e

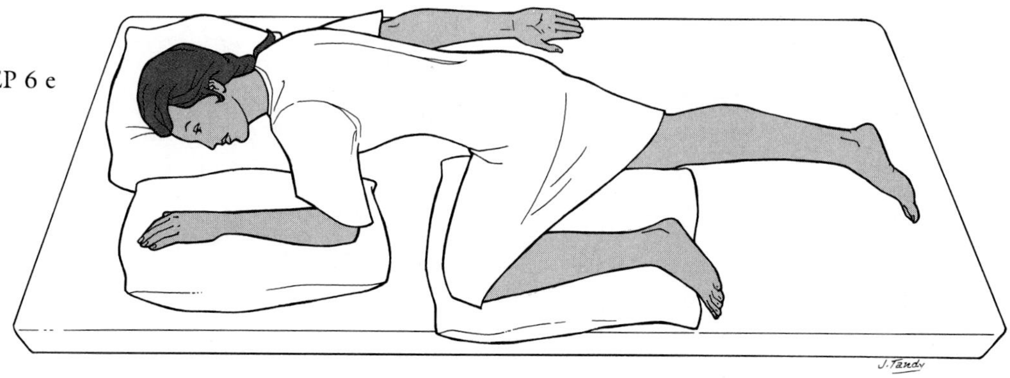

Continued.

SKILL 18-4 MOVING THE PATIENT—cont'd

Nursing action	Rationale
Implementation—cont'd	
7. Dangling the patient:	
a. Assess pulse and respirations.	Provides baseline for assessing patient's reaction to dangling.
b. Move patient to side of bed toward nurse.	Makes it easier for patient to sit up.
c. Lower bed to lowest position.	Provides patient safety when getting up.
d. Raise head of bed.	Easier for patient to swing around to sitting position.
e. Support patient's shoulders and help to swing legs around and off bed; do this all in one motion; feet must touch floor.	Prevents strain on patient, especially if has an incision.
f. Help patient don slippers; cover legs.	Protects from chilling.
g. Assess patient's pulse and respiration.	Determines patient's response to dangling.
8. Logrolling the patient:	
a. Three nurses stand by side of bed.	Use of three nurses provides safety.
b. One nurse places arms under patient's legs; second nurse places arms under patient's buttocks; third nurse places arms under patient's chest, shoulders, and neck.	Ensures that patient is turned like log is rolled (as a unit).
c. The nurse nearest head of patient gives prearranged signal to turn patient simultaneously.	Ensures appropriate logrolling.
d. Make patient comfortable.	Provides comfort.
9. Transferring the patient from bed to straight chair and wheelchair:	
a. Lower bed to lowest position.	Provides patient safety when getting up.
b. Raise head of bed.	Makes it easier for patient to swing around to sitting position.
c. Support patient's shoulder and help to swing legs around and off bed; perform all in one motion.	Prevents strain on patient, especially if patient has incision.
d. Help patient don robe and slippers.	Prevents chilling.

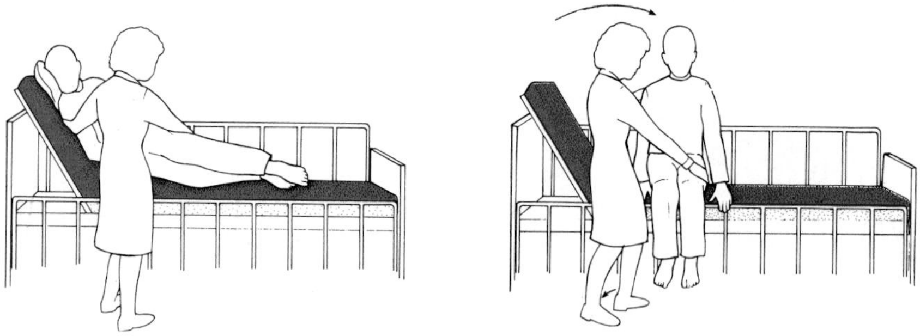

STEP 7 e

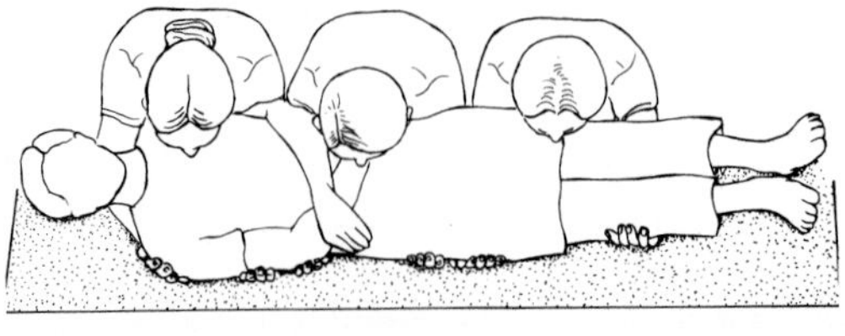

STEP 8 b

SKILL 18-4

MOVING THE PATIENT—cont'd

Nursing action	Rationale
Implementation—cont'd	
e. Have chair placed beside bed with seat facing foot of bed:	Provides easy access to chair.
1) Lock wheels of wheelchair.	Provides safety.
2) Place straight chair against wall.	Provides safety.
f. Stand in front of patient, and place hands under patient's axillae.	Prepares patient for movement to chair.
g. Assist patient to stand and swing around with back toward seat of chair.	Provides patient safety.
h. Help patient to sit down as nurse bends knees to assist process.	Prevents patient from slipping and falling.
i. Apply blanket for legs.	Provides extra warmth.
10. Wash hands.	Helps prevent cross-contamination.
11. Document.	Records procedure and patient's response.

DOCUMENTATION

1. Report and record movement of patient. — Provides information regarding improvement.

Sample charting

DATE	TIME	NOTES
12/5/90	1000	Moved up to head of bed. Placed in appropriate body alignment. ____________ *(nurse's signature)*
12/5/90	1100	Repositioned to L side. ____________ *(nurse's signature)*
12/5/90	0800	Dangled at side of bed 10 minutes. Tolerated well. p. 74, with regular rate and rhythm. Respirations 18 and regular. ____________ *(nurse's signature)*

FOLLOW-UP

1. Assess that wheelchair locks are in working order. — Provides patient safety.
2. If patient begins to fall, protect by holding patient and allow patient to sit down on floor. — Prevents patient injury.

EVALUATION

1. Assess for appropriate body alignment after patient movement. — Determines safety and comfort.

SPECIAL CONCERNS

- Do not overtire patient during ambulation.
- Give patient time to talk about ambulation needs.
- Children on bed rest may be irritable because of restrained activity.
- Older patients on bed rest are at risk for impairment.

PATIENT TEACHING

- Explain the importance of physical movement.

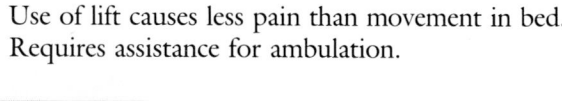

SKILL 18-5: USING THE LIFT FOR MOVING THE PATIENT

Guidelines

Mechanical devices, such as the hydraulic lift used with a Hoyer sling (see Fig. 18-26), are used for moving patients safely, for protecting the nurse's back, and for full-weight lifting of patients who cannot assist. Agency policy is followed for use of the lift.

Purposes

The nurse uses the lift for moving the patient for the following reasons:

- to place patient in chair
- to place patient on gurney
- to place patient in tub

SUPPLIES/EQUIPMENT

2 cotton blankets
sling hydraulic lift, such as the Hoyer

Related Knowledge and Skills

Before moving a patient in a lift, the nurse should understand the following:

- communication (Chapter 4)
- documentation (Chapter 6)
- physical assessment (Chapter 13)
- vital signs (Chapter 14)
- safety measures (Chapter 17)

SKILL 18-5

USING THE LIFT FOR MOVING THE PATIENT

Nursing action	Rationale
Assessment	
1. Assess need for using hydraulic lift, such as a Hoyer sling.	Determines mobility.
Nursing diagnosis	
1. Cluster assessment data to reveal actual or potential nursing diagnoses:	
a. Activity intolerance.	Use of lift causes less pain than movement in bed.
b. Impaired physical mobility.	Requires assistance for ambulation.

STEP 1

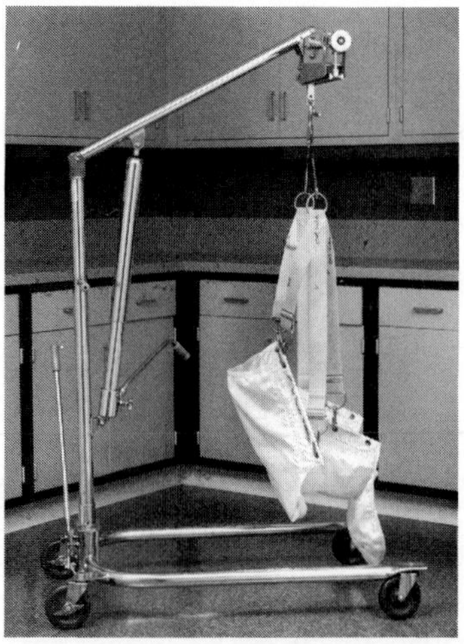

SKILL 18-5 USING THE LIFT FOR MOVING THE PATIENT—cont'd

Nursing action	Rationale
Planning	
1. Read physician's order.	Provides basis for care.
2. Wash hands.	Helps prevent cross-contamination.
3. Obtain supplies.	Organizes procedure.
4. Develop individualized patient goals based on nursing diagnoses, including:	
a. Pressure areas will be avoided.	Immobility causes skin impairment.
b. Patient injury will not occur.	Prevents injury.
Implementation	
1. Introduce self.	Decreases anxiety level.
2. Identify patient by identification band.	Identifies correct patient for procedure.
3. Explain procedure to patient.	Seeks cooperation, and decreases anxiety.
4. Wash hands.	Helps prevent cross-contamination.
5. Secure appropriate number of personnel to assist.	Provides patient safety.
6. Place chair near bed.	Prepares seat for patient.
7. Raise bed to maximum height.	Helps using of appropriate body mechanics.
8. Place canvas seat under patient appropriately.	Helps in lifting safely.
9. Slide horseshoe-shaped bar under bed on one side.	Places lift close to bed.
10. Lower horizontal bar to level of sling by releasing hydraulic valve, and lock valve.	Places lift close to patient.
11. Fasten hooks on chain to openings in sling.	Places lift to sling seat.
12. Raise head of bed.	Places patient in sitting position.
13. Fold patient's arms over chest.	Prevents patient injury.
14. Pump lift handle until patient is raised off bed.	Ensures patient safety.
15. With steering handle, pull lift off bed and down to chair.	Places patient safely.
16. Release valve slowly to left, and lower patient to chair.	Places patient appropriately in chair.
17. Close off valve, and release straps.	Prevents patient injury from boom.
18. Remove straps and hydraulic lift.	Provides safety and comfort.
19. Wash hands.	Helps prevent cross-contamination.
20. Document.	Records procedure and patient's response.

DOCUMENTATION

1. Record procedure.	Documents procedure.
2. Report patient's response.	Documents and reports patient's response.

Sample charting

DATE	TIME	NOTES
12/29/90	1000	Sat in chair by use of lift.
	1030	Returned to bed. No skin impairment. Tolerated well.

____

(nurse's signature)

Continued.

SKILL 18-5 USING THE LIFT FOR MOVING THE PATIENT—cont'd

FOLLOW-UP

1. Assess for skin impairment.	Prevention is best treatment.
2. Assess effects of procedure on patient.	Ensures assistance if needed.

EVALUATION

1. Assess for body alignment.	Helps prevent skin impairment.
2. Assess patient's response to movement.	Helps determine patient's mobility potential.

SPECIAL CONCERNS

- Explain procedures thoroughly to patient to help prevent fear of lift.
- Praise patient's progress regarding mobility.

PATIENT TEACHING

- Explain the importance of mobility.
- Explain the effects of immobility.
- Consider the older patient who has hearing loss when explaining.
- Explain how to secure lift for home care.

REFERENCES AND SUGGESTED READINGS

1. Mosby's medical, nursing, and allied health dictionary, ed 3, St Louis, 1990, The CV Mosby Co.
2. Perry AG and Potter PA: Clinical nursing skills and techniques, ed 2, St Louis, 1990, The CV Mosby Co.
3. Potter PA and Perry AG: Basic nursing: theory and practice, St Louis, 1987, The CV Mosby Co.
4. Potter PA and Perry AG: Fundamentals of nursing: concepts, process, and practice, ed 2, St Louis, 1989, The CV Mosby Co.
5. Sorrentino SA: Mosby's textbook for nursing assistants, ed 2, St Louis, 1987, The CV Mosby Co.

CHAPTER CHALLENGE

STUDY QUESTIONS

1. Before placing a patient in any position, the nurse should use appropriate body mechanics. The nurse should *first:*
   a. Wash hands
   b. Obtain all necessary equipment
   c. Check the physician's orders
   d. Begin with a wide base of support
2. When placing a patient in Fowler's position, the nurse should:
   a. Elevate the head of the bed to a 90-degree angle
   b. Lower the head of the bed
   c. Elevate the head of the bed to a 45-degree angle
   d. Adjust the head of the bed as desired by the patient
3. The position of the patient's body in Fowler's position is:
   a. Prone
   b. Supine
   c. Side lying
   d. Semiprone
4. In passive range-of-motion exercises:
   a. The nurse exercises the joints of a patient
   b. The patient exercises his/her own joints
   c. The patient assists the nurse
   d. The nurse assists the physical therapist
5. When the nurse performs range-of-motion exercises, it is important to:
   a. Massage each joint vigorously before beginning
   b. Apply warm compresses to "limber up" the joints before beginning
   c. Work quickly to avoid tiring the patient
   d. Refrain from taking the joint beyond its normal range of mobility
6. When helping a patient to get up for the first time, the nurse should:
   a. Ask for assistance
   b. Check the pulse and respirations
   c. Support the feet
   d. Lift the patient from bed to chair
7. The primary purpose for a log-rolling technique is to:
   a. Make it easier to turn a patient
   b. Prevent trauma or injury to the spinal cord
   c. Provide a change in positioning
   d. Avoid using supports for body parts

19

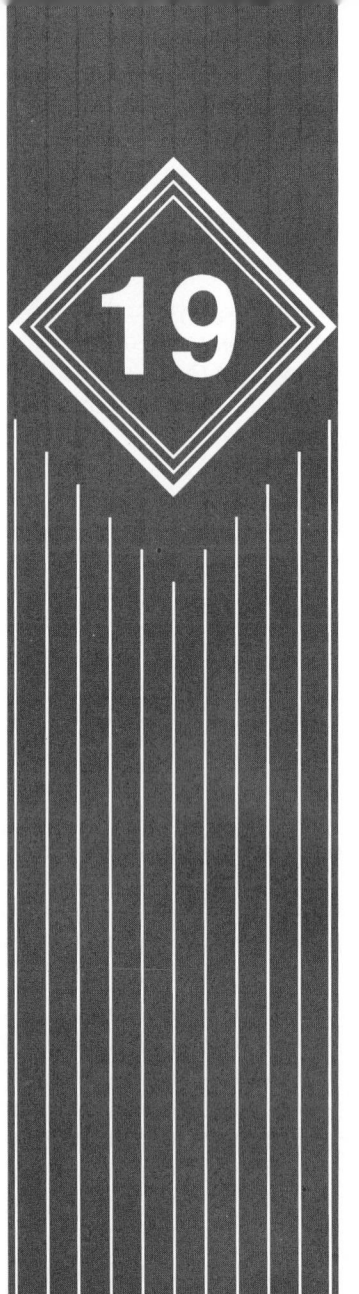

Comfort, Rest, and Sleep

BARBARA LAURITSEN CHRISTENSEN

LEARNING OBJECTIVES

After reading this chapter, the student should be able to do the following:

- Define the key terms.
- List six possible causes of discomfort.
- Give McCaffery's description of pain.
- Explain the relationship of the gate control theory to selecting nursing interventions for pain relief.
- Identify subjective and objective data in pain assessment.
- Explain two recently developed tools to identify intensity of pain.
- Discuss the responsibilities of the nurse in pain control.
- List six methods for pain control.
- Identify nursing interventions to control painful stimuli in the patient's environment.
- Describe the difference and similarities between sleep and rest.
- Outline nursing interventions that promote rest and sleep.
- Discuss the sleep cycle, differentiating between NREM and REM sleep.
- List six signs and symptoms of sleep deprivation.
- Identify two nursing diagnoses related to sleep problems.

RELATED TOPICS OF INTEREST

- Signs, symptoms, and physical assessment (Chapter 13)
- Hygiene and care of the patient's environment (Chapter 20)
- Principles and practice of medication administration (Chapter 25)
- The surgical patient (Chapter 26)
- Care of the patient with a neurological disorder (Chapter 38)

KEY TERMS

Define the following:

- acute pain
- chronic pain
- endorphin
- gate control theory
- nonrapid eye movement (NREM)
- noxious
- patient-controlled analgesia (PCA)
- placebo
- rapid eye movement (REM)
- referred pain
- transcutaneous electrical nerve stimulation (TENS)
- visual analog scale

THE MEANING OF COMFORT

One of the greatest challenges of the nurse is to provide comfort to the patient. *To comfort* means to give strength and hope, to cheer, and to ease the grief or trouble of another. Promoting physical and psychological comfort is a vital part of the role of a nurse.

For the patient, the lack of comfort can be the result of many factors and can take many forms, including the following:

pain	singultus
nausea	hypothermia
vomiting	hyperthermia
thirst	fatigue
dry mouth	pruritus
dyspnea	diaphoresis
sadness	constricting edema
depression	muscle cramping
distention	headache
anxiety	hopelessness
fear	incontinence

The nurse should pursue methods to assist the patient in achieving relief from discomfort.

It is important to explore with the patient what constitutes comfort to him. By actively listening to the patient, the nurse will be better prepared to plan nursing interventions. The nurse who knows what might constitute patient discomfort will recognize discomfort signals even when the patient cannot verbalize, as in the case of a patient who is aphasic or one who is semicomatose.

The nurse must be diligent in her efforts to relieve patients' discomfort. If interventions are not successful, alternative interventions should be pursued.

Regardless of age, patients receive comfort and a sense of well-being from gentle touch and eye contact (Fig. 19-1). The following depicts the nurse's role in bringing physical and psychological comfort to the patient.

PATIENT EXAMPLE: DISCOMFORT TO COMFORT

Mr. P.D. is a 91-year-old patient hospitalized for pneumonia and COPD. The night nurse reported that he had been belligerent and occasionally combative.

Upon entering Mr. P.D.'s room, the nurse sees a pale, thin, and slightly dyspneic patient. He appears fragile and vulnerable. Mr. P.D. complains of pain and tenderness on his lower left gum line. He also states, "I can't hear without my hearing aids, and I am cold."

The nurse acknowledges Mr. P.D.'s complaints of oral discomfort, inability to hear, and being cold. Immediate nursing interventions are to place a warm bath blanket over him, put his hearing aids in place, encourage him to cough, and assist in repositioning. The nurse assesses his oral cavity, using

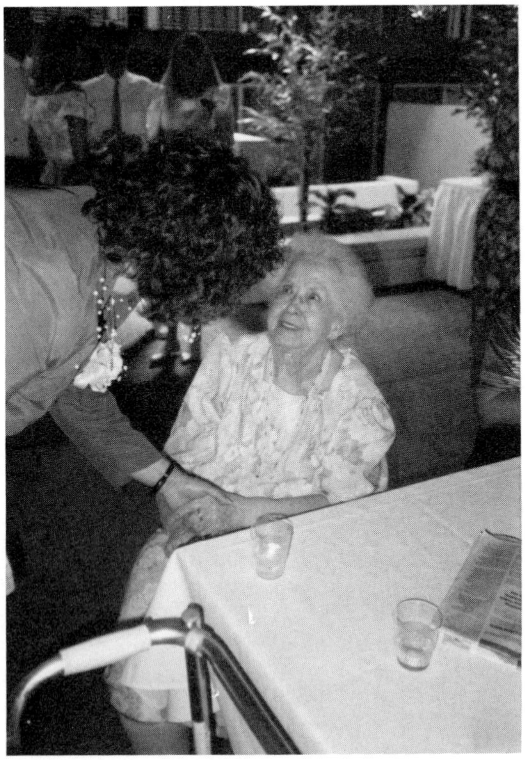

FIG. 19-1 Comfort and well-being can be promoted with eye contact and gentle touch.

a flashlight for better visualization; an erythematous area is noted. She gently cleanses the area with a soothing mouthwash applied with Toothettes and gives him a glass of apple juice to sooth his erythematous and tender mouth. These interventions are followed with a warm towel bath to enhance his well-being. The nurse speaks slowly and distinctly while facing Mr. P.D. to improve his ability to hear. Gentle touch, eye contact, and a projection of concern are employed during the interventions.

Mr. P.D. is more comfortable and verbalizes this. He then makes a significant comment: "I have very little jaw bone left, and I drool; the nurses have to wipe it off my face and that makes me feel like a bum." The nurse listens to this revealing statement and acknowledges his feelings of loss of control over his ability to contain his saliva. After providing opportunity for Mr. P.D. to verbalize his feelings of powerlessness, the nurse places facial tissues within his reach to assist him in wiping secretions from his face. Mr. P.D. has a comfortable morning and does not display belligerent or combative behavior.

The interventions addressed the patient's discomfort, physically as well as psychologically, and comfort was established.

NATURE OF PAIN

Pain is a complex, abstract, personal experience. It is an unpleasant sensation caused by **noxious** stimulation of the sensory nerve endings. Pain cannot be seen. It serves as a warning to the body because it often occurs where there is actual or potential tissue damage. Pain can also occur when there is no tissue damage. Examples of this are the pain of grief at the death of a loved one or the pain of migraine headaches, in which there is no tissue damage.

Pain is subjective; the interpretation and significance of pain depend on the individual's learned experiences and involves psychosocial and cultural factors. Only the person who is bearing the pain is an expert about that pain. McCaffery has a realistic description of pain: "Pain is whatever the experiencing person says it is, existing whenever he says it does." According to McCaffery's definition of pain, the nurse must believe every patient who says he has pain. The nurse should remember also that some patients may deny pain for a variety of reasons and that this situation must be explored as well.

Because so many health care providers have difficulty with the concept of pain, it must be emphasized that *there is no test for pain*. Even though some nurses with years of experience think they can identify all patients in pain, it is not always possible. Lack of pain expression does not mean lack of pain.[8]

Function and Types of Pain

Pain may be a cardinal symptom of inflammation and is valuable in the diagnosis of many disorders and conditions. There are many types of pain: mild or severe, chronic or acute, intermittent or intractable (constant), burning, dull, or sharp, precisely or poorly localized, or referred. **Referred pain** is felt at a site other than the injured or diseased organ or part of the body. An example of referred pain is angina: the pain of coronary artery insufficiency may be felt in the left shoulder, arm, or jaw.

Acute and chronic pain. Acute pain is intense and of short duration; the pain lasts less than 6 months. Generally acute pain provides a warning to the individual of actual or potential tissue damage. It creates an autonomic response commonly referred to as the *fight-or-flight* response. When healing occurs, the pain also resolves. There is usually anxiety associated with the pain. Because the pain is of short duration, physicians are more likely to prescribe narcotics and analgesics.

Chronic pain is generally characterized by pain lasting longer than 6 months. The pain can be continuous or intermittent and can be as intense as acute pain. The fight-or-flight response is no longer present. Chronic pain does not serve as a warning of tissue damage. In rheumatoid arthritis, for example, joint pain may continue when the disease process is no longer active, because of the structural damage that has already occurred in the joint.[17] The reason for some forms of chronic pain may not be known. Because of the prolonged time involved in chronic pain, the patient often develops chronic low self-esteem, change in social identity, changes in role and social interaction, depression, anxiety, and irritability.

Because of the general differences between acute and chronic pain, some aspects of nursing interventions for these conditions may differ. The nurse must remember the realness of the pain, whether acute or chronic, and use appropriate measures to relieve that pain.[17]

Behavioral Characteristics of Pain

The defining characteristic of pain is the verbal or nonverbal communication by the patient of the presence of pain. Behavioral characteristics of pain are noted in Box 19-1.

BOX 19-1 BEHAVIORAL CHARACTERISTICS OF PAIN

1. Is self-protective; guards the painful area—places hands over the area
2. Has narrowed focus; cannot think of anything but the pain
3. Withdraws from social contact
4. Has impaired thought processes
5. Demonstrates distraction behavior, which includes moaning, crying, pacing, restlessness, or seeking out other people or activities
6. Presents facial mask of pain, recognized by eyes that appear dull or lusterless, fixed or scattered facial movements, or grimace
7. Experiences alterations in muscle tone, ranging from lassitude to rigidity
8. Exhibits diaphoresis, changes in blood pressure and pulse rate, pupillary dilation, and increased or decreased rate of respiration
9. May demonstrate no outward expressions of pain. However, the nurse must remember that lack of pain expression does not mean lack of pain. There is no specific "picture" of a patient in pain

Theories of Pain Transmission

The gate control theory of pain, proposed by Melzack and Wall,[11] suggests that pain impulses can be regulated or even blocked by gating mechanisms located along the central nervous system. The proposed location of the gates is in the dorsal horn of the spinal cord. Pain and other sensations of the skin and muscles travel the same pathways through the large nerves in the spinal cord. If other cutaneous stimuli besides pain are transmitted, the "gate" through which the pain impulse must travel is temporarily blocked by the stimuli. The brain cannot determine the pain while it is interpreting the other stimuli. When gates are open, pain impulses flow freely. When gates are closed, pain impulses become blocked. Partial openings may occur. A bombardment of sensory impulses, such as those from the presssure of a backrub, the heat of a warm compress, or the cold from ice applications, will close the gates to painful stimuli. Some patients can be distracted from pain by removing the sensation of pain from their center of attention. Auditory or visual stimuli can distract patients and help make pain more tolerable[16] (Fig. 19-2).

Gating mechanisms can also be altered by thoughts, feelings, and memories. The cerebral cortex and thalamus can influence whether pain impulses reach a person's conscious awareness. There is conscious control over how pain is perceived, and this helps explain the various ways people react and adjust to pain.

Endorphins. The body contains a natural supply of morphine-like substances called **endorphins.** Stress and pain

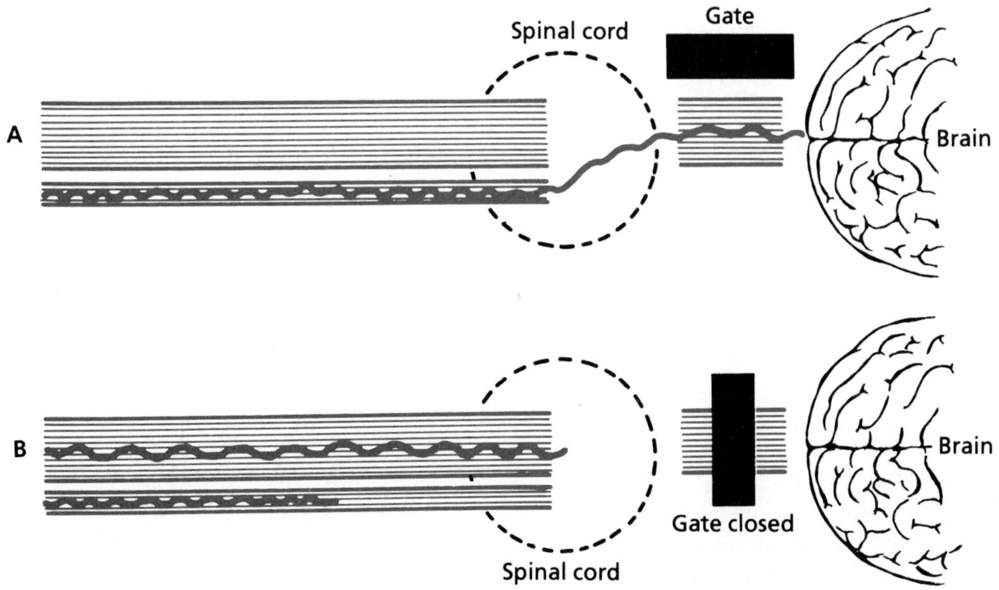

FIG. 19-2 Diagrammatic sketch of gate control theory.

activate endorphins. Analgesia results when certain endorphins attach to opiate receptors in the brain. People who have less pain than others from a similar injury have higher endorphin levels. Pain relief measures, such as **transcutaneous electrical nerve stimulation (TENS)** and acupuncture, are believed to cause release of endorphins.

NURSING ASSESSMENT OF PAIN

Collection of Subjective Data

It is important for the nurse to obtain accurate information from the patient concerning his pain, including characteristics and description of the pain. The characteristics may include the site, severity, duration, and location of pain. When documenting the presence of pain, the nurse should describe the specific location and intensity. Charting "patient complains of pain" provides no useful information. It is necessary to ask the patient what relieves the pain and what does not relieve the pain. Sociocultural information includes identifying usual coping mechanisms and the patient's, family's, and friends' expectations of appropriate behavior when in pain. If medications are taken for pain, the name, dose, frequency, and effect of the drugs must be determined.

The nurse must be sensitive to the patient's condition. Obviously, patients who are critically ill or in excruciating pain should be asked only a few key questions at any given time rather than be subjected to a long list of questions. The nurse must project an interest and concern for the patient so he will openly discuss his pain.[15]

There has been interest recently in developing tools specifically for assessment of pain. Nurses who are frequently faced with difficulties in assessing pain may wish to use one of the currently available tools or to develop one of their own. One effective method of identifying intensity is the McGill Pain Scale.[11] The person is asked to rate the pain on a scale of 0 to 5 as described below:

0 No pain
1 Mild pain
2 Discomforting pain
3 Distressing pain
4 Horrible pain
5 Excruciating pain

Visual analog scales may be used (Fig. 19-3) and may be helpful for comparison of a person's concept of the pain intensity over time.

Collection of Objective Data

The nurse must carefully observe the patient. Some objective signs may be tachycardia, increased rate and depth of respirations, diaphoresis, increased systolic or diastolic blood pressure, pallor, dilated pupils, and increased muscle tension. The patient may complain of nausea or weakness.[15]

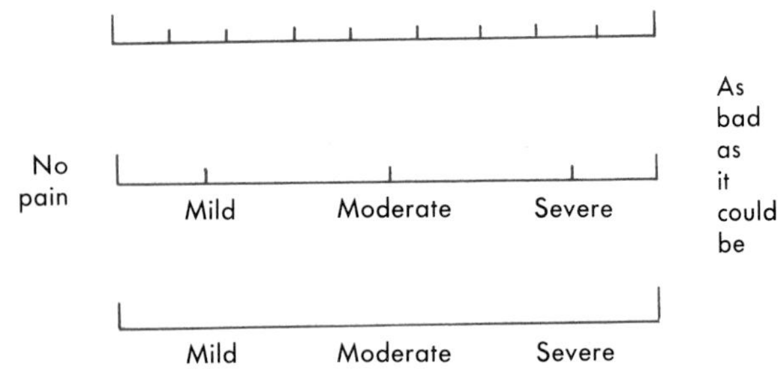

FIG. 19-3 Visual analog pain scales. Person marks line describing intensity of pain.

If the pain is chronic or less severe, the physiological changes may be less prominent. The nurse may notice changes in facial expressions, such as frowning or gritting of teeth. Some persons clench their fists and withdraw when in pain. Others may complain bitterly, cry, moan, toss about in bed, assume a fetal position, or clutch at the affected body part. Still others will pace if they have energy to do so. Some patients in pain want someone in constant attendance, whereas others want to be left alone.[15]

Nurses must be nonbiased and nonjudgmental when gathering objective data: the patient is doing the best he can at the given moment. The immediate intervention by the nurse is to relieve or decrease the pain. It should be remembered that pain is what the patient says it is. The nurse should not expect the patient to behave in any set manner when in pain.

NURSING DIAGNOSES FOR PAIN

The following nursing diagnoses are directly associated with the care of patients with pain:

- Chronic pain
- Pain

Possible other nursing diagnoses that may be appropriate because of the effects of pain on other aspects of a patient's life include the following:

- Anxiety
- Body image disturbance
- Colonic constipation
- Ineffective family coping: disabling
- Ineffective individual coping
- Altered family processes
- Fatigue
- Fear
- Anticipatory grieving
- Knowledge deficit (specify)
- Altered nutrition: less than/more than body requirements
- Impaired physical mobility

NURSING CARE PLAN: THE PATIENT WITH CHRONIC PAIN

The patient is a 45-year-old man with a 15-year history of severe, crippling rheumatoid arthritis. He has had numerous joint replacements, has had a weight loss of 40 pounds in the past year, and has developed corneal ulcers from the presence of Sjögren's syndrome. He is in constant chronic pain and has limited mobility. He states he has difficulty accomplishing home care instructions.

Nursing diagnoses	Patient goals	Nursing interventions
Chronic pain related to joint/muscle inflammation and degeneration manifested by complaints of pain, narrow focus of interest, guarded movement, and social withdrawal	Patient and/or family will verbalize a reduction in anxiety and pain when using relaxation massage, cutaneous stimulation, and analgesias.	Teach relaxation exercises. Perform massage to relieve pain and to enhance nurse/patient communications. Administer analgesics as ordered; apply cold/heat applications as ordered. Maintain transcutaneous electrical nerve stimulation (TENS) as ordered.
Impaired physical mobility, related to musculoskeletal degeneration, pain and edema manifested by slow, painful movements, decreased range of motion, and loss of muscle strength	Patient will demonstrate increase in mobility of joints.	Place patient in position of comfort, support joints anatomically with pillows or pads, and change position every hour. Assist with ROM exercise. Avoid restrictive clothing. Assist to ambulate as tolerated. Maintain a safe environment: handrails in shower, tub, and toilet; raised toilet seat; and rubber-tipped cane or walker.
Dressing/grooming self-care deficit, related to pain, decreased vision, lack of range of motion, and weakness manifested by increasing difficulties in performing activities of daily living	Patient's independence in self-care activities will increase within parameters of disability.	Teach self-care activities. Establish and teach routine plan for ADLs. Set goals with patient: encourage short-term, easily accomplished goals. Discuss use of snaps on clothing and slip-on shoes.
Chronic low self-esteem, related to inability to work, and body image change manifested by preoccupation with body changes and verbalization of powerlessness	Patient will verbalize understanding of changes in body image caused by disease process and will begin to exhibit increased confidence in dealing with self-esteem.	Encourage verbalization about fears and anxiety of disease process. Deal with behavioral changes, denial, powerlessness, anxiety, and dependence. Be supportive and kind in setting goals. Encourage independence, and give praise for tasks accomplished. Modify environment, and allow time for patient to accomplish goals.
Knowledge deficit, related to home care management manifested by statements of concern/misconceptions about medication regimen, exercise program, and diet	Patient and/or significant others will demonstrate understanding of home care follow-up instructions through interactive discussion and actual demonstration.	Stress importance of maintaining prescribed exercise, activities, rest, diet, and medication regimen. Reinforce physician's explanation of disease process, expectations, and limitations. Discuss diet management; stress importance of balanced diet. Provide medication schedule, including name, dosage, purpose, and side effects. Promote follow-up visits with physician.

- Powerlessness
- Altered role performance
- Bathing/hygiene self-care deficit
- Dressing/grooming self-care deficit
- Toileting self-care deficit
- Sexual dysfunction
- Sleep pattern disturbance
- Social isolation
- Altered thought processes

The extensiveness of the list alerts the nurse to the numerous problems that may develop because of pain.

THE RESPONSIBILITY OF THE NURSE IN PAIN CONTROL

The nurse can assist the patient in pain relief by telling the patient, "I believe that you are in pain, and I will assist you in whatever way I can to relieve your pain." This reduces the patient's anxiety level. A patient should not be required to use his energies to convince the nurse that his pain is real. The nurse should begin pain intervention as soon as the patient states he is in pain.

The founding principle of effective pain management is Meinhart and McCaffery's statement that "the failure to treat pain is inhumane and constitutes professional negligence."[9] Every patient has the right to be free of pain; it is the nurse's responsibility to do everything possible to alleviate the patient's pain.

GUIDELINES FOR INDIVIDUALIZING PAIN THERAPY

In providing pain relief measures it is important for the nurse to choose therapies suited to the patient's unique pain experience. McCaffery suggests patient's unique guidelines for individualizing pain therapy[9]:

1. Use different types of pain relief measures—using more than one therapy has an additive effect in reducing pain. In addition, the character of pain may change throughout the day, requiring several different therapies. Combining physical and psychological approaches (e.g., analgesics and relaxation) controls all components of the pain experience.
2. Provide pain relief measures before pain becomes severe—an ounce of prevention is worth a pound of cure (it is easier to prevent severe pain than to relieve it). Giving an analgesic 30 minutes before a patient must walk or perform an activity is an example of controlling pain early.
3. Use measures the patient believes are effective—the patient is the expert on his own pain. He may have ideas about what measures to use (e.g., rubbing lotion on an edematous finger) and when to use them that will make pain therapy successful.
4. Consider the patient's ability or willingness to participate in pain relief measures—some patients cannot actively assist with pain therapy because of fatigue, sedation, or altered levels of consciousness. However, there are variations of pain relief measures that require little effort, such as relaxation exercises in bed or listening to music as a distraction. The nurse will not relieve pain by forcing an unwilling patient to participate in therapy. The depressed patient with chronic pain has little motivation to participate.
5. Choose pain relief measures appropriate to the severity of the pain as reflected by the patient's behavior—it would be poor judgment to administer a potent narcotic to a patient who is displaying only mild pain. The nurse carefully assesses what the patient says and how he behaves before choosing pain therapy. Some patients acquire relief from severe pain after using only mild analgesics. Only the patient can determine the degree of effectiveness of a therapy.
6. If a therapy is ineffective at first, encourage the patient to try it again before abandoning it—often anxiety or doubt prevents patient from gaining relief from therapy. Some approaches, such as distraction, require practice. Some measures that seem ineffective may merely require adjustment to become effective. For example, the dosage of an analgesic may be increased if severe pain is initially unrelieved. The nurse should be persistent and understanding in helping the patient learn to use measures that do not afford immediate relief.
7. Keep an open mind about what may relieve pain—new ways are found to control pain. There is much to be learned about the pain experience. Rejecting a patient's nonconventional therapies will lead to mistrust. It is, however, the nurse's responsibility to monitor therapies to ensure the patient's safety and well-being.
8. Keep trying—the nurse can easily become frustrated when efforts at pain relief fail. It is important not to abandon the patient when pain persists. The patient in severe chronic pain who is ignored may choose suicide as an alternative. If the patient gains no relief, the nurse should reassess the situation and consider whether alternative therapies are needed.
9. Protect the patient—pain therapy should not cause more distress than the pain itself. The nurse always observes the response to therapy. Any pain relief measure may cause side effects, such as fatigue, anxiety, or additional pain. The nurse's aim is to relieve pain without disabling the patient mentally, emotionally, or physically.

NURSING INTERVENTIONS TO CONTROL PAINFUL STIMULI IN PATIENTS' ENVIRONMENT

The following measures can be performed by the nurse to assist in pain control[16]:

- Tighten wrinkled bed linens
- Reposition drainage tubes or other objects on which patient is lying
- Place warm bath blankets for coldness
- Loosen constricting bandages
- Change wet dressings
- Position patient in anatomical alignment
- Check temperature of hot and cold applications, including bath water
- Lift, not pull, patient up in bed; handle gently
- Position patient correctly on bedpan
- Avoid exposing skin or mucous membranes to irritants (e.g., diarrheal stool or wound drainage)
- Prevent urinary retention by ensuring patency of Foley catheter
- Prevent constipation by encouraging appropriate fluid intake, diet, and exercise

Noninvasive Pain Relief Techniques

Noninvasive pain relief measures can be helpful alone or in conjunction with other methods of management of pain. These approaches include cutaneous stimulation (heat, cold, massage, and TENS), distraction, relaxation, imagery, hypnosis, and biofeedback.

Whether these techniques work because of the gate control theory or because they decrease anxiety, they undoubtedly have many advantages for pain control; most are inexpensive and easy to perform, have low risk and few side effects, and may not require a physician's order. Probably the greatest advantage of these techniques is the patient's ability to have some control over the treatment of his pain. Although not everyone will react successfully to these pain relief measures, it is worthwhile to attempt any of them before advancing to more invasive techniques. It also enables the nurse to offer options for pain relief to patients.[1]

Transcutaneous electrical nerve stimulation (TENS). This pocket-sized, battery-operated device provides a continuous, mild electrical current to the skin via electrodes (see Fig. 26-5). Generally the electrodes are placed on or near the painful site. As with other forms of cutaneous stimulation, it is thought the TENS works by stimulating large nerve fibers to "close the gate" in the spinal cord. In addition, TENS may stimulate endorphin production.

Invasive Approach to Pain Management

Invasive means anything that enters the body. Examples of invasive techniques are nerve blocks, neurosurgical procedures, and acupuncture. Certain invasive techniques can be helpful for the patient with pain. However, careful patient selection and proper technique are essential, because the costs and risks are high.

Medication Approach to Pain Management

Analgesics can provide patients effective pain relief. Nurses and physicians frequently have misconceptions about the dangers and effects of analgesics. They often undertreat patients because of (1) incorrect pharmacological information, (2) concerns about contributing to addiction, (3) anxiety over errors in judgment while using a narcotic analgesic, and (4) administering less medication than is ordered. Often because of a nurse's uncertainty about the correct administration of analgesics, pain is only reduced, not relieved.

Nurses must understand the medications available for pain relief and their effects. A drug may act at the peripheral receptor level or at the central nervous system level. The most common peripheral analgesics include acetylsalicylic acid (aspirin), acetaminophen (Tylenol), and the nonsteroidal antiinflammatory drugs, ibuprofen (Motrin) and naproxen (Naprosyn) PO and ketorolac tromethamine (Toradol) IM. These drugs act primarily as peripheral receptors to diminish reception of pain stimuli.

Narcotic analgesics, such as morphine, meperidine (Demerol), and codeine, act on higher centers of the brain to modify perception and reaction to pain. The danger of morphine and other narcotic analgesics is the potential for depression of vital nervous system functions. Opiates cause respiratory depression by depressing the respiratory center within the brainstem.[16]

The nurse must learn what is the most effective analgesic and means of administration for the patient's specific need. It takes skill to determine if the medication should be given orally, IM, or IV (see Chapter 25).

Because nurses sometimes fear overtreating patients' pain, a helpful rule is that severe pain requires a greater amount of analgesic to relieve it. Dosages at the upper end of normally prescribed ranges are usually safe. If a well-meaning nurse administers a low dose that proves ineffective, the patient may suffer until the required time interval has passed before a drug can again be given.[16]

The patient should be an active participant by telling the nurse when pain perception occurs. The nurse also assesses the patient for nonverbal expressions of pain. If any pain-producing procedure, such as walking, sitting up, or a dressing change, is scheduled, the nurse should give an analgesic before the activity. The drug should be administered so that its peak effect is reached during the patient's most active time.

Patient-controlled analgesia. A drug delivery system called **patient-controlled analgesia (PCA)** allows patients to administer pain medications when they need them. The PCA is a portable, computerized pump with a chamber for a syringe. The pump intravenously delivers a small, preset dose of medication, usually morphine or meperidine (Demerol). To receive a dose, the patient pushes a button on a cord attached to the pump (see Fig. 25-16). A timer prevents the system from delivering more than a specified number of doses every hour, to avoid overdoses. Each dose may be as small as 1 ml or 1 mg of morphine every 6 to 12 minutes. It has a locked safety system that prevents tampering.

Placebos. A **placebo** is an inactive substance or procedure that is given to a patient for its suggestive effect. A placebo is any treatment that produces an effect because of its intent and not its physical or chemical properties, according to McCaffery.[9] An inactive substance, such as injectable normal saline or an oral preparation of sugar, is often prescribed as if it were medication. Some researchers believe that placebos increase endorphin levels. Others believe they create a psychological sense of pain relief, lowering a patient's pain perception. The patient's belief that a placebo is a real form of therapy may be the necessary factor in relieving pain.

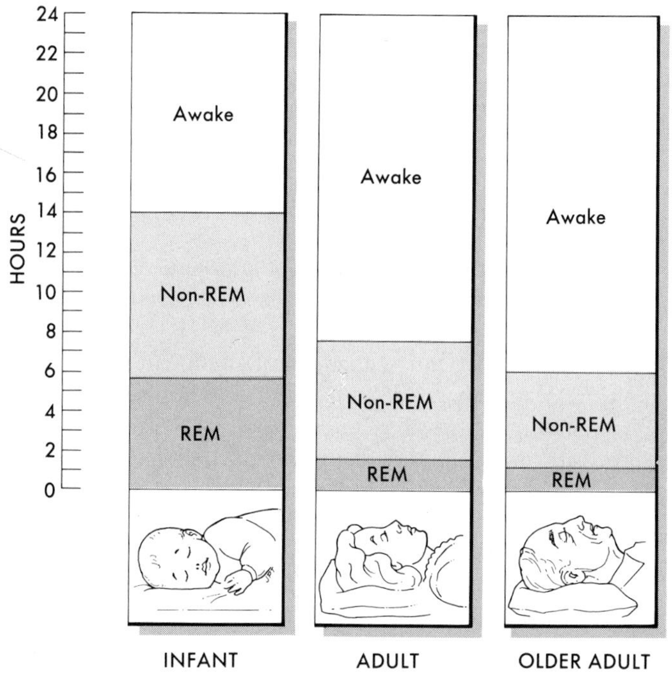

FIG. 19-4 Sleep-wake cycles across the life span. Infants: approximately 40% of total sleep time is REM. Adults: 20% of total sleep time is REM. Older adults: total sleep time is slightly reduced, REM remains 20% of total.

SLEEP AND REST

A patient at rest feels mentally relaxed, free from worry, and physically calm. A patient at rest is free from physical or mental exertion. All persons have their own method of obtaining rest and can usually adjust to new environments or conditions that affect the ability to rest.

Nurses frequently care for patients for whom bed rest has been prescribed. This treatment confines patients to bed to decrease physical or psychological demands on the body. Bed rest does not necessarily mean a patient is resting. Emotional or metabolic stressors may cause the patient to be restless.

Sleep is a state of rest that occurs for a sustained period. The reduced consciousness during sleep provides time for repair and recovery of body systems for the next period of wakefulness. Sleep restores a person's energy and feeling of well-being.

When the patient enters the hospital or other health care facility, his rest and sleep habits can easily be disrupted by hospital routines. The extent of the change depends on the gravity of the illness, as well as the environment in which the patient is placed. The nurse must remain aware of the patient's need for rest. Without rest, the patient becomes fatigued and irritable and has a decreased ability to cope with stressors.[16]

Sleep Cycle

Sleep involves two phases: **rapid eye movement (REM)** and **nonrapid eye movement (NREM).** NREM sleep is further divided into four stages, through which a sleeper progresses during a typical sleeping cycle. The sleeping states are highly individualized (Fig. 19-4 and Box 19-2).

Normally in an adult the routine sleep pattern begins with a presleep period during which the person is aware only of a gradually developing drowsiness. This period normally lasts 10 to 30 minutes, but if a person has difficulty falling asleep, it may last an hour or longer.

As adults fall asleep, they progress through the four stages of NREM sleep. At the end of the fourth stage, they come out of a deep sleep, go back to stage 2, and then enter a period of REM. A person reaches REM sleep in about 90 minutes (average). Each person differs, but a typical night's sleep consists of four to six such cycles. People on the average awaken five times during the night and are twice as likely to awaken from REM sleep as any other stage.

Dreams occur during both the NREM and REM stages. The dream of REM sleep is believed to be functionally important, more vivid, and elaborate.[16] Dreaming allows a person to clarify emotions and prepare the mind for events of the next day. Most medications used to promote sleep, relieve anxiety, and overcome depression interfere with REM sleep. The person may sleep, but not feel rested.

BOX 19-2 STAGES OF SLEEP

STAGE 1: NREM

Lightest level of sleep
Lasts a few minutes
Decreased physiological activity begins with gradual fall in vital signs and metabolism
Person easily aroused by sensory stimuli, such as noise
If person awakes, feels as though daydreaming

STAGE 2: NREM

Period of sound sleep
Relaxation progresses
Arousal is still easy
Lasts 10 to 20 minutes
Body functions continue to slow

STAGE 3: NREM

Initial stages of deep sleep
Sleeper is difficult to arouse and rarely moves
Muscles completely relax
Vital signs decline but remain regular
Lasts 15 to 30 minutes

STAGE 4: NREM

Deepest stage of sleep
Very difficult to arouse sleeper
If sleep loss has occurred, sleeper will spend considerable portion of sleep in this stage
Stage responsible for restoring and resting body
Vital signs significantly lower than during waking hours
Lasts approximately 15 to 30 minutes
Sleepwalking and enuresis may occur

REM SLEEP

Stage of vivid, full-color dreaming (less vivid dreaming may occur in other stages)
Usually begins every 50 to 90 minutes after sleep has begun
Typified by autonomic response of rapidly moving eyes, fluctuating heart and respiratory rates, and blood pressure
Loss of skeletal muscle tone
Responsible for mental restoration
Sleeper most difficult to arouse
Duration of REM sleep increases with each cycle and averages 20 minutes

Sleep Deprivation

Sleep deprivation is a problem many patients experience as a result of hospitalization. Sleep deprivation involves decreases in the amount, quality, and consistency of sleep. When sleep is interrupted or fragmented, changes in the normal sequence of sleep stages occur, and cycles cannot be completed.[6] Gradually a cumulative deprivation develops.

Patients may experience a variety of physiological and psychological signs and symptoms. Physiological signs and symptoms include hand tremors, decreased reflexes, slowed response time, reduction in word memory, decreased reasoning and judgment, and cardiac dysrhythmias. Psychological signs and symptoms include mood swings, disorientation, irritability, decreased motivation, fatigue, sleepiness, and hyperexcitability.[16]

Promoting Rest and Sleep

The nurse should determine the patient's usual rest and sleep patterns, decide if they are sufficient, and note why the patient is not getting sufficient rest. A plan should be developed with the patient and family to provide for more rest. The plan might include limiting interruptions during the night for vital sign checks and other procedures, providing a quiet environment, limiting the number of visitors and the duration of visits, and carrying out all procedures within a given time frame.

In preparing the patient for sleep, the nurse should wash the patient's back if he is on bed rest, gently massage it, freshen the linens, make certain the patient is warm enough, offer a noncaffeine beverage, such as milk, change soiled dressings, and have the patient void. Environmental stimuli should be decreased by dimming the lights and decreasing the noise level. The nurse should direct the patient to assume a comfortable position and assist if needed. The patient should be instructed to concentrate on each extremity, one at a time, to focus on how light and relaxed each extremity is, and to begin to breathe slowly, but carefully, allowing no other thoughts to enter the mind. With practice, this approach can be used by the patient when going to sleep. A sleeping medication or analgesic may be administered if the patient cannot sleep.[15]

Nursing diagnoses and nursing interventions for the patient with sleep disturbance are as follows:

NURSING DIAGNOSES	NURSING INTERVENTIONS
Sleep pattern disturbance, related to illness and psychological stress manifested by change in behavior performance and increasing irritability and listlessness	Encourage patient to ambulate 15 min if able, 1 to 2 hr before bedtime. Provide glass of milk 30 min before bedtime unless contraindicated. Perform all necessary procedures before 9 PM to ensure uninterrupted sleep. Massage back, freshen linens, reduce noise, and dim lights. Administer hypnotic as ordered.
Altered thought processes, related to sleep deprivation manifested by slower reaction time, altered attention span, and disorientation.	Maintain periods of uninterrupted rest. Provide safe environment. Close door to patient room. Orient to reality. Administer analgesic and/or sedative about 30 minutes before bedtime, if ordered.

REFERENCES AND SUGGESTED READINGS

1. Beare PG and Meyers JL: Principles and practices of adult health nursing, St Louis, 1990, The CV Mosby Co.
2. Cancer pain relief, Geneva, 1986, World Health Organization.
3. Donovan MI, Dillon P, and McGuire L: Incidence and characteristics of pain in a sample of medical-surgical inpatients, Pain 30:69, 1987.
4. Funk SG and others: Key aspects of comfort: management of pain, fatigue, and nausea, New York, 1989, Springer Publishing Co, Inc.
5. Hood GH and Dincher JR: Total patient care: foundations and practice, ed 7, St Louis, 1988, The CV Mosby Co.
6. Fisher ME: ICU syndrome, Crit Care Nurse 4:39, 1984.
7. Lewis LW and Timby BK: Fundamental skills and concepts in patient care, ed 4, Philadelphia, 1988, JB Lippincott Co.
8. McCaffery M and Beebe A: Pain: clinical manual for nursing practice, St Louis, 1989, The CV Mosby Co.
9. McCaffery M: Nursing management of the patient with pain, ed 2, Philadelphia, 1979, JB Lippincott Co.
10. Meinhort NT and McCaffery M: Pain: a nursing approach to assessment and analysis, New York, 1983, Appleton-Century-Crofts.
11. Melzack R: Pain measurement and assessment, New York, 1983, Raven Press.
12. Moorehouse MF and Doenges ME: Nurses' clinical pocket manual: nursing diagnosis, care planning, and documentation, ed 10, Philadelphia, 1990, FA Davis Co.
13. Mosby's medical, nursing, and allied health dictionary, St. Louis, 1990, The CV Mosby Co.
14. Parce JA: The phenomenon of analgesic tolerance in cancer pain management, Oncol Nurs Forum 15(4):455, 1988.
15. Phipps WJ, Long BC, and Woods NF: Medical-surgical nursing: concepts and clinical practice, St Louis, 1987, The CV Mosby Co.
16. Potter PA and Perry AG: Fundamentals of nursing: concepts, process, and practice, ed 2, St Louis, 1989, The CV Mosby Co.
17. Thompson JM and others: Mosby's manual of clinical nursing, ed 2, St Louis, 1989, The CV Mosby Co.
18. Watt-Watson JH: Nurses' knowledge of pain issues: a survey, Pain and Symptom Manage 2(4):207, 1987.

CHAPTER CHALLENGE

STUDY QUESTIONS

1. The most accurate description of pain is:
   a. Pain is whatever the experiencing person says it is, existing wherever he says it does
   b. Pain is an unpleasant sensation caused by noxious stimulation of motor nerve endings
   c. Pain is a cardinal sign of inflammation
   d. Pain always results in specific behavioral characteristics
2. All of the following are correct behavioral characteristics of pain except:
   a. Self-protective, guarding the painful area
   b. A broad focus—patient is able to think of several topics of interest
   c. Alterations in muscle tone, ranging from lassitude to rigidity
   d. Lack of pain expression does not mean lack of pain
3. The gate control theory of pain suggests that:
   a. The body contains a natural supply of morphine-like substance called endorphins
   b. Pain is a specific modality and that there are specific nerve fibers that transmit pain impulses to the brain
   c. Pain impulses can be regulated or even blocked by mechanisms located along the central nervous system
   d. Pain is a manifestation of an intricate chain of electrochemical events
4. Pain is:
   a. Subjective
   b. Objective
5. Referred pain is:
   a. Constant, unremitting
   b. Precisely localized
   c. At a site different from that of an injured or diseased organ
   d. None of the above
6. The most frequently quoted authority on pain is:
   a. Wiese
   b. Champagne
   c. Hood
   d. McCaffery
7. The ongoing collection of subjective data concerning pain should include:
   a. Duration
   b. Location
   c. Intensity
   d. All of the above
8. A visual analog scale may be helpful for:
   a. Comparison of a person's concept of pain intensity over time
   b. Rating the pain on a scale of 0 to 5
   c. Determining the proposed location of pain in the dorsal horn of the spinal cord
   d. None of the above
9. People who have less pain than others from a similar injury have a:
   a. Higher level of endorphin levels
   b. Lower level of endorphin levels
10. Examples of cutaneous stimulation for relief of pain are all of the following except:
    a. Heat, cold
    b. TENS
    c. Massage
    d. PCA
11. A common central nervous system analgesic is:
    a. Aspirin
    b. Tylenol
    c. Morphine
    d. Motrin
12. Research shows nurses have a tendency to overtreat pain or undertreat pain:
    a. Overtreat
    b. Undertreat
13. A drug delivery system that allows patients to administer their own pain medications via a portable computerized pump with a chamber for a syringe is called:
    a. Patient-controlled analgesia
    b. Transcutaneous electric nerve stimulation
    c. Venous access device
    d. Placebo
14. Which of the following are helpful nursing interventions to control painful stimuli in the patient's environment:
    a. Tighten wrinkled bed linens
    b. Loosen constricting bandages
    c. Position patient in anatomical alignment
    d. All of the above
15. Most medications used to promote sleep, relieve anxiety, and overcome depression:
    a. Enhance REM sleep
    b. Interfere with REM sleep
16. The following nursing intervention(s) is(are) helpful to promote rest and sleep:
    a. Decrease noise level
    b. Cleanse and massage the back
    c. Direct the patient to assume a comfortable position; assist if needed
    d. All of the above

20

Hygiene and Care of the Patient's Environment

ELAINE ODEN KOCKROW

LEARNING OBJECTIVES

After reading this chapter, the student should be able to do the following:

- Define the key terms.
- Discuss variations of the bath procedure determined by the patient's condition and physician's orders.
- Demonstrate the correct procedure for administering the bed bath.
- Identify nursing interventions for the prevention and treatment of decubitus ulcers.
- Describe components of the bath procedure: oral hygiene, shaving, hair care, nail care, eye, ear, and nose care.
- Demonstrate the correct procedure for administering the back rub.
- Demonstrate the correct procedure for administering perineal care to the male and female.
- Demonstrate the correct procedure for administering skin care.
- Demonstrate the correct procedure for making the unoccupied bed: open, closed, and surgical.
- Demonstrate the correct procedure for making the occupied bed.
- Discuss measures to assist the patient in the use of the bedpan, urinal, and bedside commode.

RELATED KNOWLEDGE AND SKILLS

- Communication (Chapter 4)
- Documentation (Chapter 6)
- Signs, symptoms, and physical assessment (Chapter 13)
- Medical asepsis (Chapter 16)
- Safety (Chapter 17)
- Body mechanics (Chapter 18)
- Comfort, rest, and sleep (Chapter 19)
- Care of the patient with an integumentary disorder (Chapter 29)
- Care of the patient with a urinary disorder (Chapter 33)
- Care of the patient with an eye or ear disorder (Chapter 37)

SKILLS

20-1 Administering a bed bath/partial bath
20-2 Administering a towel bath
20-3 Assisting the patient to take a tub bath or shower
20-4 Administering a tepid sponge bath for temperature reduction
20-5 Administering a medicated bath
20-6 Administering oral hygiene
20-7 Cleaning dentures
20-8 Shaving the patient
20-9 Administering a bed shampoo
20-10 Caring for the hands and feet
20-11 Administering perineal care for male and female patients
20-12 Administering perineal care for the patient with an indwelling catheter
20-13 Administering the back-rub
20-14 Making the occupied bed
20-15 Making the unoccupied bed
20-16 Positioning the bedpan

KEY TERMS

Define the following:

- axilla
- bedpan
- canthus
- cerumen
- Chux
- circumorbital
- denture
- erythema
- flatus
- hygiene
- labia majora
- labia minora
- medical asepsis
- microorganisms
- oral hygiene
- perineal care
- prone
- range of motion
- sanguineous
- Sims'
- supine
- syncope
- umbilicus
- urinal
- vertigo

GUIDELINES

When providing the patient's hygiene needs, the nurse has an opportunity to observe the patient's ability to perform self-care.

During the bath the nurse notes the patient's physical and emotional state. All body systems can be assessed during the patient's bath. Because the bath, especially the bed bath, involves close contact with the patient, the nurse can use communication skills to enhance the therapeutic relationship, thereby learning about the emotional needs of the patient.

Patients are often placed in a dependent role, dependent on the nurse to assist them in carrying out personal hygiene. The nurse should preserve the patient's well-being, encourage as much of the patient's independence as possible, and respect the patient's privacy.

At times the nurse will need to teach health promotion practices, and hygiene care provides an excellent opportunity for this. The nurse must project an attitude of acceptance when caring for a patient whose hygiene is obviously poor. Many factors influence the practice of an individual's personal hygiene: (1) physical condition; (2) personal preferences; (3) cultural variables; (4) knowledge; (5) socioeconomic status; (6) social practices; and (7) body image. The prudent nurse will consider all of these factors when assisting the patient with personal hygiene.

Hygiene includes care of not only the skin but also the hair, hands, feet, eyes, ears, nose, mouth, back, and perineum. This chapter will include the bath, components of the bath, bed making, and assisting the patient in the use of the bedpan, urinal, and bedside commode.

BATHING

The extent of the patient's bath and methods used for bathing depend on the patient's capabilities, the degree of hygiene required, and the physician's order, as in the case of therapeutic baths (Box 20-1).

A complete bed bath is for patients who are totally dependent and require total hygiene (Skill 20-1).

The seriously or critically ill patient may need a towel bath (Skill 20-2).

As the patient improves, only partial assistance may be required. The nurse assists the patient to bathe those body parts that are inaccessible to the patient.

Self Care

If the patient's condition warrants and ambulation has been ordered, the patient may be allowed to take a tub bath or shower (Skill 20-3).

A sitz bath may be ordered for the patient who has undergone rectal or vaginal surgery. This bath promotes healing and pain relief (see Box 20-1).

Text continued on p. 308.

BOX 20-1 SPECIAL BATHS

SITZ BATH

This bath cleanses and aids in reducing inflammation of the perineal and anal areas of the patient who has undergone rectal or vaginal surgery or childbirth. Discomfort from hemorrhoids or fissures is relieved by a sitz bath also.

Appliances for the sitz bath are shown in Figs. 20-1 and 20-2. Depending on the patient's diagnosis and the physician's order, the desired results could be obtained from a tub bath. However, the tub is the least desirable method because heat is also applied to the legs, thus reducing the effects on the pelvic region.

The nurse maintains a water temperature of 110° F (about 43° C) if the purpose is to apply heat to the affected area. If the purpose is to promote healing or to produce relaxation, a water temperature of about 98° to 102° F (34° to 39° C) is used. The nurse also should remember to prevent chilling by covering the patient's legs with a bath blanket and his shoulders with a towel. A towel may be placed behind the patient's back for comfort.

The sitz bath should last from 20 to 30 minutes. If the patient has reading material, the time will seem to pass more quickly.

The patient should be observed for signs and symptoms of weakness, such as rapid, weak pulse, tachypnea, and dizziness (**vertigo**) or fainting (**syncope**). The patient should never be left alone unless the nurse is sure the patient is safe; then a call signal should be placed within easy reach.

The patient should be instructed to stay out of drafts and to rest after a sitz bath.

COOL WATER TUB BATH

This bath may be given to relieve tension or lower body temperature. The nurse must institute measures to prevent the patient from chilling. The water temperature is tepid, not cold (98.6° F [37° C]).

WARM WATER TUB BATH

This bath is given chiefly to reduce muscle tension. The recommended water temperature is 109.4° F (43° C).

HOT WATER TUB BATH

This bath is given to assist in relieving muscle soreness and muscle spasms. This procedure is not recommended for children. The water temperature for adults should be 113° to 115° F (45° to 46° C). The nurse should remember that danger of burns exists and should take precautions to avoid this.*

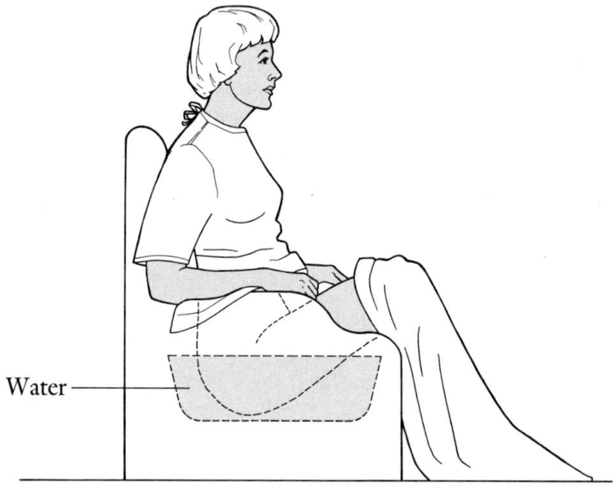

FIG. 20-1 The built-in sitz bath.

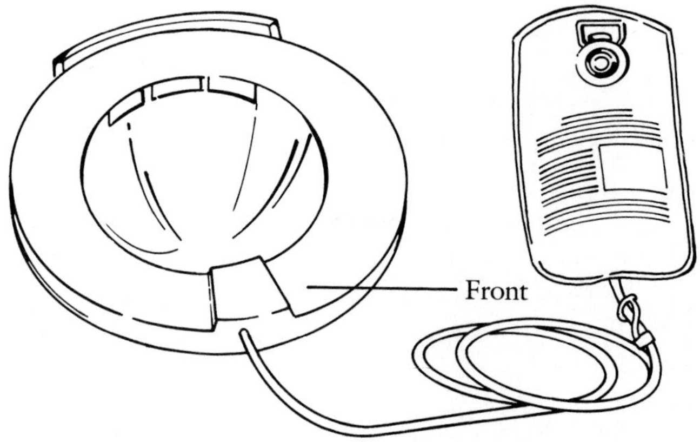

FIG. 20-2 The disposable sitz bath.

*Not used for patients with neurological disorders or circulatory impairment because of the danger of burning.

SKILL 20-1 ADMINISTERING A BED BATH/PARTIAL BATH

Nursing action	Rationale
1. Check physician's orders.	Provides a basis for care.
2. Introduce self, and explain procedure.	Promotes cooperation.
3. Adjust room temperature, and provide privacy.	Prevents chilling, and encourages relaxation.
4. Prepare supplies: ■ bath towels (2) ■ wash cloths (2) ■ wash basin ■ soap and soap dish ■ bath blanket ■ gown ■ hygiene articles, such as lotion, powder, and deodorant ■ laundry bag or hamper ■ disposable gloves	Promotes organization.
5. Suggest use of bedpan/urinal/bathroom.	Prevents interruptions during procedure, and provides for patient comfort.
6. Wash hands.	Prevents spread of **microorganisms.**
7. Lower side rail, position patient on side of bed closest to nurse, and raise bed to working level.	Ensures good body mechanics.
8. Loosen top linens from the foot of the bed; place bath blanket over the top linens. Ask patient to hold bath blanket while nurse removes top linens. If patient is unable, nurse will need to hold bath blanket in place while removing linens.	Provides warmth and privacy.
9. Place soiled laundry in laundry bag—do not touch uniform with soiled laundry.	Prevents spread of microorganisms.
10. Assist patient with oral hygiene. If patient is unable, the nurse performs procedure (see Skills 20-6 and 20-7).	Prevents mouth diseases, improves self-image, and improves appetite.
11. Remove patient's gown, all undergarments and jewelry.	Facilitates more effective bed bath.
12. Raise side rail, and fill water basin ⅔ full with water at 110° to 115° F (43° to 46° C).	Maintains patient's safety.
13. Remove pillow, and raise head of bed to semi-Fowler's position if patient can tolerate it.	Patient's face, ears, and neck are more accessible to wash.

Continued.

SKILL 20-1

ADMINISTERING A BED BATH/PARTIAL BATH—cont'd

Nursing action	Rationale
14. Form mitt with bath cloth around your hand; dip mitt and hand into bath water. Squeeze out excess water.	Easier to handle bath cloth, and prevents corners from brushing against patient.
15. Wash around patient's eyes using a different portion of wash cloth for each eye. Cleanse from inner to outer **canthus** (corner of eye). Dry gently.	Prevents irritation, spread of infection, and injury.
16. Rinse bath cloth (continue to use as mitt), and finish washing face. (Ask patient about using soap on face.) Ears and neck are washed at this time. Cleanse pinna with cotton-tipped applicators.	Some patients, especially female patients, do not use soap on face.
17. Expose arm farthest from nurse. Place towel lengthwise under patient's arm. Place wash basin on towel, and place patient's hand in basin of water. Bathe arms using long, firm strokes. Supporting arm, raise it above patient's head to bathe **axilla.** Rinse and dry well. Nail care is done at this time (see Skill 20-10). Deodorant may be applied.	Beginning on far side prevents reaching over clean area; long, firm strokes stimulates circulation. Raising arm promotes range of motion, as well as exposes axilla. (Axilla should be bathed last because it is considered less clean than arm.)

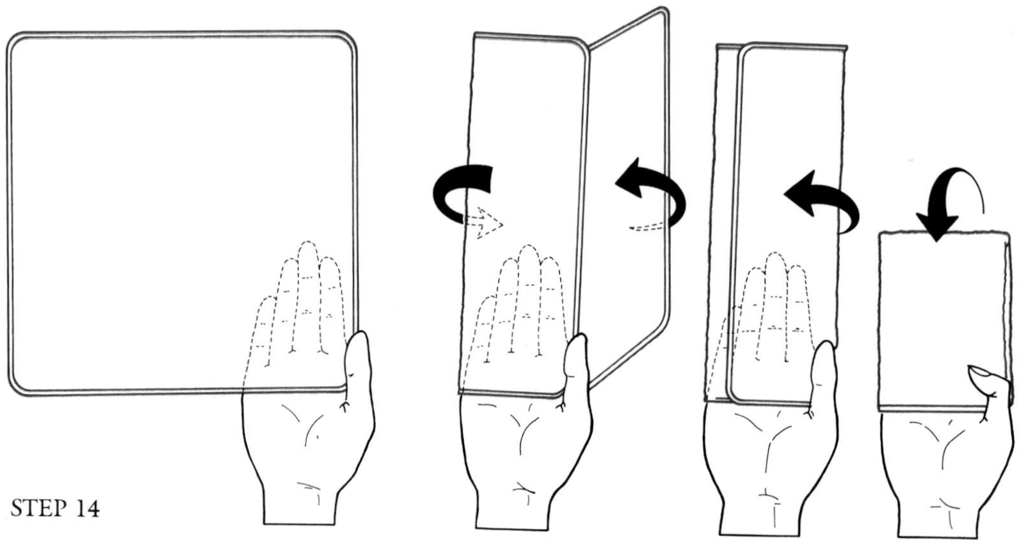

STEP 14

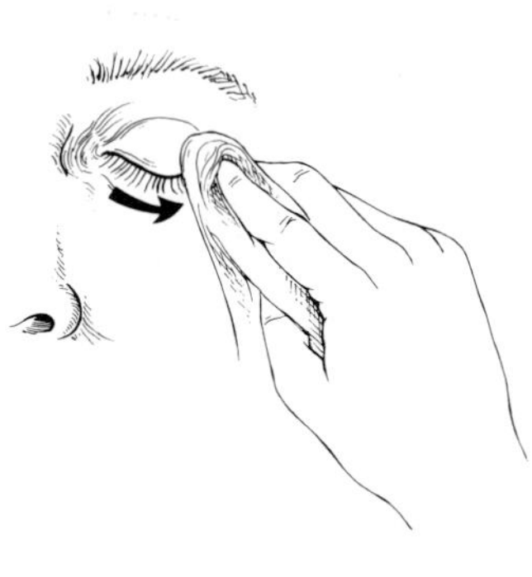

STEP 15

SKILL 20-1 ADMINISTERING A BED BATH/PARTIAL BATH—cont'd

Nursing action	Rationale
18. When doing nail care, allow hand to soak for 3 to 5 min; push back cuticles gently with wash cloth. Clean under nails, and file smoothly as needed. Dry thoroughly.	Enhances feeling of self-worth and decreases spread of infection. Soaking softens cuticles and loosens debris under nails.
19. Bathe arm closest to nurse. Follow steps 17 and 18.	
20. Cover patient's chest with bath towel; fold bath blanket down to waist, and wash chest with circular motion. Be certain to cleanse and dry well in skin folds and under breasts.	Using circular motion while bathing chest prevents injury to delicate breast tissue. Covering chest with towel prevents unnecessary exposure. Cleansing well in skin folds and under breasts maintains skin integrity.
21. Fold bath blanket down to pubic area, keeping chest covered with dry towel. Wash abdomen including **umbilicus** (using cotton-tipped applicators) and skin folds. Dry thoroughly.	Maintains patient's privacy. Prevents unnecessary exposure. Prevents skin impairment.
22. Raise side rail; empty basin into hopper or stool. Rinse basin and wash cloth. Refill basin ⅔ full with water at 110° to 115° F (43° to 46° C).	Promotes patient safety and comfort.
23. Expose leg farthest away from nurse, keeping perineum covered. Place bath towel lengthwise on bed under patient's leg. Place wash basin on towel, and place foot in basin. (Make certain to support patient's leg properly; flex knee and grasp heel.)	If patient is unable to place foot in wash basin, wash leg and foot with mitted wash cloth.
24. Using long, firm strokes, bathe leg. After soaking, do nail care (see Skill 20-10). If skin is dry, lotion may be applied. Do not massage legs.	Promotes circulation. Lower extremities are never massaged, to prevent possible embolus (a moving blood clot).
25. Bathe other leg and foot as in steps 23 and 24.	
26. Raise side rail. Make sure patient is covered with bath blanket. Change water (see step 22).	Maintains patient's safety and privacy.
27. Lower side rail. If patient tolerates, position in **prone** (on abdomen) or in **Sims'** (side-lying) position. Place towel lengthwise on bed along back. Wash and dry back from neckline down to buttocks.	If patient can tolerate a massage action, while washing back, do so to promote circulation, thus preventing skin impairment.
28. Reposition patient in **supine** (face up) position. Provide basin of water, soap, wash cloth, and towel, and instruct patient to cleanse perineal area. (Give patient privacy while this is done.)	If patient is unable to finish bath, nurse will don gloves and complete this aspect of patient care (see Skill 20-11).

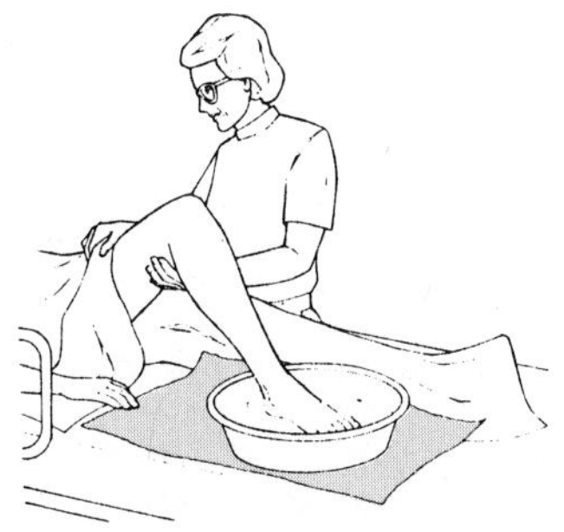

STEP 23

Continued.

SKILL 20-1 ADMINISTERING A BED BATH/PARTIAL BATH—cont'd

Nursing action	Rationale
29. Make certain patient is covered with blanket. Raise side rail. Empty basin, and wash and rinse basin. Replace basin in bedside stand. Place wash cloth in laundry bag for soiled linen.	Prevents patient from chilling. Promotes safety. Maintains **medical asepsis.**
30. Position patient in Sims' or prone position close to nurse. Place towel lengthwise along patient's back. Give back rub (see Skill 20-13).	Facilitates back care. Back care provides comfort and promotes skin integrity.
31. Assist patient into clean gown. If ordered, ambulate patient to chair, place towel over shoulders, and comb hair.	Promotes positive self-image. Women may wish to apply makeup at this time.
32. While patient is in chair, make unoccupied bed (see Skill 20-15). If patient is not ambulatory, nurse must make occupied bed (see Skill 20-14).	Maintains clean environment.
33. Place all soiled linen into laundry bag. Make certain all bath equipment is clean and replaced as necessary. Place call light, over-bed table, night stand, and telephone within easy reach.	Prevents the spread of microorganisms. Promotes safety.
34. Wash hands.	Prevents spread of microorganisms.

The partial bed bath differs from the bed bath only in that the patient can bathe various anatomical regions himself. The nurse then assists to bathe those areas which the patient cannot reach. All steps of the bath are followed, and the same considerations prevail. Supplies are placed within easy reach. Water is changed as noted in the bed bath skill, and back care, skin care, nail care, and hair care are given.

DOCUMENTATION

1. Record procedure.	Proves performance.

Sample charting

DATE	TIME	NOTES
12/30/90	0830	Awake but lethargic. Complains of "muscle soreness." Cast to right forearm clean and dry. Slight digital edema noted. Fingers pale but mobile. Bed bath given. Noted small, intact, erythematous area over coccyx. Massage given. States "that felt good." Positioned for comfort. Reported to P. Shahan, RN. ________ *(nurse's signature)*
	1000	Asleep
12/30/90	0830	Awake. Denies discomfort. Left leg cast clean and dry. Left toes pink, warm, and mobile. Capillary refill is prompt. States "I hope to go home this evening." Partial bed bath given. This nurse assisted with back, legs, feet, and nail care. Color pink, and skin warm and dry. Respirations unlabored. Very talkative this AM. Reported to E. Maseburg, RN. ________ *(nurse's signature)*

SKILL 20-1 ADMINISTERING A BED BATH/PARTIAL BATH—cont'd

SPECIAL CONCERNS

- Do not place soap in bath water—too much suds will prevent adequate rinsing.
- The nurse observes the condition of the patient's skin, degree of mobility, and behavior. She encourages the patient to verbalize his concerns.
- Patients with diabetes mellitus require special foot care.
- Be certain to expose only those body parts being bathed.
- If danger of contact with body fluids exists, don gloves.
- A firm stroke rather than a light stroke prevents a tickling sensation.
- Maintain a neat, clean work area.

PATIENT TEACHING

- When appropriate, the nurse should take the opportunity to instruct the patient in personal hygiene and skin care.

SKILL 20-2 ADMINISTERING A TOWEL BATH

Nursing action	Rationale
1. Check physician's order. Confer with charge nurse to determine need for towel bath.	Ensures accuracy of procedure.
2. Explain procedure.	Reduces anxiety.
3. Adjust room temperature, and provide privacy.	Prevents chilling, and encourages relaxation.
4. Obtain supplies: ■ concentrate/solution (e.g., Septi-Soft) ■ measuring device, such as plastic medication cup or liter-calibrated container ■ towel-bath towel (3 ft × 7½ ft) ■ large plastic bag ■ bath towel ■ wash cloths (2) ■ bath blankets (2 or 3) ■ disposable gloves ■ linens for bedmaking ■ articles for personal hygiene—comb, tooth brush, lotion, toothpaste, and mouthwash	Promotes orderly procedure.
5. Prepare patient. a. Remove patient's clothing and excess bedding (top linens, bedspread). Place patient on bath blanket, and cover patient with bath blanket.	Preparing patient ensures bath towel will be warm enough for patient's comfort, as well as for effective towel bath.
b. Cover with plastic any surgical dressings, casts, or areas that should not be wet.	Prevents contamination of dressing or cast.
c. Fan fold a clean bath blanket at foot of the bed.	
d. Position patient supine (lying on back with legs partially separated and arms loosely at sides).	

Continued.

SKILL 20-2 ADMINISTERING A TOWEL BATH—cont'd

Nursing action	Rationale
6. Prepare towel. a. Fold towel in half, top to bottom; fold in half again, top to bottom; now half again, side to side. Then roll towel-bath towel, with bath towel and wash cloth inside, beginning with folded edge. b. Place rolled-up towel-bath towel (with bath towel and wash cloths inside) in plastic bag with selvage edges toward open end of bag. c. Draw 2000 ml of water at 115° to 120° F into plastic pitcher. Measure 30 ml of concentrate or 90 ml of solution. (If using dispenser with a pump, single stroke measures [30 ml].) Mix 2000 ml of water and Septi-Soft. d. Pour mixture over towel in plastic bag. e. Knead the solution quickly into towel, position plastic bag with open end in sink, and squeeze out excess water, giving added wringing twist to selvage edges of towel.	Preparing towel prevents unnecessary cleanups and promotes effective procedure.

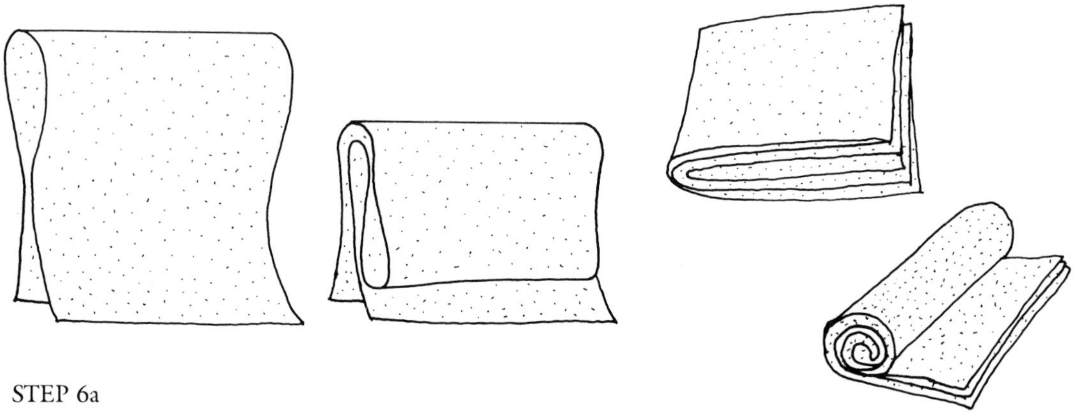

STEP 6a

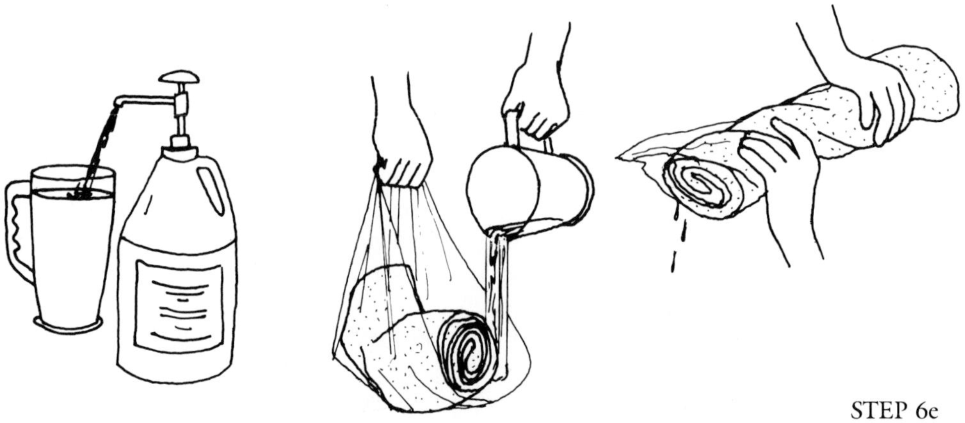

STEP 6e

SKILL 20-2 ADMINISTERING A TOWEL BATH—cont'd

Nursing action

7. Bathe patient.
   a. Fold bath blanket down to waist. Remove warm, moist towel from plastic bag and place on patient's right or left chest with open edges up and outward. (Unroll towel across chest.)
   b. Open towel to cover entire body while removing top bath blanket. Tuck towel-bath towel in and around body (leave bath towel and wash cloths in plastic bag to keep warm).
   c. Begin bathing at feet, using gentle, massaging motion. Employ clean section of towel for each part of body as nurse moves toward patient's head.
   d. Fold lower part of towel upward away from feet as bathing continues.
   e. Put clean bath blanket up over patient as nurse moves upward. Leave 3 in of exposed skin between towel and bath blanket. Skin will dry in 2 or 3 sec.
   f. Wash face, neck, and ears with one of prepared wash cloths.
   g. Turn patient onto side.
   h. Use bath towel for back care.
   i. Use second wash cloth for perineal care (don disposable gloves).
   j. When bath is completed, remove towel and place with soiled linens in plastic laundry bag.
   k. If top bath blanket is not soiled, fold and use later.

Rationale

Bathing patient following these steps promotes effective towel bath, provides warmth, and keeps bed dry, avoiding causing the patient to chill.

STEP 7b

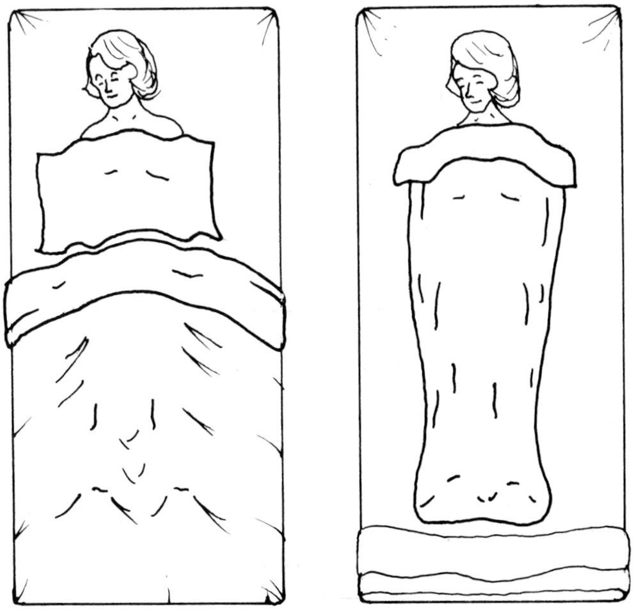

Continued.

SKILL 20-2 ADMINISTERING A TOWEL BATH—cont'd

Nursing action	Rationale
8. Make occupied bed (see Skill 20-14).	Provides comfort, and promotes practices of medical asepsis.
9. Document procedure and any abnormal findings, such as skin impairment.	Records patient care in timely fashion.

DOCUMENTATION

Many agencies have flow sheets for recording the type of bath; if the facility requires narrative charting, see example.

Proves performance.

Sample charting

DATE	TIME	NOTES
12/4/90	0900	Color pale. Respirations 30 and labored. Complains of weakness. Towel bath given. A harsh, nonproductive cough noted at infrequent intervals. Positioned for comfort. Sleeping. Reported to C. Homan, RN.

____
(nurse's signature)

SPECIAL CONCERNS

- The patient must be readied before the bath towel is prepared—the temperature cools down quickly.
- If the towel is not warm, saunalike effect will not be produced and the patient will chill.
- A basin of warm water, soap, wash cloth, towel, and gloves may be necessary to perform perineal care.
- If the towel bath is given properly, the patient will be refreshed and relaxed.
- If the nurse has an assistant, the bath is given more efficiently.

SKILL 20-3

ASSISTING THE PATIENT TO TAKE A TUB BATH OR SHOWER

Nursing action	Rationale
1. Determine if activity is allowed: consult with RN in charge, and check physician's order.	Provides a basis for patient care.
2. Make certain tub or shower appliance is clean. See agency's policy. Place nonskid mat on tub or shower floor and disposable mat outside of tub or shower.	Promotes patient safety.
3. Gather all items necessary for bathing: ■ towel ■ washcloth ■ soap ■ deodorant ■ lotion ■ clean gown	Prevents unnecessary interruptions.
4. Assist patient to tub or shower. Be certain patient wears robe and slippers.	Promotes patient safety. Prevents patient from chilling.
5. Instruct patient on how to use call signal and place "in use" sign on tub or shower door if private bath is not being used.	Provides for patient safety and privacy.
6. If tub is used, fill with warm water: 109° F (43° C). Have patient test water, and adjust temperature. Instruct patient on use of faucets—which is hot and which is cold. If shower is used, turn water on and adjust temperature.	Prevents accidental burns and promotes safety.
7. Caution patient to use safety bars, and discourage use of bath oil in water. Check on patient q 5 min. Do not allow patient to remain in tub more than 20 min.	Maintains patient safety. Prevents vertigo and syncope.
8. Return to room when patient signals, to assist from tub. Knock before entering.	Provides privacy.
9. Assist patient out of tub and with drying. If patient complains of weakness, vertigo, or syncope, drain tub before patient gets out and place towel over patient's shoulder.	Prevents falls.
10. Assist patient into clean gown, robe, and slippers. Accompany to room, and position for comfort, in either chair or bed.	Maintains warmth.
11. Make unoccupied bed if patient can tolerate sitting in chair. Perform back, hair, nail, and skin care.	Maintains clean environment. Promotes positive self-image and promotes medical asepsis.
12. Return to shower or tub. Clean according to agency policy. Place all soiled linens in laundry bag and return all articles to patient's bedside.	Promotes orderly environment.
13. Wash hands.	Reduces spread of microorganisms.

Continued

SKILL 20-3

ASSISTING THE PATIENT TO TAKE A TUB BATH OR SHOWER—cont'd

DOCUMENTATION

1. If hospital policy requires, record procedure. — Proves performance.

Sample charting

DATE	TIME	NOTES
12/4/90	1000	Color pink. Skin warm and dry. NPO for upper GI series. Denies discomfort. Up to shower assisted by this nurse. Respirations even and unlabored. Ambulated down to end of west hall and returned to bed assisted by this nurse. Denies abdominal pain. Reported to A. McCance, RN.

____
(nurse's signature)

SPECIAL CONCERNS

- Safety must be maintained at all times.
- An unoccupied bed may be made while the patient bathes unless patient condition is such that the nurse should remain with the patient.
- Return to the tub or shower room, and offer to wash the patient's back.
- Observe the patient for signs and symptoms of weakness, which are rapid pulse, pale color, diaphoresis, unsteady gait, tachypnea, vertigo, and syncope.
- Shower chairs are available in most facilities. The patient may be transported from the bedside to the shower, bathed, dried, and returned to bed.

PATIENT TEACHING

- The nurse should emphasize to the patient the importance of safety.

A tepid sponge bath is administered to reduce an elevated temperature. This procedure is commonly used for patients who are febrile (Skill 20-4).

A medicated bath may be ordered. This bath may include agents such as oatmeal, cornstarch, Burow's solution, and soda bicarbonate (alkaline bath). The medicated bath is ordered to reduce tension and relax the patient and to relieve pruritus or certain skin disorders (Skill 20-5).

Purposes

The nurse provides or facilitates a patient's bath for the following reasons:

- to cleanse the skin
- to apply medication
- to stimulate circulation
- to improve self-image
- to reduce body odors
- to promote range of motion
- to demonstrate caring—an important aspect of the nurse/patient relationship

SKILL 20-4

ADMINISTERING A TEPID SPONGE BATH FOR TEMPERATURE REDUCTION

Nursing action	Rationale
1. Observe patient for elevated temperature. Review physician's orders.	Provides basis for care.
2. Explain to patient: outline steps of the procedure.	Reduces anxiety.
3. Prepare equipment: ▪ bath basin ▪ tepid water (37° C or 98.6° F) ▪ wash cloths (4) ▪ bath thermometer ▪ bath blanket ▪ patient thermometer	Promotes organization.
4. Provide privacy, and wash hands.	Promotes relaxation. Prevents spread of microorganisms.
5. Cover patient with bath blanket, remove gown, and close widows and doors.	Prevents chilling.
6. Test water temperature. Place wash cloths in water, and then apply wet cloths to each axilla and groin. If patient is in tub, allow to stay in water for 20 to 30 min.	Promotes cooler temperature. Allows for more effective heat loss because blood vessels are close to the surface of the body in the axilla and groin.
7. Gently sponge an extremity for about 5 min. If patient in tub, gently sponge water over upper torso, chest, and back.	Prevents sudden drop in body temperature.
8. Continue sponge bath to other extremities, back, and buttocks for 3 to 5 min each. Determine temperature q 15 min.	Minimizes risk of patient chilling.
9. Change water, and reapply freshly moistened wash cloths to axilla and groin as necessary.	Maintains tepid water temperature.
10. Continue with sponge bath until body temperature falls to slightly above normal. Discontinue procedure according to agency's policy.	Prevents body temperature from falling below normal.
11. Dry patient thoroughly, and cover with light blanket or sheet.	Prevents patient from chilling.
12. Return equipment to storage, clean area, and change bed linens as necessary. Wash hands.	Prevents spread of microorganisms.
13. Record time procedure was started, when ended, vital signs, and patient's response.	Temperature and pulse indicate patient's response to treatment.

Continued.

SKILL 20-4

ADMINISTERING A TEPID SPONGE BATH FOR TEMPERATURE REDUCTION—cont'd

DOCUMENTATION

1. Record procedure. — Proves performance.

Sample charting

DATE	TIME	NOTES
12/4/90	0230	Color flushed. Skin very warm and moist. C/o headache. Temperature 102.2° F, pulse 100, respirations 28, BP 160/92. Sponge bath for temperature reduction performed for 15 minutes. Temperature 101.6° F. Reported to N. Hudson, RN. _(nurse's signature)_
12/4/90	0250	Sponge bath continued for 15 minutes. Temperature 100.8° F.
	0310	Sponge bath continued for 15 minutes. Temperature 99.6° F. States "I'm feeling better." Sponge bath continued for 15 minutes. Temperature 99° F, pulse 88, respirations 20, BP 138/82. Denies headache. Skin cool; color pink. Reported to J. Peterson, RN. _(nurse's signature)_
12/4/90	0350	Sponge bath discontinued. Complete bed change done. Fluids encouraged. Reported to R. Trumbull, RN. _(nurse's signature)_

SPECIAL CONCERNS

- Measure temperature and pulse every 15 minutes.
- Keep body parts covered that are not being sponged.
- Observe patient's response to therapy and document accurately.
- Avoid rubbing the skin too vigorously, because this may cause an increase in heat production.

PATIENT TEACHING

- Remind patient to call for assistance when getting up; the combination of the elevated temperature and sponge bath could weaken the patient.

SKILL 20-5 ADMINISTERING A MEDICATED BATH

Nursing action	Rationale
1. Prepare tub bath (see Skill 20-3).	Promotes an orderly procedure.
2. Add appropriate agent as ordered by physician.	Follows physician's orders.
3. Assist patient to tub.	Maintains patient safety.
4. Allow patient to remain in tub for required time.	Promotes effective procedure.
5. Assist patient out of tub.	Maintains patient's safety.
6. Gently pat dry.	Allows medication to remain on patient's skin.
7. Assist patient into gown or pajamas.	Prevents patient from chilling.
8. Assist patient to return to bed, and position for comfort.	Allows patient to rest and relax.
9. Wash hands.	Prevents spread of microorganisms.

DOCUMENTATION

1. Record procedure.	Proves performance. Communicates patient care.

Sample charting

DATE	TIME	NOTES
12/4/90	0830	Alkaline bath with soda bicarbonate 1:5 solution administered as tub bath for 30 minutes. Patted dry gently. Assisted to bed and positioned for comfort. States "the itching is not quite as bad." Edematous, erythematous patches over lower extremities are not as prominent as yesterday. Reported to D. Hoffmann, RN.
		____________________ *(nurse's signature)*

PATIENT TEACHING

- Teach patient not to scratch the lesions to avoid further irritation and to prevent infection.

COMPONENTS OF THE PATIENT'S HYGIENE

Care of the Skin

When a person's physical condition changes, the skin often reflects this by alterations in color, thickness, texture, turgor, temperature, and hydration (see Chapter 29). As long as the skin remains intact and healthy, its physiological function remains optimal.

Collection of data. The nurse will determine the condition of the skin by observing its color, texture, thickness, turgor, temperature, and hydration (Box 20-2).

The nursing diagnosis of impairment of skin integrity, either actual or potential, applies to every patient with whom the nurse has contact. Prevention and treatment of skin impairment are often responsibilities of the nurse. Prevention is the ultimate goal, but when this is not possible, good nursing interventions can result in (1) optimal healing of the impaired skin without complications, (2) a decrease in the patient's discomfort, (3) a decrease in length of hospitalization, and (4) a decrease in the cost of ongoing care.

A major manifestation of impairment of skin integrity is decubitus ulcers (pressure sores). A patient who stays in one position without relief of pressure, especially over bony prominences, can develop a decubitus ulcer. Patients especially at risk are those who are chronically ill, debilitated, elderly, or disabled or who have a spinal cord injury.

Decubitus ulcers occur when there is sufficient pressure on the skin to cause the blood vessels in an area to collapse. The flow of blood and fluid to the cells is impaired, resulting in ischemia, or lack of oxygen and nutrients, to the cells. If the pressure continues without relief for more than 2 hours, cell necrosis may occur in the layers of skin involved. Pressure is usually most severe over bony prominences, for example, the sacrum, ischial tuberosities, trochanteric areas of the hips, heels, and malleoli of the ankles.

BOX 20-2 NORMAL SKIN CHARACTERISTICS

Intact, without abrasions
Warm
Localized changes in texture across surface
Good turgor (elastic and firm) and generally smooth and soft
Color variations from body part to body part

In addition to unrelieved pressure, two mechanical factors can result in decubitus ulcers. The first is *shearing force*. This occurs when the tissue layers of skin slide on each other, resulting in kinking or stretching of subcutaneous blood vessels, which results in an interruption of blood flow to the skin (Fig. 20-3).

The second mechanical factor is *friction*. The rubbing of skin over a surface produces friction, which may remove layers of tissue. Examples of when this might occur are (1) moving the patient in bed by sliding him over the linen, (2) improper lifting of the patient, or (3) improper placement of the bedpan.

The first goal in the care of the patient's skin is to prevent skin impairment. A critical factor in achieving this goal is careful observation of each patient to determine who is at increased risk for impairment in skin integrity. The six areas to include in the data collection are as follows:

1. General physical condition
2. Level of consciousness
3. Level of activity
4. Mobility
5. Presence of continence or incontinence
6. Nutritional state

The patients at highest risk are those who are confined to a bed or chair, who have limited mobility, who are incontinent, or who have poor overall nutrition. Those who are incontinent are at risk because continual contact of the skin with urine and feces may cause chemical irritation, resulting in skin impairment. Nutritional factors are pertinent for those who are overweight and those who are underweight. Obesity increases the risk because fat tissue has decreased vascularity and resilience, and

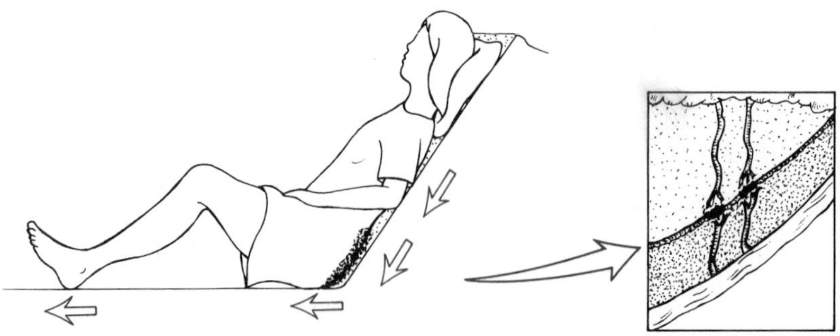

FIG. 20-3 Diagrammatic sketch of shearing force exerted against sacral area.

increases weight and pressure on bony prominences. Underweight increases the risk because of a lack of cushion over the bones and muscles. In addition, any condition that results in a decrease in oxygen and nutrients to the cells, such as anemia, atherosclerosis, or edema, increases the risk of skin impairment, because the cells are not adequately nourished.

Patients who are at increased risk for any reason will need careful, ongoing observation and a plan of care aimed at the prevention of skin impairment.

NURSING DIAGNOSIS	NURSING INTERVENTIONS
Potential impaired skin integrity, related to immobilization	Inspect skin for presence of pressure points at least TID. Provide daily baths. Provide perineal care after each voiding and defecation. Apply skin lotion to areas of skin that become easily erythematous (coccyx, heels, scapulae, and greater trochanteric regions). Keep bed linen clean, dry, neat, and wrinkle-free as possible. Encourage a nutritious diet. Encourage adequate fluid intake. Perform **range-of-motion** exercises. Use mechanical means, such as sheepskin pads, Eggcrate mattress, heel and elbow protectors, and foam- or water-filled chair cushions. Turn q 2 hr.

Nursing diagnoses are formulated, goals are determined by stages of the decubitus ulcer (Fig. 20-4), and interventions are implemented.

If the patient already has a skin impairment, it is necessary to assess the severity of the decubitus ulcer. A commonly accepted system of classifying decubitus ulcers divides them into five stages (Box 20-3).

Nursing interventions for these patients include ongoing assessment for evaluating whether improvement is occurring. Assessment data include the size and depth of

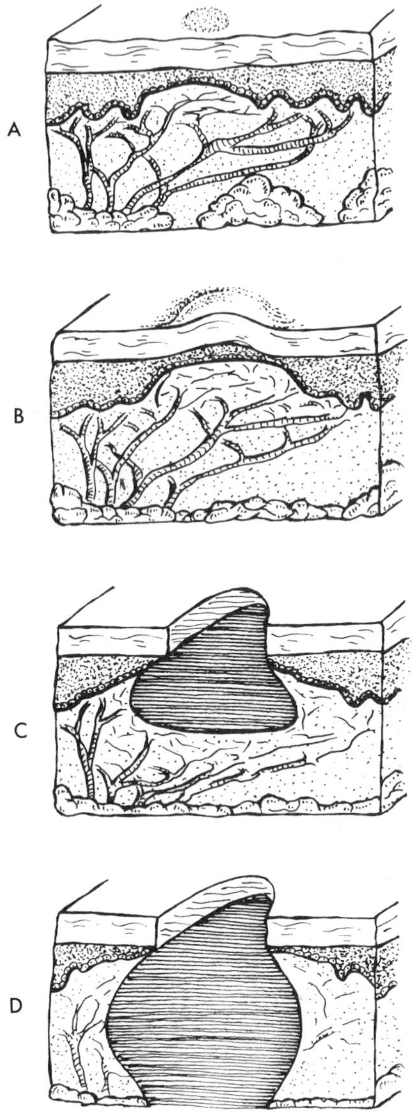

FIG. 20-4 **A,** Stage I decubitus ulcer. **B,** Stage II decubitus ulcer. **C,** Stage III decubitus ulcer. **D,** Stage IV decubitus ulcer.

BOX 20-3 **FIVE STAGES OF DECUBITUS ULCERS**

Stage I	Transient circulatory disturbance: **erythema** or blanching with pressure that disappears when pressure is removed. The signs are the result of a compensatory mechanism. When pressure is released, circulation is restored to the area. With prolonged pressure, estimated to be more than 2 hours, this compensatory mechanism may not be able to respond and the skin at the site suffers ischemia and necrosis.
Stage II	Erythematous or blanched area with no impairment of skin integrity. Patient may complain of pain at the site.
Stage III	Erythema and edema with vesicle and/or impairment of skin integrity.
Stage IV	Full-thickness lesion extending to subcutaneous fat with or without serosanguineous exudate (drainage).
Stage V and beyond	Full-thickness lesion extending to deep fascia, muscle, and bone.

the ulcer, the amount and color of any exudate, the presence of pain or odor, and the color of the exposed tissue. Healing is a long-term process; therefore the plan of care should be consistent over time and evaluated for effectiveness.

Nursing interventions are aimed at preventing, as well as healing, the ulcers. Specific interventions are determined by the stage of the ulcer.

Many kinds of topical agents are available for application to the wound and edges of the wound to facilitate healing. Care should be used to evaluate the effectiveness of any product used on the ulcer. Products that might damage fragile skin and prevent epithelialization, such as hydrogen peroxide or alcohol, should be used with caution.

NURSING DIAGNOSES	NURSING INTERVENTIONS
Impaired skin integrity, related to pressure ulcer (stages I, II, and III)	Assess skin, and identify stage of ulcer development. Eliminate causative factors, and initiate appropriate ulcer care. Cleanse area at least q 4 hr with mild soap and water, and pat dry. Massage area gently to increase circulation; avoid vigorous rubbing. If possible, expose area to sunlight and air q 2 to 4 hr or to heat lamp every day for 15 minutes; observe area frequently to prevent burning. Position patient on unaffected areas. Protect skin surface and affected area with one or combination of the following: ■ Apply karaya powder lightly; dust off excess. ■ Apply skin prep or skin gel. ■ Cover area with moisture-permeable adhesive or wafer barrier. ■ Apply Granulex spray q 8 hr or commercial fat pad, according to manufacturer's directions. ■ Continue one type of application or combination for 48 to 72 hr; if improvement is apparent, continue applications; if no improvement is noted, begin another type of treatment.
Impairment of skin integrity, related to pressure ulcer (stages IV and V)	Assess ulcer for size, color, odor, and amount and type of drainage. Monitor temperature for elevation. Culture ulcer as needed. Continue applications to promote healing. If healing is not evident, prepare for débridement as ordered. After débridement, change dressings as ordered. Administer antibiotics as ordered. If available, consult enterostomal therapist.

Oral Hygiene

Oral hygiene helps maintain a healthy state of the mouth, teeth, gums, and lips. Brushing the teeth removes food particles, plaque, and bacteria, massages the gums, and relieves discomfort resulting from unpleasant odors and tastes. Complete oral hygiene gives a sense of well-being and thus can stimulate appetite.

Certain patients are at risk for oral disorders because of (1) a lack of knowledge about oral hygiene, (2) an inability to perform oral care, or (3) an alteration in the integrity of teeth and mucosa resulting from disease or treatments.

Patients who are particularly at risk are those who (1) are paralyzed, (2) are seriously ill, (3) have upper extremity activity limitations, (4) are unconscious, (5) are confused, (6) are diabetic, or (7) are NPO status. Patients who are undergoing radiation therapy, receiving chemotherapeutic drugs, or undergoing oral surgery also are at risk.

The nurse will allow the patient to brush his own teeth whenever possible. When the patient is unable to do so, the nurse will need to perform this procedure for him (Skill 20-6).

SKILL 20-6

ADMINISTERING ORAL HYGIENE

Nursing action	Rationale
1. Position patient's head to side toward nurse (dependent side if possible) as close to nurse as possible.	Prevents aspiration.
2. Explain procedure even to unconscious patient.	Unconscious patients may be able to hear.
3. Prepare equipment: ■ cleansing solution, such as diluted hydrogen peroxide, toothpaste, normal saline, soda solution, or mouthwash ■ Toothette, toothbrush, or tongue blade wrapped with gauze ■ towel ■ emesis basin ■ disposable wash cloths ■ water glass filled with cool water ■ water-soluble lubricant ■ disposable gloves ■ flashlight	Organizes procedure.
4. Wash hands, and don gloves.	Prevents spread of microorganisms.
5. Provide privacy, and arrange equipment.	Promotes an orderly procedure.
6. Raise bed to working level, and lower side rail.	Enables good body mechanics.
7. Place towel under patient's face and emesis basin under patient's chin.	Facilitates procedure. Prevents soiling bed.
8. Carefully separate patient's jaws.	Protects nurse's fingers.
9. Cleanse mouth using brush, tongue blade, or Toothette moistened with cleansing agent. Clean inner and outer teeth surfaces. Swab roof of mouth and inside cheeks. Use flashlight for better visualization of oral cavity. Gently swab tongue. Rinse and repeat. Rinse several times.	Removes food particles, secretions, and dried exuade and moistens mucosa. Leaves mouth fresh.
10. Apply lubricant to lips.	Provides moisture to prevent drying and cracking.
11. Remove gloves, and dispose of properly.	Prevents spread of microorganisms.
12. Position patient for comfort, raise side rail, and lower bed.	Promotes comfort and safety.
13. Clean and return equipment to storage. Place soiled linen in laundry bag.	Maintains clean environment.
14. Wash hands.	Prevents spread of microorganisms.
15. Record procedure. Include any pertinent observations, such as gum bleeding or ulcerations.	Documents patient response—any unusual findings may indicate more serious problems.

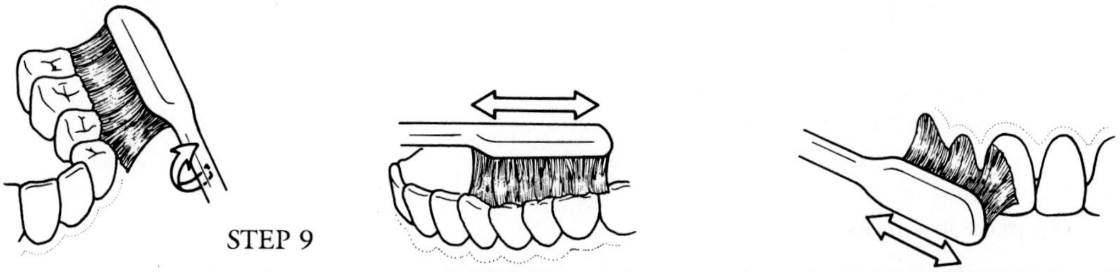

STEP 9

Continued.

SKILL 20-6 ADMINISTERING ORAL HYGIENE—cont'd

SPECIAL CONCERNS

- Good oral hygiene requires preventive and therapeutic measures. Proper care will prevent oral disease and tooth destruction.
- Patients in hospitals or long-term care facilities often do not receive the aggressive care they need.
- Oral care must be provided on a regular basis; frequency of hygiene measures will depend on the condition of the patient's mouth.
- The beneficial outcomes of oral hygiene may not be seen for several days.
- Repeated cleansing is often needed to remove tenacious, dried exudate of the tongue and to restore the mucosa's hydration to normal.

DENTURE CARE

- Patients should be encouraged to care for their own **dentures** as often as for natural teeth to prevent infection and irritation.
- If the patient becomes disabled, incapacitated, or confused, the nurse must assist with denture care. (See Skill 20-7.)
- Dentures are expensive and easily broken and are the patient's personal property; therefore they must be handled with care.
- Dentures should be stored in an enclosed and labeled cup during soaking or when not worn; patients should be discouraged from wrapping them in tissue or placing them on meal trays, since the dentures may be accidentally discarded.

SKILL 20-7 CLEANING DENTURES

Nursing action	Rationale
1. Explain procedure to patient.	Promotes cooperation.
2. Prepare equipment: ■ soft-bristled toothbrush ■ denture brush ■ emesis basin or sink ■ cleansing agent ■ water glass ■ wash cloth ■ 4 × 4 gauze ■ denture cup ■ disposable gloves	Promotes orderly procedure.
3. Wash hands.	Prevents spread of microorganisms.
4. Arrange supplies close by.	Promotes organized procedure.
5. Fill emesis basin ½ full of tepid water.	Acts as a cushion for the dentures if accidentally dropped, preventing damage to dentures.
6. Don gloves.	Prevents spread of microorganisms.
7. Ask patient to remove dentures and place in emesis basin. If patient is unable to remove own dentures, break suction that holds upper denture in place by using thumb and finger. With gauze apply gentle downward tug and carefully remove from patient's mouth. Next remove lower denture by carefully lifting up and turning sideways. Remove and place in emesis basin.	Prevents slipping while handling dentures.

CLEANING DENTURES—cont'd

Nursing action	Rationale
8. Cleanse biting surfaces. Cleanse outer and inner teeth surfaces. Be certain to cleanse under surface of dentures.	Cleansing prevents food, bacteria, odor, and stain formation.
9. Rinse dentures thoroughly with tepid water.	Warm water is more effective than cold water.
10. Replace dentures either in patient's mouth or in container of solution placed in safe place.	Dentures may become brittle and warped if not kept moist.
11. Before replacing dentures in patient's mouth or after storing dentures properly, gently brush patient's gums, tongue, and inside of cheek, and rinse thoroughly.	Oral cavity needs cleansing also to promote healthy gums and mucosa.
12. Remove gloves, and discard appropriately. Clean and store equipment. Wash hands.	Prevents spread of microorganisms.

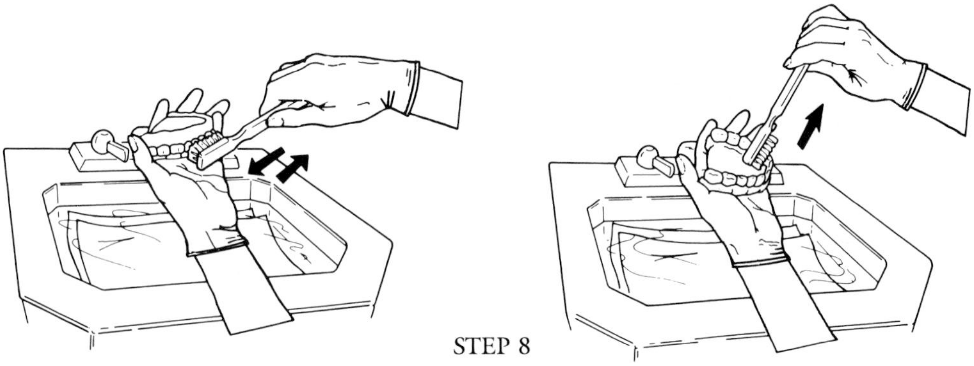

STEP 8

DOCUMENTATION

1. Record procedure.	Proves performance. Communicates patient care.

Sample charting

DATE	TIME	NOTES
12/4/90	0935	Oral care given. Dentures cleaned. Tongue, gums, and mucosa cleaned. Slight **sanguineous** exudate noted. Dentures replaced in patient's mouth. Lubricant applied to lips. Patient states, "Oh, that feels better." Reported to L. Stebbins, RN.

____

(nurse's signature)

Continued

SKILL 20-7

CLEANING DENTURES—cont'd

SPECIAL CONCERNS

- Dentures are expensive and easily broken; care must be taken to prevent breakage or loss. Hold over a basin or sink of water or over a soft cloth while cleaning.
- When reinserting the dentures, replace the upper denture first if patient has both dentures. Apply gentle pressure to reestablish the suction. Moisten dentures for easier insertion. Make certain dentures are comfortably situated in patient's mouth before leaving the bedside.
- Observe dentures for a loose fit. Observe the gums and mucous membrane for tenderness and irritation. These areas may need special care.
- Report any unusual findings.

PATIENT TEACHING

- Teach patient proper method of caring for dentures, including storage and avoiding damage to dentures.

Shaving the Patient

Many patients prefer to shave at the time of bathing. The nurse should remember that those patients who have a bleeding disorder or are taking anticoagulants (medications that increase the tendency to bleed) should use electric razors. The nurse will not allow a confused or depressed patient to use a razor with a blade, to prevent accidental or self-inflicted injury. Patient's beard, mustache, or sideburns are never removed without written consent, except for emergency purpose.

The nurse will need to shave the patient when he is unable to, e.g., because he is too ill or an arm is immobilized in traction or a cast. (See Skill 20-8.)

Hair Care

Proper hair care is important to the patient's self-image. Combing, brushing, and shampooing are basic hygiene measures for all patients. Illness or disability may prevent patients from performing their own daily hair care. A bedfast patient's hair may soon become tangled. It is important for the nurse to remember that most patients are aware of their appearance at all times. Therefore good hair care must be performed routinely, at least daily, to meet the hygiene needs of the patient. If the patient cannot carry out this part of his personal hygiene, the nurse will be required to give assistance. If the patient can take a shower or tub bath, the hair can be shampooed easily. A portable chair may be used in the shower, or a chair may be placed in front of a sink.

For the helpless, bedfast patient, the shampoo must be done in bed. A physician's order may or may not be necessary. Most facilities have portable blow dryers and curling irons available, as well as shampoo boards. (See Skill 20-9).

SKILL 20-8

SHAVING THE PATIENT

Nursing action	Rationale
1. Determine patient's usual shaving method. Explain procedure.	Attempt to follow patient's pattern as much as possible.
2. Wash hands.	Prevents spread of microorganisms.
3. Assemble equipment: ■ razor with sharp blade ■ shaving cream/soap/brush ■ bath towel ■ face towel ■ wash cloth ■ bath blanket ■ basin with hot water ([46° C] 115° F) or as patient prefers ■ after-shave lotion/powder ■ mirror	Organizes procedure. Choose equipment with safety in mind.
4. Assist patient to sitting position if patient is able. Provide privacy. Drape patient with bath blanket.	Similar to normal position. Some patients prefer privacy. Keeps patient warm.
5. Observe face and neck for lesions, moles, or birthmarks.	Cutting could cause infection, bleeding, or irritation.
6. Use shaving cream or soap.	Lathering will soften beard and facilitate shave.
7. Shave in direction hair grows. Use short strokes. Start with upper face and lip, and then extend to neck. If patient is able, it will help if he will hyperextend his head to help shave curved areas.	Provides for closer shave without irritation.
8. Pull skin taut with nondominant hand below the area being shaved.	Promotes uniform shaving.
9. Rinse razor after each stroke.	Keeps cutting edge clean.
10. Rinse and dry face.	Removes remnants of lather and shaved hair.
11. If patient desires, apply lotion or cologne.	Will cause cooling sensation that feels refreshing.
12. Clean and store equipment. Dispose of used blades in safety container.	Protects others from accidental injury.
13. Wash hands.	

STEP 8

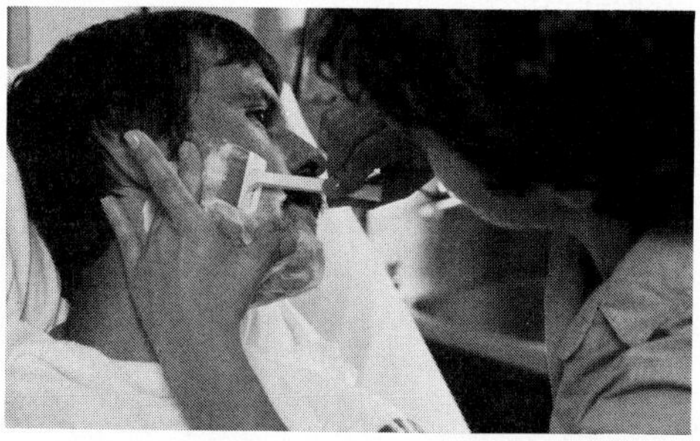

SKILL 20-9 ADMINISTERING A BED SHAMPOO

Nursing action	Rationale
1. Review physician's order.	Special shampoos may be ordered.
2. Explain procedure.	Patient may be anxious.
3. Prepare equipment: ■ bath towels (2) ■ wash cloth or hand towel ■ water pitcher ■ shampoo ■ shampoo board ■ wash basin ■ bath blanket ■ comb and brush ■ hair dryer and curling iron if needed	Promotes an orderly procedure.
4. Wash hands.	Prevents spread of microorganisms.
5. Arrange equipment conveniently.	Prevents interruptions during procedure.
6. Position patient close to one side of bed. Place shampoo board under patient's head and wash basin at end of spout. Make sure spout extends over edge of mattress.	Prevents getting bed linens wet.
7. Position rolled-up bath towel under patient's neck.	Minimizes discomfort.
8. Brush and comb patient's hair.	Removes tangles and loosens dried secretions.
9. Obtain water in pitcher about 110° F (43° C).	Prevents burns.
10. If patient is able, instruct patient to hold wash cloth over eyes. Completely wet hair, and apply small amount of shampoo.	Prevents water and shampoo from getting into eyes.
11. Massage scalp with fingertips, not nails. Shampoo hairline, back of neck (lift head slightly), and sides of hair.	Ensures thorough cleansing and increases scalp circulation.
12. Rinse thoroughly and apply more shampoo, repeating steps 10 and 11. Rinse, and repeat rinsing until hair is free of shampoo.	Prevents scalp irritation.
13. Wrap dry towel around patient's head. Dry patient's face, neck, and shoulders. Dry hair and scalp using second towel if necessary.	Prevents patient from chilling.

SKILL 20-9

ADMINISTERING A BED SHAMPOO—cont'd

Nursing action	Rationale
14. Comb hair and/or dry with blow dryer as quickly as possible.	Prevents patient from chilling.
15. Complete styling hair, and position patient for comfort.	Promotes sense of well-being.
16. Place soiled linens in hamper. Clean and store equipment. Wash hands.	Prevents spread of microorganisms.

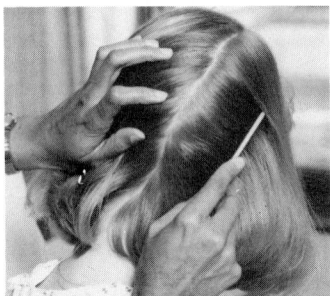

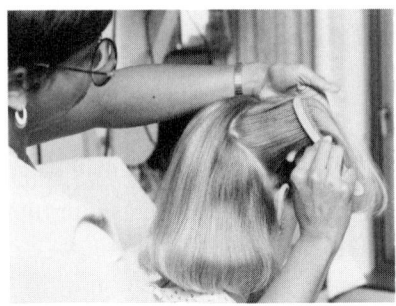

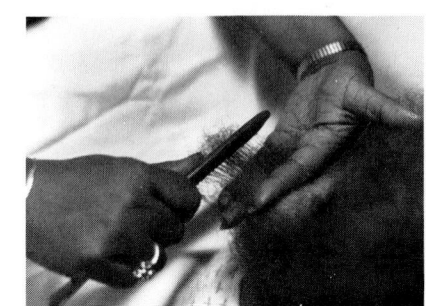

STEP 14

DOCUMENTATION

1. Record procedure.	Proves performance.

Sample charting

DATE	TIME	NOTES
12/9/90	0920	Bed shampoo given. Scalp pink and intact. Denies discomfort. Dried hair immediately with hair dryer and styled. States "I'm so glad to have that done." Reported to H. Tufts, RN.

____
(nurse's signature)

SPECIAL CONCERNS

- Certain conditions, such as cervical neck injuries, open incisions, or a tracheostomy, may place the patient at risk for injury.
- In extreme cases a physician's order may be necessary.
- If hair is matted with blood, hydrogen peroxide is effective as a cleansing agent.
- Inspect condition of scalp; report any unusual findings.
- Make every effort to prevent the patient from chilling.
- Document procedure according to agency policy.

PATIENT TEACHING

- It may be necessary to teach a significant other shampooing techniques.

Hands and Feet Care

Hands and feet often require special attention to prevent infection, odors, and injury. Problems arise from abuse or poor care of the hands and feet, for example, biting the nails or wearing ill-fitting shoes.

Assessment of the feet involves a thorough examination of all skin surfaces. The area between the toes should be carefully checked. Patients with diabetes mellitus or peripheral vascular disease should be observed for adequate circulation to the feet. The elderly also are at risk for foot disorders, because of poor vision or decreased mobility.

Care of the hands and feet can be administered during the morning bath or at another time. (See Skill 20-10.)

SKILL 20-10 CARING FOR THE HANDS AND FEET

Nursing action	Rationale
1. Obtain physician's order if necessary.	The patient's physical condition may place him at risk for infection.
2. Explain procedure.	Patient may be anxious or fatigued.
3. Prepare equipment: ▪ wash basin ▪ emesis basin ▪ wash cloth ▪ hand towel ▪ nail clippers, emory board, and orangewood stick ▪ lotion ▪ disposable bath mat ▪ disposable gloves (optional)	Prevents interruptions during procedure.
4. Wash hands. Arrange supplies within easy reach.	Prevents spread of microorganisms.
5. Provide privacy. Position patient in chair. If possible place disposable mat under patient's feet.	Protects patient's bare feet from floor.
6. Fill basin with water at 100° to 110° F (43° to 44° C). Place basin on disposable mat, and assist patient to place feet into basin. Allow to soak 10 to 20 min. Rewarm water as necessary.	Soaking in warm water will soften nails and ensures easy manipulation of cuticles.
7. Place overbed table in low position in front of patient. Fill emesis basin with water at 100° to 110° F (43° to 44° C). Place basin on table, and place patient's fingers in basin. Allow fingernails to soak 10 to 20 min. Rewarm water as necessary.	Soaking loosens foreign particles under nails and ensures easy manipulation of cuticles.

STEP 6

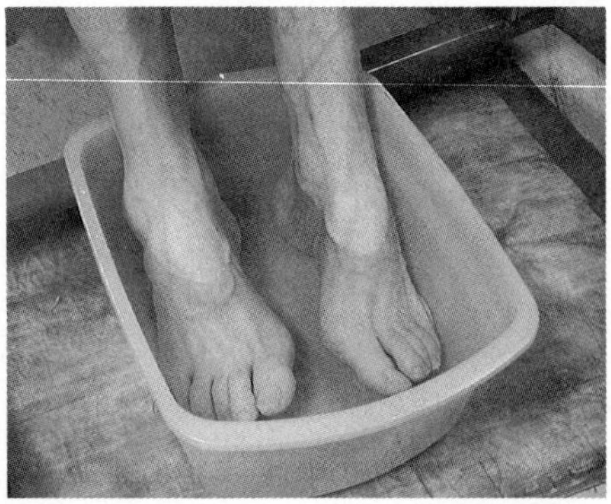

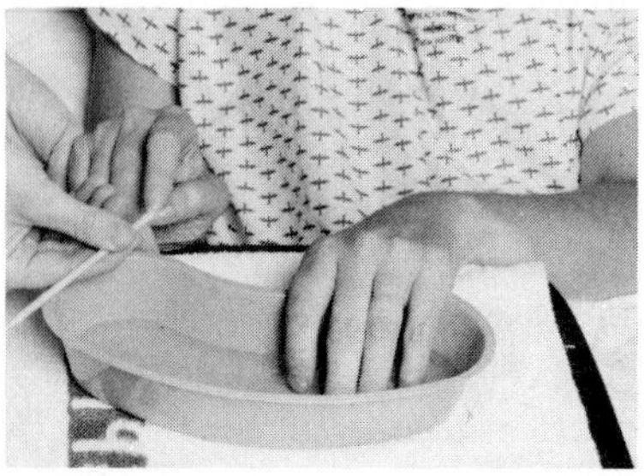

STEP 7

SKILL 20-10 CARING FOR THE HANDS AND FEET—cont'd

Nursing action	Rationale
8. Using orange stick, gently clean under fingernails. With clippers, trim nails straight across and even with tip of fingers. With emory board shape fingernails. Push cuticles back gently with wash cloth or orange wood stick.	Prevents injury to delicate nail beds.
9. Don gloves, and with wash cloth scrub areas of feet that are calloused.	Prevents spread of microorganisms.
10. Trim and clean toenails following step 8.	

STEP 8

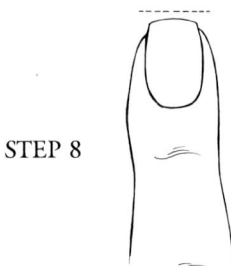

Nursing action	Rationale
11. Apply lotion or cream to hands and feet. Return patient to bed, and position for comfort.	Creams and lotions lubricate dry skin.
12. Remove and dispose of gloves in proper container. Clean and store equipment. Place soiled linen in laundry bag. Wash hands.	Prevents spread of microorganisms.

DOCUMENTATION

1. Record procedure.	Proves performance. Communicates patient care.

Sample charting

DATE	TIME	NOTES
12/4/90	1015	Hands and feet soaked for 15 minutes. Nails trimmed straight across. Hands and feet dried thoroughly. Skin areas dry and intact. Lotion applied. Reported to S. Lauritsen, RN.

____

(nurse's signature)

Continued.

SKILL 20-10 CARING FOR THE HANDS AND FEET—cont'd

SPECIAL CONCERNS

- Care of the feet and nails may be accomplished during the bath procedure, especially the bed bath. However, for those patients who have special problems, such as the elderly patient or the patient with diabetes mellitus, special attention must be given to this important part of the patient's hygiene.
- Other health disorders that put the patient at risk for foot and/or nail problems are heart failure, renal disease, cerebral vascular accident (CVA), and peripheral vascular conditions.
- On completion of procedure, observe the nails and surrounding tissue for condition of skin and any remaining rough edges.
- If a patient's nails are extremely hard or if a patient is unable to perform personal nail care, a podiatrist (a person trained in the treatment of nail and foot problems) can provide nail care.

PATIENT TEACHING

- The nurse must take time during the procedure to teach the patient the appropriate techniques for cleaning and trimming the nails.

Eye, Ear, and Nose Care

Special attention is given to the cleansing of the eyes, ears, and nose during the patient's bath. The nurse often has the responsibility of assisting patients in the care of eye glasses, contact lenses, or artificial eyes. For patients who wear eye glasses, contact lenses, artificial eyes, or hearing aids, the nurse will assess the patient's knowledge and methods used to care for the aids, as well as any problems caused by the aids. Patients who cannot grasp small objects, have limited mobility in the upper extremities, have reduced vision, or are seriously fatigued will require assistance from the nurse.

The eyes, ears, and nose are sensitive, and therefore extra care should be taken to avoid injury to these tissues (see Chapter 37).

Care of the eyes. Cleansing of the **circumorbital** (circular area around the eye) area of the eyes is usually performed during the bath and involves washing with a clean wash cloth moistened with clear water. The use of soap is generally omitted because it may cause burning and irritation. The eye is cleansed from the inner to outer canthus. A separate section of the wash cloth is used each time to prevent spread of infection. If the patient has dried exudate that is not removed easily with gentle cleansing, the nurse may first place a damp cotton ball or gauze on the lid margins to loosen secretions. Never apply direct pressure over the eyeball, because this may cause serious injury. Exudate from the eyes should be removed carefully and as often as necessary to keep the eye clean.

The eyes are well protected with eyelashes, tearing, and a split-second blink reflex and usually do not require special care. However, the unconscious patient may need frequent special eye care. Secretions may collect along the margins of the lid and inner canthus when the blink reflex is absent or when the eyes do not completely close. Lubricating eye drops may be ordered by the physician. Sometimes the eyes may be medicated and covered to prevent corneal drying and irritation.

Many patients wear eye glasses. This represents a large financial investment for them. Therefore the nurse will use care when cleaning glasses and should protect them from breakage or other damage when not worn.

Eye glasses should be stored in the case and placed in the drawer of the bedside stand when not in use to avoid accidental damage. Glasses are made of hardened glass or plastic that is impact resistant to prevent shattering but can be easily scratched. Plastic lenses require special cleansing solutions and drying tissues. Warm water is adequate to clean glass lenses, and the use of a soft cloth to dry is best to prevent scratching of the lenses.

Most patients prefer caring for their own contact lenses. A contact lens is a small, round, sometimes colored disk that fits on the cornea of the eye over the pupil. If the patient's condition does not permit him to remove the lenses, the nurse should seek assistance from someone who is familiar with the procedure. The lenses need not be reinserted until the patient is more capable of caring for the lenses himself. It is important that the nurse protect those patients who are unable to care for their lenses properly, because prolonged wearing of contact lenses may cause serious damage to the cornea. There is a large variety of products available for lens care. Each type of lens (hard, soft, or rigid gas-permeable) requires a different cleansing technique. Each set of lenses is stored in a case with solution according to manufacturer's directions.

Care of the ears. The ears are cleansed by the nurse during the bed bath. A clean corner of a moistened wash cloth rotated gently into the ear canal works best for cleaning. Also, a cotton-tipped applicator is useful for cleansing the pinna. The nurse should teach patients never to use bobby pins, toothpicks, or cotton-tipped applicators to clean the external auditory canal. These objects may damage the tympanic membrane (eardrum) or cause wax **(cerumen)** impacted within the canal.

Hearing aids. Hearing loss is a common health problem. The ability to hear enables patients to communicate and react appropriately within their environment. There are several types of hearing aids available (see Chapter 37). The care of the hearing aid involves routine cleanings, battery care, and proper insertion technique. The nurse will assess the patient's knowledge of and routines for cleaning and caring for the hearing aid. The nurse will determine whether the patient can hear clearly with the use of the aid by talking slowly and clearly in a normal voice tone. The nurse should have the patient suggest any additional tips for care of the hearing aid. When not in use, the hearing aid should be stored where it will not become damaged. The hearing aid should be turned off when not in use to prolong the life of the battery. The outside of the hearing aid should be cleaned with a dry, soft cloth.

Care of the nose. The patient can usually remove secretions from the nose by gently blowing into a soft tissue. This could be the only daily hygiene necessary. The nurse should teach the patient that harsh blowing causes pressure capable of injuring the eardrum, nasal mucosa, and even sensitive eye structures. If the patient is not able to clean his nose, the nurse will assist using a saline-moistened wash cloth or cotton-tipped applicator. The applicator should not be inserted beyond the cotton tip. If nasal secretions are excessive, suctioning may be necessary. When patients receive oxygen per nasal cannula or have a nasogastric tube, the nurse should cleanse the nares every 8 hours with a cotton-tipped applicator moistened with saline. Because secretions are more likely to collect and dry around the tube, the nurse will also need to gently cleanse the tube with soap and water.

Perineal Care

Perineal care (pericare) is part of the complete bed bath. Those patients most in need of scrupulous pericare are those at risk for acquiring an infection, for example, patients with indwelling catheters, patients recovering from rectal or genital surgery, or postpartum patients. If patients are able to do their own pericare, they should be allowed to do so. Embarrassment should never cause the nurse to overlook this nursing intervention. A professional, dignified attitude can diminish embarrassment and put patients at ease. (See Skill 20-11.)

The nurse should be alert for signs of vaginal or urethral discharge, skin impairment, unpleasant odors, complaints of burning during urination, or localized tenderness or pain of the perineum. The nurse should also observe for skin impairment in the perineal area in those patients with urinary or fecal incontinence, rectal and perineal surgical dressings, and indwelling urinary catheters (see Skill 20-12).

Perineal care for the patient with an indwelling catheter. Catheter care is to be performed twice daily on all patients with indwelling catheters unless otherwise ordered by the physician. Daily catheter care should include cleansing of the meatal-catheter junction with soap and water and application of a water-soluble microbicidal ointment (Betadine, unless other ointment or cream is ordered by physician). If possible, the patient should perform the procedure, but the nurse should observe for proper technique.

Indwelling urinary catheters should never be used solely as a matter of convenience and should be discontinued promptly when they are no longer necessary. Insertion of an indwelling urinary catheter should be done only by adequately trained personnel using sterile technique, including gloves, catheter, microbicidal antiseptic solution (Betadine) and a water-soluble microbicidal ointment (Betadine), or as ordered.

A sterile, closed-drainage system with disposable, clear plastic bag and connecting tubes should be used. The system should provide for removal of urine without break in sterile continuity and should be changed if sterility is compromised by a break in tubing or technique. Drainage bags should never be inverted or elevated to or above the level of the patient's bladder.

Back Care/Backrub

The backrub is usually administered after the patient's bath. It should be offered to the patient because it promotes relaxation, relieves muscular tension, and stimu-

Text continued on p. 330.

SKILL 20-11

ADMINISTERING PERINEAL CARE FOR MALE AND FEMALE PATIENTS

Nursing action	Rationale
1. Explain procedure.	Minimizes anxiety.
2. Prepare equipment: ▪ soap dish/soap ▪ wash basin ▪ wash cloths (2) ▪ bath towel ▪ bath blanket ▪ bedpan ▪ toilet tissue ▪ disposable gloves When perineal care is given other than routinely during the bath, the nurse will need perineal bottle (peribottle) filled with cleansing solution.	Promotes organization.
3. Provide privacy. Arrange supplies within easy reach.	Reduces anxiety. Ensures orderliness.
4. Raise bed to working height, and lower the side rail. Assist patient to the dorsal recumbent position for females or supine position for males.	Enables good body mechanics.
5. Female perineal care	
a. Drape patient with bath blanket.	Prevents unnecessary exposure.
b. Raise side rail, and fill basin ⅔ full with water at 105° to 109° F (41° to 43° C).	Promotes patient safety.
c. Wash hands, and don gloves.	Prevents spread of microorganisms.
d. Wash and dry patient's upper thighs.	Surrounding skin surfaces need cleansing also.
e. Wash both **labia majora** and **labia minora.** Wash carefully in skin folds. Cleanse in direction anterior to posterior.	Use separate corner of wash cloth for each skin fold. Prevents spread of microorganisms.
f. Separate labia to expose the urinary meatus and vaginal orifice. Wash *downward* toward rectum with smooth strokes.	Use separate corner of wash cloth for each smooth stroke. Prevents spread of microorganisms.
g. Cleanse, rinse, and dry thoroughly. (If patient is on bedpan and peribottle is used, direct flow of cleansing solution down over perineal area and dry thoroughly.)	Retained moisture harbors microorganisms.
h. Assist patient to side-lying position, and cleanse rectal area with toilet tissue, if necessary. Wash area by cleansing from perineal area toward anus. (Several wash cloths may be needed.) Wash, rinse, and dry thoroughly.	Prevents spread of microorganisms. Prevents skin impairment.

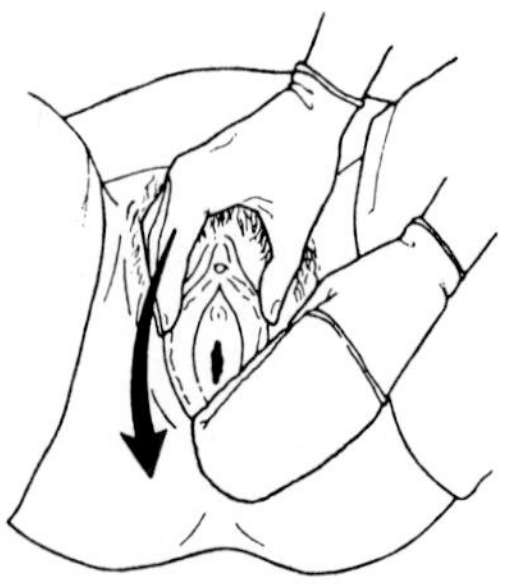

STEP 5g

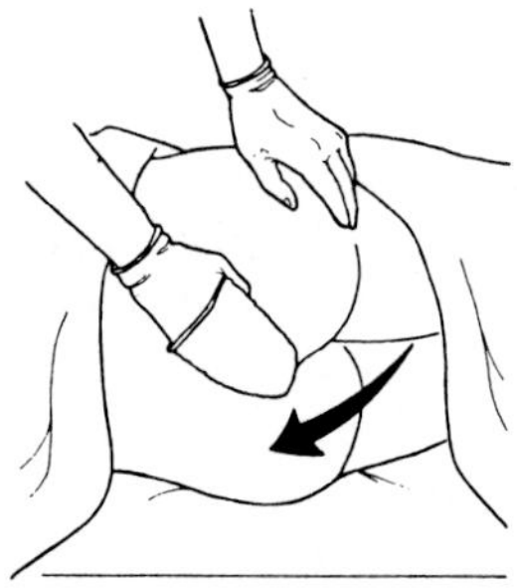

STEP 5h

SKILL 20-11

ADMINISTERING PERINEAL CARE FOR MALE AND FEMALE PATIENTS—cont'd

Nursing action	Rationale
i. Remove and discard gloves properly.	Prevents spread of microorganisms.
j. Position patient for comfort, and provide warmth.	Promotes patient's comfort.
k. Clean and store equipment. Place soiled linen in laundry bag.	Promotes an orderly environment.
l. Wash hands.	Prevents spread of microorganisms.
6. Male perineal care	
a. Position patient.	Facilitates procedure.
b. Raise bed to working height.	Enables good body mechanics.
c. Drape patient.	Provides privacy.
d. Raise side rail, fill basin ⅔ full with water 105° to 110° F (41° to 43° C).	Provides for patient safety.
e. Wash hands, and don gloves.	Prevents spread of microorganisms.
f. Gently grasp shaft of penis. Retract foreskin of uncircumcised patient.	Secretions collect under foreskin.
g. Wash tip of penis with circular motion. Cleanse from meatus outward. Two wash cloths may be necessary. Wash, rinse, and dry gently.	Prevents microorganisms from entering urethra.

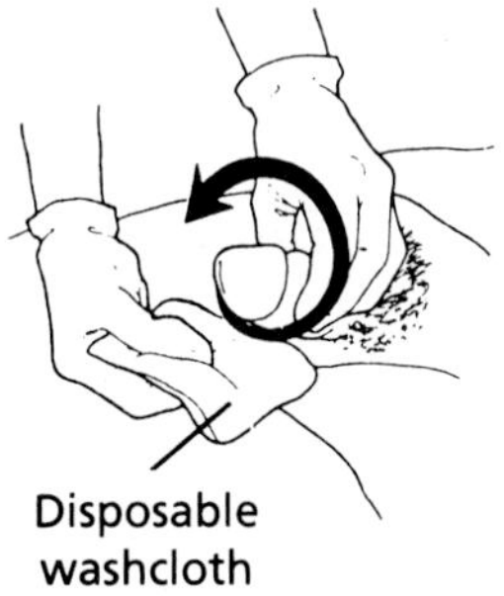

STEP 6g

Nursing action	Rationale
h. Replace foreskin, and wash shaft of penis with a firm but gentle downward stroke. Rinse and dry thoroughly.	Retained moisture harbors microorganisms.
i. Cleanse scrotum gently. Cleanse carefully in underlying skin folds. Rinse and dry.	Pressure on scrotal tissue can be very painful.
j. Assist patient to a side-lying position. Cleanse anal area following step H of female perineal care.	Facilitates procedure.
k. Follow steps i-l of female perineal care.	

Continued.

SKILL 20-11 ADMINISTERING PERINEAL CARE FOR MALE AND FEMALE PATIENTS—cont'd

DOCUMENTATION

1. Record procedure and any abnormal findings. — Proves performance. Communicates patient care.

Sample charting

DATE	TIME	NOTES
12/4/90	1000	Noted moderate amount of tenacious, white, odorless vaginal exudate. Perineal care given. Vulva area erythematous and edematous. Complains of burning on urination. Fluids encouraged. Reported to L. Zlomke, RN.
		_______________ *(nurse's signature)*

SPECIAL CONCERNS

- The foreskin of the uncircumcised male patient must be replaced after thorough cleansing to prevent edema and discomfort.
- If the patient has an indwelling catheter, the nurse should make certain the catheter is cleansed thoroughly and should apply antibacterial ointment if ordered (see Skill 20-12).
- Patients with indwelling catheters or surgical incisions and patients with fecal or urinary incontinence are at risk for developing infection of the urinary or reproductive tract. Perineal care twice daily decreases this risk.
- Careful observation can assist in determining the need for additional therapy.

SKILL 20-12 ADMINISTERING PERINEAL CARE FOR THE PATIENT WITH AN INDWELLING CATHETER

Nursing action	Rationale
1. Check physician's orders.	Provides basis for care.
2. Introduce self, and explain procedure.	Promotes cooperation.
3. Provide privacy.	Encourages relaxation.
4. Obtain supplies: ■ Betadine (or ointment of physician's choice) ■ soft wash cloth ■ soap and water ■ sterile cotton-tipped applicator and gloves	Promotes orderly procedure.
5. Wash hands, and don gloves.	Prevents cross-contamination.
6. Position patient for comfort.	Promotes ease of procedure.
7. Cleanse around urethral meatus and adjacent catheter. Cleanse entire catheter with soap and water.	Prevents urinary tract infections.
8. Repeat cleansing to remove all exudate from meatus and catheter.	Exudates can be irritating and serve as good medium for infectious organisms.
9. Open package of sterile cotton-tipped applicators. Do not touch cotton tip. Apply Betadine ointment to applicator. Do not touch wrapper to cotton tip.	Maintains sterility.
10. Apply ointment to junction of catheter and urethral meatus.	Reduces irritation and prevents spread of microorganisms.
11. Remove gloves. Clean and store equipment. Dispose of contaminated supplies in proper receptacle.	Prevents spread of microorganisms.
12. Wash hands.	Prevents spread of microorganisms.
13. Position patient for comfort.	Promotes relaxation.

DOCUMENTATION

Record any unusual findings.	Communicates patient care in timely fashion.

Sample charting

DATE	TIME	NOTES
12/4/90	1015	Perineal care with catheter care performed. Genitalia pink and moist. Betadine ointment applied. Catheter draining clear, amber urine. Fluids encouraged.

____
(nurse's signature)

SPECIAL CONCERNS

- Catheter care is to be done three times daily on all patients with indwelling catheters unless ordered otherwise by the physician.

PATIENT TEACHING

- Teach patient importance of washing hands before and after performing catheter care.

lates circulation. During the backrub the nurse is able to observe the patient's skin. To give an effective backrub, the nurse will massage the back for 3 to 5 minutes (see Skill 20-13).

SKILL 20-13 ADMINISTERING THE BACKRUB

Nursing action	Rationale
1. Explain procedure.	Promotes relaxation.
2. Prepare equipment: ▪ bath blanket (optional) ▪ bath towel ▪ skin lotion, alcohol, or powder	Lotion lubricates skin, whereas alcohol has drying effect.
3. Adjust bed height to working level.	Ensures proper body mechanics.
4. Provide privacy and quiet environment.	Promotes relaxation.
5. Lower side rail. Position patient with back toward nurse. Cover patient so that only parts to massage are exposed.	Prevents unnecessary exposure.
6. Wash hands, and warm if necessary. Warm lotion by holding some in hands. Explain that lotion may feel cool.	Enhances relaxation.
7. Begin massage by starting in sacral area using circular motions. Stroke upwards to shoulders. Use firm, smooth strokes to massage over scapulae. Continue to upper arms with one smooth stroke and down along side of back to iliac crests. Do not break contact with patient's skin. Complete massage in 3 to 5 min.	Firm, gentle pressure provides relaxation. Using firm pressure prevents tickling sensation. Continuous contact with skin surface is soothing and stimulates circulation.

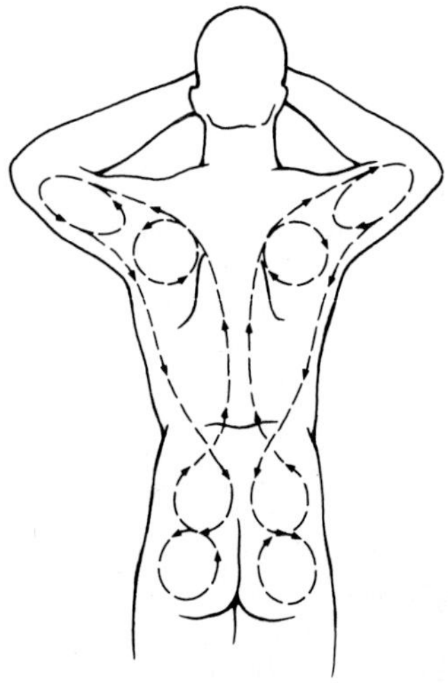

STEP 7

SKILL 20-13

ADMINISTERING THE BACKRUB—cont'd

Nursing action	Rationale
8. Gently but firmly knead skin by grasping area between thumb and fingers. Work across each shoulder and around nape of neck. Continue downward along each side to sacrum.	Increases circulation. Is soothing and relaxing.
9. With long, smooth strokes, end massage. Remove excess lubricant from patient's back with towel, and retie gown. Position for comfort. Lower bed, and raise side rail as needed.	Most soothing of all massage movements. Promotes patient safety.
10. Place soiled laundry in proper receptacle. Wash hands.	Prevents spread of microorganisms.

STEP 8

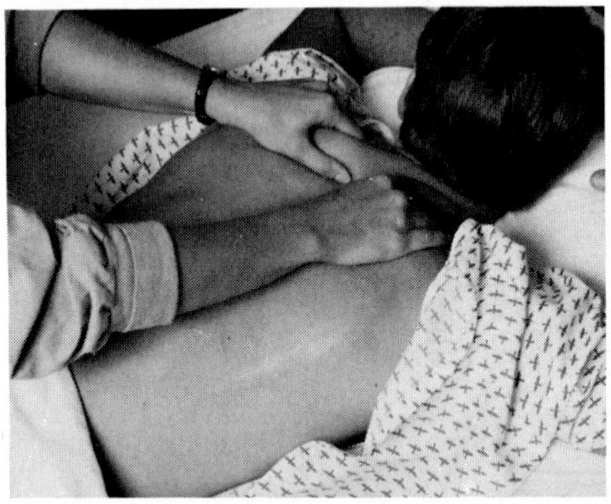

DOCUMENTATION

1. Record procedure, condition of skin, and patient's response.	Proves performance. Communicates patient care and condition.

Sample charting

DATE	TIME	NOTES
12/4/90	2250	Complaining of generalized fatigue. Restless. Expressing concerns over financial matters. Back rub given with lotion. Noted several small erythematous areas over both scapulae. Special massage given to these areas. Denies discomfort. Positioned for comfort.
12/4/90	2330	Asleep. Reported to L. Chia, RN.

____
(nurse's signature)

SPECIAL CONCERNS

- The backrub is contraindicated if the patient has such conditions as fractures of the ribs or vertebral column, burns, pulmonary embolism, or open wounds.
- Monitor pulse and blood pressure of those patients with a history of hypertension or dysrhythmias.

PATIENT TEACHING

- Perhaps a significant other can be taught how to perform the backrub. A backrub could become part of the patient's sleep routine.

Bedmaking

The patient's bed is usually made in the morning after the bath. When possible the bed is made while not occupied. The patient may be in the tub, showering, or out of the room for a diagnostic examination or procedure. When the patient is unable to be out of bed, the nurse will make an occupied bed.

The patient's safety is always foremost in the nurse's mind. Comfort and privacy are also important. The nurse remembers to use side rails, to keep the call light within easy reach, and to maintain the bed in the proper position: high position while working at the bedside, and low position when work is completed, to prevent the patient from accidental falls.

It is the nurse's responsibility to keep the bed as clean and comfortable as possible. This may require frequent inspections to make certain bedding is clean, dry, and wrinkle-free. The nurse will check the linens for food particles after meals and for urine incontinence or involuntary stool. If linens are soiled with urine, feces, blood, or emesis, they should be changed.

The nurse will follow basic principles of asepsis. These principles are the following:

1. Keep soiled linens away from uniform.
2. Place soiled linens in hamper or plastic bag.
3. Never fan linens in the air. (This causes air currents, which spread microorganisms.)
4. Never place soiled linens on the floor. If clean linens touch the floor, place in laundry hamper immediately.

The nurse must use proper body mechanics while making the bed, such as raising the bed to a working level to avoid bending down or stretching. Also, the principles of body mechanics should be applied while turning and repositioning the patient.

An occupied bed is made with the patient in it (see Skill 20-14). An unoccupied bed may be made open or closed. In the open bed the top linens are fan folded toward the foot of the bed to allow the patient to return to bed more easily. A closed bed is prepared after the patient is dismissed, transferred, or dies, before another patient is admitted to the room (see Skill 20-15).

Text continued on p. 338.

SKILL 20-14 MAKING THE OCCUPIED BED

Nursing action	Rationale
1. Explain procedure.	Patient could be feeling anxious if uncomfortable or fatigued.
2. Prepare supplies: ▪ laundry bag ▪ mattress pad (optional) ▪ bottom sheet—many facilities use the contour/fitted sheet ▪ protective draw sheet (optional) ▪ linen draw sheet ▪ top sheet, flat ▪ blanket ▪ spread ▪ **Chux** or bath blanket (2) ▪ pillow case(s) ▪ bedside chair or table	Organizes procedure.
3. Wash hands.	Prevents spread of microorganisms.
4. Assemble equipment, and arrange conveniently.	Provides for smooth procedure.
5. Provide privacy, lower side rail, remove call light, and adjust bed height.	Ensures proper body mechanics.
6. Remove spread and blanket separately, and if soiled, place in laundry bag or if to reuse, fold neatly and place over back of chair. (Keep linens away from uniform.) Do not fan or shake linens.	Prevents spread of microorganisms.

SKILL 20-14 MAKING THE OCCUPIED BED—cont'd

Nursing action	Rationale
7. Place bath blanket over patient on top of sheet. Request patient to hold onto bath blanket while nurse removes top sheet by drawing sheet out from under bath blanket at foot of bed. If patient is unable to assist, nurse will need to hold bath blanket in place while removing sheet. Place soiled sheet in laundry bag.	Provides unnecessary exposure.
8. With assistance from coworker, slide mattress to top of bed.	If mattress has shifted to foot of bed, it will be difficult to tuck in linens.
9. Position patient to far side of bed with his back toward nurse. Adjust pillow for comfort. Be sure side rail is up.	Provides patient safety.
10. Beginning at head and moving toward foot, loosen bottom linens. Fan fold linen draw sheet, protective draw sheet, and bottom sheet, tucking edges of linens under patient.	Provides maximum work space.
11. Apply clean linens to bed by first placing mattress pad (if used). Fold lengthwise, making sure crease is in center of bed. Likewise, unfold bottom sheet and place over mattress pad. Hem of bottom sheet should be placed with rough edge down and just even with bottom edge of mattress.	Minimizes energy and time needed by nurse for bed-making.
12. Miter corners (if flat sheet) at head of bed. Continue to tuck in sheet along side toward front, keeping linens smooth.	Prevents linens from becoming easily loosened.

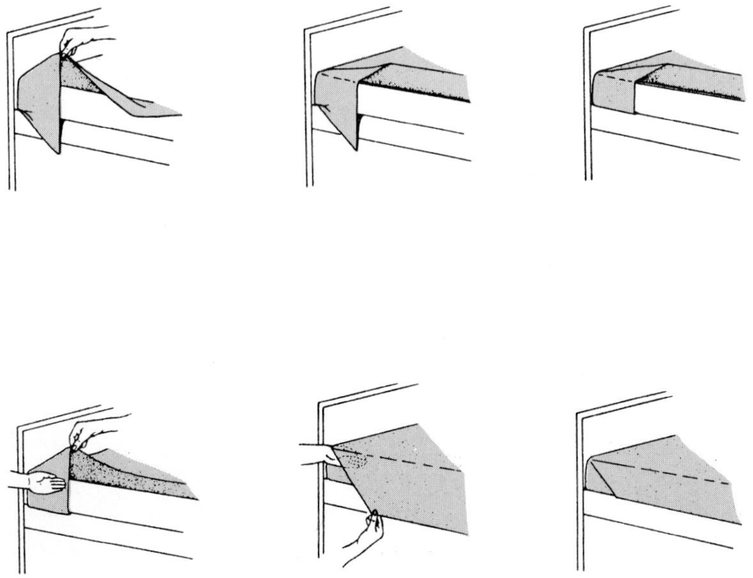

STEP 12

Continued.

SKILL 20-14

MAKING THE OCCUPIED BED—cont'd

Nursing action	Rationale
13. Reach under patient to pull out protective draw sheet (if used), and smooth out over clean bottom sheet. Tuck in. Unfold linen draw sheet, and place center fold along middle of bed, smooth out over protective draw sheet, and tuck in. Tuck in folded linens in center of bed so they are under patient's buttocks and torso. Keep palms down as linens are tucked under mattress.	Provides for patient's comfort.
14. Raise side rail, and assist patient to roll slowly toward nurse over folds of linen. Go to opposite side of bed and lower side rail.	Maintains patient's safety.
15. Loosen edges of all soiled linens. Remove by folding into a bundle, and place in laundry bag.	Prevents spread of microorganisms.
16. Spread clean linens including protective draw sheet out over mattress, and smooth out wrinkles. Assist patient to supine position, and position pillow for comfort.	Maintains patient's comfort.
17. Miter top corner of bottom sheet, pulling sheet taut (see step 12). Tuck bottom sheet under mattress all the way to foot of bed.	Maintains smooth linens. Avoid lifting mattress too far, to ensure tight fit.
18. Smooth out draw sheets. Pulling sheet taut, tuck in protective draw sheet and then tuck in linen draw sheet, first in center, then top, and last, bottom.	Ensures tight fit.
19. Place top sheet over bath blanket that is over patient. Request patient to hold top sheet while nurse removes bath blanket. Place blanket in laundry bag. (Make sure center fold of sheet is in center of bed.) If blanket is used, place over sheet and place spread over blanket. Form cuff with top linens under patient's chin.	Provides for patient comfort and warmth.

STEP 15

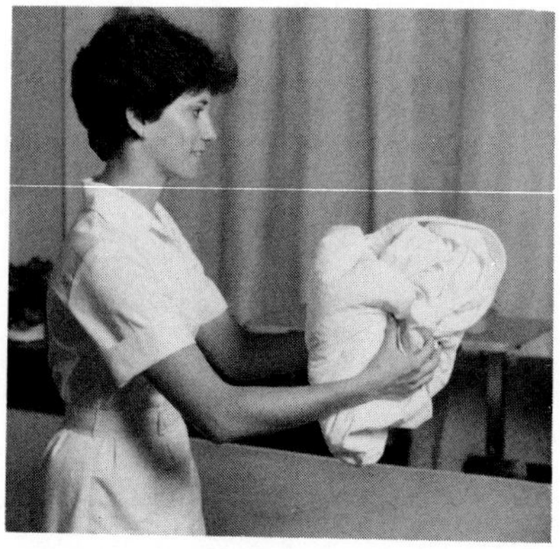

SKILL 20-14

MAKING THE OCCUPIED BED—cont'd

Nursing action	Rationale
20. Tuck in all linens at foot of bed, making modified miter corner. See illustration. Raise side rail and make opposite side of bed. Remember to allow for toe pleat. Make toe pleat by placing fold either lengthwise down center of bed or across foot of bed.	Prevents unnecessary pressure on patient's feet, possibly causing footdrop.
21. Change pillow case. Remove case by grasping pillow through opened end, and draw pillow out through case. Grasp closed end of pillow case, turning case inside out over hand. Now grasp one end of pillow with hand in the case. With other hand pull pillow case over pillow and smooth out wrinkles, making sure pillow corners fit into pillow case corners.	As pillow is removed from under patient, support neck muscles to prevent injury. Nurses should never hold pillow under their chin (risk of spreading microorganisms).
22. Place call light within easy reach, and lower bed. Place personal items within easy reach on bedside stand or table.	Provides safety and comfort.
23. Remove all soiled linens, and place in proper receptacle. Wash hands.	Prevents spread of microorganisms.

STEP 20

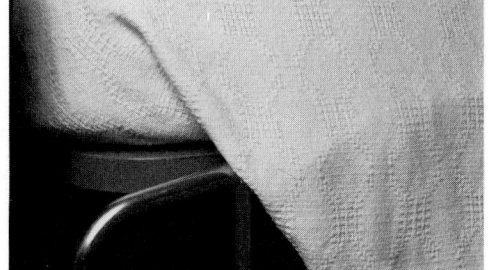

STEP 21

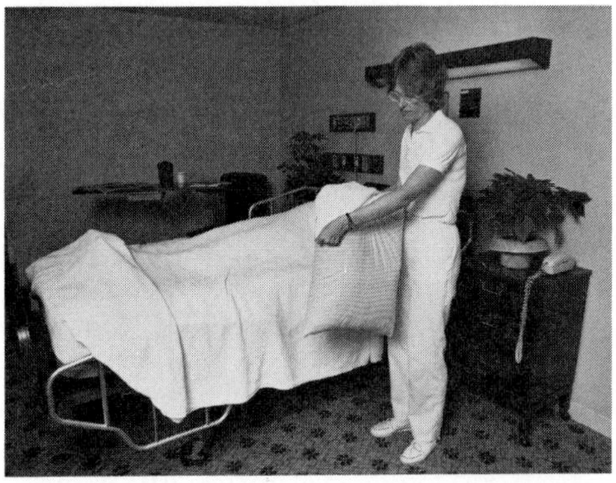

SPECIAL CONCERNS

- If patient is incontinent or if there is excessive drainage, waterproof pads or an extra bath blanket may be necessary.
- Check physician's order for any precautions in moving or positioning the patient.
- Remove all unnecessary equipment, and maintain a neat work area.
- Rough hem edges should be away from the patient to prevent skin impairment.
- All linens should be smooth and wrinkle free to promote patient's comfort.
- Assure patient that he will not fall out of bed.
- Patients with certain conditions, such as a respiratory disorder, may not be able to tolerate lying flat.

PATIENT TEACHING

- Explain steps of procedure in which patient will be participating.

SKILL 20-15

MAKING THE UNOCCUPIED BED

Nursing action	Rationale
1. Prepare supplies: ▪ laundry bag ▪ mattress pad (optional) ▪ bottom sheet (may be contoured) protective draw sheet (optional) linen draw sheet top sheet (flat) blanket spread Chux or bath blanket (optional) pillow case(s) bedside chair or table	Ensures orderly procedure.
2. Wash hands.	Prevents spread of microorganisms.
3. Assemble equipment, and arrange conveniently.	Provides for a smooth procedure.
4. Lower side rail. Adjust bed level, and remove call light.	Ensures good body mechanics.
5. Starting at head of bed, loosen linens all the way to foot. Go to opposite side of bed, loosen linens, roll all linens up in ball (see Skill 20-14, step 15), and place in soiled laundry bag. Do not permit linens to come in contact with uniform. Do not shake or fan linens.	Linen is easier to remove. Prevents spread of microorganisms.
6. If blanket and spread are to be reused, fold neatly and place over back of chair. Remove soiled pillow case as in Skill 20-14, step 21.	Facilitates replacement, and prevents wrinkles.
7. Slide mattress to head of bed.	Easier to tuck in linens.
8. If necessary, cleanse mattress with moistened cloth with antiseptic solution and dry thoroughly.	Prevents spread of microorganisms.
9. Begin to make bed standing on side where linens are placed. Unfold bottom sheet, placing fold lengthwise down center of bed. Make certain rough edge of hem lies down away from patient's heels and even with edge of mattress. Smooth out sheet over top edge of mattress, and miter corner. (See illustration, Skill 20-14.) Tuck remaining sheet under mattress all the way to foot. Keep linens smooth.	Time is saved if one side of bed is made at a time. Fan folding all linen lengthwise down bed promotes neatness and prevents wrinkling.

STEP 9

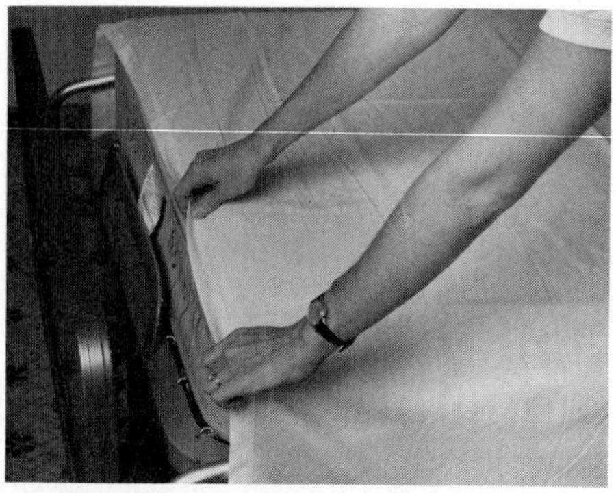

SKILL 20-15 MAKING THE UNOCCUPIED BED—cont'd

Nursing action	Rationale
10. Place draw sheet on bed so that center fold lies down middle of bed. If protective draw sheet is to be used, place it on first. Smooth out over mattress, and tuck in. Keep palms down.	Prevents loosening and wrinkling.
11. Place top sheet over bed, and smooth out. Place blanket over top sheet. Smooth out. Place spread over blanket, and smooth out. Make cuff with top linens.	Provides for patient's comfort.
12. Allow for toe pleat. Make modified mitered corner by not tucking tip of triangle under mattress (see Skill 20-14, step 20).	Provides for patient comfort.
13. Move to opposite side of bed, and complete making bed as described in steps 9 to 12. Pull linens tight, and keep taut as linens are tucked in.	Saves nurse's time and energy.

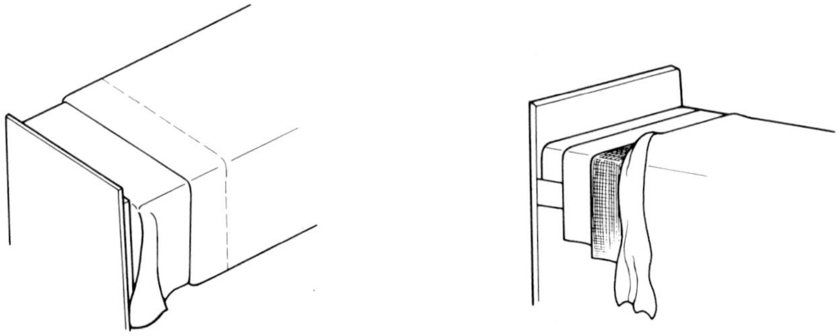

STEP 11

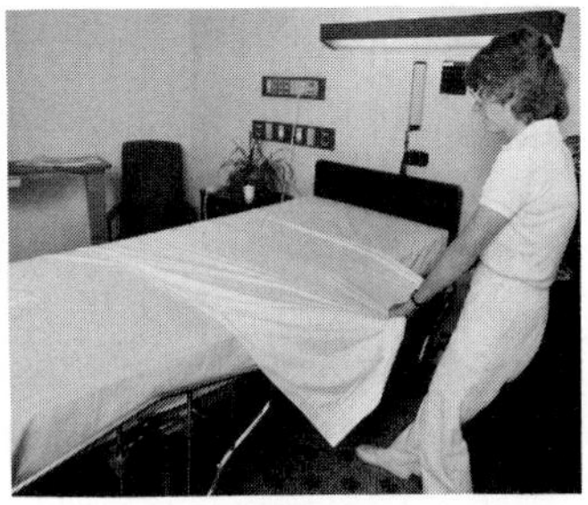

STEP 13

Nursing action	Rationale
14. Put on clean pillow case (see Skill 20-14, step 21). Position pillow at head of bed. Place call light within easy reach, and lower bed level.	Makes it easy to slide case over pillow.
15. If patient is to return to bed, fan fold top linens down to foot of bed. Make sure cuff at top of linens is easily accessible to patient.	Makes it easier for patient to return to bed.
16. Arrange personal items on bed table or bedside stand, and place within patient's easy reach. Leave area neat and clean.	Promotes sense of well-being.
17. Place all soiled linens in proper receptacle. Wash hands.	Prevents spread of microorganisms.
18. Assist patient to bed, and position for comfort.	Provides safety and patient's comfort.

The postoperative bed is a form of the open bed. The top sheet and spread are not mitered or tucked in at the corners. The top linens may be fan folded lengthwise or crosswise at the foot of the bed. The top bed linens should be arranged in such a way as to allow easy transfer of the surgical patient from the gurney to the bed. A complete linen change is done if the patient is returning from surgery.

A complete linen change is done when the patient is discharged. The mattress and bed are cleaned by housekeeping personnel, and fresh linens are applied.

Assisting the Patient with Elimination

The bedpan or urinal is used when a patient is unable to get up to the bathroom for the purpose of urination (the act of emptying the urinary bladder) or of defecation (the act of eliminating feces [BM]). This procedure is personal, and the patient should be afforded as much privacy as his condition allows.

The nurse should offer the bedpan or urinal frequently, because patients may accidentally soil bedclothes if their elimination needs are not met. It is not unusual for a patient to procrastinate using a bedpan because it is uncomfortable and embarrassing. Patients may try to get to the bathroom unassisted even if their condition prohibits ambulation. The nurse should remind patients of the possibility of accidents or falls.

Characteristics of normal urine are as follows:

1. Ranges from a pale, straw color to amber (depends on its concentration)
2. Is transparent at the time of voiding
3. Has a characteristic odor—faintly aromatic
4. Is negative for protein, glucose, ketone bodies, red blood cells, and white blood cells

The nurse notes any abnormality (see Chapter 33).

Characteristics of normal stool are as follows:

1. Is brown in color
2. Odor is affected by food types
3. Has soft, formed consistency
4. Frequency ranges from 1/day to 2 or 3/week
5. Resembles the shape of the rectum
6. Contains undigested food, dead bacteria, fat, bile pigment, living cells, intestinal mucosa, and water

The nurse notes any abnormality (see Chapter 31).

The **bedpan** is made of metal or plastic. There are two types of bedpans. One type has a high back. The second type is flat and smaller and is called a *fracture pan* (Fig. 20-5).

A **urinal** is made of metal or plastic. There are two types of urinals. One type is used by the male for voiding (Fig. 20-6). The other type is called a *female urinal* and has a different shape than the male urinal. The metal urinal may be warmed by running warm water over its surface.

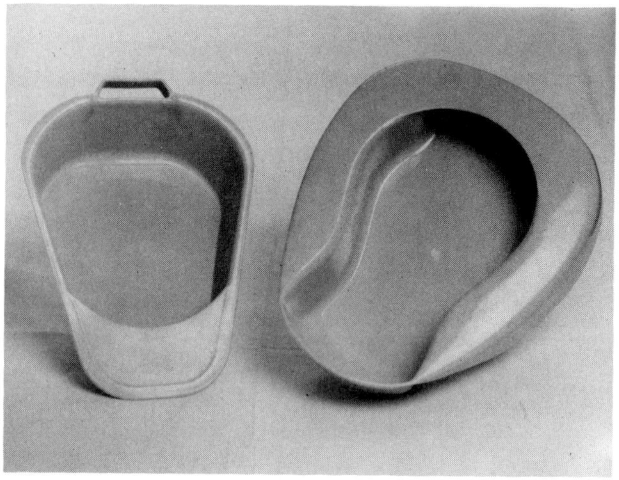

FIG. 20-5 Types of bedpans. *Left,* Fracture bedpan; *right,* regular bedpan.

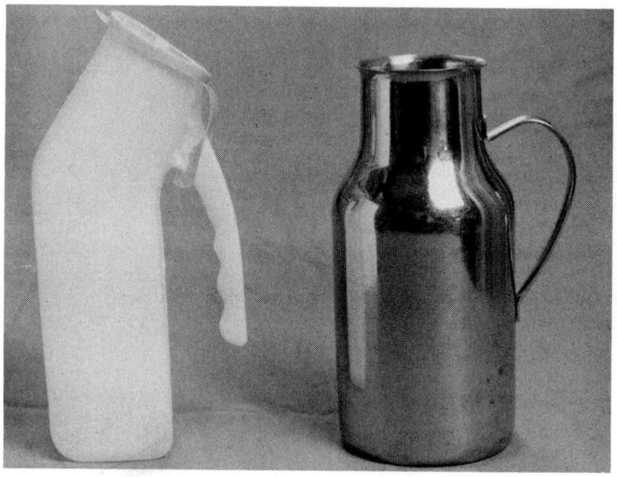

FIG. 20-6 Types of male urinals.

If the patient is unable to place the urinal for himself, the nurse will need to assist him:

1. Request the patient to abduct his legs a slight distance.
2. Holding the urinal by the handle and directing the urinal at an angle, place the urinal between the patient's legs, making certain the bottom of the urinal is resting on the bed.
3. Gently raising the penis, place it fully within the urinal.

The bedpan and urinal should be emptied immediately after use, cleansed, and stored properly. If the patient's intake and output are being monitored, urine should be measured and recorded. Liquid stool is estimated on the appropriate form according to agency's policy. The nurse will remember to wear gloves if soiling is likely. See Skill 20-16: Positioning the Bedpan.

SKILL 20-16 POSITIONING THE BEDPAN

Nursing action	Rationale
1. Assess patient's needs.	Allows nurse to note any potential problems in elimination.
2. Check physician's order.	Provides basis for care.
3. Wash hands.	Prevents cross contamination.
4. Gather supplies.	Organizes procedure.
5. Introduce self.	Decreases anxiety level.
6. Explain procedure to patient.	Encourages cooperation.
7. Provide privacy.	Promotes relaxation.
8. Don gloves if soiling is likely.	Protects the nurse from patient's body fluids.
9. Place protector under patient if necessary.	Provides protection for bed.
10. Warm metal bedpan under running warm water.	Provides for patient comfort.
11. When patient is able to assist self onto bedpan, nurse will position patient in supine position with knees flexed and bottom of feet flat on bed surface. As patient raises hips, nurse supports patient's lower back with her arm and slides bedpan under patient. When patient has finished with elimination, nurse removes bedpan in same manner.	Allows for some measure of independence.
12. For patient unable to assist self on bedpan:	
▪ Turn patient away from nurse toward opposite side rail, moving linens out of way.	Provides for patient safety.
▪ Fit bedpan to patient's buttocks.	Prevents injury to patient's skin.
▪ Assist patient to turn over onto bedpan while nurse secures bedpan.	Allows nurse to use appropriate body mechanics.
▪ Raise head of bed 30 degrees.	Promotes patient comfort.
▪ Place toilet tissue and call light within easy reach.	Patient convenience. Promotes certain measure of independence.

STEP 12

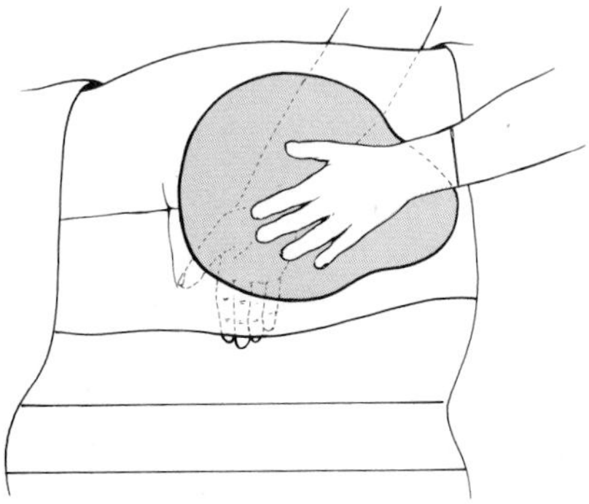

Continued.

SKILL 20-16

POSITIONING THE BEDPAN—cont'd

DOCUMENTATION

1. Record amount, color, and consistency of urine and feces.

Records patient's pattern of elimination.

Sample charting

DATE	TIME	NOTES
12/4/90	0920	Voided 300 ml in bedpan. Urine clear amber. Denies discomfort. Perineal care given. Fluids encouraged. _(nurse's signature)_
12/4/90	0920	Voided 500 ml in urinal. Urine red with moderate amount of sediment. Complains of urgency and frequency. Fluids encouraged. Reported to B. Anderson, RN. _(nurse's signature)_
12/4/90	1045	Up to bathroom with assistance. Large, soft, brown stool with moderate amount **flatus** expelled. Perineal care given. Returned to bed and positioned for comfort. _(nurse's signature)_
12/4/90	1045	Assisted onto bedpan. Moderate amount of green, liquid stool and much flatus expelled. Complains of abdominal cramping. Bowel sounds hyperactive. Reported to J. Gutschenritter, RN. _(nurse's signature)_

SKILL 20-16 POSITIONING THE BEDPAN—cont'd

SPECIAL CONCERNS

- Allow the patient enough time for elimination. Ignoring the urge to defecate or urinate or not taking time to eliminate completely is a common cause of constipation or urine retention.
- The nurse must be prompt to assist the patient to the bathroom or onto the bedpan or bedside commode.
- When the patient shares a room with another patient, be certain to curtain off the patient's area. This enables the patient to relax, knowing that interruptions will not occur.
- Bathroom doors must be closed. If necessary to remain nearby, stand outside door or curtains.
- For those patients unable to assume the normal squatting position, there are stool risers, which require less effort to sit or stand.
- For those patients who can be out of bed but are unable to ambulate far, there is the bedside commode (Fig. 20-7). Some are equipped with wheels, which allow the patient to be moved to the bathroom for more privacy.
- When transferring a patient to the commode, assist the patient in the same manner as if assisting to a chair.

PATIENT TEACHING

- Teach patients who have trapeze bars on their beds how to lift themselves on and off the bedpan.

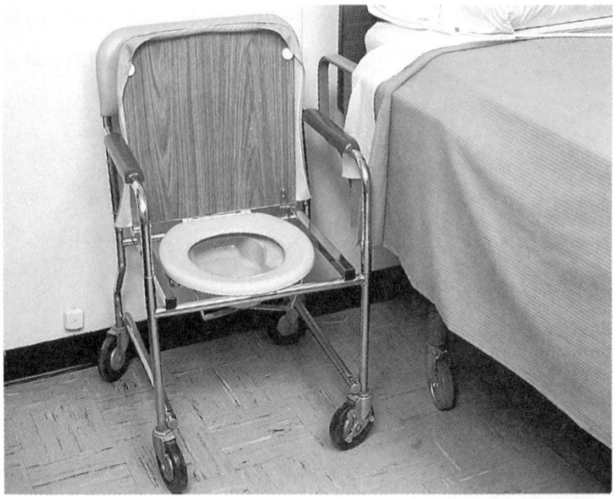

FIG. 20-7 The bedside commode has a toilet seat with a container. The container slides out from under the toilet seat for emptying.

REFERENCES AND SUGGESTED READINGS

1. Ellis JR, Nowlis EA, and Bentz PM: Basic nursing skills, ed 4, vol 2, Boston, 1988, Houghton Mifflin Co.
2. Flynn JM and Hackel R: Technological foundations in nursing, East Norwalk, Conn, 1990, Appleton & Lange.
3. Lewis LW and Timby BK: Fundamental skills and concepts in patient care, ed 4, Philadelphia, 1988, JB Lippincott Co.
4. Malasanos L, Barkauskas V, and Stoltenberg-Allen K: Health assessment, ed 4, St Louis, 1990, The CV Mosby Co.
5. Mosby's medical, nursing, and allied health dictionary, ed 3, St Louis, 1990, The CV Mosby Co.
6. Perry AG and Potter PA: Clinical nursing skills and techniques, ed 2, St Louis, 1990, The CV Mosby Co.
7. Potter PA and Perry AG: Fundamentals of nursing: concepts, process and practice, ed 2, St Louis, 1989, The CV Mosby Co.
8. Sorrentino SA: Mosby's textbook for nursing assistants, ed 2, St Louis, 1987, The CV Mosby Co.
9. Tucker SM and others: Patient care standards: nursing process, diagnosis, and outcome, ed 4, St Louis, 1988, The CV Mosby Co.

CHAPTER CHALLENGE

STUDY QUESTIONS

1. Microorganisms are spread by which of the following ways:
   a. On bedpans and urinals
   b. By fanning the clean linen over the bed
   c. By placing soiled linens on the floor
   d. All of these
2. During the bed bath the nurse covers the patient with a bath blanket for all of the following reasons except:
   a. To prevent unnecessary exposure
   b. To provide privacy
   c. To prevent the spread of microorganisms
   d. To prevent chilling
3. An erythematous and edematous area over a bony prominence that could become an open lesion is referred to as:
   a. An inflammatory ulcer
   b. A decubitus ulcer
   c. A stasis ulcer
   d. The inner canthus
4. Nursing interventions to prevent skin impairment are:
   a. Keeping skin dry and clean
   b. Maintaining clean, dry bed with wrinkle-free linens
   c. Massaging bony prominences
   d. All of these
5. Oral hygiene is performed for all of the following reasons except:
   a. To promote comfort
   b. To improve patient's appetite
   c. To prevent epidemic parotitis
   d. To prevent cavities
6. The nurse offers the patient the use of a bedpan or urinal before starting the bath procedure because:
   a. The patient will feel more comfortable after voiding
   b. It prevents interruptions during the bath
   c. Both of these
7. An important element for the nurse to consider when positioning the patient on the bedpan is preventing muscle strain and discomfort:
   a. True
   b. False
8. Perineal care includes bathing the:
   a. Back and buttocks
   b. Eyes, ears, and nose
   c. Upper torso and thighs
   d. Upper thighs, genitalia, and area around the anus
9. Which of the following statements is *not* true of bedmaking:
   a. It is essential to keep the bed as clean and comfortable as possible
   b. Any linen that becomes wet or soiled should be changed
   c. A closed bed is prepared while the patient is showering
   d. Using side rails, keeping call lights within easy reach, and maintaining proper bed position promote patient safety
10. Which of the following patients would be *most* at risk for skin impairment:
    a. Child on bed rest
    b. Infant with cool skin temperature
    c. Young man with diarrhea
    d. Elderly patient in a body cast
11. The nurse plans to give Mrs. Johnson a complete bed bath. When caring for her face, the nurse should:
    a. Use only water when washing the face
    b. Ask patient her preference for face care
    c. Use soap in all areas except the eyes
    d. Use a cleansing cream on the face

CHAPTER CHALLENGE

STUDY QUESTIONS (cont'd)

12. Proper eye care would be:
    a. To wash from outer canthus to inner canthus of eye
    b. To cleanse dried exudate off the eyelid with hot water
    c. To avoid drying circumorbital area after washing
    d. To use a different section of wash cloth for each eye
13. Proper water temperature for a tub bath is:
    a. 105° to 110° F
    b. 110° to 115° F
    c. 98° to 100° F
    d. 48° to 50° C
14. Tepid sponge bathing can be used to:
    a. Reduce temperature on febrile patient
    b. Cleanse patient's groin and axillary areas
    c. Stimulate circulation to the skin
    d. Warm hypothermic patient
15. When administering perineal care to an uncircumcised male patient, the nurse should:
    a. Retract the foreskin, wash the penis, and allow the foreskin to return to former position
    b. Sprinkle powder under foreskin
    c. Leave the foreskin slightly damp
    d. After washing under foreskin, return foreskin with a gentle forward motion
16. The proper procedure for cleaning the female perineal area is to:
    a. Cleanse the area in circular motions around the rectum
    b. Cleanse from the rectum toward the pubis
    c. Cleanse from the pubis toward the rectum
    d. Cleanse in circular motions around the vaginal area
17. Which of the following patients are most at risk for complications of the feet:
    a. Young man in a career that requires standing
    b. Confused, elderly man
    c. Person with diabetes mellitus
    d. Child with growing feet
18. The optimal position for providing oral hygiene to the unconscious patient is:
    a. High Fowler's position
    b. High Fowler's position with head hyperextended
    c. Supine with the head lowered
    d. Side-lying with head lowered
19. All of the following interventions are *contraindicated* in cleansing the ear except:
    a. Cleansing the outer ear with the wash cloth during the bath
    b. Retracting the outer ear downward to loosen visible cerumen
    c. Irrigating to remove tenacious cerumen
    d. Using cotton-tipped applicators to remove cerumen
20. Which of the following interventions is *contraindicated* in the bedmaking process:
    a. Preparing an open bed for receiving postoperative patients
    b. Shaking soiled linen before placement in the hamper
    c. Mitering the corners of the bottom sheet, if not fitted
    d. Washing hands thoroughly after handling soiled linen

21

Specimen Collection

JENANN ALLEN

LEARNING OBJECTIVES

After reading this chapter the student should be able to do the following:

- Define key terms.
- List and explain nursing interventions required for collecting specimens.
- Identify the role of the nurse when performing a procedure for specimen collection.
- Discuss patient teaching for a specimen collection.
- State appropriate labeling for a collected specimen.
- List the proper steps for teaching self–blood-glucose-monitoring.
- Demonstrate the correct procedure for the glucose/acetone determination using Ketodistik, Clinitest tablet, Tes-Tape, and Acetest tablet.
- Discuss the procedure for obtaining a stool specimen for occult blood.
- State the correct procedure for collecting a sputum specimen.
- List the proper steps when obtaining a sterile urine specimen for culture and sensitivity.
- List the nursing responsibilities for the glucose tolerance test.
- Discuss the nursing interventions necessary for proper preparations for a patient having an intravenous pyelogram.
- List the diagnostic tests in which the nurse should determine whether the patient is allergic to iodine.

SKILLS

21-1 Preparing the patient for diagnostic examinations
21-2 Collecting a midstream urine specimen
21-3 Collecting a sterile urine specimen
21-4 Collecting a 24-hour urine specimen
21-5 Performing glucose/acetone determination
21-6 Measuring blood glucose
21-7 Collecting a stool specimen
21-8 Determining presence of occult blood in stool (Hemoccult)
21-9 Collecting sputum

KEY TERMS

Define the following:

- culture
- cytological
- expectorate
- exudate
- fixative
- glucose tolerance test
- Hemoccult test
- ketone
- midstream urine
- morphology
- occult
- paracentesis
- reagent
- sensitivity
- specimen
- thoracentesis

SKILL 21-1: PREPARING THE PATIENT FOR DIAGNOSTIC EXAMINATIONS

Guidelines

Many laboratory and diagnostic examinations can be performed today, and the nurse must be aware of all aspects of the effects on the patient even though other personnel may be doing the procedures. The nurse must know how to prepare the patient for each test, the appropriate requisition form to complete and where it must be sent, the side effects of each test, nursing measures to perform, how to interpret each test in order to notify the physician, what the patient will endure during the test, the follow-up care, and how to document the test. For procedures requiring informed consent, the nurse is usually responsible for seeing that the consent is signed by the patient.

Purposes

The nurse prepares the patient for tests for the following reasons:

- to ensure the patient is ready for the test to be performed
- to avoid prolonging hospital stay because of inadequate test preparation

The nurse must inform the patient that a test is to be performed and answer questions for which the patient may need clarification. The patient needs to know if he is to have nothing by mouth (NPO) after 12 midnight or if breakfast will be held until the examination is completed. The patient needs to know if a special room or equipment is required for the test, as well as special medications needed before or during the test. The more informed the patient, the more cooperative he can be during any test.

Related Knowledge and Skills

Before preparing a patient for a diagnostic examination, the nurse should understand the following:

- documentation (see Chapter 6)
- patient teaching (see Chapter 4)
- physical assessment (see Chapter 13)
- medical asepsis (see Chapter 16)
- urinary elimination (see Chapter 33)
- bowel elimination (see Chapter 31)

SKILL 21-1 PREPARING THE PATIENT FOR DIAGNOSTIC EXAMINATIONS

Nursing action	Rationale
1. Read physician's order.	Provides basis for care.
2. Collect supplies.	Organizes procedure.
3. Introduce self.	Decreases anxiety level.
4. Identify patient by identification band.	Identifies correct patient for procedure.
5. Explain procedure to patient.	Seeks cooperation and decreases anxiety.
6. Wash hands, and don clean gloves.	Helps prevent cross-contamination.
7. Assist physician with procedure.	Provides help to physician while providing support to patient.
8. Answer questions from patient.	Provides security and emotional support to patient.
9. Ensure delivery of specimen to laboratory when applicable. Using correct protocol; be certain specimen is accurately labeled with patient's name, age, room number, physician, date, and type of specimen.	Ensures accuracy of appropriate specimen.
0. Document.	Documents procedure and patient's response.

SKILL 21-2: COLLECTING A MIDSTREAM URINE SPECIMEN

Guidelines

There are several methods for collecting a urine **specimen** for urinalysis, one of the most commonly ordered diagnostic tests. Several tests can be ordered on one sample of urine, including pH, protein, glucose, **ketones,** blood, and specific gravity. The responsibilities of the nurse are to collect and label the urine sample, to ensure its safe delivery to the laboratory, and to assess the results. The nurse also explains test collection to the patient.

The patient must be aware of the upcoming test and told to contact the nurse before the next voiding. The nurse should instruct the patient to drink extra water to assist voiding, to not put toilet tissue in container, and to not allow fecal matter to come in contact with the urine specimen. Midstream urine specimen is urine collected after voiding is initiated (midstream); this is the cleanest part of the voided specimen.

Purposes

The nurse collects a urine specimen and ensures its delivery to the laboratory for the following reasons:

- to help the physician make a diagnosis
- to evaluate the effectiveness of treatment

Related Knowledge and Skills

Before collecting a urine specimen, the nurse should understand the following:

- documentation (see Chapter 6)
- patient teaching (see Chapter 4)
- handwashing (see Chapter 16)

SUPPLIES/EQUIPMENT

gloves
sterile midstream collection kit
label
laboratory requisition

SKILL 21-2 COLLECTING A MIDSTREAM URINE SPECIMEN

Nursing action	Rationale
1. Read physician's order.	Provides basis for care.
2. Collect supplies: sterile cotton balls, antiseptic, and sterile specimen container.	Organizes procedure.
3. Introduce self.	Decreases anxiety level.
4. Identify patient by identification band.	Identifies correct patient for procedure.
5. Explain procedure to patient. Make certain patient understands how to perform procedure.	Seeks cooperation, decreases anxiety, and ensures accuracy of specimen collection.
6. Wash hands, and don clean gloves.	Helps prevent cross-contamination.
7. If patient is able, allow patient to cleanse perineum with antiseptic solution. Separate the labia well on a female patient. Retract foreskin of an uncircumcised male. Use each cotton ball that is saturated with antiseptic solution one time only. If patient is unable to cleanse area, the nurse will don gloves and assist with procedure.	Provides a cleaner specimen. Prevents organisms at or near the meatus from being washed into the specimen.
8. Request that patient (1) begin to void into container about 30 ml; then place the sterile specimen container so the sides of the labia of the female do not touch; (2) without stopping flow, void a small amount into specimen cup; and (3) without stopping flow, finish voiding into toilet seat collector.	Collects **midstream urine** specimen appropriately. The first 30 ml is discarded so that the organisms at the meatus will be washed away.
9. Secure lid on container.	Prevents spillage.
10. Cleanse and return toilet seat collector, if applicable.	Readies for next use.
11. Label specimen appropriately.	Provides accuracy.
12. Ensure that specimen is taken to laboratory with requisition.	Ensures fresh specimen for testing.
13. Document.	Documents procedure and patient's response.

DOCUMENTATION

1. Document procedure performed.	Provides communication of procedure.

Sample charting

DATE	TIME	NOTES
1/28/91	1110	Collected midstream urine specimen. Specimen sent to laboratory.

____
(nurse's signature)

Continued.

SKILL 21-2 COLLECTING A MIDSTREAM URINE SPECIMEN—cont'd

FOLLOW-UP

1. Allow patient to wash hands after procedure.	Helps prevent cross-contamination.

SPECIAL CONCERNS

- Have all supplies ready for patient to perform procedure.
- Make certain patient understands the proper procedure for collecting the urine specimen.
- Be certain specimen is labeled correctly: patient's name, room number, date, physician, and type of specimen.

PATIENT TEACHING

- Teach patient the importance of appropriate collection of urine specimen.

SKILL 21-3: COLLECTING A STERILE URINE SPECIMEN

Guidelines

A sterile urine specimen can be obtained either by inserting a straight catheter into the urinary bladder and removing urine or by obtaining a specimen from the port of an indwelling catheter using sterile technique. Urine from the dependent drainage bag should not be used for a specimen, since it is not fresh and would not reflect accurate test results. Residual urine, urine left in the bladder after voiding, can be measured at the time of catheterization. The patient voids, and catheterization is performed within 10 minutes. If more than 60 ml of urine remains in the bladder, this is *residual urine* and the patient may need to have an indwelling catheter inserted.

The nurse must prepare the patient by explaining which type of urine specimen will be collected. It is important to relieve any anxiety by assuring the patient that there should be no discomfort during the procedure if the patient will remain relaxed: the patient should experience only mild pressure as the catheter is inserted and will feel nothing when urine is collected from the catheter port.

Purposes

The nurse collects a sterile urine specimen for the following reasons:

- to prevent risk of infection to the patient
- to obtain uncontaminated urine for diagnostic testing
- to obtain uncontaminated urine to ascertain effectiveness of treatment

SUPPLIES/EQUIPMENT

Port collection
sterile specimen cup with lid
20 ml syringe
21 or 22½ inch needle
tube clamp
alcohol prep
label
requisition slip

Straight catheter collection
straight catheter tray
label
requisition

Related Knowledge and Skills

Before collecting a sterile urine specimen, the nurse should understand the following:

- documentation (see Chapter 6)
- patient teaching (see Chapter 4)
- handwashing (see Chapter 16)
- urinary disorders (see Chapter 33)

SKILL 21-3 COLLECTING A STERILE URINE SPECIMEN

Nursing action	Rationale
1. Read physician's order.	Provides basis for care.
2. Collect supplies.	Organizes procedure.
3. Introduce self.	Decreases anxiety level.
4. Identify patient by identification band.	Identifies correct patient for procedure.
5. Explain procedure to patient.	Seeks cooperation and decreases anxiety.
6. Wash hands, and don clean gloves.	Helps prevent cross-contamination.
7. Catheter port collection:	
a. Clamp just below catheter port for about 30 minutes.	Allows urine to collect for removal.
b. Return in 30 minutes, and clean port with alcohol prep.	Cleanses port for needle puncture.
c. Insert needle into port at 30-degree angle, and withdraw 5 to 10 ml of urine for a specimen.	Provides urine for testing.
d. Place urine in sterile specimen cup.	Keeps specimen sterile.
e. Unclamp catheter.	Allows continuous urine flow.
f. Label specimen, and send to laboratory with requisition.	Provides accuracy of specimen.
g. Document.	Documents procedure.

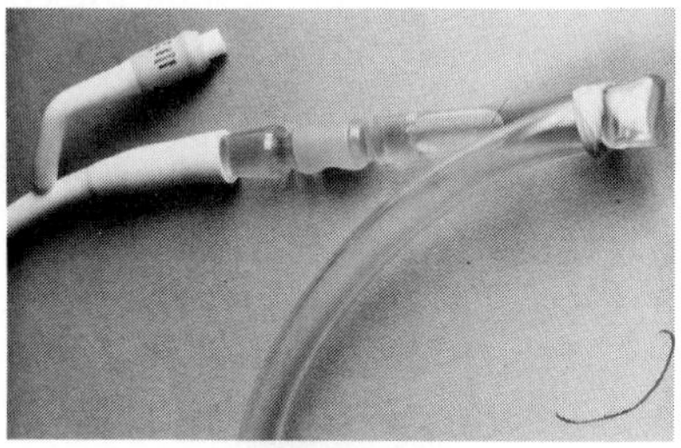

STEP 7 a

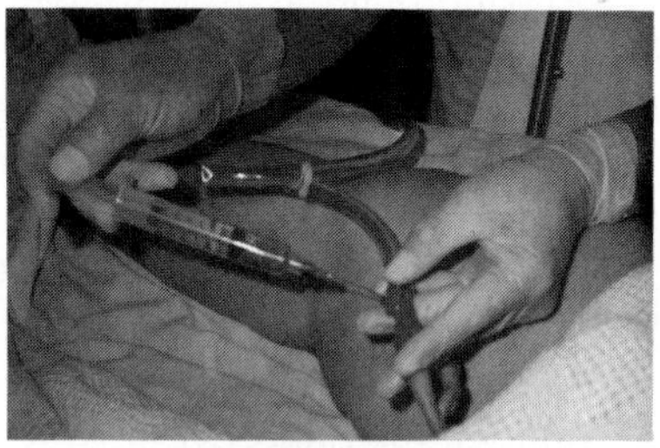

STEP 7 c

Nursing action	Rationale
8. Straight catheter collection:	
a. Wash hands.	Helps prevent cross-contamination.
b. Don sterile gloves, and prepare supplies, using sterile technique—wrap the edges of the sterile drape around the gloved hands.	Wrapping drape around the gloved hands prevents contamination.
c. Place sterile drape under patient's buttocks.	Prepares sterile fluid.
d. Open the lubricant container; add antiseptic (usually iodine solution) to the cotton balls.	All equipment inside the container is sterile, and surgical asepsis must be maintained.
e. Lubricate the catheter about 1½ to 2 inches (3.5 to 5 cm).	Lubrication facilitates easier insertion.
f. To expose the meatus, place the thumb and forefinger of the nondominant hand between the labia minora. Spread and separate upward. Consider the gloved hand that has touched the patient to be contaminated.	Separating the labia minora provides the means to differentiate the urinary meatus from the vaginal meatus.

Continued.

SKILL 21-3 COLLECTING A STERILE URINE SPECIMEN—cont'd

Nursing action	Rationale
8. Straight catheter collection—cont'd	
g. Maintain the position of the contaminated hand until urine is flowing.	If one allows the labia to drop back into position, one may contaminate the surface of the catheter as it is advanced into the bladder.
h. Pick up the forceps, and secure a cotton ball saturated with antiseptic solution—use one cotton ball for each stroke.	By using the forceps one does not contaminate the remaining sterile glove.
i. Bring the cotton ball down the center over the meatus towards the rectum; next cleanse each lateral area from superior to inferior.	Thorough cleansing helps prevent introducing organisms into the bladder.
j. Deposit used cotton balls onto plastic cover.	Used cotton balls are considered contaminated and should not be placed on the sterile field.
Male catheterization differs somewhat from the female catheterization because of anatomical differences:	
k. To cleanse the penis, swab the center of the meatus outward in a circular manner. Continue, using a new cotton ball for each progressively larger circle.	The penis is a round surface and is more easily cleansed in a circular manner to remove pathogens that may enter the bladder and contribute to an infection.
l. To insert a catheter into a male, apply gentle traction and pull the penis straight up; slightly pinch the end of the penis and insert the catheter 15 to 20 cm (6 to 8 inches). To facilitate the more difficult passage through the male urethra, ask the patient to breathe deeply; then rotate the catheter slightly. DO NOT FORCE ENTRY OF THE CATHETER. Discontinue the treatment if either the male or female patient has unusual discomfort or if there is continual resistance to the insertion of the catheter. Report the information promptly.	Holding the penis straight up with slight traction helps to straighten the urethra. Compressing the end of the penis provides a wider opening through which the catheter may be inserted. Expect the indicated distance will place the catheter tip within the bladder. Applying force is liable to injure mucous membranes.
m. To insert a catheter into a female with sterile gloves pick up catheter and insert through urinary meatus 2 to 3 inches (5 to 7.5 cm).	Female urethra is about 1½ to 2½ inches long (4 to 6.5 cm).
n. When urine flows, place end of catheter in specimen cup.	Collect urine specimen.
o. Place lid on urine cup, and label and clean up supplies.	Prevents spillage and appropriately labels specimens.
p. Send specimen to lab with requisition.	Provides accuracy of specimen.
q. Document.	Documents procedure and patient's response.

SKILL 21-3 COLLECTING A STERILE URINE SPECIMEN—cont'd

DOCUMENTATION

1. Document procedure and observations. — Communicates with others patient care administered.

Sample charting

DATE	TIME	NOTES
1/28/91	1030	10 ml sterile urine specimen collected from catheter port and sent to laboratory. *(nurse's signature)*
1/31/91	1140	Obtained 360 ml clear, yellow urine per catheterization, and specimen sent to laboratory. Tolerated well. *(nurse's signature)*

FOLLOW-UP

1. Make patient comfortable, and position appropriately. — Provides safe patient environment.

SPECIAL CONCERNS

- Use strict sterile technique to prevent infection in urinary system.
- Insert catheter gently to prevent pain or discomfort: catheterization should not be painful.

PATIENT TEACHING

- Teach patient to relax by deep breathing during a catheterization.
- Answer patient questions about the procedure.

SKILL 21-4: COLLECTING A 24-HOUR URINE SPECIMEN

Guidelines

Some tests require that the entire volume of urine from a 24-hour period be collected. The procedure for ensuring that the test can be performed accurately should be followed carefully.

SUPPLIES/EQUIPMENT

urinal/bedpan/specimen hat
specimen container with added preservative of agency's choice

SKILL 21-4 COLLECTING A 24-HOUR URINE SPECIMEN

Nursing action	Rationale
1. Read physician's order.	Verifies procedure.
2. Wash hands.	Promotes medical asepsis.
3. Identify patient.	Ensures accuracy.
4. Post signs on patient's door, bathroom door, and near patient's bed.	Alerts the staff and reminds the patient to save all urine.
5. Explain procedure.	Ensures patient's cooperation.
6. Instruct patient about the importance of collecting *all* urine for a period of 24 hours.	Ensures a valid test can be obtained of 24-hour kidney function.
7. Instruct patient not to place toilet tissue or fecal material in urine.	Prevents contamination of specimen and alterations of results.
8. Have patient void when the 24-hour specimen collection is to begin; discard this voiding.	This voiding has been formed in urinary system before the study began.
9. Place labeled container on ice if required. (Some agencies require refrigeration of all specimens. Others advocate that the urine container be placed on ice. For some collection procedures, such as the creatinine clearance test, refrigeration may not be necessary.	Keeping the specimen cool decreases decomposition and odor.
10. Save all urine for the 24-hour period; place each voided specimen into the larger container with preservative.	All urine must be saved or results will be altered.
11. Instruct patient to void a few minutes before end of 24 hours; this urine is part of the 24-hour specimen.	Empties bladder before the end of testing.
12. Send specimen to lab promptly; be certain label includes date and time specimen started, patient's name, room number, and test ordered. If more than one container is necessary, make certain both are labeled and numbered.	Ensures proper identification of specimen.

DOCUMENTATION

1. Document procedure and observations.	Communicates with others patient care administered.

Sample charting

DATE	TIME	NOTES
1/6/91	0700	Voided 300 ml light amber urine. Urine discarded; 24-hour urine specimen collection begun.

____
(nurse's signature)

SKILL 21-4

COLLECTING A 24-HOUR URINE SPECIMEN—cont'd

DOCUMENTATION—cont'd

1/7/91 0700 Voided 300 ml light amber urine. Urine added to collection specimen. The entire 24-hour urine collection sent to laboratory.

(nurse's signature)

SPECIAL CONCERNS

- Wash hands and don gloves each time a specimen is collected and transferred to the large collection container to prevent spread of microorganisms.
- If patient is menstruating, be certain to note this on requisition form to ensure accuracy of results.

SKILL 21-5: PERFORMING GLUCOSE/ ACETONE, OR CLINITEST/ACETEST, DETERMINATION

Guidelines

A glucose/acetone determination test is performed to measure the amount of sugar (glucose) and acetone in a sample of urine from the patient who is diabetic. It is one part of the diabetic regimen and must be appropriately carried out. There are several types of products used for the test, such as Clinitest tablets, Tes-Tape, Dipstick, Acetest tablets, and Ketodistiks.

The patient is taught to perform the test at certain times during the day, such as before meals and at bedtime. The specimen should be a double-voided one to ensure accurate test results. This test is done less often now for glucose determination in the urine because of availability of self–blood-glucose-monitoring or blood glucose monitoring by the laboratory personnel or the nurse. Blood glucose monitoring provides more current and accurate information on glucose levels in the body.

The patient should be informed of the times during the day the test will be performed in order to give a urine sample as needed. Test results are usually charted on a flow sheet and are reported to the medication nurse when a sliding scale for insulin is ordered. In this case, insulin is administered according to the test results. This test is simple to perform but must be done accurately, since the amount of insulin given may be determined by the results.

Purposes

The nurse performs the glucose/acetone determination test for the following reasons:

- to aid the physician in deciding the amount of insulin to order
- to assist in controlling diabetes
- to detect elevated glucose levels before the patient is given more glucose
- to help adjust food intake, exercise, and insulin requirements

SUPPLIES/EQUIPMENT

For reagent tablet testing	For reagent strip testing
bedpan or urinal	specimen container
specimen container	glucose/ketone test strip
10 ml test tube	test strip color chart
test tube holder	
medicine dropper	
clean container for water	
Clinitest tablets	
Acetest tablets	
color charts	
tissues or paper towel	

Related Knowledge and Skills

Before performing glucose/acetone determination, the nurse should understand the following:

- documentation (see Chapter 6)
- patient teaching (see Chapter 4)
- handwashing (see Chapter 16)

SKILL 21-5 PERFORMING GLUCOSE/ACETONE DETERMINATION

Nursing action	Rationale
1. Read physician's order.	Provides basis for care.
2. Collect supplies.	Organizes procedure.
3. Introduce self.	Decreases anxiety level.
4. Identify patient by identification band.	Identifies correct patient for procedure.
5. Explain procedure to patient.	Seeks cooperation and decreases anxiety.
6. Wash hands, and don clean gloves.	Helps prevent cross-contamination.
7. Obtain double-voided specimen ½ hour apart.	Provides most accurate results from freshest urine.
8. Perform glucose reagent tablet test:	
a. Drop 5 drops of urine from medicine dropper into test tube, and rinse dropper.	Provides accuracy of test results.
b. Add 10 drops water to urine in test tube.	Provides accuracy of test results.
c. Add reagent tablet to test tube.	Provides chemical reaction for test.
d. Hold test tube near top or place tube in holder.	Prevents nurse from receiving burn from chemical reaction.
e. Shake test tube gently 15 seconds after boiling action stops, and compare color of solution with color chart.	Gives results of test.
f. Cleanse test tube and rinse.	Prepares for next use of the article.
g. There is also a 2-drop method; it follows the same procedure except 2 drops of urine is used and this method has a different color chart.	
9. Perform glucose reagent tape test:	
a. Tear 1½ inches Tes-Tape from holder, and immerse end of strip in and immediately out of urine.	Helps determine accuracy of test.
b. Tap gently on side of container	Excess urine can dilute reagent.
c. After appropriate amount of time, compare with color chart.	Provides test results.
10. Perform acetone reagent tablet test:	
a. Place Acetest tablet on dry paper towel; do not touch with bare hands.	Moisture can cause inaccurate results.
b. Place 1 drop of urine from medicine dropper onto tablet.	Provides chemical reaction.
c. After appropriate amount of time, compare with color chart.	Provides test results.
11. Wash hands.	Reduces number of microorganisms.
12. Document.	Documents procedure and patient's response.

SKILL 21-5

PERFORMING GLUCOSE/ACETONE DETERMINATION—cont'd

DOCUMENTATION

1. Record glucose/acetone determination.	Documents procedure, patient's test response, and test results.

Sample charting

DATE	TIME	NOTES
1/26/91	1110	Glucose/acetone test performed. Voided 300 ml clear, yellow urine. Clinitest negative and Acetest negative. Reported to medication nurse.
		_______________ *(nurse's signature)*

FOLLOW-UP

1. Clean and replace supplies and equipment.	Prepares for next procedure to be performed and keeps environment clean.
2. Make sure bottle cap is replaced tightly.	Tablets may react to moisture in the air, which renders the tablets chemically inactive.

SPECIAL CONCERNS

- Patient must be given enough time to give a double-voided specimen.
- Offer extra water to drink to increase renal perfusion.
- Read instructions carefully on all glucose/acetone testing materials before performing tests.
- Chart glucose/acetone results on flow sheet.
- Test first specimen of urine if patient cannot give double-voided specimen, and report and record even though not considered accurate.

PATIENT TEACHING

- Teach patient to perform glucose/acetone urine tests.
- Explain results of tests where applicable.
- Teach skin puncture for blood glucose if applicable; this test is replacing urine testing and gives more accurate information.

SKILL 21-6: MEASURING BLOOD GLUCOSE

Guidelines

The use of a meter to measure blood glucose is a more meaningful test for use by diabetics than testing urine for the presence of glucose. A skin puncture can be easily performed by the patient at home.

Purposes

The nurse measures blood glucose for the following reasons:

- to monitor blood glucose levels, especially for the patient who is diabetic and the patient who is receiving IV hyperalimentation
- to formulate a nursing diagnosis
- to teach the diabetic patient how to control blood glucose levels
- to teach the diabetic patient to measure blood glucose levels to perform procedure at home

SUPPLIES/EQUIPMENT

lancet
automatic lancing device
cotton balls
vial of test strips
meter to measure glucose

Related Knowledge and Skills

Before measuring a blood glucose level, the nurse should understand the following:

- docmentation (see Chapter 6)
- patient teaching (see Chapter 4)
- handwashing (see Chapter 16)
- endocrine disorders (see Chapter 35)

SKILL 21-6

MEASURING BLOOD GLUCOSE

Nursing action	Rationale
1. Read physician's order.	Provides basis for care.
2. Collect supplies.	Organizes procedure.
3. Introduce self.	Decreases anxiety level.
4. Identify patient by identification band.	Identifies correct patient for procedure.
5. Explain procedure to patient.	Seeks cooperation and decreases anxiety.
6. Wash hands, and don clean gloves.	Helps prevent cross-contamination and protects nurse from blood and body fluids.
7. Remove cap from lancet using sterile technique.	Maintains sterility of point.
8. Place lancet into automatic lancing device according to instructions in operating manual.	Allows proper puncture of skin.
9. Select site on side of any fingertip (heel used for infant).	Side of finger less responsive to pain from puncture.
10. Wipe selected site with alcohol swab, and discard.	Prepares site.
11. Ask patient to hold arm at side 30 seconds.	Increases blood flow to site and allows site to dry.
12. Gently squeeze fingertip with thumb of same hand.	Increases blood supply to site.
13. Hold lancing device.	Provides easy access to device.

SKILL 21-6

MEASURING BLOOD GLUCOSE—cont'd

Nursing action	Rationale
14. Place trigger platform of lancing device on side of finger, and press.	Activates lancing mechanism.
15. Squeeze finger in downward motion (wipe off first drop of blood).	Obtains enough blood to cover test pad on test strip. Removes surface contaminant.
16. While holding strip level, touch drop of blood to test pad.	Enables covering of test pad without smearing.
17. Begin recommended timing. After 60 seconds blot blood off test strip (A), place reagent strip into appropriate site on meter (B), and wait for numeric readout (C).	Ensures test accuracy.
18. Remove lancet from device, and discard.	Prevents needle puncture of nurse.
19. Remove gloves, and discard.	Prevents cross-contamination.
20. Document.	Documents procedure and patient's response.

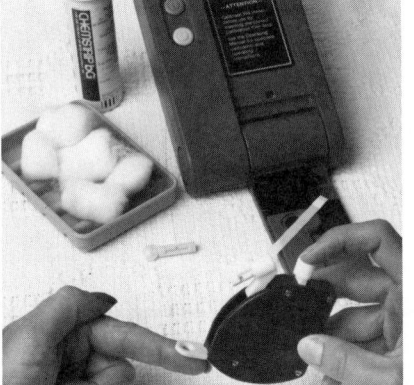

STEP 14

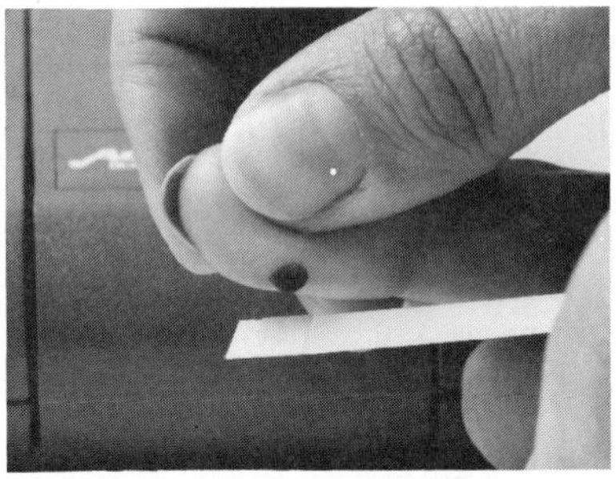
STEP 16

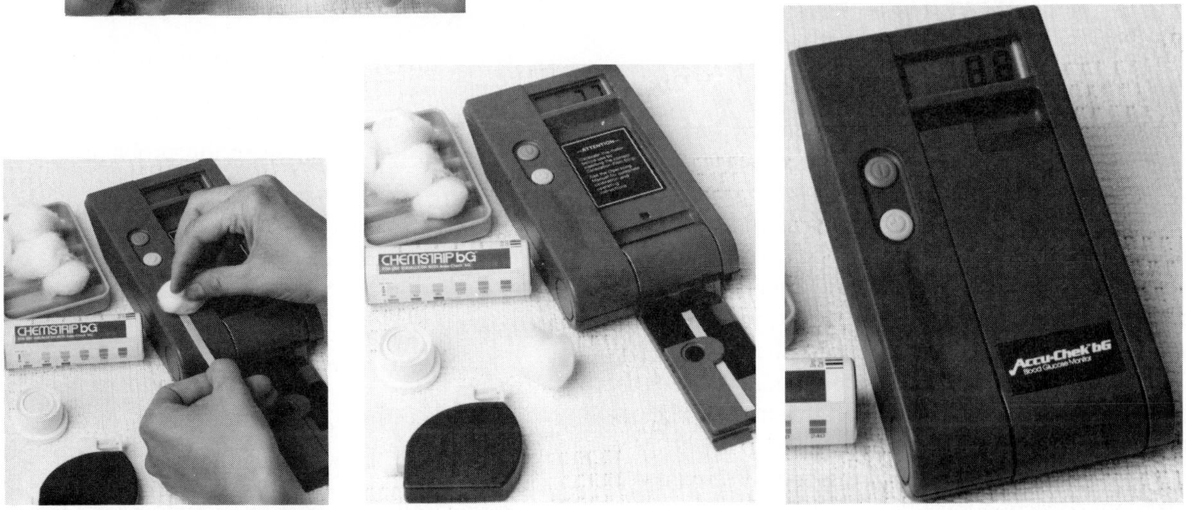

A B C

STEP 17

Continued.

SKILL 21-6 MEASURING BLOOD GLUCOSE—cont'd

DOCUMENTATION

1. Document procedure and observations.

Communicates with others patient care administration.

Sample charting

DATE	TIME	NOTES
2/20/91	1730	Skin puncture performed on left index finger for blood glucose. Results: 84 per glucometer. Tolerated well. Verbalizes understanding of blood glucose level. Dr. Smith notified per phone of test results.
		_______________ *(nurse's signature)*

SPECIAL CONCERNS

- Make certain staff is aware of what tests are scheduled for each day.
- Have all supplies available if patient is to perform procedure.
- Carry out strict sterile technique during procedure.
- Wear clean gloves when in contact with body fluids.
- Make certain patient understands how to perform procedure, to ensure patient safety and accurate test results.

PATIENT TEACHING

- Teach patient to perform a skin puncture when appropriate.
- Have patient return demonstration for a skin puncture.
- Explain normal blood glucose levels to the patient.
- Explain to patient which blood glucose levels should be reported to the physician.

SKILL 21-7: COLLECTING A STOOL SPECIMEN

Guidelines

Stool specimens are collected and examined for a variety of reasons including: to determine the presence of infection, bleeding, or hemorrhage; to observe the amount, color, consistency, and presence of fats; and to identify parasites, ova, and bacteria. The nurse collects the feces, labels the specimen appropriately, and sends the specimen and laboratory request to the laboratory. Stool to be examined for parasites must be taken immediately to the laboratory in order for parasites to be examined under the microscope while alive. A stool specimen may also be collected from a colostomy or ileostomy.

The patient must be informed that a stool specimen is needed, but collection must be carried out in such a manner that will not cause stress or make the patient feel hurried. Arrange supplies if patient will collect the stool. The nurse must understand why the stool specimen is being collected to use the appropriate supplies.

Purposes

The nurse collects stool specimens for the following reasons:

- to test for abnormal elements in the stool
- to determine malabsorption problems

SUPPLIES/EQUIPMENT

stool specimen cup
tongue depressor
bedpan, specimen device, or commode
gloves
label
laboratory requisition

Related Knowledge and Skills

Before collecting a stool specimen, the nurse should understand the following:

- documentation (see Chapter 6)
- patient teaching (see Chapter 4)
- handwashing (see Chapter 16)

SKILL 21-7

COLLECTING A STOOL SPECIMEN

Nursing action	Rationale
1. Read physician's order.	Provides basis for care.
2. Collect supplies.	Organizes procedure.
3. Introduce self.	Decreases anxiety level.
4. Identify patient by identification band.	Identifies correct patient for procedure.
5. Explain procedure to patient; make certain patient understands what is expected.	Seeks cooperation and decreases anxiety.
6. Wash hands, and don gloves.	Help prevent cross-contamination.
7. Assist to bathroom when necessary.	Provides patient safety.
8. Request patient to defecate into commode, specimen device, or bedpan, and to prevent urine from entering specimen.	Prevents contamination of specimen.
9. Transfer stool to specimen cup with use of a tongue blade, and close lid.	Protects specimen.

STEP 8

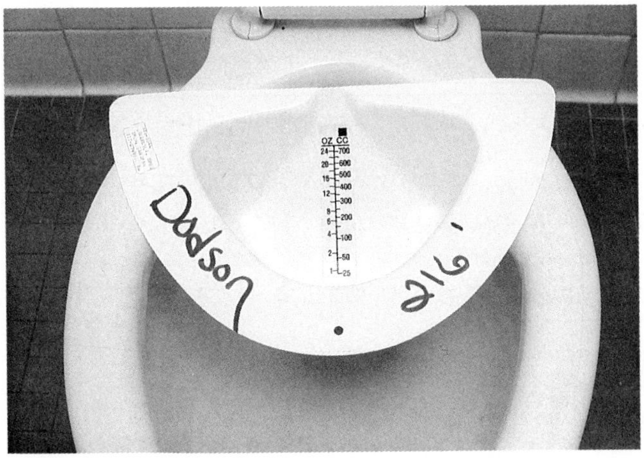

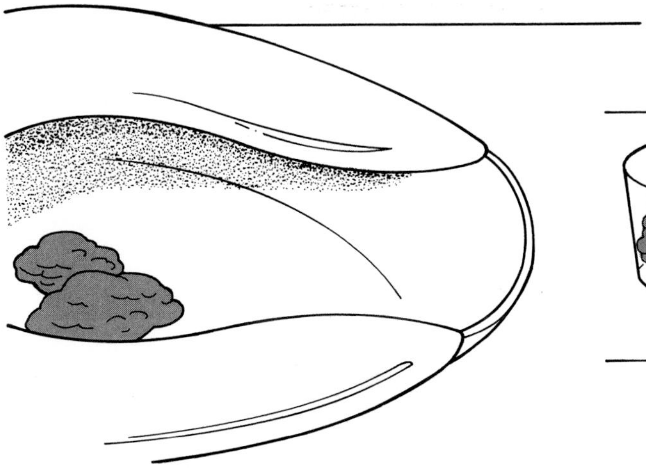

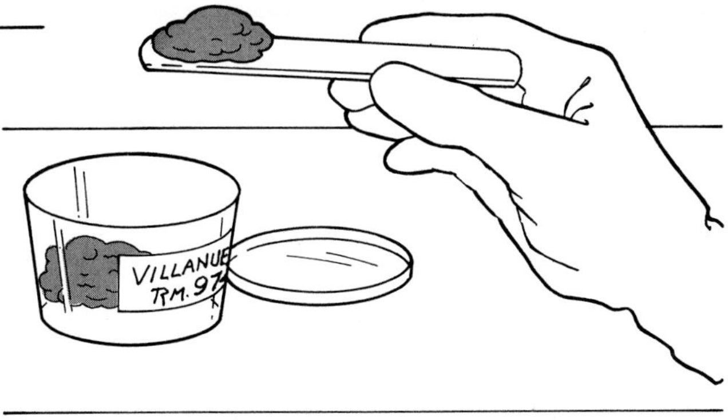

STEP 9

Continued.

SKILL 21-7 COLLECTING A STOOL SPECIMEN—cont'd

Nursing action	Rationale
10. Remove gloves, and wash hands.	Protects nurse from contamination.
11. Attach lab request, and send specimen to laboratory.	Identifies specimen for laboratory.
12. Assist patient to bed.	Provides patient safety.
13. Document.	Documents procedure and patient's response.

DOCUMENTATION

1. Document procedure and observations.	Communicates with others patient care administered.

Sample charting

DATE	TIME	NOTES
12/4/90	1040	Specimen of soft, brown stool collected and taken with requisition form to laboratory.

(nurse's signature)

SPECIAL CONCERNS

- Nurse must know what type stool specimen is ordered and how to collect the specimen.
- Make certain patient understands what is expected, to provide patient safety.
- Specimen to be examined for ova and parasites must be taken to the laboratory while still warm.
- Other stool specimens may be kept at room temperature.

PATIENT TEACHING

- Explain how to collect a stool specimen appropriately.
- Teach purpose for collecting a stool specimen.

SKILL 21-8: DETERMINING PRESENCE OF OCCULT BLOOD IN STOOL

Guidelines

The presence of blood in body waste is abnormal. Blood in the stool may be bright red, which indicates that the blood is fresh and that the site of bleeding is in the lower GI tract. On the other hand, black tarry feces means the presence of old blood and that the site of bleeding is higher in the gastrointestinal tract. When blood is present in the stool but cannot be seeen without the use of a microscope, it is referred to as **occult** or hidden. A **Hemoccult test** detects occult blood in feces.

The nurse must instruct the patient on how many stool specimens are ordered by the physician and how to collect a stool specimen. The Hemoccult card is then labeled appropriately and sent to the laboratory.

Purposes

The nurse collects a stool specimen and sends it to the laboratory for the following reasons:

- to detect the presence of blood in the stool
- to aid the physician in making a diagnosis

SUPPLIES/EQUIPMENT

Hemoccult card
wooden applicator
clean bedpan or specimen device for commode
clean gloves

Related Knowledge and Skills

Before collecting a stool specimen and taking it to the laboratory, the nurse should understand the following:

- documentation (see Chapter 6)
- patient teaching (see Chapter 4)
- handwashing (see Chapter 16)

SKILL 21-9: COLLECTING SPUTUM

Guidelines

Sputum is mucus from the lung. A sputum specimen must come from deep in the bronchial tree. Expectoration from throat and mouth secretions cannot be used as a sputum specimen. Early morning is the best time to collect a sputum specimen because the patient has not yet cleared the respiratory passages. Many tests can be performed on sputum, such as **culture** and **sensitivity, cytological** examination, and test for acid-fast bacillus. Some patients cannot **expectorate** a specimen and must have a pharyngeal suctioning to obtain sputum. Closed-method collection containers protect the nurse from contamination from body fluids. The nurse explains the procedure and prepares the patient for the test.

The nurse instructs the patient the night before the test to drink extra fluids, since this will assist loosening secretions to more easily expectorate for the specimen. Saliva cannot be used as a specimen, and the patient must be so instructed.

Purposes

The nurse collects a sputum specimen for the following reasons:

- to determine (1) if pathogenic microorganisms are present in the sputum, (2) the type of microorganism present, and (3) to what drugs it is sensitive (by doing a culture and sensitivity)
- to determine if cancer cells are present
- to determine the presence of an organism called the *tubercle bacillus,* which causes tuberculosis

SUPPLIES/EQUIPMENT

sterile sputum collector
tissues
label for specimen
laboratory requisition
gloves

Related Knowledge and Skills

Before collecting a sputum specimen, the nurse should understand the following:

- documentation (see Chapter 6)
- patient teaching (see Chapter 4)
- handwashing (see Chapter 16)
- respiratory disorders (see Chapter 34)

For a more comprehensive look at other diagnostic examinations refer to Table 21-1.

SKILL 21-8 DETERMINING PRESENCE OF OCCULT BLOOD IN STOOL

Nursing action	Rationale
1. Read physician's order.	Provides basis for care.
2. Collect supplies.	Organizes procedure.
3. Introduce self.	Decreases anxiety level.
4. Identify patient by identification band.	Identifies correct patient for procedure.
5. Explain procedure to patient.	Seeks cooperation and decreases anxiety.
6. Wash hands, and don gloves.	Helps prevent cross-contamination.
7. Collect stool specimen.	Provides stool for Hemoccult.
8. Follow steps on Hemoccult slide test:	
a. Open flap.	Begins test.
b. Smear very small amount with tongue blade (smear) in first box (A).	Prepares slide.
c. Smear very small amount with tongue blade (smear) from another part of stool, and transfer to box B.	Prepares second slide.
d. Close card, and label.	Ensures accurate identification of specimen.
e. Send specimen to lab.	Provides fresh specimen for testing.
9. Remove gloves, and wash hands.	Helps prevent cross-contamination.
10. Document.	Documents procedure and patient's response.

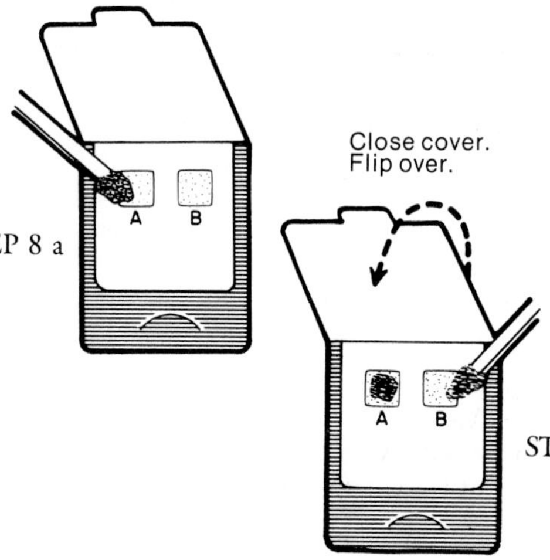

STEP 8 a

STEP 8 c

Review

DOCUMENTATION

1. Document procedure and observations.	Communicates with others collection of patient stool specimen.

Sample charting

DATE	TIME	NOTES
1/28/91	1310	Expelled large amount soft, brown stool. First specimen for occult blood collected and sent to laboratory. Instructed regarding need for total of three specimens.

____
(nurse's signature)

SKILL 21-8 DETERMINING PRESENCE OF OCCULT BLOOD IN STOOL—cont'd

FOLLOW-UP

1. Read further orders for changes in regimen after test results.	Results of tests can lead to further changes.

SPECIAL CONCERNS

- Do not confuse hemorrhoidal bleeding with upper gastrointestinal bleeding.
- Meat-free diet may be ordered 3 days before test.

PATIENT TEACHING

- Make certain patient understands test and why it is being performed.
- Teach patient how to perform procedure if discharged before three specimens are collected.

Table 21-1 Nurses' Role in Preparation of Patient for Diagnostic Examinations

Examination	Nursing Examination Responsibilities	Nursing Responsibilities After Examination
Urinalysis	Prepare requisition form. Explain purpose and specific method of urine collection. Wash perineal area, if soiled. If patient is menstruating, note this on requisition form.	Report results.
CBC	Prepare requisition form. Explain procedure.	Observe site for bleeding. Report results.
Blood chemistries	Prepare requisition form. NPO or hold meal. Explain procedure. Smoking may be prohibited.	Observe site for bleeding. Be certain patient's meal is served after test is completed. Report results.
Glucose tolerance	Prepare requisition slip. Explain procedure. NPO—encourage H_2O intake so patient can provide urine samples. Obtain urine samples at designated times. Blood and urine specimen will be collected at the same time. The procedure will be as follows: 1. Make certain the patient empties his bladder and 30 minutes later obtain a fasting UA. 2. Laboratory will administer 75 grams of dextrose orally. 3. The nurse will collect urine specimen ½ hour, 1 hour, 1½ hours, 2½ hours, 3½ hours, up to 5 hours after dextrose, depending on the physician's orders.	Observe venipuncture site for bleeding. Make certain patient received meal when test is completed. Report results: An elevated blood glucose level at the 2-hour point usually indicates some disorder of carbohydrate metabolism; depending on the elevation of the blood glucose, there may be glucose present in the urine.

Continued.

Table 21-1 Nurses' Role in Preparation of Patient for Diagnostic Examinations—cont'd

Examination	Nursing Examination Responsibilities	Nursing Responsibilities After Examination
Lumbar puncture	Explain before procedure and after procedure routine. Obtain written consent. Bladder and bowel should be empty if possible. Provide necessary equipment. Assist patient to assume appropriate position. The nurse may be asked to hold manometer straight. Label and number specimens.	Keep patient flat after procedure. Observe patient for mobility of extremities, pain, drainage, and ability to void. Notify physician if any unusual occurrences. Report results.
Chest x-ray	Prepare requisition form. Explain procedure. Be certain there are no snaps or pins on gown.	Report results.
Bone scan	Prepare requisition form. Explain procedure. Instruct patient to remove jewelry or any metal objects. Encourage patient to drink several glasses of water. Patient should void before examination.	Observe injection site for erythema or edema; if hematoma forms, apply warm soaks to the area to relieve pain.
Ultrasound/sonogram	Most of these procedures require little preparation. Prepare requisition form. Explain procedure. If a pelvic sonogram is ordered, the patient needs a full bladder. If a gallbladder sonogram is ordered, the patient needs to be NPO. Signed consent form may be required.	Because this procedure is noninvasion, no specific follow-up care is needed. Usual diet may be resumed after examination.
Bronchoscopy (Fig. 21-1)	Prepare requisition form. Explain procedure. Obtain an informed consent before patient is premedicated. Patient is NPO after midnight. Administer preoperative medication as ordered. Remove and safely store contact lenses, dentures, glasses. Reassure patient.	Do not allow patient to eat or drink after procedure until the effect of anesthesia no longer exists and gag reflex has returned—usually about 2 hours. Observe any sputum for blood. Monitor vital signs frequently: fever is normal within the first 24 hours after bronchoscopy. Observe for impaired respirations. Observe closely until effects of anesthesia no longer exist. If patient complains of sore throat, warm saline gargles and lozenges may be ordered.

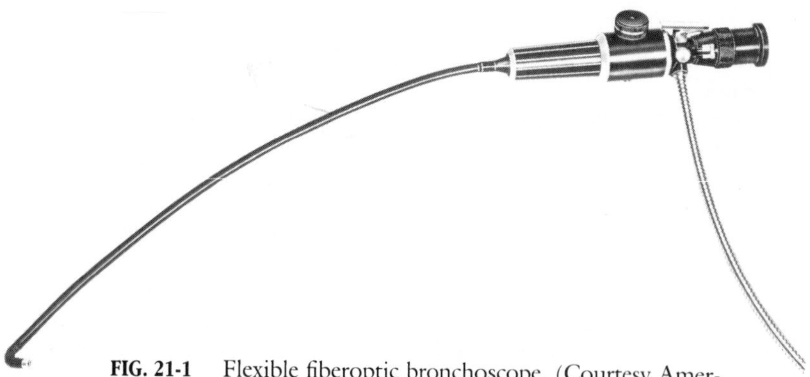

FIG. 21-1 Flexible fiberoptic bronchoscope. (Courtesy American Cystoscope Makers, Inc, Pelham, NY.)

Table 21-1 Nurses' Role in Preparation of Patient for Diagnostic Examinations—cont'd

Examination	Nursing Examination Responsibilities	Nursing Responsibilities After Examination
Myelogram	NPO for 4 hours before examination. Explain procedure. Obtain written consent.	Proper positioning will be prescribed by the physician. Observe the patient for fever, stiff neck, occipital headache, or photophobia. Monitor vital signs. Monitor ability to void. Encourage fluids so patient does not get dehydrated; this will result in a severe headache.
Mammography	Prepare requisition form. Explain procedure. If patient is embarrassed by the procedure, ask patient to verbalize her feelings. Provide emotional support. Instruct patient not to wear deodorant, powder, or lotion.	Explain how test results can be obtained.

COMPUTED TOMOGRAPHY (Fig.21-2)

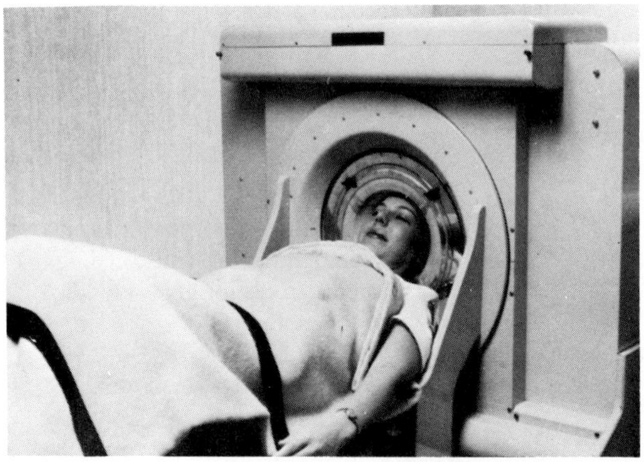

FIG. 21-2 Patient receiving CT scanning.

Examination	Nursing Examination Responsibilities	Nursing Responsibilities After Examination
Brain scan	Explain procedure. Keep patient NPO for 4 hours before examination. Instruct patient not to wear wig, hairpins, or clips. Observe patient for iodine allergies. If ordered, give sedation.	No special care required after procedure. Encourage fluid intake.
Body scan	Prepare requisition form. Explain procedure. No specific preparation.	No specific follow-up care.
Abdominal scan	Prepare requisition form. Explain procedure. Patient is NPO for 4 hours before examination.	No specific follow-up care.
Lung scan	Prepare requisition form. Explain procedure. Patient is NPO for 4 hours before examination. Observe the patient for allergies to iodine.	No specific follow-up care. Encourage fluid intake.

Continued.

Table 21-1 Nurses' Role in Preparation of Patient for Diagnostic Examinations—cont'd

Examination	Nursing Examination Responsibilities	Nursing Responsibilities After Examination
Endoscopy and gastroscopy (Fig. 21-3)	Prepare requisition form. Administer preexamination medication if ordered. Explain procedure. Obtain written consent. Keep patient NPO after midnight. Provide emotional support. Remove patient's dentures and eye glasses. Perform oral hygiene measures.	Perform oral hygiene measures. Do not allow food or drink until the gag reflex returns (2-4 hours). Explain that drinking cool fluids and gargling will help relieve some soreness. Observe the patient for bleeding, fever, abdominal pain, dysphagia, and dyspnea. Monitor vital signs. Observe safety precautions until the effects of the sedatives no longer exist.
Colonoscopy	Prepare requisition form. Explain procedure. Obtain written consent. Assist with the bowel prep. Record the results from the cathartics and enemas.	Observe the patient for abdominal pain, tenderness, and bleeding. Examine stools for gross blood. Encourage fluids. Offer normal diet. A warm bath may be soothing. Allow time for rest. Take safety precautions until the effects of the medication no longer exist.
Proctoscopy and sigmoidoscopy (Fig. 21-4)	Prepare requisition form. Explain procedure. Provide emotional support. Obtain written consent. Patient is allowed a light breakfast on day of exam. Administer enemas as ordered, and record results.	Observe the patient for fever, bleeding, abdominal distention, and unusual complaints of pain.

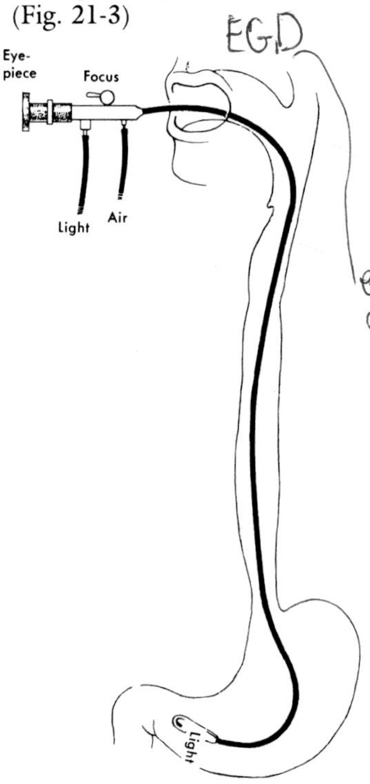

FIG. 21-3 Fiberoptic endoscope.

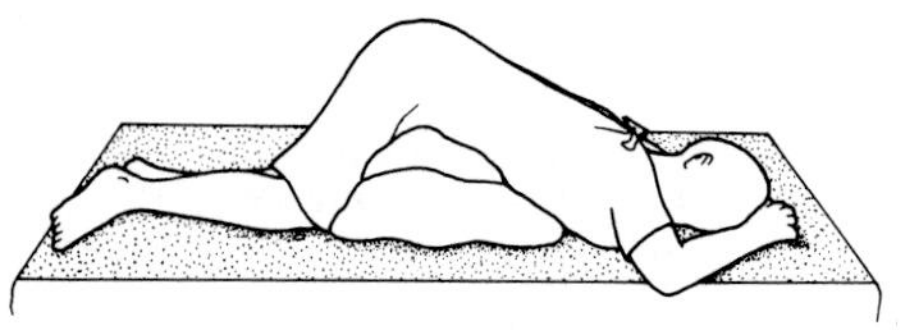

FIG. 21-4 Position for proctoscopy.

Table 21-1 Nurses' Role in Preparation of Patient for Diagnostic Examinations—cont'd

Examination	Nursing Examination Responsibilities	Nursing Responsibilities After Examination
Cystoscopy	Explain procedure. Obtain written consent. Administer enemas as ordered, and record results. If patient will be under local anesthesia, a liquid breakfast may be allowed. If patient will be under general anesthesia, keep patient NPO. Administer preprocedure medications as ordered.	Assess patient's ability to void for at least 24 hours after procedure. Record urine color—if bright red, report to physician. Warm sitz baths may be soothing. Encourage fluid intake. Observe vital signs. Observe for hemorrhage and for sepsis. Administer antibiotic as ordered.
Intravenous pyelogram	Prepare requisition form. Be certain IVP is done before barium x-rays are performed. Explain procedure. Check for allergies to iodine, since the intravenous dye usually contains iodine. Administer cathartics or laxatives as ordered (children and infants are not given cathartics or laxatives). Keep patient NPO after midnight (if an intravenous solution is infusing, ask physician if he wishes to decrease IV to a keep-open-rate to prevent hydration: in an IVP the patient needs to have fluid restricted for the dye to be taken up by the kidney).	Observe for anaphylaxis (respiratory distress, shock, and drop in blood pressure). Allow patient normal diet. Encourage fluid intake to help eliminate any dye left in body. Assess for weakness. Encourage to ambulate with assistance unless contraindicated.
Electrocardiogram	Prepare requisition form. Explain procedure.	Remove gel from patient's skin with a tissue.
Arteriogram	Explain procedure.	Keep patient at bed rest for 8 hours.
Femoral angiogram	Provide emotional support. Observe patient for allergies to iodine dye. Obtain written consent. Keep patient NPO after midnight.	Observe catheter insertion site for inflammation, hemorrhage, hematoma at the site, or absence of peripheral pulses. Observe the involved extremity for numbness, tingling, pain, or loss of function. Monitor vital signs. Cold compresses to the puncture site may reduce discomfort and edema. If patient complains of continuous, severe pain, notify physician.
Echocardiogram	Prepare requisition form. Explain procedure. Answer questions.	Remove the gel from the patient's chest with a tissue.
Electroencephalogram	Prepare requisition form. Explain procedure. Hair should be clean; administer shampoo as necessary. Confer with physician if any medications should be discontinued before examination. Administer sedatives or hypnotics as ordered. Encourage food intake but eliminate coffee, tea, and colas.	Assist the patient to remove the electrode paste. Shampoo hair. Ensure safety precautions until effects of the sedatives no longer exist.

Continued.

Table 21-1 Nurses' Role in Preparation of Patient for Diagnostic Examinations—cont'd

Examination	Nursing Examination Responsibilities	Nursing Responsibilities After Examination
Renal angiography	Explain procedure. Answer questions. Obtain written consent. Assess patient for allergy to iodine dye. Keep patient NPO after midnight. Administer cathartics as ordered. Administer preprocedure medications.	Observe arterial puncture site frequently. Monitor the extremity for adequate circulation. Monitor pedal pulses and vital signs frequently. Keep patient on bed rest for 12-24 hours. Cold compresses to puncture site will help to reduce discomfort and edema. Encourage fluids.
Amniocentesis	Explain procedure. Encourage verbalization. Obtain written consent. Monitor fetal heart tones.	Monitor fetal heart tones. If patient complains of vertigo, allow her to rest on her left side for several minutes before leaving examination room. If patient has any fluid loss or temperature elevation, instruct her to notify her physician. Inform patient to contact her physician to obtain results.
Thoracentesis (Fig. 21-5)	Explain procedure. Obtain written consent. Obtain equipment. Assist patient to assume the appropriate position (usually sitting). Offer emotional support.	Monitor vital signs. Monitor patient for coughing or for hemoptysis. Monitor patient for complications; notify physician if any unusual signs and symptoms occur. Monitor patient's lung sounds. If no complaints of dyspnea, normal activity can be resumed in an hour. Send specimen to laboratory for examination if requested.
Paracentesis	Explain procedure. Obtain written consent. Provide emotional support. Obtain equipment. Assist physician.	Observe puncture site. Observe for syncope. Monitor vital signs. Encourage a period of rest after examination. Send specimen to laboratory for examination if requested.
Upper gastrointestinal series	Prepare requisition form. Explain procedure. Answer questions. Offer emotional support. Keep patient NPO after midnight.	Patient may eat as soon as series is completed unless contraindicated. Encourage fluids. Monitor stools. Administer milk of magnesia, 2 oz., or per hospital protocol.
Barium enema	Prepare requisition form. Explain procedure. Provide needed emotional support. Assist with required preparations—monitor effects of cathartics and/or enemas. Patient is NPO after midnight. Some facilities allow liquids for breakfast.	Patient may resume regular diet as soon as exam is completed. Monitor stools—barium may cause constipation. A local anesthetic ointment may be ordered after examination to relieve anal discomfort. A warm bath may be soothing. Administer milk of magnesia, 2 oz., after examination as per hospital protocol. Allow time for rest.

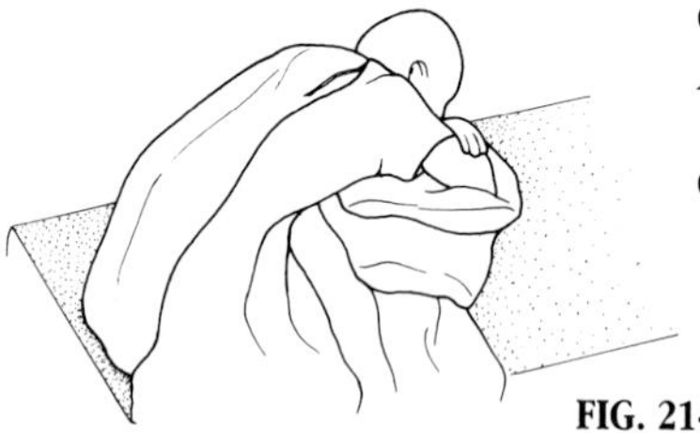

FIG. 21-5 Position for thoracentesis.

Table 21-1 Nurses' Role in Preparation of Patient for Diagnostic Examinations—cont'd

Examination	Nursing Examination Responsibilities	Nursing Responsibilities After Examination
Gallbladder series Cholecystogram	Prepare requisition form. Explain procedure. A fat-free meal is allowed the evening before examination. Assess patient for allergy to iodine. Administer the iopanoic acid tablets (Telepaque) as ordered the day before the examination—usually early evening. A number of tablets are ordered; the tablets should not be crushed and should be taken one at a time, waiting 15 minutes between each tablet.	Monitor patient for side effects to the tablets. Usual diet may be resumed as soon as series is completed.
Bone marrow aspiration (Fig. 21-6)	Prepare requisition form. Explain procedure. Obtain written consent. Assist in obtaining specimens. Provide needed emotional support.	Observe the puncture site for bleeding. Monitor patient for signs and symptoms of shock. Patient may assume normal activity 30-60 minutes after examination. Mild analgesics may be needed for complaints of tenderness at the puncture site.

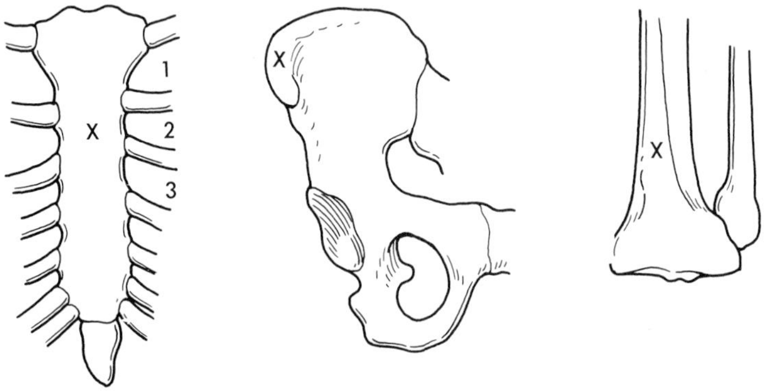

FIG. 21-6 Bone marrow is located in spongy bone.

Examination	Nursing Examination Responsibilities	Nursing Responsibilities After Examination
Hematest of stools	Explain procedure. Assist patient in obtaining specimens. Document specimens as sent to laboratory.	No specific follow-up care. Read results.
Liver biopsy	Explain procedure. Obtain written consent. NPO before examination. Assist physician. Send specimens to laboratory promptly. Have specimen placed in proper **fixative**; usually 10% formalin is used but the nurse must consult with the laboratory or pathologist. If the liver specimen is for detection of lymphoma, saline solution is used.	Keep patient at bed rest for 24 hours. Observe for hemorrhage. Monitor vital signs. Observe biopsy site.
Cardiac catheterization	Explain procedure. Obtain written consent. Provide needed emotional support. NPO for 6-8 hours. Determine if any dye allergies. Administer preexamination medications as ordered.	Monitor vital signs. Observe catheter site for bleeding. Monitor pedal pulses for adequate circulation. Encourage rest. Encourage fluids.
Exercise tolerance test	Explain procedure. Patient will be NPO until after the test except for water. Hold medications. Instruct patient not to smoke. Instruct patient to wear suitable clothing.	Diet as usual. Resume medication regime. Patient to rest several hours after examination and is not to shower immediately after examination.

SKILL 21-9 COLLECTING SPUTUM

Nursing action	Rationale
1. Read physician's order.	Provides basis for care.
2. Collect supplies.	Organizes procedure.
3. Introduce self.	Decreases anxiety level.
4. Identify patient by identification band.	Identifies correct patient for procedure.
5. Explain procedure to patient.	Seeks cooperation and decreases anxiety.
6. Wash hands, and don gloves.	Helps prevent cross-contamination.
7. Position patient in Fowler's position.	Assists coughing.
8. Instruct patient to take three breaths and force cough into sterile container.	Helps patient expectorate mucus.
9. Label specimen container.	Ensures appropriate specimen reaches laboratory.
10. Attach laboratory requisition, and immediately send specimen to laboratory.	Ensures specimen to laboratory.
11. Remove gloves, and wash hands.	Helps prevent cross-contamination.
12. Document.	Documents procedure and patient's response.

STEP 8

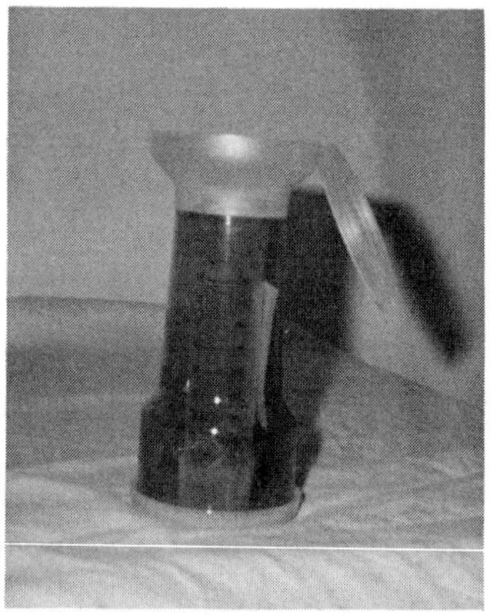

SKILL 21-9

COLLECTING SPUTUM—cont'd

DOCUMENTATION

1. Document procedure and observations.

Communicates with others patient care administered.

Sample charting

DATE	TIME	NOTES
12/4/90	0630	Sputum specimen collected and sent to lab for culture and sensitivity. Obtained moderate amount of light green, tenacious mucus. Tolerated fairly well. Respirations 22 and regular.
		_______________ *(nurse's signature)*

SPECIAL CONCERNS

- Oral hygiene should be provided after the procedure for patient comfort.
- Accuracy of test decreases if delivery of specimen to laboratory is delayed.
- Make certain patient knows how to perform sputum collection.
- The nurse must be prepared to obtain the specimen by suctioning if the patient cannot cough.

PATIENT TEACHING

- Instruct patient regarding the importance of drinking fluids to decrease thickness of mucus.
- Stress to patient the importance of coughing from deep in the bronchial tree.

REFERENCES AND SUGGESTED READINGS

1. Flynn JM and Hackel R: Technological foundations in nursing, East Norwalk, Conn, 1990, Appleton & Lange.
2. Hood GH and Dincher JR: Total patient care: foundations and practice, ed 7, St Louis, 1988, The CV Mosby Co.
3. Keans CB: Essentials of medical-surgical nursing, ed 2, Philadelphia, 1986, WB Saunders Co.
4. Lewis LW and Timby BK: Fundamental skills and concepts in patient care, ed 4, Philadelphia, 1988, JB Lippincott Co.
5. Pagana KD and Pagana TJ: Diagnostic testing and nursing implications (a case study approach), ed 3, St Louis, 1990, The CV Mosby Co.
6. Perry AG and Potter PA: Clinical nursing skills and techniques, ed 2, St Louis, 1990, The CV Mosby Co.
7. Potter PA and Perry AG: Basic nursing theory and practice, ed 2, St Louis, 1991, Mosby–Year Book, Inc.
8. Potter PA and Perry AG: Fundamentals of nursing: concepts, process, and practice, ed 2, St Louis, 1989, The CV Mosby Co.

CHAPTER CHALLENGE

STUDY QUESTIONS

1. The role of the nurse in preparing a patient for diagnostic testing includes:
   a. Assisting the physician with the test
   b. Preparing the patient and follow-up care
   c. Patient teaching and knowlege of the procedure
   d. All of these
2. Requesting the patient to hold the arm at the side for 30 seconds before obtaining blood sample to measure glucose:
   a. Increases blood flow to site
   b. Provides easy access to device
   c. Prepares site
   d. Prevents needle puncture of nurse
3. When performing glucose/acetone determination, the specimen should be a double-voided specimen to:
   a. Provide a chemical reaction
   b. Determine the insulin requirements for the patient
   c. Ensure accurate test results
   d. Obtain a pooled urine specimen
4. For patients who cannot cough up sputum from deep in the bronchial tree, the specimen must be collected by:
   a. Endotracheal suctioning
   b. Pharyngeal suctioning
   c. Oropharyngeal drainage
   d. All of the above
5. The type of blood that can be found in the stool but cannot be seen with the naked eye is called:
   a. Occult blood
   b. Hemoccult
   c. Gross blood
   d. Melena
6. The type of urine specimen that is taken after voiding has begun is called:
   a. Sterile specimen
   b. Catheterized specimen
   c. Voided specimen
   d. Midstream specimen
7. The equipment used to collect a sterile urine specimen includes:
   a. Straight catheter tray
   b. Label
   c. Requisition
   d. All of the above
8. All of the following are correct nursing responsibilities to correctly prepare a patient for an intravenous pyelogram except:
   a. Force fluids
   b. Check if patient has an allergy to iodine
   c. Cathartic or enema before examination
   d. NPO from midnight on
   e. Decrease IV to keep-open rate unless contraindicated
9. The correct preparation for a patient for a cholecystogram includes:
   a. Cathartic or enema
   b. Written consent form
   c. Iopanoic (Telepaque) tablets the evening before examination
   d. Encourage fluids
10. The postexamination responsibilities of the nurse caring for a patient having a renal angiography include:
    a. Observe puncture site for bleeding
    b. Monitor pedal pulses
    c. Apply cold compresses to puncture site
    d. All of the above
11. When a glucose tolerance test is performed, the nurse should do the following:
    a. Obtain the first urine specimen from the first voided specimen of the morning
    b. Collect urine specimens ½ hour, 1 hour, 1½ hour, and 2½ hour as ordered
    c. Maintain patient NPO from water, as well as food
    d. Obtain a written consent form
12. When assisting the physician during a liver biopsy, the nurse should be cognizant of the proper method of caring for the specimen. This includes:
    a. Taking specimen to the laboratory at the end of the shift
    b. Placing the specimen in a sterile container without fixative
    c. Having specimen placed in proper fixative—usually formalin 10%
    d. Placing specimen in sterile water fixative

VI

Nutrition

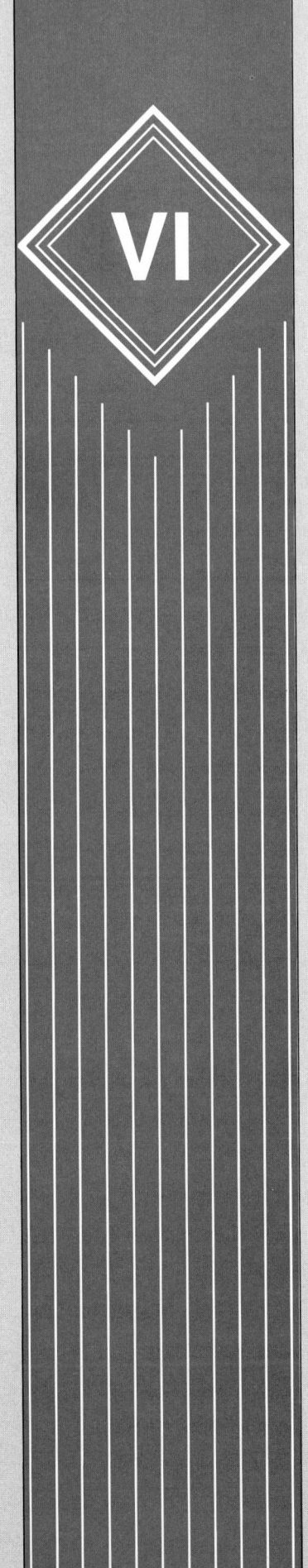

Ever since I can remember I wanted to be a nurse. Nurses are special people. Each has a unique sense of caring. It is the nurse who offers patients compassion and understanding. It is the nurse who will sit at the bedside and hold the patient's hand when he is afraid and fears the unknown. It is the nurse who bathes, feeds, and provides comfort to patients. Nursing to me is a rewarding job. Every patient's needs are different, and if I am able to make one person smile or help an ill patient to wellness, this gives me a wonderful feeling of satisfaction.

TAMI CLINE
Student Nurse

22

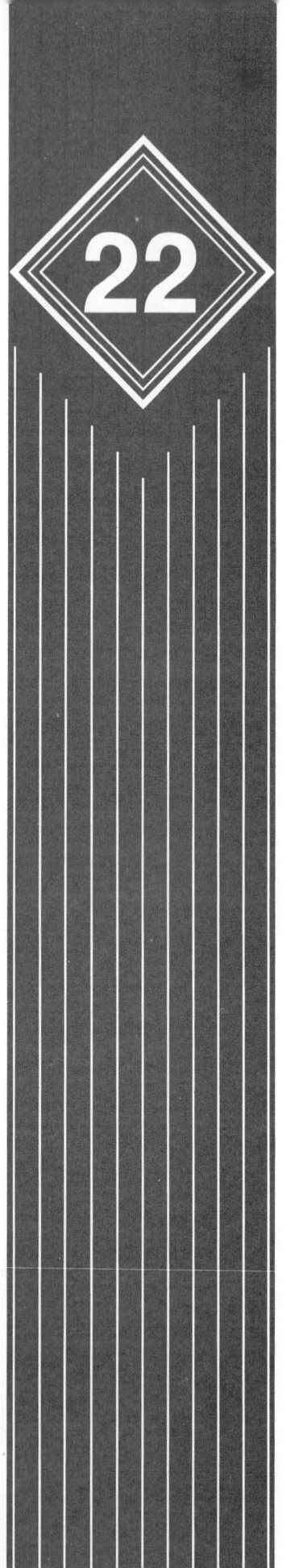

Basic Nutrition

KRISTEN KARTCHNER MAUGHAN

LEARNING OBJECTIVES

After reading this chapter, the student should be able to do the following:

- Define the key terms.
- Discuss the role of the nurse in promoting good nutrition.
- Explain how to use the Basic Four Food Groups, the Dietary Guidelines for Americans, and the Recommended Dietary Allowances (RDA) in diet planning and assessment.
- List the six classes of essential nutrients and identify those that provide energy.
- Identify the three basic functions of nutrients in the body.
- List food sources and possible health benefits of dietary fiber.
- List the functions and food sources of protein, carbohydrates, and fats.
- Discuss the difference between saturated and unsaturated fats, and explain the effect of excess fat intake on health.
- Discuss the effects of deficiencies and toxicities of vitamins and minerals.
- List food sources of each of the vitamins and minerals.
- Discuss the benefits of receiving nutrients from food rather than from dietary supplements.
- Discuss the changes in nutrient needs throughout the life cycle.
- Suggest ideas for developing sound dietary habits in children.
- Distinguish between anorexia nervosa and bulimia, and discuss the dietary treatment of these disorders.
- Identify factors that may lead to poor nutrition in the elderly.

RELATED TOPICS OF INTEREST

- Diet therapy (Chapter 23)
- The surgical patient (Chapter 26)
- Care of the patient with a gastrointestinal or accessory organ disorder (Chapter 31)
- Mental health concepts (Chapter 49)
- The patient with an addictive personality (Chapter 50)

KEY TERMS

Define the following:

- adipose tissue
- amino acids
- anorexia nervosa
- antioxidant
- beriberi
- bulemia
- carbohydrate
- cholesterol (dietary)
- cholesterol (serum)
- dietary fiber
- digestion
- electrolyte
- enzyme
- essential nutrients
- fat
- glycogen
- iron deficiency anemia
- kilocalorie
- kwashiorkor
- lipoprotein
- marasmus
- metabolism
- mineral
- nutrient dense
- nutrition
- pellagra
- pernicious anemia
- protein (food)
- satiety
- scurvy
- toxicity
- vegan
- vitamin

Prevention—perhaps this word best describes why nutrition is becoming increasingly important in health care. More and more evidence points to the fact that nutrition plays a role in many disease states and that, in many cases, proper nutrition may help prevent or delay the onset of certain diseases. It has long been known that optimal nutrition ensures proper growth in children, teens, and pregnant women. But nutrition is important at every age, not only for growth, but for quality of life. **Nutrition** is vital for the proper functioning of the cardiovascular, renal, pulmonary, nervous, digestive, and immune systems, among others. In short, nutrition plays a role directly or indirectly in all body processes. Its importance must not be overlooked.

THE ROLE OF THE NURSE IN PROMOTING NUTRITION

Because the nurse is most directly involved with the patient, the patient looks to the nurse as a source of health information. Therefore nurses should have a basic knowledge of nutrition. Although the dietitian is the nutrition expert, the nurse will have opportunities to apply nutrition knowledge in a number of ways by:

Helping the patient understand the importance of the diet
Assisting some patients with the eating process
Taking and recording patient weights
Recording patient intakes
Observing clinical signs of poor nutrition and reporting them
Serving as a communication link between the patient, dietitian, physician, or other members of the health care team.

Nurses can also apply nutrition knowledge in their personal lives. What better reason for understanding nutrition?

DIET PLANNING GUIDES

The Basic Four

A number of guidelines have been established in the United States to help in planning for optimal nutrition. Probably the Basic Four is the most widely recognized food guide. It is easy to teach and use. Foods are divided into four groups: milk, meat, fruit/vegetable, and grain. Recommendations for number of servings from each group are given for different age groups and for pregnant and lactating women. Fig. 22-1 describes the food groups and the recommended number of servings from each.

Dietary Guidelines for Americans

In 1980 the first Dietary Guidelines for Americans were published, with a subsequent revision in 1985. These guidelines, developed specifically for

Group	Serving Size	Food	Children 1-10	Teenagers and Young Adults 11-24	Adults 25+	Pregnant Women	Breastfeeding Women	Comments
Milk Group	1 cup	Milk	3	4	2	4	4	†Good sources of calcium such as milk, yogurt, and cheese are recommended daily. Cottage cheese, ice cream, ice milk, and frozen yogurt have about 1/4 to 1/3 the amount of calcium per serving as milk, yogurt, and cheese.
	1 cup	Yogurt						
	1 oz	Cheese						
	1/2 cup	Cottage cheese†						
	1/2 cup	Ice cream, ice milk, frozen yogurt†						
Meat Group	2-3 oz	Cooked, lean meat, fish, poultry	2	2	2	3	2	‡Eggs, dried beans, and peanut butter have about 1/2 the amount of protein per serving as meat.
	1	Egg‡						
	1/2 cup	Cooked, dried peas, dried beans‡						
	2 tbsp	Peanut butter‡						
	1/4 cup	Nuts, seeds‡						
Fruit-Vegetable Group	1/2 cup	Juice	4	4	4	4	4	Dark green, leafy, or orange vegetables and fruit are recommended 3 or 4 times a week for vitamin A. Good sources of vitamin C such as oranges, strawberries, tomatoes, potatoes, and green peppers are recommended daily.
	1/2 cup	Vegetable, fruit						
	1 medium	Apple, banana, orange						
	1/2	Grapefruit						
	1/4	Cantaloupe						
	1/4 cup	Dried fruit						
Grain Group	1 slice	Bread	4	4	4	4	4	Whole grain, fortified, or enriched grain products are recommended.
	1/2	English muffin, hamburger bun						
	1 oz	Ready-to-eat cereal						
	1/2 cup	Pasta, rice, grits, cooked cereal						
	1	Tortilla, roll, muffin						
Combination Foods	1 cup	Soup	These count as servings (or partial servings) from the food groups from which they are made.					Combination Foods supply the same nutrients as the foods they contain.
	1 cup	Macaroni and cheese, lasagna, stew, chili, casserole						
	1/8 15"	Pizza						
	1	Sandwich, taco						
"Others" Category	1 oz	Potato chips, pretzels	There is no recommended number of servings for foods in the "Others" category.					"Others" don't take the place of foods from the Four Food Groups in supplying nutrients. And they are often high in fat or calories.
	2	Cookies						
	1/16 9"	Layer cake						
	1 tsp	Sugar, jelly						
	12 oz	Soft drink, beer						
	1 tsp	Margarine, butter						
	1 tbsp	Salad dressing, mayonnaise						

Minimum Recommended Number of Servings*

*These servings provide the nutrients your body needs. They also supply about 1200 Calories. However most people need more than 1200 Calories. If you do, add more servings.

FIG. 22-1 The Basic Four Food Groups. (From Guide to Good Eating, Courtesy of NATIONAL DAIRY COUNCIL.®)

the U.S. population, address the prevention of overnutrition and disease. Overnutrition is evident in the typical American diet, which is rich in fat, high in sodium, and sometimes filled with excess calories and other nutrients. Since the development of the Dietary Guidelines for Americans, other reports, such as the Surgeon General's Report on Nutrition and Health, have issued similar guidelines. Box 22-1 lists the Dietary Guidelines for Americans with suggestions for their use.

Recommended Dietary Allowances (RDAs)

The RDAs are the "levels of intake of essential nutrients that . . . are judged . . . to be adequate to meet the known nutrient needs of practically all healthy persons." These guidelines are determined by a group of distinguished scientists chosen by the National Academy of Sciences. Recommendations are given for various age groups of both sexes (Table 22-1). The RDAs are not absolute requirements but are recommendations. Each person's nutrient needs are individual, so to say that everyone needs exactly what the RDAs list is unrealistic. Rather, the RDAs are better used as a guide to evaluate average intakes of groups of people.

Using Diet Planning Guides Simultaneously

There are disadvantages to using just one guide in diet planning. The Basic Four Food Group plan may not provide adequate nutrients if one uses no variety and can also be high in calories if calorie-rich foods are selected. The Dietary Guidelines for Americans focus on prevention of overnutrition but do not present a specific guide of food selection. The RDAs may be too complex for the lay public. Used as a whole, however, these guides can aid in proper food selection. By following the Basic Four pattern, using *variety* in food selection and exercising *moderation* in the intake of fat, sugar, sodium, alcohol, and calories, one can eat both well and nutritiously. Variety and moderation are the key principles in diet planning. The RDAs can further help in label reading and assessment of various nutrient intakes in the diet.

THE NUTRIENTS

The Essential Nutrients

A nutrient is a substance found in food that is necessary for good health. Nutrients may perform any or all of these basic functions: (1) provide energy, (2) build and repair tissue, and (3) regulate body processes. **Essential nutrients** are those that our bodies cannot make in amounts necessary for good health, and therefore, we

BOX 22-1 **DIETARY GUIDELINES FOR AMERICANS AND SUGGESTIONS FOR THEIR USE**

1. EAT A VARIETY OF FOODS. The Basic Four can provide a guide for eating a variety of foods. Remember to include a variety of foods from each group. For example, eat different types of vegetables rather than the same ones each day. No one food can provide all dietary needs.
2. MAINTAIN DESIRABLE WEIGHT. Use moderation in the use of high-calorie, nutrient-poor foods such as fatty foods, sweets, and alcohol. Use more nutrient-dense foods (those high in nutrients relative to calories). Include physical activity regularly.
3. AVOID TOO MUCH FAT, SATURATED FAT, AND CHOLESTEROL. Choose low-fat dairy products, lean meats, poultry, and fish. Limit the use of eggs and organ meats, and add less fat to foods. Bake, broil, or poach rather than fry. Limit rich desserts.
4. EAT FOODS WITH ADEQUATE STARCH AND FIBER. Include whole grain products, fruits and vegetables, beans, peas, nuts, and seeds. The bulk of the diet should be provided by these foods.
5. AVOID TOO MUCH SUGAR. Limit intake of sugar, honey, syrup, molasses, candy, cakes, sweetened beverages, and gelatins. Use fresh fruits or fruits canned in light syrup or their own juices.
6. AVOID TOO MUCH SODIUM. Use less salt in cooking and at the table. Limit the use of processed foods, snack foods, canned soups, and cured and pickled products. Generally, the more processed a food, the more sodium it will contain. Read labels for sodium content.
7. IF YOU DRINK ALCOHOL, DO SO IN MODERATION. Those who drink should consume no more than two alcoholic beverages per day. One alcoholic beverage is equivalent to 12 oz of beer, 4 oz of wine, or 1 oz of hard liquor. Pregnant women should refrain from drinking.

From USDA and US Department of Health and Human Services: Home and Garden Bull No 232, 1985.

must obtain them through diet or other sources. There are six classes of essential nutrients: carbohydrates, fats, proteins, **vitamins, minerals,** and water. Each is necessary for life.

Kilocalories and energy. A **kilocalorie** (kcal) is a measurement of energy, much like a pound is a measurement of weight. When we say a certain food has so many kilocalories, we are actually saying it will provide energy. The more kilocalories in a food, the greater its energy-giving potential. Of the six essential nutrients, three provide energy—carbohydrate, fat, and protein. Carbohydrate and protein provide approximately 4 kcal/g, whereas fat provides 9 kcal/g. Most authorities recommend that about 55% to 60% of daily kilocalories be supplied by carbohydrate, 25% to 30% of kilocalories from fat, and 15% to 20% of daily kilocalories from protein. This is called the caloric distribution of the diet.

Vitamins, minerals, and water do not provide energy. They have no energy or kilocalorie value.

Carbohydrates

The main function of **carbohydrates** is to provide energy. Carbohydrates should provide the bulk of the kilocalories in the diet—55% to 60%. Carbohydrates are also important in adequate amounts to spare protein from being used as an energy source. Carbohydrates may be classified as either simple or complex. Table 22-2 summarizes the classification of carbohydrates.

Simple carbohydrates. From a chemical view carbohydrates are made of molecular units called saccharides. The simple carbohydrates include the monosaccharides and disaccharides. Monosaccharides are single carbohydrate units. They include glucose, fructose, and galactose. Glucose is the main monosaccharide found in the body. It circulates in the blood stream and is used by the cells for energy. The brain derives almost all its energy from glucose. Fructose, the sweetest of all the carbohydrates, is found most commonly in fruits and honey. Galactose is not found singularly in nature; rather, it is chemically bonded to glucose in the disaccharide lactose. All other carbohydrates are made of combinations of these monosaccharides or sugar units.

Disaccharides, as indicated by the name, are sugars made from two bonded saccharide units. These include sucrose, lactose, and maltose. Sucrose is a combination of glucose and fructose. It is the common table sugar. Lactose is made of glucose and galactose and is only found in milk products. Maltose is made from two glucose units and is not as common as the other disaccharides. It may be found in products containing malted barley or other grains. Sugar consumption is high in the United States, and recommendations have been made to reduce sugar intake to less than 10% of total kilocalories. Sugar contributes to dental caries (cavities). Table sugar and sweeteners such as honey and corn syrup are high in kilocalories and virtually void of nutrients.

Complex carbohydrates. Complex carbohydrates are termed polysaccharides because they are made from many bonded glucose units. They include starch, glycogen, and dietary fiber. Starch is found in many plant foods such as grains, legumes, and vegetables, particularly starchy vegetables like corn and potatoes. **Glycogen** is not generally consumed in the diet but is the body's storage form of carbohydrate. It is found mainly in the liver, with some storage in the muscles.

Dietary fiber. Fiber is a complex carbohydrate made of long chains of bonded glucose units; however, fiber is

Table 22-1 Food and Nutrition Board, National Academy of Sciences National Research Council Recommended Dietary Allowances,[a] Revised 1989

Category	Age (years) or Condition	Weight[b] (kg)	Weight[b] (lb)	Height[b] (cm)	Height[b] (in)	Protein (g)	Fat-Soluble vitamins: Vitamin A (μg RE)[c]	Vitamin D (μg)[d]	Vitamin E (mg α-TE)[e]	Vitamin K (μg)
Infants	0.0-0.5	6	13	60	24	13	375	7.5	3	5
	0.5-1.0	9	20	71	28	14	375	10	4	10
Children	1-3	13	29	90	35	16	400	10	6	15
	4-6	20	44	112	44	24	500	10	7	20
	7-10	28	62	132	52	28	700	10	7	30
Males	11-14	45	99	157	62	45	1000	10	10	45
	15-18	66	145	176	69	59	1000	10	10	65
	19-24	72	160	177	70	58	1000	10	10	70
	25-50	79	174	176	70	63	1000	5	10	80
	51+	77	170	173	68	63	1000	5	10	80
Females	11-14	46	101	157	62	46	800	10	8	45
	15-18	55	120	163	64	44	800	10	8	55
	19-24	58	128	164	65	46	800	10	8	60
	25-50	63	138	163	64	50	800	5	8	65
	51+	65	143	160	63	50	800	5	8	65
Pregnant						60	800	10	10	65
Lactating	1st 6 Months					65	1300	10	12	65
	2nd 6 Months					62	1200	10	11	65

[a]The allowances, expressed as average daily intakes over time, are intended to provide for individual variations among most normal persons as they live in the United States under usual environmental stresses. Diets should be based on a variety of common foods in order to provide other nutrients for which human requirements have been less well defined. See text for detailed discussion of allowances and of nutrients not tabulated.
[b]Weights and heights of Reference Adults are actual medians for the U.S. population of the designated age, as reported by NHANES II. The use of these figures does not imply that the height-to-weight ratios are ideal.

bonded in such a way that the body cannot digest it. Therefore most of the fiber we consume is eventually excreted in the feces. Fiber has received much attention recently, focusing on its relationship to health and disease. There are a number of fiber types having varying effects on the body. Fiber may be categorized as either water-soluble or water-insoluble.

Insoluble fibers include cellulose, lignin, and many hemicelluloses. They are found most abundantly in vegetables, wheat, and most whole grains. Insoluble fiber appears to be effective in softening stools, speeding transit of foods through the digestive tract, and reducing pressure in the colon. Thus it may help relieve constipation and reduce the risk of certain gastrointestinal disorders such as diverticulosis or hemorrhoids.

Water-soluble fibers include pectins, gums, mucilages, and some hemicelluloses. This type of fiber is found in fruits, oats, barley, and legumes. Oat bran and beans are particularly good sources of soluble fiber. Soluble fiber binds with bile acids and cholesterol in the digestive tract, preventing their absorption and thereby helping to lower blood cholesterol. It also helps delay gastric emptying and provides a feeling of fullness, which may be beneficial in the treatment of obesity.

Both types of fiber may enhance weight reduction efforts if fiber-rich foods are included in the diet in place of high-fat or high-kilocalorie foods. Soluble and insoluble fibers seem to delay glucose absorption. This is particularly beneficial for control of blood glucose levels in diabetes and may help reduce the need for insulin. Many medical professionals now recommend a high-fiber diet for patients with diabetes.

Colon cancer incidence is lower in populations consuming a high-fiber diet. Fiber may reduce colon cancer by reducing concentration and bacterial synthesis of carcinogens (cancer-causing substances) in the bowel. It also reduces the amount of time the carcinogens are in contact with the lining of the colon. Both types of fiber appear beneficial in reducing colon cancer risk.

Because fiber research is relatively new, precise recommendations for levels of intake have not been made; however, tentative recommendations range from 25 to 50 g of dietary fiber per day. To include more fiber in the diet, consume more fruits and vegetables (taking care to eat the skins and seeds where reasonable), and include more legumes, nuts, and seeds in the diet. Box 22-2 lists the fiber content of some foods. Most individuals can receive adequate fiber in the diet without using supplements. There may be hazards to consuming too much fiber, including poor mineral absorption. Moderation should be used with fiber consumption as with any dietary component.

Water-Soluble Vitamins							Minerals						
Vitamin C (mg)	Thiamin (mg)	Riboflavin (mg)	Niacin (mg NE[f])	Vitamin B_6 (mg)	Folate (μg)	Vitamin B_{12} (μg)	Calcium (mg)	Phosphorus (mg)	Magnesium (mg)	Iron (mg)	Zinc (mg)	Iodine (μg)	Selenium (μg)
30	0.3	0.4	5	0.3	25	0.3	400	300	40	6	5	40	10
35	0.4	0.5	6	0.6	35	0.5	600	500	60	10	5	50	15
40	0.7	0.8	9	1.0	50	0.7	800	800	80	10	10	70	20
45	0.9	1.1	12	1.1	75	1.0	800	800	120	10	10	90	20
45	1.0	1.2	13	1.4	100	1.4	800	800	170	10	10	120	30
50	1.3	1.5	17	1.7	150	2.0	1200	1200	270	12	15	150	40
60	1.5	1.8	20	2.0	200	2.0	1200	1200	400	12	15	150	50
60	1.5	1.7	19	2.0	200	2.0	1200	1200	350	10	15	150	70
60	1.5	1.7	19	2.0	200	2.0	800	800	350	10	15	150	70
60	1.2	1.4	15	2.0	200	2.0	800	800	350	10	15	150	70
50	1.1	1.3	15	1.4	150	2.0	1200	1200	280	15	12	150	45
60	1.1	1.3	15	1.5	180	2.0	1200	1200	300	15	12	150	50
60	1.1	1.3	15	1.6	180	2.0	1200	1200	280	15	12	150	55
60	1.1	1.3	15	1.6	180	2.0	800	800	280	15	12	150	55
60	1.0	1.2	13	1.6	180	2.0	800	800	280	10	12	150	55
70	1.5	1.6	17	2.2	400	2.2	1200	1200	320	30	15	175	65
95	1.6	1.8	20	2.1	280	2.6	1200	1200	355	15	19	200	75
90	1.6	1.7	20	2.1	260	2.6	1200	1200	340	15	16	200	75

[c] Retinol equivalents. 1 retinol equivalent = 1 μg retinol or 6 μg β-carotene.
[d] As cholecalciferol, 10 μg cholecalciferol = 400 IU of vitamin D.
[e] α-Tocopherol equivalents. 1 mg d-α tocopherol = 1 α-TE.
[f] 1 NE (niacin equivalent) is equal to 1 mg of niacin or 60 mg of dietary tryptophan.
Recommended Dietary Allowances by the National Academy of Sciences, Washington DC, 1989, National Academy Press.

Table 22-2 Summary of Carbohydrate Classification

Chemical Class	Class Members	Dietary Sources
SIMPLE CARBOHYDRATE		
Monosaccharides	Glucose	Dextrose, corn syrup
	Fructose	Fruit, honey
	Galactose	Milk (only found in lactose)
Disaccharides	Sucrose	Table sugar, sugar cane, beet sugar, powdered and brown sugar
	Lactose	Milk
	Maltose	Malted grain products
COMPLEX CARBOHYDRATE		
Polysaccharides	Starch	Grains and grain products, i.e., cereals, breads, crackers, pasta, rice, legumes, corn, potatoes, vegetables
	Glycogen	No significant dietary source (storage form of carbohydrate in animal tissue)
	Dietary fiber	Whole grains, legumes, fruits, vegetables, nuts, seeds

Digestion and metabolism of carbohydrate. All carbohydrates are broken down in the digestive tract into monosaccharides. They are then absorbed and may be converted to glucose for energy. If energy needs are met, carbohydrate will be stored as glycogen, with any excess carbohydrate being converted to fat and stored as adipose tissue (body fat).

Fats (Lipids)

Fats, or lipids, are essential to good health. With all the attention recently given to fat and cholesterol and their relationship to disease, many erroneously believe that fat should be totally eliminated from the diet. This is incorrect. Fat performs a number of functions in the body. **Fat** provides the most concentrated source of en-

BOX 22-2 FIBER CONTENT OF SELECTED FOODS

FOOD/SERVING SIZE	FIBER (g)
Beans, Peas, Legumes (½ cup cooked)	
Pinto beans	9.5
Kidney beans	9.2
Pork and beans, Campbell's	8.7
Black-eyed peas	8.2
Navy beans	6.0
Lima beans	5.0
Lentils	3.7
Split peas	2.7
Breads	
Whole wheat (1 slice)	2.0
White (1 slice)	<1.0
Part wheat (1 slice)	1.0
Bran muffin (1)	3.0
Bagel, plain (1)	<1.0
Cereals	
Servings in parenthesis are equal to 1 oz. Hot cereal servings apply to prepared cereal.	
Fiber One (½ c)	13.0
Wheat bran (⅓ c)	12.6
All Bran (⅓ c)	10.0
100% Bran (½ c)	10.0
Bran buds (⅓ c)	8.0
Bran Chex (⅔ c)	6.1
Rice bran (⅓ c)	6.1
Fruitful Bran (⅔ c)	5.0
Raisin Bran (¾ c)	5.0
Fruit & Fibre (½ c)	5.0
Wheatena (½ c)	4.0
Oat bran, hot cereal (⅔ c)	4.0
Wheat germ (¼ c)	3.3
Grape Nuts (¼ c)	3.0
Total or Wheaties (1 c)	3.0
Shredded wheat (1)	3.0
Oatmeal, quick cooking (⅔ c)	4.0
Oatmeal, instant (⅔ c)	2.7
Corn flakes (1 c)	1.0
Cream of wheat (⅔ c)	1.0
Oat Granola (⅓ c)	1.0
Rice Krispies (1 c)	<1.0
Special K (1 c)	<1.0
Sugar Smacks (1 c)	<1.0
Snack Foods	
Wheat 'n Bran Triscuits (3)	2.0
Oat Thins (8)	1.0
Triscuits (3)	<1.0
Saltines (4)	<1.0
Popcorn (3 c)	3.9
Snickers bar (1)	1.4
Fig bars (2)	1.3
Graham crackers (4)	1.0
Potato chips (14)	1.0
Nature Valley Granola Bar	0.8
Almonds (¼ c)	3.8
Peanuts (¼ c)	2.9
Cashews (¼ c)	2.0
Peanut butter (2 Tbls)	2.0
Fruits and Vegetables	
Figs, dried (3)	5.3
Apple, large w/skin (1)	4.7
Pear (1)	4.3
Baked potato w/skin (1 med)	4.2
Orange (1)	3.5
Brussels sprouts (½ c)	3.3
Strawberries (½ c)	3.1
Corn (½ c)	3.1
Peas or winter squash (½ c)	2.9
Carrot, raw (1)	2.3
Broccoli or spinach (½ c)	2.0
Raisins (¼ c)	2.0
Banana (1 med)	1.8
Tomato (1)	1.6
Cauliflower (½ c)	1.4
Peach (1)	1.4
Green pepper, raw (1)	1.2
Cantaloupe (¼)	1.1
Grapefruit (½)	0.7
Lettuce, iceberg (1 c)	0.6
Mushrooms or cucumbers (½ c)	0.5
Orange juice (6 oz)	0.4
Grapes (10)	0.4
Pasta and Rice	
Whole wheat spaghetti (1 c)	5.9
Brown rice (1 c)	3.3
Macaroni or spaghetti (1 c)	2.1
White rice (1 c)	1.0

From Center for Science in the Public Interest (CSPI): New fiber scorecard, Nutrition Action Newsletter 17(2):8, 1990.

ergy of all the nutrients (9 kcal/g). Both the fat in foods and that stored as adipose tissue can be used for energy. **Adipose tissue** is the body's storage form of fat and helps to insulate the body from temperature extremes. It serves as a cushion to protect organs and other tissues from being bumped or jarred. Likewise, fat is a component in all cell membranes.

Dietary fat provides **satiety** or a feeling of satisfaction from food. It adds flavor and aroma to foods. Fat provides the body with the three essential fatty acids—linoleic acid, linolenic acid, and arachidonic acid. It also carries the fat-soluble vitamins, A, D, E, and K. Fat intake should comprise about 25% to 30% of daily kilocalorie intake of the adult. Most dietary fat is found in the form of triglycerides. Triglycerides are composed of glycerol, a three-carbon chain with three fatty acids attached to it, hence, the name triglyceride. Fatty acids can be classified as either saturated or unsaturated.

Saturated fatty acids. A saturated fatty acid is one whose chemical bonds are completely filled or saturated with hydrogen. Saturated fats share similar characteristics. They are generally of animal origin and solid at room temperature. Oils that have undergone hydrogenation, the process of adding hydrogen to a fatty acid, are also saturated. Those fats in which the majority of fatty acids are saturated are listed in Table 22-3. Saturated fats tend to increase blood cholesterol levels, thus increasing the risk of atherosclerosis (the buildup of fatty deposits on the artery walls).

Unsaturated fatty acids. An unsaturated fatty acid has one or more places on its chemical chain where hydrogen is missing. These are called points of unsaturation. A fatty acid with only one point of unsaturation is called a monounsaturated fatty acid. Fatty acids with two or more points of unsaturation are termed polyunsaturated. Unsaturated fats are usually from plant sources and are liquid at room temperature. Sources of monounsaturated fats and polyunsaturated fats are seen in Table 22-3. Unsaturated fats seem to have a blood cholesterol lowering effect at moderate levels of intake and in combination with lowered saturated fat intake.

Table 22-3 Summary of Fatty Acid Classification

Fatty Acid Class	Food Sources
Saturated	Coconut, palm, and palm kernel oils Beef tallow Fat in and on meats Skin on poultry Egg yolk Butter, cream, milkfat Hydrogenated oils
Monounsaturated	Olive oil, olives Canola oil Peanuts and peanut oil Most other nuts Avocados
Polyunsaturated	Safflower oil Sunflower oil Cottonseed oil Soybean oil Corn oil Most fish oils

From USDA Handbook 8-4.

Cholesterol. Cholesterol is a lipid belonging to a class of chemical substances called sterols. Cholesterol performs specific functions in the body, but it is synthesized in the liver and, therefore, does not need to be consumed in the diet. Since cholesterol is produced in the liver, it is only found in foods of animal origin. Plant foods and oils do not contain cholesterol. **Dietary cholesterol** is highest in organ meats and egg yolks. It is also found in smaller amounts in seafood, meats, poultry, and dairy products. Low-fat dairy products and lean meats have less cholesterol than their higher-fat counterparts. By decreasing intake of animal fats, dietary cholesterol intake will similarly be lowered. Dietary cholesterol seems to increase blood cholesterol levels but not as greatly as saturated fats.

The American Heart Association (AHA) and the American Cancer Society (ACS) recommend that 30% or fewer of daily kilocalories come from fat. Particular attention should be given to reducing saturated fat, since it seems to have the greatest effect on blood cholesterol levels. The AHA also recommends a dietary cholesterol intake of 300 mg or less each day. Studies indicate that diets lower in saturated fats and cholesterol, with increased complex carbohydrate intake, contribute to reduced blood cholesterol and blood pressure. These diets may also be helpful in reducing cancer risks.

Fat digestion and metabolism. For fat to be digested, it must be emulsified, or pulled into suspension with digestive juices. Bile, a secretion of the liver, is necessary to emulsify fat. Bile is stored in the gallbladder and dispensed into the duodenum when fat is present. Once emulsified, fats can be broken down and absorbed. Fat may be used for various functions mentioned previously or may be used for energy. Excess dietary fat will be stored as adipose tissue.

After absorption, fats are carried in the blood stream in packages called lipoproteins. Simply stated, **lipoproteins** are lipids wrapped in protein. Types of lipoproteins include chylomicrons, high-density lipoproteins (HDL), low-density lipoproteins (LDL), and very low-density lipoproteins (VLDL). Of particular interest in cardiovascular disease are the LDLs and HDLs. Both lipoproteins carry cholesterol in the blood stream; however, it appears that the cholesterol found in the LDLs increases the risk of atherosclerosis by contributing to plaque buildup on the artery walls. On the other hand, HDL

Table 22-4 Evaluation Criteria for Screening and Monitoring Persons for Treatment of Elevated Blood Cholesterol

Type of Test	Blood Level Classifications (mg/dl)
TOTAL PLASMA CHOLESTEROL	
Desirable level	<200
Borderline-high level	200-239
High level	≥240
LDL CHOLESTEROL	
Borderline high-risk	130-159
High-risk	≥160

cholesterol seems to have the opposite effect. It appears that HDLs carry cholesterol *from* the blood stream to the liver to be degraded and excreted. LDLs are sometimes referred to as carrying the "bad" cholesterol, whereas HDLs carry the "good" cholesterol.

Dietary goals for the American population stress reducing total serum (blood) cholesterol levels, particularly LDL cholesterol. Table 22-4 lists serum cholesterol values used to determine risk of atherosclerosis. LDL cholesterol may be reduced by implementing a fat-controlled diet that lowers total fat intake with emphasis on reduced saturated fat and dietary cholesterol intake. Regular aerobic exercise appears to both lower LDL cholesterol and increase HDL cholesterol, both beneficial effects.

Protein

The human body contains thousands of different proteins. Proteins have numerous functions in the body in comparison with either carbohydrate or fat. Proteins make up the bulk of the body's tissues and organs. They are necessary for tissue growth, repair, and wound healing. Collagen, a vital connective tissue, is made of protein. Some hormones are protein, including thyroxine and insulin. All **enzymes** are proteins and are necessary for **digestion** and **metabolism**. The plasma proteins aid in fluid balance within the body. Albumin, a plasma protein, attracts water and can pull fluid from one body compartment to another to attain balance. Immunoglobulins (antibodies) are also made of protein, emphasizing the role protein plays in immune function. If necessary, protein may be used for energy. It supplies 4 kcal/g; however, if the body uses protein as an energy source, it is rendered useless for any other function. Of the daily caloric intake in the adult, 15% to 20% should come from protein. This is more than adequate to meet the needs of most healthy individuals.

Proteins are made of smaller units called **amino acids**. There are 22 common amino acids, and they can be bonded in a variety of ways to form different proteins. The body uses all 22 amino acids, but only 9 of them are considered essential amino acids. In other words, the body does not make them in sufficient quantity to sustain health. The 9 essential amino acids must be obtained from diet. The body can manufacture adequate amounts of the other amino acids from those that are essential.

Complete proteins. Food proteins can be classified as either complete or incomplete. A complete protein is one that contains all nine essential amino acids in sufficient quantity and ratio for the body's needs. Complete proteins are generally of animal origin and are found in foods such as meat, poultry and fish, milk, cheese, and eggs.

Incomplete proteins. Incomplete proteins are those that are lacking in one or more of the essential amino acids. Incomplete proteins are of plant origin. This includes the protein in grains, legumes, nuts, and seeds. For the body to use protein for functions other than energy, all nine essential amino acids must be present at the same time. When different incomplete proteins are consumed at the same time, the body can use those incomplete proteins together to obtain a balance of the essential amino acids. Incomplete proteins consumed together are called *complementary* proteins.

Vegetarian diets. Some people choose not to consume any animal products in their diets and are called **vegans** (strict vegetarians). Others omit animal flesh but consume products such as milk and cheese (lacto-vegetarians) and eggs (lacto-ovo-vegetarians). Whatever the type of vegetarian diet, protein needs can be met. A vegan can receive adequate protein by eating a wide variety of protein-rich plant foods. Different plant foods eaten together will generally supply all nine essential amino acids. Lacto-vegetarians and lacto-ovo-vegetarians can receive adequate proteins from milk and eggs in combination with plant proteins.

Digestion and metabolism of protein. Proteins must be broken down to smaller amino acid units or individual amino acids before absorption. Once absorbed, amino acids are reassembled by the body into new proteins to be used for the various needs at hand. There are exceptions to this process. If the body has not received adequate carbohydrate and fat for energy, then dietary protein will be disassembled and used for energy rather than to build new proteins. The body can also break down its own protein stores, such as muscle, for energy if kilocalorie intake is too low. On the other hand, if protein intake exceeds the amount needed for protein functions and for energy needs, the amino acids may be chemically changed, converted to fat, and stored as adipose tissue. Therefore, more dietary protein does not necessarily make more muscle.

Protein-kilocalorie malnutrition (PCM). When individuals suffer from a lack of kilocalories or protein, the body breaks down its own protein stores for energy. When this occurs for extended periods of time, the person may suffer from PCM (sometimes referred to as protein-energy malnutrition). Two types of PCM exist. **Kwashiorkor** is malnutrition caused by a lack of dietary protein. It may occur in the presence of adequate kilocalories. It generally occurs in infancy or childhood, and onset is usually at the time of weaning from the breast. Symptoms may include retarded growth, changes in skin and hair pigmentation, diarrhea, loss of appetite, irritability, edema, dermatoses, and fatty liver (causing distended abdomen). Multiple vitamin and mineral deficiencies may also occur. **Marasmus** is malnutrition from inadequate kilocalories and protein. It is most often seen in failure-to-thrive children and in starvation. A child with marasmus will be very thin with wasted muscles and little, if any, subcutaneous fat. If marasmus occurs during the first years of life, brain development may be impaired.

Vitamins

The American population is interested in vitamins. Claims have been made that vitamins can help reduce stress, prevent colds, increase sexuality, increase energy, and improve physical performance, among others. Sometimes it is difficult to divide fact from fiction. The simple truth is that for most people vitamins are best received from a balanced, varied diet, not from pills.

Nonetheless, vitamins are important and essential. Vitamins are organic chemical compounds that perform specific roles in the body. They are noncaloric and needed in only small amounts. Vitamins are sometimes destroyed by heat, light, and exposure to air. They can also be lost when foods are cooked in water. Thus methods of preparation and storage can affect the final vitamin content of foods. Tips to preserve vitamin content of foods are found in Box 22-3. Vitamins are classified by whether they are soluble in fat or soluble in water.

The fat-soluble vitamins. Vitamins A, D, E, and K are the fat-soluble vitamins. They are usually carried in the fatty portions of food. Fat-soluble vitamins can be stored by the body, and it is possible for an excess of these to reach toxic levels in the body. Because these vitamins are stored in the body, good dietary sources may only be needed every other day.

Vitamin A. Vitamin A is necessary for vision, tissue strength, and bone and soft tissue growth. A mild deficiency of vitamin A will produce night blindness. A severe deficiency can lead to drying and hardening of the cornea producing total and permanent blindness. This condition is called xerophthalmia. Vitamin A is essential for healthy skin and mucous membranes. Deficiencies may lead to dry tissues and decreased resistance to infection. A deficiency of vitamin A may also lead to cessation of bone growth or changes in bone shape.

Foods that supply vitamin A include the dark leafy greens, such as spinach, collards, and kale, or the dark yellow or deep orange vegetables such as carrots, winter squash, and sweet potatoes. Other sources include liver, eggs, milk, and dairy products. Toxic or harmful effects from vitamin A can occur in adults with intakes of 5 to 10 times the RDA. Children may be affected by smaller dosages. **Toxicity** symptoms may include fatigue, irritability, loss of appetite, dry skin, hair loss, bone pain, and growth retardation. It generally occurs secondary to supplementation, and therefore, it is best to get vitamin A from food sources.

Vitamin D. The main function of vitamin D in the body is to aid in the mineralization of bones and teeth. Vitamin D stimulates calcium and phosphorus absorption from the intestine and regulates their action on bone tissue. Deficiency of vitamin D leads to weakening and softening of bones. In children this is called rickets (Figure 22-2). In adults it is termed osteomalacia. Children with rickets often have bowed legs because their bones become malformed under their own weight.

Vitamin D can be obtained in two ways. It is found in small amounts in liver, eggs, and some fish, but the most common dietary sources include fortified milk and milk products. Nonfortified milk is a poor source of vitamin D. The body can also make vitamin D from exposure to sunlight. But the amount produced varies depending on skin pigmentation, age, and length of exposure. Dietary vitamin D sources are particularly important for those who are confined indoors, such as nursing home residents.

Vitamin D may be toxic with intakes of only five times the RDA. Toxicity can lead to calcification of the body's soft tissues. Dietary supplements of vitamin D may be detrimental to children and adults who regularly consume fortified milk.

Vitamin E. Vitamin E functions as an **antioxidant,** that is, it helps protect cell membranes from being oxidized (being altered or destroyed in the presence of oxygen). The vitamin E will be oxidized itself to spare the cell membrane. Vitamin E exerts its protective effect on the lung tissues, body lipids, and both white and red blood

BOX 22-3 **METHODS OF PRESERVING THE VITAMIN CONTENT OF FOODS**

1. Expose food to as little water as possible; steam, microwave, stir-fry, or bake rather than boil.
2. Expose food to as little air as possible; keep prepared vegetables, fruits, and juices covered and airtight; cut and manipulate food as little as possible; keep lids on pans while cooking.
3. Keep and use the cooking water.
4. Store fruits and vegetables cold.
5. Keep milk in opaque containers.
6. Use foods in the whole form whenever possible.

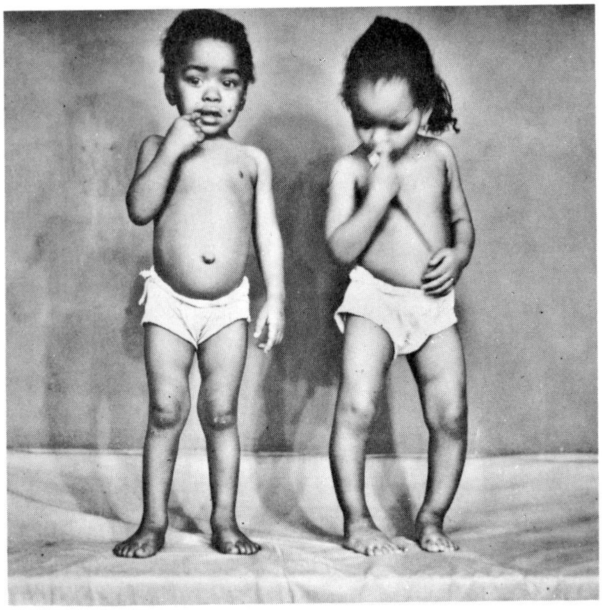

FIG. 22-2 Children with rickets.

cells. Deficiency is rarely seen except in premature infants or individuals with fat malabsorption. Deficiency is often exhibited by excessive destruction of red blood cells (erythrocyte hemolysis).

Vitamin E is found in vegetable oils and products made with them, leafy green vegetables, wheat germ, and nuts. Large amounts of vitamin E may enhance anticoagulant effects of drugs used to prevent clotting. Patients on anticoagulant therapy should not take vitamin E supplements.

Vitamin K. Vitamin K is essential to the blood clotting process. It is necessary for the formation of various blood clotting factors. Deficiency is uncommon but may occur in fat malabsorption, during prolonged antibiotic treatments, and in infants not given vitamin K injections at birth. Deficiency results in hemorrhaging (excessive bleeding).

Vitamin K is synthesized by bacteria in the intestine, and much of the daily needs can be met by bacterial synthesis. Dietarily, vitamin K is found abundantly in green leafy vegetables. It is also present in milk, meats, eggs, cereals, fruits, and other vegetables.

Water-soluble vitamins. The water-soluble vitamins include the B vitamins and vitamin C. Since they are water soluble, these vitamins are not readily stored in the body. Excesses are generally excreted in the urine. Daily intake of these vitamins is necessary since body reserves are minimal.

Thiamin (vitamin B_1). Thiamin is necessary for the metabolism of carbohydrates and the consequent release of energy. In the United States deficiency of thiamin is most commonly seen in those with alcoholism, because of both poor dietary intakes and an increased need for thiamin in alcohol metabolism. **Beriberi** is the name given the thiamin deficiency disease. Its signs and symptoms include mental confusion, peripheral paralysis, anorexia, muscle weakness and wasting, enlarged heart, and edema.

Since thiamin is needed for energy production, needs are based on energy expenditure. Requirements can easily be met by eating a varied diet. Sources include whole, unrefined grains, enriched and fortified grain products, liver, pork, legumes, and nuts.

Riboflavin (vitamin B_2). Riboflavin is also necessary for energy production as well as functioning in protein metabolism. Deficiency symptoms often involve tissue impairment. Signs of riboflavin deficiency (ariboflavinosis) include cracked lips and mouth corners (cheilosis), dermatitis, and sensitivity to light.

Riboflavin is found in milk and milk products, meats, poultry and fish, enriched or fortified cereal products, and some green vegetables. The vitamin riboflavin is destroyed in ultraviolet light. This is why milk distributors package milk in opaque containers.

Niacin. Sometimes called vitamin B_3, niacin is another vitamin that is necessary for energy production. Deficiency is not common in the United States. It results in **pellagra,** a disease characterized by dermatitis, diarrhea, and dementia (deteriorating mental state).

Niacin is found abundantly in meats and poultry. Smaller amounts are found in milk, fish, and green leafy vegetables. Niacin is added to enriched and fortified cereal products. Niacin can be made in the body from tryptophan, one of the essential amino acids. Therefore, foods with complete proteins can contribute to the niacin needs of the body.

Niacin (nicotinic acid) is sometimes used in pharmacological doses to lower blood lipids. Large doses of niacin may produce vascular dilation, or "flushing," with a feeling of burning or stinging of the hands and face. Other body systems may also be affected. Caution should be used in taking large doses.

Vitamin B_6 **(pyridoxine).** Vitamin B_6 functions in amino acid metabolism. It also plays a role in both carbohydrate and fat metabolism. Because of its role in protein metabolism, vitamin B_6 requirements are roughly based on protein intake. Deficiency of vitamin B_6 is rare and if seen, is usually accompanied by other B complex deficiencies. It may result in anemia, smooth tongue (glossitis), irritability, and convulsions.

Vitamin B_6 is widely distributed in animal and plant foods. It is most highly concentrated in meats, poultry, fish, and eggs. Other sources include brown rice, wheat, oats, soybeans, some nuts, and seeds.

Toxicity of vitamin B_6 may occur if megadoses (very large doses) are taken over a long time. Symptoms include changes in peripheral nerve sensations and muscle coordination.

Folate. Folate, folic acid, or folacin all refer to this B vitamin. Folate is necessary for the production of deoxyribonucleic acid (DNA), the nucleic acid that carries genetic information and is the basis of heredity. Deficiency of folate affects rapidly growing tissues. It is manifested by a type of anemia called megaloblastic anemia (large cell type). Folate is found in liver, green leafy vegetables, legumes, and some fruits.

Vitamin B_{12}. Vitamin B_{12} is also called cobalamin. A deficiency of vitamin B_{12} appears similar to and is related to a folic acid deficiency. These two vitamins work together in the manufacture of red blood cells. Deficiency causes macrocytic megaloblastic anemia (large, immature red blood cells). Vitamin B_{12} deficiency over time may also result in paralysis and nerve damage.

Vitamin B_{12} requires a special *intrinsic factor* produced in the lower portion of the stomach for absorption. When the intrinsic factor is missing, for example, after stomach excision, **pernicious anemia** develops. Pernicious anemia results because B_{12} is not absorbed. It manifests itself as a B_{12} deficiency. Treatment of pernicious anemia requires B_{12} injections.

Vitamin B_{12} is found in animal tissues and animal products. Dietary deficiency is uncommon and takes many years to manifest itself. Vegans (strict vegetarians) may be at risk of deficiency if they consume no animal foods over an extended time.

Biotin and panotothenic acid. Biotin and Pantothenic acid are both B vitamins with specific functions in the body. Their importance cannot be discounted; however, both are widely distributed in the food supply and deficiencies are not seen in humans consuming a normal diet.

Vitamin C (ascorbic acid). The functions of vitamin C are not completely understood, and much controversy surrounds the issue of vitamin C requirements. Vitamin C functions in the formation of collagen, the strong matrix that is necessary for wound healing and bone formation. It is also an antioxidant, similar to vitamin E. When ingested in the same meal, vitamin C enhances the absorption of iron from the gastrointestinal (GI) tract. Vitamin C can also affect the immune response. A severe deficiency of vitamin C results in a condition called **scurvy.** Early signs of vitamin C deficiency include bleeding gums, pinpoint hemorrhages, and easy bruising. Further deficiency results in rough, scaly skin, mood changes, muscle atrophy, poor wound healing, increased infections, painful joints, and fractures.

Vitamin C is found almost exclusively in the fruits and vegetables food group. The other food groups are poor sources of vitamin C. Particularly rich sources of vitamin C include citrus fruits and juices, green and red peppers, cantaloupe, strawberries, kiwi fruit, and broccoli. Table 22-5 lists the vitamin C content of some foods.

The most recent RDA for vitamin C is 60 mg/day for the adult. Regular cigarette smokers need more vitamin C because of increased metabolic turnover of the vitamin. The RDAs suggest 100 mg/day for smokers. Vitamin C requirements can easily be obtained through diet without supplement usage.

Still, vitamin C supplementation has become a common practice of many. Claims have been made that megadoses of vitamin C may prevent colds and reduce or cure cancer. Although it is true that adequate vitamin C is necessary for proper immune function and may also be beneficial in reducing cancer risk, large doses of the vitamin have not been consistently and conclusively shown to be of greater value than that which can be obtained solely through diet. And whereas moderate doses of vitamin C do not seem to be harmful, larger doses may cause cramps and diarrhea. Routine supplementation with large amounts of vitamin C (1000 mg or more) is not recommended.

Table 22-5 Vitamin C Content of Selected Foods

Food and Portion Size	Vitamin C (mg)
Orange juice, fresh squeezed (1 c)	124
Cantaloupe (½ melon)	112
Orange juice, from concentrate (1 c)	97
Strawberries, whole (1 c)	85
Grapefruit juice, from concentrate (1 c)	83
Kiwi (1 medium)	75
Green pepper (1)	70
Orange (1 medium)	70
Broccoli, cooked (½ c)	60
Brussels sprouts, cooked (½ c)	48
Grapefruit, pink (½ medium)	47
Watermelon (1 inch round)	47
Tomato juice (1 c)	45
Cauliflower, cooked (½ c)	34
Potato, baked (1)	26
Tomato (1)	22
Spinach, cooked (½ c)	20

From USDA Handbooks 456 and 8.

Minerals

Minerals differ from vitamins in that they are inorganic and they are single elements rather than compounds. Because they are elements, minerals cannot be destroyed as vitamins can. They can, however, be lost in cooking water. Similar to vitamins, minerals are needed in only small amounts in the body. Many minerals are stored in body tissues; thus excesses may lead to toxicity. The major minerals are those needed in amounts greater than 100 mg/day. The trace minerals are needed in much smaller amounts.

The major minerals. The major minerals include calcium, phosphorus, magnesium, sulfur, sodium, potassium, and chloride.

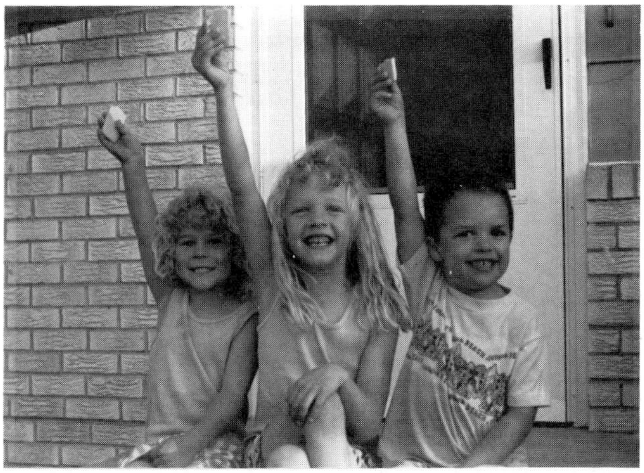

FIG. 22-3 Say cheese! A fun snack and a healthy way to help children meet their calcium requirements.

Calcium. Of the calcium in the body 99% is found in the bones and teeth. Calcium is necessary for both the formation and the maintenance of bones and teeth. it is also essential in nerve conduction, muscle contraction, and blood clotting. Calcium is found in the blood stream as well as in the bones. Generally, blood calcium levels remain constant regardless of dietary calcium intake. If diet is inadequate, calcium may be pulled from the bones to maintain blood calcium levels. Thus a low intake of calcium over a long period may contribute to osteoporosis, an abnormal reduction in bone density leading to bone pain, fractures, loss of stature, and various deformities.

The causes of osteoporosis are multiple. Growth and mineralization of bone occur from birth until approximately 25 years of age. Peak bone mass is determined not only by calcium intake, but by genetic influences, sex hormones, physical activity, and dietary intake of vitamin D, fluoride, and other trace minerals. During the fifth decade of life, bone mass begins to decline. In women menopause greatly accelerates the rate of bone loss. This results in weakened bones and a greater risk of fractures. If peak bone mass reached in young adulthood is higher, the risk of bone fractures at a given age will be reduced. Therefore calcium intake in childhood, adolescence, and young adulthood is very important (Fig. 22-3). Calcium is also necessary in adulthood for bone maintenance and to prevent excessive bone loss.

The RDA for calcium for adults is 800 mg/day. For ages 11 to 25 years, the RDA is 1200 mg/day. The best sources of calcium come from the milk group. One cup of milk, 1½ oz of cheese, or 1 cup of yogurt provides about 300 mg of calcium. Three servings of milk would easily meet the RDA for calcium for the adult. Other sources of calcium include green leafy vegetables, such as spinach or broccoli, tofu (soybean curds), and fish with bones, such as sardines and salmon.

Calcium absorption from the GI tract varies depending on circumstances surrounding its consumption. It appears that calcium in milk products is absorbed best. Calcium supplements are absorbed better when taken with milk or with a meal. Absorption is increased when body needs are great, such as during childhood, pregnancy, or lactation, and absorption decreases in old age.

Phosphorus. Phosphorus works together with calcium in bone and tooth formation. Phosphorus has many other roles in the body as well. It is part of DNA and ribonucleic acid (RNA), the genetic code material in each cell. Phosphorus is necessary for the release of energy in many chemical reactions, and phosphorus also assists in maintaining the acid-base balance of body fluids.

Phosphorus is present in nearly all foods. It is particularly abundant in protein-rich foods, such as meat and milk, and in cereal grains. Natural dietary deficiencies are not known.

Magnesium. Many body processes require magnesium. It is necessary for the release of energy, protein synthesis, transmission of genetic code, muscle contraction and relaxation, and necessary in the activation of more than 300 enzymes. Magnesium deficiency has not been reported in people consuming typical diets. When it does occur, it is usually associated with other disease states such as alcoholism, protein malnutrition, excessive vomiting or diarrhea, renal dysfunction, or long-term intravenous feedings. A severe deficiency may lead to tetany, a severe and prolonged contraction of the muscles.

Magnesium is found in nuts, legumes, and unmilled grains. Green vegetables contain magnesium, which is found in the green pigment chlorophyll.

Sulfur. Sulfur is an essential nutrient, functioning in tissue structure and some metabolic reactions; however, no dietary requirements have been set. Sulfur is found in all proteins, and dietary deficiency of sulfur by itself has never been reported. Deficiency may be seen in severe protein malnutrition.

Electrolytes. Sodium, potassium, and chloride are all major minerals. They are also the principal **electrolytes** found in the body. Other minerals such as calcium and magnesium may also serve as electrolytes in lesser capacities. An electrolyte is a compound of electrically charged particles (ions), which dissociates or separates in water. A solution containing electrolytes conducts electricity. Electrolytes function in regulating fluid and acid-base balance and in conducting electrical impulses such as those necessary for nerve conduction and muscle contraction.

Sodium. Sodium is the principal positively charged ion (cation) in the extracellular fluid. It functions as an electrolyte as previously discussed. Sodium deficiency is uncommon, possibly being seen in chronic diarrhea or renal failure or in prolonged diaphoresis (extreme perspiration).

Of more concern is the possibility that excess sodium

BOX 22-4 **SODIUM CONTENT OF FOODS**

1 tsp salt = 2100 mg sodium

800-1000+ mg/serving

Baking soda, 1 tsp
Cheeseburger, ¼ lb
Chili, canned, 1 c
Condensed canned soup, prepared, 1 c
Crab, canned, 3 oz
Dill pickle, 1 large
Ham, 3 oz
Soy sauce, 1 Tbls
Tomato juice, 6 oz

500-799 mg/serving

Frankfurter, 1
Gravy, from mix, ½ c
Nuts, roasted, salted, 1 c
Parmesan cheese, 1 oz
Sardines, 3 oz
Sauerkraut, ½ c
Tomato sauce, ½ c

300-499 mg/serving

Baking powder, 1 tsp
Bologna, 1 oz slice
Bran flakes, 1 c
Corn flakes, 1 oz
Cottage cheese, ½ c
Instant chocolate pudding, ½ c
Processed cheese, 1 oz
Tuna, canned, 3 oz

100-299 mg/serving

Bacon, 2 slices
Bread, 1 slice
Canned vegetables (corn, green beans, peas), ½ c
Catsup, 1 Tbls
Corn chips, 1 oz
French fries, 1 small bag
Lobster, 3 oz
Margarine, 1 Tbls
Milk, 1 c
Milkshake, 1 medium
Natural cheeses, 1 oz
Potato chips, 1 oz
Saltines, 4
Sweet pickle, 1

Less than 100 mg/serving

Beef round, 3 oz
Carrot, 1 raw*
Celery, 1 stalk*
Chicken breast, 3 oz
Cola, 12 oz*
Diet cola, 12 oz*
Fresh cooked vegetables, ½ c
Fruit juices, 1 c*
Rice, cooked, ½ c*
Trout, 3 oz

From USDA Handbooks 456 and 8.
*Indicates less than 50 mg/serving.

may be detrimental to health. Excess sodium intake may be related to hypertension (high blood pressure) in sensitive individuals. Sodium reduction in some people helps to reduce blood pressure. Sodium attracts water; because of this, a high-sodium diet consumed by individuals who suffer with edema (fluid retention) may exacerbate the problem.

Sodium is found naturally in practically all foods. Most processed foods contain additional sodium in the form of salt and other additives. This, combined with the salt that many people add during cooking and at the table, adds up to an abundance of dietary sodium. The AHA recommends that individuals consume less than 3000 mg of sodium per day. Other experts recommend intakes of less than 2500 mg/day. The National Research Council has set a safe *minimum* daily requirement at a much lower figure of only 500 mg/day. Almost any diet of natural foods from all of the food groups with no added salt whatsoever would easily provide 500 mg of sodium. Box 22-4 lists sodium content of some foods.

Potassium. Potassium is the major intracellular cation. It also performs the functions of an electrolyte. Potassium is particularly important in maintaining the heartbeat. Potassium deficiency may occur with use of potassium-wasting diuretics and in cases of chronic vomiting, diarrhea, or laxative use. Although dietary deficiency is uncommon, more and more evidence points to the fact that dietary potassium exerts a beneficial effect on hypertension, and recommendations have been made to increase potassium intake from foods. Potassium supplementation is not recommended except when prescribed by a physician. Toxicity may lead to cardiac arrest. The National Research Council has suggested 2000 mg potassium/day as a *minimum* requirement for adults. Box 22-5 lists potassium content of some foods.

Chloride. Chloride is a negatively charged ion or anion. It functions as an electrolyte and is also a principal component in gastric juice. Dietary deficiency of chloride does not occur; however, prolonged gastric secretion loss through nasogastric drainage may cause a decrease in

BOX 22-5 POTASSIUM CONTENT OF FOODS

(Serving size equals ½ cup unless otherwise indicated.)

601-800 mg/serving

Avocado, ½ fruit
Baked potato, 1 medium
Cantaloupe, ½ melon

401-600 mg/serving

Banana, 1 medium
Peaches, dried, 4 halves
Winter squash

301-400 mg/serving

Artichoke, 1 medium
Apricots, dried, 6 halves
Kidney beans, cooked
Lima beans, cooked
Milk, 1 cup
Spinach, cooked

201-300 mg/serving

Asparagus, cooked
Broccoli, cooked
Brussels sprouts, cooked
Chocolate pudding
Carrot, 1 whole
Meat, poultry, or fish, 3 oz
Orange, 1 medium
Orange juice
Parsnips, cooked
Peach, 1 medium
Pumpkin, mashed
Sweet potato, mashed
Tomato, 1 whole
Tomato juice

From USDA Handbooks 456 and 8.

serum chloride. The most common source of chloride is table salt.

Trace minerals. Trace minerals include iron, zinc, iodine, selenium, copper, manganese, fluoride, chromium, and molybdenum. Other trace minerals thought to be essential, but of which less is known, include arsenic, boron, nickel, and silicon.

Iron. Iron is a part of hemoglobin, myoglobin, and a number of enzymes. Hemoglobin is part of the red blood cell and carries oxygen to the cells. Myoglobin is a similar compound in the muscle tissue.

Iron deficiency manifests itself as a microcytic (small cell size), hypochromic (less cell color) **anemia.** Not all anemia is caused by a marginal intake or excess loss of iron, but iron deficiency anemia is a major health problem around the world. Symptoms include fatigue, weakness, headaches, apathy, and pale skin and mucous membranes. Immune function may also be decreased. It is difficult to measure the effects of anemia, but work capacity and job performance may be greatly diminished. In children iron deficiency has been associated with a short attention span, irritability, and a reduced ability to learn.

Children 6 months to 4 years, adolescents, menstruating women, and pregnant women are at greatest risk for iron deficiency anemia. Dietary requirements for adult women are 50% higher than for men because of the monthly blood loss of menstruation. Iron RDAs are set at 15 mg/day for adolescent girls and premenopausal adult women. Postmenopausal women, adult men, and children have an RDA of 10 mg of iron per day. Male adolescents' RDA for iron is 12 mg/day. Pregnant women have an iron requirement set at twice that for nonpregnant women—30 mg/day.

Iron is found in liver, meat, poultry, fish, legumes, whole grains, enriched grain products, green leafy vegetables, and dried fruits. Dietary iron is found in two forms—heme and nonheme. Heme iron is well absorbed. About 40% of the iron in animal tissues (meats, poultry, and fish) is heme iron, with the remaining 60% being nonheme iron. Nonheme iron is not well absorbed from the GI tract. The iron in plant products is nonheme. Supplemental iron also seems to be poorly absorbed. Iron absorption from the GI tract may be enhanced or inhibited by certain dietary factors. They are listed in Box 22-6. The use of vitamin C rich foods and meat, fish, or poultry with meals may increase iron absorption by as much as fourfold.

Iron can be toxic and even fatal. Iron poisoning is seen each year in children who overdose on iron-containing vitamin/mineral supplements. Medical attention should be immediate if a child ingests large amounts of iron-containing supplements.

Zinc. Zinc functions in a number of metabolic pathways in the body and is necessary for the functioning of over 70 enzymes. Signs of zinc deficiency include loss of appetite, decreased taste perception, growth retardation, skin changes, and immune system dysfunction. Severe dietary deficiencies in the Middle East have resulted in dwarfism and retarded sexual maturation. In persons with low blood zinc levels, increased zinc intake seems to improve wound healing and taste acuity.

The best sources of zinc include meat, liver, eggs, and seafood. Cereals, grains, and legumes also contain zinc, but in a less absorbable form. Massive doses of zinc result in gastrointestinal upset, vomiting, and diarrhea. Even moderately elevated intakes of zinc may adversely affect the immune system and impair the body's use of copper. Zinc supplementation is not recommended without medical supervision.

Iodine. Iodine is part of the thyroid hormones that regulate the basal metabolic rate. Iodine deficiency is manifest by an enlarged thyroid gland, or goiter. If the thyroid gland is unable to function, the metabolic rate is

BOX 22-6 **FACTORS AFFECTING IRON ABSORPTION FROM THE GI TRACT**

Factors that enhance iron absorption

1. Meat, fish, and poultry (MFP). Animal tissues seem to have a factor, sometimes called the MFP factor, which enhances iron absorption.
2. Vitamin C (ascorbic acid), when eaten in the same meal with iron-containing foods.
3. Physiological need. Generally when needs are greater, such as in pregnancy, more iron is absorbed.

Factors that inhibit iron absorption

1. Bran and some fibers. Phytates in some fibers bind iron in the GI tract so that it is not absorbed.
2. Tea and coffee. The tannins present inhibit absorption of iron.
3. Some medications, such as antacids.
4. Soybeans and other legumes.*

From Monsen ER: Iron nutrition and absorption: dietary factors which impact iron bioavailability, J Am Diet Assoc 88:786, 1988.
*Further research is needed for conclusive evidence.

reduced, causing sluggishness, weight gain, skin and hair changes, and intolerance to cold. Iodine deficiency in pregnancy results in severe mental and physical retardation of the newborn infant. This condition is called cretinism. Iodine deficiency is a worldwide problem, especially in underdeveloped countries.

Iodine content of foods varies widely depending on geographic area. Soils in coastal regions contain iodine, and thus the plants grown on these soils will provide iodine. Seafood is also a source of iodine. But by far the most reliable source of iodine in the United States is iodized salt, which has almost abolished goiter in this country. Most North Americans receive sufficient amounts of iodine each day.

Selenium. Selenium functions as an antioxidant in conjunction with vitamin E. Deficiency may be manifest by muscular discomfort, weakness, and cardiomyopathy (disease of the myocardium).

Selenium is found in seafood, liver, and meats. Grains and seeds contain selenium in varying amounts depending on soil content. Toxicity of selenium was seen in the United States in individuals who consumed an improperly manufactured supplement containing excess selenium. Symptoms included nausea, diarrhea, nail and hair changes, peripheral neuropathy, and fatigue.

Other trace minerals. Copper is essential for blood formation. Deficiencies are rare and result in anemia and nervous system changes.

Fluoride plays a role in increasing the strength of teeth and increasing resistance to tooth decay. It may also increase bone strength and help delay osteoporosis. Fluorine is found naturally in many water supplies and is added in small amounts of others. In areas where water is not fluoridated, fluoride supplements for children may be of benefit for dental health.

Chromium is necessary for glucose metabolism and seems to work with insulin in the regulation of blood glucose. Studies are now focusing on its relationship to diabetes mellitus. Deficiencies, although rare, produce a diabetes-like condition.

Manganese is an essential element, but deficiencies are rare. It is found abundantly in plant foods. Toxicities have been seen in miners, who inhale manganese dust on the job.

Nutrient Supplementation

The evidence regarding toxicity of some vitamins and minerals points to the fact that more is not necessarily better. Our food supply can provide adequate amounts of nutrients for health if the diet is well planned. Except in cases where nutritional needs are increased, such as during pregnancy and lactation and in certain disease states or medical/surgical conditions, supplementation is not necessary. For those who like to use a supplement as "insurance" against an imperfect diet, a simple multivitamin and mineral supplement providing about 100% of the U.S. RDA should suffice. Large doses or megadoses of nutrients and the taking of numerous types of supplements should be avoided.

Water

Water is the nutrient most vital to life. Lack of this nutrient will bring detrimental effects faster than any other. Body weight is 55% to 60% water. Water performs many functions. It provides form and structure to body tissues. It acts as a solvent and is necessary for most of the body's chemical processes to occur. Water transports nutrients and other substances throughout the body by way of the blood, body secretions, and tissue fluids. It lubricates and protects moving parts of the body such as joints. It also lubricates food and aids in digestion. Water is necessary to regulate body temperature. If fluid needs are not met, dehydration will result. This can become life-threatening when more than 10% of body weight is lost. Signs of dehydration include poor skin turgor, flushed dry skin, dry mouth, decreased urine output, irritability, and confusion.

Needs for water vary depending on factors such as activity level, metabolic needs, temperature, water losses, and age, so it is impossible to give a specific requirement. For most adults, 2 to 3 L (8 to 12 cups) of water per day is adequate. Pregnant and lactating women have increased water needs. Infants may be at a greater risk of dehydration because they have a higher percentage of water as body weight and are more susceptible to greater skin losses of water. In the young infant breast milk and formula normally provide adequate fluid, but extra fluids may be needed in warmer weather. The elderly have a decreased sensitivity to thirst and are at greater risk for dehydration. Special attention should be given to this population to make certain fluid needs are met.

LIFE CYCLE NUTRITION

Pregnancy and Lactation

Nutrient needs during periods of intensive growth, such as during pregnancy and in infancy, are greater than at any other time during the life cycle. During pregnancy a woman's need for protein, calcium, phosphorus, magnesium, and folate increase greatly. Other nutrients are also needed in greater amounts. Protein is necessary for tissue growth. Calcium, phosphorus, and magnesium contribute to skeletal development, whereas folate, iron, and vitamin B_{12} are necessary for the increase in blood volume.

Diet during pregnancy should reflect changes in nutrient needs. The RDAs suggest that pregnant women consume an additional 300 kcal/day. This is only a modest increase, and since kilocalorie needs increase less than nutrient needs, a woman should try to select **nutrient-dense** foods, that is, foods that contain large amounts of nutrients relative to kilocalories. Some nutrient-dense food choices might include skim or low-fat milk and yogurt, cottage cheese, lean meats, poultry, fish, whole grains, and fresh fruits and vegetables. The Basic Four food group plan recommends that a pregnant woman consume each day, 4 servings from the milk group, 3 servings from the meat group, 4 servings from the fruit and vegetable group, and 4 servings from the grain group (see Table 22-1). After meeting the Basic Four recommendations, women who need more kilocalories should increase consumption of foods from the fruit and vegetable group and the grain group.

Concerns of pregnancy

Weight gain. Weight gain in pregnancy is important, with an ideal weight gain being near 25 lb. Weight gain should follow the pattern of approximately 2 to 4 lb during the first trimester, and 1 lb/week thereafter. Pregnant adolescents and underweight women may need to gain more weight (30 lb or more), whereas overweight women may gain slightly less (20 lb). Under no condition should weight loss be attempted in pregnancy. Mothers who do not gain adequate weight in pregnancy may give birth to a low birth weight (LBW) infant. LBW infants have a birth weight of less than 2500 g (5½ lb). These babies have a greater risk of complications during and after birth. Mortality rates are higher for LBW infants.

Discomforts and complications. Many women experience discomforts during pregnancy. Some of these may be alleviated with dietary alterations. A few suggested nutritional aids to help relieve discomfort are listed in Box 22-7.

BOX 22-7 NUTRITIONAL AIDS FOR DISCOMFORTS OF PREGNANCY

Nausea and vomiting:	Eat soda crackers before getting out of bed. Eat smaller meals more often. Drink liquids before or after meals, rather than with them. Avoid high-fat or fried foods in excess.
Constipation:	Drink plenty of fluids. Include fiber-rich foods in each meal. Include daily exercise or physical activity.
Gastric distress:	Eat smaller, more frequent meals. Avoid high-fat and fried foods. Do not lie down after eating, and do not eat immediately before going to bed.

Occasionally, pregnancy will bring about medical conditions that may pose dangers for both the mother and the fetus. Pregnancy-induced hypertension (PIH), formerly called toxemia or preeclampsia, is a condition occurring after about the fifth month of pregnancy. It occurs more frequently in the malnourished. Symptoms include hypertension, edema, and proteinuria. Proper nutrition is vital throughout pregnancy and may help to avert this condition. Once PIH has begun, adequate nutrition should be a part of therapy. Contrary to old practices, salt should not be restricted in most cases of PIH.

Gestational diabetes is a type of diabetes mellitus that occurs only in pregnancy. It usually develops in the latter part of pregnancy. Women should be screened for diabetes in about the sixth month of pregnancy. If gestational diabetes occurs, diet is a major part of therapy. Chapter 23 discusses diabetes in more detail.

Anemia is also a common nutritional problem in pregnancy. Both iron deficiency and folacin deficiency anemia may occur. Adequate diet including meats, poultry and fish, green leafy vegetables, and a variety of other fruits and vegetables should be consumed along with a prenatal vitamin/mineral supplement.

Practices to avoid. Some dietary practices should be avoided during pregnancy, especially alcohol consumption. Alcohol contributes to an increased risk of mental and physical retardation of the fetus. Fetal alcohol syndrome (FAS) is the name given for the cluster of symptoms seen in an infant whose mother consumed excess alcohol during her pregnancy. It not only includes physical and mental retardation, but characteristic facial and other body deformities. There has been no determination of a safe level of alcohol consumption during pregnancy, and most nutrition experts seem to favor total abstinence.

Smoking, although not dietary, should be discouraged. Low birth weight occurs more frequently in infants of mothers who smoke. Drugs of any kind should be avoided, except under the advice of a physician. Also, dieting for weight reduction may be harmful during pregnancy.

Lactation. During lactation a woman would do well to follow a diet similar to that followed during pregnancy. Nutrient needs are similar and kilocalorie needs are actually higher than during pregnancy. An increase of 500 kcal extra per day is recommended. Fluid needs are increased in lactation and can be obtained through the consumption of water, milk, juices, and other beverages. Coffee, tea, and alcohol, if consumed, should be used in moderation since caffeine and alcohol can enter the breast milk.

During lactation adequate nutrition is vital. Studies show that during lactation a poor kilocalorie and nutrient intake will decrease the quantity of milk produced. Nutritional quality of the milk remains fairly constant except in cases of severe nutrient deficiency. Therefore, it is essential for the lactating mother to be properly nourished to ensure lactation continues and milk supply is adequate. If a lactating mother complains that she is unable to produce "enough" milk for the infant, a nurse would do well to ask about her dietary intake.

Infancy

The time from birth to 1 year of age is one of rapid growth and development. The average infant's birth weight triples by the first birthday. Obviously, nutrition is important for proper growth and development.

Breast milk or infant formula is generally adequate for the first 6 months of life. Breast-feeding confers several advantages on the infant as well as the lactating mother. Breast-feeding should be encouraged whenever possible; however, if a woman prefers to formula feed her infant, she should be supported in that decision. Box 22-8 lists benefits of breast-feeding.

Sometime between 4 and 6 months of age, an infant begins to need more iron in the diet. This is a good time to introduce solids into the diet. Formula-fed infants may begin drinking iron-fortified formula at this time as well. Solids generally need not be given before 4 months of age. The tendency to develop allergies is greater, and most infants are not developmentally or physiologically ready to handle solid foods.

There is no absolute guideline for the introduction of solid foods to the infant; however, a few principles should be followed. Foods should be introduced singularly at weekly intervals. This will allow sufficient time to detect any food-related allergies. Solid food should always be introduced by spoon feeding rather than in bottles or syringes, and juice should be given in a cup. This allows the infant to develop proper eating skills and may prevent overfeeding. No particular foods should be introduced first or last; however, rice cereal is usually recommended first because it is the least allergenic of any cereal. Fruits need not be given before vegetables. In fact, many mothers prefer to introduce vegetables before fruits so that the infant may enjoy their flavor before becoming accustomed to the naturally sweet taste of fruits. There is no need to introduce all of one food group before going on to another. For families with a history of food allergies, wheat cereal, wheat products, and egg whites may need to be withheld until 1 year of age. Table 22-6 gives a general guide for the introduction of solid foods. By about age 1, most children can eat many of the same foods as the rest of the family and should be consuming a wide variety of solid foods (Fig. 22-4).

Most commercially prepared baby foods in the United States are nutritious, safe, and of high quality. However, it is important to read labels and use foods without added

BOX 22-8 ADVANTAGES OF BREAST-FEEDING

ANTIINFECTIVE PROPERTIES

Immunoglobulins, lymphocytes, and other immune components are present in breast milk and provide protection against infection in the infant. The bifidus factor in breast milk encourages growth of normal bacterial flora in the infant GI tract.

NUTRITION

Breast milk is specifically made for the human infant. Its protein, carbohydrate, and fat ratio is thought to be ideal for growth and development. It is well digested and readily absorbed.

GROWTH AND DEVELOPMENT

Breast-feeding promotes better tooth and jaw alignment. It may be less likely to produce obesity in the child, and it may favor optimum bonding between mother and infant.

ALLERGY

Breast-feeding may reduce the incidence of allergies in infants at high risk for allergic conditions.

MATERNAL BENEFITS

Hormones produced in breast-feeding help contract and shrink the uterus. Breast-feeding requires no formula preparation and bottle sterilization and is more economical than formula feeding.

Table 22-6 A Guide for the Introduction of Foods to the Infant

Age	Foods Added to the Diet
4-6 months	Iron-fortified cereals for infants (rice, oats, barley)
5-7 months	Strained fruits, vegetables, and juices (from a cup)
6-8 months	Strained or ground meats, cheese, yogurt, egg yolks, cooked legumes
8-12 months	Finger foods, chopped meats, soft table foods, whole eggs, wheat cereal

- Introduce individual foods one at a time at weekly intervals. Watch for adverse affects to detect allergies. Of the cereals, introduce wheat last.
- Use a cup to introduce juices.
- Use a spoon. Do not put semisolid foods into a bottle or syringe. This may lead to overfeeding or choking and does not encourage proper development of eating skills.
- Do not use honey until after 1 year of age because of the risk of botulism.

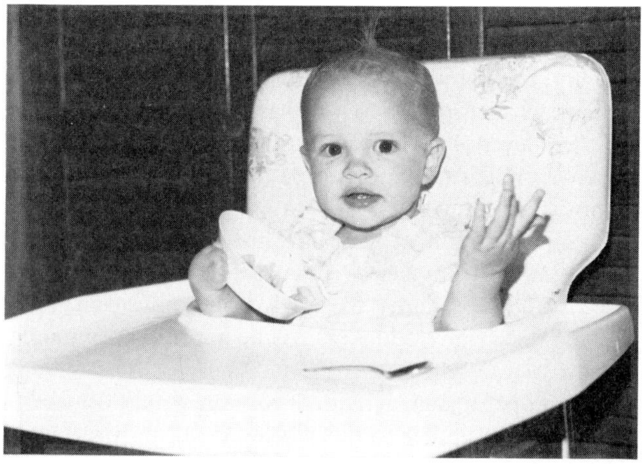

FIG. 22-4 The 1-year-old child can eat a variety of solid foods, including many of the same foods the rest of the family eats.

salt and sugar. Plain, simple foods are often better choices than the mixed dinner type of baby foods. The simple foods can be mixed to make a more nutritious meal having fewer fillers. If baby foods are prepared at home, care should be taken to reduce the risk of food poisoning by having a sanitary preparation area and proper storage conditions. Honey should not be given to infants until after the age of 1 year because it may carry botulism spores and cause food poisoning in the small body of the infant.

Controversy exists concerning the use of low-fat milk for infants. Unlike adults, infants need a higher percentage of kilocalories from fat. Therefore, milks of reduced fat content such as skim and 2% milk are not recommended until at least after 1 year of age and, preferably, not until after 2 years of age. Whole cow milk may be introduced at approximately 6 months of age, provided the infant is also consuming at least one third of its kilocalories from solid foods, including iron-fortified cereals. The best recommendation, however, is to continue with infant formula or breast milk until 1 year of age and then introduce regular cow milk. Breast milk and formula are more readily digested and put less of a physiological stress on the kidneys.

Childhood

At approximately age 1, appetite generally tapers off, and the growth rate slows from that of infancy. Children still need adequate nutrition, although nutrient needs relative to weight are generally less than in infancy. The four food group plan (see Table 22-1) recommends that children receive three servings of milk, two of meat, four of fruits and vegetables, and four of grain each day. Obviously, the younger child may need smaller serving sizes than adults, and as they grow, serving sizes will increase.

Childhood is a critical time for instilling good dietary habits. It is also a time for children to test their independence. Food is often a source of contention at mealtime, with the parents resorting to coaxing to get the child to eat or arguing with the child to gain compliance. Often, the more pressure that is placed on the child at mealtime, the more negative the experience will become, and the child may then be more resistant to developing sound eating habits. In general if children are offered nutritious foods in pleasant surroundings and in nonthreatening ways, they will most likely be adequately nourished. Ways to help make mealtimes more pleasant and food habits more appropriate are found in Box 22-9. A good rule to keep in mind is that parents and caregivers should decide which foods to serve and at what time. The child should be able to decide what and how much to eat. The development of good nutritional habits in childhood will provide a sound nutritional base with which to enter the adolescent years.

Adolescence

The adolescent years are years of both physical and emotional growth. In making food choices teenagers are influenced greatly by peer pressure and social acceptance. Their diets are often filled with kilocalorie-rich and nutrient-poor snack foods. Fast foods make up a large portion of the diet, and although these foods do not lack nutrients, the fast food diet is often void of fruits and vegetables and, sometimes, milk. Common dietary inadequacies in adolescence include iron and calcium (par-

BOX 22-9 WAYS TO ENCOURAGE SOUND DIETARY HABITS IN CHILDREN

1. Children should be encouraged to eat meals and snacks at regular times and usually at the table. By having set eating times, children will learn that they cannot eat continually all day.
2. Try to make meals relaxed and enjoyable. Children need time to eat correctly and mealtimes should be a positive experience.
3. Offer a variety of foods from all four food groups, and give children a choice of what they may eat.
4. Remember, physical growth and appetite come in spurts. Do not force children to eat more than they want to eat.
5. Give small servings, or teach children how to serve themselves small servings. Then let them have seconds if still hungry.
6. Offer new foods, but do not force children to eat foods they dislike. If the child will not eat a new food, quietly remove the food and offer it again at another time.
7. Encourage children to help with food selection and preparation.
8. Keep nutritious snacks available, such as fruit, cheese, crackers, raw vegetables, and bread. Most children need to snack.
9. Limit sweets, and do not use sweets and foods as rewards or bribes.
10. Encourage children to be physically active.

ticularly in girls) and vitamins A and C and folate. Iron needs increase with the onset of menstruation in girls, and anemia is a common problem. Boys' nutritional intakes are generally better than girls. During adolescence many teenagers experiment with alcohol and drugs, and these substances are not without detrimental effects on nutritional status.

Eating disorders. Puberty brings with it hormonal changes and the emergence of sexual characteristics. Some teenagers, particularly young women, resist these changes and turn to inappropriate dieting. Two eating disorders, anorexia nervosa and bulimia, may occur in adolescents and young adults.

Anorexia nervosa. **Anorexia nervosa** is an eating disorder characterized by self-imposed starvation. Certain features are common in individuals with this disorder. They are generally women in their midteens, although young adult women and men sometimes develop the disorder. Often, they are high achievers from educated, middle-class families. The young person with anorexia nervosa is frequently a perfectionist and uses food and exercise as a means of controlling the body. These people become obsessed with weight loss and soon develop a distorted body image, seeing themselves as "fat" even when their weight is much less than the average for their height and age. The brain's electrical activity is affected, leading to altered thinking patterns, disturbed sleep, and bad dreams. Personality changes, depression, and apathy may occur. As weight loss continues, other physical symptoms occur such as cold intolerance, heart irregularities, and hypotension. GI function is affected causing slowed peristalsis and feelings of distention. The lining of the digestive tract deteriorates so that on eating the person may experience malabsorption and diarrhea. This further compounds the negative perception of food. Amenorrhea occurs in women, whereas men experience loss of sexual interest. Loss of scalp hair may occur, and finally, a fine, downy hair (lanugo) may grow on the body and face. Death may occur in as many as 20% of those with anorexia nervosa.

Treatment requires a multidisciplinary approach involving nutritional therapy and counseling along with psychological and family counseling. Nutritional goals for treatment of anorexia nervosa are listed in Box 22-10.

Bulimia. **Bulimia** is an eating disorder characterized by periods of binge eating followed by purging. This behavior may be alternated with periods of fasting as well. The cycle may go something like this: The person may binge several times per week. The episode may last 2 hours or more, and the person will consume large amounts of easily ingested kilocalorie-dense foods such as ice cream, candies, cakes, breads, and pastries. The binge is often followed by self-induced vomiting or the use of laxatives or diuretics or a combination of these behaviors. Of course, behavior may differ among individuals with bulimia.

BOX 22-10 NUTRITIONAL GUIDELINES FOR INTERVENTION IN ANOREXIA NERVOSA

- Increase kilocalories slowly.
- Provide balanced meals, including adequate fiber to ease elimination.
- Use small frequent meals to reduce sensations of fullness and distention.
- Use finger foods (snacks) and cold or room temperature foods to reduce feelings of satiety.
- Give multivitamin and mineral supplements at RDA levels.
- Add liquid supplements when desired intake cannot be achieved with solid foods.
- Limit caffeine intake.
- In behavioral programs, link rewards to kilocalorie intake, not to weight gain.
- Provide ongoing nutritional counseling.
- Use intravenous nutrition support or tube feedings only in severe states of malnutrition or ill health.

Modified from Rock CL and Yager J: Nutrition and eating disorders: a primer for clinicians, Int J Eating Disorders 6:276, 1987.

BOX 22-11 GUIDELINES FOR DIETARY TREATMENT OF BULIMIA

- Use structured, nonflexible eating plans during the initial stages of treatment.
- Prescribe a well-balanced diet. For variety and to help prolong the meal include adequate amounts of vegetables, fruits, salads, and whole-grain and high-fiber breads and cereals.
- Avoid finger foods; plan meals requiring utensils.
- To increase satiety include warm foods rather than cold or room temperature foods.
- Provide adequate amounts of complex carbohydrates (starches and fiber) to promote satiety and adequate fat to help slow gastric emptying and enhance the feeling of fullness.
- Use foods naturally divided into portions, such as precut meats and chicken parts, individual serving size packages of yogurt, ice cream, or cottage cheese, frozen dinners and entrees, and foods such as baked potatoes (as opposed to rice or pasta or mashed potatoes).
- Require that foods be eaten while sitting down.
- Keep a food diary, requiring that food be recorded before eating.

Modified from Rock CL and Yager J: Nutrition and eating disorders: a primer for clinicians, Int J Eating Disorders 6:276, 1987.

Table 22-7 Danger Signs of Eating Disorders

Diagnostic Category	Symptom or Behavior
Eating behaviors	Caloric restriction; preoccupation with dieting and calorie counting Binge eating; secretive eating Extreme preoccupation with food—reading cookbooks, recipes, shopping and preparing food for others, exhibiting peculiar eating rituals
Purging behaviors	Evidence of forced vomiting Abuse of laxatives, diuretics, enemas, or diet pills Excessive amounts of exercise
Physiological changes	Amenorrhea in women Insomnia, constipation, hair loss, dry skin, weak and brittle nails Cold intolerance Weight loss
Psychological changes	Distorted body image (thinking they are fat when they are very thin) Depression Withdrawal from friends, family, and social activities Inability to concentrate

Bulimia occurs more frequently than anorexia nervosa and is seen most often in young women. It is thought to be prevalent among college students. Those with bulimia are often of normal weight or even overweight. Most are aware that their eating patterns are abnormal. They often experience fear of not being able to stop eating and experience depression, guilt, and remorse after a binge. Clinical symptoms of bulimia may include tooth erosion, calloused knuckles, stomach lacerations, and esophageal infections from excessive vomiting. Electrolyte imbalances may occur leading to abnormal heart rhythms and injury to the kidneys. Repeated infections of the bladder and kidney may lead to renal failure.

Treatment of bulimia, like anorexia nervosa, must be multidisciplinary. Psychological counseling and therapy are necessary. Nutrition intervention differs somewhat from that for anorexia nervosa, and guidelines are listed in Box 22-11.

Eating disorders are relatively new in medical science, and their prevalence seems to be increasing. Bulimia was first medically defined as an eating disorder in 1980. Both disorders occur almost exclusively in developed nations, and it appears obvious that our society with its focus on thinness has helped bring about their occurrence. In young adolescence, women are already concerned that they are "too fat"; many are on diets. They see magazine pictures, models, and television images of beautiful and extremely thin women. For some the quest for unrealistic thinness, beauty, and happiness leads to eating disorders.

Recognizing and treating eating disorders early may lessen their effects. Table 22-7 lists some danger signs for which to look. Above all, the greatest focus should be placed on prevention. As a society our focus should be on good health rather than on thinness. Each individual must learn to respect and value his own uniqueness.

Obesity in Childhood and Adolescence

Obesity in the young is a problem occurring frequently in our society. As previously mentioned, these years are a time of growth, and although obesity is not ideal, restrictive diets can be harmful, may suppress development, and may lead to eating disorders. Attention should be focused on good eating habits rather than restrictions and should emphasize adequate physical activity. Weight reduction diets should only be attempted under the advice of a physician and with the guidance of a dietitian.

Adulthood

During adulthood, nutrient needs change very little in comparison to the years of growth and development. Energy needs, however, decrease with age. At the same time, many adults decrease activity levels. The combined effects of decreased energy needs and reduced physical activity often result in weight gain. As adults advance in years, it is important to use nutrient-dense foods and thereby receive adequate nutrition with fewer kilocalories. Emphasis should also be placed on maintaining an active life-style.

With age comes the increasing likelihood of age-related illness. Because many older Americans suffer from heart disease, arthritis, osteoporosis, diabetes, kidney disease, and other disorders, nutrient needs vary greatly from individual to individual.

Medical conditions and disease states often require medication. Many elderly people take a number of prescription medications daily. Some of these drugs may affect appetite and nutrition. Older adults should be informed of possible nutrient interactions and side effects.

Old age also brings with it physical changes such as loss of eyesight, hearing, and teeth. Digestive function diminishes and physical stamina decreases. Psychological changes may take place, such as forgetfulness, depression, or apathy. Also, financial burdens often increase, whereas income is less. Social, psychological, physical, and financial factors can all contribute to malnutrition in the elderly. Malnutrition can then increase the likelihood of some diseases. The result is a vicious cycle. Older Americans must be encouraged to value good nutrition. They may sometimes need assistance with shopping or food preparation. Food assistance programs such as food stamps and Senior Citizen's Congregate Meals can help facilitate better nutrition.

Older Americans are particularly vulnerable to health fraud. They should be cautioned to be wary of products promoting quick and painless cures, "secret" formulas, or "scientific breakthroughs." Suspicious products and treatments should be discussed with a doctor, dietitian, nurse, or other health professional.

REFERENCES AND SUGGESTED READINGS

1. American Academy of Pediatrics, Committee on Nutrition: The use of whole cows milk in infancy, Pediatrics 72:253, 1983.
2. Anderson JW and others: Dietary fiber and diabetes: A comprehensive review and practical application, J Am Diet Assoc 87(9):1189, 1987.
3. Center for Science in the Public Interest: New fiber scorecard, Nutrition Action Newsletter 17(2):8, 1990.
4. Council on Scientific Affairs: Vitamin preparations as dietary supplements and as therapeutic agents, JAMA 257:1929, 1987.
5. Glanze WD, editor: Mosby's medical & nursing dictionary, ed 3, St Louis, 1990, The CV Mosby Co.
6. Greenwald P, Lanza E, and Eddy GA: Dietary fiber in the reduction of colon cancer risk, J Am Diet Assoc 87(9):1178, 1987.
7. Hamilton EN, Whitney EN, and Sizer FS: Nutrition: concepts and controversies, ed 4, St Paul, 1988, West Publishing Co.
8. Iacono JM: Dietary intervention studies to reduce risk factors related to cardiovascular diseases and cancer, Prev Med 16:516, 1987.
9. Klurfeld DM: The role of dietary fiber in gastrointestinal disease, J Am Diet Assoc 87(9):1172, 1987.
10. Lucas AF and Huse DM: Behavioral disorders affecting food intake: Anorexia nervosa and bulimia. In Shils ME and Young VR, editors: Modern nutrition in health and disease, ed 7, Philadelphia, 1988, Lea & Febiger.
11. McCormick DB: Niacin. In Shils ME and Young VR, editors: Modern nutrition in health and disease, ed 7, Philadelphia, 1988, Lea & Febiger.
12. Monsen ER: Iron nutrition and absorption: dietary factors which impact iron bioavailability, J Am Diet Assoc 88:786, 1988.
13. National Research Council: Recommended dietary allowances, ed 10, Washington, DC, 1989, National Academy Press.
14. Nielsen FH: Ultratrace minerals. In Shils ME and Young VR, editors: Modern nutrition in health and disease, ed 7, Philadelphia, 1988, Lea & Febiger.
15. Rock CL and Yager J: Nutrition and eating disorders: a primer for clinicians, Int J Eating Disorders 6:276, 1987.
16. Satter E: How to get your kid to eat—but not too much, Palo Alto, 1987, Bull Publishing Co.
17. US Department of Health and Human Services: The surgeon general's report on nutrition and health, DHHS (PHS) Pub No 88-50211, Washington, DC, 1989, National Academy Press.
18. USDA and US Department of Health and Human Services: Dietary guidelines for Americans, ed 2, Home and Garden Bull No 232, 1985.
19. Whitney EN, Hamilton EN, and Rolfes SR: Understanding nutrition, ed 5, St Paul, 1990, West Publishing Co.
20. Williams SR: Basic nutrition and diet therapy, ed 8, St Louis, 1988, Times Mirror/Mosby College Publishing.
21. Williams SR: Essentials of Nutrition and diet therapy, ed 5, St Louis, 1990, Times Mirror/Mosby College Publishing.

CHAPTER CHALLENGE

KEY POINTS

- Nutrients are necessary for the proper functioning of all life processes in the body.
- Nurses play an important role in promoting good nutrition.
- Food planning guides such as the Four Food Groups, the Dietary Guidelines for Americans, and the Recommended Dietary Allowances (RDAs) have been developed to plan and assess diets for nutritional adequacy.
- The six classes of essential nutrients include carbohydrates, proteins, fats, vitamins, minerals, and water.
- Kilocalories are a measure of energy. Carbohydrates, proteins, and fats provide energy.
- Dietary fiber, found abundantly in whole grains, legumes, and fruits and vegetables, may exert a protective effect against certain diseases such as diverticulosis, constipation, cancer, and heart disease. It may also help in the control of diabetes mellitus and obesity.
- Fat and cholesterol are carried in the blood stream in the form of lipoproteins. Elevated levels of low-density lipoproteins (LDL) combined with lower levels of high-density lipoproteins (HDL) may lead to heart disease. Reduced consumption of saturated fats and cholesterol may help lower LDL levels.
- The essential nutrients perform specific functions in the body. Marginal intakes and deficiencies lead to dysfunction of various body systems.
- Excesses of nutrients may lead to system dysfunction as well. Overnutrition may be related to heart disease, hypertension, cancer, obesity, and dental caries.
- For normal, healthy Americans, well-planned diets can provide adequate nutrition without supplementation.
- Nutrient needs change during pregnancy and lactation to facilitate fetal and maternal growth and milk production. Nutrient-dense foods should provide the bulk of kilocalories. Vitamin/mineral supplements are generally recommended.
- Infancy and childhood are years of rapid growth and change. Good nutrition is vital for proper development. During these years dietary habits are being formed.
- Adolescents' nutritional status may be affected by high consumption of fast foods and kilocalorie-rich snacks, the stress of puberty, alcohol and drug use, and peer pressure. The eating disorders anorexia nervosa and bulimia may appear at this age. Emphasis should be placed on promoting good health and individuality.
- Lower activity levels combined with a constant kilocaloric intake in adults often leads to obesity. Nutrient-dense foods and active life-styles should be encouraged.
- Social, physical, psychological, and financial factors can affect nutritional status of the elderly. Diet planning should be individualized, keeping these various factors in mind.

STUDY QUESTIONS

1. The main function of carbohydrate in the body is to:
   a. Provide energy
   b. Provide structure to cell walls
   c. Control digestive processes
   d. Synthesize fat
2. Most experts recommend that fat intake in adults should be at ___ of kilocalories or less:
   a. 10%
   b. 20%
   c. 30%
   d. 40%
3. The RDAs for nutrients are:
   a. The minimum amounts needed for individuals
   b. Set high enough to meet the needs of practically all healthy Americans
   c. The exact amounts of nutrients needed for each individual
   d. The same for both men and women
4. A patient with iron-deficiency anemia asks you to explain ways to increase iron absorption. Which of the following would be the best response:
   a. Consume vitamin C–rich foods and iron-rich foods at the same meal
   b. Eat more legumes
   c. Drink coffee or tea at each meal
   d. Increase bran in the diet
5. Calcium intake for the prevention of osteoporosis is most effective at what age:
   a. Before age 25
   b. Throughout adulthood
   c. After menopause in women or age 65 in men
6. The water-soluble vitamins include:
   a. Vitamins A, D, E, and K
   b. B vitamins and vitamin D
   c. Vitamins C and A
   d. B vitamins and vitamin C
7. Which of the following statements about vitamin C is true:
   a. Most people need a vitamin C supplement
   b. Vitamin C needs are decreased in smokers
   c. The only food group that contains appreciable amounts of vitamin C is the fruit and vegetable group
   d. Vitamin C prevents cancer
8. What is the appropriate age for introduction of solid foods to the infant:
   a. 2 weeks to 1 month of age
   b. 2 to 3 months of age
   c. 4 to 6 months of age
   d. Not before 9 to 12 months of age
9. Anorexia nervosa is:
   a. Binge eating alternated with self-induced vomiting
   b. Loss of appetite
   c. An eating disorder characterized by self-imposed starvation
   d. An eating disorder that can be easily treated with medication

Match each nutrient with the statement that describes it best.

10. _____ Niacin	a. Destroyed by ultraviolet light
11. _____ Vitamin B_{12}	b. Can be synthesized from exposure to sunlight
12. _____ Iron	c. A trace mineral important in dental health
13. _____ Fluoride	d. Deficiency leads to goiter
14. _____ Vitamin A	e. In those with low blood levels of this nutrient supplementation improves wound healing
15. _____ Vitamin D	f. An important component of hemoglobin
16. _____ Riboflavin	g. Necessary for the production of collagen
17. _____ Zinc	h. Deficiency leads to night blindness
18. _____ Iodine	i. Requires intrinsic factor for absorption
19. _____ Vitamin C	j. Deficiency disease of this nutrient is called pellagra

23

Diet Therapy

KRISTEN KARTCHNER MAUGHAN

LEARNING OBJECTIVES

After reading this chapter, the student should be able to do the following:

- Define the key terms.
- Discuss nurse's role in diet therapy.
- Identify standard hospital diets and modifications for texture, consistency, and meal frequency.
- List medical or surgical conditions that require a high-kilocalorie diet, and discuss ways to increase kilocalories in the diet.
- Define obesity. List the three necessary components of an effective weight management program.
- Compare the diets in the treatment of insulin-dependent diabetes mellitus (IDDM) and non-insulin-dependent diabetes mellitus (NIDDM).
- List conditions that require a fat-modified diet, and compare fat-controlled and low-fat diets.
- Identify high-fat foods and food preparation methods that should be limited in fat-controlled and low-fat diets.
- Discuss medical or surgical conditions requiring modifications in sodium, potassium, and/or fluid.
- Identify food items to avoid or limit on sodium-restricted diets.
- Discuss rationale for protein restriction in renal and liver disease.
- Identify tube feeding routes of administration, and list medical or surgical conditions that may require a tube feeding.
- Define parenteral nutrition, and describe the two methods of administration. List medical or surgical conditions where parenteral nutrition may be indicated.
- Describe the responsibilities of the nurse in monitoring the patient on nutritional support.

RELATED TOPICS OF INTEREST

- Basic nutrition (Chapter 22)
- The surgical patient (Chapter 26)
- Fluid and electrolytes (Chapter 28)
- Care of the patient with an integumentary disorder (Chapter 29)
- Care of the patient with a gastrointestinal disorder (Chapter 31)
- Care of the patient with a cardiovascular disorder (Chapter 32)
- Care of the patient with a urinary disorder (Chapter 33)
- Care of the patient with an endocrine disorder (Chapter 35)

KEY TERMS

Define the following:

- anorexia
- anuria
- atherosclerosis
- basal metabolic rate (BMR)
- diet therapy
- diverticulitis
- diverticulosis
- dumping syndrome
- enteral nutrition
- exacerbation
- hyperglycemia
- hyperlipidemia
- hypoglycemia
- inflammatory bowel disease
- ketoacidosis
- myocardial infarction (MI)
- obesity
- oliguria
- parenteral nutrition
- peptic ulcer
- peripheral parenteral nutrition (PPN)
- postprandial
- residue
- total parenteral nutrition (TPN)
- tube feeding

Diet therapy is the treatment of disease through diet. It involves modifying diets in such a way as to meet the requirements created by disease or injury. A diet used as a medical treatment is called a therapeutic diet. If a patient needs a special diet, the physician should prescribe the diet and write the diet order in the medical record. The therapeutic diet is planned by the dietitian and usually served and monitored by the nurse. Nurses and other health professionals should consult with the physician when conditions may necessitate a change in diet order.

THE NURSE AND DIET THERAPY

Hospital food service must accommodate a wide range of patients from varying backgrounds. Many different therapeutic diets must be planned, and the number and type of meals to be served changes daily. It is no wonder hospital food does not always measure up to "home cookin'." Nevertheless, hospital menus are planned to be nutritionally adequate and well balanced. Efforts are made to accommodate each individual patient. Patients sometimes have a negative perception of hospital food. If they are on a restricted diet, they may have even less of a desire to eat.

The nurse can make an impact on the patients nutritional therapy in a number of ways. First, it is imperative for the nursing and dietary department to have a working communication link. For example, if a patient who has a food allergy is admitted, the nurse should inform the dietary department promptly so as to avoid having that particular food sent to the patient. Or, if a diagnostic test is being performed that requires that the patient omit breakfast, the nurse could alert dietary the night before and ask them to withhold breakfast but send a snack at the time the patient will be back from the test. Also, the nurse works closely with the patient on a daily basis and may notice whether inappropriate foods are served or whether the patient has an inadequate intake or manifests clinical signs of malnutrition. It is essential for the nurse to report these findings to the dietitian and physician so proper nutrition intervention can occur.

Second, meal trays should be served in a positive manner. Nurses should avoid making negative statements about the food. Meal trays should be served promptly while foods are at the correct temperature. Some patients may need assistance opening milk cartons, cutting meats, or sitting up to eat. The nurse must be sensitive to these needs, for many patients will leave the food uneaten rather than ask for help.

THERAPEUTIC DIETS

Consistency, Texture, and Frequency Modifications

Often when we think of therapeutic diets we think of nutrient-modified diets, such as low-fat or low-sodium diets. But modifications in textures, consistencies, and meal frequency may also be therapeutic.

Table 23-1 Foods Included in Liquid Diets

Clear Liquid	Full Liquid
Bouillon	All clear liquids
Fat-free broth	Strained cereals
Grape,* apple, cranberry juice	Strained soups
Fruit drinks	Fruit and vegetable juices
Popsicles	Milk, milkshakes
Gelatin	Ice cream, sherbet
Tea,* coffee*	Custard
Ginger ale, lemon-lime soda	Puddings

* Some facilities restrict the use of these items.

Most hospitals have standard diets based on consistency, specifically: liquid, soft, and regular diets.

Liquid diets. The two types of liquid diets are clear liquid and full liquid. The clear liquid diet is a nonirritating diet consisting of liquids that are easily digested and absorbed and leave little residue in the gastrointestinal (GI) tract. This diet may be used before diagnostic tests, particularly tests on the GI tract, or before surgery. It is commonly used postoperatively until the bowel resumes activity and may also be used during times of vomiting or diarrhea. The clear liquid diet is low in kilocalories, protein, and most nutrients. It should be used temporarily and for less than 1 week.

The full liquid diet is used as a transition diet after a clear liquid diet. It may be used until the patient is ready for solid foods. A full liquid diet is more nutritionally complete than clear liquid but is still lacking in some nutrients, such as iron and zinc and fiber. This diet too, should only be used temporarily. Table 23-1 lists foods included in both of the liquid diets.

Soft diets. Soft diets can be used as an intermediate diet when the patient is progressing from a liquid to a regular diet. Soft diets may also be used on a long-term basis for those with conditions affecting the GI tract. A soft diet is sometimes called a low-fiber diet. It can include foods from all four food groups including meats, fish, poultry, eggs, milk, grains, and fruits and vegetables. Foods excluded are whole grains and cereals; nuts; seeds; bran; fried meats, fish or poultry; fried eggs; fried breads and pastries; legumes, peas, corn, and gas-producing vegetables such as cabbage; raw fruits (except bananas); and raw vegetables. Foods with strong spices may also be limited.

The low-residue diet is a variation of the soft diet. Its restrictions are similar to the soft or low-fiber diet, but the diet may also exclude milk and milk products because they leave more **residue** in the colon. If milk is omitted, care should be taken that the patient receives adequate calcium from other sources.

Both soft and low-residue diets are used in the treatment of diverticulitis, particularly during periods of **exacerbation.** Other GI conditions for which these diets are prescribed include **inflammatory bowel disease,** gastritis, and periods of diarrhea or indigestion. See Chapter 31 for more information on GI disorders.

The mechanical soft diet is specifically for those with chewing or swallowing difficulties. The diet eliminates foods that are difficult to chew or swallow. Other foods may be chopped, pureed, or liquified. This diet must be individualized depending on the extent of chewing or swallowing difficulties.

Bland diet. The bland diet of the past was a restrictive diet prescribed most often for patients with **peptic ulcers** (erosion of the tissue lining the stomach or duodenum). Spices and fiber were avoided, and milk and cream were consumed in excess. As long ago as 1971 the American Dietetic Association published a position paper stating that the rationale for the typical bland diet was not supported by scientific evidence. Yet these restrictive diets are sometimes still prescribed. A liberalized bland diet is now the preferred dietary treatment. Patients with peptic ulcers are instructed to individualize their diet, omitting foods that tend to bother them. In addition, all patients are to (1) eat smaller meals more often and eat in a relaxed environment, (2) avoid caffeinated beverages, such as coffee, tea, and colas (decaffeinated coffee is also restricted), (3) avoid pepper, chili powder, and cocoa, and (4) avoid alcohol. Adequate protein is necessary for the ulcer to heal. Treatment for peptic ulcer includes a combination of diet, medication, and rest.

High-fiber diets. The high-fiber diet is a variation of the regular diet and may be used therapeutically. It may be used as a treatment for some GI disorders and may induce a preventive effect against some diseases (see Chapter 22). High-fiber diets are used in the treatment of constipation. With adequate fluids, fiber can reduce constipation in the young, as well as the elderly. This diet is recommended for those with **diverticulosis** during the latent stages of the disease. Fiber seems to lessen the occurrence of **diverticulitis.** It may also help prevent diverticulitis in susceptible individuals. High-fiber diets are often used in treating diabetes, with other dietary controls to help regulate blood sugar. Complex carbohydrates and fiber seem to moderate the rise in **postprandial** blood glucose levels. High-fiber diets may also be used in the treatment of **atherosclerosis.**

The high-fiber diet uses foods with high-fiber content in place of similar foods with little, if any, fiber. For example, whole grain products, rather than refined, are used. Fresh cooked or raw fruits and vegetables, including peelings where possible, should be used, rather than canned or processed fruits and vegetables. Nurses should advise patients who are just beginning a high-fiber diet to increase intake gradually so the body can become accustomed to larger amounts of fiber. A table in Chapter 22 (Table 22-4) lists some high-fiber foods.

Meal frequency modifications. Often, especially in GI-related disorders, small, frequent meals will be used rather than three larger meals. Perhaps as many as six to eight small meals or snacks may be consumed daily. By eating smaller meals, the workload placed on the GI tract and cardiovascular system is less than that with a large meal.

Small, frequent meals may be used for GI disorders, such as hiatal hernia and epigastric distress, during periods of nausea or indigestion, for esophageal reflux, and in pancreatitis. They may also be prescribed after **myocardial infarction** (MI) and in congestive heart failure.

Kilocalorie Modifications

The body requires a specific amount of energy each day to carry out its tasks. Energy intake includes foods and beverages consumed daily. Energy output includes energy used for (1) **basal metabolic rate** (BMR), (2) physical activity, and (3) digestion of food. Energy balance is achieved when energy intake equals output. During energy balance, weight should remain constant. If energy intake is greater than output, positive energy balance results, causing weight gain. On the other hand, if intake is less than output, negative energy balance occurs leading to weight loss.

High-kilocalorie and high-protein diets. During times of physiological stress, such as after surgery, bone fractures, sepsis, burns, cancer, and some other disease states, the body's energy and protein needs are increased. Medical trauma can greatly increase the BMR, so that if energy needs are not met by diet, negative energy balance will result. The patient will lose protein stores and weight.

Many trauma and cancer patients suffer from **anorexia,** or lack of appetite, and may also have difficulty with the eating process. This further complicates the problem of nutritional inadequacies. Dietary treatment should aim at restoring energy balance in the normal weight patient or creating a positive energy balance in the underweight patient. High-kilocalorie and high-protein diets should provide increased amounts of kilocalories and protein in a small volume. Commercially prepared liquid supplements may be used. Other suggestions to help increase kilocalories and protein are listed in Box 23-1.

Of course, the diet should still provide a balance of foods from all the food groups. It should be kept in mind that the appearance of the food and how it is served may determine whether or not it is eaten. Those serving foods should do so with a positive attitude and encouragement. The meals should be as attractive as possible. Beverages, especially liquid supplements, should be served in glasses, not cans. Foods should be served at the correct temperature: meals should be served promptly, and snacks and supplements should be refrigerated if necessary.

If a patient is not able to consume adequate kilocalories or refuses to eat, nutritional support in the form of tube feedings or intravenous (IV) feedings may be considered. This is discussed later in the chapter.

BOX 23-1 SUGGESTIONS TO INCREASE KILOCALORIES AND PROTEIN

- Add extra powdered milk to milkshakes, beverages, soups, puddings, and cooked cereals
- Spread peanut butter on crackers, fruit, or celery
- Add cheese to casseroles, soups, and sauces
- Use extra meat, chicken, or fish in casseroles and soups
- Add sugar to foods where reasonable (this only adds kilocalories)
- Use generous amounts of kilocalorie-dense foods such as butter, margarine, mayonnaise, cream cheese, sour cream, and cream in recipes, as spreads, or as dips
- Add nuts and dried fruits to cereals, breads, or desserts
- Have snacks available at all times
- Encourage the patient to eat high-kilocalorie foods first and eat the lower-kilocalorie foods if still hungry

Kilocalorie-controlled and low-kilocalorie diets. Obesity is the condition of having an abnormally large amount of fat on the body. In the simplest terms, it is overfatness. Occurrence of obesity in the United States is estimated at 15% to 50% of adults, 20% to 30% of adolescents, and 6% to 15% of children.

Overweight may be defined as body weight 10% above a desirable weight, whereas obesity is a body weight 20% or more above desirable standards. These norms are roughly based on life insurance weight tables (Table 23-2) and are simple to use, but are not always accurate. Weighing more than the norm does not necessarily mean obesity. For example, a 6-foot, 225-lb male athlete, according to the weight table, is obese, but if his body composition is made up of more lean tissue and less fat, the muscles, and not the fat, account for the added weight.

Ideally, then, obesity should be determined using measures of body composition. Methods of measuring body composition include hydrostatic weighing (submerging the body in a tank of water and measuring displacement), fatfold thickness measures (measuring a pinch of skin using skinfold calipers), and electrical impedance tests (a small electrical current is transmitted through the body and its resistance measured). These methods measure percent of body fat and are better suited for determining obesity; however, they are not always available nor are they as simple as using a weight scale.

The cause of obesity is at best difficult to explain. Many factors may contribute to the positive energy balance that leads to obesity. Most experts agree that both heredity

Table 23-2 Metropolitan Life Insurance Co. Height and Weight Tables

	Weight in Pounds		
Height	Small Frame	Medium Frame	Large Frame
MEN*			
5′ 2″	128-134	131-141	138-150
5′ 3″	130-136	133-143	140-153
5′ 4″	132-138	135-145	142-156
5′ 5″	134-140	137-148	144-160
5′ 6″	136-142	139-151	146-164
5′ 7″	138-145	142-154	149-168
5′ 8″	140-148	145-157	152-172
5′ 9″	142-151	148-160	155-176
5′ 10″	144-154	151-163	158-180
5′ 11″	146-157	154-166	161-184
6′ 0″	149-160	157-170	164-188
6′ 1″	152-164	160-174	168-192
6′ 2″	155-168	164-178	172-197
6′ 3″	158-172	167-182	176-202
6′ 4″	162-176	171-187	181-207
WOMEN†			
4′ 10″	102-111	109-121	118-131
4′ 11″	103-113	111-123	120-134
5′ 0″	104-115	113-126	122-137
5′ 1″	106-118	115-129	125-140
5′ 2″	108-121	118-132	128-143
5′ 3″	111-124	121-135	131-147
5′ 4″	114-127	124-138	134-151
5′ 5″	117-130	127-141	137-155
5′ 6″	120-133	130-144	140-159
5′ 7″	123-136	133-147	143-163
5′ 8″	126-139	136-150	146-167
5′ 9″	129-142	139-135	149-170
5′ 10″	132-145	142-156	152-173
5′ 11″	135-148	145-159	155-176
6′ 0″	138-151	148-162	158-179

*Weights at ages 25 to 59 based on lowest mortality. Weight in pounds according to frame (in indoor clothing weighing 5 lb, shoes with 1″ heels).

†Weights at ages 25 to 59 based on lowest mortality. Weight in pounds according to frame (in indoor clothing weighing 3 lb, shoes with 1″ heels).

Courtesy of Metropolitan Life Insurance Company.

and life-style contribute to obesity. Regardless of cause, obesity is a major health problem, particularly in well-developed countries. Obese people have a higher incidence of non-insulin-dependent diabetes mellitus (NIDDM), high blood lipid levels, hypertension, coronary heart disease, postsurgical complications, gynecological irregularities, pregnancy-induced hypertension, and gout. Excess weight exacerbates arthritis and some respiratory problems. It can lead to varicose veins and abdominal hernias.

Obesity is resistant to treatment. Some studies have shown that if "cure" from obesity is defined as reduction to ideal weight and maintenance of that weight for 5 years, a person is more likely to recover from many forms of cancer than from obesity. Treatment of obesity has ranged from diets, medications, and psychotherapy to surgery. The goal of any treatment is to cause a negative energy balance resulting in weight loss. By far the most common treatment and probably the safest is a low-kilocalorie diet and exercise. Low-kilocalorie diets may be based on the exchange lists for meal planning discussed in the section of this chapter on diabetes mellitus. A successful weight reduction program should incorporate three major components: (1) a lower-kilocalorie diet, (2) exercise and physical activity, and (3) behavior modification and other life-style changes. The program should help prepare patients to control weight throughout life and not just on a temporary basis. Diet should be no less than 1200 kcal/day, and weight loss should occur at the rate of approximately 1 to 2 lb/week. Diets that require the purchase of specially prepared foods, supplements, or "magic" diet aides should be avoided. Persons trying to lose weight must learn to take charge of their own life and not rely on expensive products for weight control. Individuals consuming less than 1500 kcal/day may need to take a multivitamin/mineral supplement providing approximately 100% of the U.S. recommended dietary allowance (RDA).

Very-low-calorie diets (VLCD). VLCD programs, sometimes called liquid fasts, are being used increasingly in many hospital outpatient clinics and doctors' offices. These diets consist of a low-kilocalorie, nutritionally balanced, liquid diet providing 300 to 500 kcal/day. Throughout the liquid fast, patients are monitored by their physician and other health professionals. They should receive dietary and behavioral counseling and should be involved in an exercise program. The patient continues on the liquid fast for a given period, eating no other foods, and then begins a gradual refeeding program and is instructed on a diet for weight maintenance. In 1990 the American Dietetic Association issued the following statement on VLCDs:

> It is the position of the American Dietetic Association that while very-low-calorie diets promote rapid weight loss and may be beneficial for certain individuals, such diets may have health risks and should be undertaken only with the supervision of a multidisciplinary health team with monitoring by a physician and nutrition counseling by a registered dietitian.

Long-term results of VLCDs prove disappointing, showing a higher percentage of dieters regaining over half of the weight lost on the program. With VLCDs, as with any weight reduction regimen, the principles of weight management still apply. Unless exercise continues, food intake is controlled, and dietary habits are changed, weight loss will be only temporary.

Carbohydrate-Modified Diets

Diabetes mellitus. Probably the most common type of carbohydrate-modified diet is the diabetic diet used for those with diabetes mellitus. In diabetes mellitus beta cells in the pancreas do not produce enough insulin or cannot use it properly. Insulin is the hormone necessary to move glucose from the blood stream into the cells where it is used for energy. Without insulin, glucose builds up in the blood stream, leading to **hyperglycemia** (elevated blood glucose). Diabetes also may affect fat metabolism and increase levels of blood lipids (cholesterol and triglycerides). Over time, elevated blood glucose and lipid levels may cause serious long-term complications. See Chapter 35 for a discussion on diabetes mellitus.

Perhaps not enough emphasis has been placed on the role of diet in the management of diabetes. Proper diet is essential for blood glucose control and may help reduce insulin needs if strictly followed. By keeping blood glucose levels relatively constant and in an appropriate range, the risk of diabetic complications may be lessened. Persons with diabetes should continually be encouraged to follow their individualized meal plan. Dietary goals differ somewhat depending on the type of diabetes being treated.

Insulin-dependent diabetes mellitus (IDDM). IDDM occurs most often in children and adolescents. Those with IDDM do not produce insulin. The body cannot use glucose for energy and begins to burn fat. When fat is burned for energy in the absence of glucose, acid wastes called *ketones* are formed. Ketones build up in the blood and lead to a life-threatening condition called **ketoacidosis.** People with IDDM must take insulin to avoid this condition.

The most important principle for those with IDDM is consistency. Meals and snacks should be eaten at about the same time each day. The types and amounts of foods eaten should be similar from day to day. This is necessary because the carbohydrate eaten must balance the insulin administered each day. Carbohydrate intake should be distributed evenly throughout the day to provide adequate amounts of glucose for the available insulin to move from the blood stream to the cells. This is called carbohydrate distribution.

Those with IDDM should follow a diet that restricts the use of simple sugars, emphasizes adequate fiber intake, and limits dietary fat and cholesterol. The Exchange Lists for Meal Planning were developed by the American Diabetes Association and the American Dietetic Association for use in diabetic meal planning. Because of the flexibility and variation allowed in the exchange lists, they are often used in weight reduction programs as well. Foods are divided into six food groups called *exchange lists.* The foods in each group are similar in protein, carbohydrate, fat, and caloric values. Thus a serving of any food from one exchange list should have approximately the same nutrient and caloric value as another food in the same list. The six exchange lists, their nutrient values, and representative foods from each are found in Box 23-2.

The patient should be given a meal plan to follow that specifies the number of food choices (exchanges) to be consumed at each meal and snack. Carbohydrate is distributed among the meals to correspond with insulin dosage. Table 23-3 shows an example of a 1500-kcal meal plan. Although the meal plan should be followed each day, the individual can vary food choices for variety. Menu 1 and menu 2 on Table 23-3 are examples of menus that fit into the same 1500-kcal meal plan.

If a person taking insulin fails to consume adequate carbohydrate, blood glucose levels may drop, causing **hypoglycemia** (low blood glucose). Symptoms of hypoglycemia may include headache, confusion, weakness, perspiration, shallow breathing, nervousness, visual disturbances, and vertigo and may lead to unconsciousness. Sometimes the person experiencing hypoglycemia may be mistakenly judged to be intoxicated. Proper medical identification should be worn to prevent such a mistake. Hypoglycemia should be treated with immediate administration of glucose in a readily available form, such as orange juice, followed by food containing both carbohydrate and protein. If juice is not available, sugar or hard candy may be eaten. In the event unconsciousness has occurred, glucose should be administered intravenously.

In times of illness, the patient with diabetes may not want to eat the usual foods on the meal plan. In such cases, it is essential to provide carbohydrate in the diet to correspond with insulin dosage. Carbohydrate-containing beverages, such as juices and punch, should be offered. Popsicles, flavored gelatin, crackers, puddings, and ice milk provide carbohydrate and may be better accepted during illness.

Non-insulin-dependent diabetes mellitus (NIDDM). NIDDM usually occurs in adults, many of whom are overweight. People with NIDDM produce insulin, but either there is not enough insulin or the body is unable to use it properly. This type of diabetes often may be controlled by diet and exercise. Some people with NIDDM use oral hypoglycemic agents, medications that stimulate insulin production and use. In some instances insulin injections may be needed to help regulate blood glucose levels. Whenever insulin is administered, the dietary principles for IDDM should be used.

Many people with NIDDM are overweight, and one of the major dietary goals with this type of diabetes is weight control. For the obese person with NIDDM, weight reduction can help control blood glucose and reduce the need for medication. Kilocalorie control is more important than carbohydrate distribution in this type of diabetes. A diet using the exchange lists is an ideal method of weight control. As with IDDM, simple sugar should

BOX 23-2 EXCHANGE LISTS FOR MEAL PLANNING

LIST 1: STARCH/BREAD LIST

Each serving contains: 15 g carbohydrate, 3 g protein, trace of fat
80 kcal

Representative servings: ½ c cooked cereal, pasta, or starchy vegetables; 1 oz of a bread product (1 slice bread); ¾ c ready-to-eat cereal; ⅓ c cooked rice

LIST 2: MEAT LIST

Each serving contains: 7 g protein, 5 g fat, no carbohydrate 75 kcal

Representative servings: 1 oz lean meat, fish, or poultry; 1 oz low-fat cheese or ¼ c cottage cheese; 1 egg

LIST 3: VEGETABLE LIST

Each serving contains: 5 g carbohydrate, 2 g protein, no fat
25 kcal

Representative servings: ½ c cooked vegetables or vegetable juice; 1 c raw vegetables

LIST 4: FRUIT LIST

Each serving contains: 15 g carbohydrate, no protein or fat
60 kcal

Representative servings: 1 medium-sized piece fresh fruit; ½ c canned fruit or fruit juice; ¼ c dried fruit; 1 c cubed melon or berries

LIST 5: MILK LIST

Each serving contains: 12 g carbohydrate, 8 g protein, trace of fat
90 kcal

Representative servings: 1 c skim milk, 1% milk, or buttermilk; 1 c plain low-fat yogurt

LIST 6: FAT LIST

Each serving contains: 5 g fat, very little protein or carbohydrate

Representative servings: 1 tsp butter, margarine, or oil; 1 Tbls cream or salad dressings; 1 Tbls chopped nuts; 1 tsp mayonnaise; 1 slice bacon; 2 Tbls coconut

From American Diabetes Association and American Dietetic Association: Exchange lists for meal planning, 1986.

Table 23-3 1500-kcal Meal Plan and Menu Examples Using the Exchange Lists for Meal Planning

Meal	Exchange List	Number of Servings	Menu 1	Menu 2
Breakfast	Starch/bread	2	1 slice wheat toast ½ c oatmeal	1 whole wheat bagel (2 halves)
	Fruit	1	½ c orange juice	1 fresh peach
	Milk	1	1 c skim milk	1 c plain yogurt
	Fat	1	1 tsp margarine	1 Tbls cream cheese 1 c coffee, black (free)
Lunch	Starch/bread	3	2 slices wheat bread 3 gingersnaps	1 hamburger bun ½ c potato salad
	Meat	2	½ c tuna (water)	2 oz ground beef, lean
	Vegetable	1	1 c carrot & celery sticks, raw	½ c tomato juice cucumber slices (free)
	Fruit	1	1 small apple	15 grapes
	Fat	1	2 tsp salad dressing	2 tsp dressing in potato salad
Supper	Starch/bread	2	⅔ c brown rice	½ c mashed potatoes ½ c stuffing
	Meat	2	2 oz top round steak	2 oz roast turkey
	Vegetable	1	½ c mixed vegetables	½ c asparagus
	Fruit	1	¾ c fresh pineapple	1 c melon balls
	Milk	1	1 c skim milk	1 c skim milk
	Fat	1	1 tsp oil for stir-frying	¼ c turkey gravy
Snack	Starch/bread	1	½ English muffin	3 squares graham crackers
	Meat	1	1 oz mozzarella cheese melted on muffin	¼ c cottage cheese
	Fruit	1	1 c whole strawberries	½ c fruit cocktail
	Fat	1	2 Tbls whipped cream	1 Tbls sunflower seeds

be restricted and adequate fiber intake emphasized.

Exercise reduces blood glucose levels. This is helpful in the control of blood glucose and is also important for weight control. People with either type of diabetes may be able to reduce insulin or medication needs with regular exercise. Diet can also be adjusted to compensate for exercise. If a patient with IDDM is to be involved in a physical activity that he is not accustomed to, some carbohydrate-containing food (milk, fruits, vegetables, or starches) may be added to the meal just before engaging in the activity. In this way the extra carbohydrate will provide more glucose to satisfy the demands of exercise.

Dumping syndrome. Dumping syndrome may occur after surgery where a portion or all of the stomach is removed (partial or total gastrectomy). After partial or total gastrectomy, the stomach contents may empty too rapidly into the jejunum. The body reacts by sending water to the intestinal tract, thus blood pressure is reduced. The load in the intestinal tract increases peristalsis (contractions that move food through the GI tract), leading to diarrhea. Symptoms occur 15 to 30 minutes after meals and include cramping, weakness, diaphoresis, vertigo, nausea, and possibly vomiting.

Diet therapy involves giving small, frequent meals that are higher in protein and fat and lower in carbohydrates. Concentrated sweets should be avoided, and fluids should be taken 30 to 60 minutes before or after a meal. The dumping syndrome diet may be needed only temporarily until the body adjusts to the changes caused by surgery.

Lactose intolerance. Lactose intolerance occurs as a result of a lack of the digestive enzyme *lactase*. Because of this, the GI tract is unable to break down lactose, the milk sugar. Symptoms occur after ingestion of milk products and include nausea, cramps, a bloated feeling, flatulence, and diarrhea.

Diet for lactose intolerance excludes milk and milk products, such as ice cream, puddings, cheese, and powdered milk. Foods with milk added, such as biscuit or muffin mixes, some soups, and other prepared foods, may need to be avoided.

Some individuals have a deficiency rather than a total absence of lactase. These individuals may be able to tolerate small amounts of milk products. Yogurt and cheese are often well tolerated. Lactase enzyme–containing preparations are available and can be added to milk before drinking.

Fat-Modified Diets

As mentioned in Chapter 22, fat- and cholesterol-controlled diets may be beneficial in reducing the risk of atherosclerosis and certain cancers. Dietary fat intake may also be modified in the treatment of disease.

Fat-controlled diets. A fat-controlled diet is desirable for the treatment of atherosclerosis, heart disease, and **hyperlipidemias.** Diabetic diets also incorporate fat control. A fat-controlled diet limits both total fat and saturated fat intake. Usually when saturated fat intake is reduced, cholesterol intake also drops, since it is often found in foods containing saturated fat. The individual who is reducing saturated fat in the diet should choose low-fat dairy products, lean meats, skinless poultry, and fish. Eggs should be limited to three per week and organ meats, such as liver, limited to one serving per week or less. Visible fats, such as butter, margarine, mayonnaise, cream, sour cream, nuts, and rich desserts, should be limited. Cooking methods may need to be altered as well. Patients should be encouraged to bake, broil, or poach food, rather than to fry and add breading or batter to it. Foods should be eaten without the addition of sauces, gravies, or dips that are high in fat.

When fat is necessary in food preparation, unsaturated fats (monounsaturated and polyunsaturated) should be used in place of saturated fats. Table 23-4 shows dietary guidelines for implementing a fat-controlled diet.

Low-fat diets. Other medical conditions warrant the use of a low-fat diet. Low-fat diets differ from fat-controlled diets in that all fats are limited, regardless of saturation. Any time fat malabsorption occurs, dietary fat should be limited. GI diseases that involve malabsorption of fat include cystic fibrosis, inflammatory bowel disease, pancreatitis, and short-bowel syndrome (secondary to bowel resection). Gallbladder disease often requires a low-fat diet. The gallbladder stores bile and contracts whenever fat is present in the intestinal tract. If gallstones are present or inflammation of the gallbladder exists, contraction may be painful. A low-fat diet may alleviate some discomfort. After the gallbladder is removed (cholecystectomy), a low-fat diet is no longer required. Some patients with gallbladder disease may be overweight or obese. Weight reduction is indicated for these individuals and may reduce symptoms of gallbladder disease.

Protein-, Electrolyte-, and Fluid-Modified Diets

Protein-restricted diets. In disease states, increased protein needs are often considered to facilitate healing. However, in the presence of defects in protein metabolism or excretion, protein intake should be reduced or controlled. One such case is during renal failure. Renal failure can occur rapidly (acute renal failure) or may progress slowly (end-stage renal disease). Acute renal failure is often temporary, whereas end-stage renal disease is irreversible.

The kidney normally functions to excrete wastes, concentrate urine, and conserve needed electrolytes. During renal failure the nephrons (working units of the kidney) fail to maintain normal function. **Oliguria** (decreased urine output) or **anuria** (no urine output) may result. Urea and other nitrogenous wastes, the end products of protein metabolism, build up in the blood stream, leading to a condition known as *azotemia*. Many electrolytes, particularly potassium, sodium, and phosphorus, are re-

Table 23-4 Guidelines for Lowering Fat, Saturated Fat, and Cholesterol

Food Groups	Choose	Decrease
Fish, chicken, turkey, and lean meats (3-oz cooked portions)	Fish, poultry without skin, lean cuts of beef, lamb, pork, or veal, shellfish	Fatty cuts of beef, lamb, pork, spare ribs, organ meats, regular cold cuts, sausages, hot dogs, bacon, sardines, roe
Skim and low-fat milk, cheese, yogurt, and dairy substitutes	Skim or 1%-fat milk (liquid, powdered, evaporated), buttermilk	Whole milk: (4% fat) regular, evaporated, condensed; cream, half and half; 2% milk, imitation milk products, most nondairy creamers, whipped toppings
	Nonfat (0% fat) or low-fat yogurt	Whole-milk yogurt
	Low-fat cottage cheese (1% or 2% fat)	Whole-milk cottage cheese (4% fat)
	Low-fat cheeses, farmer or pot cheeses (all of these should be labeled "no more than 2 to 6 g fat per oz")	All natural cheeses (e.g., bleu, Roquefort, Camembert, cheddar, Swiss)
		Low-fat or "light" cream cheese, low-fat or "light" sour cream
		Cream cheeses, sour cream
	Sherbet, sorbet	Ice cream
Eggs	Egg whites (2 whites = 1 whole egg in recipes), cholesterol-free egg substitutes	Egg yolks
Fruits and vegetables	Fresh, frozen, canned, or dried fruits and vegetables	Vegetables prepared with butter, cream, or other sauces
Breads and cereals	Homemade baked goods using unsaturated oils sparingly, angel food cake, low-fat crackers, low-fat cookies	Commercially baked goods; pies, cakes, doughnuts, croissants, pastries, muffins, biscuits, high-fat crackers, high-fat cookies
	Rice, pasta	Egg noodles
	Whole-grain breads and cereals (e.g., oatmeal, whole wheat, rye, bran, multigrain)	Breads in which eggs are major ingredient
Fats and oils	Baking cocoa	Chocolate
	Unsaturated vegetable oils: corn, olive, rapeseed, safflower, sesame, soybean, sunflower	Butter, coconut oil, palm oil, palm kernel oil, lard, bacon fat
	Margarine or shortenings made from one of the unsaturated oils listed above	
	Diet margarine	
	Mayonnaise, salad dressings made with unsaturated oils listed above	Dressings made with egg yolk
	Low-fat dressings	
	Seeds and nuts	Coconut

tained, and increased blood levels of these nutrients may occur.

Because of the buildup of protein waste products, dietary protein should be restricted. A therapeutic diet for renal failure limits the amount of protein consumed; the degree of limitation depends on the extent of renal failure. Patients are encouarged to consume moderate amounts of only high-quality, or complete, proteins found in milk, meat, fish, poultry, and eggs. Incomplete proteins, those found in plant products, contribute to uremia and should be restricted. Other dietary modifications in renal failure include the restriction of potassium, sodium, phosphorus, and fluids. Vitamin/mineral supplements are generally prescribed.

Cirrhosis is a chronic, degenerative disease of the liver. It is most often seen secondary to alcoholism but may also be seen as a result of hepatitis A and B or other infection. Scar tissue develops in the liver, hampering its effectiveness in removing waste products from the blood stream. In this case ammonia, a waste product of protein metabolism, builds up in the blood stream. If not controlled, high ammonia levels may contribute to hepatic coma (coma secondary to liver disease), brain damage, and death. Ascites, a condition characterized by accumulation of fluid in the abdominal cavity, may occur. If the liver is unable to produce bile, fat malabsorption also may take place.

In the presence of cirrhosis, protein intake should ini-

BOX 23-3 LOW-PROTEIN DIETS: 15 g, 30 g, 40 g, and 50 g PROTEIN

GENERAL DESCRIPTION

- The following diets are used when dietary protein is to be restricted.
- The patterns limit foods containing a large percentage of protein, such as milk, eggs, cheese, meat, fish, fowl, and legumes.
- Meat extractives, soups, broth, bouillon, gravies, and gelatin desserts should also be avoided.

BASIC MEAL PATTERNS (contain approximately 15 g of protein)

Breakfast	Lunch	Dinner
½ c fruit or fruit juice	1 small potato	1 small potato
½ c cereal	½ c vegetable	½ c vegetable
1 slice toast	Salad (vegetable or fruit)	Salad (vegetable or fruit)
butter	1 slice bread	1 slice bread
Jelly	Butter	Butter
Sugar	1 serving fruit	1 serving fruit
2 Tbls cream	Sugar	Sugar
Coffee	Coffee or tea	Coffee or tea

FOR 30 g PROTEIN

Add: 1 c milk
28 g (1 oz) meat, 1 egg, or equivalent

EXAMPLES OF MEAT PORTIONS

28 g (1 oz) meat = 1 thin slice roast, 4 × 5 cm (1½ × 2 in)
1 rounded tbsp cottage cheese
1 slice American cheese

FOR 40 g PROTEIN

Add: 1 c milk
70 g (2½ oz) meat, or 1 egg and
42 g (1½ oz) meat

70 g (2½ oz) meat = Ground beef patty (5 from 448 g [1 lb])
1 slice roast

FOR 50 g PROTEIN

Add: 1 c milk
112 g (4 oz) meat, or 2 eggs and
56 g (2 oz) meat

112 g (4 oz) meat = 2 lamb chops
1 average steak

tially be at or above the RDA to facilitate healing and tissue regeneration. However, if blood ammonia levels become elevated and signs of impending coma are present, such as confusion, apathy, and drowsiness, a strict low-protein diet should be followed. The low-protein diets for cirrhosis restrict milk and milk products, meats, fish, poultry, cheese, eggs, legumes, and nuts. Box 23-3 shows examples of various levels of protein restriction. Special nutritional support formulas with modified protein content have also been developed for hepatic coma.

The veins at the lower end of the esophagus may become enlarged and tortuous during cirrhosis, a condition called *esophageal varices*. Esophageal varices are painful, and the use of a soft or liquid diet may be beneficial in this case. Other dietary modifications for cirrhosis include total abstinence from alcohol and may require restriction of sodium and fluid if ascites occurs and fat restriction if malabsorption is present. Vitamin/mineral supplements are also given.

Sodium-restricted diets. Sodium restrictions may be used to treat a number of medical conditions. Hypertension is often responsive to a lowered sodium intake. It is estimated that 20% of the population is "sodium sensitive," that is, they have a genetic sensitivity to sodium that leads to hypertension. In such individuals sodium reduction appears beneficial in controlling blood pressure.

Sodium is also restricted when water retention or edema is present. In the presence of congestive heart failure sodium intake should be decreased to alleviate pulmonary and peripheral edema. Directly after a myocardial infarction, sodium, fluid, kilocalorie, and fat restrictions may be implemented. These restrictions are to minimize the work load on the heart. As recovery progresses, the diet will be liberalized as individual condition permits. If cirrhosis is accompanied by ascites, sodium intake should be reduced, and in renal failure, if anuria or oliguria exists, sodium should be restricted.

Sodium-restricted diets vary in degree of restriction. The no-added-salt (NAS) diet is the least restrictive, allowing 2000 to 3000 mg of sodium/day. This diet allows the use of most foods with the exception of highly salted

BOX 23-4 **FOODS TO AVOID IN SODIUM RESTRICTION* (250 mg to 2000 mg)**

1. Salt in cooking or at the table
2. Salty snack foods, i.e., chips, nuts, crackers, pretzels, salted popcorn
3. Regular canned soups
4. Salty condiments, such as soy sauce, barbeque sauce, Worcestershire and steak sauces, bouillon, prepared mustard, meat tenderizers, monosodium glutamate (MSG), spice salts, and regular salad dressings
5. Regular cheese and peanut butter, smoked or cured meats, luncheon meats, canned meats, corned beef, shellfish
6. Canned vegetables with salt, pickled foods, sauerkraut, and olives
7. Leavening agents, such as baking soda and baking powder
8. Commercially prepared foods and mixes, such as pudding, instant breakfast cereals, beverage mixes, biscuit and muffin mixes, cake and pastry mixes
9. Most ready-to-eat cereals
10. Commercially prepared milk mixes, such as ice milk and milkshakes
11. Salted butter and margarine

*The diet becomes more flexible the higher the sodium limit. Very strict low-sodium diets (250-500 mg) also incorporate the use of special dietetic products, such as low-sodium milk and breads.

snack foods and prepared foods. Patients following this diet should read nutrition labels to assess the sodium content of food products and determine which would be appropriate for their diet. No salt should be added in cooking or at the table. Other sodium-restricted diets range from 2000 mg (2 g) sodium to as little as 250 mg of sodium/day. Box 23-4 lists foods restricted on low-sodium diets.

In the presence of cystic fibrosis, the sweat glands produce excessive amounts of sodium and chloride. In this special condition sodium intake is not restricted, but generous amounts of sodium and salt are encouraged to compensate for the large losses of sodium.

Potassium-modified diets. Potassium is considered to play a role in blood pressure control. Evidence indicates that populations with higher potassium intakes have less incidence of hypertension. Increased potassium intake from foods may be beneficial for blood pressure control. Many patients with hypertension or other conditions that cause water retention may take potassium-wasting diuretics. An increased intake of potassium is needed to counteract the loss of potassium caused by the diuretic. Potassium-rich foods are listed in Table 22-9 in Chapter 22.

In end-stage renal disease and other kidney disease, potassium intake may need to be restricted to as little as 1500 to 2000 mg/day. In this case the foods listed in Table 22-9 should be restricted.

Fluid-modified diets. Fluid is found in the diet in a number of forms. Of course, all beverages, milk, juices, coffee, and tea add fluid to the diet. Other dietary fluid sources include gelatins, ice cream, sherbet, puddings, popsicles, fruit ices, and soups.

During end-stage renal disease and other kidney disease with oliguria or anuria, fluid is restricted to 400 to 500 ml/day plus an amount equal to daily urine output, if any. Fluid restrictions may also be implemented during congestive heart failure, directly after an MI, or in hepatic coma or ascites.

During fluid restrictions, patients may experience excessive thirst. Some suggestions to help alleviate thirst include rinsing the mouth with cold mouthwash, putting lemon into cold water to make it more refreshing, freezing fluid so it takes longer to consume, eating cold fruits and raw vegetables, chewing gum, sucking on breath mints or hard candies (in moderation), and brushing teeth often.

Increased fluid intake is a common dietary treatment for renal calculi (kidney stones) and urinary tract infection. Additional fluid helps to dilute the urine and increase urinary output. Fluid needs are also increased during periods of diarrhea, vomiting, or malabsorption, such as in inflammatory bowel disease. Care should be taken to replace fluids that are lost, to prevent dehydration.

The burn victim loses a large volume of fluids from the wounds. Immediately after a severe burn, fluids, electrolytes, and protein are given intravenously rather than orally, because burn patients experience a temporary loss of bowel function. Once bowel activity resumes, adequate fluids should be a part of dietary treatment.

Most conditions requiring diet therapy involve combinations of therapeutic diets. As a summary, Table 23-5 lists different medical conditions and their commonly prescribed diets.

NUTRITION SUPPORT

Occasionally a patient may not be able to consume an oral diet. For whatever reason, alternative feeding methods are available in the form of tube feedings or intravenous feedings.

Tube Feedings

A **tube feeding** is often referred to as **enteral nutrition** support. Tube feedings may be indicated when a patient is unable to chew or swallow, such as after oral surgery or facial trauma; when a person has no appetite or refuses to eat; in times of great nutritional needs, such as in the burn or trauma patient; in the comatose patient; or during periods of moderate malabsorption or diarrhea. Box

Table 23-5 Summary of Diet Modifications

Condition	Possible Diet Modifications
Acquired immune deficiency syndrome (AIDS)	High kilocalorie and protein; increased fluid intake; mechanical soft; possible tube feeding or TPN
Atherosclerosis	Fat controlled; high fiber; when necessary, kilocalorie- and/or sodium-restricted diet
Burns	High kilocalorie and protein; increased fluid intake; vitamin/mineral therapy
Cancer	High kilocalorie and protein; dietary adjustments made based on symptoms; possible tube feeding or TPN
Cirrhosis/hepatic coma	Protein restricted; possible sodium and fluid restriction
Congestive heart failure	Sodium-restricted; fluid-restricted; small, frequent feedings; soft diet; possible kilocalorie restriction
Constipation	High fiber; increased fluid intake
Cystic fibrosis	High kilocalorie and protein; low fat; generous sodium; vitamin and mineral supplementation
Diabetes mellitus	
IDDM	Carbohydrate controlled; no concentrated sweets; fat controlled; high fiber
NIDDM	Kilocalorie restricted; no concentrated sweets; fat controlled; high fiber
Diverticulitis	Soft, low residue
Diverticulosis	High fiber
Dumping syndrome	Carbohydrate restricted; no concentrated sweets; small, frequent feedings; fluids before or after meals; when necessary, fluid and electrolyte replacement
Gallbladder disease	Low fat, kilocalorie restricted
Gastritis	Low residue, liberalized bland
Hepatitis	High kilocalorie and protein
Hiatal hernia	Small, frequent feedings; low fat; bland; when necessary, kilocalorie restricted
Hyperlipidemia	Fat controlled; when necessary, kilocalorie restricted; carbohydrate controlled
Hypertension	Sodium restricted; high potassium; fat controlled; when necessary, kilocalorie restricted
Hypoglycemia	No concentrated sweets; small, frequent feedings
Inflammatory bowel disease	Low residue; low fat; high kilocalorie and protein; fluid and electrolyte replacement; vitamin/mineral supplementation; possible lactose restriction, tube feeding, or TPN
Lactose intolerance	Lactose restricted
Malabsorption	Low fat; high kilocalorie and protein; fluid and electrolyte replacement
Mouth, conditions affecting	
Broken jaw/oral surgery	Mechanical soft; possible tube feeding
Dental caries/periodontal disease/ill fitting dentures/missing teeth	Mechanical soft
Dry mouth	Mechanical soft; increased fluid intake
Dysphagia (difficulty swallowing)	Mechanical soft; possible tube feeding
Ulcers of mouth or gums	Mechanical soft; bland
Myocardial infarction	Low sodium; kilocalorie restricted; soft; bland; small, frequent feedings; fat controlled; fluid restricted (temporary); moderate temperature foods
Nausea	Soft; bland; small, frequent feedings
Obesity	Kilocalorie restricted; fat controlled; high fiber
Pancreatitis	Low fat; small, frequent feedings; possible tube feedings or TPN
Peptic ulcer	Liberalized bland diet
Reflux esophagitis	Small frequent feedings; low fat; bland
Renal calculi (kidney stones)	Increased fluid intake; possible calcium controlled
Renal failure	
Acute	Protein restricted; high kilocalorie; fluid, sodium, and potassium controlled
Chronic	Protein restricted; low sodium; potassium, fluid, and phosphorus restricted; vitamin/mineral supplement
Underweight	High kilocalorie and protein
Vomiting	Fluid and electrolyte replacement

Modified from Cataldo CB, Nyenhuis JR, and Whitney EN: Nutrition and diet therapy: principles and practice, ed 2, St Paul, 1989, West Publishing Co.

23-5 lists conditions that may require a tube feeding.

Tube feedings should be used only when all or at least part of the GI tract is functioning. Tube feedings are most commonly administered by way of a nasogastric tube, that is, a tube that is passed through the nose and into the stomach (Fig. 23-1). If regurgitation is common or gastric residual is high, a nasojejunal tube (a tube that is passed through the nose and into the jejunum) may be used to reduce the risk of aspiration.

In cases where long-term tube feedings are necessary, such as in a patient with a gastrectomy or intestinal resection, or in a patient with an upper GI obstruction, feeding ostomies may be employed. Ostomies are surgical openings through which a feeding tube may pass. Ostomies may be made into the pharynx (pharyngostomy), esophagus (esophagostomy), stomach (gastrostomy), or the jejunum (jejunostomy) (see Fig. 23-1). Ostomy feeding need not be continuous, but can be given intermittently, permitting more freedom of movement.

Formulas vary in composition. If the tube feeding is the sole source of nutrition, a complete formula that provides adequate kilocalories, protein, carbohydrate, fat, vitamins, and minerals to meet RDAs should be used. Intact formulas are formulas containing proteins, carbohydrates, and fats in whole forms, as found in foods. These formulas are available with or without fiber. Elemental or hydrolyzed formulas are available for individuals experiencing malabsorption, such as in inflammatory bowel disease, or for those who experience diarrhea and malabsorption with intact formulas. Elemental formulas are predigested, that is, the nutrients are already broken down into smaller units. Therefore they require little digestive action before being absorbed.

In the hospital, tube feedings can be fed on a contin-

BOX 23-5 **INDICATIONS FOR THE USE OF ENTERAL NUTRITION SUPPORT (TUBE FEEDING)**

- Protein kilocalorie malnutrition with inadequate intake for past 5 days
- Hospitalized patient consuming less than 50% of nutritional needs for past 7 to 10 days
- Severe dysphagia (difficulty swallowing)
- Major burns
- Sustained major trauma wounds
- Liver failure
- Renal dysfunction
- Radiation therapy
- Mild chemotherapy
- As adjunctive therapy with TPN for small bowel regeneration
- Low output enterocutaneous fistulas (abnormal passage from the intestine to the body surface) that can be successfully bypassed with a tube

Modified from ASPEN Board of Directors: Guidelines for the use of enteral nutrition in the adult patient, J Parenter Enteral Nutr 11(5): 435, 1987.

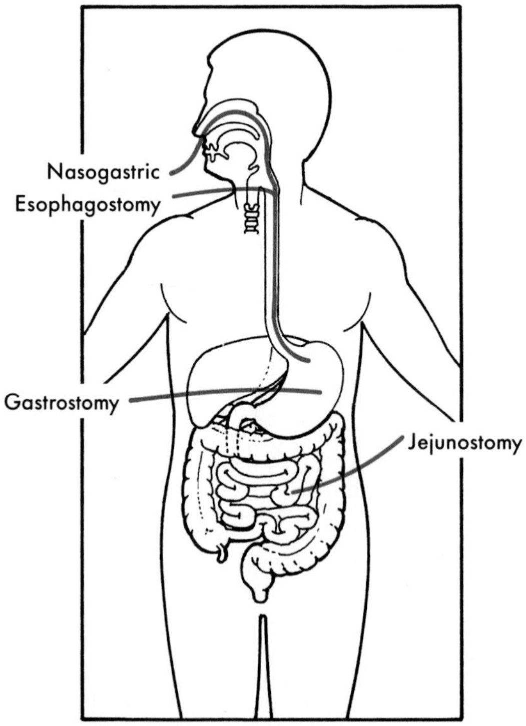

FIG. 23-1 Tube feeding sites.

uous basis, using a continuous drip pump that administers the formula slowly over 16 to 24 hours. Feedings may also be given intermittently. This involves giving a specific volume of formula over a short time, about 20 to 30 minutes. This may be done four to six times daily. Intermittent feeding is preferred by many long-term tube-fed patients. Bolus feedings (giving a 4- to-6-hour volume of formula in a matter of minutes) may also be given but are poorly tolerated in most patients.

Tube feedings should always be started slowly, and most formulas should be diluted to one third to one half of regular strength. The strength and the amount of formula can then be increased at different intervals until the full prescription is given. Distention, diarrhea, and nausea may indicate that the formula strength and/or volume is too great. Dumping syndrome may also occur with rapid and concentrated formula delivery.

Tube feeding is considered to be aggressive nutritional therapy. Complications may arise, including diarrhea; contamination of formula; infection; aspiration; overhydration or dehydration; abnormalities of blood concentrations of electrolytes, glucose, and other nutrients; and development of liver abnormalities. The patient should be monitored closely. A monitoring checklist for the tube-fed patient is found in Table 23-6.

Parenteral Nutrition Support

Parenteral nutrition is the term used to describe intravenous feedings. Parenteral nutrition may be administered through peripheral veins, such as those in the arms or legs. This administration route is called **peripheral parenteral nutrition (PPN).** The term **total parenteral nutrition (TPN)** usually refers to administration into a large central vein (most often the superior vena cava), by way of the subclavian vein, or by way of the internal jugular vein (Fig. 23-2). TPN and PPN formulas are composed of glucose, amino acids, vitamins, minerals, and electrolytes. Fat, in the form of triglycerides, is also given as a supplement to the main formula. It is administered separately through a Y-connector tube.

Parenteral nutrition support is indicated for the patient with a nonfunctioning or dysfunctioning GI tract. Many

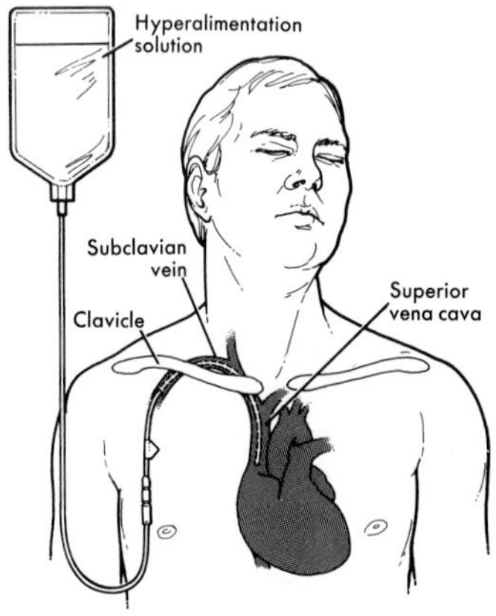

FIG. 23-2 Administration of total parenteral nutrition.

Table 23-6 Guidelines for Monitoring the Tube-Fed Patient

Frequency	Procedure
Before starting a new or intermittent feeding	Review nutritional assessment; check tube placement; check residual formula in stomach (if 150 ml, consider reasons for delayed gastric emptying)
Every ½ hour	Check gravity drip rate when applicable
Every hour	Check pump drip rate when applicable
Every 2 to 4 hours of continuous feeding	Check residual
Every 4 hours	Check vital signs, including blood pressure, temperature, pulse, and respiration; monitor blood glucose (may be discontinued after 48 hours if glucose is consistently normal in the nondiabetic patient)
Every 8 hours	Check intake and output Chart patient's acceptance of and tolerance to tube feeding
Every day	Weigh patient; change feeding bag and tubing (except portion of tube in GI tract); monitor electrolytes, blood urea nitrogen, and blood glucose until stabilized
Every 7 to 10 days	Check all laboratory findings; review current nutritional assessment and dietary goals
As needed	Observe patient for any undesirable responses to tube feeding, for example, nausea, vomiting, or diarrhea; check tube placement (nasogastric only); chart significant details

Modified from Cataldo CB, Nyenhuis JR, and Whitney EN: Nutrition and diet therapy: principles and practice, ed 2, St Paul, 1989, West Publishing Co.

patients with nonfunctioning GI tracts can be maintained on saline solutions for 5 to 7 days, but if the digestive tract is still nonfunctioning after that time, PPN or TPN should be initiated.

When intravenous nutrition is necessary, PPN should be the first choice of administration where possible. PPN carries less risk of complications, requires less monitoring, and costs less than the central venous route. Candidates for PPN are those needing 3000 or fewer kilocalories/day, those needing supplementation to oral diet, or those requiring short-term therapy (less than 3 weeks).

Total parenteral nutrition is indicated for patients needing a highly concentrated formula, such as those who need more kilocalories than can be administered peripherally or those requiring a fluid restriction—a concentrated formula delivers more kilocalories and nutrients in a smaller volume. Other candidates for TPN include those who must be on IV feedings for more than 3 weeks and those with unsuitable or unavailable peripheral veins. Box 23-6 identifies conditions requiring TPN.

TPN requires constant medical care. Central venous administration requires surgical placement of a catheter in one of the central veins. This imposes significant risks on the patient, including sepsis (major infection), pneumothorax (air in the pleural cavity), hemothorax (blood in the pleural cavity), phlebitis (inflammation of the vein), or thrombosis (blood clots). The catheter site must be kept aseptic, and feeding solutions must be sterile. Biochemical and clinical status of the patient must be constantly monitored.

The patient receiving TPN may experience fluid and electrolyte imbalances, hyperglycemia or hypoglycemia, metabolic disturbances, and bone disorders, such as osteomalacia (softening of the bones). For this reason blood chemistries should be monitored frequently. Blood glucose should be checked several times each day. Regular insulin may be administered on a sliding scale to maintain blood glucose levels below 200 mg/dl.

BOX 23-6

POSSIBLE INDICATIONS FOR THE USE OF TOTAL PARENTERAL NUTRITION

- Bone marrow transplantation
- Chronic intractable vomiting (such as hyperemesis gravidarum, the severe nausea and vomiting of pregnancy)
- Severe malabsorption and diarrhea
- Inflammatory bowel disease
- Enterocutaneous fistulas (abnormal passage from the intestine to the body surface)
- Small bowel obstruction or surgical resection
- Moderate to acute pancreatitis
- High-dose chemotherapy
- High-dose radiation therapy affecting the GI tract
- Preoperative therapy when intensive medical or surgical intervention is used in the malnourished
- Severe malnutrition in the face of a nonfunctioning GI tract
- Hospitalization, when adequate enteral nutrition cannot be established within 7 to 10 days

In any condition, TPN should not be used for those patients whose dependence on parenteral nutritional support is expected to be shorter than 5 days.

Modified from ASPEN Board of Directors: Guidelines for use of total parenteral nutrition in the hospitalized adult patient, J Parenter Enteral Nutr 10(5):441, 1986.

REFERENCES AND SUGGESTED READINGS

1. American Dietetic Association: Position of the American Dietetic Association: Very low calorie weight loss diets, J Am Diet Assoc 90(5):722, 1990.
2. ASPEN Board of Directors: Guidelines for the use of enteral nutrition in the adult patient, J Parenter Enteral Nutr 11(5):435, 1987.
3. ASPEN Board of Directors: Guidelines for use of total parenteral nutrition in the hospitalized adult patient, J Parenter Enteral Nutr 10(5):441, 1986.
4. Cataldo CB, Nyenhuis JR, and Whitney EN: Nutrition and diet therapy: principles and practice, ed 2, St Paul, 1989, West Publishing Co.
5. Council on Scientific Affairs: Treatment of obesity in adults, JAMA 260(17):2547, 1988.
6. Glanze WD, editor: Mosby's medical & nursing dictionary, ed 3, St Louis, 1990, The CV Mosby Co.
7. Khaw KT and Barrett-Connor E: The association between blood pressure, age, and dietary sodium and potassium: a population study, Circulation 77:53, 1988.
8. National Research Council: Recommended dietary allowances, ed 10, Washington, DC, 1989, National Academy Press.
9. Pi-Sunyer FX: Obesity. In Shils ME and Young VR, editors: Modern nutrition in health and disease, ed 7, Philadelphia, 1988, Lea & Febiger.
10. Shils ME: Enteral (tube) and parenteral nutrition support. In Shils ME and Young VR, editors: Modern nutrition in health and disease, ed 7, Philadelphia, 1988, Lea & Febiger.
11. Smoller JW, Wadden TA, and Brownell KD: Popular and very low-calorie diets in the treatment of obesity. In Frankle RT and Yang M, editors: Obesity and weight control, Rockville, 1988, Aspen Publications.
12. Wadden TA and Stunkard AJ: Controlled trial of very low calorie diet, behavior therapy, and their combination in the treatment of obesity, J Consult Clin Psychol 54:482, 1986.
13. Williams SR: Basic nutrition and diet therapy, ed 8, St Louis, 1988, Times Mirror/Mosby College Publishing.
14. Williams SR: Essentials of nutrition and diet therapy, ed 5, St Louis, 1990, Times Mirror/Mosby College Publishing.

CHAPTER CHALLENGE

KEY POINTS

- Diet therapy involves using the diet as medical treatment for disease or injury.
- Diets may be altered in consistency when GI function prohibits the use of a regular diet. Liquid diets are not nutritionally adequate and should only be used temporarily.
- In some GI disorders, in hypoglycemia, after MI, or in congestive heart failure, small frequent feedings are used as diet therapy.
- High kilocalorie and protein diets are used when patients need to gain weight or maintain present weight in the face of increased metabolic needs.
- Low-kilocalorie diets are used in conjunction with exercise and life-style changes in the treatment of obesity.
- Carbohydrate-controlled diets are used in diabetes, hypoglycemia, and lactose intolerance.
- Fat-controlled diets are prescribed in atherosclerosis, heart disease, hyperlipidemias, and diabetes. Attention should focus on reducing both total fat and saturated fat intake.
- Low-fat diets restrict all fats and are used to treat malabsorption syndromes and gallbladder disease.
- Reduced dietary sodium and increased dietary potassium seem to help lower
- Electrolyte and protein restrictions apply in many forms of renal disease including end-stage renal disease. They often apply in cirrhosis of the liver.
- Fluid restrictions may be necessary during heart failure, edema, and reduced urine output. Kidney stones and urinary tract infections necessitate the use of high fluid intakes.
- Nutritional support (tube feedings or total parenteral nutrition) may be necessary when oral intake is impossible or inadequate to meet needs. GI function usually indicates which type of feeding is to be used.

STUDY QUESTIONS

1. Consistency modifications are often prescribed for:
   a. Patients with atherosclerosis
   b. Patients with renal disease
   c. GI dysfunction
   d. Diabetic patients
2. The purpose of small, frequent feedings is to:
   a. Decrease the amount of stress placed on the GI tract and circulatory system at a given time
   b. Help regulate blood pressure
   c. Help keep the patient awake all day
   d. Alleviate constipation
3. For patients on fluid-restricted diets who experience excess thirst, the nurse could recommend:
   a. Eating ice, since it would not count as fluid
   b. Chewing gum or brushing teeth frequently
   c. Drinking ice tea, since it is low kilocalorie
   d. Eating low-sodium bread products
4. A child with IDDM is ill and refuses to eat lunch. She has already had her full insulin dosage for the day. You should:
   a. Give her less insulin in the next injection
   b. Encourage her to eat the protein-rich foods
   c. Offer some carbohydrate-containing beverages or snacks
   d. Force her to eat lunch
5. Weight management programs should incorporate a low-kilocalorie diet with:
   a. Exercise
   b. Behavior modification
   c. Avoidance of all sweets
   d. a and b
   e. a and c
6. The exchange lists for meal planning divide foods into groups based on:
   a. Their origin (plant vs animal)
   b. The amount of saturated fat vs unsaturated fat
   c. Vitamin and mineral content
   d. Kilocalorie, protein, carbohydrate, and fat content
7. Often, in protein-controlled diets, incomplete proteins should be avoided and only complete proteins consumed. Which foods would not be appropriate on a protein-controlled diet:
   a. Eggs
   b. Milk
   c. Legumes
   d. Beef
8. A cancer patient is suffering from anorexia and weight loss. Which of the following suggestions may help the patient consume a higher kilocalorie diet?
   a. Discourage between-meal snacks
   b. Encourage eating high-kilocalorie foods first in each meal
   c. Tell the patient to eat larger portions
   d. Serve liquid supplements at room temperature
9. Total parenteral nutritional support may be preferred over tube feeding in which of the following conditions:
   a. GI fistulas
   b. Facial trauma resulting in inability to chew or swallow
   c. Anorexia
   d. Long-term feeding after gastrectomy
10. Mark whether the following foods should be restricted or allowed on a low-sodium diet:

Food Item	*Restrict*	*Allow*
a. Olives	R	A
b. Bananas	R	A
c. Coffee	R	A
d. Potato chips	R	A
e. Instant chocolate pudding	R	A
f. Cheese	R	A
g. Frankfurters	R	A
h. Fresh broccoli	R	A
i. Baked potato	R	A
j. Canned soup	R	A

11. Mark whether the following foods should be restricted or allowed on a low-fat diet:

Food Item	*Restrict*	*Allow*
a. Bacon	R	A
b. Potato chips	R	A
c. Bananas	R	A
d. Angel food cake	R	A
e. Skim chocolate milk	R	A
f. Cheese, cheddar	R	A
g. Peanut butter	R	A
h. Orange juice	R	A
i. Cola drinks	R	A
j. Prime rib of beef	R	A

VII

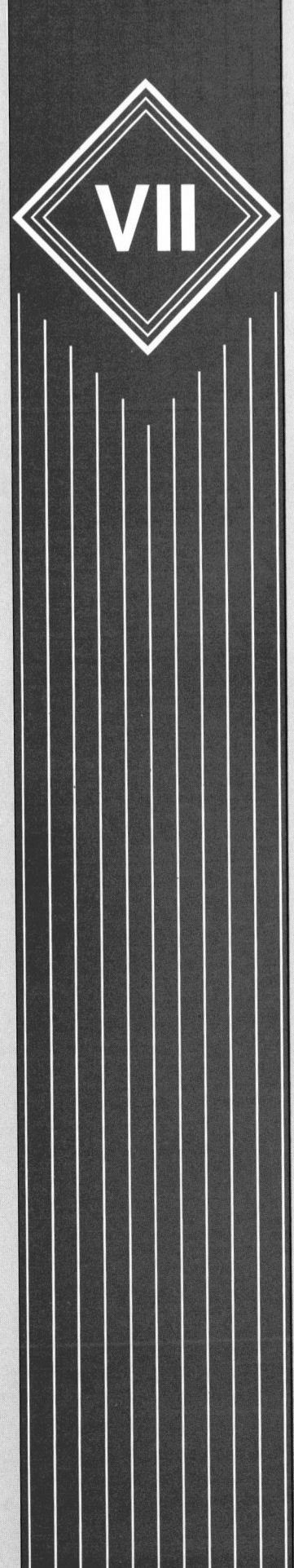

Medication Administration

My love of nursing is extremely rewarding. I always receive more from each of my patients than I could ever hope to give. They and their families are brave, lovely people, who many times are enduring great pain and fear, yet manage to express gratitude for the smallest service. It is a privilege to be a member of the team, which is continuously discovering new techniques and drugs to provide relief for the suffering and cures for the incurable. Nursing is love, learning, growing, rewarding, and a privilege.

MARGERET HARTER
Student Nurse

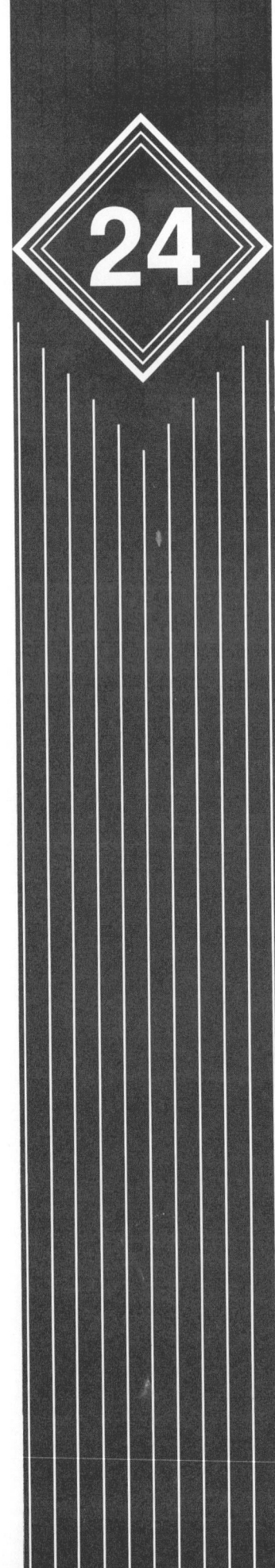

24

Mathematics Review

CYNTHIA M. DAVIS

LEARNING OBJECTIVES

After reading this chapter, the student should be able to do the following:

- Define key terms.
- Confidently use basic mathematical skills to solve dosage problems accurately.
- Set up and work problems using the formula:

$$\frac{\text{Desired dose}}{\text{Available dose}} \times \text{Amount}$$

- Set up and work problems using the proportion method.
- Use "key" equivalents of metric and apothecary measurement systems in dosage problems.
- Convert measurement units within the metric system.
- Convert between measurement units of the metric system and the apothecary system.
- Determine the appropriateness of dosage orders for children by the use of Young's, Clark's, and Fried's rule and the body surface area nomogram.

KEY TERMS

Define the following:

- denominator
- extremes
- means
- numerator

The practical/vocational nurse must accurately calculate drug dosages to provide safe medication administration to each patient. The review of basic mathematics section of this chapter will provide the LPN/LVN with a review of basic math, three measurement systems, two methods of solving dosage problems, and methods of determining the appropriateness of children's drug orders.

FRACTIONS

Are you afraid of fractions? Many students are. What *is* a fraction? A fraction is a "part" of a whole number. For example:

Fraction **Whole**

½ of a pie 1 whole pie

Definitions

numerator the "top" number of a fraction.
denominator the "bottom" number of a fraction.

Types of fractions

Proper fractions—the numerator is less than the denominator.

EXAMPLE: $\frac{1}{2}$ Numerator / Denominator

Improper fractions—the numerator is larger than the denominator.

EXAMPLE: $\frac{2}{1}$ Numerator / Denominator

Mixed fractions—consist of a whole number plus a fraction.

EXAMPLE: $1\frac{1}{2}$ 1 is the whole number; $\frac{1}{2}$ is the fraction

Changing an improper fraction to a whole or mixed number

RULE 1: Divide the denominator (bottom number) into the numerator (top number).

EXAMPLE: Change $\frac{10}{5}$ to a ***whole*** number.

$10 \div 5 = 2$ (a WHOLE number)

Change $\frac{40}{5}$ to a ***whole*** number.

$40 \div 5 = 8$ (a WHOLE number)

EXAMPLE: Change $\frac{20}{7}$ (an improper fraction) to a ***mixed*** number.

$$20 \div 7 = 7\overline{)20} = 2\frac{6}{7} \text{ (a MIXED number)}$$

(quotient 2; 20 − 14 = 6; remainder $\frac{6}{7}$)

Change $\frac{54}{5}$ to a ***mixed*** number.

$$54 \div 5 = 5\overline{)54} = 10\frac{4}{5} \text{ (a MIXED number)}$$

(quotient 10; 54 − 5 … remainder 4; $\frac{4}{5}$)

Changing a mixed number to an improper fraction

RULE 1: Multiply the denominator (bottom number) by the whole number.

RULE 2: Add numerator to the product; the sum is now the new number.

EXAMPLE: Change $2\frac{6}{7}$ (a mixed number) to an improper fraction.

Multiply the denominator 7 by the whole number 2.

$7 \times 2 = 14$ (The answer from numbers multiplied is called the *product*.)

Add the numerator to the product.

$6 + 14 = 20$ (The answer from numbers added is called the *sum*.)

Place the sum, 20, over the original denominator, 7, to have an improper fraction.

$$\frac{20}{7}$$

The mixed number $2\frac{6}{7}$ is now the improper fraction $\frac{20}{7}$.

Reducing fractions to the lowest term

Fractions are commonly reduced to the lowest term in which they can be expressed, because it is easier to work with smaller numbers. For example, $\frac{20}{80}$ or $\frac{25}{100}$, which can both be reduced to $\frac{1}{4}$, become more convenient to use in calculation.

RULE 1: Find a number that will evenly divide into the numerator *and* the denominator.

EXAMPLE: $\frac{2}{10}$

What number will divide into the numerator, 2?

2 will divide evenly into the numerator, 2, one time.

2 will divide into the denominator, 10, five times.

$\frac{2}{10} = \frac{1}{5}$ (Reduce all fractions to their lowest terms.)

EXAMPLE: $\frac{16}{60} = \frac{4}{15}$ (The number, 4, divides evenly into both the numerator and the denominator.)

Determining which fraction is larger

RULE 1: If the denominators are the *same,* the fraction with the *larger numerator* is the larger fraction.

Which is larger? $\frac{4}{6}$ or $\frac{2}{6}$

$\frac{4}{6}$ is larger

RULE 2: If the denominators are *different,* such as $\frac{2}{5}$ and $\frac{1}{3}$, you must find a "common denominator." (Finding a common denominator means to find a number into which both denominators can be divided.) A common, or equivalent, will also be found.

PROBLEM: Find a common denominator for $\frac{2}{5}$ and $\frac{1}{3}$.

(Try multiplying the denominators to get a common denominator.)

EXAMPLE: $\frac{2}{5} = \frac{}{15}$ $\frac{1}{3} = \frac{}{15}$

PROBLEM: Which is larger? $\frac{2}{3}$ or $\frac{6}{8}$

$\frac{2}{3} = \frac{16}{24}$ $\frac{6}{8} = \frac{18}{24}$

$\frac{6}{8}$ is larger

RULE 3: After the common denominator is found, an equivalent numerator for each fraction must be found.

$\frac{2}{5} = \frac{?}{15}$ $\frac{1}{3} = \frac{?}{15}$

Find an equivalent numerator by dividing the first denominator into the equivalent denominator; multiply the answer by the first numerator.

EXAMPLE:

$\frac{2}{5} = \frac{6}{15}$ $(15 \div 5 = 3; 3 \times 2 = 6)$

$\frac{1}{3} = \frac{5}{15}$ $(15 \div 3 = 5; 5 \times 1 = 5)$

RULE 4: Compare the two fractions.

PROBLEM: Which is larger? $\frac{6}{15}$ or $\frac{5}{15}$

$\frac{6}{15}$ is larger

Adding fractions that have the same denominator

RULE 1: *Add* the numerators and place the sum of the numerators over the denominator.

EXAMPLE:

$$\begin{array}{r} \frac{1}{6} \\ + \frac{1}{6} \\ \hline \frac{2}{6} = \frac{1}{3} \end{array}$$

Adding fractions that have different denominators

RULE 1: Find common denominators for all fractions in the problem.

EXAMPLE:

$$\begin{array}{r} \frac{1}{3} = \frac{}{12} \\ + \frac{2}{4} = \frac{}{12} \end{array}$$

(3 and 4 will divide into 12; 12 is the common denominator.)

RULE 2: Find the equivalent numerators.

$$\begin{array}{r} \frac{1}{3} = \frac{4}{12} \ (12 \div 3 = 4;\ 4 \times 1 = 4) \\ + \frac{2}{4} = \frac{6}{12} \ (12 \div 4 = 3;\ 3 \times 2 = 6) \\ \hline \frac{10}{12} = \frac{5}{6} \end{array}$$

$$\begin{array}{r} \frac{6}{20} = \frac{6}{20} \\ + \frac{12}{20} = \frac{12}{20} \\ \hline \frac{18}{20} = \frac{9}{10} \end{array}$$

Adding mixed numbers

RULE 1: Add the fractions of the mixed number. Then, add the sum of the fractions to the whole numbers.

EXAMPLE:

$$\begin{array}{r} 1\frac{2}{3} \\ + 2\frac{1}{3} \\ \hline 3\frac{3}{3} = 4 \end{array}$$

$$\begin{array}{r} 1\frac{3}{5} = 1\frac{6}{10} \\ + 4\frac{5}{10} = 4\frac{5}{10} \\ \hline 5\frac{11}{10} = 5 + 1 \text{ whole} + \frac{1}{10}, \end{array}$$

$$\text{which} = 6\frac{1}{10}$$

Subtracting fractions with the same denominator

RULE 1: Subtract the numerator and place it over the denominator in the answer.

EXAMPLE:

$$\begin{array}{r} \frac{3}{5} \\ - \frac{1}{5} \\ \hline \frac{2}{5} \end{array} \qquad \begin{array}{r} \frac{4}{7} \\ - \frac{2}{7} \\ \hline \frac{2}{7} \end{array}$$

Subtracting fractions with different denominators

RULE 1: Find a common denominator, then subtract. Hint: Try multiplying the two denominators as a way to find a common denominator.

EXAMPLE:

$$\begin{array}{r} \frac{3}{4} = \frac{9}{12} \\ - \frac{1}{3} = \frac{4}{12} \\ \hline \frac{5}{12} \end{array} \qquad \begin{array}{r} \frac{1}{2} = \frac{3}{6} \\ - \frac{2}{3} = \frac{4}{6} \\ \hline \frac{7}{6} = 1\frac{1}{6} \end{array}$$

Subtracting mixed numbers

RULE 1: When the numerator of the top fraction is smaller than the bottom fraction, borrow one whole number from the whole number of the mixed fraction and express it as a fraction.

PROBLEM:

$$\begin{array}{r} 3\frac{9}{15} \\ - 2\frac{10}{15} \\ \hline \end{array}$$

EXAMPLE: $3 = 2\frac{15}{15}$

RULE 2: Add the fraction of the original mixed number to the new fraction.

$$3\frac{9}{15} = 2\frac{15}{15} + \frac{9}{15} = 2\frac{24}{15}$$

RULE 3: Subtract fractions and whole numbers, if any.

$$\begin{array}{r} 2\frac{24}{15} - 2\frac{10}{15} \\ \hline \frac{14}{15} \end{array}$$

EXAMPLE:

$$\begin{array}{r} 5\frac{6}{10} = 4\frac{10}{10} + \frac{6}{10} = 4\frac{16}{10} \\ - 3\frac{8}{10} = 3\frac{8}{10} \qquad - 3\frac{8}{10} \\ \hline 1\frac{2}{10} \text{ or } 1\frac{1}{5} \end{array}$$

Multiplying fractions

RULE 1: Multiply the numerators; multiply the denominators.

EXAMPLE: $\frac{1}{2} \times \frac{3}{4} = \frac{1 \times 3}{2 \times 4} = \frac{3}{8}$

$\frac{4}{8} \times \frac{1}{3} = \frac{4 \times 1}{8 \times 3} = \frac{4}{24} = \frac{1}{6}$

Multiplying fractions and mixed numbers

RULE 1: Change the mixed number to an improper fraction. (See the section on changing mixed numbers to improper fractions, p. 422.)

RULE 2: Multiply.

PROBLEM: Multiply $3\frac{1}{2}$ by $1\frac{2}{3}$

EXAMPLE: a. Change $3\frac{1}{2}$ and $1\frac{2}{3}$ to improper fractions.

$3\frac{1}{2} = \frac{7}{2}$ $\quad 1\frac{2}{3} = \frac{5}{3}$

b. Multiply.

$\frac{7 \times 5}{2 \times 3} = \frac{35}{6} = 6\overline{)35} = 5\frac{5}{6}$ (quotient 5; 30; remainder $\frac{5}{6}$)

PROBLEM: Multiply $1\frac{2}{3}$ by $2\frac{3}{4}$

EXAMPLE: $1\frac{2}{3} = \frac{5}{3}$ $\quad 2\frac{3}{4} = \frac{11}{4}$

$\frac{5}{3} \times \frac{11}{4} = \frac{55}{12} = 4\frac{7}{12}$

Dividing fractions

RULE 1: Write the problem down *correctly;* invert the second fraction.

RULE 2: Multiply.

PROBLEM: Divide $\frac{1}{2}$ by $\frac{3}{4}$

EXAMPLE: a. Write the problem down *correctly*.

$\frac{1}{2} \div \frac{3}{4}$

b. Invert the second fraction; change the division sign to a multiplication sign; multiply.

$\frac{1}{2} \times \frac{4}{3} = \frac{4}{6}$

c. Reduce to the lowest terms.

$\frac{4}{6} = \frac{2}{3}$

Dividing fraction and whole numbers

RULE 1: Change the whole number to a fraction.

RULE 2: Divide.

PROBLEM: Divide 4 by $\frac{3}{5}$.

EXAMPLE: a. Change 4 to a fraction. Make 4 the numerator and use 1 as the denominator.

$\frac{4}{1}$

b. Invert second fraction; multiply.

$\frac{4 \times 5}{1 \times 3} = \frac{20}{3}$

c. Reduce to lowest terms.

$\frac{20}{3} = 6\frac{2}{3}$ $\quad 3\overline{)20}$ (quotient 6; 18; remainder $\frac{2}{3}$)

DECIMAL FRACTIONS

The decimal fraction is a type of fraction that uses a decimal to indicate the denominator of the fraction. The placement or position of the decimal point determines whether the denominator is 10, multiples of 10, or divisions of 10.

Names of Decimal Places

.00001	One-hundred thousandths
.0001	Ten thousandths
.001	Thousandths
.01	Hundredths
.1	Tenths
1.	Unit (whole numbers)
10	Tens
100	Hundreds
1,000	Thousands
10,000	Ten thousands
100,000	One-hundred thousands

RULE 1: A decimal point found left of a whole number means that the number is a *fraction* of a whole number.

EXAMPLE: 0.1 "Point one" is $\frac{1}{10}$ of the whole number, 1.

Hint: Place a zero left of the decimal point to avoid mistaking .1 with 1.
Correct placement of decimal points in drug dosages is *critical.*

RULE 2: A decimal point found *after* a number means that it is a whole number.

EXAMPLE: 5. = 5

RULE 3: A number *without* a decimal point is understood to have an "invisible" decimal point behind it.

EXAMPLE: 1 = 1.0

Adding decimals

RULE 1: Align the decimal point of each decimal fraction in a column.

RULE 2: Add.

PROBLEM: Add 3.34 and 0.6

EXAMPLE:
```
   3.34  Align decimal point in column; add.
 + 0.6
 -----
   3.94
   ↑ Make sure that the decimal point is
     aligned properly in the answer.
```

Hint: Zeroes may be added to the right of the decimal point if needed to help align the column. The value of the number is *not* changed by adding zeroes.

EXAMPLE: 1.00 = 1   5.0 = 5

Subtracting decimals

RULE 1: Align the decimal points of each decimal fraction in a column.

RULE 2: Subtract.

PROBLEM: Subtract 7.45 from 15.

EXAMPLE: a. Align decimal points in column; subtract.
```
   15.00  (Note zeroes used to align the
 -  7.45   two columns.)
 -------
    7.55
```

Rounding a number

RULE 1: Numbers found after the decimal point that are 5 or larger can increase the number before it by one whole number.

EXAMPLE: 7.55 = 7.6 or 8

Hint: There are times when it is practical to round a volume of medication.

PROBLEM: How can 7.55 minims easily be given?

EXAMPLE: Round 7.55 to 8; give 8 minims.

Note: Minims are very small units of measurement. Milliliters/cubic centimeters are not rounded in this manner, since drug dosage would be altered.

Multiplying decimals

RULE 1: Multiply. Decimal points in the problem *do not* have to be aligned.

RULE 2: The decimal place in the answer is determined by how many numbers are found right of the decimal points in the numbers multiplied.

EXAMPLE:
```
      5.50
  ×   2.15     (There are 4 numbers found
  --------     after the decimal points; 2 on
      2750     the top and 2 on the bottom.)
      550
    1100
  --------
   11.8250x
     ↑____| x = 11.8250 or 12 (rounded)
```

Note: A small "x" hereafter indicates the unexpressed decimal after a whole number or a decimal point that has been moved from one place to another.

Dividing decimals

RULE 1: Change a decimal fraction in the divisor to a whole number by moving the decimal point *all* the way to the right.

PROBLEM: Divide 2.5 by 1.5.

EXAMPLE: a. (divisor) 1.5 |2.5 (dividend)

b. 1.5x |2.5 (15 |2.5)

RULE 2: Move the decimal point in the dividend the *same number of places* moved in the divisor.

EXAMPLE: 1.5x |2.5x The decimal point in the divisor is unexpressed after it is moved.

RULE 3: Place the decimal point in the answer directly over the decimal point in the dividend after moving the decimal point in the dividend.

EXAMPLE: 15 |25.

RULE 4: If a decimal point is in the divisor, but not in the dividend (such as .5 |15), move it the same number of places as the divisor. Remember there is an unexpressed decimal point at the right of all whole numbers. Add zeroes after the decimal point in the dividend as needed.

EXAMPLE: .5x |15.0x   5 |150.0

RULE 5: If the dividend contains a decimal fraction and the divisor does not, leave the divisor as it is.

EXAMPLE: 5 |2.5 would remain unchanged.

Changing fractions to decimals

RULE 1: Divide the numerator (the top number) by the denominator (the bottom number).

PROBLEM: Change $\frac{3}{4}$ to a decimal fraction.

EXAMPLE:
```
         .75
 3/4 = 4|3.00
         28
          20
          20
```

Changing a decimal fraction to a common fraction

Decimal fractions are based on 10's, multiples of 10, and divisions of 10. The position or place of the decimal point indicates the denominator.

RULE 1: To change a decimal fraction to a common fraction, give the decimal fraction a denominator according to the position of the decimal point in the decimal fraction.

PROBLEM: Change .1 to a common fraction.

EXAMPLE: a. .1 (The decimal point is in the "tens" place; 10 is the denominator.)

$$\frac{}{10}$$

b. Now that the denominator is 10, place the 1 over it to make a common fraction.

$$\frac{1}{10}$$

PERCENTS

The word *percent,* and its symbol, %, mean "hundredths." A hundredth is a fraction of a whole number; therefore a number followed by % is a *fraction*. The denominator of the fraction is understood to be 100.

EXAMPLE: 25% is the same as $\frac{25}{100}$

$\frac{25}{100}$ can be reduced to $\frac{1}{4}$

Changing percent to a decimal fraction

RULE 1: Remove %; move the decimal point two places to the left to indicate "hundredths."

PROBLEM: Change 25% to a decimal fraction.

EXAMPLE: .25

Changing a fraction to a percent

RULE 1: Change a fraction to a percent by dividing the numerator by the denominator.
RULE 2: Multiply the answer by 100.
RULE 3: Label the answer with the percent symbol.

EXAMPLE: $\frac{3}{4} = 4\overline{)3.00}$ = .75

```
     .75
 4 ) 3.00
     28
      20
      20
```

```
   100
 ×  .75
   500
   700
  75.00x
```

(There are two decimal places in this problem; move the decimal point in the answer 2 places to the left.)

75% Therefore ¾ = 75%

Multiplying by percent

RULE 1: Change percent to a decimal (move decimal point 2 places to the left).
RULE 2: Multiply.

PROBLEM: Multiply 80 by 7.5%.

EXAMPLE: 7.5% is .075

```
    80
 × .075
   400
   560
   00
  6.000x
```

(Move decimal point 3 places to the left = 6)

RATIO

Ratio shows the relationship of one number or quantity to another number or quantity. Numbers of a ratio are separated by a colon. Ratio is also a fraction. The value of a ratio is not changed if both terms are multiplied or divided by the same number.

EXAMPLE: 2:4 is the same as 1:2 or 4:8

When numbers are written in ratio, they must all be expressed in the same units.

EXAMPLE: 1 liter, 2 ounces, and 30 milliliters (ml) must all be expressed in the same way, as:

1000 ml:60 ml:30 ml

A fraction may be written as a ratio.

EXAMPLE: $\frac{1}{25} = 1:25$ $\frac{3}{4} = 3:4$

Ratio is an important concept that is used in the following methods of calculating dosages.

PROPORTION

Proportion shows that the relationship between two ratios has equal value.

EXAMPLE: 1 is to 2 as 4 is to 8 or 1:2 :: 4:8

Definitions

extremes the outer terms of the proportion.
means the inner terms of the proportion.

EXAMPLE: 1:2 :: 4:8 (means: 2 and 4) 1:2 :: 4:8 (extremes: 1 and 8)

Set up the left side of the proportion as the "known" side using information that is known or given. The known information will be:

EXAMPLE: a. An equivalent such as 60 milligrams = 1 grain (60 mg: 1 gr)

or

b. A doctor's medication or IV order, such as "give 1000 ml in 8 hr" (1000 ml: 8 hr)

or

c. A drug dosage you have on hand or available, such as information on a drug label that reads "50 mg/ml (50 mg: 1 ml)"

PROBLEM: The doctor orders Demerol 25 mg q 3-4 hr prn for pain. On hand is a vial labeled "50 mg/1 ml."

RULE 1: Set up the known side.

EXAMPLE: 50 mg: 1 ml (given on the label)

RULE 2: Set up the unknown side. Use *x* for what you are trying to find, such as "How many milliliters are needed to give 25 mg?"

	Known		*Unknown*
EXAMPLE:	50 mg: 1 ml	::	25 mg: x ml

RULE 3: Set up the units, such as milligrams and milliliters, in the *same position on each side* of the problem.

EXAMPLE: ___ mg: ___ ml :: ___ mg : ___ ml

RULE 4: Multiply the means.
RULE 5: Multiply the extremes.

PROBLEM: 50 mg: 1 ml:: 25 mg: x ml

EXAMPLE: Multiply the means.

50 mg: 1 ml:: 25 mg: x ml
= 25

Multiply the extremes.

50 mg: 1 ml:: 25 mg: x ml
50x = 25

RULE 6: Solve for *x* (divide the number with the *x* into the number on the opposite side of the problem).

EXAMPLE: 50 mg: 1 ml:: 25 mg: x ml
50x = 25 = $50\overline{)25.0}$ = .5
x = .5

RULE 7: Label the answer with the unit of measurement that accompanies the *x* in the problem.

EXAMPLE: 50 mg: 1 ml:: 25 mg: x ml
50x = 25
x = .5 ml

Review of proportion method

1. Set up problems in the *same order* on both sides.
2. Multiply the means; multiply the extremes.
3. The number multiplied with the *x* is always that number with the *x* to the right of it.

   EXAMPLE: 2 mg: ml: 5 mg: *x* ml

4. Divide the number with the *x* into the number on the other side of the problem.
5. Label the problem by looking to see what unit of measurement the *x* is with the proportion.

$\frac{\textbf{Desired dosage}}{\textbf{Available dosage}}$ × Amount method

Many nurses use the following method of solving dosage problems.

RULE 1: Place the dose that the doctor wants given over the dose that the nurse has available (on hand).

PROBLEM: The physician orders 40 mg of furosemide (Lasix). The nurse has an ampule of furosemide labeled Lasix 20 mg/ml.

EXAMPLE:

$$\frac{\text{(Desired dosage) } 40 \text{ mg}}{\text{(Available dose) } 20 \text{ mg}} \times \frac{1 \text{ ml}}{1} = \frac{40}{20} =$$
$$40 \div 20 = 2 \text{ ml}$$

PROBLEM: The physician orders 15 mg of diazepam (Valium). The nurse has Valium tablets that contain 5 mg/tablet.

EXAMPLE:

$$\frac{\text{(Desired dosage) } 15 \text{ mg}}{\text{(Available dose) } 5 \text{ mg}} \times \frac{1 \text{ Tab}}{\text{x tab}} = \frac{15}{5\text{x}} = \text{x} =$$
$$15 \div 5 = 3 \text{ Tablets}$$

NURSE ALERT

- There is no room for error in calculating dosages.
- Check math work with another nurse.
- Work problems systematically and carefully *on paper*.
- Reduce distractions while working problems.
- Recheck calculations.
- Is the answer reasonable?

THE METRIC SYSTEM

The metric system is the preferred system of weights and measures. It is more accurate and easier to use in calculating dosage problems.

Similar to the U.S. monetary system, which is based on the dollar, the metric system is also based on the decimal system. The decimal system uses division and multiples of a unit, which is always in ratios of tens.

EXAMPLE: 1 dollar = 10 dimes
10 dimes = 20 nickles
20 nickles = 100 pennies
All of these units are multiples or divisions of tens.

The metric system uses the following basic units of volume, weight, and length:

liter (L) volume (amount) of fluids.
gram (g) weight of solids.
meter (m) measure of length.

Smaller units of the system are designated by the following prefixes:

deci 0.1 of the unit; tens (liter, gram, meter)
centi 0.01 of the units; hundredths
milli 0.001 of the unit; thousandths

Larger units of the system are designated with the following prefixes:

Deka = 10 times the unit (liter, gram, meter)
Hecto = 100 times the unit
Kilo = 1000 times the unit

Units of weight

1 Gram (g) = 1000 milligrams (mg)
0.001 Gram (g) = 1 milligram (mg)
1 Kilogram (kg) = 1000 grams (g)
0.001 Kilogram (kg) = 1 gram (g)

Units of volume

1 Liter (L) = 1000 milliliters (ml)
0.001 Liter (L) = 1 milliliter (ml)
1 Milliliter (ml) = 1 cubic centimeter (cc)

Approximate Equivalents of the Metric System and the Apothecary System

The apothecary system is a system of measurement that is still used by some physicians and hospitals. It is being replaced slowly by the metric system. Since it continues to be used, the following equivalents are needed to convert dosages from one system to another. The conversions are approximations only but are acceptable equivalents with which to work.

Volume

METRIC		APOTHECARY
1 milliliter (ml)	=	16 minims (♏ XVI)
4 milliliters (ml)	=	1 fluid dram (fʒ ṫ)
30 milliliters (ml)	=	1 fluid ounce (f℥ ṫ)
500 milliliters (ml)	=	1 pint (O ṫ)
1000 milliliters (ml) or 1 Liter (L)	=	1 quart (1 Qt.)

The symbols for the above apothecary units are:

Minim = ♏
Fluid dram = ʒ
Fluid ounce = ℥
Pint = O or pt
Quart = Qt

The symbols appear in front of the number (which is written in roman numerals).

EXAMPLE: 16 minims is written ♏ XVI

Weight

METRIC		APOTHECARY
60 milligrams (mg)	=	1 grain (the symbol is gr. for grain)
1000 milligrams (mg)	=	15 grains (gr. XV)
4 grams (g or Gm)	=	1 dram (ʒ ṫ)
30 grams (g)	=	1 ounce (℥ ṫ)
0.45 kilogram (kg)	=	1 pound (lb)
1 kilogram (kg)	=	2.2 pounds (lb)

Convert from one system to another to work dosage problems in the same measurement units.

Metric Measurements of Length

The basic unit of length in the metric system is the meter. The meter is equal to 39.37 inches, about 3½ inches longer than 1 yard (36 inches). Some of the tasks that the nurse will perform using the metric measurements of length will be to:

Measure area size for topical applications.
Measure results of intradermal skin tests (size of drug or allergen reaction on the skin).
Measure wound size.
Measure decubiti.
Measure height, length, and head circumference (such as is common in pediatrics).
Measure abdominal girth (obstetrics).

Length

0.001 meter	=	1 millimeter (mm)
0.01 meter	=	1 centimeter (cm)
0.1 meter	=	1 decimeter (dm)
10 meters	=	1 dekameter (dam)
100 meters	=	1 hectometer (hm)
1000 meters	=	1 kilometer (km)

Most frequently used equivalents are:

1 meter (m)	=	1000 millimeters (mm)
0.001 meter (m)	=	1 milliliter (mm)
1 meter (m)	=	100 centimeters (cm)
1 centimeter (cm)	=	10 millimeters (mm)
1 millimeter (mm)	=	0.1 centimeter (cm)

BIG TO SMALL RULE

Whatever method is used to solve dosage problems, the units of measurement in the problem must *always* be converted to the same unit of measurement.

Some students find it difficult to convert dosages that contain decimal fractions. Discussed here is a quick and easy method called the "big to small" rule. It is useful in converting dosages within the same system (the metric system).

Because there are 1000 ml in 1 L (and 1000 mg in 1 g), milliliters can be converted to liters (and milligrams to grams) by this method. Likewise, liters can be converted to milliliters (and grams to milligrams) by this method.

Converting larger units of measurement to smaller units of measurement (grams to milligrams; liters to milliliters)

RULE 1: Write down BIG → SMALL.

RULE 2: Place the large unit under the word BIG and the small unit under the word SMALL.

EXAMPLE: BIG ————→ SMALL
2.5 g = ________ mg

RULE 3: Move the decimal point 3 places in the direction of the arrow; add zeroes.

EXAMPLE: BIG → SMALL
2.5 g = 2 × 500 mg

Converting smaller units of measurement to larger units of measurement (milligrams to grams; milliliters to liters)

RULE 1: Write down the big to small rule formula.

EXAMPLE: BIG → SMALL

RULE 2: Reverse the direction of the arrow.

EXAMPLE: BIG ← SMALL

RULE 3: Place the large unit under the word BIG and the small unit under the word SMALL.

EXAMPLE: BIG → SMALL
x g = 2500 mg

RULE 4: Move the decimal point 3 places in the direction that the arrow points.

EXAMPLE: BIG ← SMALL
2.5 g = 2500x mg

PEDIATRIC CONSIDERATIONS

Pediatric dosage refers to the determination of the correct amount, frequency, and total number of doses of a medication to be administered to a child or infant.

Age, weight, body surface area, and the ability of the child to absorb, metabolize, and excrete medication must be considered when administering medication to a child.

It is the physician's responsibility to determine medication orders and dosage for a pediatric patient, but the nurse must be able to recognize appropriate and inappropriate drug dosages and orders.

The nurse must be knowledgeable about the four standard formulas for calculating children's dosages. These are Young's rule, Clark's rule, Fried's rule, and the body surface area method.

Young's rule

Young's rule is as follows:

$$\frac{\text{Age of child}}{\text{Age of child} + 12} \times \text{Average adult dose} = \text{Child's dose}$$

This rule applies to children up to the age of 12.

PROBLEM: The average adult dose of a particular medication is 50 mg. What is an appropriate dose of this medication for an 8-year-old child?

EXAMPLE:

$$\frac{8 \text{ yr}}{8 + 12} \times 50 \text{ mg} = \frac{8}{20} \times \frac{50}{1} = \frac{400}{20} = 20 \overline{)400} \quad (\text{quotient } 20;\ 40,\ 0,\ 0)$$

ANSWER: 20 mg is an appropriate dose.

Clark's rule

Clark's rule is as follows:

$$\frac{\text{Weight of child}}{150} \text{ in pounds} \times \text{Average adult dose} = \text{Child's dose}$$

This rule uses the child's weight to determine dosage.

PROBLEM: The average adult dose of a particular medication is 25 mg. What is an appropriate dose of this medication for a child who weighs 40 pounds?

EXAMPLE:

$$\frac{40 \text{ lb}}{150} \times 25 \text{ mg} = \frac{40}{150} \times \frac{25}{1} = \frac{1000}{150} = 150 \overline{)1000.00} \quad (\text{quotient } 6.66;\ 900,\ 1000,\ 900,\ 1000)$$

ANSWER: 6.7 mg is an appropriate dose.

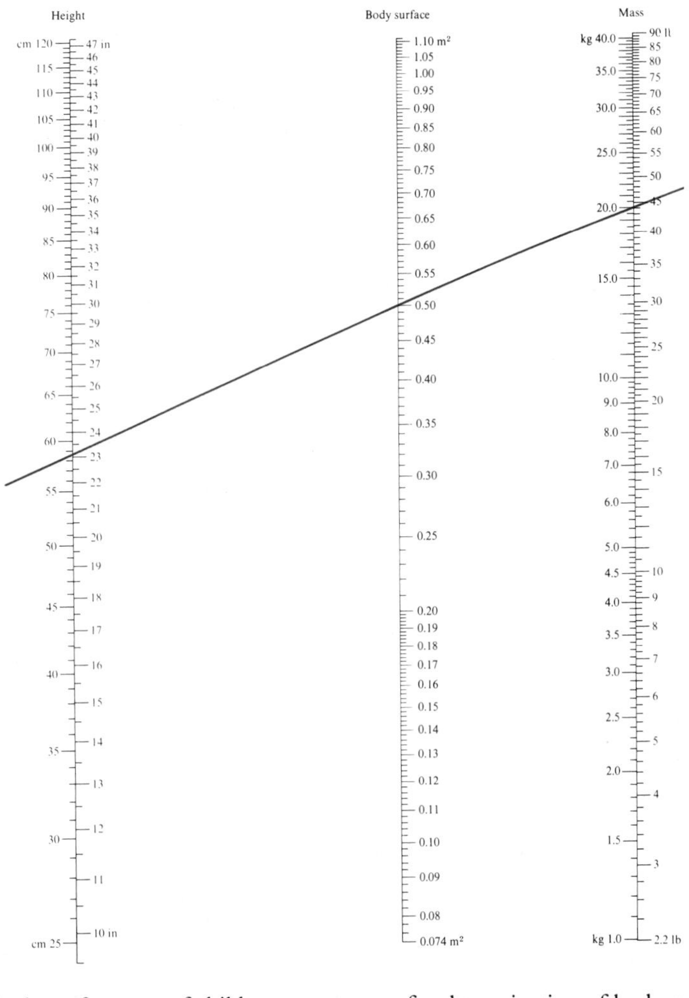

FIG. 24-1 Body surface area of children: nomogram for determination of body surface from height and mass, based on the formula of DuBois and DuBois, Arch Intern Med 17:863, 1916: $S = M^{0.425} \times H^{0.725} \times 71.84$, or $\log S = \log M \times 0.425 \times \log H \times 0.725 \times 1.8564$ (*S,* body surface in cm^2; *M,* mass in kg; *H,* height in cm). Courtesy CIBA-GEIGY, Ltd, Basel, Switzerland.

Fried's rule

Fried's rule is as follows:

$$\frac{\text{Age in months}}{150} \times \text{Average adult dose} = \text{Child's dose}$$

This rule is used for infants less than 2 years of age.

PROBLEM: The average adult dose of a particular medication is 25 mg. What is an appropriate dose of this medication for a child who is 22 months of age?

EXAMPLE:

$$\frac{22\text{ mo}}{150} \times 25\text{ mg} = \frac{550}{150} = 150\overline{)550.00}$$

```
       3.66
150 | 550.00
      450
      1000
       900
      1000
```

ANSWER: 3.7 mg is an appropriate dose.

Body surface area method

LaRocca and Otto give the formula and nomogram for determining dosage for a child based on height, weight, and body surface area (Fig. 24-1). Height is correlated with the weight of the child to determine the body surface area of the child. The drug dose is then ordered as mg/m^2.

EXAMPLE: Child's height = 23 inches; weight = 44 pounds

Plot the height and weight of the child on the nomogram (which is a graphic representation of a numeric relationship) to determine the body surface area (BSA). Multiply the BSA (which is given in square meters on the nomogram) by mg/m^2.

EXAMPLE: The drug literature recommends 1 mg/m^2.
$0.50 \times 1\text{ mg} = x\text{ dose}$
$x = 0.50\text{ mg of drug}$

REFERENCES AND SUGGESTED READINGS

1. Dison N: Simplified drugs and solutions for nurses including mathematics, ed 9, St Louis, 1988, The CV Mosby Co.
2. Lannon MC and Arcangelo VP: Essentials of clinical pharmacology and dosage calculation, ed 2, Philadelphia, 1986, JB Lippincott Co.
3. LaRocca JC and Otto SE: Pocket guide to intravenous therapy, St Louis, 1989, The CV Mosby Co.

STUDY QUESTIONS

CHAPTER CHALLENGE

Work the following problems. Use the **proportion method** or $\frac{\textbf{desired dose}}{\textbf{available dose}}$ formula, **key equivalents,** and the **big to small rule.**

Section I

1. The physician has ordered 0.5 g of ampicillin. You have available a vial labelled 250 mg/ml. How many milliliters will you give your patient:
   a. 2 ml c. 0.05 ml
   b. 0.2 ml d. 0.5 ml
2. Digoxin (Lanoxin) 0.125 mg is ordered. On hand is Lanoxin 0.5 mg/ml. How many milliliters will be given:
   a. 3 ml c. 2.5 ml
   b. 0.25 ml d. 0.025 ml
3. Mrs. Brown is to give her child 30 ml of a liquid medication. Her only measuring tool in her new apartment is a tablespoon. How many tablespoons of the medication should she give:
   a. 1 Tbsp c. 3 Tbsp
   b. 2 Tbsp d. 1/2 Tbsp
4. The pediatrician has requested Tim's weight in kilograms. Your scales say that Tim weighs 30 lb. How many kilograms will be reported to the physician:
   a. 20.6 kg c. 13.6 kg
   b. 15 kg d. 22 kg

Section II

Work these problems using the **proportion method.** Multiply milliliters by the drip factor to convert milliliters to drops.

1. Ordered is 1 L of D5W to run over 8 hours. The drip factor stated on the IV tubing is 15 gtt/ml. How many milliliters will be infused every hour:
   a. 100/hr c. 150/hr
   b. 125/hr d. 175/hr
2. An IV of 1 L D_5 1/2 NS is to run at 150 ml/hr. How many hours will this IV run:
   a. 6 hr c. 7.5 hr
   b. 6.6 hr
3. At 3 PM an 8-hour bag of 1L D_5LR, which was started at 9 AM, has 100 ml left in the bag. Does this infusion need to run slower: Faster: Or is it running at the correct rate:
   a. Needs to infuse slower
   b. Needs to infuse faster
   c. It is at the correct rate
   d. Needs to be discontinued

Section III

Insulin may be given in a tuberculin syringe if there are no insulin syringes available or if the dose to be given is extremely small. All insulin is now 100 units per milliliter. Use the **proportion method** to work these problems. (Hint: 100 U:1 ml. is the "known" in every problem.)

1. The physician orders 30 units of insulin. Using a tuberculin syringe, you will give how much of a milliliter:
   a. 0.03 ml c. 0.3 ml
   b. 3.0 ml d. 0.003 ml
2. The physician orders 50 units of insulin given. What part of a milliliter will be given:
   a. 5/100 of 1 ml c. 5/10,000 of 1 ml
   b. 5/1000 of 1 ml d. 5/10 of 1 ml
3. How many minims will be given in problem number 2:
   a. 6 ♏ c. 8 ♏
   b. 5 ♏ d. 16 ♏
4. The nurse calculates that 8 ♏ is the correct amount that the physician has ordered. Cathy asks another LPN, "What part of a milliliter is 8 minims?" The correct answer given by the LPN was:
   a. 0.5 ml
   b. More than 0.5 ml
   c. 1 ml
   d. More than 1 ml
5. Dr. Wertz wants 15 units of insulin given. What part of a milliliter is this:
   a. 0.015 ml c. 1.5 ml
   b. 0.15 ml d. 15 ml

STUDY QUESTIONS (cont'd)

CHAPTER CHALLENGE

Section IV

Are the following doses appropriate for these children:

1. Dr. Green orders 50 mg of meperidine HCl (Demerol) for Andrea, an 8-year-old. Is 50 mg appropriate for her age (the average adult dose of Demerol is 75 mg):
   a. 10 mg is appropriate
   b. 20 mg is appropriate
   c. 30 mg is appropriate
   c. 50 mg is appropriate
2. Dr. Jones orders 500 mg of acetaminophen (Tylenol) for a 2-month-old infant. Is this appropriate (the average adult dose of Tylenol is 500 mg):
   a. It is appropriate
   b. It is a little too much
   c. It is an extreme overdose
   d. It is not enough
3. The average dose of a medication is 0.4 mg (gr 1/150) for an adult. What is the dosage for a 12-year-old:
   a. 2 mg
   b. 0.002 mg
   c. 0.02 mg
   d. 0.2 mg
4. An adult dose of diazepam (Valium) is 5 mg. John weights 27 kilograms. How many milligrams is appropriate for John:
   a. 2 mg
   b. 1.5 mg
   c. 3 mg
   d. 2.5 mg

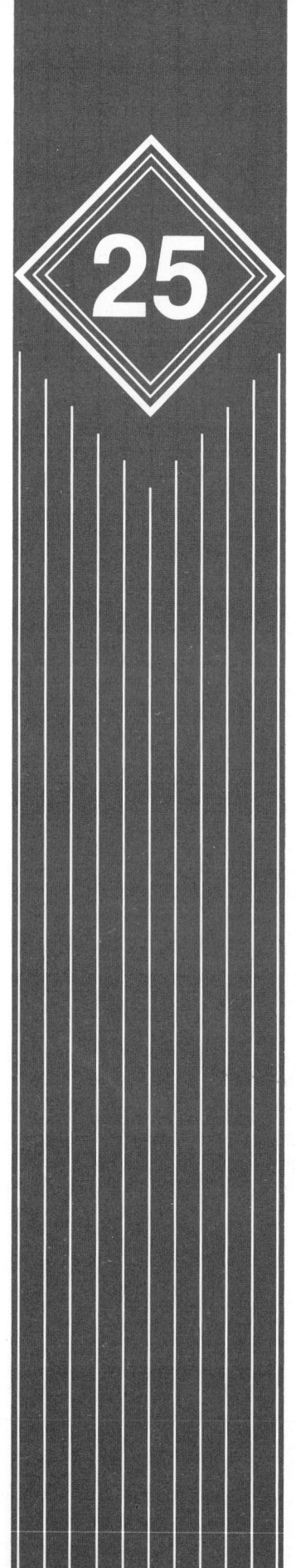

25

Principles and Practice of Medication Administration

CYNTHIA M. DAVIS

LEARNING OBJECTIVES

After reading this chapter, the student should be able to do the following:

- Define the key terms.
- Define each phase of drug action.
- Explain the importance of decreased hepatic and renal functioning.
- Define drug dosage.
- Define therapeutic dosage.
- Define minimal dosage.
- Define maximal dosage.
- Define toxic dosage.
- Define lethal dosage.
- Define potentiation.
- Define cumulative effect.
- Define tolerance.
- Define idiosyncratic response.
- Explain the importance of an antagonist counteracting an agonist.
- Describe five factors that affect drug action in patients.
- Describe the importance of the accurate transcription of medication orders.
- Give the order of priority in the following terms: stat, ASAP, SOS, now, and prn.
- Explain what is meant by a controlled substance.
- List three ways medication orders are given.

RELATED TOPICS OF INTEREST

- Legal Aspects of Nursing (Chapter 2)
- Documentation (Chapter 6)
- Mathematics Review (Chapter 24)

KEY TERMS

Define the following:

- adverse drug reaction
- agonist
- anaphylactic shock
- antagonist
- buccal
- compatibility
- cumulative
- drip factor
- enteral
- enteric coated
- gauge
- graduated
- heparin lock
- idiosyncratic
- interactions
- lumen
- meniscus
- metabolites
- parenteral
- patient-controlled analgesia (PCA)
- pharmacology
- potentiation
- pulverized
- souffle cup
- sublingual
- therapeutic
- tolerance
- topical

Learning objectives are provided at the beginning of each section of this chapter.

PRINCIPLES OF PHARMACOLOGY

Pharmacology is the study of drugs and their action on the living body. Substances derived from plants and animals, from vitamins and minerals, and from synthetic (manmade) sources can be used as drugs in the treatment and prevention of disease; in the restoration and maintenance of the healthy functioning of body tissues, organs, and systems; and in diagnostic procedures.

The action of any drug on the body is a complicated process. This process begins with the pharmaceutical phase—the making of the drug until absorption of the drug takes place in the patient's body. Absorption occurs when the active ingredient of the drug enters the body fluids.

The pharmacokinetic phase involves the movement or distribution of the drug's active ingredients from the body fluids to the site where the intended action of the drug takes place.

In the pharmacodynamic phase the drug's active ingredient interacts with the intended body tissues. The body's cells respond to the action of the drug and change as the drug is metabolized.[13]

The liver is the main organ that inactivates and metabolizes drugs; the kidneys are the principal organs that eliminate the metabolites of drugs from the body. **Metabolites** are substances produced by metabolic action.[9]

The nurse must understand the process of drug action and elimination from the body, because each patient will be affected differently by the drugs they are given. Each patient's hepatic (liver) and renal (kidney) functions must be assessed and considered, because decreased hepatic and/or renal function may prolong the length of time a drug stays in the body.

Drugs that are not excreted in the urine, feces, sweat, tears, breast milk (in lactating mothers), and expired air may build up in the body. A drug that builds up in the body is said to have a **cumulative** effect, which can lead to *toxic* (harmful) or even lethal (deadly) effects.

Drug Dosage

Dosage is the amount of a drug prescribed for the patient by the physician (e.g., "Give 300 mg Dilantin po tid").

Three hundred milligrams is the dosage ordered in the example. The nurse will give three doses of Dilantin po three times a day. Each dose contains 100 mg per capsule. A *dose* of medicine refers to a single prescribed amount

BOX 25-1 DOSAGE TERMS

Minimal dose	The smallest amount of a drug that produces a therapeutic effect
Maximal dose	The largest amount of a drug that can be given safely
Toxic dose	The amount of a drug that produces symptoms of poisoning
Lethal dose	The amount of a drug that will cause death

From Asperheim M: Pharmacology: an introductory text, ed 6, Philadelphia, 1987, WB Saunders Co.

of drug given at one time. Nurses must become familiar with **therapeutic** (helpful) dosages of frequently used drugs to confidently administer doses of medication to each patient (Box 25-1).

Drug Actions and Interactions

There are two general types of drug action—local and systemic. Drugs that produce a local action affect only the area where the drug is placed. Systemic drug action affects the entire body, because the drug enters the systemic circulation.

When one drug alters the action of another drug, it is called a *drug interaction*. When two or more drugs are given together, the combined actions of the drugs may produce a totally different effect than the expected effect of either drug. These effects can be beneficial or harmful. When one drug increases the action or the effect of another drug, it is called **potentiation** or synergism. This is often done purposely to "boost" the action of one or the other of the drugs administered.

Some drugs *do not* combine chemically with other drugs. This is called drug *incompatibility*. For example, when two drugs are mixed and the solution changes color, becomes cloudy, or forms a precipitate (solid mass), incompatibility is suspected. **Compatibility** charts allow quick reference to determine whether one drug may be given along with another drug in the same syringe or intravenous infusion.

Knowledge of agonistic and antagonistic drug action is helpful to the nurse and physician. A drug that produces a response at the intended site of action is called an **agonist**. An **antagonist** is a drug that will block the action of another drug. Antagonistic drugs are used to counteract the effects of a previously given drug. For example, naloxone HCl (Narcan) works against the central nervous system depressant effects of meperidine HCl (Demerol) or other central nervous system depressants by blocking the action of the depressants.

Because each patient responds differently to medications, the nurse must be alert to the possibility of idiosyncratic drug reactions. An **idiosyncratic** response to a drug is an unexpected response to a medication. Idiosyncratic reactions are thought to have a genetic basis.[12] An idiosyncratic reaction to a sedative that was given to produce calmness in a patient may unexpectedly cause him to become agitated and restless. For this reason, it is important to observe and assess patients for signs of overdose, toxicity, and unexpected drug reactions even though they are receiving the correct therapeutic dose.

A patient may be hypersensitive or allergic to a drug. The nurse should assess the patient's drug history *before* giving a drug. Has the patient taken the drug before? Does the patient have any known allergies to medications? If so, the drug should be withheld and this information reported to the RN. When in doubt, "Don't."

A reduced response to a drug is called drug **tolerance**. The patient who has developed tolerance to a drug requires a larger dose of the drug to achieve the same effect that a smaller therapeutic dose once gave. Drug tolerance may either be acquired from taking increasing dosages of the drug over a period of time or result from genetic factors unique to the individual.

Drug administration is a tremendous nursing responsibility. The nurse must not give any unfamiliar medication and should look up the medication in a drug reference book *before* giving it to the patient.

Each patient's reaction to drug therapy must be observed, particularly when he is given a drug for the first time. The patient's mental and physical status must be assessed before a new medication is started to establish a baseline reference. Changes in mental or physical status should be reported to the RN. The change may be caused by **adverse drug reaction,** drug hypersensitivity, or drug intolerance.

The *Physicians' Desk Reference* is a book usually found in the nurses' station. It can be used to find therapeutic dosage, indications for use of the drug, contraindications (conditions in which the drug should *not* be used), side effects, routes, generic and trade names, a list of poison control centers, and information for managing overdosages.

Drug **interactions** are more likely to occur with drugs that are especially potent (strong), such as digitalis. The cardiotonics (drugs that slow and strengthen the heart), antihypertensives (drugs that lower blood pressure), hypoglycemic agents (oral medications that lower blood glucose [sugar]), insulin (injectable medication that lowers blood glucose), and heparin (medication that decreases the clotting of blood) are all powerful agents that the nurse must be familiar with *before* giving.

Clayton[4] states that drug interactions are a frequent cause of adverse effects, decreased patient compliance, and prolonged hospitalizations. Continual awareness of the possibility of interactions and observation for these complications are the responsibility of all health professionals. The nurse should watch for changes in level of consciousness such as slurred speech or ataxia (unsteady gait) and for changes in vital signs. The nurse should *listen* to what the patient says about how his medication is affecting him. The LPN/LVN reports observations to the RN and documents these observations objectively in the nurse's notes. Physicians depend on the ongoing nursing assessment of each patient's response to drug therapy.

The following factors affect how patients respond to medication and must be considered in assessment:

- *Age*: Very young and very old people generally react more acutely to drugs than others. Elderly persons tend to have a higher ratio of fat tissue to muscle tissue, and the higher fat percentage may affect the distribution and accumulation of fat-soluble drugs. Prolonged drug action is likely to occur in older adults, because renal and hepatic function may be decreased. The very young do not have fully developed renal and hepatic functions; therefore drugs are inefficiently metabolized and excreted.
- *Weight*: Overweight persons may require higher drug dosages than those of average weight. Underweight individuals usually require lower drug dosages. Body surface area, height, and weight are important factors in determining drug dosages in children.
- *Physical health*: Persons in poor physical health do not tolerate average dosages as well as those in good health. Disease processes alter dosage requirements, particularly in patients with renal, hepatic, cardiovascular, and gastrointestinal dysfunctions.
- *Psychological status*: Stress, emotional conflict, anxiety, and fear may alter response to drug therapy. If the patient has faith in the drug, the hospital, the physician, and the nurse, he is more likely to adhere to his medication therapy. The nurse's actions, attitudes, and skills also affect the patient's response to drug therapy.
- *Environmental temperature*: Heat may increase the metabolism of a drug; cold may decrease the metabolic rate.
- *Sex*: Women tend to have a higher percentage of body fat than men, whereas men have a higher percentage of body fluid. Since some drugs are fat soluble, females with high body fat percentage may accumulate fat-soluble drugs in their body. Pregnant and lactating women must be advised that the substances taken during pregnancy may pass through the placenta and adversely affect the fetus. Drugs may also be passed to infants through breast milk.
- *Amount of food in the stomach*: Drugs taken on an empty stomach reach the bloodstream faster than those taken on a full stomach. Irritating drugs are given after or with meals so that they will not irritate the gastrointestinal tract.
- *Dosage forms*: Dosage forms influence the onset, intensity, and duration of a drug. Intravenous and intramuscular drugs react more quickly than drugs taken orally.

It is important to continually assess and evaluate drug action in each individual patient. The nurse must use judgment before giving medications, because any drug can be harmful.

The nurse must be knowledgeable about the basics of drug action, how drug orders are written, how to interpret them, and how they are transcribed. The basic practices and principles of safe medication administration must *always* be followed. High personal and professional standards protect the patient and prevent the nurse from making medication errors.

Medication Orders

The nurse is ethically and legally responsible for ensuring that the patient receives the correct medication ordered by the physician. Physicians write medication orders during patient admissions, during morning and evening rounds, after surgery, and any other time throughout the day or night as needed. As soon as possible after a physician writes an order, the nurse should read and interpret the order. The nurse then transcribes the drug order to the Medex (or Kardex, depending on the facility) *exactly* the same way that the order appears on the order sheet. If the handwriting is illegible, another nurse should be asked to help or the physician called for clarification.

The medication request for the patient's medications is sent to the pharmacy. The pharmacist will prepare and send the medications to the patient's unit.

Some drugs come in multidose vials or bottles; others come in unit dose (one dose per vial or package). The unit dose system was instituted to reduce medication errors and to make it easier to keep accurate records of medications used and not used. For example, if a patient goes home or dies, the unused unit dose medications are returned to the pharmacy for credit to the patient's account.

Whether unit dose or multidose is used, it is the nurse's responsibility to properly store medications on the ward. The storage instructions of each drug must be followed; some must be refrigerated, whereas others must be kept in a dark or cool area. Narcotics, barbiturates, and other controlled drugs that have a high potential for abuse must be safely and securely stored.

Frequently the drug received on the ward has a different name than that ordered by the physician. Each drug has several names; the two most commonly used are the trade name and the generic name. The *trade name* is the brand name given to it by the manufacturer. It is followed by the symbol ®. The trade name is short and easy to spell and to pronounce, such as "Demerol." It is capitalized. The generic name, frequently used, is usually longer, is not capitalized, and is used by the manufacturer. The generic name for Demerol is meperidine.

The nurse must make certain that the drug received is the same drug that was ordered. The pharmacist should be consulted if there is a question about the identity of a drug. Once assured that the medication is the correct one, the nurse clearly and accurately transcribes the medication name, dosage, times, and stop date on the Medex. In many facilities unit clerks transcribe drug orders. The RN or LPN/LVN who transcribes or verifies the order writes his or her signature and title and the time and date immediately after the last order on the order sheet. The nurse draws a line after the last order to indicate the end of that physician's particular order.

Medication orders should include the following:

1. Patient's name (on physician's order sheet)
2. Date and time of the order (usually on the left side of the order sheet); written by the physician
3. Name of drug
4. Dosage of the drug (e.g., give ASA grains [gr] X prn q 3-4 hr)
5. Route of administration (if none is given, it is understood to be by mouth)
6. Time or frequency drug is given (e.g., give bid [two times a day])
7. Signature of the physician
8. Any special instructions regarding any aspect of administering the drug (e.g., give ASA grains [gr] X q 3-4 hr if temp >101° F)

See Box 25-2 for common terms used with medication orders.

One-time-only orders, such as stat, now, ASAP, or SOS, are signed off on the physician's order sheet by the RN as soon as possible after the medication has been given. Doing so prevents another nurse from "double-dosing" the patient as a result of poor communication between nurses. If the order is written on the Medex (Fig. 25-1), the nurse must properly transcribe the order and discontinue the order immediately after giving the medication. (See Medex examples.)

Controlled substances. Narcotics, barbiturates, and other controlled drugs that have a high possibility for abuse or addiction are double-locked. The "narcotic keys" are kept by one designated nurse per shift. It is that nurse's responsibility to see that each controlled drug used that shift is logged in the narcotic log book. At the end of each shift controlled drugs in the locker are carefully counted by the key-holding nurse of the outgoing shift and the nurse of the incoming shift. The number of drugs given, according to the log book, and the actual number of medications contained in the locker *must* be exactly the same. The staff are *not* dismissed until the narcotic count is done. If the count is incorrect, the error or the missing drug must be found before anyone is dismissed. The nurse *must not* take the keys home.

The nurse should always have a witness to the "wasting" (disposal) of part of a controlled medication. The witness and the person wasting the medication must sign the log book to indicate that the medication was wasted. Controlled substances are handled only by people with licenses, such as an RN or an LPN, or a student nurse under the supervision of the nurse educator.

BOX 25-2 COMMON TERMS USED WITH MEDICATION ORDERS

STAT	Immediately; number one priority; give before any other type of order. Be careful to document that the medication was given to avoid mistakes. A "Stat" order is a one-time only dose.
Now	Give now; number two priority; give before orders of lower priority. Cancel order after giving.
ASAP	As soon as possible; number three priority; give before orders of lower priority. Cancel order after giving.
SOS	One time only, if needed; may be given *only* one time, *and if* it is needed according to the patient's wishes or according to the nurse's assessment of the patient's need. Cancel order after giving.
PRN	Give as necessary; the patient may request prn medication, or the nurse may offer a prn medication; prn medications should have a definite time interval within which the medication is to be given.

Types of Orders

Standing orders. Standing orders are already written by a physician for all his or her patients on a particular unit or area. They are carried out without having to call the physician and without the presence of the physician. A copy of the orders is kept on the unit. The nurse should know where the orders are located, be knowledgeable about standing orders, and use assessment and judgment skills in implementing these orders. A patient may be unnecessarily stressed or uncomfortable if the nurse is unaware that the physician has left standing orders. If there is *any* question about a standing order, the nurse should get verification or clarification from the physician who wrote them. Each physician leaves different standing orders; the nurse *must know* the physicians' orders.

There are two types of standing orders:

Standing order with expiration: The order is written and kept in a folder at the nurses' station. The order

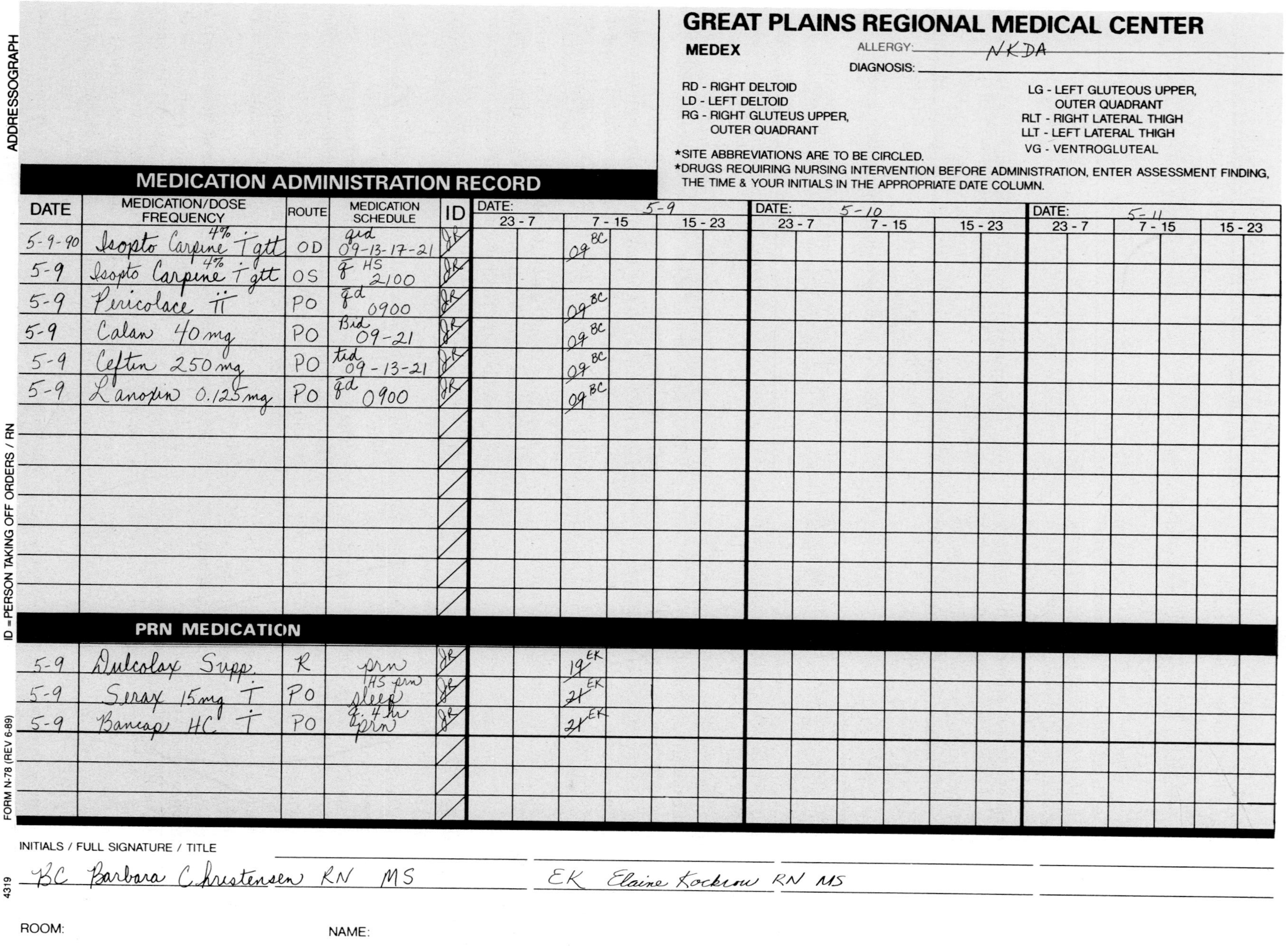

ADDRESSOGRAPH

GREAT PLAINS REGIONAL MEDICAL CENTER

MEDEX

ALLERGY: NKDA

DIAGNOSIS:

RD - RIGHT DELTOID
LD - LEFT DELTOID
RG - RIGHT GLUTEUS UPPER, OUTER QUADRANT
LG - LEFT GLUTEOUS UPPER, OUTER QUADRANT
RLT - RIGHT LATERAL THIGH
LLT - LEFT LATERAL THIGH
VG - VENTROGLUTEAL

*SITE ABBREVIATIONS ARE TO BE CIRCLED.
*DRUGS REQUIRING NURSING INTERVENTION BEFORE ADMINISTRATION, ENTER ASSESSMENT FINDING, THE TIME & YOUR INITIALS IN THE APPROPRIATE DATE COLUMN.

MEDICATION ADMINISTRATION RECORD

DATE	MEDICATION/DOSE FREQUENCY	ROUTE	MEDICATION SCHEDULE	ID	DATE: 5-9 23-7	7-15	15-23
5-9-90	Isopto Carpine 4% İ gtt	OD	qid 09-13-17-21	JR		09 BC	
5-9	Isopto Carpine 4% İ gtt	OS	q HS 2100	JR			
5-9	Pericolace ïï	PO	qd 0900	JR		09 BC	
5-9	Calan 40 mg	PO	Bid 09-21	JR		09 BC	
5-9	Ceftin 250 mg	PO	tid 09-13-21	JR		09 BC	
5-9	Lanoxin 0.125 mg	PO	qd 0900	JR		09 BC	

PRN MEDICATION

DATE	MEDICATION/DOSE FREQUENCY	ROUTE	MEDICATION SCHEDULE	ID	DATE: 5-9 23-7	7-15	15-23
5-9	Dulcolax Supp.	R	prn	JR		19 EK	
5-9	Serax 15 mg İ	PO	HS prn sleep	JR		21 EK	
5-9	Bancap HC İ	PO	q 4 hr prn	JR		21 EK	

DATE: 5-10 (23-7, 7-15, 15-23) DATE: 5-11 (23-7, 7-15, 15-23)

ID = PERSON TAKING OFF ORDERS / RN

FORM N-78 (REV 6-89)

INITIALS / FULL SIGNATURE / TITLE
BC Barbara Christensen RN MS
EK Elaine Kockrow RN MS

4319

ROOM: NAME:

ORIGINAL - PLACE IN CHART 3rd DAY, DISCARD COPY 2

FIG. 25-1 Medication record.

must be discontinued or reordered on the expiration date.

Standing order without expiration: The order is written and kept in a folder at the nurses' station, but no expiration date is given.

Verbal orders. A verbal order from a physician may be given in the presence of an LPN/LVN or an RN directly or over the telephone. Hospital policy for LPNs taking verbal and telephone orders should be observed. Verbal orders are written on the physicians' order sheet exactly as the physician gave them. The physician should sign the order as soon as possible. The nurse should be alert and careful when taking verbal orders. If the order is unclear or confusing, the nurse should not hesitate to ask the physician about the order. The nurse should always repeat the order to the physician to make sure that what was heard is what the physician actually said.

LEARNING OBJECTIVES

After reading this section, the student should be able to do the following:

- Give the five "rights" of drug administration and describe the nursing responsibilities involved in each "right."
- Describe when a medication label is read (or checked) three times.
- Define qid, tid, bid, hs, ac, pc, and qd.
- Explain "universal precautions."
- List 13 safety rules for preventing medication errors.

GENERAL PRINCIPLES AND PRACTICES OF MEDICATION ADMINISTRATION

The nurse employs each step of the nursing process in carrying out the responsibilities of drug administration.

Drugs are administered in a variety of ways. Regardless of the route by which a drug enters the body, the same practices and principles of medication administration apply.

Following the "five rights," performing the "three label checks," using universal precautions, and practicing good handwashing and aseptic technique ensure excellent drug administration practice.

The "five rights" are followed every time a drug is given (Box 25-3).

The Right Medication

The nurse must make sure the drug to be given is the correct drug, checking the label on its container three times (Box 25-4).

BOX 25-3 THE FIVE RIGHTS OF MEDICATION ADMINISTRATION

1. Give the *right medication* in the
2. *Right dose* to the
3. *Right patient* at the
4. *Right time* by the
5. *Right route*

BOX 25-4 THE THREE LABEL CHECKS OF MEDICATION ADMINISTRATION

1. Check the label when taking the medication from its storage area.
2. Check the label when removing the medication from its container.
3. Check the label when discarding or replacing the medication container.

The nurse should *never* give a medication that has been prepared by another person and *never* prepare or use a medication that is not labelled. In both cases it is impossible to know for sure what medication was prepared or what medication was in the unlabelled container.

The nurse should check the physician's order to verify the Medex if there is a question about a medication. The nurse must become familiar with generic and trade names of frequently used medications. Consult the *PDR* or the pharmacist if necessary.

The Right Dose

The nurse should check the Medex to verify the dosage of a drug. If there is a question, then the physician's order should be checked. The nurse always checks the label on the container for the dose per milliliter or dose per tablet and consults with another nurse to check calculations or clarify a dosage.

The appropriateness of the dose must be assessed: Is the dose consistent with the age of the patient, the diagnosis of the patient, the sex of the patient? The nurse looks at the number of tablets that constitute the dose or the number of milliliters that make the dose. Does the number of tablets or the number of milliliters in the syringe "look" or "sound" reasonable? The decimal place in the dosage ordered and the nurse's calculations must be checked; a decimal in the wrong place can cause a serious drug error.

Table 25-1 Commonly Used Abbreviations

Abbreviation	Meaning	Example
bid	Two times a day	9 AM—9 PM
tid	Three times a day	9 AM—1 PM—5 PM
qid	Four times a day	8 AM—12 N—4 PM—8 PM
qd	Every day	9 AM
ac	Before eating	Varies with hospital or unit
pc	After eating	Varies with hospital or unit
hs	Hours of sleep	Varies with hospital or unit

The Right Time

The nurse is responsible for placing the drug order on the right time schedule. A standardized schedule is generally specified by the hospital. A medication should be worked into the standardized schedule as soon as possible. Table 25-1 lists commonly used abbreviations.

Medications should be given on time. If it is impossible to give a medication exactly at the scheduled time, the nurse should give it at least within 30 minutes of the scheduled time. Antibiotics in particular should be given on time to maintain therapeutic blood levels.

Medications to be administered prn should not be given before the time specified by the physician's order. The nurse should check the date that the drug order was written to be sure that the drug, intravenous infusion, or blood product is started and given on the right day and at the right time. The order sheet and/or the Medex should be checked for dates and times to be sure that the medication has not been discontinued (d/c).

The Right Route

The drug order should indicate the preferred route of administration. If no route is given, it is understood that the route is *po* (per os; by mouth). If there is doubt, the nurse should verify the order with the physician.

If the medication is parenteral (intramuscular, IM; subcutaneous, SQ; intradermal, ID; and intravenous, IV), the nurse must be certain to inject the drug into the tissue specified.

The Right Patient

The nurse makes sure the medication is given to the right patient by systematically identifying the patient in every situation by checking the name, room number, and bed number of the patient against the drug order. Once in the patient's room, the nurse asks the patient to state his full name. The patient may also be asked to spell his name as the nurse checks his identification band.

An unconscious patient cannot identify himself; his safety depends on the nurse. A family member or visitor may be at the bedside, but do not rely on others to identify the patient. The nurse should *always* check the identification band on conscious or unconscious patients and *never* give medications or perform procedures on a patient who does not have an ID band.

After the five rights have been observed and the three label checks have been done, the nurse employs universal precautions (Box 25-5).

BOX 25-5 **UNIVERSAL PRECAUTIONS TO MINIMIZE TRANSMISSION OF AIDS**

1. Gloves are worn for touching body fluids, mucous membranes, or nonintact skin of all patients.
2. Gloves are worn for handling items or surfaces soiled with blood or body fluids.
3. Gloves are worn when a staff member has a break in his or her skin.
4. Gloves are *not* worn when 1, 2, or 3 above is not present or likely (e.g., when transporting patients).
5. Gloves are worn for performing venipuncture and other vascular access procedures.
6. Hands are washed immediately after gloves are removed.
7. Hands or other skin surfaces are washed immediately and thoroughly if contaminated with blood or other body fluids.
8. Used sharps, such as needles or scalpels, are placed in a biohazard needle box.
9. Needles are *not* purposely bent, broken, or re-capped.
10. The needle container is not overfilled.
11. Disposable wastes and articles contaminated with blood or large amounts of body fluids are placed in impervious (no holes present) containers for a trash pickup.
12. Spills of blood or body fluids are cleaned up with a 1:10 solution (prepared daily) of Clorox and water.
13. Masks and protective eyewear are worn during procedures that are likely to generate droplets of blood or body fluid (e.g., nasotracheal suctioning) to prevent exposure of mucous membrane.
14. Gowns are worn during procedures that are likely to generate splashes of blood or other body fluids (e.g., wound irrigation, cleansing a patient with bowel or bladder incontinence).
15. Reusable items (e.g., suction bottles and oxygen setups) are emptied with care to avoid splashing.
16. *All* soiled linen is placed in a laundry bag, and the bag is *not* overfilled.
17. For patients with diarrhea—there is no change in practice by a staff member, whether a patient has been diagnosed as having AIDS or not.
18. For patients who are coughing—there is no change in practice by a staff member, whether a patient has been diagnosed as having AIDS or not.

Important Considerations of Medication Administration

While handling equipment during medication administration, the nurse must always think, "sterile to sterile and clean to clean." Hands must be washed between each patient. Work spaces and equipment must be kept clean and orderly, and practices should be established that will keep staff members and patients safe. Short cuts should not be taken, and staff should never deviate from principles that are effective. The following rules should be applied:

1. If you did not pour it, do not give it.
2. If you gave it, chart it.
3. Do not chart for someone else or have someone chart for you.
4. Do not transport or accept a container that is not labeled.
5. Do not put down an unlabeled syringe; keep it in your hand or label it before you put it down.
6. If given a verbal order, repeat the order to the physician.
7. If you make an error, report it *immediately* to the charge nurse or supervisor, or if you are in charge notify the physician.
8. *Never* leave a medication tray or cart unattended or unlocked.
9. *Do not* leave a medication with a patient or family member. *Watch* the patient take and swallow the medication.
10. *Always return* to assess the patient's response to the medication.
11. Chart as soon as possible after giving medication.
12. If a patient refuses medication do not force it; chart "Refused medication because of . . . ."
13. If you elect to omit a dose based on your nursing judgment, let another nurse help make the decision. If medication is not given, document "Dose omitted because of . . . . " Be objective and exact in charting. Report your decision to the physician.

LEARNING OBJECTIVES

After reading this section, the student should be able to do the following:

- List and define the three general routes of administration.
- Define enteral, enteric-coated, enteric, and gastrointestinal tract.
- Define parenteral, intramuscular, intradermal, subcutaneous, intravenous, percutaneous, sublingual, and topical.
- List five solid dosage forms.
- List two types of glass containers of injectable liquids.
- Name four enteral routes.
- Name four percutaneous routes.
- Name four parenteral routes.
- Describe the difference between a tablet and a pill, and a capsule and a tablet.

INTRODUCTION TO THE ROUTES OF ADMINISTRATION

Drugs enter the body through three general routes—enteral, parenteral, and percutaneous. The drugs that enter the body by these routes come in various forms.

Drugs that enter through the **enteral** (by the gastrointestinal tract) routes are given in these forms:

1. Powders: Often mixed with a liquid (diluent) before administration
2. Pills: Round, solid drug form that must be broken down into solution form (dissolution) in the stomach
3. Tablets: Round, spherical, or oddly shaped forms that dissolve in the stomach
   Types of tablets
   a. Scored: Indented to allow tablet to be broken in half
   b. **Enteric-coated:** Candylike coated shell encases tablet to keep tablet from being absorbed in the stomach; absorption takes place in the intestine
   c. Capsule: Powders or pellets enclosed in a gelatin-like, elongated, spherical form; encapsulated because (1) substance may be bad tasting, or (2) substance may be a spansule with time-released pellets to delay the action of the drug
   d. Lozenge/troche: A sweet mucilage-type tablet that dissolves in the mouth to release medication

4. Suspensions: Solid particles and liquid that must be *shaken to disperse* solid particles throughout the liquid portion *before* absorption can occur
5. Suppositories: Drugs mixed with lubricated substance molded to insert into body cavities such as the rectum; *must melt* at body temperature to be absorbed

The above dosage forms are given by the enteral routes. The enteral routes are as follows:

1. po: by mouth
2. Tubal: by nasogastric tube (Levin tube) into the stomach
3. Suppository: by rectum, vagina, or urethra
4. Enema: by rectum

Dosage forms used by the percutaneous route (through the skin or mucous membranes) include lotions, ointments, creams, and powders.

The percutaneous routes are as follows:

1. Topical: Applied to the skin
2. Instillation: To the mucous membranes of the mouth:
   a. **Sublingual** (under the tongue)
   b. **Buccal** (in the cheek)
   c. To the mucous membranes of the:
      eye
      ear
      nose
      vagina
3. Inhalation: Aerosolized liquids, gases

Parenteral means by any method other than the enteral route. It is usually thought of as the "needle" route.

Ampules. Ampules are glass containers that are opened by snapping off the top part of the ampule. They are intended for unit dose use.

Vials. Vials are glass containers that are sealed with a metal cap with a rubber diaphragm in the middle of the cap. The rubber diaphragm permits a needle to enter the vial for either unit dose or multidose use (depending on the contents of the vial).

Large volumes of fluids are contained in plastic or glass containers, such as intravenous fluid bags. IV fluid bags or bottles range in amounts from 50 ml to 1,000 ml.

The parenteral routes are as follows:

IM: Intramuscular (within the muscle)
SC, SQ, or Subq: Subcutaneous (under the dermis; fatty tissue)
ID: Intradermal (within the dermis)
IV: Intravenous (within the vein)

LEARNING OBJECTIVES

After reading this section, the student should be able to do the following:

- Administer medications by the enteral routes.
- Describe how to properly pour a tablet, pill, or capsule.
- Explain how to set up a medication tray for several patients.
- Explain why po medications must not be given to unconscious patients.
- Describe in detail how to pour a liquid medication.
- Describe how to protect the label of a liquid medication and what to do if the label becomes soiled.
- Define meniscus.
- Give two reasons why a patient would receive a rectal suppository rather than a medication by mouth.
- Describe in detail how to check the position of an NG tube.

ADMINISTERING THE ENTERAL ROUTES

Preparation of Tablets, Pills, and Capsules

Tablets, pills, and capsules that enter the gastrointestinal tract are absorbed more slowly into the bloodstream than by any other route. The slow absorption rate makes the po (by mouth; oral) route relatively safe.

If an error is made, report it immediately to the RN. An incident report should be done to document the error. The nurse should not hesitate to report an error, because prompt intervention may prevent adverse effects on the patient.

Nurses must also be aware that some po medications are irritating to the gastrointestinal tract and that larger tablets may be difficult for some patients to swallow. See Skill 25-1.

SKILL 25-1 ADMINISTERING TABLETS, PILLS, AND CAPSULES

1. Follow the five rights (Box 25-3).
2. Perform the three label checks (Box 25-4).
3. Follow universal precautions (Box 25-5).
4. Wash hands.
5. If using unit dose package, place unopened package in medicine cup.
6. If using a multidose bottle, pour tablet, without touching it, into cap of bottle.
7. Pour tablet from cap into medicine cup.
8. If using medicine tray (for several patients), set it up from left to right, front to back.
9. If pouring from multidose bottle and patient is to receive several tablets, use separate cup for medications such as digitalis. If the patient's pulse is less than 60/min, withhold the medication and report this to the RN. By placing digitalis in a separate cup marked with a red heart it will be identified easily.
10. Do not replace pills, tablets, or capsules that come from multidose bottles if they have been handled or dropped on the floor.
11. Take medication to the room.
12. Follow procedure for room, bed, and patient identification (p. 441).
13. Explain procedure to patient.
14. Document administration of medication on the Medex with time, date, and initials.
15. Return to assess patient's response to medication.
16. Document assessment in nursing notes.

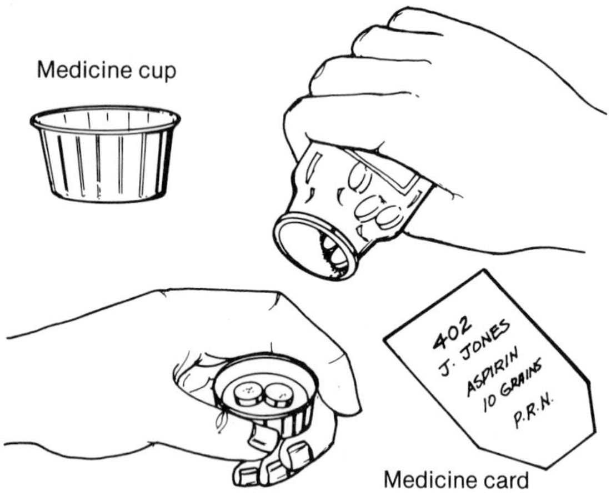

STEP 6

Preparation of Liquid Medications

Liquid medication is often given to children, to patients who cannot swallow tablets, pills, or capsules, and to geriatric patients. Liquids may be given po or via a nasogastric tube or gastrostomy tube.

Liquids must *not* be given to unconscious patients because of the possibility of aspirating (inhaling) the medication into the respiratory tract.

The nurse must be aware that some liquid medications are *not* to be followed with water and that some medications, such as iron, may stain the teeth. The nurse should look for and follow any instructions on the label. See Skill 25-2.

Suppositories

A suppository is a cone-shaped, egg-shaped, or spindle-shaped medication made for insertion into the rectum, urethra, or vagina. Suppositories dissolve at body temperature and are absorbed directly into the bloodstream. Suppositories are useful for babies, patients who cannot take oral preparations, and patients with nausea and vomiting.

Suppositories should be stored in a cool place to avoid melting; they may be placed in the refrigerator. See Skill 25-3.

SKILL 25-2 ADMINISTERING LIQUID MEDICATIONS

1. Follow the five rights (Box 25-3).
2. Perform the three label checks (Box 25-4).
3. Follow universal precautions (Box 25-5).
4. Wash hands.
5. Remove liquid preparation from patient's drug box/bin (or from medication cabinet).
6. Check dosage per milliliter and total volume of medication in container.
7. Calculate dosage; if the dosage ordered is different from the dosage per milliliter stated on the label, calculate correct dose; if ordered medication is labeled in a different measurement system, convert by using appropriate equivalent. Work problem on paper.
8. Check calculations with another nurse.
9. Obtain **graduated** (has markings indicating amount) medicine cup (total volume of cup is 30 ml or 1 oz).
10. Face label of bottle toward palm of hand to avoid soiling label; if label becomes soiled, return the bottle to the pharmacy; do not give medication if label is unreadable.
11. Place medicine cup on flat surface or hold at eye level while pouring.
12. Place cap of bottle with inner rim up to avoid contaminating inside of cap (which would contaminate remaining contents of bottle).
13. Read dosage amount at lower level of **meniscus** (curve formed by liquid's upper surface).
14. Transport medication to patient's room.
15. Follow procedure for room, bed, and patient identification (p. 441).
16. Explain procedure to patient.
17. Document administration on Medex with time, date, and initials.
18. Return to assess patient's response to medication.
19. Document assessment in nursing notes.

SKILL 25-3 ADMINISTERING RECTAL SUPPOSITORIES

1. Follow the five rights (Box 25-3).
2. Perform the three label checks (Box 25-4).
3. Follow universal precautions (Box 25-5).
4. Wash hands.
5. Obtain suppository from refrigerator or from patient's medication bin.
6. Place unopened suppository into medicine cup or **souffle cup** (ungraduated disposable paper cup).
7. Take disposable, unsterile gloves or finger cot (single-digit plastic finger cover) to room.
8. Follow procedure of room, bed, and patient identification (p. 441).
9. Explain procedure to patient.
10. Gain patient's cooperation.
11. Provide privacy.
12. Position patient in Sims' position (on left side with upper leg flexed at knee).
13. Unwrap suppository.
14. Maintain privacy; expose buttocks.
15. Don gloves.
16. Apply lubricant, such as KY jelly, to tapered end of suppository.
17. Ask patient to take deep breath; insert beyond internal anal sphincter. Insert suppository as patient exhales to relax anal sphincter.
18. Ask patient to retain suppository as long as possible to allow the medication to completely dissolve and absorb through mucous membranes of rectum into capillaries of systemic circulatory system. Hold the buttocks together to help patient to retain suppository.
19. Discard gloves.
20. Help patient assume comfortable position.
21. Document administration of suppository in Medex with time and initials.
22. Return to assess patient's response to medication.
23. Document assessment in nurse's notes.

Tubal Medications

Nasogastric (NG) tubes are used to administer liquid medications to unconscious patients, dysphagic patients (who have difficulty in swallowing), and those who are too ill to eat. A gastrostomy tube (placed through the abdominal wall and into the stomach) is also used in the same manner as the NG tube.

Many medicines come in liquid form. If they do not, solid tablets may be crushed or **pulverized** in a mortar and pestle. Mix the crushed tablet with 30 ml of water and give through the tube. Capsules can also be opened, mixed with 30 ml of water, and administered. See Skill 25-4.

SKILL 25-4 ADMINISTERING TUBAL MEDICATIONS

1. Follow the five rights (Box 25-3).
2. Perform the three label checks (Box 25-4).
3. Follow universal precautions (Box 25-5).
4. Wash hands.
5. Prepare medication using the same procedure as for liquid medications.
6. Gather equipment: 10 ml syringe, towel, stethoscope, bulb or Asepto syringe, tap water.
7. Take equipment and medication to patient's room.
8. Follow procedure of room, bed, patient identification (see p. 441).
9. Explain procedure; answer questions patient may have about the procedure.
10. Place patient in high Fowler's position.
11. Put towel over patient's chest (to protect clothing and bed linen).
12. Don disposable, unsterile gloves.
13. Check and recheck placement and patency of tube with at least two methods to ensure that tube is in the stomach and *not* in the respiratory tract.
    Method A: Attach bulb or Asepto syringe to end of NG tube. Pull plunger back or release suction of bulb syringe to aspirate stomach contents. If stomach contents are seen, proceed with medication.
    Method B: Place stethoscope over stomach. Push 10 ml of air through NG tube with syringe. The rush of air is heard in stomach with stethoscope if tube is in stomach. Proceed with medication.
14. Clamp tube with rubber-tipped hemostats or other clamping device.
15. Attach syringe to end of tube (with plunger out of syringe).
16. Pour medication into syringe.
17. Unclamp tubing to allow medication to slowly flow by gravity.
18. Follow medication with 30 to 50 ml of water to flush the medication into stomach. Water is essential to enhance absorption of medication and is also used to clean and maintain patency of NG tube.
19. Clamp tubing; secure tube after medication is given.
20. If NG tube is attached to suction, do *not* reconnect suction for 30 minutes. The medication will then have time to absorb, since medication will not be aspirated through tube.
21. Remove towel from patient.
22. Remove gloves.
23. Leave patient in comfortable position.
24. Gather equipment; clean up patient and area.
25. Document administration of NG medication in Medex with time, date, and initials.
26. Return to assess patient's response to medication.
27. Document assessment in nursing notes.

LEARNING OBJECTIVES

After reading this section, the student should be able to do the following:

- Administer medication by the percutaneous routes.
- Define and list the percutaneous routes.
- Define ointment, cream, lotion, buccal, sublingual, and topical.
- Describe the procedure for instilling ophthalmic ointments and ophthalmic drops.
- Describe the methods of instilling eardrops to an adult and to a child.
- Describe the position a patient should be placed in while instilling nose drops, and explain why this position is used.
- List four medications that may be administered by inhalation.
- Explain why the sublingual route is the preferred route for patient self-administration of nitroglycerine (NTG).

ADMINISTERING PERCUTANEOUS ROUTES

The percutaneous routes are those routes by which medications are absorbed through the skin or the mucous membranes. Most percutaneous medications produce a local action, but there are some that produce a systemic action.

The percutaneous routes include **topical** applications (applied to the skin), instillations, and inhalations. Absorption is rapid, but of short duration.

Topical medications include ointments, creams, powders, and lotions.

Ointments. An ointment is an oil-based semisolid medication; it may be applied to the skin or a mucous membrane. Nitroglycerin (NTG) is a commonly used ointment that produces an effect of longer duration than the sublingual form. NTG ointment is applied topically by using applicator paper and is placed on the skin with the ointment side on the skin. The topical disk is a transdermal patch that provides controlled release of NTG through the semipermeable membrane of the disk. The adhesive side of the system is placed on a selected body site where there is little hair, and the disk is pressed into the site. The nurse should not touch the NTG side of the applicator paper or the NTG side of the disk.

Sites commonly used for NTG applications are the chest, flank, and upper arm. Ointments are removed with cottonseed oil and gauze.

Creams. Creams are semisolid, nongreasy emulsions that contain medication for external application. Creams are gently rubbed into the area and are easily removed with water and gauze.

Lotions. Lotions are generally aqueous preparations that are used as soothing agents that relieve pruritus, protect the skin, cleanse the skin, or act as astringents. Lotions contain suspended particles that must be brought into solution by shaking before application. Lotions are gently patted (not rubbed) onto the skin, and they may be removed with soap and water. See Skill 25-5.

SKILL 25-5 APPLYING TOPICAL AGENTS

1. Follow the five rights (Box 25-3).
2. Perform the three label checks (Box 25-4).
3. Follow universal precautions (Box 25-5).
4. Wash hands.
5. Transport medication to room.
6. Identify room, bed, and patient (p. 441).
7. Introduce yourself; explain procedure to patient.
8. Provide privacy; place patient in comfortable position that allows exposure of selected site.
9. Cleanse site with appropriate materials (according to whether application is oil or water based).
10. Don gloves.
11. Prepare medicinal agent (ointments, creams, and lotions may have to be squeezed or removed with a tongue blade, depending on preparation used).
12. Apply paper applicator, disk, lotion, ointment, or cream.
13. Remove gloves.
14. Leave patient properly draped or clothed in comfortable position.
15. Answer patient's questions, and teach patient to perform self-applications if appropriate.
16. Clean work area.
17. Record administration in Medex with initials, date, and time.
18. Return to assess patient's response to medication.
19. Document assessment in nursing notes.

SKILL 25-6

ADMINISTERING EYE DROPS AND EYE OINTMENTS

1. Follow the five rights (Box 25-3).
2. Perform the three label checks (Box 25-4).
3. Follow universal precautions (Box 25-5).
4. Wash hands.
5. Transport medications to room.
6. Identify room, bed, and patient (p. 441).
7. Introduce yourself; explain procedure.
8. Provide privacy; position back of patient's head on pillow; direct patient's face upward toward ceiling.
9. Don gloves.
10. Remove exudate; clean eye as needed using sterile solution of saline; use cotton balls to wipe away exudate; use one cotton ball per stroke, wiping from inner canthus outward.
11. *To apply drops,* expose lower conjunctival sac by having patient look upward while gentle traction is applied to lower eyelid.
12. Put prescribed number of drops into conjunctival sac, *not* onto eyeball.
13. Using a cotton ball or tissue, apply gentle pressure above bone at inner corner of eyelid for 1 and 2 minutes.
14. Apply sterile dressing, if ordered.
15. *To apply ointment,* expose lower conjunctival sac by having patient look upward while gentle traction is applied to lower eyelid.
16. Squeeze ointment into lower conjunctival sac.
17. Ask patient to close eye; and move it around in circular motion to spread medication.
18. Apply sterile dressing, if ordered.
19. After applying drops or ointment to an eye, leave patient in comfortable position; clean up the work area.
20. Answer patient's questions and if appropriate, teach patient to perform self-care.
21. Record administration of medications in Medex with initials, date, and time.
22. Return to assess patient's response to medication.
23. Document assessment in nursing notes.

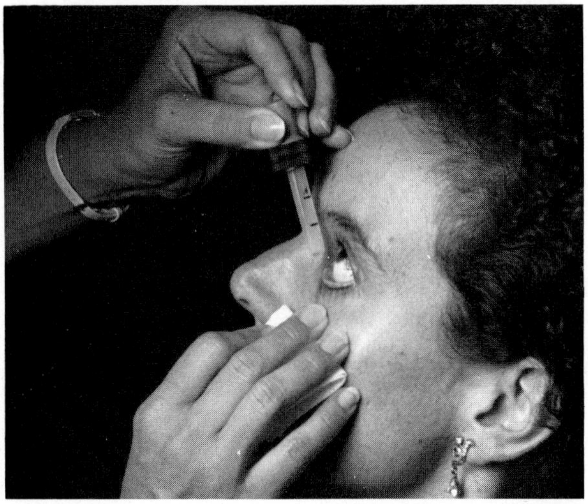

STEP 11

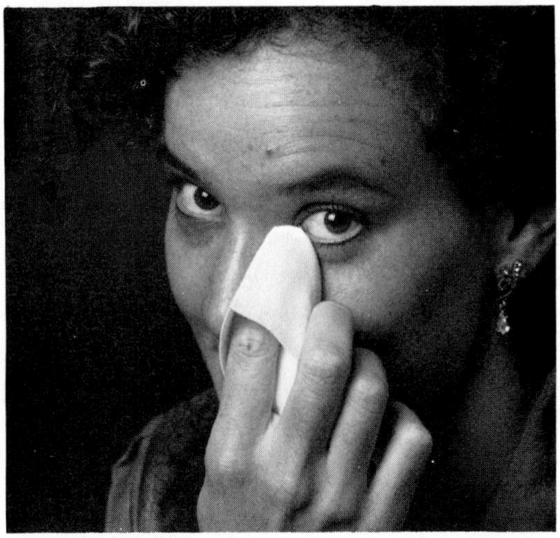

STEP 13

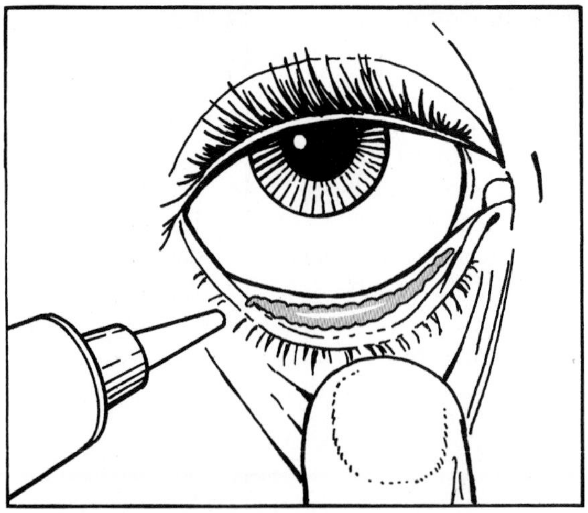

STEP 15

Eyedrops and Eye Ointments

Eyedrops and ointments are sterile. Care should be taken to keep all ophthalmic (eye) preparations sterile by not touching the dropper or the tube of ointment to the eye. The container should be checked to ensure that the medication is marked "for ophthalmic use." Ophthalmic medications are used for only one patient and are not shared. See Skill 25-6.

Eardrops

Containers of solutions to be used as eardrops will be labeled "otic." They must be at room temperature when applied. Individual bottles are used for each patient. See Skill 25-7.

SKILL 25-7 ADMINISTERING EARDROPS

1. Follow the five rights (Box 25-3).
2. Perform the three label checks (Box 25-4).
3. Follow universal precautions (Box 25-5).
4. Wash hands.
5. Transport medication to room.
6. Identify room, bed, and patient (p. 441).
7. Introduce yourself; explain procedure.
8. Provide privacy; position patient with affected ear upward.
9. Don gloves.
10. Remove external exudate from ear; an order must be obtained before irrigating the ear.
11. Draw medication into dropper.
12. For adults and for children over 3 years old, turn head with affected side up; pull ear lobe *upward* and *back* to straighten external auditory canal; give drops without touching ear with dropper.
13. For children under 3 years old, turn head with affected side up; pull earlobe *downward* and *back*; instill drops without touching ear with dropper.
14. Tell patient to remain in same position for a few minutes to allow medication to drain into ear by gravity.
15. A cotton ball may be placed loosely into ear as needed.
16. Leave patient in comfortable position; clean work area.
17. Answer patient's questions and if appropriate, teach patient self-care.
18. Record administration in Medex with initials, date, and time.
19. Return to assess patient's response to medication.
20. Document assessment in nursing notes.

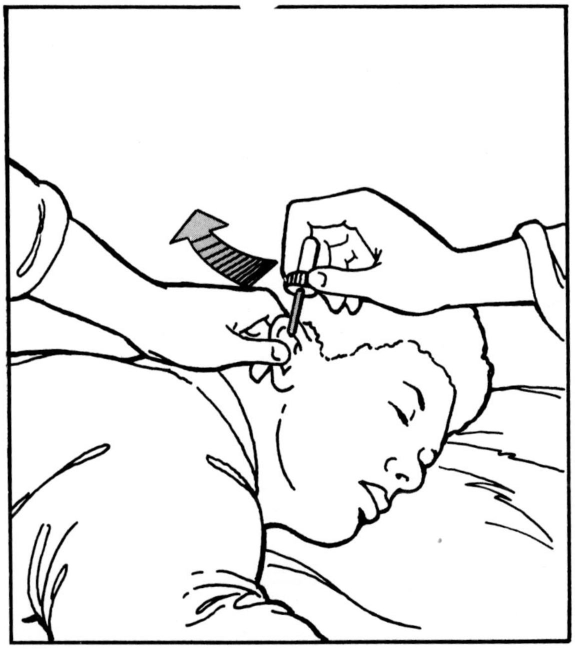

STEP 12

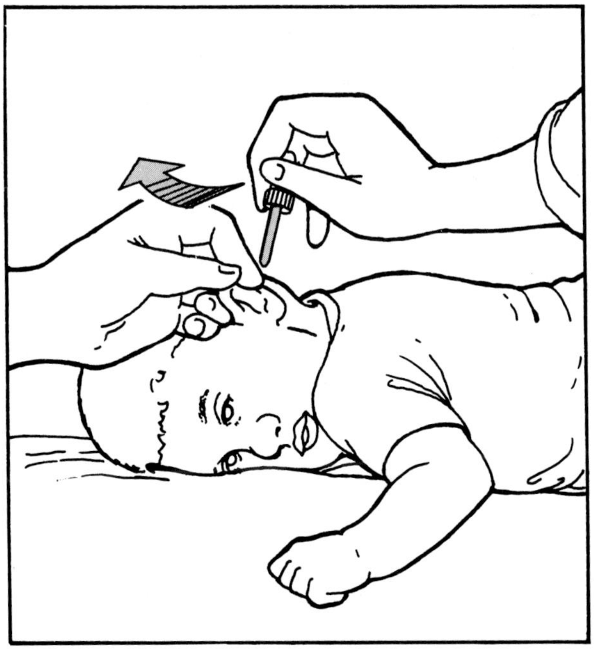

STEP 13

Nosedrops

Nosedrops are for individual use *only*. See Skill 25-8.

SKILL 25-8

ADMINISTERING NOSEDROPS

1. Follow the five rights (Box 25-3).
2. Perform the three label checks (Box 25-4).
3. Follow universal precautions (Box 25-5).
4. Wash hands.
5. Transport medication to room.
6. Identify room, bed, and patient (p. 441).
7. Introduce yourself; explain procedure.
8. Provide privacy.
9. Don gloves.
10. Ask adult or older child to clear nose of accumulations by blowing gently into tissue.
11. Have patient lie down, hanging head backward over edge of bed or with pillow under shoulders to hyperextend the neck if patient can tolerate it.
12. After drawing medication into dropper, instill medication while holding dropper above nostril being treated.
13. If ordered, repeat procedure to instill drops in other nostril.
14. Tell patient to hold position for a few minutes to allow medication to remain in place.
15. Administer nosedrops to a younger child after positioning him on bed with head backward and downward, or to an infant while holding him with head backward and downward.
16. Administer drops in same way as to an adult.
17. Tell patient to refrain from blowing nose immediately after instillation.
18. Offer tissues for later use.
19. Leave patient in comfortable position; clean work area.
20. Answer patient's questions and if appropriate, teach patient self-care.
21. Record administration in Medex with initials, date, and time.
22. Return to assess patient's response to medication.
23. Document assessment in nursing notes.

STEP 12

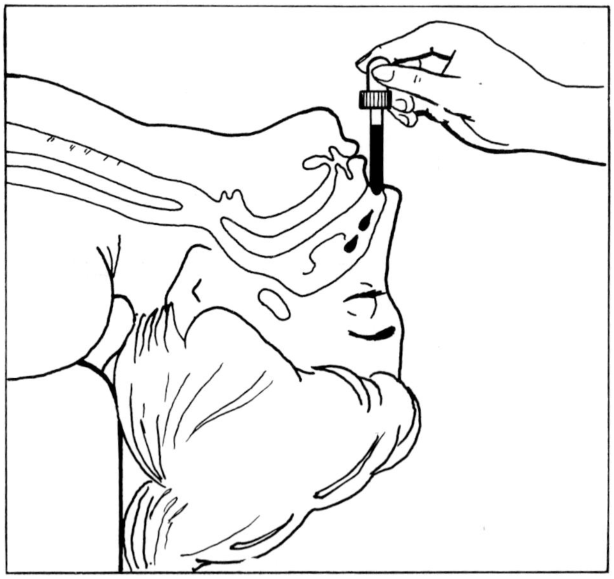

Nasal Sprays

Because nasal sprays are absorbed quickly, less medication is used and wasted when administered in this manner. Nasal sprays are for individual use *only*. See Skill 25-9.

Administering Medications by Inhalation

Drugs may be absorbed through the mucous membranes of the respiratory tract. They may produce a relatively limited effect or a systemic effect. The inhalation route is accessible to the bloodstream for vapors such as ammonia, anesthetic gases (such as chloroform, nitrous oxide, and halothane), and for respiratory therapy agents (such as acetylcysteine [Mucomyst] and Alevaire).

Respiratory therapy departments actively use the inhalation route, as do anesthesiologists and nurse anesthetists.

The nurse's participation in inhalation therapy may be limited to helping patients use metered-dose inhalers that contain bronchodilators or corticosteroids. Directions for use of these inhalers should be read and followed thoroughly, because methods of use may vary among manufacturers.

SKILL 25-9

ADMINISTERING NASAL SPRAYS

1. Follow the five rights (Box 25-3).
2. Follow the three label checks (Box 25-4).
3. Follow universal precautions (Box 25-5).
4. Wash hands.
5. Transport medication to patient.
6. Identify room, bed, and patient (p. 441).
7. Introduce yourself; explain procedure.
8. Provide privacy; position patient upright.
9. Have patient gently blow nose to clear nasal passages of accumulations.
10. Compress one nostril.
11. Shake bottle while holding it upright.
12. Insert tip of spray bottle into patient's patent nostril.
13. Instruct patient to inhale; while he inhales, squeeze bottle.
14. If ordered, repeat procedure for other nostril.
15. Tell patient to refrain from blowing nose for a few minutes; offer tissues for later use.
16. Answer patient's questions and if appropriate, teach self-administration.
17. Record administration in Medex with initials, date, and time.
18. Return to assess patient's response to medication.
19. Document assessment in nursing notes.

Sublingual Administration

Sublingual administration of a drug (usually in tablet form) is achieved by placing the tablet beneath the tongue until the tablet dissolves. After dissolution, the active ingredient, such as nitroglycerin (NTG), is rapidly absorbed into the bloodstream. Drugs given by sublingual routes bypass the liver, which reduces the time it takes for the drug to produce its desired action.

Nitroglycerin is a common sublingual medication. It is usually ordered to be left at the bedside so the patient may take it ad lib (as desired). The patient is allowed to take the NTG tablets to the x-ray department or to any other diagnostic testing area in case a tablet is needed for anginal pain.

The administration of sublingual tablets follows the same procedure as the preparation of solid oral medication, with the exceptions noted in Skill 25-10.

Buccal Administration

Buccal administration is achieved by placing a tablet between the cheek and the teeth, or between the cheek and the gums. It is left there until it dissolves. Absorption into the capillaries of the mucous membranes of the cheek gives rapid onset of the drug's active ingredient because of its direct entry into the systemic circulation.

Buccal administration is accomplished by the same procedure as solid tablet administration or sublingual administration See Skill 25-11.

SKILL 25-10 ADMINISTERING SUBLINGUAL MEDICATIONS

1. Follow the five rights (Box 25-3).
2. Perform the three label checks (Box 25-4).
3. Follow universal precautions (Box 25-5).
4. Wash hands.
5. Follow procedure for room, bed, and patient identification (p. 441).
6. Wear gloves to place tablet under patient's tongue.
7. *Do not* follow with water.
8. Instruct patient *not* to swallow tablet.
9. Explain to patient how to place medication under tongue. Instruct him to let it dissolve.
10. Document sublingual administration in Medex with time, date, and initials.
11. Return to assess patient's response to medication.
12. Document assessment in nursing notes.

SKILL 25-11 ADMINISTERING BUCCAL MEDICATIONS

1. Follow the five rights (Box 25-3).
2. Perform the three label checks (Box 25-4).
3. Follow universal precautions (Box 25-5).
4. Wash hands.
5. Follow procedure for room, bed, and patient identification (p. 441).
6. Wear gloves to place medication between patient's cheek and gum.
7. *Do not* follow with water.
8. Instruct patient *not to swallow* tablet; let it dissolve.
9. Explain to patient how to place medication between gum and cheek.
10. Document buccal administration in Medex with time, date, and initials.
11. Return to assess patient's response to medication.
12. Document assessment in nurse's notes.

LEARNING OBJECTIVES

After reading this section, the student should be able to do the following:

- Administer medication by the parenteral routes.
- Give five reasons for the use of the parenteral routes.
- Accurately describe the components of syringes and needles.
- Describe the parenteral dosage forms and the procedures used to prepare and administer parenteral medications using aseptic techniques.
- Identify the anatomical landmarks for intramuscular, intradermal, and subcutaneous injections.
- Accurately perform the procedures and techniques of administering intramuscular, intradermal, and subcutaneous injections.
- State five purposes of intravenous therapy.
- Give five methods of administering intravenous medication.
- Accurately calculate intravenous flow rates.
- Identify four factors that must be monitored by the nurse during intravenous infusion.
- Withdraw medication from a vial or ampule accurately using aseptic technique.
- Identify four complications of intravenous therapy.
- Competently inject a medication intramuscularly by the Z-track method.
- Appropriately select the correct syringe and needle for IM, ID, and SC (SQ) injections.
- Prepare a solution for injection using aseptic technique.

ADMINISTERING THE PARENTERAL ROUTES

The intramuscular, subcutaneous, intradermal, and intravenous routes are called the *parenteral routes;* "parenteral" actually refers to all routes other than the gastrointestinal, or enteral, routes. Parenteral routes are used for the following reasons:

1. Some medications, such as insulin, are altered by the secretions of the gastroinestinal tract.
2. Some patients cannot take medications by mouth, such as those who are intubated, severely dysphagic (unable to eat), have full-thickness burns, shock, nausea, and/or vomiting.
3. The parenteral route gives a more rapid onset of action than the oral route.
4. The *duration* of the effects of parenteral administration is shorter than by the oral route.
5. Smaller doses of parenteral drugs may be used, because active drug ingredients are not changed or lost in the GI tract and liver.
6. Intravenous administration of a drug can be carefully regulated. Immediate entry into the bloodstream gives immediate onset of the drug's action.

Hands should be thoroughly washed before selecting and handling syringes, needles, and other equipment. Aseptic technique is used, because the skin is penetrated (which makes a portal of entry into the body for pathogenic organisms).

Parenteral medication administration must be performed skillfully and accurately. Dosages must be exact and proper site selected for the injection.

Equipment

Syringes. A syringe consists of a barrel, a plunger, and a tip (Fig. 25-2). The outside part of the barrel is calibrated in milliliters, minims, insulin units, or heparin units.

Barrels range in size from 1 ml to 50 ml. The outside of the barrel is not sterile, but the inside is. The tip of the barrel may be the plain or Luer-Lok. The needle slips directly onto the plain barrel tip, whereas the Luer-Lok needle must be turned to the right as it is placed onto the barrel tip.

The plunger inside of the barrel is also sterile; the nurse should avoid touching the plunger anywhere except the tip. The plunger is used to draw up and inject medication from the syringe. The plunger has a black rubber stopper on the end that is inside the barrel. The volume of a medication is read at the point of the black rubber stopper nearest the needle.

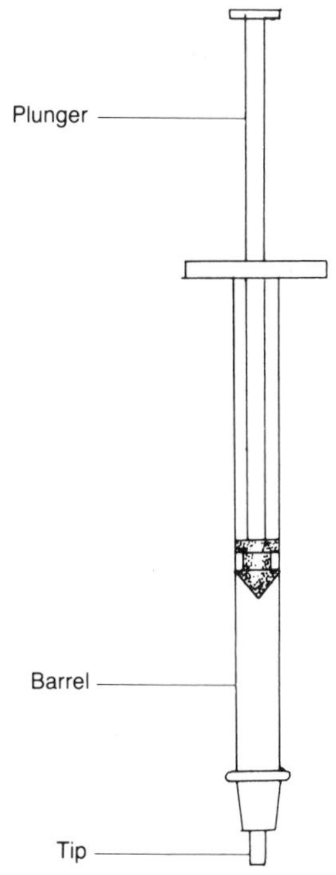

FIG. 25-2 Parts of a syringe.

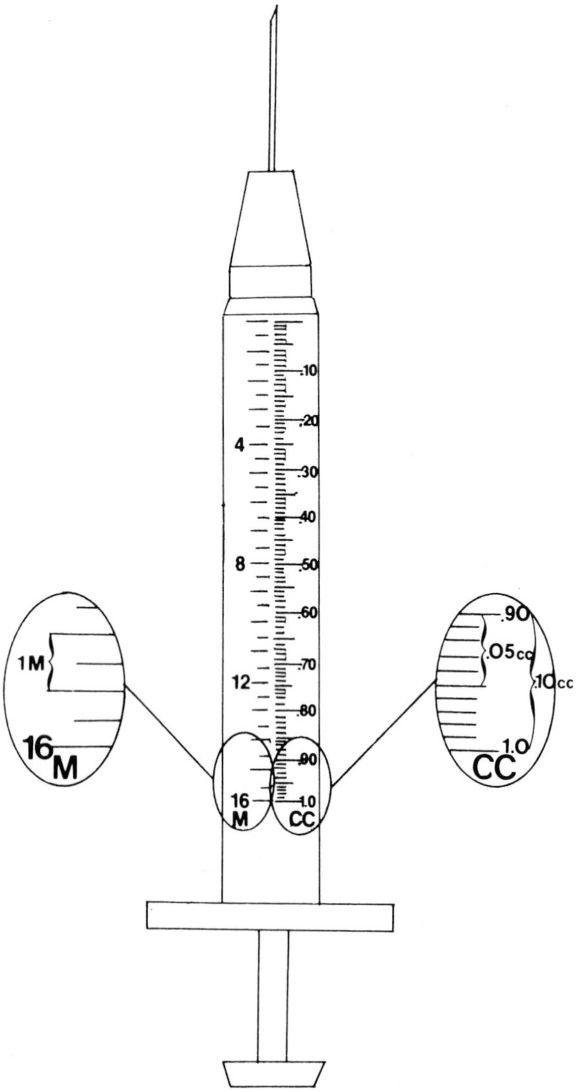

FIG. 25-3 Tuberculin syringe calibration.

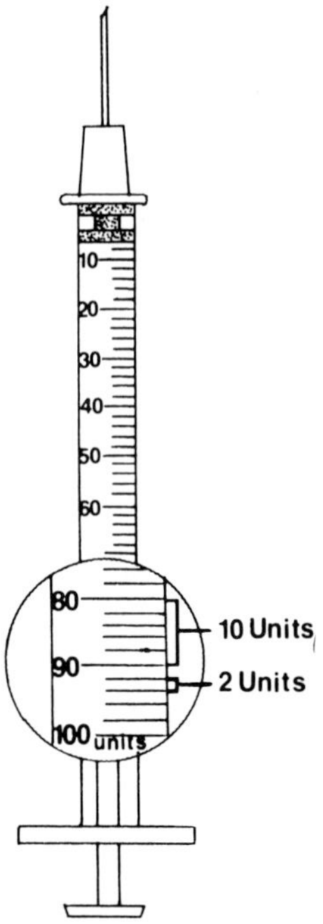

FIG. 25-4 Calibration of U-100 insulin syringe.

The most commonly used syringes are the 1 ml (tuberculin syringe), 3 ml, and 5 ml.

Tuberculin syringe. The tuberculin syringe (Fig. 25-3) holds a total of 1 ml or 16 minims (♏) (1 ml = 16 ♏). It is used to give volumes of medication of 1 ml volume or less. It is used for giving small doses of epinephrine, intradermal skin tests, insulin (U100, when no insulin syringe is available), and subcutaneous medication.

One side of the tuberculin syringe is measured in minims. The long line of the minim scale represents 1♏; the shorter lines represent 0.5 (5/10 or ½ ♏).

The other side is measured in milliliters (ml). The long lines represent 0.1 (1/10) ml, the shorter lines represent 0.05 (5/100) ml, and the shortest lines represent 0.01 (1/100) ml.

Insulin syringe. The insulin syringe is used only for insulin, because it is calibrated in units (Fig. 25-4). Most insulin is made in the concentration of U-100. The U-100 syringe holds 100 units of insulin per 1 ml. All insulin dosages should be checked with another nurse before administering to the patient.

Three-milliliter syringe. The most frequently used syringe is the 3 ml syringe (Fig. 25-5). The 3 ml syringe is chosen for giving volumes of medication of 1 ml to 3 ml. It is used for most intramuscular injections. The 3 ml syringe is calibrated in milliliters (ml) or cubic centimeters (cc), which are equivalent units. The short lines represent 0.1 ml; the longer lines represent 0.5 ml.

Syringe selection is based on the volume of medication that is to be given.

Needles. The parts of a needle are the hub, shaft, and beveled tip (Fig. 25-6). The opening at the needle's beveled tip is the **lumen.** The size of the diameter of the inside of the needle's shaft determines the **gauge** of the needle (Fig. 25-7). The smaller the gauge, the larger the diameter of the needle. Needle gauge selection is based on the viscosity (thickness) of the medication. The thicker the medication, the smaller the gauge required. A 20- to 22-gauge needle is usually adequate for most nonviscous intramuscular injections. A 16- to 18-gauge intravenous needle is appropriate for blood administration, emergency IV routes, and for surgical cases. A 23- to 26-gauge is frequently used for infants and children and for intradermal injections.

Needle length. Needle length is selected based on the depth of the tissue into which the medication is to be injected. Intradermal injections require only ⅜ to ½ inch needle length, whereas an intramuscular injection may

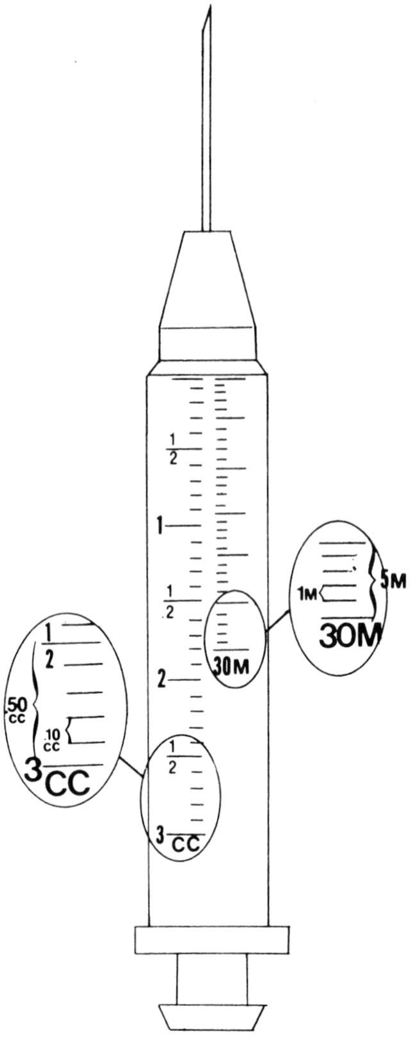

FIG. 25-5 Reading the calibrations of a 3 ml syringe.

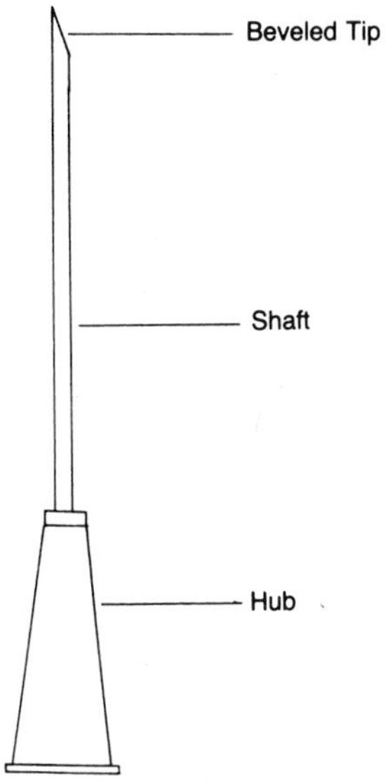

FIG. 25-6 Parts of a needle.

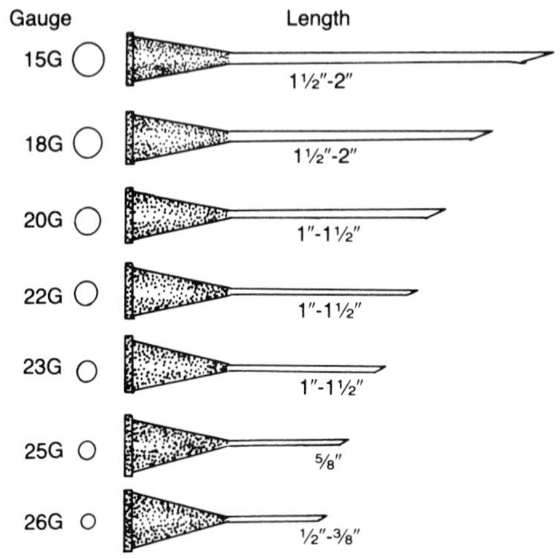

FIG. 25-7 Needle length and gauge.

require ½ to 1¼ inch needle length, depending on the amount of muscle tissue the patient has. Needle length for subcutaneous injections is based on depth of appropriate tissue.

Intravenous needles. Two types of needles made especially for intravenous (IV) use are the butterfly and the over-the-needle catheter.

The butterfly (also called a scalp needle or a wing-tipped needle) is useful in administering intravenous fluids on a short-term basis. They are used in pediatric cases in which veins are sometimes hard to find except in the scalp. Butterflies are easy to put in, but some hospitals or doctors prefer over-the-needle catheters.

Over-the-needle catheters (Fig. 25-8) are called *Angiocaths, Jelcos,* or *Abbocaths,* according to the manufacturer of the needle.

Over-the-needle catheters are preferred for emergency situations, surgery cases, blood and blood product transfusion, intensive care cases, transporting situations such as in helicopters or ambulances, and thick, intravenous infusions or hyperalimentation.

Angiocaths are plastic catheters over a stainless steel needle *stylet.* A stylet is a sharp, bevel-tipped metal guide that is used to pierce the skin and vein. Once the catheter is in the vein, blood return is seen and the stylet is removed. The plastic catheter is left in the vein. The catheter is preferred for long-term IV use, because it is more flexible and can withstand patient movement.

Butterflies (Fig. 25-9) and angiocaths cannot be used for an indefinite length of time and should be assessed for patency (openness) and intactness or complications every shift.

Intracaths are similar to angiocaths, except that they are much longer. Physicians insert intracaths for long-term intravenous administration or for intravenous nutritional feedings (hyperalimentation). See Skill 25-12 for preparation of parenteral medications.

SKILL 25-12

PREPARING PARENTERAL MEDICATIONS

1. Follow the five rights procedure (Box 25-3).
2. Perform the three label checks (Box 25-4).
3. Follow universal precautions (Box 25-5).
4. Wash hands before handling equipment; prepare medication in clean area; reduce distractions.
5. Keep sterile parts of syringe and needle sterile. Use aseptic technique throughout preparation.
6. Compare drug and dosage ordered with drug and dosage on hand; check expiration date, dosage per milliliter, total volume of solution in vial/ampule. Look for contaminants or defects in vial or ampule.
7. Calculate drug dosage and check calculations with another nurse.
8. Check compatibility chart or consult pharmacy if mixing two medications.

Withdrawing medication from a vial

1. Remove metal cap from top of vial; wipe rubber diaphragm briskly with alcohol sponge.
2. Pull plunger of syringe back to aspirate air into syringe equal to amount of drug to be withdrawn.
3. Insert needle into inverted vial; inject air and withdraw volume of solution to be given. Keep needle under solution to prevent aspiration of air into syringe.
4. Push plunger gently to disperse solution to tip of needle. Remove air bubbles by gently tapping syringe.

Withdrawing medication from an ampule

1. Tap the top of ampule to move solution from top of ampule to bottom of ampule.
2. Cover neck of ampule with an alcohol sponge; break off top of ampule; deposit top of glass ampule in "sharps" container.
3. Use a filter needle to aspirate medication from ampule. Filter or aspiration needles catch particles of glass that may be in the solution from the broken ampule.
4. Insert filter needle into open neck of ampule; invert ampule to withdraw correct dose.
5. Replace filter needle with needle appropriate for purpose of and viscosity of solution.
6. Push plunger gently until the medication is at tip of needle.

STEP 1

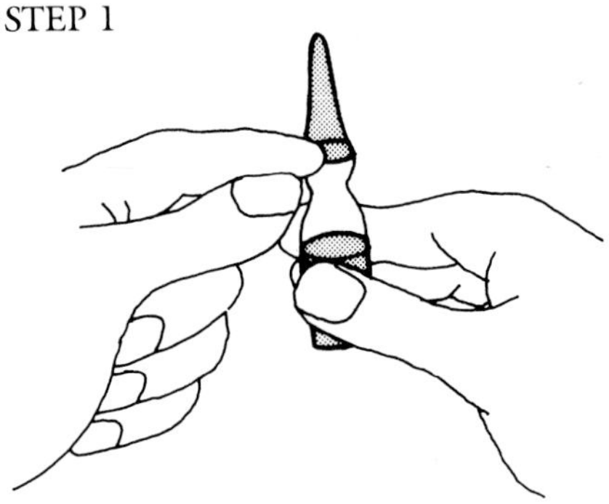

STEP 2

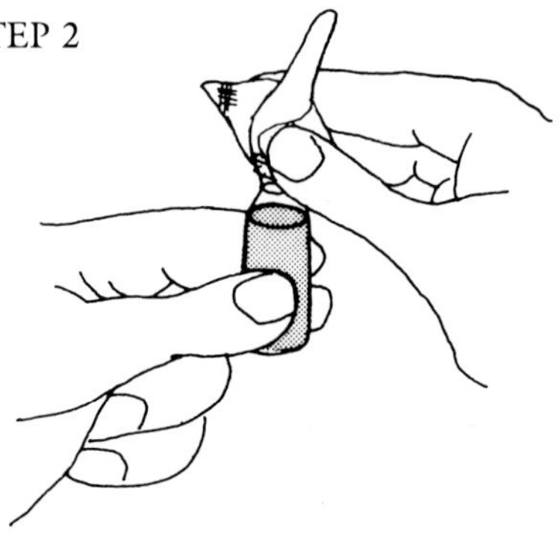

STEP 3

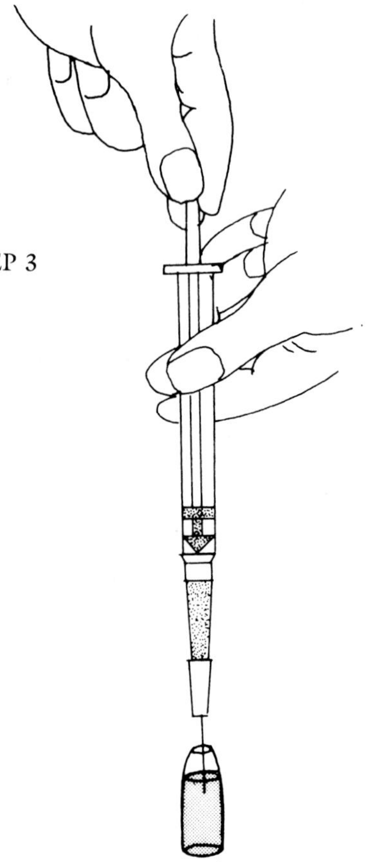

SKILL 25-12 PREPARING PARENTERAL MEDICATIONS—cont'd

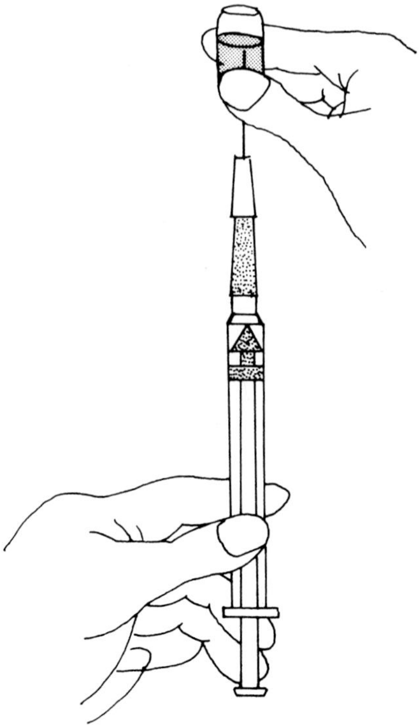

STEP 4

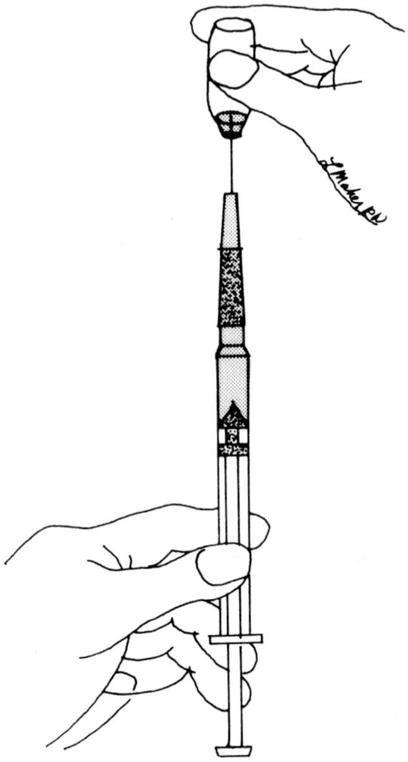

Reconstituting a powdered dosage form

1. Follow instructions on manufacturer's box and drug insert. The instructions will specify the type and amount of diluent to use (e.g., add 10 ml bacteriostatic saline to prepare a ratio of 500 mg/ml).
2. Remove the protective cap from diluent; withdraw diluent using sterile technique.
3. Withdraw needle from diluent vial.
4. Inject diluent into vial of powdered drug; gently shake and tap vial to dissolve powder into solution.
5. Label solution with:
   a. Date and time mixed
   b. Name of person who mixed drug and diluent
   c. Dosage per milliliter obtained (concentration)
   d. Amount and type of diluent used
6. Withdraw correct dose; select appropriate needle gauge and length for patient.

Placing two medications into one syringe (insulin example used)

1. Check compatibility of two drugs with a compatibility chart or call pharmacy.
2. Check and compare label of each drug ordered with label of each drug on hand.
3. Compare each label with medication order.
4. Roll long- and intermediate-acting insulin between the palms; do not shake any insulin.
5. Briskly wipe tops of both vials with separate alcohol swab.
6. Pull back plunger of syringe to amount equal to volume of longer-acting insulin to be given.
7. Insert needle and inject air into vial of longer-acting insulin.
8. Withdraw needle from vial; *do not* remove insulin.
9. Pull back plunger of syringe to amount equal to volume of shorter-acting (regular) insulin to be given.
10. Insert needle through rubber stopper of second vial; inject air into vial.
11. Invert vial; withdraw volume of shorter-acting (regular) insulin.
12. Check dosage in syringe against medication order.
13. Wipe rubber stopper of longer-acting insulin; insert needle of the syringe containing shorter-acting insulin and withdraw ordered dose of longer-acting insulin.
14. Remove needle/syringe from vial.
15. Check labels of both vials against medication order; check order/dosage with another nurse.
16. Pull plunger back enough to allow space in barrel of syringe for insulin to be gently mixed. Mix by tilting syringe back and forth; remove air.
17. Change needles; inject subcutaneously.

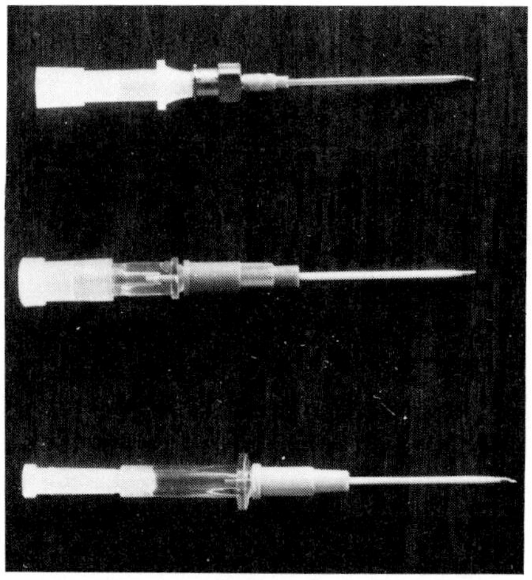

FIG. 25-8 Over-the-needle cannulae. (Courtesy Alton Ochsner Medical Foundation, New Orleans.)

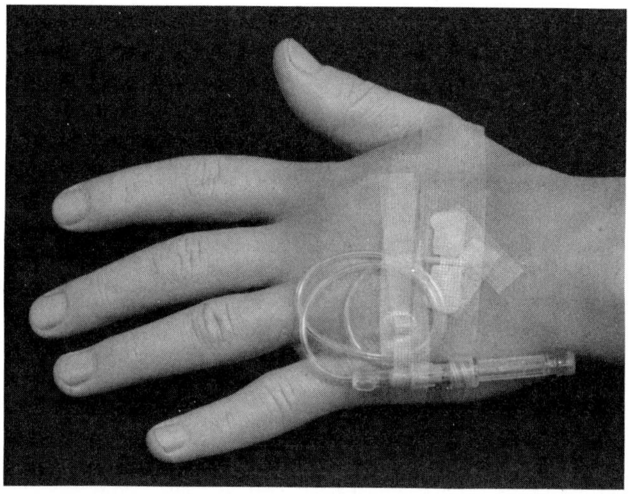

FIG. 25-9 Butterfly, scalp, or wing-tipped needle in place as a heparin lock.

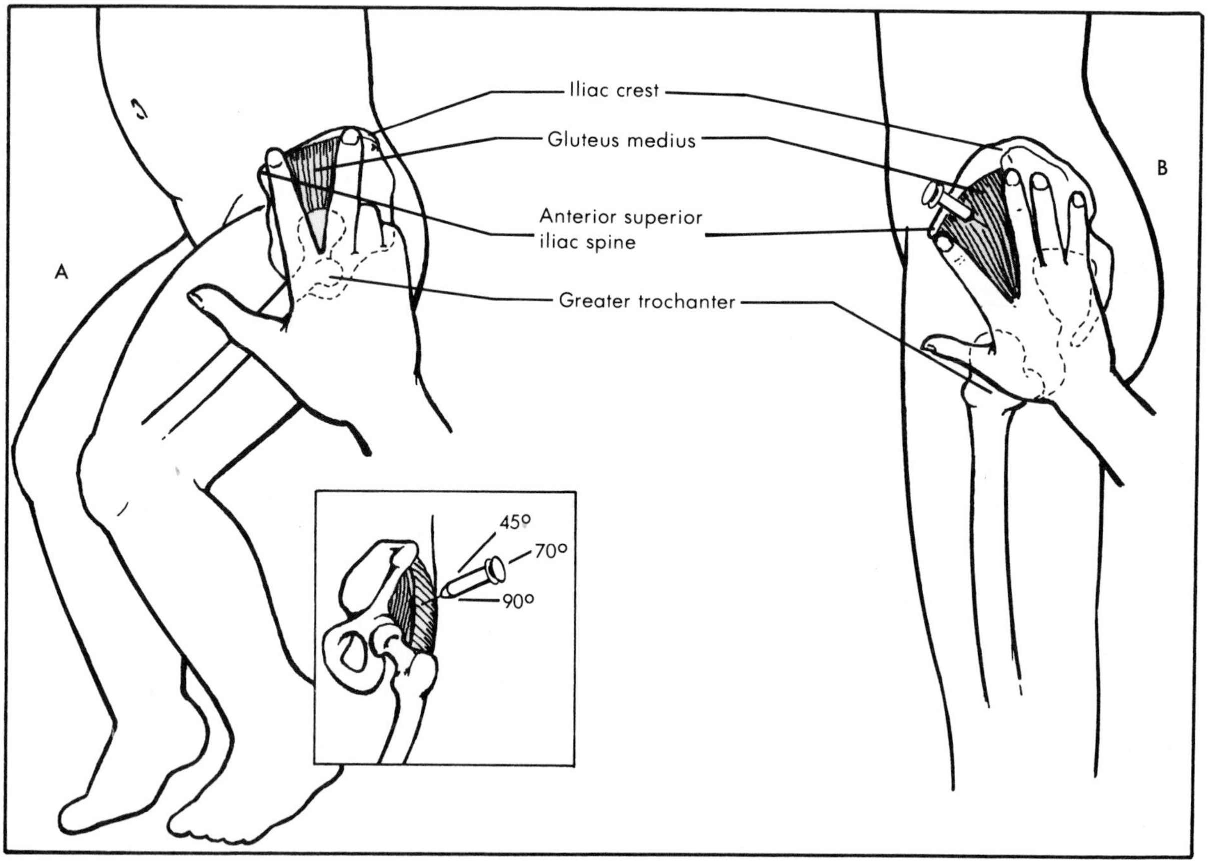

FIG. 25-10 Ventrogluteal site. **A,** Child/infant. **B,** Adult.

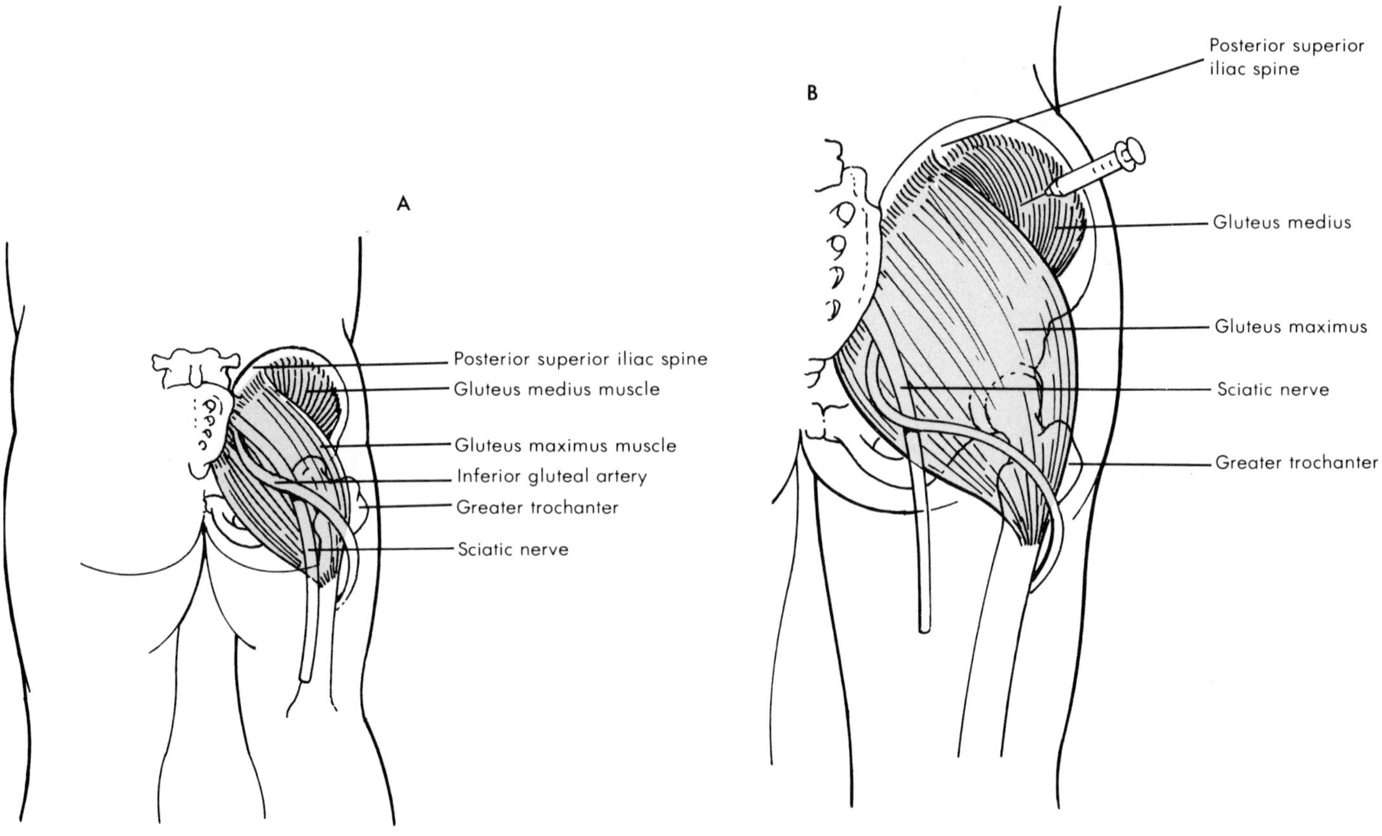

FIG. 25-11 Dorsogluteal site. **A,** Child/infant. **B,** Adult.

Intramuscular Injections

An intramuscular (IM) injection involves inserting a needle into the muscle tissue to administer medication. Since muscle tissue has a large blood supply, absorption of an IM medication is faster than a subcutaneous injection. The most commonly used sites are the upper, outer quadrant of the gluteal area, the ventrogluteal area, and the vastus lateralis of the thigh, and the deltoid muscle of the arm.

Site selection is based on the amount and type of medication to be injected, the size of the individual's muscle mass and the integrity of the individual's tissue. Damage to nerves or blood vessels may result from improper site selection.

Site selection

Gluteal sites. The gluteal sites are the ventrogluteal and the dorsogluteal. The ventrogluteal site (Fig. 25-10) is located by using three landmarks—the greater trochanter, the anterior iliac spine, and the iliac crest (the hip bone).

With the palm of the hand on the lateral portion of the greater trochanter and the index (pointer) finger on the anterior superior iliac spine, the nurse extends the middle finger to the iliac crest. Medication is injected into the V formed by the index and middle fingers.

The best position for the patient is prone. Muscle relaxation is promoted by turning the patient's toes inward. A side-lying position may also be used, with muscle relaxation promoted by flexing the upper leg.

The dorsogluteal site (Fig. 25-11) is located by using the posterior superior iliac spine and the greater trochanter. An imaginary line is drawn between these two landmarks, and medication is injected at any point along the imaginary line and below the curve of the iliac crest.

The patient should be in a prone position with the toes turned inward to promote muscle relaxation.

The gluteal sites are used commonly for IM preoperative medications or analgesic, because the gluteal muscles are large enough in most patients to inject up to 3 ml in one site. The gluteal muscles should not be used in children under 3 years of age, because their gluteal muscles are not developed from walking.

The sciatic nerve and superior gluteal artery are bypassed when proper site selection is carried out.

A second method is to visualize imaginary lines that divide the buttocks into a square box with four equal quadrants. The top of the square begins at the iliac crest; the bottom of the square is the gluteal fold where the buttocks join the thigh. The upper outer quadrant is the site for injection.

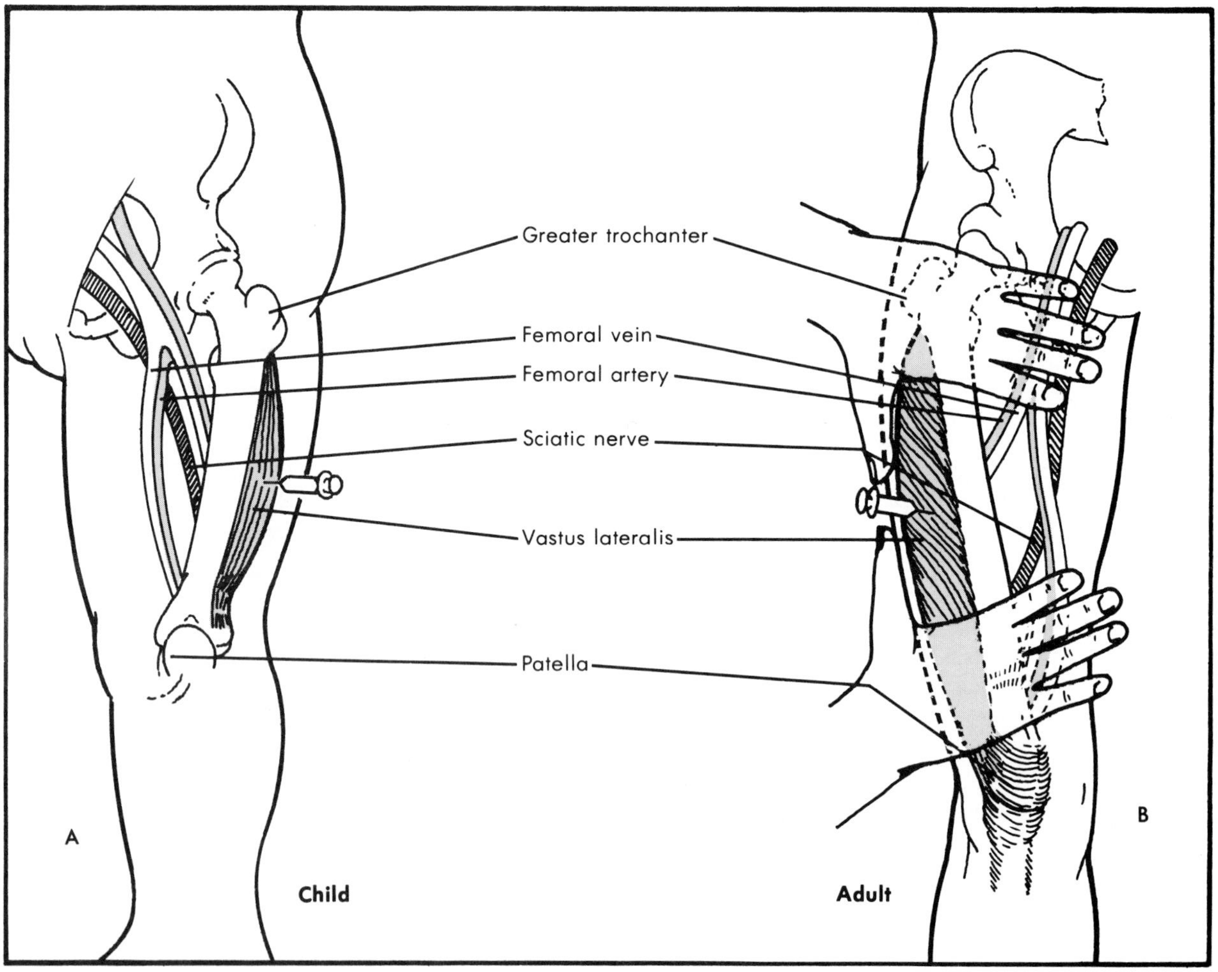

FIG. 25-12 Vastus lateralis muscle. **A,** Child/infant. **B,** Adult.

The vastus lateralis muscle (Fig. 25-12) is the preferred site for children under 3 years of age, because it is free of nerves and blood vessels. It is also used in adults when other sites are not accessible. The vastus is located on the anterior *lateral* thigh.

The patient should be in a supine or sitting position. One hand is placed above the patient's knee and one hand below the greater trochanter. The IM injection is made in the area between the two hands.

Depending on development of this muscle, up to 3 ml of medication may be injected.

The rectus femoris muscle (Fig. 25-13) is located by the same manner as the vastus lateralis. The rectus femoris is *medial* to the vastus lateralis. It is the common site for self-administration of medication. The sciatic nerve lies close to this muscle, and major blood vessels are also present in this area, making the site potentially dangerous to use.

The deltoid muscle (Fig. 25-14) of the upper arm is a relatively small area. No more than 2 ml should be injected into this muscle. The patient may be positioned in a sitting, standing, prone, or supine position. The patient is asked to relax his arm during the injection to decrease discomfort.

The landmarks for locating the proper area for injection are the acromion process of the scapula and the axillary fold. An imaginary line can be drawn that extends from the axillary fold across the lateral aspect of the arm; the center of this area is the thicker midportion of the muscle, where the injection is given.

Generally, the deltoid is too small in children and the elderly. Also the brachial vein and artery and the radial nerve are in this area. See Skill 25-13.

Z-track method. Z-track is used for injecting medications that are irritating to the tissues. Z-track IM administration seals medication deep within muscle tissue. Z-track does not allow staining or tracking of the medication into the tissue as the needle is withdrawn. This method is used when giving Inferon (iron). See Skill 25-14.

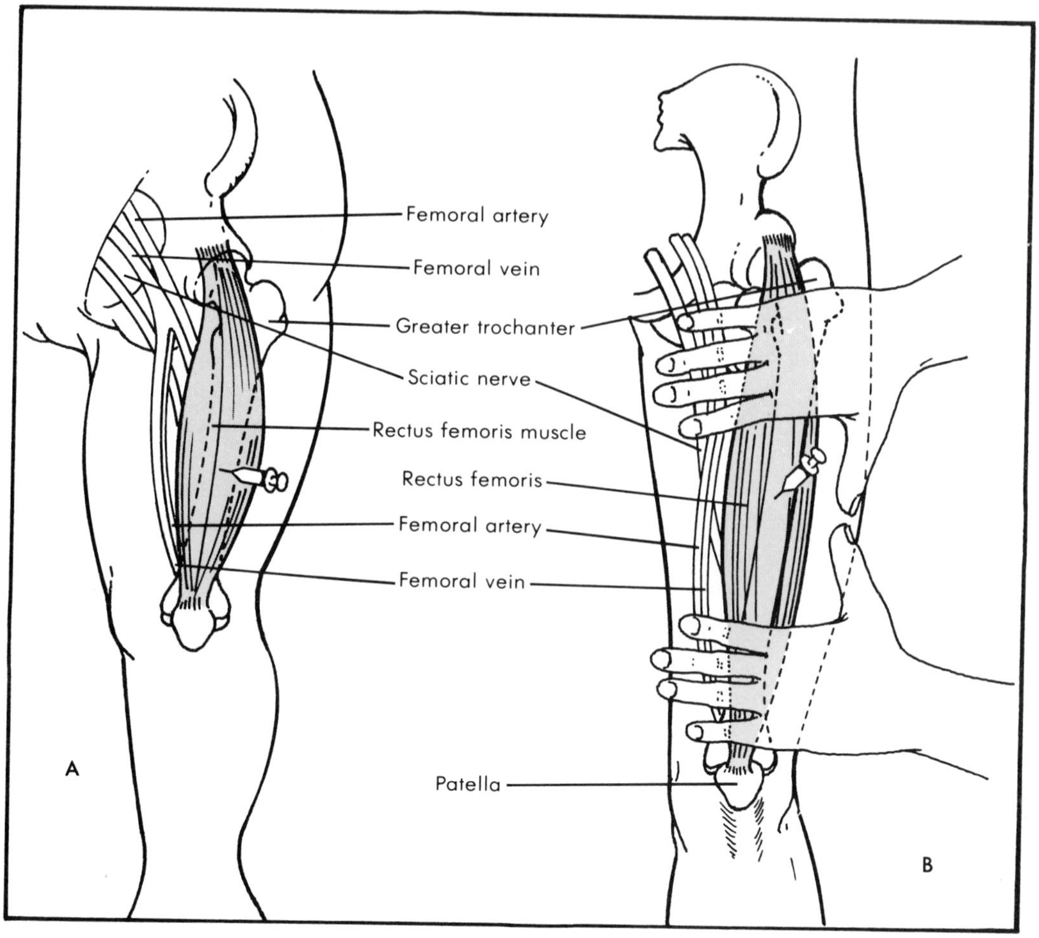

FIG. 25-13 Rectus femoris muscle. **A,** Child/infant. **B,** Adult.

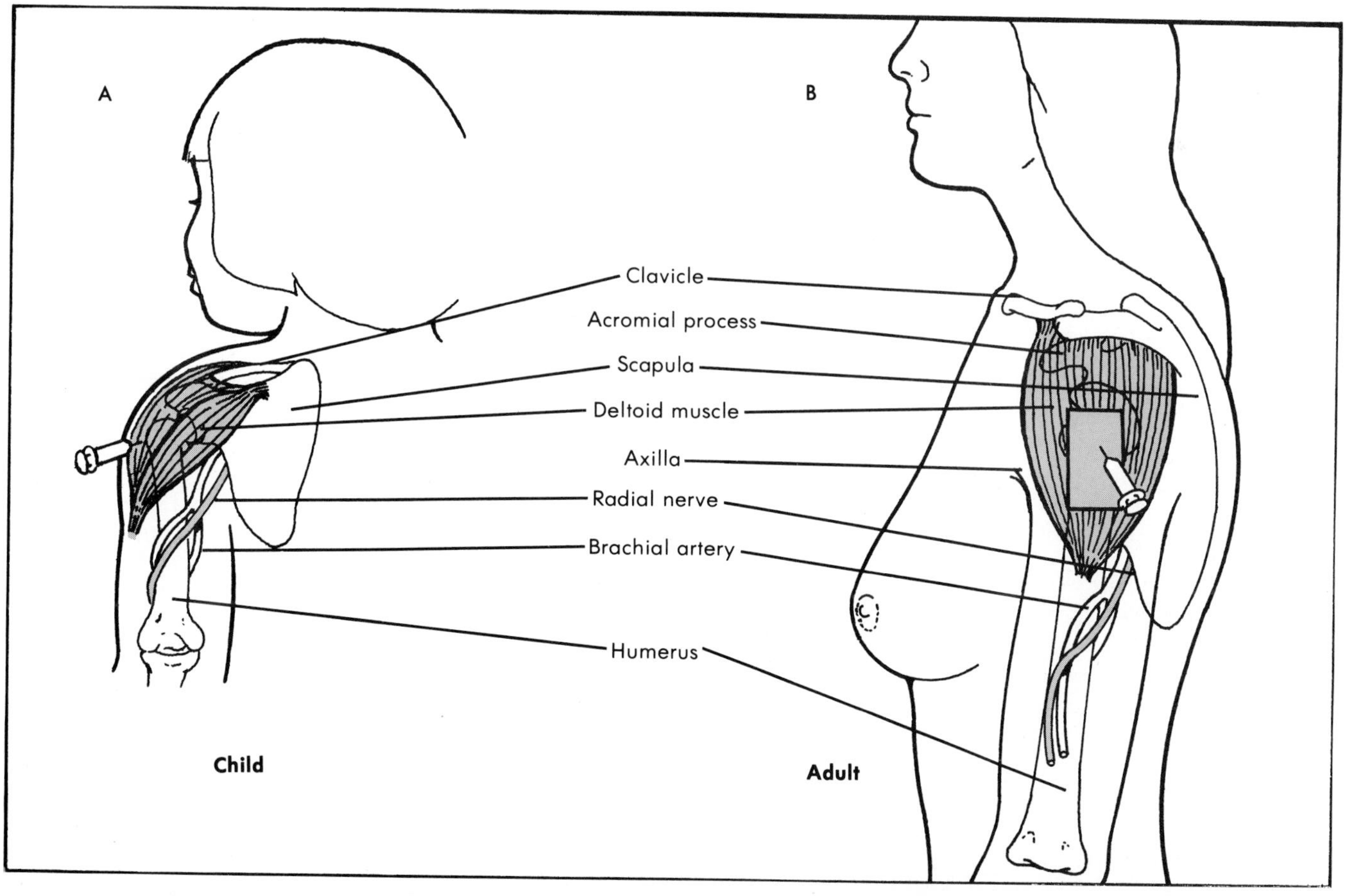

FIG. 25-14 Deltoid muscle site. **A,** Child/infant. **B,** Adult.

SKILL 25-13

GIVING AN INTRAMUSCULAR INJECTION

1. Follow the five rights procedure (Box 25-3).
2. Perform the three label checks (Box 25-4).
3. Follow universal precautions (Box 25-5).
4. Wash hands
5. Prepare medication according to standard procedure for injectables.
6. Don gloves.
7. Identify patient and explain the procedure.
8. Select and expose site (according to IM site selection procedure); provide privacy.
9. Clean skin with alcohol swab (from center outward), spread skin tight with thumb and index finger; let dry.
10. Ask patient to take a deep breath and exhale slowly to relax muscle as needle is inserted (lessens pain from injection).
11. Insert needle at a 90-degree angle quickly in a dartlike motion. Quickness reduces discomfort.
12. Maintain needle in muscle; gently aspirate (pull back plunger) to be certain needle is in muscle (and not in a vein or an artery).
13. If blood is seen, needle is in a vein or artery; withdraw needle; prepare new medication. Select another site.
14. Slowly inject medication into muscle to lessen discomfort.
15. Withdraw needle quickly without bending or twisting it.
16. Use pressure and gauze (2 × 2) to stop any bleeding.
17. *Do not* recap needle; dispose directly into sharps container.
18. Chart site used and amount and type of medication (e.g., Demerol 50 mg given IM Ⓛ ventrogluteal). Remember a quick, dartlike insertion followed by slow injection of the medication is much less painful to the patient.

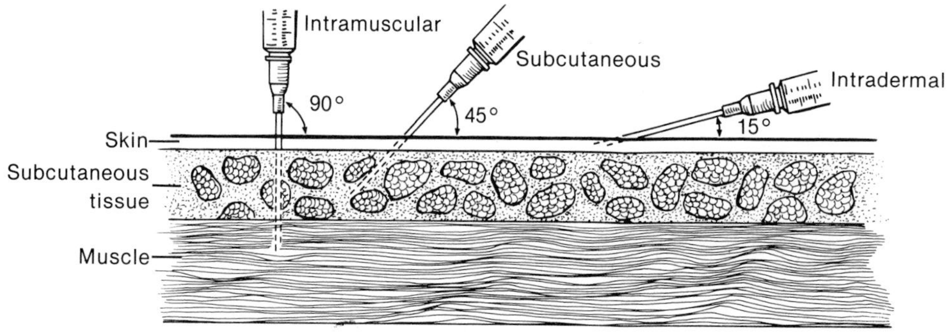

SKILL 25-14 GIVING A Z-TRACK INJECTION

1. Follow the five rights procedure (Box 25-3).
2. Perform the three label checks (Box 25-4).
3. Follow universal precautions (Box 25-5).
4. Wash hands.
5. Prepare medication according to standard procedure for injectables.
6. Don gloves.
7. Use one needle to withdraw dose from container. Use another needle (1½ to 2 inches) to inject medication.
8. Expose and locate dorsogluteal site according to IM site selection procedure; provide privacy.
9. Clean site with an alcohol swab.
10. Ask the patient to take a deep breath and to slowly exhale (to relax the muscle). Pull skin tightly in a lateral direction (move skin at least 1 inch to one side). Continue to hold the tissue in this same manner.
11. Insert needle at a 90-degree angle; aspirate; if no blood is seen, inject medication slowly; wait 10 seconds.
12. Withdraw needle quickly; allow skin to return to its normal position.
13. Use a 2 × 2 or Band-Aid as needed.
14. *Do not* massage.
15. *Do not* recap needle; dispose directly into sharps container.
16. Chart site used, Z-track method used, amount and type of medication given.

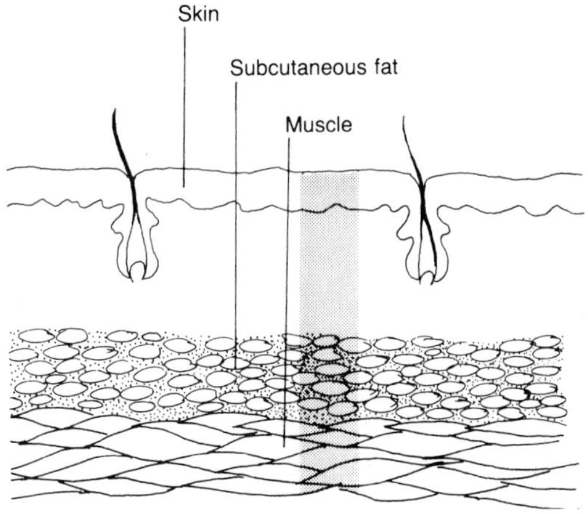

STEP 8

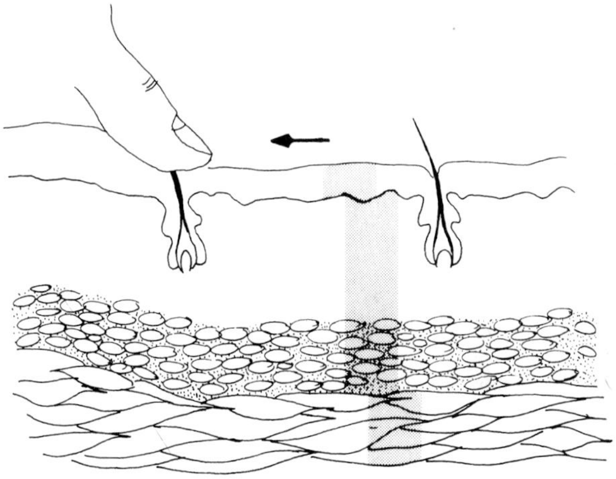

STEP 10

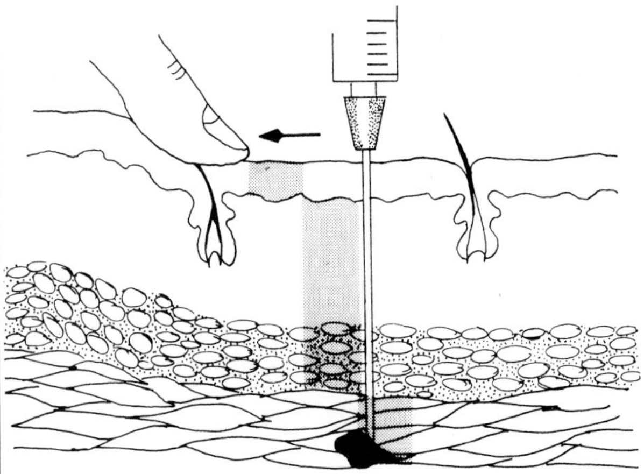

STEP 11

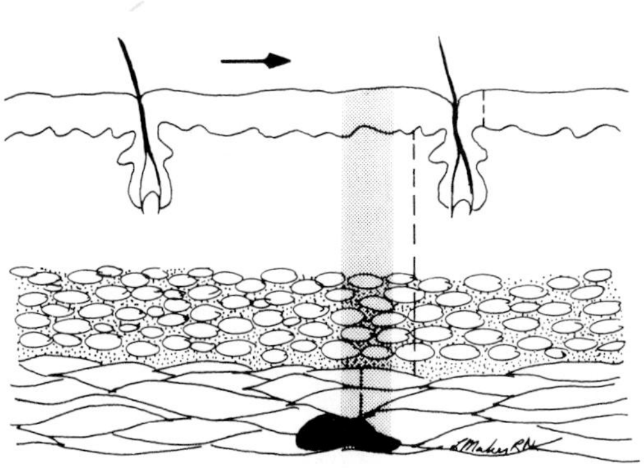

STEP 12

Intradermal Injections

An intradermal (ID) injection is the introduction of a hypodermic needle into the dermis for the purpose of instilling a substance such as a serum, vaccine, or skin test agent. Intradermals are not aspirated.

Small volumes such as 0.1 ml are injected to form a small bubblelike wheal just under the skin. Absorption is slow, which makes it the best route for allergy sensitivity tests, desensitization injections, local anesthetics, and vaccinations.

A tuberculin syringe is used to give intradermals because the tuberculin syringe only holds a maximum of 1 ml or 16 ♏. A 25-gauge, ⅝ inch needle is used.

The upper chest, inner aspect of the lower arm, and the scapular area are used for intradermal injections. See Skill 25-15.

SKILL 25-15

GIVING AN INTRADERMAL INJECTION

1. Follow the five rights procedure (Box 25-3).
2. Perform the three label checks (Box 25-4).
3. Follow universal precautions (Box 25-5).
4. Wash hands.
5. Prepare medication according to standard procedure for injectables.
6. Don gloves.
7. Identify patient and explain procedure (see p. 441).
8. Select and expose inner aspect of lower arm.
9. Clean site gently with alcohol swab from center outward; let dry.
10. Two injections are made if test is for sensitivity. One injection is a control using sterile water or bacteriostatic saline; the other is substance that is to be tested.
11. Insert a 25-gauge needle with bevel up directly under skin to make a small bleb (bubble) with test solution. Insert needle at approximately a 15-degree angle (see p. 462). *Do not* inject into subcutaneous tissue. Inject control of saline into another site for comparison with test substance at designated time interval.
12. *Do not* massage.
13. Draw a circle around skin test with a marker; label area with date, time, and name of test. Another method is to make a diagram in patient's chart to indicate location of site.
14. If an elevated, erythematous area is observed, measure and record results in millimeters with metric ruler.
15. Compare control with agent; document results in chart.

Subcutaneous Injections

Insulin and heparin are given by the subcutaneous route. Injections are made into the tissue between the dermis and the muscle layer. The outer aspect of the upper arms, the abdomen, thighs, and the scapula are sites used for subcutaneous (SQ, SC, Subq) injections. The site of subcutaneous injections should receive no more than 1 ml of solution, and location should always be carefully charted. Sites are rotated to prevent damage to the tissue and to prevent discomfort.

Subcutaneous injections are given at a 45-degree angle if the patient is thin or at a 90-degree angle if the patient has ample subcutaneous tissue. Judgment is used in selecting sites for injection and in determining the angle of injection. Needle length is selected so that the medication will be injected into subcutaneous tissue and not muscle tissue. Usual needle length is ½ to ⅝ inch, and a 25-gauge needle is the one of choice. See Skill 25-16.

SKILL 25-16 GIVING A SUBCUTANEOUS INJECTION

1. Follow the five rights procedure (Box 25-3).
2. Perform the three label checks (Box 25-4).
3. Follow universal precautions (Box 25-5).
4. Wash hands.
5. Prepare medication according to standard procedure for injectables.
6. Don gloves.
7. Identify patient and explain procedure (see p. 441).
8. Select and expose site (check which site was used previously and rotate site). The abdomen is the usual preferred site when administering heparin.
9. Clean site with an alcohol swab from center outward in circular motion; let dry.
10. *Method A:* Spread skin of selected site taut and hold firmly; insert needle at 45-degree angle (see p. 462) and aspirate; inject medication. ~~Do not aspirate if heparin is being administered.~~
    Method B: Grasp and press together skin of selected site so that it forms roll between fingers. Insert needle at a 90-degree angle and aspirate. ~~Do not aspirate if heparin is being given.~~ Inject medication.
11. Withdraw needle quickly and apply an antiseptic swab or a 2 × 2 gauze sponge. Do not massage the site if heparin is administered, because this will increase local bleeding and ecchymosis will occur.
12. *Do not* recap needle; dispose directly into sharps container.
13. Chart site used and amount and type of medication.

Intravenous Therapy

The intravenous route of administration is used more frequently as nurses assume more responsibility in IV therapy. Advances in technology of IV equipment also enable nurses and physicians to deliver intravenous fluids and medications more safely (Fig. 25-15).

The intravenous route is used to (1) provide fluid and electrolyte maintenance, restoration, and replacement, (2) administer medications and nutritional feedings, (3) administer blood and blood products, (4) administer chemotherapy to cancer patients, and (5) administer patient-controlled analgesics.

Methods of IV administration. Intravenous medications may be administered by several methods, discussed below.

IV push. The medication is given directly into a vein or by means of a heparin or saline lock or injection port of an existing IV tubing set.

Heparin locks. Heparin locks are devices that attach onto the needle hub. Once attached, the heparin lock is filled with the anticoagulant heparin; thus the name. Heparin locks revolutionized intravenous therapy and heparin therapy. They are also used in a wide variety of diagnostic tests. Heparin locks make intravenous antibiotic therapy and other IV drug therapies readily accessible without causing the unnecessary pain of a restick with every dose.

Diluted heparin is used in the lock to keep the vein open; therefore IV medication can be administered at intervals without requiring a continuous infusion of fluid to ensure patency. A patient is able to receive IV medication without the necessity of running a fluid. This procedure is done by an RN.

The heparin lock, when ready for use, is flushed with 3 ml of normal saline before and after the medication. The lock is then injected with diluted heparin. This procedure is done by an RN. Flushing the heparin lock prevents drug incompatibility from occurring between two incompatible drugs or fluids.

Intermittent infusion (or piggyback). IV piggybacks (IVPB) are drug infusions that are given at intervals, such as qid (four times a day). They may be connected to heparin or saline locks or to the injection port of the IV tubing. Once the medication has infused, the piggyback is removed from the heparin or saline lock or IV tubing. Antibiotics are frequently given in this manner.

Continuous infusions. Medication is added to a bag of IV fluid and is infused over the time that the IV fluid infuses.

Electronic pumps and controllers. Pumps and controllers regulate the flow rate of infusions. Pumps deliver the fluid via pressure while controllers deliver the infusion with the aid of gravity. Controllers monitor the flow rate of fluid by a photoelectric eye.

Patient-controlled analgesia (PCA). Patient-controlled analgesia (PCA) (Fig. 25-16) is administered by a programmable pump that is controlled by the patient. The patient presses a button that triggers the pump to deliver a set amount of analgesic agent to the patient via the vein. The nurse programs the pump according to the physician's order, which specifies the amount of narcotic the patient receives per each dose. The pump also controls the total amount of drug that may be received over a specific period.

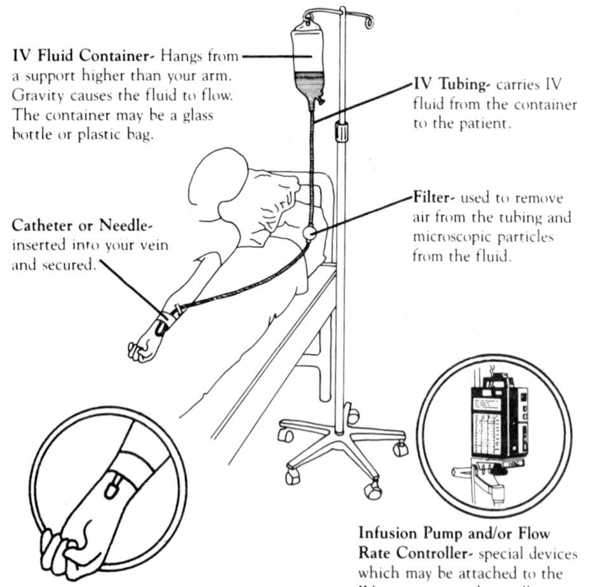
IV Fluid Container- Hangs from a support higher than your arm. Gravity causes the fluid to flow. The container may be a glass bottle or plastic bag.
IV Tubing- carries IV fluid from the container to the patient.
Catheter or Needle- inserted into your vein and secured.
Filter- used to remove air from the tubing and microscopic particles from the fluid.
IV Lock- a small, plastic tube with a rubber seal on one end which allows IV medications to be given intermittently.
Infusion Pump and/or Flow Rate Controller- special devices which may be attached to the IV system to mechanically control and maintain a precise rate of flow. If your pump or controller alarm sounds, your nurse will attend to the device.

FIG. 25-15 Intravenous therapy.

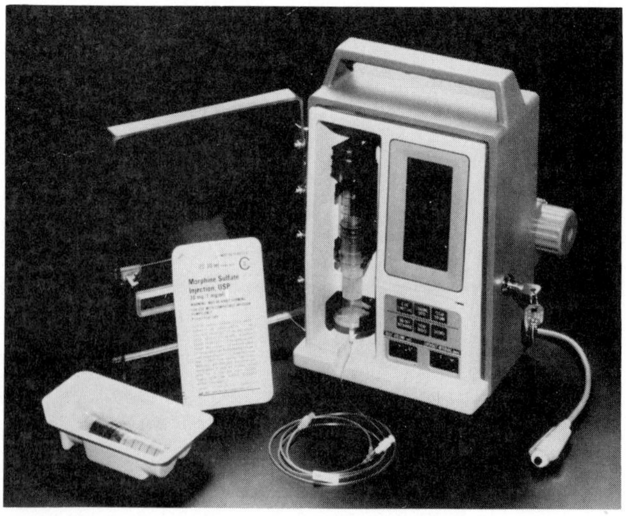

FIG. 25-16 Patient-controlled analgesia (PCA). (Courtesy Abbott Laboratories, Abbott Park, Ill.)

Volumetric chambers. A volumetric chamber consists of IV tubing with a chamber that holds a prescribed amount of fluid; it is separate from the drip chamber. Medication may be added to the fluid in the chamber such as Pitocin or lidocaine. The delivery of the medication to the patient is carefully controlled by this method.

The nurse's responsibility in maintaining IV infusions. The physician orders the amount (see Fig. 24-1) and type of IV fluid and length of time that the infusion is to run. The nurse ensures that the ordered type and amount of fluid is started and that it is regulated to infuse over the period ordered by the physician. An IV infusion is regulated by knowing the number of drops per minute that it will take for the entire volume of fluid to infuse over the specified time ordered by the physician.

To find the number of drops per minute (the *drip rate*), one must know which type of IV tubing will be used with the infusion. The nurse must look on the IV tubing box for the **drip factor.** The box will indicate whether the IV tubing is calibrated to deliver macrodrops or microdrops. Macrodrop sets will deliver 10, 15, or 20 drops per 1 ml of fluid while microdrop, or minidrop, sets will deliver 60 drops per 1 ml of fluid. The drip factor must be known to change milliliters to drops when calculating IV flow rates.

For example, a physician orders 1000 ml of D_5 ½ NS with 20 mEq KCl to be infused over an 8-hour period. How will the nurse know how many drops must drip from the drip chamber every minute for 8 hours to make the fluid run out in 8 hours? To find drops per minute, milliliters must be changed to drops by multiplying milliliters by the drip factor on the tubing set; 1000 milliliters times 15 (the drip factor on the box) = 15,000 drops; thus 15,000 drops will drip over an 8-hour period. How many drops will drip over a 1-minute period? (8 hours = 480 minutes.)

EXAMPLE: 15,000 drops : 480 minutes : : X drops : 1 minute

$$480X = 15{,}000$$
$$X = 15{,}000 \div 480$$
$$X = 31 \text{ drops/min}$$

The rate of fluid flow is regulated by adjusting the volume control clamp until 31 drops drip from the chamber in 1 minute. In 8 hours the infusion should be completed as ordered.

EXAMPLE: The physician orders 1000 ml D_5W with 1 ampule of multiple vitamins to be infused over an 8-hour period. The drip factor on the box is 10 drips per 1 ml of fluid. Divide the amount to infuse (1000 ml) by the time period (8 hours). This will give the milliliters per hour.

$$8 \text{ hours}\overline{)1000 \text{ ml}} = 125 \text{ ml/hour}$$

To reduce the milliliters per hour to drops per minute, compute the following formula:

$$\frac{\text{Amount} \times \text{Drip factor}}{\text{Time}}$$

$$\frac{(\text{amount})\ 125(\text{ml}) \times 10\ (\text{drip factor})}{60\ \text{sec (time)}}$$

$$\frac{1250}{60} \qquad 60\ \text{sec}\overline{)1250} = 20/21\ \text{drops/min}$$

ANSWER: 20/21 drops/min

Monitoring IV therapy. The nurse should check the infusion and the IV needle site at least every hour, looking at the flow of fluid, which may be altered or stopped by air in the tubing, kinked tubing, or by clotted blood in the tubing. The tubing must be kept patent (open) to keep the venous site open. If the fluid flow is obstructed or significantly slowed, the needle will become occluded with coagulated blood. Another IV site will have to be selected and another venipuncture will have to be performed. The tubing must not be allowed to get air in it as a result of an IV bag running dry. If bags are near completion, this should be reported to the RN.

The nurse observes the IV site every time the infusion is checked, looking for erythema, wetness, and edema. Inflammation may mean the onset of phlebitis (inflamed vein), edema may be an extravasation (fluid infusing outside of the vein) or an infiltration of fluid into the tissue. These conditions should be reported. In addition, the following should be reported:

- A patient with sudden onset of chills, fever, headache, nausea, and vomiting
- An anxious, dyspneic patient with a weak and rapid pulse

These factors may indicate complications of IV therapy that require immediate medical intervention.

Allergic reactions may occur as a result of IV medication administration. Reactions range from a mild rash to **anaphylactic shock** (a severe, life-threatening allergic reaction). Symptoms may appear suddenly or may appear as long as 30 to 60 minutes after an infusion of an IV medication. The following should be reported:

1. Respiratory distress such as restlessness, dyspnea, wheezing, and cyanosis (bluish coloration of the skin)
2. Skin reactions such as pruritus (itching) or urticaria (hives)
3. Signs of circulatory collapse, such as rapidly falling blood pressure and weak and rapid (thready) pulse, vertigo
4. Gastrointestinal symptoms such as nausea, vomiting, and diarrhea

Anaphylactic shock requires immediate intervention. The LPN/LVN should notify the RN immediately if any allergic symptoms are observed.

GERIATRIC CONSIDERATIONS

There is an increased risk of drug interactions in older adults. Because they are more likely to have at least one chronic illness such as hypertension, diabetes, cardiovascular disease, or renal disease, geriatric patients may be taking several medications every day.

Metabolic changes that occur as people age may make the older adult overly sensitive to the action of certain drugs. The actions of potent drugs such as cardiotonics, anticoagulants, CNS depressants, and even antihistamines may be significantly enhanced when combined.

Age-related changes in absorption, distribution, metabolism, and excretion also increase the possibility of adverse drug reactions and drug interactions.

The older adult *must* be monitored closely. The nurse should make an effort to identify potential problems by assessing the medications prescribed for each patient, and intervening quickly and accurately when a potential or actual adverse drug interaction occurs. The nurse should know each patient and each patient's level of consciousness before and after medications are administered.

The nurse, who is often the first to recognize adverse medication interactions, should assess each patient when giving medications and return to evaluate the response of the patient to the medication. The patient's level of consciousness should be assessed each shift and observed for changes.

The prevention of drug-related problems is the combined responsibility of the nurse, physician, pharmacist, and others who care for the patient. Communication between the health care team, the patient, *and* the patient's family must be strengthened to medicate the elderly safely and effectively.

REFERENCES AND SUGGESTED READINGS

1. Asperheim M: Pharmacology: an introductory test, ed 6, Philadelphia, 1987, WB Saunders Co.
2. Berkow R and Fletcher A: The Merck manual of diagnosis and therapy, ed 15, Rahway, NJ, 1987, Merck, Sharp & Dohme Research Laboratories.
3. Campbell R: Clinical use of insulin: its types and characteristics (part I), Pract Nurs 39(2):17, 1989.
4. Clayton B: Mosby's handbook of pharmacology in nursing, ed 3, St Louis, 1986, The CV Mosby Co.
5. Clayton B and Stock Y: Basic pharmacology for nurses, ed 9, St Louis, 1989, The CV Mosby Co.
6. Cooper J: Patient counseling drug information guide (handout), Athens, 1986, The University of Georgia College of Pharmacology.
7. Glanzw W, editor: Mosby's medical and nursing dictionary, ed 3, St Louis, 1989, The CV Mosby Co.
8. Hussar D: Geriatric drug interactions, East Hanover, NJ, 1986, Sandoz Pharamceutical Corporation.
9. Kennewill P and Taylor J: Introductory medicinal chemistry, Chichester, England, 1985, Ellis Horwood Publishers.
10. LaRocca C and Otto S: Pocket guide to intravenous therapy, St Louis, 1989, The CV Mosby Co.
11. Deleted in proofs.
12. Medcom: Basic clinical skills diabetic procedures: mixing insulin, blood and urine glucose monitoring, program mo44, 1986, Garden Grove, Calif, Medcom, Inc.
13. NPH ILETIN I: information for the patient (drug insert), Indianapolis, 1987, Eli Lilly & Co.
14. Reiss B and Melick M: Pharmacological aspects of nursing care, ed 2, Albany, NY, 1987, Delmar.
15. Rutherford C: Fluid and electrolyte therapy: considerations for patient care, Intravenous Nurs 12(3):173, 1989.
16. Ryan K: Standardized care plans for IV therapy, Intravenous Nurs 12(2):94, 1989.
17. Sewester S: Facts and comparisons drug information, Philadelphia, 1989, JB Lippincott Co.
18. Swonger A and Matejski M: Nursing pharmacology: an integrated approach to drug therapy and nursing practice, Glenview, Ill, 1988, Scott Foresman Co.
19. Thompson D and Jowett N: A trial povidone-iodine antiseptic solution for the prevention of cannula-related thrombophlebitis, Intravenous Nurs 12(2):99, 1989.
20. Wieck L, King E, and Dyer M: Illustrated manual of nursing techniques, ed 3, Philadelphia, 1986, JB Lippincott Co.
21. Yannes-Eyles M: Mosby's comprehensive review of practical nursing, ed 9, St. Louis, 1990, The CV Mosby Co.

CHAPTER CHALLENGE

STUDY QUESTIONS

1. Mr. Brown receives the following medications at 8 AM. Which drug would be given last:
   a. Sublingual nitroglycerin
   b. Capoten tablet
   c. Robitussin cough syrup
   d. Librium capsule
2. You are asked to take an unlabeled container of solution to the operating room. Your response is:
   a. Of course, right away!
   b. What is in the container?
   c. I will have the orderly take it.
   d. I cannot transport an unlabeled container.
3. Skin testing is performed by this type of injection:
   a. Intramuscular
   b. Subcutaneous
   c. Intradermal
   d. Intravenous
4. A subcutaneous injection is ordered for Mr. Brown. Which needle gauge is best for this form of injection:
   a. 21-gauge
   b. 25-gauge
   c. 18-gauge
   d. 22-gauge
5. The above subcutaneous injection may be given at an angle of:
   a. 45 degrees or 90 degrees
   b. 45 degrees only
   c. 90 degrees only
   d. 15 degrees only
6. The angle of the above injection will be determined by:
   a. The amount of solution in the syringe
   b. The length of the needle
   c. The amount of subcutaneous tissue of the patient
   d. The needle length and the amount of subcutaneous tissue available
7. An intramuscular injection is generally performed with a needle that is:
   a. 1 to 3 inches long
   b. ⅜ inch long
   c. ⅝ inch long
   d. ¼ inch long
8. The best site for an IM injection for an infant is:
   a. The deltoid
   b. The ventrogluteal site
   c. The gluteus maximus
   d. The vastus lateralis
9. 0.3 ml of drug is ordered subcutaneously. The best syringe with which to administer a small amount of solution such as 0.3 ml is:
   a. A 1 ml tuberculin syringe
   b. A 100 U per 1 ml insulin syringe
   c. A 3 ml syringe
   d. Any of the above may be used
10. Elderly patients generally require drug dosages that are:
    a. The same for pediatric patients
    b. The same as average adult dosages
    c. Higher than average adult dosages
    d. Lower than average adult dosages
11. After performing an intramuscular injection:
    a. Recap the needle; dispose in sharps container
    b. Do *not* recap the needle; dispose in sharps container
    c. Bend the needle; dispose in sharps container
    d. Remove the needle from the syringe; dispose in sharps container
12. Regular insulin may be given by:
    a. IM and PO
    b. SC and IV
    c. ID and SC
    d. IV and IM
13. Two IM preop drugs are to be drawn up and given in the same syringe. Before giving the nurse should *first:*
    a. Check a drug compatibility chart
    b. Refuse to do so
    c. Select an appropriate IM site
    d. Select the appropriate syringe and needle
14. It is important to know that:
    a. All patients respond to drugs in the same way
    b. Each patient will respond in his own unique way
    c. A drug only produces one desired effect
    d. One drug's action does not affect another drug's action

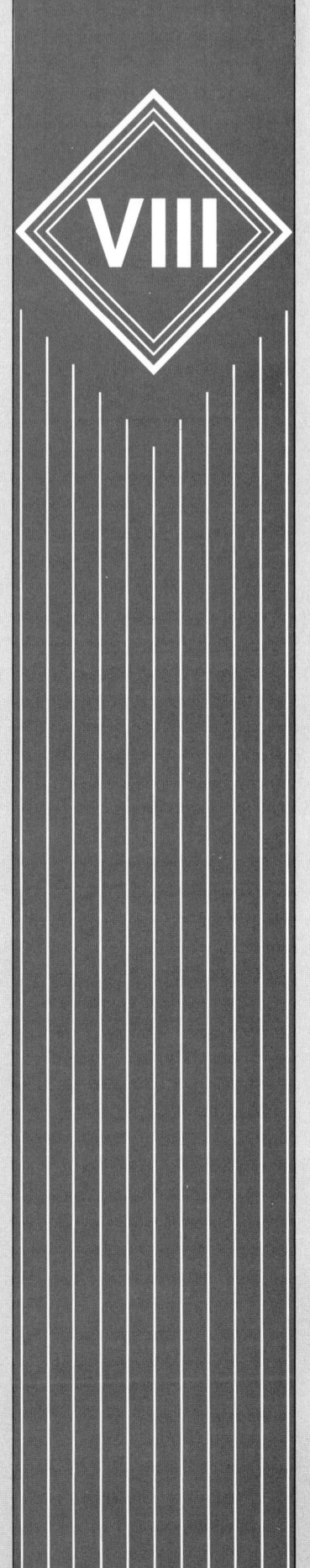

VIII

The Surgical Patient

I have always wanted to be a nurse. I have a need for caring for others who need a helping hand, a shoulder, and a smile. I crave the knowledge and technology of modern medicine. I strive for the comfort and caring warmth of my patient. Everyone is special and treated as a person, flesh and blood, rich and poor, young and old. I am always willing to help other patients, as well as fellow staff. I believe nursing is teamwork, and I want to be a part of that team. It is wonderful to see a new family leave for home or surgical patients on their feet. Caring for dying patients is one of love and caring even after they have past this world. Support for the family is always required of a caring nurse. I have a willingness to learn and want the chance to care for others.

PAULETTE WORTH
Student Nurse

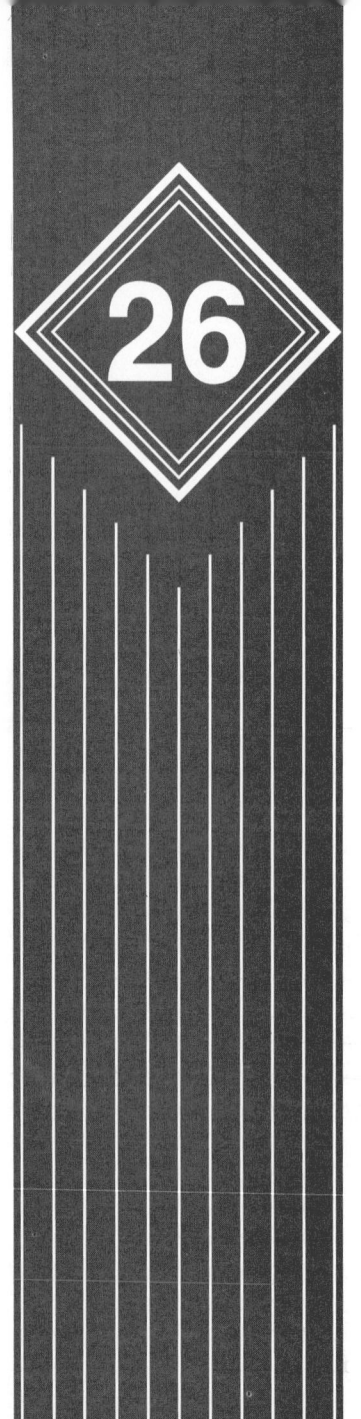

26

The Surgical Patient

JEANETTE M. JEFFERS

LEARNING OBJECTIVES

After reading this chapter, the student should be able to do the following:

- Define the key terms.
- Identify assessment factors and interventions to use in caring for the patient preoperatively.
- Examine the effects of the intraoperative and recovery room on the patient's postoperative recovery.
- State observations, complications, and interventions in the postoperative period.
- Describe implications for parenteral fluids and assessment factors to implement for patients receiving intravenous therapy.
- Explain complications and interventions associated with blood therapy.
- State five assessments and interventions to implement when evaluating surgical wounds.
- Identify types of wounds and the factors that inhibit and promote healing.
- Define the terms inflammation and infection, noting assessments and interventions to implement.
- List five assessments and nursing interventions to complete when evaluating drainage from the surgical wound.
- Consider assessment factors and resources to use in planning for discharge needs postoperatively.

RELATED TOPICS OF INTEREST

- Cultural aspects of nursing care (Chapter 12)
- Signs, symptoms, and physical assessment (Chapter 13)
- Admission, transfer, and discharge (Chapter 15)
- Medical asepsis (Chapter 16)
- Basic nutrition (Chapter 22)
- Diet therapy (Chapter 23)
- Mathematics review (Chapter 24)
- Principles and practice of medication administration (Chapter 25)
- Fluids and electrolytes (Chapter 28)
- Care of the patient with a respiratory disorder (Chapter 34)

KEY TERMS

Define the following:

- anesthesia
- asepsis
- atelectasis
- contamination
- dehiscence
- drainage
- evisceration
- exudate
- fibroblast
- granulation
- incision
- intraoperative
- major surgery
- patency
- pathological
- phagocytosis
- prostheses
- purulent
- sanguineous
- scar
- serosanguineous
- serous
- stasis
- sterile
- surgery
- suture
- traumatic
- wound

Throughout history surgery has held a mysterious aura. Ancient surgical procedures were performed by medicine men, shamans, or priests as part of healing rituals or ceremonies. Gradually, physicians became responsible for treating disease and trauma through surgical interventions. Primitive Babylonian medicine divided the practice of medicine into either surgery or internal medicine, with surgery considered the more advanced field as depicted in early writings.[5] Although modern-day surgical suites have moved surgery from the Dark Ages, patients often view the surgical process as mysterious and frightening.

PREOPERATIVE AND POSTOPERATIVE CARE: OVERVIEW

Surgery is performed for many reasons. It may be used to cure, restore function, provide relief, or diagnose. In recent years, transplant operations have also become important surgical interventions. Surgery is classified as elective, urgent, or emergent. Elective surgery is not necessary to preserve life and may be performed when the patient chooses (e.g., excising a benign cyst). Urgent surgery is required to keep additional health problems from occurring (e.g., removal of the gallbladder because of calculi). Emergency surgery is performed immediately to save the individual's life or preserve the function of a body part (e.g., perforated ulcer).[18] Although a surgical procedure may also be labeled as either **major surgery** or minor surgery, all surgeries have an element of risk.

See Table 26-1 for frequently used surgical terminology.

Traditionally surgical procedures were performed in a hospital setting. With the discovery of new technologies and today's emphasis on decreasing health care costs, the surgical suite may now be in a variety of settings. Although each community may use different terms for its surgery setting and process, common variations follow:

Inpatient: Patient hospitalized for surgery

One-day (same-day) surgery: Patient is admitted the day surgery is scheduled and dismissed the same day

Outpatient: Patient, not hospitalized, who is being treated; individual is either admitted to a short-stay unit or directly to the surgical suite

Short-stay surgical center ("surgicenter"): Independently owned agency; surgery performed when overnight hospitalization is not required; also called ambulatory surgical center or one-day surgery center[25]

Short-stay unit: Department or floor where a patient's stay does not exceed 24 hours (sometimes referred to as outpatient)

Table 26-1 Surgical Terminology

Term	Interpretation with Example
Anastomosis	Surgical joining of two ducts or blood vessels to allow flow from one to another; to bypass an area (e.g., Billroth I—joins together stomach and duodenum)
-ectomy	Surgical removal of (e.g., cholecystectomy—removal of the gallbladder)
lysis	Destruction or dissolution of (e.g., lysis of adhesions—removal of adhesions)
-orrhaphy	Surgical repair of (e.g., herniorrhaphy—repair of a hernia)
-oscopy	Direct visualization by a scope (e.g., cystoscopy—direct visualization of the urinary tract by means of a cystoscope)
-ostomy	Opening is made to allow the passage of drainage (e.g., ileostomy—formation of an opening of the ileum onto the surface of the abdomen for passage of feces)
-otomy	Opening into (e.g., thoracotomy—surgical opening into the thoracic cavity)
-pexy	Fixation of (e.g., ceopexy—fixation or suspension of the cecum to correct its excessive mobility)
-plasty	Plastic surgery (e.g., mammoplasty—reshaping of the breasts to reduce, lift, reconstruct)

Influencing Factors

Regardless of the surgical procedure scheduled, the process is a stressful experience for the patient. Observing a patient's mannerisms and listening to questions helps identify the patient's feelings and concerns. Fear of the unknown can best be addressed by providing information and support; the nurse should assist patients to express their concerns so that support and reassurance can be offered.

Numerous factors affect the individual's ability to tolerate surgery.

Age. The young and the old do not tolerate major surgical treatment as well as other age-groups. Their altered metabolic needs may not respond to physiological changes quickly. Of specific concern in these age-groups is the body's response to temperature changes, cardiovascular shifts, respiratory needs, and renal function. To help patients return to their maximal level of health, nursing assessments and actions should be ongoing.

Physical condition. Healthy patients have smoother and faster recovery periods than patients who have coexisting health problems. The nurse assesses each body system to identify actual and potential problems. Once problems are identified, the nurse selects measures to lessen potential postsurgical complications.

Nutrition factors. The body uses carbohydrates, proteins, and fats to supply energy-producing glucose to its cells. Whereas carbohydrates and fats are the primary energy producers, protein is essential to build and repair body tissue.[9] During stressful conditions, the body's need for energy and repair increases. Nutritional needs vary with a patient's age and physical requirements; patients who maintain a sound, nutritional diet tend to recover more quickly.

A completed diet history identifies the patient's usual eating habits and nutritional patterns. Because dietary practices are influenced by a patient's ethnic, cultural, religious, and socioeconomic background, the history highlights food preferences and dislikes (see Chapter 12). With this information, foods high in energy-producing nutrients can be offered. Because surgery may decrease a patient's appetite and alter metabolic functions, the nurse observes the patient for signs of malnutrition. If malnutrition is promptly identified, tube feedings, intravenous therapy, or parenteral hyperalimentation can be initiated.

Emotional and mental needs. As patients and families plan for surgery, they frequently express concern about possible outcomes. Although improved health is the ultimate goal, there may be fears not easily identified or understood. Many patients worry about possible postoperative complications: pain, disfigurement, change in body image, loss of control, disabilities, detection of cancer, and the concern that the surgery will not be successful. For some, there is a fear of dying. These concerns are normal; preoperative teaching lessens the fear of the unknown.

While the patient attempts to understand the approaching surgery, family members and support persons are also trying to cope. Besides the pending surgery, families may have additional burdens: financial obligations, living changes, and added personal responsibilities. The patient often expresses a feeling of helplessness. In addition to nursing and medical personnel, support can be provided to patients and their families by ministerial staff, social workers, or patient advocates during this stressful time.

Socioeconomic and cultural needs. Rearing practices influence an individual's behaviors and beliefs. Because the United States is a nation of diverse individuals, patient reactions are influenced by social, economic, religious, ethnic, and cultural values. Even geographical locations affect the way an individual responds. Therefore it is important to allow patients and families to express themselves openly. By allowing each patient to share personal needs, the nurse allows the total person to be treated.

Education and experience. As individuals age, life experiences influence problem-solving abilities and coping methods. Tailoring information to a patient's educational level permits fear to be replaced with accurate knowledge. The nurse can encourage patients to repeat or summarize what has been presented. This process validates not only what the patient heard, but also how the information was interpreted (see Chapter 4).

PREOPERATIVE PERIOD

A thorough health assessment is needed before surgery. Acute or chronic diseases hinder the body's ability to repair itself or adjust to surgical treatment. Disorders of the systems identified in Table 26-2 present high-risk conditions for surgery. Each system is further affected by the patient's age, health condition, nutritional status, and mental state.

Assessment questions to ascertain the patient's use of chemicals, alcohol, and abusive substances assist the health team to select medications tolerated by the body. Postoperative care is also adjusted to compensate, when possible, for potential complications. If a patient has been a heavy smoker, alveoli may be impaired and the patient's lung capacity reduced. Mucus and anesthesia by-products may be trapped in the lung, causing atelectasis and pneumonia. Breathing exercises and treatments for the smoker postoperatively aid in lung expansion and decrease the risk of respiratory complications.

Additional preoperative questions identify the patient's allergies, past surgeries, and infection and disease history. When questioning the patient about medication practices, the nurse asks the patient to name prescription drugs currently taken, as well as over-the-counter drugs and home remedies used. The nurse also records the patient's vital signs and height and weight before surgery to have a baseline for postoperative comparisons.

Table 26-2 Surgical Effects on Body Systems

Body System	Disease/Disorder	Surgical Effect
Cardiovascular	Heart diseases Hypertension Blood dyscrasias Peripheral vascular disease	Stress on the system increases workload and output
Endocrine	Liver diseases Diabetes mellitus Thyroid disorders Adrenal insufficiency	Increases the metabolic needs and the system becomes taxed
Immune	Allergies Immune deficiency Radiotherapy effects Chemotherapy effects	Slows the body's ability to fight infection
Respiratory	Emphysema Asthma Tumors Cystic fibrosis Pulmonary obstructive disease	Decreases lung motility and slows gas exchange
Urinary	Nephritis Polycystic disease Renal failure Tumors	Impaired kidney function decreases excretion of anesthesia; alters acid-base balance

Preoperative Teaching

Patient teaching before surgery helps decrease the stress that patients feel. Because fear of the unknown is a primary stressor of preoperative patients, providing information lessens stresses associated with not knowing. Preoperative information helps to (1) lessen anxiety, (2) reduce the amount of anesthesia needed, (3) decrease postsurgical pain, and (4) reduce corticosteroid production.[3] Although some patients ignore preoperative instruction, most patients want to help themselves deal with the situation. By decreasing postsurgical complications through preoperative teaching, wound healing occurs more rapidly.[3]

In providing preoperative teaching, the nurse should include the patient and family and remember that basic terminology and information are easier to understand than complex explanations. The nurse should frequently stop to verify the patient's understanding of information shared, ask questions, and encourage responses. Questions that can be answered "yes" or "no" should be avoided. "Do you have any questions?" is not as clarifying as "What questions do you have?" If printed materials or videotapes are routinely used in preoperative teaching sessions, it is important to document what the patient read, heard, or saw. Older adults may have difficulty reading small print or hearing taped messages. If the patient is not a native speaker of English, an interpreter may be needed to explain information presented.

Ideally, preoperative teaching is provided 1 or 2 days before surgery, when anxiety is not as high. Although preoperative preparation varies, most institutions have an established teaching program. Preoperative teaching is began by clarifying the sequence of preoperative and postoperative events. Generally, the nurse should instruct the patient about the surgical procedure, informed consent, the method of skin preparation, and gastrointestinal cleanser to be used. The nurse reviews the time of the surgery and information about the recovery area. Although most patients return to their previously assigned units after surgery, a few may be transferred to an intensive care area, specialty unit, or outpatient area. If a transfer will occur, it is helpful to take the patient and family on a tour of the new unit. The nurse reinforces that vital signs, dressings, and tubes are checked every 15 to 30 minutes until the patient is awake and stable. A checklist frequently is used to provide a systematic preoperative teaching plan.

Preparation

Preparation for surgery depends on the patient's age, physical and nutritional status, type of surgery, and the preference of the surgeon. When the surgery is performed in a short-stay or ambulatory setting, the workup normally occurs a few days in advance. If a patient is admitted to the hospital, testing may be conducted to assess for potential problems. If the presenting problem has been diagnosed, preparation frequently includes both in-hospital testing and evaluation of test results previously completed in the physician's office.

Laboratory and radiography. Testing before surgery depends on the institution's policies, physician's directives, and condition of the patient. The nurse follows standing orders to complete this overall process. Laboratory tests commonly reviewed before surgery include a urinalysis and complete blood count to assess kidney and cardiovascular functions. Serum electrolytes are evaluated if extensive surgery is planned or the patient has extenuating problems. One of the essential electrolytes examined is potassium; if potassium is not available in adequate amounts, dysrhythmias can occur during anesthesia and the patient's postoperative recovery may be slowed by general muscle weakness. A chest x-ray evaluation and electrocardiogram are used to identify disease processes or previous respiratory or heart damage. Additional tests are conducted to assess the organ being evaluated. Blood chemistry tests (LDH, gamma GT, alkaline phosphatase, total bilirubin) and urine bilirubin levels verify the liver's functioning ability.

Informed consent. The Patient's Bill of Rights (p. 12) affirms that patients be given informed consent before the beginning of any procedure. In signing the consent form, the patient is competent and agrees to have the procedure that is stated on the form. Information is to be clear, the risks explained, expected benefits identified, and consequences or alternatives for the presenting problem stated. Witnesses are required, to meet the legal requirements of the state. Ideally, the surgeon discusses the surgical procedure with the patient in advance. In some institutions the surgical consent is completed in the physician's office or in the admissions department before the patient is admitted to the unit (Fig. 26-1).

If the patient does not see or hear well, the nurse should allow additional time to explain the surgery. For individuals who are not native speakers of English, an interpreter may be used if necessary. The patient should never be coerced into signing a consent that is not understood or that contains information that differs from what was originally explained.

In an emergency the patient may not be able to give consent for surgery. Every effort is made to locate family members to assume this responsibility. Occasionally telephone permission may be obtained. In cases in which verbal consent is received, the hospital will have standard guidelines. If the patient's life is in danger and family members cannot be located, the surgeon may legally perform surgery. In cases in which family members object to surgery that the physician believes is essential, a court order may be obtained for the procedure. This practice is used very carefully, for example, when a child's life is in danger. The consent cannot be signed by the patient if he has taken a narcotic within the previous 4 hours.

Gastrointestinal preparation. At midnight before surgery, the patient is usually placed on NPO status (i.e., receives nothing by mouth); this keeps the gastrointestinal tract empty when the patient is anesthesized, thereby decreasing the chance of his vomiting or aspirating emesis after surgery. An NPO sign is posted over the patient's bed, and all fluids are removed from the room. The nurse should reinforce with both the patient and family the importance of not ingesting foods or fluids. If the patient breaks the fast, the physician is notified.

While NPO, patients can be provided oral care. The nurse should caution the patient not to swallow fluids used during care. A wet cloth on the lips helps relieve dryness. If patients need to be hydrated or if special IV medications are needed, parenteral fluids or medication may be ordered. Depending on the nature of the surgery, many patients postoperatively resume foods and fluids the day of their surgeries.

Because anesthesia relaxes the bowel, a bowel cleanser may be ordered to evacuate fecal material and lessen postoperative gastrointestinal problems (ileus). Frequently used evacuates are the cleansing enema or a general laxative. A gastrointestinal lavage solution, GoLYTELY, an isosmotic solution, rapidly evacuates the bowel. GoLYTELY is contraindicated, however, in patients with gastrointestinal obstruction, gastric retention ,bowel perforation, toxic colitis, or megacolon. If a bowel preparation is used, the nurse charts the type of preparation used, the patient's tolerance to the procedure, and results. Before bowel surgery, medication (neomycin, sulfonamides) may be given over a period of days to detoxify and sterilize the gastrointestinal tract. This lessens the chance of fecal contamination during surgery.

Skin preparation. Preoperatively the patient takes a shower, unless contraindicated, using an antiseptic soap, such as Hibiclens®, followed by hair removal at the surgical site. There is debate about what is the best method to remove hair. A lower rate of infection occurs with either no shave or a hair clip than with any other method (electric shave, no shave but hair clipped, and razor shave). Use of a depilatory agent has also proved to have a low wound infection rate. Maintaining the skin's integrity is more important than removing hair. If shaving is used, it should be performed as close to the actual time of the surgical procedure as possible (Skill 26-1). Some surgical departments prepare the patient either in a surgical holding room or in the operating room itself.

CONSENT TO OPERATION, ADMINISTRATION OF ANESTHETICS AND THE RENDERING OF OTHER MEDICAL SERVICES

GREAT PLAINS REGIONAL MEDICAL CENTER HOSPITAL

Date January 31, 1991

Hour 10 A. M.

Amy Hartman
(NAME OF PATIENT)

1. I authorize and direct Dr. Jennifer Christensen
my surgeon and/or associates or assistants of his choice to perform the following operation or procedure upon me:

panhysterosalpingoophorectomy
OK to receive blood transfusion if absolutely necessary.
(LIST PROCEDURE(S))

I further consent to the performance of operations and procedures in addition to or different from those now contemplated, whether or not arising from presently unforeseen conditions, which the above-named doctor or his associates or assistants may consider necessary or advisable in the course of the operation.

2. The procedure(s) in paragraph 1 has (have) been explained to me by my physician and I understand the intended nature and consequences of the procedure(s) to be as follows:
Dr. Christensen will remove my ovaries, tubes and uterus
(Designation of procedure(s) in terms of what will be done to the patient's body and intended consequences)

3. I confirm the following: That my physician has explained to me the nature, purpose, and possible consequences of the procedure(s) as well as the risks involved, and the possible complications and/or alternative methods of treatment. I understand that the explanation I have received is not exhaustive because of unforeseen circumstances that may arise and I have been advised that a more detailed and complete explanation of the preceding matter will be given to me if I so desire. Upon reading the previous statement, I do not desire such further explanations. Furthermore, I acknowledge that I have received no guarantees or assurances as to the results that may be obtained from the performance of this operation or procedure.

4. I hereby authorize and direct the above-named surgeon and/or his associates or assistants to provide such additional services for me as he or they may deem reasonable and necessary, including but not limited to, the administration and maintenance of anesthesia, and the performance of services involving pathology and radiology, and I hereby consent thereto.

5. I understand that the above-named surgeon and his associates or assistants will be occupied solely with performing such operation, and that persons in attendance at such operation for the purpose of administering anesthesia, and the persons performing services involving pathology and radiology may not be the agents, servants or employees of the hospital nor of any surgeon, but may be independent contractors.

6. I hereby authorize the hospital pathologist to use his discretion in the disposal of any severed tissue or member, except ____________

Patient's Signature Amy Hartman

Witness Lynn Huffman LPN

(If patient is a minor or unable to sign, complete the following)

Patient is a minor ____________, or is unable to sign,

because ____________

Witness: ____________ Authorized Representative Signature ____________

Relationship to Patient ____________

Witness: ____________

PHYSICIAN'S STATEMENT

I certify that I am the physician of the above-named patient and that I have explained the nature, purpose, and possible consequences of the procedure(s) as well as the risks involved, and the possible complications and/or alternative methods of treatment.

Date: January 31, 1991 Dr J. H. Christensen
Physician's Signature

N-1 2728

FIG. 26-1 Patient consent form for surgery.

SKILL 26-1 PERFORMING SURGICAL PREP

1. Wash hands.
2. Refer to procedure manual to verify anatomical area to be shaved according to surgery to be performed.
3. Close door, and pull curtains.
4. Explain procedure to patient.
5. Position bed and patient.
6. Place towel or waterproof pad under area to be shaved.
7. Fill basin with warm water.
8. Use bath blanket to drape patient appropriately to limit exposure.
9. Adjust lighting.
10. Don gloves.
11. Lather skin well with antiseptic soap or lather and warm water, using gauze squares.
12. Hold razor at a 30- to 45-degree angle to skin.
    a. Shave small area at a time while holding skin taut.
    b. Use short, smooth strokes.
    c. Shave hair in direction it grows.
13. Rinse razor frequently.
    a. Change blade as needed. Replace razor, if disposable razor is used.
    b. Change water as needed.
    c. Cleanse navel area with sterile cotton-tipped applicators.
14. When entire area is shaved, use washcloth and clean, warm water to cleanse area; dry skin.
15. Reassess skin for cuts or abrasions.
16. Return patient to comfortable status.
17. Clean and dispose of equipment.
18. Remove gloves.
19. Wash hands.
20. Often a patient is asked to shower with an antiseptic soap, such as Hibiclens®, after the surgical shave or prep to remove any hair and for further cleansing.

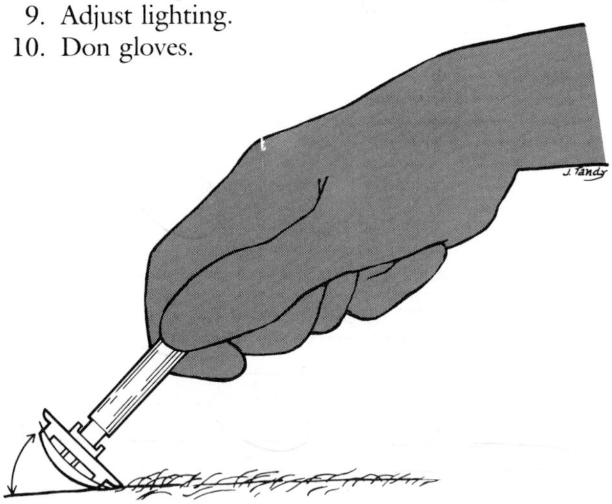

STEP 12

DOCUMENTATION

Sample charting

DATE	TIME	NOTES
12/8/90	8:30	Skin at surgical site shaved, including entire abdomen from nipple line to pubis. Skin intact and has no cuts or abrasions. Several small, brown nevi noted to right of umbilicus. Procedure tolerated well.

____

(nurse's signature)

SPECIAL CONCERNS

- Small children may be easily frightened by this procedure, and it may need to be done in the operating room.
- Older adults will need detailed explanation to relieve their anxiety.
- Older adults have less subcutaneous tissue, less skin elasticity, and more delicate skin tissue. Extreme care will need to be taken when shaving the older adult.
- Older adults are usually more susceptible to infections.

SKILL 26-2

TEACHING CONTROLLED COUGHING

1. Wash hands.
2. Don gloves.
3. Assist patient to upright position. Place pillow between bed or chair and patient.
4. Demonstrate coughing exercise for patient.
   a. Take several deep breaths.
   b. Inhale through nose.
   c. Exhale through mouth with pursed lips.
   d. Inhale deeply again and hold breath for count of 3.
   e. Cough two or three consecutive coughs without inhaling between coughs.
5. Abdominal or thoracic incision can be splinted before coughing with hands, pillow, towel, or rolled bath blanket.
6. Encourage patient to practice coughing while splinting the incisional area once or twice an hour during waking hours. Assist patient as indicated.
7. Provide tissues and emesis basin for any mucus expectorated.
8. Provide washcloth and warm water for washing hands and face and return patient to comfortable position.

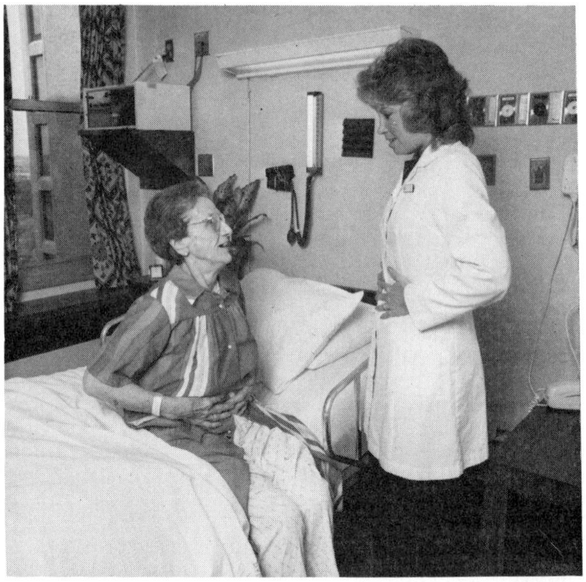

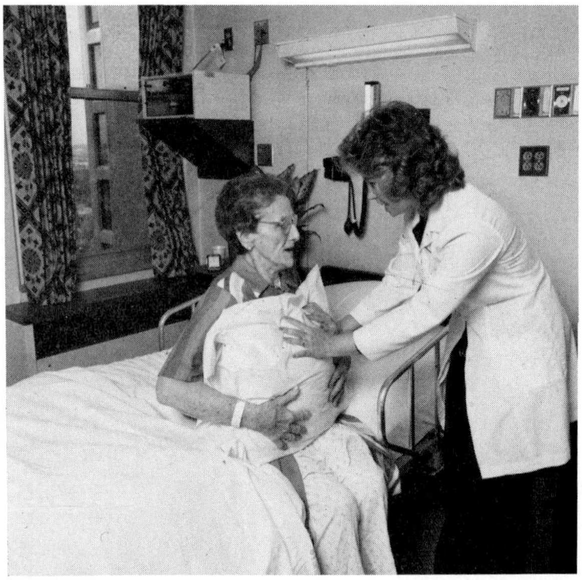

STEP 4

DOCUMENTATION

Sample charting

DATE	TIME	NOTES
12/8/90	2:00	Assisted to full Fowler's position. Controlled coughing completed with pillow splinting the abdominal incision. Small amount of tenacious, white mucus expectorated. No complaints of pain or discomfort noted during procedure. Oral hygiene given and returned to side-lying position.

(nurse's signature)

Continued.

SKILL 26-2 TEACHING CONTROLLED COUGHING—cont'd

SPECIAL CONCERNS

- Young children or older adults may not fully understand the importance of controlled coughing, and continuous reinforcement of teaching and assistance may be needed.
- Family members of a young child should be taught the procedure to assist the child. This will also help family members in meeting their needs by assisting in the care of the child.

PATIENT TEACHING

The patient should be instructed on the following:

- For the patient entering the hospital for same-day surgery, the teaching of controlled coughing may need to be taught in the physician's office, in the preoperative area, or postoperatively before being discharged.
- The home health nurse may need to reinforce the importance of coughing two to three times an hour for the first few days postoperatively.

Respiratory preparation. If a general anesthesic is administered, ventilating the lungs is vital postoperatively to prevent atelectasis and pneumonia. Because the lungs do not expand fully during surgery, mucus and gases remain in the lungs until expelled. Lung exercises can assist in expanding the lungs and removing these byproducts. Before surgery the nurse should assist the patient to practice turning, coughing (Skill 26-2), and deep breathing (Skill 26-3). Since coughing increases intracranial pressure, it is usually contraindicated in cranial-related surgeries. Patients are frequently ambulated within a few hours after surgery to return cardiovascular and respiratory functions to normal more quickly.

Accompanying the need to turn, cough, and deep breathe is the need to practice leg exercises (Skill 26-3). Because blood stasis occurs when the patient is lying flat, leg exercises should be encouraged to assist venous blood flow. With the venous blood slowing, thrombi may form. If a thrombus is dislodged, it can travel as an embolus to the lungs, heart, or brain where the vessel can be occluded. Without an adequate blood supply, an infarct can occur. Antiembolic stockings or Jobst pumps may be ordered to provide support for the lower extremities (Skill 26-4).

Genitourinary concerns. After general anesthesia, the urinary bladder's tone is decreased. Therefore the nurse should know the patient's normal bladder habits and be able to identify when the bladder is full and distended. The nurse informs the patient preoperatively that the lower part of the abdomen will be palpated at intervals to check for bladder fullness. Once patients are awake and tolerating fluids, the nurse should encourage them to maintain an adequate intake. Occasionally a urinary catheter is inserted to monitor urinary output. This procedure is normally reserved for patients undergoing urinary surgery or who may have difficulty voiding. If a catheter is inserted, it is usually removed 1 to 3 days postoperatively to reduce the chance of bladder infection. Once it is removed, the nurse should encourage the patient to drink 8 ounces of fluids per hour while awake unless contraindicated. The nurse also monitors intake and output values until voiding returns to the patient's normal pattern.

Vital signs. Vital signs mirror the body's response to anesthesia and surgery. The nurse instructs the patient before surgery that it is normal for the blood pressure, temperature, pulse, and respiration to be monitored until stable. The schedule for monitoring vital signs depends on the protocol of the hospital and the stability of the patient. Preoperative vital signs serve as the baseline for deciding when stability has returned. Guidelines for monitoring postoperative vital signs are identified under the Postoperative Period, Immediate Assessment (p. 486).

SKILL 26-3

TEACHING POSTOPERATIVE BREATHING TECHNIQUES AND LEG EXERCISES

1. Wash hands.
2. Assist patient to comfortable position—sitting or standing.
3. Place pillow between patient and bed or chair.
4. Sit or stand facing patient.
5. Demonstrate taking slow, deep breaths. Avoid using shoulder and chest while inhaling. Inhale through nose.
6. Hold breath for count of 3, and slowly exhale through pursed lips.
7. Repeat exercise three to five times.
8. Have patient practice exercise.
9. Instruct patient to take 10 slow, deep breaths every 2 hours postoperatively during waking hours until up and around.
10. If patient has an abdominal or thoracic incision, instruct patient to splint incisional area, if desired, during breathing exercises.

Leg exercises

11. Lifting one leg at a time and supporting joints, gently flex and extend the leg five to ten times. Encourage medial and lateral movement of ankles 5 to 10 times.
12. Repeat on opposite leg. Lifting the leg and supporting the joints, gently flex and extend the leg five to ten times. Encourage medial and lateral movement of ankles 5 to 10 times.
13. Document procedure.

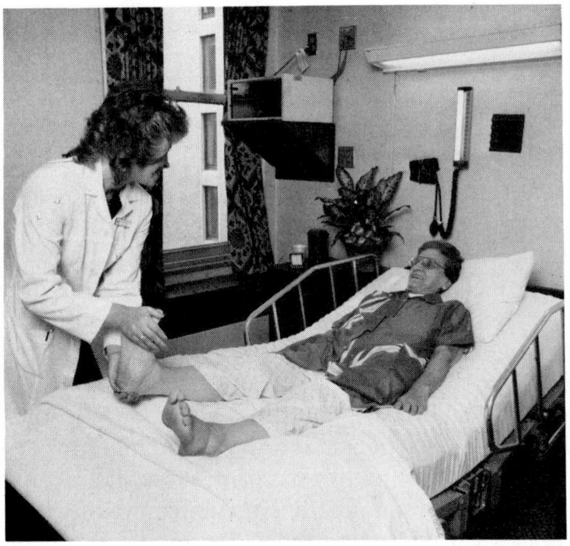

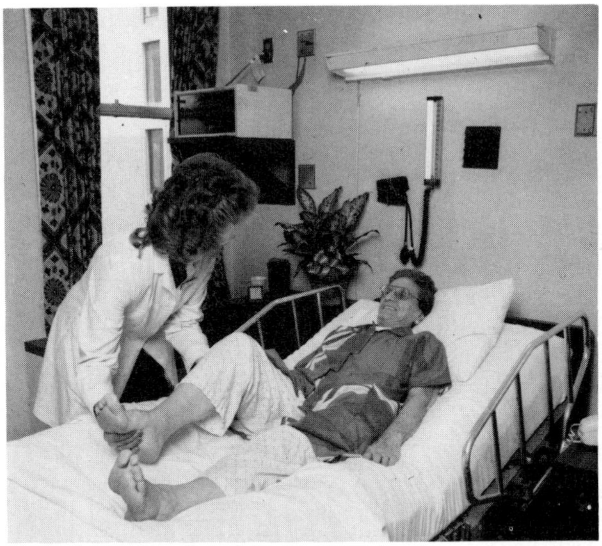

STEP 11

DOCUMENTATION

Sample charting

DATE	TIME	NOTES
4/8/90	1:00	Deep breathing and leg exercises taught. Return demonstration satisfactorily performed. No evidence of dyspnea noted. Instructed to practice exercises at least three more times before surgery in the AM.

____
(nurse's signature)

Continued.

SKILL 26-3 TEACHING POSTOPERATIVE BREATHING TECHNIQUES AND LEG EXERCISES—cont'd

SPECIAL CONCERNS

- Special care should be taken in teaching children deep breathing exercises. Be sure to teach the family members for reinforcement.
- Elderly patients may need to be encouraged to practice the breathing and leg exercises; they may not fully understand the importance of the procedure.
- Patients who have chronic respiratory conditions may need assistance and encouragement in car-

PATIENT TEACHING

The following should be considered for the patient who requires instruction on postoperative exercise and breathing techniques:

- For the patient entering the hospital for same-day surgery, deep breathing and leg exercises may need to be taught in the physician's office, in the preoperative area, or postoperatively.
- The home health nurse may need to reinforce the importance of the deep breathing and leg exercises

Surgical wound. With today's technologies, incisions are closed in a variety of ways: suture, staples, Steri-Strips, or transparent strips. If the nurse knows the type of closure, its appearance can be explained to the patient. Some surgeries require the removal of exudate. For these patients, a drain may be in place. The nurse can explain the purpose of the drain and the need for close monitoring. Although not all incisions require dressings, the nurse will observe the wound's appearance. Wounds and drainage are described in more detail later in this unit.

Pain. Patients fear pain more than any other postsurgical complication. A variety of methods are used to reduce discomfort. If the patient considers nontraditional analgesia (imagery, biofeedback, relaxation), the nurse should review these techniques and allow practice time. The majority of patients elect to obtain comfort through traditional analgesia. Postoperative pain is real, so it is important to reassure patients that addiction to analgesics rarely occurs in the time frame needed for comfort. For the patient who is apprehensive about injections and is allowed oral intake, oral analgesics coupled with nontraditional methods are often effective.

Tubes. Depending on the surgery, patient teaching includes information about nasogastric tubes, wound evacuation units, and intravenous and oxygen therapy. Allowing patients to view these items and understand their purposes lessens the fear associated with each.

Preoperative medication. Preoperative medication reduces the patient's anxiety, decreases the amount of anesthetic needed, and reduces respiratory tract secretions. Barbiturates and tranquilizers (phenobarbital and diazepam [Valium]) are sometimes given for sedation. Narcotic analgesics (meperidine and morphine) may be administered if the patient has pain before surgery; this too reduces the amount of anesthetic required. Anticholinergics, such as atropine, reduce spasms of smooth muscles and decrease gastric, bronchial, and salivary secretions. The patient frequently becomes drowsy, notices a dry mouth, and may experience vertigo after the preoperative medication is given.[18]

If preoperative medication is given on the nursing unit, the patient must remain in bed, and the nurse raises side rails and monitors the patient every 15 to 30 minutes until the patient leaves for surgery. In many institutions the preoperative medication is given by the anesthesiologist in the preoperative holding area. These patients should be reassured and provided a quiet environment on the nursing unit while they are waiting to be transported to the surgical suite.

SKILL 26-4

APPLYING ANTIEMBOLISM STOCKINGS

1. Wash hands.
2. Measure thigh and calf circumference and length from groin to plantar area for full-length antiembolism stockings; measure calf circumference for knee-length antiembolism stockings; secure correct size according to measurements.
3. Assist patient to supine position.
4. Turn stockings inside-out, grasp foot and heel of the stocking, and invert sock over your hand—turn leg and foot of stockings inside-out to the heel portion.
5. Remove hand and slip foot portion over patient's toes, foot, and heel, fitting patient's foot into heel and toe appropriately.
6. Pull leg portion of stocking over foot and up as far as it will go.
7. Adjust stocking to fit evenly and smoothly with no wrinkles.
8. Repeat procedure for opposite leg.
9. Assess patient periodically.
10. Assess stocking at regular intervals.
11. Document procedure.

DOCUMENTATION

Sample charting

DATE	TIME	NOTES
12/8/90	7:00	Knee-high antiembolism stockings applied to both legs. Skin is pink and warm, and pedal pulses are present bilaterally.

(nurse's signature)

SPECIAL CONCERNS

- Postoperative patients with abdominal or thoracic incisions will not be able to bend and pull on own stockings.
- Stockings may be hard to apply for the elderly patients; the nurse or family members will assist the patient.
- Stockings may be hard to fit and maintain in the obese patient and the very thin patient.

PATIENT TEACHING

The patient who will be applying antiembolism stockings should be instructed on the following:

- Patients will need to be instructed on procedure to appropriately apply antiembolism stockings.
- Nurse can teach patient appropriate care of the stockings.
- Nurse should instruct patient not to massage legs because of the risk of dislodging a blood clot.
- Patient may need to continue to apply stockings at home, if ordered by the physician, and will need to know the procedure for applying and caring for the stockings and signs of possible complications.

Great Plains Regional Medical Center
Box 1167 - 601 West Leota
North Platte, Nebraska 69101
308-534-9310

ADDRESSOGRAPH

(Please check carefully and initial)

Date January 15, 1991

1. Medical Admission Permit Signed ✓ L.H.
2. Surgical Permit Signed & Witnessed ✓ L.H.
3. Blood Transfusion Permit ✓ L.H.
4. Sterilization Permit Signed & Witnessed ✓ L.H.
5. Bone Bank Protocol 0 Recipient 0 Donor 0
6. Authorization for Partial Abortion 0
7. Allergies, list: penicillin
8. Identification Band ✓ L.H. Blood Bracelet ✓ L.H. Medex ✓ L.H.
9. Pre-Op Prep Done ✓ L.H. Checked By RN Fran Ranck RN.
10. Pre-Op Bath ✓ L.H. Hospital Gown ✓ L.H. Bath Blanket ✓ L.H.
11. Remove: Dentures 0 Glasses/Contacts ✓ L.H. Jewelry/Nail Polish/Hair Pins/Make-up ✓ L.H.
12. TED stockings when ordered ✓ L.H. Side Rails Up ✓ L.H. Addressograph ✓ L.H.
13. Pre-Op Vital Signs (T 98⁶ P 80 R 20 BP 120/80
14. Pre-Op Medications Demerol 50 mgm + atropine 0.3 mgm Im 0900
15. Insert Foley Catheter ✓ L.H.
16. Physical Disability, such as Amputations, Glass Eye, Etc. 0
17. Systemic Diseases NIDDM
18. History and Physical ✓ L.H.
19. Lab Reports:
    A. Hgb on all Menstrual Age Females ✓ L.H.
    B. All Patients Age 40-60 Hgb and EKG 0
    C. All Patients Over 60 Hgb, EKG and Chest X-ray 0
    D. Type and Crossmatch ✓ L.H.

NURSING STAFF IDENTIFICATION

L. H. - Lynn Huffman LPN

20. Infectious Process Present ____ Yes X No
    Type of Infection ————
21. Additional Comments pre + post op. nursing interventions explained
22. Chart Signed Off Lynn Huffman LPN

PRE-OP ASSESSMENT FORM

FIG. 26-2 Preoperative assessment form.

Preoperative check list. The nurse completes the preoperative check list before the patient leaves the nursing unit (Fig. 26-2). If the preoperative medication is to be given on the nursing unit, the nurse completes the preoperative check list before administering the medication. **Prostheses,** contact lenses, dentures, jewelry, and other valuables are removed and either given to family members or placed in a secure area. If rings are worn, they should be secured with tape and the disposition of personal items charted. The patient should void before the preoperative medication is administered, or 1 hour before surgery is scheduled. Although the majority of patients become drowsy after administration of a preoperative medication, a few will either become hyperactive or demonstrate no side effects. The patient should be reminded to remain in bed and the side rails raised. The call light should be placed within reach and its location identified for the patient.

The patient is transported to the surgical area approximately 30 to 60 minutes before the scheduled procedure. Once the patient is admitted to the surgical suite, final preoperative measures are completed: the skin is prepared, an intravenous needle is inserted, vital signs are assessed, and chart data are reviewed. If intravenous therapy was not previously started, fluids are begun. An IV site is needed not only for the administration of the anesthetic, but also to hydrate body cells. The intravenous site is kept patent until the patient has reached a satisfactory recovery period on the surgical unit.

The type of **anesthesia** chosen depends on the surgery performed and level of unconsciousness desired. During the time the patient is anesthetized, care is taken by the surgical team to provide a safe surgical environment. Local or regional anesthesia may be the choice for some patients. Regional anesthesia is classified according to its induction method: nerve block, spinal anesthesia, or epidural anesthesia. Although the patient is awake with local or regional anesthesia, a tranquilizer may be ordered to help the patient relax. If the patient is awake, the environment must be carefully monitored to prevent the patient from becoming frightened.

Intraoperative care centers around the care and protection of the patient. Maintaining a sterile environment in the surgical suite is crucial if the wound is to remain free of contamination. A primary step in promoting wound healing in the operating room is skin preparation. Because skin cannot be sterilized, maintaining strict aseptic technique in the surgical suite is imperative.

Once surgery is completed, the patient is transported to the recovery room (or postanesthesia care unit) or the intensive care area. Evaluation of the patient follows the ABCs of immediate postoperative observation: airway, breathing, consciousness, and circulation. Table 26-3 lists interventions associated with the ABCs. Vital signs are assessed every 15 minutes during the recovery period, and respiratory, circulatory, and gastrointestinal functions are monitored. The wound is evaluated for any **drainage.** When the patient has a patent airway and stable vital signs, is conscious, and responds to stimuli, the anesthesiologist or surgeon approves the transfer of the patient back to the nursing unit. As the patient regains consciousness, relief of pain is often the first need expressed; frequently, medication is given in the recovery area. Documentation from the surgical suite and recovery room is reviewed by staff on the nursing unit to assess how well the patient tolerated the surgical process.

Table 26-3 Interventions Associated with the ABCs of Immediate Recovery ✓

Assessment Mode	Intervention
A—Airway	Maintain patency: keep head tilted up and back; may position on side with the face down and neck slightly extended Note presence or absence of gag/swallowing reflex Suction until awake and alert Provide oxygen if necessary
B—Breathing	Evaluate depth, rate, sounds, rhythm, and chest movement Assess color of mucous membranes Place hand above nose to detect respirations if shallow Initiate coughing and deep breathing exercises as soon as able to respond Chart time oxygen is discontinued
C—Consciousness	Able to extubate airway Responds to commands Verbalizes responses Reacts to stimuli
C—Circulation	Monitor T, P, R every 10 to 15 minutes; take axillary or rectal temp if warranted Assess rate, rhythm, quality of pulse Evaluate color and warmth of skin and nail beds Check peripheral pulses if indicated Assess incision/dressing Monitor IVs: solution, rate, site
S—System review	Assess neurological functions Monitor drains, tubes, color and amount of output Evaluate pain response; may need to give analgesic Observe for allergic reactions Assess urinary output if Foley catheter is in place

Table 26-4 Temperature Assessment and Intervention

Temperature Alterations Postoperatively	Rationale	Assessment and Intervention
Within first 12 hr	Response to surgery, anesthesia, and body exposure	Check for warmth Provide warm blankets Do not expose for long periods Check orientation
24 to 48 hr	Dehydration Decreased lung activity Inflammatory response to surgery	Monitor IV rate Encourage fluids Assess I&O Turn, cough, and deep breathe Use spirometer Assess lung sounds Observe incision
After day 2	Infection: respiratory, wound, urinary, or circulatory	Assess lung sounds and expectoration Evaluate incision and drainage Monitor I&O Encourage fluids of 6-8 oz/hr unless contraindicated Note urine color, odor, amount, and consistency, and patient's complaints of burning Do leg exercises q2h, and ambulate q4h

POSTOPERATIVE PERIOD

Immediate assessments. When the patient returns to the nursing unit, a thorough postsurgical assessment follows. Vital signs, the intravenous and incisional sites, any tubes, and postoperative orders are reviewed. A review of each body system identifies when body functions return and provides a guideline for further assessments. Unless otherwise indicated, the nurse monitors vital signs and makes general assessments using the "times four" factor—every 15 minutes times 4; every 30 minutes times 4; every hour times 4; then every 4 hours, or until assessments are within expected ranges. The times four gauge is the maximal time that should elapse between assessments. Table 26-4 details body temperature responses to surgery. A postoperative flow sheet (Fig. 26-3) is frequently used to assess the patient's progress.

Significant observations are critical for the patient after surgery. Although the patient may respond, the level of functioning is impaired. Side rails should be kept in the up position and the call light within reach. Until the patient is fully conscious, a pillow should not be placed under his head. The nurse should either position him on the side or raise the head of the bed to a 45-degree angle. By positioning the head higher than the chest, the chance of the patient's aspirating vomitus lessens. Because nausea and vomiting are normal in the first 12 to 24 hours, the emesis basin should remain at the bedside. If the patient vomits, the amount should be measured and carefully described in the charting. Any emesis that is red should be reported immediately. Frequently, the patient remains on NPO status for the first few hours after surgery. Fluids are introduced gradually. The usual fluid regimen ordered by the physician includes ice chips followed by clear or full liquids.

Postoperative complications can occur suddenly; therefore any change should be noted. Because the patient is often cold, additional blankets should be provided for comfort; however, sweating should not be induced. Vital signs, coupled with the patient's behavior, are first-line observations. A pulse that increases and becomes thready, coupled with a declining blood pressure, cool and clammy skin, reduced urine output, and restlessness may signal hypovolemic shock. Hypovolemic shock in the postoperative period is frequently caused by internal hemorrhage—a life-threatening emergency.

Incision. The incisional dressing is monitored, because bleeding or excessive drainage may also signal postoperative hemorrhage. Normally dressings are not changed but are reinforced during the first 24 hours. To accurately measure the amount of drainage, the nurse circles the drainage markings on the dressing and writes the time and date. A surgical incision may separate; this action of **dehiscence** may occur within 3 days to over 2 weeks postoperatively. Wound separation that occurs in the first 3 days is usually related to technical factors, such as the sutures. Separation from 3 to 14 days postoperatively is usually associated with postoperative complications, such as distention, vomiting, excessive coughing, dehydration, or infection. Wound separation after 2 weeks is usually associated with metabolic factors, such as cachexia, hypoproteinemia, increased age, or malignancy. If internal organs protrude through the incision, wound **evisceration** has occurred. Both wound dehiscence and evisceration require prompt attention (See Fig. 26-7). If the patient feels a sudden "give," sutures may have broken.

Ventilation. Because lung ventilation is vital, the nurse assists the patient to turn, cough, and deep breathe every 1 to 2 hours until the chest is clear. Having practiced this combination preoperatively, the patient is usually able to adequately remove trapped mucus and surgical gases. To ease the pressure on the incision, the nurse

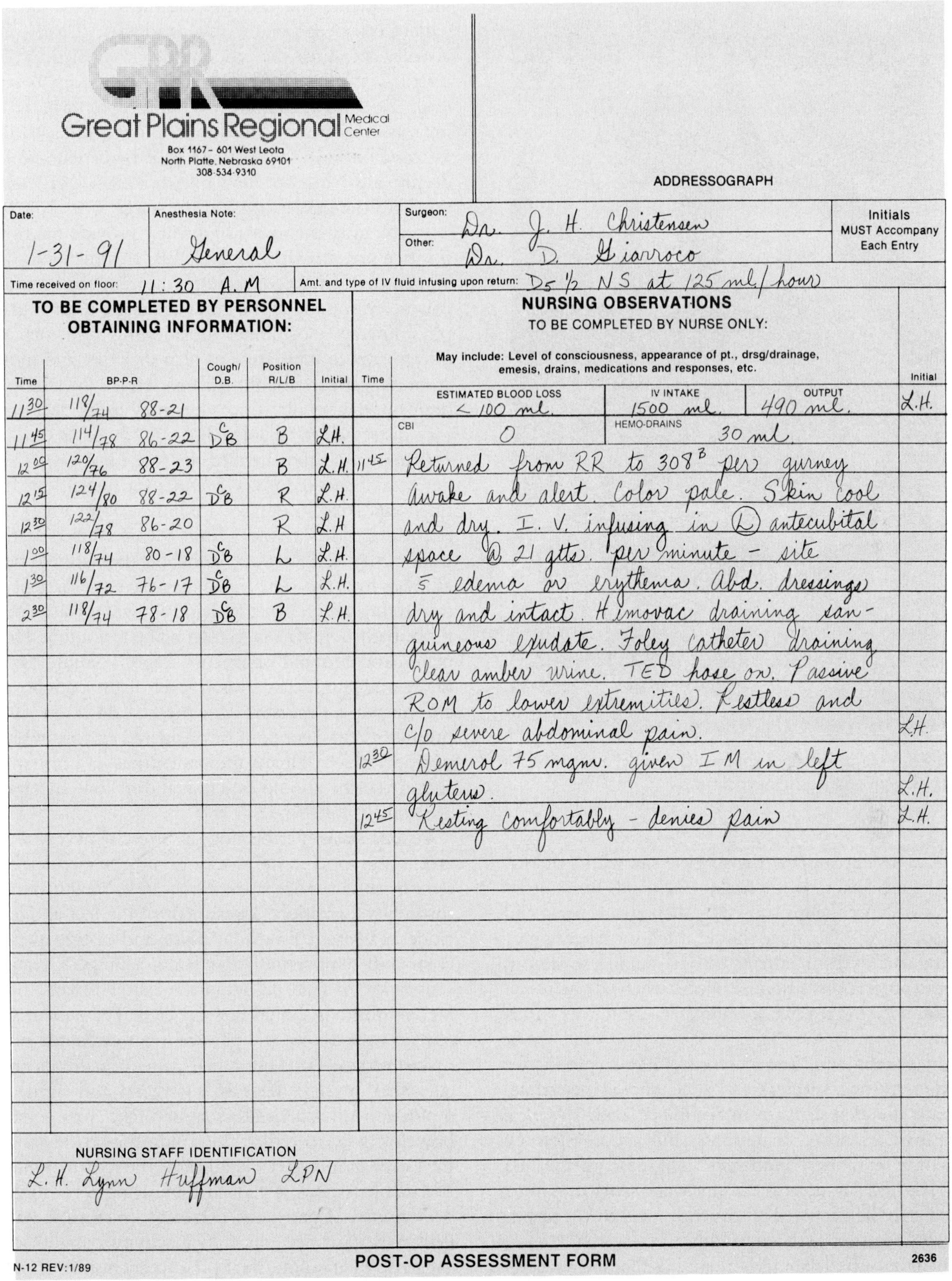

Great Plains Regional Medical Center
Box 1167 - 601 West Leota
North Platte, Nebraska 69101
308-534-9310

ADDRESSOGRAPH

RECOVERY ROOM REPORT

Date:	Anesthesia Note:	Surgeon: / Other:	Initials MUST Accompany Each Entry
1-31-91	General	Surgeon: Dr. J. H. Christensen Other: Dr. D. Giarroco	

Time received on floor: 11:30 A.M Amt. and type of IV fluid infusing upon return: D5 ½ NS at 125 ml/hour

TO BE COMPLETED BY PERSONNEL OBTAINING INFORMATION:

Time	BP-P-R		Cough/ D.B.	Position R/L/B	Initial
11[30]	118/74	88-21			
11[45]	114/78	86-22	c̄ DB	B	LH.
12[00]	120/76	88-23		B	L.H.
12[15]	124/80	88-22	c̄ DB	R	L.H.
12[30]	122/78	86-20		R	L.H
1[00]	118/74	80-18	c̄ DB	L	L.H.
1[30]	116/72	76-17	c̄ DB	L	L.H.
2[30]	118/74	78-18	c̄ DB	B	L.H.

NURSING OBSERVATIONS
TO BE COMPLETED BY NURSE ONLY:
May include: Level of consciousness, appearance of pt., drsg/drainage, emesis, drains, medications and responses, etc.

ESTIMATED BLOOD LOSS	IV INTAKE	OUTPUT	Initial
< 100 ml.	1500 ml.	490 ml.	L.H.
CBI: 0	HEMO-DRAINS: 30 ml.		

Time		Initial
11[45]	Returned from RR to 308B per gurney. Awake and alert. Color pale. Skin cool and dry. I. V. infusing in (L) antecubital space @ 21 gtts. per minute - site s̄ edema or erythema. Abd. dressings dry and intact. Hemovac draining san-guineous exudate. Foley catheter draining clear amber urine. TED hose on. Passive ROM to lower extremities. Restless and c/o severe abdominal pain.	L.H.
12[30]	Demerol 75 mgm. given IM in left gluteus.	L.H.
12[45]	Resting comfortably - denies pain	L.H.

NURSING STAFF IDENTIFICATION
L.H. Lynn Huffman LPN

N-12 REV:1/89 **POST-OP ASSESSMENT FORM** 2636

FIG. 26-3 Postoperative assessment form.

A

B

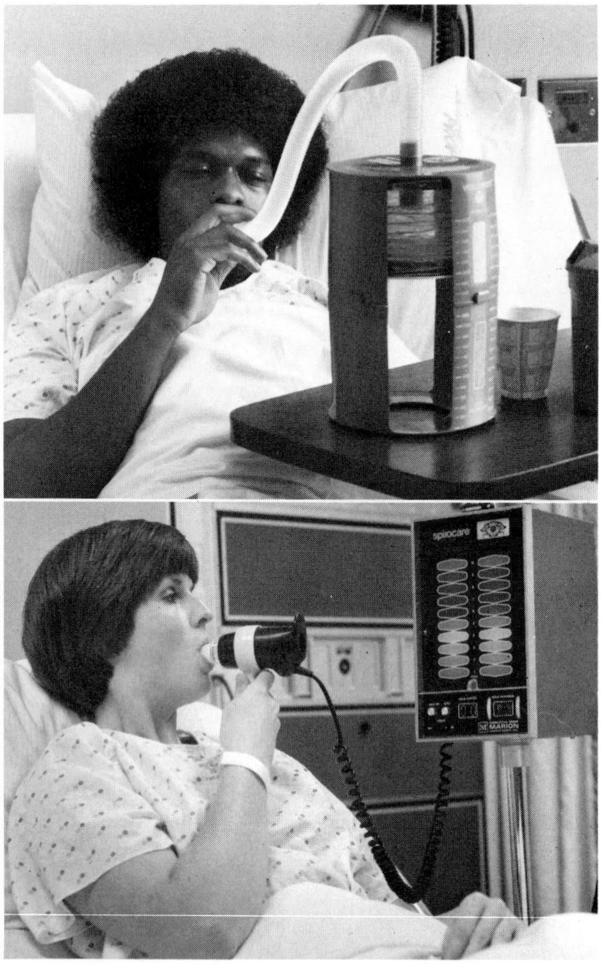

FIG. 26-4 Volume-oriented spirometer. **A,** Bellows visible to patient. **B,** Achievement light indicator.

helps the patient support the surgical site with a pillow, rolled bath blanket, or the heel of the hand. Respiratory infections are frequently caused by shallow breathing and poor coughing. The nurse should listen for wheezing or crowing sounds from patients who have undergone head or neck surgery; this response occurs when edema places pressure over the trachea, resulting in respiratory insufficiency.

If the patient feels chest pain or has a fever, productive cough, or dyspnea, **atelectasis** or pneumonia may be developing. Sudden chest pain combined with dyspnea, tachycardia, cyanosis, diaphoresis, and hypotension are signs of a pulmonary embolism. The head of the bed should be raised to decrease dyspnea, and symptoms must immediately be reported. Frequently oxygen therapy is instituted to assist with respirations.

Whenever air exchange is reduced, postoperative recovery slows. Medication, suctioning, and oxygen therapy may be needed to assist the patient with respiratory distress. Mechanical devices, such as incentive spirometers and blow bottles, are also used to stimulate deep breathing. Frequently the incentive spirometer is used when the patient can deep breathe independently; the instrument visually measures the amount of air inhaled. Volume-oriented spirometers assist patients in deep breathing (Fig. 26-4). Patients are encouraged to take 10 deep breaths every hour while awake. Blow bottles, while not as common as in the past, are used by patients to inhale deeply and blow out air while moving water from one bottle to the next to expand the lungs.

Respiratory therapists frequently provide intermittent positive pressure breathing (IPPB) treatments to deliver a mixture of air and oxygen; medication can be added to enhance respirations. Postural drainage, a form of chest physiotherapy, combines positioning and percussion movements to lung areas to help dislodge and move secretions. Patients are not left unattended during postural drainage treatments, since they may experience respiratory distress (See Chapter 34).

Urinary. Anesthesia retards urinary function. The bladder area is checked every 2 hours for distention. It routinely takes 6 to 8 hours for voiding to occur after surgery. If patients do not void within 8 to 12 hours, catheterization may be necessary. Catheterization should be used as a last measure. The nurse may have the patient listen to running water, place his hands in warm water, or walk to the bathroom if he is able, to facilitate voiding. Helping male patients stand often encourages voiding. To accurately evaluate the hydration level of the patient, intake and output are measured for the first 24 hours. A urine output of 30 ml per hour is considered an acceptable level postoperatively. Unless the patient has had urinary tract surgery, urine should be clear and yellow and have an ammonia odor.

Venous stasis. Performing leg exercises every 2 hours and using antiembolic stockings aid the circulatory system, because venous **stasis** is the underlying cause of the thrombus formation. Assessment of the feet and legs includes palpating for pedal pulse and noting the skin's color and temperature. If edema, aching or cramping, sensitivity, or pain occurs in the calf (Homans' sign) or leg, a thrombus should be suspected. The patient should remain in bed until the physician has evaluated him.

Gastrointestinal. Abdominal distention frequently occurs after surgery. Because anesthesia and surgical manipulation slow peristalsis, it may take 3 to 4 days for bowel activity to return. Listening for bowel sounds in the lower abdomen can help gauge the return of function. Normal peristalsis is gauged by hearing 5 to 30 gurgles per minute. If peristalsis decreases or stops, a paralytic ileus may have developed. If inactivity continues, a nasogastric or nasointestinal tube to suction is usually ordered to help remove the gas formed in the stomach and small intestine. When listening for bowel sounds in patients who have a nasogastric or nasointestinal tube, the nurse should turn off the suction machine but should *never* leave the room without turning the machine on.

Abdominal distention can be verified by measuring the patient's abdominal girth. Accurate measurement is ensured by marking on the skin the placement for the tape measure. The nurse should assess and chart the expelling of flatus, bowel sounds, and abdominal girth. Occasionally, analgesics (meperidine) and other medications may slow peristalsis; charting the patient's gastrointestinal habits aids in identifying etiological factors.

Encouraging activity (turning every 2 hours, early ambulation) assists gastrointestinal activity. A rectal tube or up-and-down flush (a 250 ml tap water enema instilled into the colon; enema container lowered to withdraw air from colon; and repeat) may be ordered for ongoing distress. For the patient who has difficulty with flatus, limiting iced beverages and encouraging warm liquids may help resolve the discomfort. The patient may have fluids and food withheld until flatus is expelled. As patients return to previous eating habits, bowel function slowly resumes its preoperative state. Constipation is also a frequent problem after surgery. The same aids for abdominal distention assist in alleviating constipation. If feces are not passed within 2 to 3 days after the patient has resumed solid foods, a suppository or tap water enema may be ordered. Ambulation is encouraged to promote peristalsis.

Hiccups (singultus) are involuntary contractions of the diaphragm followed by rapid closure of the glottis. Singultus results from irritation of the phrenic nerve. Since abdominal distention may be the cause, the nurse assesses the patient's abdomen for proper GI function. Although abdominal distention usually occurs from gas in the intestinal tract, the cause may be internal bleeding. The nurse should evaluate the patient for signs of shock: vital signs, skin condition, and level of consciousness.

Pain. Although internal organs do not have many nerve endings, a skin incision does produce painful responses. Because pain is normal postoperatively, the nurse should offer patients ordered analgesics. Within 24 to 48 hours, acute pain begins to subside. Pain medication is subsequently adjusted to meet the patient's need. In the early stages of recovery, comfort interventions help ease pain (Table 26-5). After the acute phase ends, comfort measures may be the only interventions required.

A patient's level of pain can be difficult to evaluate. There are standard pain indexes (restlessness, moaning, grimacing, diaphoresis), but some patients may not outwardly exhibit symptoms. Objective pain factors are detectable signs that the body is responding to "pain": vital sign changes (BP lowers and pulse increases), restlessness, diaphoresis, pallor. The patient's description of discomfort represents subjective pain factors. The way the pain is affecting the patient emotionally is termed *suffering*. Pain behaviors are influenced by the patient's culture and past experiences. Behaviors include moaning, grimacing, and favoring a body area.

Table 26-5 Postoperative Comfort Measures for Pain

Decrease external stimuli	Darken room: close drapes Keep TV/radio off or low Monitor hall traffic/noise Assess staff interruptions Check room for noise—dripping water, buzzing lights
Reduce interruptions	Plan care to allow rest Post do not disturb sign Unplug telephone Restrict visitors Pull curtains around bed
Eliminate odors	Discuss offending odors and assess elimination Remove from room all dressings that are soiled with exudate Post no smoking sign Alert housekeeping—omit room-cleaning products Install air circulating unit Alert dietary department to reduce foods with odors
Nursing interventions	Question normal relaxation patterns/practices Practice deep breathing and relaxation techniques Plan rest periods Provide back rub Provide conversation and ask about concerns/fears Encourage diversional activities Reposition and support with pillows, bed rolls. Check tube placement Offer warm fluids if indicated Reduce room clutter Provide restful environment

The effectiveness of analgesic measures differs with each person; if relief is not obtained, changing the medication or administration schedule may provide effective pain control. Each patient interprets pain differently and has a personal pain tolerance level; therefore, if a patient expresses pain, it is real for that person. Patients experiencing chronic pain may have more difficulty obtaining relief than individuals with acute episodes.

The success of pain managment depends on the nature of the surgery, emotional state of the patient, and postoperative complications. Commonly used analgesic measures are nurse-administered narcotics, self-controlled intravenous medication administration (patient-controlled analgesia [PCA] system), and pain control via the trans-

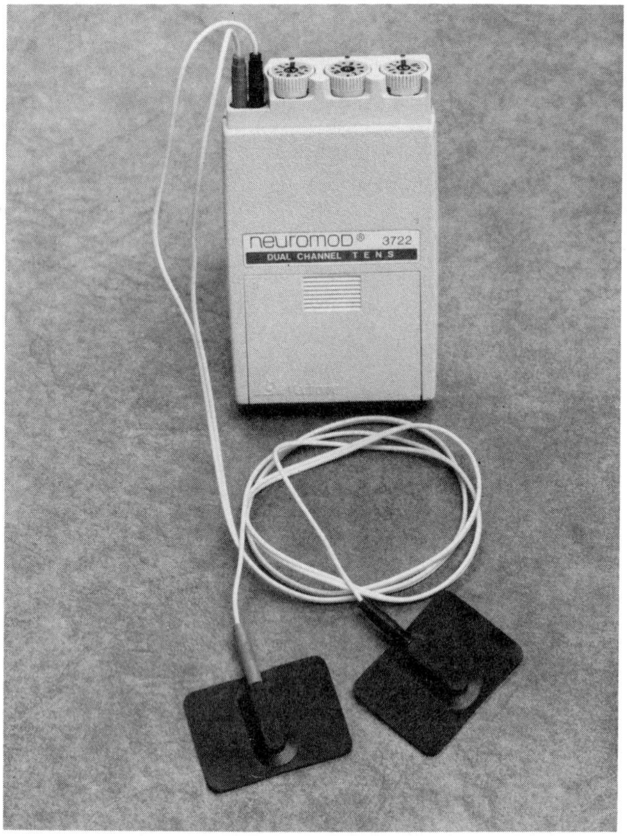

FIG. 26-5 TENS.

cutaneous electric nerve stimulation (TENS) unit (Fig. 26-5). The PCA system is a pump that has a predetermined amount of analgesic contained within the unit; the system is programmed to allow only a given amount of medication to be dispensed. The patient can self-administer an analgesic by pressing a control button. Attached to the skin, the TENS unit applies electric impulses to the nerve endings and blocks transmission of pain signals to the brain.

Fluids and electrolytes. Fluid tolerance and electrolyte values are closely monitored during the postoperative period. When the patient returns from the recovery room, intravenous therapy will be in progress. Until the patient is past the nausea and vomiting period and can tolerate oral fluids, parenteral therapy should be maintained. The intravenous line is observed for patency and ordered fluid rate, and the intravenous site is monitored for erythema, edema, heat, and pain. Because intravenous therapy may become infiltrated because of movement or inadvertently dislodging the needle when ambulating, the site should be assessed every 30 to 60 minutes. The assessment for rate of infusion is extremely important for elderly patients, who may experience fluid overload and pulmonary edema very quickly.

Muscles and nerves require ongoing nourishment to function adequately, and parenteral fluids contain the necessary glucose and electrolytes. Depending on the type of surgery and nutritional needs of the patient, intravenous therapy lasts from a few hours to a few days. As long as parenteral fluids are received, the nurse should record the patient's intake and output. If there is concern about the patient's overall nutritional state, the patient should be weighed daily.

As oral fluids are introduced, patients should be encouraged to drink small amounts frequently (6 to 8 ounces per hour). The nurse reviews the diet history to note fluids normally enjoyed. Unless otherwise ordered, patients usually begin by ingesting clear liquids (7-Up, water, tea, broth, gelatin) and progress as their gastrointestinal system returns to normal functioning. If the patient has difficulty drinking the amount of fluid recommended, fluids can be offered more frequently and without a straw. (A straw, while convenient, reduces the amount of fluids ingested.) Unless there are other problems (decreased renal excretion because of renal failure, age), patients should be encouraged to drink 2000 to 2400 ml in 24 hours. Because iced and carbonated beverages cause gastrointestinal disturbances in some individuals, these fluids should be avoided until active peristalsis is noted. If nausea and vomiting persist, an antiemetic, such as promethazine (Phenergan), benzquinamide (Emete-Con), or prochlorperazine (Compazine), is usually ordered to be administered IM, IV, or rectally. (See the nursing care plan for the postoperative patient.)

PARENTERAL FLUIDS

Healing is directly associated with well-nourished body cells. Without adequate electrolytes and nutrients, healing is hindered. For surgical patients, a patent intravenous site is maintained for the administration of nutrients, fluids, medications, and blood. The overall goal of intravenous fluid administration is to correct or prevent fluid and electrolyte imbalances. Poor tissue absorption, inadequate gastrointestinal tract function, and the need for maintaining medications at optimum levels are indicators for intravenous therapy. Intravenous therapy continues postoperatively until the patient tolerates fluids and oral nutrients.

Solutions. Parenteral fluids are selected for the electrolytes and nutrients provided. Three basic types of fluids exist: isotonic, hypotonic, and hypertonic. Each fluid is categorized by its total electrolyte amount and whether total osmolarity is less than, greater than, or equal to that of blood.

Parenteral solutions are chosen for their actions. *Isotonic* solutions have the same concentration of solutes (substances dissolved in a solution) as another solution. Isotonic solutions do not expand or shrink cells. Dextrose 5% in water or lactated Ringer's solution and 0.9% sodium chloride (normal saline) are examples of isotonic

NURSING CARE PLAN: THE POSTOPERATIVE PATIENT

Forty-six-year-old obese woman admitted for a cholecystectomy.
Patient has no preexisting health problems.

Nursing diagnoses	Patient goals	Nursing interventions
Ineffective airway clearance, related to inability to cough deeply and retention of secretions	Patient will cough deeply with splinting of incision. Patient will expectorate mucus. Patient's temperature will be normal. Patient's lung sounds will clear after coughing.	Raise head of bed to full Fowler's position during exercises. Splint incision with rolled bath blanket. Turn, cough, and deep breathe q1h while awake. Use spirometer hourly. Take VS q4h and note evidence of dyspnea or restlessness. Offer 8 oz fluid qh if permissible.
Ineffective breathing pattern, related to poor body mechanics and incisional pain	Patient will deep breathe effectively q 1 to 2 h. Patient will effectively use incentive spirometer. Patient will not demonstrate dyspnea or restlessness. Patient's respirations will be even and unlabored.	Encourage deep breathing q1-2h while awake. Reposition q2h; support joints and incision. Continue oxygen @ 2 L per cannula; cleanse nares q4h; post no smoking sign. Encourage use of incentive spirometer. Record R q4h, noting depth, rate, quality. Assess skin and nail beds; report slow blanching color and condition q4h. Darken room; decrease stimuli, monitor pain and offer analgesic prn.
Potential for infection, related to open surgical incision and draining wound.	Patient's wound will not be erythematous or produce purulent exudate. Patient's temperature will remain within normal range. Patient will not complain of pain or tenderness from wound site. Patient's WBC will remain within normal range.	Use good handwashing technique. Monitor wound q4h, noting amount and color of drainage; skin for armth, color, and sensation. Mark drainage on dressing q4h; reinforce prn. Report irritability, weakness, or irregular pulse. Use surgical asepsis when changing dressing. Monitor temperature q4h. Monitor WBC as ordered.

solutions. Their primary use is to replace fluids and provide calories. Normal saline is used to expand plasma volume and replace sodium losses, such as gastrointestinal fluid loss.

Fluids that have less solute than another solution are called *hypotonic;* cells expand in a hypotonic solution. Hypotonic fluids are used to replace cellular fluids and provide water to remove body wastes. Sodium chloride (NaCl) 0.45% is an example of a hypotonic fluid. *Hypertonic* fluids have a greater concentration of solute than body fluids; fluids are pulled out of cells, causing the cells to shrink. If 5% dextrose is added to normal saline or Ringer's solution (5% dextrose and 0.9% NaCl), a hypertonic solution is created. Frequently a hypertonic solution is given to provide extra calories. To help the body dilute the heavy solute concentrations found in hypertonic fluids, fluids are often administered into central veins.

Parenteral therapy is also used to administer amino acids, high concentrations of calories (hyperalimentation solutions), fat emulsions, blood products, and medications. Potassium is commonly added to the IVs of patients who have nasogastric tubes or drainage (from ostomies or wounds) and thereby lose potassium chloride.

Regardless of the solution administered, the nurse should observe the following three guidelines: (1) monitoring the solution drip rate at the ordered infusion rate, (2) infusing the amount of prescribed solution, and (3) maintaining the patency of the intravenous needle.[15] Monitoring the site every 1 to 2 hours is recommended, and an intravenous line should be assessed at least every 4 hours. During parenteral therapy, the patient's intake and output should be recorded.

Hyperalimentation, or total parenteral nutrition (TPN), provides the patient with glucose, essential amino acids, vitamins, and minerals. Roughly 1000 calories per liter of TPN therapy is supplied to patients who are unable to tolerate nutrients in the normal manner. Because of the overload TPN can exert on body systems, measurement of intake and output is essential. Because hypoglycemia or hyperglycemia can occur with the high concentration of glucose, blood glucose levels should be assessed, using the Accucheck unit (glucose monitoring unit) every 4 to 6 hours. Occasionally regular insulin is ordered to help assimilate infused glucose. The jugular or subclavian vein is used as the infusion site, because TPN is highly concentrated and requires a large blood volume to help dilute it. **Sterile** technique (surgical asepsis) is critical whenever the site or solution is handled, to prevent the introduction of pathogens. The infusion rate of TPN solution should never be changed unless the physician orders it. To ensure a constant flow rate, TPN is administered by an infusion pump.

Intravenous monitoring. Intravenous sites are selected to accommodate the intended solution. Most insertion sites for postoperative patients are located in the hand or arm. Foot veins can be used if the patient is not ambulatory. A central vein, such as the subclavian vein, is used to deliver large amounts of fluids or concentrated solutions directly into the bloodstream.

Assessment of the intravenous site centers on the **patency** of the system. A routine should be established for checking the intravenous site, beginning at the solution container and ending at the site. The flow rate should be checked against the physician's order. Tubing is assessed for kinks or obstructions, and the position of the patient's hand or arm is checked. If the extremity is flexed, the vein may become occluded. Patients should be reminded to keep extremities extended. The nurse inspects and palpates the site for edema, erythema, induration (hardness), heat, and discomfort. A burning sensation can mean the solution is irritating the vein; the infusion rate should be slowed and monitoring should be continued. The extremity is compared with the opposite hand or arm if the site seems edematous. Edema may indicate an infiltration has occurred. It is incorrect to assume that obtaining a blood return at the IV site indicates a patent vein. Although an infiltrated IV routinely is discontinued, each institution has policies for monitoring and discontinuing intravenous therapy.

The flow rate is monitored according to the physician's orders. If the patient is dehydrated, in shock, or critically ill, a slow infusion rate does not provide the cardiovascular system with enough fluid. By contrast, an infusion rate that is too rapid can place too much fluid into the circulation and overload the cardiovascular, neurological, and urinary systems. Fluid overload can be fatal. Signs and symptoms associated with fluid overload include dyspnea, a rapid, weak pulse, cough, confusion, increased or decreased blood pressure, rales, pitting edema, weight gain, and decreased urine output. If an overload is suspected, the nurse should immediately slow the infusion rate and contact the charge nurse.

Infiltration. If edema is detected, the nurse should first loosen the tape over the insertion point. Edema that does not subside generally indicates that the catheter is out of the vein and infiltration has occurred. Discomfort or dysfunction may also indicate the solution has infiltrated. With an infiltration, the drip rate decreases in patients who have good skin turgor. When palpating the site, the nurse will find that an infiltrated area feels cool, and the skin may have a blanched appearance. If fluid seeps into the tissue and infiltration is confirmed, the solution is discontinued and another site is used to continue therapy. The site of the infiltration is monitored; usually fluid reabsorbs within 24 hours. Warm compresses should not be applied to infiltrations caused by blood and vesicants (medication that induces blistering); the institution's policy on care to be provided should be followed.

Phlebitis. Phlebitis results from mechanical irritation (the needle moves inside the vein, injuring the vessel), the low pH of some IV solutions, and highly concentrated additives. Erythema, warmth, edema, and discomfort are classic signs of phlebitis. The IV is discontinued and restarted in a different site. Reducing injurious agents, maintaining sterile technique when beginning an IV, and using in-line filters decrease vein irritation and trauma. Applying warm compresses to the inflamed area lessens discomfort.

Septicemia. If a systemic infection occurs from pathogens introduced into the circulating blood stream, septicemia (blood poisoning) results. Signs and symptoms include a fever, chills, prostration, pain, headache, nausea, and vomiting. Antibiotic therapy is vigorously initiated if blood cultures verify a septicemic condition. Using sterile technique reduces the potential for introduction of pathogenic organisms through IV therapy.

Blood therapy. Blood replacement therapy is most commonly used postoperatively to replace blood losses. Individuals who have personal concerns about receiving another person's blood may store their own blood with the American Red Cross before the anticipated surgery for infusion during hospitalization. The fear of receiving the HIV virus has led patients to refuse blood products (see Chapter 40 for information on AIDS). Testing procedures used to collect blood products by the American Red Cross to detect the HIV virus have dramatically reduced the incidence of its being transmitted. Plasma expanders (Plasmanate, Dextran) can be used for patients who refuse blood transfusions because of personal or religious beliefs. A drainage/reinfusion system (See Fig. 26-9), Solcotrans, permits a patient's blood to be collected and reinfused after surgery.[20] The Solcotrans system is connected to a closed wound drain intraoperatively. With a vacuum, blood is aspirated; after a maximum of 500 ml is collected, reinfusion can be done following blood transfusion procedures.

Blood transfusion reactions. If the infused blood is not compatible with the patient's blood type, a reaction results. Close monitoring is therefore crucial in assessing the patient's tolerance to the infusing blood. Vital signs are taken before beginning a blood transfusion, 15 minutes into the transfusion, and on completion. Patients experiencing tranfusion reactions frequently say they are "not feeling right." They may have chills, fever, low back pain, pruritus, hypotension, nausea and vomiting, decreased urine output, chest pain, and dyspnea. Frequently symptoms occur within the first 15 minutes. Because symptoms vary, the nurse should report any change in the patient. If the patient is unconscious, the nurse should closely assess vital signs, urine output, and skin appearance. If a transfusion reaction is suspected, the transfusion should be stopped. The vein is kept open with 0.9% sodium chloride solution, and the physician and blood bank are notified. The nurse monitors the patient's vital signs and urine output every 15 minutes.[15] Because transfusion reaction can be frightening, the nurse should reassure and support the patient.

If the patient is experiencing a hemolytic reaction, transfused blood is incompatible with the patient's blood type and death can occur. Although a reaction normally occurs within the first 15 minutes, it can occur any time during the infusing process. If the reaction is severe, the patient could go into shock and die. Other types of blood transfusion reactions are febrile nonhemolytic, allergic, and anaphylactic reactions. In each type of reaction, a component within the unit of blood is incompatible with the patient's blood. The reaction can occur immediately (febrile nonhemolytic and anaphylactic) or any time during the transfusion.

After any blood transfusion reaction, remaining blood should be returned to the blood bank for analysis. The nurse should comply with the institution's policies for monitoring blood transfusions and reactions.

WOUND CARE

Promoting wound healing is the focus during the postsurgical recovery phase. Various stresses affect the wound's ability to repair itself. Stress and strain (nausea, vomiting, abdominal distention, coughing, respiratory efforts) place tension against the surgical incision.[17] During this phase, the abdominal muscles contract and cause intraabdominal pressure; if the incisional area is weak, dehiscence may occur. As the postoperative period lengthens, patient-related factors influence wound healing: age, nutritional status, physical condition, preexisting health problems, and medication habits. Other factors that may affect wound healing include preoperative skin preparation, type and severity of the surgical procedure, environment within the surgical suite, and postoperative wound care.

Surgical wound. Wound categories result from their cause, severity of injury, amount of **contamination,** or the skin's integrity. For planned surgery, a wound is made by an **incision** or puncture (stab wound for a drainage system). In unplanned or emergency surgeries (**traumatic** injury from a knife stabbing), wound edges are brought together to aid healing. Unless a "dirty surgery" is performed (e.g., a perforated bowel, ruptured appendix), a surgical incision is cleaner than a traumatic wound.

The Centers for Disease Control[4] classifies wounds according to the amount of contamination involved: clean, clean-contaminated, contaminated, dirty, or infected. A *clean* wound is an uninfected surgical wound; the chance of an infection occurring postoperatively is less than 5%. A surgical incision made into the respiratory, gastrointestinal, or genitourinary tract after special presurgical preparation is called a *clean-contaminated* wound. The likelihood that an infection will occur postoperatively in a clean-contaminated wound is between 3% and 11%. A *contaminated* wound results from the presence of gastrointestinal products (feces with *Escherichia coli* in the colon), an acute, nonpurulent inflammation (inflamed appendix), or when aseptic technique is broken during surgery (scalpel is reused after incising a contaminated area). A wound infection occurs 10% to 17% of the time from a contaminated wound. *Dirty* or *infected* wounds have a 27% chance of causing a wound infection. Wounds in this category (e.g., gangrenous toe) are infected before surgery.

Wound healing begins immediately after an injury and may continue for a year or longer. Although the healing process follows the same pattern, the type of wound and tissue, severity, and overall condition of the patient influence the overall process. Wound healing follows four phases: hemostasis, inflammatory, reconstruction, and maturation.[17]

Hemostasis begins as soon as the injury occurs. As blood platelets adhere to the walls of the injured vessel, a clot begins to form. Fibrin in the clot begins to hold the wound together, and bleeding subsides.

During the inflammatory phase an initial increase in blood elements (antibodies, electrolytes, plasma proteins) and water flow out of the blood vessel into the vascular space. This process causes the cardinal signs and symptoms of inflammation: redness (rubor), heat (calor), edema (tumor), pain (dolor), and tissue dysfunction. Leukocytes appear and begin to engulf bacteria, fungi, viruses, and toxic proteins. If an infection is not present, the number of leukocytes decreases. During the inflammatory phase, cells migrate, divide, and form new cells. Slowly, blood clots dissolve and the wound fills; the sides of the wound usually meet in 24 to 48 hours. As the inflammatory phase ends, new cells and capillaries fill the wound from the underlying tissue to the surface. This process seals the wound to protect it from contamination.

Collagen formation occurs during the reconstruction phase. **Fibroblasts** produce collagen, a gluelike protein substance that adds tensile strength to the wound and tissue. Collagen formation increases rapidly between postoperative days 5 and 25. During this phase the wound's appearance changes to an irregular, raised, purplish, immature scar. Foods rich in protein and vitamins A and C, which assist in wound repair, are encouraged during this time. If a patient is not well nourished, nutrient supplements may be ordered. Wound dehiscence most frequently occurs during the reconstructive phase.

Approximately 3 weeks after surgery, fibroblasts begin to exit the wound. The wound continues to gain strength, although healed wounds rarely return to the strength the tissue had before surgery. Although tissue heals at varying speeds, internal wounds (stomach, colon) regain strength faster than skin wounds. Occasionally a keloid, which is an overgrowth of collagenous scar tissue, may form during this phase. The keloid's color ranges from red to pink to white. African Americans and dark-complexioned Caucasians have a higher incidence of keloid formation than other races.

Forms of wound healing. Three types of wound healing occur: first intention (primary union), second intention (granulation), and third intention (secondary suture).[17] Wounds that are made surgically and that have little tissue loss heal by first intention; skin edges are close together, and minimal scarring results. First intention healing begins during the inflammatory phase of healing (Fig. 26-6).

Second intention occurs when skin edges are not close together (approximated) or when pus has formed. If the wound has a **purulent exudate** that forms when injured or diseased tissue dies, the surgeon provides a means for its release. This is accomplished through a drainage system or by packing the wound with gauze. Slowly the necrotized tissue decomposes and escapes; the cavity begins to fill with soft, pink, fleshy projections consisting of capillaries surrounded by fibrous collagen, or **granulation** tissue. The amount of granulation tissue required depends on the size of the wound; scarring is greater in a large wound.

Healing by third intention results if there is a delay in closing the wound and two close, granulated areas are brought together. This frequently occurs when a deep wound was not sutured or the wound breaks down. The wound is resutured when infection is no longer present.

Factors affecting healing. To promote healing the nurse should closely monitor fluid and nutritional needs of the patient. If the patient cannot tolerate food or fluids, parenteral fluids or nasogastric feedings can be provided. Because patients may not be able to tolerate large meals or solid foods, dietary services can provide small, frequent feedings. Fluids, when tolerated, should be offered hourly. Unless contraindicated, the nurse should encourage an intake of 2000 to 2400 ml in 24 hours. As the patient progresses from clear to full liquids, fluids the patient enjoys should be provided. Until the patient's hydration level is stable (usually 24 to 72 hours), the patient's intake and output is monitored.

The nurse assists the patient to achieve a balance between time to rest as a means to facilitate healing and activity to decrease venous stasis. When the patient is confined to bed, moving one body section at a time—head, chest, hip, legs—should be encouraged. To sit up, the patient should roll to the side and, using the elbow as a lever, push to a sitting position; this reduces the stress placed on the incision. If coughing occurs, the nurse can apply a pillow, rolled bath blanket, or the palms of the hands to the incisional area to lessen intraabdominal pressure. Visitors may be restricted if the patient tires too easily.

Preexisting conditions, such as heart murmurs, and chronic diseases (arthritis, diabetes mellitus, hypertension) add stress to the recovering body and require ongoing monitoring. Treatment addresses both the postoperative healing process and management of influencing problems. Nursing assessments are heightened by the need to observe symptoms associated with incisional healing, as well as accompanying disorders.

Surgical site. The selection of the site is based on the tissue and organ involved, nature of the injury or disease process, presence of inflammation or infection, and strength of the site. If surgical procedures require a drainage system, the position of the drain also influences the placement of the incision. The surgeon's goal is to enter the cavity involved, repair the injured or diseased area, and minimize trauma as quickly as possible. Patients may be placed in positions that add stress to the tissue to

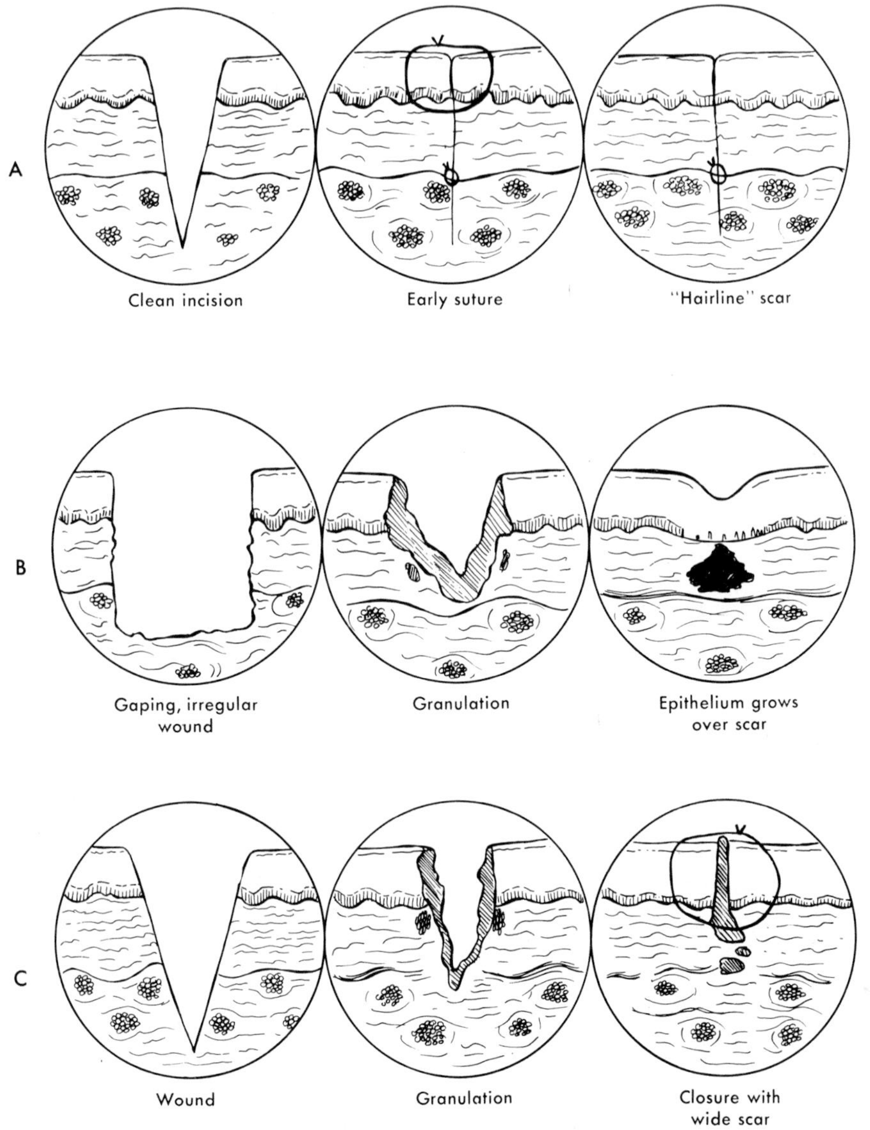

FIG. 26-6 Types of wound healing. **A,** First intention, primary union. **B,** Second intention, granulation. **C,** Third intention, secondary suture. (From Hardy JD, editor: Rhoads textbook of surgery: principles and practice, ed 5, Philadelphia, 1977, JB Lippincott Co.)

facilitate the surgery. Therefore pain after surgery may be caused from strained muscles and ligaments, as well as from the surgical process.

Many options are available to the surgeon for closing the surgical **incision.** Common closures are **sutures,** staples, Steri-Strips, butterfly strips, and transparent sprays and films. A binder or bandage may be used to support the incision or secure dressings without using adhesive materials (Skills 26-5 and 26-6). The nurse inspects dressing every 2 to 4 hours for the first 24 hours. The day of surgery, most wounds produce either **sanguineous** or **serosanguineous** drainage.[11] Because pressure to the surgical wound is desired to retard bleeding, wounds are usually covered by a gauze dressing. It is imperative that the nurse inspect both the dressing or incisional area and the area *under* the patient. Drainage follows the flow of gravity; therefore, depending on the contour of the body, the dressing may remain dry while blood flows under the body, and hemorrhaging might go undetected.

Incisional care. If a closed wound is covered by a dressing, the dressing is observed but not changed until an order is issued. Should a dressing become saturated with drainage before the order is given, the dressing over the incisional area can be reinforced by placing sterile gauze on top of the original dressing and anchoring it securely. The nurse should record and report any dressing that is reinforced. The amount of drainage observed and dressings applied are charted.

There is a trend either to leave sutured, clean wounds not dressed after surgery or to use loose dressings. These methods allow atmospheric oxygen to circulate above the wound, aiding in the healing process. In many cases if a dressing has been used for closed wounds, it is removed within 24 hours postoperatively to allow air circulation.[13] Within 24 hours enough fibrin has usually been produced at the wound site to stop the entry of microorganisms.

An open wound, while generally covered by a dressing, has packing or dressings within the cavity. Open wounds occur when an infection is present and the surgeon wants to promote drainage. As granulation takes place and the infection is treated, healing by second or third intention results. Open wounds frequently leave large, uneven **scars.**

Sterile technique is followed whenever the wound or dressing is handled (Skills 26-7, 26-8, and 26-9). Sterile asepsis not only protects the nurse against wound drainage, but also decreases the introduction of **pathological** organisms into the wound. Using sterile **asepsis** lessens the chance of the patient's acquiring a nosocomial (hospital-acquired) infection. Universal precautions should be employed when handling body secretions.[24] Good handwashing technique and the use of sterile aseptic procedures are essential when providing surgical wound care. A gown, mask, and protective goggles are worn if soiling or splashing of wound exudate is expected.

SKILL 26-5

APPLYING A BANDAGE

1. Wash hands.
2. Position patient in comfortable position, arranging support for area to be bandaged.
3. Provide privacy.
4. Ensure that skin and/or dressing is clean and dry.
5. Separate any adjacent skin surfaces.
6. Align part to be bandaged, providing slight flexion if appropriate and not contraindicated.
7. Apply the bandage from the distal to the proximal part.
8. Apply bandage with even distribution of pressure.
9. Use proper bandage turns:
   a. Circular
      (1) Apply bandage so that each round overlaps the previous turn.
      (2) Secure in place, if appropriate.
   b. Spiral
      (1) Make two circular turns.
      (2) Continue so that each round of bandage slightly overlaps the previous round by about two thirds, progressing up the limb.
      (3) End with two circular turns, and secure with pins, tape, or clips.
   c. Spiral-reverse
      (1) Make two circular turns.
      (2) Bring bandage upward at 30-degree angle.
      (3) Place thumb of free hand on upper edge of bandage.
      (4) Fold bandage back on itself.
      (5) Continue to bandage limb, overlapping the previous turn by two-thirds the width of bandage.
      (6) Perform reversal of bandage at same spot on each turn.
      (7) End with two circular turns, and secure with safety pins, tape, or clips.
   d. Recurrent
      (1) Make two circular turns with bandage.
      (2) Fold bandage back on itself, and bring it centrally over distal end to be bandaged.
      (3) Holding it with other hand, bring bandage back over the distal end to the right of center bandage.
      (4) Pass bandage from front to back and right to left, overlapping until entire area is covered.
      (5) Make two circular turns over initial turns.
   e. Figure-eight
      (1) Make two circular turns.
      (2) Carry bandage above joint and around it, then below joint and around it.
      (3) Continue above and below joint, overlapping previous turn by about two-thirds width of bandage.
      (4) End bandage above joint, making two circular turns.
10. Assess tension of bandage and circulation of extremity.
11. Position patient for comfort.
12. Document procedure.

Wound complications. Impaired wound healing, regardless of the cause, requires accurate observation and ongoing interventions. Because wound complications can be life threatening, recognizing the seriousness of symptoms is vital throughout the patient's recovery phase (Table 26-6). Additional costs of medical treatment and hospitalization for patients with wound complications increase the total cost of health care. Complications frequently result with patients who are aged, malnourished, or obese or who have infections or coexisting health conditions.

Wound bleeding may indicate a slipped suture, dislodged clot, coagulation problem, or trauma placed on blood vessels or tissue.[17] Inspection of the wound and dressing aids in detecting increased drainage and color changes. If hemorrhage results internally, the dressing may remain dry while the abdominal cavity collects blood. The patient with increased thirst, restlessness, rapid, thready pulse, decreased blood pressure, decreased urinary output, and cool, clammy skin may be hemorrhaging. Thus monitoring vital signs, intake and output, skin condition, wound site, and overall patient responses hastens the identification of hemorrhage and hypovolemic shock. Internal abdominal bleeding, if allowed to continue, causes the abdomen to become rigid and distended. If hemorrhage is not detected and stopped, hypovolemic

Text continued on p. 504.

SKILL 26-5 APPLYING A BANDAGE—cont'd

DOCUMENTATION

Sample charting

DATE	TIME	NOTES
12/5/90	8:30	Elastic spiral bandage applied to right lower leg. Toes warm to touch, pink and nails blanch well. Pedal pulse strong and regular. Tolerated procedure well.

____

(nurse's signature)

SPECIAL CONCERNS

- Children will require smaller bandages.
- Elderly persons must be reassessed more often, because circulatory complications occur more frequently.

PATIENT TEACHING

When applying a bandage, the patient should be instructed on the following:

- Patient will need to be instructed on functions of bandaging.
- Patient should be taught to elevate extremity or body part if signs of impaired circulation occur (e.g., edema, decreased capillary refill).
- If bandage is applied over sterile dressing, patient must be taught procedure for changing dressing also.
- Patient and family will need to be taught the technique for applying the bandage.
- Teach family how to care for bandage.
- Patient and family will need to be taught to report changes in the affected part to the physician. Signs and symptoms of complications will need to be identified for the family.

SKILL 26-6

APPLYING A BINDER

1. Provide privacy for patient.
2. Assist patient to comfortable position.
3. Wash hands.
4. Change dressing if appropriate; cleanse skin if needed.
5. Separate skin surfaces, or pad bony prominences.
6. Apply binder:
   a. Triangular binder (sling) (see Skill 54-2)
      (1) Have patient flex arm at approximately 80-degree angle, depending on purpose of binder.
      (2) Place end of triangular binder over shoulder of injured side (anterior to posterior).
      (3) Grasp other end of binder, and bring it up and over injured arm to shoulder of injured arm.
      (4) Use square knot to tie two ends together at lateral area of neck on injured side.
      (5) Support wrist well with binder; do not allow it to extend over end of binder.
      (6) Fold third triangle end neatly around elbow, and secure with safety pins.
   b. T-binder
      (1) Provide privacy
      (2) Using appropriate binder, place the waistband smoothly under patient's waist; tails should be under patient.
      (3) Secure two ends of waistband together with safety pin.
      (4) Single tail—bring the tail up between legs to secure dressing in place.
      Two-tail—bring tails up one on each side of penis or large dressing.
      (5) Bring tails under and over waistband, and secure with safety pins.
   c. Elastic abdominal binder
      (1) Center binder smoothly under appropriate part of patient.
      (2) Bring ends around patient and overlap away from incision.
      (3) Secure binder with Velcro or safety pins placed horizontally on abdomen.
7. Note comfort level of patient. Smooth binder to prevent wrinkles.
8. Document procedure.

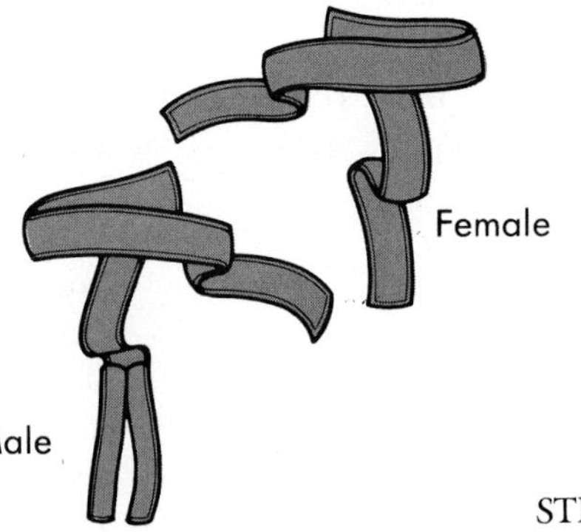

STEP 6b

SKILL 26-6

APPLYING A BINDER—cont'd

DOCUMENTATION

Sample charting

DATE	TIME	NOTES
12/5/90	8:45	Incisional dressing dry and intact. Abdominal binder applied as ordered. Patient states, "I feel much better about getting out of bed now."
		____________ *(nurse's signature)*

SPECIAL CONCERNS

- Patients with tubes or drains who have binders applied will need to be assessed frequently to ensure patency of tubes and drainage.

PATIENT TEACHING

When applying a binder, the patient should be instructed on the following:

- Teach function of the binder to patient and family.
- Teach patient to report if binder is loose or causing pain or discomfort.
- Patient should report any breathing restrictions if binder is too tight.
- Patient will need to be taught proper application if binder will need to be applied at home.
- Patient will need to know proper care of the binder.

SKILL 26-7

APPLYING A WET-TO-DRY DRESSING

1. Identify patient.
2. Wash hands.
3. Provide for patient privacy.
4. Explain procedure to patient.
5. Position patient.
6. Place waterproof pad appropriately.
7. Place refuse container appropriately.
8. Set up sterile field:
   a. Open barrier drape.
   b. Add sterile dressing and gauze.
   c. Add sterile basin.
   d. Pour sterile solution into basin.
   e. Add sterile instrument set if needed.
   f. Add antiseptic swabs.
9. Loosen tapes by pulling toward incision and gently pulling skin away from tape.
10. Don clean gloves, and remove dressing and discard into refuse bag. (Refuse bag may be used for additional soiled material.)
11. Assess status of the wound.
12. Don sterile gloves.
13. Cleanse wound from incision outward, one stroke per swab, and discard.
14. Place gauze into basin.
15. Wring excess solution from dressing.
16. Place sterile (4 inch by 4 inch) gauze over open wound surfaces and press into any depressed areas.
17. Apply dry, sterile dressing (4 inch by 4 inch) over wet gauze.
18. Cover with additional dressing as needed, usually 8 inch by 10 inch abdominal dressing.
19. Secure with tape or Montgomery straps.
20. Remove gloves, and discard.
21. Reposition patient.
22. Discard refuse appropriately.
23. Wash hands.
24. Document status of wound, description of exudate, dressing, and solution applied, and patient response.

DOCUMENTATION

Sample charting

DATE	TIME	NOTES
12/5/90	11:00	Wet-to-dry dressing on left lower quadrant of abdomen removed. 2 × 3 cm of serosanguineous exudate noted on dressing. Skin around wound is pink and intact. Wet-to-dry dressing applied using ¼ strength H_2O_2 solution and normal saline. Covered with 4 × 4s and ABD pads. Patient states, "The pill before this dressing change really helped."

____
(nurse's signature)

SPECIAL CONCERNS

- Appropriately assess all wounds to prevent infection.
- Infected wounds cause longer hospitalization for the patient, resulting in higher cost and longer recovery time.
- It is vitally important that the nurse continually carry out appropriate technique in all patient care.

PATIENT TEACHING

- Teach the patient about healing by secondary intention.

SKILL 26-8

CHANGING A STERILE DRESSING

1. Identify patient.
2. Wash hands.
3. Provide for patient privacy.
4. Explain procedure to patient.
5. Position patient.
6. Place refuse container in convenient location away from sterile field.
7. Set up sterile field.
   a. Open sterile dressings.
   b. Use barrier drape if needed.
   c. Open sterile gloves.
   d. Dressing set if needed.
   e. Antiseptic swabs.
8. Loosen tapes by pulling toward incision and gently pulling skin away from tape.
9. Don clean gloves, and remove dressing; note color and amount of exudate, and discard soiled dressing. (Refuse bag may be used for additional soiled material.)
10. Assess status of wound.
11. Don sterile gloves.
12. Cleanse wound and surrounding area with antiseptic swab, starting from incision outward, one stroke per swab.
13. Use sterile gauze to swab in same manner or let antiseptic air dry.
14. Cleanse drain site if applicable.
15. Apply special-order ointment, antibiotic, debridement granules, etc., if applicable.
16. Cover wound with appropriately sized dry sterile dressing and use drain dressing, if applicable.
17. Secure dressing with tape, Montgomery straps, or binder.
18. Remove gloves appropriately.
19. Discard refuse in appropriate manner.
20. Reposition patient.
21. Wash hands.
22. Document status of wound, description of drainage, if any, dressings applied, and patient response to procedure.

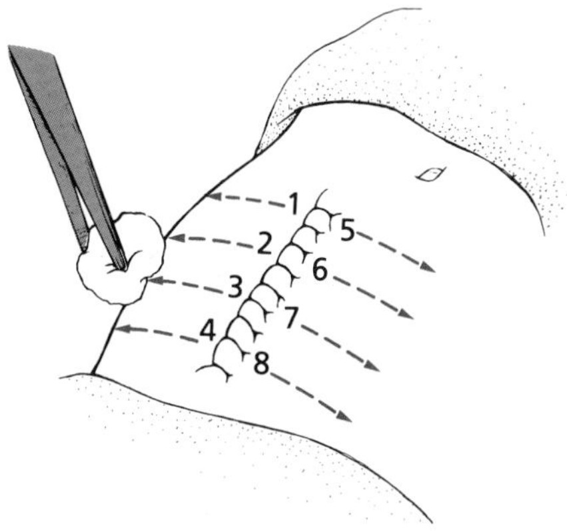

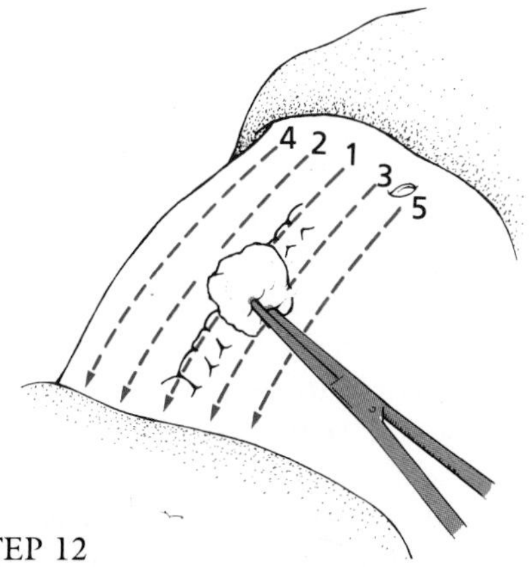

STEP 12

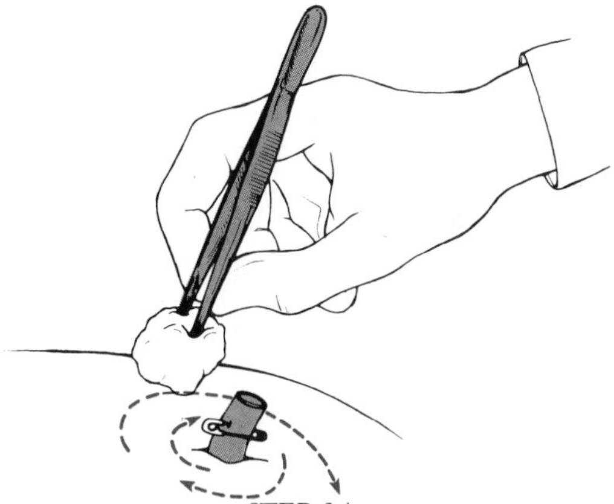

STEP 14

Continued.

SKILL 26-8

CHANGING A STERILE DRESSING—cont'd

STEP 17

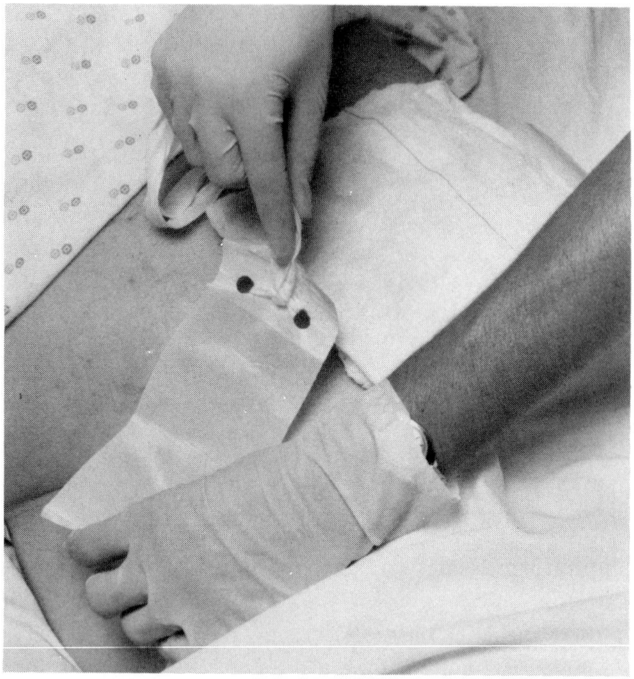

DOCUMENTATION
Sample charting

DATE	TIME	NOTES
12/5/90	10:00	Abdominal dressing removed, 3 × 4 cm of dry, sanguineous exudate noted on dressing. Sutures remain intact with wound edges well approximated. Cleansed with Betadine swab. Sterile dressing applied. Patient stated, "I have less pain in my incision today."

____

(nurse's signature)

SPECIAL CONCERNS

- Include specific interventions or techniques of dressing changes in nursing care plan to provide continuity.
- Skin surrounding wound should be protected from drainage to prevent tissue breakdown.
- Consider use of Montgomery straps when dressing requires frequent changing to prevent tape irritation of skin.
- Assess need for and provide patient teaching during dressing change.

PATIENT TEACHING

When changing a dressing, the patient should be instructed on the following:

- Assist patient to accept the surgical wound by stating the progress of the wound and how healing is occurring.
- Teach the patient the importance of early ambulation after surgery.
- Teach the patient the importance of a nutritious diet in wound healing.
- Explain to patient that dressings may be required at home and how to purchase what will be needed. Inform patient of home health services if dressings need to be changed when patient is discharged per physician's order.

SKILL 26-9

STERILE IRRIGATION OF A WOUND

1. Identify patient.
2. Wash hands.
3. Provide for patient privacy.
4. Explain procedure to patient.
5. Position patient and waterproof pad appropriately.
6. Place refuse container in convenient location away from sterile field.
7. Set up sterile field:
   a. Sterile basin.
   b. Add sterile, warmed irrigation solution to basin.
   c. Open sterile dressings.
   d. Add antiseptic swabs.
   e. Open sterile gloves.
   f. Dressing set (optional).
   g. Add sterile syringe and catheter if necessary.
8. Don gown and goggles if appropriate.
9. Don clean gloves, and remove dressing; assess dressing for color and amount of exudate, and discard dressing.

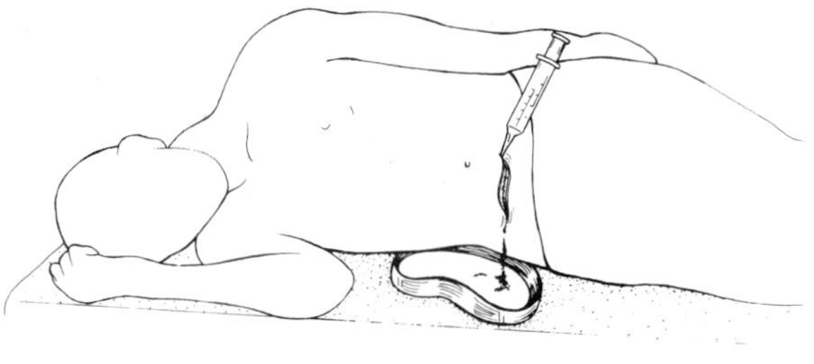

STEP 5

10. Assess status of the wound.
11. Place collection basin appropriately.
12. Don sterile gloves.
13. Cleanse area around wound with antiseptic swabs.
14. Fill irrigating syringe with solution; attach soft catheter if irrigating a deep wound with small opening.
15. Instill solution gently into wound, holding syringe approximately 1 inch above wound. (If using catheter, gently insert into wound opening until slight resistance is met, pull back, and gently instill solution.)
    a. Solution must flow from clean area of wound to contaminated area.
    b. Pinch off catheter during withdrawal from wound.
16. Refill syringe, and continue irrigation as above until solution returns clear or prescribed amount is used.
17. Blot wound edges with sterile gauze.
18. Redress wound, if applicable, following sterile dressing change procedure.
19. Remove gloves.
20. Discard soiled material and contaminated solution appropriately.
21. Reposition patient.
22. Wash hands.
23. Document status of wound, description of exudate, type and amount of irrigating solution, equipment used, results of irrigation, dressings used, and patient response.

DOCUMENTATION

Sample charting

DATE	TIME	NOTES
12/6/90	12:00	Right buttock dressing removed; purulent drainage 2 cm in diameter noted. Wound remains 4 cm × 1 cm, approximately 2 cm deep. No erythema noted at wound edge. Wound irrigation with Asepto syringe using 250 ml of half-strength hydrogen peroxide solution and normal saline. Return solution clear. Temp 99.8, P 86, R 22, B/P 180/98. Patient states, "There is less pain."

(nurse's signature)

SPECIAL CONCERNS

- Patient comfort should be provided, since an irrigation can cause pain. Patient may need to be medicated before performing procedure.
- Gentleness is important in performing any type of irrigation to avoid tissue damage and pain.

PATIENT TEACHING

When performing sterile irrigation of a wound, the patient should be instructed on the following:

- Explain why wound is being allowed to heal by secondary intention.

Table 26-6 Terms Associated with Wound Complications

Term	Definition
Abscess	Cavity containing pus and surrounded by inflamed tissue, formed as a result of suppuration in a localized infection
Adhesion	Band of scar tissue that binds together two anatomical surfaces normally separated; most commonly found in the abdomen
Cellulitis	Infection of the skin characterized by heat, pain, erythema, and edema
Dehiscence	Separation of a surgical incision, or rupture of a wound closure
Eviseration	Protrusion of an internal organ through a wound or surgical incision
Extravasation	Passage or escape into the tissues; usually of blood, serum, or lymph
Hematoma	Collection of extravasated blood trapped in the tissues or in an organ resulting from incomplete hemostasis after surgery

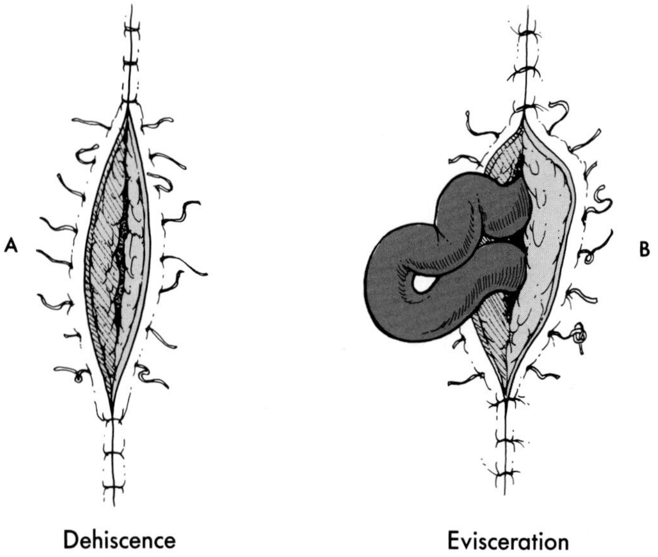

FIG. 26-7 **A,** Wound dehiscence. **B,** Evisceration.

shock can cause the circulatory system to collapse, causing death.

When wound layers separate, the patient may say that something has given way. This feeling may result after periods of sneezing, coughing, or vomiting. Evidence of serosanguineous drainage on the dressing is an important sign to assess. Dehiscence may be preceded by serosanguineous drainage. If the wound is not covered and dehiscence occurs, the patient should remain in bed and be kept NPO, told not to cough, and be reassured, and the nurse should place a sterile dressing over the area until the physician evaluates the site. When a skin suture breaks and dehiscence occurs, Steri-Strips or a butterfly strip may close the wound effectively. Dehiscence most frequently occurs between the fifth and twelfth postoperative day. Because many patients have been dismissed from the hospital by day twelve, patient teaching should include identification of dehiscence and the care to provide.

If an evisceration follows the dehiscence (Fig. 26-7), the wound and contents should be covered with warm, sterile saline dressings. The surgeon is notified immediately. This is a medical emergency, and the wound requires surgical repair.

Wound infection, or wound sepsis, results when the surgical wound becomes contaminated. The Centers for Disease Control[4] labels a wound infected when it contains purulent (pus) drainage. A surgical wound infection may develop by the fourth or fifth postoperative day, whereas a contaminated wound may show an infectious process in 2 or 3 days.[18] A patient with an infected wound displays a fever, tenderness and pain at the wound, edema, and an elevated WBC. Purulent drainage has an odor and is brown, yellow, or green, depending on the pathogen.

A *Staphylococcus aureus* infection is the most common type of wound infection. Its incubation period is from 4 to 6 days. *Staphylococcus aureus* tends to have yellow drainage and is localized. When infection is localized, an abscess forms. In addition to experiencing the classic symptoms of an infection, the patient reports a localized, throbbing pain. Treatment consists of antibiotic therapy, surgical opening (incision and drainage) of the wound, rest, heat, and elevation of the affected part. Drainage and secretion isolation usually is initiated if *S. aureus* is the causative organism.

Pathogens that live in the presence of oxygen (gram-negative bacilli) have become ubiquitous. The more common gram-negative bacilli are *Escherichia coli, Enterobacter, Proteus,* and *Pseudomonas aeruginosa.* Gram-negative bacilli have incubation periods of 7 to 14 days. Adequate drainage of the wound and antibiotic therapy are the primary treatments.

Streptococcal infections materialize with local tissue breakdown, gangrene, or necrotizing fasciitis. This infection produces a thin, watery pus. Symptoms associated with streptococci include elevated temperature and pulse, perspiration, exhaustion, and chills. Cellulitis is an example of a streptococcal infection. Treatment consists of an antibiotic (penicillin is the medication of choice), wet compresses, rest, and elevation of the infected area.

Gas gangrene and clostridial wound infections usually occur with extensive muscle damage. Amputation of a gangrenous limb may result because of necrosis accompanied by gas bubbles in the soft tissue; this condition (gas gangrene) is caused by the exotoxins of the pathogen. Cellulitis and tetanus may also result from these pathogens. In infections, exudate cultures confirm the presence of the pathogenic organism, so that the appropriate medical therapy can follow.

DRAINAGE SYSTEM

During surgery, tissue may be injured in a variety of ways. Not only is the diseased organ repaired or removed, but blood vessels are also cut and sutured. In addition, organs and vessels are retracted out of the surgeon's operative field during the surgical procedure. Because vessels are fragile, bruising and injury may occur. As cells are injured, inflammation begins.

Inflammation is the protective response of tissue to irritation or injury. Although this process may be chronic or acute, during surgery acute inflammation occurs. Inflammation begins as soon as the cell is traumatized by handling or cutting. As inflammation occurs, large amounts of histamine, bradykinin, and serotonin are released and vascular permeability takes place.

Gradually fluid from the cells cluster with leukocytes along the vessel walls, so that fibrin walls off the injury and begins to build a new cell. The amount of inflammation depends on the level of injury inflicted, size of the area involved, and physical condition of the patient. With repair, leukocytes attempt to rid the tissue of exudate from the injured cells. This process, phagocytosis, is an important function of leukocytes. **Phagocytosis** occurs when exudate from the injured cell is surrounded, engulfed, and digested by leukocytes. The leukocyte becomes the body's vacuum cleaner by removing its debris. Evidence of leukocyte action can be observed through WBC changes.

Cardinal signs of inflammation. Tissue involved in the inflammation process responds by becoming erythematous, hot, edematous, and painful. As the injured cell's fluid presses against surrounding tissue, there is frequently a loss of function in that area. Function generally returns when inflammation subsides. The inflammatory process normally occurs within the first 1 to 4 days after surgery. This process is the first phase in wound healing.

Drainage. Drainage is described as serous, sanguineous, or serosanguineous. **Serous** drainage is a clear, watery fluid that has been separated from its solid elements (e.g., the exudate from a blister). Serous fluid has the characteristics of serum. Serum is the clear, thin, sticky fluid portion of blood that remains after coagulation. In contrast, sanguineous drainage is fluid that contains blood. Thus serosanguineous drainage is exudate that is thin and red (usually described as pink), because it is composed of both serum and blood. If the tissue is infected, drainage may be purulent or a brown-green color. Drainage from organs has its own particular color, i.e., bile from the liver and gallbladder is green or green-brown.

The type and amount of drainage produced depends on the tissue and organs involved. Normally drainage begins as sanguineous and progresses to serosanguineous. Drainage greater than 300 ml in the first 24 hours should be treated as abnormal. By the second or third postoperative day, drainage becomes serous. When patients first ambulate, a slight drainage increase may occur. However, if drainage increases after it has decreased or the exudate becomes red or brown after it has been serosanguineous or serous, infection or wound complications should be suspected. If sanguineous drainage continues, small blood vessels may be oozing.

Not all surgical wounds drain. If drainage does occur, accurate assessments are vital. The following drainage characteristics are important to note and chart: color, amount, consistency (thick/thin), and odor. Drainage may be contained either in a drainage system or on a dressing. If a dressing is used, the amount of drainage can be monitored either by weighing the soiled dressing or by circling and dating the drainage area. Until the surgeon orders a dressing change, the soiled dressings should be reinforced.

Drainage system. Frequently surgical procedures are performed to remove or repair organs that lie within the body (e.g., removing the gallbladder). In these cases a mechanism is needed to assist gravity in removing exudate from the cavity. If a gastrectomy were performed using an upper abdominal midline incision, fluid would collect and remain at the surgical site. To facilitate drainage, an incision, or stab wound, is made close to the incision. The site for the stab wound is planned deliberately. It is the intent of the surgeon to drain exudate away from the incision, not toward it. If the exudate were to enter the surgical incision, contamination and infection could follow.

Gentle suction is needed in some surgeries to help gravity move the exudate. As drainage is removed, the chance of infection decreases and healing occurs more rapidly. A drainage system is chosen to fit the area to be drained, type of exudate, and amount of drainage expected (Fig. 26-8). A rubber or plastic drain may be used to remove exudate from the wound and deposit it on the skin (open drain system) or may be situated through the surgical incision or stab wound. The Penrose drain is commonly used for this purpose. When it is inserted, a safety pin is placed through the drain to keep it from sliding into the wound. When the surgeon wants a gentle vacuum, a closed drainage system can be used. The portable vacuum container (e.g., Hemovac, Redi-Vacettem Snyder, Solcotrans [Fig. 26-9], Surgivac) is an expandable unit that is connected by tubes to the drainage site (Skill 26-10). As gentle suction is provided, exudate is collected in the drainage unit. The Jackson-Pratt and Davol evacuators are other types of closed drainage sys-

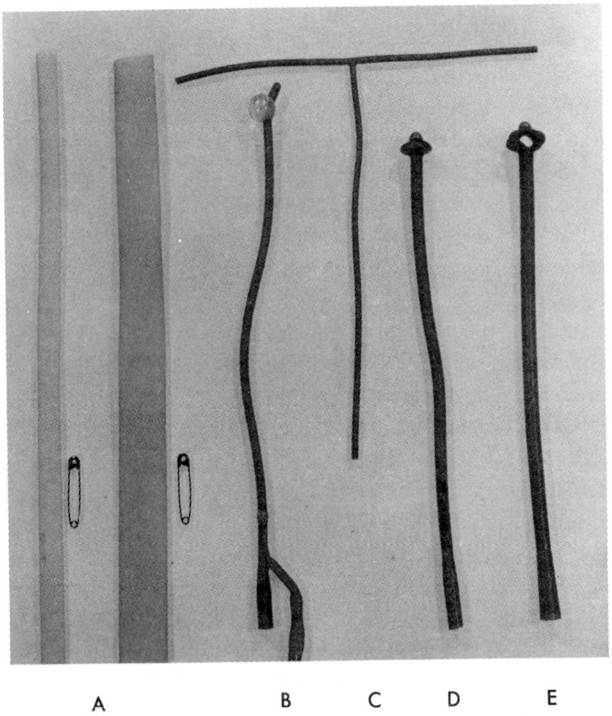

FIG. 26-8 Commonly used surgical drains. **A,** Penrose drains. **B,** Foley catheter. **C,** T-tube. **D,** Mushroom, or Pezzer. **E,** Bat-wing, or Malecot.

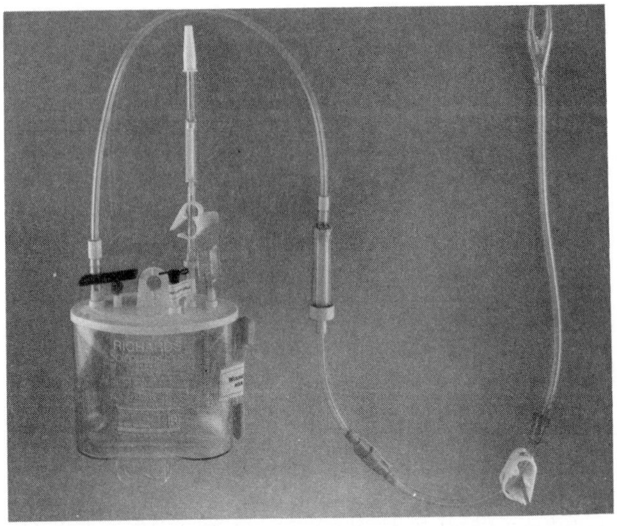

FIG. 26-9 The Solcotrans unit serves a twofold purpose: it permits drainage from the surgical site and allows for reinfusion of the patient's own blood—a plus in this day of widespread communicable diseases such as AIDS. (Courtesy Smith & Nephew Richards, Inc, Memphis, Tenn.)

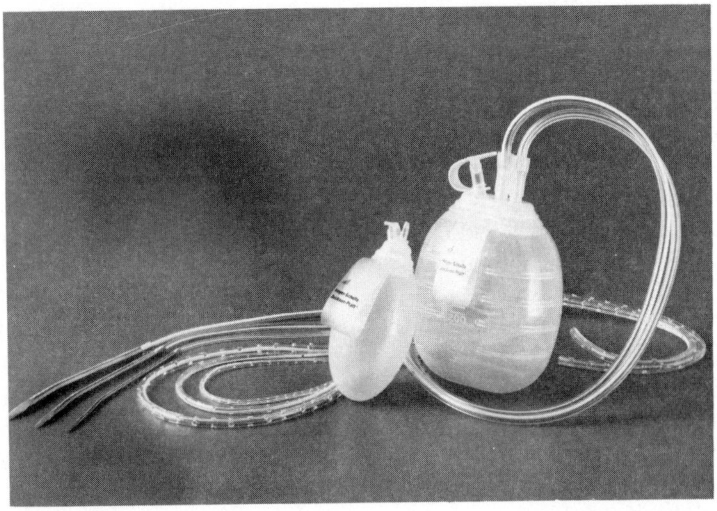

FIG. 26-10 Closed wound drainage system: Jackson-Pratt 100 ml and 400 ml reservoirs with round silicone drains and attached trocars. (Courtesy American V Mueller, American Hospital Supply Corp, Chicago.)

tems that use a bulb to provide the needed vacuum (Fig. 26-10).

Special drainage systems frequently are used for more difficult sites. Thoracic surgery requires negative pressure to remove drainage from the pleural space. Water-sealed systems (Emerson, Pleur-evac) are used after chest surgery to reexpand the lung and remove exudate and air. There are various water-sealed arrangements: single-bottle, two-bottle, or three-bottle systems. Regardless of the system used, the tube from the pleural space extends

SKILL 26-10 MAINTAINING HEMOVAC SUCTION AND DAVOL

1. Wash hands.
2. Check patient's care plan/physician order.
3. Identify patient, explain procedure, and give patient time to ask questions.
4. Bring supplies to bedside.
5. Provide for comfort and privacy.
6. Elevate bed to convenient height.
7. Drape patient, exposing only the area necessary—exposing catheter insertion site. Place the Hemovac/Davol on the absorbent pad.
8. Examine drainage system (pump and tubing) for seal, patency, and stability. If not working, notify head nurse/physician.
9. Don disposable gloves.
10. Remove Hemovac/Davol plug labeled "pouring spout."
11. Empty drainage into measuring device.
12. When emptying Hemovac, compress device by pushing top and bottom together with your hands.
13. Hold pump of Hemovac tightly compressed, and reinsert plug to reestablish closed drainage system. When caring for a Davol, reestablish suction by pumping bulb until balloon is completely inflated—recap drainage port. For both Hemovac and Davol keep plug out of drainage stream—hold the plug by stem—maintain sterility.
14. Observe the drainage for color, consistency, and odor.
15. Measure and record amount of drainage—rinse measuring container.
16. Position drainage system on bed, and secure system.
17. Dispose of drainage, and rinse container.
18. Remove gloves, and wash hands.
19. If specimen is ordered, send to laboratory.
20. Observe Davol/Hemovac every 2 to 4 hours to ascertain integrity of suction. Measure drainage every 8 hours or as ordered.

DOCUMENTATION

Sample charting

DATE	TIME	NOTES
9/8/90	7:00	Davol emptied from right lower quadrant stab wound site. 75 ml serosanguineous exudate. Balloon reinflated. Suction reestablished. Patient states, "I am not in any discomfort at present time."

(nurse's signature)

SPECIAL CONCERNS

- Davol/Hemovac should be observed every 2 to 4 hours to note color and amount of exudate; output should be measured and recorded every 8 hours as ordered.
- An accurate output of exudate must be recorded so the physician can determine any decrease or increase in wound exudate.
- Observe suction system to be certain Hemovac is compressed and Davol balloon is inflated to maintain proper suctioning.

PATIENT TEACHING

- Explain purpose of wound drainage system.
- Inform patient of importance of nurse measuring output.
- Instruct patient to keep Hemovac/Davol tubing clipped/pinned to gown to prevent accidental dislodgment.

SKILL 26-11 T-TUBE DRAINAGE COLLECTION

1. Wash hands.
2. Check patient's care plan/physician's order.
3. Identify patient, and explain procedure—give patient time to ask questions.
4. Bring supplies to bedside.
5. Provide for comfort and privacy.
6. Elevate bed to convenient height.
7. Drape patient, exposing only area necessary—place drainage bag on absorbent pad.
8. Examine drainage system for patency and for leakage.
9. Don disposable gloves.
10. Remove plug, holding drainage spout over calibrated container.
11. Empty drainage into the measuring container—recap the drainage bag—maintain sterility.
12. Measure and record amount of drainage.
13. Rinse and replace measuring container.
14. Remove gloves, and wash hands.
15. If dressing change is required, do so at this time.
16. Position patient for comfort.

DOCUMENTATION

Sample charting

DATE	TIME	NOTES
12/21/90	0935	Abdominal dressings changed. Moderate amount of serosanguineous exudate. T-tube in place and draining dark green liquid. 60 ml emptied from drainage bag. Incision approximated. No erythema noted. Staples in place. Assisted to bathroom. Voided 200 ml clear amber urine. Expelled moderate amount of yellow, semiformed stool. Reported to H. Christensen, RN.

____
(nurse's signature)

SPECIAL CONCERNS

- Normal bile drainage for 24 hours is 500 ml to 1000 ml of viscous, green-brown liquid.
- Always keep the drainage bag below the level of the common bile duct to prevent contamination from backflow.
- Excessive bile leakage from wounds can indicate an occluded system; notify the physician.

under the water in one of the bottles. This allows drainage and air from the lung to be expelled under water without air moving back into the lung. In time the lung reexpands. The Pleur-Evac is a commercial drainage system that has three bottles (chambers) self-contained in one compartment. The system functions like a three-bottle system in that the unit collects drainage, maintains a seal to prevent air from entering the pleural cavity, and prevents excessive buildup of negative pressure. (See Chapter 34.)

Various surgical drains are commonly used to facilitate drainage (Fig. 26-8). A T-tube drain is used when the common bile duct has been explored for cholelithiasis. Because edema occurs after the common bile duct is manipulated, a tube is placed in the duct to allow bile to drain (Skill 26-11). Gastric drainage can be obtained through a Levin, Salem sump, Sengstaken-Blakemore, or similar decompression tube. Similarly, the Malecot and Pezzer drains can be attached to continuous or intermittent suction to facilitate internal drainage. Intestinal decompression is accomplished by using the Cantor, Miller-Abbott, or Baker tube. While gastrointestinal decompression is occurring, the patient remains NPO. Nursing interventions consist of nasal care, oral and lip care, bowel assessments, and monitoring of intake and output. To ease the discomfort associated with the tube, mouth washes, ice chips, or hard candy, if allowed, is offered. When peristalsis and normal gastrointestinal functions return, gastric and intestinal tubes are discontinued. (See Chapter 31.)

A drainage system requires close monitoring. In addition to noting the color, consistency, and amount of drainage, the tube's patency is important. A tube should not be kinked or occluded; if blood clots or exudate has slowed drainage, this should be recorded and reported. The nurse should follow hospital protocol if nasogastric tube (NG) irrigation is indicated. If a patient has nausea, the nurse first assesses the NG tube's patency. When continuous or intermittent suctioning is attached to the drainage system, the unit should be observed for proper functioning: connections tight, machine on, visible drainage. The nurse should not disconnect, change the suction speed, or turn off a machine unless an order is received. Occasionally a drainage tube will be clamped; the nurse should report discomfort, distention, or pain experienced. It is important to properly anchor the NG tube to the patient's nose to prevent dislodgment or unnecessary discomfort. Tube guards are available that anchor the tube securely to the nose to prevent unnecessary movement of the tube. When possible, this device should be used for patient comfort rather than adhesive tape.

Containing drainage is paramount; drainage that enters a surgical incision is likely to cause an infection of the operative area. To minimize this possibility, soiled dressings should be changed. If bed clothing or linen becomes soiled, gloves should be worn during the handling of contaminated materials. Using sterile asepsis during dressing changes is vital to help decrease the chance of an infection. In caring for all postsurgical patients, good handwashing technique is the nurse's first line of defense; gloves, gown, and eye protectors are necessary if secretions cannot be contained. Universal precautions assist in protecting both the patient and nurse. If an infection is suspected, a wound culture is ordered to identify the bacterial agent.

Nosocomial infections are a continual threat to the postsurgical patient. The virulence of the bacterial contamination and the resistance of the patient are the two major factors in determining whether a wound becomes infected. Because wound infections usually have an incubation period of 4 to 6 days, some patients may have been discharged when problems are noted. Patient teaching should include observations to be made so that medical treatment can be obtained if needed. Although drainage is a sign of healing, accurate assessments can signal potential wound complications.

DISCHARGE PLANNING

Patients are discharged either the day of surgery or as soon postoperatively as their condition permits.

The nurse should review with the patient how to do incisional care, evaluate drainage, and change the wound dressing. The importance of identifying signs and symptoms of a wound infection should be reinforced so prompt medical treatment is obtained. The nurse can discuss (1) how to use comfort measures and analgesics for postoperative discomfort and (2) common side effects. If gastrointestinal functions have not become regular, the medical plan provided by the physician can be reviewed. Once discharge information has been discussed, the nurse evaluates the patient's comprehension by asking questions, requesting a return demonstration, or posing problems (for example, "If you feel a 'give' in the incisional area, what would you do?"). The patient's responses are charted on the discharge summary form.

REFERENCES AND SUGGESTED READINGS

1. Bennett JV and Brachman PS: Hospital infections, ed 2, Boston, 1986, Little, Brown & Co.
2. Braintree: GoLYTELY fact sheet: Braintree, Mass, 1985, Braintree Laboratories, Inc.
3. Bysshe JE: The effect of giving information to patients before surgery, Nurs 88 3(30):36, 1988.
4. Centers for Disease Control: Guidelines for prevention of surgical wound infection, Washington, DC, 1985, US Department of Health and Human Services.
5. Donahue MP: Nursing: the finest art, St Louis, 1985, The CV Mosby Co.
6. Geach B: Pain and coping, Image J Nurs Sch 19(1):12, 1987.
7. Gioiella EC and Bevil CW: Nursing care of the aging client, Norwalk, Conn, 1985, Appleton-Century-Crofts.
8. Great Plains Regional Medical Center: Admission of the patient to the recovery room policy, N. Platte, Neb, 1987.
9. Green ML and Harry J: Nutrition in contemporary nursing practice, ed 2, New York, 1987, John Wiley & Son.
10. Gruendemann BJ and Meeker H: Alexander's care of the patient in surgery, ed 8, St Louis, 1987, The CV Mosby Co.
11. LaRocca JC and Otto SE: Pocket guide to intravenous therapy, St Louis, 1989, The CV Mosby Co.
12. Lewis SM and Collier IC: Medical-surgical nursing, ed 2, New York, 1987, McGraw-Hill Book Co.
13. Neuberger GB: Wound care—what's clean, what's not, Nurs 87 17(2):34, 1987.
14. Olsson G and Parker G: A model approach to pain assessment, Nurs 87 17(5):52, 1987.
15. Peck NL: Action stat! Blood transfusion reaction, Nurs 87 17(1):33, 1987.
16. Perry AG and Potter PA: Clinical nursing skills and techniques, ed 2, St Louis, 1990, The CV Mosby Co.
17. Potter PA and Perry AG: Basic nursing: theory and practice, ed 2, St Louis, 1991, Mosby–Year Book, Inc.
18. Potter PA and Perry AG: Fundamentals of nursing: concepts, process, and practice, ed 2, St Louis, 1989, The CV Mosby Co.
19. Quaschnick MS: Discharge planning in a small hospital, Cont Care Coord 4(4):25, 1985.
20. Raffensperger EB, Zusy ML, and Marchesseault LC: Clinical nursing handbook, Philadelphia, 1986, JB Lippincott Co.
21. Selco Basie, Inc: Solcotrans-orthopaedic drainage/reinfusion system, Rockland, Mass, 1988.
22. Thompson JM et al: Clinical nursing, ed 2, St Louis, 1989, The CV Mosby Co.
23. Tinning R: Safe intravenous practice, Nurs Times 82(30):40, 1986.
24. Universal precautions, Salt Lake City, 1987, Brevis Corp.
25. Wilson FA and Neuhauser D: Health services in the United States, ed 2, Cambridge, Mass, 1985, Ballinger Publishing Co.

CHAPTER CHALLENGE

KEY POINTS

- Surgery is a highly stressful experience.
- Preoperative teaching is an individualized process and helps to reduce concerns and fears.
- Patients fear that postoperative pain will not be controlled.
- Preoperative assessments serve as postoperative guidelines.
- A consent form cannot be signed after the patient receives preoperative medication or has had a narcotic during the previous 4 hours.
- Maintaining a patent airway is the most vital postoperative assessment.
- Postoperative complications have objective assessments.
- Pain management is individually managed with analgesics and comfort measures.
- Hemorrhage and shock are life-threatening conditions.
- Healing is affected by a patient's life-style, physical and mental condition, and preexisting health problems.
- Good handwashing technique and sterile asepsis reduce wound infections.
- Wound dehiscence usually occurs after the third postoperative day.
- Wound drainage enhances postoperative healing but is a medium for infection.
- Discharge planning identifies home care measures to promote recovery.

STUDY QUESTIONS

1. Preoperatively, what is the patient's greatest fear:
   a. Disfigurement
   b. Dying
   c. Hemorrhage
   d. Pain
2. A woman of what age would be *most at risk* for major surgery:
   a. 35 years old
   b. 45 years old
   c. 55 years old
   d. 65 years old
3. What is the primary reason for assessing vital signs before surgery:
   a. To examine the patient's level of health
   b. To identify the patient's stress level
   c. To obtain the patient's baseline levels
   d. To provide the patient time to ask questions
4. Which of the following preoperative interventions is correctly related to its postoperative concern:
   a. NPO: prevent aspiration
   b. Turn, cough, and deep breathe: overexpand lungs
   c. Bowel prep: lessen constipation
   d. Skin shave: decrease irritation
5. Why is preoperative medication given:
   a. To put the patient to sleep before leaving the unit
   b. To slow mental and emotional responses before surgery
   c. To decrease respiratory tract secretions
   d. To tone the circulatory tract for surgery
6. Jasper Browne, age 75, has returned to his room after abdominal surgery; which of the following is the *first* assessment to make:
   a. Abdominal dressing
   b. Airway for patency
   c. Intravenous site
   d. Urinary output
7. Two hours after Mr. Browne returns to his room from surgery, he is restless, his systolic blood pressure has decreased 20 points, his pulse is thready, and his skin is cool and clammy. Which of the following problems is most likely:
   a. Acute postsurgical pain
   b. Body adjustment to surgery
   c. Hypovolemic shock
   d. Pulmonary embolism
8. Mr. Browne has an elevated temperature on his first postoperative day. He probably has which of the following:
   a. Congested lungs
   b. A wound infection
   c. Urinary infection
   d. Venous stasis
9. One day postoperatively, Mr. Browne states that his analgesic is not relieving his "severe, radiating" pain. He probably:
   a. Has become addicted to the medication
   b. Does not want to ambulate as requested
   c. Has an abnormally low pain threshhold
   d. Is not receiving enough medication
10. Which signs or symptoms represent a blood transfusion reaction:
    a. Rapid pulse and hot, dry skin
    b. Nausea, chills, and chest pain
    c. Vomiting, cyanosis, and clammy skin
    d. Back pain and increased urine output
11. An infected wound shows what signs:
    a. Edema and purulent exudate
    b. Open edges and yellow-red exudate
    c. Separated edges and serosanguineous exudate
    d. Clear, brown-red exudate
12. Which of the following hinders healing:
    a. Obesity and hydration
    b. Malnourishment and good skin turgor
    c. Chronic disease and extended bed rest
    d. Dirty wound and antibiotics

Match the terms in the first column with the descriptions in the second column. Each description may be used once or not at all.

C 13. -ectomy
___ 14. lysis
___ 15. -orrhaphy
___ 16. -otomy
___ 17. -pexy

a. Opening into
b. Joining of two ducts
c. Surgical removal of
d. Destruction of
e. Surgical repair of
f. Fixation of
g. Opening for drainage

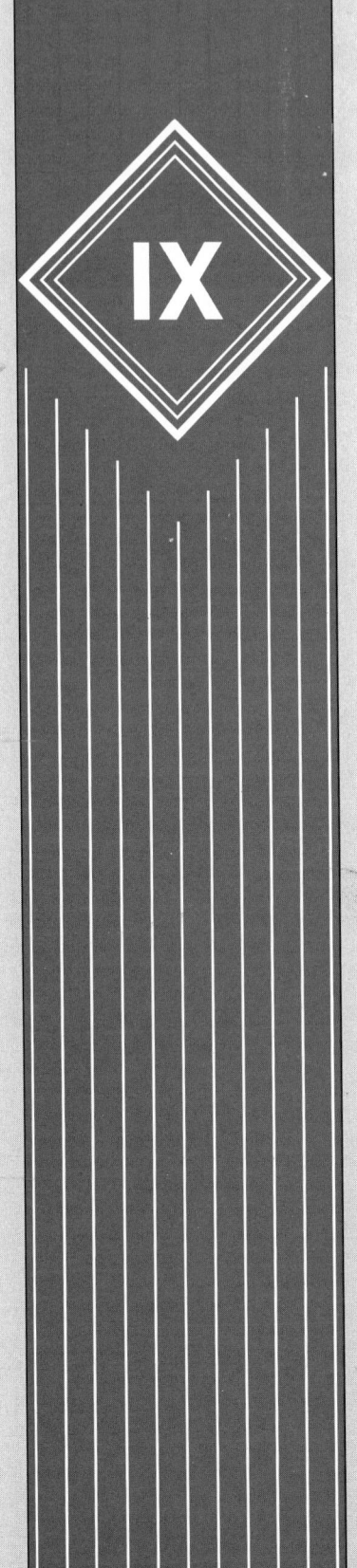

IX

Therapeutic Management of Adult Health Disorders

Nursing has been a dream of mine for a long time—one I thought I would never accomplish. I find joy in helping and caring for those who are ill become well again. It is a feeling that comes from way down deep inside—a feeling that is so very hard to explain. Working in the hospital, giving that extra special touch, or going the extra mile—it is all worth it to see the faces light up or to know that whatever I did helped that person feel better. That means the world to me. A nurse is there to lend a hand before it is asked, and help in any way just when it is needed most. Just giving a little touch may sometimes make a world of difference. I believe a nurse can be many things: kind, reliable, gentle, companion to the lonely or elderly, compassionate, self-confident, enthusiastic, and above all, dedicated and true with a warm smile. Nursing to me is a very rewarding career. I find such joy and contentment in helping others, feeling satisfied when what I have done has helped. A nurse should start out the day with a heart full of hope and sprinkle that hope as she goes on her way.

PEG MIESBAUER
Student Nurse

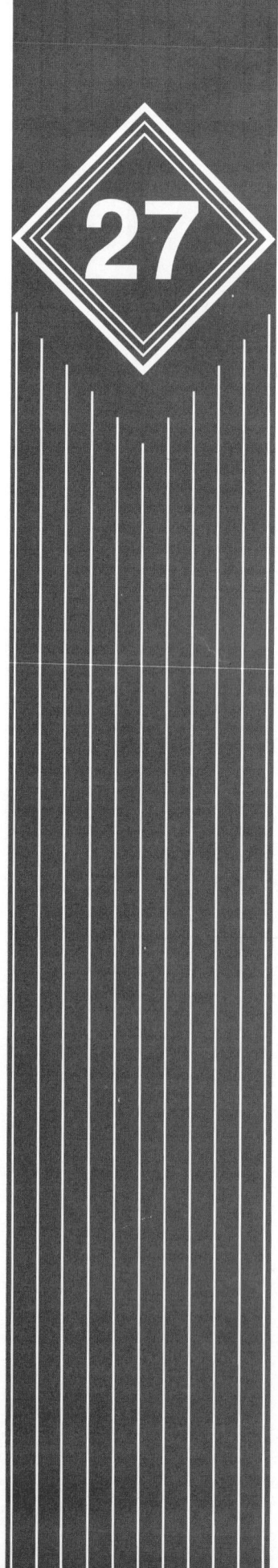

27

Cells, Tissues, and Membranes

CHRISTINE NEFF

LEARNING OBJECTIVES

After reading this chapter, the student should be able to do the following:

- Define the key terms.
- Use each word of a given list of anatomical terminology in a sentence.
- Define the difference between anatomy and physiology.
- Demonstrate an understanding of the body planes by labeling a diagram appropriately.
- Identify and define the most common parts of the cell.
- Discuss the stages of mitosis and explain the importance of cellular reproduction.
- Describe the four types of body tissues.
- List the body systems, and give an example of their functions.
- Explain what will happen if cells are placed in solutions with the same or different concentrations than the cells.
- Differentiate between active and passive transport processes.

RELATED TOPICS OF INTEREST

- Fluids and electrolytes (Chapter 28)
- Anatomy and physiology of all body systems (Chapters 29 to 38)

KEY TERMS

Define the following:

- active transport
- anatomy
- cell
- centriole
- chromatin
- connective tissue
- diffusion
- epithelial tissue
- Golgi apparatus
- homeostasis
- lysosome
- membrane
- mitochondria
- passive transport
- phagocytosis
- physiology
- pinocytosis
- ribosomes
- tissues

To care for an individual with a disease process, the nurse must understand the normal functioning of the human body. To accomplish this task, the nurse must study basic human anatomy and physiology.

Anatomy explains the shape and structure of the body. **Physiology** explains the functions of the various structures and how they interrelate with one another. The normal, healthy human body can be compared with a finely tuned machine with each part performing a special function to accomplish a given goal; and as with the machine, when the human body malfunctions, the repairer must understand how it functions internally.

ANATOMICAL TERMINOLOGY

To study the human body, certain terms must be mastered to specifically locate a structure. To understand the following terms, the student should consider the body in a normal anatomical position, that is, standing erect with the face and palms of the hands facing forward (Fig. 27-1).

Anterior (or ventral): to face forward; the front of the body. The nose is located on the anterior of the head.

Posterior (or dorsal): toward the back. The heel is located on the posterior portion of the foot.

Cranial: toward the head. The brain is located in the cranial portion of the body.

Caudal: toward the "tail"; the distal portion of the spine. A caudal anesthetic may be given to a patient.

Superior: toward the head or above. The neck is superior to the shoulders.

Inferior: lower; below another. The foot is inferior to the ankle.

Medial: toward the midline. The sternum (breastbone) is located in the medial portion of the chest.

Lateral: toward the side. The ribs are lateral to the heart.

Proximal: nearest the origin of the structure; nearest the trunk. The elbow is proximal to the forearm.

Distal: farthest from the origin of the structure; farthest from the trunk. The fingers are distal to the hand.

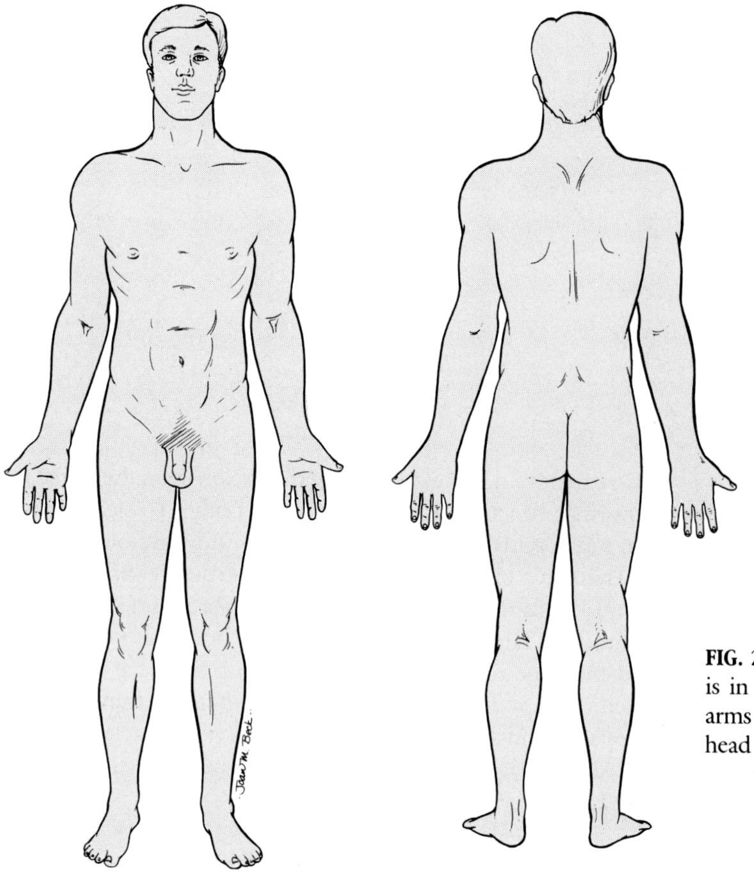

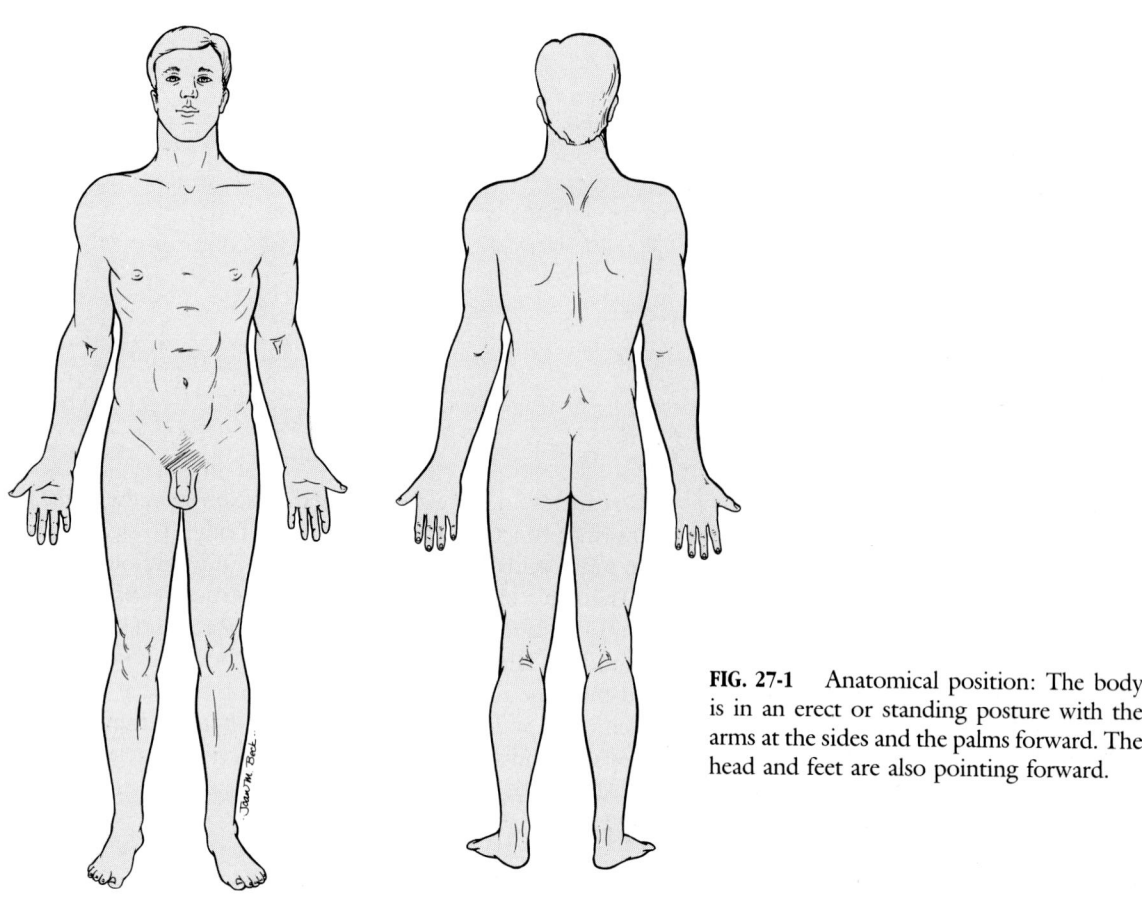

FIG. 27-1 Anatomical position: The body is in an erect or standing posture with the arms at the sides and the palms forward. The head and feet are also pointing forward.

BODY PLANES

To facilitate the study of the human body, it is helpful to divide it into three imaginary planes: the sagittal, the coronal, and the transverse.

1. The sagittal plane runs lengthwise from the front to the back. A sagittal cut gives a right and left portion of the body. A midsagittal cut gives two equal halves.
2. The coronal (frontal) plane divides the body into a ventral (front) and dorsal (back) section.
3. The transverse plane cuts the body horizontally and yields a superior (upper) and inferior (lower) portion.

BODY CAVITIES

The body may be divided into two major portions: axial and appendicular. The axial portion contains the head, neck, and trunk. The appendicular portion contains the upper and lower extremities.

The internal body is composed of open areas, or cavities, which allow for systematic organization of the internal organs. The body cavities are divided into two large groups: the dorsal and ventral cavities. The dorsal cavity is smaller than the ventral cavity.

The dorsal cavity is composed of the cranial and spinal cavities. The cranial cavity houses the brain, whereas the spinal cavity contains the spinal cord.

The diaphragm (a muscle directly beneath the lungs) separates the ventral cavity into the thoracic (chest) and abdominal cavities (see Fig. 31-1). The thoracic cavity contains the heart and lungs. The lungs are situated in the pleural cavity (a subdivision of the thoracic cavity).

The abdominal cavity contains the stomach, kidneys, liver, gallbladder, spleen, pancreas, and a large portion of the intestines. A subdivision called the pelvic cavity contains the lower portion of the intestines, the urinary bladder, and the internal structures of the reproductive system.

The abdominal and pelvic cavities are not separated by any structures and therefore may be referred to as the abdominopelvic cavity.

ABDOMINAL REGIONS

To simplify the study and location of the abdominal organs, the abdomen has been divided into nine regions.

1. *Superior regions:* are above the level of the ninth rib and include the right hypochondriac region, epigastric region, and the left hypochondriac region.

2. *Midregion:* extend inferiorly from the ninth rib to the level of the hip bones and include the right lumbar region, the umbilical region, and the left lumbar region.
3. *Inferior regions:* are below the level of the hip bones and include the right iliac (inguinal) region, the hypogastric region, and the left iliac (inguinal) region.

STRUCTURAL UNITS

Cells

Nearly 300 years ago Robert Hooke discovered the first cell while examining plant fragments under the microscope. The structures reminded him of tiny, individual rooms or cells, hence, the name **cell** (Fig. 27-2).

All **cells** are microscopic but differ widely in size and shape. Regardless of size or shape, they exhibit five unique characteristics of life—growth, metabolism, responsiveness, reproduction, and **homeostasis.** The human body contains trillions of these tiny powerhouses of life.

Each cell is surrounded by a thin membrane called the plasma, or cytoplasmic, membrane. The exterior walls of the cells are bathed in a special fluid (tissue fluid), which is composed of a weak salt solution.

The cell membrane is selectively permeable. This means the membrane permits certain substances to enter and leave at will, while not allowing other substances to cross.

Cell structures

Cytoplasm. Cytoplasm (protoplasm) is a sticky fluidlike substance that lies between the cytoplasmic membrane

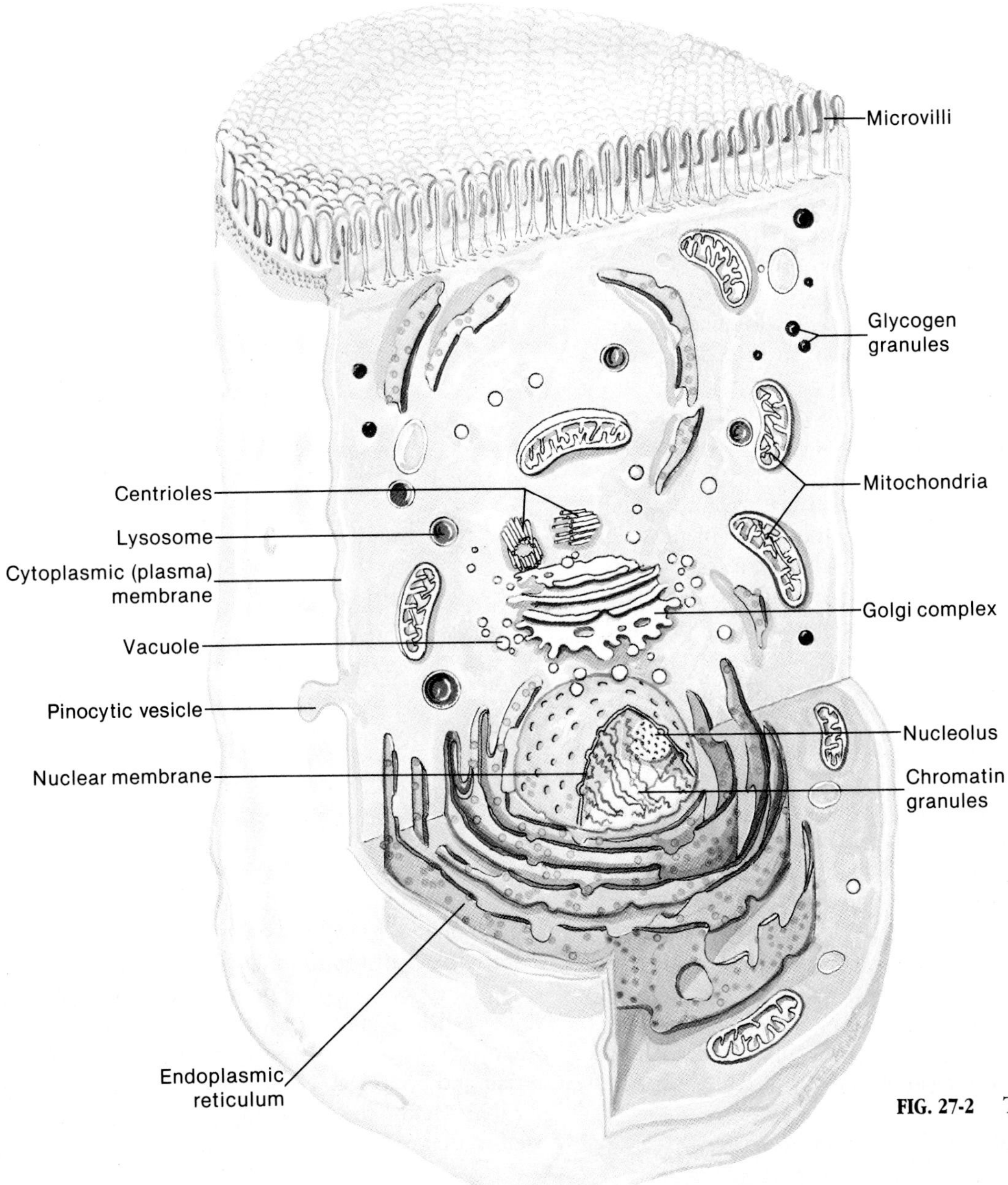

FIG. 27-2 Typical cell structure.

and the nucleus of the cell. Situated within the cytoplasm are numerous organelles (tiny functioning structures). These organelles were not discovered until the development of the powerful electron microscope.

Cytoplasm is composed of 70% water with traces of proteins, lipids, carbohydrates, minerals, and salts.

Nucleus. The nucleus is the largest organelle within the cell. It is responsible for cell reproduction and control of the other organelles. The nucleus is surrounded by a membrane called the nuclear membrane. It contains nucleoplasm, a refined form of cytoplasm. The nucleus contains two specialized structures, the nucleolus and **chromatin** granules. The nucleolus is critical in the formation of protein. The chromatin granules are composed of protein and DNA (deoxyribonucleic acid). DNA contains the genetic code, or blueprint, of the body.

Endoplasmic reticulum. Throughout the cytoplasm lies a system of membranes, or canals, called the endoplasmic reticulum (ER). ER functions as a minicirculating system for the cell by carrying substances from one part of the cell to another. There are two types of ER: (1) smooth, found in cells that deal with fatty substances, and (2) rough, found in cells that manufacture proteins.

Ribosomes. **Ribosomes** are tiny structures floating free in the cytoplasm or attached to the rough ER. They are called protein factories because they are responsible for the production of enzymes and other proteins.

Mitochondria. The **mitochondria** are the powerhouses of the cells. They are bean-shaped with a foldlike interior membrane. They take food and convert it to the energy form adenosine triphosphate (ATP) for use by the cell.

Lysosomes. **Lysosomes** are small saclike structures containing enzymes that digest food compounds and microbes that have invaded the cell.

Golgi apparatus. The **Golgi apparatus** is usually located near the nucleus. It is the "packaging plant" of the cell. It packages certain carbohydrate and protein compounds into globules. Then, it moves outward toward and through the cell membrane where it breaks open and releases its contents.

Centrioles. The **centrioles** are paired, rod-shaped organelles. During cell division (mitosis), they aid in the formation of the spindle, a structure necessary for cell reproduction.

Protein synthesis. Protein is a vital component of every cell in the body. To produce protein, nucleic acids exist in the cytoplasm and the nucleus of the cell.

Two important nucleic acids are: (1) deoxyribonucleic acid (DNA) (Fig. 27-3), which is located in the nucleus, and (2) ribonucleic acid (RNA), which is located in the cytoplasm. The DNA encodes the message for protein synthesis and sends it to the RNA, which transports it to the ribosomes where the protein is produced. Hence, DNA is called the chemical blueprint and RNA is called the chemical messenger.

Cell division. All cells in the body (except sex cells) reproduce by mitosis (cell division) (Fig. 27-4). The original cell divides to form two daughter cells that retain the characteristics of the original cell.

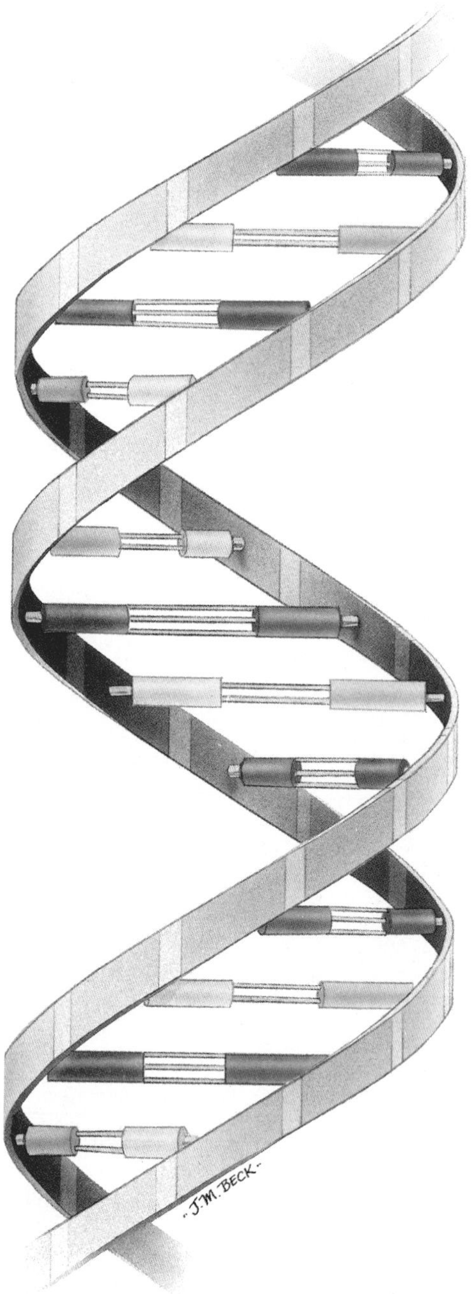

FIG. 27-3 DNA structure.

The chromosomes (spindle-shaped rods) in the nucleus of the cell carry the genes that are responsible for the organism's traits. The traits carry such hereditary factors as hair and eye color. These chromosomes are composed of DNA. Before the cell divides, the DNA must replicate itself so that each new daughter cell contains the original

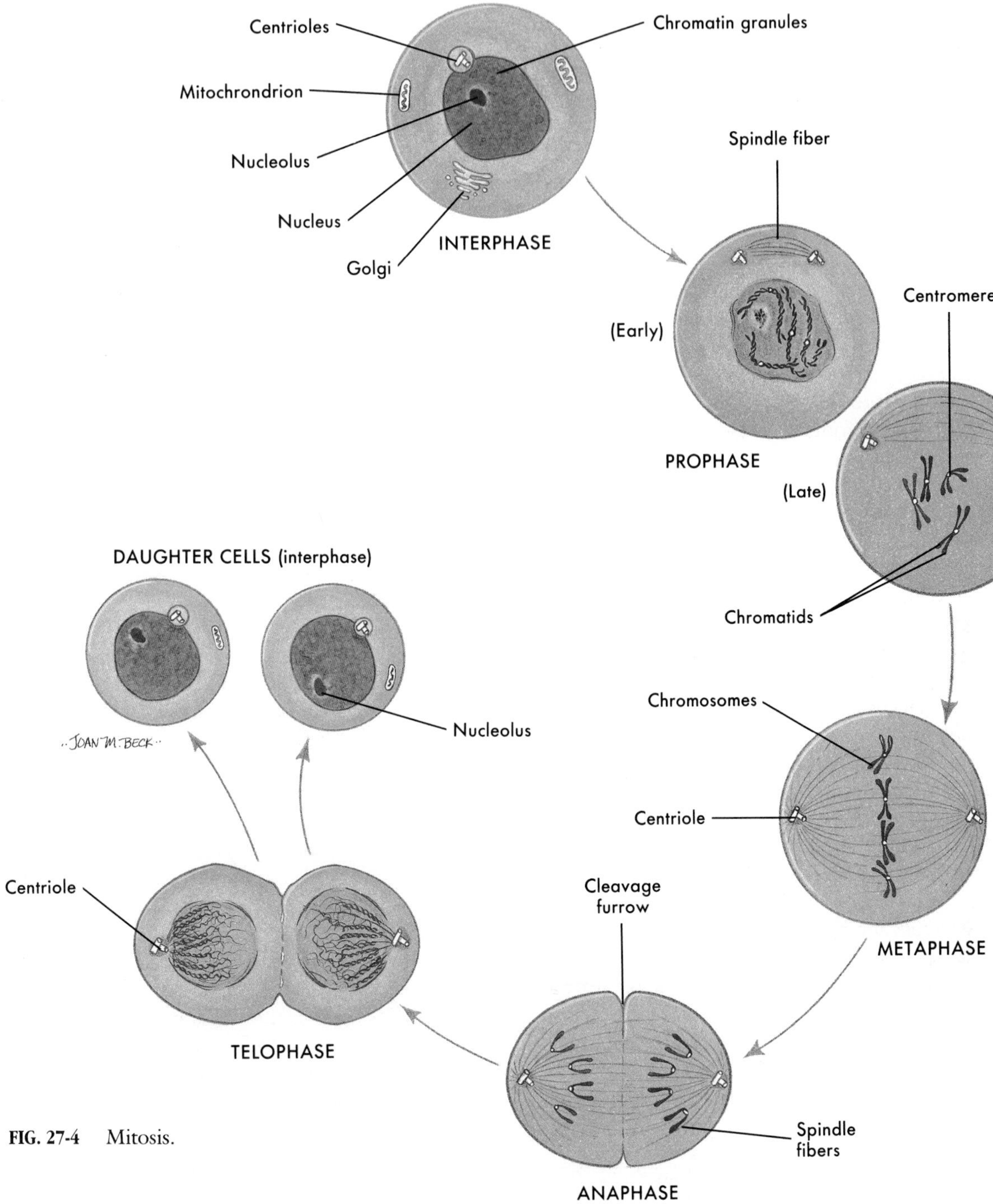

FIG. 27-4 Mitosis.

DNA. At the completion of cell division, the daughter cells contain both the nucleus and cytoplasm of the original cell. Each body cell in humans contains 46 chromosomes. These chromosomes exist in pairs. One member of each pair was received from the father of the offspring at the time of fertilization, and one was received from the mother. These paired chromosomes, except for the pair that determines sex, are alike in size and appearance and carry genes for the same traits.

During mitosis, the cell goes through four phases: prophase, metaphase, anaphase, and finally, telephase.

Prophase: In the nucleus the chromosomes form two strands called chromatids. In the cytoplasm the centrioles form a network of spindle fibers.

Metaphase: The nucleus membrane and nucleolus disappear and the chromosomes are aligned across the center of the cell. The centrioles are at the opposite ends of the cell and spindle fibers are attached to each chromatid.

Anaphase: The chromosomes are pulled to the opposite ends of the cell and cell division begins.

Telephase: At this final phase of cell division, the two nuclei appear and the chromosomes disperse. At the end of this phase, two new daughter cells appear.

Movement of materials across cell membranes. For a cell to survive, it must receive food and oxygen and must secrete its waste products. To accomplish this task, a number of processes allow for this mass movement of substances into and out of the cells. These transport processes are classified under two general headings: passive transport and active transport.

The difference between the two categories is based on whether energy is required to effect the movement of something through the cell membrane. **Active transport** processes require the expenditure of energy by the cell, and passive transport processes do not. The energy required for active transport processes is obtained from an important chemical substance called adenosine triphosphate, or ATP. ATP is produced in the cell from nutrients and is capable of releasing energy that in turn enables the cell to do work. The breakdown of ATP and use of the energy that is released are required for active transport processes to occur. In **passive transport** processes no cellular energy is required to move substances from a high concentration to a lower concentration; in active transport processes cellular energy is required to move substances from a low concentration to a high concentration.

Passive transport processes. The primary passive transport processes that move through the cell membrane include the following:

1. ***Diffusion:*** a process in which solid particles in a fluid move from an area of higher concentration to an area of lower concentration, which results in an even distribution of the particles in the fluid (see Fig. 28-3).
2. ***Osmosis:*** the diffusion of water across a semipermeable membrane. The water molecules travel from an area of greater water-molecule concentration (less substance dissolved) to an area of lesser water-molecule concentration (more substance dissolved) (see Fig. 28-4).
3. ***Filtration:*** the movement of water and particles through a membrane by a force from either pressure or gravity. The movement is from an area of greater pressure to an area of lesser pressure.

Use the information concerning filtration, diffusion, and osmosis to understand what would occur if red blood cells were placed in isotonic, hypotonic, and hypertonic solutions (Fig 27-5).

Active transport processes. *Active transport* is the movement of material across the membrane of a cell by means of a chemical activity that allows the cell to admit larger molecules than would otherwise be able to enter. Certain enzymes play a role in active transport, providing a chemical "pump" that helps move substances through the cell membrane. For example, insulin binds with glucose and transports the glucose into the cell. Two other active transport processes that move an object or substance through the plasma membrane and into the cytoplasm are:

1. ***Phagocytosis:*** (Greek for "cell-eating") permits a cell to engulf or surround foreign material and digest it. The function is often performed by white blood cells in the human body.
2. ***Pinocytosis:*** the process by which extracellular fluid is taken into the cell. The cell membrane develops a saclike indentation filled with extracellular fluid, then closes around it, and digests it.

Tissues

Tissues are groups of similar cells that work together to perform a specific function. The body is composed of four main types of tissues: epithelial, connective, muscle, and nervous tissues. Consult Table 27-1 for a summary of their locations and functions.

Epithelial tissue. Epithelial cells are packed closely together and contain no blood vessels. The **epithelial tissue** covers the outside of the body and some of the internal structures. There are four types or forms of epithelial tissue: simple squamous, stratified squamous, simple columnar, and stratified transitional. Table 27-1 gives the

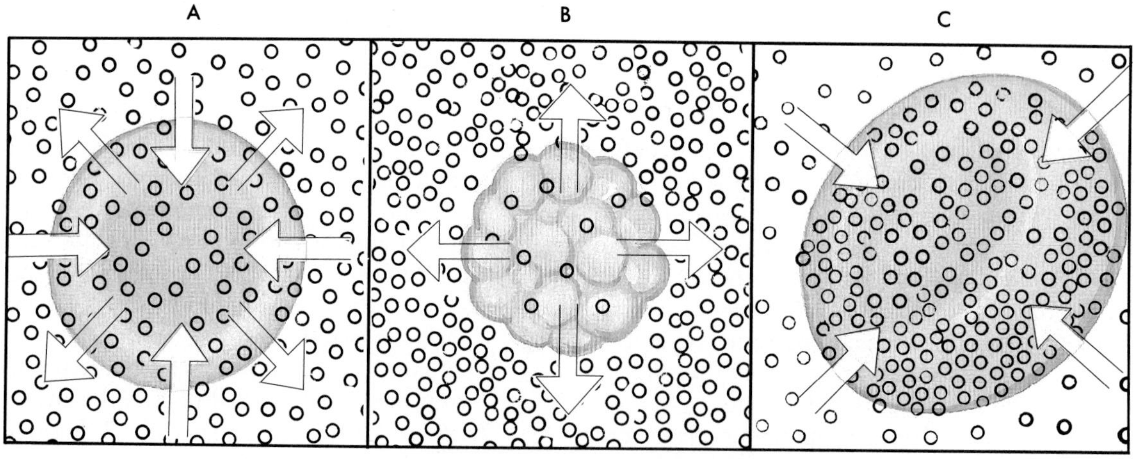

FIG. 27-5 Types of salt solutions. **A,** Isotonic. **B,** Hypertonic. **C,** Hypotonic.

locations and functions of each of these types.

Epithelial tissue serves several important functions in the body. Some of the more important are listed in the following:

1. *Protection:* Covering the body and many of its organs, it serves as a protective barrier against invasion.
2. *Absorption:* Certain specialized epithelial cells can absorb material in the body, e.g., the lining of the small intestine can absorb digested nutrients.
3. *Secretion:* Mucus is secreted in areas such as the respiratory and digestive tracts.

Connective tissue. As the name suggests, **connective tissue** "connects," or joins, tissues or structures of the body. It also supports and protects body structures and exists in varying forms. It can be thin and delicate or

Table 27-1 Tissues

Tissue	Location	Function
EPITHELIAL		
Simple squamous	Alveoli of lungs	Absorption by diffusion of respiratory gases between alveolar air and blood
	Lining of blood and lymphatic vessels	Absorption by diffusion, filtration, and osmosis
Stratified squamous	Surface of lining of mouth and esophagus	Protection
	Surface of skin (epidermis)	Protection
Simple columnar	Surface layer of lining of stomach, intestines, and parts of respiratory tract	Protection; secretion; absorption
Stratified transitional	Urinary bladder	Protection
CONNECTIVE*		
Areolar	Between other tissues and organs	Connection
Adipose (fat)	Under skin	Protection
	Padding at various points	Insulation; support; reserve food
Dense fibrous	Tendons; ligaments	Flexible but strong connection
Bone	Skeleton	Support; protection
Cartilage	Part of nasal septum; covering articular surfaces of bones; larynx; rings in trachea and bronchi	Firm but flexible support
	Disks between vertebrae	
	External ear	
Blood	Blood vessels	Transportation
MUSCLE		
Skeletal (striated voluntary)	Muscles that attach to bones	Movement of bones
	Eyeball muscles	Eye movements
	Upper third of esophagus	First part of swallowing
Cardiac (striated involuntary)	Wall of heart	Contraction of heart
Visceral (nonstriated involuntary or smooth)	In walls of tubular viscera of digestive, respiratory, and genitourinary tracts	Movement of substances along respective tracts.
	In walls of blood vessels and large lymphatic vessels	Changing of diameter of blood vessels
	In ducts of glands	Movement of substances along ducts
	Intrinsic eye muscles (iris and ciliary body)	Changing of diameter of pupils and shape of lens
	Arrector muscles of hairs	Erection of hairs (gooseflesh)
NERVOUS		
	Brain; spinal cord; nerves	Irritability; conduction

*Connective tissues are the most widely distributed of all tissues.

tough and cord like; it also exists in liquid form (blood). Unlike the closely packed epithelial tissue, the connective tissue cells are spaced among varying amounts of intercellular fluid, which is composed of protein complexes and tissue fluid.

Some of the most important forms of connective tissue are areolar connective tissue, adipose (fat) tissue, bone, cartilage, and blood. Consult Table 27-1 for the locations and functions of these tissues.

Muscle tissue. Muscle tissue is composed of cells that contract in response to a message from the brain or spinal cord. There are three types of muscle cells: (1) skeletal (striated, voluntary), (2) cardiac (striated, involuntary), and (3) visceral (smooth, involuntary).

1. Skeletal muscle cells are striated (have a striped appearance) and attach to bones to produce voluntary movement.
2. Cardiac muscle cells are striated with fibers that branch to form networks, or webs. They are found only in the walls of the heart and generally do not function at will (involuntary).
3. Visceral muscle cells are nonstriated and have a smooth appearance. These cells appear in the viscera, or internal organs, such as the walls of the blood vessels, intestines, and uterus. Generally, they are involuntary, but some control can be exerted through the use of biofeedback techniques.

Nervous tissue. Nervous tissue is composed of two types of cells: neurons and glial cells. The neurons are the nerve cells and are responsible for the transmission of impulses or messages. The glial cells are support cells; they support and nourish the neurons.

Neurons have three parts: (1) dendrites, which carry impulses toward the cell body; (2) cell body; and (3) axons, which carry impulses away from the cell body (see Fig. 38-2).

Membranes

Membranes are thin sheets of tissue that serve many functions in the body. They cover body surfaces, line and lubricate hollow organs, and protect and anchor organs and bones.

The two major types of membranes are the epithelial and the connective tissue membranes.

Epithelial membranes. Epithelial membranes are usually composed of a thin layer of epithelial cells with an underlying layer of connective tissue for strength. Epithelial membranes may be divided into two subgroups: mucous membranes and serous membranes.

1. Mucous membranes secrete mucus (a thick, slippery material) that keeps the membranes moist and soft and protects against bacterial invasion. They line the body surfaces that open to the outside environment. Examples include the nose, mouth, urinary, and reproductive tracts.
2. Serous membranes secrete a thin, watery fluid that prevents friction when organs rub against one another. They line the body surfaces that do not open to the outside environment. Examples include the lungs (pleura), intestines (peritoneum), and heart (pericardium).

Connective tissue membranes. Connective tissue membranes are smooth, slick, and secrete synovial fluid (a thick, lubricating fluid). These membranes line the joint spaces between bones and prevent friction between the ends of the bones, thus allowing free movement of the joints.

Organs/systems. When several kinds of tissues are united to form a special function, they are called organs. Examples are the heart, stomach, and kidneys. These organs are arranged to perform complex functions in the body and are then called systems.

The following is a list of the ten major systems of the body with a brief description of their function.

1. *Integumentary (skin) system:* covers the body and is the body's first line of defense
2. *Musculoskeletal system:* provides the body's framework and allows for movement
3. *Circulatory system:* is the major transportation system for nutrition, water, oxygen, and wastes
4. *Digestive system:* processes food and water and removes waste products
5. *Respiratory system:* delivers oxygen and removes carbon dioxide
6. *Urinary system:* removes excess water and waste products
7. *Nervous system:* contains the body's control center and is responsible for the coordination of all the body's activities
8. *Endocrine system:* releases chemicals that regulate the body's activities.
9. *Reproductive system:* enables the procreation of life
10. *Sensory system:* protects the individual by detecting changes in the environment.

REFERENCES AND SUGGESTED READINGS

1. Anagnostakos NP and Tortora GJ: Principles of anatomy and physiology, ed 5, New York, 1987, Harper & Row, Publishers, Inc.
2. Caldwell E and Hegner BR: Geriatrics: a study of maturity, ed 4, New York, 1986, Delmar Publishers, Inc.
3. Fong E, Ferris EB, and Skelly EG: Body structures and functions, ed 7, New York, 1989, Delmar Publishers, Inc.
4. Hood GH and Dincher JR: Total patient care, ed 7, St Louis, 1988, The CV Mosby Co.
5. Long BC and Phipps WJ: Medical-surgical nursing, ed 2, St Louis, 1989, The CV Mosby Co.
6. Marieb EN: Essentials of human anatomy and physiology, Reading, Mass, 1984, Addison-Wesley Publishing Co.
7. Memmler RL and Wood DL: Structure and function of the human body, ed 4, Philadelphia, 1987, WB Saunders Co.
8. Solomon EP and Phillips GA: Understanding human anatomy and physiology, Philadelphia, 1987, WB Saunders Co.
9. Thibodeau GA and Anthony CP: Structure and function of the body, ed 8, St Louis, 1988, Times Mirror/Mosby College Publishing.

CHAPTER CHALLENGE

KEY POINTS

- Anatomy is the study of the shape and structure of the body, whereas physiology explains the function of the various structures and how they relate to one another.
- The normal anatomical position of the body is standing erect with the face and the palms of the hands forward.
- To study the body, it is divided into three imaginary planes: the sagittal, the coronal, and the transverse.
- The body can be divided into two large groups of cavities, the dorsal and the ventral. The dorsal cavity contains the cranial and spinal cavities. The ventral cavity contains the thoracic cavity, the abdominal cavity, and the pelvic cavity.
- To study the abdominal region, it is divided into nine regions: right hypochondriac region, epigastric region, and left hypochondriac region; right lumbar region, umbilical region, and left lumbar region; and right iliac region, hypogastric region, and left iliac region.
- Cells are the smallest units of life and contain five characteristics: growth, metabolism, responsiveness, reproduction, and homeostasis.
- The major structures of the cell are: the cytoplasm, the nucleus, the endoplasmic reticulum, the ribosomes, the mitochondria, the lysosomes, the Golgi apparatus, and the centrioles.
- To receive nutrition and oxygen and to rid itself of wastes, the cell performs these processes: passive transport (diffusion, osmosis, filtration) and active transport (phagocytosis and pinocytosis).
- The body is composed of four main types of tissues: epithelial, connective, muscle, and nervous tissues.
- The ten major systems of the body are: integumentary, musculoskeletal, circulatory, digestive, respiratory, urinary, nervous, endocrine, reproductive, and sensory.

STUDY QUESTIONS

1. The axial portions of the body contain:
   a. The neck only
   b. The trunk only
   c. The head, neck, and trunk
   d. The upper and lower extremities
2. The left lower quadrant of the body is:
   a. The left hypochondriac region
   b. The left iliac region
   c. The left hip
   d. None of the above
3. The sticky fluidlike substance that lies between the cell membrane and the nucleus is called:
   a. Golgi apparatus
   b. Cell substance
   c. Cytoplasm
   d. Tissue
4. Another name for the powerhouse of the cell is:
   a. Golgi apparatus
   b. Mitochondria
   c. Lysosomes
   d. Nucleus
5. A process in which solid particles in a fluid move from an area of greater concentration to an area of lesser concentration, resulting in an even distribution of the particles in the fluid, is called:
   a. Phagocytosis
   b. Pinocytosis
   c. Osmosis
   d. Diffusion
6. What type of tissue contains closely packed cells and no blood vessels:
   a. Epithelial
   b. Connective
   c. Nervous
   d. Muscle
7. What type of muscle cells are found only in the walls of the heart:
   a. Visceral
   b. Skeletal
   c. Epithelial
   d. Cardiac
8. What system is the body's first line of defense:
   a. Endocrine
   b. Nervous
   c. Integumentary
   d. Respiratory
9. All of the following processes are examples of passive transport except:
   a. Diffusion
   b. Osmosis
   c. Filtration
   d. Phagocytosis
10. What is produced in the cell from nutrients and is capable of releasing energy that allows the cell to work:
    a. ATP
    b. Pinocytosis
    c. Membrane
    d. Oxytocic

28

Fluids and Electrolytes

GEORGEANNA TEMRES SMITH

LEARNING OBJECTIVES

After reading this chapter, the student should be able to do the following:

- Define the key terms.
- Describe the distribution of fluid compartments.
- Describe the daily balance of intake and output.
- Explain the mechanisms by which body fluids move.
- Discuss the role of specific electrolytes in maintaining homeostasis.
- Describe the cause and effect of deficits and excesses of sodium, potassium, chloride, calcium, magnesium, phosphorus, and bicarbonate.
- Explain the role of the buffers, lungs, and kidneys in maintenance of acid-base balance.
- Describe the four major types of acid-base imbalances.

RELATED TOPICS OF INTEREST

- Basic nutrition (Chapter 22)
- Diet therapy (Chapter 23)
- Cells, tissues, and membranes (Chapter 27)
- Care of the patient with a gastrointestinal or accessory organ disorder (Chapter 31)
- Care of the patient with a urinary disorder (Chapter 33)
- Care of the patient with a respiratory disorder (Chapter 34)
- Care of the patient with an endocrine disorder (Chapter 35)

KEY TERMS

Define the following:

- active transport
- anion
- bicarbonate
- buffer
- calcium
- cation
- chloride
- diffusion
- electrolyte
- extracellular
- filtration
- homeostasis
- hypertonic
- hypotonic
- interstitial
- intracellular
- intravascular
- isotonic
- magnesium
- milliequivalent
- osmosis
- passive transport
- phosphorus
- potassium
- sodium

FLUIDS (WATER)

Water has many functions. It provides an extracellular transportation route to deliver nutrients to the cells and carry waste products from the cells. Once inside the cells, it provides a medium in which chemical reactions, or metabolism, can occur. Water also acts as a lubricant for tissues. Two other important functions of water are to aid in the maintenance of acid-base balance and to assist in heat regulation by evaporation.

Water is critically important to the body. The major percentage of body weight is water. This percentage depends on several factors and varies with each individual. First, age affects the amount of water in the body. A newborn has a water content of 70% to 80% of its body weight. That percentage increases in a premature infant to as high as 90%. The infant begins to lose body fluid most rapidly in the first 6 months, and by 12 years, the proportion approaches that of an adult. The percentage of water content in the body declines from that highest percentage at birth to 50% to 60% as adults and 45% to 55% in the elderly person.

Another important influence on the amount of water in the body is the amount of fat in the individual. There is a correlation between water content and fat content; fat contains relatively little water. The female has proportionately more body fat than the male, which means the female has less body fluid than the male. The more obese an individual, the smaller the percentage of body water. Both obese and elderly persons are at risk for complications of illness from dehydration or fluid shifts because of less fluid reserve in their bodies. Infants are also at a risk for dehydration. Over one half of an infant's fluid is **extracellular** fluid (outside the cells) (Fig. 28-1). Extracellular fluid is lost from the body more rapidly than **intracellular** fluid (inside the cells).

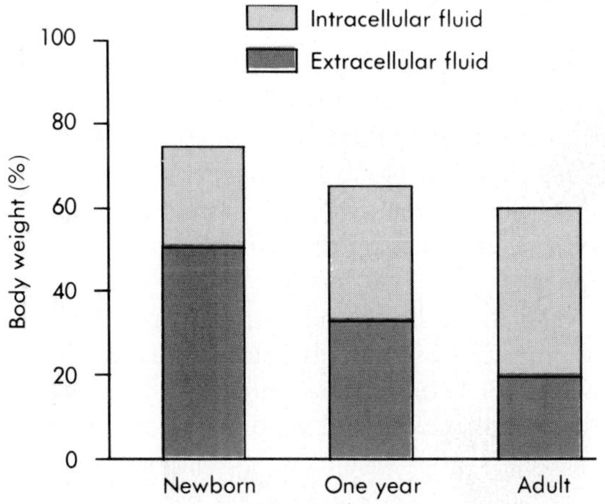

FIG. 28-1 In the newborn, more than half of total body fluid is extracellular. As the child grows, proportions gradually approximate adult levels.

Table 28-1 Body Fluid Distribution

Compartment	Description	Fluid
Intracellular	Fluid within cells	Intracellular fluid (ICF)
Extracellular	Fluid outside cells	Extracellular fluid (ECF)
Intravascular	Fluid within blood vessels	Plasma
Interstitial	Fluid in tissues (between cells or in body spaces)	Examples: interstitial fluid, lymph, cerebrospinal fluid, intraocular fluid, GI secretions, urine, sweat, exudates

The very young, the very old, and the obese patients are at a higher risk for developing a fluid volume deficit. A loss of 10% of body fluid is serious in an adult, and a 20% loss is fatal. In an infant, those figures are even more significant. A loss of 5% is mild, 10% is moderate, and 15% is very serious.

FLUID COMPARTMENTS

Identifying the location of fluids in the body is done by categorizing them into compartments. However, it is an abstract term, because rather than being contained in a compartment in a specific area, the fluids are in constant motion throughout the body to carry out their functions.

The body has two fluid compartments: intracellular and extracellular (Fig. 28-2). Even though each is specific in its location and functions, there is constant interaction between the compartments.

The fluid compartments (Tables 28-1 and 28-2) are as follows:

1. Intracellular
2. Extracellular
   a. Interstitial
   b. Intravascular

The intracellular fluid compartment is the larger of the two compartments. It contains the fluid inside the billions of cells within the body.

The extracellular compartment contains any fluid outside the cells. This compartment is further divided into the interstitial and intravascular fluid compartments.

Interstitial fluid is between the cells or in the tissues. It accounts for approximately 27% of the fluid in the body. Examples of interstitial fluid include lymph, cerebrospinal fluid, and gastrointestional secretions.

Intravascular fluid is the plasma within the vessels. The cells of the blood are considered solid particles. After the cells are removed, the liquid that remains is the plasma. It makes up the remaining 7% of our fluid volume.

The intracellular and extracellular compartments are separated by a semipermeable membrane. This membrane allows for a constant back and forth flow as nutrients are taken into the cell and waste products are carried out of the cell.

INTAKE AND OUTPUT

As water moves through all parts of the body, it is constantly being lost. Fluid leaves the body through the kidneys, lungs, skin, and GI tract. To maintain **homeostasis,** the normal daily loss must be met by the normal daily intake. Homeostasis is a relative constancy in the internal environment of the body, naturally maintained by adaptive responses that promote healthy survival. Daily water intake and output is about 2500 ml (Table 28-3).

Water loss is replenished in two ways—first, by inges-

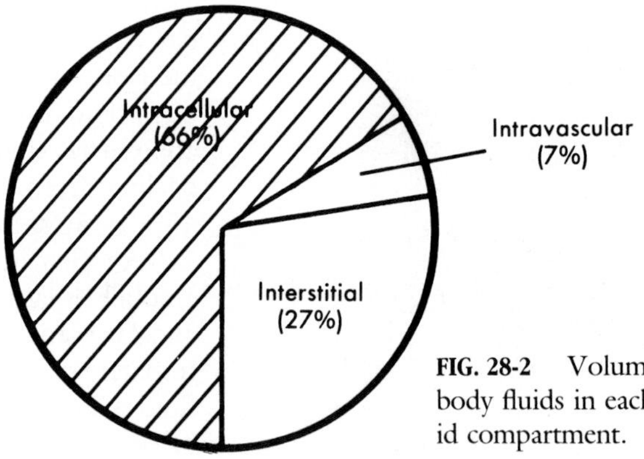

FIG. 28-2 Volumes of body fluids in each fluid compartment.

Table 28-2 Body Fluid Distribution

Compartment	Percent of Total Body Weight	Fluid Volume (liters)
Extracellular fluid		
Interstitial fluid	16	11.2
Plasma	4	2.8
Intracellular fluid	80	42.0

Table 28-3 Normal Fluid Intake and Loss in an Adult Eating 2500 Calories Per Day (Approximate Figures)

Intake		Output	
Route	Gain (ml)	Route	Amount of Loss (ml)
Water in food	1000	Skin	500
Water from oxidation	300	Lungs	350
Water as liquid	1200	Feces	150
		Kidney	1500
TOTAL	2500	TOTAL	2500

tion of liquids and food and, second, by metabolism, both of food and in our body tissues. The determination of exact amounts of fluid loss and fluid replacement is not possible as part of nursing care, so approximations are used. Because fluid intake and urine output can be measured, the importance of accurate record keeping cannot be overstressed when determining a patient's fluid needs. A simple and accurate method of determining water balance is by weighing the patient under exact conditions, for example, same time of day, same amount of bed clothing, same type of gown, and same attached equipment, such as electrodes. Because 1 liter of fluid equals 1 kilogram (2.2 pounds), a weight change of 1 kilogram will refect a loss or gain of 1 liter of body fluid.

MOVEMENT OF FLUID AND ELECTROLYTES

Substances entering the body begin their journey in the extracellular fluid. However, to carry out their functions, they must cross the semipermeable membrane surrounding each body cell to enter the cell. The fat and protein molecules that make up the membrane are arranged so that some substances can enter the cells and others cannot. There are several methods used to move fluids, electrolytes and other solutes, or dissolved substances from one compartment to the other.

DIFFUSION

Water can move freely from one compartment to another by diffusion. **Diffusion** is the movement of particles in all directions through a solution or gas (Fig. 28-3). Diffusion occurs when ink is dropped into a glass of water. The ink will disperse in all directions until it is evenly distributed throughout the fluid. When diffusion occurs in the body, the molecules have the same action as the ink spreading through the water. With each inhalation oxygen enters the lungs and moves into the intravascular compartment and into the cells by diffusion. Oxygen can diffuse easily across the cell membrane.

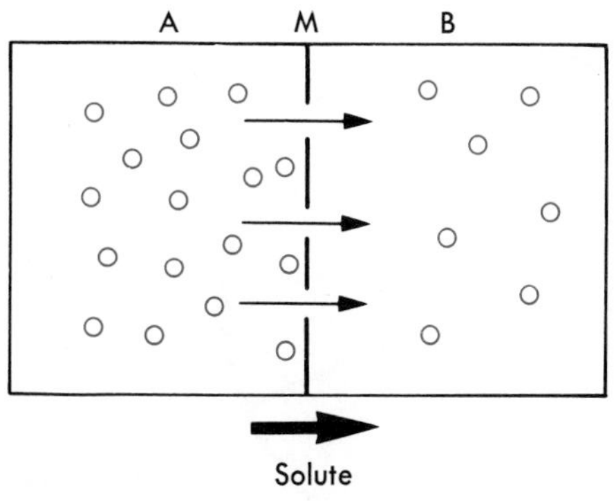

FIG. 28-3 Diffusion: solute moves through membrane *(M)* from area of greater concentration *(A)* to area of lesser concentration *(B)* until concentration on both sides is equal.

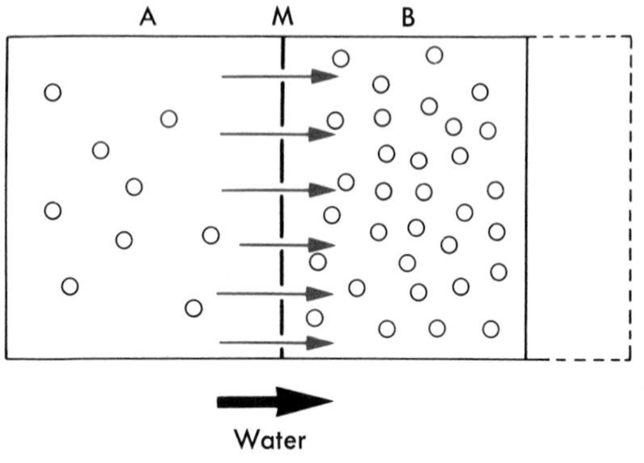

FIG. 28-4 Osmosis: water moves from area of lesser solute concentration *(A)* through a membrane *(M)* to area of greater solute concentration *(B)* until concentration of solute on both sides of the membrane is equal. Compartment *(B)* will have to expand *(as shown by dotted lines)* to accept the additional water.

OSMOSIS

Osmosis is the movement of water from an area of lower concentration to an area of higher concentration (Fig. 28-4). Osmosis equalizes the concentration of ions or molecules on each side of the membrane. The flow of water will continue until the number of ions or molecules on both sides of the membrane is equal. Boiling a hot dog in water is an example of osmosis. The concentration of molecules inside the hot dog is greater than in the water. The water passes through the hot dog skin, which is a semipermeable membrane, in an attempt to equalize the number of molecules on both sides of the membrane. Finally, when the hot dog can hold no more water, the skin, or semipermeable membrane, ruptures.

The red blood cells offer an example of the osmotic process in the body. If extracellular fluid is more concentrated than intracellular fluid, the fluid from the cell moves out to the extracellular fluid, causing the red blood cell to shrink. If the fluid among the compartments is in equilibrium, fluid will enter and leave the cell at the same rate and the cell size will not change. Another example is when extracellular fluid is less concentrated than the fluid in the red blood cells. Fluid moves into the cell, causing it to enlarge. The process can continue until the cell ruptures.

Solutions are classified as hypertonic, isotonic, or hypotonic according to the electrolyte concentration. The concentration of the solution will cause the cells of the body to react the same as the red blood cell. **Hypertonic** solutions pull fluid from the cells, **isotonic** solutions expand the body's fluid volume without causing a fluid shift from one compartment to another, and **hypotonic** solutions move into the cells, causing them to enlarge. Each of these actions occurs through osmosis.

FILTRATION

Filtration is the transfer of water and dissolved substances from an area of higher pressure to an area of lower pressure. An example of filtration occurs at the capillary level of the circulation. There is a force behind filtration called hydrostatic pressure, which is the force of fluid pressing outward on a vessel wall. The pumping action of the heart is responsible for the amount of force of the hydrostatic pressure that causes water and electrolytes to move from the capillaries to the interstitial fluid.

ACTIVE TRANSPORT

The fluid movements discussed to this point have required no energy expenditure by the body; they have been examples of **passive** transport. **Active transport** requires energy; it is a force that moves molecules into cells without regard for their positive or negative charge and against concentration factors that would prevent entry into the cell via diffusion. Active transport moves fluid and electrolytes from an area of lower concentration to an area of higher concentration. Adenosine triphosphate (ATP) is the energy source used to accomplish active transport. ATP energy is released in a complex metabolic process within the body's cells known as the Krebs cycle. (Krebs cycle is a sequence of enzymatic reactions involving the metabolism of carbon chains of sugars, fatty acids, and amino acids to yield carbon dioxide, water, and high-energy phosphate bonds.)

Substances actively transported through the cell membrane include sodium, potassium, calcium, iron, hydrogen, and amino acids. The movement of glucose into the cells occurs through the process of active transport. Insulin provides the transport for glucose to leave the intravascular compartment and move into the cells, where the glucose can then be used for energy.

ELECTROLYTES

As water moves through the compartments of the body, it contains substances that are sometimes called minerals or salts, but are technically known as **electrolytes.** Electrolytes develop tiny electrical charges when they dissolve in water and break up into particles known as ions. Ions develop either a positive or negative electrical charge. Ions with a positive charge are called cations. Ions with a negative charge are called anions.

Examples of cations:

1. Sodium Na^+
2. Potassium K^+
3. Calcium Ca^{++}
4. Magnesium Mg^{++}

Examples of anions:

1. Chloride Cl^-
2. Bicarbonate HCO_3^-
3. Sulfate SO_4^-
4. Phosphate HPO_4^-

A balance exists between the electrolytes. For each positively charged cation, there must be a negatively charged anion.

A sample of plasma is used to measure the electrolytes. The measurement is done in milliequivalents (mEq). Rather than electrolytes being measured by their weights, they are measured by their electrical activity. A **milliequivalent** is a measure of the chemical activity or chemical combining power of an ion. The chemical activity of an electrolyte is compared with the chemical activity of hydrogen. One milliequivalent of any electrolyte has the same chemical combining power as 1 mEq of hydrogen. In each fluid compartment in the body, the cations and anions balance each other with their chemical combining power to maintain electrical neutrality, which, again, keeps the body in homeostasis.

Although the electrolytes move freely among the fluid compartments, each has a primary location. The location and function of each electrolyte becomes important in understanding disease processes. The body maintains homeostasis by correcting any excesses or deficiences of the electrolytes.

Sodium

The normal blood level of **sodium** (Na^+), the most abundant electrolyte in the body, is 134 to 142 mEq/L. It is the major extracellular electrolyte, and because the plasma sample used to measure electrolyte levels comes from the extracellular fluid, the level is high. In contrast, the intracellular level of sodium is approximately 10 mEq. The major source of sodium comes from the diet. That is true of all the electrolytes. However, unlike the other electrolytes, sodium is a substance that frequently needs to be limited in the diet rather than encouraged. The kidneys are the primary excretion route for sodium. It is important to know that many electrolytes, such as sodium, not only pass into and out of the body, but also move back and forth between a number of body fluids during each 24-hour period. Fig. 28-5 shows the large

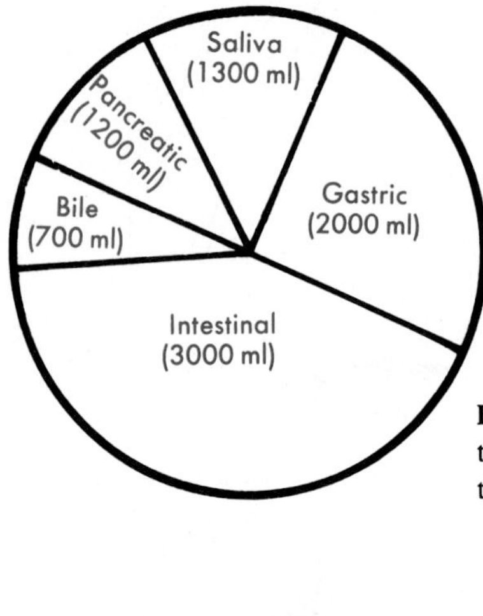

FIG. 28-5 Sodium-containing internal secretions produced every day.

volumes of sodium-containing internal secretions that are produced each day. During a 24-hour period, more than 8 L of fluid containing 1000 to 1300 mEq of sodium is poured into the digestive system. This sodium, along with most of that contained in the diet, is almost completely reabsorbed. Precise regulation and control of sodium levels are required for survival.

The functions of sodium include regulation of the water balance. Sodium controls the extracellular fluid volume mainly through osmotic pressure, because water follows the sodium in the body. It also increases cell membrane permeability. Sodium stimulates conduction of nerve impulses and helps maintain neuromuscular irritability. Sodium is important in controlling contractility of muscles, especially the heart.

Hyponatremia. A less than normal concentration of sodium in the blood is called hyponatremia. This condition can occur when there is a sodium loss or a water excess (Box 28-1). Hyponatremia occurs when the sodium drops below 135 mEq/L in the extracellular fluid.

BOX 28-1 CAUSES AND SYMPTOMS OF HYPONATREMIA

CAUSES

- Loss of GI fluids
  - Vomiting
  - Diarrhea
  - GI or biliary drainage via nasogastric tube or T-tube
  - Fistulas
- Loss through skin
  - Diaphoresis
  - Large open lesions (burns)
- Shifting of body fluids
  - Massive edema
  - Ascites
  - Burns
  - Small bowel obstruction

SYMPTOMS

- Headache
- Muscle weakness
- Fatigue
- Apathy
- Postural hypotension
- Nausea/vomiting
- Abdominal cramps
- Severe or Prolonged Deficit
  - Shock
  - Mental confusion
  - Coma

When a deficiency results from sodium loss, the body attempts to compensate by decreasing water excretion. If hyponatremia occurs because of water excess, the result has a diluting effect on all of the blood components because water is being retained in the body. The signs and symptoms of hyponatremia depend on the cause and also on how rapid and severe the sodium loss. As sodium levels decrease in the extracellular fluid, water is pulled into the cells, causing them to swell, and as the fluid moves into the cells, potassium is shifted out; therefore the patient is likely to also have a potassium imbalance.

Hypernatremia. Hypernatremia is a greater than normal concentration of sodium. The sodium level exceeds 145 mEq/L. It is caused by an excess of sodium or a decrease in body water (Box 28-2). The body attempts to correct the imbalance by conserving water through renal reabsorption. Hypernatremia causes fluid to shift from the cells to the interstitial spaces, resulting in cellular dehydration and an interruption in cellular processes. Again, a potassium imbalance frequently occurs. In sodium retention, potassium is excreted.

Potassium

The normal blood level of potassium (K^+), the dominant intracellular cation, is 3.5 to 5.5 mEq/L. The level of potassium in the extracellur fluid is low because **potassium** is an intracellular electrolyte. Intracellular levels of potassium are 150 mEq/L. Of the body's potassium, 98% is in the cells and 2% is in the extracellular fluid.

A well-balanced diet usually provides adequate potassium. Approximately 65 mEq of potassium is required

BOX 28-2 CAUSES AND SYMPTOMS OF HYPERNATREMIA

CAUSES

- More water than sodium is lost from the body
- An abnormally large intake of sodium
  - Taking too many salt tablets
  - IV saline infused too rapidly

SYMPTOMS

- Dry, tenacious mucous membranes
- Low urinary output
- Firm, rubbery tissue turgor
- Severe or Prolonged Excess
  - Manic excitement
  - Tachycardia
  - Death

each day. Leading food sources include bananas, melons, raisins, dates, white beans, orange juice, tomato juice, and vegetables.

The routes of potassium excretion are the kidneys (80% to 90%) and in the feces and perspiration (10% to 20%). The kidneys control the excretion of potassium. Sodium and potassium seem to pair off against one another, and the kidneys prefer to conserve sodium, even when both electrolytes are depleted. In both normal and abnormal situations, sodium will be reabsorbed and potassium will be excreted. Because the major route of excretion of potassium is the kidneys, any condition that causes a decrease in urine output also causes a retention of potassium. A rise in potassium requires continuous monitoring. An important consideration in homeostasis is that kidney function will determine the potassium level in the body. Too little or too much potassium affects the heart muscle and can be life threatening.

The main function of potassium is regulation of water and electrolyte content within the cell. With sodium and calcium, it promotes transmission of nerve impulses and also skeletal muscle function. Potassium assists in the cellular metabolism of carbohydrates and proteins. Another function of potassium is to control the hydrogen ion concentration. When potassium moves out of the cell, sodium and hydrogen ions move in. The result is the regulation of acid-base balance.

Hypokalemia. A decrease in the body's potassium to a level below 3.5 mEq/L is known as hypokalemia. The major cause of potassium loss is renal excretion (Box 28-3). The kidneys do not conserve potassium and excrete it even when the body needs the potassium. The use of diuretics, such as thiazides or furosemide (Lasix), promotes hypokalemia. Conditions that cause injury to the cells, in turn, cause the release of potassium from the cells to the interstitial spaces and ultimately to the kidneys. If renal function is normal, the potassium will be excreted. Because the normal amounts of potassium are so small, fluctuations have the potential to develop into serious problems. Hypokalemia can affect skeletal and cardiac function. The resulting muscle weakness causes life-threatening cardiac conduction abnormalities.

Hyperkalemia. An increase in the body's serum potassium level above 5.5 mEq/L is known as hyperkalemia. This condition is not as common as hypokalemia when renal function is normal. The major cause of potassium excess is renal disease, in which potassium cannot be excreted adequately (Box 28-4). When severe tissue damage occurs, potassium is released from the cells. Shock often accompanies this damage, resulting in reduced kid-

BOX 28-3 CAUSES AND SYMPTOMS OF HYPOKALEMIA

CAUSES

Decreased potassium intake
Increased potassium loss
  Increased aldosterone activity
  GI losses
  Potassium-losing diuretics
  Loss from cells, as in trauma, burns
Conditions causing very large urine output
Potassium shift into cells
  Treatment of acidosis
  Metabolic alkalosis

SYMPTOMS

Muscle weakness
Anorexia, nausea/vomiting
Diminished deep tendon reflexes, lethargy
Cardiac dysrhythmias
ECG changes
Severe or Prolonged Deficit
  Flaccid paralysis
  Kidney damage
  Paralytic ileus
  Cardiac/respiratory arrest

BOX 28-4 CAUSES AND SYMPTOMS OF HYPERKALEMIA

CAUSES

Potassium intake (parenteral or oral) in excess of kidney's ability to excrete
Renal failure
Adrenal insufficiency
Potassium enters bloodstream, from injured cells with extensive trauma
Metabolic acidosis

SYMPTOMS

Nausea, vomiting
Diarrhea, colic
Cardiac dysrhythmias
ECG changes
Numbness, tingling
Severe or Prolonged Excess*
  Flaccid paralysis
  Cardiac arrest
  Anuria

*Prolonged potassium excess results in symptoms similar to those of hypokalemia.

ney output. The result is an elevated potassium level. Although hyperkalemia is less common than hypokalemia, it is often more dangerous, because of cardiac arrest, which is caused by overstimulation of the cardiac muscle.

Chloride

The normal blood level of **chloride** (Cl^-), an extracellular anion, is 96 to 105 mEq/L. It is the chief anion in interstitial and intravascular fluid. Even though chloride accounts for more than two thirds of the anions in the body, it is usually not considered alone. Chloride has the ability to diffuse quickly between the intracellular and extracellular compartments and combines easily with sodium to form sodium chloride or with potassium to form potassium chloride. It is more often linked with sodium.

The daily requirement of chloride is equal to that of sodium (3.65 g to 10.85 g per day). Foods containing sodium also contain chloride. The main route of excretion is through the kidneys.

Chloride is necessary for the formation of hydrochloric acid in gastric juice. It is also a valuable electrolyte in regulating osmotic pressure between the compartments and assisting in regulation of acid-base balance.

Hypochloremia. Hypochloremia usually occurs when sodium is lost, because sodium and chloride are frequently paired. The most common causes of hypochloremia are vomiting and prolonged nasogastric or fistula drainage.

Hyperchloremia. Hyperchloremia rarely occurs but may be seen when bicarbonate levels fall. The chloride anions attempt to compensate to maintain equal numbers with the cations in the body fluid. Because chloride imbalances rarely occur independently of other electrolytes, there are no specific signs and symptoms to identify a chloride imbalance.

Calcium

The normal blood level of calcium (Ca^{++}) is approximately 4.5 mEq/L. Of the 1200 g of calcium in the body, 99% is concentrated in the bones and teeth, where it is physiologically inactive. The remaining 1% is found in the soft tissue and the extracellular fluid. Calcium is deposited in the bones and mobilized as needed to keep the blood level constant during any period of insufficient intake. Three considerations are important in the blood calcium level:

1. The deposition and resorption of the bone
2. The absorption of calcium from the gastrointestinal tract
3. The excretion of calcium in the urine and feces.

Vitamin D, calcitonin, and parathyroid hormones are necessary for the absorption and utilization of calcium.

The best food sources of calcium are milk and cheese. Other sources include beans, nuts, cauliflower, lettuce, and egg yolks. The average daily intake is 200 to 2500 mg. The recommended daily allowances vary from 360 mg for infants to 1200 mg for females 15 to 18 years of age. During pregnancy, 1300 mg is required. Calcium is removed from the body via the urine and feces.

Calcium is required for the formation and maintenance of strong bones and teeth. It is also necessary for normal blood clotting. Calcium has a depressing or sedative effect on neuromuscular irritability and thus promotes normal transmission of nerve impulses, as well as helps to regulate normal muscle contraction and relaxation. It helps hold body cells together by establishing the thickness and strength of cell membranes. One of its most important functions is to act as an enzyme activator for chemical reactions in the body.

Hypocalcemia. Hypocalcemia develops when the serum level is below 4.5 mEq/L. A deficiency may be caused by a variety of problems:

1. Infusion of excess amounts of citrated blood (citrates bind to the calcium)
2. Excessive loss through diarrhea
3. Inadequate dietary intake of calcium or vitamin D
4. Decreased parathyroid function
5. Pancreatic disease
6. Small bowel disease (Box 28-5)

The signs and symptoms of hypocalcemia are neuromuscular irritation and increased excitability. As neuromuscular signs and symptoms increase, tetany can occur. Tetany is a condition characterized by excessive muscle cramps, laryngeal spasms, stridor, and carpal pedal spasms.

Hypercalcemia. Hypercalcemia occurs when calcium levels exceed 5.8 mEq/L. It may occur when calcium stored in the bone enters the circulation, for example, in patients who are immobilized (Box 28-6). An increased intake of calcium or vitamin D also causes hypercalcemia. Neuromuscular activity is depressed, and renal calculi may develop because of the excretion of high levels of calcium by the kidneys.

Phosphorus

The normal blood level of **phosphorus** (HPO_4), chiefly an intracellular anion, is approximately 4 mEq/L. Phosphorus and calcium have an inverse relationship in the body: an increase in one causes a decrease in the other.

BOX 28-5 CAUSES AND SYMPTOMS OF HYPOCALCEMIA

CAUSES

Excess binding of calcium ions
Large amount of citrated blood
Alkalosis
Dietary deficiency of calcium
Chronic renal failure
Pancreatic disease
Disease of small bowel
Draining intestinal fistulas
Deficiency of parathyroid hormone or vitamin D
Increased magnesium

SYMPTOMS

Osteoporosis, pathological fractures
Tingling around nose, mouth, ears, fingers, toes
Muscle spasm of feet and hands
Tetany
Nausea, vomiting
Diarrhea
Cardiac dysrhythmias, cardiac arrest
Calcium deposits in body tissues

BOX 28-6 CAUSES AND SYMPTOMS OF HYPERCALCEMIA

CAUSES

Loss from bone
  Immobilization
  Metastatic bone cancer
  Multiple myeloma
Excess intake
  Dietary
  Antacids containing calcium
Increased absorption
  Increased parathyroid hormone
  Increased vitamin D

SYMPTOMS

Thirst, polyuria
Renal stones
Decreased deep tendon reflexes
Lethargy, coma
Cardiac dysrhythmias, cardiac arrest
Decreased muscle tone
Decreased GI motility

As blood calcium levels increase, phosphorus levels must decrease, and vice versa. The majority (70% to 80%) of phosphorus is found in bones and teeth combined with calcium, 10% is in the muscle, and the remaining 10% is in the nerve tissue of the body.

Dietary intake of phosphorus is usually 800 mg to 1500 mg per day. The minimum daily requirement is 800 mg. Intake should be increased during pregnancy and lactation. An adequate intake of vitamin D is necessary for the absorption of both calcium and phosphorus. Because there is a generous amount of phosphorus in many foods, a deficiency seldom occurs. Foods especially high in phosphorus include beef, pork, fish, poultry, milk products, and legumes. The kidneys are responsible for approximately 90% of the excretion of phosphorus. The remainder is excreted in the feces.

With calcium, phosphorus contributes to the support and maintenance of bones and teeth. It is important in many chemical reactions and acts as a buffer to regulate the body's acid-base balance. It promotes the effectiveness of many of the B vitamins, assists in normal nerve and muscle activity, and participates in carbohydrate metabolism.

Hypophosphatemia. Hypophosphatemia can occur from a dietary insufficiency, impaired kidney function, or maldistribution of phosphate in the body. Muscle weakness, especially affecting the respiratory muscles, may occur.

Hyperphosphatemia. Hyperphosphatemia most commonly occurs as a result of renal insufficiency. Another cause is increased intake of phosphate or vitamin D. Symptoms of tetany, numbness and tingling around the mouth, and muscle spasms develop.

Magnesium

The normal blood level of **magnesium** (Mg^{++}), the second most abundant cation in the intracellular fluid, is 1.5 to 2.4 mEq/L. Although there are only small amounts of magnesium in the blood, it is important in maintaining normal body function. The majority (60%) is found in the bone, 39% in the muscle and soft tissue, and 1% in the extracellular fluid, most of which is in the cerebrospinal fluid.

Dietary intake is usually 200 to 400 mg daily. The minimum daily requirement is 250 mg for the average adult, 150 mg for an infant, and 400 mg for a female during pregnancy and lactation. Magnesium is another electrolyte commonly distributed in foods. Whole grains, fruits, vegetables, meat, fish, legumes, and dairy products are dietary sources.

The major route of magnesium excretion is the kidneys. There is a correlation between the amount of magnesium and the amount of potassium excreted. The kidneys do not conserve potassium, but they do conserve magnesium; therefore if a magnesium deficiency develops, the body will conserve magnesium at the expense of excreting potassium.

Magnesium has not been a widely recognized electrolyte until recently. It is now linked as a cofactor in the activation of many enzymes. It also promotes regulation of serum calcium, phosphate, and potassium levels and is essential for integrity of nervous tissue, skeletal muscle, and cardiac functioning.

BOX 28-7 **CAUSES AND SYMPTOMS OF HYPOMAGNESEMIA**

CAUSES

- Decreased intake
  - Prolonged malnutrition
  - Starvation
- Impaired absorption from GI tract
  - Alcoholism
  - Hypercalcemia
  - Diarrhea
  - Draining intestinal fistulas
- Conditions causing large losses of urine

SYMPTOMS

- Mental changes
  - Agitation, depression, confusion
- Paresthesias
- Tremors
- Ataxia
- Cramps, spasticity, tetany
- Tachycardia
- Hypotension
- Dysrhythmias

BOX 28-8 **CAUSES AND SYMPTOMS OF HYPERMAGNESEMIA**

CAUSES

- Renal failure
- Diabetic ketoacidosis with severe water loss

SYMPTOMS

- Hypotension
- Vasodilation
  - Heat
  - Thirst
  - Nausea/vomiting
- Loss of deep tendon reflexes
- Respiratory depression

Prolonged or Severe Excess

- Coma
- Cardiac arrest

Hypomagnesemia. Hypomagnesia develops when blood levels fall below 1.5 mEq/L. A decrease in magnesium often parallels decreased potassium, because if the magnesium level is low, the kidneys tend to excrete more potassium. Hypomagnesemia presents signs and symptoms of increased neuromuscular irritability similar to those observed with hypocalcemia (Box 28-7). The major causes of low magnesium are increased excretion by the kidneys, impaired absorption from the GI tract, and prolonged malnutrition.

Hypermagnesemia. Hypermagnesemia develops when blood levels exceed 2.5 mEq/L. It rarely occurs when kidney function is normal. The three major causes are impaired renal function, excess magnesium administration, and diabetic ketoacidosis when there is severe water loss (Box 28-8). An excess of magnesium severely restricts nerve and muscle activity.

Bicarbonate

The normal level of **bicarbonate** (HCO_3), a main anion of the extracellular fluid, is 22 to 24 mEq/L. It is an alkaline electrolyte whose major function is the regulation of the acid-base balance, also called acid-alkaline balance. Bicarbonate acts as a buffer to neutralize acids in the body and maintain the 20:1 bicarbonate:carbonic acid ratio needed to keep the body in homeostasis. The kidneys selectively regulate the amount of bicarbonate retained or excreted.

ACID-BASE BALANCE

Acid-base balance means homeostasis of the hydrogen ion (H^+) concentration in the body fluids. The hydrogen ion concentration is determined by the ratio of carbonic acid (H_2CO_3) to bicarbonate (HCO_3) in the extracellular fluid. The ratio needed for homeostasis is 1 part carbonic acid to 20 parts bicarbonate. The symbol used to indicate hydrogen ion balance is pH. When pH is measured, it is the hydrogen ion concentration in the body that is measured. A sample of extracellular fluid, specifically arterial blood, is used to measure pH.

Arterial blood gases will determine if a solution is acid, neutral, or alkaline. The more hydrogen ions in a solution, the more acid the solution. The fewer hydrogen ions in a solution, the more alkaline the solution. The terms *base* and *alkaline* are interchangeable: a base is an alkaline substance. An inverse relationship exists between hydrogen ion concentration and the pH level: as the hydrogen ion numbers increase, the acidity of the solution increases and the pH decreases. The opposite happens with alkalinity: the number of hydrogen ions decreases and the pH increases. A pH of less than 7.35 is acid. A pH of greater than 7.45 is alkaline. The normal pH of arterial blood is approximately 7.45, whereas the normal pH of

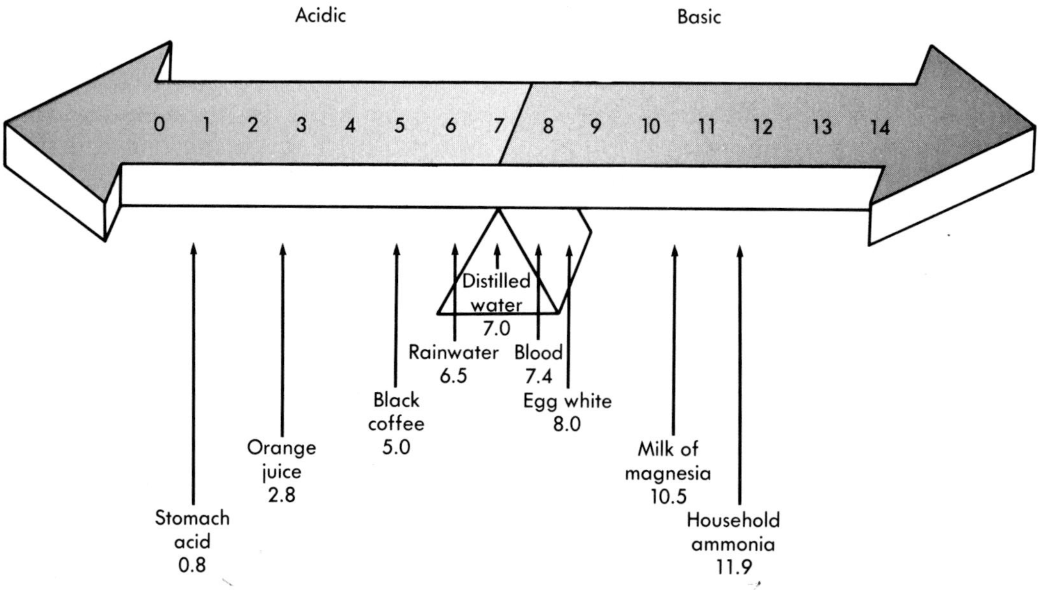

FIG. 28-6 The pH scale. A pH of 7 is considered neutral, so the scale is depicted as balancing at that point. Values to the left (below 7) are acidic (the lower the number, the more acidic). Values to the right (above 7) are basic (the higher the number, the more basic). Representative fluids and their approximate pHs are listed below the figure.

venous blood and interstitial fluid is approximately 7.35. Between 7.35 and 7.45 is considered normal blood pH (Fig. 28-6).

There are two general types of disturbances that can cause a pH imbalance. One imbalance adds or subtracts the base substance—bicarbonate. The other imbalance adds or subtracts the acid substance—carbonic acid. The body's metabolism affects the base side of balance, so a bicarbonate imbalance causes metabolic acidosis or alkalosis. The body's respiratory system affects the acid side of the balance, so a carbonic acid imbalance causes respiratory acidosis or alkalosis. Fig. 28-7 shows carbonic acid/bicarbonate ratio and pH.

The body has three systems that work to keep the pH in the narrow range of normal: the blood buffers, the respiratory system, and the kidneys. These systems are

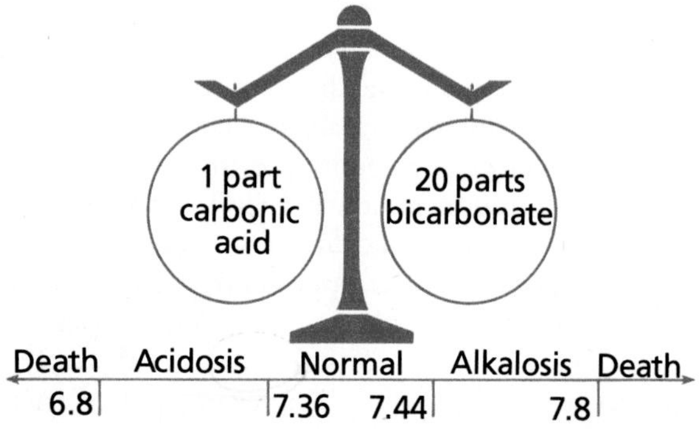

FIG. 28-7 Carbonic acid/bicarbonate ratio and pH.

the body's three lines of defense that are constantly working to maintain a normal pH.

The blood **buffers** can be considered chemical sponges. They circulate throughout the body in pairs, neutralizing excess acids or alkalines by contributing or accepting hydrogen ions. One buffer will dominate if the solution is too acid; the other if the solution is too alkaline. They work within a fraction of a second to prevent an excessive change in the hydrogen ion concentration. There are four major buffer systems in the body. The bicarbonate/carbonic acid system is the most important. Others are the phosphates, proteins, and hemoglobin buffer systems.

For every 1 million hydrogen ions that enter the body, the buffer systems can neutralize all but five! Once they are exhausted, they call on the second line of defense: the lungs. By speeding up or slowing down respirations, the lungs can increase or decrease the amount of carbon dioxide in the blood. When carbon dioxide is removed from the blood, the carbonic acid level is lowered. Where it took seconds for the buffer systems to work, it takes minutes for the lungs to begin to adjust the pH. Even though the respiratory system is slower than the buffers, the lungs can eliminate large amounts of acid from the body in the form of carbon dioxide. The respiratory system regulates pH by removing carbon dioxide from the blood. Just enough carbon dioxide is retained in the blood to maintain a normal pH level. If the pH drops suddenly from the normal range of 7.35 to 7.45 to 7.0, the respiratory system can return the pH to about 7.2 to 7.3 within 1 minute. The respiratory center in the brain provides the stimulus to increase respirations; however, as the hydrogen ion concentration approaches normal, the stimulus is lost. The buffers will assist in returning the level to the normal range.

The third line of defense is the kidneys. The role of the lungs in coping with an imbalance is simple: we breathe either slower or faster. The kidneys have much selective control. They can excrete varying amounts of acid or base. If the acidity of blood rises above normal, the kidneys will selectively eliminate more acids so the hydrogen ion concentration increases in the blood. If the blood becomes too alkaline, the kidneys will selectively eliminate more bases, especially bicarbonate. Normal urine is acidic because the body produces excess acids in the metabolic processes that occur continuously in the body. The kidneys are the slowest of the systems, but they are efficient enough to return the pH to exactly normal. Their response takes hours to days.

The three systems work closely together to maintain a normal hydrogen ion concentration. The buffers are immediate and continuous in contributing or accepting hydrogen ions. The respiratory system can come into play within minutes, regulating the carbon dioxide level in the blood and thus controlling carbonic acid. The kidneys are the third line of defense, and although they work more slowly than the other two systems, they can eliminate either hydrogen ions or bicarbonate ions, which means they can either increase or decrease pH.

ACID-BASE IMBALANCES

Acid-base balance means homeostasis of the hydrogen ion concentration. An upset in acid-base balance results in either acidosis or alkalosis. When blood pH is below 7.35 acidosis exists; when blood pH is above 7.45, alkalosis exists. The lungs and the kidneys are the two major organs responsible for regulation of the acid and base substances in the body. When imbalances occur, they represent an imbalance in the function of the lungs, kidneys, or both.

There are four primary types of acid-base imbalances: respiratory acidosis, respiratory alkalosis, metabolic acidosis, and metabolic alkalosis.

Respiratory Acidosis

Any condition that impairs a normal ventilation causes respiratory acidosis (Box 28-9). A retention of carbon dioxide occurs with a resultant increase of carbonic acid in the blood. As pH falls and the normal 1:20 carbonic acid:bicarbonate ratio is upset, the PCO_2 (partial carbon dioxide) level increases. Shallow respirations result because of the retained carbon dioxide. The patient will also experience a depression of central nervous system activity. Because the lungs are responsible for the respiratory parameters of the acid-base balance, the kidneys, which are responsible for the metabolic parameters, will attempt to compensate by retaining the base substance bicarbonate.

Treatment for respiratory acidosis is aimed at improving ventilation. The primary goal is to support the patient's respirations. Intermittent positive-pressure breathing (IPPB) to assist in exhaling carbon dioxide, antibiotic for any respiratory infection, adequate hydration (2 to 3 L/day) to keep the mucous membranes moist and aid in removal of secretions, and bronchodilators to help reduce bronchial spasms may be part of the treatment regimen. Therapy is also directed at correcting the primary condition responsible for the imbalance.

BOX 28-9 CAUSES AND COMMON CLINICAL SIGNS AND SYMPTOMS OF RESPIRATORY ACIDOSIS

CAUSES

- Pneumonia
- Respiratory failure
- Atelectasis
- Drug overdose
- Paralysis of respiratory muscles (Guillain-Barré syndrome, poliomyelitis, myasthenia gravis)
- Traumatic injuries to the thorax (flail chest)
- Obesity
- Airway obstruction
- Head injuries
- Cerebrovascular accident (stroke)
- Drowning
- Cystic fibrosis

COMMON CLINICAL SIGNS AND SYMPTOMS

Central Nervous System
- Lethargy
- Confusion
- Occipital headache
- Dizziness
- Decreasing level of consciousness

Cardiopulmonary System
- Dyspnea
- Tachycardia
- Hypertension
- Cardiac dysrhythmias

Musculoskeletal System
- Tremors
- Weakness

LABORATORY DATA

- pH less than 7.36
- $PaCO_2$ greater than 44 mm Hg (unless the patient has chronic obstructive pulmonary disease)
- PaO_2 normal or below 80 mm Hg, depending on severity of acidosis
- O_2 saturation normal or below 95%, depending on severity of acidosis
- HCO_3 normal in early respiratory acidosis
- K^+ above 5.5 mEq/L

BOX 28-10 **CAUSES AND COMMON CLINICAL SIGNS AND SYMPTOMS OF RESPIRATORY ALKALOSIS**

CAUSES

- Anxiety
- Fear
- Anemia
- Hypermetabolic states
- Disorders of the central nervous system (head injuries, infections)
- Drugs (aspirin overdose)
- Asthma
- Pneumonia
- Inappropriate mechanical ventilator settings

COMMON CLINICAL SIGNS AND SYMPTOMS

Central Nervous System
- Anxious appearance
- Irritability
- Tingling of the extremities
- Fainting
- Dizziness

Cardiopulmonary System
- Tachypnea
- Cardiac dysrhythmias

Musculoskeletal System
- Tetany
- Muscle weakness

LABORATORY DATA

- pH 7.44 or greater
- $Paco_2$ less than 36 mm Hg
- Pao_2 normal
- O_2 saturation normal
- HCO_3 normal
- K^+ below 3.5 mEq/L

Respiratory Alkalosis

Respiratory alkalosis is caused by hyperventilation (Box 28-10). Respirations that increase in rate, depth, or both can result in the loss of excessive amounts of carbon dioxide with a resultant lowering of the carbonic acid level in the blood. The pH rises because of the decrease in carbonic acid being "blown off" with each exhalation.

The common treatment for respiratory alkalosis is sedation and reassurance. If the cause is anxiety, the patient should be made aware of his abnormal breathing pattern. The patient should be instructed to breathe slowly to retain and accumulate carbon dioxide in the body. Another effective treatment is for the patient to breathe into a paper bag, which will cause rebreathing of the exhaled carbon dioxide.

BOX 28-11 **CAUSES AND COMMON CLINICAL SIGNS AND SYMPTOMS OF METABOLIC ACIDOSIS**

CAUSES

- Starvation
- Dehydration
- Diabetic ketoacidosis
- Renal failure
- Shock
- Diarrhea
- Drugs (methanol, ethanol, formic acid, paraldehyde, aspirin)
- Renal tubular acidosis

COMMON CLINICAL SIGNS AND SYMPTOMS

Central Nervous System
- Lethargy
- Headache
- Decreasing level of consciousness

Cardiopulmonary System
- Kussmaul respirations
- Cardiac dysrhythmias

Gastrointestinal System
- Anorexia
- Nausea
- Vomiting
- Diarrhea

Musculoskeletal System
- Weakness

LABORATORY DATA

- pH less than 7.36
- $Paco_2$ normal, or less than 36 mm Hg if lungs are compensating
- Pao_2 normal, or less than 36 mm Hg if lungs are compensating
- O_2 saturation normal
- HCO_3 below 22 mEq/L
- K^+ above 5.5 mEq/L

Metabolic Acidosis

Metabolic acidosis can result from a gain of hydrogen ions or a loss of bicarbonate; in other words, retaining too many acids (H^+ ions) or losing too many bases (HCO_3^-) (Box 28-11). Without sufficient bases, the pH of the blood falls below the normal 7.35 to 7.45. With the loss of base substances, the bicarbonate level will also drop. The effect of metabolic acidosis is hyperventilation, as the lungs attempt to compensate by blowing off carbon dioxide to lower the Pco_2 level. There are many causes of metabolic acidosis. Administration of sodium bicarbonate is the usual treatment for acidosis.

BOX 28-12

CAUSES AND COMMON CLINICAL SIGNS AND SYMPTOMS OF METABOLIC ALKALOSIS

CAUSES

- Excessive vomiting
- Prolonged gastric suctioning
- Electrolyte disturbance
- Cushing's disease
- Drugs (steroids, sodium bicarbonate, diuretics)
- Hyperaldosteronism

COMMON CLINICAL SIGNS AND SYMPTOMS

Central Nervous System

- Headache
- Irritability
- Lethargy
- Decreases in level of consciousness

Cardiopulmonary System

- Atrial tachycardia
- Slow, shallow respirations with periods of apnea
- Bradycardia

Gastrointestinal System

- Nausea
- Vomiting

Musculoskeletal System

- Numbness and tingling of extremities
- Hypertonicity of muscles
- Tetany

LABORATORY DATA

- pH greater than 7.44
- $Paco_2$ normal or greater than 44 mm Hg if lungs are compensating
- Pao_2 normal
- O_2 saturation normal
- HCO_3 above 26 mEq/L
- K^+ less than 3.5 mEq/L

Metabolic Alkalosis

Metabolic alkalosis results when a significant amount of acid is lost from the body or an increase in the bicarbonate level occurs (Box 28-12). The most common cause of metabolic alkalosis is vomiting gastric content, normally high in acid. Metabolic alkalosis can occur also in patients who ingest excess amounts of alkaline agents, such as bicarbonate-containing antacids, for example, Alka-Seltzer or soda bicarbonate. Metabolic alkalosis depresses the central nervous system. Again, as with the other acid-base imbalances, treatment is aimed at the cause.

REFERENCES AND SUGGESTED READINGS

1. Barta MA: Correcting electrolyte imbalances, RN 2:30, 1987.
2. Brunner LS: Textbook of medical-surgical nursing, ed 6, Philadelphia, 1988, JB Lippincott Co.
3. Calloway C: When the problem involves magnesium, calcium, or phosphate, RN 5:30, 1987.
4. Chambers JK: Common fluid and electrolyte disorders, Nurs Clin North Am 22(4):749, 1987.
5. Groer MW: Basic pathophysiology: a holistic approach, ed 3, St Louis, 1989, The CV Mosby Co.
6. Long BC: Medical-surgical nursing: nursing process approach, ed 2, St Louis, 1989, The CV Mosby Co.
7. Metheney NM: Fluid and electrolyte balance: nursing considerations, Philadelphia, 1987, JB Lippincott Co.
8. Potter PA and Perry AG: Fundamentals of nursing: concepts, process, and practice, ed 2, St Louis, 1989, The CV Mosby Co.
9. Weldy NJ: Body fluids and electrolytes: a programmed presentation, ed 5, St Louis, 1988, The CV Mosby Co.

CHAPTER CHALLENGE

KEY POINTS

- Water is the primary fluid in the body.
- The two fluid compartments are the intracellular and extracellular compartments. The extracellular compartment is composed of the interstitial and intravascular areas.
- Fluid movement takes place by means of three passive transport systems: diffusion, osmosis, and filtration; and one active transport system: active transport by ATP energy.
- Electrolytes are chemical compounds that carry either a positive or negative charge. Positive ions are called cations; negative ions are called anions. To maintain homeostasis, the cations and anions must balance each other in the body fluids.
- Sodium is the major extracellular cation in the body. Water follows sodium as it moves from one fluid compartment to another.
- Potassium is the major intracellular cation in the body. Imbalances in potassium, either high or low levels, may cause life-threatening cardiac conditions.
- The four acid-base imbalances are respiratory acidosis, respiratory alkalosis, metabolic acidosis, and metabolic alkalosis.
- Any process that interferes with normal ventilation and causes a decrease or increase in the excretion of volatile acids can cause respiratory acidosis or respiratory alkalosis.
- Any process that interferes with normal production or excretion of nonvolatile hydrogen ions can cause metabolic acidosis or metabolic alkalosis.
- The lungs are responsible for the regulation of respiratory acidosis or alkalosis. The kidneys are responsible for the regulation of metabolic acidosis or alkalosis.
- When an imbalance causes respiratory acidosis or alkalosis, the kidneys attempt to compensate. When an imbalance causes metabolic acidosis or alkalosis, the lungs attempt to compensate.

STUDY QUESTIONS

1. The major percentage of body weight is:
   a. Muscle mass
   b. Water
   c. Adipose tissue
   d. Bone
2. Which is the larger of the two fluid compartments in the body:
   a. Intracellular
   b. Extracellular
3. All of the following patients are at a higher risk for developing a fluid volume deficit except:
   a. Obese patient
   b. Elderly patient
   c. Infant patient
   d. Thin patient
4. The movement of glucose into the cells occurs through the process of:
   a. Active transport
   b. Passive transport
5. Diffusion, osmosis, and filtration are all examples of:
   a. Active transport
   b. Passive transport
6. A relative constancy in the internal environment of the body, naturally maintained by adaptive responses that promote healthy survival, is called:
   a. ATP (adenosine triphosphate)
   b. Hydrostatic pressure
   c. Hypotonic solution
   d. Homeostasis
7. The electrolytes sodium, potassium, calcium, and magnesium are examples of:
   a. Cations
   b. Anions
8. The symbol used to indicate hydrogen ion concentration in the body that is measured is called:
   a. mEq
   b. ATP
   c. pH
   d. Krebs cycle
9. If acidosis develops in a patient, the hydrogen ion would be represented as:
   a. 7.35
   b. 7.10
   c. 7.48
   d. 7.50
10. Which of the three regulatory systems is the third line of defense to keep the body's pH level within the normal range:
    a. Buffers in the blood
    b. Respiratory system
    c. Kidneys
11. Hypokalemia or hyperkalemia is serious because it affects the:
    a. Heart muscle
    b. Lungs
    c. Nervous system
12. List the fluid compartments in the body, from the largest to the smallest.
13. Why is an infant or a geriatric patient at a higher risk for developing a fluid imbalance?
14. How does the movement of fluids and electrolytes via active transport differ from the other fluid movement methods?
15. How does glucose enter the peripheral tissue cells?
16. What effect on the cell does a hypertonic solution have? a hypotonic solution? an isotonic solution?
17. What is the symbol for the measurement of hydrogen ions?
18. What happens to the H^+ ion concentration when acidosis develops? when alkalosis develops?
19. Which of the three regulatory systems is the first line of defense to keep the body's pH level within the normal range? What happens when that regulatory system needs help?
20. Name five foods high in potassium.
21. What would you teach a patient experiencing respiratory alkalosis?

29

Care of the Patient with an Integumentary Disorder

LINDA NORTH

LEARNING OBJECTIVES

After reading this chapter, the student should be able to do the following:

- Define the key terms.
- List and discuss the three functions of the skin.
- Describe the differences between epidermis and dermis.
- List the three major types of glands located in the skin and discuss their functions.
- State general nursing interventions for the patient with a skin disorder.
- Identify the nursing interventions needed to meet the emotional needs of a patient with a skin disorder.
- Differentiate between type I and type II herpes.
- Discuss nursing interventions for the patient with impetigo contagiosa.
- List three nursing diagnoses for the patient with acne.
- State five important interventions in order of priority in the emergent phase of a major burn.
- State how to classify burns according to depth and surface body area involved.
- Identify the nursing interventions for each phase of burn care to prevent complications and promote homeostasis.
- List the primary patient and family education areas in discharge planning for the burn patient.

RELATED TOPICS OF INTEREST

- Signs, symptoms, and physical assessment (Chapter 13)
- Diet therapy (Chapter 23)
- Cells, tissues, and membranes (Chapter 27)
- Fluids and electrolytes (Chapter 28)
- Care of the patient with a urinary disorder (Chapter 33)
- Care of the patient with an immune disorder (Chapter 39)

KEY TERMS

Define the following:

- alopecia
- autograft
- ceruminous gland
- contracture
- corium
- corticosteroid
- Curling's ulcer
- débridement
- epidermis
- eschar
- excoriation
- exudate
- heterograft (xenograft)
- homograft (allograft)
- integument
- keloids
- macule
- melanin
- nevi
- papule
- pediculosis
- pruritus
- pustulant vesicles
- rule of nines
- scale
- sebaceous
- sebum
- sudoriferous
- suppuration
- urticaria
- verruca
- vesicle
- wheal

The skin, or **integument,** is the outer covering of the body, and together with its appendages—the hair, nails, and special glands—makes up the integumentary system. Society has long held healthy skin in high esteem, probably because it is so easily viewed by others. People spend many hours grooming their hair, cleansing their skin, and manicuring their nails. A closer look reveals that the integument is really the body's protector—its first line of defense against infection and injury. It is pliable yet tough, it resists abrasions, and as it wears, it is constantly renewed from layers directly beneath it. It also insulates and cushions deeper organs. It functions in the prevention of loss of body fluids and in the regulation of body temperature. The skin also is the sensory contact with the environment: it is sensitive to heat, cold, touch, pressure, and pain.

ANATOMY AND PHYSIOLOGY

Functions of the Skin

Even though the skin covers the outside of the body, its main function is homeostasis and protection of the internal organs (Box 29-1). Daily it is subjected to temperature and humidity changes, trauma, ecchymosis, abrasions, contact with pathogens, and wear and tear. In an attempt to protect and maintain the body, the skin carries out the following functions.

Protection. Within the skin are sensory receptors that receive information about the environment. Messages about heat, cold, pain, pressure, and touch are received and relayed to the central nervous system for interpretation. As long as the skin remains intact it is resistant to many bacteria and fungi present in the environment. Healthy skin also protects the body from absorbing many chemicals and foreign substances. A layer of adipose tissue (fat) cushions internal organs and provides reserve energy sources.

Temperature regulation. Skin assists the body to maintain a constant temperature under varying internal and external conditions. It accomplishes this by allowing blood vessels near the surface to constrict when the environment is cold to preserve heat and allowing them to dilate when it is hot to release excess body heat. Sweat glands release moisture, which results in cooling as the moisture is evaporated. A layer of adipose tissue works as an insulator by retaining heat.

Vitamin D synthesis. Cholesterol compounds located in the skin are converted to vitamin D when exposed to the ultraviolet rays of the sun. This vitamin is necessary for healthy bone development. Prolonged exposure to the sun's rays should be avoided because of the increased possibility of development of skin cancer.

BOX 29-1 FUNCTIONS OF THE SKIN

Protection from environment: pathogenic organisms, foreign substances, heat rays

Heat regulation

- Conduction: transfer of heat by direct contact to other objects or air
- Convection: removal of heat by air currents on skin
- Evaporation: removal of heat by water loss from skin surface

Sensory perception: sensory receptors in skin
Excretion: removal of water and electrolytes
Production of vitamin D: effect of sunlight

Basic Structure of the Skin

Skin consists of two layers: the outermost epidermis and the inner dermis or corium. Beneath these layers of skin lies the subcutaneous layer, or superficial fascia (Fig. 29-1).

Epidermis. The **epidermis** is composed of stratified squamous (from Latin *squama,* scale) epithelium. It is divided into layers, or strata. The cells of the epidermis are tightly packed without any distinct blood supply. The innermost layer is called the *stratum germinativum;* it is the only stratum of the epidermis that is able to undergo cell division and reproduce itself. It receives its blood supply and nutrition from the underlying dermis through the process called diffusion. This provides a constant new supply of cells for the upper strata and also enables the skin to repair itself from injury. As these cells are pushed to the surface, they undergo a series of changes. The internal structures of the cells are destroyed and the cells die. When they reach the outermost layer, called the *stratum corneum,* they have become flat and the cell structure

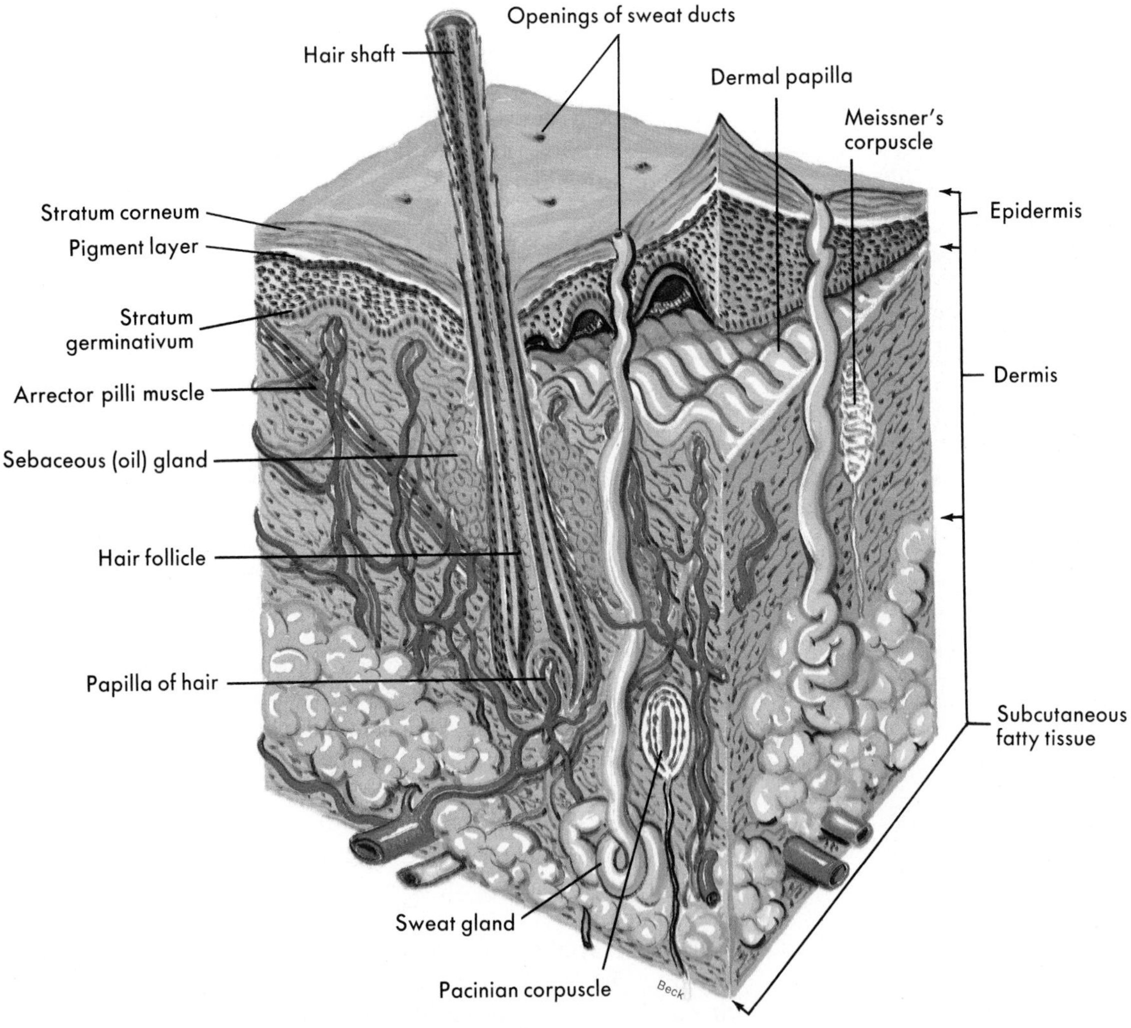

FIG. 29-1 Microscopic view of the skin in longitudinal section. The epidermis is shown raised at one corner to reveal the ridges in the dermis.

has become filled with a protein called *keratin* (horn), sometimes referred to as the horny layer. The keratin makes the cells dry, tough, and somewhat waterproof. There are several layers of these cells, and they are continually sloughing off, only to be replaced by new ones. From the birth of the new cell in the stratum germinativum to the death and sloughing off in the stratum corneum, the cell undergoes many changes. This whole process takes approximately 1 month. Another stratum in the epidermis contains highly specialized cells called *melanocytes;* these cells give rise to the pigment called **melanin,** which is responsible for skin color. The greater the concentration of melanin, the darker the color of the skin. Sometimes irregular patches of concentrations of melanin occur producing "freckles." The amount of melanin a person has is inherited from his parents. Although skin color is inherited, exposure to the sun and other extraneous factors can influence skin color.

Occasionally an individual has an inherited inability to produce melanin. This results in a condition called *albinism.* An individual who has this condition is called an *albino* and has an absence of color in the skin, hair, and eyes.

Carotene, another pigment, can be found in the stratum corneum in persons of Asian descent. Carotene, along with melanin, gives rise to the yellow hue of the skin.

On the soles of the feet, palms of the hands, and tips of fingers and toes, there is a series of ridges and grooves that develop in utero, during the third and fourth month of fetal development. These grooves and ridges are genetically determined and unique to each individual. Their function is to increase gripping ability. Because they are unique, footprints and fingerprints may be used for identification purposes.

Dermis. The dermis or **corium** is often referred to as the true skin. It is well supplied with blood vessels and nerves and also contains glands and hair follicles. It varies in thickness throughout the body but tends to be very thick in the palms and soles. The dermis is composed of connective tissue with the cells scattered among collagen and elastic fibers. The collagen gives strength to the dermis, while the elastic connective fibers give it flexibility. The cells throughout this layer are bathed in tissue fluid called interstitial fluid. With the normal aging process the dermis loses some of its elastic connective fibers, and the subcutaneous tissue directly beneath it loses some of its adipose tissue: wrinkling of the skin results. Located in the upper portion of the dermis are small, fingerlike projections called *papillae* that actually project into the lower epidermal layer. They contain many capillaries that allow oxygen and nutrient exchange within the epidermal layer. Without the dermal papillae, the epidermal layer would be unable to survive.

Subcutaneous layer. The subcutaneous layer, sometimes called the *superficial fascia,* is the layer of tissue directly beneath the dermis that connects the skin to the muscle surfaces. This layer is composed of adipose tissue and loose connective tissue. It serves several important functions:

1. It stores water and fat.
2. It insulates the body by virtue of its composition.
3. It serves as a shock absorber, protecting tissues and organs lying beneath it.
4. It serves as a pathway for nerves and vessels.

The distribution of subcutaneous tissue throughout the body provides shape and contour. A woman's body usually contains more subcutaneous tissue than a man's; thus her body is softer and more rounded.

Glands of the skin. There are two basic types of glands associated with the integumentary system: sudoriferous and sebaceous gland.

Sudoriferous glands. The **sudoriferous** (sweat) glands are coiled, tubelike structures located in the dermis and subcutaneous layers. The tubes open into pores on the surface of the skin. There are approximately 3 million sweat glands located throughout the body. These glands excrete sweat, resulting in cooling of the body surface. Sweat is composed of water, salts, urea, uric acid, ammonia, sugar, lactic acid, and ascorbic acid. These glands can be classified in two groups according to location and secretion. *Eccrine* glands are the most numerous and are located throughout the body. They secrete a clear, watery sweat through pores on the surface of the body. *Aprocrine* glands are located in the axillary and genital region and secrete a more milky-type secretion through excretory ducts that open into the hair follicles.

Ceruminous glands are modified sudoriferous glands. They secrete a waxlike substance called *cerumen* and are located in the external ear canal. It is thought that cerumen protects the canal from foreign body invasion.

Sebaceous glands. The **sebaceous** (oil) glands secrete their oily substance, **sebum,** through the hair follicles distributed over the body. Their function is to lubricate the skin and hair covering the body. Sebum also inhibits the growth of bacteria. During puberty, as blood levels of sex hormones increase, the amount of sebum secreted also increases.

Skin Appendages

Hair. Hair is composed of modified dead epidermal tissue, mainly keratin. It is distributed all over the body in varying amounts. The root of the hair is enclosed in a follicle deep in the dermis. The shaft of the hair protrudes from the skin. Surrounding the hair follicle is a band of muscle tissue called *arrector pili* (Fig. 29-2). A sensation of cold or fear causes these muscles to contract; the hair stands upright, and the skin surrounding it be-

FIG. 29-2 Hair follicle. Relationship of a hair follicle and related structures to the epidermal and dermal layers of the skin.

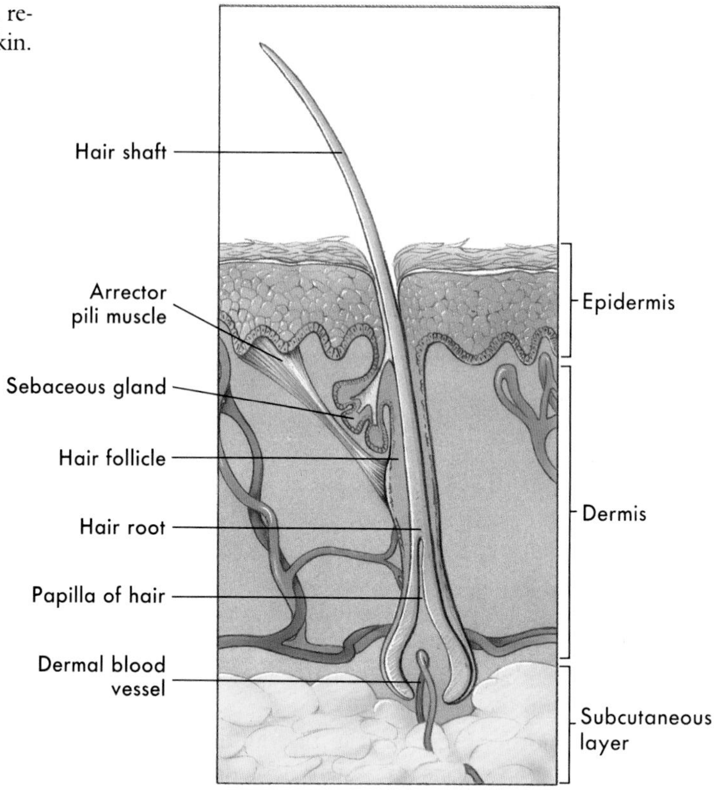

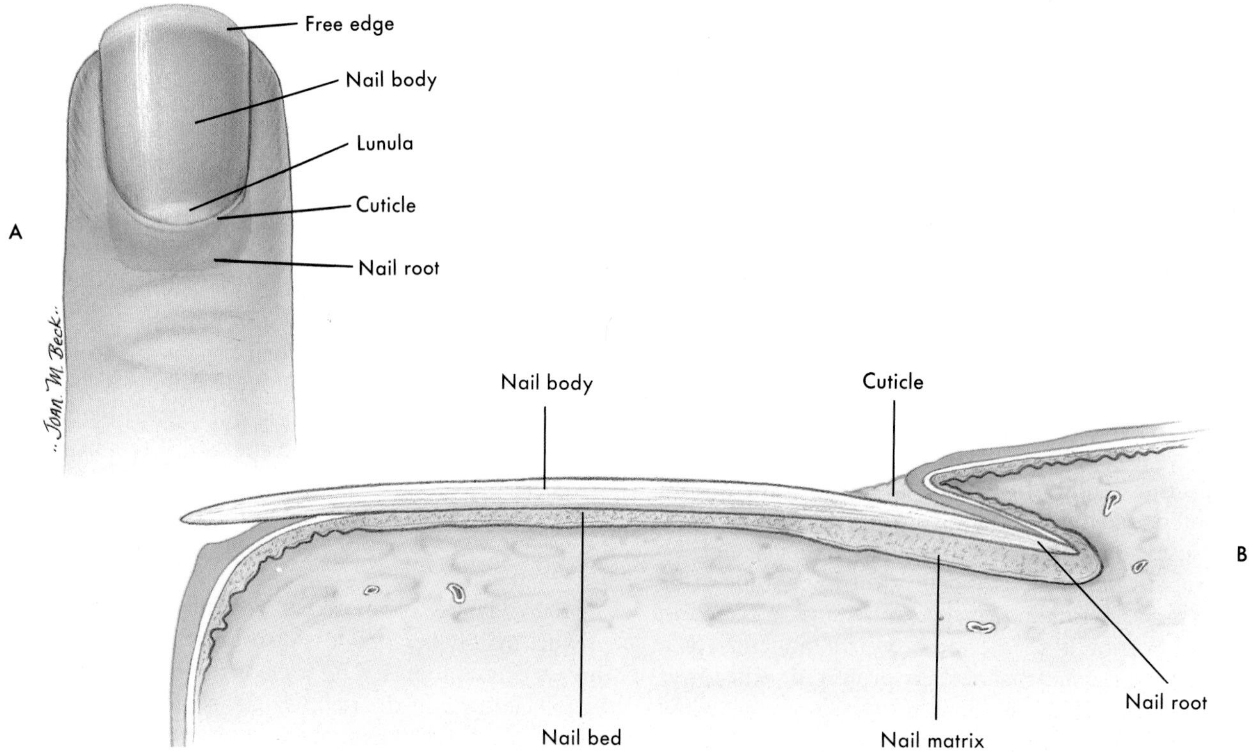

FIG. 29-3 Structure of nails. **A,** Fingernail viewed from above. **B,** Sagittal section of fingernail and associated structures.

comes dimpled. This effect is described as "hair standing on end" and "goose flesh."

Nails. Nails are also composed mainly of keratin, but it is more closely compressed. The base of the nail, the root, is composed of living cells and is mostly covered by the cuticle. Part of the root, the lunula, is exposed and looks like a white crescent. The remainder of the nail is called the *nail body*. It appears pink because of the blood vessels lying immediately beneath it (Fig. 29-3).

GENERAL ASSESSMENT

Assessment of the skin is an important nursing skill, because the skin is a patient's primary defense mechanism. The nurse needs to be aware of normal functions to accurately assess nursing problems.

The nurse should use all senses to assess the patient's skin, using the skills of inspection and palpation. Morning care (the bath) provides an excellent opportunity for the nurse to assess the skin without exposure or embarrassment of the patient.

Nurses should observe the skin for color. The color of the skin depends on many physiological factors including the following:

1. The amount of hemoglobin in the blood
2. The oxygen saturation in the blood
3. The amount of such substances as bilirubin, urea, or other chemicals in the blood
4. The quality of blood circulating in the superficial blood vessels
5. The amount of melanin in the epidermis

Assessment also includes the presence of rashes, scars, lesions, or ecchymoses, and distribution of hair. Temperature and texture should be assessed by touch using the palms of the hands to compare opposite body areas. For example, the nurse should feel both legs before stating that the left leg is cold. Using a sharp needle to touch the sole of the foot provides a means to assess sensation. The nails should be inspected for normal development, color, shape, and thickness. Clubbing (broadening) of the fingertips indicates decreased oxygen and should be reported. The hair should be inspected for thickness, dryness, or dullness. Assessment also includes inspecting the mucous membranes for pallor or cyanosis. Profuse sweating or any sign of impaired skin integrity needs to be documented. The ceruminous and sebaceous glands should be inspected for overactivity or underactivity using appropriate questions, such as "Tell me how often the physician has had to remove the wax from your ears."

If lesions are found, the exact location, length, width, and general appearance should be documented. Proper identification serves as a baseline for making evaluations of nursing interventions.

Specific types of skin lesions, their appearance, location, and duration also assist the dermatologist to diagnose a skin disorder. Primary signs and symptoms should be evaluated to identify (1) provocative and palliative factors, (2) the quality or quantity (characteristics and size) of the lesion, (3) specific region of the body, (4) severity of the signs and symptoms, and (5) the length of time the patient has had the disorder. A simple way to remember this assessment technique is to remember these letters:

P Provocative/palliative
Q Quality or quantity
R Region
S Severity
T Time

The aim of skin care should be prevention through patient teaching. (Box 29-2)

Well-cared-for skin is a physiological, psychological, and social asset. Well-groomed skin supports self-esteem, social acceptance, and adjustment to life in society. How a person perceives himself is important to the development of a healthy personality.

BOX 29-2 PREVENTION OF SKIN DISORDERS

MAINTAINING HEALTHY SKIN

1. Avoid strong or harsh soaps or detergents.
2. Keep skin well hydrated; apply lubricating lotion or cream to dry areas after bathing.
3. Avoid scraping or stripping skin surface by dry razors or removal of tape.
4. Dry damp areas (such as between toes) well to prevent maceration of skin.
5. Wear loose clothing on hot days to permit loss of heat by evaporation.

AVOIDING CAUSATIVE AGENTS

1. Avoid agents that cause skin disorders in most persons, for example, poison ivy, excessive sunlight.
2. Avoid specific agents known to cause a skin disorder in self.
3. Use protective skin lotions when exposed to excessive sunlight.

OBSERVING SKIN CHANGES

1. Note and report changes in size, color, or general appearance of pigmented skin areas, particularly nevi.
2. Note and report changes in size and appearance of existing skin lesions.

AVOIDING SELF-TREATMENT

1. Do not use previously prescribed prescriptions on new or different skin lesions.
2. Seek medical advice when skin conditions develop.

Types of Skin Lesions

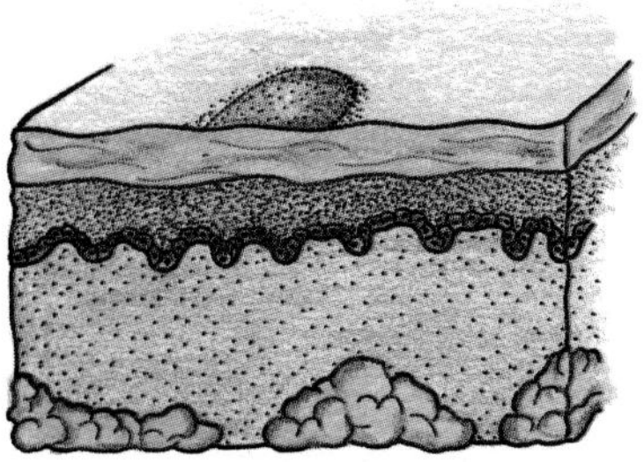

Macule flat, nonpalpable, change in skin color, smaller than 1 cm (for example, freckle, petechia).

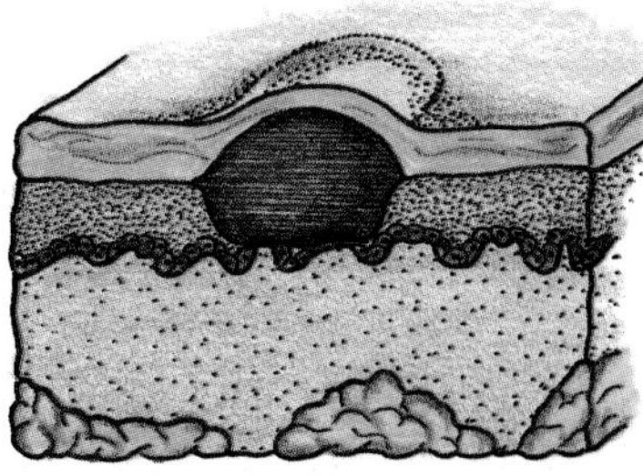

Papule: palpable, circumscribed, solid elevation in skin, smaller than 0.5 cm (for example, elevated nevus).

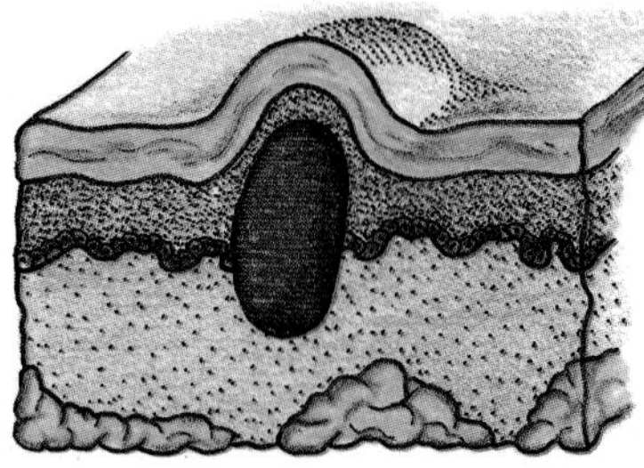

Nodule: elevated solid mass, deeper and firmer than papule, 0.5-0.2 cm (for example, wart).

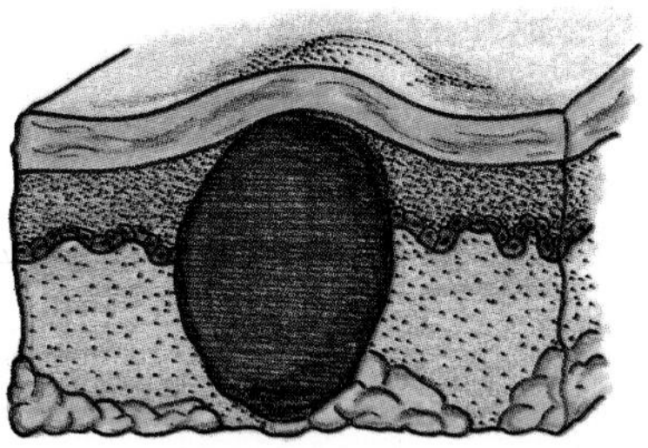

Tumor: solid mass that may extend deep through subcutaneous tissue, larger than 1-2 cm (for example, epithelioma).

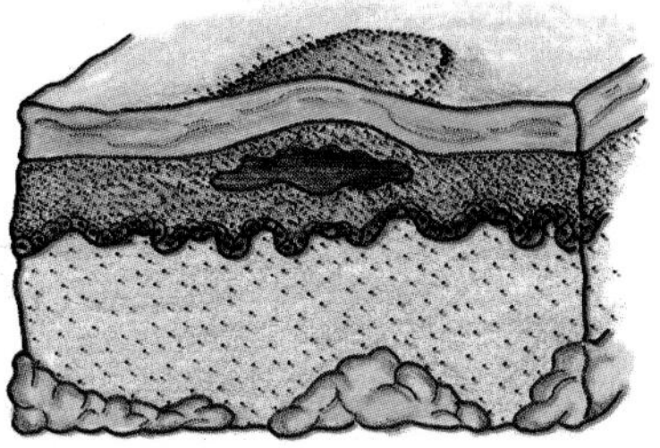

Wheal: irregularly shaped, elevated area or superficial localized edema, varies in size (for example, hive, mosquito bite).

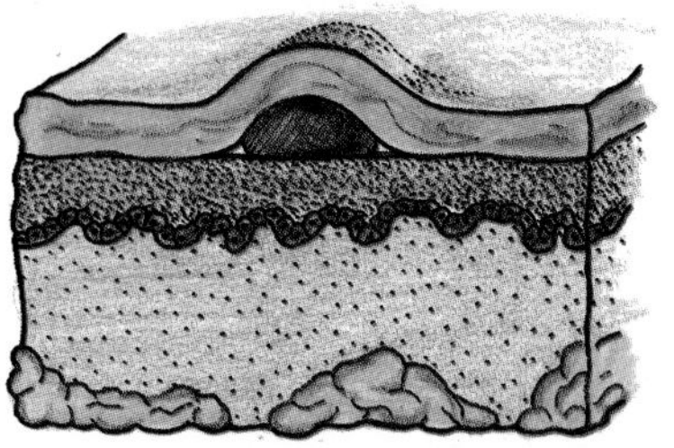

Vesicle: circumscribed elevation of skin filled with serous fluid, smaller than 0.5 cm (for example, herpes simplex, chickenpox).

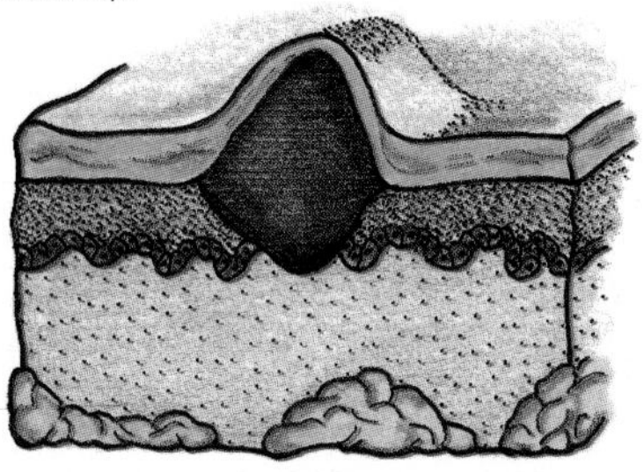

Pustule: circumscribed elevation of skin similar to vesicle but filled with pus, varies in size (for example, acne, staphylococcal infection).

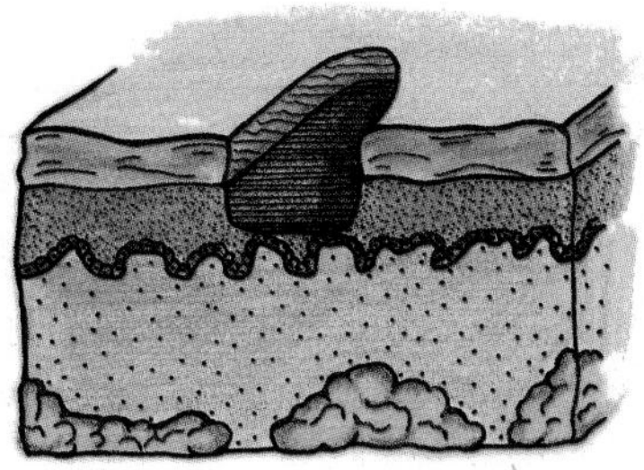

Ulcer: deep loss of skin surface that may extend to dermis and frequently bleeds and scars, varies in size (for example, venous stasis ulcer).

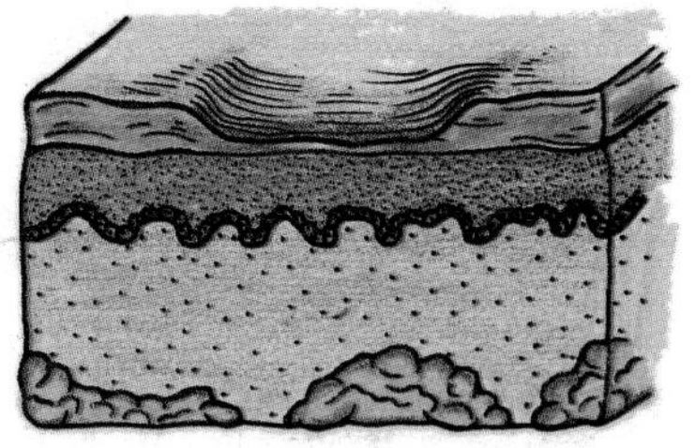

Atrophy: thinning of skin with loss of normal skin furrow with skin appearing shiny and translucent, varies in size (for example, arterial insufficiency).

Assessment and Description of Skin Lesions

Assessment of specific skin lesions, their appearance, and location assist the dermatologist to diagnose skin disorders and the nurse to provide care. Most disorders have only one or two types of lesions. Some of the typical clinical manifestations of skin disorders are shown and additional ones are listed below:

Atrophy: wasting or shrinkage of body tissue
Bleb: irregular, raised area of the skin filled with serous or seropurulent fluid; blebs can vary in size
Bulla: vesicle larger than 1 cm in diameter
Crust: dry area several layers thick; commonly called a **scale**
Fissure: crack or slit in the skin
Gumma: tumorlike lesion that resembles an abscess and is seen in late stages of syphilis
Nodule: raised, solid lesion

OVERVIEW OF NURSING INTERVENTIONS FOR THE SKIN

Nursing interventions for the patient with a skin disorder involve several basic nursing procedures. The principles involved in good hygiene are the foundation for skin care. Therapeutic baths, application of hot and cold, aseptic technique, sterile technique, surgical dressing changes, and application of topical medications are used.

Therapeutic baths (Table 29-1) are used to stimulate

Table 29-1 Preparations Commonly Used for Baths or Soaks

Substance	Effect	Suggested Actions
Colloids: oatmeal, cornstarch, soybean powder	Antipruritic, drying	Tub surfaces become very slippery; support person to prevent falls
Potassium permanganate	Antifungal, drying, deodorizing	Strain pulverized tablet through cheesecloth to prevent irritation; stains surfaces and linens
Burow's solution (aluminum acetate)	Antibacterial, drying	Commonly used for soaks
Sulfur bath suspension	Antibacterial	Rinse body with tepid water after bath to remove residual sulfur particles
Tar preparations	Antipruritic, moisturizing	Do not use soap with tar baths
Bath oils: Alpha-Keri, Jeri-Bath, Domol	Antipruritic, moisturizing	Tub surfaces may become slippery

circulation, remove transient bacteria, increase suppuration, or improve self-esteem. Specifically for the patient requiring skin care, the bath may be performed to cleanse, disinfect, deodorize, soften, lubricate, remove parasites, or soothe **pruritus** (the symptom of itching). Special soaps, oils, medications, and other substances are used, including oatmeal, starch, baking soda, vinegar, and bran.

The nurse responsible for bathing the patient needs to understand the rationale before the procedure is performed. Specific directions may need to be followed, such as adding the oatmeal directly under running water or to a gauze bag and placing it in the tub. The nurse's assessment of the situation is imperative if the goals of treatment are to be met.

The optimal temperature of the water ranges from 95° to 100° F (35° to 37.8° C). The tub should be thoroughly clean and full enough to cover the involved body area. Most therapeutic baths are done two to four times a day, lasting from 20 minutes to 1 hour each. When the bath is completed, the skin is patted dry, not rubbed. Safety measures should be followed to protect the patient from falling, chilling, or burning himself (Box 29-3).

Applications of hot and cold are used in the form of wet dressings. Wet dressings are used in skin diseases primarily to promote healing. The temperature of the solution needs to be monitored carefully to prevent further skin damage.

Wet dressings are used for a variety of reasons. The physician determines the type of wet dressing based on the goal to be achieved. Open wet dressings should be made from muslin, gauze, or fluffs (gauze that has been folded loosely to absorb exudate). Open lesions require sterile technique and proper wound management. Solutions that are frequently used are diluted sodium hypochlorite (Dakin's solution), 5% aluminum acetate (Burow's solution), and isotonic saline. Continuous wet dressings should be removed once every 6 to 8 hours to let the skin dry.

Soaks can be used to increase or decrease circulation, loosen or soften tissue, or promote **suppuration** (to produce purulent material). These are done three to four times a day. The solution and temperature will be determined by the physician.

BOX 29-3 GUIDELINES FOR BATHS AND SOAKS

1. The water temperature should be of comfort to patient—usually 90° to 100° F (32° to 38° C).
2. Medication should be completely dissolved while tub is filled.
3. The soak should last 20 to 30 minutes.
4. Persons are assisted out of the water when oils are added, to prevent slipping.
5. A rubber mat will help prevent slipping.
6. Skin is *patted* dry, not rubbed, to avoid skin irritation.
7. Creams or ointments are applied immediately after the bath to retain moisture.
8. After a medicated bath, pour 1 cup bleach into used tub water; let stand 5 minutes; wipe sides and bottom of tub; drain tub and clean as usual.

Emotional Aspects of Care

The person with a skin disorder may have a chronic or acute condition. Regardless of the severity, recovery may be a lengthy process that is visible to the patient—and others. The person's body image and self-esteem are affected. Society's reaction to a person has significant impact on him. Personal appearance is a primary concern to many individuals, and others may think the person is infectious and isolate him because of his appearance. The impact of a skin disease on a patient's self-concept can be detrimental because of the value society places on a person's physical characteristics.

The nurse needs to assess the patient's coping abilities

by encouraging him to talk and ventilate his feelings. Open-ended questions are used to facilitate communication. The nurse should validate and/or correct a patient's knowledge base. Rarely are skin diseases fatal, and very few are contagious. Nurses need to have worked through their own feelings about a patient's skin appearance before they can be a source of encouragement. The nurse's attitude and interventions should be nonjudgmental, warm, and accepting. The nurse must be skilled and knowledgeable about skin care.

VIRAL DISORDERS OF THE SKIN

Herpes Simplex

Etiology/pathophysiology. The herpetovirus *Herpesvirus hominis* is the cause of herpes simplex. Two types of the virus are known. Type 1, the most common, causes the common cold sore; type 2 is found in lesions in the genital area and is known as genital herpes. The viruses are self-limiting, and there is no cure. Type 1 is usually associated with febrile conditions.

Genital herpes can be transmitted by the mother to the baby during vaginal deliveries, causing death of the neonate. Transmission of the virus may occur by direct contact with any open lesion. The lesions are usually present for 2 to 3 weeks. The pain is most severe during the first week. Complications can be severe if the disease spreads to other body areas. The primary mode of transmission is unclean hands.

Clinical manifestations. Type 1 herpes simplex is characterized by a **vesicle** at the corner of the mouth, on the lips, or on the nose. It is commonly known as a "cold sore." The involved area is usually erythematous and edematous. The vesicle then appears, ulcerates, and encrusts. When the vesicle ruptures, a burning pain is felt. General malaise and fatigue are expressed by the patient. Usual occurrence is during an acute illness or infection.

Type 2, genital herpes, produces various types of vesicles that rupture and encrust, causing ulcerations. The cervix is the most common site in women, and the penis is the most common area in men. Flulike symptoms occur 3 to 4 days after the vesicles erupt. Headache, fatigue, myalgia, elevated temperature, and anorexia are common.

Assessment. Assessment primarily involves inspection of the skin. The nurse must obtain a good health history to support assessment data. Collection of *subjective data* will include complaints of fatigue; pruritus in the mouth for herpes simplex type 1, and in the genital area for herpes simplex type 2 (genital herpes); and complaints of a burning pain in the involved area.

Collection of *objective data* for herpes simplex type 1 will include an edematous, erythematous area at the corner of the lip. In herples simplex type 2 the labia, vulva, or penis will appear edematous and erythematous. The vesicular lesions may rupture and develop a dried **exudate.**

Diagnostic tests. Diagnosis of the herpes virus is made by laboratory assessment of cultures from the lesion. Inspection and health history also support the diagnosis.

Medical management. There is no cure for the herpes virus, but treatment is aimed at relieving symptoms. Acyclovir (Zovirax) is an antiviral agent that can alter the course of the disease. It can be administered orally, topically, or intravenously.

Nursing interventions. Nursing interventions are primarily directed toward treatment of symptoms and prevention of the spread of the disease. Hot, warm compresses can be used to relieve the pain and severe pruritus. The lesions should be kept dry and direct contact avoided. Analgesics such as acetaminophen (Tylenol) are effective in pain control. The specific nursing diagnoses for herpes are based on assessment data gathered.

NURSING DIAGNOSES	NURSING INTERVENTIONS
Pain, related to pruritus	Assess factors that precipitate pruritus. Apply local anesthetic, such as Orabase, for pain. Apply drying agent to lesions. Apply warm compresses. Patient should wear loose-fitting cotton clothing that will not constrict movement or occlude circulation.
Impaired skin integrity, related to open lesions	Inspect lesions for drainage, color, and location. Wash hands before and after contact. Keep area dry. Administer antiviral agents as ordered. In genital herpes use of a hair dryer can promote drying of the lesions and patient comfort.
Potential for infection, related to break in the skin	Assess for signs of infection, such as pyrexia. Practice aseptic handwashing and meticulous personal hygiene. Avoid use of occlusive ointments that prevent drying.
Knowledge deficit, related to cause and spread of the disease	Assess patient's level of understanding of the cause, treatment, and spread of the condition by using open-ended questions. Teach aseptic personal hygiene techniques. Instruct the patient that contact with the open lesions should be avoided. Stress the importance of proper follow-up care.

Patient teaching. The patient should be taught techniques to prevent the spread of the disease. He should be taught to use good hygiene in all areas of care. The complications and precipitating factors should be included in discharge planning.

Herpes Zoster (Shingles)

Etiology/pathophysiology. Herpes zoster is caused by the same virus that causes chicken pox (varicella) *(Herpes varicellae)*. The lesions are located along the nerve fibers of spinal ganglia.

Herpes zoster is commonly known as *shingles*. The virus causes an inflammation of the spinal ganglia. It is believed that the virus responsible for shingles lies dormant in patients until their resistance to infections has been lowered. The virus then advances to the skin by way of the peripheral nerves. At the skin surface, the virus multiplies and forms an erythematous rash of small vesicles along a spinal nerve pathway.

Clinical manifestations. The eruption of the vesicles is proceeded by pain. The rash generally occurs in the thoracic region; the vesicles erupt in a line along the involved nerve. The vesicles rupture and form a crust, and the serous fluid in the vesicle may become purulent. The virus can also effect the lumbar, cervical, or cranial areas. The course of this painful condition is from 7 to 28 days.

The pain associated with herpes zoster is severe; most patients describe the pain as burning and knifelike. Extreme tenderness and pruritus in the area are assessed. Patients with herpes zoster will request analgesic medications at frequent intervals.

Herpes zoster (shingles) is usually not permanently disabling to healthy adults. The greatest risk occurs to patients who have a lowered resistance to infection, such as those on chemotherapy or large doses of prednisone, in which the disease could be fatal.

Assessment. The assessment of the patient should include both the subjective and objective data. A good health history and thorough inspection skills are necessary to gather relevant data.

Collection of *subjective data* will include these symptoms: (1) sharp, burning pain, usually on one side only, (2) severe pruritus of the lesions, (3) general malaise, and (4) a history of chicken pox (varicella).

Collection of *objective data* includes: (1) evidence of skin excoriation related to scratching, (2) patches of vesicles on erythematous skin following a peripheral nerve pathway, and (3) demonstration of tenderness to touch.

Diagnostic tests. The diagnostic test for herpes zoster is a culture to isolate the virus. Other diagnostic measures are physical examinations and a thorough history obtained at admission.

Medical management. Medical interventions are directed at controlling the pain and preventing secondary complications. Analgesics are given for the pain; many times the pain requires narcotic analgesics such as codeine. Steroids may be given to decrease inflammation and edema. Lotions may be used to relieve pruritus and **corticosteroids** to relieve the pruritus and inflammation. Oral and intravenous acyclovir (Zovirax), administered early, has been found to reduce the pain and duration of the virus.

Nursing interventions. Nursing interventions are directed at relieving the patient's symptoms. Pain, pruritus, and the prevention of secondary complications are the primary concerns. Tranquilizers such as lorazepam (Ativan) and hydroxyzine HCl (Atarax) may be given to decrease the anxiety associated with severe pain. Analgesics are given to control pain. The nurse needs to understand and be able to apply the principles of pain management to provide nursing care. Medicated baths and warm compresses may be ordered to soothe the skin. The nurse will use aseptic technique when caring for open lesions.

NURSING DIAGNOSES	NURSING INTERVENTIONS
Pain, acute, related to pruritus	Assess pain and pruritus for relief measures necessary. Administer medications for pain and pruritus. Stress relaxation techniques and diversional activities.
Impaired skin integrity, related to break in skin	Assess the skin for open lesions. Assess skin for **excoriation** (an injury to the surface of the skin caused by a scratch or abrasion). Keep patient's fingernails short, and/or apply mittens. Plan a balanced diet with increased protein.
Potential for infection, related to tissue destruction	Assess factors that contribute to infection, such as compromised patient (one who has low resistance). Monitor for signs of infection, such as pyrexia and leukocytosis. Stress aseptic handwashing technique. Maintain aseptic technique when providing care. Limit visitors. Don gloves when caring for lesions.
Knowledge deficit, related to disease process	Assess patient's knowledge of disease and ability to learn. Identify support persons, and include them in patient's care. Provide relevant information.

Patient teaching. Patient teaching should begin with an assessment of the knowledge and readiness of the patient. Areas to cover include (1) methods for controlling the pain, (2) application of medication and wet dressings, (3) methods for inhibiting the spread of the disease, (4) techniques to prevent secondary infections, and (5) proper diet with added vitamin C to promote healing.

BACTERIAL DISORDERS OF THE SKIN

Impetigo Contagiosa

Etiology/pathophysiology. Impetigo is caused by *Staphylococcus aureus,* by streptococci, or a mixed bacterial invasion of the skin. The result is a highly contagious inflammatory disorder. Impetigo is seen at all ages but is particularly common in children.

The bacteria invade the skin. The lesions start as **macules** (small, flat blemishes that are flush with the skin surface) that develop into **pustulant vesicles** (small, circumscribed elevations of the skin, containing pus) that rupture and form a dried exudate. The crust is honey colored and easily removed. Under the dried exudate is smooth, red skin.

Clinical manifestations. The exposed areas of the body most often affected are the face, hands, arms, and legs. The pustulant lesions are distributed randomly over the involved area. The honey-colored dried exudate ranges in size from pinpoint to the size of a nickel or larger. Impetigo is highly contagious to a person who directly contacts the exudate of a lesion. The disease may be spread by touching personal articles, linens, and clothing of the infected person.

Assessment. Collection of *subjective data* will include symptoms of (1) pruritus, (2) pain, (3) malaise, (4) spreading of the disease to different body parts, and (5) other diseases present.

Collection of *objective data* will reveal all or part of the following: (1) focal erythema, (2) pruritic areas, (3) honey-colored crust over dried lesions, (4) smooth red skin under the crust, (5) low-grade fever, (6) leukocytosis, (7) positive culture for streptococcus or staphylococcus, and (8) purulent exudate.

Diagnostic tests. The diagnosis is made from a culture of the exudate. The specific bacterium is identified from this culture. Inspection and symptoms make the diagnosis complete.

Medical management. Medical treatment emphasizes the use of antiseptic soaps and cleansing agents to thoroughly clean the involved area. Systemic antibiotics are administered either orally or by injection. Penicillin or one of its synthetic forms is commonly used. The goal is to prevent glomerulonephritis (inflammation of the glomerulus of the kidney), which has been known to occur after streptococcal infections.

Nursing interventions. Interventions are aimed at disrupting the course of the disease and preventing the spread of infection. Antibiotics are used to arrest the disease process. Systemic parenteral penicillin is one of the most commonly used antibiotics. The nurse should don gloves and administer special cleansing agents to wash the lesions. Antiseptics such as povidone-iodine solution (Betadine) and chlorhexidine gluconate (Hibiclens) are examples.

The lesions are usually soaked with an antiseptic solution and the dried exudate is removed using special instruments. Topical antibiotics using sterile technique are applied several times a day.

NURSING DIAGNOSES	NURSING INTERVENTIONS
Impaired skin integrity, related to crusted, open lesions	Inspect the lesions every day for drainage, size, and extent of body area covered. Keep area clean and dry. Don gloves when giving direct patient care.
Pain, related to pruritus	Assess pain, identifying contributing factors. Administer analgesics, hot compresses, and antibiotics as directed.
Potential for infection, related to break in skin	Assess skin for signs of infection. Identify interventions to prevent/reduce the risk of infection. Monitor vital signs; assess for elevated temperature. Stress medical aseptic handwashing. Keep involved areas dry when providing care.
Knowledge deficit, related to the cause and spread of the disease	Assess the patient's knowledge level and readiness to learn. Demonstrate appropriate care and application of topical medications. Stress importance of individual personal items, such as linens and towels. Involve family in patient teaching.

Patient teaching. The patient and family members should be instructed in the principles of hygiene. The nurse assesses the patient's level of knowledge. When demonstrating home care techniques, reinforcement of correct information is recommended. It is imperative to stress the importance of preventing the spread of the disease by contact.

Folliculitis, Furuncles, Carbuncles, and Felons

Etiology/pathophysiology. Folliculitis is an infection of a hair follicle, generally from *Staphyloccus aureus* bacteria. The infection may involve one or several follicles. It often occurs after men or women shave. A stye is an example of folliculitis.

A furuncle (boil) is an inflammation that begins deep in the hair follicles and spreads to the surrounding skin. Irritation is a common predisposing factor to a furuncle. Common locations are the posterior area of the neck, the buttocks, and the axillae.

A carbuncle is a cluster of furuncles. It is an infection of several hair follicles that spreads to surrounding tissue. Obesity, poor nutrition, untreated diabetes mellitus, and poor hygiene contribute to the formation of carbuncles.

Felons occur when the soft tissue under and around an area such as the fingernail becomes infected. The involved finger becomes erythematous, edematous, and tender to touch.

Clinical manifestations. The involved area is usually edematous, erythematous, and painful, with pruritus commonly occurring. After several days the infected area will become localized. The exact area may get shiny, point up, and if a furuncle or carbuncle, the center will turn yellow. Carbuncles can have four to five cores with spontaneous rupture of the core. The pain stops immediately upon rupture of the core. A surgical incision and drain (I & D) can be performed if the core does not rupture.

Assessment. Collection of *subjective data* will include asking questions to ascertain the patient's general symptoms. Common symptoms are tenderness and pain with movement. The nurse should question the patient about a family history of diabetes mellitus or the wearing of improperly fitting clothing.

Collection of *objective data* includes noting erythema and edema in the involved area. The patient is often overweight and may use poor body hygiene techniques.

Diagnostic tests. Diagnosis is based primarily on a thorough physical examination, health history, and inspection of the area. A culture may be done of the drainage.

Medical management. Medical treatment is aimed at preventing the spread of the infection. Patients in the hospital are isolated, using drainage and secretion precautions. Surgical treatment may include draining the lesion and applying topical antibiotics.

Nursing interventions. Warm soaks, two to three times a day, can be used to speed the process of suppuration. When the lesion ruptures, the hot soaks are discontinued to prevent damage of the surrounding skin and spread of the infection. Good medical asepsis should be used by the nurse while caring for these patients. In the hospital, isolation procedures for drainage and secretion should be followed. If the lesion is incised and drained, sterile technique should be used to apply topical antibiotics. The affected part needs to be immobilized to prevent pain and elevated to decrease edema.

NURSING DIAGNOSES	NURSING INTERVENTIONS
Impaired skin integrity, related to exudate from wound	Assess wound daily for exudate and excoriation. Don gloves when providing care; use correct isolation technique. Apply skin protectant to opening.
Pain, related to edema	Assess area for edema and tenderness. Elevate involved body part above the level of the heart. Apply hot soaks, and immobilize affected part.
Knowledge deficit, related to the disease process	Assess patient's level of knowledge and ability to learn through the use of open-ended questions. Discuss and provide written material related to the disease. Demonstrate appropriate home care.

Patient teaching. Patients should be taught not to touch the exudate. Meticulous handwashing is a must before and after contact with the lesions. Good hygiene practices should be demonstrated and return demonstrations done by the patient and family. The entire family needs their own toilet items and bath linens, including encouraging the use of bacteriostatic soap and shampoo. Proper disposal and cleaning of contaminated articles needs to be demonstrated by the nurse.

FUNGAL INFECTIONS OF THE SKIN

Fungal infections are known as *dermatophytosis,* which are superficial infections of the skin. The most common types are tinea capitis, tinea corporis, tinea cruris, and tinea pedis.

Etiology/pathophysiology. Tinea capitis is commonly known as ringworm of the scalp. *Microsporum audouinii* is the major fungal pathogen. The fungus is spread by contact with infected articles. Trauma or irritation breaks the skin and facilitates spread of the infection.

Tinea corporis is known as ringworm of the body. It occurs on parts of the body with little or no hair.

Tinea cruris is known as jock itch. It is found in the groin area.

Tinea pedis is the most common of all fungal infections. Commonly known as athlete's foot, it is seen between the toes of persons whose feet perspire in hot weather. The fungus can also be spread from contaminated public bathroom facilities and swimming pools.

Clinical manifestations. Tinea capitis (ringworm of the scalp) is usually an erythematous, round lesion with pustules around the edges. Temporary alopecia occurs at the site, and infected hairs will turn a blue-green under a Wood's light.

Tinea corporis (ringworm of the body) produces flat lesions that are clear in the center with erythematous borders. Scaliness may also be found, and pruritus is severe.

Tinea cruris (jock itch) has brownish-red lesions that migrate out from the groin area. Pruritus and skin excoriation from scratching are found.

Tinea pedis (athlete's foot) produces more skin maceration than the others. Commonly seen are fissures and vesicles around and below the toes, with occasional discoloration of the infected area.

Assessment. Collection of *subjective data* will include symptoms of extreme pruritus and tenderness.

Collection of *objective data* for tinea capitis should include an inspection and location of a round lesion that is scaling and has pustules around the edges of the scalp. The involved area is erythematous and has no hair. In tinea corporis the nurse will find flat lesions with clear centers and erythematous borders on nonhairy body parts. In tinea cruris the groin area will reveal brown to red lesions that radiate outward, with skin excoriation from intense scratching. In tinea pedis, the nurse will find fissures between the toes and soft skin accompanied by vesicular lesions and thick toenails.

Diagnostic tests. The diagnosis is primarily by visual inspection. A Wood's light or Wood's lamp is an ultraviolet light used to diagnose tinea capitis. The light causes hairs infected by the fungus to become brilliantly fluorescent. No other tests are performed, but a thorough health history supports the diagnosis of all fungal infections of the skin.

Medical management. Medical treatment involves the use of topical and/or oral antifungal drugs. Griseofulvin (Fulvicin, Grifulvin) is the most common oral drug given. Antifungal soaps and shampoos are recommended. Antifungal agents such as tolnaftate 1% (Tinactin) or Desinex can be applied directly. Treatment may last from 2 to 6 weeks.

Nursing interventions. Nursing interventions for fungal infections involves two primary principles. The first is to protect the involved area from trauma and irritation by keeping it clean and dry; the second is the proper application of medications and warm compresses to alleviate the fungus.

Tinea pedis should be treated with warm soaks using Burow's solution and topical antifungal agents. Excellent foot care is stressed. The feet should be cleaned and dried thoroughly, paying special attention to the toes. Wearing sandal-type shoes or going barefoot helps decrease foot moisture. Footwear, such as stockings, needs to be of an absorbent material.

NURSING DIAGNOSIS	NURSING INTERVENTIONS
Impaired skin integrity, related to increased moisture and pruritus	Keep involved area clean and dry. Patient should wear loose-fitting clothing and shoes. Apply medications as directed.

Patient teaching. Patient education involves teaching proper skin care and comfort measures to relieve pruritus. The nurse should review the medications to be taken and the procedures to be done at home by the patient, emphasizing that fungal skin disorders may take months to cure. General education about athlete's foot should be stressed and the many misconceptions clarified, such as wearing white socks to treat the disease.

INFLAMMATORY DISORDERS OF THE SKIN

Superficial infection of the skin is known as dermatitis. It can be caused from numerous agents, such as drugs, plants, chemicals, metals, and food. Regardless of the precipitating factor, the lesions associated with dermatitis develop along the same pattern. The nurse first observes erythema and edema, followed by the eruption of vesicles that rupture and encrust. Pruritus is always present, which promotes further skin excoriation.

Contact Dermatitis

Etiology/pathophysiology. Contact dermatitis is caused by direct contact with agents in the environment to which a person is hypersensitive. The epidermis becomes inflamed and damaged by the repeated contact with the physical and chemical irritants. Common causes of dermatitis are detergents, soaps, industrial chemicals, and plants such as poison ivy.

Clinical manifestations. Lesions appear first at the point of contact with the irritant. Usually the patient feels burning, pain, pruritus, and edema. The involved area is soon erythematous, with **papules** (small, raised, solid skin lesions less than 1 cm in diameter) and vesicles appearing most often on the dorsal surfaces.

Assessment. The nurse needs to thoroughly research the history of the patient's activities. The nurse may ask the patient to write a log of his activities for the past 48 hours before development of symptoms.

Collection of *subjective data* usually reveals that the patient has (1) tried a new soap, (2) been traveling and using different personal items, (3) working with plants or flowers, (4) severe pruritus, and (5) difficulty moving the involved area.

Collection of *objective data* by the nurse should find (1) erythema, (2) papules and vesicles that generally ooze and weep a clear fluid, (3) scratch marks resulting from intense pruritus, and (4) edema of the area.

Diagnostic tests. The primary diagnostic test is accurate collection of a health history to identify the agent. Intradermal skin testing may be done to identify plants and environmental agents and elimination diets are used to identify food allergies.

Medical management. Medical intervention is directed at identifying the cause of the hypersensitive reaction. Symptomatic treatment for the inflammation, edema, and pruritus may include application of corticosteroids and the oral administration of antihistamines such as Benadryl.

Nursing interventions. The primary goal is to identify the offensive agent so as to rest the involved skin and protect it from further damage. To help identify the cause, the nurse needs to describe the pattern of the reaction.

Wet dressings, using Burow's solution, help promote

the healing process. To prevent infection, aseptic technique is used to apply the corticosteroids to the open lesions.

Pruritus is responsible for most of the discomfort. A cool environment with increased humidity decreases the pruritus. Cold compresses may be applied to decrease circulation to the area (vasoconstriction). Daily baths to cleanse the skin should be taken with an application of oil. Fingernails should be cut at the level of the fingertips to decrease excoriation from scratching. Clothing should be lightweight and loose to decrease trauma of the involved area.

NURSING DIAGNOSES	NURSING INTERVENTIONS
Impaired skin integrity, related to scratching	Assess for signs of scratching. Patient should keep fingernails short and wear mittens. Apply medications as directed.
Pain, related to pruritus	Assess degree of pruritus and discomfort every shift. Keep environment cool. Apply cold compresses.
Potential for infection, related to scratching and excoriation	Assess for signs of infection. Describe extent and location of trauma.

Patient teaching. The patient should be taught to keep an accurate history of possible predisposing offensive agents. As soon as the primary irritant has been identified, it should be avoided, as well as soaps, excessive heat, and rubbing of the area. Any time the skin is exposed to the primary irritant, the affected area should be washed thoroughly. Topical creams may be applied only as directed by a physician.

Dermatitis Venenata, Exfoliative Dermatitis, and Dermatitis Medicamentosa

Etiology and clinical manifestations. Dermatitis venenata results from contact with certain plants. Common terms used are *poison ivy* and *poison oak*. The symptoms include mild to severe erythema with pruritus. In this condition, on first exposure the body undergoes a sensitizing antigen formation. This results in an immunological change in certain lymphocytes. Subsequent exposure to the antigen causes the lymphocytes to release irritating chemicals, leading to inflammation, edema, and vesiculation. The lesions are mainly found on the body part exposed to the sensitizing agent.

Exfoliative dermatitis is caused by the ingestion of certain heavy metals, such as arsenic and mercury, which can be fatal. The skin sloughs off and the area becomes edematous and erythematous. Severe pruritus with fever occurs, and most patients require hospitalization. Treatment is individualized, but care is essential to prevent secondary infection, to avoid further irritation, and to maintain fluid balance.

Dermatitis medicamentosa occurs when a person is given a medication to which he is hypersensitive. Any drug can cause a reaction, but the common agents are penicillin, codeine, and iron.

Clinical manifestations. The clinical manifestations range from mild to severe erythema with vesicular eruptions. In severe reactions respiratory distress may occur. Any type of lesion may be found.

Assessment. Collection of *subjective data* for dermatitis is pruritus and a burning pain in the involved area.

Collection of *objective data* reveals lesions that are white in the center and red on the periphery. Vesicles are common in dermatitis venenata. In dermatitis medicamentosa, severe dyspnea caused by respiratory distress may be noted.

Medical management. The medical treatment for dermatitis ranges from therapeutic baths to administrations of corticosteroids. The medical treatment is directed at the cause.

Nursing interventions. In dermatitis venenata the patient should wash the affected part immediately after contact with the offending allergen. After the lesions appear, only cool, open, wet dressings should be used. However, calamine lotion is a common over-the-counter medication for pruritus.

Pruritus is the primary symptom in all dermatitis. Therapeutic baths using colloid solution, lotions, and ointments are used to help relieve the pruritus. Emotional support is necessary. The physical appearance of the patient is difficult for the patient and family members to accept.

In dermatitis medicamentosa, interventions revolve around identifying the drug and discontinuing its use. If the specific drug that is the offending allergen cannot be pinpointed, no drugs should be given. The physician must be notified. The lesions will disappear after the medication is discontinued. More specific nursing intervention is directed by individual patient symptoms. It is important to educate the patient to wear a Medic-Alert bracelet or necklace showing the name of the allergen; the patient should be instructed to notify all health care personnel of the medication allergy.

NURSING DIAGNOSES	NURSING INTERVENTIONS
Impaired skin integrity, related to crusted, open lesions	Inspect the lesions every day for exudate, size, and specific body area involved. Keep area clean and dry. Don gloves when giving direct patient care.
Pain, related to pruritus	Assess pain, identifying contributing factors. Administer analgesics, hot compresses, and antibiotics as directed.

NURSING DIAGNOSES	NURSING INTERVENTIONS
Potential for infection, related to break in skin	Assess skin for signs of infection. Identify interventions to prevent or reduce the risk of infection. Monitor vital signs; assess for elevated temperature. Stress medical aseptic handwashing technique. Use aseptic technique, and keep involved areas dry when providing care.
Knowledge deficit, related to the cause and spread of the disease	Assess the patient's knowledge level and readiness to learn. Demonstrate appropriate care and application of topical medications. Stress importance of individual personal items, such as linens and towels. Involve family in patient teaching.

Urticaria

Etiology/pathophysiology. Urticaria is the term applied to the presence of wheals or hives in an allergic reaction commonly caused by drugs, food, insect bites, inhalants, emotional stress, and exposure to heat or cold. The wheals of urticaria appear suddenly.

Urticaria or hives is caused by the release of histamine in an antigen-antibody reaction.

Clinical manifestations. The increased histamine causes the capillaries to dilate, resulting in increased permeability.

Assessment. Collection of *subjective data* includes pruritus and a burning pain.

Collection of *objective data* will identify transient wheals of varying shapes and sizes with well-defined erythematous margins and pale centers. Intense scratching may be seen, and in some cases respiration may be compromised.

Diagnostic tests. A detailed history is the primary tool to identify the cause of hives. An allergy skin test may be performed using minute quantities of the antigen to identify the allergic substances.

Medical management. Relief from urticaria can be achieved by administering an antihistamine and sometimes epinephrine. Identification of the cause of the urticaria is important to prevent recurrence.

Nursing interventions. Nursing interventions are directed at helping the patient identify the cause and decreasing the discomfort from the pruritus (see p. 547).

Patient teaching. The patient should be taught possible causes and prevention methods. Medications should be explained thoroughly and therapeutic baths demonstrated. The signs and symptoms of an anaphylactic reaction should be covered, such as shortness of breath, wheezing, and cyanosis.

Eczema (Atopic Dermatitis)

Etiology/pathophysiology. Eczema is primarily a disease of infants and is associated with allergies. The common allergies are to chocolate, eggs, wheat, and orange juice.

The allergen causes histamine to be released and an antigen-antibody reaction occurs.

Clinical manifestations. Papular and vesicular lesions appear, surrounded by erythema. The vesicles generally rupture, discharging a yellow, tenaceous exudate that dries and encrusts. If the lesions become infected, the skin may depigment and become shiny with dry scales.

Assessment. Collection of *subjective data* includes pruritus and scratching. Children are generally more fussy and irritable, and anorexia is commonly found. The skin is very sensitive to touch.

Collection of *objective data* will include vesicles and papules found on the scalp, forehead, cheeks, neck, and the surfaces of the extremities. The involved area is erythematous and very dry. Tiny cracks in the epithelium allow fluid to escape and further promote dryness. The primary symptoms result from the scratching because of pruritus.

Diagnostic tests. The diagnosis is generally made during a thorough history because heredity is a prominent factor in eczema. Diet elimination and skin testing may be used to identify the specific hypersensitive substance.

Medical management. The medical treatment is concerned with reducing the amount of allergen exposure. No definite cure exists for eczema, but the eruptions and pruritus can be relieved if the aggravating factor is identified and controlled. The primary goal is to break the inflammation cycle. Hydration of the skin is the key to treatment. The skin is dry because of tiny cracks that allow body fluids to escape.

The skin may be hydrated by soaking the affected area in warm water for 15 to 20 minutes and then applying an occlusive ointment to retain the water. Examples of occlusive preparations are petrolatum, corticosteroid ointments, and vegetable shortenings. The skin should be patted dry after the bath and the occlusive preparation applied immediately to the damp skin.

Nursing interventions. Nursing interventions are directed toward treatment of symptoms for the eczema patient. The nurse is responsible for administering the therapeutic bath and occlusive preparations as directed. Wet dressings may be used to maximize hydration of the skin. Topical steroids may be applied to relieve the discomfort of the lesions. The emotional impact experienced by eczema patients ranges from anger to depression. The nurse must provide an emotional outlet for these patients.

When the lesions begin to heal, lotions such as Eucerin, Alpha-Keri, Lubriderm, and Curel should be applied three to four times a day to add moisture to the skin. Wet wraps and occlusive preparations only hold water already present.

Before the development of steroids, coal tar products

were used to reduce skin inflammation. Coal tar products do not decrease inflammation as quickly as steroids, but they last longer and have fewer side effects. Therefore, coal tar preparations are recommended for chronic eczema. Coal tar preparations are applied once a day at bedtime with a moisturizer. Examples of coal tar preparations are Estar-Gel and Psori-Gel.

NURSING DIAGNOSES	NURSING INTERVENTIONS
Pain, related to pruritus	Assess comfort by evaluating behavior. Apply topical medications as directed. Patient should keep fingernails short and wear cotton clothing. Administer baths, and apply occlusive preparations.
Social isolation, related to alteration in physical appearance	Assess factors that contribute to social isolation. Identify support systems for patient. Establish therapeutic relationship. Discuss situation with patient, listening carefully to expressions of concern.

Patient teaching. Patient teaching for eczema patients should stress (1) avoidance of the agent, (2) avoidance of extreme changes in temperature, (3) how to handle dry skin, (4) no strenuous exercise in hot weather, (5) dangers of self-treatment, and (6) application of medications as directed.

The patient and family should be involved in the care; the primary concern is the chronic nature of the disease and the effect it may have on the patient's self-image and personality.

Acne Vulgaris

Etiology/pathophysiology. Acne is an inflammatory papulopustular skin eruption that involves the sebaceous glands; it occurs primarily in adolescents. The exact cause is unknown. However, several factors that have been considered are diet, stress, heredity, and overactive hormones. Hygiene has not been found to be a significant factor in the development of acne.

Acne develops when the oil glands become occluded. At puberty androgens secreted increase the size of the oil glands, causing the sebum to combine more readily with epithelial cells and bacteria. Sebum may then occlude a hair follicle, forming a *comedo* (plural, comedones). A comedo is a whitehead if it is located at the surface of the skin and becomes a blackhead if it occurs below the skin surface.

Clinical manifestations. Acne is found most often on the face, neck, upper chest, shoulder, and back. The first symptom is usually tenderness and edema in the area, followed by the comedo. The skin is oily and shiny with the lesions lasting up to 10 days. Scarring results from large lesions that are traumatized when the individual tries to rupture the comedo.

Assessment. Collection of *subjective data* includes asking the adolescent how the acne affects his life-style: Does it affect participation in activities or group communication? Most patients will acknowledge that acne affects their self-image. Common locations are the face and chin. Lesions increase with emotional upsets and stress.

Collection of *objective data* will include noting the presence of edema in the involved area. Whiteheads (closed comedones) and blackheads (open comedones) are found on the face, back, and/or chest. The nurse will also observe that patients with acne do not take part in many group activities.

Diagnostic tests. The medical diagnosis is primarily made by inspection of the lesions and a health history that supports the diagnosis. Sometimes blood samples are drawn to measure hormone levels.

Medical management. The medical management can involve topical, systemic, or intralesional medications. Topical therapy peels away the superficial skin layer to prevent sebum occlusions. A common topical medication is benzoyl peroxide gel. Effective topical therapy requires the use of special cleansing agents followed by applications of vitamin A acids, antibiotics, and sulfur-zinc lotions.

Systemic therapy may be combined with topical therapy. Systemic antibiotics such as tetracyline are used. A new drug, isotretinoin (Accutane), a form of vitamin A, is used frequently. Accutane reduces the sebum production and abnormal keratinization of gland ducts. Accutane must be prescribed with extreme caution in adolescent females, because it is destructive to fetal development during pregnancy.

Nursing interventions. In planning nursing interventions, the nurse needs to be aware that most adolescents do not comply with long-term treatment regimens. The nurse must assess and consider what acne means to them. The actual extent of the condition is not as important as the adolescent's feelings. When his face constantly has ugly black and white lesions, it is very hard for the adolescent to like himself.

In addition to psychological concerns the nurse should focus toward preventive nursing interventions. The important areas are skin care, compliance, and emotional support. Prevention stresses identification of factors that directly increase acne. Although poor hygiene may not be a cause, cleanliness decreases infection and promotes healing. The patient's hands and hair should be kept away from the face. Clothes should not restrict affected areas, and hair should be washed daily. The skin should be washed two or three times a day with a medicated soap. Cosmetics need to be water based, and products that have wax esters should be avoided. Compliance is difficult, because improvement is slow. Often 3 weeks of treatment is required before any noticeable improvement is seen by the family or friends.

NURSING DIAGNOSES	NURSING INTERVENTIONS
Impaired skin integrity, related to occluded oil glands	Assess extent of occluded oil glands by inspecting lesions for size, color, and location. Monitor for signs of infection. Wash involved areas three to four times a day. Apply medications to decrease occlusion of oil glands.
Self-esteem disturbance, related to physical appearance	Assess primary cause of low self-esteem and extent of feelings. Assess family support. Assess patient awareness and ways to deal with the situation. Note nonverbal language to discover patient's perception of the illness. Stress the importance of not comparing oneself with others. Have patient list current successes and strengths. Give positive reinforcement.
Social isolation, related to decreased self-esteem	Assess extent and feelings of isolation. Assess factors that contribute to sense of helplessness. Listen to and spend time with patient. Involve patient in support group. Focus on patient's strengths.

Patient teaching. Patient education should include the physical and emotional needs of the patient. The nurse should address diet, hygiene, stress reduction, makeup, and medications. Coping skills may need to be retaught and counseling referrals made. The extensive treatment time should be covered in minute detail, because this disease is chronic and exacerbations will occur. Keeping the adolescent communicating about his feelings will decrease any long-term affects acne may have on his personality.

Psoriasis

Etiology/pathophysiology. Psoriasis is a noninfectious skin disorder; it is a hereditary, chronic, proliferative disease involving the epidermis and can occur at any age. No specific predisposing factors are known. The skin cells divide much more rapidly than normal. The normal time for the entire skin to be replaced, through sloughing and generation of new cells, is 28 days; in psoriasis the time may decrease to 7 days. The severe scaling is a result of the rapid cell division.

Clinical manifestations. The lesions appear as raised, erythematous, circumscribed, silvery, scaling plaques. The primary lesion is papular. The papules become plaques located on the scalp, elbows, chin, and trunk.

Assessment. Collection of *subjective data* initially will reveal only mild pruritus. Sometimes feelings of depression, frustration, and loneliness are expressed. The disease causes observers to stare and avoid contact with the patient.

Collection of *objective data* includes observing dull, erythematous, sharply outlined plaques covered with silvery scales on the elbows, knees, and scalp. Fingernails can be affected and will show pitting with yellowish discoloration.

Diagnostic tests. No specific diagnostic tests exist for psoriasis. Primary diagnosis is made by observation of the patient and the symptoms displayed.

Medical management. Medical management is aimed at slowing the proliferation of epithelial layers of the skin. Topical steroids and keratolytic agents are used in occlusive wet dressings to decrease inflammation. Keratolytic agents such as tar preparations, anthralin, and salicylic acid decrease the shedding of the outer layer of the skin. Topical steroids used are hydrocortisone and Valisone.

Photochemotherapy may also be used. This treatment involves the use of a drug that is enhanced by exposure to light. PUVA therapy combines the use of methoxsalen (Psoralen), which is given orally, and the concurrent use of ultraviolet light A (uva); hence the name PUVA.

Nursing interventions. Nursing interventions include proper administration of the treatment modality. Additional rest and measures to promote psychological well-being, such as counseling, are necessary. The emotional needs of this patient are as important as the physical needs. Because of the chronic nature of this disease, the patient should be encouraged to focus on positive attributes.

NURSING DIAGNOSES	NURSING INTERVENTIONS
Impaired skin integrity, related to proliferation of epithelial cells	Assess extent of the scaliness. Administer treatment method correctly. Use medical aseptic technique.
Self-esteem disturbance, related to appearance	Assess patient's concept of body. Help patient to focus on positive aspects. Discuss with patient ways to conceal obvious lesions.
Social isolation, related to decreased self-esteem	Assess activity pattern and social outlets. Demonstrate ways to conceal lesions with clothes. Involve patient in support group.
Potential for infection, related to open lesions	Assess skin for open lesions. Use surgical asepsis when caring for open lesions.

Patient teaching. The primary points should include the nature of the disease, the correct application of the treatment modality, and compliance with medical care. It should be stressed that the patient should not treat himself. The patient should be informed that the disease is not curable.

PARASITIC DISEASES OF THE SKIN

Pediculosis

Etiology/pathophysiology. Pediculosis (lice infestation) is a parasitic disorder of the skin that is usually associated with poor living conditions and poor personal hygiene. This is not always the case, however; pediculosis can occur in any life-style. Lice obtain their nutrition from the blood of their victims. They leave their eggs (nits) on the skin surface attached to the shaft of the hair.

Humans have three types of lice: the head louse, the body louse, and the pubic louse. In pediculosis capitis, the head louse attaches itself to the hair shaft and lays 8 to 16 eggs per day. The eggs can be seen best at the back of the neck as gray, shiny, oval bodies.

In pediculosis corporis, the body louse is found around the neck, waist, and thighs. The louse is spread in the seams of clothing. Severe pruritus and pinpoint hemorrhages are caused from the bite of the louse.

The pubic louse, the parasite involved in pediculosis pubis, does not resemble the head or body louse. It looks like a crab with sharp pincers that attach to the pubic hair. Transmission can be by sexual contact, bed clothing, or bath towels.

Clinical manifestations. Nits or lice can be seen on the body. Pinpoint raised red macules, pinpoint hemorrhages, and severe pruritus confirm the diagnosis. Skin excoriation is very common because of the intense pruritus.

Assessment. Collection of *subjective data* will include complaints of pruritus in the area involved. Tenderness and difficulty wearing clothes are also noted.

Collection of *objective data* will reveal erythema, petechiae, and skin excoriation in the area.

Diagnostic tests. The diagnostic test is a physical examination of the involved area. A health history supports the diagnosis.

Medical management. The topical application of a pediculicide such as lindane (Kwell) or pyrethrin (Rid) is used in any area the contaminated patient has contacted. The specific technique for applying these products varies but should be followed very closely to control the lice.

Nursing interventions. The primary nursing interventions involves the application of the medication to rid the patient of the lice. Every place the patient has had contact needs to be cleaned. Health teaching stresses the transmission of the disease by contact. Assessment of the patient's emotional needs is important. Having a lice infestation carries a negative implication by society that the patient has poor hygiene practices.

Patient teaching. Nursing care focuses on identifying involved persons and appropriate health teaching. The nature and transmission of the disease are stressed. Each family member should be assessed for nits and taught measures to reduce pruritus, such as cool compresses and corticosteroid ointments.

Scabies

Etiology/pathophysiology. The cause of scabies is the female itch mite *(Sarcoptes scabiei)*. The mite penetrates the skin and makes a burrow. Once under the skin, the mite lays eggs that mature and rise to the skin surface. Scabies is transmitted by prolonged contact with an infected area. Overcrowded conditions, poverty, changing sexual behaviors, and world travel have increased the incidence of scabies. Scabies now occurs in all age-groups and socioeconomic classes.

Clinical manifestations. Scabies causes wavy, brown, threadlike lines on the body. Pruritus is severe and secondary infections are common from the excoriation caused by scratching. Locations for the threadlike lines are hands, arms, body folds, and genitalia.

Assessment. Collection of *subjective data* includes the severe pruritus associated with scabies and the skin excoriation resulting from the scratching.

Collection of *objective data* includes finding the wavy brown lines on the body and severe erythema from the scratching.

Diagnostic tests. Identification can be confirmed by microscopic examination of infected skin. A health history and characteristic signs and symptoms support the diagnosis.

Medical management. Medical treatment is aimed at the elimination of the mite and prevention of complications. Drug therapy is basically the same as for pediculosis. Two additional drugs used are crotamiton (Eurax) and a 4% to 8% solution of sulfur in petrolatum.

Nursing interventions. Nursing interventions are directed at improving skin integrity by using medical aseptic techniques to provide hygiene and to apply medications. Proper application of medication is essential to destroy the parasite. The nurse must also consider the emotional well-being of the patient. Using open-ended questions and listening skills helps the nurse to identify potential problem areas for the patient.

Patient teaching. The primary concern is to educate the family members about the transmission of scabies. Each family member needs to treat the whole body with a scabicide. Clothing, linens, and bath articles should be washed in hot water and dried in a dryer. If clothes are line dried, they should be ironed. Each member should realize the importance of compliance with the treatment. It is important that the nurses teach the family that scabies infestations can happen to anyone. The nurse must be able to use and convey a nonjudgmental attitude toward these patients.

TUMORS OF THE SKIN

Overgrowth of the skin cells can develop from any layer or its appendages. The majority of skin tumors are benign. Many can be predisposing factors for skin cancer.

Clinical Manifestations

The specific symptoms of skin tumors relate to the type of tumor. Keloids, which originate in scars, are hard and shiny. Angiomas resemble birthmarks, and warts (verrucae) are unattractive and located on the arms and hands. Nevi are considered to be predisposers to cancer and create anxiety in the patient when a color change is noted. Skin cancers are life threatening and occur wherever exposure to the sun may have been the greatest. Any time a patient has a change in a skin lesion, a physician should be consulted.

Assessment

Collection of *subjective data* includes a good health history. The patient's risk factors should be assessed first. Life-style, occupation, family history, and geographic location are important.

Collection of *objective data* includes describing the lesion in detail. The size, location, and any pain are significant factors in determining the type of skin tumor. The appearance of the lesions can take several forms.

Diagnostic Tests

The diagnostic test for tumors of the skin is biopsy of the lesion. A health history and visual inspection support the diagnosis.

Medical Management

The primary medical intervention for skin tumors is surgical removal. Other treatment modalities are radiation therapy to decrease the size of the tumor and application of topical medications such as corticosteroids to decrease the size and inflammation.

Nursing Interventions

The potential threat of malignancy causes great concern for the patient. Careful explanations of treatments, medications, and tests help decrease anxiety. If surgery is the treatment of choice, the patient will need to prepared for surgery.

Nursing intervention revolves around preparing the patient for the treatment needed. Most skin tumors are a threat to the patient's self-concept. Emotional care is important; the nurse should encourage the patient to verbalize feelings of fear or anxiety.

The nursing diagnoses and interventions for malignant melanoma are applicable. Although the skin tumors previously mentioned are not all malignant, the potential problems posed are the same until a definite diagnosis is made.

Patient teaching. Discharge instructions include skin care, dressing changes, and follow-up care. The nurse should involve the family in patient teaching to support the patient. The signs and symptoms of an infection should be covered for patients who have had tumors surgically removed.

Keloids

Keloids are seen more often in African-Americans than Caucasians. Collagen tissue becomes raised, hard, and shiny. Keloids usually originate from a scar and can be located anywhere on the body. The sternum, ears, neck, and arms are common locations. Keloids are usually surgically excised but may recur. Steroids and radiation therapy are two treatment measures.

Angiomas

An angioma develops when a group of blood vessels dilate and form a tumorlike mass. A common angioma is a birthmark, such as the port-wine birthmark. This stain is not elevated and may be found on one side of the face. Treatment involves electrolysis and/or x-ray therapy.

A spider angioma or telangiectasis is associated with liver disease. A group of venous capillaries dilate and branch out like a spider. Spider angiomas will usually resolve as the disease improves.

Verruca (Wart)

A **verruca** is a benign, viral, warty skin lesion with a rough, papillomatous (nipplelike) growth occurring in many forms. Verrucas may occur singularly or in groups and are thought to be contagious. Common locations are the hands, arms, and fingers, but warts can occur anywhere on the body. The plantar wart develops on the sole of the foot and is extremely painful. Treatment of a wart depends on the type, location, and number. Cauterization, solid carbon dioxide, liquid nitrogen, and preparations of salicylic acid are used to remove warts.

Nevi (Moles)

Nevi (singular, nevus) or moles are described as nonvascular tumors. Many are pigmented and present at birth. There are many types of nevi, and several may become malignant, especially if traumatized. The raised, black nevus is considered to be one of the most threatening, and removal is recommended to prevent its becoming malignant.

Basal Cell Carcinoma

Basal cell carcinoma is one type of skin cancer. Related factors to the development of skin cancer include frequent contact with certain chemicals, overexposure to the sun, and radiation treatment. Fair-skinned people are more likely to develop skin cancer, possibly because less melanin is distributed on their skin surface.

Basal cell carcinoma is found on the face and upper trunk. It may be superficial or nodular. The nodular form is raised, firm to touch, ulcerated in the center, and has a waxy pearly border. The superficial type is raised and crusted with a raised pearly border.

Squamous Cell Carcinoma

Squamous cell carcinoma occurs in body areas that have been exposed or treated with radiation. Usually the hands and head develop cancer first. The lesions are flat, nodular, and large, with some desquamation noted. It spreads more rapidly than other skin cancers.

Malignant Melanoma

Etiology/pathophysiology. A malignant melanoma is a cancerous neoplasm in which pigment cells (melanocytes) invade the epidermis, dermis, and sometimes the subcutaneous tissue. Several types of melanoma are known and are categorized by location and description.

Most melanomas arise from melanocytes in the epidermis, but some may appear in preexisting moles. Heredity is a factor, and any person who has a large number of moles with a variety of sizes and colors should be monitored.

The occurrence of melanoma has doubled over the past 2 decades, a fact associated with increased recreational exposure to the sun. The person who has a history of skin cancer is at greater risk.

Clinical manifestations. Basically, there are four types of malignant melanomas: (1) superficial spreading melanomas, (2) malignant lentigo melanomas, (3) nodular melanomas, and (4) acral lentiginous melanomas. The superficial spreading is the most common and occurs anywhere on the body. These melanomas are slightly elevated, irregularly shaped lesions, in a varying combination of hues (Fig. 29-4); common colors are tan, brown, black, blue, gray, and pink. The lentigo melanomas are usually found on the heads and necks of elderly persons. Characteristically these appear as tan, flat lesions that undergo changes in shape and size. The nodular melanoma grows and metastasizes faster than the other types. Nodular melanomas appear as a blueberry-type growth, varying from blue-black to pink. The patient often describes the lesion as a blood blister that fails to resolve.

The last type of melanomas occurs in areas not exposed to sunlight and where no hair follicles are present. Common locations are the hands, soles, and mucous membranes of dark-skinned people.

Prognosis depends on the kind, size, and location of the melanoma; metastasis can occur.

Assessment. The collection of *subjective data* should include a thorough history related to skin cancer. Patients at greatest risk have fair complexions, blue eyes, red or blond hair, and freckles. The collection of *objective data* includes the location, color, and appearance of the lesions.

Diagnostic tests. Diagnosis primarily depends on the biopsy of the tissue. The patient is also examined thoroughly for suspicious lesions. Any lesion that is varigated

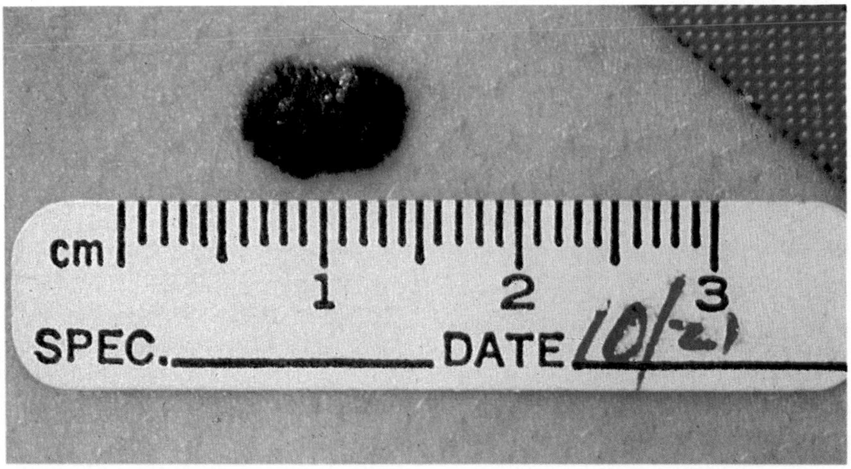

FIG. 29-4 Malignant melanoma.

in color, has an irregular border, or has an irregular surface should be monitored.

Medical management. Medical management depends on the level of invasion and the thickness of the melanoma. Small superficial lesions are treated by local excision, and large areas are widely excised and skin grafted. Sometimes antineoplastic drugs are used to disrupt cell division.

Nursing interventions. The major goals of nursing care include relief of pain, reduction of anxiety, and remission of the disease. The nurse needs to be aware that fear of the unknown is a major concern of the patient with a melanoma. Explaining procedures and diagnostic tests in terms that the patient can understand may help to decrease his anxiety.

NURSING DIAGNOSES	NURSING INTERVENTIONS
Pain, related to lesion	Assess pain using the five PQRST variables of the chief complaint. Provide nursing comfort measures, such as back rubs, to decrease pain. Administer pain medications as needed. Teach relaxation techniques.
Anxiety, related to fear of the unknown	Assess patient's coping mechanisms. Explain all procedures. Encourage patient to verbalize fears, using open-ended questions. Explain grieving process to patient. Use unhurried manner in patient care.

Patient teaching. Discharge instructions include wound care, medication, cleansing, and follow-up care. The nurse needs to assess the family's knowledge base about the seriousness and treatment of the disease. Medical aseptic techniques are stressed to prevent a secondary infection.

DISORDERS OF THE APPENDAGES

Alopecia

Alopecia is the loss of hair. The cause can be aging, drugs such as antineoplastics, anxiety, or disease processes. Alopecia is usually not permanent unless the loss is from aging; the hair will usually grow back but can take several months. Any time that a patient loses hair, the body image and self-esteem are threatened.

Hypertrichosis (Hirsutism)

Hypertrichosis is an excessive growth of hair in a masculine distribution. It can be hereditary or acquired as a result of hormone dysfunction and medications. The treatment is removal by dermabrasion, electrolysis, chemical depilation, shaving, plucking, or rubbing with pumice. Treatment of the specific cause will usually stop growth of more hair.

Hypotrichosis

Hypotrichosis is the absence of hair or a decrease in hair growth. Skin disease, endocrine problems, and malnutrition are associated factors. Treatment involves identifying and removing the cause.

Paronychia

Paronychia is a disorder of the nails. The nails get soft or brittle and the shape can change as they grow into the soft tissue (ingrown nails). In paronychia, an infection of the nail develops and spreads around the nail, thus giving it the nickname "runaround." Involved nails become painful as the nail loosens and separates from the tissue. Application of wet dressings or topical antibiotics may be used. Sometimes a surgical incision and drainage of the infected area is performed.

BURNS

Etiology/pathophysiology. Each year more than 2 million people are burned. Usually 250,000 require outpatient treatment and 80,000 require hospitalization. The most significant factor is that at least half of these burns could be prevented.

Burns result from radiation, thermal energy (heat), electricity, or chemicals. Skin destruction depends on the burning agent, the temperature of the burning agent, and how long a person is in contact with the agent.

Burns first cause the capillaries in the damaged area to dilate, resulting in capillary hyperpermeability. The increased cell permeability causes the fluid to move out of the cells into the surrounding tissues, resulting in edema and vesiculation (blistering). The larger the burned area, the greater the fluid loss. The fluid loss from the intravascular area to the interstitial area poses the greatest threat to life, because the cells become dehydrated. The blood pressure drops and blood flow to the kidneys is decreased. Symptoms of hypovolemic shock and renal failure may develop.

The pathophysiology and care of burns may be divided into three stages. The emergent phase, stage 1, is from the onset of the injury until the patient is stabilized. In the emergent phase hypovolemia is a major concern for up to 48 hours after a major burn. Stage 2, the intermediate/acute phase or diuretic stage, begins 48 to 72 hours after the burn injury. At this time the greatest concern is circulatory overload. The fluid shifts back from the interstitial spaces to the cells. The kidneys begin to excrete large volumes of urine; hence it is called the diuretic stage. Stage 3, the long-term rehabilitation phase, begins when the burn has been treated. The aim of care in this phase is to return the patient to normal status.

Usually the greatest fluid loss in a burn occurs in the first 12 hours. The proteins, plasma, and electrolytes shift from the vascular compartment to the interstitial compartment. Red blood cells tend to remain in the vascular system, causing increased viscosity of the blood and a falsely elevated hematocrit level. Acute dehydration is present, and renal perfusion is seriously compromised. Fluid loss causes the person to develop burn shock. Hypotension, a decreased urine output, an increased pulse, rapid, shallow respirations, and restlessness develop. The heart can no longer supply enough blood to perfuse the vital organs. The body responds by increasing the peripheral resistance. A decreased pulse pressure and an increased pulse (tachycardia) and respiratory rate (tachypnea) exemplify this. Most deaths from burns result directly from burn shock.

Fluids start to return to the vascular compartment in 48 to 72 hours. Fluid return denotes the end of the hypovolemic stage and the beginning of the diuretic stage. Reabsorption of the interstitial fluid causes an increased blood volume. As the blood volume increases, the cardiac output increases to increase renal perfusion. The result is diuresis. The patient now is at a great risk for fluid overload. The patient's vital signs, urinary output, and consciousness must be carefully monitored.

A burned victim may also have experienced smoke inhalation. Inhalation damage results from breathing the chemicals produced by the burn. The fumes produce damage to the cilia and mucosa of the respiratory tract. Alveolar surfactant is decreased, and atelectasis can occur. Breathing difficulties are not usually seen immediately but may take several hours to occur. The nurse needs to consider a patient who has sustained any burn to the upper chest, neck, and face at high risk for respiratory distress. Symptoms that signify respiratory difficulty are a hoarse voice or a productive cough. Other physical findings suggesting respiratory tract injury in inhalation burns include the following:

- Singed nasal hairs
- Agitation, tachypnea, flaring nostrils, or intercostal retractions
- Brassy cough, grunting, or guttural respiratory sounds
- Erythema or edema of the oropharynx or nasopharynx
- Sooty sputum

Clinical manifestations. Burns are classified (Table 29-2) as superficial partial-thickness injuries, deep partial-thickness injuries, and full-thickness injuries (Fig. 29-5). Corresponding terms are first-, second-, and third-degree

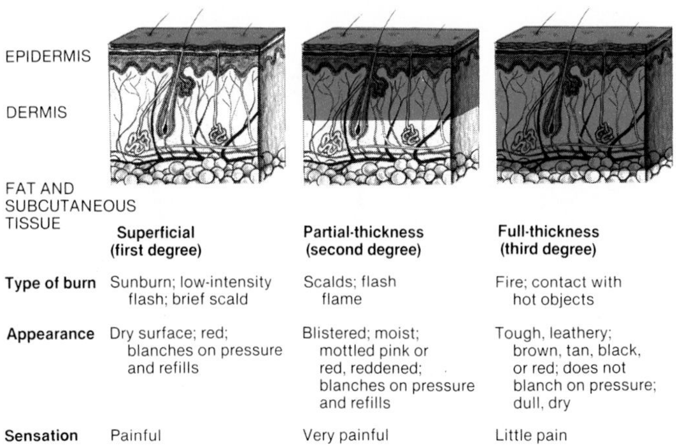

FIG. 29-5 Classification of burn depth.

Table 29-2 Causes and Factors Determining Depth of Burn Injury

Depth	Cause	Appearance	Color	Sensation
Superficial partial-thickness (first-degree)	Flash flame, ultraviolet light (sunburn)	Dry, no vesicles Minimal or no edema Blanches with fingertip pressure and refills when pressure removed	Increased erythema	Painful
Deep partial-thickness (second-degree)	Contact with hot liquids or solids Flash flame to clothing Direct flame Chemicals Ultraviolet light	Large, moist vesicles that will increase in size Blanches with fingertip pressure and refills when pressure removed	Mottled with dull, white, tan, pink, or cherry red areas	Very painful
Full-thickness (third-degree)	Contact with hot liquids or solids Flame Chemicals Electrical contact	Dry with leathery eschar Charred vessels visible under eschar Vesicles rare but thin-walled vesicles that do not increase in size may be present No blanching with pressure	White, charred, dark tan Black Red	Little or no pain Hair easily pulls out

burns. The amount of tissue destruction determines the classification.

Assessment. Factors to include in the assessment are (1) the depth of the burn, (2) the causative agent, (3) the temperature and duration of contact, and (4) the skin thickness. The patient's age and other disease processes present are equally important. The **rule of nines** is used to determine the total body surface area (BSA) involved (Fig. 29-6). The rule of nines divides the body into multiples of nine. The entire head is 9%; the anterior and posterior aspects of the arms are a total of 9% each; the legs are 9% anterior and 9% posterior; the chest and back are 18% each, and the perineum is 1%. The rule of nines does not take into account the different levels of growth and development and is not accurate for children.

The rule of nines for calculating percentage of body area burned for infants and child differs from the adult because the surface area of the child's head is greater (relative to his body) than in an adult. The child's body part and percentage total body surface are calculated as follows:

Arm (shoulder to fingertips), 9% each
Head to neck, 18%
Anterior trunk, 18%
Posterior trunk, 18%
Leg (groin to toe), 14% each

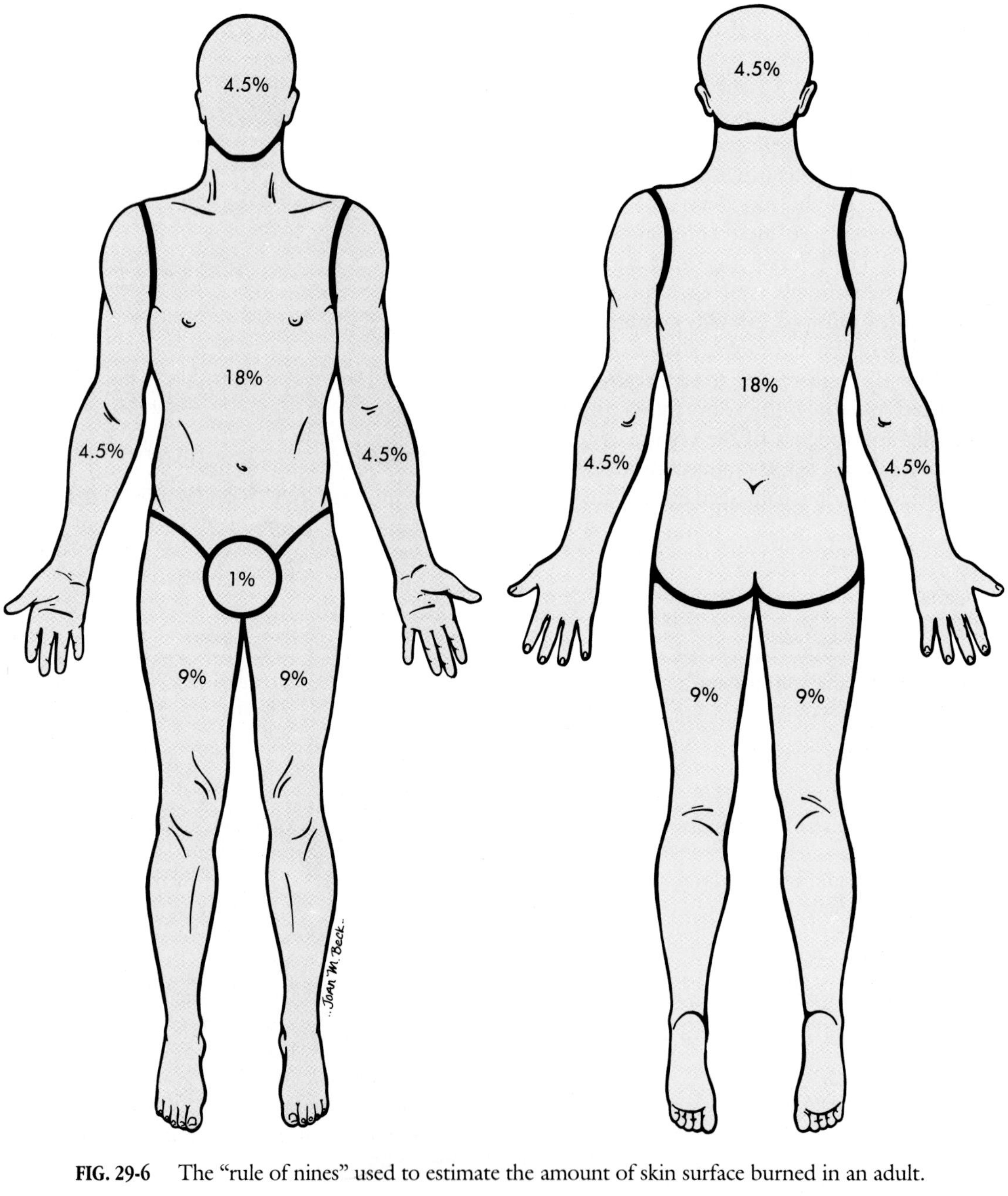

FIG. 29-6 The "rule of nines" used to estimate the amount of skin surface burned in an adult.

Collection of *subjective data* will reveal the causative agent, other diseases present, the temperature and duration of contact, and patient age.

Collection of *objective data* includes the depth of the burn, the skin thickness involved, the percentage of body surface area burned, the specific location, and any other injuries sustained. Any time a patient has a burn that involves the face, neck, or chest, the nurse needs to be observant for respiratory difficulty. It is important to identify whether the victim has had a tetanus booster in the past 10 years to prevent complications.

The severity of the burn depends on several factors. Major burns are those that require the most skilled nursing interventions. Moderate and minor burns require fewer nursing interventions. Factors determining a major, moderate, or minor burn are (1) the percentage of the body surface area burned, (2) the age of the victim, (3) the specific location of the burn, (4) the cause of the burn, (5) other diseases present, (6) the depth of the burn, and (7) injuries sustained during the burn (Box 29-4).

Diagnostic tests. The primary diagnostic test is a physical examination to determine the amount of burned area.

BOX 29-4 CLASSIFICATION OF SEVERITY OF BURNS

MAJOR BURN INJURIES

Greater than 25% BSA (greater than 20% in children under 10 years and adults over 40 years of age)

Greater than 10% BSA, full-thickness

Involvement of face, eyes, ears, hands, feet, perineum

Electrical burns

Burns complicated by inhalation injury or major trauma

Burns in patients with preexisting disease (diabetes, congestive heart failure, or chronic renal failure)

MODERATE BURN INJURIES

15% to 25% BSA in adults, partial-thickness (10% to 20% BSA in children under 10 years and adults over 40 years of age)

Less than 10% BSA full-thickness

Burns with no concurrent injury

Burns in patients with no preexisting disease

MINOR BURN INJURIES

Less than 15% BSA in adults (10% in children or the elderly)

Less than 2% BSA full-thickness injury

Burns in patients with no preexisting disease

Blood assessments, such as electrolytes, CBC, serum chemistries, and ABGs, may be done to establish the severity of the dehydration. In inhalation burns, carboxyhemoglobin level is evaluated. Among survivors with severe asphyxiation or carbon monoxide intoxication, most fatalities occur. Carbon monoxide binds to hemoglobin with greater affinity than oxygen, and therefore tissue hypoxia results.

Medical management. The medical treatment of burns is divided into three phases. Priorities exist in each phase. It is important to remember that these phases are not always clearly defined and may overlap.

Phase 1, the immediate or emergent phase, is the first 48 to 72 hours. Phase 2, the acute phase, begins with the end of the emergent phase and lasts until the burns are covered with grafts, if needed. Phase 2 ends when partial-thickness burns are healed. Phase 3, the rehabilitation phase, lasts until the person can function productively. This phase may take years.

Emergent Phase

The primary concern in the emergent phase is to stop the burning process by removing clothing and shoes from the victim and the source of the burn to arrest skin damage. Ice should not be applied; this causes vasoconstriction and can cause further injury. Step two is to provide an open airway and to control bleeding. Third, all nonadhered clothing and jewelry (rings, watches) should be removed. Fourth, the victim should be covered with a clean sheet or cloth. Fifth, the victim should be transported to the hospital. In the case of a chemical burn, it is important to rinse the skin generously with water to remove all chemicals. Electrical burns have an entry and exit point that needs to be identified. Most electrical burns result in cardiac arrest, and the patient will require CPR (see Chapter 53).

In the hospital, the severity of the burn dictates the care given. The nurse should perform a thorough assessment every hour in the emergent phase. Patients with major burns are transferred to burn care centers or units for treatment. Patients with moderate to severe burns are treated using the following steps:

1. Establish airway—administer oxygen as ordered. Often the physician will insert an endotracheal tube to ensure a patent airway (Fig. 29-7).
2. The RN will initiate fluid therapy—intravenous fluid therapy of Ringer's lactate is begun immediately. The amount of fluid given is in accordance with the percentage of body surface area burned. The patient is weighed so the physician can determine the amount of fluids needed.
3. Insert Foley catheter for hourly output—an hourly urine output of 30 to 50 ml is recommended. Intravenous fluids are given to maintain renal perfusion.

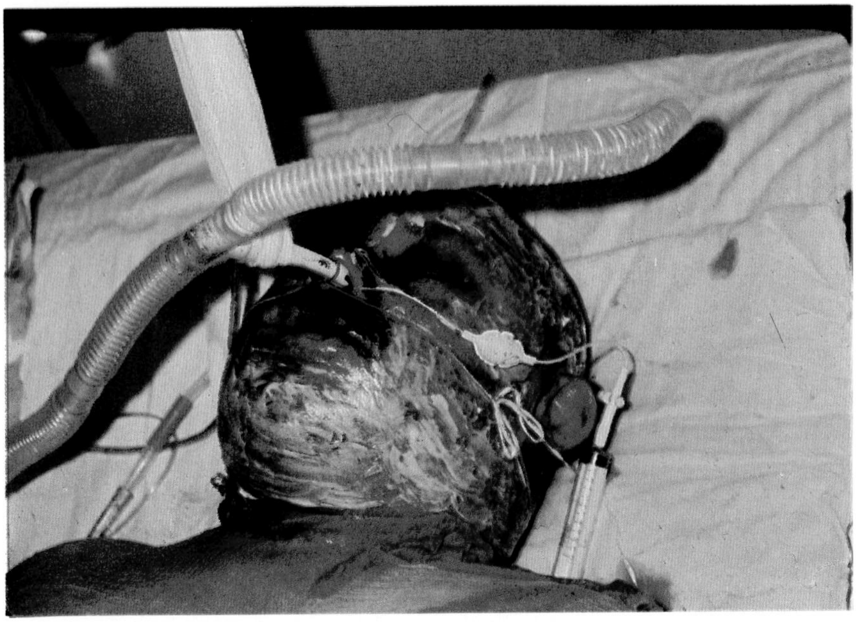

FIG. 29-7 Endotracheal intubation for patient with severe edema 5 hours after a burn injury.

4. The RN will insert a nasogastric tube to prevent aspiration. Severe burn patients often develop a paralytic ileus as a result of trauma.
5. The RN will administer pain medication in small, frequent intravenous doses. Never give any medications intramuscularly in major burn victims because of poor absorption.
6. Stabilize victim, and monitor vital signs.
7. Give tetanus as needed.

The first 72 hours require diligent medical care to prevent death. Intravenous fluids are ordered to maintain the urine output at 30 to 50 ml per hour (Boxes 29-5, 29-6, and 29-7).

Acute Phase

The acute phase begins when fluids begin to shift back to the intravascular compartment, usually 72 hours after the burn. The acute phase varies in time from 10 days to months. The two primary goals in treatment are treatment of the burn and prevention and management of complications. The most common complication and cause of death after the first 72 hours is infection. Other complications are heart failure, renal failure, **contractures** (shortening or tension of muscles that affects extension), and **Curling's ulcer** (an erosion in the lining of the stomach occurring 10 to 14 days after the burn injury); the first symptom is usually vomiting of bright red blood.

Nursing interventions. The data gathered should include: (1) respiratory pattern, (2) vital signs, (3) circulation, (4) intake and output, (5) patient movement, (6) bowel sounds, (7) inspection of the wound itself, and (8) mental status. Any signs of an infection should be reported immediately. The primary goals in the emergent phase are to maintain respiratory integrity and to prevent

BOX 29-5 INITIAL TREATMENT OF MAJOR BURNS IN THE EMERGENCY ROOM

1. Establish airway.
2. Initiate fluid therapy by intravenous catheters.
3. Insert indwelling Foley catheter for hourly urine measurement.
4. Do circulatory assessment for circumferential occlusion resulting from eschar.
5. Insert nasogastric tube to remove stomach contents and prevent gastric distention.
6. Insert central intravenous catheter, if appropriate.
7. Manage pain by intravenous narcotics in small, frequent doses.
8. Provide tetanus prophylaxis.

BOX 29-6 INDICATIONS FOR FLUID RESUSCITATION

- Burns greater than 20% BSA in adults
- Burns greater than 10% BSA in children
- Patient older than 55 or younger than 4 years of age
- Patient with preexisting disease that would reduce normal compensatory responses to minor hypovolemia (cardiac or pulmonary disease, diabetes)
- Electrical burns

BOX 29-7 **POTENTIAL NURSING DIAGNOSES FOR THE EMERGENT PHASE OF BURNS**

- Ineffective airway clearance, related to edema of the respiratory passages
- Fluid volume deficit (dehydration), related to shift of body fluids
- Fluid volume deficit, related to capillary hyperpermeability with fluid moving out of the cells into the interstitial area
- Anxiety, acute, related to injury
- Pain, acute, related to nerve injury
- Hypothermia, related to loss of skin
- Potential for infection, related to break in skin
- Impaired skin integrity, related to damage by the burns
- Decreased cardiac output, related to hypovolemia
- Sensory/perceptual alterations (tactile), related to loss of skin
- Potential for aspiration, related to decreased peristalsis
- Impaired swallowing, related to mucosal edema
- Impaired verbal communication, related to breathing difficulties
- Sleep pattern disturbance, related to hospital environment

hypovolemic shock, which may cause death.

Once the patient's condition has stabilized and the diuretic or acute phase begins, a nutritional assessment should be done. Provision for adequate nutrition is the cornerstone of burn care during the acute phase. The diet needs to include increased amounts of protein, calories, and vitamins to help repair the damaged tissue. Oral intake of nutrients should be encouraged as soon as possible. The nurse monitors nutritional improvement through daily measurement of weight, serum electrolytes, and a urinalysis. Adequate nutrition decreases healing time. Skin grafts will not be successful unless nutrition is adequate. It is important that the burn patient not lose weight, because this will increase healing time.

Nursing interventions should include measures to support the patient's psychological well-being. Pain must be controlled by intravenous narcotics in small, frequent doses to ease discomfort, but not jeopardize respiratory integrity. Specific interventions include verbal support, unhurried care, truthful explanations, and effective listening. The nurse's communication skills must be excellent.

Infection is a primary complication that should be treated at the time of the burn. Local and systemic infections are common complications at this time (Fig. 29-8). Cultures of the burn should be done at admission and periodically during care.

The burn patient does not have an intact first line of defense; the protective mechanisms are not functioning normally. The nurse should protect the patient from the environment by using protective isolation. Gowns, masks, caps, and gloves should be worn during each contact with a major burn victim. Strict surgical aseptic technique is followed during dressing changes. Use of proper equipment-cleaning procedures is imperative. Hydrotherapy (whirlpool) can be a source of infection.

Wound care involves the removal of the eschar that forms. **Eschar** is the protective cover that the body forms over burned tissue, which can harbor microorganisms and cause infection. It may also compromise circulatory status, and an escharotomy is often done to relieve the circulatory constriction (Fig. 29-9). Daily **debridement** and special cleansing help to support regeneration of the tissues. Hydrotherapy softens the eschar with water to make removal less painful. It also promotes range of motion to decrease contractures.

The specific treatment method depends on the severity of the burn. The open or exposure method is used for burns of the face, neck, ears, and perineum. The area is cleaned and exposed to air. A hard crust forms, and the regeneration of tissue occurs.

Proper positioning and range-of-motion (ROM) exercises by the physical therapist and the nurse are vital for the well-being of the burn patient (Table 29-3).

Special bed equipment is needed to prevent the burn from touching the linens. A bed cradle, a Circoelectric bed, or a Clinitron bed (Fig. 29-10) is recommended. Lights or heat lamps are used to provide additional warmth.

Advantages to the open method include the following: (1) the wound can be observed more easily, (2) movement in bed is less restricted, and (3) circulation of the body part is not restricted. Disadvantages to the open method are pain and chilling. The pain can be controlled with intravenously administered narcotics. However, considering the long-term nature of a burn, addiction is a potential problem. Diazepam (Valium) has been found to be effective. Chilling can be controlled by keeping the room temperature 85° F (24.4° C). Humidity should be between 40% and 50%.

The closed or occlusive method involves cleaning the burn, applying the medication and dressing the wound as ordered. Circulation checks are important with pressure dressings.

The topical medications used to hasten healing and prevent infection vary. Topical administration is preferred, because the capillaries are coagulated by the burn. Systemic antibiotics cannot reach the burn.

Mafenide (Sulfamylon), silver sulfadiazine (Silvadene), povidone-iodine solution (Betadine) 10%, and silver nitrate are the most common drugs used in burn care. Each drug has specific advantages and disadvantages (Table 29-4).

Burns are not dressed in large, bulky dressings; the

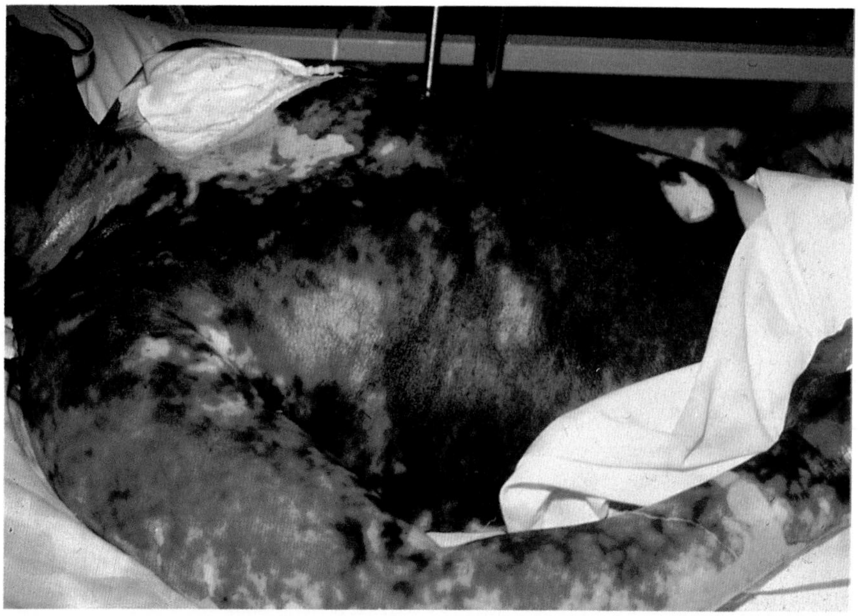

FIG. 29-8 Postburn *Pseudomonas* infection.

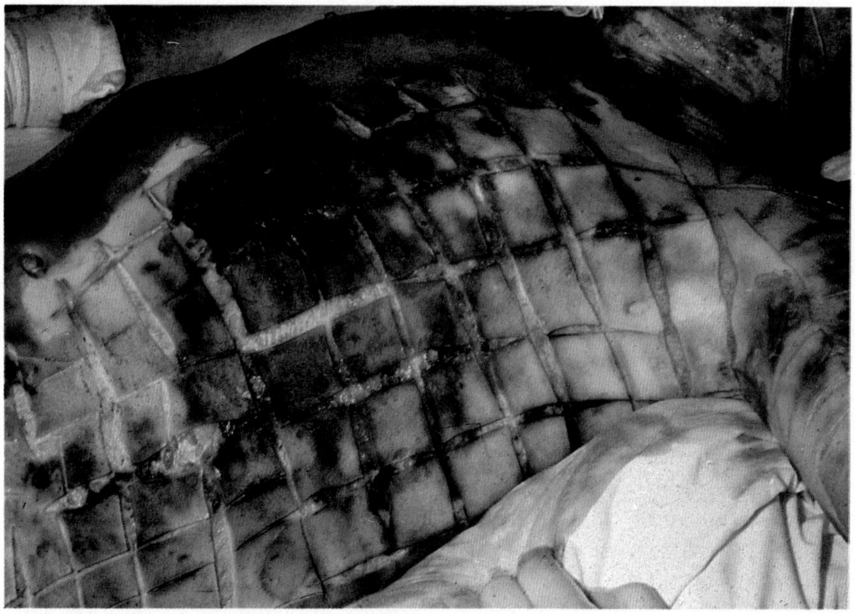

FIG. 29-9 Grid escharatomy used to alleviate circulatory and pulmonary constriction.

dressing needs to be lightweight. A single layer of gauze covered with medication and a single wrap of Kerlix are suggested.

Because changing the dressing is very painful, pain medication should be given 30 minutes before the procedure. Most dressings are changed after hydrotherapy. An important principle to follow is to remove all old medication and eschar before new medication is applied. Failure to debride promotes infection, delays healing, and increases scarring.

Skin grafts are used as soon as possible to cover the burns. Grafting promotes healing and prevents infection. The usual timespan is during the first 3 weeks of care. There are four types of grafts. An **autograft** comes from the burn victim. A **homograft** comes from another person such as a cadaver. A **heterograft** comes from another

Table 29-3 Therapeutic Positioning for the Burn Patient

Area Burned	Description of Position
Neck	No pillow Towel roll under cervical spine Neck splint
Shoulder	90 degrees' abduction, neutral rotation Elbow splint may be used to aid in maintaining position
Axilla	Abduction with 10 to 15 degrees' forward flexion and external rotation Support abducted arm by suspending from IV pole, or place on bedside table Axilla splint
Elbow	Extension Support extended arm on bedside table, foam trough Elbow splint
Hand	Hand splint
Dorsal surface	Flexion
Palmar surface	Hyperextension
Hip	Extension with neutral rotation Supine with lower extremity extended Prone lying (if medically appropriate) Trochanter roll Foam wedge along lateral aspect of thigh Knee or long leg splint
Knee	Extension Prone lying (if medically appropriate) Patient out of bed with lower extremities extended and elevated Knee splint
Ankle	Dorsiflexion Padded footboard with heels free of pressure Ankle splint

species such as a pig or a cow. Synthetic graft substitutes are now available. The autograft is permanent, whereas the other types are temporary.

Graft sites are a nursing challenge. The graft area needs as little movement as possible so as not to tear the graft. Dressings are not changed until ordered. Any movement that results in pulling the graft area can dislocate the graft. The donor site resembles a partial-thickness burn after the graft. Donor site care is as important as care of the burn site. Pain is a primary complaint after the graft and

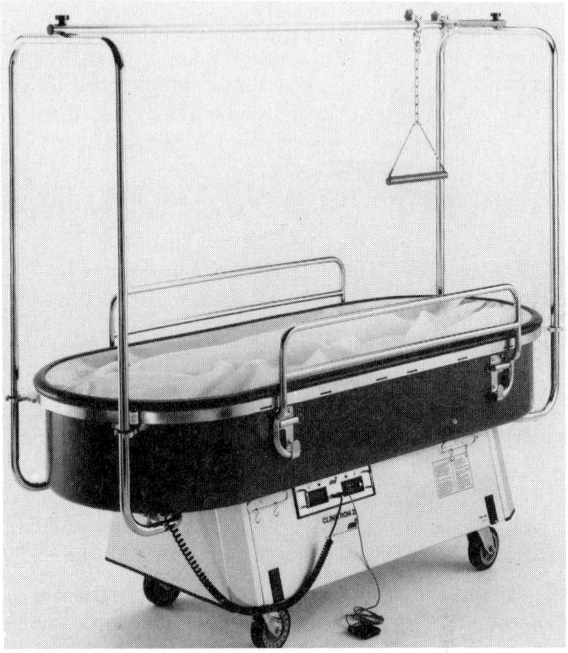

FIG. 29-10 Clinitron therapy unit.

Table 29-4 Topical Medications Used in Burn Therapy

Topical Medication	Advantages	Disadvantages
Mafenide (Sulfamylon)	Bacteriostatic against gram-negative and gram-positive organisms Penetrates thick eschar	Metabolic acidosis Pain on application Allergic rash
Silver sulfadiazine (Silvadene)	Broad antimicrobial activity against gram-negative, gram-positive, and Candida organisms No electrolyte imbalances Painless and somewhat soothing Not nephrotoxic	Repeated application may develop slimy, grayish appearance, simulating an infection despite negative cultures Prolonged use may cause skin rash and depress granulocyte formation
Povidone-iodine (Betadine)	Broad antimicrobial activity against gram-positive and gram-negative bacteria, fungi, yeasts, viruses, protozoa	Metabolic acidosis resulting from elevated serum iodine levels Stains clothing and linen Dry, crusting, scabbing wound Skin rash in unaffected area

Continued.

Table 29-4 Topical Medications Used in Burn Therapy—cont'd

Topical Medication	Advantages	Disadvantages
Silver nitrate	Bacteriostatic effect Lessens pain and eliminates odor Reduces evaporative water loss from burns	Electrolyte imbalances Stains everything it comes into contact with Does not penetrate eschar Pain on application
Nitrofurazone (Furacin)	Inhibits enzymes necessary for bacterial metabolism Broad spectrum of activity Effective against *Staphylococcus aureus* Not absorbed systemically Low incidence of sensitivity	Contact dermatitis in unaffected skin Urine turns a reddish color
Gentamycin sulfate (Garamycin)	Broad antimicrobial activity Painless	Ototoxicity Nephrotoxicity Development of resistant bacterial stains
Neomycin	Broad antimicrobial activity Causes miscoding in the messenger RNA of bacterial cells	Serious toxic effects Ototoxicity Nephrotoxicity
Scarlet red	Nonantiseptic (applied to gauze soaked with oil-base red dye) Drying agent Applied to donor site Promotes epithelialization	No antimicrobial effects Stains and irritates skin Infection may develop beneath scarlet red gauze, which may have systemic effects
Xeroform	Nonantiseptic Debrides and protects donor site Protects graft	Removal may be painful, because it sometimes adheres to wound Neither antiseptic nor antimicrobial
Sodium hypochlorite (Dakin's solution)	Chlorine-based solution that is bactericidal Aids in debriding wounds Aids cleaning and draining "soupy" wounds	Dissolves blood clots May inhibit clotting May irritate the skin
Sutilains ointment (Travase)	Topical enzymatic agent Dissolves necrotic tissue by proteolytic action Facilitates removal of eschar and purulent drainage	Mild, transient pain on application Paresthesia, bleeding, dermatitis Dressing must be kept moist at all times

should be treated. The nurse should inspect the donor site for signs of infection, such as erythema and malodor (Box 29-8).

The nutritional aspect of burn care is very important. Body proteins are destroyed and fluid loss occurs. The body tries to compensate by increasing metabolism to meet the body's extra demands. Enough energy is needed to maintain homeostasis, plus meet the increased need for repairing the injury.

The burn patient should eat by mouth as soon as possible. Intake needs to be enough to meet the caloric and protein requirements. Protein requirements are greater than normal. Normal protein intake is 0.8 g/kg of body weight. The burned patient needs 1.5 to 3.2 g/kg of body weight (a normal 150-pound man needs 55 g of protein a day; if burned he will need 102 to 158 g of

BOX 29-8 **TEACHING THE PATIENT WITH A SKIN GRAFT**

1. Keep surface of healed graft moistened daily with a skin lotion for 6 to 12 months. (Grafted skin does not perspire; it dries and cracks easily.)
2. Protect grafted skin from direct sunlight with a sunscreen lotion for at least 6 months.
3. Wear a strong elastic stocking for 4 to 6 months with grafts on lower extremities.
4. Report changes in the graft (hematoma, fluid collection) to physician.

CHAPTER CHALLENGE

KEY POINTS

- The skin, including nails, hair, and glands, makes up the integumentary system.
- The main functions of the integumentary system are protection, temperature regulation, and vitamin D synthesis.
- The two layers of true skin are the epidermis and the dermis.
- The layer of tissue directly beneath the skin is the subcutaneous layer; it is composed of adipose tissue and loose connective tissue.
- The sudoriferous (sweat) glands release perspiration through the skin.
- The sebaceous (oil) glands secrete sebum, which lubricates the skin and prevents invasion of bacteria through the skin.
- Any injury to the skin poses a threat to a person's self-concept.
- It is important to establish a therapeutic relationship to meet the psychological needs of the patient.
- Most skin disorders are not contagious and are rarely fatal. They are often chronic in nature.
- Sterile technique and isolation techniques are required with any open, draining lesion.
- Wet dressings need to be checked frequently. Constant moisture softens the skin and contributes to skin maceration.
- Application of medications must be done to clean skin.
- The nursing interventions of a skin disorder depend on the cause; however, common problems are decreased skin integrity, potential for infection, and lack of knowledge concerning the disease.
- A primary nursing intervention is patient teaching to alert the patient about the mode of transmission of the particular disease.
- The assessment of patients with skin disorders includes collection of both subjective and objective data.
- Wet dressings and baths may be done to soothe, vasoconstrict, debride, or decrease pruritus.
- Malignant skin diseases need to be prevented by educating the public about causes.
- Burns can be classified by depth and body surface area involved. The pathophysiology and care of burns involve three stages, the hypovolemic/emergent phase, the diuretic/acute phase, and the long-term/rehabilitation phase.
- The three phases of burn care are overlapping, with different goals and nursing interventions in each.
- The first priority in nursing intervention for the burn patient in phase 1 is to establish and maintain an open airway.
- The treatment method of a burn patient depends on age, body surface area involved, location, depth, and other diseases present.
- The primary causes of death in burn victims are hypovolemic shock in the first 72 hours and infection during the acute phase.

STUDY QUESTIONS

1. The layer of skin that contains blood vessels and nerves is:
   a. Epidermis
   b. Dermis
   c. Subcutaneous tissue
   d. Melanin
2. The type of gland that secretes mainly water and salts through the pores is:
   a. Sudoriferous
   b. Ceruminous
   c. Sebaceous
   d. Arrector
3. A papular lesion is described as a:
   a. Small sac containing serous fluid
   b. Small elevation of skin filled with purulent matter
   c. Firm, raised, deep lesion of the skin
   d. Small, solid elevation of the skin
4. When a patient is first admitted with lesions of the skin, the nurse should:
   a. Give the patient a disinfecting tub bath during that shift
   b. Carefully observe and record the patient's skin condition
   c. Clean the affected area carefully with soap and water
   d. Apply a comforting lotion until the physician writes the medical orders
5. Your nurse coworker has complained recently of a "fever blister" on her upper lip. You know she is probably using this common expression to describe:
   a. Shingles
   b. Herpes simplex
   c. Impetigo
   d. Epidermophytosis
6. The most important aspect of nursing intervention for the patient with impetigo is:
   a. Prevention of scarring
   b. Psychological support
   c. Prevention of spread of the disease
   d. Medical treatment
7. While one is caring for a patient with extensive burns, it is important that efforts be made to decrease the likelihood of the patient's developing which complication during the acute period:
   a. Decubitus ulcer
   b. Contractures
   c. Fecal impactions
   d. A wound infection
8. The highest priority in the initial care of the burn patient is to:
   a. Prevent infection
   b. Prevent eschar formation
   c. Assess, establish, and maintain adequate airway
   d. Restore fluid loss
   e. Maintain urinary output
9. The burn patient may be given small amounts of morphine to relieve pain. The most effective route would be:
   a. Subcutaneous
   b. Intramuscular
   c. Intravenous
   d. Oral
10. Silvery, scaling, thickened lesions of the skin describe which skin disorder:
    a. Eczema
    b. Acne vulgaris
    c. Lupus erythematosus
    d. Psoriasis

STUDY QUESTIONS (cont'd)

11. Burns are usually classified by:
    a. Location
    b. Cause
    c. Size
    d. Depth
    e. Extent of shock present
12. Using the "rule of nines," determine the burned area of a patient with burns on the back and front of one leg and the back of one arm:
    a. 13.5%
    b. 18%
    c. 22.5%
    d. 27%
13. Burn patients may have respiratory problems from smoke inhalation. Which of the following signs and symptoms warns of impending laryngeal edema:
    a. Blood-tinged sputum
    b. Carbon particles in sputum
    c. Restlessness
    d. Hypotension
14. An infection of the scalp caused by a fungus is:
    a. Tinea circinata
    b. Tinea sycosis
    c. Tinea capitis
    d. Scabies
15. The most important passive function of the skin is:
    a. Protection
    b. Excretion
    c. Secretion
    d. Heat regulation
16. The physician has ordered a high-protein, high-calorie diet for Mr. White. The high-protein diet is given because protein:
    a. Replaces sodium lost through the burned area
    b. Replaces lost body fat
    c. Builds and repairs body tissues
    d. Provides a source of quick energy
17. If a severely burned patient becomes restless, thrashes about, and complains of pain, the best initial response by the nurse would be:
    a. Give morphine sulfate gr ⅙ intramuscularly for pain
    b. Assess airway and respiratory status
    c. Gently restrain patient to prevent injury
    d. Give diazepam (Valium) 5 mg intravenously for restlessness
18. A burn patient with 30% of body surface area burned and partial-thickness to full-thickness depth has a urine output of 20 ml per hour. Would the physician be likely to order the intravenous fluid rate to be increased or decreased:
    a. Increased
    b. Decreased
19. The severity of a burn injury is determined by all of the following factors *except*:
    a. Extent of body surface area involved
    b. Depth of a burn
    c. Age
    d. Presence of concurrent medical or surgical problems
    e. Socioeconomic status

30

Care of the Patient with a Musculoskeletal Disorder

MARTHA E. SPRAY

LEARNING OBJECTIVES

After reading this chapter, the student should be able to do the following:

- Define the key terms.
- List the five basic functions of the skeletal system.
- Describe the difference between a ligament and a tendon.
- Describe three vital functions muscles perform when they contract.
- Describe the location of the major muscles of the body.
- Define the term "oxygen debt."
- List the types of body movements.
- Describe the following conditions: lordosis, scoliosis, and kyphosis.
- List at least five diagnostic procedures pertinent to musculoskeletal function.
- Compare methods for assessing circulation, nerve damage, and infection in a patient who has received a traumatic insult to the musculoskeletal system.
- List at least four healthy life-style measures a person can practice to reduce the risk of developing osteoporosis.
- List at least two types of skin and skeletal traction.
- List four nursing interventions appropriate for patients with bone cancer.
- Describe the phenomenon of "phantom pain."
- Compare the medical regimen for patients suffering from "gouty arthritis," rheumatoid arthritis, and osteoarthritis.
- Discuss the nursing intervention appropriate for patients with rheumatoid arthritis.
- Describe the nursing intervention appropriate for degenerative joint disease (osteoarthritis and ankylosing spondylitis).
- Describe the surgical intervention for arthritis of the hip and knee.
- Describe the symptoms of compartment syndrome.
- List at least three nursing interventions appropriate for a patient with fat embolism.
- Discuss the physiology of fracture healing (hematoma, granulation tissue, and callus formation).
- Discuss nursing interventions appropriate for a patient with a fractured hip.

RELATED TOPICS OF INTEREST

- Body mechanics (Chapter 18)
- Comfort, rest, and sleep (Chapter 19)
- The surgical patient (Chapter 26)
- Care of the patient with a neurological disorder (Chapter 38)
- Rehabilitation nursing (Chapter 52)
- First aid (Chapter 54)

KEY TERMS

Define the following:

- abduction
- acetabulum
- Achilles
- acromion
- adduction
- ankylosis
- arthrocentesis
- arthrodesis
- arthroplasty
- arthroscopy
- articulation
- blanching
- bursae
- calcaneus
- callus
- crepitus
- diaphysis
- epiphysis
- fat embolism syndrome (FES)
- fibula
- foramen
- foramen magnum
- fossa
- gait
- hemopoiesis
- ilium
- innominate
- insertion
- involuntary
- ischium
- joint
- kyphosis
- ligaments
- lordosis
- manubrium
- olecranon
- origin
- paresthesia
- patella
- periosteum
- phalanges
- pubis
- scoliosis
- subluxation
- synovitis
- synovectomy
- tendons
- tibia
- tophi
- traction
- vomer
- xiphoid

Bones and joints form the framework of the body, but the contraction and relaxation of the muscles allow movement. All movement of the body is orchestrated by the functioning of the bones, joints, and the muscles attached to the bones. This chapter will discuss the structure and function of bones and muscles and how they serve the body.

ANATOMY AND PHYSIOLOGY

Functions of the Skeletal System

The skeletal system has five basic functions: support, protection, movement, mineral storage, and hemopoiesis.

Support. The skeleton provides the body framework that supports internal tissues and organs.

Protection. The skeleton forms a firm, cagelike structure that protects many internal structures. The cranium (skull) protects the brain, and the ribs and sternum (breastbone) protect the lungs and heart.

Movement. Because the skeletal muscles are attached to the bones, the bones provide leverage for movement. As a muscle contracts, it exerts pull on the bone and movement occurs.

Mineral storage. The bones serve as a storage area for various minerals, particularly calcium and phosphorus. When the body does not receive adequate intake of these minerals, the minerals are released by the bones.

Hemopoiesis. Hemopoiesis (blood cell formation) takes place in the red bone marrow. The red bone marrow is spongy bone found in the ends of the long bones. A child's bones contain a proportionally larger amount of red bone marrow than an adult's. As one ages, much of the red bone marrow converts to yellow bone marrow, which is composed of fat cells.

Structure of Bones

The skeletal system is composed of 206 bones. In some areas, such as the nose, the framework is composed of both bone and cartilage. There are two basic types of bone tissue, compact and spongy. Compact bone is hard and dense; it looks smooth. Spongy bone has open areas surrounded by needlelike projections of bone tissue. These small projections contain red bone marrow.

There are four classifications of bones, based on their form and shape: long, short, flat, and irregular. Long bones are found in the extremities, short bones are found in the hands and feet, flat bones are found in the skull and sternum, and irregular bones comprise the vertebrae (backbone).

Bone markings. In the structure and shape of bones there are various raised areas, openings, and ridges. These sites mark the areas where muscles, tendons, and ligaments are attached and where blood vessels and nerves pass. These landmarks are divided into two categories: processes (projections or prominences), which grow out from the surface of the bone, and depressions (cavities), which are indentations of the bones.

Table 30-1 identifies the bone markings. Briefly, the major structures are as follows:

1. **Acromion** process: a slightly flaring projection at the lateral end of the scapula; it forms the highest point of the shoulder
2. Mastoid process; a protuberance just behind the ear
3. **Olecranon:** the upper end of the ulna, which forms the point of the elbow
4. Iliac crest: the upper curving boundary of the ilium; it can be felt by placing the hands at the level of the waist and exerting a slight downward pressure
5. Ischial tuberosity: the large posterior part of the ischium; in erect sitting position the body rests on these tuberosities
6. Ischial spine: a small prominent area on either side of the ischium, anterior to the ischial tuberosity
7. **Acetabulum:** the hip socket, formed by the hip bones, the ilium, the ischium, and the pubis
8. Greater trochanter: a protuberance of the femur located interiorly and laterally to the head of the femur

Other important structures include the following:

1. Crests: narrow ridges of bone
2. Spines: sharp, slender projections
3. **Foramen:** round openings through a bone; of particular importance is the **foramen magnum,** located at the base of the occipital bone, which allows the spinal cord to communicate with the brain
4. **Fossa:** a shallow depression in a bone
5. Sinus: a depression filled with air and lined with mucous membrane
6. Grooves: shallow depressions that are long and narrow, which allow the passage of nerves and blood vessels

Table 30-1 Identification of Bone Markings

Bone	Marking	Description
Frontal	Supraorbital margin	Arched ridge just below eyebrows
	Frontal sinuses	Cavities inside bone just above supraorbital margin; lined with mucosa; contain air
Temporal	Mastoid process	Protuberance just behind ear
	Mastoid air cells	Air-filled, mucosa-lined spaces within mastoid process
	External auditory meatus (or canal)	Opening into ear and tube extending into temporal bone
	Zygomatic process	Projection that articulates with malar (or zygomatic) bone
Occipital	Foramen magnum	Opening through which spinal cord enters cranial cavity
Sphenoid	Body	Hollow, cubelike central portion
	Sella turcica (or Turkish saddle)	Saddle-shaped depression on upper surface of sphenoid body; contains pituitary gland
	Sphenoid sinuses	Irregular, air-filled, mucosa-lined spaces within central part of sphenoid
Ethmoid	Horizontal (cribriform) plate	Olfactory nerves pass through numerous openings in this plate
	Ethmoid sinuses	Honeycombed, mucosa-lined air spaces within lateral masses of bone
Mandible	Body	Main part of body; forms chin
	Alveolar process	Teeth set into this arch
Maxilla	Alveolar process	Arch containing teeth
	Maxillary sinus	Large, air-filled, mucosa-lined cavity within body of each maxilla; largest of sinuses
Special features of skull	Sutures	Immovable joints between skull bones
	1. Sagittal	1. Joint between two parietal bones
	2. Coronal	2. Joint between parietal bones and frontal bone
	3. Lambdoidal	3. Joint between parietal bones and occipital bone

Table 30-1 Identification of Bone Markings—cont'd

Bone	Marking	Description
	Fontanels	"Soft spots" where ossification is incomplete at birth; allow some compression of skull during birth; also important in determining position of head before delivery; six such areas located at angles of parietal bones
	1. Anterior (or frontal)	1. At intersection of sagittal and coronal sutures (juncture of parietal bones and frontal bone); diamond shaped; largest of fontanels; usually closed by 1½ years of age
	2. Posterior (or occipital)	2. At intersection of sagittal and lambdoidal sutures (juncture of parietal bones and occipital bone); triangular in shape; usually closed by second month
Sternum	Body	Main central part of bone
	Xiphoid process	Projection of cartilage at lower border of bone
Scapula	Spine	Sharp ridge running diagonally across posterior surface of shoulderblade
	Acromion process	Slightly flaring projection at lateral end of scapular spine; may be felt as tip of shoulder; articulates with clavicle
	Glenoid cavity	Arm socket
Humerus	Head	Smooth, hemispherical enlargement at proximal end of humerus
Ulna	Olecranon process	Elbow
Radius	Head	Disk-shaped process forming proximal end of radius; articulates with capitulum of humerus and with radial notch of ulna
Innominate (hip)	Ilium	Upper, flaring portion
	Ischium	Lower, posterior portion
	Pubic bone or pubis	Medial, anterior section
	Acetabulum	Hip socket; formed by union of ilium, ischium, and pubis
	Iliac crests	Upper, curving boundary of ilium
	Anterosuperior spine	Prominent projection at anterior end of iliac crest; can be felt externally as "point" of hip
	Ischial tuberosity	Large, rough, quadrilateral process forming posterior part of ischium; in erect sitting position body rests on these tuberosities
	Symphysis pubis	Cartilaginous, amphiarthrotic joint between pubic bones
	Obturator foramen	Large hole in anterior surface of os coxae; formed by pubis and ischium; largest foramen in body
	Pelvic brim (or inlet)	Boundary of opening leading into true pelvis; size and shape of this inlet has great obstetrical importance, since if any of its diameters is too small, infant skull cannot enter true pelvis for natural birth
	True (or lesser) pelvis	Space below pelvic brim; true "basin" with bone and muscle walls and muscle floor; pelvic organs located in this space
	False (or greater) pelvis	Broad, shallow space above pelvic brim inlet; name "false pelvis" is misleading, since this space is actually part of abdominal cavity, not pelvic cavity
Femur	Head	Rounded, upper end of bone; fits in acetabulum
	Greater trochanter	Protuberance located interiorly and laterally to head
	Lesser trochanter	Small protuberance located inferiorly and medially to greater trochanter
Tibia	Medial malleolus	Rounded, downward projection at distal end of tibia; forms prominence on outer surface of ankle
Fibula	Lateral malleolus	Rounded prominence at distal end of fibula; forms prominence on outer surface of ankle
Tarsals	Calcaneus	Heel bone
	Talus	Uppermost of tarsals; articulates with tibia and fibula; boxed in by medial and lateral malleoli

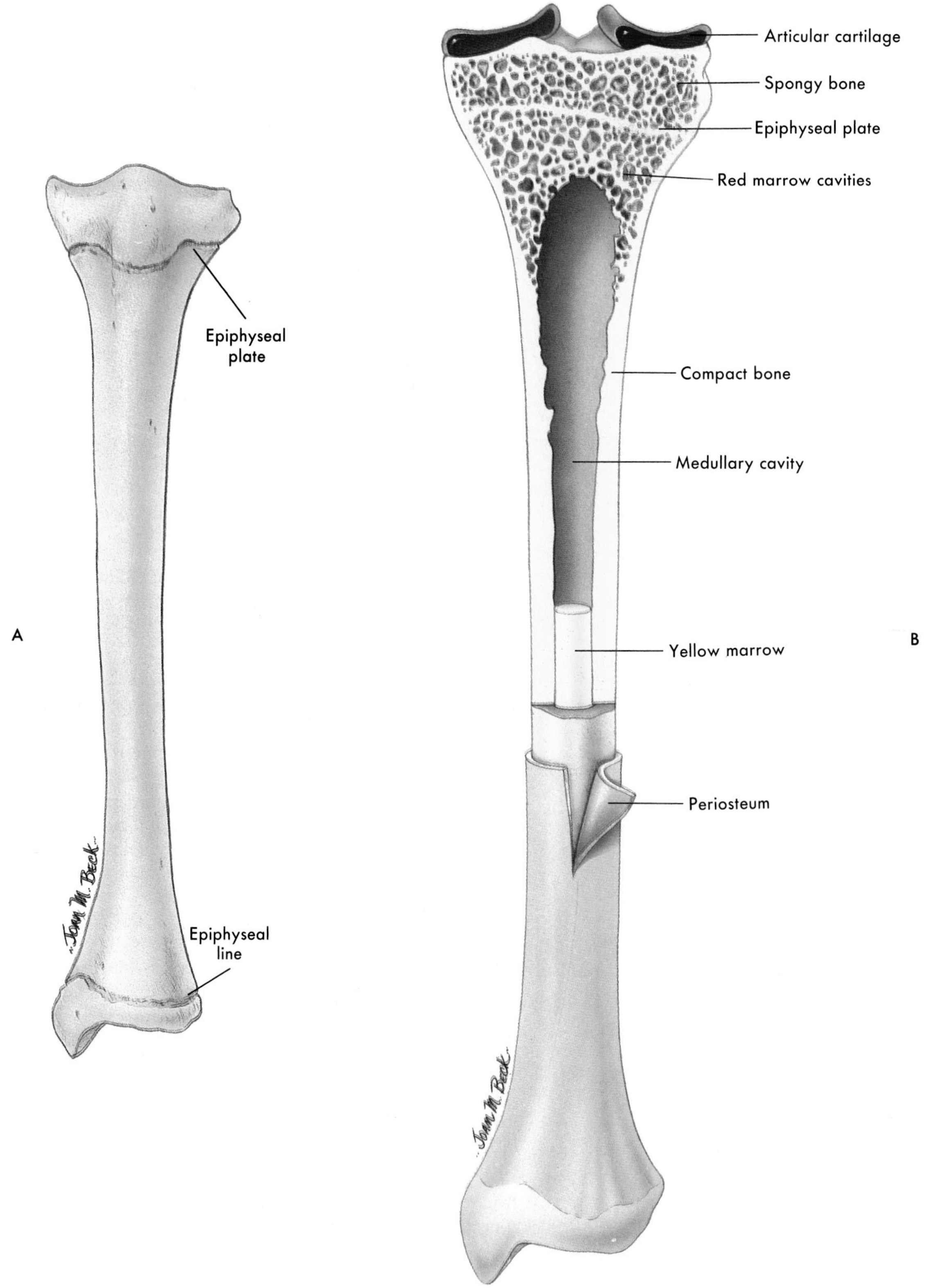

FIG. 30-1 **A,** External view of epiphyseal lines on a juvenile long bone. The area between the epiphyses is the diaphysis. **B,** Longitudinal section of long bone showing structural details.

Structure of a long bone. Fig. 30-1 shows a long bone; the following structures can be identified:

1. **Diaphysis:** composed of compact bone, yet shaped like a long, hollow tube; a strong structure but lightweight to allow movement
2. Medullary cavity: the hollow center of the bone shaft; contains the yellow bone marrow
3. **Epiphysis:** the ends of the long bones; composed of spongy bone and contains the red bone marrow
4. Articular cartilage: a thin, external covering of cartilage on each epiphysis; cushions the joint
5. **Periosteum:** a protective fibrous membrane that covers the diaphysis of the bone

Articulations (Joints)

Bones cannot bend without damage. To allow movement, individual bones articulate (move) at joint sites. Bones are held together by flexible connective tissue. The **joint** is the point of contact between the individual bones. The structure of the individual bones depends on the function of the area. Every bone in the body (except the hyoid bone, which anchors the tongue) connects or articulates with at least one other bone.

Joints perform two important functions: they hold the bones together to form the skeleton, and they allow movement and flexibility of the skeleton.

Types of joints. The most common way to classify joints is according to the degree of movement they permit. There are three types:

1. Synarthrosis: no movement
2. Amphiarthrosis: slight movement
3. Diarthrosis: free movement

Synarthrosis. These immovable joints are held together by fibrous connective tissue. An example is the suture lines of the skull, where the irregular edges of the bone are bound together by fibrous connective tissue.

Amphiarthrosis. These slightly immovable joints are connected by a disk of cartilage. Two examples of this type of joint are the pubic bones of the pelvis and the intervertebral joints of the spinal column.

Diarthrosis (synovial joints). These freely movable joints contain a joint capsule, joint cavity, and a layer of cartilage over the ends of the two bones (Fig. 30-2). The capsule fits over the ends of the two bones like a sleeve. It is composed of fibrous connective tissue and lined with synovial membrane, which is smooth and slippery. This membrane secretes synovial fluid, which allows free movement. Fig. 30-3 shows examples of diarthrotic joints: the hinge, pivot, condyloid, saddle, ball and socket, and gliding.

Ligaments (bands of connective tissue) anchor bones together, whereas **tendons** (also bands of connective tissue) anchor muscles to the bones. The articular cartilage covering the ends of the bones acts as a shock absorber.

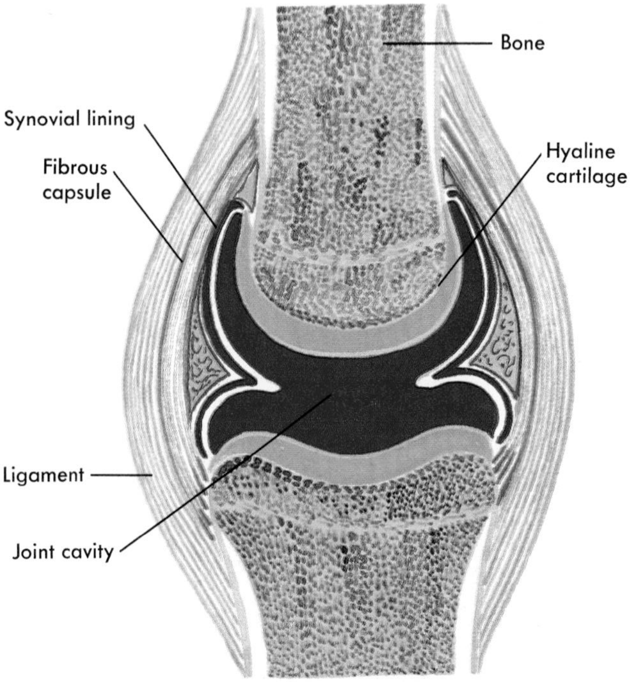

FIG. 30-2 Structure of a freely movable (diarthrotic) joint. Note these typical features: joint capsule, joint cavity lined with synovial membrane, and articular (hyaline) cartilage covering the end surfaces of the bones within the joint capsule.

Bursae (small sacs of connective tissue) also cushion shock. They are located wherever pressure is exerted (e.g., between skin and bone, between tendons and bone, and sometimes between muscles). They are lined with synovial membrane and thus contain synovial fluid.

Divisions of the Skeleton

The skeleton is divided into the axial and the appendicular skeleton. The axial skeleton is composed of the skull, the vertebral column, and the thorax (chest) (Table 30-2). The appendicular skeleton contains 126 bones and is composed of the upper extremities, the lower extremities, the shoulder girdle, and the pelvic girdle (excluding the sacrum) (Figs. 30-4 and 30-5).

Axial skeleton

Skull. The skull contains 22 bones and sits on the superior portion of the vertebral column. Eight cranial bones enclose and protect the brain: frontal bone, parietal bones (2), temporal bones (2), occipital bone, sphenoid bone, and ethmoid bone. The remaining 14 bones are the facial bones. They are the nasal bones (2), the maxillae (2), the zygomatic bones (2), the mandible, the lacrimal bones (2), the palatine bones (2), the inferior nasal conchae (2), and the **vomer** (Fig. 30-6). Table 30-3 briefly describes each bone.

Text continued on p. 585.

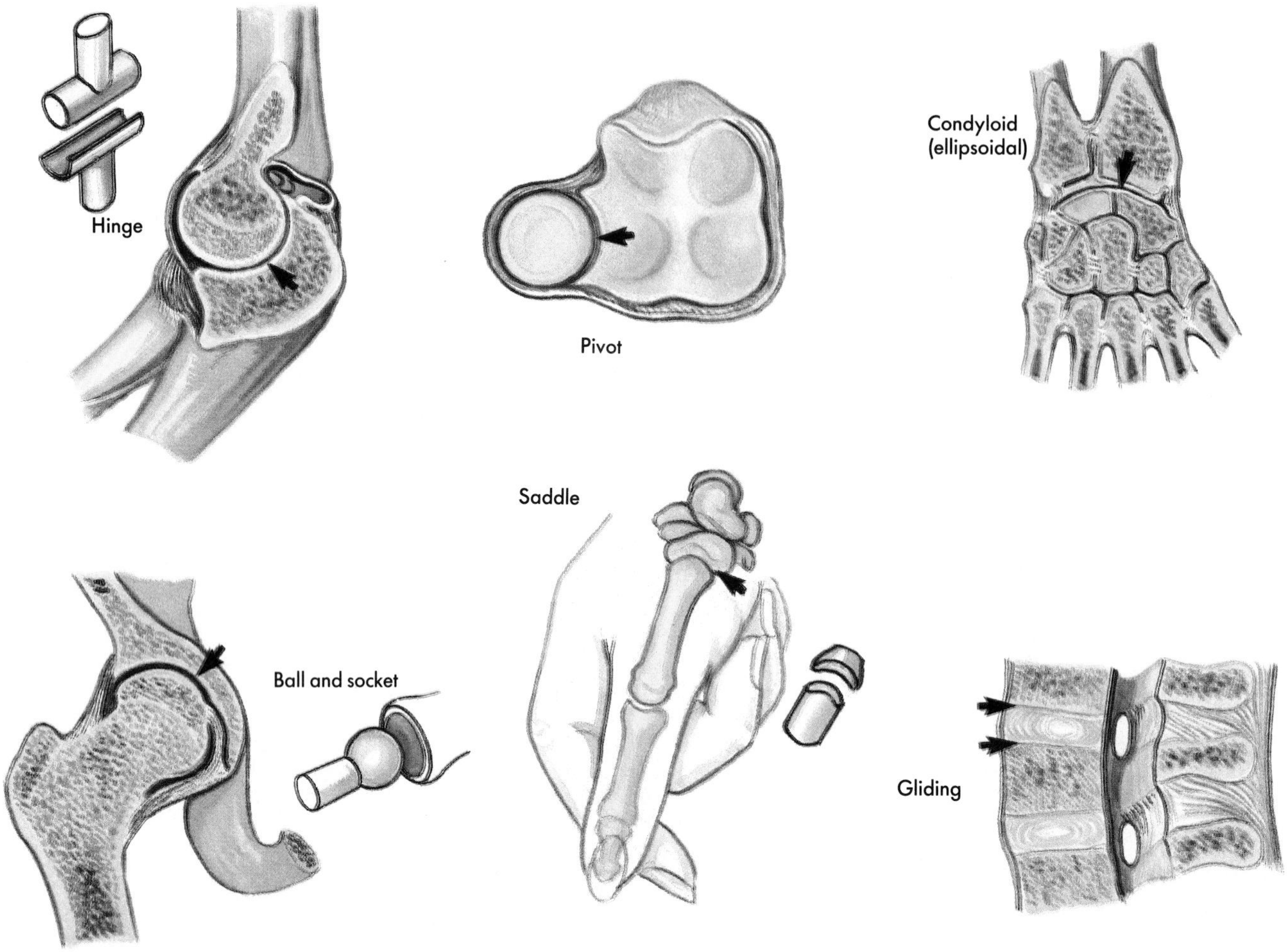

FIG. 30-3 Diarthrotic joints.

Table 30-2 Main Parts of the Skeleton

Axial Skeleton	Appendicular Skeleton
SKULL	**UPPER EXTREMITIES**
Cranium	Shoulder (pectoral) girdle
Ear bones	Arms
Face	Wrists
	Hands
SPINE	**LOWER EXTREMITIES**
Vertebrae	Hip (pelvic) girdle
THORAX	Legs
Ribs	Ankles
Sternum	Feet

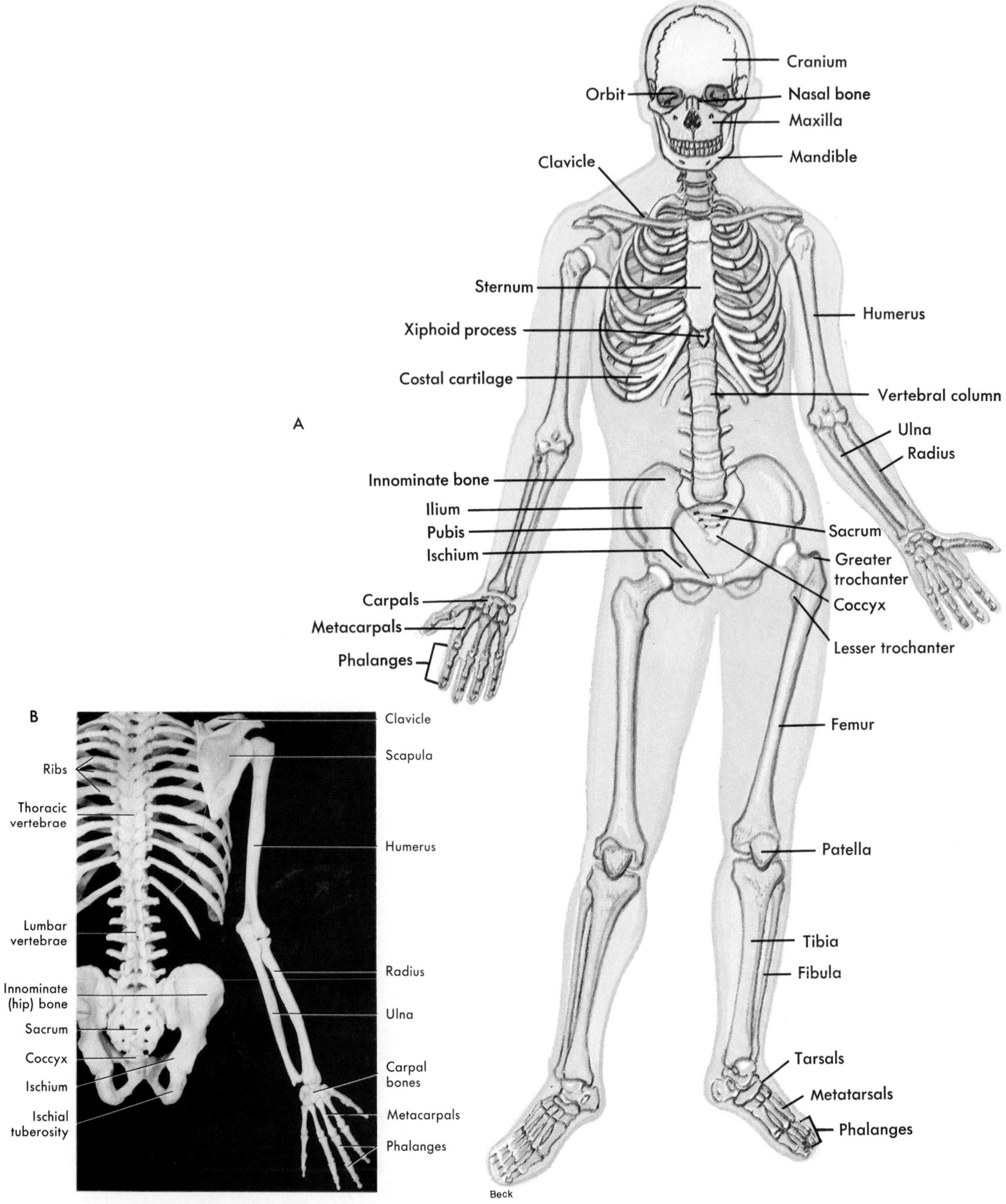

FIG. 30-4 **A,** Skeleton, anterior view. Axial skeleton is shown in blue. Appendicular system is bone colored. **B,** Photograph showing anterior aspect of the right half of the thoracic, upper limb, abdominal, and pelvic skeleton.

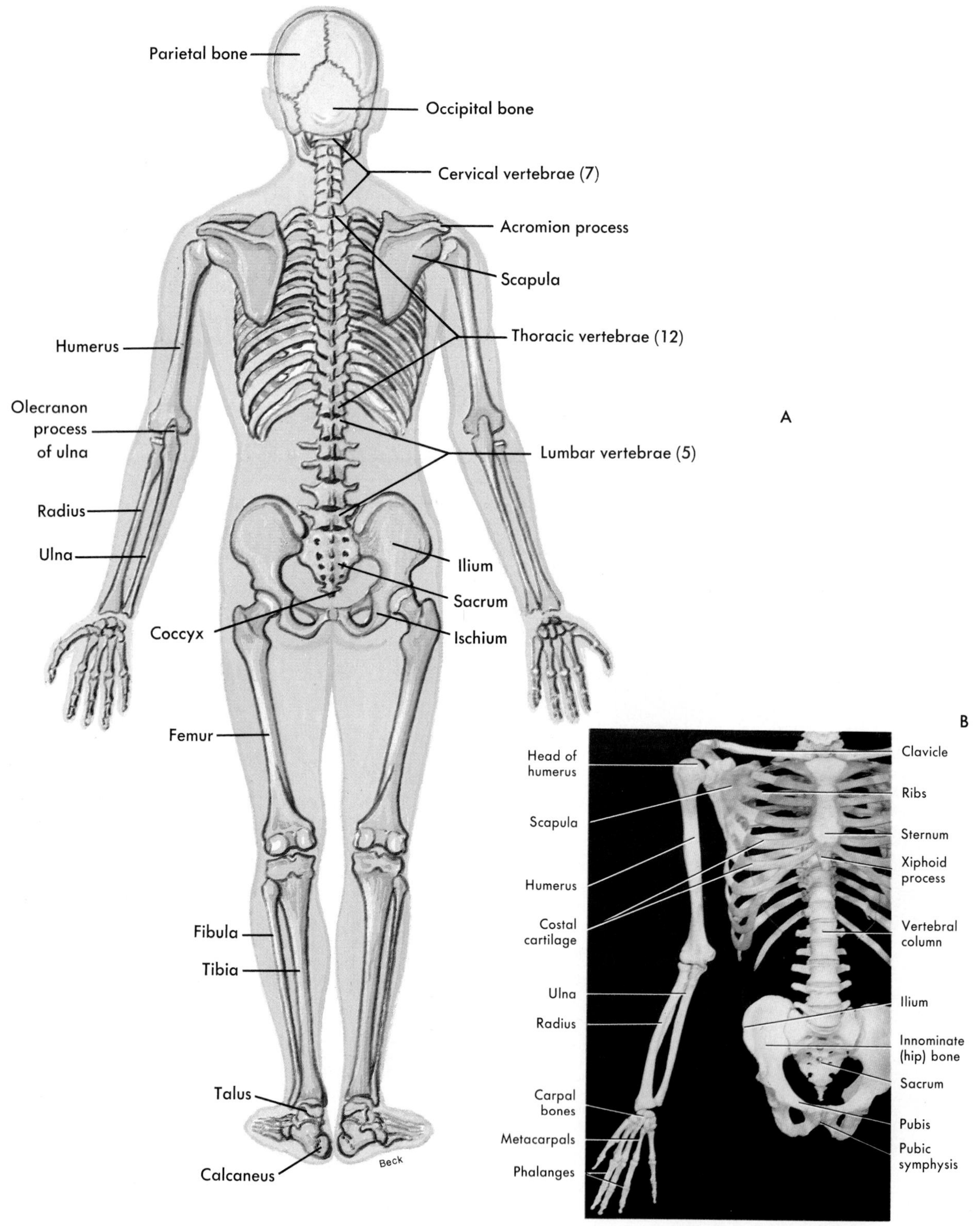

FIG. 30-5 **A,** Skeleton, posterior view. Axial skeleton is shown in blue. Appendicular system is bone colored. **B,** Photograph showing posterior aspect of the right half of the thoracic, upper limb, abdominal, and pelvic skeleton.

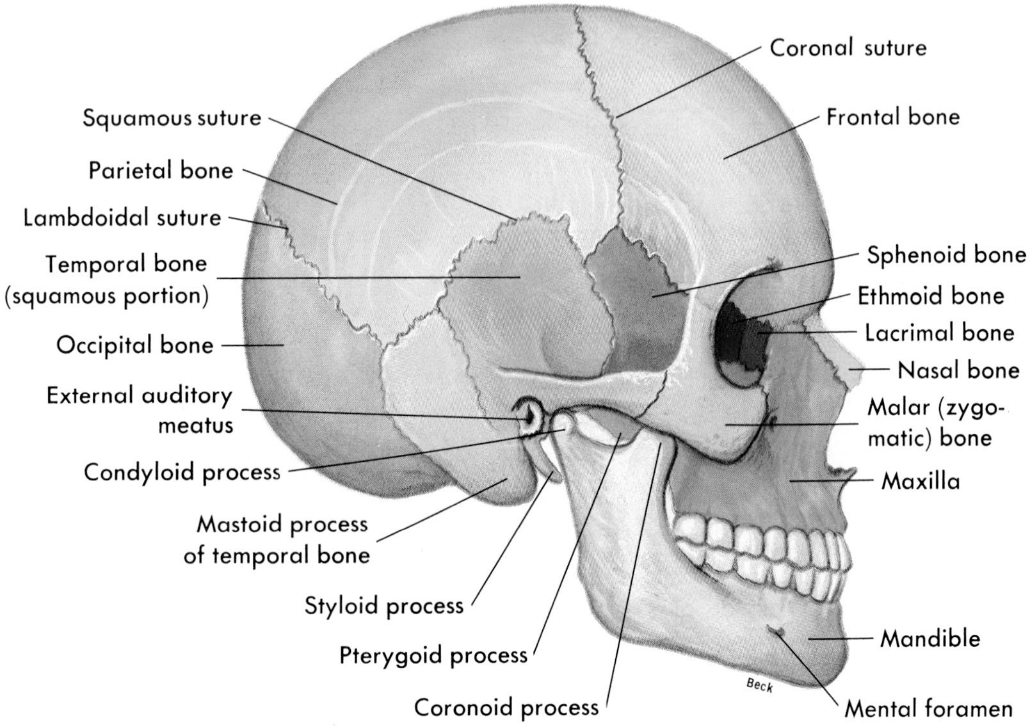

FIG. 30-6 Skull viewed from the right side.

Table 30-3 Bones of the Skeleton

Name	Number	Description
CRANIAL BONES		
Frontal	1	Forehead bone; also forms front part of floor of cranium and most of upper part of eye sockets; cavity inside bone above upper margins of eye sockets (orbits) called *frontal sinus;* lined with mucous membrane
Parietal	2	Form bulging topsides of cranium
Temporal	2	Form lower sides of cranium; contain *middle* and *inner ear structures; mastoid sinuses* are mucosa-lined spaces in *mastoid process,* the protuberance behind ear; *external auditory canal* is tube leading into temporal bone
Occipital	1	Forms back of skull; spinal cord enters cranium through large opening *(foramen magnum)* in occipital bone
Sphenoid	1	Forms central part of floor of cranium; pituitary gland located in small depression in sphenoid called sella turcica *(Turkish saddle)*
Ethmoid	1	Complicated bone that helps form floor of cranium, side walls and roof of nose and part of its middle partition (nasal septum), and part of orbit; contains honeycomb-like spaces, the *ethmoid sinuses*
FACE BONES		
Nasal	2	Small bones that form upper part of bridge of nose
Maxillary	2	Upper jawbones; also help form roof of mouth, floor, and side walls of nose and floor of orbit; large cavity in maxillary bone is *maxillary sinus*
Zygoma	2	Cheek bones; also help form orbit
Mandible	1	Lower jawbone
Lacrimal	2	Small bone; helps form medial wall of eye socket and side wall of nasal cavity
Palatine	2	Form back part of roof of mouth and floor and side walls of nose and part of floor of orbit
Vomer	1	Forms lower, back part of nasal septum

Continued.

Table 30-3 Bones of the Skeleton—cont'd

Name	Number	Description
EAR BONES		
Malleus	2	Malleus, incus, and stapes are tiny bones in middle ear cavity in temporal bone; malleus means "hammer"—shape of bone
Incus	2	Incus means "anvil"—shape of bone
Stapes	2	Stapes means "stirrup"—shape of bone
HYOID BONE	1	U-shaped bone in neck at base of tongue
VERTEBRAL COLUMN		
Cervical vertebrae	7	Upper seven vertebrae, in neck region; first cervical vertebra called *atlas;* second called *axis*
Thoracic vertebrae	12	Next twelve vertebrae; ribs attach to these
Lumbar vertebrae	5	Next five vertebrae; those in small of back
Sacrum	1	In child, five separate vertebrae; in adult, fused into one
Coccyx	1	In child, three to five separate vertebrae; in adult fused into one
THORAX		
True ribs	14	Upper seven pairs; attach to sternum by way of *costal cartilages*
False ribs	10	Lower five pairs; lowest two pairs do not attach to sternum, therefore, called *floating ribs;* next three pairs attach to sternum by way of costal cartilage of seventh ribs
Sternum	1	Breastbone; shaped like a dagger; piece of cartilage at lower end of bone called *xiphoid process*
UPPER EXTREMITIES		
Clavicle	2	Collarbones; only joints between shoulder girdle and axial skeleton are those between each clavicle and sternum
Scapula	2	Shoulder bones; scapula plus clavicle forms *shoulder girdle; acromion process*—tip of shoulder that forms joint with clavicle; *glenoid cavity*—arm socket
Humerus	2	Upper arm bone
Radius	2	Bone on thumb side of lower arm
Ulna	2	Bone on little finger side of lower arm; *olecranon process*—projection of ulna known as elbow or "funny bone"
Carpal bones	16	Irregular bones at upper end of hand; anatomical wrist
Metacarpals	10	Form framework of palm of hand
Phalanges	28	Finger bones; three in each finger, two in each thumb
LOWER EXTREMITIES		
Pelvic bones	2	Hipbones; *ilium*—upper flaring part of pelvic bone; *ischium*—lower back part; *pubic bone*—lower front part; *acetabulum*—hip socket; *symphysis pubis*—joint in midline between two pubic bones; *pelvic inlet*—opening into *true pelvis,* or pelvic cavity; if pelvic inlet is misshapen or too small, infant skull cannot enter true pelvis for natural birth
Femur	2	Thigh or upper leg bones; *head of femur*—ball-shaped, upper end of bone; fits into acetabulum
Patella	2	Kneecap
Tibia	2	Shinbone; *medial malleolus*—rounded projection at lower end of tibia commonly called *inner anklebone*
Fibula	2	Long slender bone of lateral side of lower leg; *lateral malleolus*—rounded projection at lower end of fibula commonly called *outer anklebone*
Tarsal bones	14	Form heel and back part of foot; anatomical ankle
Metatarsals	10	Form part of foot to which toes attach; tarsal and metatarsal bones so arranged that they form three arches in foot
Phalanges	28	Toe bones; three in each toe, two in each great toe
TOTAL	206	

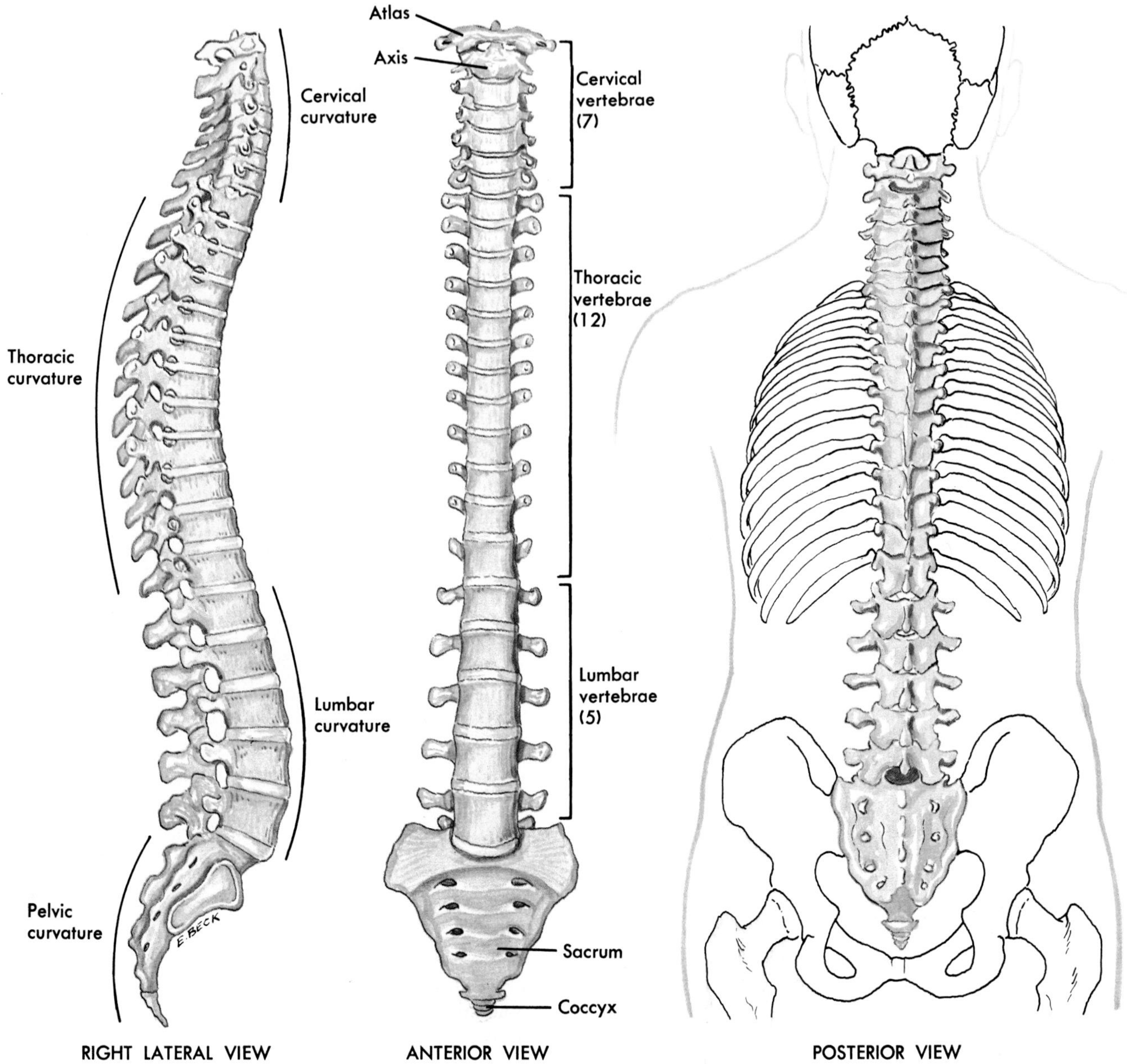

FIG. 30-7 The spinal column from three views.

Vertebral column. The vertebral column (Fig. 30-7) supports the body and is strong and flexible. It contains a total of 26 bones: 24 single bones (vertebrae), and 2 fused bones (the sacrum and the coccyx). It is composed of five sections: cervical, thoracic, lumbar, sacral, and coccyx. The column is S-shaped and contains four curves, which develop before birth. This pattern gives flexibility and strength to the column. The first seven vertebrae are the cervical vertebrae and form the neck region. The first vertebra is called the *atlas* and allows the head to nod in a "yes" motion. The second vertebra is called the *axis* and allows the head to turn in a "no" motion. Progressing in a distal fashion, the next 12 vertebrae are called the *thoracic vertebrae*. They form the chest portion of the column, where the 12 pairs of ribs attach, and they are convex (curve outward). The next five vertebrae, the lumbar vertebrae, are the largest and heaviest of the column. They are concave (curve inward) and form the lower back. The spinal cord, which continues from the brain through the vertebral column, ends at the second lumbar vertebra. The sacrum is formed by five fused vertebrae and forms the posterior pelvis. The last section of the vertebral column is the coccyx, which is composed of four or five fused bones. It is commonly called the *tailbone*.

A single vertebra is composed of three basic parts: the body, the foramen, and the processes. The large, solid structure is the body, the opening through which the spinal column passes is the foramen, and the winglike structures are the processes.

Thorax. The thorax, or rib cage, is composed of the sternum, ribs, and the thoracic vertebrae. This cagelike structure protects the heart, lungs, and great vessels.

Sternum. The sternum (breastbone) is a flat bone formed by the fusion of three bones—manubrium (upper region), body (midportion), and **xiphoid** process (distal portion). The first seven pairs of ribs are attached to it with costal cartilage. The clavicles (collar bones) are attached to it with ligaments.

Ribs. The ribcage is composed of 12 pairs of ribs. Each rib attaches posteriorly to the vertebral column. The first 10 pairs attach anteriorly to the ribcage. The remaining two pairs seem to float free; hence the name *floating* ribs. The first 7 pairs of ribs attach directly to the sternum with costal cartilage; they are called true ribs. The eighth, ninth, and tenth pairs attach to the seventh rib, therefore attaching indirectly to the sternum. They are called *false ribs*.

Appendicular skeleton

The appendicular skeleton contains 126 bones. It is composed of the bones of the limbs and the pectoral and pelvic girdles, which attach the limbs to the axial skeleton.

Pectoral girdle. The pectoral girdle is composed of the two clavicles (collar bones) and the two scapulae (shoulder-blades). It is responsible for the attachment of the upper extremities to the sternum; there is no articulation with the vertebral column. The clavicle attaches to the superior portion of the sternum, the **manubrium.** The distal portion of the clavicle attaches to the scapula. The scapulae are flat, triangular bones that resemble wings. The enlarged end of the spine of the scapula, the acromion process, connects with the clavicle. These articulations allow a wide range of motion.

Bones of the upper extremities. The upper arm is formed by a single long bone, the humerus. It is the second longest bone in the body. It attaches to the scapula at its proximal end. This rounded head has two bony projections that are sites for muscle attachments.

The forearm is formed by two bones, the radius and the ulna. They articulate with each other and the humerus, forming the elbow. Fig. 30-8 shows the large bony process, the olecranon process; this is commonly called the *funny bone*. Distally the radius and ulna articulate the bones of the wrist. In the anatomical position (arms at the side of the body with palms facing forward), the ulna lies medially, extending toward the little finger. The radius extends laterally, extending toward the thumb.

The wrist is formed by 8 irregular bones called the *carpals*. The palm of the hand is formed by 5 metacarpal bones that join the 14 finger bones, *phalanges*. Each finger contains 3 **phalanges:** proximal, middle, and distal. The thumb contains 2 phalanges: proximal and distal.

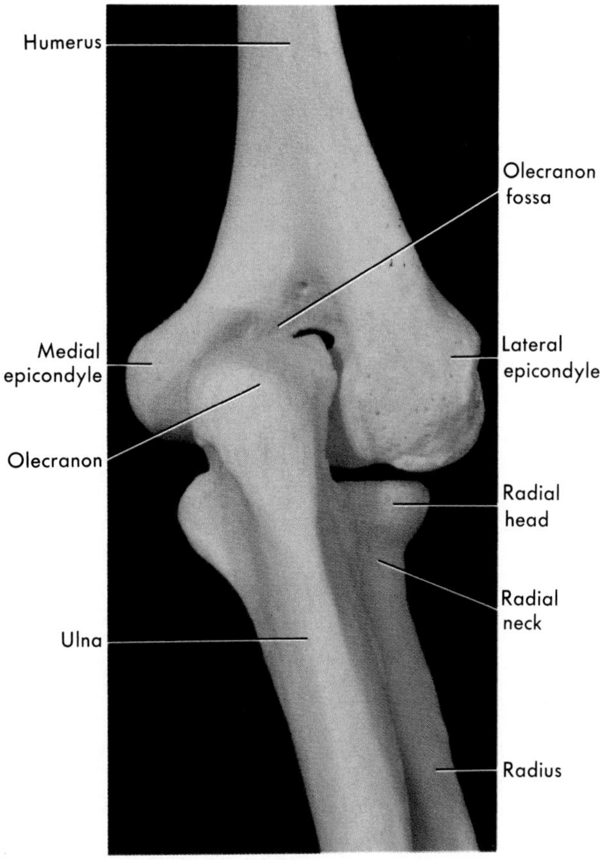

FIG. 30-8 Right elbow skeleton.

Pelvic girdle (pelvis). The pelvis is composed of the two large hipbones (innominate), the sacrum, and the coccyx. In infancy the innominate bones are composed of three separate bones: the ilium, the ischium, and the pubis. In later years these bones fuse and become one (Fig. 30-9). The ilium is the upper, flared portion. The upper rim is called the iliac crest and is an important anatomical landmark for injection technique. It connects posteriorly with the sacrum to form the sacroiliac joint. The **ischium** is the strongest section and holds the body weight when the body is in a sitting position. The **pubis** forms the anterior section of the pelvis and fuses to form the pubis symphysis, a cartilaginous joint.

Bones of the lower extremities. The upper leg bone, the femur (Fig. 30-10, *A*), is the strongest and heaviest bone in the body. The head of the femur articulates with the hip bone in a deep socket—the acetabulum. This is an excellent example of a ball and socket joint. Distally the femur articulates with the tibia (shin). Each femur angles medially; this results in the knee joints being nearer the body's line of gravity (see Fig. 30-5). Anterior to the articulation of the upper and lower leg is the **patella** (kneecap), a small, triangular bone. The patella is surrounded by four bursae, which cushion it.

The lower leg is composed of two bones, the **tibia** and the fibula (Fig. 30-10, *B*). As stated, the tibia articulates

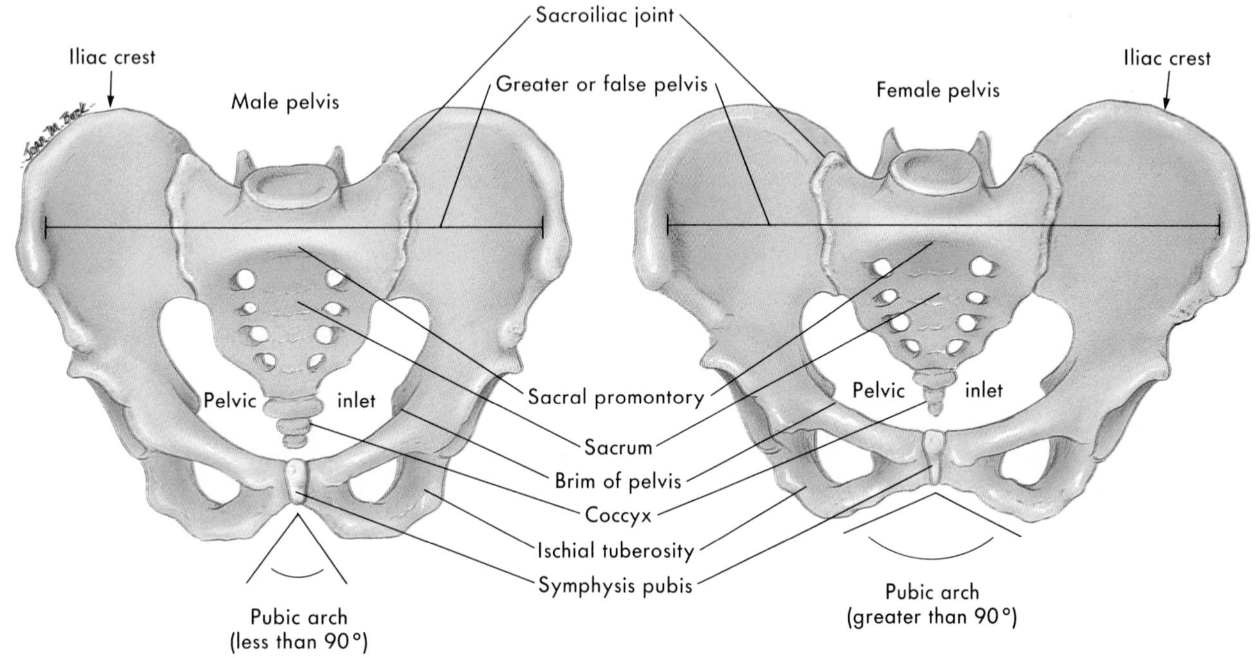

FIG. 30-9 Comparison of male and female bony pelvis.

with the femur. It is the larger of the two bones and lies medially. It bears the major portion of the body weight, and the **fibula,** which is thin and sticklike, lies beside it. The bulge on the inner aspect of the ankle is formed by the medial malleolus of the tibia; the fibula's lateral malleolus forms the lateral bulge. The length of the tibia can be easily felt along the anterior surface of the lower leg, since it is unprotected by any major muscle group.

The ankle (tarsus) is composed of seven tarsal bones. The two largest tarsals, the **calcaneus** (heelbone) and the talus (also posterior) carry most of the body weight. The talus articulates with the tibia and fibula. As a step is taken, the weight is initially carried by the talus; the weight is then transferred to the calcaneus. The foot is composed of 5 metatarsal bones (which form the instep) and 14 phalanges. There are some similarities between the feet and the hands. The great toe, like the thumb, has two bones, whereas the fingers and remaining toes have three bones. Because the foot is designed for weight bearing, it contains ligaments to bind the bones together and tendons to hold the foot in an arched position. The longitudinal arch runs from the calcaneus to the heads of the metatarsals. The transverse arch extends across the ball of the foot. These arches provide flexibility and spring motion to the gait.

The Muscular System

The bones and joints provide the framework of the body, but the muscles are necessary for movement. This motion results from contraction and relaxation of the individual muscles.

The body is composed of more than 600 muscles. They usually act in groups to execute a body movement. They comprise approximately 40% to 50% of the total body weight.

Functions. As muscles contract they perform three vital functions: motion, maintenance of posture, and production of heat.

All body movements rely on the integrated functioning of the bones, joints, and muscles. Certain involuntary kinds of motion include activities conducted by the internal organs, such as the heart beating, the gallbladder releasing bile, and the stomach churning food. Muscle tissue is under voluntary or involuntary control. Voluntary muscle is under conscious control, whereas involuntary muscle tissue responds to internal commands without any conscious control of it.

The contraction of certain skeletal muscles gives the body proper posture. These muscles exert a pull on various bones, which allows the body to maintain a sitting or standing position.

As skeletal muscles contract they produce body heat. It is estimated that approximately 85% of all body heat is generated by the contraction of skeletal muscles.

Types of muscle tissue. Muscle tissue is categorized by location, structure, and type of nervous system control. There are three types of muscle tissue: skeletal, cardiac, and smooth muscle.

1. Skeletal muscle tissue attaches to the bones to produce movement. It is called *striated* because under the microscope it appears to have stripes running perpendicular to the length of the muscle. It is also voluntary muscle tissue because it can be consciously made to contract.

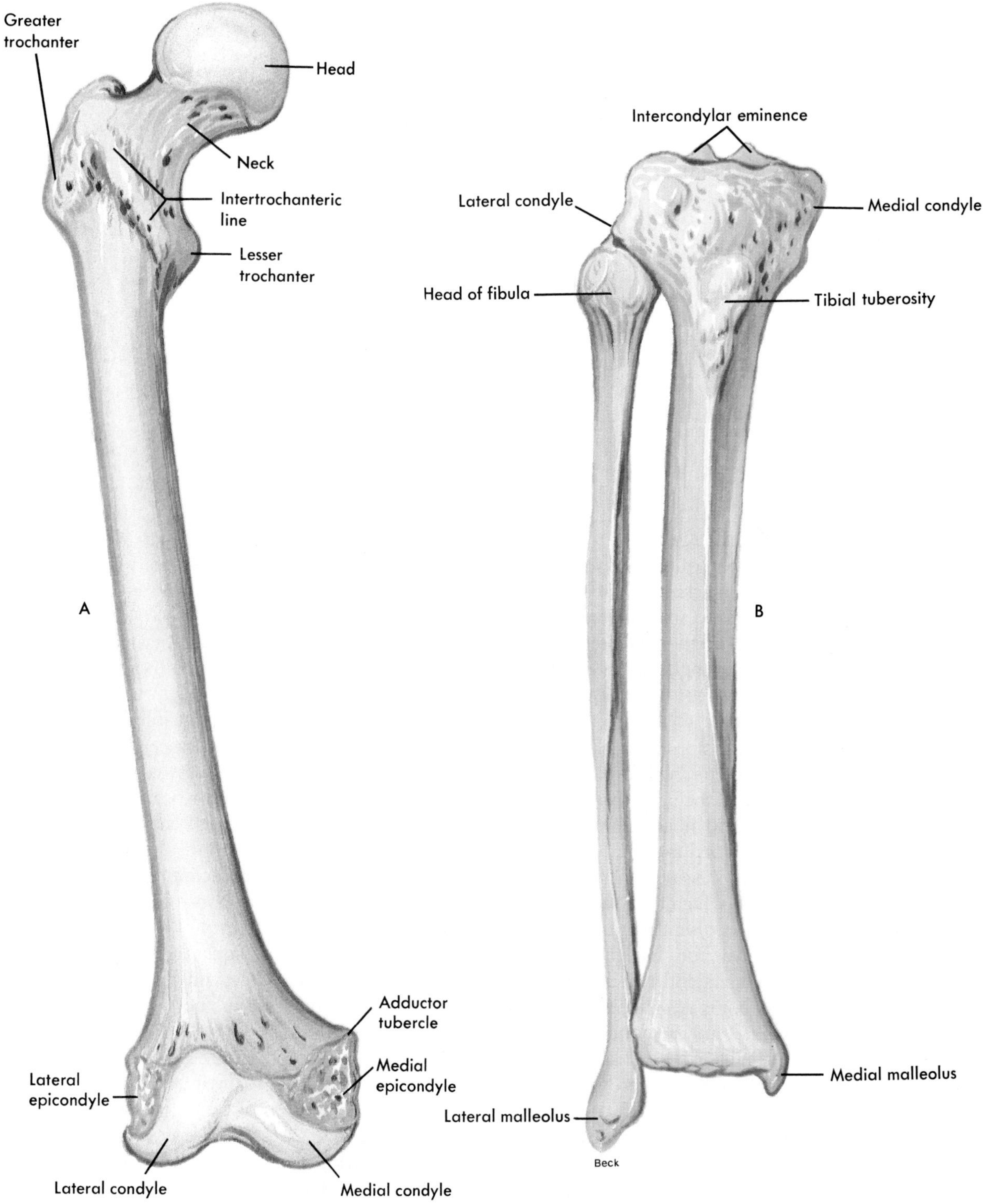

FIG. 30-10 **A,** Right femur. **B,** Right tibia and fibula.

2. The heart is composed of cardiac muscle tissue, which forms the bulk of the walls of the heart. It is also striated but is under **involuntary** control. The heart beats 24 hours a day and does not require a conscious decision about its rate.

3. Smooth muscle tissue is composed of small, spindle-shaped cells and is nonstriated. It is responsible for the maintenance of the processes within the internal environment of the body, such as the stomach and the intestines. This muscle tissue is also involuntary.

Characteristics. Muscle tissue possesses four principal characteristics: excitability, contractility, extensibility, and elasticity.

1. Excitability is the ability of muscle tissue to respond to a stimulus. A stimulus is a change in the internal or external environment that is strong enough to initiate a nerve impulse. The point at which the nerve fiber relays the message to the muscle cell is called the *neuromuscular junction*.

2. Contractility is the ability of the muscle to be extended (stretched). The muscle actually shortens and becomes thicker.

3. Extensibility is the ability of the muscle to be extended (stretched). Many muscle groups of the body are arranged in opposing pairs. For example, when the forearm is flexed (bent), the anterior group of muscles is contracted and the posterior group is extended.

4. Elasticity is the ability of the muscle to return to its former shape after repeated contraction or extension.

Skeletal muscle structure. A skeletal muscle is composed of hundreds of muscle fibers (cells). Each skeletal muscle is surrounded by a covering of connective tissue called the *epimysium*. The epimysium joins with two other inner coverings, the perimysium and the endomysium, to extend beyond the muscle to form a tough cord of connective tissue known as a *tendon*. Tendons anchor muscles to bones. As a muscle contracts, the tendon and bone corresponding to that particular muscle are pulled toward the muscle. This is how movement occurs. Tendons in the ankle and wrist are enclosed in sleeves or tubelike structures of connective tissue known as tendon sheaths. These tendon sheaths contain synovial fluid and permit the tendons to slide easily; the sheaths also keep the tendons in place. Sometimes the tendon is formed of flat, strong bands of connective tissue; it is then called an *aponeurosis*. All the tendons, ligaments, and aponeuroses of the body are composed of various sizes, shapes, and densities of connective tissue. These are collectively known as *fasciae*.

Nerve and blood supply. Because of the physical demands placed on the skeletal muscles, they need a constant supply of oxygen and nutrition. They are well supplied with blood vessels that carry oxygen and nutrition to the area and remove the waste products of metabolism.

Because the skeletal muscles are voluntary, they need a constant source of "information," which is supplied by nerve cells or fibers. These nerve cells continually send impulses that stimulate the muscle cells. These impulses enter at the neuromuscular junction, the point of contact between the nerve ending and the muscle fiber. As a nerve impulse passes through this junction, chemicals are re leased that cause the muscle to contract.

Usually one artery, two veins, and one nerve penetrate a particular muscle. Each muscle cell comes in contact with several capillaries and a portion of a nerve cell. The muscle cells, in union with the nerve cell that controls them, are called a *motor unit*.

The impulse from the nerve cell must travel across a small gap, since the nerve cell and the muscle cell do not directly touch one another. This small gap is called a *synaptic cleft* and is filled with tissue fluid. A special chemical (neurotransmitter) travels through the fluid to stimulate the muscle fiber. Acetylcholine is the specific neurotransmitter for skeletal muscle tissue. An enzyme called cholinesterase breaks down the acetylcholine once it has transferred the message. This allows the muscle cell to relax between impulses.

Muscle contraction

Muscle stimulus. Muscle cells are governed by the "all or none" law, which states that when a muscle cell is adequately stimulated or shocked, it will contract completely. Because each skeletal muscle is composed of thousands of muscle cells that react to many different nerve cells, the muscle as a whole contracts according to the "principle of graded response." The strength of the contraction of the muscle, therefore, depends on the number of individual muscle cells responding. These muscle responses allow us to tenderly brush a baby's cheek or destroy an irritating mosquito.

Muscle tone. The skeletal muscles are in a constant state of readiness for action. At any given time several muscle cells within a certain muscle are contracted; the remainder of the muscle cells are relaxed. The muscle tone provided is necessary for good posture but does not provide movement of the body. To understand the importance of muscle tone, one can observe an extremity that has become paralyzed—the muscles are flaccid, limp, or atrophied (wasted) and incapable of producing movement because the cells are no longer receiving stimuli from the nerve fibers.

Energy for contraction. An energy source is necessary for the contraction of muscle tissue. The muscle cell derives this energy from adenosine triphosphate (ATP), an energy-carrying molecule contained in all muscle tissue. When the muscle continues to contract and depletes the store of ATP, another energy source, glycogen, may be used. Glycogen (stored glucose) is found in small amounts in the skeletal muscles and in large amounts in the liver. The use of the energy sources must take place in the presence of oxygen. As the muscle contraction continues and the oxygen supply decreases, a waste product called *lactic acid* accumulates. The muscle tissue may continue to contract anaerobically (without oxygen), but the lactic acid by-product continues to accumulate. The muscle is then in a state of oxygen debt. The lactic acid that has built up causes muscle soreness. To replenish the oxygen debt, the brain stimulates the respiratory system and rapid, deep breathing occurs. This breathing pattern continues until the body has enough oxygen reserve to reverse the process.

Types of skeletal muscle contraction. The partial contraction of the muscles to maintain muscle tone has been discussed. The following is a discussion of the other major types of contraction that occur. They are isometric, isotonic, twitch, and tetanic (tetanus) contractions.

Isometric contraction. A skeletal muscle can contract without producing movement. The contraction increases the tension within the muscle but does not shorten it. The term *isometric* comes from the Greek words *isos* and *metron,* meaning equal pressure. This term refers to the fact that during relaxation and contraction the muscle length stays the same. This may be accomplished by opposing different muscles (e.g., pressing the hands together). There is no joint movement and the length of the muscle remains unchanged, but muscle strength and tone are improved. Repetition of isometric muscle contraction causes the muscles to become larger and stronger. Often, the patient who has had knee surgery is taught to use isometric exercise on the quadriceps femoris. This group of muscles covers the anterior and lateral areas of the femur and allows the individual to extend the leg.

Isotonic contraction. In an isotonic contraction the muscle shortens and can produce movement of a joint. Some examples of this type of contraction are sitting, walking, and bending the knees. Repetition of this type of contraction improves joint mobility and helps to improve muscle strength and tone.

Twitch contraction. A quick, jerky contraction in response to a single stimulus produces a muscle twitch contraction. A twitch response does not occur at the instant of the stimulation, but a fraction of a second later. It actually occurs in three phases: the latent phase, the contraction phase, and the relaxation phase. The whole process lasts less than 1⁄10 of a second. The phenomenon does not occur often but can be simulated in a laboratory setting to study muscle physiology.

Tetanic contraction (tetanus). When a series of stimuli bombard the skeletal muscle tissue (20 to 30 per second), a sustained contraction will result. Normal movement is produced by incomplete, short-term tetanic contractions. The word *tetanus* comes from the Greek word *tetanos,* meaning extreme tension.

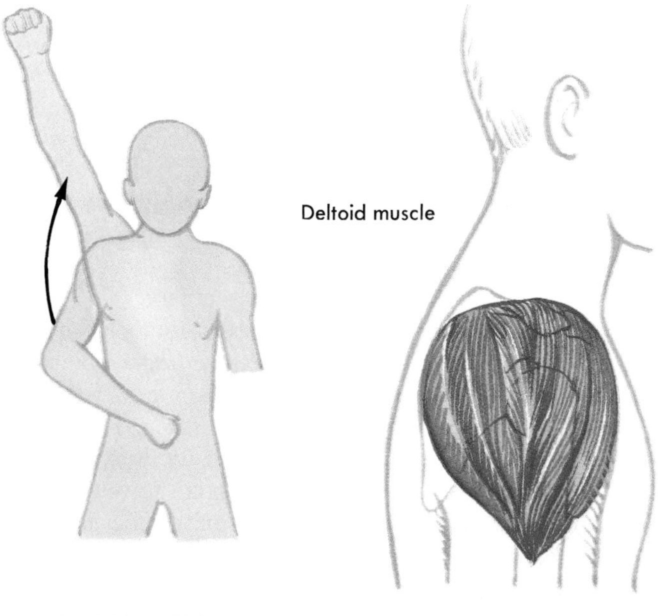

FIG. 30-11 When the deltoid muscle (shown on the figure at right) contracts, it abducts the upper arm at the shoulder joint (figure at the left).

Muscle and body movements

Origin and insertion. Muscles are attached, usually at a joint, to the bones by a tendon. The less movable, or fixed, end is called the **origin.** The more movable end is called the **insertion.** The fleshy part of the muscle, between the origin and insertion, is called the *belly* of the muscle. In the extremities the origin of the muscle is usually proximal and the insertion is usually distal. When muscles contract, the insertion moves toward the origin (Fig. 30-11).

Muscle action. Muscles have only one action—they pull. They are unable to push. Skeletal muscles are therefore arranged in groups and in opposing pairs at joints. The muscle that produces action is called the *prime mover.* The opposite muscle, the *antagonist,* is relaxed. For example, to touch the shoulder the biceps muscle contracts (prime mover) and pulls the radius bone upward. The triceps is relaxed (antagonist). To lower the arm, the triceps muscle contracts (prime mover) and pulls on the ulna. The biceps is relaxed and is the antagonist. Each muscle group may be either the prime mover or antagonist, depending on the desired movement. The antagonist will always relax and yield to the movement of the prime mover.

As the prime movers and antagonists perform their movements, certain muscles called *synergists* assist by steadying the movement. This helps the prime mover to function more efficiently. In some areas (e.g., the wrist), a muscle crosses two or more joints, and the contraction of the muscle will cause movement in all joints involved unless the synergists stabilize them.

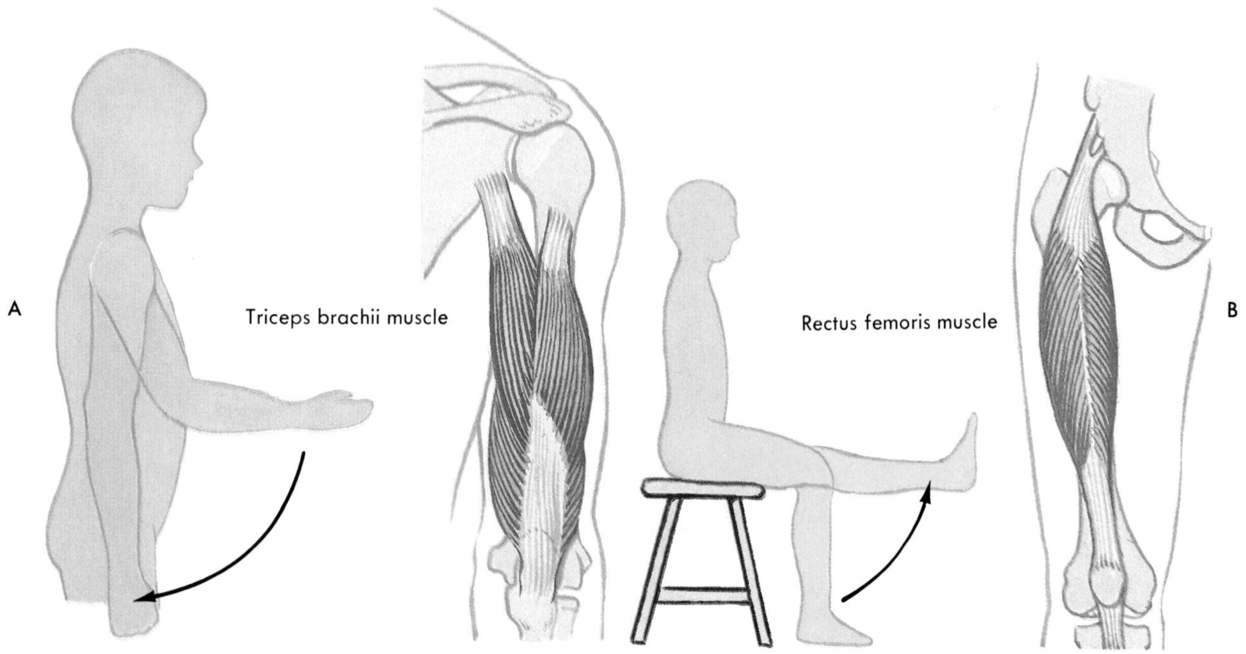

FIG. 30-12 Extension of the lower arm and lower leg. **A,** When the triceps brachii muscle (shown at the right) contracts, it extends the lower arm at the elbow joint (shown at the left). **B,** When the rectus femoris muscle (part of the quadriceps femoris muscle group) (shown at the right) contracts, it extends the lower leg at the knee joint (shown at the left).

Fixators stabilize the origin of a prime mover so that all the tension can be used to move the insertion bone. The fixators are specialized synergists. A prime example of a group of fixator muscles is the muscles that hold the scapula firmly against the posterior of the chest.

Types of body movements. Some muscles can move some body parts in only two directions, whereas others can move certain body parts in several directions. Some of the more common movements that the body is capable of producing are flexion, extension, **abduction, adduction,** rotation, supination, pronation, dorsiflexion, and plantar flexion.

Flexion: a movement that is allowed by certain joints of the skeleton that decreases the angle between two adjoining bones. For example, if the arm is bent at the elbow, the angle between the humerus and the ulna is decreased.

Extension (Fig. 30-12): a movement that is allowed by certain joints of the skeleton that increases the angle between two adjoining bones. For example, if the leg is extended, the angle between the femur and the tibia is increased. If the extension angles more than 180 degrees, the extremity is *hyperextended.*

Abduction: a movement of an extremity away from the midline of the body.

Adduction: a movement of an extremity toward the axis of the body.

Rotation: a movement of the bone around its longitudinal axis (e.g., a pivot motion, such as shaking the head "no").

Supination: a movement of the hand and forearm that causes the palm to face upward or forward.

Pronation: a movement of the hand and forearm that causes the palm to face downward or backward.

Dorsiflexion: a movement that causes the top of the foot to elevate or tilt upward.

Plantar flexion: a movement that causes the bottom of the foot to be directed downward.

Skeletal muscle groups. Skeletal muscles are usually classified into two broad categories: axial and appendicular. The axial muscle groups are those muscles located on the head, face, neck, and trunk. The appendicular muscle groups are all the muscles of the extremities. Figs. 30-13 and 30-14 show the location of muscles of the anterior and posterior trunk and extremities of the body. Fig. 30-15 shows the location of facial muscles.

Muscles of the head. The muscles of the head include the facial muscles, which are responsible for facial expression, and the mastication (chewing) muscles, which prepare our food for swallowing.

Facial muscles

Frontalis muscle: covers the frontal bone and inserts at the eyebrow. It gives movement to the forehead and permits the raising of the eyebrows.

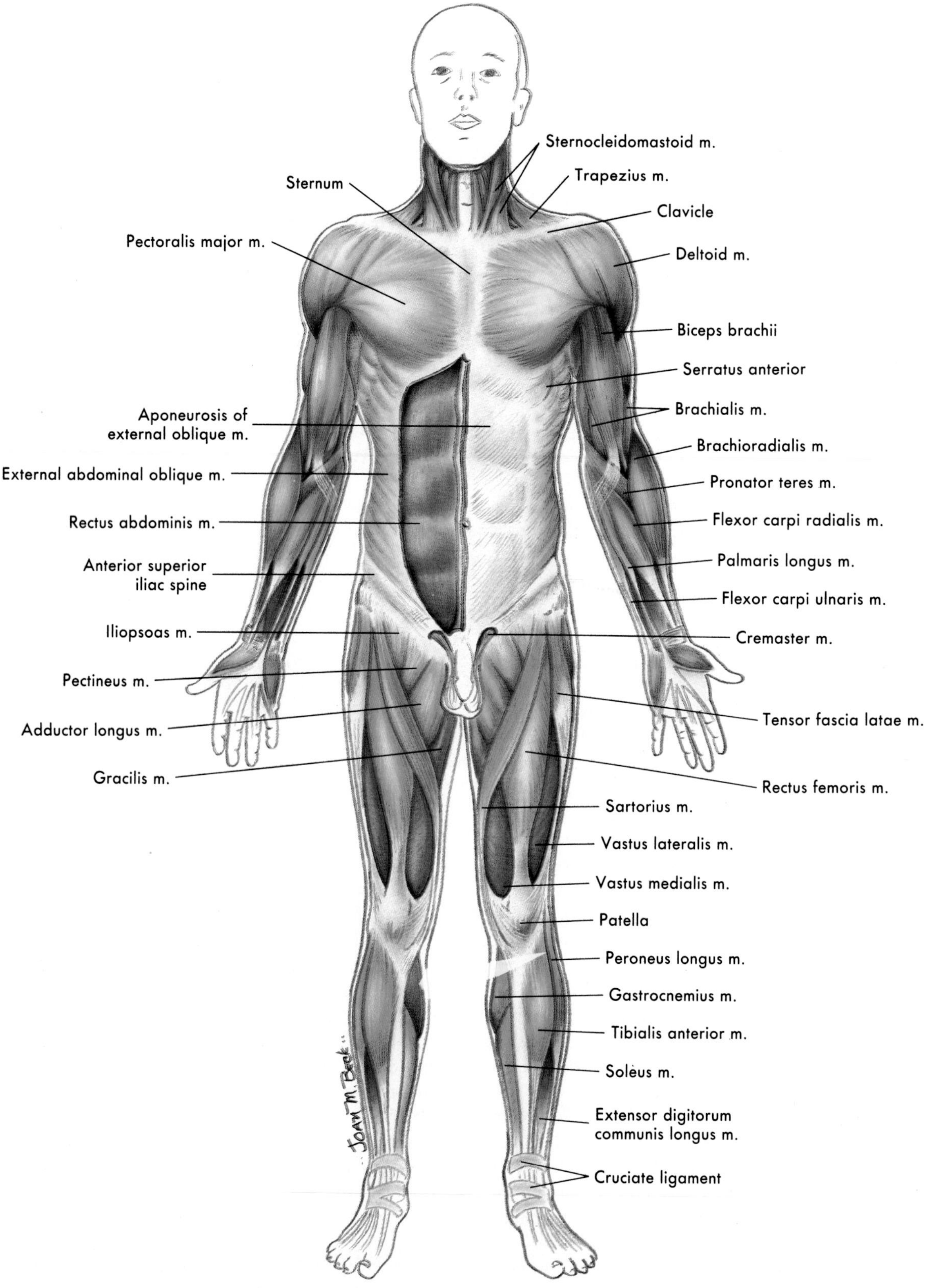

FIG. 30-13 Outer layer of the muscles of the anterior surface of the trunk and extremities.

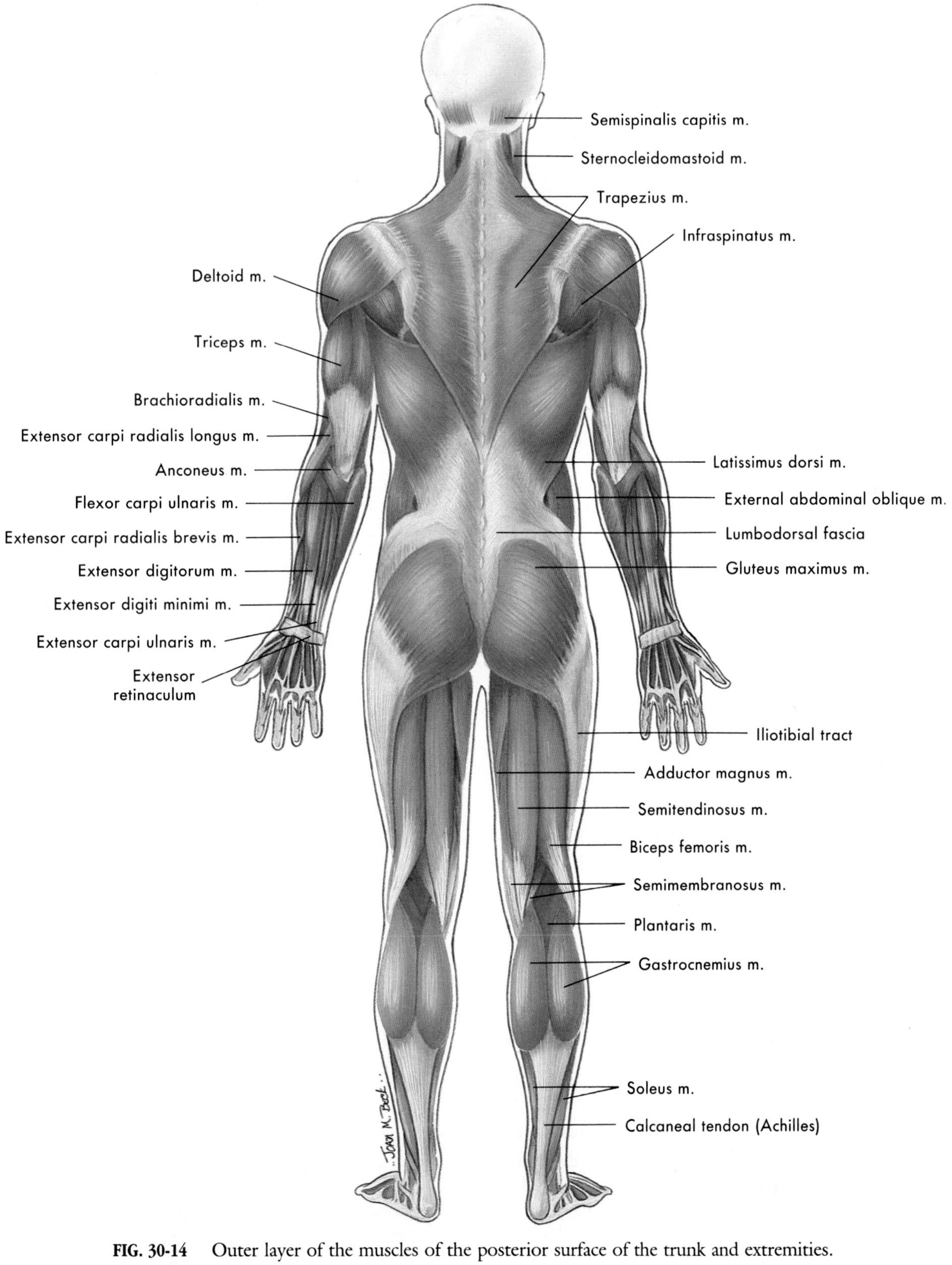

FIG. 30-14 Outer layer of the muscles of the posterior surface of the trunk and extremities.

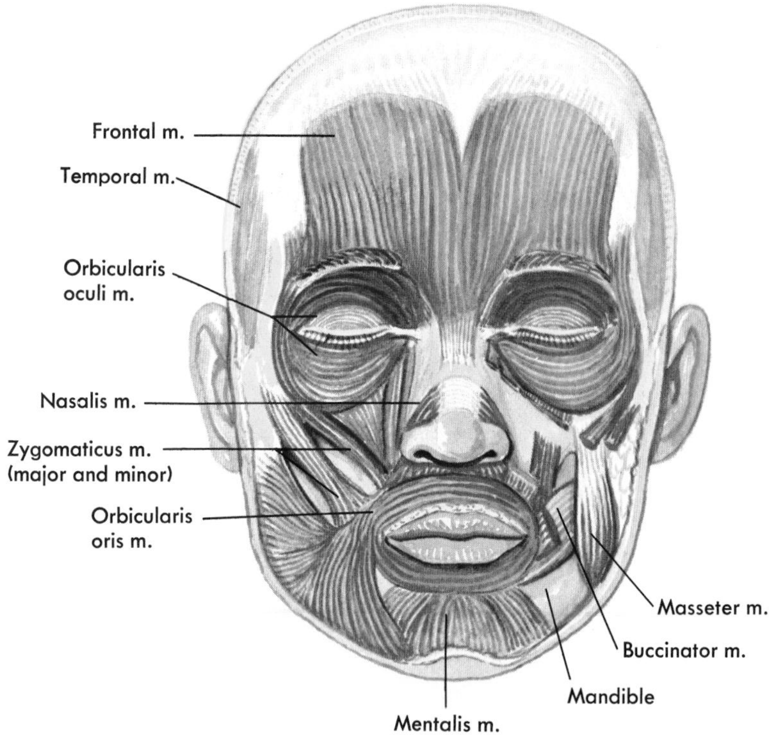

FIG. 30-15 Muscles of facial expression. Most muscles of facial expression surround the eyes, nose, and mouth. Contraction of these muscles can produce a variety of facial expressions and convey numerous emotions.

Orbicularis oculi: encircles the eyes and permits winking, blinking, and closing of the eyes.

Orbicularis oris: encircles the lips and allows the closing of the mouth. It has been referred to as the *kissing* muscle.

Buccinator: forms the fleshy part of the cheeks. It compresses the cheek to hold food for chewing. It is referred to as the *trumpeter's* muscle, because it is the muscle used for whistling and blowing.

Zygomaticus: extends from the cheekbone to the corners of the mouth. It is referred to as the *smiling* muscle, because it draws the angle of the mouth upward.

Mastication muscles

Masseter: extends across the angle of the jaw. It elevates the mandible during mastication.

Temporalis: extends from the temporal bone to the mandible. During mastication it elevates and retracts the mandible.

Muscles of the neck and trunk. The neck muscles are responsible for the support and movement of the neck and shoulder girdle. They are mostly strong, cordlike structures that extend inferiorly, superiorly, and obliquely.

The trunk muscles are responsible for the support and movement of the vertebral column, ribs, arms, and abdominal region.

The following is a brief discussion of the most important muscles, beginning with the anterior muscles and followed by the posterior muscles.

Anterior muscles

Sternocleidomastoid: a pair of muscles that extend on either side of the neck from the mastoid to the sternum. As these muscles contract, the head is flexed (moved toward the chest). Contraction of one muscle rotates the head to the opposite side.

Pectoralis major: a large, fan-shaped muscle that covers the anterior chest from the sternum to the proximal end of the humerus. It acts on the joint of the shoulder to flex, adduct, and medially rotate it.

Diaphragm: a thin, dome-shaped muscle that separates the thoracic and abdominal cavities. The aorta, esophagus, and vena cava pass through it. It aids in respiration. During inspiration it drops down and increases the volume or space within the thoracic cavity. During expiration it moves upward and decreases the space.

Serratus anterior: a thin chest wall muscle that extends from the ribs under the arm to the scapula. The serratus anterior permits rotation of the scapula and the raising of the arm (full flexion and abduction of the arm).

Intercostal muscles: located between the individual

ribs. The external intercostals raise the ribcage during inspiration, and the internal intercostals depress the ribcage during expiration. They function as secondary ventilatory muscles.

Transversus abdominis: the most interior layer of abdominal muscle. It lies horizontally across the abdomen from the iliac crests to the pubis. Constriction of this muscle compresses the abdominal contents, which assists with defecation, urination, and emesis and forces expiration.

Internal and external obliques: form the middle and outer layers of the abdominal wall. Their muscle fibers criss-cross to form a strong abdominal wall. Constriction of these muscles also compresses the abdomen with the same results as the transversus abdominis. Constriction of the one side allows the lateral movement of the vertebral column.

Rectus abdominis: a pair of superficial abdominal muscles that extend from the pubis to the sternum. They assist the transversus abdominus and the internal and external obliques with their functions.

Posterior muscles

Trapezius: paired, fan-shaped muscles that cover the posterior neck and upper back. They are responsible for extension of the head and adduction and stabilization of the scapula. In addition, they abduct and flex the arm. The origin is the occipital bone and thoracic vertebrae; the insertion is the scapula.

Latissimus dorsi: large, flat, paired muscles that extend across the thoracic and lumbar regions of the back. They provide for extension and adduction of the humerus. They provide the power and strength for the upper arms. They are often referred to as the "swimmer's muscle." The origin sites are the spines of the thoracic vertebrae, the ilium, and the ribs; the insertion site is the humerus.

Upper extremity muscles

Deltoid: a triangular, fleshy, muscular cap of the shoulder and upper arm. Intramuscular injections are commonly given in this muscle (see Fig. 30-11). Contraction of this muscle abducts, flexes, extends, and rotates the arm. The origin is the clavicle and scapula; the insertion site is the humerus.

Biceps brachii: the long muscle of the upper arm on the anterior surface of the humerus. It flexes the arm and supinates the hand. In addition, it strengthens the shoulder joint. The origin is the scapula; the insertion site is the radius.

Triceps brachii: often called the *boxer's muscle* because it straightens the elbow when a blow is delivered (see Fig. 30-12, *A*). It is opposite the biceps brachii on the dorsal surface of the humerus. The origin is the scapula and humerus; the insertion is the ulna.

Lower extremity muscles

Muscles located in the lower extremities are the longest and strongest in the body. They are responsible for locomotion and balance.

Gluteus maximus: forms the large fleshy portion of the buttocks. It is responsible for the extension and lateral rotation of the thigh. It is a common site for intramuscular injections. Its origin is the sacrum, coccyx, and ilium; the insertion is the femur.

Gluteus medius: lies interior to the gluteus maximus. It extends from the ilium (insertion) to the femur (origin). It is responsible for abduction of the hip and the rotation of the thigh medially.

Quadriceps femoris: a four-part muscle group that is located in the anterior area of the thigh. This group is responsible for the extension of the knee, particularly powerful extension, such as a kicking motion. The origin is the ilium and femur; the insertion is the tibia (see Fig. 30-12, *B*).

Hamstring group (posterior biceps and the biceps femoris): the posterior thigh muscles; their tendons can be palpated posterior to the knee bilaterally. They allow the leg to flex toward the thigh.

Adductor muscles: located on the inside, or medial, part of the thigh. They serve to press the thighs together.

Adductor longus: the most superficial of the adductor muscles. It is a triangular muscle with its origin located at the pubis and the insertion site at the femur. It adducts and flexes the thigh.

Tibialis anterior: situated on the lateral side of the tibia. It is a thick, fleshy muscle. Its origin is the lateral side of the tibia with an insertion at the first metatarsal bone. It dorsiflexes and supinates the foot.

Iliopsoas: a short muscle that is located high on the thigh extending from the lumbar vertebrae and ilium to the head of the femur. It is a flexor muscle of the thigh.

Gastrocnemius: a large muscle located in the calf of the leg. It arises from the distal femur and its tendon (Achilles) attaches to the calcaneus. It is often called the *toe dancer's muscle* because it is used to stand on tiptoe. The **Achilles** tendon is the largest tendon in the body. If it is severed, walking becomes very difficult because the heel cannot respond and this results in footdrop.

ASSESSMENT OF MUSCULOSKELETAL FUNCTION

The musculoskeletal system provides protection, support, and movement for the body. Orthopedics is the branch of medicine that deals with the prevention or correction of disorders involving locomotor structures of the body. Permanent disability and crippling will result

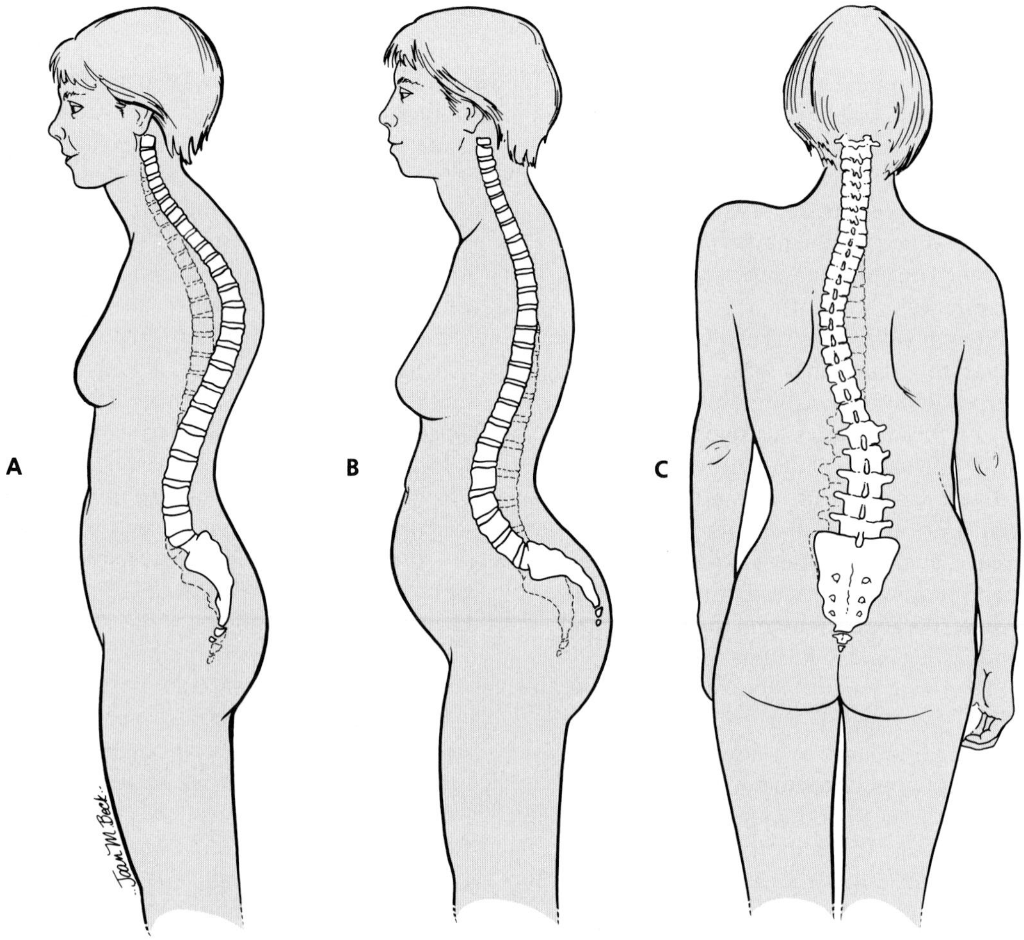

FIG. 30-16 Abnormal spinal curvatures. **A,** Kyphosis. **B,** Lordosis. **C,** Scoliosis.

if prompt treatment is not given to patients with musculoskeletal dysfunction. The ability to perform these functions is closely associated with the proper functioning of the nervous and circulatory systems.

Assessment of orthopedic function is necessary on all patients, but especially on those individuals who are (1) having difficulty with gait, (2) experiencing muscle weakness, (3) suffering from trauma of soft tissue and bone, (4) unable to produce movement that will enable activities for personal, economic, and social fulfillment, (5) experiencing diseases of the musculoskeletal system, and (6) chronically ill.

Assessment of posture and **gait** is made easily by observing the patient walking. Common posture deformities include lateral (or S) curvature of the spine known as **scoliosis;** a rounding of the thoracic spine (humpbacked appearance) known as **kyphosis;** and an increase in the curve at the lumbar space region that throws the shoulders back, making the appearance "lordly or kingly" known as **lordosis** (Fig. 30-16). Rigidity of the spine can result from ankylosing spondylitis, whereby the vertebrae are actually fused with loss of mobility, producing a rigid gait or "poker spine" appearance.

Assessment of neurological and circulatory function is important if the patient has experienced a traumatic injury; damaged blood vessels and nerves can cause permanent disabilities.

Assessing the skin for signs of coolness, pallor, or cyanosis can help the nurse determine the patient's circulatory status. A faint or absent pulse in an extremity indicates impaired circulation. Palpating the femoral, popliteal, and dorsalis pedis pulses on both extremities provides data pertinent to the lower extremities. If the pulse is not readily palpated with a light touch of the finger, a Doppler instrument can be used, which will enable the listener to hear a magnified sound of the pulsation. The absence of a pulse is serious and must be reported to the charge nurse immediately. The brachial and radial pulses are assessed to determine circulation in the upper extremities. It may be difficult to palpate a pulse when a cast or bandage makes the extremity inaccessible. It is important to reach under the cast or bandage if possible. An assessment of the pulse in the unaffected extremity is made for a comparison.

Blanching (meaning to whiten or pale) is a test of the rate of capillary refill, which signals circulation status. The nurse compresses each fingernail or toenail of the affected extremity (noting the white color as pressure is applied), releases the pressure, and notes how quickly the pink color returns to the nail bed. If the color is slow to return, this indicates impaired circulation, and prompt attention is needed to improve the circulation.

Neurovascular assessments are made on patients with musculoskeletal trauma, damage to nerves and blood vessels resulting from surgery, or tightness of bandages, splints, or casts. Impaired circulation or nerve function can cause loss of the use of an extremity; this impairment is seen more often in the extremities. Neurovascular assessment is always included as a nursing measure when caring for a patient with a cast. Immediately after a traumatic injury, postoperatively, or after casting, a neurovascular assessment is made every 15 to 30 minutes for several hours and every 3 to 4 hours thereafter, with proper documentation of the findings. Verbal complaints of numbness or tingling may result from general decreased mobility and may be relieved by flexing the fingers and toes and repositioning the extremity. However, if the numbness and tingling are not relieved by these measures and the extremity feels cool to touch, is slow in capillary refill, has diminished or absent pulses, and appears pale or cyanotic, these are significant symptoms of neurovascular impairment and the findings must be reported immediately.

Remember the 5 *P*'s when completing this assessment:

- **Pulselessness**
- **Paresthesia** (numbness or tingling sensation)
- **Pallor**
- **Puffiness** (edema)
- **Pain**

Effects of Bed Rest on Mineral Content in Bone

Studies done on persons confined to bed rest reveal a loss of body calcium. Men and women patients ages 18 to 80 years who were confined to bed rest for an average of 27 days because of musculoskeletal disorders of lumbar disk protrusion averaged 0.9% loss in mineral content per week from the lumbar vertebrae. This rate of loss over several weeks is a serious concern for an elderly individual in terms of regaining mobility; it also increases the risk of fracture. Studies done on astronauts have shown that they experienced rates of bone loss similar to bed rest rates in a weightless environment.

DIAGNOSTIC TESTS

Radiographic Studies

The diagnostic study most often used for determining musculoskeletal system integrity is the radiographic, roentgenographic, or as it is more commonly known, x-ray examination.

An x-ray examination of a joint reveals the presence of fluid, irregularity of the joint with spur formation, and changes in the size of the joint contour. It is important before x-ray examinations to ask women of child-bearing age if there is any possibility that they are pregnant, because pregnant women should not be exposed to x-ray unless in an emergency situation because of potential damage to the fetus.

Laminography or planography is also called "body section roentgenography." This x-ray procedure is useful in locating small cavities, foreign bodies, and lesions that are overshadowed by opaque structures.

Scanography (a method of producing a radiogram of internal body organs by using a series of parallel beams that eliminate size distortion) is an x-ray procedure that allows accurate measurement of bone length.

Myelogram. Myelogram examination involves injection of a radiopaque dye into the subarachnoid space at the lumbar spine to determine the presence of herniated disk syndrome (herniated nucleus pulposus) or tumors. The test involves the same procedure as a lumbar puncture (spinal tap) as is discussed in Chapter 38. Radiographic dye will cause allergic reactions in patients with allergies to iodine and seafood or who have hay fever, asthma, or eczema. It is important that the physician be notified about such allergies so that a nonionic contrast agent be used or medications such as steroids and/or antihistamines be given before the examination to minimize any reaction to the radiographic dye. This exam may involve the entire spine or just the cervical or lumbar area. After the myelogram, oil-based dye is removed through the spinal needle to prevent meningeal irritation. Water-soluble dye is used most often and does not need to be removed; it will be absorbed by the body and excreted in the urine.

The most common discomfort after a myelogram is headache. If water-soluble dye is used, the patient should lie quietly in a semi-Fowler's position for about 8 hours. The positioning of the patient is important to keep the dye in the lower spine. During this time, forcing fluids will help the body absorb the dye from the spinal column. If oil-based dye is used, the patient will need to rest in a flat position for as long as 12 hours. It is important to instruct the patient to inform the nurse if he experiences headache, stiff neck, leg weakness, or difficulty voiding. Rare complications include seizure, infection, drowsiness, severe headache, numbness, and paralysis.

Patients needing a myelogram fear the needle will be inserted into the spinal canal and damage the cord. It is important that the nurse inform the patient that the tap is done in the lumbar region of the spine at about the fourth or fifth lumbar (L_4/L_5) space. The spinal cord starts at the level of the foramen magnum and ends at the second lumbar (L_2) space (lower border of ribcage).

Nuclear scanning. Tests in which nuclear scanning is used are done in the nuclear medicine department, which has scanners or camera detectors that record the images on x-ray film. The dosages of radioactive isotopes are low for diagnostic tests; precautionary measures that are required for radium therapy are not necessary.

Nursing measures required when patients are scheduled for nuclear scanning procedures involve (1) obtaining written consent from the patient, (2) informing the patient that the radioactive isotopes will not affect family or visitors, and (3) following instructions as outlined by the nuclear medicine department as to special preparations for specific scans.

Magnetic resonance imaging. Magnetic resonance imaging (MRI) is used to detect pathological conditions of the cerebrum and spinal cord. It is currently used to detect herniated nucleus pulposus. The test involves the use of magnetism and radio waves to make images of cross sections of the body. MRI can give much more detailed pictures of fluid-filled soft tissue and blood vessels than any other test.

Patient preparation involves having the patient remove any metal, such as jewelry, clothing with metal fasteners, glasses, and hair clips. Patients with metal prostheses, such as heart valves, orthopedic screws, or cardiac pacemakers, cannot undergo MRI.

The machine looks like a narrow tunnel, and patients are required to lie still in this machine for 45 to 60 minutes. The patient enters the tunnel head first. This may cause anxiety and a feeling of claustrophobia. The procedure is painless; however, if the patient is extremely anxious, a sedative is given. Patients are encouraged to use relaxation techniques, such as imagery, during the test. Because the procedure requires the patient to be motionless, relaxation techniques that require flexing and relaxing the muscles are not appropriate.

After the test, routine vital sign measurements are taken and pretest activities can be resumed. There are no adverse effects.

Computed axial tomography (CT or CAT scan). Body sections can be examined from many different angles using a CT scanner that produces a narrow x-ray beam. Consequently, a three-dimensional picture of the structure being studied is made. The CT scanner is approximately 100 times more sensitive than the x-ray machine and should not be used unnecessarily, because of radiation exposure. Iodine contrast dye is sometimes used. CT scan is used for the head and body. It is useful in locating injuries to the ligaments or tendons and tumors of the soft tissue, and in identifying fractures in areas difficult to define by other means. Patient preparation includes (1) having the patient sign a consent form authorizing the examination if not included on the initial hospital consent form, (2) questioning the patient regarding allergies (iodine and seafood), (3) keeping the patient on NPO status (nothing by mouth) 3 to 4 hours before the test (necessary in case contrast dye is used, because the dye can cause nausea and vomiting), (4) measuring vital signs to be used as a baseline, (5) having the patient void before the test, (6) removing such articles as jewelry and hairpins, and (7) instructing the patient that he must lie still during the test and may feel warm and slightly nauseated for a few minutes when dye is injected.

Sometimes an enema to clear the colon of gas and feces is required before body scans.

After the test, the patient is observed for delayed allergic reactions (if contrast dye was used). Fluids are encouraged unless contraindicated. Pretest diet and activity can usually be resumed.

Bone scan. The bone scan test is especially valuable in detecting metastatic and inflammatory bone disease (osteomyelitis). This test involves the intravenous administration of nuclides (atomic material) approximately 2 to 3 hours before the test is scheduled. There are no food or fluid restrictions, and patients are encouraged to take liquids before and after the test to help in the elimination of the nuclides. The test takes approximately 30 to 60 minutes and requires the patient to lie still. Patients are instructed to void before the examination.

Endoscopic Examination

For an endoscopy, a lighted tube is used to visualize inside a body cavity. Although some procedures require general anesthesia, most require only local anesthesia. Emotional support and complete explanations help relieve the patient's anxiety. Preparation for an endoscopic examination is similar to surgical preparation: (1) a consent form is signed, (2) a preoperative checklist is completed with special attention to removing jewelry, dentures, and contact lenses, (3) an NPO status is initiated for 6 to 12 hours before the examination, (4) premedications are given, such as atropine and a sedative, (5) the patient is encouraged to void, (6) vital signs are taken and recorded, and (7) bed rest with side rails up is maintained after the premedication is given.

Arthroscopy. Arthroscopy is an endoscopic examination that enables direct visualization of a joint. The procedure is used to accomplish the following: (1) exploration of the joint to determine the presence of a disease process, (2) drainage of fluid from the joint cavity, and (3) removal of damaged tissue or foreign bodies from the joint.

This examination is most commonly done on the knee joint, with the synovium, articular surfaces, and meniscus (a curved, fibrous cartilage in the knee)visualized through the scope. The procedure involves insertion of a large-bore needle into the suprapatellar pouch and saline instillation into the joint. The patient may be given a general or local anesthetic agent. After the arthroscopic examination, the patient may be advised to limit activities for several days.

Aspiration

An aspiration procedure is done to obtain a specimen of body fluid. A needle is inserted into a cavity after a

Table 30-4 Laboratory Tests for Musculoskeletal Disorders

Test	Normal Value	Possible Cause for Increase/Decrease
Calcium	8.5-11.0 mg/dl	Increased in acute osteoporosis, hyperparathyroidism, and vitamin D intoxication Decreased in acute pancreatitis, hypoparathyroidism, and vitamin D deficiency
Erythrocyte sedimentation rate (ESR)	Males: less than 10 mm/hr; slightly higher in females	Indicates the presence of inflammation as seen in rheumatoid arthritis One of the most objective measurements of rheumatoid arthritis severity ESR increases as the disease worsens
Lupus erythematosus (LE) preparation	No LE cells seen	Lupus erythematosus and rheumatoid arthritis
Rheumatoid factor		An immunoglobulin found in 50% to 95% of adults with rheumatoid arthritis

local anesthetic agent is administered to the site. This procedure is performed using sterile technique. It is fairly common for the physician to take a biopsy of tissue at the same time the aspiration procedure is done. Nursing interventions are similar for all aspiration tests, with special emphasis on (1) having the consent form signed, (2) reinforcing the physician's explanation of the procedure, (3) encouraging the patient to remain immobile during the procedure, (4) having the patient void before the procedure, (5) maintaining sterile technique, (6) supporting the patient emotionally, (7) applying a sterile pressure dressing to the puncture site and maintaining the dressing until bleeding has stopped, (8) assisting with collecting, labeling, and transporting a specimen to the laboratory immediately, and (9) observing for emotional and physical distress after the procedure.

Synovial fluid aspiration. Synovial fluid examination **(arthrocentesis)** is helpful in diagnosing trauma, systemic lupus erythematosus, gout, osteoarthritis, and rheumatoid arthritis. Normally synovial fluid is straw colored, clear, or slightly cloudy. If trauma or a disease process is present, the fluid will appear cloudy, milky, sanguineous, yellow, green, or gray.

After the procedure, proper support should be given to the affected extremity. Placing the extremity on a pillow and maintaining joint rest for approximately 12 hours may be indicated. It may be necessary to apply ice to the affected joint for 24 to 48 hours unless otherwise ordered. The nurse will assess the patient for signs of infection. After the removal of the pressure dressing from the site, a Band-Aid can be used.

Electrographic Procedure

For electrographic procedures, electrodes are used to measure electrical activity in specific areas of the body.

Electromyogram (EMG). An electromyogram is a procedure that involves the insertion of needle electrodes into the skeletal muscles so that electrical activity can be heard, seen on an oscilloscope (an instrument that displays a graphic representation of electron beams on a screen), and recorded on paper at the same time. Muscles do not produce an electrical charge at rest, but with neuromuscular disorders, unusual patterns can be observed. Nerves can be observed for neuropathy and muscles for myopathy with this procedure.

Laboratory Tests

Specific laboratory tests are ordered when musculoskeletal disorders are suspected (Table 30-4).

INFLAMMATORY DISORDERS

Arthritis

Arthritis is a type of disease in which there is an inflammation of the joint. There are an estimated 50 million Americans affected by arthritis, and 4 million of these are dependent and unable to work, attend school, or participate in social functions. There are many types of arthritis, but the most common are rheumatoid arthritis, rheumatoid spondylitis, osteoarthritis (degenerative joint disease), and gout (gouty arthritis).

Rheumatoid arthritis

Etiology/pathophysiology. Rheumatoid arthritis (RA) is the most serious form of the disease and leads to severe crippling. It is a chronic, systemic disease that affects 3% of the general population. RA can strike anyone; however, certain factors make some people more prone than others. RA usually develops between the ages of 30 and 55 years, and women seem more prone than men. There is some evidence that RA has a familial tendency.

RA can affect many organ systems (lungs, heart, blood vessels, muscles, eyes, and skin). RA is characterized by a chronic inflammation of the synovial membrane **(sy-**

Table 30-5 Medications Prescribed in the Treatment of Rheumatoid Arthritis

Medication	Action	Side Effects/Toxic Effects	Precautions
SALICYLATES			
Example: acetylsalicylic acid	Analgesic, antipyretic, antiinflammatory	Gastric irritation; dose-related salicylism; skin rash; hypersensitivity	Take with food, milk, or antacid; space q 4-6 hr to maintain antiinflammatory effect
NONSTEROIDAL ANTIINFLAMMATORY AGENTS (NSAIAs)			
Indomethacin (Indocin)	Analgesic, antiinflammatory	Headache; vertigo; insomnia; confusion; gastrointestinal irritation	Take with food, milk, or antacid; discontinue if CNS symptoms develop and notify physician
Ibuprofen (Motrin)	Same as indomethacin	Same as indomethacin but believed less irritating to GI tract; fluid retention	Delayed absorption if taken with food
Tolmetin sodium (Tolectin)	Same as ibuprofen	Same as ibuprofen	Take with food or milk
Naproxen (Naprosyn)	Same as ibuprofen	Same as ibuprofen; also drowsiness	Take with food, milk, or antacid; avoid driving until dosage effect established
Diflunisal (Dolobid)	Analgesic, antiinflammatory	Gastric irritation; headache; vertigo; skin rash; tinnitus; fluid retention	Take with food or milk; not to be used with salicylates or other antiinflammatory medications
Piroxicam (Feldene)	Analgesic, antiinflammatory	Gastric irritation; anemia; skin rash; fluid retention; vertigo; headache	Take with food or antacid
POTENT ANTIINFLAMMATORY AGENTS			
Adrenocorticosteroids (for example, prednisone)	Interfere with body's normal inflammatory response	Fluid retention, sodium retention, potassium depletion; hypertension; decreased healing potential; increased susceptibility to infection; gastrointestinal irritation; hirsutism; osteoporosis; fat deposits; diabetes mellitus; myopathy; adrenal insufficiency or adrenal crisis if abruptly withdrawn	Take with food, milk, or antacid; dosage not to be increased or decreased without physician supervision; take in morning if taken on a once-a-day basis
Phenylbutazone (Butazolidin)	Antiinflammatory; analgesic at subcortical site in brain	Gastrointestinal irritation; hematologic toxicity; hypertension; impaired renal function	Used for a short term (7-10 days); take with food or milk
SLOW-ACTING ANTIINFLAMMATORY AGENTS			
Antimalarials			
Hydroxychloroquine (Plaquenil)	Antiinflammatory (mechanism unknown); effect not expected to be noted for 6-12 mo after beginning therapy	Gastrointestinal disturbances; retinal edema that may result in blindness	Eye examination before beginning therapy and every 6 mo thereafter
Gold salts—IM			
Gold sodium thiomalate (Myochrysine)	Antiinflammatory; effect not noted for 3-6 months after beginning therapy	Renal and hepatic damage; corneal deposits; dermatitis; ulcerations in mouth; hematologic changes	Urinalysis and CBC before each injection; report dermatitis, metallic taste in mouth, or lesions in mouth to physician

novitis) of the diarthrodial joints (also called synovial joints: freely movable joints in which continuous bony surfaces are covered by cartilage and connected by ligaments lined with synovial membrane).

Clinical manifestations. RA is believed to involve an immune reaction that won't shut off because of some failure in the immune system; agents that should protect the body attack joint tissues instead and cause a chronic inflammatory reaction in the synovial membrane. This in turn results in damage to the affected joint and surrounding tissue, possibly leading to gross deformity and loss of function.

RA is characterized by periods of remission and exacerbation. During remission, the symptoms actively cease. The inflammation, pain, stiffness, and edema subside, and progression of tissue damage is halted. (The patient may experience residual joint dysfunction even with remission.)

Assessment. Collection of *subjective data* includes noting the patient's complaints of malaise, muscle weakness (especially grip strength), loss of appetite, and generalized aching.

Collection of *objective data* includes observing the joints for edema, tenderness, subcutaneous nodules, limitation in range of motion (morning stiffness especially), symmetrical joint involvement, and fever.

Diagnostic tests. There is no single definite test for RA. Diagnosis is based on the patient history and findings during a physical examination. The four classic symptoms most frequently reported are morning stiffness, joint pain, muscle weakness, and fatigue. X-ray studies reveal loss of articular cartilage and change in subchondral bone. Laboratory tests are often used in confirming a diagnosis and in ruling out the presence of other diseases. They are as follows:

- Erythrocyte sedimentation rate: an increase indicates presence of inflammatory reaction somewhere in body
- Rheumatoid factor (RF): an elevation of this titer indicates abnormal serum protein concentration is present
- Latex agglutination test: detects presence of IgM version of rheumatoid factor, the anti-IgG antibodies
- Red cell count: detects anemia, often present during chronic infection
- Synovial fluid aspiration: normal fluid usually clear and highly viscous; however, when inflammation present, fluid is cloudy, yellow, less viscous, and contains increased protein
- Synovial fluid biopsy: shows changes in tissue

Medical management. The physician will order a medical regimen based on the patient's age, occupation, lifestyle, and joints affected. The goal of treatment is directed toward relieving pain and inflammation (see Table 30-5 for medications), preventing joint damage and deformities (physical therapy, traction, and splints are often used), and promoting activities of daily living by restoring or maintaining function of the affected part.

Nursing interventions. Nursing intervention is aimed at patient education to help the patient and family understand what is happening and what to expect as the disease progresses. Rest is important, since fatigue is a major problem. Sleeping 8 to 10 hours a night and taking a 2-hour nap during the day are recommended. Exercise helps prevent the joints from "freezing" and the muscles from weakening. A typical exercise program calls for two or three 10- to 15-minute daily sessions of "quiet" exercise that puts joints gently through range of motion. Heat is often used to relax and soothe muscles. Hot packs, heat lamps, and applications of hot paraffin wax are helpful. Rehabilitation is aimed at helping the patient learn ways of adapting to physical limitations and promote normal daily activities.

NURSING DIAGNOSES	NURSING INTERVENTIONS
Pain, related to joint inflammation	Maintain bed rest as ordered; maintain proper body alignment. Assist and teach patient to extend joints as possible and to avoid external rotation of extremities; use sand bags or trochanter rolls. Avoid use of pillows under knees. Immobilize and/or support joints. Administer treatments as ordered: hot packs, tub baths, ice packs, paraffin, or whirlpool. Administer acetylsalicylic acid as ordered.
Impaired physical mobility, related to joint inflammation, edema, and pain	Assist with and teach active and/or perform passive ROM exercises after heat treatments, or apply passive ROM machine as ordered. Maintain planned rest periods. Maintain a safe environment: 1. Handrails in shower, tub, and toilet. 2. Raised toilet seat and chairs. 3. Rubber-tipped walker or cane. 4. Wheelchair in locked position when stationary.
Feeding, bathing/hygiene, and dressing/grooming self-care deficits	Teach self-care activities. Establish and teach routine plan for ADLs. Assist with feeding prn; have patient use large-grip handles for utensils as needed. Set goals with patient; encourage short-term, easily accomplished goals. Discuss use of slip-on shoes and snaps on clothing.

Patient teaching. As with any chronic illness, patient teaching is perhaps the most important aspect of nursing care of patients with rheumatoid arthritis. Patient teaching should include information about the following:

- Joint protection and energy conservation techniques
- Proper balance of rest and activity
- Proper use of medications, that is, names of drugs, dosages, precautions in administration, and side effects or toxic effects
- Plans for implementation of the exercise program prescribed by the physician or physical therapist
- Proper application of heat and/or cold packs
- Proper use of walking aids
- Safety measures to prevent injury
- Basics of good nutrition and importance of avoiding weight gain
- Danger of following programs that promise a "cure"

Ankylosing Spondylitis

Etiology/pathophysiology. Ankylosing spondylitis (AKS) is a chronic, progressive disorder of the sacroiliac and hip joints, the synovial joints of the spine, and the adjacent soft tissues. It can affect both sexes but is seen more often in young men. Women develop a milder form of AKS, and fusion of the spine is rarely seen. It is sometimes referred to as *rheumatoid spondylitis*.

Clinical manifestations. AKS involves inflammation of the spine, and as a result, the bones of the spine grow together (**ankylosis,** fuse). AKS involves inflammation where the ligament or tendon attaches to the bone and does not affect the synovial membrane, as seen in rheumatoid arthritis. AKS can affect joints, such as the neck, jaw, shoulders, knees, and hips. The disease process causes the ligaments to become ossified (hardened). The cardiovascular system can be involved, and heart enlargement and pericarditis can occur. If the thoracic joints are affected, kyphosis can occur and alter respirations. Vision loss occurs with chronic AKS, and blindness may result from glaucoma and pupil damage.

Assessment. Collection of *subjective data* includes patient complaints of low backache, stiffness, and alternating or bilateral "sciatica pain" that lasts for a few days at a time and then subsides. Pain is more pronounced when an erect position is maintained. Inactivity causes the pain to exacerbate, and exercise gives relief. Complaints of weight loss, abdominal distention, visual problems, and fatigue are common.

Collection of *objective data* includes assessment for tenderness over the spine and sacroiliac region. Peripheral joint edema and decreased range of motion may be seen. Assessment of the vital signs may indicate elevated temperature, tachycardia, and hyperpnea. Respiratory difficulties will arise if there is limited expansion of the chest as is often seen in kyphosis.

Diagnostic tests. Patients with AKS will often have the following laboratory test results:

- Low hemoglobin and hematocrit, indicative of anemia
- Elevated erythroctye sedimentation rate, common in chronic inflammatory disease
- Elevated serum alkaline phosphatase levels, seen in patients who are immobilized or have bone resorption

X-ray examination often reveals sacroiliac joint and intervertebral disk inflammation with bony erosion and joint space fusion.

Medical management. The physician usually prescribes oral analgesics and nonsteroidal antiinflammatory drugs (NSAIDs). Exercise programs (swimming and walking) are important to prevent demineralization of bone.

Surgery may be necessary to replace fused joints (hip or knee is most common). Cervical or lumbar osteotomy can be done for severe kyphosis.

Nursing interventions. Nursing intervention is aimed at maintaining alignment of the spine. Providing a firm mattress, bed board, and back brace helps provide support. Postural and breathing exercises help compensate for the possibility of impaired gas exchange caused by the changes in posture and chest cavity size. Encouraging the patient to lie on the abdomen at least 15 to 30 minutes qid helps to extend the spine. Turning and positioning q 2 hours helps to prevent decubitus ulcers.

NURSING DIAGNOSIS	NURSING INTERVENTIONS
Self-esteem disturbance, related to body image change	Encourage verbalization about fears and anxiety of disease process. Deal with behavior changes: denial, powerlessness, anxiety, and dependence. Be supportive but kindly firm in setting goals. Encourage independence, and provide for tasks accomplished. Be aware of limitations, and encourage discussion of feelings and concerns.

Patient teaching. The patient should be taught the appropriate use of prescribed medications, prescribed postural exercises, and methods of applying heat to back and hips. Correct posture and prevention of complications should be promoted by the following:

- Encouraging the use of a firm mattress
- Encouraging the patient to sleep without a pillow under the head
- Encouraging respiratory exercises

Degenerative joint disease (osteoarthritis)

Etiology/pathophysiology. Degenerative joint disease (DJD) is also known as osteoarthritis, hypertrophic arthritis, osteoarthrosis, or senescent arthritis. Almost everyone past 40 years of age has hypertrophic changes in the joints. There are two forms of osteoarthritis: primary (cause is unknown) and secondary (caused by trauma, infections, previous fractures, rheumatoid arthritis, stress on weight-bearing joints from obesity, or such occupations as coal mining or boxing).

Osteoarthritis is a nonsystemic, noninflammatory disorder that progressively causes bones and joints to degenerate.

Clinical manifestations. This disorder affects the joints of the hand, knee, hip, and cervical and lumbar vertebrae. Osteoarthritis appears to be related to aging, but researchers are unclear as to the cause. Nearly all persons older than 60 years will show osteoarthritic changes, with women being affected more often than men. The disease affects the hands in women more often, whereas in men the hips are affected.

Assessment. Collection of *subjective data* involves questioning the patient about complaints of pain and stiffness (rest usually relieves the pain in the early stages). Past illnesses, surgical procedures, or trauma may be relative, and information about excessive weight gain and occupation may be significant. Complaints of muscle spasms and reduced grip strength are common.

Collection of *objective data* includes assessment for joint edema, tenderness, instability, and deformity. Heberden's nodes appear on the side of the distal joints of fingers, and Bouchard's nodes appear on the proximal joints of fingers—these are hard, bony, and cartilaginous enlargements. The patient's gait will reveal a limp, especially if the hips or legs are affected.

Diagnostic tests. There is no specific test to diagnose osteoarthritis. However, x-ray studies, arthroscopy, synovial fluid examination, and bone scans are used to provide information.

Medical management. The physician will order an exercise plan that is balanced with rest periods. Physical therapy using heat application helps reduce stiffness, pain, and muscle spasms. Gait enhancers, such as canes, walkers, and shoe inserts, help relieve discomfort while using weight-bearing joints. Drug therapy involves using large dosages (10 to 15 gr three to four times daily after meals) of salicylates (aspirin) or nonsteroidal antiinflammatory drugs (such as Motrin 400 mg, four times a day). Steroids (cortisone) are sometimes used in low dosages or injected into joints to produce immediate pain relief and temporarily halt the destructive process.

Surgical intervention, such as osteotomy, may help correct malalignment. Joint replacement may be necessary to replace all or part of the joint's articulating surface. Hip and knee arthroplasty are the most common surgical interventions.

Nursing interventions. Nursing intervention involves encouraging the patient to maintain activities of daily living and adapt to limitations of the disease. Encouraging the patient to alternate sitting, walking, and standing with periods of rest can help reduce joint discomfort and deterioration. Elderly patients may be physically capable of turning and moving in bed but may forget to do so because of alteration in their level of orientation. Assisting the patient with a weight-reduction plan may be necessary if obesity is a problem. If splints are needed to support a painful joint, the nurse needs to assess for neurovascular impairment above and below the site of application. Gait enhancers should be checked for safety considerations, such as rubber tips on ends, proper size, and patient knowledge about use. If the patient has been taking aspirin over a period of time, GI bleeding may occur. It may be necessary for the nurse to perform a guaiac test on stool and emesis to determine the presence of occult blood.

Patient teaching. As with rheumatoid arthritis, teaching the person with osteoarthritis about the disease process and the steps to control that process is the most important aspect of nursing interventions. Patient teaching should include the same information as for rheumatoid arthritis, pp. 601 and 602.

Gout (Gouty Arthritis)

Etiology/pathophysiology. This is a metabolic disease resulting from an accumulation of uric acid in the blood. It is an acute inflammatory condition associated with ineffective metabolism of purines. Gout can be primary (linked with hereditary factors), secondary (resulting from use of certain drugs or complication of another disease), or idiopathic (unknown origin). It affects men 8 to 9 times more frequently than women and usually occurs in middle life. It does not occur before puberty in the male or before menopause in the female. It takes about 20 years for sufficient urates to accumulate in the body before causing symptoms when the disease is primary. Of all persons with gout, 85% have a genetic tendency to develop the disease.

Uric acid crystals form in the synovial tissue, resulting in inflammation of the joint; it is unclear why this occurs. Typically the big toes are involved, but other joints can also be affected.

Clinical manifestations. The onset occurs at night, with excruciating pain, edema, and inflammation in the affected joint. The pain may be of short duration, returning at intervals, or it may be severe and continuous for 5 to 10 days. The patient may have repeated attacks or only one attack during his life. **Tophi** (deposits of monosodium urate in the tissue) are seen around the rim of the ear and can disfigure the ear. Surgical removal may be necessary.

Assessment. Collection of *subjective data* involves noting a complaint of pain occurring at night involving the great toe. Data collection involves a dietary history, with specific questions concerning consumption of alcohol and foods high in purine, such as organ meats (brain, kidney, liver, and heart), anchovies, yeast, herring, mackerel, and scallops.

Collection of *objective data* includes assessment of joints (especially the great toe) for signs of edema, heat, discoloration (may appear erythematous or purple), and limited movement. Vital sign data may reveal an elevated temperature and hypertension, tachycardia, and tachypnea. Careful assessment of urinary output is necessary, because tophi can form in the kidneys and alter kidney function. The patient should be assessed for the presence of tophi (typically seen on the earlobes, fingers, hands, and toes).

Diagnostic tests. Laboratory tests used to diagnose gout include serum and urinary uric acid levels (elevation is significant); complete blood count (leukocytosis and anemia may be present); and elevated erythrocyte sedimentation rate. X-ray studies reveal cysts and toe bone pockets. Synovial fluid will contain urate crystals.

Medical management. Several drugs are used in the treatment of the disease. For acute attacks colchicine is administered orally or may be given intravenously. When administered orally, 0.5 mg may be given hourly for 12 doses. The drug is discontinued if gastrointestinal symptoms develop or the patient has not been relieved of pain. Phenylbutazone (Butazolidin) and indomethacin (Indocin) are effective antiinflammatory drugs in treating gout. Corticosteroids can be administered orally, intravenously, or intraarticularly and will relieve symptoms within 12 hours. The physician may order allopurinol (Zyloprim) to decrease the production of uric acid; probenecid (Benemid) to increase secretion of uric acid by the kidneys; and sulfinpyrazone (Anturane) to prevent the development of tophi in various parts of the body, including the kidneys.

Nursing interventions. Nursing intervention is aimed at giving medications prescribed by the physician for relief of pain and inflammation. When giving colchicine it is important to observe for side effects, such as diarrhea, nausea, and vomiting. Increasing the patient's fluid intake to at least 2000 ml daily helps eliminate the excess urinary urates. About 10% to 20% of patients with gouty arthritis have uric acid kidney stones. Careful documentation of intake and output is necessary. Bed rest and joint immobilization are maintained during the time the patient is symptomatic. Bed cradles prevent pressure from bed linens on the affected great toe.

NURSING DIAGNOSES	NURSING INTERVENTIONS
Pain, related to disease process	Maintain patient in position of comfort with foot supported and in alignment; place bed cradle over foot; no weight bearing. Apply cold packs as ordered, keeping pressure off joint. Administer analgesics and antigout and antiinflammatory agents as ordered; observe for side effects.
Knowledge deficit regarding medications and home care management	Provide medication schedule, including name, dosage, purpose, and side effects. Discuss importance of diet, exercise, and rest program. Encourage follow-up visits with physician.

Patient teaching. Patient teaching is aimed at giving information about the disease and stressing the importance of keeping the serum uric acid levels within normal range by taking the prescribed medications, following the prescribed diet, and avoiding infections, lack of sleep, and stress. Cochicine, Benemid, Zyloprim, and Anturane are drugs that the patient may need to take for several years, even when the symptoms are not present.

OTHER DISORDERS

Osteoporosis

Etiology/pathophysiology. The cause of osteoporosis has not been completely identified. Women between the ages of 55 and 65 years are identified as a high-risk group for postmenopausal osteoporosis, and many researchers believe that this is related to the loss of the female hormone *estrogen*. Studies of postmenopausal osteoporosis suggest estrogen deficiency is connected with increased bone reabsorption and sensitivity to parathyroid hormone (substance that weakens bone by increasing calcium movement from bone into extracellular fluid). Senile osteoporosis is seen in persons between ages 70 and 85 years and affects twice as many women as men. Other factors that may contribute to the condition include immobilization, use of steroids, and high intake of caffeine. Genetic (small bone structure) and environmental factors (limited exercise) can contribute to the rate of bone loss. Osteoporosis affects the vertebrae, neck of the femur, pelvis, hands, and wrists.

Clinical manifestations. The disorder develops slowly and the first sign is a complaint of backache. As the disease progresses, the bones become porous and brittle, which is caused by a lack of calcium.

Assessment. Collection of *subjective data* includes questioning the patient about life-style practices and complaints of pain (low thoracic and lumbar) that worsens with sitting, standing, coughing, sneezing, and straining.

Collection of *objective data* involves assessing the patient for dowager's hump (spinal deformity and height loss that develops from repeated spinal vertebral fractures) and increased lordosis, scoliosis, and kyphosis. Assessment should be done for gait impairment associated with inability to maintain erect posture.

Diagnostic tests. The physician will order a complete blood count, serum calcium, phosphorus, and alkaline phosphatase, blood urea nitrogen, creatinine level, urinalysis, liver and thyroid function tests, and x-ray studies.

Medical management. The physician will order a treatment regimen aimed at promoting the increase of bone density and retardation of bone loss. Calcium supplements that bring the total calcium intake to 1000 mg for men and 1500 mg for postmenopausal women are recommended. Exercise programs to improve muscle tone, such as walking, have been effective in preventing further bone loss and stimulating new bone formation. Treatment may include adequate doses of estrogen. Estrogen will not correct the condition but will help to prevent fractures.

Nursing interventions. Nursing intervention is aimed at preventing further bone loss and fractures. A diet rich in milk and dairy products provides most of the calcium in the diet. Food and beverages that contain caffeine also contain phosphorus, which contributes to bone loss. Teaching patients relaxation techniques and encouraging them to stop smoking are recommended. Estrogen therapy is not without risk, and patients who take estrogen need information about the higher risk for thromboembolism, endometrial cancer, and possibly breast cancer. Safety measures, such as siderails, handrails, bedside commodes with seat elevators, and rubber mats in showers can prevent falls in the elderly patient.

NURSING DIAGNOSES	NURSING INTERVENTIONS
Impaired physical mobility, related to disease process	Provide firm mattress. Encourage ambulation with walker or cane if indicated. Assist and teach active ROM exercises q 4 hr. Monitor and maintain body alignment; fractures can occur without patient's knowledge. Handle patient carefully, and assist with and teach correct body mechanics. Administer analgesics, estrogen, calcium, and vitamin D as ordered. Provide diet high in calcium and vitamins C and D. Monitor serum calcium levels.
Knowledge deficit regarding home care management	Stress importance of diet, activity, and rest; provide written aerobic exercise schedule; caution patient to avoid jogging. Provide medication schedule, including name, dosage, purpose, and side effects. Discuss importance of safe environment to prevent falling. Encourage reduction of caffeine, alcohol intake, and smoking.

Patient teaching. To prevent osteoporosis, young women are advised to have an adequate daily intake of calcium and vitamin D, to exercise regularly, and to avoid smoking. After menopause the usual recommended daily allowance of 800 mg of calcium should be increased to 1500 mg. Vitamin D, which increases calcium absorption, may also need to be added to the daily regimen of postmenopausal women as per physician's orders. Follow-up visits to the physician are encouraged for direction as to medication, diet, and exercise regimen.

Osteomyelitis

Etiology/pathophysiology. Osteomyelitis (inflammation of the bone) can occur from bacteria introduced through wounds, as in the case of a compound fracture. Also, bacteria may travel by the bloodstream from another site in the body to a bone, causing the bone to become infected.

Bacteria invade the bone, and degeneration of bone tissue occurs. If osteomyelitis becomes chronic, the bone tissue affected often will be weakened and predisposed to spontaneous fractures.

Clinical manifestations. The patient with osteomyelitis is subject to contractures in the affected extremity if positioned incorrectly. It is not unusual for a new focus of infection to develop months and sometimes years after the initial infection is diagnosed.

Assessment. Collection of *subjective data* includes a complete history of injuries, surgical procedures, and diseases. An assessment includes patient's complaints of pain. An assessment of allergies should be done, especially to medications, since antibiotics are given long term.

Collection of *objective data* includes careful inspection of any wounds. The drainage is assessed for color, amount, and presence of odor. Vital signs are assessed for signs of infection (temperature elevation, tachycardia, and tachypnea). Assessment for edema is noted, especially in the joints with limited mobility.

Diagnostic tests. A complete history is taken, along with physical examination. The physician will order x-ray studies and bone scan, complete blood count (leukocytosis may be present), erythrocyte sedimentation rate, and cultures of blood and drainage (if present).

Medical management. Intravenous antibiotic therapy is ordered; a broad-spectrum antibiotic, such as Keflin, is used. For some patients surgery may be performed to remove a fragment of necrotic bone that is partially or entirely detached from the surrounding or adjacent healthy bone (sequestrum).

Nursing interventions. Nursing intervention includes gentleness in moving the diseased extremity. Often wounds are irrigated with hydrogen peroxide or other antiseptic or antibiotic solution and then covered with a sterile dressing, using strict surgical asepsis. Patients are placed on drainage and secretion precautions. Dietary planning is done with emphasis on a diet high in calories, protein, and vitamins.

Patient teaching. This includes information about the signs of infection, such as elevated temperature. Because chronic osteomyelitis may last a lifetime, it is important for the patient to be aware of the recurrence of signs and symptoms. Patients must avoid trauma to the affected bone, since pathological fractures are common in bones affected by osteomyelitis.

NURSING DIAGNOSES	NURSING INTERVENTIONS
Potential for injury, related to decreased mobility and/or decrease in level of orientation	Maintain bed in low position. Keep siderails up. Maintain protective gentle restraints. Leave night-light on. Orient patient to surroundings.

NURSING DIAGNOSES	NURSING INTERVENTIONS
	Assist patient in ambulation with assistive devices as needed. Maintain safe environment.
Impaired skin integrity, related to immobility	Identify skin areas at risk, particularly areas over bony prominences (heels, sacrum, elbows, and ischial tuberosities). Regularly inspect (at least q 4 hr) for signs of pressure (for example, erythema or induration). Regularly turn patient (at least q 2 hr) within limits of immobilization. Use sheepskin pads, flotation pads, Eggcrate mattress, or Clinitron or CircOlectric bed. Assist patient to keep skin clean and dry, especially under casts. Massage skin with lotion q 2 to 4 hr. Encourage nutritious diet to maintain skin integrity.

Herniation of Intervertebral Disk (Herniated Nucleus Pulposus)

Etiology/pathophysiology. Herniated nucleus pulposus can occur suddenly (from lifting, twisting, or trauma) or gradually (from degenerative changes [as seen with degenerative joint disease, osteoporosis, aging, and chronic diseases affecting bones]). Herniations of the lumbar spine usually affect persons 20 to 45 years old; cervical herniations are seen most in persons 45 years old and older. Men are more prone to this disorder than women.

Herniation occurs when the central portion of the intervertebral disk (nucleus pulposus) slips through the anulus fibrosus (surrounding the disk) into the spinal canal. This displacement puts pressure on nerve roots. Lumbar and cervical herniations are most common (Fig. 30-17).

Clinical manifestations. Low back pain that occurs with the slightest movement is the most common symptom. The pain radiates over the buttock and down the leg, following the sciatic nerve pathway (radicular pain), causing numbness and tingling in the affected leg.

Assessment. Collection of *subjective data* involves pain assessment and patient-stated relief measures. Pain is often exacerbated with activity. Complaints of pain in the back radiating down the leg (sciatica) are common. Complaints about activity intolerance and alteration in bowel and bladder elimination (constipation and urinary retention) are significant.

Collection of *objective data* includes observing for signs of limited spinal flexibility (limited forward bending) and gait alteration (patient may favor supporting weight on one extremity). An ineffective breathing pattern may be present and result from pain and decreased mobility. Assessment includes determination of bowel and bladder elimination and maintenance of traction equipment.

Diagnostic tests. Complete history and physical examination is obtained. The physician will order x-ray studies, computed tomography, myelography, and electromye-

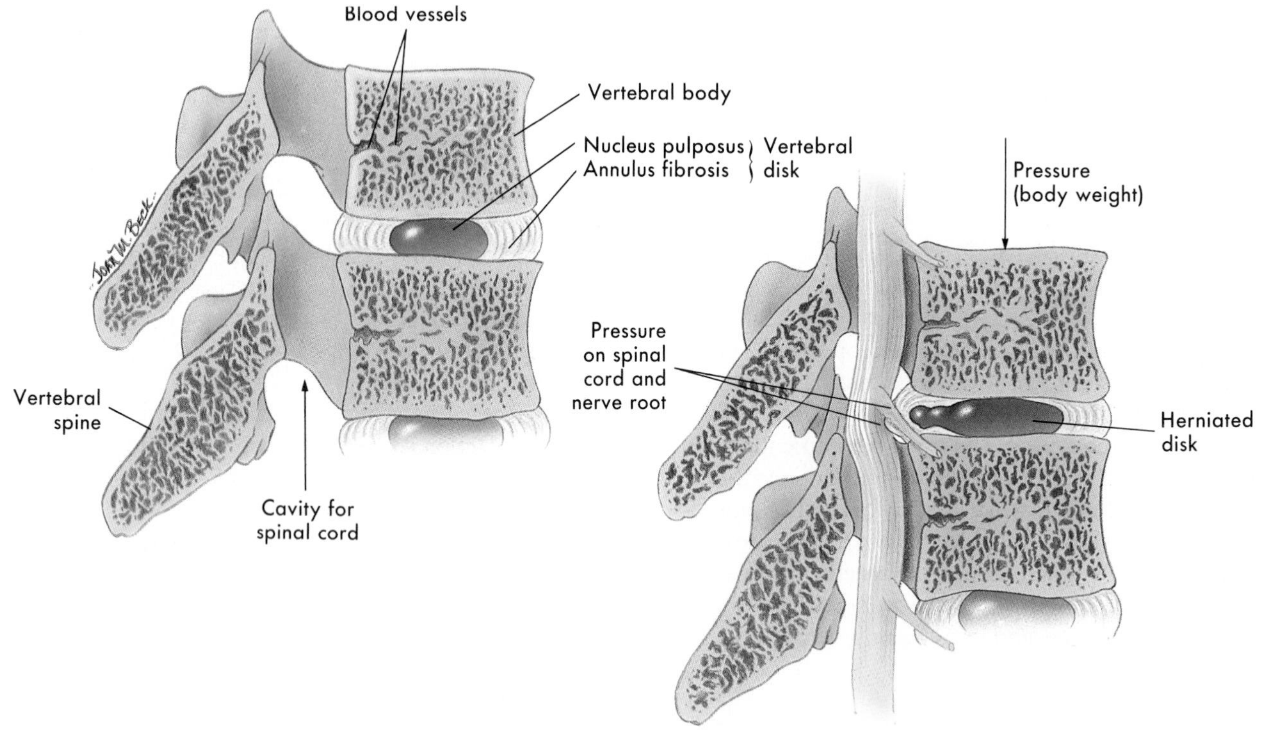

FIG. 30-17 Sagittal section of vertebrae showing both normal and herniated disks.

lography (to determine nerve involvement).

Medical management. The physician will order bed rest, pain control, physical therapy (aimed at muscle strengthening and comfort), and skin traction (may be pelvic or cervical). If the patient demonstrates neurological deterioration or continued pain, a surgical procedure may be required, such as the following:

- Laminectomy: partial or total removal of the lamina and removal of the herniated nucleus pulposus.
- Spinal fusion (arthrodesis): removal of the lamina and removal of several herniated nucleus pulposus. A portion of bone taken from the patient's iliac crest or from a bone bank is used as a bone graft in the vertebral spaces.
- Diskectomy: often done with a microscope. Only the extruded disk material is removed. Percutaneous lateral diskectomy is performed under local anesthesia with the surgeon cutting a window around the anulus fibrosus.
- Chemonucleolysis: can be done on patients who have no nerve involvement. The procedure involves administering a local anesthetic agent and then guiding a needle into the nucleus pulposus to inject chymopapain (drug which dissolves the nucleus pulposus).

Postoperative laminectomy care includes assessing the incision site for signs of infection, such as drainage, edema, odor, and temperature elevation. After a chemonucleolysis, careful assessment is noted for signs of allergic reactions to chymopapain, such as urticaria and respiratory difficulties.

Nursing interventions. Nursing intervention is aimed at providing nursing care appropriate for the following nursing diagnoses:

- Anxiety, related to discomfort, fear of unknown, and life-style changes
- Pain (back), related to muscle spasms and painful diagnostic tests
- Colonic constipation and altered patterns of urinary elimination, related to pain, pain medications, immobility, and neurological involvement

Nursing intervention involves giving the patient and the family information about procedures and hospital protocol to help reduce their anxiety. It is important to administer the medications prescribed on schedule and document the effectiveness of the medication. Distraction, heat or ice application (if ordered), and moving (by log rolling) and positioning the patient q 2 hr (if not contraindicated because of maintaining traction) can help promote patient comfort. Careful documentation of intake and output provides information about bowel and bladder function. The nurse should encourage the patient to sit in a straight, firm chair for no longer than 20 to 30 minutes at one time. It is important to monitor the patient for evidence of respiratory distress and paralytic ileus and for complications seen in laminectomy patients.

NURSING DIAGNOSES	NURSING INTERVENTIONS
Knowledge deficit regarding home care management	Stress importance of prescribed rehabilitation plan of activity, rest, and, exercise. Provide diet instructions as to type and amount, and weight maintenance (no gain) if applicable. Discuss medications: name, purpose, schedule, dosage, and side effects. Discuss signs and symptoms to report to physician: severe pain; changes in temperature, color, or sensation in extremity; and malodorous drainage from wound. Encourage follow-up visits with physician.
Powerlessness, related to decreased mobility/pain	Use active listening, and permit verbalization of anger and helplessness. Assist patient with identifying coping mechanisms that will reduce feeling of powerlessness; use those that have been successful in past. Offer positive recognition for increased activity level. Assist patient in identifying areas over which he has control. Involve patient in decision-making process for own care.
Altered nutrition: less than body requirements; more than body requirements	Encourage diet high in protein: 150 to 300 g/day unless contraindicated. Teach patient to avoid weight gain, especially if in a molded brace. Encourage patient to eat regular meals. Give patient ample time to eat. Encourage self-feeding, but help patient or provide special assistive utensils as necessary. Attend to patient's need for roughage and fluid as noted, and encourage iron and vitamins for bone repair. Position patient to facilitate comfortable intake of food and fluids.
Potential for infection, related to immobility and/or surgical intervention	Assess wound integrity, and observe for signs of infection or drainage. Monitor and change dressings prn; cleanse with hydrogen peroxide, using surgical asepsis at least q 8 hr or per physician's protocol. Monitor temperature. Encourage coughing, turning, and deep breathing q 2 hr as indicated. Encourage ambulation as permitted.

Patient teaching. Activity out of bed may begin as early as 1 day after a simple laminectomy or 2 to 4 days after a laminectomy and fusion. The nurse should transfer the patient out of bed with as little time spent in the sitting position as possible. The patient may be permitted to walk as much as tolerated, with assistance if necessary. Braces or corsets, if prescribed, are applied before the patient gets out of bed. The nurse should encourage the patient to participate in ADLs within prescribed limits of mobility.

The patient should be instructed not to lift or carry anything heavier than 2.25 kg (5 lb), not to drive a car until permitted by the surgeon, and to avoid twisting motions of the trunk.

Tumors of the Bone

Etiology/pathophysiology. Tumors of the bone may be primary or secondary and may be benign or maligant. As with other types of tumors, the cause of bone tumors is not always known. Carcinoma of the prostate, lung, breast, thyroid, and kidney may metastasize to the bones. Osteogenic sarcoma is a primary malignant bone tumor that is seen most often in young people. Osteogenic sarcoma can metastasize to the lungs and to the rest of the body via the bloodstream. Osteochondroma is a type of benign tumor.

Osteogenic sarcoma is a fast-growing and aggressive tumor that affects the long bones of the body. About 50% of these tumors occur in the femur (at the distal end), affecting males between the ages of 10 and 25 more often than females.

Osteochondroma is the most common benign osteogenic tumor. This tumor is seen more often in males between the ages of 10 and 30. Osteochondromas can occur as a single tumor or as multiple tumors. They usually affect the humerus, tibia, and femur.

Clinical manifestations. When healthy bone cells are replaced by cancer cells, the strength of the bone is altered and spontaneous fractures can occur. Anemia occurs when cancer invades the long bones and interrupts the manufacturing of red blood cells in the bone marrow. Cancerous bone tumors metastasize and invade other bones and lung tissue.

Benign bone tumors can grow large enough to put pressure on blood vessels and nerves. Benign tumors do not spread. However, they may undergo cancerous changes and become malignant.

Assessment. Collection of *subjective data* includes an awareness that malignant and benign bone tumors will cause pain in the affected bone site. Complaints of pain, especially with weight bearing, are common. The pain may result from a spontaneous fracture. The patient may also complain of tenderness at the affected side.

Collection of *objective data* includes assessment of the painful part, which may reveal edema and discoloration of the skin.

Diagnostic tests. Diagnosis is confirmed with x-ray studies, bone scan, bone biopsy, and laboratory studies, such as: complete blood cell count and platelet count (relative to bone marrow involvement); serum protein levels (elevated in multiple myeloma); and serum alkaline phosphatase level (elevation may indicate osteogenic sarcoma).

Medical management. The physician will evaluate the tumor type, size, and location and plan the treatment accordingly.

Larger, symptomatic, benign tumors and malignant tumors require surgical intervention. The surgical procedure depends on the tumor size, location, and extent of tissue involvement. The surgery may involve (1) wide excision or resection, (2) bone curettage, or (3) leg or arm amputation.

Treatment is aimed at destroying or removing the malignant lesion. Amputation of the affected extremity followed by chemotherapy or radiation is the widely accepted protocol for treatment of malignant bone tumors.

Chemotherapy is aimed at destroying cancer cells at both primary and metastatic sites. Patients usually receive chemotherapy in cycles of 3- or 4-week intervals. Radiation therapy may be given internally and externally. It is important for the nurse to know the safety precautions and side effects of both chemotherapy and radiation therapy. (See Chapter 41 for a discussion of care of the patient with cancer.)

Nursing interventions. Preoperatively the patient and family need complete and concise information about procedures and postoperative expectations.

Postoperative nursing interventions will include the following:

- Performing a neurovascular assessment
- Monitoring vital signs
- Administering analgesics and evaluating the effectiveness
- Providing cast care and/or dressing changes with careful documentation of drainage, odors, and signs of circulation impairment
- Cooperating with physical and occupational therapists to promote mobility and activities of daily living
- Educating the patient and family about home health care and early detection of tumor recurrence

NURSING DIAGNOSES	NURSING INTERVENTIONS
Anxiety, related to fear of cancer, body image change, life-style change, and possible death	Establish therapeutic relationship: acknowledge fear and encourage patient to acknowledge and express feelings. Give accurate information about condition and therapies. Refer to resources when necessary (e.g., social worker and religious counselor).
Pain, related to soft tissue trauma, edema, and compression of nerve tissue in affected extremity	Assess type and location of pain; observe for increasing pain or dysfunction. Assist patient with changing position frequently; administer back rubs.

NURSING DIAGNOSES	NURSING INTERVENTIONS
	Administer analgesics as ordered; assess effectiveness of pain relief measures. Provide diversional activities.
Impaired physical mobility, related to surgical and medical intervention, pain, and weakness	Maintain bed rest in correct body alignment as ordered with splint and/or pillows. Assist with activity as tolerated and ordered. Ambulate with assistance if tolerated; assist to use crutches, cane, or walker if needed. Maintain planned rest periods.

TRAUMATIC INJURIES

Traumatic injuries to the musculoskeletal system can occur in all age groups. However, aged persons may have disorders that predispose to musculoskeletal injuries. The more serious injuries involving fractures will be treated in a hospital, whereas the less serious, such as contusions, sprains, or strains, may be treated in an outpatient facility.

Contusions

Etiology/pathophysiology/clinical manifestations. Contusions are the most common soft tissue injury. An injury from a blow or blunt force will cause local bleeding under the skin and possibly a hematoma (sac filled with blood). Contusions can be serious, depending on the part of the body affected. A contusion of the brain is very serious, whereas a contusion of the arm is less serious. Large areas affected by soft tissue bleeding with slow absorption of the blood have a higher potential of developing into cellulitis (an infection of the subcutaneous tissue).

Medical management. Most contusions are treated by applying ice bags or cold compresses for 15 to 20 minutes intermittently for 12 to 36 hours for the vasoconstricting effects of cold. The involved extremity is elevated to reduce edema and suppress pain.

Sprains

Etiology/pathophysiology/clinical manifestations. This injury can result from a wrenching or hyperextension of a joint, tearing the capsule and ligaments. A sprain can involve bleeding into a joint (hemarthrosis). Common sites include the knee, ankle, and cervical spine (whiplash). Sprains are often the result of a sudden, twisting injury. Medical management is similar to that for contusions.

Whiplash

Etiology/pathophysiology/clinical manifestations. Injury at the cervical spine is known as *whiplash* and is classified under cervical disk syndrome.

Whiplash is caused by an injury that involves hyperextension, which results in compression of the anatomical structures. This type of injury usually occurs as a result of sudden acceleration or deceleration, such as rear-end car collisions that cause violent back and forth movements of the head and neck. Symptoms of a whiplash may not be obvious for a few days or even a week after the injury. Cervical fractures can accompany a whiplash injury.

Assessment. Collection of *subjective data* includes the patient's complaint of pain (the most common symptom), which usually begins in the cervical area but may radiate down the arm to the fingers and increase with cervical motion. The pain may increase sharply with coughing, sneezing, or any radical movement. Other signs and symptoms may be paresthesia (numbness or tingling), headache, blurred vision, decreased skeletal function, and weakened hand grip.

Collection of *objective data* includes edema in the cervical spine region with tightening of the muscles. Vital signs are usually within normal ranges. However, if the assessment findings indicate hypertension with widened pulse pressure and bradycardia, increased intracranial pressure (IICP) should be suspected; the findings should be reported and documented immediately. A neurological assessment is done q 15 to 30 minutes to rule out IICP. (Refer to Chapter 38 for a discussion on the care of the patient with a neurological disorder.)

Diagnostic tests. Physical examination and x-ray studies are used to confirm the physician's diagnosis.

Medical management. The prognosis for this type of injury is good, but recurrence of symptoms is common. A medical approach is most often used for treatment of whiplash. Analgesics and muscle relaxants are prescribed, along with intermittent cervical traction. Surgery may be necessary if cervical fracture with displacement occurs. (See the discussion of herniated nucleus pulposus, p. 607.)

Nursing interventions. Nursing intervention involves care of the patient with restricted activity to immobilize the cervical vertebrae to decrease irritation and provide rest for the traumatized area. This is accomplished with cervical traction. Proper assessment of traction includes the following:

- Maintaining the patient's body in proper alignment; the force or pull should be in alignment with the long axis of the bone.
- Ensuring that weights are hanging freely from the bed and are *never* removed without a physician's order.
- Observing the condition of the traction cords, making sure they are not weakened or frayed.
- Ensuring that all knots that are used on the rope or cord are square knots.
- Ensuring that the ropes are centered on the traction pulley.
- Ensuring that the correct weights are used, as ordered by the physician.

- Carefully observing the skin for signs of pressure and decubitus ulcer formation.

Other treatments include special exercises, heat therapy, and administration of mild analgesics as ordered by the physician to control the pain. A soft, foam rubber neck brace collar may be used for whiplash injuries to limit head movement. Careful inspection of the skin around the neck and chin is made for signs of excoriation.

Ankle Sprains

Etiology/pathophysiology. An ankle sprain is often referred to as a *twisted ankle* and is caused by a wrenching or twisting of the foot and ankle.

Clinical manifestations. The ankle area will become edematous very quickly, with spasms of the muscles and pain on passive movement of the joint.

Assessment. Collection of *subjective data* includes assessment of pain and tenderness in the affected ankle that intensifies with movement of the foot or ankle.

Collection of *objective data* includes assessment of the traumatized ankle for signs of edema, limited movement and function of the joint, and ecchymosis of the soft tissue around the ankle.

Diagnostic tests. An x-ray examination of the injured area is the only accurate way to ensure there is no bone injury.

Medical management. Surgery may be indicated for severe sprains. The physician will suture torn ligament fibers together. If the ligaments have been torn from the bone, the surgeon will reattach them by drilling small holes in the medial malleolus (rounded bony protrusion on the medial area of the ankle).

Nursing interventions. The injured area must be elevated and kept at rest. Application of ice for 15 to 20 minutes intermittently for 12 to 36 hours, followed after 24 hours with the application of mild heat for 15 to 30 minutes, four times daily, will promote absorption of blood and fluid from the area. Compressive dressings and splinting are used to help support the injured area. A neurovascular assessment is necessary to detect impaired tissue perfusion.

Strains

Etiology/pathophysiology/clinical manifestations. This injury is characterized by microscopic muscle tears as a result of overstretching muscles and tendons. An acute strain results when the muscles and tendons are overstretched in a forceful movement, such as unaccustomed vigorous exercise.

Assessment. Collection of *subjective data* involves noting the patient's complain of sudden and severe pain away from the joint, which increases with activity. Chronic muscle strain can occur from repeated muscle overuse, and the pain may not appear for several hours after the patient has used the muscles. The patient typically complains of soreness, stiffness, and tenderness in the area.

Collection of *objective data* includes observation of stiffness, ecchymosis, and slight edema over the injury site. The most common sites are calf muscles, hamstrings, quadriceps, and the lumbosacral area. Edema can occur very rapidly in the muscle and tendon area.

Diagnostic tests. An x-ray study is necessary to rule out bone trauma.

Medical management. It is important to encourage exercises of the legs to prevent thrombosis development.

Surgical repair will be necessary if the muscle is completely ruptured. Analgesics and muscle relaxants are ordered by the physician. An exercise program is almost always prescribed if the strain is in the lumbosacral region. The exercises are aimed at strengthening the lower abdominal muscles.

Nursing interventions. Nursing intervention for a strain is similar to that for a sprain. Ice application helps relieve pain, but some physicians prefer heat application rather than ice. Back strains are among the most common strains, and during exacerbation of symptoms, the patient is advised to avoid strenuous activities, use a firm chair with rigid back support, avoid wearing high heels, use a firm mattress for sleep, never sleep on the abdomen, and place a pillow under the knees to take pressure off the back.

IMPORTANT NURSING POINT

A strain and sprain are not the same. Strains are produced by minute muscle tears and overstretching of tendons, whereas sprains are caused by a twisting of the joint.

Dislocations

Etiology/pathophysiology. Dislocations usually involve tearing of the joint capsule; **subluxations** (partial dislocations) involve stretching of the joint capsule. Both are temporary displacements of bones from their normal position within joints. A dislocation may be (1) congenital (e.g., congenital hip displacement); (2) caused by a disease process; or (3) caused by trauma. Stretching and tearing of ligaments and tendons, as well as fractures, can accompany a dislocation or subluxation. The displaced bone may rupture blood vessels. When subluxation occurs, the joint's articulating (moveable) surfaces are partially separated.

Clinical manifestations. Dislocations may or may not be visible. Sometimes a dislocation will change the length of an affected extremity. Pain and loss of function may be similar to that occurring with a fracture. However, dislocation partially immobilizes a joint, whereas a fracture site typically has abnormal free movement. Common dislocation sites include the shoulder, hip, and knee.

Assessment. Collection of *subjective data* includes the patient's description of the injury and pain. When the dislocation is of the shoulder, the nurse should assess for complaints of sensation loss and paresthesia.

Collection of *objective data* includes the assessment of any erythema, discoloration, edema, pain, tenderness, limitation of movement, and deformity or shortening of the extremity. The nurse should compare both sides for validation. Neurovascular assessment is important to determine if vascular or nerve injury is present in the affected area. For shoulder dislocation, the nurse should assess for an absent radial pulse, hypothermia of the hand, and wrist drop.

Diagnostic tests. The diagnosis is based on the present complaints of discomfort, physical examination, and diagnostic x-ray examination of the injured site.

Medical management. The physician may perform a closed reduction, which corrects the deformity through manipulation of the extremity. Surgical intervention to restore joint articulation is sometimes required.

Nursing interventions. Nursing intervention includes measures for (1) reduction of edema and discomfort, (2) immobilization of the injured part to promote healing, and (3) patient education. Ice application is recommended for the first 24 hours after trauma. After 24 hours, heat may be used if there are no indications of bleeding. Elevation of the injured extremity on pillows and the application of elastic bandages help relieve edema. Immobilization of joints may involve application of a splint, sling, or elastic bandage. The air cast or air splint brace is an immobilization device. It is inflatable and lightweight and conforms to the extremity's size and shape. When immobilization devices are used, a neurovascular assessment is done frequently. (See neurovascular assessment in box, upper right). Analgesics should be administered as prescribed by the physician as needed. Asking the patient to rate the pain on a scale from 0 to 10 is helpful in determining pain severity. For control of extreme pain, the physician may order a narcotic, such as Demerol or Dilaudid. For moderate to mild pain, Motrin or Tylenol may be prescribed. Positioning and repositioning the injured part can help reduce discomfort.

Patient teaching. Promoting an accident-free environment is essential. The nurse can explore areas of preventive medicine with patients. They are as follows:

- Environmental safety can include grab bars mounted in the bathroom near the toilet or tub and rubber mats or slip guards in the tub and shower. Removing throw rugs and obstacles from the floor can prevent falls. If the patient is using a gait enhancer, such as a cane, crutches, or a walker, it is important that he knows how to use them correctly and takes safety precautions, such as using rubber tips on the points that make contact with the floor, to prevent slippage.
- Patients in the hospital are at risk of falling out of bed if their disease condition or medication results in confusion. These patients need a careful assessment of their level of orientation, siderails applied to their beds, and safety restraints to prevent self-injury. Using a safe ladder when climbing can help prevent a fall. Wearing protective clothing while engaging in dangerous work or contact sports is also recommended.
- Appropriate health teaching should be targeted for persons at risk for musculoskeletal diseases, such as osteoporosis, which can predispose to pathological or nontraumatic fractures.

NEUROVASCULAR INTEGRITY

NURSING DIAGNOSES

Alteration in peripheral tissue perfusion, related to injury/treatment
Potential for injury, related to neurovascular impairment

NURSING INTERVENTION

Position extremities in alignment; elevate affected extremity
Compare affected extremity with unaffected extremity, using same hand for palpation
Test capillary refill
Check *each* digit for sensation and motion
Document location and characteristics of pain
Palpate pedal, tibial, or radial pulses and compare to unaffected extremity
Look for edema with pallor, cyanosis, and coldness
Elicit description of sensations from patient

Carpal Tunnel Syndrome

Etiology/pathophysiology. Carpal tunnel syndrome results from pressure on the median nerve of the wrist. The symptoms of paresthesia (sensation as of pricks of pins and needles) and hypesthesia (an abnormal weakness of sensation in response to stimulation of the sensory nerves) of the thumb, index, and middle fingers may develop spontaneously or occur as a result of disease or injury. There is a higher incidence of this condition in obese, middle-aged women and individuals employed in occupations involving repetitious motions of the fingers and hands, for example, basket weaving, meat carving, and typing. Edema of the tendon sheaths caused by rheumatoid arthritis can predispose to carpal tunnel syndrome.

Clinical manifestations. Anatomically the median nerve passes through a tunnel surrounded by the carpal bones and ligaments. When inflammation and edema of the synovial lining of the tendon sheaths occur, the tunnel space is narrowed, resulting in compression of the median nerve. The affected hand has altered ability to grasp or hold small objects. Atrophy of the thenar eminence (the padded area of the palm below the base of the thumb) is noted as the disease progresses.

Assessment. Collection of *subjective data* includes the patient's description of discomfort, such as complaints of burning pain or tingling in the hands relieved with vigorous shaking or exercising of the hands; numbness (hypesthesia) of the thumb, index, and ring fingers especially after prolonged flexion of the wrist; and inability to grasp or hold small objects.

Collection of *objective data* includes assessment of the hand, wrist, or fingers for edema, muscle atrophy, or a depressed appearance of the soft tissue at the base of the thumb on the palmar surface.

Diagnostic tests. A conduction block at the wrist confirmed by motor nerve volicity studies is used to confirm the diagnosis.

Medical Management. If the symptoms are mild and surgery is not a desirable option, an immobilizer such as a splint can be used. Hydrocortisone acetate suspension injections can be given into the carpal tunnel for relief of mild symptoms. Surgery is indicated for severe symptoms with the occurrence of muscle atrophy. The standard surgical treatment is decompression of the median nerve by section of the transverse carpal ligament.

Nursing intervention. If surgery is not required, the nurse will be involved with the application of an immobilizer to promote comfort. If surgery is required, the postoperative interventions will include the following: (1) elevating the hand and arm for 24 hours; (2) implementing and evaluating active thumb and finger motion within limits imposed by the dressing; (3) administering prescribed analgesics as needed; (4) monitoring vital signs (temperature elevation could indicate infection); and (5) checking fingers for circulation, sensation, and movement q 1-2 hr × 24 hr.

Patient teaching. Patients are encouraged to use the affected hand in normal activities as soon as 2 to 3 days after surgery.

FRACTURES

Etiology/pathophysiology. A fracture is a traumatic injury to a bone in which the continuity of the tissue of the bone is broken. Descriptions of fractures by appearance can be seen in Fig. 30-19. Most fractures result from an insult to the bone, such as a forceful blow (twisting or crushing), which places more stress on the bone than it can absorb. Fractures that occur without trauma are referred to as pathological or spontaneous fractures and can be caused by a weakening of the bone because of osteoporosis, metastatic cancer and tumors of the bone, Cushing's syndrome, malnutrition, and complications of long-term steroid therapy.

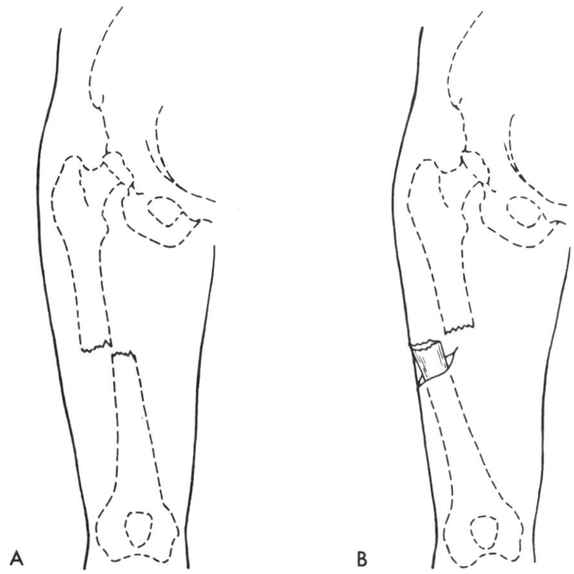

FIG. 30-18 **A,** Closed fracture. **B,** Open fracture with bone protruding through skin.

Fractures may result from (1) direct force, which results in a fracture at the site of the trauma; (2) torsion, which is seen in a twisting injury where the fracture occurs at a point remote from the trauma (e.g., a forceful twisting of the wrist may cause a fracture of the arm); or (3) violent contractions involving highly developed muscles (e.g., severe muscle spasms may cause a fracture in a paraplegic patient).

There are more than 150 types of fractures, which can be classified in various ways. First, they are described as either open (compound) or closed (simple) (Fig. 30-18), meaning that the fracture has occurred with protrusion of the bone through the skin or the fractured bone has not protruded through the skin. Open fractures are more serious, because they involve more soft tissue damage, require surgical treatment to repair, and are prone to infections. A bullet wound (injury is directed inward) that has fractured a bone is another example of an open fracture. A closed fracture does not involve a break in the skin. These fractures can usually be realigned by external manipulation and seldom require surgical intervention.

A description of a fracture can be given in terms of appearance (Fig. 30-19), such as greenstick, complete, comminuted, impacted, transverse, oblique, and spiral. They are briefly described as follows:

Greenstick fracture Incomplete fracture in which the fracture line extends only partially through the bone. The bone is broken and bent but still secured at one

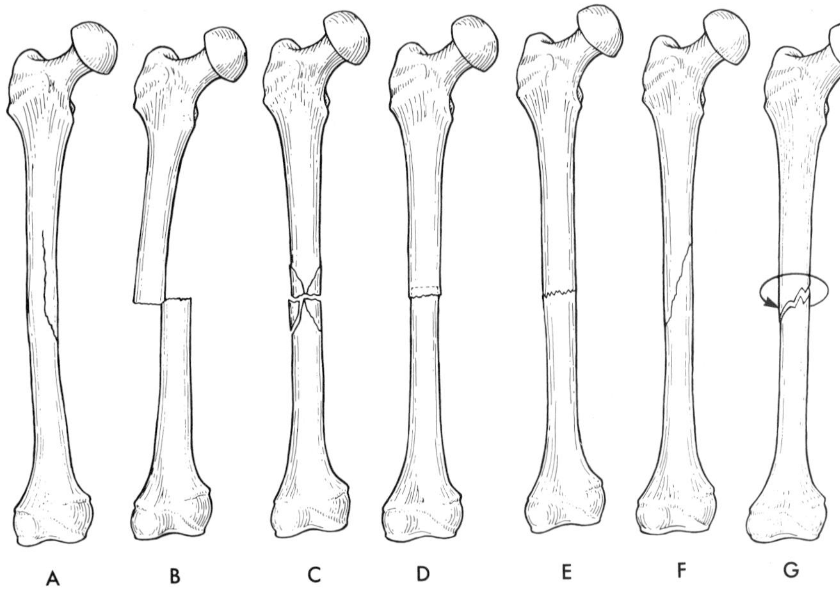

FIG. 30-19 Description of fracture by appearance. **A,** Greenstick. **B,** Complete. **C,** Comminuted. **D,** Impacted. **E,** Transverse. **F,** Oblique. **G,** Spiral.

side. This fracture is common in children, since their bones are softer and more flexible than those of adults.

Complete fracture Fracture line extends entirely through the bone with the periosteum disrupted on both sides of the bone.

Comminuted fracture Bone is splintered into three or more fragments at the site of the break. There is more than one fracture line. A butterfly fracture is a type of comminuted fracture.

Impacted fracture Sometimes called a *telescoped* fracture, because one bone fragment is forcibly wedged into another bone fragment. In long bones this can create a shortening of the extremity.

Transverse fracture Break runs directly across the bone; it is at a right angle of the bone's axis.

Oblique fracture Break runs along a slant to the length of the bone; it is at about a 45-degree angle to the shaft of the bone.

Spiral fracture Break coils around the bone. It is sometimes called a *torsion* fracture and will result from a twisting force.

Fractures are described as to their location on the bone, e.g., proximal, midshaft, or distal. Fractures can also be classified as to the force that caused the break. An example of this is the *marching* fracture, which can occur in the metatarsals as a result of a long march.

Physicians who have been the first to describe a type of fracture have given their names to fractures. Examples of this include the following:

- Colles' fracture: fracture in the distal portion of the radius that commonly occurs when a person attempts to break a fall by putting the hands down

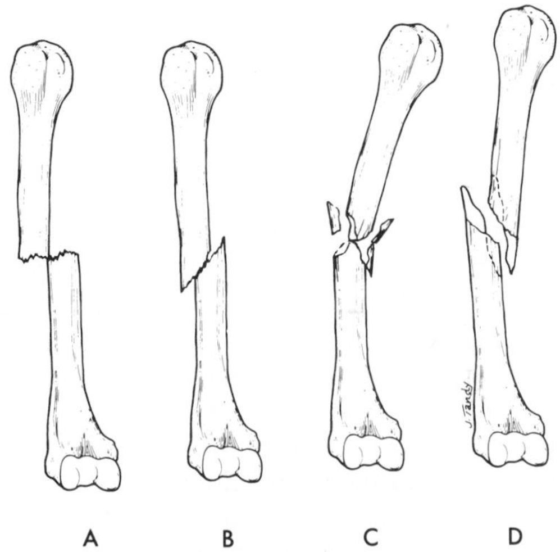

FIG. 30-20 Displacement of fragments. **A,** Sideways. **B,** Override. **C,** Angulate. **D,** Rotate.

- Pott's fracture: occurs at the distal end of the fibula and is characterized by chipping off of a piece of the medial malleolus with a displacement of the foot outward

Fractures are sometimes referred to as *joint* fractures if they involve or are close to a joint. *Articulation* fracture involves the surface of a joint. *Extracapsular* fracture involves a fracture near the joint but one that has not entered the joint capsule. *Intracapsular* fracture is a fracture within the joint capsule.

Fractures can also be described as to their displacement. Fig. 30-20 shows that fragments may be displaced sideways, can override the opposite fractured surface, may

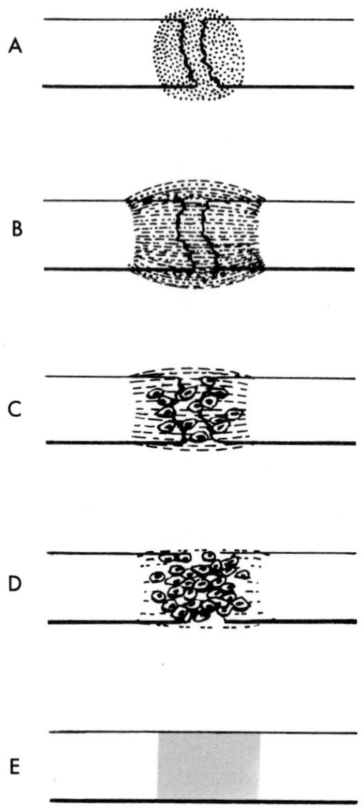

FIG. 30-21 Bone healing *(schematic representation)*.

angulate or create a bend in the bone, and may rotate away from the fracture site. When a bone is displaced, the bone fragments can cause soft tissue damage. The patient will consequently experience severe pain, edema, and muscle spasms in the early stages of healing.

The bone is vascular; therefore when a fracture occurs, there is bleeding at the site of the fracture. A clot will form at the ends of the fractured bone (Fig. 30-21, *A*). The next phase of healing occurs when the hematoma becomes organized as fibroblasts invade the area and a fibrin meshwork is formed (Fig. 30-21, *B*). Inflammation is localized as the white cells wall off the area. Osteoblasts enter the fibrous area to help hold the union firm (Fig. 30-21, *C*). Blood vessels develop, and collagen strands start to incorporate calcium deposits. **Callus** formation occurs when the osteoblasts continue to lay the network for bone buildup and osteoclasts destroy dead bone (Fig. 30-21, *D*). The collagen strengthens and continues to incorporate calcium deposits. Remodeling is the final step and occurs when the excess callus is reabsorbed and trabecular bone is laid down along the lines of stress (Fig. 30-21, *E*).

Clinical manifestations. The signs and symptoms of fractures vary according to the location and function of the involved bone, the strength of its muscle attachment, the type of fracture sustained, and the amount of related damage. Signs and symptoms are as follows:

1. Pain.
2. Loss of normal function: the injured part is incapable of voluntary movements.
3. Obvious deformity.
4. Excessive motion at site: there is motion where motion does not usually occur.
5. **Crepitus** or grating sound if limb is moved gently; no attempt should be made to determine this sign when fracture is suspected, since it may cause further damage and increase pain.
6. Soft tissue edema in area of injury.
7. Warmth over injured area.
8. Ecchymosis of skin surrounding injured area; it may not be present for several days.
9. Loss of sensation or paralysis distal to injury: indicative of nerve constricture.
10. Signs of shock, related to tissue injury, blood loss, and severe pain.

Assessment. Collection of *subjective data* includes the following:

- Pain at site of injury
- Loss of sensation or movement of affected part
- Determine cause of injury

Collection of *objective data* includes the following:

- Warmth, edema, and ecchymosis
- Obvious deformity
- Loss of normal function in the injured part
- Signs of systemic shock
- Signs of circulatory, motor, or sensory impairment

Diagnostic tests. An accurate diagnosis of the fracture is made by x-ray examination or fluoroscopy.

Medical management. Immediate management includes:

1. Splinting to prevent edema of the affected part
2. Preservation of body alignment
3. Elevation of body part to limit edema
4. Application of cold packs (during first 24 hours) to reduce hemorrhage, edema, and pain
5. Administration of analgesics
6. Observation for change in color, sensation, or temperature
7. Observation for signs of shock

Secondary management is outlined as follows:

I. Simple fracture—Optimal reduction: replacing bone fragments in their correct anatomical position
   A. Closed reduction: manual manipulations, moving bony fragments into position by applying distraction and pressure to distal fragments
   B. Traction
   C. Open reduction: surgical intervention that may use an internal fixation device
   D. Immobilization
      1. External fixation: cast or splint
      2. Traction
      3. Internal fixation, such as pins, plates, screws, wires, and prostheses
      4. Combination of the above

II. Compound fracture
  A. Surgical débridement of wound to remove dirt, foreign materials, devitalized tissue, and necrotic bone
  B. Administration of tetanus toxoid
  C. Culture of wound
  D. Treatment with antibiotics
  E. Observation for signs of osteomyelitis, tetanus, and/or gangrene
  F. Closure of wound when there is no sign of infection
  G. Reduction of fracture
  H. Immobilization of fracture
  I. Treatment of complications

Nursing interventions. The nursing intervention of patients with fractures is essentially that given any surgical patient. The care of the patient in traction and in a cast will be discussed later in this chapter. The patient needs a well-balanced diet, and opinions differ on the value of vitamin and mineral supplements in hastening bone repair. Fluids should be encouraged. Exercise of the unaffected joints, muscle-setting exercises, skin care, and elimination are important considerations in patient care. Internal fixation has simplified nursing intervention for many patients with fractures and shortened the period of hospitalization, but many patients will require longer periods of hospitalization. If activity is restricted, the complications that result from immobility must be anticipated and prevented.

NURSING DIAGNOSES	NURSING INTERVENTIONS
Pain, related to fracture and/or trauma	During initial stages of treatment, administer prescribed narcotic and nonnarcotic analgesic in appropriate dosages at timely intervals.
	Administer prescribed agents, such as diazepam (Valium), to reduce muscle spasm.
	Apply ice compresses as ordered to affected part.
	Reposition patient frequently within restrictions of the prescribed treatment.
	Instruct patient how to use relaxation techniques (deep breathing and imagery) to reduce tension.
	As pain subsides, decrease the strength and/or frequency of analgesics.
Impaired physical mobility	Allow and encourage the patient to move about to the greatest extent possible within the restrictions of the fracture reduction and the immobilizing devices.
	Allow and encourage the patient to accomplish as much self-care as possible.
	Encourage the patient to perform muscle-toning (isometric) exercises on a regular basis, for example, quadriceps setting and gluteal setting.
	Encourage and assist the patient to follow through with exercise program (including ambulation) prescribed by the physician and taught by the physical therapist.
	Encourage and assist patient to resume normal functioning of all ADLs (within limits of immobilization and fixation device) as soon as possible; for example, using bedside commode or toilet instead of bedpan.

Patient teaching. Patient teaching should include the following:

- How to move comfortably in bed
- How to transfer safely in and out of bed
- What weight-bearing restrictions to observe and for how long
- What activity limitations to observe and for how long
- How to properly use ambulatory assistive devices
- How to avoid edema in the affected part by proper elevation
- How to control pain or discomfort in the affected part
- What exercises to perform to maintain strength and enhance circulation
- Proper method to cleanse pins, using surgical asepsis per physician's protocol

Fracture of the Hip

Etiology/pathophysiology. Hip fractures are the most common type of fracture treated in the hospital. Complications of hip fractures are the most common cause of death after the age of 75 and occur more often in women. Women may be at a higher risk because of the potential for developing osteoporosis and because they have a longer life expectancy than men. Hip fractures in the elderly are often complicated by the presence of other medical conditions, such as diabetes mellitus; cardiac problems, e.g., congestive heart failure; and neurological disorders, e.g., cerebral vascular accidents.

Fractures of the hip include the less common *intracapsular* fracture, when the femur is broken inside the joint in addition to the subcapital, transcervical, and basal neck. The more common type of hip fracture is an extracapsular fracture, one that occurs outside the hip joint capsule. An intertrochanteric fracture occurs below the lesser trochanter and is frequently seen in younger patients suffering from hip trauma (Fig. 30-22).

Clinical manifestations. Signs and symptoms of hip fracture are severe pain at the fracture site, inability to move the leg voluntarily, and shortening or external rotation of the leg.

A large bone such as the hip heals slowly in an elderly

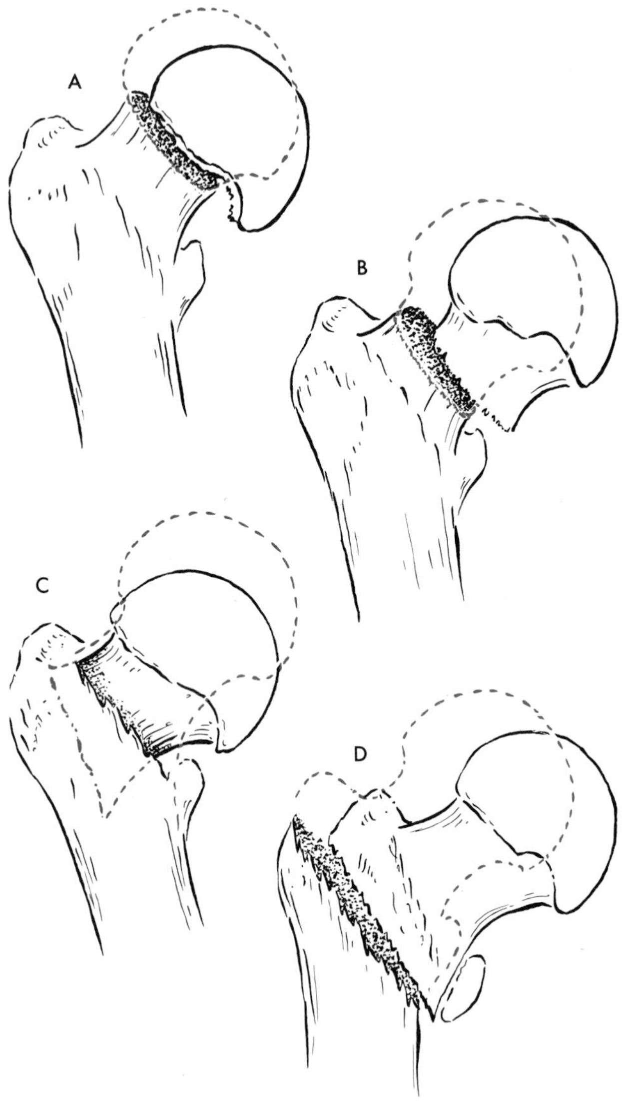

FIG. 30-22 Fractures of the hip. **A,** Subcapital fracture. **B,** Transcervical fracture. **D,** Impacted fracture of the base of the neck. **D,** Intertrochanteric fracture.

patient, and this predisposes them to various complications. They are at high risk for pneumonia, deep vein thrombosis, fat embolus, pulmonary embolus, decubitus ulcers, urinary retention, constipation, mental confusion, and depression.

Assessment. Collection of *subjective data* includes an accurate history of the events before the injury. It is important to assess the patient's level of orientation. Disorientation can occur especially in the elderly when they are in pain and anxious or are placed in an unfamiliar environment. The patient's medical and surgical history is significant, as well as any family history of bone disease. Signs and symptoms of a fracture will vary with the type and location of the break. There is usually some degree of discomfort. It may be more pronounced with slight movement of the affected part. Most patients will complain of pain in the affected leg after sustaining a fractured hip, although patients suffering from an impacted intracapsular fracture have very little pain, if any, immediately after the fracture. The nurse assesses edema, tenderness, muscle spasms, deformity, and loss of function. Patients may say they heard a "snap" or "pop" at the time the bone was injured. Impaired sensation may indicate nerve damage from the bone fragments "pinching" or severing the nerve.

Collection of *objective data* includes assessment for soft tissue injury with erythema or ecchymosis noted. When the injured limb is compared with the uninjured limb, obvious differences may be apparent. A change in the curvature or length of bone may indicate fracture. The nurse notes the affected leg is shorter, usually externally rotated about 90 degrees, and slightly flexed after an extracapsular hip fracture. With an intracapsular fracture the nurse notes the upper thigh is more edematous than the area below and the affected leg is shortened with external rotation. Subtrochanteric fractures cause excessive bleeding into the soft tissue, and the affected leg is shortened and rotated anteriorly. Crepitus is a grating sensation that may be felt or heard as the broken bone ends rub together. Neurovascular status of the extremity is assessed (see box). It is most important that the nurse keep the injured part at rest, because movement of a fractured bone can cause additional damage and may cause a closed fracture to become an open fracture. The data should also include an assessment of the patient's nutritional status. Both thin and obese patients are at risk for impaired skin integrity if bed rest is ordered. After the fracture is reduced, regular inspection of skin areas in contact with cast edges or traction apparatus to assess for signs of neurovascular compromise is necessary. It is also important for the nurse to note that patients suffering from any trauma are at risk for shock. Treating the shock condition will take precedence over treatment of the fracture.

Diagnostic tests. Diagnosis is confirmed by x-ray examination of the injured part. Blood tests, such as hemoglobin determination, often show decreased laboratory values because of bleeding at the fracture site; the blood glucose level may be elevated because of the trauma.

Medical management. Fracture reduction is the method of realigning the bone segments. This is necessary only when the bones are displaced. Fractures are reduced by closed or open reduction methods. Both methods are painful, and some type of anesthesia is recommended. Anesthesia also helps to relieve muscle spasms. Closed reduction involves the external manipulation of the bone fragments into position and the immobilization with external devices, such as casts, splints, or traction, as was discussed earlier in this chapter. Open reduction involves

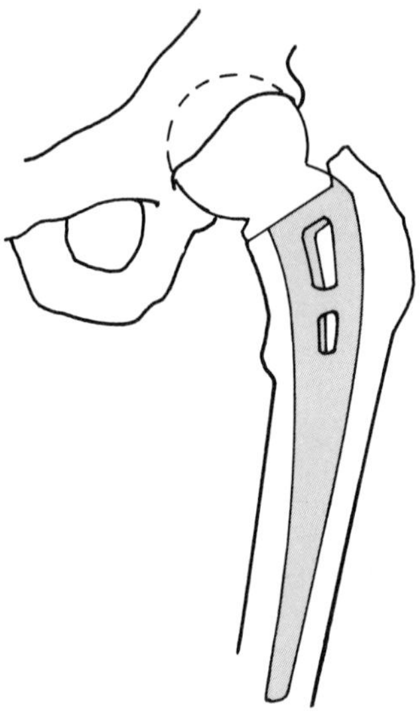

FIG. 30-23 Austin Moore prosthesis.

a surgical procedure in which the bone is exposed through a skin incision and the bone fragments are fixed in position with wires, nails, plates, screws, bolts, or a combination of these. The use of these devices is called *internal fixation*. Prosthetic implants, such as the Austin Moore prosthesis, are used to replace the femoral head and neck in fractures when the vascular supply to the femoral head may eventually be compromised (Fig. 30-23). Neufeld nail and screws are used in the repair of intertrochanteric fractures. A Küntscher nail (intramedullary rod) is used to repair midshaft femoral fractures. Sliding nails are used in repair of intertrochanteric fractures. Sliding nails will usually permit the patient to bear weight to some degree, because these nails will "give" slightly when subjected to weight-bearing forces without shifting their placement or penetrating through the femur. Bone grafts, either autograft (patient's own bone) or allograft (cadaver bone) may be used with internal fixation devices when excessive bone is lost at the fracture site. If a stable reduction cannot be achieved, the physician may elect to do an arthroplasty (surgical reconstruction of a joint). Immobilization devices, such as casts or splints, may also be used with open reduction. An x-ray or fluoroscopic examination is needed to make an accurate diagnosis of a fracture.

Nursing interventions. Nursing intervention involves stabilizing the injured limb with a splint so that movement of the bone is limited. Open fracture will require cleansing and applying a sterile bandage to the altered skin site. Elevation of the splinted extremity will reduce edema. Tetanus immunization is given if a compound fracture is present. It is most important that the nurse remain calm and reassuring to the patient. The patient may fear severe impairment of mobility as a result of the fracture. Monitoring the vital signs at least q 4 hr will enable the nurse to detect signs of infection and shock. It is important to educate the patient to turn self (if able) frequently (q 2 hr) to prevent complications of bed rest. Encouraging the patient to help himself as much as possible can prevent a feeling of powerlessness. If the patient cannot assist himself, a turn schedule should be established (q 2 hr). Nursing intervention specific for fractured hip is concerned with prevention of shock and further complications. A major emphasis is placed on maintaining proper alignment through traction and abduction of the hip when turning a patient with a fractured hip from side to side. Some physicians do not want patients turned onto their sides for several days after surgery; others may order the patient be turned only on the unoperated side. It is important to know what has been ordered. Educating patients about activity restrictions is most important. Patients who have had an internal fixation for a fractured hip should avoid elevating their affected extremity when sitting. The head of the bed is elevated a maximum of 45 degrees to avoid acute flexion of the hip and strain on the fixation device. Instructing the patient NOT to cross the legs is important, because crossing the legs can adduct the affected extremity and dislocate the hip.

The postoperative interventions of a patient with hip fracture repair include wound assessment with special attention to color, amount, and odor of exudate. Vital signs are assessed, as well as the suture line for approximation of skin edges and intact sutures or staples at least q 8 hr. Jackson Pratt drainage tubes or Hemovacs are often used and must be assessed for amount and color of wound drainage at least q 4 hr. Accurate intake and output findings are documented to help the physician establish the need for intravenous fluid therapy. The use of incentive spirometers is valuable in assisting the patient to perform adequate respiratory ventilation to prevent pneumonia. Turning and moving the patient on schedule will maintain skin integrity and promote circulation. A nursing care plan for the patient with a fractured hip is presented on pp. 618 and 619.

Patient teaching. Activity is restricted according to the fractured hip fixation device used. If a patient has a hip prosthetic implant, teaching includes the following:

- to avoid hip flexion beyond 60 degrees for approximately 10 days
- to avoid hip flexion beyond 90 degrees from the tenth day to 2 months
- to avoid adduction of the affected leg beyond midline for 2 months
- to maintain partial weight-bearing status for approximately 2 months
- to avoid positioning on the operative side in bed
- to maintain abduction of the hip by using a wedge-shaped foam bolster or pillows arranged in a wedge; this will require nursing assistance

NURSING CARE PLAN: THE PATIENT WITH A FRACTURED HIP

Nursing diagnoses	Patient goals	Nursing interventions
Knowledge deficit, related to home care management	Patient and/or significant other will demonstrate understanding of home care and follow-up instructions through interactive discussion and actual return demonstration.	Stress importance of prescribed rehabilitation plan of activity, rest, and exercise. Provide diet instructions as to type and amount, and to avoid weight gain if applicable. Discuss medications: name, purpose, schedule, dosage, and side effects. Discuss signs and symptoms to report to physician: severe pain, changes in temperature, color or sensation in extremity, malodorous drainage from wound. Encourage follow-up visits with physician.
Pain (acute), related to loss of skeletal integrity and soft tissue trauma	Patient will express minimal discomfort or absence of pain.	Ask patient to rate pain/discomfort on a scale of 0-10 (0 = no pain/discomfort, 10 = worst pain). Help patient identify comfort measures that have worked in the past, such as analgesics, distraction, and relaxation. Convey acceptance of patient's report of discomfort by a willingness to provide comfort measures. Administer pain medications before activities/procedures. Offer position change, back rub, and relaxation techniques as supplements or alternatives to medication for pain relief. Provide care in an unhurried, supportive manner. Position patient toward unoperative side.
Impaired physical mobility, related to neuromuscular/skeletal impairment, pain, and discomfort	Patient's mobility will be restored to optimal level.	Instruct and encourage the patient in active and/or passive range-of-motion exercises to maintain or develop muscle strength and endurance. Instruct the patient in safe transfer from bed to wheelchair or commode; get patient up on noninjured side. Instruct patient in correct body alignment. Encourage patient in use of trapeze. Praise efforts at mobility activities.
Altered peripheral tissue perfusion, related to vascular injury or interruption of arterial/venous flow secondary to edema	Patient's circulation will be maintained to fulfill body requirements.	Palpate site for warmth. Observe site for color. Apply moderate pressure to nail bed and subsequently observe speed of capillary refill. Question patient regarding pain and paresthesia in injured part. Assist and teach patient to turn and cough q 2 hr and deep breathe q 1 hr. Apply antiembolic stockings as ordered. Monitor vital signs q 2-4 hr.

NURSING CARE PLAN: THE PATIENT WITH A FRACTURED HIP—cont'd

Nursing diagnoses	Patient goals	Nursing interventions
Impaired skin integrity, related to immobility	Patient's skin integrity will be maintained clean, dry, and intact.	Identify early skin areas at risk, particularly areas over bony prominences (heels, sacrum, elbows, and ischial tuberosities). Regularly inspect (at least q 4 hr) for signs of pressure (for example, erythema or induration). Regularly turn (at least q 2 hr) within limits of fracture immobilization. Use sheep skin pads, flotation pads, Eggcrate mattress, Clinitron, or CircOelectric bed. Assist patient to keep skin clean and dry. Massage skin with lotion q 2-4 hr. Encourage nutritious diet to maintain skin integrity.

If a stable plate and screw fixation is used to repair the fractured hip, the patient should not bear weight for 6 weeks to 3 months, to protect the fracture site.

A telescoping nail fixation allows minimal to partial weight bearing during the first 6 weeks to 3 months.

Fracture of the Vertebrae

Etiology/pathophysiology. Injuries such as diving accidents or blows to the head or body can result in fractures of the vertebrae. Patients with osteoporosis and metastatic cancer are at risk for vertebral fractures. Motorcycle and car accidents (especially head-on collisions) occur more frequently with young men (ages 16 to 30 years).

Fractures of the vertebrae may involve the vertebral body, lamina, and articulating processes and may occur with or without displacement. If the fracture has displaced the vertebral structures, pressure may be placed on spinal nerves. The sharp bone fragments may also sever the spinal cord nerves, causing permanent paralysis from the point of injury downward.

Clinical manifestations. Signs and symptoms of vertebral fracture include the following:

1. Pain at site of injury
2. Partial or complete loss of mobility or sensation below level of injury
3. Evidence of fracture/fracture dislocation on routine x-ray examination, myelography, and/or computerized axial tomography (CAT) scans.

Assessment. Collection of *subjective data* includes assessment for pain (if fracture has altered the spinal cord, pain may not be present), numbness, tingling, and inability to move extremities from below the level of the trauma site.

Collection of *objective data* involves careful assessment of neurological function, such as pupillary reaction to light, hand grip, ability to move extremities, level of orientation, vital signs, and reaction to painful stimulation (see Chapter 38). The nurse should observe for fecal and urinary retention. The nurse should observe for signs of hemorrhage, such as hypotension, tachycardia, tachypnea, and decreased renal functioning. The continuity of traction (e.g., weights hanging free and ropes not twisted) and skin integrity (e.g., erythema, tenderness, and edema) surrounding traction equipment should be assessed.

Diagnostic tests. X-ray studies are done to determine if there is compression of the vertebral bodies. A spinal cord injury may result from a fracture or dislocation of a vertebra, and if this is suspected, the physician performs a spinal tap for evaluation of the spinal fluid (presence of blood indicates trauma). Spinal fluid is normally clear in color (see Chapter 38).

Medical management. Stable injuries to the vertebrae (that are not a threat to spinal cord integrity) are treated with pain medication and muscle relaxants. Anticoagulant therapy may be ordered as a prophylaxis for thromboembolic complications. Maintaining erect posture can be enhanced by the use of a back support, corset brace, or a cast. The patient may be allowed to ambulate with assistance (gait enhancers) when discomfort subsides.

Unstable fractures that involve a degree of displacement are more serious, and treatment is aimed at fracture reduction. The fracture may be reduced by postural positioning and traction. Cranial skeletal traction is used with cervical spine fractures. A halo brace (Fig. 30-24), an external immobilization device in which a plaster or plastic brace that incorporates metal struts attached to

A

B

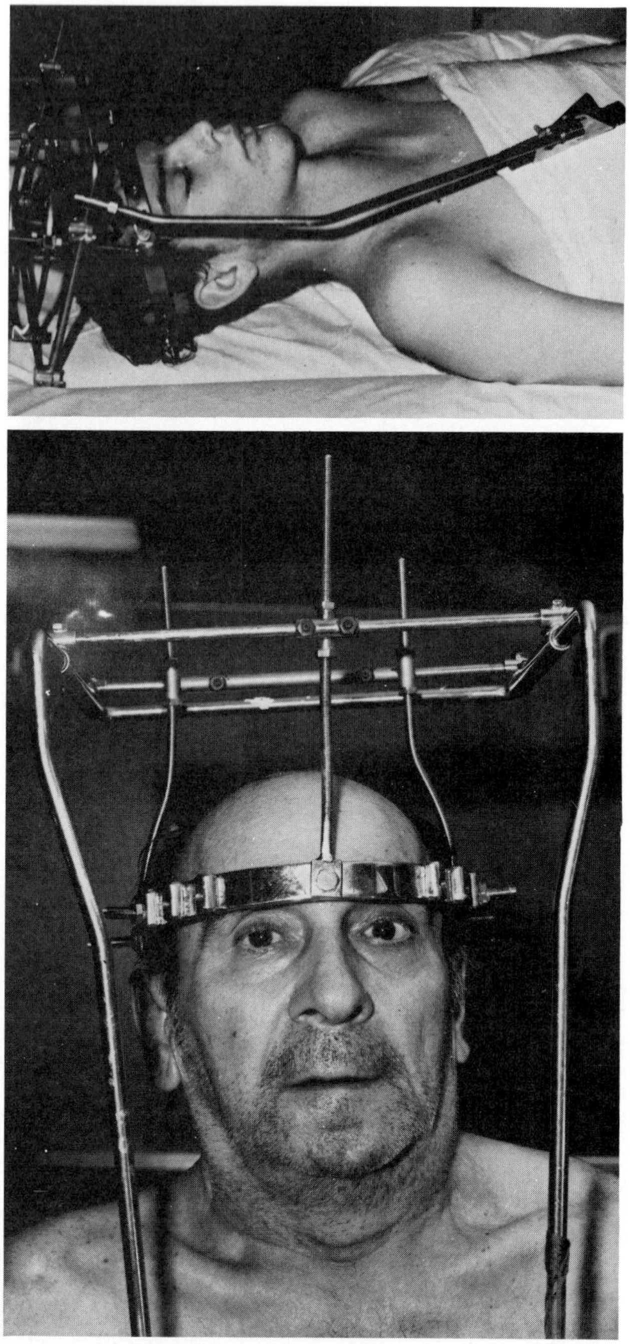

FIG. 30-24 **A,** Halo attached to body cast. Metal strut will be anchored firmly into body cast with additional plaster. **B,** Metal ring, or halo, that attaches to skull.

pins is inserted into bone, is used to allow mobility of the patient. Pelvic traction is used for lumbar spinal fractures. An open reduction may be necessary with internal fixation using a Harrington rod. After this surgical procedure the patient is placed in a body cast. A laminectomy (surgical removal of the vertebra) may be necessary (see Chapter 38).

Nursing interventions. Nursing intervention is aimed at maintaining the stability of the fracture fixation by (1) log rolling the patient for position changes; (2) following the correct procedure for turning a patient in a special bed, such as a Stryker frame or Foster bed; (3) elevating the head of the bed no more than 30 degrees; and (4) using mobilization devices for the head and back.

NURSING DIAGNOSES	NURSING INTERVENTIONS
Powerlessness, related to decreased mobility/pain	Use active listening, and permit verbalization of anger and helplessness. Assist patient with identifying coping mechanisms that will reduce feeling of powerlessness; use those that have been successful in past. Offer positive recognition for increased activity level. Assist patient in identifying areas over which he has control. Involve patient in decision-making process for own care.
Potential for infection, related to immobility and/or surgical intervention	Monitor patient for signs and symptoms of infection (elevated temperature, increased pulse rate, malodorous exudate, erythema, cloudy urine, diminished breath sounds, and presence of rales, rhonchi). Monitor laboratory values, such as CBC, and blood and wound cultures. Protect patient from cross-contamination by practicing good handwashing techniques, maintaining surgical asepsis when changing dressings, and using strict surgical asepsis with catheter care. Encourage coughing, deep breathing, and leg exercises. Prevent persons with infectious processes from contact with patient.
Impaired physical mobility, related to neuromuscular/skeletal impairment, pain, and discomfort	Maintain bed rest in correct body alignment; avoid lifting or twisting body. Place patient in immobilization device as ordered, such as cervical head halter, skeletal traction, Stryker frame, or CircOlectric bed; maintain cervical spine in extension. Assess neurovascular status q 2 hr; monitor pulse, color, temperature, sensation, and mobility of all extremities. Perform passive or assist with and teach active ROM exercises for all extremities q 2 hr. As fracture heals, traction is replaced with cast. Ambulate with assistance when ordered; monitor for vertigo and weakness; progress slowly.

NURSING DIAGNOSES	NURSING INTERVENTIONS
Ineffective breathing pattern, related to location of fracture and inactivity	Assess respiratory status q 2 hr; observe for dyspnea, cyanosis, and decreased breath sounds. Auscultate chest for breath sounds q 2 hr. Provide incentive spirometer. Reposition patient q 2 hr.
Potential fluid volume deficit, related to decrease of fluid intake and trauma	Monitor parenteral fluids as ordered. Monitor vital signs 2 to 4 hr. Measure intake and output q 8 hr; observe urine output for suppression or retention. Encourage oral fluids. Auscultate bowel sounds q 4 hr; monitor for diminished sounds.

Patient teaching. Patient teaching involves teaching the patient to support the back by (1) using a firm mattress, (2) sitting in straight, firm chairs (for no longer than 20 to 30 minutes), when allowed, (3) using proper lifting techniques (using the leg muscles, not the back), and (4) doing back exercises to strengthen spinal extensor muscles.

Fracture of the Pelvis

Etiology/pathophysiology. Most pelvic fractures result from trauma involving great force, such as falls from extreme heights, automobile accidents, or crushing accidents.

When trauma is severe enough to fracture the pelvis, vital abdominal organs may also be damaged, such as the bladder, vagina, uterus, liver, spleen, intestines, or kidneys. Because the pelvis has a rich blood supply, a fracture of the pelvis can result in extensive blood loss (as much as 2 to 8 pints).

Clinical manifestations. The patient with a fractured pelvis will be unable to bear weight without discomfort. Local tenderness and edema are common at the trauma site. Hematuria (blood in the urine) may result from trauma to the bladder. Hemorrhage is by far the most life-threatening complication to a patient with a pelvic fracture.

Assessment. Collection of *subjective data* involves complaints of pelvic pain or tenderness and backache. Complaints of restlessness, anxiety, and progressive confusion may indicate signs of shock.

Collection of *objective data* involves assessment of muscle spasms in the pelvic region; ecchymosis over the pelvis, perineum, groin, or suprapubic area; inability to raise the legs when supine; and external foot rotation on the affected side with noticeable shortening of one leg. Vital sign assessment may indicate shock (hypotension, tachycardia, tachypnea, oliguria, and diaphoresis). Careful observation for fat embolism syndrome (FES) is especially pertinent for patients with pelvic fractures. Assessing bowel sounds in all four quadrants and documenting the findings is important; large bowel and rectal lacerations are possible in patients with pelvic fractures. Assessing color and amount of urine output is necessary because of the possibility of *laceration* of the bladder.

Diagnostic tests. Abdominal x-ray studies are done in the supine and lateral positions. Computed tomography provides an evaluation of both the bony pelvis and intraabdominal contents. Intravenous pyelogram is performed to determine kidney damage. Interpretation of laboratory values for hemoglobin, hematocrit, urinalysis, and stool for occult blood helps determine if the patient is bleeding and if anemia is present.

Medical management. The patient will remain on bed rest for 3 weeks and then walk with crutches for about 6 weeks. If the patient has a symphysis pubis fracture and an iliac fracture on the same side, the physician will perform surgery. After surgery skeletal traction is applied for about 6 weeks to maintain the leg's position. When traction is released, the patient may ambulate without weight bearing for about 3 months. For a bilateral fracture of the pelvis, the physician may order a pelvic sling to support the fracture. To treat severe fractures that totally disrupt the pelvic ring and dislocate the sacroiliac joints, the physician may apply an external skeletal fixation device. He may also apply a spica or body cast to support the fracture.

Nursing interventions. Nursing intervention involves monitoring the patient for signs of progressive shock (hypotension, tachycardia, tachypnea, and decreased urinary output). Measuring the abdominal girth for signs of increased abdominal pressure that could result from internal hemorrhaging is done at least q 8 hr. Intake and output are accurately monitored for signs of hypovolemia, laceration of the bladder, and potential kidney trauma. A Foley catheter is inserted for careful monitoring of urine output and color. Nursing interventions appropriate for patients with impaired mobility, impaired skin integrity, fluid volume deficit, and pain management are implemented.

NURSING DIAGNOSIS	NURSING INTERVENTIONS
Potential altered peripheral tissue perfusion, related to hemorrhage, hypovolemia, and/or shock.	Assess for ecchymosis over pelvis and perineum. Monitor vital signs q 15 min for evidence of shock until stable. Insert Foley catheter per physician's order to monitor color and amount of urine output. Monitor parenteral fluids per physician's order. Provide quiet, therapeutic environment. Administer oxygen per physician's order. Maintain bed rest per physician's order. Monitor bowel sounds and measure abdominal girth to ascertain possible lacerated bowel.

Complications of Fractures

Compartment syndrome. Compartment syndrome is the progressive development of arterial vessel compression and reduced blood supply to an extremity. Fractures of the forearm or tibia usually precede the onset of muscle edema within the fasciae, which form compartments for the muscles of the forearm and lower leg. When there is severe trauma, such as fractures, or compression of blood vessels as a result of a tight cast or dressing, muscle ischemia (decreased blood supply to the muscles) can occur. Irreversible muscle ischemia can occur within 6 hours as a result of compression of the arteries, nerves, and tendons entering the compartment. Paralysis and sensory loss follows, with contracture and permanent disability of the extremity seen within 24 to 48 hours.

Assessment. Collection of *subjective data* includes pain assessment. Usually the patient will complain of sharp pain, which increases with passive movement of the hand or foot. The patient will experience deep, unrelenting, progressive, and poorly localized pain, which is unrelieved by analgesics or elevation of the extremity. A complaint of numbness or tingling in the affected extremity is common.

Collection of *objective data* involves assessment of the patient's inability to flex the fingers or toes, coolness of the extremity, and absence of pulsation in the affected extremity. Assessment of skin color for signs of pallor or cyanosis is made. Gentle palpation of the extremity will reveal slowing of the capillary refilling time (blanching). Close monitoring and proper documentation of vital signs is essential (especially temperature to detect signs of tissue necrosis).

Medical management. The majority of these cases require surgical intervention of fasciotomy (incision into the fascia) to relieve pressure and allow return of normal blood flow to the area. This will be done immediately (within 30 minutes). The incision is often left open to heal by granulation (healing by second intention).

Nursing interventions. Nursing intervention includes administration of analgesics with careful documentation of relief obtained. To slow further circulatory compromise, the affected limb can be elevated, but no higher than heart level, to maintain arterial pressure. Application of cold packs and removal of any constricting material, such as an elastic bandage, are necessary. The most common complication when decompression is delayed is infection as a result of tissue necrosis. Purulent drainage from the dressing is a sign of infection and must be reported immediately. If drainage and secretion isolation is required, careful instructions should be given to the patient, who may feel isolated. Patients are encouraged to express their fears and emotional needs to the nurse. Volkmann's contracture is a permanent contracture (with clawhand, flexion of wrist and fingers, and atrophy of the forearm) that can occur as a result of compartment syndrome. Proper positioning and alignment can reduce the risk of this complication.

Shock. Shock can occur as a result of blood loss from a fractured bone (bone is vascular) or from severed blood vessels, seen especially in compound fractures. Pain and fear can also cause shock. Shock can be fatal within a few hours after injury, so immediate attention is required.

Assessment. Collection of *subjective data* includes monitoring the patient's level of consciousness. Restlessness or complaints of anxiety may suggest a decrease in cerebral perfusion, resulting in brain hypoxia. Complaints of weakness and lethargy are common.

Collection of *objective data* includes monitoring vital signs. Typical shock symptoms include hypotension, tachycardia, and tachypnea. As shock progresses, hypothermia will occur. There may be pallor and cool, moist skin. Oliguria (diminished urinary output) is present with shock.

Medical management. The physician's main concern will be to restore blood volume so that there can be a rapid return of oxygen to the tissues. Blood volume can be expanded with intravenous fluids (lactated Ringer's solution or 5% dextrose in saline). Whole blood, plasma, and plasma substitutes may also be given. Respiratory assistance may be given by administering oxygen. A central venous catheter may be inserted for accurate monitoring of vital signs to prevent pulmonary edema. Shock trousers may be applied. These are pneumatic trousers designed to counteract hypotension associated with internal or external bleeding and hypovolemia.

Nursing interventions. Nursing intervention includes the nurse's responsibilities in intravenous fluid administration. These include checking (1) the contents and intravenous flow rate against the physician's orders and (2) the infusion site for signs of infiltration (erythema, edema, pain, and induration [hardening of tissue]). The patient's vital signs are monitored q 15 minutes until stable. Urinary output is monitored q 1 hour. Less than 30 ml of urine per hour is indicative of decreased renal perfusion. The patient should remain flat in bed. If there are no head injuries, the lower extremities can be raised slightly to improve venous return. The Trendelenburg position should be avoided, because it tends to push the abdominal organs against the diaphragm, reducing the effectiveness of heart and lung functions. The patient must be kept warm, but external heat should be avoided. Nothing should be given by mouth, and sedatives, tranquilizers, and narcotics should be avoided. The nurse should be aware of the anxieties of the patient's family and provide them with brief explanations of the patient's condition.

Fat embolism. Fat embolism syndrome (FES) involves the embolization of tissue fat with platelets and circulating free fatty acids within the pulmonary capillaries. Fat embolism is rare, but if it occurs, it can be life threatening because the fat droplets can effectively occlude capillaries of the pulmonary circulation, causing brain hypoxia and tissue death. Fat embolism should be suspected if the patient has multiple fractures or fractures of long bones and pelvis. The onset may occur within 48 hours of the injuries. FES is the most serious complication of long bone fractures.

Assessment. Collection of *subjective data* includes assessment of mental disturbances, such as irritability, restlessness, confusion, disorientation, stupor, and coma. These symptoms can result from effects of severe hypoxemia. There may be complaints of chest pain, especially on inspiration, and complaints of localized muscle weakness, spasticity, and rigidity.

Collection of *objective data* includes assessing for tachypnea, dyspnea, hypoxemia, and auditory rales and rhonchi (crackles and wheezes) in the lung field. As the lung filters and traps embolic material, ventilation is disturbed. Assessment of the apical pulse is performed to detect dysrhythmias. Patients will be placed on cardiac monitoring for observation of dysrhythmias and cardiovascular collapse. The nurse assesses the patient for petechiae (especially in the buccal membranes, conjunctival sacs, hard palate, chest, and anterior axillary folds) caused by occlusion of capillaries.

Diagnostic tests. The diagnosis is made on clinical signs and symptoms. These occur within 24 to 48 hours of injury. Blood gases are indicative of hypoxemia. Hemoglobin and hematocrit laboratory values are decreased. Fat will be present in the blood and urine. The sedimentation rate is increased, and the platelet count is decreased.

Medical management. The physician will order the administration of intravenous fluids to prevent shock and dilute free fatty acids. Steroid therapy is recommended to counteract the inflammatory response to the free fatty acids. Digoxin is often ordered to increase the patient's cardiac output. Oxygen will be administered if the PaO_2 is below 70 mm Hg.

Nursing interventions. Nursing intervention includes close monitoring of the patient's blood gases. Normal values include the following:

pH	7.35 to 7.45 mm Hg
$PaCO_2$	38 to 42 mm Hg
PaO_2	80 to 100 mm Hg
SaO_2	95% to 98%

Arterial hypoxia is present with fat emboli and may not be recognized clinically. If hypoxia is present, the physician will order the administration of oxygen. It is important for the nurse to check the liter flow of oxygen and educate patients and their families as to safety precautions necessary when oxygen is administered (e.g., no smoking or use of electrical equipment). Respiratory failure is the most common cause of death. Careful stabilization and immobilization of long bone fractures is an important step in preventing FES. Careful support when turning and positioning the patient can prevent the manipulation of the fracture and reduce the risk of FES. An accurate record of intake, output, and daily weights is essential to monitor fluid balance.

Gas gangrene. Gas gangrene is a severe infection of the skeletal muscle caused by Gram-positive clostridia bacteria, which may occur in the presence of compound fractures and lacerated wounds. These injuries can produce exotoxins that destroy tissue. The onset is usually sudden and may occur 1 to 14 days after injury. These organisms are anaerobic (grow and function without oxygen) and spore formers. They are normally found in soil and the intestinal tract of man. As the clostridia bacteria invade devitalized tissue (especially where blood supply is diminished), they multiply and produce toxins that cause (1) hemolysis (breakdown of red blood cells and release of hemoglobin), (2) vessel thrombosis, and (3) damage to the myocardium, liver, and kidneys.

Assessment. Collection of *subjective data* includes observation of pain, which is usually sudden and severe at the site of the injury. A characteristic finding is toxic delirium.

Collection of *objective data* includes careful inspection of the skin for gas bubbles, which may be seen at the site of the wound. The various species of clostridia bacteria produce a characteristic cellulitis, in which gas is present under the skin. This causes a crepitation (crackling sensation when the skin is touched). Signs of infection may be apparent with elevated temperature, tachycardia, tachypnea, and edema around the wound. The skin around the wound becomes necrotic and ruptures, revealing necrotic muscle. There will be a foul odor from the wound discharge, which is thin and watery. Careful documentation of the patient's progress relative to antibiotic therapy is made (e.g., decline in temperature and decrease in amount of wound drainage.)

Medical management. Treatment of gas gangrene involves establishing a larger wound opening to admit air and promote drainage. Antibiotics, such as Penicillin G or Keflin, will be ordered intravenously and must be administered as scheduled. The patient should be observed for adverse reactions. If massive gangrene develops, amputation is necessary.

Nursing interventions. Nursing intervention includes wound care using strict medical asepsis. Spore-forming bacteria are not destroyed by ordinary disinfecting methods. Therefore all contaminated equipment and linens must be autoclaved. Drainage and secretion isolation procedures are necessary to prevent the spread of the infection to other patients.

Thromboembolus

Etiology/pathophysiology. Thromboembolus is a condition in which a blood vessel is occluded by an embolus carried in the bloodstream from the site of formation. The person suffering from pelvic and hip fractures is at high risk for this complication.

Clinical manifestations. The area supplied by an obstructed artery may tingle and become cold, numb, and cyanotic.

Assessment. Collection of *subjective data* includes careful investigation of the patient's complaints of pain in the lower extremities (especially the calf of the leg). A complaint of tenderness over the area is common.

Collection of *objective data* includes assessing for a positive Homan's sign, which is indicative of thromboembolus. Homan's sign is pain in the calf of the affected leg upon dorsiflexion of the foot. The affected area may be erythematous, warm to touch, and edematous. When anticoagulant therapy is ordered, the nurse will assess for signs of bleeding, such as petechiae, epistaxis, hematuria, hematemesis, and occult or gross blood in the stool.

Diagnostic tests. A complete history is taken and a physical examination is performed. In addition to checking Homan's sign, a prothrombin time and complete blood count are obtained.

Medical management. Treatment will include administration of anticoagulants, such as heparin or Coumadin. A surgical procedure known as *thrombectomy* (removal of a thrombus from a blood vessel) may be done.

Nursing interventions. Nursing intervention involves caring for the patient on activity restriction. Many times this involves bed rest with the foot of the bed elevated to aid venous return. The nurse should teach the patient to do active exercise, such as dorsiflexion (pointing backward) and plantar flexion (pointing forward) of the toes, several times each hour. This exercise is effective in stimulating circulation to the legs. Continuous hot, moist compresses are usually ordered. Antiembolic stockings are ordered while the patient is on bed rest and are maintained even after the patient is ambulatory. It is important that the nurse adhere to the activity ordered. Close monitoring of the patient's prothrombin time is necessary when he is receiving anticoagulants.

Delayed Complications

Delayed complications deal with fracture healing. *Delayed union* implies the fracture has not healed in the time frame expected. *Nonunion* is failure of the ends of the fractured bone to unite.

> NEVER MASSAGE A PATIENT'S LOWER EXTREMITIES
> Thromboembolus can be present without clinical symptoms.

NONSURGICAL INTERVENTIONS FOR MUSCULOSKELETAL DISORDERS

External Fixation Devices

External fixation devices are used to hold bone fragments in normal position. Casts, skeletal and skin traction, braces, and metal pins are examples of these devices.

Skeletal pin external fixation. One external fixation technique immobilizes fractures by the use of pins inserted through the bone and attached to a rigid external metal frame (Fig. 30-25). This technique is becoming more popular because it provides rigid support of comminuted open fractures, infected nonunions, and infected unstable joints. However, an advantage to having the fracture open to air is the visibility of the area and accessibility for wound care. The patient can use the muscles and joints above and below the fixation and experiences less discomfort.

This procedure is performed with the patient under general anesthesia. Patients need to be reassured that the pain after the insertion of the pins is minimal. Immediately after the procedure, the extremity is placed in bal-

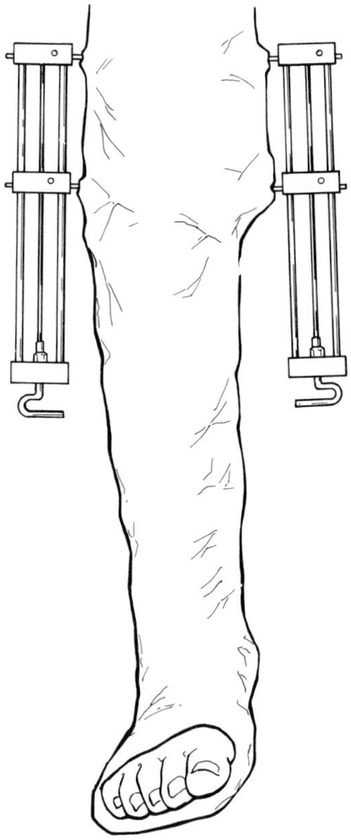

FIG. 30-25 Example of an external fixator, in this case a Charnley compression apparatus. Skeletal pins through bone above and below the area of fracture or repair attach to the external metal supports to maintain rigid fixation. This particular device is equipped with hand screws that allow the pins to be brought closer together, thus providing increased compression.

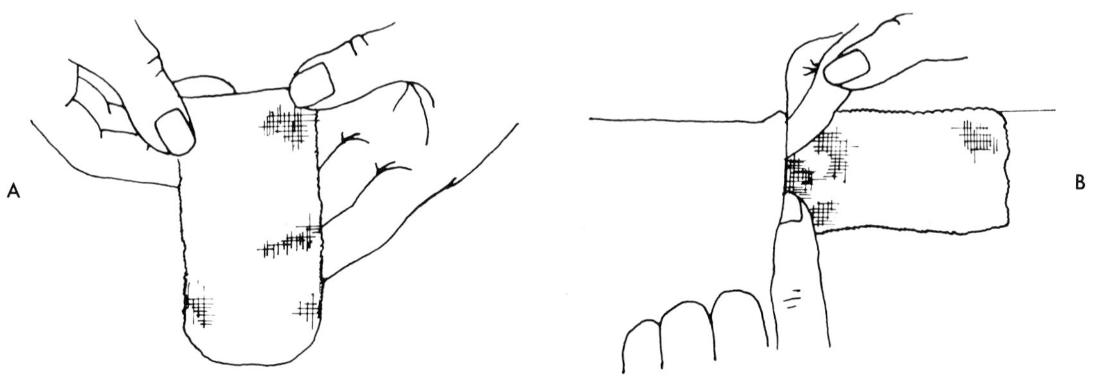

FIG. 30-26 Cast petaling. **A,** A petal is shaped from a strip of adhesive. **B,** The rounded edge of the petal is placed under the edge of the cast, and the opposite end is brought up over the edge of the cast.

anced suspension traction to help relieve the edema. Pins that are inserted through the bone are assessed at least q 8 hr with careful observation of signs of infection and loose pins. Removing dried exudate from around the pins is done 1 or 2 times daily with hydrogen peroxide or alcohol, using surgical asepsis. Patients are permitted to ambulate on crutches when soft tissue edema is relieved. They are permitted to shower when the wounds have healed but must avoid salt or chlorinated water to prevent fixator corrosion.

Casts. Casts are immobilization devices made up of layers of plaster of paris, fiberglass, or plastic roller bandages. The application is similar to that for an elastic bandage. Types of casts are indicative of the part of the body immobilized. Examples include (1) short arm cast—extends from below the elbow to the proximal palmar crease; (2) long leg cast—extends from the upper thigh to the base of the toes; (3) spica cast or body cast—covers the trunk of the patient and one or both extremities.

Casts are applied after the physician has properly aligned the bone through either external or internal fixation. Cast application is relatively painless except for the manipulation of the traumatized extremity. The casting procedure involves the application of a piece of Stockinette that covers the length of the extremity and area to be casted, followed by sheet wadding (pressed cotton that comes in rolled bandages), followed by the casting material. Most physicians will bring the Stockinette up and over the distal and proximal edge of the cast. It is important to assess these edges for rough pieces of casting that may irritate the skin. A nursing intervention to smooth out the rough edges is to "petal" the edges of the cast by placing pieces of adhesive tape (paper tape does not adhere as well as adhesive tape) cut in the shape of petals over the dried cast edges to provide a smooth surface (Fig. 30-26).

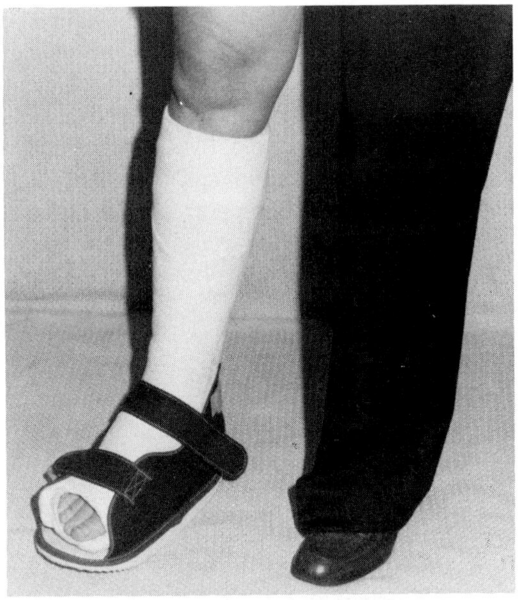

FIG. 30-27 Short leg walking cast with cast shoe.

Cast brace. The cast brace is an alternative appliance to the traditional leg cast. It provides support and stability of the plaster cast, with additional support and mobility provided by a hinged brace. The appliance is most effective for fractures of the shaft of the femur and permits early ambulation and weight bearing. It is used approximately 2 to 6 weeks after fracture reduction.

Cast bracing is based on the concept that limited weight bearing helps promote the formation of bone. A problem encountered frequently with cast bracing is edema around the knee. Patients are instructed to elevate the leg when sitting to promote venous return. A cast shoe or walking heel incorporated into a lower extremity cast will permit weight bearing without damaging the cast (Fig. 30-27).

Assessment. Nursing assessment will be similar regardless of what kind of casting material is used. A neurovascular assessment is done q 15 to 30 minutes for several hours after casting and every 4 hours the first few days. The skin at the cast edges is observed for erythema and irritation. It is important to note any odor or drainage coming from under the cast and document the findings. Both of these signs indicate infection. The nurse should assess the patient's ability to use crutches using a three-point gait to establish normal gait and rhythm and she should assess crutches for safety concerning proper fit and presence of large, rubber, suction tips on the ends.

Nursing interventions. Nursing intervention for the patient in a cast (Skill 30-1) includes patient education concerning the prevention of infection, irritation, neurovascular pressure, and misalignment of bone ends. A wet cast must be handled gently and supported with the flat of the hand or on pillows to avoid indentations that will cause pressure on the skin and lead to skin impairment. Turning the patient frequently will aid the drying process. If a cast dryer is used, the setting should be on warm and never hot (drying a plaster of paris cast too quickly from the outside may weaken the cast). Elevating the casted extremity will reduce edema (usually elevation is recommended for 24 to 48 hours). Patients using crutches should be instructed to support their weight on the hands; weight borne on the axillae can damage the brachial plexus nerves (crutch paralysis).

Cast syndrome can occur after the application of a spica (body) cast and involves acute obstruction of the duodenum. If symptoms of nausea occur, place the patient prone to relieve pressure symptoms and alert the charge nurse. Gastric decompression may be necessary, and if conventional measures fail, surgical intervention (duodenojejunostomy—making an opening into the small intestine) may be necessary.

Patient teaching. Patient teaching includes information about cleaning around the cast site with a mild soap and rinsing excessive soap so that it does not accumulate around the cast and impair the skin. A synthetic cast can be flushed with water if it becomes soiled. It must be dried afterwards to prevent skin impairment and maceration (softening of the skin). Drying a synthetic cast can be accomplished by blotting it with a towel and then using a blower hairdryer on cool or warm setting in a sweeping motion across the cast. Proper drying may take as long as 1 hour.

Patients often complain of pruritus (itching) of the skin that is covered by a cast (especially after having the cast for a few weeks). The nurse can recommend diversional activities when the pruritus begins in addition to having the patient gently rub the area below and above the cast to retard the desire to scratch. It is important to warn patients not to stick sharp objects underneath the cast to relieve the pruritus. This may cause impairment of the skin, and serious complications can occur.

SKILL 30-1 CARE OF THE PATIENT IN A CAST

1. Patient teaching
   a. Explain why the cast is being applied and how it will be applied
   b. Advise the patient that the plaster cast will feel warm as it dries
   c. Explain the extent of immobilization
   d. Explain care of the cast and expectations after discharge
   e. Instruct patient not to insert sharp objects (coat hangers or pencils) under the cast, because these may abrade the skin and lead to infection
2. Handling the new cast
   a. Support wet cast with the flat of the hands or on pillows to avoid indentations that will cause pressure on underlying skin
   b. Place cotton blankets or other absorbent material under the cast to aid drying
   c. Expose the cast to air as much as possible to aid drying
   d. Turn the patient frequently to aid drying
   e. Use a cast dryer or hair dryer on a warm, not hot, setting to circulate air over the cast
   f. Do not apply paint, varnish, or shellac to the cast; plaster is a porous material that allows air to circulate to the skin
3. Skin care
   a. Inspect skin at edges of cast and underlying cast for erythema or skin impairment; apply petal-shaped strips of adhesive tape or moleskin around rough edges of cast
   b. Remove plaster crumbs from skin with a washcloth moistened with warm water

SKILL 30-1

CARE OF THE PATIENT IN A CAST—cont'd

   c. Use creams and lotions sparingly as they may soften the skin and cause the cast to stick to the skin
   d. Apply waterproof material around perineal area to prevent soiling of and damage to cast and skin impairment
   e. Attend to patient's complaint of pain under the cast, particularly over bony prominences, because this may indicate pressure on the skin. If discomfort is not relieved by repositioning, report to physician. Cast pressure may need to be relieved by windowing or bivalving (cutting into halves)
4. Turning—turning to any position is generally permitted as long as the integrity of the cast is not compromised and the patient is comfortable
5. Toileting—for a long leg or hip spica cast
   a. Use a fracture pan with blanket roll or padding as support under the small of the back
   b. Elevate the head of the bed, if permitted, or place the bed in reverse Trendelenburg position
6. Abdominal discomfort—cast may be "windowed" (an opening cut into it) to provide relief of abdominal distention or a port for checking bladder distention
7. Mobilization
   a. Weight bearing is at the discretion of the physician, and the amount of weight bearing will be prescribed
   b. A cast shoe or a walking heel incorporated into a lower extremity cast will permit weight bearing without damaging the cast
8. Prevention of neurovascular problems
   a. Perform neurocirculatory checks every hour for at least 24 hours after cast application to detect difficulty from edema or pressure of cast on nerves or vessels. Notify physician of color changes, alterations in sensation, or motion unrelieved by position change. Cast may need to be bivalved (cut in two) to relieve pressure
   b. Elevate affected extremity on pillows until danger of edema is over (usually 24-48 hr)
   c. After mobilization of patient with lower extremity or upper extremity cast, avoid keeping extremity in dependent position for prolonged periods
   d. After lower extremity cast is removed, encourage patient to wear elastic stocking and elevate affected leg at rest until full mobility is regained

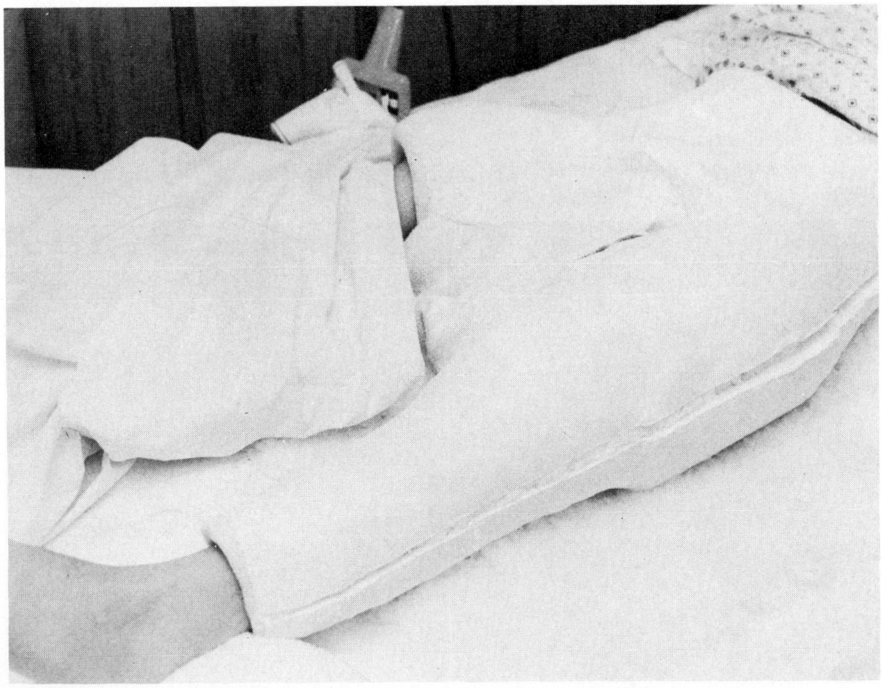

STEP 8a

Cast removal. Cast removal is done with an electric vibrating rather than cutting saw. Bivalving a cast may be done to relieve cast pressure. This involves splitting the cast down both sides and securing the cast pieces so that the extremity is supported. Patients should be reassured that the saw poses very little risk to injuring the skin beneath the cast, even though it is noisy and has the appearance of a cutting saw.

After the removal of a cast, the buildup of secretions and dead skin on the affected extremity can be removed by gently washing and applying lotion or cream to the area. This may take several days, but the patient should be cautioned against trying to remove the devitalized material rapidly for fear of causing skin impairment. Muscle atrophy is common, especially if the extremity has been casted for several weeks. Patients should be reassured that the muscle will regain strength and size with proper exercise through either physical therapy or home exercise programs.

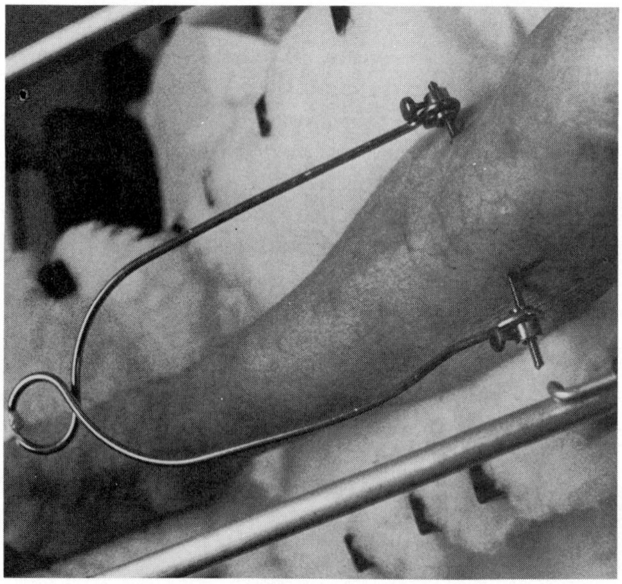

FIG. 30-28 Skeletal traction.

Traction. Traction is the process of putting an extremity, bone, or group of muscles under tension by means of weights and pulleys to (1) align and stabilize a fractured site by reducing the fractured part; (2) relieve pressure on nerves as in the case of herniated disk syndrome; (3) maintain correct positioning; (4) prevent deformities; and (5) relieve muscle spasms. The two general types of traction are *skeletal* (Fig. 30-28) and *skin* (Fig. 30-29). Traction applied for the purpose of stabilizing a fracture will be continuous traction and must not be disconnected unless ordered by the physician. It will be easier to make the patient's bed from top to bottom when bed rest is maintained. Cervical and pelvic traction are sometimes ordered as intermittent traction to be applied as ordered by the physician.

Skeletal traction. Skeletal traction is applied directly to a bone. Wires and surgical pins are inserted through the bone distal to the fracture site while the patient is under local or general anesthesia. The pin protrudes through the skin on both sides of the extremity, and weights are attached to a rope that is tied to a spreader bar for the purpose of traction. Skeletal traction can be used for fractures of the tibia, femur, humerus, and cervical spine.

Skin traction. Skin traction is accomplished by using weight that pulls on sponge rubber, moleskin, elastic bandage with adherent, or plastic materials attached to the skin below the site of the fracture, with the pull exerted on the limb. Buck's, Russell, and Bryant's are types of skin traction.

Buck's traction. Buck's traction (Fig. 30-29, *A*) is a form of traction used as a temporary measure to provide support and comfort to a fractured extremity until a more

A

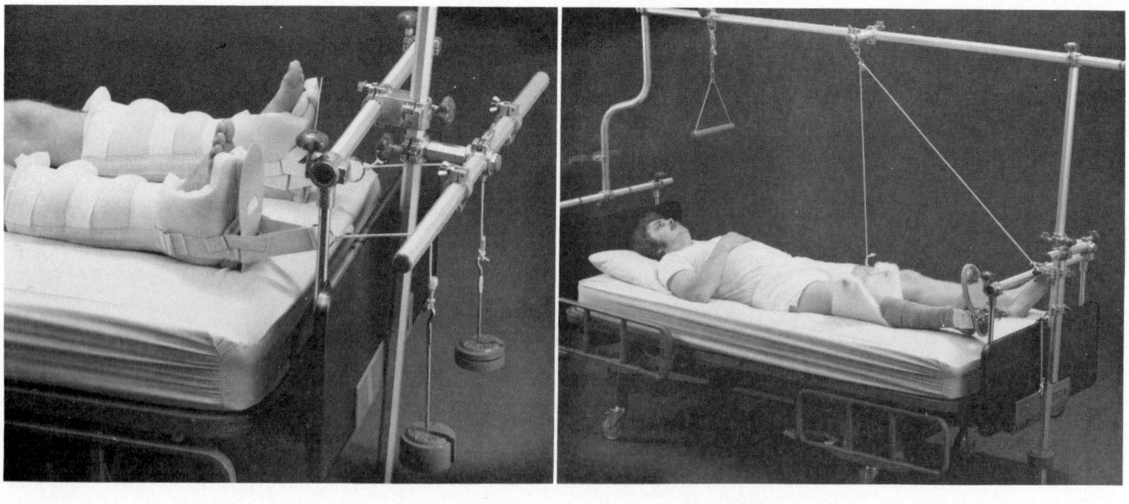

B

FIG. 30-29 Types of skin traction. **A,** Buck's traction. **B,** Russell's traction.

definite treatment is initiated. This traction is frequently used to maintain the reduction of a hip fracture before surgery. It can also be used to treat muscle spasms and minor fractures of the lower spine.

Russell traction. Russell traction (Fig. 30-29, *B*) is set up similar to Buck's traction. However, a knee sling is used to provide support of the affected leg. It allows more movement in bed and permits flexion of the knee joint. Russell traction is commonly used to treat hip and knee fractures.

Bryant's traction. Bryant's traction is used in pediatrics for small children with fractured femurs. Both legs are suspended at a 90-degree angle to the trunk of the body, and the weight of the lower body pulls the bone fragments of the fractured leg into alignment.

Nursing interventions. Nursing intervention of patients in traction includes the following measures:

- Maintain the patient's body in proper alignment. The force or pull on the extremities should be in alignment with the long axis of the bone.
- Ensure that weights hang freely from the bed and are *never* removed without a physician's order.
- Question patients as to their understanding of the purpose of the traction, and assess their ability to use a trapeze bar for self-movement. Elevate the foot of the bed to help prevent the patient from sliding down toward the foot of the bed.
- Observe the condition of the traction cords, making sure they are not weakened or frayed. All knots used on the rope or cord are to be square knots.
- Center the ropes on the traction pulley.
- Assess, document, and report neurovascular impairment.
- Ensure that weight used is the correct weight as ordered by the physician.
- Carefully observe the skin for signs of pressure decubitus ulcer formation. Use sheepskin heel protectors and bed pads to reduce impairment.
- If skeletal traction is used, assess the pin site for signs of infection. Cleanse the pin site q 8 hr with hydrogen peroxide or alcohol if ordered.
- Assess the dorsalis pedis pulses bilaterally for circulatory integrity of the lower extremities.
- Inspect for loss of sensation in the dorsal area of the foot with weakness and inversion of the foot (inside surface turned outward).

Orthopedic Devices

Frames can be used for orthopedic patients to assist with turning and positioning while maintaining proper alignment. The Balkan frame is a wooden or steel attachment to the regular hospital bed. The frame has adjustable pulleys and a trapeze bar attached to an overhead bar.

The Bradford frame is made of rectangular steel with two pieces of canvas stretched tightly and laced to the frame. A space is left in the buttocks area for toileting and hygiene.

The Stryker wedge turning frame and Foster bed are similar and assist in changing the patient's position from supine to prone. Patients may become apprehensive when turned on a frame for fear of falling, so thorough explanations and reassurances are helpful.

The CircOlectric bed is a vertical turning bed that can be operated electrically by one person and can be placed in a variety of positions. Side-to-side movement can be accomplished while maintaining proper positioning if traction is ordered.

RotoRest bed can rock a patient as much as 62 degrees, 17 times an hour. The electric-powered bed can promote decubiti healing, prevent venous thrombosis, and reduce kidney stone formation. Orthopedic traction can be attached to the bed, as well as a television set for diversional activity.

Splints, crutches, and braces are used to immobilize and assist with ambulation. There are numerous types of splints and braces, and it is important that the nurse understand the procedure for proper application.

Safety is the first concern when ambulatory devices are used. Crutch safety involves (1) proper measurement (weight must be on hands, not axillae, to avoid brachial plexus paralysis), and proper measurement involves a 2-inch width between the axillary fold and the arm piece on the crutches; (2) rubber tips on the ends of the crutches to prevent slippage; and (3) adequate muscle strength in the upper extremities to support the patient's weight. The nurse should encourage the patient to do push-ups to gain strength.

Types of crutch walking depend on the number of points making contact with the floor (Fig. 30-30). For example, three-point gait involves two crutch points plus one leg making contact with the floor (patient must have strong arms to support body weight). In addition to three-point gait, there are four-point gait (slower, but stable) and two-point gait (faster; requires balance). Another type of crutch walking is swing-to or swing-through gait. This involves the patient swinging the body up to or beyond the two points of the crutch tips. Most crutch walking is taught by a physical therapist. However, it is important for the nurse to monitor the patient's progress.

Cane walking is more popular with elderly patients and is used for balance and support. The patient is instructed to hold the cane in the opposite hand of the affected extremity and advance the cane at the same time the affected leg is advanced forward. An effective rubber tip on the point will help prevent slippage. Walkers are also used by the elderly and will assist the patient to maintain balance. Safety concerns are the same as for the cane.

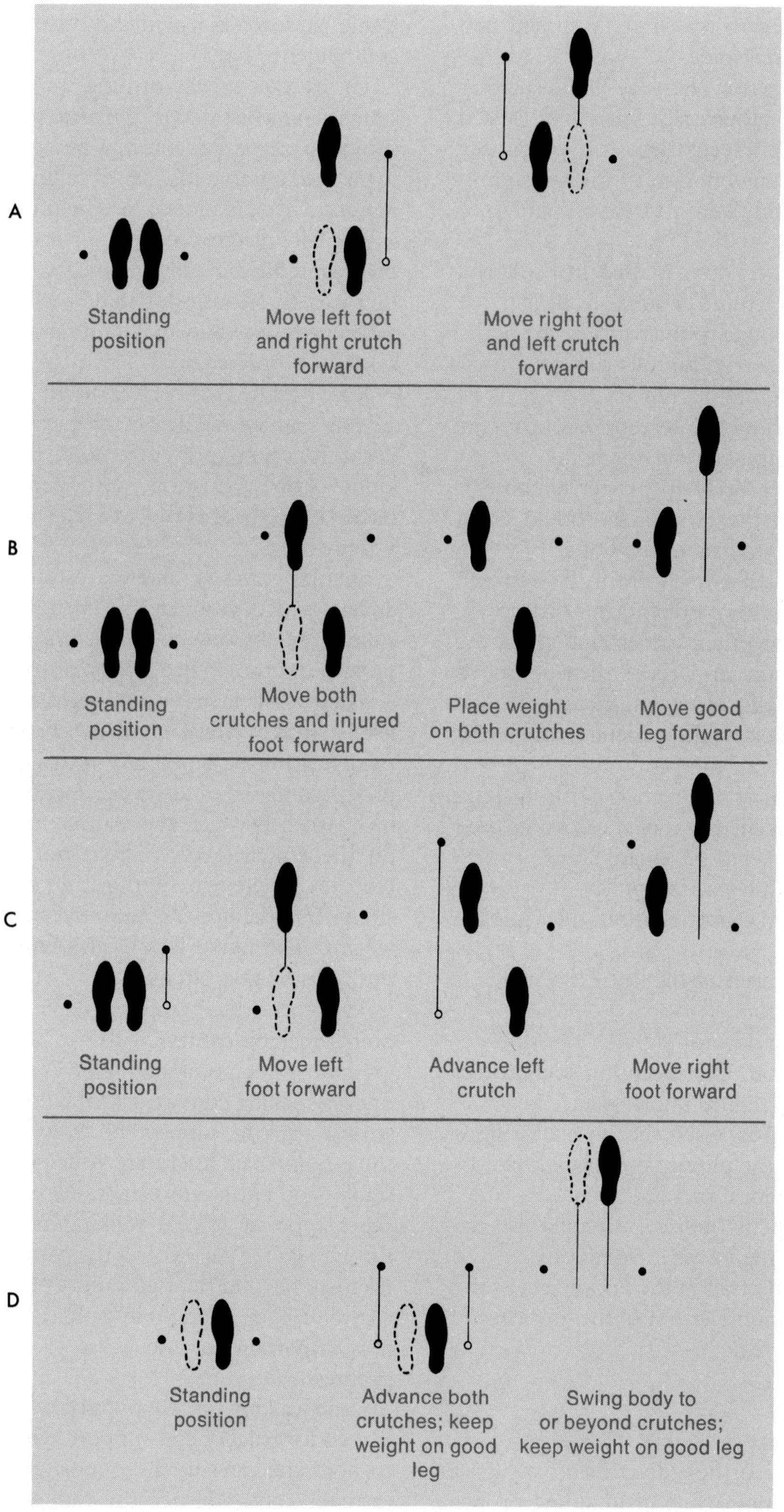

FIG. 30-30 Crutch walking. **A,** Two-point gait. **B,** Three-point gait. **C,** Four-point gait. **D,** Swing-through gait.

SURGICAL INTERVENTION FOR MUSCULOSKELETAL DISORDERS

Surgical procedures can prevent progressive deformities, relieve pain, improve function, and correct deformities resulting from rheumatoid arthritis, osteoarthritis, and other disorders. Tendon transplants can be done to replace damaged muscles. Patients with rheumatoid arthritis may need a **synovectomy** (excision of synovial membrane) to maintain joint function. An osteotomy (cutting into bone to correct bone or joint deformities) can help to improve function and relieve pain. **Arthrodesis** (surgical fusion of a joint) can be performed when severe joint destruction has occurred. **Arthroplasty** (plastic surgery) is often required on the elbow, hip, knee, or shoulder joint to restore or increase mobility.

Knee Arthroplasty

Replacement of the knee joint may be necessary to restore motion of the joint, relieve pain, or correct deformity. Fig. 30-31 shows the tibial and femoral components of a knee prosthesis. Nursing intervention of the patient undergoing total knee replacement is shown in Box 30-1.

Hip Arthroplasty

A hip arthroplasty is a commonly performed procedure when arthritis involves the head of the femur and acetabulum. A Vitallium cup is cemented into the arthritic acetabulum to receive the head of the femur. Total hip replacement is a recent development and was originally developed by Dr. John Charnley, a British orthopedic surgeon. There are several variations, but similar equipment is used. The Bechtol total hip system involves the use of a white plastic cup cemented in place to replace the damaged acetabulum. A stainless steel or Vitallium ball on a stem replaces the head of the femur, which is surgically removed. The stem is cemented into the femoral canal, and the new head fits precisely into the plastic acetabulum, providing friction-free movement in the joint. The cement used is a soft, surgical bone cement that hardens quickly and stabilizes the prosthesis to prevent future erosion of surrounding bone (Fig. 30-32).

Assessment. Collection of *subjective data* involves assessing the patient's level of orientation, since confusion can be present in the elderly resulting from a change in the environment (home to hospital setting). Complaints of pain and numbness, tingling, or paresthesia indicate neurovascular impairment.

Collection of *objective data* includes assessment of the patient's compliance with nursing interventions to promote circulation, prevent impairment of skin integrity, and prevent hypostatic pneumonia by such means as coughing, turning (to the unaffected side, additional pillows are used to keep the affected leg abducted), and deep breathing q 2 hr. Assessment of vital signs for evidence of excessive bleeding includes hypotension, tachycardia, and tachypnea. Decreased urinary output is indicative of hypovolemia. A careful assessment of the surgical wound for drainage is made at least q 4 hr. Hemovacs or other suction devices are placed in the wound during surgery to provide closed-wound suction. Assessing approximation of incision line and signs of inflammation (erythema, edema, fever, and pain) is necessary. Also included is assessing traction (if used) for correct amount of weight and proper alignment, main-

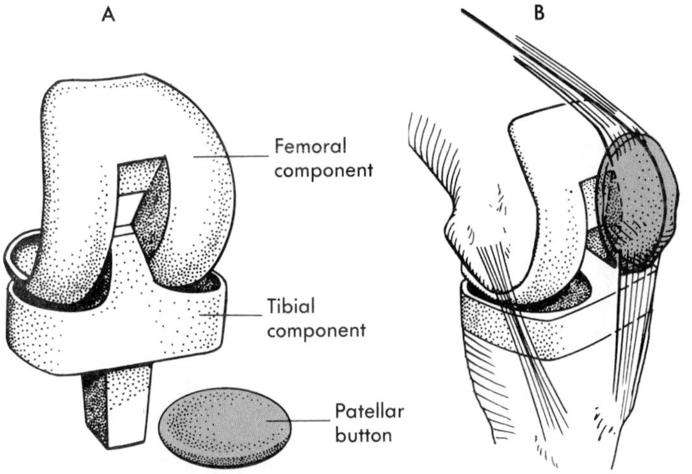

FIG. 30-31 **A,** Tibial and femoral components of total knee prosthesis. Patellar button, made of polyethylene, protects the posterior surface of the patella from friction against the femoral component when the knee is moved through flexion and extension. **B,** Total knee prosthesis in place.

BOX 30-1 NURSING INTERVENTION OF THE PATIENT UNDERGOING TOTAL KNEE REPLACEMENT

PREOPERATIVE INTERVENTIONS

Same as for any major surgery (see Chapter 26).

POSTOPERATIVE INTERVENTIONS

1. Positioning
   a. The operative leg is elevated on pillows to enhance venous return for the first 48 hours. Pillows are placed with caution not to flex the knee.
   b. The patient may be turned from side to back to side.
2. Wound care
   a. Care of drains as for total hip replacement.
   b. Patient is assessed for systemic evidence of loss of blood (hypotension, tachycardia) if bulky compression dressing is used as it may hold large quantities of drainage before drainage is visible.
   c. Bulky dressings are removed before the patient begins active flexion.
3. Activity
   a. Passive flexion in a continuous passive motion machine (CPM) within prescribed flexion-extension limits may be started in the recovery room. Patient's leg should remain in machine as much as tolerated (up to 22 hours per day) to facilitate even healing of tissue.
   b. Patient is encouraged to perform active dorsiplantar flexion of the ankles, quadriceps setting, and, after the drain is removed, straight leg raising exercises.
   c. Patient begins active flexion exercises three to four times a day about the fifth postoperative day.
   d. Light weight bearing with an assistive device may be started as early as the first postoperative day and increased as the patient tolerates.
   e. Sitting in a chair with the leg elevated may be started on the first postoperative day.
   f. Patient is encouraged to wear a resting knee extension splint (immobilizer) on the operated leg until able to demonstrate quadriceps control (independent straight leg raising).
4. Pain control
   a. Initial control of pain with narcotics, positioning; gradual decrease of medication to nonnarcotic analgesics as patient tolerates.
   b. Patient is encouraged to use ice to knee for 20-30 minutes before and after active flexion exercise.
5. Discharge instructions
   a. Patient must observe partial weight-bearing restriction and use ambulatory aid for approximately 2 months following discharge.
   b. Patient should continue active flexion and straight leg raising exercises at home.

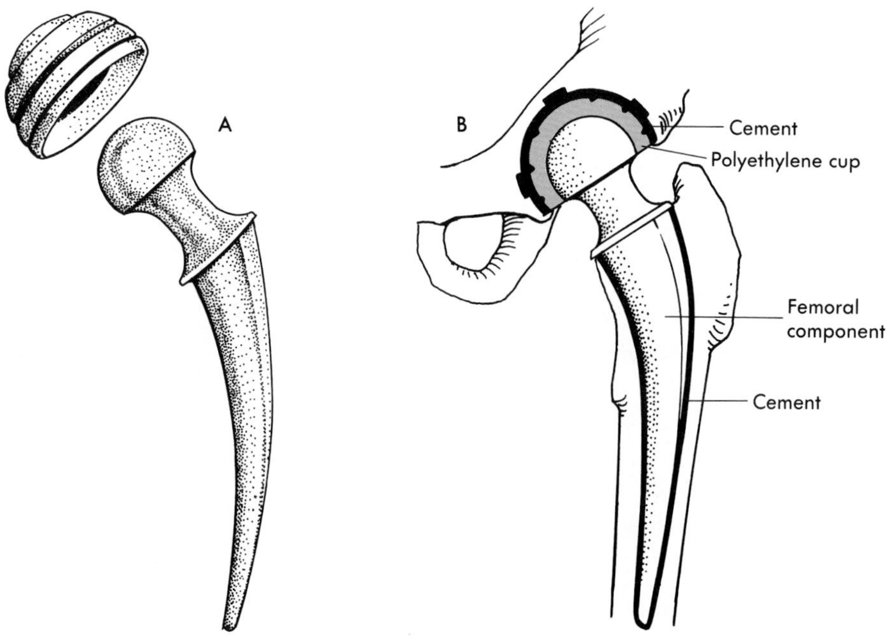

FIG. 30-32 **A,** Acetabular and femoral components of total hip prosthesis. **B,** Total hip prosthesis in place.

taining the affected leg in an abducted position, and carefully observing for any reaction to the cement, signs of phlebitis (edema, erythema, and pain), and urinary retention (indwelling catheters may be used for the first 48 hours postoperatively).

Nursing interventions. Nursing intervention is aimed at promoting healing and facilitating mobility. The patient is taught to do isometric exercises on the quadriceps and gluteal muscles of the affected extremity by keeping the toes pointed up, flexing the ankles, and flexing and extending the knee of the unaffected extremity. Careful documentation of the patient's intake and output is needed. Thigh-high antiembolism stockings are applied before or during surgery. A plan of weight bearing and physical therapy will be ordered by the physician and must be explained to the patient.

NURSING DIAGNOSES	NURSING INTERVENTIONS
Pain, related to preoperative arthritic pain necessitating surgery and postoperative hip incisional pain caused by bone and soft tissue trauma of surgery	Explain analgesic therapy, including medication, dose, and schedule. If patient is candidate for patient-controlled analgesic (PCA), explain concept and routine. Administer analgesics as ordered and per hospital policy/procedure. Respond quickly to pain complaints. Instruct patient to request analgesic before pain is severe. Encourage use of analgesics 30 to 45 min before therapy. Unrelieved pain hinders rehabilitation progress. Provide Eggcrate mattress. Change position (within hip precautions) q 2 hr. Document all responses to analgesics.
Potential for injury: hip dislocation, related to improper hip joint positioning	Frequently instruct/reinforce hip positions: ■ Abduction of legs. ■ Flexion of hip <90 degrees. ■ Neutral or external rotation of affected leg. Constantly practice precautions essential to prevent dislocation of new hip joint. Dislocation can occur easily, necessitating further hospitalization and possible surgery. Maintain abduction of legs and abduction splint (in and out of bed). Abduction splint between patient's legs prevents adduction of legs. Instruct patient on use of raised toilet seat (prevents hip flexion >90 degrees). Turn patient side to side in bed with abduction splint between legs (may turn on to affected hip unless contraindicated by physician).
Potential altered peripheral tissue perfusion, related to surgery intervention	Encourage patient to be out of bed as soon as ordered. Maintain total hip arthroplasty precautions and weight-bearing status. Encourage incentive spirometry q 1 hr while awake to increase lung expansion and prevent atelectasis, hypoxemia, pneumonia, and pulmonary embolism. Institute antiembolic devices as ordered (sequential compression device or TED hose). Antiembolic devices increase venous blood flow to heart and decrease risk of deep vein thrombosis and pulmonary embolism. Encourage leg exercises, including quadriceps sets and active ankle ROM.
Impaired physical mobility, related to surgical procedure and discomfort	Allow patient to dangle feet at bedside several minutes before getting patient out of bed. Reinforce physical therapist's instructions for exercises and ambulation techniques and devices. Maintain weight-bearing status on affected extremity as prescribed. Consistent instructions from interdisciplinary team members promote safe, secure rehabilitation environment. Keep abduction pillow between legs while turning in bed. May turn on to operative side unless otherwise specified. Use trapeze in bed to assist in mobility.

Patient teaching. Discharge instructions include the following:

1. Patient must use ambulatory aid and should avoid adduction.
2. Home environment should be altered to facilitate flexion restriction.
3. Patient must be aware that antibiotic prophylaxis may be necessary before invasive procedures such as dental work (e.g., tooth extraction or root canal procedure) to protect the prosthesis from bacterial infection.

Amputation

The amputation of a portion of or an entire extremity may be necessary because of malignant tumors, injuries, impaired circulation (caused by diabetes mellitus or arteriosclerosis), congenital deformities, and infections. Most amputations are elective surgery unless the amputation is necessary because of trauma. Advances in microsurgery techniques have made it possible for surgeons to reattach severed extremities. Therefore traumatic amputations can sometimes be reversed by replantation of the part if the severed limb is kept sterile and moist in a plastic bag filled with ice water. (The part should be protected from direct contact with ice, and dry ice should not be used.)

Amputation of long bones can result in postoperative anemia. A traumatic or surgical amputation of an extremity can cause serious blood loss. Malignant bone tumors can metastasize via the bloodstream to other body systems.

Preoperative assessment. Collection of *subjective data* includes questioning the patient to determine his understanding of the nature of the injury or disease process. Assessment of complaints of pain and symptoms of neurovascular impairment is made and documented. Assessment of the patient's level of orientation is important, since many amputations occur in the elderly population as a result of medical conditions that impair circulation.

Collection of *objective data* includes assessment of vital signs (temperature elevation, tachycardia, and hyperpnea indicate infection). Arterial blood flow is assessed by palpation of bilateral pedal pulses and Doppler pressure measurements. Assessment is done of wound drainage for color, amount, and presence of odor. Evaluation of upper body muscle strength and nutritional status is important.

Postoperative assessment. Collection of *subjective data* involves careful assessment of pain. Phantom pain (pain felt in the missing extremity as if it were still present) may occur and be frightening to the patient. Phantom pain occurs because the nerve tracks that register pain in the amputated area continue to send a message to the brain—this is normal.

Collection of *objective data* includes observing for signs of hemorrhage, such as hypotension, tachycardia, hyperpnea, pallor, decreased urinary output, restlessness, and progressive loss of consciousness. Monitoring suction drainage and documenting it is important as are assessing and protecting the remaining extremity. The nurse should observe for neurovascular impairment (done hourly in the immediate postoperative period) from tightly applied elastic wraps, dressings, or casts.

Diagnostic tests. A complete blood count is done to determine blood dyscrasias, such as anemia and bleeding tendencies, that would influence the surgical outcome and increase postoperative complications (such as hemorrhage, delayed wound healing, and disorientation). Laboratory studies, such as blood urea nitrogen (BUN), potassium levels, and routine urinalysis, are ordered. An electrocardiogram (ECG) is ordered to detect cardiac dysrhythmias that are often present in the elderly patient.

Medical management. When the amputation results from traumatic injury to an extremity, the physician's interventions will include measures to restore circulating blood volume, control pain, prevent infection in the wound, perform a plastic surgical repair at the amputation site to facilitate the use of a prosthesis, and maintain adequate urinary output.

If the amputation is an elective surgical procedure, the physician makes an assessment of the patient's physiological, psychological, and emotional status. If there is any infection present in the body (gangrene may occur in the presence of impaired circulation), treatment will include administration of antibiotics and every attempt will be made to control the infection before surgery is performed. The physician will discuss the possibility of the patient using a prosthesis. Much of the preoperative preparation will focus on the patient attaining a physical and emotional status conducive to wearing a prosthesis or achieving mobility through the use of a wheelchair or a gait enhancer, such as crutches or a walker.

Postoperative nursing interventions. Nursing intervention is aimed at prevention of deformities (contractures, especially in the joint above the amputation, or abduction deformities are common). Flexion hip contractures can be prevented postoperatively by raising the foot of the bed slightly to elevate the residual extremity (care should be taken not to flex the patient's hips by elevating the stump on a pillow), encouraging movement from side to side, and placing the patient in a prone position at least twice a day. This will stretch the flexor muscles. The nurse will be involved with teaching the patient how to strengthen remaining muscles to facilitate mobility and prevent muscle atrophy (push-ups from a prone position and sit-ups from a seated position). The application of elastic wraps to shrink and reshape the residual extremity into a cone is necessary to facilitate the proper fit and subsequent use of a prosthesis. A prosthesis may be fitted as early as 2 or 3 weeks postoperatively. Because many amputations are performed in persons between 60 and 70 years of age, the patient must be observed carefully for pulmonary complications (such as pulmonary embolus) and cardiovascular collapse. Suction equipment and oxygen should be at the bedside. Patient education concerning the phenomenon of phantom-limb sensation can help relieve patient fears if patients know it is a normal physiological response. The response may be one of pain or other sensations, such as burning, tingling, throbbing, or pruritus in the amputated extremity. These sensations can last for months or decades on a consistent or intermittent basis. It is recommended that patients gently rub the residual extremity for relief. Pain medication may be necessary.

The patient should be encouraged to ventilate his feelings over the loss of the extremity. The loss of an extremity results in a grieving process. The patient should be taught the importance of allowing the grieving process to occur.

For persistent, severe phantom pain, the following measures may be employed:

- Stump revision with reamputation at a higher level
- Local infiltration of the stump with procaine
- Mechanical percussion by striking the sensitive digital stump against a solid object—believed to shrink neuromas (small tumors that form in the scar tissue of the stump)
- Sympathetic nerve block

REFERENCES AND SUGGESTED READINGS

1. Aisenbrey J: Exercise in the prevention and management of osteoporosis, Phys Ther 67:1100, 1987.
2. Anagnostakos NP and Tortora GJ: Principles of anatomy and physiology, ed 5, New York, 1987, Harper & Row Publishers, Inc.
3. Berg E: Hemi-arthroplasty in femoral neck fractures, Orthop Nurs 8(3):62, 1989.
4. Caldwell E and Hegner BR: Geriatrics: a study of maturity, ed 4, New York, 1986, Delmar Publishers, Inc.
5. Cochran S: Action stat! Open fracture, Nurs '87 17 (5):33, 1987.
6. Cress M and Schultz E: Aging muscle: functional, morphologic, biochemical, and regenerative capacity, Geriatr Rehab 1:11, 1985.
7. Fong E, Ferris EB, and Skelly EG: Body structures and functions, ed 7, New York, 1989, Delmar Publishers, Inc.
8. Frontera W and Evans W: Exercise performance and endurance training in the elderly, Geriatr Rehab 2:17, 1986.
9. Gamron R: Taking the pressure out of compartment syndrome, Am J Nurs 8:1076, 1988.
10. Gose J: Continuous passive motion in the postoperative treatment of patients with total knee replacement, Phys Ther 67:39, 1987.
11. Henning L and Burrows S: Keeping up on arthritis meds, RN 2:32, 1986.
12. Hood G and Dincher J: Total patient care: foundations and practice, ed 7, St Louis, 1988, The CV Mosby Co.
13. Jensen TS and others: Immediate and long-term phantom limb pain in amputees: incidence, clinical characteristics, and relationship to preamputation limb pain, Pain 21:267, 1985.
14. Lederer J and others: Care planning pocket guide: a nursing diagnosis approach, ed 3, Reading, Mass, 1990, Addison-Wesley Publishing Co, Inc.
15. Liddel DR: An in-depth look at osteoporosis, Orthop Nurs 4(3): 23, 1985.
16. Long B and Phipps W: Medical-surgical nursing: a nursing process approach, ed 2, St Louis, 1989, The CV Mosby Co.
17. Marieb EN: Essentials of human anatomy and physiology, Reading, Mass, 1984, Addison-Wesley Publishing Co, Inc.
18. McFarland G: Nursing diagnosis and intervention: planning for patient care, St Louis, 1989, The CV Mosby Co.
19. Memmler RL and Wood DL: Structure and function of the human body, ed 4, Philadelphia, 1987, WB Saunders Co.
20. Mims B: Fat embolism syndrome: a variant of ARDS, Orthop Nurs 8(3):22, 1989.
21. Monroe D: Patient teaching for x-ray and other diagnostics, RN 9:50, 1989.
22. Morris L and others: Special care for skeletal traction, RN 2: 24, 1988.
23. Mosby's medical nursing & allied health dictionary, ed 3, St Louis, 1990, The CV Mosby Co.
24. Raab D and Smith E: Exercise and aging effects on bone, Geriatr Rehab 1:31, 1985.
25. Smithmather, ML: The secret to life in a spica, Am J Nurs 87:56, 1987.
26. Solomon EP and Phillips GA: Understanding human anatomy and physiology, Philadelphia, 1987, WB Saunders Co.
27. Stotts K: Action stat! Traumatic amputation, Nurs '88 18:50, 1988.
28. Thibodeau GA and Anthony CP: Structure and function of the body, ed 8, St Louis, 1988, Times Mirror/Mosby College Publishing.
29. Thomas DF: An ambulation assessment system you can count on, Nurs '86 16(11):58, 1986.
30. Tucker S and others: Patient care standards, ed 4, St Louis, 1988, The CV Mosby Co.
31. Unkle D and DeLong W: Abdominal trauma associated with pelvic fractures, Orthop Nurs 8(4):27, 1989.

CHAPTER CHALLENGE

KEY POINTS

- The skeletal system has five basic functions: support of the body, protection of internal organs, movement of the body, storage of minerals, and blood cell formation.
- Joints hold the bones together and allow movement and flexibility. Differences in the structure determine the amount of mobility.
- A long bone is composed of the epiphysis (end) and the diaphysis (shaft). The medullary cavity (interior of the diaphysis) contains yellow bone marrow. The epiphysis contains red bone marrow.
- The periosteum is a strong membrane that covers the bone and nourishes it.
- The skeleton is composed of two main divisions:
  1. The axial skeleton—containing the skull, vertebrae, and thorax.
  2. The appendicular skeleton—containing the upper and lower extremities.
- Some of the more freely movable joints are the ball and socket, hinge, pivot, and saddle.
- Bones are classified according to their shape and bone composition. They are long, short, flat, and irregular.
- The three types of muscle tissue are:
  1. Smooth (involuntary) muscles, usually in the internal organs.
  2. Skeletal (voluntary) muscles, attached to the bones and allow movement.
  3. Cardiac (involuntary) seen only in the heart and responsible for the contraction of the chambers of the heart.
- Muscle cells are governed by the "all or none" law, which states that when a muscle cell is adequately stimulated, it will contract; otherwise there is no response.
- Muscle tissue possesses four principal characteristics:
  1. Excitability—capacity to respond to a stimulus.
  2. Contractility—ability to shorten and become thicker.
  3. Extensibility—ability to be stretched.
  4. Elasticity—ability to return to normal shape.
- The muscle tissue keeps a temporary energy store called *adenosine triphosphate (ATP)*, which is released chemically in times of need.
- Most muscles extend over a joint and attach at the origin (an immovable bone) and at the insertion (a bone that moves readily).
- Tendons attach muscles to bone, whereas ligaments attach bones to bones; both are composed of fibrous connective tissue.
- An erythrocyte sedimentation rate (ESR) is the most objective laboratory test for determining the severity of rheumatoid arthritis.
- External fixation devices (such as casts, braces, metal pins, and skeletal and skin traction) are used to hold bone fragments in normal position.
- Regardless of whether the casting material is plaster of paris or a synthetic material, proper drying, cleansing, handling, and assessing are required to prevent patient complications.
- The nurse caring for a patient in traction is responsible for knowing (1) the purpose of the traction (traction applied for fractures must be continuous); (2) the equipment needed and appropriate safety measures; (3) the amount of weight ordered; and (4) the patient's knowledge regarding the traction.
- Crutches, canes, and walkers are used as gait enhancers for patients with altered mobility.
- Crutch walking involving the three-point gait is most commonly used for patients wearing leg casts.
- Osteogenic sarcoma is a common primary malignant tumor seen in young people; it can metastasize to the lungs.
- A significant postoperative nursing intervention for a patient with an amputation is proper care of the stump to facilitate the use of a prosthetic device.
- Rheumatoid arthritis affects a young population (ages 30 to 55) with crippling changes in the synovial membrane of the joints.
- Salicylates and nonsteroidal antiinflammatory agents (NSAIAs) are used to treat rheumatoid arthritis and osteoarthritis.
- Osteoarthritis is a degenerative joint disease (DJD) that affects the population over 40 years of age and causes articular cartilage degeneration.
- Arthroplasty procedures (such as hip and knee arthroplasty) are commonly performed on patients suffering from severe arthritis.
- Porous and brittle bones caused by a lack of calcium is one of the physiological changes noted in osteoporosis.

CHAPTER CHALLENGE—cont'd

KEY POINTS (cont'd)

- Nursing intervention specific to the care of a patient suffering from a fractured hip involves maintaining abduction of the affected leg.
- Fractured hip fixation devices, such as hip prosthetic implant, plate and screw fixation, and telescoping nail fixation, require some degree of non–weight bearing for 6 weeks to 3 months.
- Compartment syndrome, shock, fat embolism, gas gangrene, thromboembolus, and osteomyelitis are complications resulting from a fractured bone.
- Herniated nucleus pulposus is seen most often in the cervical and lumbar spinal region and can be treated surgically (laminectomy and spinal fusion) or medically (medication, traction, and physical therapy).

STUDY QUESTIONS

1. The end of a long bone is called:
   a. Medullary cavity
   b. Diaphysis
   c. Epiphysis
   d. Olecranon process
2. The heaviest and strongest bone in the body is the:
   a. Tibia
   b. Femur
   c. Patella
3. What type of muscle tissue is voluntary:
   a. Cardiac
   b. Smooth
   c. Internal
   d. Skeletal
4. The largest tendon in the body is the:
   a. Achilles
   b. Metacarpal
   c. Prime mover
   d. Trapezius
5. What is the anatomical name for the "swimmer's muscle":
   a. Latissimus dorsi
   b. Patella
   c. Deltoid
   d. Hamstring
6. What is the name of the muscle in the upper arm that is often used for intramuscular injections:
   a. Biceps
   b. Deltoid
   c. Patella
   d. Gluteus maximus
7. Red blood cells are manufactured in the:
   a. Epiphysis
   b. Diaphysis
   c. Periosteum
   d. Tendons
8. An example of a ball and socket joint is:
   a. Knee
   b. Hip
   c. Wrist
   d. Ankle
9. Another name for the breast bone is the:
   a. Tibia
   b. Zygomaticus
   c. Mandible
   d. Sternum
10. Mrs. Smith is 24 years old and has been admitted to the medical unit for complaints of malaise, pain, edema, tenderness in her joints, loss of appetite, and muscle weakness (especially grip strength). Based on the symptoms, the diagnosis most suspected would be:
    a. Osteoarthritis
    b. Rheumatoid arthritis
    c. Gouty arthritis
    d. Spondylitis
11. Mr. Jones is a 75-year-old retired construction worker seen in the clinic. He has been seeing the physician for complaints of osteoarthritis. Today he is discussing concerns over his condition and asks what has caused osteoarthritis. An appropriate response would be:
    a. You have osteoarthritis because of the difficult construction work you did for so many years.
    b. Everybody your age has arthritis; you are fortunate you are still able to walk.
    c. The cause of osteoarthritis is unknown. However, almost all persons past 40 years of age have some changes in their joints.
    d. You probably did not exercise as much as you should have, and you should start vigorous exercising now to prevent further complications.
12. The most common type of fracture treated in the hospital is:
    a. Hip
    b. Greenstick
    c. Spiral
    d. Subluxation

STUDY QUESTIONS (cont'd)

13. Mr. Spray has recently been diagnosed as having gouty arthritis. The medication that is most effective for this type of arthritis is:
    a. Enteric-coated aspirin
    b. Colchicine
    c. Keflin
    d. Motrin
14. Mrs. Benedict is a 72-year-old widow who has fallen off a small step ladder. She is admitted to the hospital with complaints of pain in her left leg. She stated she heard a "snap" after falling. Her left leg is shortened with external rotation. The nurse's assessment reveals edema in the upper left thigh. The patient's age and symptoms suggest she suffered a:
    a. Fractured pelvis
    b. Fractured spine
    c. Fractured hip
    d. Fractured femur
15. The surgical intervention for a fractured hip includes ALL of the following EXCEPT:
    a. Hip prosthetic implant
    c. Stable plate and screw fixation
    c. Telescoping nail fixation
    d. Crutchfield tong skeletal fixation
16. An appropriate nursing intervention for a hip fracture patient is:
    a. Maintain proper alignment and abduction of the affected hip
    b. Ambulate as soon as the patient's pain subsides
    c. Elevate both legs to prevent edema of the lower extremities
    d. Explain the dynamics of phantom pain
17. Heidi Michaels is 23 years old and suffers from a traumatic injury to her left lower leg that involves a compound fracture of the tibia. A serious complication seen approximately 48 hours after long bone fracture is:
    a. Thrombopblebitis
    b. Fat embolism
    c. Osteomyelitis
    d. Hemorrhage
18. A common complication after compartment syndrome is:
    a. Osteomyelitis
    b. Thromboembolus
    c. Volkmann's contracture
    d. Fat embolism

STUDY QUESTIONS (cont'd)

19. Mr. Wallace was injured in a car accident and is admitted to the orthopedic unit with a diagnosis of whiplash injury to the cervical spine. Nursing assessment includes the following:
    a. Complaints of headache
    b. Limited mobility of head and neck
    c. Pain radiating from neck into jaws and facial area
    d. All of the above
20. You are assigned to care for Mrs. Chris, who has a newly applied cast to her right arm. The following objective data are significant of impaired circulation:
    a. Complaints of pain and tingling
    b. Pallor, pulselessness, and puffiness
    c. Warm and pink fingers on the right hand
    d. Hypertenstion, tachycardia, and tachypnea
21. An appropriate nursing intervention for a patient in skeletal traction is:
    a. Prevent callus formation at fracture site
    b. Prevent muscle atrophy of affected extremity
    c. Encourage ambulation
    d. Cleanse pin sites with hydrogen peroxide, and observe for signs of infection
22. Mr. West has recently undergone an amputation of his left foot. He often complains of pain in his left foot. An appropriate response to this complaint would be:
    a. Your foot has been surgically removed. Therefore it is not possible to have pain in this area!
    b. You are most likely experiencing phantom pain. This can occur and will most likely disappear in a short time. While you are experiencing the symptoms, medication may be necessary.
    c. You will need to talk with your physician about this.
    d. I will elevate your stump and document your complaint.
23. Uric acid crystal formations seen in patients with gouty arthritis and found around the rim of the ear are called:
    a. Heberden's nodes
    b. Valgus deformity
    c. Tophi
    d. None of the above
24. The surgical intervention for herniated nucleus pulposus is:
    a. Neufeld nail and screws
    b. Austin Moore prosthesis
    c. Buck's extension
    d. Laminectomy

31

Care of the Patient with a Gastrointestinal or Accessory Organ Disorder

M. LYNNE ACHESON

LEARNING OBJECTIVES

After reading this chapter, the student should be able to do the following:

- Define the key terms.
- Identify the parts of the digestive system.
- Discuss the function of each digestive and accessory organ.
- Describe the process of digestion of fats, carbohydrates, and protein.
- Discuss nursing interventions for six diagnostic examinations for patients with disorders of the gastrointestinal tract.
- List the medication therapy for the patient with a peptic ulcer.
- List five signs and symptoms of gastrointestinal bleeding.
- Differentiate between ulcerative colitis and Crohn's disease.
- Identify nursing interventions for preoperative and postoperative care of the patient with gastric resection.
- Identify five nursing interventions for the patient with a colostomy.
- State the purpose of nasogastric suctioning.
- Discuss the nursing interventions of a patient with a cholecystectomy.
- List the subjective and objective data for the patient with viral hepatitis.
- State the signs and symptoms caused by the liver's inability to metabolize bilirubin.
- Discuss specific teaching content for the patient with cirrhosis of the liver.
- Describe the medical management of the patient with acute pancreatitis.

RELATED TOPICS OF INTEREST

- Signs, symptoms, and physical assessment (Chapter 13)
- Specimen collection (Chapter 21)
- Basic nutrition (Chapter 22)
- Diet therapy (Chapter 23)
- The surgical patient (Chapter 26)
- Care of the patient with cancer (Chapter 41)

KEY TERMS

Define the following:

- achalasia
- achlorhydria
- adenosine triphosphate (ATP)
- alimentary canal
- amino acid
- anabolism
- anastomosis
- ascites
- bolus
- cachexia
- carcinoembryonic antigen (CEA)
- catabolism
- chyme
- deciduous
- dehiscence
- dentin
- digestion, mechanical and chemical
- dysphagia
- enamel
- evisceration
- exacerbation
- flatulence
- gingivae
- hematemesis
- impaction
- intussusception
- jaundice
- leukoplakia
- lumen
- mastication
- morbidity
- melena
- mesentery
- occlusion
- occult blood
- parasite
- parenchyma
- pathognomonic
- pepsin
- peristalsis
- pruritus
- pyrosis
- regurgitation
- remission
- rugae
- steatorrhea
- stoma
- tenesmus
- villi
- viscus
- volvulus

ANATOMY AND PHYSIOLOGY

Digestive System

Although it is understood that food is necessary for existence, not everyone understands (1) what happens to food once it is chewed and swallowed, (2) how food is prepared for its trip to each individual cell, and (3) the many changes that food undergoes, both chemically and physically. This chapter will discuss these changes and their impact on the body.

The digestive tract, or **alimentary canal,** is approximately 30 feet long. During **peristalsis** (wavelike, rhythmic contractions) the tract shortens to approximately 15 feet. The tract begins at the mouth and continues through the body trunk to exit at the anus. It consists of the mouth, pharynx, esophagus, stomach, small intestine, large intestine, and anus (Fig. 31-1).

The alimentary tract is composed of four layers of specialized tissue. They are as follows:

1. Mucosa (mucous membrane): innermost layer, which secretes mucus
2. Submucosa: layer of connective tissue rich in blood vessels and nerves, which plays a regulatory role
3. Smooth muscle layer: circular and longitudinal layer, which aids in peristalsis
4. Fibrous connective tissue with a thin outer serous membrane

Accessory organs aid in the digestive process but are not considered part of the digestive tract. They release chemicals into the system through a series of ducts. The liver, gallbladder, and pancreas are considered accessory organs. These will be discussed in detail later in the chapter.

Organs of the digestive tract (Table 31-1)

Mouth. The mouth (buccal cavity) marks the entrance to the digestive system. The roof of the mouth is composed of the hard and soft palates. The hard palate is

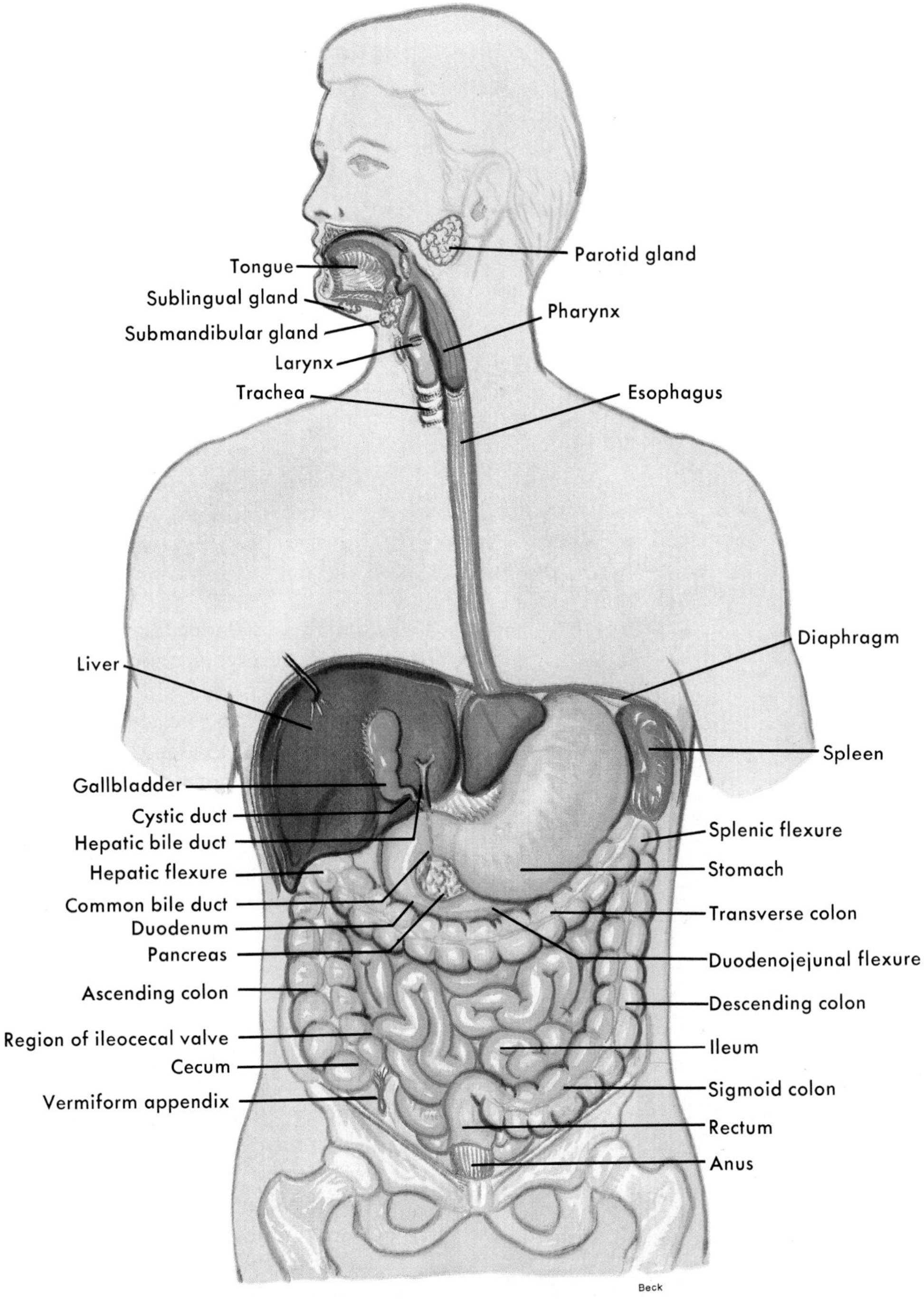

FIG. 31-1 Location of digestive organs.

formed by bony structures; the soft palate is composed of muscle and covered by mucous membrane. The soft palate is posterior to the hard palate and contains muscle, blood vessels, nerves, and mucous glands. The uvula, a small tag of tissue, extends from the middle of the posterior edge of the soft palate. It protects the entrance to the nasal cavity upon swallowing. The lateral walls of the mouth are formed by the cheeks.

The floor of the mouth contains a muscular appendage, the tongue. The anterior portion of the tongue is attached to the floor of the mouth by the frenulum, a fold of mucous membrane. The tongue is involved in chewing, swallowing, and the formation of speech. Tiny elevations, papillae, contain the taste buds. They differentiate between bitter, sweet, sour, and salty sensations.

Digestion begins in the mouth. Here the teeth mechanically shred and grind the food and the enzymes begin the chemical breakdown of carbohydrates. In addition, the oral cavity, the tongue, and the teeth play a role in speech production.

Table 31-1 Organs of the Digestive System

Main Organs	Accessory Organs
Mouth	Teeth and tongue
Pharynx (throat)	Salivary glands
Esophagus (foodpipe)	Parotid
Stomach	Submandibular
Small intestine	Sublingual
Duodenum	Liver
Jejunum	Gallbladder
Ileum	Pancreas
Large intestine	Vermiform appendix
Cecum	
Colon	
Ascending colon	
Transverse colon	
Descending colon	
Sigmoid colon	
Rectum	
Anal canal	

Teeth. Everyone has two sets of teeth during his lifetime. The first set (**deciduous,** baby teeth) begins to erupt at 6 months of age; the deciduous teeth continue to appear until 2 years of age, when a total of 20 teeth are in place. These remain until the age of 6 years. By this time the jawbone has grown sufficiently to accommodate the larger, permanent teeth that replace the deciduous teeth.

The permanent teeth are structured to last a lifetime. Generally, by 12 years of age all the deciduous teeth have been replaced by permanent teeth. By adulthood, permanent teeth will number 32. Each tooth is designed to carry out a specific task. Immediately to the center of the mouth lie the incisors, which are structured for biting and cutting. Posterior to the incisors are the canines, pointed teeth used for tearing and shredding food. The molars are to the rear of the jaw (Fig. 31-2). These teeth have four cusps (points) and are used for **mastication** (to crush and grind food). The last set of molars to erupt,

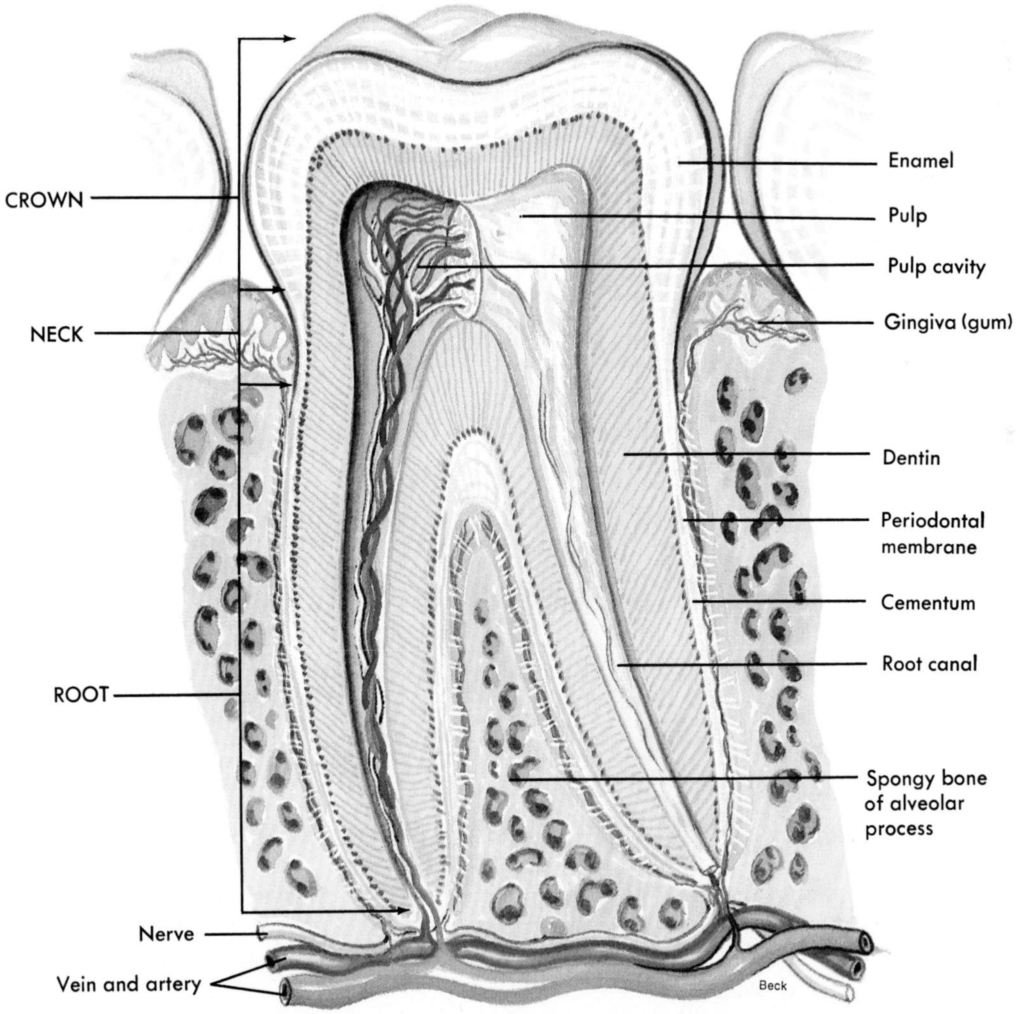

FIG. 31-2 A molar tooth sectioned to show its bony socket and details of its three main parts: crown, neck, and root. Enamel (over the crown) and cementum (over the neck and root) surround the dentin layer. The pulp contains nerves and blood vessels.

one superior and one inferior bilaterally, is referred to as *wisdom teeth*. They usually do not erupt until age 18. Often the jaw will not accommodate the extra molars and they remain imbedded in the jawbone. This results in a condition called **impaction,** and the wisdom teeth must be surgically removed.

Tooth construction. Each tooth develops in a socket (alveolus) deep in the jaw, which is really an extension of the mandible and maxilla. The **gingivae** (gums) cover the area and extend partially into the socket. The portion of the tooth above the gum line is the crown; the portion below the gum line is the root. The neck of the tooth is the junction between the crown and the root.

The centermost part of the tooth is the pulp cavity; it contains the blood vessels and nerves. Surrounding the pulp is the **dentin,** a calcified tissue that gives shape and structure to the tooth. The outer covering of the tooth is the **enamel,** the strongest material in the body. It protects the inner structures of the tooth from wearing away and from exposure to the many acids in foods.

Salivary glands. There are three pairs of salivary glands (Fig. 31-3). They secrete a fluid called *saliva,* which is approximately 99% water with enzymes and mucus. The largest pair, the parotid glands, lies just anterior to the ear near the jawline. These are the glands that become edematous and hurt with epidemic parotitis (mumps). Their ducts (Stensen's ducts) open into the oral cavity just superior to the upper second molars. The second set, the submandibular glands, is found inferior to the tongue in the posterior part of the mouth. Their ducts (Wharton's ducts) are found posterior to the lower central incisors bilateral to the frenulum. The third set of glands, the sublingual glands, lies immediately anterior to the submandibular glands. Their ducts open onto the floor of the mouth directly inferior to the tongue.

Normally these glands secrete enough fluid (saliva) to keep the mucous membrane of the mouth moist. Once food enters the mouth, the secretion increases to lubricate, dissolve, and begin the chemical process of digestion. The salivary glands secrete about 1000 to 1500 ml daily. The major enzyme is salivary amylase (ptyalin), which is responsible for the initiation of carbohydrate metabolism. Another enzyme, lysozyme, destroys bacteria, which protects the mucous membrane from infections and protects the teeth from decay. After food has been ingested, the salivary glands continue to secrete saliva, which cleanses the mouth.

Esophagus. The esophagus is a muscular, collapsible tube, which is approximately 10 inches long. It articulates the laryngopharynx with the opening to the stomach. It passes through the diaphragm via an opening called the *esophageal hiatus* (a weakness in this area results in a condition called *hiatal hernia*). The esophagus is a passageway for the **bolus** (food broken down and mixed with saliva) to pass to the stomach. No digestion takes place here. Peristalsis moves the bolus through the tube in approximately 5 to 6 seconds.

Stomach. The stomach is located in the left upper quadrant of the abdomen, directly inferior to the diaphragm (Fig. 31-4). When the stomach is empty, the inner lining

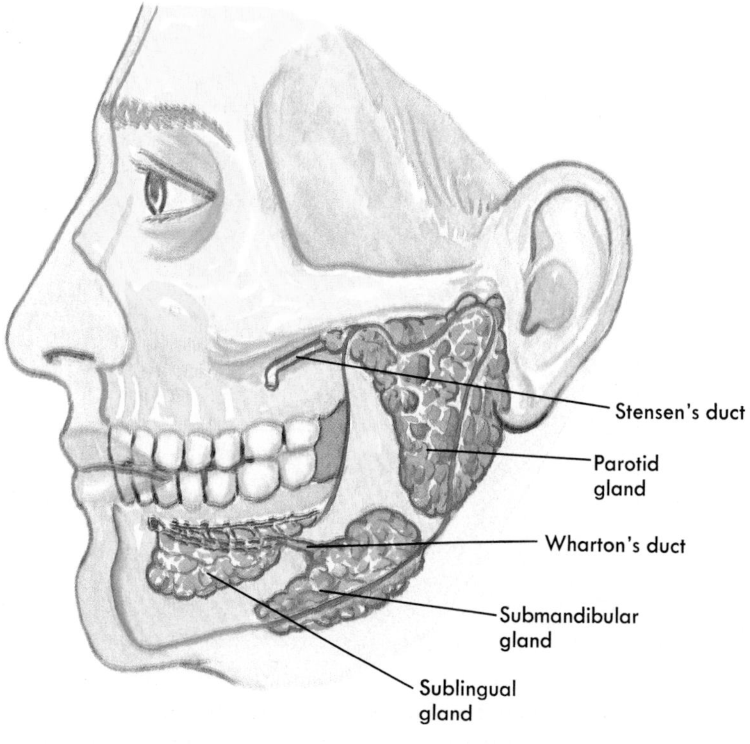

FIG. 31-3 The salivary glands.

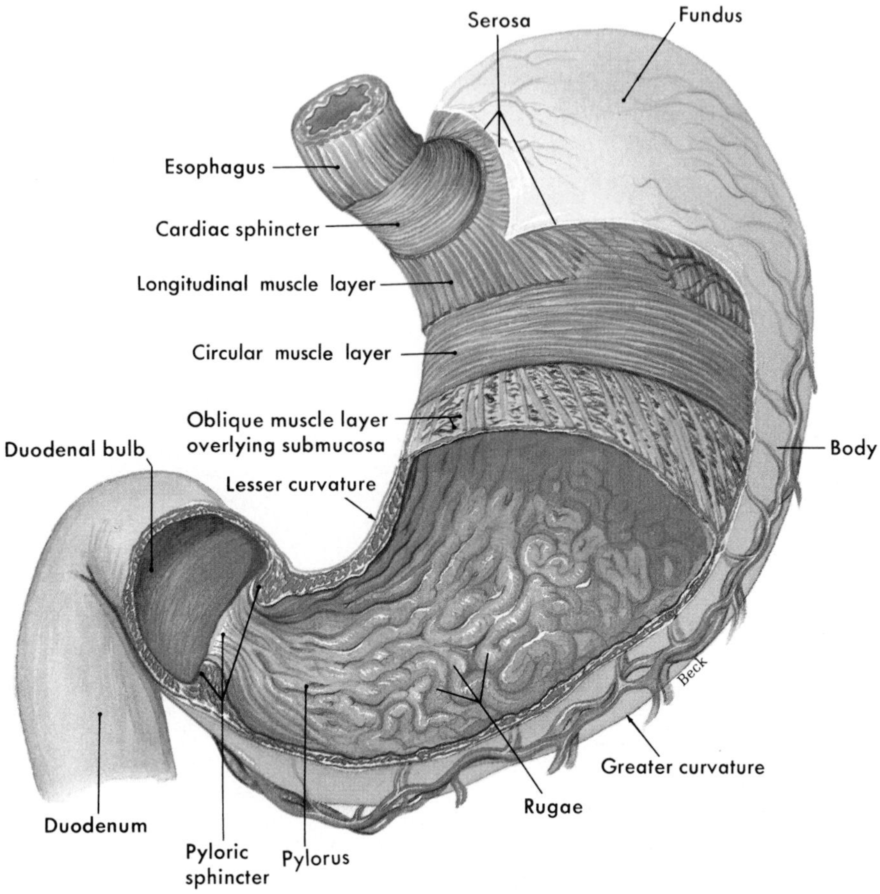

FIG. 31-4 Stomach. Cutaway section shows muscle layers and interior mucosa thrown into folds called *rugae*.

collapses into folds called **rugae.** When the stomach is filled, it stretches to the size of a football and holds approximately 1 liter. It receives its blood supply from the celiac artery. The stomach is divided into three major sections: (1) fundus—superior section, (2) body—middle section, and (3) pyloric portion—inferior section. The outer angle of the stomach is called the *greater curvature,* and the inner angle is called the *lesser curvature.* The entrance to the stomach is the *cardiac sphincter;* the exit is the *pyloric sphincter.*

As the food leaves the esophagus, it enters through the relaxed cardiac sphincter. The sphincter then contracts, preventing esophageal reflux (splashing, or return flow), which can be irritating. This condition is sometimes referred to as *heartburn.*

Once the bolus has entered the stomach, the muscular layers of the stomach churn and contract to mix and compress the contents with the gastric juices and water. The gastric juices are a group of secretions that are released by the gastric glands. Digestion of protein begins in the stomach. Hydrochloric acid softens the connective tissue in meat, kills bacteria, and activates **pepsin,** an enzyme that digests protein. Mucin is released to protect the stomach lining. Intrinsic factor is produced to allow absorption of vitamin B_{12}. After the stomach has completed its work, the food has been broken down into a semiliquid substance called **chyme.** The chyme is then sent through the pyloric sphincter to the small intestine for the next phase of digestion.

Small intestine (Fig. 31-5). The small intestine is a 20-foot-long tube; it is 1 inch in diameter. It starts at the pyloric valve and ends at the ileocecal valve. It is divided into three major sections: duodenum, jejunum, and ileum. The inner mucous membrane lining contains the intestinal glands, which secrete the intestinal juices (enzymes). Most of digestion is accomplished here—as much as 90%. The intestinal juices finish the metabolism of carbohydrates and proteins. Bile and pancreatic juices enter the duodenum. The bile from the liver breaks fat molecules into smaller droplets, which enables the digestive juices to complete their process. Pancreatic juices finish the metabolism of the protein, fats, and carbohydrates.

The inner surface of the small intestine falls into numerous folds called *plicae.* These folds contain millions of tiny, fingerlike projections called **villi.** They are responsible for the absorption of the products of digestion into the bloodstream. They increase the absorption area

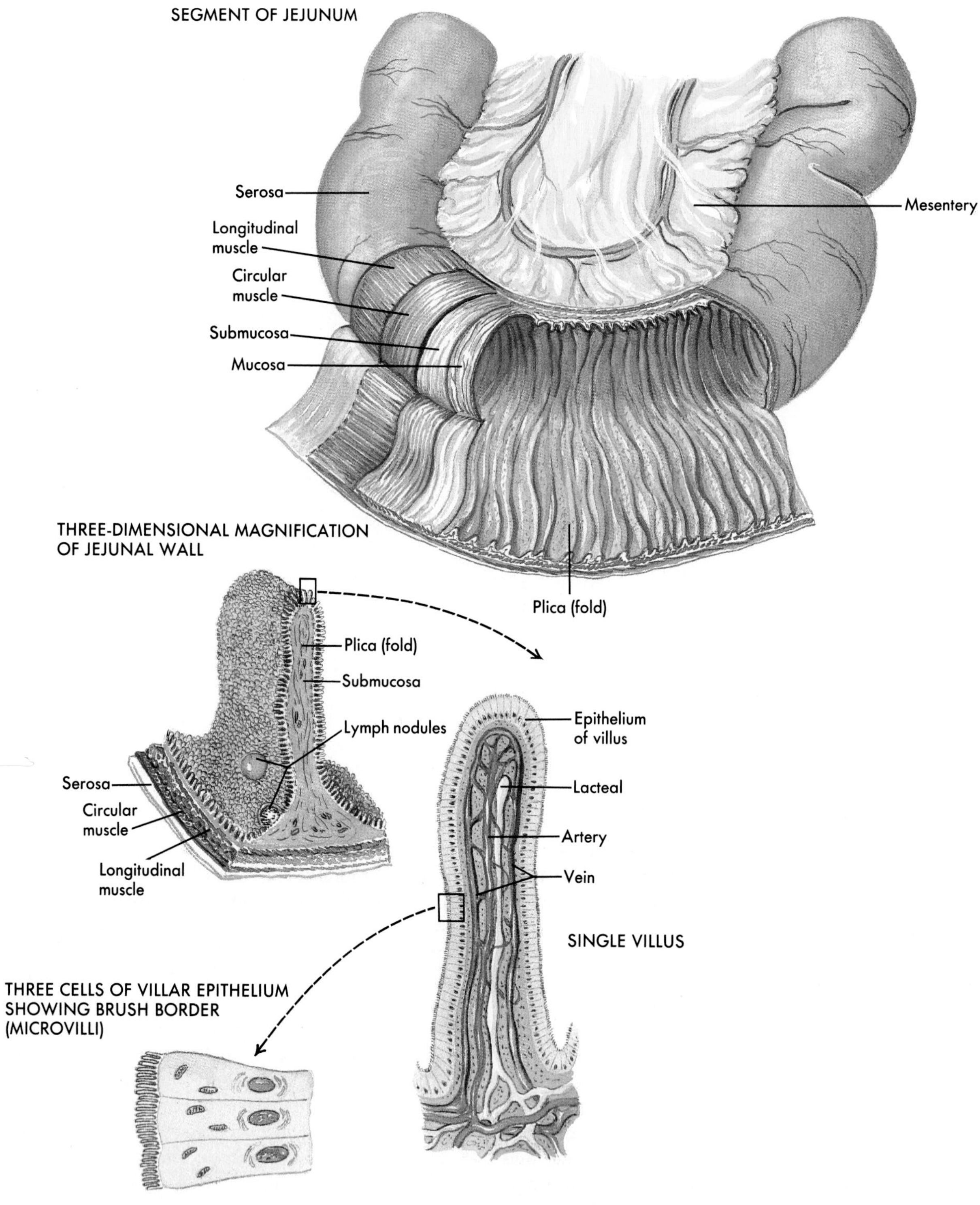

FIG. 31-5 The small intestine. Note that the folds of mucosa are covered with villi and that each villus is covered with epithelium, which increases the surface area for absorption of food.

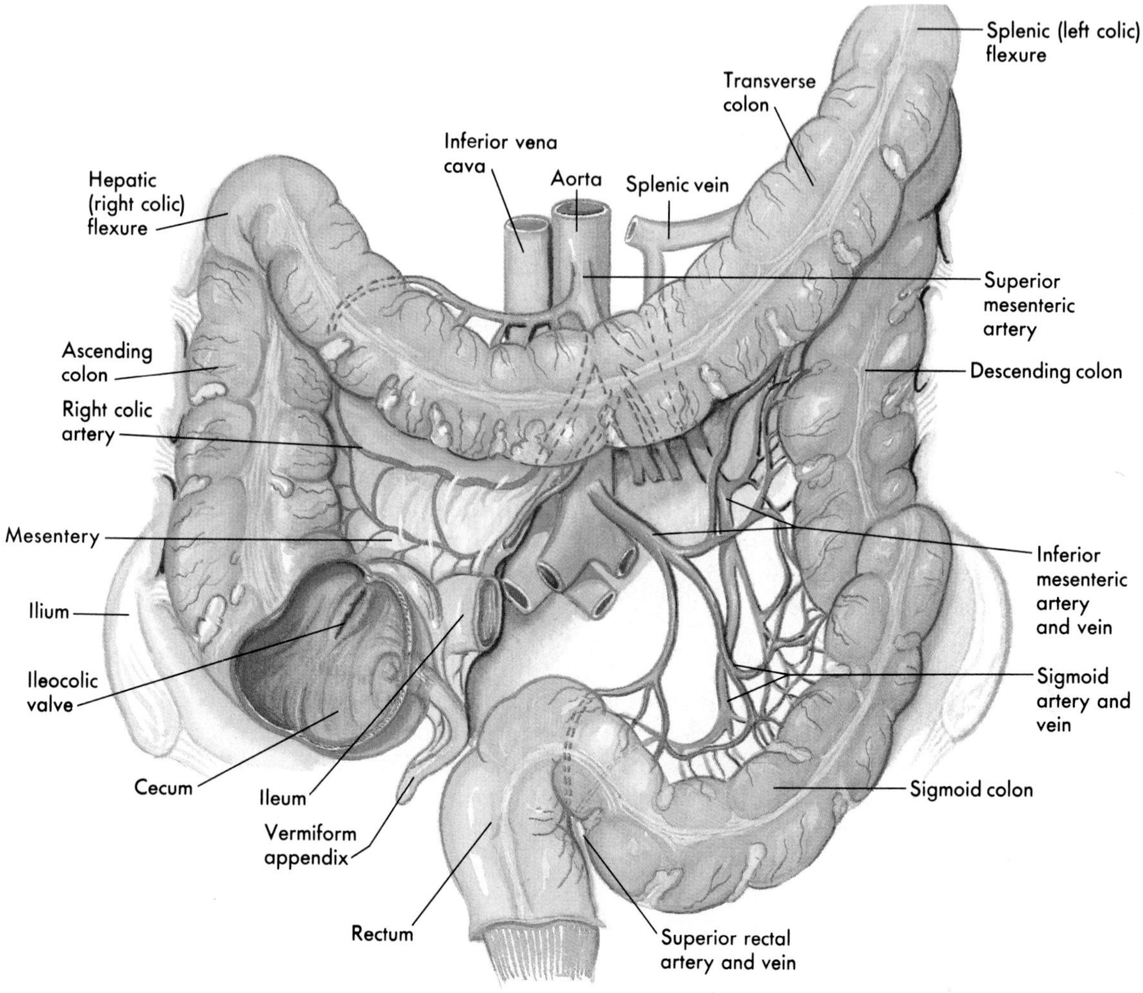

FIG. 31-6 Divisions of the large intestine.

of the small intestine 600 times. Inside each villus is a rich capillary bed, along with modified lymph capillaries called *lacteals*. The lacteals are responsible for the absorption of metabolized fats.

Large intestine. Once the small intestine has finished with its specific tasks, the ileocecal valve opens and releases the contents into the large intestine. This tube is larger in diameter (2 inches) but shorter (5 feet). It is composed of the cecum, appendix, colon, rectum, and anus (Fig. 31-6). The process of digestion is completed here in the terminal portion of the digestive tract. Basically the large intestine has four major functions: (1) completion of absorption; (2) manufacture of certain vitamins; (3) formation of feces; and (4) expulsion of feces.

Just inferior to the ileocecal valve is the cecum, a blind pouch approximately 2 to 3 inches long. Dangling from the cecum is a small, wormlike structure, the vermiform appendix. It is composed of lymphoid tissue. To date there is no known function for the appendix. It is common for the appendix to become inflamed, resulting in a condition known as *appendicitis,* which requires prompt surgical attention to prevent infection of the surrounding tissues. The open end of the cecum connects the small and large intestine. The colon is divided into four portions: (1) ascending; (2) transverse; (3) descending; and (4) sigmoid. The ascending colon continues upward on the right side of the abdomen to the inferior area of the liver. It crosses to the left side of the abdomen, forming the transverse colon. The transverse colon continues inferior to the spleen. The descending colon passes downward on the left side of the abdomen to the level of the iliac crest. The sigmoid colon begins here and continues toward the midline to the level of the third sacral vertebra. The last 8 inches forms the rectum, which appends to the exit—the anal canal, which terminates with the anus. Under usual conditions the anus remains closed. It contains an internal sphincter composed of smooth muscle (involuntary) and an external sphincter composed of skeletal muscle (voluntary). With the urge to defecate, these sphincters relax and feces is expelled.

Bacteria in the large intestine change the chyme into fecal material by releasing the remaining nutrients. The bacteria are also responsible for the synthesis of vitamin K and the production of some of the B-complex vitamins. Only mucus is secreted by the large intestine, since most of the digestive process has already taken place in the small intestine. As the fecal material continues its journey, the remaining water is absorbed into the bloodstream by osmosis. Sodium and other salts are absorbed by active transport.

Rectum. Finally, the waste products have been prepared for expulsion from the body, metabolism and absorption have been completed, and feces has been formed. The rectum carries the feces from the colon to the anal canal and functions as an excretory canal. It is approximately 4 to 6 inches long. It contains muscular rings, sphincters, that are under the control of the nervous system. As the rectum becomes distended with stool, the urge to defecate becomes apparent. The brain sends a message to the anal sphincters, they relax, and stool is expelled.

Accessory organs of digestion

Liver. The liver is the largest glandular organ in the body. In the adult it weighs 3 pounds. It is located just inferior to the diaphragm, covering most of the right upper quadrant and extending into part of the left epigastrium. It is divided into the right and left lobes. Approximately 1500 ml of blood is delivered to the liver every minute by the portal vein and the hepatic artery. Oxygenated blood is carried by the hepatic artery, and the portal vein delivers deoxygenated blood that is rich in nutrients that have been absorbed from the small intestine.

The cells of the liver produce a product called *bile,* a yellow-brown or green-brown liquid. It consists mostly of water, salts, cholesterol, and bile pigments. Bile is necessary for the metabolism of fats. The liver releases 500 to 1000 ml of bile daily. The bile travels to the gallbladder through the right and left hepatic ducts. If it is not needed, it backs up into the cystic duct to be stored in the gallbladder for later use.

Bilirubin is the main bile pigment. It is released as red blood cells are broken down by the liver. When it reaches the intestines, the bilirubin is broken down and its products give feces its color.

In addition to the production of bile, some of the many other functions of the liver are the following:

1. It manufactures heparin, prothrombin, and fibrinogen—all necessary for blood coagulation management.
2. It manufactures albumin, which helps maintain normal blood volume.
3. It filters out old red blood cells and detoxifies certain bacteria.
4. It detoxifies alcohol and certain drugs.
5. It stores iron, copper, and certain vitamins.
6. It stores sugar in the form of glycogen for later use by the body.
7. It participates with the kidneys to activate vitamin D.
8. It breaks down nitrogenous wastes (from protein metabolism) to urea, which the kidneys can then excrete from the body.

Gallbladder (Fig. 31-7). The gallbladder is an oval, muscular sac, about 3 to 4 inches long. It is located on the right inferior surface of the liver. Because the small intestine needs bile only a few times a day, the gallbladder stores and concentrates it. When chyme, containing fat, enters the first portion of the small intestine (duodenum), the gallbladder contracts and releases bile through the cystic duct into the common bile duct, which empties into the duodenum under the influence of cholecystokinin, an enzyme.

If a stone occludes the common bile duct, bile refluxes into the hepatic ducts and then into the liver. This puts pressure on the liver to release it into the bloodstream. This results in **jaundice** (yellow skin, sclerae, and mucous membranes).

It is important to remember that bile is produced by the liver and stored and concentrated by the gallbladder. It is then released into the duodenum for the metabolism of fats. It travels from the liver through the right and left hepatic ducts through the cystic duct to the gallbladder. Once the gallbladder contracts, bile travels down the cystic duct to the common bile duct and then into the duodenum. The system of passageways is referred to as the *biliary ductal system* or *biliary apparatus.*

Pancreas. The pancreas is an elongated gland that lies posterior to the stomach (see Chapter 35). It is an active organ that is involved in both endocrine and exocrine duties. In this chapter the discussion of the pancreas is limited to the exocrine activities. It involves the production of digestive enzymes that are transported through ducts to the duodenum. The pancreatic duct connects to the common bile duct from the liver and gallbladder and empties through a small orifice in the duodenum called the *ampulla of Vater.*

Each day the pancreas produces 1000 to 1500 ml of pancreatic juice to aid in digestion. This pancreatic juice contains the most important digestive enzymes because of their ability to digest the three major components of chyme—fats, carbohydrates, and proteins. In addition, it contains an alkaline substance, sodium bicarbonate, which has the ability to neutralize the hydrochloric acid in the gastric juices that enter the small intestine from the stomach.

Occasionally the pancreas becomes diseased, resulting in pancreatic digestive juices actually digesting the pancreas. This serious condition is called *acute pancreatitis.*

Peritoneum. The peritoneum is a serous membrane that

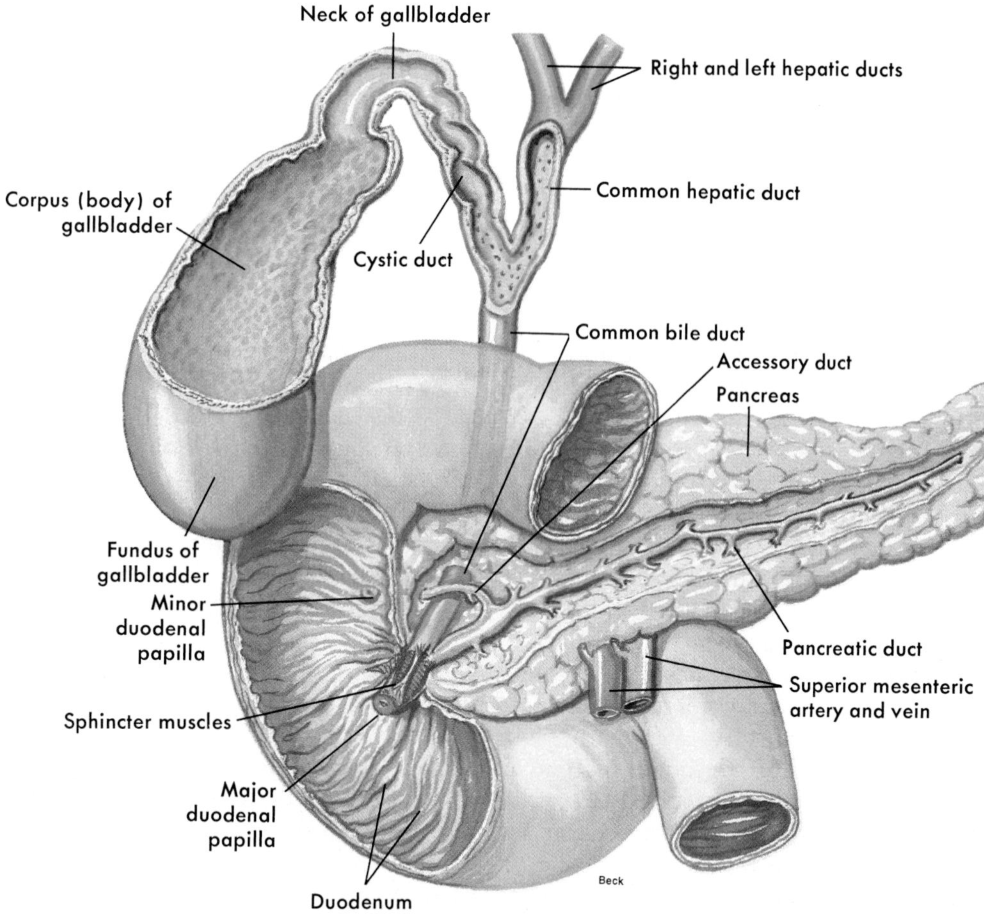

FIG. 31-7 The gallbladder and bile ducts. Obstruction of either the hepatic or common bile duct by stone or spasm occludes the exit of the bile from the liver, where it is formed, and prevents bile from being ejected into the duodenum.

covers most of the abdominal organs. It is the largest membrane in the body; the heart and lungs are also covered with serous membrane. The peritoneum is composed of squamous epithelium with a supportive layer of connective tissue. The walls of the abdominal cavity are covered with the parietal peritoneum, and the abdominal organs are covered with visceral peritoneum. The space between these two layers is called the *peritoneal cavity*. It has a thin coating of serous fluid. This allows the two layers of the membranes to slide against each other. Some organs that lie on the posterior wall of the abdomen have only an anterior covering of peritoneum; the kidneys and pancreas are examples. They are referred to as *retroperitoneal* organs. If an organ within the abdominal cavity becomes infected, the infection can spread easily to the membrane, resulting in a condition called *peritonitis*. Usually it can be resolved with antibiotic therapy, but the individual is very ill with severe abdominal pain and elevated temperature.

Extensions. The peritoneum lies in large folds throughout the abdominal cavity, surrounding the various organs. These large folds contain blood vessels, lymph vessels, and the nerves that supply the abdominal organs. The peritoneum anchors the organs to each other and also to the abdominal walls. The first extension of the peritoneum, which is called the **mesentery,** anchors the small intestine to the posterior abdominal wall. The mesocolon attaches the large intestine to the posterior abdominal wall. The mesocolon carries the blood supply to the intestines.

Two other extensions are called the *lesser* and *greater omenta*. They too arise from the peritoneal folds. The lesser omentum arises from the lesser curvature of the stomach and suspends the stomach and duodenum from the liver. The greater omentum arises from the greater curvature of the stomach and is attached to the duodenum, stomach, and large intestine. It contains large quantities of adipose tissue and is often referred to as a "fatty apron." The greater omentum also contains many lymph nodes, which, in the presence of infection, will attempt to resolve the infection and prevent its spread to the peritoneum.

Regulation of Food Intake

The hypothalamus contains two centers that have an impact on eating habits. The first area is called the *feeding center.* When it is stimulated, an individual will eat even if he is not hungry. The second center is the *satiety center*, and when stimulated it signals the individual to stop eating. These centers work in conjunction with other areas of the brain to balance eating patterns. Many other factors also impact eating styles. For example, distention of the stomach activates the satiety center, decreasing the appetite. Cool temperatures increase appetite. Warm temperatures decrease it. In addition to the many controls within our bodies, life-styles, eating habits, and genetic factors all blend together to give each individual his body build.

Digestion. Once food is ingested into the digestive system, two major types of processes take place to prepare the food for use by the cells. The first is **mechanical digestion**. The food is broken into smaller particles and propelled through the system to become mixed with the various enzymes. It is important to remember that in mechanical digestion the chemical structure of the food is not altered—it changes the physical size of the product to prepare it for chemical digestion.

The second process is **chemical digestion** (Table 31-2). It is the series of reactions that breaks the proteins, fats, and carbohydrates into molecules that the cells can readily use. The speed of the process is enhanced by the presence of the various enzymes throughout the digestive tract. It starts with the enzyme in saliva and ends with the intestinal enzymes.

Metabolism. Metabolism refers to the total of all the changes, both physical and chemical, that prepare the food for ingestion within the system. It can be divided into two phases. The first is **catabolism**, in which chemical compounds are broken into simpler forms with the release of energy. This energy provides the cells strength to perform their various activities. Catabolism is the destructive phase of metabolism; it releases usable forms of energy. The second phase, **anabolism**, is the building aspect, in which the energy released from catabolism allows the cells to build more complex, usable forms of nutrients. For example, fats are converted to phospholipids, which in turn form the plasma membrane. Anabolism is the building and repairing phase of metabolism.

The amount of energy used by the body at rest is called the *basal metabolic rate (BMR)*. It is the amount of energy necessary for vital body functions, such as respiration and circulation, to continue. When foods are metabolized, they give off different amounts of energy. This energy value is measured in units called *kilocalories (kcal)*. The more active the body is, the more kilocalories it needs to maintain homeostasis. Any excess is stored for later use.

Fats yield 9 kcal per gram, proteins yield 4 kcal per gram, and carbohydrates also yield 4 kcal per gram. If the number of grams of a specific food is determined, this number is easily converted to caloric value. For example, a banana contains 25 grams of carbohydrates. Because carbohydrates contain 4 kcal per gram, multiplying 4×25 shows that a banana contains 100 calories. Many books and pamphlets are available that list caloric value of foods.

Carbohydrate digestion and metabolism. Most carbohydrates that are ingested are in the form of complex sugars (polysaccharides). They must be converted to simple sugars (monosaccharides) to be absorbed and used

Table 31-2 Chemical Digestion

Digestive Juices and Enzymes	Enzyme Digests (or Hydrolyzes)	Resulting Product*
Saliva		
Amylase (ptyalin)	Starch (polysaccharide)	Maltose (a disaccharide, or double sugar)
Gastric juice		
Protease (pepsin) plus hydrochloric acid	Proteins, including casein	Proteoses and peptones (partially digested proteins)
Lipase (of little importance)	Emulsified fats (butter, cream, and so on)	**Fatty acids and glycerol**
Pancreatic juice		
Protease (trypsin)†	Proteins (either intact or partially digested)	Proteoses, peptides, and **amino acids**
Lipase (steapsin)	Bile—emulsified fats	**Fatty acids and glycerol**
Amylase (amylopsin)	Starch	Maltose
Intestinal juice (succus entericus)		
Peptidases	Peptides	**Amino acids**
Sucrase	Sucrose (cane sugar)	**Glucose and fructose‡** (Simple sugars of monosaccharides)
Lactase	Lactose (milk sugar)	**Glucose and galactose** (simple sugars)
Maltase	Maltose (malt sugar)	**Glucose** (grape sugar)

* Substances in boldface type are end products of digestion; that is, completely digested foods ready for absorption.
† Secreted in inactive form (trypsinogen); activated by enterokinase, an enzyme in the intestinal juice.
‡ Glucose is also called *dextrose;* fructose is called *levulose.*

by the cells. This process begins in the mouth with the enzyme *salivary amylase*. Because food passes quickly through the mouth, salivary amylase (ptyalin) only initiates the process of conversion. It continues to work on carbohydrates in the stomach for 15 to 20 minutes until hydrochloric acid, released by the stomach, stops the process. As chyme passes to the small intestine, the process begins again with the release of pancreatic amylase from the pancreas and the three major enzymes from the small intestine—maltase, sucrase, and lactase. Once the carbohydrates have been changed to glucose, they can enter the cell wall. Once inside the cell, a series of processes takes place that releases energy for cell use. Approximately one half of the energy is stored as **adenosine triphosphate (ATP)**, which can be released instantaneously by the cell as needed. A certain amount of glucose is stored in the liver in the form of glycogen. When the body needs this reserve, the liver breaks the glycogen down to glucose and releases it into the bloodstream for immediate use.

Fat digestion and metabolism. Most fat (lipid) digestion and metabolism occur in the small intestines. Bile, which is produced by the liver and stored in the gallbladder, is released through the cystic duct into the duodenum. It mechanically breaks the large fat globules into small droplets. Pancreatic lipase, an enzyme found in pancreatic juice, chemically converts the droplets into a usable form of fatty acids and glycerol. The fatty acids and glycerol are then absorbed into the lymph system through the lacteals in the villi of the small intestine and are then transported to the liver. The liver uses some of the lipids for energy and releases the rest for use by the cells.

Lipids are necessary for the proper absorption of the fat-soluble vitamins (A,D,E,K), for cushioning of the internal organs, as a reserve energy source, and as part of many cell structures.

Protein digestion and metabolism. Protein breakdown begins in the stomach with the release of the enzyme *pepsin*. It converts the protein to a usable form called **amino acids**. Protein conversion is completed in the small intestine where the enzymes *trypsin* and *chymotrypsin* are found in the pancreatic juice. As the amino acids are freed, they are absorbed by the villi of the small intestine and sent to the liver for dispersal throughout the body. Amino acids (protein) are the chief structural components of the body. Muscle tissue, some chromosomes, enzymes, and some hormones are composed of amino acids.

ASSESSMENT OF THE GASTROINTESTINAL SYSTEM AND ACCESSORY ORGANS

Laboratory and Diagnostic Examinations

Upper gastrointestinal study (upper GI series, UGI)

Rationale. The upper GI study consists of a series of x-ray films of the lower esophagus, stomach, and duodenum, using barium sulfate as the contrast medium. A UGI series will detect any abnormal conditions of the upper gastrointestinal tract, any tumors, or other ulcerative lesions.

Nursing interventions. The patient should maintain NPO status after midnight. The nurse should explain to the patient the importance of rectally expelling all the barium after the examination. Stools will be light in color until all of the barium is expelled. Eventual absorption of fecal water may cause a hardened barium impaction. Increasing fluid intake is usually effective. Milk of Magnesia (60 ml) is commonly given after the examination unless contraindicated.

Tube gastric analysis

Rationale. The contents of the stomach are aspirated to determine the amount of acid produced by the parietal cells in the stomach. The analysis is done to determine the completeness of a vagotomy, confirm hypersecretion or **achlorhydria**, estimate acid secretory capacity, or assay for intrinsic factor.

Nursing interventions. The patient should receive no anticholinergic medications for 24 hours before the test and should maintain NPO status after midnight so the gastric acid secretion will not be altered. The nurse should inform the patient that smoking is prohibited before the test because nicotine stimulates the flow of gastric secretions.

The nurse or radiology personnel will insert a nasogastric tube into the stomach to aspirate gastric content. Specimens should be labeled properly and sent to the laboratory immediately. The nasogastric tube is removed as soon as specimens are collected. The patient may then eat if indicated.

Esophagogastroduodenoscopy (UGI endoscopy, gastroscopy)

Rationale. Endoscopy enables direct visualization of the upper GI tract by means of a long, fiberoptic, flexible scope. The esophagus, stomach, and duodenum are examined for tumors, varices, mucosal inflammations, hiatal hernias, polyps, ulcers, and obstructions. Also, the endoscopist can remove polyps and coagulate sources of active gastrointestinal bleeding through endoscopy. Areas of narrowing can be dilated by the endoscope itself or by passing a dilator through the scope. Camera equipment may be attached to the viewing lens, and the existing pathological condition can be photographed.

Not only can the esophagus, stomach, and duodenum be evaluated by endoscopy, but by the use of a longer fiberoptic scope, the upper small intestine can be evaluated. This is referred to as *enteroscopy*.

Nursing interventions. The nurse should explain the procedure to the patient. The patient should maintain NPO status after midnight. The nurse should obtain the patient's signature on a consent form for the endoscopic examination. Because the patient's pharynx has been anesthetized (by spraying) with Xylocaine, the nurse should not allow the patient to eat or drink until the gag reflex returns (usually about 2 to 4 hours).

Barium swallow

Rationale. This barium contrast study is a more thorough study of the esophagus than that provided by most UGI examinations. As in most barium contrast studies, defects in luminal filling and narrowing of the barium column indicate tumor, scarred stricture, or varix. With a barium swallow, anatomical abnormalities, such as hiatal hernia, are easily recognized. Left atrial dilation, aortic aneurysm, and paraesophageal tumors (such as bronchial or mediastinal tumors) may cause extrinsic compression of the barium column within the esophagus.

A product called Gastrografin is now used in place of barium for patients where bleeding from the gastrointestinal system may occur and surgery is being considered. Gastrografin facilitates imaging through x-ray, but if the product escapes from the gastrointestinal tract, unlike barium, it is absorbed by the surrounding tissue. Complications can occur if barium leaks from the GI tract.

Nursing interventions. The patient should maintain NPO status after midnight. Food and fluid in the stomach will prevent the barium from accurately outlining the GI tract, and the radiographical results may be misleading. The nurse should explain to the patient the importance of rectally expelling all barium. Stools will be light in color until this occurs. Eventual absorption of fecal water may cause a hardened barium impaction. Increasing fluid intake is usually effective. Milk of Magnesia (60 ml) is usually given after the examination unless contraindicated.

Esophageal function studies

Rationale. The Bernstein test, an acid-perfusion test, is an attempt to reproduce the symptoms of gastroesophageal reflux. It aids in differentiating esophageal pain caused by esophageal reflux from that caused by angina pectoris. If the patient suffers pain with the instillation of hydrochloric acid into the esophagus, the test is positive and indicates reflux esophagitis.

Nursing interventions. The nurse should avoid sedating the patient, because the patient's participation is essential for swallowing the tubes, swallowing during acid clearance, and describing any discomfort during the instillation of hydrochloric acid. The patient is NPO for 8 hours before the examination, and any medications that may interfere with the production of acid, such as antacids and analgesics, are withheld.

Examination of stool for occult blood

Rationale. Tumors of the large intestine grow into the **lumen** and are subjected to repeated trauma by the fecal stream. Eventually the tumor ulcerates and bleeding occurs. Usually the bleeding is so slight that gross blood is not seen in the stool. If this **occult blood** is detected in the stool, a benign or malignant gastrointestinal tumor should be suspected.

Occult blood in the stool may occur also in ulceration and inflammation of the upper or lower gastrointestinal system. Other causes include swallowing blood of oral or nasopharyngeal origin.

Stool may be obtained by digital retrieval by the nurse or physician. However, the patient is usually asked to collect stool in a container.

Nursing interventions. The nurse should instruct the patient to keep the stool specimen free of urine or toilet paper, because either can contaminate the specimen and alter the test results. The nurse or patient should don gloves and use tongue blades to transfer the stool to the proper receptacle.

Sigmoidoscopy (lower GI endoscopy)

Rationale. Endoscopy of the lower GI tract allows visualization and, if indicated, access to obtain biopsy specimens of tumors, polyps, or ulcerations of the anus, rectum, and sigmoid colon. Because the lower GI tract is difficult to visualize radiographically, the direct visualization afforded through sigmoidoscopy is beneficial. Microscopic review of tissue specimens obtained using this procedure can provide the diagnoses of many lower bowel disorders.

Nursing interventions. The nurse should explain the procedure to the patient. The patient should sign a consent form for the procedure. The nurse administers enemas as ordered on the evening before and/or the morning of the examination to ensure optimum visualization of the lower GI tract. After the examination the nurse observes the patient for evidence of bowel perforation (abdominal pain, tenderness, distention, and bleeding).

Barium enema study (lower GI series)

Rationale. The barium enema (BE) study consists of a series of x-ray films of the colon used to demonstrate the presence and location of polyps, tumors, and diverticula. Positional abnormalities (such as malrotation) can also be detected. Therapeutically, the BE study may be used to reduce nonstrangulated ileocolic **intussusception** (infolding of one segment of the intestine within another) in children.

Nursing interventions. The nurse may administer castor oil (60 ml) the evening before the BE or administer a cleansing enema (Skill 31-1) the evening before or morning of the BE if directed by the physician's order or hospital policy. Milk of Magnesia (60 ml) may be ordered after the BE to stimulate evacuation of the barium.

After the BE study, the patient should be assessed for complete evacuation of the barium. Retained barium may cause a hardened impaction. Stool will be light in color until all of the barium has been expelled.

SKILL 31-1 ADMINISTERING AN ENEMA

1. Introduce self.
2. Identify patient.
3. Wash hands.
4. Explain procedure.
5. Arrange equipment at bedside.
6. Pull curtain and close door to provide privacy.
7. Place patient in left Sims' position.
8. Place waterproof pad under patient.
9. Place bath blanket over patient, and fanfold linen to foot of bed; place patient gown out of way yet providing privacy.
10. Don gloves.
11. Clamp tubing 7 inches (28 cm) from end; fill container with correctly warmed solution (usually 1000 ml at 105° F) and any additive (read disposable package instructions). Release clamp, allowing solution to flow through tubing; reclamp.
12. Lubricate 4 inches (10 cm) of end of the tubing; spread patient's buttocks to expose anus; while rotating tube, gently insert it 3 to 4 inches (7 to 10 cm).
13. Elevate container 12-18 inches (30-45 cm) above level of patient's anus to allow solution to flow at adequate rate.
14. Release clamp; allow solution to flow slowly while holding clamp; solution should flow over 5-10 minutes.
15. Lower container or clamp tubing if patient complains of cramping; encourage slow, deep breathing.
16. Clamp and remove tube when enough solution has been administered; encourage patient to retain solution at least 5 minutes—retention of solution promotes peristalsis and enhances defecation.

For commercially prepared enema

- Remove cover from tip of enema (tip is prelubricated); insert entire tip into anus.
- Squeeze container until it is empty.

For both forms of enemas

17. When patient can no longer retain solution, assist to bedpan, bedside commode, or bathroom; remind patient not to flush toilet.
18. Provide for patient hygiene; assist patient to bed or chair.
19. Dispose of equipment and supplies; remove gloves; wash hands.
20. Record procedure and observations.
21. Report abnormalities.

Colonoscopy

Rationale. With the development of the fiberoptic colonoscope, the entire colon from anus to cecum can be examined in a high percentage of patients. Therefore with colonoscopy the detection of lesions in the proximal colon, which would otherwise be undetected by sigmoidoscopy, is possible. As with sigmoidoscopy, benign and malignant neoplasms, mucosal inflammation or ulceration, and sites of active hemorrhage can be visualized. Also, biopsy specimens can be obtained and small tumors removed through the scope with the use of cable-activated instruments. Actively bleeding vessels can be coagulated.

Patients who have had cancer of the colon are at high risk for developing another colon cancer. For this patient population colonoscopy allows early detection of any secondary tumors.

Nursing interventions. The patient signs a consent form. The nurse explains the procedure to the patient. The patient is instructed regarding dietary restrictions, usually a clear liquid diet is permitted 1 to 3 days before the procedure, and then NPO status is maintained for 8 hours before the procedure. The nurse administers a cathartic, enemas, and premedication as ordered.

After colonoscopy, the nurse checks for evidence of bowel perforation (abdominal pain, distention, tenderness, and bleeding) and examines stools for gross blood.

Stool culture (stool for culture and sensitivity [C & S]; stool for ova and parasites [O & P])

Rationale. The feces (stool) can be examined for the presence of bacteria, ova, and **parasites**. Many bacteria (such as *Escherichia coli*) are indigenous in the bowel. Bacterial cultures are usually done to detect enteropathogens (such as *Staphylococcus aureus*, *Salmonella*, and *Shigella*).

When a patient is suspected of having a parasitic infection, the stool is examined for ova and parasites (O & P). Usually at least three stool specimens are collected on subsequent days.

Nursing interventions. If an enema must be administered to collect specimens, only normal saline or tap water should be used. Soapsuds or any other substance could affect the viability of the organisms collected.

Stool samples for ova and parasites are obtained before barium examinations. The patient is instructed not to mix urine with feces. The nurse dons gloves to collect the specimen. The specimen should be taken to the laboratory within 30 minutes of collection.

Obstruction series (flat plate of the abdomen)

Rationale. The obstruction series is a group of x-ray studies performed on the abdomen of patients who have suspected bowel obstruction, paralytic ileus, perforated viscus, or abdominal abscess. This series usually consists of at least two x-ray studies. The first is an erect abdominal x-ray study that should include visualization of both diaphragms. X-ray images are examined for evidence of free air under either diaphragm, which is **pathognomonic** (sign or symptom specific to a disease condition) of a perforated **viscus**. This x-ray study is used also to detect air fluid levels within the intestine.

Nursing interventions. For adequate visualization, the nurse should ensure that this study is scheduled before any barium studies.

Diagnostic studies used in the assessment of the hepatobiliary and pancreatic systems

Serum bilirubin test. Normal values are as follows:
Direct bilirubin: 0.1-0.3 mg/dl
Indirect bilirubin: 0.2-0.8 mg/dl
Total bilirubin: 0.1-1.0 mg/dl
Total bilirubin in newborns: 1-12 mg/dl

Rationale. Total serum bilirubin determination measures both direct, or conjugated (water-soluble), and indirect, or unconjugated (water-insoluble), bilirubin. Total serum bilirubin level is the sum of the direct and indirect bilirubin levels. Testing for bilirubin in the blood provides valuable information for diagnosis and evaluation of liver disease, biliary obstruction, and hemolytic anemia.

Nursing interventions. The nurse should keep the patient on NPO status until after the blood specimen is drawn.

Liver enzymes tests. The normal values are as follows:
AST (formerly serum glutamic oxaloacetic transaminase [SGOT]): 0-41 U/L
ALT (formerly serum glutamic pyruvic transaminase [SGPT]): 0-45 U/L
LDH: 60-200 U/L
Alkaline phosphatase: 50-150 U/L (alkaline phosphatase level is elevated in obstructive disorders of the biliary tract)
Gamma GT: 0-45 U/L (this test is elevated in liver cell dysfunction and alcohol ingestion)

Rationale. The liver is a storehouse of many enzymes. Injury or diseases affecting the liver will cause release of these intracellular enzymes into the bloodstream, and their levels will be elevated. Some of these enzymes are produced also in other organs, and injury or disease affecting these other organs will also cause an elevated serum level. Therefore although elevation of these serum enzymes is found in pathological liver conditions, the test is not specific for liver diseases alone.

Nursing interventions. The nurse should assess the venipuncture site for bleeding.

Serum protein test. The normal values are as follows:
Total protein: 6-8 g/dl
Albumin: 3.2-4.5 g/dl
Globulin: 2.3-3.4 g/dl
Albumin globulin (A/G ratio): 1.2-2.2 g/dl

Rationale. One way to assess the functional status of the liver is to measure the products that are synthesized there. One of these products is protein, especially albumin. When disease affects the liver cell, the hepatocyte loses its ability to synthesize albumin and the serum albumin level is markedly decreased.

Low serum albumin levels may result also from (1) excessive loss of albumin into urine (as in nephrotic syndrome) or into third-space volumes (as in ascites) or (2) from protein-caloric malnutrition.

Nursing interventions. The nurse should assess the venipuncture site for bleeding.

Oral cholecystography (gallbladder series, GB series, cholecystogram)

Rationale. The oral cholecystogram provides x-ray visualization of the gallbladder after the oral ingestion of a radiopaque, iodinated dye. Adequate visualization of the gallbladder requires concentration of the dye within the gallbladder. The following factors are necessary for adequate dye concentration:

1. Ingestion by the patient of the correct number of dye tablets the evening before the examination
2. Adequate absorption of the dye from the GI tract; vomiting or diarrhea will preclude absorption of the dye
3. Abstinence from food (especially a fatty meal) on the morning of the test
4. Uptake from the portal system and excretion of the dye by the liver
5. Patency of the cystic duct
6. Concentration of the dye within the gallbladder

Nursing interventions. Before the administration of the dye, the nurse should make certain the patient is not allergic to iodine, to prevent anaphylaxis. If no allergy to iodine is present, the nurse administers six iopanoic acid (Telepaque) tablets orally, one at 5-minute intervals after the evening meal. The patient is on NPO status from midnight. The patient is informed that he may be given a high-fat meal or beverage to stimulate emptying of the gallbladder after the test has begun. No other food or fluids will be allowed until the examination is complete.

Intravenous cholangiography (intravenous cholangiogram, IVC)

Rationale. In this study intravenously administered radiographical dye is concentrated by the liver and secreted into the bile duct. IVC allows visualization of the hepatic and common bile ducts and also the gallbladder if the cystic duct is patent. IVC is used to demonstrate stones, stricture, or tumor of the hepatic duct, common bile duct, and gallbladder.

Operative cholangiography. In operative cholangiography, the common bile duct is directly injected with radiopaque dye. Stones appear as radiolucent shadows, and tumors cause partial or total obstruction of the flow of dye into the duodenum. By visualization of the biliary duct structures, the surgeon is provided with a "road map" of a commonly difficult anatomical area. This reduces the possibility of inadvertently injuring the common duct.

If common duct stones are suspected, not only must a cholecystectomy be performed, but also a common duct exploration (CDE). When intraoperative cholangiography is used routinely, CDE is performed only on those with positive cholangiography.

T-tube cholangiography (postoperative cholangiography)

Rationale. T-tube cholangiography is performed to diagnose retained ductal stones postoperatively in the patient who has had a cholecystectomy and a common bile duct exploration. The test is performed through the use of a T-shaped rubber tube that the surgeon places in the bile duct during the operation. Through the end of the T-tube that exits through the abdominal wall, dye can be injected and x-ray films taken.

Nursing implications. The nurse should protect the patient from sepsis by connecting the T-tube (if left in place) to a sterile closed-drainage system. If the T-tube is removed, the T-tube tract site should be kept covered with a sterile dressing to prevent bacteria from entering the ductal system.

Nursing interventions. Before the administration of the dye, the nurse should ensure that the patient is not allergic to iodine. Preparation of the patient also includes NPO after midnight and until the examination is completed. The nurse administers a cleansing enema on the morning of the examination, if ordered.

Ultrasound examination of the liver and biliary system (echogram of the liver and biliary system)

Rationale. Ultrasound is used with increasing frequency to corroborate data already obtained by "questionable positive" cholangiograms, liver scans, and oral cholecystograms.

Nursing interventions. The patient is NPO from midnight. If the patient has had recent barium contrast studies, the nurse should request an order for cathartics. Ultrasound cannot penetrate barium, and the study will not be adequate.

Gallbladder scanning (hepatobiliary imaging, HIDA scanning)

Rationale. Through the use of technetium (Tc) (technetium 99), the biliary tract can be evaluated in a safe, accurate, and noninvasive manner. The primary use of this study is in the diagnosis of acute cholecystitis. This procedure is superior to oral cholecystography, ultrasonography, and CT scanning of the abdomen for the detection of acute cholecystitis.

Nursing interventions. The nurse should assure the patient that exposure to radioactivity is minimal because only tracer doses of the radioisotopes are used. The patient is NPO from midnight until the examination is complete.

Liver biopsy

Rationale. Liver biopsy is a safe, simple, and valuable method of diagnosing pathological liver conditions. For this study a specially designed needle is inserted through the skin and abdominal wall and into the liver. A piece of liver tissue is removed for microscopic examination. Percutaneous liver biopsy is used in the diagnosis of various liver disorders, such as cirrhosis, hepatitis, drug reactions, granuloma, and tumor.

Nursing interventions. The nurse should explain the procedure to the patient and obtain the patient's signature on a consent form. Food and fluids are withheld 4 to 8 hours before the test. The nurse ensures that platelet and prothrombin tests have been ordered and any abnormal values are reported to the physician. After the procedure the nurse observes the patient for symptoms of bleeding. Vital signs are monitored every 15 minutes for 1 hour, then every 30 minutes for 4 hours, and then every 4 hours for 24 hours.

Some pain is common. When leakage involves a large quantity of blood or bile, the peritoneal reaction is great and the resulting pain is severe. The nurse should report these symptoms immediately to the physician. The patient should remain on bed rest for 24 hours.

Liver scanning (radioisotope liver scanning)

Rationale. This radionuclide procedure is used to outline and detect structural changes of the liver. A radionuclide is given intravenously. Later, a gamma ray detecting device (Geiger counter) is passed over the patient's abdomen. This records the distribution of the radioactive particles in the liver. The spleen can also be visualized by the detector when technetium 99 sulfur is used.

Nursing interventions. The patient should be NPO from midnight. The nurse should assure the patient that he will not be exposed to a large amount of radioactivity, because only tracer doses of isotopes are used.

Blood ammonia. The normal laboratory value for adults is 15-55 μmol/L.

Rationale. Ammonia, a by-product of protein metabolism, is normally converted by the liver into urea and then secreted by the kidneys (see BUN). With severe liver dysfunction or when the blood flow to the liver is altered, the blood ammonia level rises and the BUN level decreases. The blood ammonia level is primarily used as an aid in diagnosing hepatic encephalopathy or coma. Elevated blood ammonia levels suggest liver dysfunction as the cause of these symptoms.

Nursing interventions. The nurse should list on the laboratory requisition any antibiotics the patient is currently taking. Certain antibiotics can cause a decreased ammonia level, thus giving inaccurate test results.

Hepatitis virus studies (hepatitis-associated antigen [HAA]). A normal laboratory test result will be negative for the presence of the antigen.

Rationale. Hepatitis is an inflammation of the liver caused by a virus. Three common viruses are now recognized that can cause this disease: hepatitis A virus; hepatitis B virus; and hepatitis non-A–non-B virus (also called hepatitis C virus). The individual hepatitis viruses can be detected by different antigen and antibody levels, and different incubation periods must be considered.

Nursing interventions. The nurse should use universal precautions and should handle the serum specimen as if it were capable of transmitting viral hepatitis. Health care personnel will don gloves when handling any blood or body fluids and will wash hands carefully after handling all equipment.

Serum amylase test. The normal value for this test is 5-81 U/L.

Rationale. The serum amylase test is an easily and rapidly performed test for pancreatitis. Damage to pancreas cells (as in pancreatitis) or obstruction to the pancreatic ductal flow (as in pancreatic carcinoma) will cause an outpouring of this enzyme into the intrapancreatic lymph system and also into the free peritoneum. Blood vessels draining the free peritoneum and absorbing the lymph pick up this excess amylase. An abnormal rise in the serum level of amylase is the result, and it will occur within 12 hours of the onset of pancreatic disease. Because amylase is rapidly cleared by the kidney, serum levels may return to normal within 48 to 72 hours.

Nursing interventions. The nurse should note on the laboratory requisition if the patient is receiving IV dextrose or any medications, because these can cause a false negative result.

Urine amylase test. The normal value for this study is 50-300 IU/L per 24 hours.

Rationale. Because the kidney rapidly clears amylase, disorders affecting the pancreas will cause elevated amylase levels in the urine. Levels of amylase in the urine remain elevated for 7 to 10 days after the onset of disease. This fact is important if the diagnosis of pancreatitis is to be made in patients who have had symptoms for 3 days or longer.

Nursing interventions. The nurse should record the exact times of the beginning and end of the collection period. A 6-hour, 12-hour, or 24-hour collection can be perfomed, depending on the physician's order. The collection begins after the patient empties the bladder and discards that specimen. All subsequent urine is collected, including the voiding at the end of the collection period. The specimen should be kept on ice or refrigerated until it is sent to the laboratory.

Ultrasound examination of the pancreas

Rationale. Through the use of reflected sound waves, ultrasonography of the pancreas provides diagnostic information of this rather inaccessible abdominal organ. Ultrasound examination of the pancreas is mainly used to establish the diagnosis of carcinoma, pseudocyst, pancreatitis, and pancreatic abscess. Because ultrasound abnormalities persist from several days to weeks, the diagnosis of pancreatitis can be supported by this study even after the serum amylase and lipase levels have returned to normal. Furthermore, follow-up ultrasound study can be used to monitor the resolution of pancreatic inflammation and the response of a tumor to therapy.

Nursing interventions. Fluids and foods are withheld for 8 hours before the examination. If the patient's abdomen is distended with gas or if the patient has had a recent barium examination, this study should be postponed, because gas and barium will interfere with sound wave transmission.

Computed tomography of the abdomen (CT scan of the abdomen)

Rationale. CT scan of the abdomen is a noninvasive, accurate x-ray procedure used to diagnose pathological pancreatic conditions, such as inflammation, tumor, cyst formation, ascites, aneurysm, and cirrhosis of the liver. The recognizable cross-sectional image produced by a CT scan is especially important for studying the pancreas, because this organ is retroperitoneal and well hidden by the overlying peritoneal organs.

Nursing interventions. Fluids and food are withheld from midnight until the examination is complete. If possible, the nurse should show the patient a picture of the machine and encourage the patient to verbalize fears, since some patients suffer claustrophobia when enclosed in the machine.

Endoscopic retrograde cholangiopancreatography of the pancreatic duct (ERCP of the pancreatic duct)

Rationale. Not only can the biliary system be visualized by ERCP, the pancreatic duct can be seen also. During the test a fiberoptic duodenoscope is inserted through the oral pharynx, through the esophagus and stomach, and into the duodenum. Dye is injected for radiographic visualization of the common bile duct and pancreatic duct. ERCP of the pancreas is a sensitive and reliable procedure for detecting clinically significant degrees of pancreatic dysfunction. Localized pancreatic duct narrowing indicates tumor. Chronic pancreatitis is demonstrated by multiple areas of ductal narrowing, which can be visualized by ERCP.

Nursing interventions. Food and fluids are withheld for 8 hours before the examination, and the patient's signature on a consent form is obtained. The nurse should tell the patient that the test takes approximately 1 hour, during which time he must lie completely motionless on a hard x-ray table. Remaining still for this period of time may be uncomfortable for the patient.

DISORDERS OF THE MOUTH

Common disorders of the mouth and esophagus that interfere with adequate nutrition include poor dental hygiene, infections, inflammation, and cancer.

Dental Plaque and Caries

Etiology/pathophysiology. Dental decay is an erosive process that results from the action of bacteria on carbohydrates in the mouth, which in turn produces acids that dissolve tooth enamel. Most Americans (95%) experience tooth decay sometime in their life span. Dental decay can be caused by one of several factors:

- The presence of dental plaque, a thin film on the teeth made of mucin and colloidal material found in saliva and often secondarily invaded by bacteria
- The strength of acids and the ability of the saliva to neutralize them
- The length of time the acids are in contact with the teeth
- Susceptibility of the teeth to decay

Medical management. Interventions include treatment of dental caries by removal of affected areas of the tooth and replacement with some form of dental material. Treatment of periodontal disease centers on removal of plaque from the teeth. If the disease has advanced, surgical interventions of the gingivae and alveolar bone may be necessary.

Nursing interventions and patient teaching. Proper technique for brushing and flossing the teeth at least twice a day is the nurse's primary focus of teaching for this patient. Plaque forms continuously and must be removed periodically through regular visits to the dentist. The patient must understand the importance of prevention through continuous care. Because carbohydrates create an environment where caries develop and plaque accumulates more easily, proper nutrition is included in patient teaching. When the patient is ill, the normal cleansing action of the mouth is impaired. Illnesses, drugs, and irradiation all interfere with the normal action of saliva. If the patient is unable to perform his own oral hygiene, the nurse must assume this responsibility.

NURSING DIAGNOSES	NURSING INTERVENTIONS
Knowledge deficit, related to inability to prevent dental caries and periodontal disease	Assess and observe the oral cavity for moisture, color, and cleanliness. Stress importance of meticulous oral hygiene. Explain need to see dentist at least yearly for examination.
Noncompliance, related to hygiene and dietary restrictions	Brush teeth bid and prn with toothpaste or powder, baking soda, or mouthwash. Rinse with water or mouthwash. Cleanse mouth with equal parts of hydrogen peroxide and water prn for halitosis. Teach oral hygiene to patient.

Candidiasis

Etiology/pathophysiology. This condition is any infection caused by a species of *Candidia*, usually *Candida albicans. Candida* is a fungal organism normally present in the mucous membranes of the mouth, intestinal tract, and vagina and is also found on the skin of healthy people. This infection is also referred to as *thrush* and *moniliasis*.

This disease appears more commonly in the newborn infant who becomes infected in passing through the birth canal. In the older individual, candidiasis may be found in those with leukemia, diabetes mellitus, and alcoholism, and in the person who has been on antibiotics (chlortetracycline or tetracycline) or steroids for long periods or is in a general weakened state.

Clinical manifestations. Candidiasis appears as small white patches on the mucous membrane of the mouth and tongue. There may be one or more lesions on the mucosa, depending on duration of infection. If the patch or plaque is removed, painful bleeding can occur.

Medical management. Treatment may include 1 to 4 ml of nystatin (Mycostatin) dropped in the infected infant's mouth several times a day. For the adult, half-strength hydrogen peroxide/saline mouth rinses may provide some relief. Nystatin vaginal tablets (100,000 units dissolved) inserted into the vagina BID has proven to be effective. Ketoconazole taken systemically appears to be equally effective.

Nursing interventions. The nurse must use meticulous handwashing to prevent spread of infection. The infection may be spread in the nursery by carelessness of nursing personnel. Handwashing, care of feeding equipment, and cleanliness of the mother's nipples are important to prevent spread. The nurse should cleanse the mouth of any foreign material, rinsing the mouth and lubricating the lips. The mouth should be inspected using a flashlight and tongue blade.

Carcinoma of the Oral Cavity

Etiology/pathophysiology. The lips, the oral cavity, the tongue, and the pharynx are prone to develop malignant lesions. The largest number of these tumors are squamous cell epitheliomas that grow rapidly and metastasize to adjacent structures more quickly than do most malignant tumors of the skin. In the United States oral cancer accounts for 4% of the cancers in males and 2% in females.

Tumors of the salivary glands occur primarily in the parotid gland and are usually benign. Tumors of the submaxillary gland have a high incidence of malignancy. These malignant tumors grow rapidly and may be accompanied by pain and impaired facial function.

Kaposi's sarcoma is a malignant skin tumor that occurs primarily on the legs of men between 50 and 70 years of age. Recently it has been seen with increased frequency as a nonsquamous tumor of the oral cavity in patients with AIDS. The lesions are purple and nonulcerated. Irradiation is the treatment of choice.

Cancer or neoplasm is characterized by the uncontrolled growth of anaplastic cells that tend to invade surrounding tissue and to metastasize to distant body sites.

The tumor seen with cancer of the lip is usually called an *epithelioma*. It occurs most frequently as a chronic ulcer of the lower lip in men. The cure rate for cancer of the lips is high because the lesion is easily apparent to the patient and to others. Metastasis to regional lymph nodes has occurred in only 10% of persons when diagnosed. In some instances a lesion may spread rapidly and involve the mandible and the floor of the mouth by direct extension. Occasionally the tumor may be a basal cell lesion that starts in the skin and spreads to the lip.

Cancer of the anterior tongue and floor of the mouth may seem to occur together because their spread to adjacent tissues is so rapid. Metastasis to the neck has already occurred in more than 60% of patients when the diagnosis is made because of the tongue's abundant vascular and lymphatic drainage. Recent investigation has revealed a higher incidence of cancers of the mouth and throat among persons who are heavy drinkers and smokers. Also, data show that the mortality for young males between the ages of 10 and 20 has doubled over the past 30 years as a result of the use of smokeless tobacco (snuff). This combination of high alcohol consumption and smoking or chewing tobacco causes an apparent breakdown in the body's defense mechanism. Predisposing factors include exposure to the sun and wind, but more important is the progression of leukoplakia to an epidermoid lip cancer.

Clinical manifestations. Leukoplakia is a white patch on the mouth or tongue mucosa that cannot be classified as another disease. These nonsloughing lesions cannot be rubbed off by simple mechanical force. They can be benign or malignant. A small percentage develop into squamous cell carcinomas, and biopsy is recommended if the lesions persist for longer than 2 weeks. They occur most frequently between the ages of 50 and 70 years and appear more commonly in men.

Assessment. Collection of *subjective data* includes understanding that malignant lesions of the mouth are usually asymptomatic. The patient may feel only a roughened area with his tongue. As the disease progresses, the first complaints may be (1) difficulty in chewing, swallowing, or speaking; (2) edema, numbness, or loss of feeling in any part of the mouth; and (3) earache, faceache, and toothache, which may become constant. Cancer of the lip is associated with discomfort and irritation caused by the presence of a nonhealing lesion that may be raised or ulcerated. Malignancy at the base of the tongue produces less obvious symptoms: slight dysphagia, sore throat, and salivation.

Collection of *objective data* includes observing for premalignant lesions, including leukoplakia (white patches). Unusual bleeding in the mouth, some blood-tinged sputum, lumps or edema in the neck, and hoarseness may be observed.

Diagnostic tests. Indirect laryngoscopy is an important diagnostic test for examination of the soft tissue. This procedure is especially important for men 40 years of age or older who have dysphagia and a history of smoking and alcohol ingestion. Radiographical evaluation of the mandibular structures is also an essential part of the head and neck examination to rule out the presence of cancer. Excisional biopsy is the most accurate method for a definitive diagnosis. Oral exfoliative cytology is a means of screening intraoral lesions. A scraping of the lesion provides cells for cytological examination. The chance for a false negative finding is about 26%.

Medical management. Treatment depends on the location and staging of the malignant tumor. Stage I oral cancers are treated by surgery or radiation. Stages II and III cancers require both surgery and radiation. Treatment for stage IV cancer is usually palliative. The survival rate for patients with oral cancers averages less than 50%.

Small, accessible tumors can be excised surgically and include a glossectomy, removal of the tongue; hemiglossectomy, removal of part of the tongue; mandibulectomy, removal of the mandible; and total or supraglottic laryngectomy, removal of the entire larynx or the portion above the true vocal cords.

Large tumors usually require more extensive and traumatic surgery. In a functional neck dissection of neck cancer with no growth in the lymph nodes, the lymph nodes are removed but the jugular vein, sternocleidomastoid muscle, and spinal accessory nerve are preserved. In radical neck dissection, all of these structures are removed and reconstructive surgery is necessary after tissue resection. These patients may have drains in the incision sites that are connected to suction to aid healing and reduce hematomas. A tracheostomy may also be performed, depending on the degree of tumor invasion.

Because of the location of the surgery, complications can occur. These include airway obstruction, hemorrhage, tracheal aspiration, facial edema, fistula formation, and necrosis of the skin flaps. Neurological complications can occur because of nerves being severed and manipulated during surgery.

Radiation may be in the form of external radiation by use of roentgenograms or other radioactive substances or in the form of internal radiation by means of needles or seeds. The purpose of radiation therapy is to shrink the tumor. It can be given preoperatively or postoperatively, depending on the physician's preference and the patient's disease process. In more advanced cases, chemotherapy may be combined with radiation postoperatively to make the patient more comfortable. Options of treatment other than radiation and surgery include laser excision.

Nursing interventions. It is important that the nurse have a holistic approach to the patient. This includes being aware of the patient's level of knowledge regarding the disease, the emotional response and coping abilities, and the spiritual needs. The nursing interventions must be individualized to the patient, beginning with the preoperative stage, through the postoperative stage, and is complete after the patient's rehabilitation in his home environment. Family members, hospice members, close friends, social workers, and pastoral care staff may be necessary for information and support during this potentially fatal disease.

NURSING DIAGNOSES	NURSING INTERVENTIONS
Altered nutrition: less than body requirements, related to oral pain or postoperative tissue loss (mucous membranes)	Monitor the patient for changes in the character and quantity of mucus after radiation therapy. Provide meticulous oral hygiene. Observe for temporary or permanent loss of taste and the need for alternative routes for nutrition by monitoring daily weights.
Body image and personal identity disturbance, related to disfiguring appearance of an oral lesion or reconstructive surgery	Provide alternative methods for communication of dysarthria results from radiation treatment. Provide information to the patient and family to help with difficult decisions related to surgery, radiation, or chemotherapy. Be a support person to the patient and family.

Patient teaching. Prevention centers on avoidance of predisposing factors: excess exposure to sun and wind on the lips, elimination of smoking or chewing tobacco, and maintenance of good oral and dental care. There is a high correlation between the incidence of cancer of the mouth and cirrhosis of the liver associated with alcohol intake. Early detection of oral cancer can help increase the patient's chance of survival. Any person with a mouth lesion that does not heal within 2 to 3 weeks is urged to seek immediate medical care. Preoperative and postoperative care must be taught to the surgical patient, with full explanations regarding speech loss and alternate methods of nutritional intake. Explanation of tracheostomy care and other tubes the patient may be discharged with will relieve anxiety and encourage the patient's control over the situation.

DISORDERS OF THE ESOPHAGUS

Carcinoma of the Esophagus

Etiology/pathophysiology. This disorder is a malignant epithelial neoplasm that has invaded the esophagus and has been diagnosed for the presence of a squamous cell carcinoma or an adenocarcinoma.

Of esophageal cancers, 90% are squamous cell carcinomas, which are associated with both alcohol intake and tobacco use and possibly long-standing **achalasia** (an abnormal condition characterized by the inability of a muscle to relax, particularly the cardiac sphincter of the stomach). Of cancers of the esophagus, 6% are adenocarcinomas and are associated with reflux esophagitis. Environmental carcinogens, nutritional deficiencies, chronic irritation, and mucosal damage have all been considered as causes of esophageal cancer. Unfortunately, because of the location, esophageal cancer is usually at a late stage when discovered and treatment is aimed toward comfort and control rather than cure. The prevalent age group for esophageal cancer is 55 to 70 years. It occurs more commonly in men.

The esophagus with its extensive lymphatic network facilitates the rapid spread of malignant cells to varying local and distant sites. Carcinoma of the esophagus carries a general survival rate of 1% to 5%, with an overall 5-year survival rate of less than 4%.

Clinical manifestations. The most common clinical symptom is progressive dysphagia over a 6-month period, with the sensation of food sticking in the throat.

Assessment. Collection of *subjective data* includes noting that initially the patient may have difficulty in swallowing solid foods and then become unable to swallow semisolid or soft foods. Eventually the patient may not be able to swallow liquids and saliva. Another symptom is *odynophagia* (painful swallowing).

Collection of *objective data* includes the nurse observing the patient for **regurgitation**, vomiting, hoarseness, chronic cough, and iron-deficiency anemia. Weight loss may be directly related to the tumor or a side effect of treatment or the inability to swallow.

Diagnostic tests. A barium swallow examination with fluoroscopy and endoscopy is used to detect esophageal cancer. A biopsy and cytological examination provide a high degree of accuracy in the final diagnosis.

Medical management. Tumor staging must be addressed to determine tumor size and patient management. In advanced cases, surgery is offered for palliative purposes to relieve dysphagia and restore continuity of the alimentary tract. Even patients who seem free of metastasis at the time of surgery have a mean survival rate of only 13 months.

Radiation therapy may be curative and/or palliative. Special problems associated with radiation therapy include the development of fistulas (an abnormal passage between two internal organs). Aspiration from the fistula and edema from the radiation must be anticipated. Chemotherapy using a single drug or a combination of drugs is considered a palliative treatment of advanced cancer of the esophagus. Because of the extreme toxicity of these drugs, side effects of respiratory and liver dysfunction, nausea and vomiting, leukopenia, and sepsis can be anticipated.

Four types of surgical procedures can be performed:

1. *Esophagectomy*—Removal of all or part of the esophagus, using a synthetic graft to replace the parts resected
2. *Esophagogastrostomy*—Resection of the lower portion of the esophagus and anastomosis of the remaining portion of the stomach
3. *Esophagoenterostomy*—Resection of the esophagus and anastomosis to a portion of the colon
4. *Gastrostomy*—Insertion of a catheter into the stomach and suture to the abdominal wall; performed when it is assumed the patient will not be able to take food orally because of inoperable cancer of the esophagus interfering with swallowing

Nursing interventions. Following are nursing diagnoses and interventions for the patient with esophageal carcinoma.

NURSING DIAGNOSES	NURSING INTERVENTIONS
Ineffective breathing pattern, related to incisional pain and proximity to the diaphragm	Monitor respirations carefully because of proximity of incision to diaphragm and difficulty in carrying out breathing exercises.
Altered nutrition: less than body requirements, related to dysphagia, decreased stomach capacity, gastrostomy tube	Monitor intake and output and daily weights to determine adequate nutritional intake.
Potential for infection, related to poor nutritional status, weakness, and impaired healing process	Assess for signs of infection: low-grade temperature, abnormal breath sounds, and increased pulse and respiratory rates.
Potential impaired skin integrity, related to gastrostomy tube or fistula output	Inspect skin frequently for leakage from gastrostomy tube or from fistula formation.

Patient teaching. The nurse should discuss with the patient and family all aspects of care, including surgery, radiation, and chemotherapy if necessary. Psychological adjustment of the patient who cannot ingest food orally, whether temporary or permanent, is difficult. Step-by-step explanations of all diagnostic tests, medications, procedures, and the treatment plan will help to decrease the patient's anxiety. The nurse should support the patient with this serious diagnosis by allowing time for questions.

Achalasia

Etiology/pathophysiology. Achalasia, also called *cardiospasm*, is an abnormal condition characterized by the inability of a muscle to relax, particularly the cardiac sphincter of the stomach.

Although the cause is unknown, nerve degeneration, esophageal dilation, and hypertrophy are thought to contribute to the disruption of the normal neuromuscular activity of the esophagus. This results in decreased motility of the lower portion of the esophagus, absence of peristalsis, and dilation of the lower portion. Thus little or no food can enter the stomach, and in extreme cases, the dilated portion of the esophagus can hold as much as a liter or more of fluid. This disease may occur in persons of any age, but it is more prevalent in those between 20 and 50 years.

Clinical manifestations. The primary symptom of achalasia is **dysphagia** (difficulty in swallowing both liquids and solids). The patient has a sensation of food sticking in the lower portion of the esophagus. As the condition progresses, the patient complains of regurgitation of food, which relieves prolonged distention of the esophagus. There may be some occurrence of substernal chest pain.

Assessment. The nurse should observe for loss of weight, poor skin turgor, and weakness.

Diagnostic tests. Radiological studies show esophageal dilation above the narrowing at the cardioesophageal junction. The diagnosis is confirmed by manometry, which shows the absence of primary peristalsis. Esophagoscopy is also used to confirm the diagnosis.

Medical management. The conservative treatment of achalasia includes drug therapy and forceful dilation of the narrowed area of the esophagus. Anticholinergics, nitrates, and calcium channel blockers reduce lower esophageal sphincter pressure.

Dilation is done by first emptying the esophagus. Then a dilator with a deflated balloon is passed down to the sphincter. The balloon is inflated and remains so for 1 minute; it may need to be reinflated one or two times. Esophageal motility is not restored, but the open sphincter relieves the dysphagia in about 80% of the cases and the esophageal lumen is reduced in size.

A cardiomyotomy is the preferred surgical approach. In this procedure the muscular layer is incised longitudinally, down to but not through the mucosa. Two thirds of the incision is in the esophagus, and the remaining one third is in the stomach; this permits the mucosa to expand so that food can pass more easily into the stomach.

Nursing interventions. Following are nursing diagnoses and interventions for the patient with achalasia. Nursing

BOX 31-1 NURSING INTERVENTIONS OF THE PERSON EXPERIENCING ESOPHAGEAL SURGERY

PREOPERATIVE NURSING INTERVENTIONS

1. Encourage improved nutritional status.
   a. High-protein, high-calorie diet if oral diet is possible.
   b. Total parenteral nutrition may be necessary for severe dysphagia or obstruction.
2. Give meticulous oral hygiene; breath may be malodorous.
3. Give preoperative preparation appropriate for thoracic surgery.
4. Give prescribed antibiotics before esophageal resection or bypass, as ordered.

POSTOPERATIVE NURSING INTERVENTIONS

1. Promote good pulmonary ventilation.
2. Maintain chest drainage system as prescribed.
3. Maintain gastric drainage system.
   a. Small amounts of blood may drain from nasogastric tube for 6 to 12 hours after surgery.
   b. Do not disturb nasogastric tube (to prevent traction on suture line).
4. Maintain nutrition.
   a. Start clear fluids at frequent intervals when oral intake is permitted.
   b. Introduce soft foods gradually to several small meals of bland foods.
   c. Have patient maintain semi-Fowler's position for 2 hours after eating and while sleeping if heartburn (pyrosis) occurs.

interventions of the person experiencing esophageal surgery is presented in Box 31-1.

NURSING DIAGNOSES	NURSING INTERVENTIONS
Altered nutrition: less than body requirements, related to difficulty in swallowing both liquids and solids	Encourage fluids with meals to increase lower esophageal sphincter pressure and push food into stomach. Monitor liquid diet for 24 hours after dilation procedure.
Anxiety, related to continuous dilation process with threat of complications	Monitor for signs of esophageal perforation (chest pain, shock, dyspnea, fever) after dilation. Provide calm, nonstressful environment. Reinforce physician's explanation of disease process. Encourage verbalization of fears; assist patient with identifying stressors and positive coping behaviors.

Patient teaching. Home care and follow-up care should be discussed in preparation for dismissal. A family member or support person should be included if possible, and the patient should be an active participant in the planning.

The following teaching should be included:

1. Explain need for high-calorie, high-protein diet, and provide printed material with same.
2. Explain need to elevate head while sleeping and to avoid bending and stooping.
3. Discuss medications if prescribed: name, dosage, time of administration, purpose, and side effects.
4. Discuss methods of avoiding constipation by using high-fiber foods if tolerated and natural laxatives.
5. Explain importance of follow-up care with physician.
6. Discuss symptoms of recurrence or progression of disease and need to report these to physician.

DISORDERS OF THE STOMACH

Gastritis (Acute)

Etiology/pathophysiology. Gastritis is an inflammation of the lining of the stomach. Acute gastritis refers to a temporary inflammation associated with alcoholism, smoking, and stressful physical problems, such as burns, major surgery, food allergens, presence of viral, bacterial, or chemical toxins, chemotherapy, or radiation therapy. Changes occur in the mucosal lining that interfere with acid and pepsin secretion. Acute gastritis is often a single occurrence that resolves when the offending agent is removed.

Clinical manifestations. If the condition is acute, fever, epigastric pain, nausea, vomiting, headache, coating of the tongue, and loss of appetite may occur. If the condition results from ingestion of contaminated food, the intestines are usually affected and diarrhea may occur.

Assessment. Collection of *subjective data* involves observing for anorexia, nausea, discomfort after eating, and pain, although some patients with gastritis have no symptoms.

Collection of *objective data* includes observing for vomiting, hematemesis, and melena caused by gastric bleeding.

Diagnostic tests. Testing the stools for occult blood, noting WBC differential increases related to certain bacteria, evaluating serum electrolytes, and observing for elevated hematocrit related to dehydration all aid in the diagnosis.

Medical management. If medical treatment is required, antiemetics, such as prochlorperazine (Compazine) or trimethobenzamide (Tigan), may be prescribed. Antacids and cimetidine (Tagament) or ranitidine (Zantac) may be given in combination. Antibiotics are given if the cause is a bacterial agent. Intravenous fluids are used to correct fluid and electrolyte imbalances. Patients who experience gastrointestinal bleeding from hemorrhagic gastritis require fluid and blood replacement and nasogastric lavage.

Nursing interventions. The nurse records the patient's intake and output. Foods and fluids are withheld orally as prescribed until the signs and symptoms subside. The nurse should monitor the patient's tolerance to oral feedings. The nurse will monitor the intravenous feedings as prescribed.

NURSING DIAGNOSIS	NURSING INTERVENTIONS
Fluid volume deficit, related to vomiting, diarrhea, and blood loss	Keep patient NPO or on restricted food and fluids as ordered, and advance as tolerated. Monitor laboratory data for fluid and electrolyte imbalances (potassium, sodium, and chloride). Record intake and output.

Patient teaching. Patient education should include an explanation of (1) the effects of stress on the mucosal lining of the stomach, (2) how salicylates and nonsteroidal antiinflammatory medications and particular foods may be irritating; and (3) how life-styles that include alcohol and tobacco may be harmful. The nurse should be able to assist the patient in locating self-help groups in the community to deal with these stressful behaviors.

Peptic Ulcers

Peptic ulcers are ulcerations of the mucous membrane or deeper structures of the gastrointestinal tract. They most commonly occur in the stomach and duodenum. The term *peptic ulcer* refers to ulcers that are the result of acid and pepsin imbalances.

Peptic ulcer disease remains a major health problem and affects more men than women. The elderly reflect an increase in this disease, perhaps as a result of the use of nonsteroidal antiinflammatory drugs. Symptoms are common between the ages of 25 to 50, with the peak occurrence at age 40. Peptic ulcers require the presence of gastric acid and result from two major causes: an excess of gastric acid (duodenal ulcers) or a decrease in the natural ability of the gastrointestinal mucosa to protect itself from acid and pepsin (gastric ulcers).

Types of peptic ulcers

Gastric ulcers

Etiology/pathophysiology. The most common site of a gastric ulcer is in the distal half of the stomach. The cause of gastric ulcers is not clear. There is a relationship between diet, genetic predisposition, ingestion of excessive amounts of salicylates, and use of tobacco and increased incidence of gastric ulcers. Once the gastric mucosal barrier is damaged, acid secretion is stimulated. Without intervention, the cells die, erosion occurs, and ulcers develop. Gastric mucosal damage can occur in some individuals within 1 hour after the ingestion of acetylsalicylic acid. Reflux of duodenal contents (bile acids) also causes severe gastric mucosal damage. Gastric ulcers may occur on the surface of a gastric tumor because of interference with the blood supply.

Duodenal ulcers

Etiology/pathophysiology. The term *duodenal ulcer* is given to a group of disorders that may or may not be caused by hypersecretion. Excessive production or excessive release of gastrin and/or increased sensitivity to gastrin is found in 40% of people with these ulcers. In the other 60%, the amount of acid produced is normal but perhaps the buffering ability is lacking in the duodenum. Ulceration occurs when the acid secretion exceeds the buffering factors.

Clinical manifestations. Both gastric and duodenal ulcers may have similar symptoms but differ in timing, degree, or factors that worsen or alleviate the symptoms. Pain is the characteristic symptom and is described as dull, burning, boring, or gnawing; it is located in the midline of the epigastric region.

Assessment. Collection of *subjective data* requires an awareness that in gastric ulcer patients, the pain is closely associated with food intake and usually does not awaken the patient at night like the pain experienced by those with duodenal ulcers. Nausea, eructation, and distention are common complaints, termed *dyspepsia.* All of these subjective symptoms intensify if the complications of perforation and obstruction are manifested.

Collection of *objective data* includes observing for hemorrhage, a common complication with gastric ulcers; more gastric ulcers bleed than do duodenal ulcers. Duodenal ulcers are more apt to have chronic bleeding and are more prone to perforate than gastric ulcers.

When GI bleeding occurs, one sign is vomiting blood (**hematemesis**) that has a coffee grounds appearance as a result of action of the gastric acid on the hemoglobin molecule. There may be presence of **melena**, when the blood becomes black and tarry as it passes through the digestive tract. In extreme cases, bright red blood may be passed rectally. Both salicylates and alcohol aggravate bleeding in patients with a history of peptic ulcers.

Bleeding from a gastric ulcer is more difficult to control compared with bleeding from a duodenal ulcer. Hemorrhage, with accompanying symptoms of shock, occurs when the ulcer erodes into a blood vessel. Surgical intervention is indicated if the patient remains unstable after receiving blood over several hours.

Perforation occurs when the ulcer crater penetrates the entire thickness of the wall of the stomach or duodenum. The release of gastric acid, pancreatic enzymes, or bile causes signs and symptoms of pain, emesis, fever, hypotension, and hematemesis.

Diagnostic tests. Fiberoptic endoscopy can detect both gastric and duodenal ulcers. The lesion can be viewed, biopsy performed, and cell washings taken for cytological examination. Radiological studies (UGI) are not as specific for small lesions but are still commonly used. Hematest of feces for detecting occult blood in the intestinal tract may also be used for diagnosis.

Medical management. The physician may order a nasogastric tube to be inserted to remove gastric content and blood (see p. 664 for a discussion of nursing interventions for nasogastric tubes). Treatment may also include gastric resection with removal of the ulcer, with or without vagotomy.

Scar tissue builds up with repeat episodes of ulceration and healing, causing obstruction, particularly at the pylorus. The patient may present with gastric dilation, vomiting, and distention. When fluid and electrolyte balance is achieved, surgical intervention is possible.

The primary treatment for peptic ulcers is to reduce signs and symptoms by decreasing or neutralizing the normal gastric acidity with drug therapy. The types of drugs most commonly used include the following:

- Antacids: neutralize or reduce the acidity of the stomach contents; these are Maalox, Gaviscon, Rolaids, Tums, Mylanta, and Riopan.
- Histamine H_2 receptor blockers: decrease acid secretions by blocking the histamine H_2 receptors; these include cimetidine (Tagamet) and ranitidine (Zantac).
- Mucosal healing agents: heal ulcers without antisecretory properties, possibly by adhering to the proteins in the ulcer base; this includes sucralfate (Carafate).

Diet therapy to promote healing includes diets high in fat and carbohydrates and low in protein and milk products. However, most patients do not understand or choose not to follow this regimen. Therefore it is recommended that smaller meals taken more frequently throughout the day decrease the degree of gastric motor activity. Bland diets do not promote patient compliance. Because both caffeinated and decaffeinated coffee, tobacco, alcohol, and aspirin aggravate the mucosal lining of the stomach and duodenum, an effort should be made to change the life-style of the patient with ulcers.

The most commonly used surgical procedures include the following:

- Antrectomy: removal of the entire antrum, the gastric-producing portion of the lower stomach, to eliminate the main stimuli to acid production.
- Gastroduodenostomy (Billroth I) (Fig. 31-8, *A*): fundus of the stomach is directly anastomosed to the duodenum; used to remove ulcers or cancer located in the antrum of the stomach.
- Gastrojejunostomy (Billroth II) (Fig. 31-8, *B*): duodenum is closed, and the fundus of the stomach is anastomosed into the jejunum; used to remove ulcers or cancer located in the body of the fundus.
- Total gastrectomy: removal of the entire stomach; is rarely used for patients with gastric cancer.
- Vagotomy: removal of the vagal innervation to the fundus, decreasing acid produced by the parietal cells of the stomach. (Fig. 31-9)

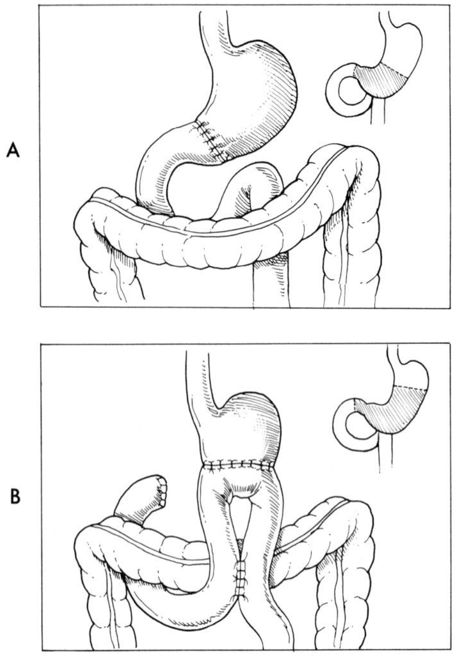

FIG. 31-8 Types of gastric resections with anastomoses. **A,** Billroth I. **B,** Billroth II.

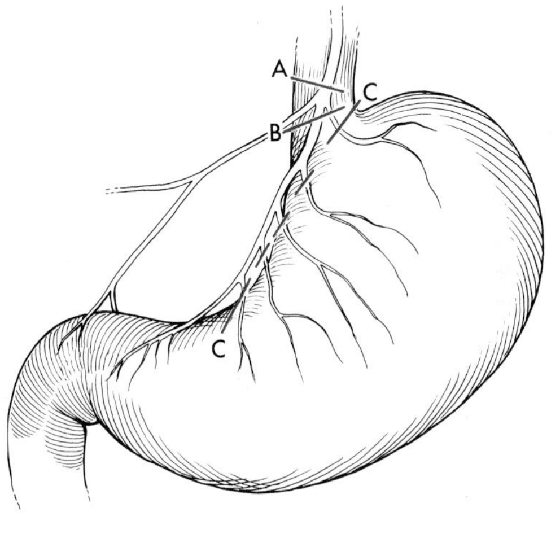

FIG. 31-9 Different types of vagotomies: truncal (*A*), selective (*B*), proximal or parietal cell (*C*).

- Pyloroplasty: surgical enlargement of the pylorus to provide drainage of the gastric contents.

The decision as to which procedure to use is difficult; the choice depends on physician preference and results of diagnostic testing. Regardless of the procedure selected, postoperative complications can occur.

Bleeding may occur up to 7 days after gastric surgery. Abdominal rigidity, abdominal pain, restlessness, an elevated temperature, increase in pulse, decrease in blood pressure, and leukocytosis are all possible indication of postoperative bleeding. The amount and type of drainage from the incision must be noted. Surgical intervention may be necessary to correct the bleeding.

The *dumping syndrome* is a rapid gastric emptying causing distention of the duodenum or jejunum produced by a bolus of hypertonic food. Increased intestinal motility and peristalsis and changes in blood glucose levels occur. Diaphoresis, nausea, vomiting, epigastric pain, explosive diarrhea, borborygmi (noises made from gas passing through the liquid of the small intestine), and dyspepsia may be reported by patients. The dumping syndrome can occur after gastric resection procedures. Treatment includes eating six small meals daily that are high in protein and fat and low in carbohydrates, eating slowly, and avoiding fluids during meals. This complication is treated with (1) anticholinergic agents to decrease stomach motility and (2) reclining for approximately 1 hour after meals.

There are several other complications after gastric surgery that present serious health threats. Diarrhea is common and usually responds to conservative treatment of controlled diet and antidiarrheal agents. Lomotil, Imodium, paregoric, or codeine is often used. Reflux esophagitis and nutritional deficits, including weight loss, malabsorption, anemia, and vitamin deficiency, can also be life threatening.

Pernicious anemia is a serious potential complication in any patient who has had a total gastrectomy or extensive resections. This is caused by a deficiency of the intrinsic factor, produced exclusively by the stomach, that aids intestinal absorption of vitamin B_{12}. It is recommended that all patients with a partial gastrectomy have vitamin B_{12} levels measured every 1 to 2 years so that replacement therapy can be instituted before anemia appears. The most common cause of anemia after gastric surgery is iron deficiency. Iron-deficiency anemia is caused by impaired absorption in the duodenum and proximal jejunum as a result of rapid gastric emptying. Replacement therapy consists of oral iron in the ferrous form.

Nursing interventions. Nasogastric tube insertion, irrigation, and gastrointestinal suctioning are often performed while a patient is feeling ill and uncomfortable. In addition to being skilled and knowledgeable in performing these procedures, the nurse is responsible for allaying the patient's fears and anxieties. Eliciting patient cooperation not only makes the procedures easier but also helps reduce patient discomfort.

Patients often are discharged home with gastrostomy tubes. As early as possible after insertion, the patient must be taught and encouraged to participate in care of the tube to be prepared for discharge.

An understanding of the following points will enable the nurse to help patients through the experience of gastrointestinal intubation:

- For most patients, gastrointestinal intubation is a new and frightening experience.
- Inability to chew, taste, and swallow food and liquids may contribute to patient anxieties during gastrointestinal intubation.
- A patient with a nasogastric (NG) or intestinal tube is usually on NPO status.
- The presence of a nasogastric or intestinal tube is a constant irritant to the nasopharynx and nares, requiring frequent care to the mouth and nose.
- A patient with a gastrointestinal tube may be afraid that moving about will dislodge the tube. The nurse must implement frequent position changes to enhance tube functioning and prevent complications of immobility.

An NG tube is inserted through the nose and passes through the pharynx and esophagus into the stomach. Various tubes are available, depending on the purpose (Fig. 31-10).

During insertion the tube may enter the trachea rather than the stomach. Before either instilling liquids through

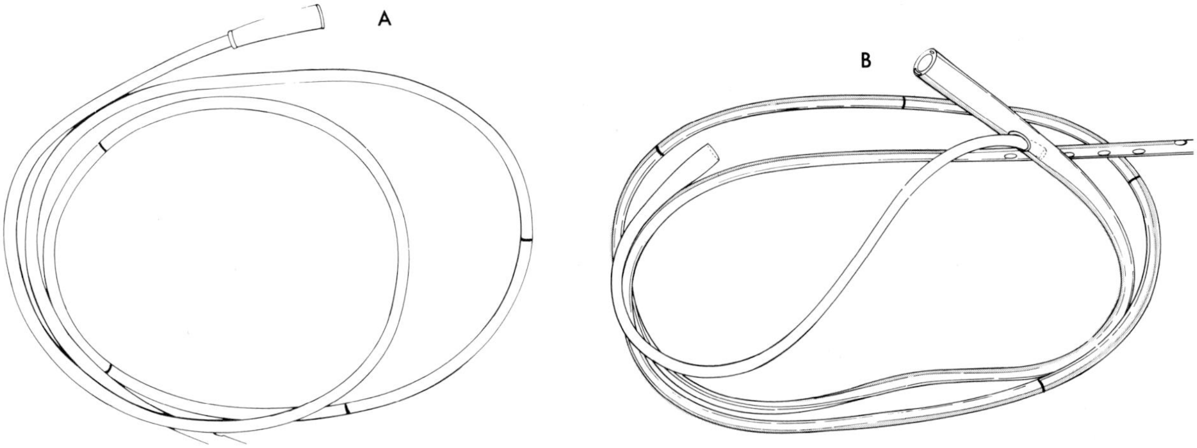

FIG. 31-10 Nasogastric tubes. **A,** Levin tube. **B,** Salem sump tube.

SKILL 31-2 GASTRIC AND INTESTINAL SUCTIONING CARE

1. Introduce self.
2. Identify patient.
3. Wash hands.
4. Explain procedure.
5. Check suction apparatus:
   a. For suction machine (Gomco)
      1. Machine is plugged in securely.
      2. Light is blinking on and off.
      3. Tubing connections are tight.
      4. Setting is correct.
   b. For wall suction
      1. Pressure gauge connections are tight.
      2. Pressure indicated on gauge is as ordered or according to agency policy.
      3. Suction is set at *intermittent* or *continuous* as ordered.
6. Ensure that tubing is not kinked and that patient is not lying on tubing.
7. Pin NG tube to patient's gown with enough slack to allow movement.
8. Verify that drainage is moving through tubing to drainage collection bottle.
9. For Salem sump tube, see that vent is pointing upward; vent pointing downward could promote drainage through vent via gravity.
   Listen at opening of blue air vent; hissing sound indicates air vent is patent.
10. Don gloves, and measure amount of drainage in bottle, noting color; empty if becoming full and at end of each shift.
11. Remove gloves, and wash hands.
12. Record procedure and observations.
13. Report abnormalities.

SKILL 31-3 NASOGASTRIC TUBE IRRIGATION

1. Introduce self.
2. Identify patient.
3. Wash hands.
4. Explain procedure.
5. Arrange equipment at bedside.
6. Pull curtain and close door to provide privacy.
7. Don gloves.
8. Verify that tube is in stomach:
   a. Attach syringe to tube, and aspirate gastric contents.
   b. If no gastric contents are aspirated, place stethoscope over epigastric area; while auscultating, inject 10 to 20 ml of air into tube.
9. Pour normal saline into container; draw up 30 ml (or amount ordered) into bulb or piston syringe.
10. Connect syringe to NG tube; keeping syringe in upright position, gently instill 30 ml saline (or ordered amount); do not use force.
11. If resistance is met, change patient's position and repeat attempt; if resistance continues, check with RN or physician.
12. Withdraw fluid into syringe, and measure; continue irrigating with ordered amount of saline until purpose of irrigation has been accomplished.
13. Reconnect NG tube to suction.
14. Note amount of saline instilled and withdrawn.
15. Dispose of equipment.
16. Remove gloves; wash hands.
17. Record procedure and observations.
18. Report abnormalities.

the tube or attaching the tube to suction, the nurse should determine that the tube is in the stomach (see Skill 31-3, Step 8). Skills 31-2 to 31-4 present various aspects of NG tube care.

Nursing interventions depend on the stage of the ulcer disease. The emphasis on patient care should always be on prevention and early detection of pain in the epigastric region, hematemesis, melena, or tenderness and rigidity of the abdomen. Nursing diagnoses and interventions follow for specific stages of ulcer care. See sample therapeutic dialogue (p. 666) and nursing care plan (p. 667) for the patient with gastrointestinal bleeding.

SKILL 31-4 NASOGASTRIC TUBE REMOVAL

1. Introduce self.
2. Identify patient.
3. Wash hands.
4. Explain procedure.
5. Arrange equipment at bedside.
6. Pull curtain and close door to provide privacy.
7. If tube is attached to suction, turn off suction machine and disconnect tubing; remove nose guard, and unfasten pin from gown.
8. Place towel or waterproof pad across patient's chest, and give patient tissues.
9. Don gloves.
10. Have patient take deep breath and hold breath; pinch tube with fingers or clamp; quickly and smoothly remove tube while patient is holding breath.
11. Place tubing in plastic bag or towel.
12. Provide oral and nasal care; make patient comfortable.
13. Dispose of tube and equipment; measure drainage; note color; write down for documentation later.
14. Remove gloves; wash hands.
15. Record procedure and observations.
16. Report abnormalities.

THERAPEUTIC DIALOGUE

NURSE: You look like you are resting better, Mrs. Snodgrass. How have you been feeling? *(Reaffirming a relationship that was begun yesterday.)*

PATIENT: Hello, Mrs. Brown. My stomach pain is much better. The medicine helped.

NURSE: If you are comfortable, perhaps you and your husband have some questions about why you are here. *(Trying to determine if the patient is receptive to patient teaching. A knowledge deficit was suspected on admission.)*

PATIENT; I was scared when I started to vomit blood. It has happened before but not this much. Where does the blood come from?

NURSE: The doctor has admitted you with a diagnosis of GI bleed with questionable duodenal ulcer. That means you have bleeding in the gastrointestinal system, either in the stomach or some part of the intestine. *(The nurse begins with the admitting diagnosis and explains one thing at a time, making sure the patient verbalizes understanding before continuing.)*

Do you understand what I have said so far?

PATIENT: Well, I understand where the bleeding is coming from, but why am I bleeding there?

NURSE: We are not sure yet, Mrs. Snodgrass, but you are scheduled for a procedure that will allow the doctor to actually look at the surface of the stomach and a portion of the intestine. It is called an endoscopy, and it will be done tomorrow morning. Did someone explain this to you?

(The nurse answers the question openly and honestly and uses the answer to lead into further patient education.)

NURSING DIAGNOSES	NURSING INTERVENTIONS
Peptic ulcer disease	
Knowledge deficit, related to medications, diet, and signs and symptoms of bleeding or perforation	Provide verbal and written instruction on exact dosage and time intervals for medications and if medication is taken with or without food. Have dietician provide instructions on therapeutic diet. Explain that repeat episodes are not uncommon; listen carefully for aggravating factors.
Pain, related to ulceration of gastric or duodenal mucosa	Instruct patient on side effects of antacid drugs (constipation or diarrhea) and importance of contacting physician if this occurs.
Altered nutrition: less than body requirements, related to pain, dyspepsia	Explain to patient reason for six meals and avoidance of foods that irritate mucosa lining.
Noncompliance with treatment and behavior modification	Teach patient to report pain of sudden and severe onset and passage of blood by emesis or rectally.
Anxiety, related to disease process	Help patient identify risk behaviors: anxiety, restlessness, and insomnia; and available resources for behavior modification.
Gastric surgery	
Potential fluid volume deficit, related to hemorrhage	Monitor for hypotension and tachycardia, sudden and severe abdominal pain, shallow respirations, vomiting, rigid and tender abdomen, and diminished bowel sounds. Monitor vital signs; record accurate intake and output; note weight gain or loss.

NURSING CARE PLAN: THE PATIENT WITH GASTROINTESTINAL BLEEDING

Nursing diagnoses	Patient goals	Nursing interventions
Impaired gas exchange, related to weakened condition, hemorrhage	Patient will demonstrate normal respiratory rate. Patient will breathe deeply and cough with assistance. Patient will not demonstrate rales or rhonchi.	Assess emergency ABCs of Airway, Breathing, and Circulation.
Potential fluid volume deficit, related to hemorrhage, vomiting, and diarrhea	Patient will have normal fluid balance as evidenced by balanced intake and ouput within 48 hr, including stable weight. Blood pressure, pulse, and respiratory rate will be within normal limits. Patient will have normal tissue turgor.	Accurately record intake and output q 1 hr until stable: emesis, urine, and stool. Document fluid losses for possible imbalance; urine output less than 30 ml/hr may indicate hypovolemia. Monitor for signs and symptoms of dehydration and fluid electrolyte imbalance (dry mucous membranes, poor skin turgor, thirst, decreased urinary output, and changes in behavior) q 15 min until stable, then q 2 hr. Document characteristics of output. Test all emesis and fecal output for presence of blood. Prepare to assist with inserting an NG tube. Irrigate NG tube with cool saline as ordered to promote clotting; irrigation removes old blood from the stomach.
Altered tissue perfusion, related to blood and fluid loss	Patient will demonstrate adequate renal perfusion as evidenced by urine output greater than 30 ml/hr. Patient will have normal blood pressure, pulse, and respirations. Patient will be oriented $\times 3$.	Assess for signs and symptoms of hypoxia continually: cyanosis, dyspnea, and confusion. Assess for urine output less than 30 ml/hr; insert Foley catheter as ordered. Monitor hemoglobin and hematocrit values on each laboratory report; normal ranges are: Hgb: 12-14 g/dl Hct: 37%-49% Assess vital signs q 15 min or q 1-2 hr if stable.
Anxiety, related to hospitalization and illness	Patient will demonstrate decrease in anxiety as evidenced by ability to sleep and/or rest at frequent intervals, verbalization of feelings, and blood pressure and pulse within normal limits.	Assess physiological components of anxiety: restlessness, increased pulse and respirations, diaphoresis, and elevated blood pressure at least q 8 hr. Provide concise explanations for all procedures; prepare patient for surgery if indicated. Develop rapport with patient and family members with each contact.

NURSING DIAGNOSES	NURSING INTERVENTIONS
Gastric surgery—cont'd Potential fluid volume deficit, related to hemorrhage—cont'd	Monitor temperature and oral mucous membranes for dryness; provide oral hygiene (toothbrushing or mouthwash); apply lubricant to lips and nares prn. Monitor parenteral fluids as ordered.
Noncompliance, related to risk behaviors (use of tobacco/alcohol) and dietary patterns	Assess patient's level of knowledge regarding food and other irritants to mucosal lining. Teach preventive measures. Explain need for small frequent meals. Caution to avoid high-fiber foods, sugar, salt, caffeine, alcohol, and milk. Remind to ,take fluids between meals, not with meals. Explain to eat slowly and chew food well. Discuss importance of adequate rest and exercise.
Altered nutrition: less than body requirements, related to preoperative and postoperative food and fluid restrictions	Maintain NPO status. Connect nasogastric tube to intermittent suction apparatus. Note color and amount of gastric output q 4 hr. Do not reposition tube. Maintain patency of tube by irrigation with measured amounts of saline *only* if ordered; NOTE: After gastrectomy, exudate will be minimal. Monitor parenteral fluids with electrolyte additives as ordered. Measure intake and output. When bowel sounds return, administer clear liquids as ordered. Progress to small, frequent meals of soft food as ordered; avoid milk, since it may cause dumping syndrome.

Patient teaching. It is necessary for the nurse to form a trusting relationship with the patient because of the severity and long-term treatment of the ulcer patient. The family should be included with the patient for understanding and support, and the patient should be involved in goal setting if compliance is to be obtained.

The patient should be aware that if severe and sudden pain occurs, medical attention should be sought immediately. Assistance should be given to the patient in describing his signs and symptoms of weakness, anorexia, nausea, diarrhea, constipation, anxiety, or restlessness. When medications are prescribed, the patient must fully understand (1) why the drugs are taken in large doses (30 ml), seven times daily (1 and 3 hours after a meal and at bedtime) or the specific times ordered and (2) the side effects that are known (diarrhea and constipation). Preventive teaching includes identifying risk behaviors in the patient's life-style, such as the use of tobacco and alcohol and engaging in stress-related activities. Dietary needs should emphasize six smaller meals daily and avoidance of any foods that cause noticeable stomach discomfort.

If surgery is required, procedures should be explained thoroughly, including the reasons for them. The nurse should explain immediate postoperative care, including deep breathing, coughing, position changes, the need for frequently monitoring vital signs, intravenous tubing, nasogastric tubing, catheters, and other drainage tubes, and the use of patient-controlled analgesia or other medications for pain relief. The ability of the patient to eat normally after healing will depend on the type of surgery and when peristalsis returns. The nurse should help the patient to realize that repeat episodes of symptoms are not unusual and to seek medical care if they recur.

Cancer of the Stomach

Etiology/pathophysiology. The most common neoplasm or malignant growth in the stomach is an adenocarcinoma. The primary location is in the pyloric area. Because of the location, the tumor may metastasize to lymph nodes, liver, spleen, pancreas, or esophagus.

The cause is not known, but numerous factors are associated with the disease. These include history of polyps, pernicious anemia, gastrectomy, chronic atrophic gastritis, and gastric ulcer. Because the stomach has prolonged contact with food, an association exists between cancer in this part of the body and diets high in salt, preservatives, and carbohydrates and low in fresh fruits and vegetables.

Clinical manifestations. The patient may be asymptomatic in early stages of the disease.

Assessment. Collection of *subjective data* may include a patient complaint of an ulcerlike pain that does not respond to therapy. Anorexia, weakness, and indigestion are also common.

Collection of *objective data* may include weight loss, bleeding in the stools, hematemesis, and vomiting that results from a feeling of fullness after drinking fluids or eating meals.

Diagnostic tests. The tumor is diagnosed by x-ray studies (gastrointestinal series), endoscopic/gastroscopic examinations with biopsy, and gastric analysis. Carcinoembryonic antigen (CEA) is usually elevated in advanced gastric cancer.

Medical management. The most therapeutic management of stomach cancer is surgical removal. With early detection, cure is possible. Unfortunately, the purpose of the surgery may be exploratory to determine involvement or to make the patient more comfortable. A partial or total resection is the choice for an extensive lesion. Surgery for advanced gastric cancer carries high **morbidity** and mortality. At this time, patients with no intervention have a longer survival rate (approximately 11 months) than patients who have exploratory or palliative surgical procedures (4 or 5 months).

Wound healing may be disrupted by **dehiscence**, a partial or complete separation of the wound edges, or by **evisceration**, when the patient's viscera protrude through the disrupted wound (see Fig. 26-7). Dehiscence and evisceration may be caused by problems in suturing the wound or by poor tissue integrity. Some of the factors that may predispose a wound to dehiscence are excessive coughing, straining, malnutrition, obesity, and infection. Nursing interventions of the patient who has experienced dehiscence include instructing the patient to remain quiet and to avoid coughing or straining. The patient should be positioned to remove further stress on the wound. If evisceration occurs, the patient is kept on bed rest and the protruding viscera is loosely covered with a warm, sterile saline dressing. The surgeon should be notified immediately, since treatment consists of reapproximating the wound edges (see Chapter 26).

Chemotherapy has greater response rates and survival time than radiation. Radiation when combined with chemotherapy has been more effective. These two treatment modalities are often used in conjunction with surgery.

Nursing interventions. The nurse should provide further clarification of the disease and the surgical intervention to the patient and family. The preoperative preparation includes improving the patient's nutritional status by monitoring hyperalimentation and providing supplemental diet feedings. Postoperative teaching is necessary to relieve anxiety and promote understanding of drainage tubes, feeding tubes, dressing changes, weakness, medications, and other routine care.

NURSING DIAGNOSES	NURSING INTERVENTIONS
Ineffective breathing pattern, related to pain, exploration of chest and abdominal cavities, and abdominal distention	Place patient in semi-Fowler's position to aid ventilation. Encourage and assist with gentle turning and repositioning. Encourage patient to turn, breathe deeply, and cough at least q 2 hr until patient is ambulating well; splint incision before patient coughs; encourage ambulation.
Potential for injury, related to aspiration, infection, hemorrhage, anastomotic leak into abdominal cavity, and anemia/vitamin deficiency	Monitor closely for elevated temperature, bleeding from incision, pallor, dyspnea, cyanosis, tachycardia, increased respirations, and chest pain. Monitor laboratory results and activity tolerance because of possible anemia. Change dressings, using sterile technique.

Patient teaching. Because care encompasses so many areas, instruction should be (1) planned according to the patient's needs and level of understanding, (2) given when the patient is free of pain and rested, and (3) communicated both verbally and in print. Surgery, chemotherapy, radiation therapy, continued nutritional needs, pain relief, and support groups for psychosocial needs should be explained.

Weight loss will indicate the need for additional caloric intake and can be measured by daily weights compared with the patient's normal weight before illness. Prevention of skin excoriation around the feeding tube is important. Hypermotility or diarrhea that follows radiation therapy can be treated with medication. Alternative methods of care for the debilitated patient and family may include referral for hospice care.

PATIENTS WITH INTESTINAL DISORDERS

Intestinal Infections

Etiology/pathophysiology. Intestinal infections are the invasion of the alimentary canal (both the small and large intestine) by pathogenic microorganisms that reproduce and multiply. The infectious agent can enter the body by several routes. The most common entry is through the mouth by contaminated food or water. Some intestinal infections occur as a result of person-to-person contact. Fecal-oral transmission occurs through poor handwashing after elimination. In active homosexual males, "gay bowel syndrome" is introduced by single-cell protozoal infections.

There are bacterial flora indigenous to the intestines to combat infection. Their presence can be altered through long-term antibiotic therapy. The impaired immune response in some individuals delays the body's attempt to destroy invading pathogens.

Infectious diarrhea causes secretion of fluid into the intestinal lumen. Clostridial and *Salmonella* bacteria are associated with intestinal infections. These bacteria produce toxic substances, and the mucosal cells respond by secreting water and electrolytes, causing an imbalance. The amount of fluid secreted exceeds the ability of the large intestine to reabsorb the fluid into the vascular system.

Clinical manifestations. Diarrhea is the most common manifestation of an intestinal infection. The fecal output has increased water content, and if the intestinal mucosa is directly invaded, the feces may contain blood and mucus.

Assessment. Collection of *subjective data* includes noting complaints of diarrhea, rectal urgency, ineffective and painful straining with defecation (**tenesmus**), nausea, and abdominal cramping.

Collection of *objective data* may include a fever greater than 102° F and vomiting. History taking will provide useful information regarding number and consistency of bowel movements, recent use of antibiotics, recent travel, food intake, and exposure to noninfectious causes of diarrhea. Noninfectious diarrhea may be caused by heavy metal poisoning, shellfish allergy, and ingestion of toxic mushrooms and fish toxins. Diarrhea from noninfectious causes is usually characterized by a short incubation period (minutes to hours after exposure).

Diagnostic tests. The key laboratory test for patients with intestinal infections is a stool culture. Other laboratory tests that may be included are blood chemistry studies to monitor changes in fluid and electrolyte status.

Medical management. Usually the treatment of intestinal infections is conservative, letting the body limit the infection. Antibiotics may be given in cases of prolonged or severe diarrhea with a stool positive for leukocytes. If fluid and electrolyte replacement is necessary to offset the losses from diarrhea, the oral route is usually sufficient. The intravenous route is indicated if the patient cannot take sufficient fluids orally.

The use of antidiarrheals and antispasmodic agents may actually increase the severity of the infection by prolonging the contact time of the microbe with the intestinal wall. Kaolin and pectin (Kaopectate) may be used to increase stool consistency. Bismuth subsalicylate (Pepto-Bismol) can effectively decrease intestinal secretions and decrease the diarrhea volume. These medications require large doses to be effective (30 to 60 ml every 30 minutes to 1 hour), and their use remains controversial.

Nursing interventions. The nurse must do a thorough assessment to determine the seriousness of the intestinal infection. Determining the onset of the disease and the number of people exposed is important, because the majority of GI infections are communicable and represent a community health problem. The nurse must also assess for fluid imbalance. This assessment should include measurement of postural changes in blood pressure, skin turgor, mucous membrane hydration, and urine output.

NURSING DIAGNOSES	NURSING INTERVENTIONS
Fluid volume deficit, related to excessive losses from diarrhea and vomiting	If oral intake can be tolerated, apple juice, clear carbonated beverages, clear broth, plain gelatin, and water should be offered. If intravenous feedings are required, these fluids should have electrolytes added.
Pain: abdominal, related to intestinal inflammation and diarrhea	Discontinue oral feedings if intestinal stimulation occurs. Bed rest may decrease abdominal peristalsis.
Altered nutrition: less than body requirements, related to decreased intake and decreased absorption	Monitor for decreasing episodes of diarrhea. Monitor blood pressure, mucous membranes, and urinary output. Monitor weight loss if symptoms are severe.
Impaired skin integrity: anal, related to excoriation from diarrhea	Promote hygiene and prevent additional excoriation by offering soothing ointments, sitz baths, and perineal washes after bowel movements.

Patient teaching. The nurse should instruct the patient to report the number, color, and consistency of bowel movements, abdominal cramping, and pain. The patient and family should understand the importance of handwashing after bowel movements to interrupt the fecal-oral route of transmission. Those family members responsible for food preparation should be made aware of the importance of proper methods of food preparation and storage to reduce the growth of infecting organisms.

Chronic Inflammatory Bowel Disease

Ulcerative colitis and Crohn's disease

Etiology/pathophysiology. Ulcerative colitis and Crohn's disease are chronic, episodic, inflammatory diseases and have many common features. Because the nursing interventions of these patients are similar, these conditions are discussed together. These disorders afflict young adults with education, careers, and the raising of families ahead of them. The two diseases are difficult to differentiate. It becomes necessary only if surgical intervention is considered, because the two require different interventions.

The causes of ulcerative colitis and Crohn's disease are unknown, although theories exist. These include viral infection, allergies to certain foods, immunological factors, and psychosomatic disorders. There seems to be a stronger association between Crohn's disease and altered immune mechanisms. In ulcerative colitis, the common enteric bacterium *E. coli* may play a role. Psychosomatic factors may cause, aggravate, or be a result of inflammatory bowel disease. The chronic illness, social isolation, and frustration cause difficulties in effective coping.

Ulcerative colitis and Crohn's disease appear more often in women, in the Jewish population, and in the nonwhite population; there seems to be a familial tendency.

The two diseases demonstrate different pathological features. The disease is confined to the mucosa and submucosa of the colon in ulcerative colitis. In Crohn's disease, the inflammatory process involves all layers of the bowel and can occur throughout the GI tract. Patients have been known to present features of both diseases, making a definite diagnosis difficult.

Ulcerative colitis can affect segments or the entire colon, depending on the staging. This disease usually starts on the left side of the colon and progresses to the right side. Tiny abscesses form, which grow and produce purulent drainage, sloughing of the mucosa, and subsequent ulceration. Capillaries become friable and bleed, causing the characteristic diarrhea containing pus and blood. Pseudopolyps are common in chronic ulcerative disease.

In Crohn's disease, all layers of the bowel are involved and the disease process can occur in any area of the GI tract. Again, segments or the entire colon may be involved. This disease usually starts at the right side of the colon in the area of the ileocecal valve and moves left. The disease progresses from granulomas of the mucosa and is characterized by cobblestone ulcerations along the mucosa, a thickening of the intestinal wall, and the formation of scar tissue. As the granulomas increase, deeper layers of the bowel wall are affected. The ulcers are likely to perforate and form fistulas that connect with the colon, bladder, or vagina. Scar tissue that forms prevents the normal absorption of food, and strictures may cause intestinal obstruction.

Clinical manifestations. The pathological findings of the two diseases differ in clinical manifestations and in particular individuals. Inflammatory bowel disease is characterized by **exacerbations** and **remissions**. Diarrhea is a predominant symptom.

Complication of ulcerative colitis includes toxic megacolon (toxic dilation of the large bowel). This life-threatening complication of inflammatory bowel disease occurs in less than 5% of patients. The bowel becomes distended and so thin that perforation could happen at any time. Clinical manifestations include a temperature of 104° F or more and abdominal distention. Carcinoma of the colon in patients who have had chronic ulcerative colitis for 10 to 15 years occurs in 40% to 50% of patients with total colonic involvement. Surgical intervention for treatment of this complication is usually necessary.

Assessment. Collection of *subjective data* for the patient with Crohn's disease includes noting the patient's list of vague complaints, possibly including abdominal, colicky pain, lethargy, and loss of appetite.

Collection of *objective data* for the patient with Crohn's disease includes complaints of diarrhea—three or four semisolid stools daily, containing mucus and pus but no blood. **Steatorrhea** may also be present if the ulceration extends high in the small intestine. Intestinal fistulas or poor absorption of bile salts by the ileum may cause stools to become watery. Fever and unexplained anemia may also occur. Anal diseases, such as fissures or fistulas in the anus, are common manifestations.

Collection of *subjective data* for the patient with ulcerative colitis includes complaints of rectal bleeding and abdominal cramping. Lethargy, a sense of frustration, and loss of control result from painful abdominal cramping and the unpredictable bowel movements.

Collection of *objective data* for the patient with ulcerative colitis includes weight loss, abdominal distention, fever, tachycardia, and leukocytosis. There may be as many as 15 to 20 liquid stools a day.

Diagnostic tests. Barium studies of the intestine, sigmoidoscopy and colonoscopy with possible biopsy, and checking the stool for melena aid the physician in diagnosis. Additional studies include radiological examination of the abdomen, determination of serum electrolytes, albumin, and liver function, and other hematological studies.

Medical management. The medical interventions chosen depend on the phase of the disease, whether the patient has ulcerative colitis or Crohn's disease, and the individual response to therapy. There are common treatment modalities for both diseases, including medication, diet intervention, and stress reduction.

Drug therapy. The four major categories of drugs used are (1) those that affect the inflammatory response, (2) antibacterial drugs, (3) drugs that affect the immune system, and (4) antidiarrheal preparations.

- Sulfasalazine (Azulfidine) containing acetylsalicylic acid is the drug of choice for mild chronic ulcerative colitis. It affects the inflammatory response and provides some antibacterial activity.
- Non-sulfa drugs include Dipentum, given orally, and Rowasa, given by retention enema.
- Corticosteroids are antiinflammatory drugs effective in relieving symptoms of moderate and severe colitis; they can be given systemically or topically.
- Flagyl is used in Crohn's perianal disease to treat bacterial infections caused by anaerobic microorganisms; it can be given orally or infused intravenously.
- Antidiarrheal agents are recommended over anticholinergic agents because anticholinergic drugs can mask obstruction or contribute to toxic colonic dilation. Loperamide (Imodium) may be used to treat cramping and diarrhea of chronic ulcerative colitis and Crohn's disease. Azathioprine (Imuran) is efficacious for treating the chronic ulcerative colitis patient also.

Diet therapy. Diet therapy that excludes milk products and highly spiced foods has been effective in approximately 20% of the patients. A high-protein, high-calorie diet is recommended for persons who are nutritionally deficient. Hyperalimentation may be used for nutrition, fluid, and electrolyte replacement in severe cases.

Stress control. Both ulcerative colitis and Crohn's disease are aggravated by stress. Identifying the factors that cause stress is the first step in controlling the disease. Working with the patient to find healthful coping mechanisms is part of the holistic approach in nursing interventions.

Surgical intervention. If an acute episode does not respond to treatment, if complications occur, or if the risk of cancer becomes greater because of the presence of chronic ulcerative colitis, surgical intervention is indicated (Box 31-2). Most surgeons prefer a conservative approach, removing only the diseased portion of the colon. The operations of choice may be a single-stage total proctocolectomy with construction of internal reservoir and valve (Kock's pouch, or Kock's continent ileostomy) (Fig. 31-11), total proctocolectomy with ileoanal anastomosis with or without construction of an internal reservoir, and temporary ileostomy. In the case of a poor-risk patient, a subtotal colectomy may be performed with ileostomy (Fig. 31-12). After the patient's recovery (approximately 2 to 4 months), removal of the rectum or construction of an internal reservoir can be done.

Today some patients view a permanent ileostomy as more forbidding than the disease itself. These surgical procedures are not without risk, and the patient may want to live with the disease and long-term risk of cancer rather than undergo the procedure.

Nursing interventions. Areas of nursing intervention in-

BOX 31-2 SURGICAL INTERVENTIONS

Colon resection: Removal of a portion of the large intestine and anastomosis of the remaining segment
Ileostomy: Surgical formation of an opening of the ileum onto the surface of the abdomen, through which fecal matter is emptied
Ileoanal anastomosis: Removal of the colon and rectum but the anus is left intact along with the anal sphincter; anastomosis is formed between the lower end of the small intestine and the anus
Proctocolectomy: Removal of anus, rectum, and colon; ileostomy is established for the removal of digestive tract wastes
Kock's pouch (Kock's continent ileostomy): Surgical removal of the rectum and colon (proctocolectomy) with formation of a reservoir by suturing loops of adjacent ileum together to form a pouchlike structure, nipple valve, and stoma.

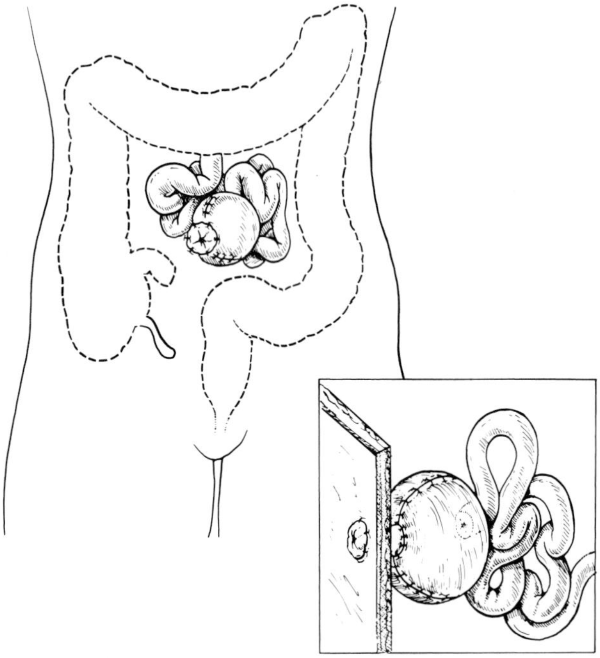

FIG. 31-11 Kock's pouch (Kock's continent ileostomy).

clude a thorough assessment of the patient's bowel elimination, knowledge level, support systems, coping abilities, nutritional status, pain, and ability to understand the disease process and treatment required. The patient needs a complete understanding of the plan of care so he can make informed choices. Prevention of future episodes is a goal for the ulcerative colitis patient. There is no known therapy that will maintain a patient with Crohn's disease in remission.

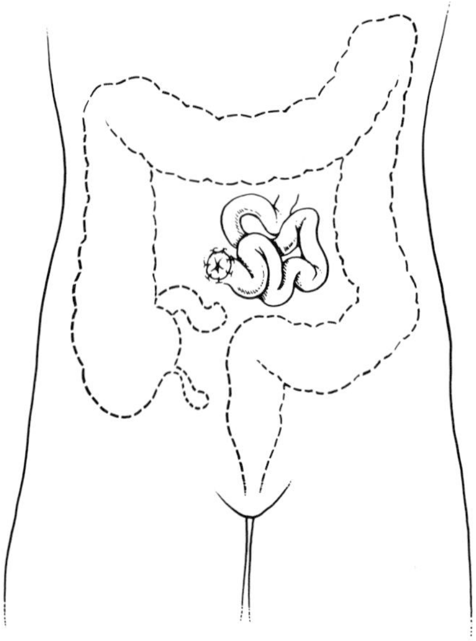

FIG. 31-12 Ileostomy with absence of resected bowel.

Preoperative care for these patients includes (1) selection of stoma site, (2) performing additional diagnostic tests if cancer is suspected, (3) allocation of time to accept that previous treatments were unsuccessful in curing the disease, and (4) preparation of the bowel for surgery. The bowel is prepared 2 or 3 days preoperatively. A bland to clear liquid diet is ordered, and a bowel prep of laxatives, GoLYTELY (an oral or NG colonic lavage/electrolyte solution [see Chapter 26]), and enemas as ordered (see Skill 31-1). Antibiotics, such an erythromycin and neomycin, are given to decrease the number of bacteria in the bowel.

Postoperative nursing interventions depend on the type of procedure performed and the individual's response. Areas of concern are bowel and urinary elimination, fluid and electrolyte balance, tissue perfusion, comfort/pain, nutrition, gas exchange, infection, and in the case of ostomy construction, assessment of the ileostomy and peristomal skin integrity.

NURSING DIAGNOSES	NURSING INTERVENTIONS
Knowledge deficit, related to lack of information about disease and treatment	Actively listen for 15 minutes daily. Explain disease process to patient and/or family. Instruct patient on dosage of medications and side effects.
Anxiety, related to unknown disease outcome	Examine stressors in patient's life and realistic ways to reduce them. Use regularly scheduled pain medication rather than PRN administration to manage pain.
Altered nutrition: less than body requirements, related to bowel hypermotility and decreased absorption	Provide small frequent meals, which will help patients with poor appetite or intolerance to larger amounts. Eliminate foods that aggravate condition.

NURSING DIAGNOSES	NURSING INTERVENTIONS
Diarrhea, related to bowel irritability	Keep bedpan or commode nearby; use room deodorizer to control odor. Offer support to patient during diagnostic and treatment phase.
Powerlessness, related to loss of control of body function	Assist weakened patient with activities of daily living (bathing, oral hygiene, shaving, and other grooming needs). Offer choices to patient, when possible, to facilitate patient control.

Nursing diagnoses for the surgical patient may be focused on potential ineffective individual coping, disturbance in self-esteem, and body image disturbance. Nursing interventions include reinforcement of the physician's explanation of the surgical procedure and expected outcomes. Providing reading material and demonstrating the care of an ostomy pouch when the patient demonstrates readiness will reduce anxiety. A visitor from the United Ostomy Association can provide hope, as a recovered and productive role model. The nurse should not expect *immediate* patient acceptance of the stoma; acceptance will be gradual. The nurse should be supportive and should encourage the patient to verbalize fears. See Box 31-3 for postoperative nursing interventions.

Peristomal area integrity. The nurse should assess the peristomal skin for impairment of integrity. Four primary factors contributing to loss of peristomal skin integrity are allergies, mechanical trauma, chemical reactions, and infection.

Allergies to pouches, adhesives, skin barriers, powders and paste, or belts are evident at areas of contact. The skin may appear erythematous, eroded, weeping, and bleeding. Avoidance of the irritant by changing the type of pouch, tape, or adhesive may resolve the problem.

Mechanical trauma caused by pressure, friction, or stripping of adhesives and skin barriers can be avoided by less frequent changes of the pouch, using adhesive tape sparingly, and wearing a belt only when the patient feels it is necessary. The skin must be protected when the pouch is removed.

The most common chemical irritant is the stool from the stoma. The skin must be protected from these digestive enzymes by using skin barriers before applying the pouch. Skin barriers include adhesives (Stomahesive), powders (Stomahesive power), liquid skin barriers (Skin Prep), and caulking paste (Stomahesive paste).

A common cause of infection of the peristomal skin is *Candida albicans*. Persons who have been on antibiotics for 5 or more days may be prone to this problem. Treatment is application of nystatin powder or cream, by physician order. A skin barrier should be applied over the medicated area to ensure adherence of the adhesive.

Patient teaching. The patient or significant other must be taught the appropriate care of the ileostomy or colostomy to foster independence (Skill 31-5). This includes pouch change, cleansing, irrigation, and skin care. A list of foods that are known to commonly cause problems of constipation, diarrhea, blockage, odors, and flatus is helpful. A list of resource people, phone numbers, where to obtain supplies, and what to ask for should be sent home with the patient.

BOX 31-3

POSTOPERATIVE NURSING INTERVENTIONS

1. Monitor nasogastric suction for patency until bowel function is resumed. Accurately record color and amount of output. Irrigate NG tube PRN. Apply water-soluble lubricant to nares. Assess bowel sounds, being certain to turn off NG suction when auscultating bowel sounds.
2. Initiate ostomy care and teaching when bowel activity begins. Nurse should be sensitive to patient's pain level and readiness for teaching of ostomy care.
3. Observe stoma for color and size (should be erythematous and slightly edematous).
4. Select pouch that has skin-protective barrier, accordion flange to ease pressure applied to new incisional site, adhesive backing, and pouch opening no more that 1/16 inch larger than stoma. Stomas change in size over time and should be measured before new supplies are ordered.
5. Empty pouch when it is approximately one-third full to prevent breaking seal, resulting in pouch leakage.
6. Explain that initial dark green liquid will change to yellow-brown as patient is allowed to eat.
7. Teach patient to care for his stoma; this includes having patient look at stoma and gradually assist with emptying, cleaning, and changing pouch; teach patient that normal grieving occurs after loss of rectal function. Be supportive of patient's concerns.
8. Promote independence and self-care to decrease state of denial.
9. Instruct on follow-up home care, including changing pouch every 5 to 7 days. Using antacids, skin protective paste, and liquid skin barrier may be appropriate if skin excoriation is observed.
10. Patient may shower or bathe with or without pouch on.
11. Patient should avoid lifting objects over 10 lb.
12. A special diet is not necessary, but should include 8 to 10 glasses of water, food should be chewed well, and certain gas-forming foods should be limited or avoided.
13. Sexual relationships can be resumed when physician feels it is not harmful to the surgical area. Counseling may be appropriate if patient has fear of resuming this activity.

SKILL 31-5 PERFORMING COLOSTOMY/ILEOSTOMY CARE

1. Introduce self.
2. Identify patient.
3. Wash hands.
4. Explain procedure.
5. Arrange supplies/equipment at bedside or in bathroom.
6. Pull curtain and close door to provide privacy.
7. Position patient so that stoma is easily accessible and patient is comfortable.
8. Don gloves.

NOTE:
As many of the following steps as possible should be performed by the patient with the nurse teaching and assisting as needed. Independence will come. Be alert to signs of patient readiness.

9. Unfasten and remove belt; carefully remove wafer seal from skin (adhesive solvent may be needed).
10. Place reusable pouch in bedpan or disposable pouch in plastic bag.
11. Cleanse skin with warm water; pat dry to avoid rubbing and skin impairment.
12. Measure stoma using measuring device.
13. Place toilet tissue over stoma; use gauze for ileostomy to prevent expelled stool from causing skin impairment; note color and viability of stoma. If using Skin Prep, apply to skin and allow to dry.
14. Apply protective stoma paste about 1/16 inch from stoma.
15. Apply protective wafer with flange, cutting an opening in the center of wafer 1/16 inch larger than stoma.
16. Gently attach pouch to flange by compressing the two together.
17. If Karaya seal pouch is used, moisten seal with a few drops of warm water until seal is sticky.
18. Remove tissue or gauze from stoma and backing from protectant; center opening over stoma, and press against skin for 1 to 2 minutes, smoothing outward with fingers.
19. If belt is used, attach at this time.
20. Assist patient to comfortable position in bed or chair; remove equipment from bedside.
21. Empty, wash, and dry reusable pouch.
22. Dispose of soiled supplies in plastic bag; remove gloves; wash hands.
23. Record procedure and observations.
24. Report abnormalities.

SKILL 31-6 PERFORMING UROSTOMY CARE

1. Introduce self.
2. Identify patient.
3. Wash hands.
4. Explain procedure.
5. Arrange supplies at bedside or in bathroom.
6. Pull curtain and close door to provide privacy.
7. Position patient so that stoma is easily accessible and patient is comfortable.
8. Don gloves.

NOTE:
As many of the following steps as possible should be performed by the patient with the nurse teaching and assisting as needed. Independence will come. Be alert to signs of patient readiness.

9. Empty urine into graduated pitcher; write down amount for later documentation.
10. Carefully remove wafer seal from skin (adhesive solvent may need to be used) and place pouch in plastic bag.
11. Cleanse skin with warm water, and pat dry to avoid rubbing and causing skin impairment.
12. Measure stoma using measuring device; note color and viability of stoma.
13. Place gauze over stoma to prevent urine from contacting skin.
14. If using Skin Prep, apply to skin and allow to dry; apply protective stoma paste about 1/16 inch from the stoma.
15. Apply protective wafer with flange, cutting an opening in the center of wafer 1/16 inch larger than stoma.
16. Gently attach pouch to flange by compressing the two together.
17. If belt is used, attach at this time.
18. Attach pouch to gravity drainage tubing if ordered.
19. Assist patient to comfortable position.
20. Clean and store equipment.
21. Dispose of soiled supplies in plastic bag; remove gloves; wash hands.
22. Record procedure and observations.
23. Report abnormalities to RN or physician.

Because of the similarities of nursing interventions for a patient with a urostomy, ileostomy, and colostomy, the skill of performing urostomy care is included in this chapter (Skill 31-6).

Acute Abdominal Inflammations

Appendicitis

Etiology/pathophysiology. Appendicitis is the inflammation of the vermiform appendix, usually acute, which if undiagnosed leads rapidly to perforation and peritonitis.

Appendicitis is most apt to occur in teenagers and young adults and is more common in males.

The vermiform appendix is a small tube in the right lower quadrant of the abdomen. The lumen of the proximal end is shared with that of the cecum, whereas the distal end is closed. The appendix fills and empties regularly in the same way as the cecum. However, the lumen is tiny and is easily obstructed. If it becomes obstructed and inflammation occurs, pathogenic bacteria (*Escherichia coli*) begin to multiply in the appendix and infection develops with the formation of pus. If distention and infection are severe enough, the appendix may rupture, releasing its contents into the abdomen. The infection may be contained within an appendiceal abscess or may spread to the abdominal cavity, causing generalized peritonitis.

Clinical manifestations. Light palpation of the abdomen will elicit rebound tenderness. The abdomen musculature overlying the right lower quadrant may feel tense as a result of voluntary rigidity. The patient will often be lying on his back or side with knees flexed in an attempt to decrease muscular strain on the abdominal wall.

Assessment. Collection of *subjective data* includes the most common complaint of constant pain in the right lower quadrant of the abdomen around McBurney's point (exactly halfway between the umbilicus and the crest of the right ilium). The pain may be accompanied by nausea and anorexia.

Collection of *objective data* includes vomiting, a low-grade fever (99° to 102° F), an elevated white blood count, rebound tenderness, a rigid abdomen, and decreased or absent bowel sounds.

Diagnostic tests. A white blood count with differential will be ordered. Approximately 90% of persons will have a WBC above 10,000/mm^3 and approximately 75% will have a neutrophil count above 75%. A flat film of the abdomen is helpful for diagnosis. When diagnosis is difficult, Hypaque contrast studies, ultrasound, and laparoscopy may be used.

Medical management. Emergency surgical intervention is the treatment of choice for acute appendicitis. It may be performed as an incidental procedure when a patient is having another abdominal surgical procedure. Because mortality correlates with perforation and perforation correlates with duration of symptoms, early diagnosis and appendectomy are essential for the lowest acceptable morbidity and mortality. Antibiotic therapy is given both prophylactically and when perforation is likely. Complications that can occur include infection, intraabdominal abscess, and mechanical small bowel obstruction.

Nursing interventions. The nursing interventions of the patient include following general preoperative procedure. The nurse should explain diagnostic tests and possible surgical procedures to relieve anxiety. Other interventions include bed rest, NPO status, comfort measures for pain relief so that symptoms will not be masked by medication, and the need for fluid and electrolyte replacement. The temperature, blood pressure, pulse, and respirations are monitored and documented every hour because of the threat of perforation with peritonitis.

No narcotics are given during diagnosis to prevent masking of symptoms; sedatives may be given if necessary. In some cases an ice bag to relieve pain is given; *no* heat is applied, since this may increase circulation to the appendix and lead to rupture. A cleansing enema is usually not ordered because of the danger of rupture. Postoperatively, a rectal tube may be inserted for relief of flatus (Skill 31-7). General postoperative care is performed (see Chapter 26).

NURSING DIAGNOSES	NURSING INTERVENTIONS
Knowledge deficit, related to disease process and surgery	Explain definition of diagnosis, diagnostic tests as they are ordered, and possible surgical intervention.
Fluid volume deficit, related to vomiting	Monitor patient for signs of dehydration and fluid and electrolyte imbalance (poor skin turgor, flushed dry skin, coated tongue, oliguria, confusion, and abnormal sodium, potassium, and chloride levels).
Pain, related to inflammation	Provide support to patient and family through listening and explanation of tests and procedures; explain need to withhold medications. Monitor increase in amount of pain experienced, rebound tenderness, and abdominal rigidity. Take vital signs frequently (q 15 min).
Potential for infection, related to rupture of appendix	Monitor incision site for pain, tenderness, and edema. Maintain sterile asepsis for dressing changes. Monitor temperature for elevation q 4 hr.

Patient teaching. Patient teaching may include the reason for intravenous fluids with gradual advancement of diet from clear liquids to general as peristalsis returns. If antibiotics or oral medications are continued postoperatively, the patient should understand the name, purpose, and side effects of each medication. If complications occur necessitating an NG tube or drainage tubes, the nurse should ensure the patient understands the reason for these interventions.

SKILL 31-7 INSERTING A RECTAL TUBE

1. Introduce self.
2. Identify patient.
3. Wash hands.
4. Explain procedure.
5. Arrange equipment at bedside.
6. Pull curtain and close door to provide privacy.
7. Have patient assume side-lying position, and arrange gown and top linens out of the way yet covering patient.
8. Place waterproof pad under buttocks.
9. Don gloves, and lubricate tube well with petrolatum or water-soluble lubricant.
10. Expose anus, and insert tube 4 to 6 inches (10 to 15 cm).
11. Insert drainage end into receptacle, or use commercially prepared set.
12. Instruct patient to lie quietly to prevent dislodgement of tube; leave tube in place no more than 30 minutes or as ordered.
13. Remove tube and assist patient to bedpan, bedside commode, or toilet as necessary; stimulation of peristalsis may result in bowel movement.
14. Provide for patient hygiene; assist patient to bed or chair.
15. Dispose of equipment and supplies; remove gloves, and wash hands.
16. If flatulence, abdominal discomfort, or distention continues, reinsert tube PRN or as ordered by physician.
17. Record procedure and observations.
18. Report abnormalities.

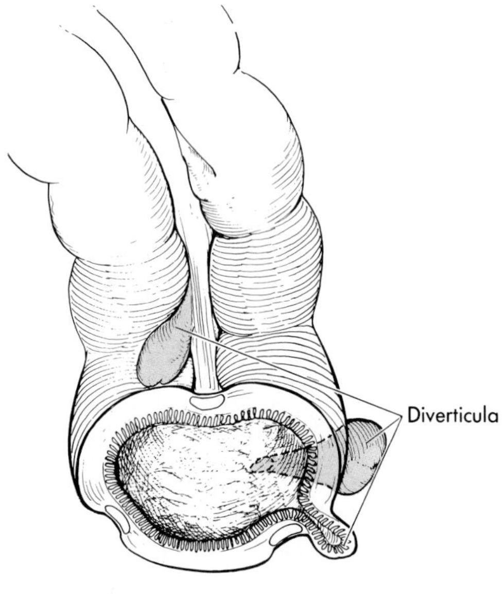

FIG. 31-13 Diverticuli of colon.

Diverticular disease of colon

Etiology/pathophysiology. Diverticular disease has two clinical forms, *diverticulosis* and *diverticulitis*. Diverticulosis is the presence of pouchlike herniations through the muscular layer of the colon, particularly the sigmoid colon (Fig. 31-13). Diverticulitis is the inflammation of one or more diverticula.

Diverticulosis affects increasing numbers of people over 50 years of age and may be the result of the modern, highly refined, low-residue diet. The penetration of fecal matter through the thin-walled diverticula causes inflammation and abscess formation in the tissues surrounding the colon. With repeated inflammation, the lumen of the colon narrows and may become obstructed. When one or more diverticula become inflamed, diverticulitis results, which is a complication of diverticulosis. This inflammation can lead to perforation, abscess, peritonitis, obstruction, and hemorrhage.

Clinical manifestations. When diverticula perforate and diverticulitis develops, the patient will complain of mild to severe pain in the lower left quadrant of the abdomen and will have fever and an elevated white blood cell count and sedimentation rate. If the condition goes untreated, septicemia and septic shock can develop. This patient will be hypotensive and have a rapid pulse. Intestinal obstruction can occur, and the patient will experience abdominal distention, nausea, and vomiting.

Assessment. Collection of *subjective data* includes an awareness that the patient with diverticulosis may not display any problematic symptoms. Subjective complaints of constipation and diarrhea accompanied by pain in the left lower quadrant are common to some. Other common symptoms include increased flatus and chronic constipation alternating with diarrhea, anorexia, and nausea.

Collection of *objective data* may include abdominal distention, low-grade fever, vomiting, and blood in the stool.

Diagnostic tests. Hypaque contrast studies are preferred over barium enema for diagnostic studies because there is less chance of bowel rupture. Both will visualize the outpouchings along with the distortions and narrowing of the lumen. Colonoscopy may be beneficial in diagnosing certain cases and is especially helpful in ruling out carcinoma.

Medical management. The treatment of diverticulosis depends on the cause. If muscle atrophy is responsible for the disease, a low-residue diet, stool softeners, and bed rest are traditional interventions. When increased intracolonic pressure and muscle thickening are causes, a high-fiber diet of bran, fruits, and vegetables is recommended. Sulfa drugs have been used to treat uncomplicated signs of inflammation. Microperforation resulting in localized abscess is treated with a combination of antimicrobials effective against Gram-negative, Gram-positive, and anaerobic organisms. Analgesics are given intramuscularly for pain. Patients with acute attacks of diverticulitis that do not respond to antibiotics and bed rest may require hospitalization with nasogastric drainage, parenteral fluids, and intravenous antibiotics.

Surgical treatment is advised if long-term problems do not respond to medical management and is mandatory if complications, such as hemorrhage, obstruction, abscesses, or perforation, occur. In elective surgery a thorough bowel preparation is most important. Laxatives, enemas, or intestinal lavage by GoLYTELY, as discussed, are given to cleanse the bowel, depending on the surgeon's preference. Antibiotics are given orally and parenterally.

In cases of perforation, abscess, peritonitis, or fistula, resection of the bowel with a temporary colostomy is needed. Either the one-stage procedure (resection of the affected bowel with **anastomosis** and no diverting colostomy) or the two-stage procedure (resection of the diseased bowel with diverting colostomy) is performed.

The bowel diversion can be accomplished by the Hartmann's procedure (Fig. 31-14) where the descending colon is resected, the proximal end is brought to the abdominal wall surface, and the distal bowel is sealed off for later anastamosis. The second procedure is the double-barrel colostomy, where the bowel is brought up through the abdominal surface, or loop colostomy (Figs. 31-15 and 31-16). The bowel can be opened at the time of surgery or postoperatively. Removal of the affected bowel segment and reanastomosis of the bowel are done during the initial procedure.

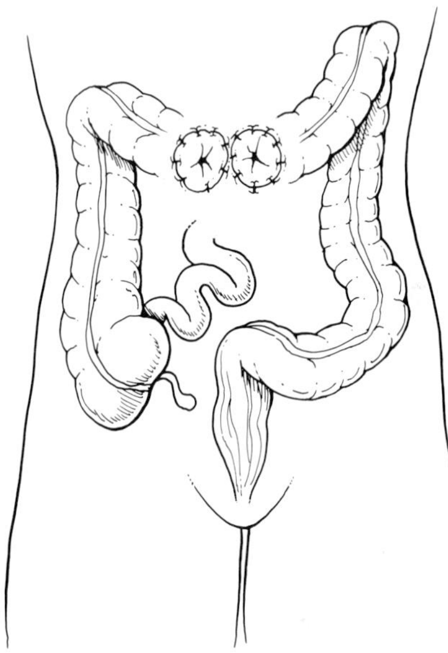

FIG. 31-15 Double-barrel transverse colostomy.

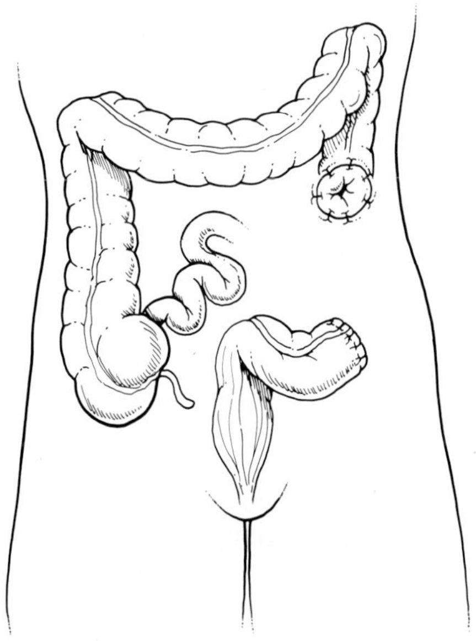

FIG. 31-14 Hartmann's pouch.

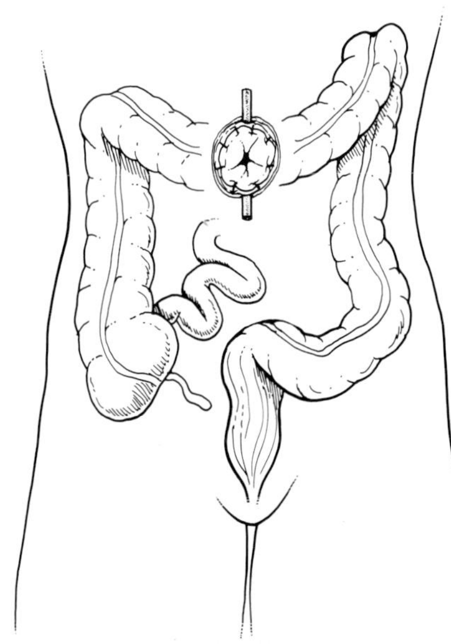

FIG. 31-16 Transverse loop colostomy with rod/butterfly.

Closure of the temporary colostomy is the desired goal in the case of diverticular disease. Usually this is done from 6 weeks to 3 months after the initial surgical procedure. Again, the bowel must be prepared for closure by a liquid diet, laxatives, antibiotics, intestinal lavage as mentioned, and a cleansing colostomy irrigation of the proximal and, in the case of the loop or double-barrel colostomy, distal end of the stoma.

Nursing interventions. Nurses should remember that when the distal loop is irrigated, irrigating solution and bowel contents will usually return from both the distal opening and rectum, so placement of the patient on the toilet or bedpan is important during the procedure.

The return of bowel activity after closure may take several days. The patient will again have intravenous fluids and a nasogastric tube for the first few days postoperatively.

Nursing interventions include patient teaching of the disease process and surgery, if planned. The nutritional status must be assessed and discussion and reinforcement given as needed. The nurse should determine the nature of the pain the patient is having so that interventions of comfort measures or medication can be administered to provide relief. The patient and family should be included in the goals of the teaching plan.

NURSING DIAGNOSES	NURSING INTERVENTIONS
Knowledge deficit, related to disease process and treatment	Instruct patient and significant others in disease process and signs and symptoms of acute diverticulitis attack.
Altered nutrition: less than body requirements, related to decreased oral intake	Instruct in dietary roughage (for prevention) or bland, low-residue diet (for inflammatory phase).
Pain, related to inflammation of bowel	Administer proper diet to prevent aggravation; administer analgesics as ordered for pain. Provide uninterrupted periods of rest.
Anxiety, related to concerns about surgery	Explain diagnostic tests, reason for surgery if necessary, and possibility of temporary colostomy and what this means. Spend additional time listening to patient.
Potential for infection, related to abscesses, perforation, purulent drainage, and fecal material	Observe wound and drain sites frequently for signs of infection. Perform meticulous wound care if wound is left open for drainage. Monitor for elevated temperature q 4 hr.

Patient teaching. When a colostomy is performed, the patient or significant other should be able to verbalize and demonstrate understanding of the ostomy care to the nurse. The teaching of colostomy care should not be rushed and must be done when the patient is free of pain and receptive to learning. A family member may be taught to help the patient until he is able to assume self-care, keeping in mind that the ultimate goal is patient independence. A home care referral may be needed so that the teaching process can continue after discharge.

Peritonitis

Etiology/pathophysiology. Peritonitis is an inflammation of the abdominal peritoneum. This condition occurs after fecal matter seeps from the rupture site, causing bacterial contamination of the peritoneal cavity. Some examples may be diverticular abscess and rupture, acute appendicitis with rupture, and strangulated hernia. Chemical irritation can also cause peritonitis. Blood, bile, necrotic tissue, pancreatic enzymes, or foreign bodies are examples of these chemical irritants.

Clinical manifestations. Generalized peritonitis is an extremely serious condition characterized by severe abdominal pain. The patient usually lies on his back with the knees flexed to relax the abdominal muscles; any movement is painful. The abdomen is usually tympanic and extremely tender to the touch.

Assessment. Collection of *subjective data* includes observing for severe abdominal pain; any movement is painful. Nausea and vomiting occur, and as peristalsis ceases, constipation occurs with no passage of flatus. Chills, weakness, and abdominal tenderness (local and diffuse, often rebound) are also subjective data manifested.

Collection of *objective data* includes noting a weak and rapid pulse, fever, and lowered blood pressure. Leukocytosis and marked dehydration occur, and the patient can collapse and die.

Diagnostic tests. A flat plate of the abdomen is ordered to ascertain if free air is present under the diaphragm as a result of visceral perforation. A CBC with differential is ordered to determine the degree of leukocytosis present. A blood chemistry profile to determine renal perfusion and electrolyte balance is done.

Medical management. Aggressive therapy includes correction of the contamination or removal of the chemical irritant by surgery, and parenteral antibiotics. Nasogastric intubation is ordered to prevent gastrointestinal distention. Intravenous fluids and electrolytes will prevent or correct imbalances.

Nursing interventions. Nursing interventions for the patient with peritonitis include the following:

1. Place patient on bed rest in semi-Fowler's position to help localize purulent exudate in lower abdomen or pelvis.
2. Give oral hygiene to prevent drying of mucous membranes and cracking of lips from dehydration.
3. Monitor fluid and electrolyte replacement.
4. Encourage deep breathing exercises; patient tends to have shallow respirations as a result of abdominal pain or distention.
5. Use measures to reduce anxiety.
6. Use meticulous surgical asepsis for wound care.

Patient teaching. The nurse should instruct the patient of the importance of ambulation, coughing, deep breathing, and leg exercises. If the patient has a draining wound at discharge, he should be taught surgical asepsis for dressing changes. A nutritious diet is encouraged. The patient should be instructed not to lift more than 10 pounds until instructed by the physician to do so. The importance of the patient keeping physician follow-up appointments is stressed.

Hernias

Abdominal hernia

Etiology/pathophysiology. Most hernias result from congenital or acquired weakness of the abdominal wall or postoperative defect, coupled with increased intraabdominal pressure from coughing, straining, or an enlarging lesion within the abdomen.

The different types of hernias include abdominal, femoral or inguinal, hiatal, and umbilical. A femoral or inguinal hernia is caused by a weakness in the lower abdominal wall opening through which the spermatic cord emerges in men and the round ligament emerges in women. A hiatal hernia (esophageal hernia or diaphragmatic hernia) results from a weakness of the diaphragm (see discussion on hiatal hernia). An umbilical hernia is when the rectus abdominis muscle is weak, and the bowel protrudes against the umbilicus.

A hernia may be reducible (i.e., can be returned to its original position by manipulation) or irreducible (cannot be returned to its body cavity). An incarcerated hernia is when the intestinal flow is obstructed. The hernia is strangulated when the blood supply is occluded. Immediate surgical intervention is performed when a hernia strangulates, to prevent anaerobic infection in this affected area.

Factors such as age, wound infection, malnutrition, obesity, increased intraabdominal pressure, or abdominal distention affect formation of hernias after surgical incisions. Fewer hernias occur with transverse incisions than with longitudinal incisions. Also, upper abdominal incisions are associated with fewer hernias than lower abdominal incisions.

Assessment. Collection of *subjective data* includes palpation of the hernia area, revealing the contents of the sac as soft and nodular (omentum) or smooth and fluctuant (bowel). At no time should the nurse attempt to reduce the sac in the ring, since this can lead to complications, such as rupture of the strangulated contents.

Both subjective and objective signs and symptoms depend on where the hernia occurs. With an inguinal hernia, the patient may complain of pain, urgency, and the presence of a mass in the groin region.

Collection of *objective data* includes visibility of a protruding mass or bulge around the umbilicus, in the inguinal area, or near an incision; this is the most common objective sign. If complications such as incarceration or strangulation follow, there may be bowel obstruction, vomiting, and abdominal distention.

Diagnostic tests. The diagnosis is aided by palpation of the weakened wall. X-ray films of the suspected area are diagnostic tests that may be ordered.

Medical management. Hernias that cause no discomfort can be left unrepaired unless strangulation or obstruction follows. The patient should be taught to seek medical advice promptly if abdominal pain, distention, changing bowel habits, temperature elevation, nausea, and/or vomiting occurs. If the hernia can be reduced manually, a truss or firm pad placed over the hernia site and held in place with a belt prevents the hernia from protruding and holds abdominal contents in place.

Elective surgery for hernia repair may be done because of the inconvenience to the patient or constant risk of strangulation. A procedure to close the hernia defect by approximating adjacent muscles or using a synthetic mesh is done either on an inpatient or outpatient basis.

Nursing interventions. The nursing interventions of the patient with an abdominal hernia require observation of the hernia's location and size; the patient may be limited in activity and the type of clothing he can wear. Tissue perfusion to the area should be observed.

Open abdominal surgery may be necessary for the patient with a strangulated hernia. The patient should be prepared for a longer hospitalization, which may include nasogastric suctioning, intravenous antibiotics, fluid and electrolyte replacement, and parenteral pain medication until peristalsis returns.

Postoperatively the patient should be monitored for urinary retention, wound infection at the incision site, and with inguinal hernia repair, scrotal edema. If scrotal edema is present, it may be decreased by elevating the scrotum on a rolled pad, applying an ice pack, and providing a supportive garment (jockstrap or Jockey shorts). The patient should deep breathe every 2 hours, but many physicians discourage coughing. The nurse should verify the postoperative orders. The patient should be taught support of the incision by splinting the area with pillow or pad. This support along with analgesics will help to relieve pain.

NURSING DIAGNOSES	NURSING INTERVENTIONS
Knowledge deficit, related to disease process	Instruct patient to observe and report hernias that become nonreducible, begin to become edematous, or produce increased pain. Abdominal distention and change in bowel habits should be reported also.
Pain, related to tissue edema	Explain reason to avoid prolonged standing, lifting, or straining. Instruct patient to support weakened area by use of truss or manually as needed (as when coughing).

NURSING DIAGNOSES	NURSING INTERVENTIONS
Altered tissue perfusion, related to strangulation/incarceration of hernia	Monitor patient for increased pain, distention, changing bowel habits, temperature elevation, nausea, and vomiting. Report changes in appearance and signs and symptoms to physician.

Patient teaching. Follow-up care includes teaching the patient to limit activities and avoid lifting heavy objects or straining with bowel movements for 5 to 6 weeks. Also the patient should immediately report to the physician any erythema or edema of the surgical area or increased pain or drainage.

Hiatal hernia. Hiatal hernia is a protrusion of the stomach and other abdominal viscera through an opening in the membrane or tissue of the diaphragm (Fig. 31-17). A hiatal hernia is the most common problem of the diaphragm that affects the alimentary tract. A hiatal hernia is an anatomical condition and not a disease. This condition occurs in about 40% of the population, and most people display few, if any, symptoms. The major difficulty in symptomatic patients is gastroesophageal reflux, and these patients present with complaints of pyrosis (heartburn) after overeating. Complications of strangulation, infarction, or ulceration of the herniated stomach are serious and require surgical intervention. Factors contributing to the development of these hernias include obesity, trauma, and a general weakening of the supporting structures as a result of aging.

Medical management. The physician may select one of the following procedures:

- A posterior gastropexy, where the stomach is returned to the abdomen and sutured in place.
- Transabdominal or transthoracic fundoplication, where the fundus is wrapped around the lower part of the esophagus and sutured in place (Fig. 31-18).

Nursing interventions. Nursing care of the patient after surgery is similar to that after gastric surgery or thoracic surgery, depending on the procedure performed (see Chapter 26).

Intestinal Obstruction

Etiology/pathophysiology. An intestinal obstruction is any obstruction that results in failure of the contents of the intestine to pass through the lumen of the bowel (Fig. 31-19). Some conditions do not cause occlusion, but decrease peristalsis. This is referred to as *paralytic ileus.*

Most obstructions occur in the ileum, which is the narrowest segment of the small intestine. Adhesions or incarcerated hernias cause 90% of all obstructions. Other causes include impacted feces, tumor of the bowel, intussusception (prolapse of one segment of bowel into the lumen of another segment), **volvulus,** (a twisting of bowel onto itself), or the strictures of inflammatory bowel disease. Residues from foods high in fiber, such as raw coconut or fruit pulp, can also obstruct the small bowel.

When the small intestine becomes obstructed, the normal process of secretion and reabsorption of 7 to 8 liters of electrolyte-rich fluid is interrupted. Large amounts of fluid, bacteria, and swallowed air build up in the bowel proximal to the obstruction. Water and salts shift from the circulatory system to the intestinal lumen, causing distention and further interference with absorption. Increased capillary permeability results, allowing bacterial movement across the bowel.

Clinical manifestations. The signs and symptoms of intestinal obstruction vary with the site and degree of obstruction. During partial or early phases of mechanical obstruction, auscultation of the abdomen will reveal loud, frequent, high-pitched sounds, but when smooth muscle atony (weak, lacking normal tone) occurs, bowel sounds will be absent.

Assessment. Collection of *subjective data* should include information about the pattern of the patient's pain, including onset, frequency, and characteristics. Complaints of early intestinal obstruction of the small intestine include spasms of cramping abdominal pain as peristaltic activity increases proximal to the obstruction. As the obstruction progresses, the intestine becomes fatigued and there may be periods of decreased or absent bowel sounds and complaints of increased abdominal pain. Any history

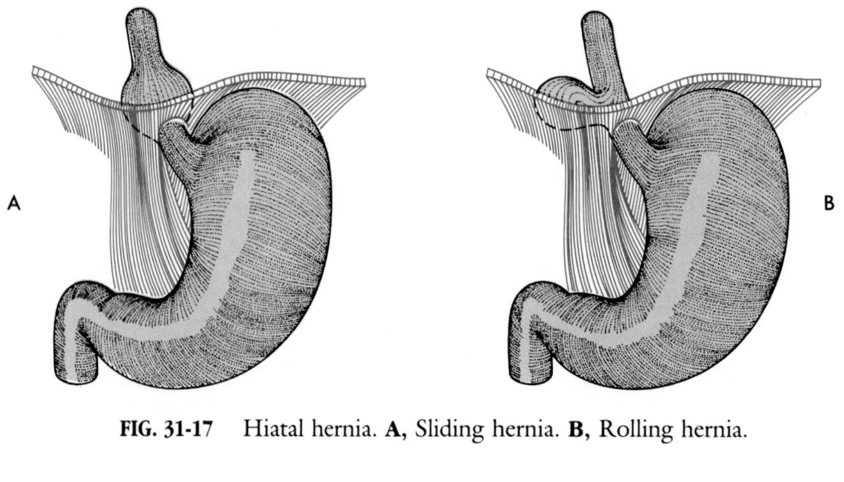

FIG. 31-17 Hiatal hernia. **A,** Sliding hernia. **B,** Rolling hernia.

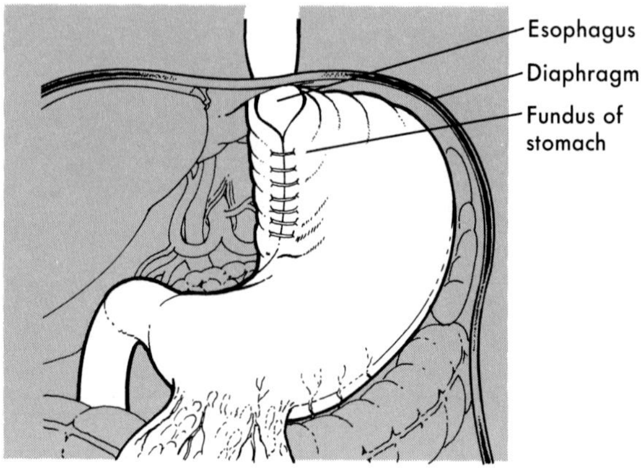

FIG. 31-18 Nissen fundoplication for hiatal hernia showing fundus of stomach wrapped around distal esophagus and sutured to itself.

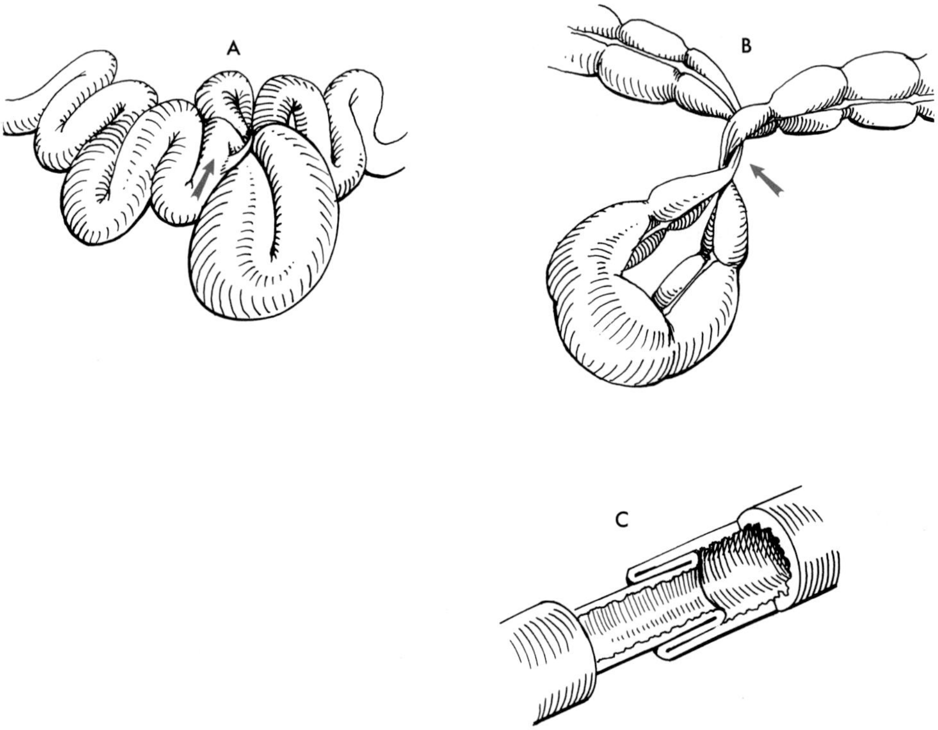

FIG. 31-19 Some causes of intestinal obstruction. **A,** Constriction by adhesions. **B,** Volvulus. **C,** Intussusception.

of previous bowel disorders or abdominal surgeries and changes in bowel elimination should be noted.

Collection of *objective data* begins with assessment of the patient's abdomen. The abdominal surface is inspected for evidence of distention, hernias, scars indicating previous surgeries, or visible peristaltic waves. The increased peristaltic activity produces an increase in auscultated bowel sounds. Other objective data include vomiting, signs of dehydration caused by the fluid shift, abdominal tenderness and muscle guarding, and decreased blood pressure.

Obstruction of the colon causes less severe pain than obstruction of the small intestine, marked abdominal distention, and constipation. The patient with a bowel obstruction may continue to have bowel movements. The colon distal to the obstruction continues to empty.

Diagnostic tests. X-ray examination reveals the level of obstruction and its cause. The fluid and electrolyte balance can be monitored through laboratory test results. Elevated blood urea nitrogen (BUN) and decreased serum sodium, potassium, and magnesium are common. The patient's hemoglobin and hematocrit may be in-

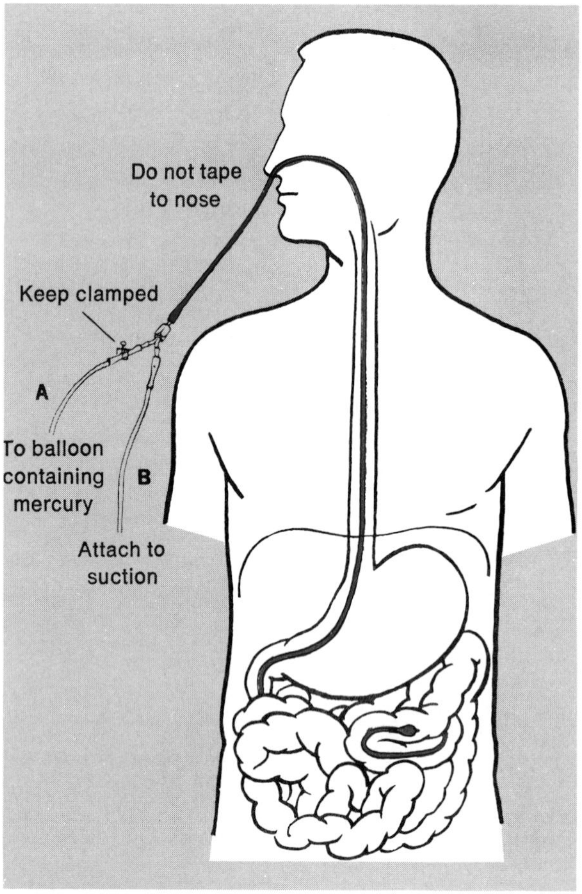

FIG. 31-20 Intestinal decompression tube in place. Note that tube is not taped to nose. **A,** Arm of Y-tube leading to balloon containing mercury or air must be kept clamped. **B,** Arm of Y-tube is attached to rubber tubing leading to suction.

creased because of hemoconcentration associated with the fluid volume deficit.

Medical management. Treatment includes the evacuation of intestinal contents by means of an intestinal tube. A nasogastric or nasojejunal tube will be inserted to decompress the intestine. The use of a long nasointestinal tube with a mercury weight at the distal portion of the tube helps relieve an obstruction (Fig. 31-20). Surgical repair is necessary to relieve mechanical obstructions caused by adhesions and hernias. Fluid and electrolyte balances are restored by carefully monitored intravenous infusion. Nonnarcotic analgesics are usually prescribed to avoid the decrease in intestinal motility that often accompanies the administration of narcotic analgesics.

Nursing interventions. Unless surgery is indicated, the nursing intervention consists of careful monitoring of fluids and electrolytes, observation of the function of tubes used to decompress and relieve distention, and the administration of analgesics.

For the patient with intestinal obstruction undergoing surgery, the preoperative preparation will include explanations of the procedure at a level the patient can understand. Emotional support for the patient will be important because the patient is experiencing not only the stressors of pain and vomiting, but also the added stressor of emergency surgery.

The postoperative nursing interventions are similar to those for any patient who has had abdominal surgery (see Chapter 26). The nurse should place the patient in Fowler's position for greater diaphragm expansion and should encourage the patient to breathe through the nose and not swallow air, which would increase distention and discomfort. She should encourage deep breathing and coughing. Nasointestinal suctioning will be continued until bowel activity returns. The nurse should assess for bowel sounds and abdominal girth to help to determine the return of peristalsis. Some patients may require temporary bowel diversion in the form of a double barrel or loop colostomy to manage the obstruction.

NURSING DIAGNOSES	NURSING INTERVENTIONS
Pain, acute, related to increased peristalsis	Reposition patient frequently to help intestinal tube advance. Irrigate suction tubing with sterile saline to keep tube patent. Explain purpose of all procedures. Provide comfort measures. Administer analgesics as ordered.
Fluid volume deficit, related to increased losses from vomiting and shift of fluids	Monitor for signs of dehydration, decreased blood pressure, change in laboratory values, and decreased urine output. Record and report frequency, amount, and nature of emesis. Record urine output.
Impaired gas exchange, related to abdominal distention	Observe for changes in size, tenderness, and bowel sounds in abdomen. Note any change in respiratory pattern and increased anxiety. Monitor arterial blood gas returns, reporting changes as they occur.

Patient teaching. Follow-up teaching focuses on prevention and includes dietary management, prevention of constipation, and recognition of early symptoms of recurrence and the need to seek prompt medical care. For the patient with a temporary ostomy, follow-up care will be necessary as plans are made for closure of the stoma.

Cancer of the Colon

Etiology/pathophysiology. Malignant neoplasms that invade the epithelium and surrounding tissue of the colon and rectum are the second most prevalent internal cancers in the United States. Colon cancer has an estimated 50% cure rate.

In the colon, 45% of growths are seen in the sigmoid and rectal areas, 25% in the cecum and ascending colon, and the remaining 30% are in the transverse splenic flexure, hepatic flexure, and descending colon. Cancer occurs with the same frequency in men and women, with the highest incidence in the ages of 60 years and older.

The cause of colorectal cancer remains unknown, but certain conditions appear to be more prone to malignant changes. These conditions are termed *predisposing* or *risk factors*. Particular diseases over time, including ulcerative colitis and diverticulosis, increase the risk of colorectal cancer. Neoplastic polyps or adenomas may undergo malignant change and become frank carcinomas. There are stronger tendencies in certain families, making history taking and regular check-ups important preventive measures. Other factors implicated in colorectal cancer include lack of bulk in the diet, high fat intake, and high bacterial counts in the colon. It is theorized that carcinogens are formed from degraded bile salts, and the stool that remains in the large bowel for a longer period as a result of too little fiber to stimulate its passage may overexpose the bowel to these carcinogens. There is also a theory that the increased transit time for low-fiber diets to pass through the intestine is related to malignancy. These factors have encouraged diet changes, with decreased animal fat and increased complex carbohydrates and dietary fiber as a primary preventive measure.

Clinical manifestations. Symptoms of cancer of the colon vary with the location of the growth.

Assessment. Collection of *subjective data* includes complaints of a change in bowel habits alternating between constipation and diarrhea. Constipation is more likely produced by descending colon cancer, while ascending colon cancer may occur with no change in bowel habits (Skill 31-8). The other complaint may be rectal bleeding, with the color varying from dark to bright red, depending on the location of the neoplasm. Later stages of colon cancer may include subjective symptoms of abdominal pain, nausea, and **cachexia** (weakness and emaciation associated with general ill health and malnutrition).

Collection of *objective data* includes observing for vomiting, weight loss, abdominal distention or ascites, and test results that are compatible with the diagnosis.

Diagnostic tests. Early diagnosis of the tumor, including identifying the type of cells involved, is the most important factor in treating the disease. Digital examination can identify 15% of colorectal cancers. Proctosigmoidoscopy can enable detection of 66% of these tumors. The fecal occult blood examination followed by proctosigmoidoscopy remains the most reliable tool for screening. Other laboratory and diagnostic studies include an upper GI series, radiological abdominal series, barium enema, CBC, electrolytes, and the blood test for **carcinoembryonic antigen (CEA).** Active malignancy growth within the body can be assayed by a blood test when cancer and metastasis are suspected. The CEA is a specific glycoprotein antigen in adenocarcinomas of the GI tract. Antibodies to this antigen are measured.

Medical management. Medical treatment includes radiation, chemotherapy, and surgery. Radiation therapy is often used before surgery to decrease the chance of cancer cell implantation at the time of resection. Radiation can both reduce the size of the tumor and decrease the rate of lymphatic involvement. There are few side effects from radiation before surgery, but there are complications.

Postoperatively those patients at high risk for recur-

SKILL 31-8

DIGITAL EXAMINATION WITH REMOVAL OF FECAL IMPACTION

1. Introduce self.
2. Identify patient and explain procedure.
3. Wash hands.
4. Arrange equipment at bedside.
5. Pull curtain and close door to provide privacy.
6. Place patient in left Sims' position, and place waterproof pad under patient's buttocks.
7. Place the bedpan on the bed close to the patient's buttocks.
8. Arrange patient's gown and top linen out of the way yet exposing only what is necessary.
9. Don gloves; lubricate forefinger well with petrolatum or water-soluble lubricant to reduce irritation.
10. Insert finger gently; slowly but gently move finger into and around the fecal mass; as pieces of the mass are broken off, remove them to bedpan.
11. Continue procedure until impaction is removed.
12. Stop procedure for a few minutes if patient complains of severe discomfort, to give patient opportunity to rest.
13. After removal is complete, wash and dry perineal area.
14. Remove waterproof pad and equipment; reposition patient.
15. Dispose of supplies; clean and return equipment.
16. Remove gloves; wash hands.
17. Record procedure and observations.
18. Report abnormalities.

rence or persons whose disease has progressed may receive radiation administered over 4 to 6 weeks (see Chapter 41 for a discussion of radiation).

Chemotherapy is given to patients (1) with systemic disease that is incurable by surgery or radiation alone, (2) in whom undetectable metastasis is suspected, or (3) for palliative therapy to reduce tumor size or relieve symptoms of the disease, such as obstruction or pain. Physician opinion and individual patient response regarding use of chemotherapy for colorectal cancer vary (see Chapter 41 for a discussion of chemotherapy).

Surgical interventions for treatment depend on the location of the tumor, presence of obstruction or perforation of the bowel, possible metastasis, the patient's health status, and the surgeon's preferences. When obstruction has not occurred, a portion of the bowel on either side of the tumor is removed and an end-to-end anastomosis is done between the divided ends. When obstruction of the bowel occurs, the commonly used procedures are as follows:

- One-stage resection with anastomosis.
- Two-stage resection with either (1) resection by bringing the ends of the bowel to the surface and creating a temporary colostomy and mucus fistula or Hartmann's pouch (see Fig. 31-14), (2) a double-barrel colostomy (see Fig. 31-15), or (3) a temporary loop colostomy (see Fig. 31-16), for closure later.

Surgical procedures for colorectal cancer include the following:

- Right hemicolectomy: resection of ascending colon and hepatic flexure (Fig. 31-21, *A*); ileum anastomosed to transverse colon.
- Left hemicolectomy: resection of splenic flexure, descending colon, and sigmoid colon (Fig. 31-21, *B*); transverse colon anastomosed to rectum.
- Anterior rectosigmoid resection: resection of part of

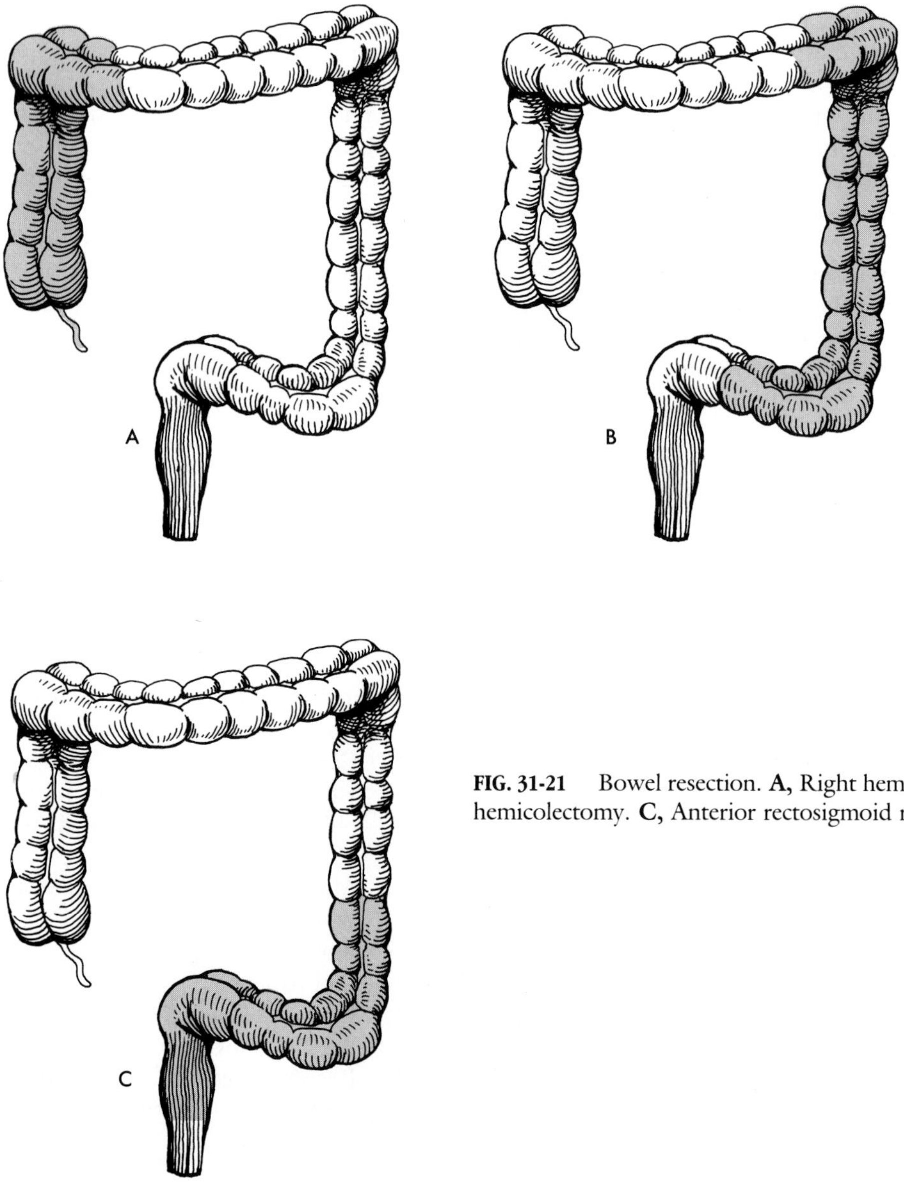

FIG. 31-21 Bowel resection. **A,** Right hemicolectomy. **B,** Left hemicolectomy. **C,** Anterior rectosigmoid resection.

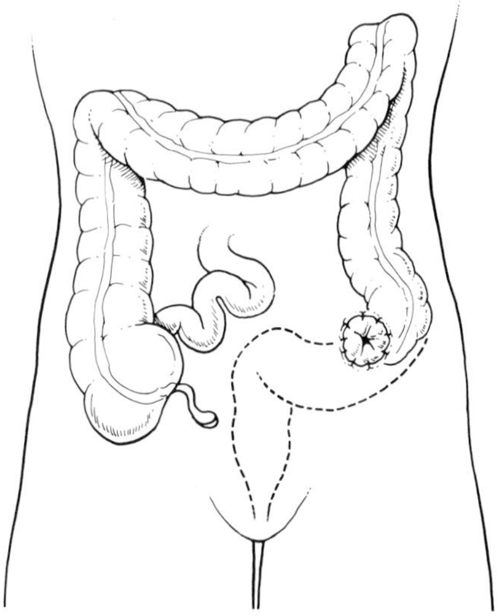

FIG. 31-22 Descending/sigmoid colostomy.

descending colon, the sigmoid colon, and upper rectum (Fig. 31-21, *C*); descending colon anastomosed to remaining rectum.

In carcinoma of the rectum every effort is made by the surgeon to preserve the sphincter. An end-to-end anastomosis is often used. If the surgeon is unable to do an anastomosis, an abdominoperineal resection may be done. This refers to removal of the colon and rectum by way of the abdomen and the perineum. The proximal end of the descending colon is brought through the abdominal wall to form a permanent colostomy (Fig. 31-22).

Nutritional status is important because of the threat of infection and the postoperative healing process that may follow an already compromised state as a result of constipation, diarrhea, nausea, vomiting, and possible obstruction.

Nursing interventions. The assessment of bowel and urinary elimination, fluid and electrolyte balance, tissue perfusion, nutrition, comfort/pain, gas exchange, infection, and peristomal skin integrity was discussed previously in the chapter. Long-term complications of abdominal resection with permanent colostomy are urinary retention or incontinence, pelvic abscess, failure of perineal wound healing or wound infection, and sexual dysfunction.

In addition to monitoring the **stoma** for color, size, location, and the condition of the peristomal skin, the nurse must watch for possible complications. Common stoma complications in the immediate postoperative period are necrosis and abscess. Necrosis results from a compromised blood flow to the stoma, causing the stoma to appear pale and dusky to black. Abscess caused by stoma placement too close to the wound, retention sutures, and drains must be assessed promptly. All complications must be reported promptly to the surgeon and documented in the medical record.

NURSING DIAGNOSES	NURSING INTERVENTIONS
Altered nutrition: less than body requirements, related to vomiting and/or anorexia, surgical intervention, and depression	Maintain NPO status as ordered. Monitor parenteral fluids. Monitor patency and function of nasogastric tube. Measure intake and output. Monitor vital signs and serum electrolytes, Hct, and Hgb. Provide high-protein, high-carbohydrate, high-calorie, low-residue diet as allowed and tolerated.
Powerlessness, related to loss of control of bowel elimination	Involve the patient in decision making where possible. Foster independence in daily activities as soon as possible. Explain if surgical procedure is temporary.
Ineffective individual/family coping, related to illness/surgery and prognosis	Plan time for patient's verbalization. Listen carefully. Involve significant other in health teaching and decision making. Explain all procedures and treatments. Reinforce physician's explanations of disease process and prognosis. Assess present coping patterns, and identify strengths and weaknesses.
Knowledge deficit, related to home care needs and chemotherapy and/or radiotherapy	Provide information about diet, activity, and rest. Discuss medications: name, dosage, purpose, time of administration, and side effects. Explain side effects of chemotherapy and ways of managing them using other members of health team. Encourage follow-up visits with physician. Refer to community resource agencies as necessary.
Body image disturbance, related to loss of normal body function (colostomy)	Allow time for grieving. Assist patient and significant other in accepting ostomy. Allow time for and encourage verbalization. Answer all questions, and explain treatment and procedure. Provide care in positive manner; always avoid facial expressions connoting distaste. Observe for signs of denial, grief, or anger. Provide privacy and safe environment. Encourage self-care and independence when patient demonstrates readiness.

Patient education. The patient with a permanent end colostomy can be taught two forms of colostomy management: (1) emptying and cleansing the pouch as needed and (2) managing colostomy irrigation (Skill 31-9). Factors to consider in planning patient teaching are past bowel habits, location of colostomy, age of the patient,

SKILL 31-9 PERFORMING A COLOSTOMY IRRIGATION

1. Introduce self.
2. Identify patient.
3. Wash hands and explain procedure.
4. Pull curtain and close bathroom door to provide privacy.

NOTE:
As many of the following steps as possible should be performed by the patient with the nurse teaching and assisting as needed. Independence will come. Be alert to signs of patient readiness.

5. Arrange equipment at bedside or in bathroom.
6. Position patient:
   In bathroom—have patient sit on toilet or on chair in front of toilet.
   In bed—have patient lie comfortably with head elevated slightly.
7. Don gloves.
8. Remove pouch, cleanse skin, and place irrigation sleeve over stoma; attach belt if using; place end of sleeve in toilet.
9. Close clamp on irrigating tubing; fill irrigating container with 1000 ml tepid water (or as otherwise ordered). Container may be hung on a hook at patient's shoulder level. Allow a small amount of water to flow through tubing.
10. Attach cone to tubing; lubricate cone; insert cone into stoma through top of sleeve.
11. While holding cone in place, allow solution to flow slowly into colon. If patient complains of cramping, stop flow without removing cone until cramps subside.
12. After all solution is instilled, remove cone and close top of sleeve.
13. Instruct patient to sit about 15 minutes while returns flow into toilet.
14. Drain sleeve; rinse and remove it.
15. Observe patient and results of irrigation; flush toilet.
16. Perform colostomy care (see Skill 31-5).
17. Clean and dry irrigation equipment; dispose of nonreusable supplies; remove gloves, and wash hands.
18. Assist patient to comfortable position.
19. Record procedure and observations.
20. Report abnormalities.

general health of the patient, and the patient's personal preference.

Nerves that control the bladder may be damaged when a large amount of tissue is removed in the abdominoperineal resection. After the Foley catheter is removed after surgery, the patient may be unable to void or empty the bladder completely. If the problem does not resolve, the patient may need a Foley catheter and a urology consultation.

When a large amount of tissue is removed, as in the abdominoperineal resection, and a cavity is left as sanctuary for bacteria, there is increased risk of infection. The drain site is monitored for increased pain, erythema, and purulent drainage, and body temperature is monitored for elevation. The perineal wound may be closed in one of three ways. The closed wound with a drain to suction has a high risk for abscess formation. The semiclosed wound is partially closed with either a Davol or Penrose drain that is left in place longer, with the drain shortened over time by the physician. The open wound, where packing is used and later removed, may need irrigating and sitz baths may be required to facilitate healing. Changes in exudate color and odor and temperature elevation should be reported to the physician and documented.

Sexual dysfunction by both men and women is related to removal of the rectum. Contributing factors may be partial to complete disruption of the nerve's supply to the genital organs, psychological factors, or decreased activity associated with age. When a comfortable relationship exists between the nurse and the patient, the topic of sex can be introduced more effectively. Exploring the patient's and the partner's fears and providing information on penile prosthesis surgery and simple suggestions to both partners will help decrease anxiety concerning intercourse. Counseling may be necessary if the patient's and spouse's perceptions of body image have been altered. Support groups are available to the cancer patient in most communities. Above all, the nurse's silent communication of touch and eye contact can give the patient a message that he is accepted and valued.

Hemorrhoids

Etiology/pathophysiology. Hemorrhoids are varicosities (dilated veins) that may occur outside the anal sphincter as external hemorrhoids or inside the sphincter as internal hemorrhoids. This condition is one of the most common health problems seen in humans, with the greatest incidence from ages 20 to 50 years. Etiological factors include straining at stool with increased intraabdominal and hemorrhoidal venous pressures. With repeated increased pressure and obstructed blood flow, permanent dilation occurs. Factors causing hemorrhoids are constipation, diarrhea, pregnancy, congestive heart failure, portal hypertension, and prolonged sitting and standing.

Clinical manifestations. The most common symptoms associated with enlarged, abnormal hemorrhoids are prolapse and bleeding. The bright red bleeding and prolapse usually occur at time of defecation.

Assessment. Collection of *subjective data* includes noting the patient's complaints of constipation, **pruritus,** severe pain when dilated veins become thrombosed, and bleeding from the rectum that is not mixed with feces.

Collection of *objective data* includes observing external hemorrhoids and palpating internal hemorrhoids on examination. Because bleeding and constipation are signs of cancer of the rectum, all patients with these symptoms should have a thorough examination to rule out cancer.

Medical management. Conservative interventions include the use of bulk stool softeners, such as Metamucil, bran, and natural food fibers, to relieve straining. Topical creams with hydrocortisone relieve pruritus and inflammation, and analgesic ointments, such as dibucaine (Nupercainal), relieve pain. Sitz baths are usually given to relieve pain and edema and promote healing.

The rubberband ligation is a popular and easy method of treatment. Tight bands are applied with a special instrument in the physician's office, causing constriction and necrosis. The destroyed tissue sloughs off in about 1 week, and discomfort is minimal. Sclerotherapy (a needle is inserted at the apex of the hemorrhoid column and a sclerosing agent is injected), cryotherapy (another method of tissue destruction by freezing), infrared photocoagulation (destruction of tissue by creation of a small burn), laser excision, and operative hemorrhoidectomy are additional interventions.

Hemorrhoidectomy, the surgical removal of hemorrhoids, can be performed if other interventions fail to relieve the distressing signs and symptoms. After removal of the hemorrhoid, wounds can be left open or closed, although closed wounds are reported to heal faster. Although this surgery is not considered a major procedure, pain may be acute, requiring narcotics and analgesic ointments. Complications of hemorrhoidectomy include hemorrhage, local infection, pain, urinary retention, and abscess.

Nursing interventions. Rectal conditions can be embarrassing to the patient, and the nurse's direct but concerned attitude can decrease this embarrassment. The nurse can assess the knowledge level by asking the patient about the condition, what he has been told about treatment, and what treatments have been done before surgery and why.

The nurse should assess the patient with a prolapsed hemorrhoid for edema, thrombosis, and ischemia. Ischemic tissue will be dark red to necrotic (black). A low-bulk diet can produce chronic constipation, and this should be explained to the patient.

For the surgical patient, vital signs should be taken frequently for the first 24 hours to rule out internal bleeding. Early ambulation and a soft diet facilitate bowel elimination. The patient may have a great deal of anxiety concerning the first defecation, and this should be discussed.

NURSING DIAGNOSES	NURSING INTERVENTIONS
Pain, related to edema, prolapse, and surgical intervention	Instruct patient to wash anal area after defecation and pat dry. Sitz baths or local heat applied to site may be soothing. Use of local anesthetics (Nupercainal ointment or Tucks pads) may give relief. Reinforce need for high-residue diet. Instruct patient on manual reduction of external hemorrhoids. Apply ice packs to hemorrhoids if thrombosed to prevent edema and pain. Use a cushion for sitting postoperatively.
Altered tissue perfusion, related to postoperative hemorrhage	Inspect site frequently first 24 hours. Check vital signs on regular postoperative routine. Avoid rectal tubes and rectal temperatures. Assess Hgb and Hct levels.
Anxiety, related to previous experiences, fear of first bowel movement postoperatively, and lack of knowledge regarding diet	Establish a supportive relationship with patient. Explain need for high-residue diet. Administer laxatives and oil retention enema as ordered. Give analgesic before first bowel movement and a sitz bath after for pain relief.

Patient teaching. The patient is advised to include bulk-forming foods, such as fresh fruit, vegetables, and bran cereals, as well as 8 to 10 glasses of fluid a day unless contraindicated. If the patient is anemic, discussion of foods high in iron, such as red meats, liver, and dark green leafy vegetables, can be included. Moderate exercise and establishing a routine time for a daily bowel movement should be emphasized. The patient should also be instructed to report any signs of infection or delayed healing.

Anal Fissure and Fistula

Anal fissure is a linear ulceration or laceration of the skin of the anus. Usually it is the result of trauma caused by hard stool that overstretches the anal lining. The fissure is aggravated by defecation, which initiates spasm of the anal sphincter, pain, and at times, slight bleeding. If the lesion does not heal spontaneously, the tract is excised surgically.

An anal fistula is an abnormal opening on the cutaneous surface near the anus. Usually this is from a local crypt abscess and also is common in Crohn's disease. A perianal fistula may or may not communicate with the rectum. It results from rupture or drainage of an anal abscess. This chronic condition is treated by a fistulectomy (removal) or fistulotomy (opening of the fistula tract).

The postoperative care required for repair of an anal fissure or fistula is similar to that for the patient who has had a hemorrhoidectomy.

DISORDERS OF THE LIVER, BILIARY TRACT, AND EXOCRINE PANCREAS

The liver, gallbladder, and exocrine pancreas are all organs that help with digestion.

Disorders of the Liver

Cirrhosis

Etiology/pathophysiology. Cirrhosis is a chronic, degenerative disease of the liver in which the lobes are covered with fibrous tissue, the **parenchyma** (tissue of the organ) degenerates, and the lobules are infiltrated with fat. The fibrous (scar) tissue restricts the flow of blood to the organ, which contributes to its destruction. Hepatomegaly (enlargement of the liver) and, later, liver contraction cause loss of the organ's function.

There are several forms of cirrhosis, caused by different factors. Laennec's cirrhosis, more commonly found in the Western world, affects more men than women and is found in patients with a history of chronic ingestion of alcohol. Postnecrotic cirrhosis, found worldwide, is caused by viral hepatitis, exposure to hepatotoxins (i.e., industrial chemicals), or infection. Primary biliary cirrhosis is found more often in women and results from destruction of the bile ducts. Secondary biliary cirrhosis is caused by chronic biliary tree obstruction caused by gallstones, a tumor, or biliary atresia in children. There are other types of cirrhosis, some of which may or may not have known causes.

With repeated insults, the liver can progress through the following stages: destruction, inflammation, fibrotic regeneration, and hepatic insufficiency. Although the liver cells have a great potential for regeneration, repeated scarring decreases their ability to be replaced. As the blood supply continues to be diminished and the scar tissue increases, the organ atrophies.

Functions of the liver are altered in several ways. The liver's ability to synthesize albumin is reduced as a result of liver cell damage. The obstruction of the portal vein as it enters the liver results in portal hypertension, or increased pressure in the veins that drain the gastrointestinal tract. This increased pressure forces fluid and albumin into the peritoneal cavity, which is called **ascites.** The damaged liver cannot metabolize protein in the usual manner; therefore protein intake may result in an elevation of blood ammonia levels. Reduced synthesis of protein and the leaking of existing protein result in hypoalbuminemia (reduced protein or albumin level in the blood), which reduces the blood's ability to regain fluids through osmosis. Protein must be present in adequate amounts to create colloidal osmotic pressure and "attract" the fluid to pass back into the blood vessels after it escapes in the capillaries. As fluid leaves the blood and the circulating volume decreases, the receptors in the brain signal the adrenal cortex to increase secretion of aldosterone to stimulate the kidneys to retain sodium and water. The normal liver inactivates the hormone *aldosterone,* but the damaged liver allows its effect to continue (hyperaldosteronism). Retention of fluid and sodium then results in increased pressure in the blood vessels and lymphatic channels, adding to the problem of portal hypertension. Ascites is therefore a result of portal hypertension, hypoalbuminemia, and hyperaldosteronism.

Hepatic insufficiency gradually causes veins in the upper part of the body to distend, including the esophageal vein. Esophageal varicosities develop, which may rupture, causing severe hemorrhage.

Clinical manifestations. Clinical manifestations of cirrhosis of the liver differ, depending on whether the patient is in the early stages of disease or the later stages. In early stages, the liver is firm and therefore easier to palpate, and abdominal pain may be present because of rapid enlargement that produces tension on the fibrous covering of the organ. Later stages of the disease present manifestations of dyspepsia, changes in bowel habits, gradual weight loss, ascites (accumulation of fluid in the peritoneal cavity), enlarged spleen, and spider telangiectases (dilated superficial arterioles). These later manifestations are the result of scarring of liver tissue that produces chronic failure of liver function and also fibrotic changes that cause obstruction of the portal circulation.

When enough cells of the liver become involved to interfere with its function and obstruct its circulation, the gastrointestinal organs and the spleen become congested and cannot function properly. Anemia occurs because of the body's decreased ability to produce RBCs and platelets. The cirrhotic liver cannot absorb vitamin K or produce the clotting factors VII, IX, and X. This causes the patient with cirrhosis to have bleeding tendencies.

Assessment. Collection of *subjective data* in *early stages* may include the patient describing his symptoms as "flulike," including loss of appetite, nausea and vomiting, general weakness, fatigue, indigestion, abnormal bowel function (either constipation or diarrhea), flatulence, and abdominal discomfort. The anatomical area most commonly affected is in the epigastric region or the right upper quadrant of the abdomen.

Collection of *subjective data* in *later stages* includes noting those subjective symptoms listed under early stages but they are more intense. The patient may complain of dyspnea and severe fatigue that interfere with the ability to carry out routine activities.

Collection of *objective data* in *early stages* may include observing low hemoglobin, fever, jaundice, and loss of weight.

Collection of *objective data* in *later stages* may include noting epistaxis, purpura, hematuria, spider hemangioma, and bleeding gums. Late symptoms are ascites, hematological disorders, splenic enlargement, and hemorrhage from esophageal varices or other distended gastrointestinal veins. The patient may also appear mentally disoriented, unable to understand, and display different behaviors or speech patterns. Prolonged interference with gas exchange leads to hypoxia, coma, and ultimately death.

Diagnostic tests. There are many diagnostic tests to aid in the diagnosis of cirrhosis. Abnormal electrolyte values, elevated serum bilirubin, AST (SGOT), ALT (SGPT), LDH, and Gamma GT, decreased serum albumin, elevated ammonia, abnormal CBC, prolonged prothrombin time, and abnormal urinalysis may give evidence of poor liver functioning. Visualization through endoscopic retrograde cholangiopancreatography (to detect common bile duct obstruction), esophagoscopy with barium esophagography to visualize varices, scans and biopsy of the liver, and ultrasonography, are used to diagnose cirrhosis. Paracentesis, a procedure in which fluid is withdrawn from the abdominal cavity, will relieve ascites and also provide fluid for laboratory examination.

Medical management. When possible causes have been identified, the initial treatment is to eliminate these causes, decrease the buildup of fluids in the body, prevent further damage to the liver, and provide individual supportive care to the patient. Eliminating alcohol, hepatotoxins (i.e., acetaminophen [Tylenol]), or environmental exposure to harmful chemicals is essential to prevent further damage to the liver. Diet therapy is aimed at correcting malnutrition, promoting the regeneration of functional liver tissue, and compensating for the liver's inability to store vitamins, while avoiding fluid retention and hepatic encephalopathy. A well-balanced, high-calorie (2500 to 3000 calories/day), moderate-high-protein (75 g of high-quality protein/day), low-fat, low-sodium (200 to 1000 mg/day) diet with additional vitamins and folic acid will usually meet the needs of the patient with cirrhosis and improve deficiencies that exist.

Antiemetics may be prescribed to control nausea or vomiting. The patient must be monitored closely for toxicity that develops quickly when the poorly functioning liver cannot clear these drugs from the system. Diphenhydramine (Benadryl) or dimenhydrinate (Dramamine) may be given, whereas prochlorperazine maleate (Compazine), hydroxyzine pamoate (Vistaril), or hydroyzine hydrochloride (Atarax) should be avoided.

Complications and treatment of cirrhosis. Ascites is the presence of excessive fluid in the peritoneal cavity. The severity of fluid retention will determine the treatment. Initially the patient will be placed on bed rest with accurate monitoring of intake and output. The patient's diet will be restricted for amount of fluid (500 to 1000 ml) and sodium (200 to 1000 mg). Diuretic therapy may be added if the diet does not control the ascites and edema. Spironolactone (Aldactone) 300 to 1000 mg/day may be used to obtain the desired diuresis. Other diuretics may be added, including furosemide (Lasix) or hydrochlorothiazide (HydroDIURIL). Salt-poor albumin may be administered in attempt to restore plasma volume if the intravascular volume is decreased significantly. Complications of diuretic therapy include plasma volume deficit, decreased renal function, and electrolyte imbalance.

Another method of treatment for ascites and edema is the LeVeen continuous peritoneal jugular shunt, introduced in 1962 (Fig. 31-23). This procedure allows the continuous shunting of ascitic fluid from the abdominal cavity through a one-way, pressure-sensitive valve into a silicone tube that empties into the superior vena cava. The patient with this shunt must be monitored carefully for complications, which include congestive heart failure, leakage of the ascitic fluid, infection at the insertion sites, peritonitis, septicemia, and shunt thrombosis.

Paracentesis is a temporary method of removing fluid by withdrawing fluid from the abdominal cavity by either gravity or vacuum. An incision is made in the skin, and a hollow trocar, cannula, or catheter is passed through the incision and into the cavity. The fluid is removed over a period of 30 to 90 minutes to prevent sudden changes in blood pressure, which could lead to syncope. The patient is monitored closely for signs of hypovolemia and electrolyte imbalances. A dressing is applied over the insertion site, and the nurse observes for bleeding and drainage.

Portal hypertension is an increased venous pressure in the portal circulation caused by compression or by occlusion in the portal or hepatic vascular system. In most instances, portal hypertension that develops from cirrhosis is irreversible.

Esophageal varices are a complex of longitudinal, tortuous veins at the lower end of the esophagus. These vessels enlarge and become edematous as the result of portal hypertension. They are especially susceptible to ulceration and hemorrhage. Varices can rupture as a result of anything that increases the abdominal venous pressure, such as coughing, sneezing, vomiting, or the Valsalva maneuver. Rupture may occur slowly over several days or suddenly and without pain. An endoscopy may be performed to identify the varices or to rule out bleeding from other sources.

Therapeutic management of a ruptured esophageal varix is a medical emergency. The patient's airway must be maintained, the bleeding varix controlled, and IV lines established for fluids and blood replacement as needed. The hormone *vasopressin*, administered intravenously or directly into the superior vena cava, is used to decrease or stop the hemorrhaging. If the vasopressin drip does not stop or control bleeding, a Sengstaken-Blakemore

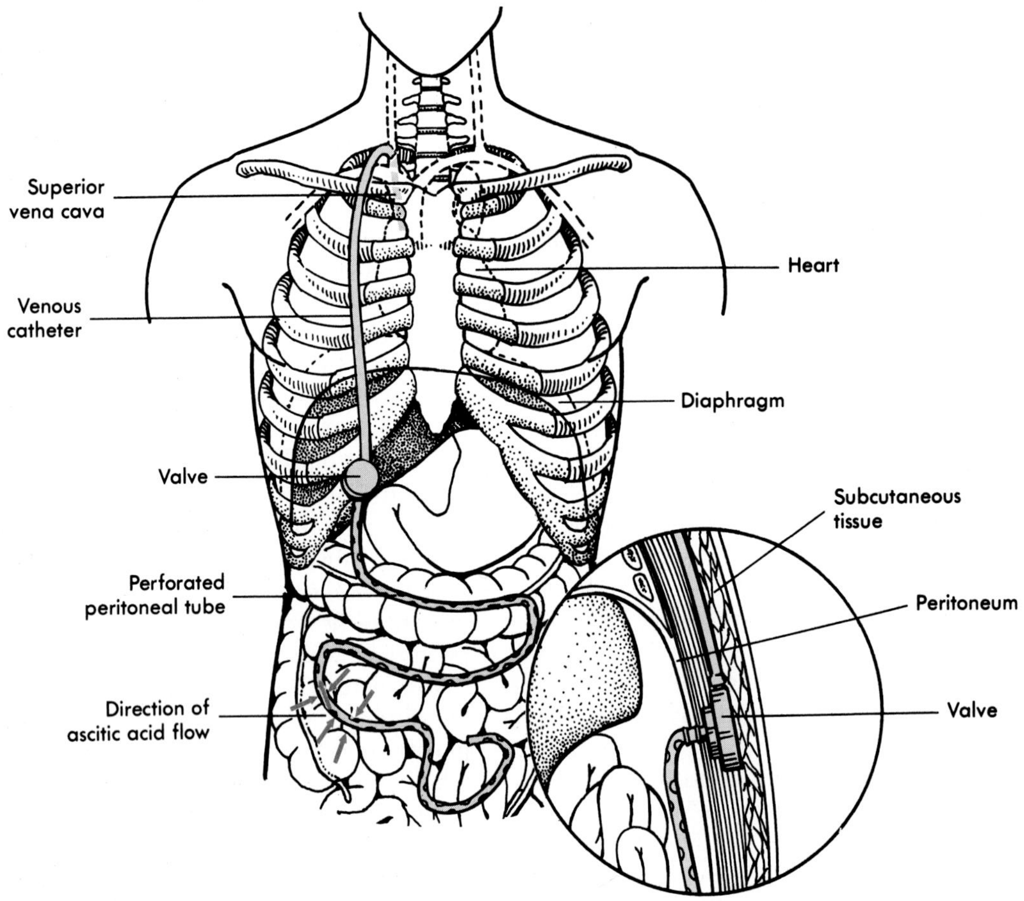

FIG. 31-23 LeVeen shunt showing placement of catheter.

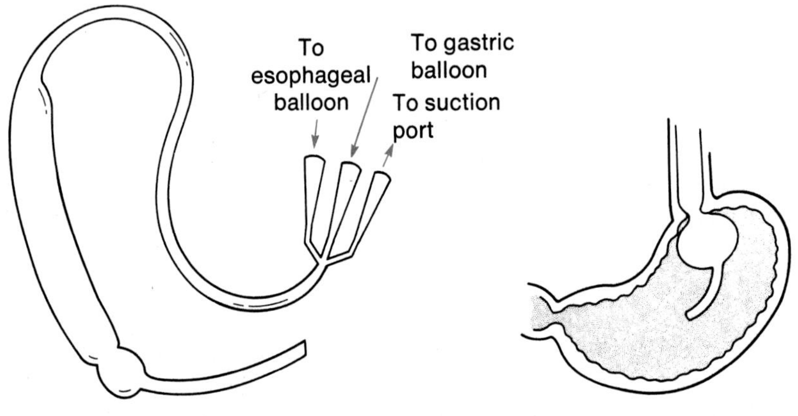

FIG. 31-24 Sengstaken-Blakemore tube.

tube with openings at the tip may be inserted. This triple-lumen tube has a lumen for inflating the esophageal balloon, one for inflating the gastric balloon, and one for gastric lavage (Fig. 31-24). The tube is passed through the nose, and when it is in place, the balloon in the stomach or the one in the esophagus or both are inflated to press against the bleeding vessels and control the hemorrhage. The gastric aspiration is attached to low intermittent suction. When either balloon is inflated, a Levin tube is passed into the esophagus through the mouth and attached to low suction to drain the saliva that cannot drain into the stomach. The balloon must be deflated periodically to prevent necrosis. The patient is allowed nothing by mouth, and the head of the bed should be elevated 30 to 45 degrees to help prevent aspiration of stomach contents and help the patient breathe.

Gastric lavage will be performed to remove any swallowed blood from the stomach. Iced, isotonic saline solutions for the lavage are used by some to facilitate vasoconstriction. Endoscopic sclerotherapy may also be used to control the bleeding.

Patients suffering from portal hypertension and esophageal varices may benefit from surgical shunting procedures that divert blood from the portal system to the venous system. The portacaval shunt diverts blood from the portal vein to the inferior vena cava. The splenorenal shunt requires the removal of the spleen, and the splenic vein is anastomosed to the left renal vein. The mesocaval shunt involves anastomosis of the superior mesenteric vein to the inferior vena cava. These procedures have a high mortality. They may be performed in an emergency situation to control acute esophageal varix bleeding or in a therapeutic situation when a patient has already bled. Complications of surgical shunting procedures are hepatic encephalopathy, gastrointestinal bleeding, ascites, and liver failure.

Care of the patient who has hemorrhaged from an esophageal varix includes maintenance of oxygen content levels within the blood, blood transfusions with fresh whole blood to supply the body with more clotting factors, and electrolyte replacements as needed without fluid overload. The buildup of ammonia can be prevented with the use of cathartics and enemas to remove any blood that has entered the intestinal tract. Antibiotics are given to destroy colonic bacteria.

Hepatic encephalopathy is a type of brain damage caused by liver disease and consequent ammonia intoxication. It is thought to be the result of a damaged liver being unable to metabolize substances that can be toxic to the brain, such as ammonia. The patient presents symptoms that progress from inappropriate behavior, confusion, flapping tremors, and twitching of the extremities to stupor and coma. Treatment of the patient with hepatic encephalopathy is to give supportive care that will prevent further damage to the liver. Protein in the diet and drugs that are normally detoxified by the liver are avoided until the liver regains adequate function. Medications may be given to cleanse the bowel and help decrease the serum ammonia. Lactulose (Chronulac) decreases the bowel's pH, thus decreasing the production of ammonia by bacteria within the bowel. It also functions as a cathartic. Neomycin inhibits protein synthesis in bacteria, thereby decreasing the production of ammonia. Flapping tremor (asterixis) is when the patient stretches out his arm and hyperextends his wrist with his fingers separated, relaxed, and extended. A rapid, irregular flexion and extension (flapping) of the wrist will occur in the acutely ill patient.

Nursing interventions. The nurse should check vital signs every 4 hours and more often if evidence of hemorrhage is present. The patient should be observed for gastrointestinal hemorrhage as evidenced by hematemesis, melena, anxiety, and restlessness.

Most patients will require a well-balanced, protein-adequate high-carbohydrate diet with adequate vitamins. Sodium restriction is frequently necessary, and this can make providing a palatable diet more difficult. Frequent oral hygiene and a pleasant environment should be provided to help increase food intake.

A major nursing focus for many patients is helping them to deal with alcoholism. This requires trust that the health team is interested in their well-being. Patients must admit that they have drinking problems. Confrontation may sometimes be used to help patients accept the problems. Patients are often referred for counseling for their alcoholism.

Because of pruritus, malnutrition, and edema, the patient with cirrhosis is prone to skin lesions and decubitus formation. Preventive nursing interventions to avoid impairment of skin integrity, such as Eggcrate mattresses, frequent turning, back rubs, and massage of bony prominences, should be initiated. The nurse should apply soothing lotion to relieve pruritus.

The nurse should observe the patient's mental status and report changes, such as confusion, headache, or lethargy. It is important for the nurse to assist in activities of daily living as needed to promote good hygiene while conserving energy. The nurse observes for edema by measuring ankles daily and observes for ascites by measuring abdominal girth. An accurate intake and output is recorded, as well as daily weight.

NURSING DIAGNOSES	NURSING INTERVENTIONS
Alteration in tissue perfusion, related to impaired blood coagulation or hemorrhage from portal hypertension	Monitor patient for signs of bleeding: gums, injection sites, decrease in BP, increase in pulse, hematemesis, and melena. Monitor Hgb and Hct. Monitor parenteral fluids and/or blood transfusions. Administer vitamin K and neomycin as ordered. Instruct patient to avoid straining with stools and to avoid vigorous toothbrushing. Monitor gastric output—color and consistency.
Altered thought processes, related to potential increase of serum ammonia and hepatic coma	Observe frequently for changes in mental status: lethargy, drowsiness, and confusion. Monitor neurological status for decreased motor ability. Provide safe environment; side rails up, bed in low position, and restraints if necessary. Avoid use of sedatives, tranquilizers, and narcotics.
Altered nutrition: less than body requirements, related to inadequate diet, vomiting, or anorexia	Provide small, frequent feedings of prescribed diet; the amount of protein, carbohydrates, and fat will depend on the patient's ability to metabolize these nutrients; salt may be restricted. Assist and encourage patient to eat, and consider preferences in food choices.

Patient teaching. The patient with cirrhosis must understand the need for adequate rest and avoiding infections. His activity must be planned around complete bed rest until he regains strength. Turning the patient at least every 2 hours and providing range-of-motion exercises will help avoid infection and prevent thrombophlebitis. The nurse should instruct the patient to use a soft-bristled toothbrush, use an electric razor, blow nose cautiously, and avoid straining at stools to prevent bleeding as a result of a lack of vitamin K and certain clotting factors. Soap, perfumed lotion, and rubbing alcohol should be avoided because they will cause further drying of the skin. If pruritus and dryness of skin are present, diphenhydramine (Benadryl) may be administered. The nurse should explain the relationship of the therapeutic diet to the patient's diagnosis and ability of the liver to function.

Community resources for home health care and detoxification programs may help the patient and family deal with problems that arise after discharge. Because of the seriousness of the disease, the patient and family need understanding and support throughout the treatment.

Hepatitis

Etiology/pathophysiology. Hepatitis is an inflammation of the liver resulting from several causes, including viral agents, bacterial agents, or exposure to toxic substances.

The three types of viral hepatitis are caused by distinct but similar viruses that produce almost identical signs and symptoms but vary in their incubation period and mode of transmission. Hepatitis A, formerly called *infectious hepatitis,* is the most common form today and is a short-incubation virus (10 to 40 days). Hepatitis B, formerly called *serum hepatitis,* is a long-incubation virus (28 to 160 days). A third virus not yet positively identified, known as *non-A–non-B (also known as hepatitis C),* has an incubation period similar to type B. Health officials are required by law to report all cases of viral hepatitis to the Centers for Disease Control (CDC) in Atlanta.

The mode of transmission of the three types of viral hepatitis are:

- Hepatitis A spreads by direct contact, through fecal-contaminated food or water, or parenterally
- Hepatitis B is transmitted by the oral-fecal route, in contaminated serum by blood transfusion, by the use of contaminated needles and instruments, and by direct contact with body fluids from the infected persons, such as breast milk and sexual contact
- Non-A–non-B hepatitis is transmitted in the blood and is a major cause of transfusion-related viral hepatitis; it is also transmitted by sexual contact.

The basic pathological findings in the three forms of viral hepatitis are identical. A diffuse inflammatory reaction occurs, and liver cells begin to degenerate and die. As the liver cells degenerate, the normal functions of the liver slow down. The outcome of the disease may be affected by the virulence of the virus, the preexisting condition of the liver, and the health care given when the disease is diagnosed.

Clinical manifestations. The clinical manifestations for viral hepatitis vary greatly: some patients are asymptomatic, whereas others develop hepatic failure or hepatic encephalopathy. Usually recovery can be expected with only mild liver damage.

Assessment. Collection of *subjective data* includes patients' reports of general malaise, aching muscles, photophobia, lassitude, headaches and chills. Abdominal pain, dyspepsia, nausea, diarrhea, and constipation are reported also. The patient may complain of pruritus from the presence of bile on the skin. The patient will complain of tenderness in the liver and will remain fatigued for several weeks.

Collection of *objective data* includes observing hepatomegaly (enlarged liver), enlarged lymph nodes, weight loss, and rhinitis. Jaundice appears because of the damaged liver's inability to metabolize bilirubin; the resultant signs noted are yellow skin, sclera, and mucous membranes, as well as dark amber urine, and clay-colored stools. It is not uncommon for relapses to occur in the convalescent stage.

Diagnostic tests. Changes in the liver caused by viral hepatitis cause elevated direct bilirubin, gamma GT, AST (SGOT), ALT (SGPT), and alkaline phosphatase, prolonged prothrombin time, and a decreased serum albumin. Leukopenia is common in these patients, and hypoglycemia is present in approximately 50% of the patients with hepatitis. Serum is examined for the presence of HAA (hepatitis-associated antigen) A, B, or non-A–non-B.

Medical management. There is no specific treatment for patients with viral hepatitis other than supportive therapy for existing signs and symptoms and preventing the transmission of the disease. The patient's care can be in the hospital when signs and symptoms are acute, but usually the patient is cared for at home. Bed rest for several weeks is commonly prescribed.

Alcohol in the diet is not allowed for at least 1 year, and the patient may need supportive care from the community to facilitate compliance. Most patients will tolerate a low-fat, high-carbohydrate diet, with the largest meal taken in the morning. If the patient is anorexic, smaller meals with adequate fluid and caloric intake are helpful. Hydroxyzine (Atarax) or trimethobenzamide (Tigan) may be given 30 minutes before meals for patients with nausea. If the patient is dehydrated, intravenous fluids will be given with additions of vitamin C for healing, vitamin B complex to assist the damaged liver's inability to absorb fat-soluble vitamins, and vitamin K to combat prolonged coagulation time.

Gamma globulin or immune serum globulin should be given as soon as possible to persons who have been in direct contact with a person with hepatitis A during the infectious period (2 weeks before and 1 week after onset of symptoms). The dosage of 0.02 ml/kg of body weight, given intramuscularly, is effective in preventing hepatitis A in 80% to 90% of the cases.

Individuals who have been exposed to hepatitis B virus via a needle puncture, contact with feces or oral secretions, or sexual contact should be protected with hepatitis B immune globulin (HBIG). A dose of 0.06 ml/kg of body weight is administered intramuscularly as quickly after exposure as possible. This dose is repeated 1 month later.

Persons identified as being at high risk for developing hepatitis B may be vaccinated if they are not already immune. These persons include the following:

- High-risk health care personnel (emergency room, operating room, intensive care unit, and dialysis personnel, phlebotomists, and laboratory technicians)
- Persons with high-risk life-styles (drug addicts, homosexuals, and prostitutes)
- Infants born to mothers who are hepatitis B surface antigen (HBsAg)–positive

The protection program consists of three vaccinations: an initial vaccination, a vaccination 1 month later, and a third vaccination 6 months after the first injection. The hepatitis B vaccine has been shown to provide protection for 3 to 5 years in approximately 90% of the persons treated.

Because non-A–non-B hepatitis is spread mainly through blood transfusions, blood products should be used only when necessary. The blood used should be screened for elevated SGPT and anti-hepatitis B core (anti-HBC).

Nursing interventions. The care of the patient with viral hepatitis includes ensuring rest, maintaining adequate nutrition, and caring for the skin. The care of the patient with hepatitis continues over time, and support and patient education are necessary throughout the entire illness.

Preventing the transmission of the disease is of primary importance in caring for the patient with viral hepatitis. The patient, family, and health care providers must be knowledgeable about routes of transmission of the virus and take steps to avoid such transmission. Proper personal hygiene and good sanitation will help prevent the spread of hepatitis A. Patients should be given a thorough explanation of the reasons for the precautions and should be instructed in the proper handling of their own secretions and body wastes and in thorough methods of handwashing. Gown and gloves should be worn when handling excreta, giving enemas, taking rectal temperatures, handling food wastes, handling needles, disposing of urine, or carrying out any other procedure or hygiene measure that involves direct contact with the patient's body fluids.

When the patient has hepatitis B, utmost care must be taken in handling syringes, needles, and other instruments that are contaminated with the patient's serum. Disposable equipment and dishes should be used and isolation precautions taken. Special handling of blood, oral secretions, and excreta is essential to prevent the transmission of both viruses.

NURSING DIAGNOSES	NURSING INTERVENTIONS
Potential for injury, related to poor nutrition and prolonged clotting times	Pad side rails if necessary. Assist weakened patient with activities. Encourage use of electric razors and soft toothbrush.
Altered nutrition: less than body requirements, related to inadequate intake associated with current anorexia, nausea, vomiting, and altered metabolism of nutrients by the liver	Provide diet high in carbohydrates and low in fats, and encourage total fluid intake of 2500 to 3000 ml daily. Monitor intake and output. Monitor daily weight. Note color and consistency of stool and color and amount of urine. Administer antiemetics as ordered. Offer support and understanding. Promote adequate rest.
Pain, related to pruritus as a result of elevated bilirubin levels	Avoid soap and rubbing alcohol on patient's skin. Pat skin dry; use soft clothes, bed linens, and towels. Provide moisturizing lotions. Administer antihistamines for severe pruritus as ordered.

Patient teaching. When the patient with viral hepatitis can be cared for at home, the family will need to be taught necessary precautions. Intimate contact should be avoided during the infectious period. If possible, separate bathroom facilities should be used by the patient. Personal care items and drinking glasses should not be shared. The patient's clothes should be laundered separately in hot water. Contaminated items should be disposed of properly.

The patient and family should be aware of signs and symptoms associated with hepatitis, including light-colored stools, dark-colored urine, jaundice, fever, gastrointestinal disturbances, unusual bleeding that might be indicative of a prolonged prothrombin time, and tenderness or pain in the abdomen. The danger of alcohol use and its effect on the liver should be clearly understood.

Cholecystitis and Cholelithiasis

Etiology/pathophysiology. Disorders of the biliary system are common in the United States and are responsible for the hospitalization of more than one-half million people per year. The two most common conditions are cholecystitis and cholelithiasis. These two diseases are seen more commonly in women than men, in Native Americans and Caucasians than in Orientals and African-Americans, and in obese people, pregnant women, people with diabetes, multiparous women, and women who use birth control pills.

Cholecystitis can be caused by an obstruction, a gallstone, or a tumor. More than 90% of the cases of cho-

BOX 31-4 DEFINITIONS

chole pertaining to bile
cholang pertaining to bile ducts
cholangiography x-ray examination of bile ducts
cholangitis inflammation of bile duct
cholecyst pertaining to gallbladder
cholecystectomy removal of gallbladder
cholecystitis inflammation of gallbladder
cholecystography x-ray examination of gallbladder
cholecystostomy incision and drainage of gallbladder
choledocho pertaining to common bile duct
choledocholithiasis stones in common bile duct
choledochostomy exploration of common bile duct
cholelith gallstone
cholelithiasis presence of gallstones

lecystitis are caused by gallstones. The exact cause of stone formation in the gallbladder and the common bile duct is not known. However, an alteration in lipid metabolism and the role of female sex hormones are related to the disease.

When an obstruction, gallstone, or tumor prevents bile from leaving the gallbladder, the trapped bile acts as an irritant, causing cellular infiltration of the gallbladder wall after 3 to 4 days. A typical inflammatory response occurs, and the gallbladder becomes enlarged and edematous. The vascular occlusion along with bile stasis causes the mucosal lining of the gallbladder to become necrotic. Initially the bile in the gallbladder is sterile. The bacterial growth is caused by the ischemia and occurs usually within a few days. There is danger of rupture of the gallbladder and spread of infection to the hepatic duct and liver. When the disease is severe enough to interfere with the blood supply, the gallbladder wall may become gangrenous.

Clinical manifestations. The condition may be acute, with a sudden onset of nausea and vomiting and severe pain in the right upper quadrant of the abdomen, or chronic, evidenced by several milder attacks of pain and a history of fat intolerance. Many patients with gallstones are asymptomatic, and the gallstones are discovered only during an examination for another problem.

Assessment. Collection of *subjective data* includes complaints of indigestion after eating foods high in fat, pain and tenderness in the right subcostal region or in the epigastric region, radiation of pain to the back or shoulder, anorexia, nausea, vomiting, and **flatulence**. The patient may experience increased heart and respiratory rates and become diaphoretic, leading the individual to think he is having a heart attack. These symptoms are decreased or absent in the patient with chronic cholecystitis.

Collection of *objective data* may include a low-grade fever and an elevated leukocyte count, as well as mild jaundice, stool that contains fat (steatorrhea), and clay-colored stool caused by a lack of bile in the intestinal tract. The urine may be dark amber and contain urobilinogen as the kidneys try to remove the excess bilirubin from the bloodstream.

Diagnostic tests. There are a number of diagnostic studies that are performed to confirm a diagnosis of cholecystitis and cholelithiasis. Fecal studies, oral cholecystogram, x-ray, serum bilirubin tests, and ultrasound of the biliary system may be done. Operative cholangiography is when the common bile duct is directly injected with the radiopaque dye and is most commonly done at the time of gallbladder surgery.

Medical management. If the attack of cholelithiasis is mild, the patient is treated conservatively. Bed rest is prescribed, a nasogastric tube is inserted and connected to low suction, and the patient is placed on no fluids by mouth (NPO). This allows the gastrointestinal tract and thus the gallbladder to rest. Intravenous fluids are given to rehydrate the patient and replace drainage from the nasogastric tube.

Antispasmodic and analgesic drugs may be given to decrease the patient's pain. Meperidine (Demerol) is commonly used, because there is decreased incidence of spasms of the sphincter of Oddi with this drug. Antibiotics may be given (1) prophylactically to prevent infection, (2) to treat an already present infection, and (3) after perforation, should it occur. A diet that is low in fat and cholesterol may be prescribed. Avoidance of foods that are spicy is also suggested.

Lithotripsy. Extracorporeal shock wave lithotripsy (ESWL) is used to treat a patient who has mild or moderate symptoms caused by a few stones. The patient is treated by a machine that discharges a series of shock waves through water or a cushion that breaks the stone into fragments. The natural flow of bile carries the stone fragments out of the gallbladder into the intestine for eventual excretion. Nursing intervention after the procedure is similar to that for patients undergoing liver biopsy.

Surgical intervention. A cholecystectomy (removal of the gallbladder) is usually the treatment of choice. The gallbladder is removed, and the cystic duct, vein, and artery are ligated. A Jackson-Pratt drain, Hemovac, or a Penrose drain may be inserted. If the stones are in the common bile duct and edema is present, a biliary drainage tube, or T-tube, will be inserted to keep the duct open and allow drainage of the bile until the edema resolves. The short end of the tube is placed in the common bile duct, and the longer end of the tube is brought to the surface through a stab wound. The long end is attached

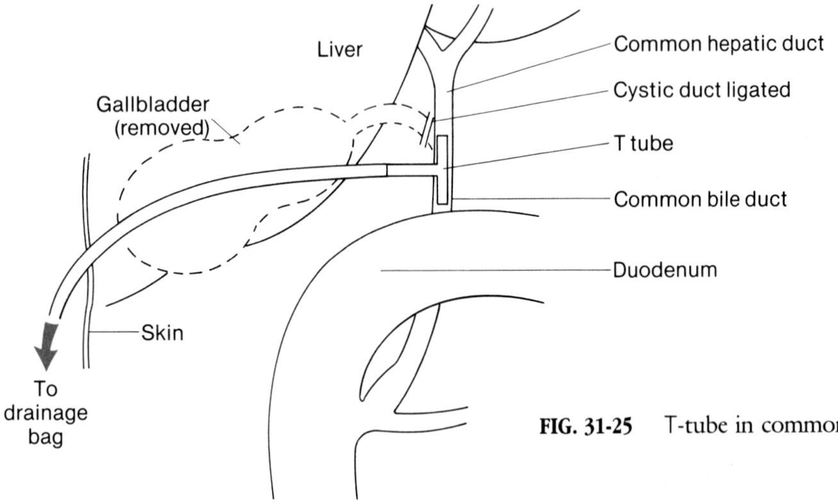

FIG. 31-25 T-tube in common bile duct.

to a closed drainage system (bile bag) that is placed below the level of the common bile duct (Fig. 31-25).

The T-tube also provides a route for postoperative cholangiography if desired (T-tube cholangiogram). The cholangiogram assesses the patency of the common bile duct. The T-tube will be removed 24 hours after the cholangiogram if the edema is resolved and the common bile duct appear normal. The 24-hour period allows the dye to drain out of the common bile duct. If the edema does not resolve in this time, the patient may be discharged with the T-tube in place.

A new operative procedure gaining in popularity for the removal of the gallbladder is done by way of endoscopy, called a laparoscopic cholecystectomy. This procedure is more comfortable for the patient postoperatively, and it is possible for the patient to be discharged within 1 or 2 days compared with 5 to 7 days after conventional surgery.

Nursing interventions. Nursing interventions begin with careful assessment of the characteristics of pain if present and any signs of jaundice of the skin, sclera, and mucous membrane. The urine and stool should be observed for alterations in the presence of bilirubin.

When the patient is treated conservatively, the nursing interventions center on keeping the patient comfortable by carefully administering the medications prescribed and monitoring the patient's response to the medication. The patient on NPO status because of the presence of a nasogastric tube must be monitored closely for amount, color, and consistency of output. The nasogastric tube should be connected to low suction, and the nasal area should be inspected for irritation and necrosis from the tube. Antiemetics may be administered if nausea persists.

IV infusions are observed for patency, correct rates, and entry sites that are free from erythema and edema. Intake and output are measured and described carefully.

Preoperative care includes teaching the patient to turn, cough, and deep breathe and to use an incentive spirometer to facilitate air movement in and out of the lungs to prevent pneumonia. By understanding how to splint the abdomen with the hands or a bath blanket before attempting a cough, practicing repositioning in the hospital bed, and assuming a sitting position from a standing or lying position, the patient will be able to follow postoperative instructions more easily. Explaining the nasogastric tube, intravenous tubing, and urinary catheter and their functions will help relieve patient anxiety. The patient should be familiar with any medications that may be used to relieve pain and nausea, and should understand that vitamin K and antibiotics are given preoperatively to prevent hemorrhage and infection.

Postoperative care includes monitoring vital signs and observing dressings frequently and carefully for exudate or hemorrhage. The dressings will usually require reinforcement at the drain site. The patient is placed in semi-Fowler's position to facilitate drainage. A Jackson-Pratt or Penrose drain or Hemovac, which promote bile drainage and prevent pressure and fluid accumulation under the diaphragm, must be monitored for patency. Initially there should be less than 50 ml of serosanguineous exudate during an 8-hour period. The surgeon should be notified if the drainage is excessive, contains bile, or is bright red.

The patient will need encouragement to perform deep breathing and coughing because of the location of the incision. Pain medication should be given frequently in the early postoperative period to facilitate movement and deep breathing. The patient is usually dangled the night of surgery and ambulated the first postoperative day. The patient's neurological status is monitored by checking his ability to be aroused easily, his orientation to the environment and family, and his ability to move extremities equally on command.

Fluid balance is maintained with intravenous therapy; potassium is usually added to compensate for loss from surgery. The nurse should check the nasogastric tube for proper drainage and may irrigate with physiological saline solution. Usually 30 ml of solution is sufficient to determine the tube's patency. The patient is given nothing by mouth while the nasogastric tube is in place, although sips of water or ice chips may be allowed to keep the mouth moist. The nurse should check the physician's order before giving ice or fluids to the patient, and the patient should be allowed to rinse the mouth frequently. Glycerin or petroleum jelly should be applied to the lips, and the nostril through which the tube is passed should be cleansed and lubricated. A tube guard is placed on the nose and to the nasogastric tube to maintain tube placement.

The nurse will be responsible for the care of the T-tube if one is placed. The drainage bag for the T-tube is placed below the level of the common bile duct to prevent the reflux of bile. The bag must be positioned so the tube is not kinked or bile cannot drain from the liver. The position of the bag and tube and the color and amount of exudate must be checked frequently during the first 24 hours and recorded. A gauze roll should be placed under the tube, anchoring it to the patient's abdomen and preventing tension and pull on the tube caused by the weight of the bag. The tube will drain as much as 500 ml during the first 24 hours. The amount should decrease as the edema resolves and bile begins flowing through the common bile duct. The nurse must be careful not to dislodge the T-tube when the patient's dressings are changed as prescribed by the physician.

After oral intake is resumed, the physician may order the tube clamped for 1 to 2 hours before meals and unclamped 1 to 2 hours after the patient eats, to aid in the digestion of fat. The patient may show signs of distress while the tube is clamped, which include abdominal pain, nausea, vomiting, light brown urine, and clay-colored stools. If distress occurs, the tube should be unclamped immediately. The time that the T-tube remains clamped will be increased as the patient tolerates the procedure. The tube may be left in place for as long as 10 days. The physician will remove the tube when the common bile duct is patent for drainage of bile.

Bowel sounds should be checked every 8 hours to determine the return of peristalsis. A clear liquid diet is usually ordered 24 to 48 hours postoperatively and increased as tolerated. When solid food is started, it will usually be low in fat. Flatulence or nausea after eating certain foods may persist after surgery, and the patient should be instructed to experiment with different foods.

The patient who undergoes a cholecystectomy must be observed for complications. These include jaundice, from an occluded common duct, and hemorrhage, indicated by a decrease in blood pressure, a rise in pulse, and increased exudate at the dressing site. An elevated temperature could indicate peritonitis or wound infection. Pancreatitis may occur after cholecystectomy.

Patients at high risk of not surviving a cholecystectomy may need a cholecystostomy (forming an opening into the gallbladder through the abdominal wall). This can be done using a local anesthetic. The opening will provide a means of removing purulent exudate and possibly the stone. It also allows drainage of the bile.

NURSING DIAGNOSES	NURSING INTERVENTIONS
Ineffective breathing pattern, related to pain of high abdominal incision and failure to splint area with coughing and movement	Assist patient to cough and to take 10 deep breaths hourly; instruct patient on splinting techniques. Turn q 2 hr. Administer analgesics as ordered to facilitate deep breathing and movement. Ambulate as early as possible.
Potential impaired skin integrity, related to wound drainage and accidental obstruction of bile drainage	If T-tube is present: Maintain patency and prevent tension on tube. Promote drainage by placing patient in low- to semi-Fowler's position. Observe, describe, and record amount and character of exudate at least q 8 hr. Empty bag when half full. Clamp tube as ordered by physician 3 to 4 days postoperatively. Reinforce primary dressing, and observe exudate; change and apply sterile, dry dressing as ordered; use Montgomery straps to secure if drainage is profuse. Cleanse skin thoroughly at insertion site before applying sterile dressing. Apply skin barriers for added protection PRN; Betadine ointment may be used as antimicrobial agent.
Potential fluid volume deficit, related to intolerance for diet, nausea and vomiting, presence of nasogastric tube, and amount of bile drainage	Maintain intravenous fluid therapy as ordered. Maintain patency of nasogastric tube if present. Record intake and output. Monitor drainage on dressings if present. Reinforce dietary instruction for fat-restricted diet. Observe color of skin, sclera and mucous membrane for jaundice, and signs of bile flow obstruction. Administer bile or bile salts if ordered.

Patient teaching. Dietary teaching is necessary for the patient who is treated conservatively for cholecystitis, as well as the patient who undergoes surgery. The patient who is treated conservatively must remain on continuous dietary restrictions of fatty foods. Foods to avoid include fried foods, cream, whole milk, butter, margarine, peanut butter, nuts, chocolate, pastries, and gravies. For the post-surgical patient, instruction is given to try small amounts of foods that previously caused discomfort and gradually eliminate those that continue to do so. The patient can usually resume a normal diet without difficulty once he is able to tolerate a regular diet.

The patient should understand that stones may recur elsewhere in the biliary system. The patient should be able to identify the signs of complications that should be reported. These include jaundice caused by occlusion or stricture of a duct, hemorrhage and/or leakage of bile, elevated temperature, pain, and dietary intolerance associated with another attack. The patient should also be able to demonstrate care of the T-tube, if present on discharge, identify activity restrictions, and identify a date for return visit to the physician.

Pancreatitis

Etiology/pathophysiology. Pancreatitis is an inflammatory condition of the pancreas that may be acute or chronic. Although the exact cause of pancreatitis remains unknown, many predisposing factors have been identified. Acute or chronic pancreatitis is generally the result of damage to the biliary tract, as by alcohol, trauma, infectious disease, or certain drugs. Alcoholism and biliary tract disease are the two factors most commonly associated with pancreatitis. Acute pancreatitis is associated with a mortality of 50%.

In the pathophysiological process of pancreatitis, the enzymes cannot flow out of the pancreas because of **occlusion** of the duct by edema, stones, or scar tissue. The pancreatic enzymes build up and cause an increase in pressure within the duct. The duct ruptures, releasing the enzymes, and the enzymes begin digesting the pancreas (autodigestion). In chronic pancreatitis, actual atrophy of the acinar tissue allows replacement of fibrotic tissue and necrosis of the pancreas occurs.

The development of pseudocysts or abscesses in pancreatic tissue is a serious complication. After autodigestion occurs, the pancreas and occasionally surrounding organs form walls around cystic fluid, including pancreatic enzymes, and necrotic debris. These pseudocysts can develop into an abscess.

Clinical manifestations. Clinical manifestations include severe abdominal pain radiating to the back. The pain is sometimes relieved by the patient assuming a forward position, taking the weight of the stomach off of the pancreas. Jaundice may be noted if the common bile duct is obstructed.

Assessment. Collection of *subjective data* may include noting that patients exhibit extreme symptoms or none at all. When symptoms are evident, it is difficult to distinguish the symptoms of pancreatitis from other abdominal disorders. The most specific complaint is abdominal pain that radiates to the back. The pain can be excruciating. This pain is caused by the enlargement of the pancreatic capsule, an obstruction, or the chemical irritation from the enzymes. The pain is usually decreased by flexing the trunk or assuming the fetal position and is aggravated by eating. Other subjective complaints include anorexia, nausea, malaise, and restlessness.

Collection of *objective data* may include noting the presence of low-grade fever, vomiting in 70% to 90% of patients, jaundice if the common bile duct is obstructed, steatorrhea, and tachycardia.

Diagnostic tests. Both acute and chronic pancreatitis are diagnosed by radiological studies (abdominal CT scan and ultrasound), endoscopy, and laboratory analysis of the amount of pancreatic enzymes in the blood. Laboratory tests will reveal an increased serum amylase during the first few days and then increased urine amylase thereafter. Leukocytosis, an elevated hematocrit, hypocalcemia, and hypoalbuminemia may also be present. Pancreatic insulin production may be diminished if the islets of Langerhans become infected, and some patients develop diabetes mellitus.

Medical management. The treatment of patients is medical unless the precipitating cause is biliary tract disease; then surgery may be indicated. Food and fluids are withheld to avoid stimulating pancreatic activity, and intravenous fluids are administered. The patient is kept on NPO status, and a nasogastric tube is inserted to decrease pancreatic stimulation, treat or prevent nausea and vomiting, and decrease abdominal distention. The most common complaint is constant, severe pain, and meperidine (Demerol) 50 to 100 mg every 3 to 4 hours is administered. Morphine may cause spasms of the sphincter of Oddi and should be avoided.

Parenteral anticholinergic medication, such as atropine or propantheline (Pro-Banthine), will help decrease pancreatic activity. Antacids or antihistamine–H_2 receptor antagonists, such as cimetidine (Tagamet), may be given to prevent the development of stress ulcers caused by decreased gastric pH. Antibiotics are used by some but usually only to counteract secondary infections.

If the patient has severe acute pancreatitis, hyperalimentation may be required to maintain an adequate state of nutrition. As the patient improves, further attacks may be prevented by maintaining a bland, low-fat, high-protein, high-carbohydrate diet. The diet must be free of alcohol and gastric stimulants, such as coffee. Oral hypoglycemic agents or insulin may be needed if there is destruction of the islets of Langerhans.

A partial or total pancreatectomy, surgical removal of part or all of the pancreas, may be performed to remove a cyst or tumor, treat pancreatitis, or repair trauma. If it is necessary to remove the entire pancreas, the secretion of insulin will be eliminated, and it will be necessary for the patient to take insulin for the rest of his life. The preoperative preparation of the patient is the same as that for other abdominal surgery. Postoperatively, the patient should be monitored for complications of peritonitis, jaundice, and intestinal obstruction.

Nursing interventions. The presence and location of

pain is important to determine, as well as what aggravates or relieves the pain. Keeping the patient as comfortable as possible involves proper administration of pain medications. The patient is usually on bed rest with bathroom privileges to decrease the flow of pancreatic enzymes. Nutritional needs are met by intravenous feedings as long as necessary. The patient who is addicted to alcohol may go through withdrawal while in the hospital. The nurse must be prepared to protect the patient from injury and provide supportive care to the patient and his family. All replacement fluids and medications must be monitored carefully for proper administration.

NURSING DIAGNOSES	NURSING INTERVENTIONS
Pain, related to stimulation of nerve endings caused by enlargement of pancreatic capsule, obstruction, or chemical irritation from enzymes	Administer medications as prescribed, and monitor relief. Restrict diet as necessary to prevent aggravation of pain (free from fats, alcohol, caffeine). Use alternative comfort measures: repositioning, positive imagery, and providing time for listening. Monitor nasogastric tube for functioning to prevent abdominal distention.
Altered nutrition: less than body requirements, related to inadequate intake associated with current anorexia, nausea, vomiting, and loss of enzymes necessary for the digestive process	Administer intravenous fluids or hyperalimentation as ordered. Weigh patient daily at same time and using same scale. Record intake and output, including nasogastric tube output. Administer antacids and antiemetics as prescribed. Instruct patient in a diet that is bland, low in fat, and high in protein and carbohydrate.

Patient teaching. The patient will remain on a bland, low-fat, high-calorie, high-carbohydrate diet after discharge. Alcohol and beverages or foods containing caffeine will not be allowed if full recovery is desired. The patient should also understand the disease process and the severity of the disease and related complications.

REFERENCES AND SUGGESTED READINGS

1. Anagnostakos NP and Tortora GJ: Principles of anatomy and physiology, ed 5, New York, 1987, Harper & Row, Publishers, Inc.
2. Beare PG and Myers JL: Principles and practice of adult health nursing, St Louis, 1990, The CV Mosby Co.
3. Billings DM and Stokes LG: Medical-surgical nursing, ed 2, St Louis, 1987, The CV Mosby Co.
4. Boyer MJ: Study guide to Brunner/Suddarth's testbook of medical-surgical nursing, ed 6, Philadelphia, 1988, JB Lippincott Co.
5. Brunner LS and Suddarth DS: Textbook of medical-surgical nursing, ed 6, Philadelphia, 1988, JB Lippincott Co.
6. Eisenberg P: Enteral nutrition: indications, formulas, and delivery techniques, Nurs Clin North Am 24(2):315, 1989.
7. Fong E, Ferris EB, and Skelley EG: Body structures and functions, ed 7, New York, 1989, Delmar Publishers, Inc.
8. Greifzu S: Colorectal cancer: when a polyp is more than a polyp, RN 49(9):23, 1986.
9. Hennessy K: Nutritional support and gastrointestinal disease, Nurs Clin North Am 24(2):373, 1989.
10. Hood G and Dincher J: Total patient care: foundations and practice, ed 7, St Louis, 1988, The CV Mosby Co.
11. Jermier BJ and Treloar DM: Bringing your patient through gallbladder surgery, RN 49(11):18, 1986.
12. Johnson S: A safer gastrostomy for the high-risk patient, RN 49(3):29, 1986.
13. Kearns PC: Exercises to ease pain after abdominal surgery, RN 49(7):45, 1986.
14. Kohn CL and Keithley JH: Enteral nutrition: potential complications and patient monitoring, Nurs Clin North Am 24 (2): 1989.
15. Marieb EN: Essentials of human anatomy and physiology, Menlo Park, Calif, 1984, Addison-Wesley Publishing Co, Inc.
16. McFarland L and Stamm W: Review of *Clostridium difficile*–associated diseases, Am J Infect Control, p 99, June 1986.
17. Memmler RL and Wood DL: Structure and function of the human body, ed 4, Philadelphia, 1987, JB Lippincott Co.
18. Monroe D and Jaffe E: Patient teaching for x-ray and other diagnostics, RN 53(4):52, 1990.
19. Pagana K and Pagana T: Diagnostic testing and nursing implications: a case study approach, ed 3, St Louis, 1990, The CV Mosby Co.
20. Rhosdahl CB: Textbook of basic nursing, ed 4, Philadelphia, 1985, JB Lippincott Co.
21. Schaefer KM: Easing the torment of an irritable bowel, RN 49(4):34, 1986.
22. Seidel HM and others: Mosby's guide to physical examination, St Louis, 1987, The CV Mosby Co.
23. Solomon EP and Phillips GA: Understanding human anatomy and physiology, Philadelphia, 1987, WB Saunders Co.
24. Thibodeau GA and Anthony CP: Structure and function of the body, ed 8, St Louis, 1988, Times Mirror/Mosby College Publishing.
25. Tucker SM and others: Patient care standards: nursing process, diagnosis, and outcome, ed 4, St Louis, 1988, The CV Mosby Co.
26. Willis D and others: Gallstones: alternatives to surgery, RN 15(4):44:, 1990.

CHAPTER CHALLENGE

KEY POINTS

- The digestive tract begins with the mouth, extends through the thoracic and abdominal cavities, and ends with the anus.
- The major processes of digestion and absorption take place in the small intestine.
- The large intestine is responsible for the preparation and evacuation of the waste products—feces.
- Mechanical digestion is the physical breakup of large particles of food.
- Chemical digestion refers to the series of reactions that breaks the protein, fats, and carbohydrates into simpler chemical forms.
- Diet therapy has an important role in the treatment of gastrointestinal disorders.
- Treatment of esophageal disorders often involves providing the patient with a means of eating, in addition to treating the disorder.
- Common causes of gastric disorders are alcohol, tobacco, aspirin, and antiinflammatory agents.
- Duodenal ulcers are the most common type of peptic ulcer disease.
- New surgical procedures are available to create alternatives to the traditional ileostomy and colostomy.
- A nursing goal for the patient with an ileostomy or colostomy is fostering patient independence in daily care when the patient demonstrates readiness.
- Keeping the surgical area free of contamination is of primary importance after rectal surgery.
- The approximate location of gastrointestinal bleeding may be determined by the characteristics of the emesis or fecal material.
- The nurse explains the purpose of any diagnostic procedure, how the procedure is performed, and the preparation necessary for the procedure and assists in the patient's understanding of the results.
- Individuals with inflammatory bowel disease have a greater risk of developing cancer of the bowel.
- Early detection of cancer in the gastrointestinal system facilitates early treatment and a better prognosis.
- A nasogastric tube is inserted to keep the stomach empty until peristalsis is resumed after a general anesthetic or any condition that interferes with peristalsis.
- Effective postoperative care begins with patient teaching during the preoperative period.
- Cholecystectomy (removal of the gallbladder) is one of the most commonly performed surgical procedures.
- The most common cause of cirrhosis of the liver is alcohol ingestion.
- Pancreatic disorders may cause diabetes mellitus because of interference with insulin production.
- The nurse must be aware of the effect of medications on the gastrointestinal system and how this may affect the patient.
- Planned nursing interventions must be individualized according to each patient's and family's unique needs.
- Prevention of the spread of hepatitis is a primary concern of health care professionals.
- An important aspect of nursing interventions in patients with hepatitis and cirrhosis of the liver is the relief of pruritus.

STUDY QUESTIONS

1. Bile is stored in the:
   a. Pancreas
   b. Gallbladder
   c. Liver
   d. Small intestine
2. The majority of digestion and absorption takes place in the:
   a. Gallbladder
   b. Mouth
   c. Small intestine
   d. Large intestine
3. The following are all correct nursing interventions for the patient having an endoscopic examination except:
   a. Keep the patient NPO after midnight
   b. Have the patient sign a consent form
   c. Allow the patient to drink fluids as soon as the examination is complete
   d. Notify the appropriate personnel
4. The nursing interventions necessary when caring for a patient with a liver biopsy include:
   a. Ensure platelet and prothrombin tests have been ordered
   b. Keep patient on bed rest for 24 hours after biopsy
   c. Take vital signs every 15 minutes for 1 hour, then every 30 minutes for 4 hours
   d. All of the above
5. The drugs most commonly used to treat peptic ulcers include:
   a. Maalox, Kayexalate
   b. Tagamet and Zantac
   c. Erythromycin and Flagyl
   d. Dyazide and Carafate
6. Both ulcerative colitis and Crohn's disease are aggravated by:
   a. Stress
   b. Azulfidine
   c. High-carbohydrate, high-protein diet
   d. High fluid intake
7. For prophylaxis to be effective for hepatitis B:
   a. Prophylaxis must be instituted before exposure
   b. Prophylaxis can be instituted either before exposure for persons at high risk or after exposure
   c. Prophylaxis must be instituted after exposure
   d. None of the above
8. Usually the first symptom associated with esophageal disease is:
   a. Dysphagia
   b. Malnutrition
   c. Pain
   d. Regurgitation of food
9. A hiatal hernia involves a(n):
   a. Extension of the esophagus through the diaphragm
   b. Involution of the esophagus, which causes a severe stricture
   c. Protrusion of the upper stomach into the lower portion of the thorax
   d. Twisting of the duodenum through an opening in the diaphragm
10. A common complication of esophageal cancer after radiation surgery is:
    a. Aspiration from fistula formation
    b. Hemorrhage
    c. Incompetence of the suture line, resulting in fluid seepage
    d. The dumping syndrome
11. Intrinsic factor is a gastric secretion necessary for the intestinal absorption of vitamin:
    a. B_1
    b. B_{12}
    c. C
    d. K

STUDY QUESTIONS (cont'd)

12. Before a gastroscopy, the nurse should inform the patient that:
    a. He must fast for 6 to 8 hours before the examination
    b. His throat will be sprayed with a local anesthetic
    c. After gastroscopy, he will not be given anything to eat or drink until his gag reflex returns
    d. All of the above will be necessary
13. The dumping syndrome after Billroth II surgery occurs when high-carbohydrate foods are administered over a period of less than 20 minutes; a nursing measure that will prevent or minimize the dumping syndrome is to administer the feeding:
    a. In six small meals daily, high in protein and fat
    b. By bolus to prevent continuous intestinal distention
    c. With about 100 ml of fluid to dilute the high carbohydrate concentration
    d. With the patient in semi-Fowler's position to decrease transit time influenced by gravity
14. The best time to administer an antacid is:
    a. With the meal
    b. 30 minutes before the meal
    c. 1 to 3 hours after the meal
    d. Immediately after the meal
15. A nursing intervention(s) associated with peptic ulcer bleeding is (are):
    a. Checking the blood pressure and pulse rates every 15 minutes to 1 to 2 hours
    b. Frequently monitoring hemoglobin and hematocrit levels
    c. Observing stools and vomitus for color, consistency, and volume
    d. All of the above
16. Pulmonary complications frequently follow upper abdominal incisions because:
    a. Aspiration is a common occurrence
    b. Pneumothorax is a common complication of abdominal surgery when the chest cavity has been entered
    c. The patient tends to have shallow respirations in an attempt to minimize incisional pain
    d. All of the above are true
17. Diverticulitis is clinically manifested by:
    a. A low-grade fever
    b. A change in bowel habits
    c. Left lower quadrant pain
    d. All of the above
18. A problem in all patients with an ileostomy is that:
    a. Regular bowel habits cannot be established
    b. Sexual activity is restricted
    c. Skin excoriation can occur
    d. The collecting applicance is bulky and large
19. Preoperatively, intestinal antibiotics are given for colon surgery to:
    a. Decrease the bulk of colon contents
    b. Reduce the bacteria content of the colon
    c. Soften the stool
    d. Do all of the above
20. Clinical manifestations of common bile duct obstruction include all of the following except:
    a. Amber urine
    b. Clay-colored feces
    d. Pruritus
    d. Jaundice

32

Care of the Patient with a Cardiovascular or Blood Disorder

PHYLLIS J. TURNER

LEARNING OBJECTIVES

After reading this chapter, the student should be able to do the following:

- Define the key terms.
- Describe the components of blood.
- List the functions of the various components of blood.
- Describe the blood clotting process.
- List the names of the basic blood groups.
- Identify the chambers of the heart.
- List the functions of the chambers of the heart.
- Identify the valves of the heart and their locations.
- Trace a drop of blood through the heart and lungs.
- Trace a drop of blood through the hepatic system.
- Describe the difference between veins and arteries.
- Describe the difference between lymph and blood.
- Describe the function of the lymphatic system.
- List common diagnostic tests for evaluation of blood and lymph disorders, and discuss the significance of the results.
- Compare uncontrollable risk factors in coronary artery disease with factors that are controllable in life-style and health management.
- Identify differences in the pain process of angina pectoris and myocardial infarction.
- Outline educational points for rehabilitation of an individual recovering from myocardial infarction.
- Compare nursing observations and interventions indicated for a patient with congestive heart failure and pulmonary edema.
- Differentiate various types of inflammatory heart diseases.
- Explain the effects of exercise on the cardiovascular system, outlining points in support of activity related to health promotion.
- Participate in the development of nursing diagnoses and interventions for the various types of anemia.
- List various cardiovascular medication classifications, and identify examples of each.

RELATED TOPICS OF INTEREST

- Basic nutrition (Chapter 22)
- Diet therapy (Chapter 23)
- Care of the patient with a gastrointestinal or accessory organ disorder (Chapter 31)
- Care of the patient with a respiratory disorder (Chapter 34)
- Cardiopulmonary resuscitation (Chapter 53)

KEY TERMS

Define the following:

- antibody
- antigen
- aorta
- aplasia
- arteriole
- arteriosclerosis
- artery
- atheroma
- atherosclerosis
- atria
- atrioventricular valve
- bruit
- capillary
- cardiovascular
- coronary
- diastole
- dysrhythmia
- embolus
- erythrocyte
- extravasation
- fibrin
- hemoglobin
- heterozygous
- homozygous
- infarct
- intermittent claudication
- ischemia
- leukocyte
- lumen
- lymphocyte
- mediastinum
- monocyte
- myocardium
- occlusion
- orthopnea
- patent
- rubor
- semilunar valves
- septum
- stasis
- systole
- thrombocyte
- universal donor
- valve
- vein
- vena cava
- ventricle
- venule

ANATOMY AND PHYSIOLOGY

The cardiovascular (circulatory) system is the transportation system of the body. It delivers oxygen and nutrition to the cells for their individual activity and transports the cells' waste products to the appropriate organ for disposal. In ancient times the blood was referred to as the "river of life," or "fluid of life." Some even believed it had magical properties. All knew it was necessary to maintain life.

In this chapter the composition of blood and the structure and function of the blood vessels, the heart, and the lymphatic system will be discussed.

Characteristics of Blood

Blood is a viscous (thick), red fluid that contains red blood cells, white blood cells, and platelets, which are suspended in a light yellow fluid called *plasma* (Fig. 32-1). Plasma constitutes 55% of the blood's volume; the remaining 45% is composed of the blood cells and platelets.

Blood is slightly alkaline, with a pH range of 7.35 to 7.45. It has a sodium chloride (Na, salt) concentration of 0.9%. The average adult blood volume is 5 to 6 quarts (liters), or 10 to 12 pints.

The blood performs three critical functions. First, as stated, it transports oxygen and nutrition to the cells and waste products away from the cells. Second, it regulates the acid-base balance (pH) with buffers, aids with body temperature because of its water content, and controls the water content of its cells as a result of dissolved sodium ions. Third, it protects the body against infection with special cells and prevents blood loss with special clotting mechanisms.

The individual components of the blood are discussed in the following text.

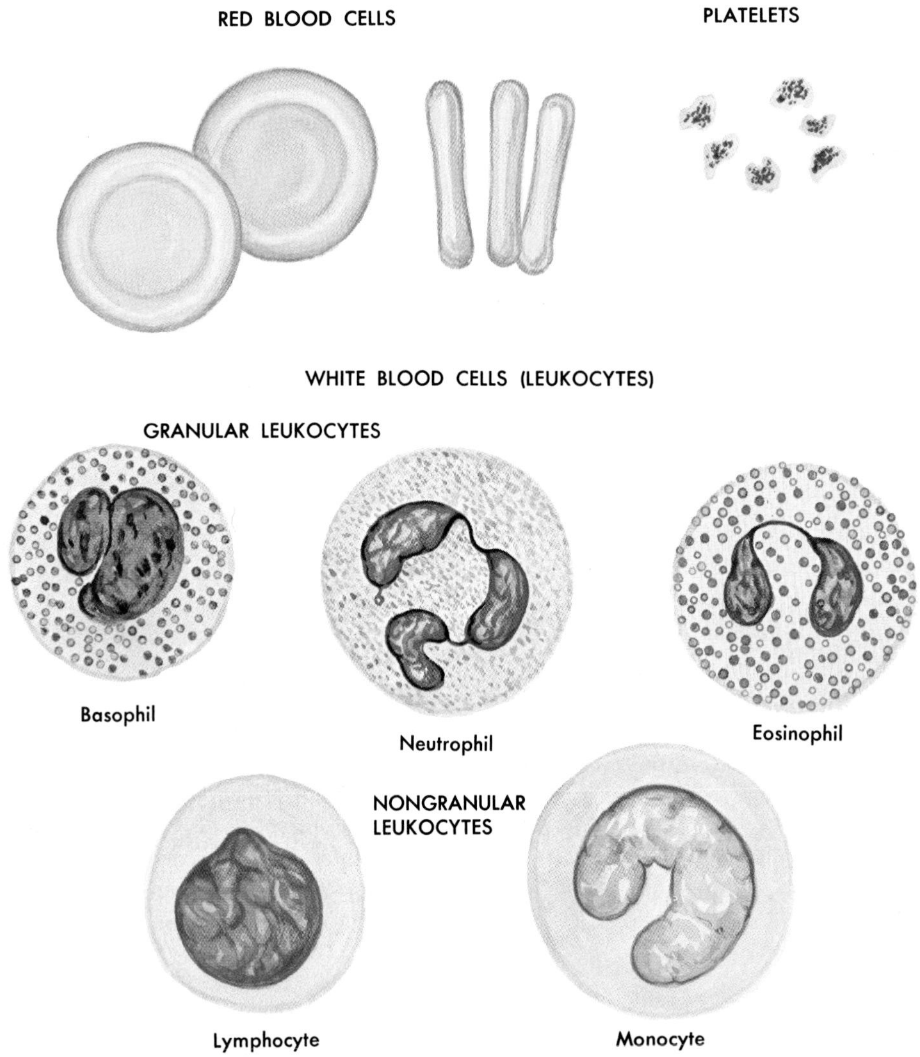

FIG. 32-1 Human blood cells. There are approximately 30 trillion blood cells in the adult. Each cubic millimeter of blood contains from 4½ to 5½ million red blood cells, 7500 white blood cells, and an average of 300,000 platelets.

Red Blood Cells

Erythrocytes (red blood cells, RBCs) give blood its rich red color. The mature RBC contains cytoplasm and the red pigment, **hemoglobin** (Hg), but no nucleus. Its average life span is 120 days. The hemoglobin molecule is composed of globin surrounded by 4 iron compounds called *heme*. When the RBC passes through the lung, the hemoglobin combines chemically with the oxygen to form *oxyhemoglobin,* which travels to the body cells where the oxygen is released. The hemoglobin, in turn, picks up carbon dioxide and chemically forms carboxyhemoglobin, which it returns to the lungs where it releases the carbon dioxide and picks up more oxygen to repeat the cycle.

Erythrocytes are continuously produced in the red bone marrow. They number 4.5 to 5 million per cubic millimeter (mm^3) of blood. As they age and are no longer useful, they are destroyed by the liver and the spleen.

White Blood Cells

Unlike the erythrocytes, the **leukocytes** (white blood cells, WBC) have nuclei, are colorless, and live from a few days to several years. They are primarily involved in body defenses, such as destruction of bacteria and viruses. They number 5000 to 10,000 per cubic millimeter of blood. Some WBCs can actually leave the bloodstream and move through tissue spaces to fight foreign invaders, such as bacteria.

There are two broad categories of white cells: granulocytes (granule-containing) and agranulocytes (granule-free). The three types of granulocytes are neutrophils, eosinophils, and basophils. The agranulocytes include the lymphocytes and monocytes.

The granulocytes develop from the red bone marrow and contain granules in their cytoplasm. The granules are demonstrated when the cells are stained with Wright's stain (a chemical solution). Neutrophils ingest bacteria and dispose of dead tissue by the process of phagocytosis (engulfing and digesting). They also release lysozyme, an enzyme that destroys certain bacteria. Eosinophils play a role in allergic reactions and are effective against certain parasitic worms. Basophils release histamine (vasodilator) and heparin (anticoagulant) during tissue damage or invasion. **Monocytes** function similarly to neutrophils, with phagocytosis of dead or injured cells. They are useful in removing dead bacteria and cells in the recovery stage of acute bacterial infections. The lymphocytes are responsible for **antibody** formation, a special protein that combats foreign invaders, or **antigens.** They set up the antigen-antibody process, which protects our body. There are two groups of lymphocytes, B cells and T cells. The function of the B cells is to search out, identify, and bind with specific antigens. T cells, when exposed to an antigen, divide rapidly and produce large numbers of new T cells that are sensitized to that antigen. They work together with the B cells to destroy the foreign antigen.

Platelets

Thrombocytes (platelets) are small, circular cell fragments, which do not contain nuclei. They have a life span of 5 to 9 days and number 200,000 to 400,000 per cubic millimeter of blood. They are produced in the red bone marrow and function in hemostasis (prevention of blood loss). They assist in clotting formation, which seals off a break in the continuity of the walls of the blood vessels.

Hemostasis

Hemostasis is a body process that prevents hemorrhage. Three actions take place: (1) vessel spasm, (2) platelet plug formation, and (3) clot formation (Fig. 32-2). When a vessel has a tear or rupture, the smooth muscle in the walls of the vessel causes it to contract. Platelets rush to the area and attempt to seal the area, which is effective in small vessel tears. The third process, clot formation, is more detailed and occurs in larger injuries.

Once the platelets reach the injured area and attempt to plug it, a series of reactions involving clotting factors (proteins in the blood) takes place (Fig. 32-3). Thromboplastin is released by the injured tissues and initiates a series of chemical reactions that lead to clot formation. The thromboplastin chemically reacts, along with calcium ions (present in the blood), to convert prothrombin (manufactured in the liver and present in the blood) to thrombin. The thrombin links with fibrinogen (present in the blood) to form **fibrin.** Fibrin molecules are long, thin strands that collect red blood cells and platelets at the injury site. This action forms a clot. Vitamin K stimulates the liver cells to increase the synthesis of prothrombin. This causes faster thrombin formation, which results in faster clotting time (Fig. 32-4).

Summary of this process:
Injury . . . hemorrhage . . . grouping of platelets . . . thromboplastin released . . . (reacts along with calcium ions) . . . converts prothrombin . . . to thrombin . . . links with fibrinogen . . . forms fibrin . . . traps RBCs and platelets . . . FORMS CLOT

Blood Types (Groups)

A person's blood group or type is determined genetically and inherited from the parents. Blood types are determined according to the presence or absence of specific proteins (antigens) on the outer surface of the RBCs. In certain types of blood the antigens on the RBCs are accompanied by other proteins found in the blood plasma (antibodies).

The four major types of blood are *A, B, AB,* and *O.* Type *A* blood contains the antigen *A* on the surface of its RBCs, type *B* contains the antigen *B* on its RBCs, type *AB* contains both *A* and *B* on its RBCs, and type *O* contains *no* antigens.

Circulating in the plasma of the various types are the antibodies A, B, and AB. Type A blood has B antibodies, type B contains A antibodies, type AB contains no antibodies, and type O contains AB antibodies. It is important to remember that antibodies are capable of destroying certain antigens. For example, type A blood con-

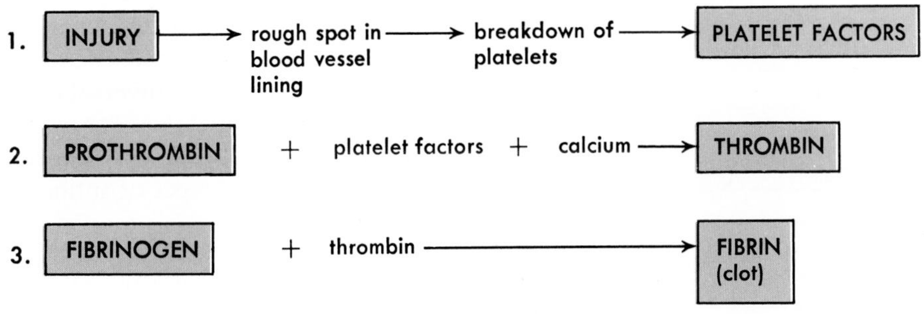

FIG. 32-2 Diagram showing the main steps in blood clotting—a process far more complex than is indicated here.

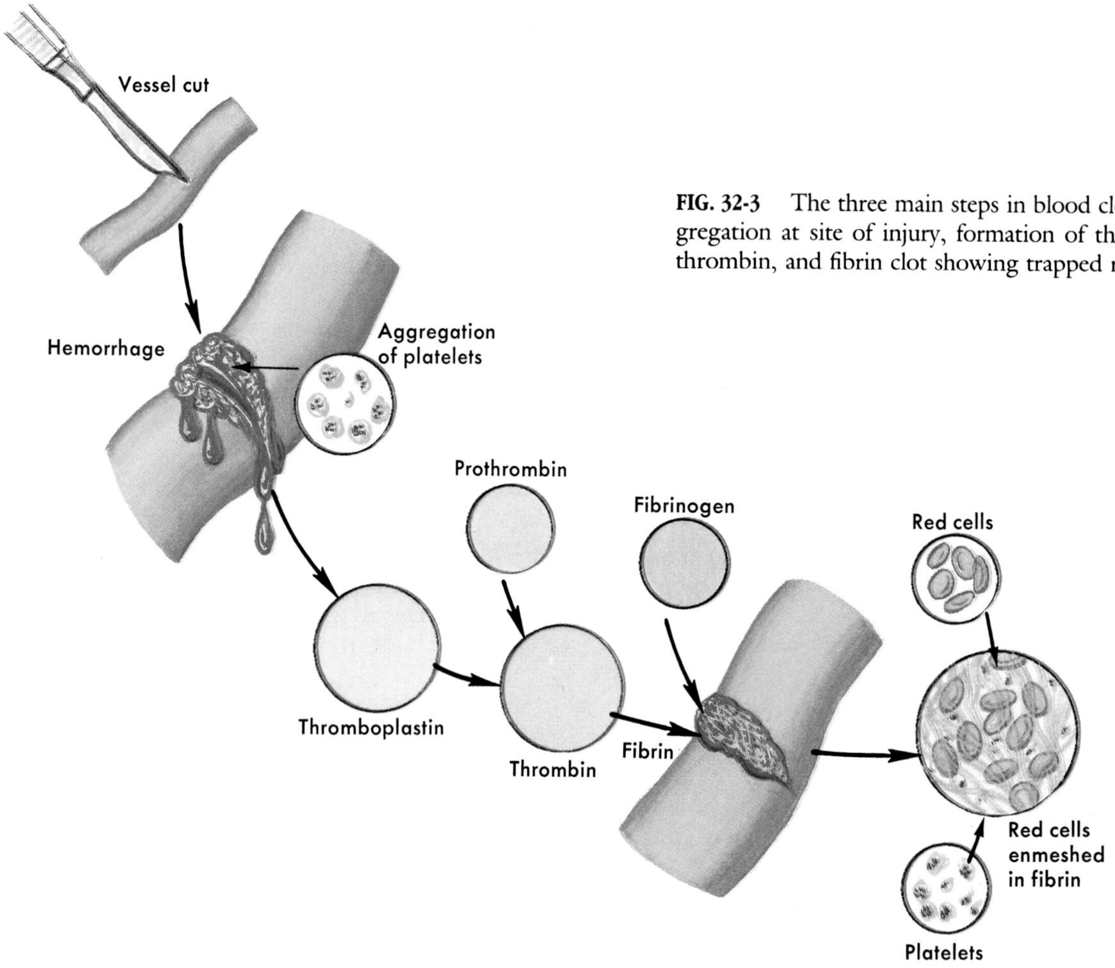

FIG. 32-3 The three main steps in blood clotting: platelet aggregation at site of injury, formation of thrombin from prothrombin, and fibrin clot showing trapped red cells.

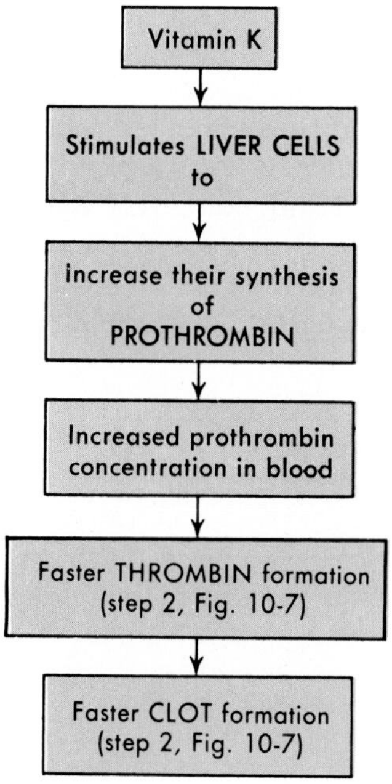

FIG. 32-4 How vitamin K acts to accelerate blood clotting.

tains type B antibodies—if a person had type A blood and received type B blood, the B antibodies would set up a sensitivity reaction (fight). Typing is necessary because these antibodies actually destroy the RBCs of the recipient. Thus the donor blood and the recipient blood must be the same type.

There are two types of reactions that can occur: *agglutination* and *hemolyzation*. In agglutination the donor cells clump together because of the antibodies; this occludes the arteries and can result in death. In the second process, hemolyzation, the antibodies cause the RBCs of the recipient to rupture and release their cell contents; this can also lead to death.

Type O blood is the **universal donor** (can be donated to all types), because it does not contain antibodies. Type AB is the universal recipient (can receive all types), because it contains all types of antibodies.

Rh Factor

In 1940 a genetic factor was discovered when research was being conducted on the blood of the Rhesus monkey, hence the name *Rh factor*. People who have the Rh factor, which is located on the surface of the RBCs, are said to be Rh positive; people who do not have the factor are said to be Rh negative. Of the population, 85% have the factor; 15% do not.

Normally human plasma does not contain Rh antibodies. They develop in response to an individual receiving the wrong type of blood. This occurs if an Rh-negative person receives a transfusion of Rh-positive blood. In approximately 2 weeks, Rh antibodies are produced and remain in the blood. If the person then receives more Rh-positive blood, a severe reaction occurs because the Rh-positive antibodies react with the donor blood. It hemolyzes the red blood cells, causing them to rupture and lose their contents.

Rh incompatibility is seen more commonly in pregnancy. For example, the father has Rh-positive blood, the mother has Rh-negative blood, and the baby has inherited Rh-positive blood from the father. At birth a small amount of blood from the baby can intermingle with the blood of the mother (transplacental bleeding). If she should become pregnant again and carry another Rh-positive baby, the antibodies that she has produced could cross to the baby and cause hemolysis of the baby's RBCs. This condition in the baby is known as *erythroblastosis fetalis*.

Fortunately there is a means to prevent this sequence of events. The mother's blood can be tested for antibodies, and she can receive an intramuscular dose of RhoGAM—a desensitization drug. This enables her to carry the next infant without Rh incompatibility.

The Heart

The heart is a remarkable organ that is not much bigger than the fist (Fig. 32-5). It is responsible for pumping 1000 gallons of blood every day. It beats 100,000 times a day and transports the blood 60,000 miles through a network of blood vessels. It is a hollow organ composed mainly of muscle tissue with a series of one-way valves.

It is located in the chest cavity between the lungs in a region called the **mediastinum.** Two thirds of the heart

A

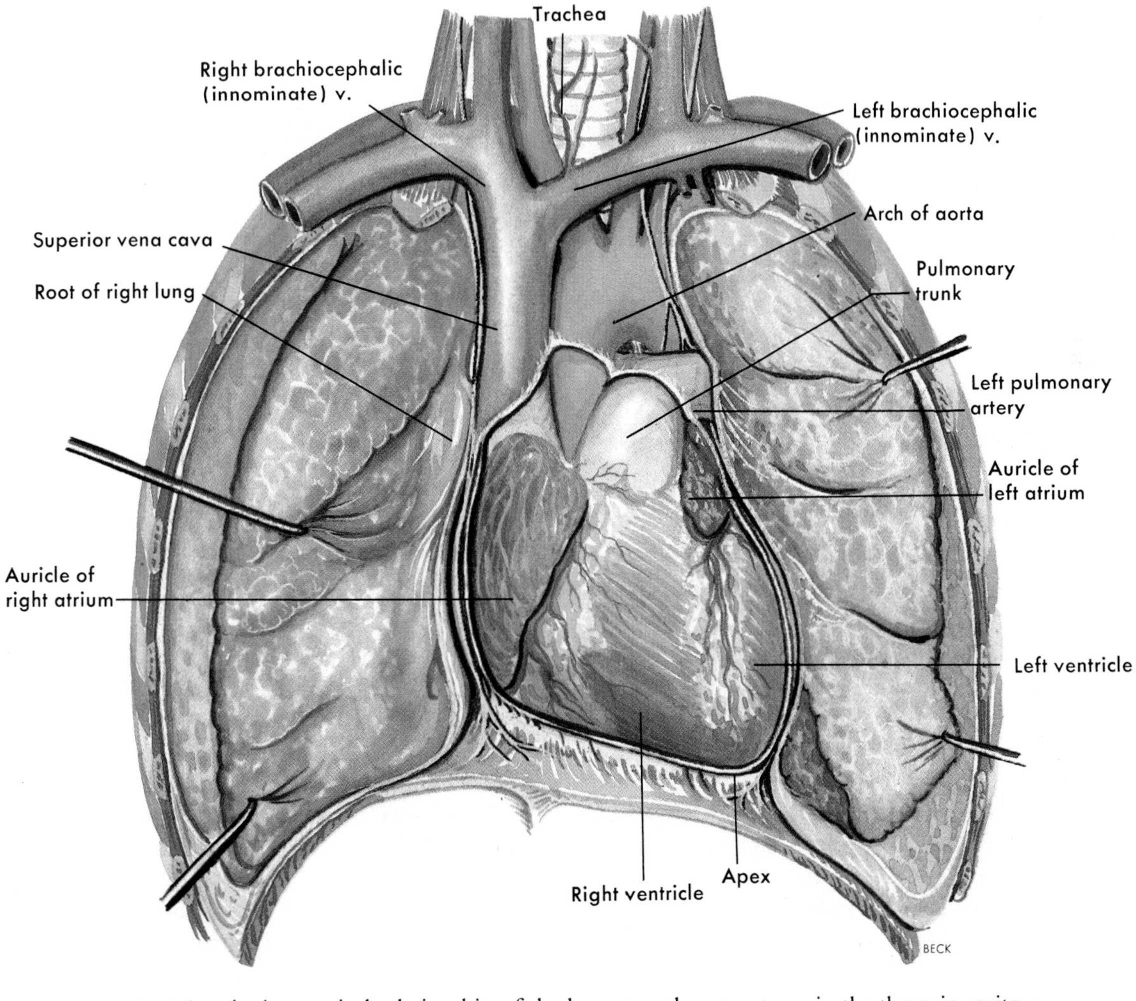

FIG. 32-5 **A,** Anatomical relationship of the heart to other structures in the thoracic cavity.
Continued.

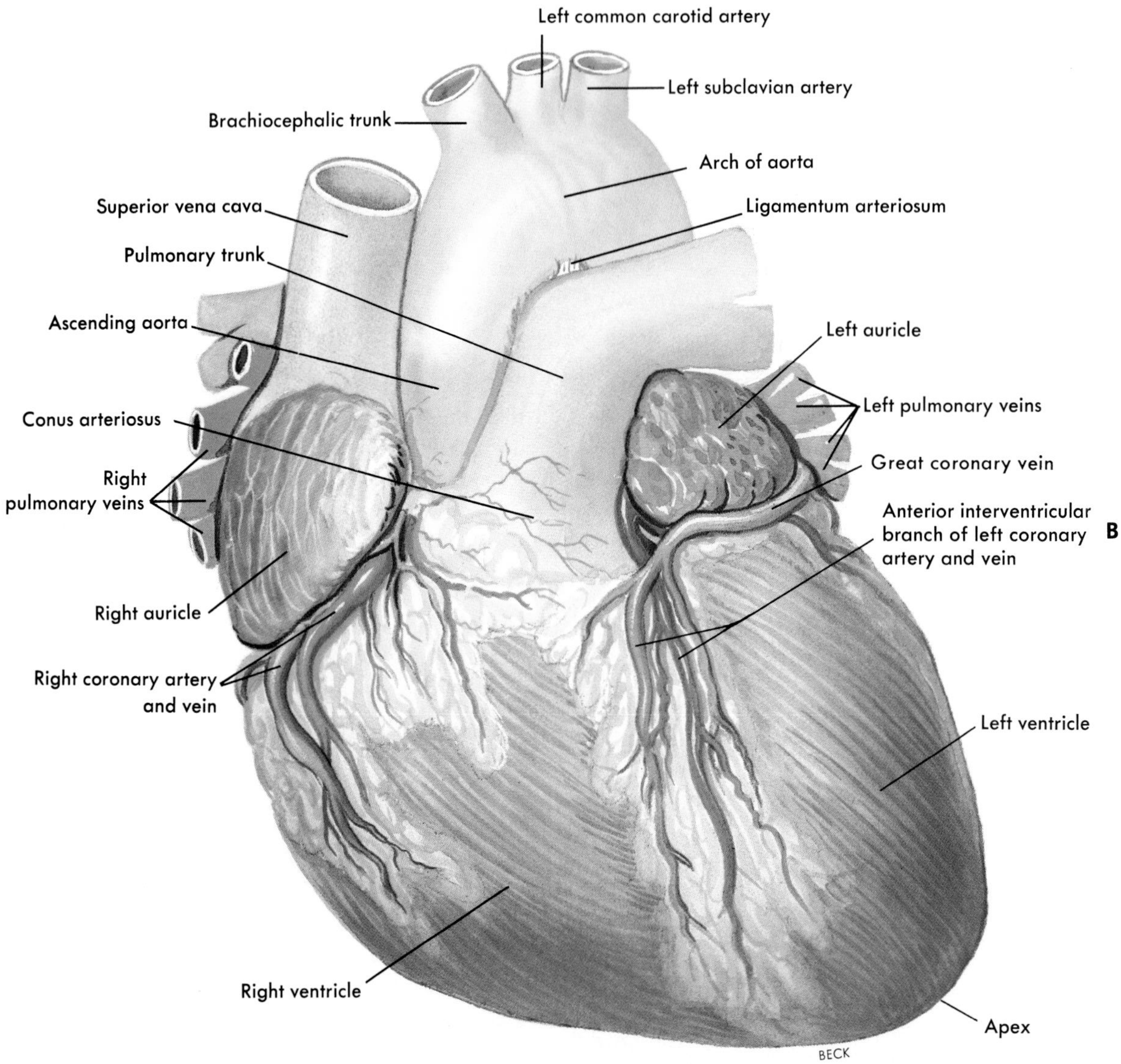

FIG. 32-5, cont'd **B,** Heart and major blood vessels viewed from the front (anterior).

lies left of the midline (Fig. 32-5, *A*). The lungs lie to either side of it. The wider base of the heart lies superiorly and beneath the second rib. The apex, or narrow part, of the heart lies inferiorly, slightly to the left between the fifth and sixth ribs near the diaphragm.

Heart wall. The heart is composed of three layers: epicardium, myocardium, and endocardium. The total structure is covered by a two-layered serous membrane called the *pericardium*. The inner layer is the *epicardium*, or *visceral pericardium*. It adheres to the heart, whereas the outer layer, the parietal pericardium, anchors the heart within the chest wall. Between the two thin membranes is a serous fluid that allows friction-free movement of the heart as it contracts and relaxes.

The **myocardium** (middle layer) is the thickest and strongest layer of the heart. It is composed of cardiac muscle tissue. The contraction of this tissue is responsible for the pumping of the blood.

The endocardium (innermost layer) is composed of a thin layer of connective tissue. It lines the interior of the heart, the valves, and the large vessels of the heart.

Heart chambers. The heart is divided into a right and left half by a muscular partition called the **septum** (Fig. 32-6). There are four chambers: two **atria** and two **ventricles.** The upper chambers are the right and left atria, and the lower chambers are the two ventricles. The septum dividing the atria is called the *interatrial septum,* and the septum dividing the ventricles is called the *interventricular septum.* In the normal healthy heart there is no opening between the right and left sides of the heart. Each chamber of the heart and its function will be discussed in the text that follows.

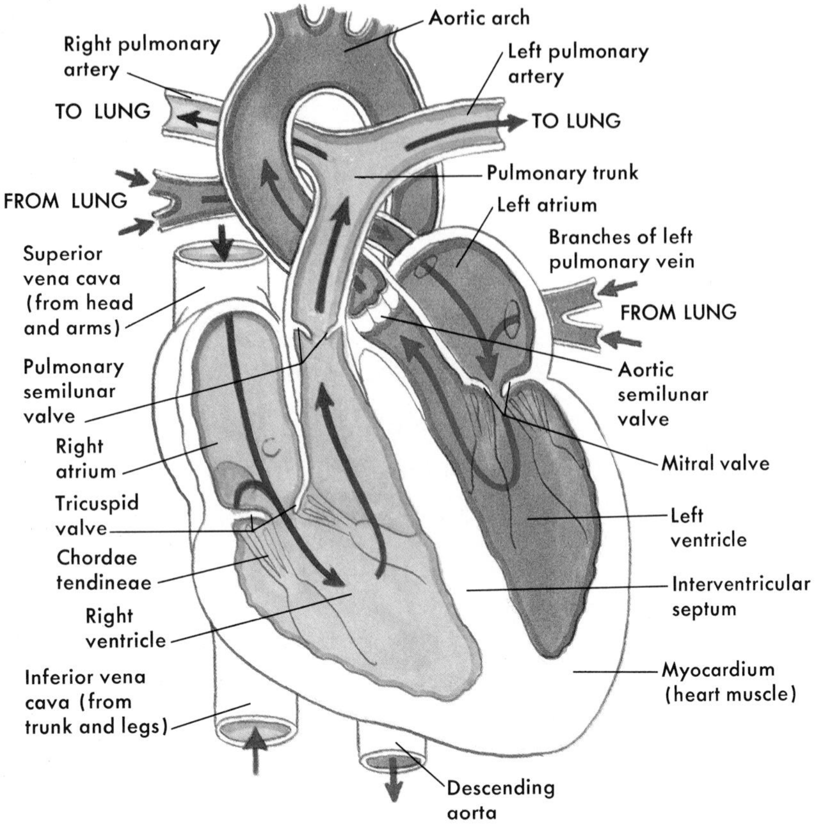

FIG. 32-6 Cutaway view of the front section of the heart showing the four chambers, the valves, the openings, and the major vessels. Arrows indicate the direction of blood flow: the blue areas represent unoxygenated blood and the red areas represent oxygenated blood.

The right atrium. The upper right chamber, the right atrium, receives deoxygenated blood from the entire body. The superior vena cava returns blood from the head, neck, arms, and trunk. The inferior vena cava returns blood from the lower body. The coronary sinus returns it from the heart muscle.

The right ventricle. The right ventricle is the lower right chamber, and it receives blood from the right atrium. It should be remembered that this blood is deoxygenated. The right ventricle pumps it to the lungs via the pulmonary artery to release carbon dioxide and receive oxygen.

The left atrium. The left atrium is the upper left chamber of the heart. It receives the oxygenated blood from the lungs via the four pulmonary veins.

The left ventricle. The left ventricle is the lower left chamber of the heart. It receives the oxygenated blood from the left atrium. It is the thickest, most muscular section of the heart and pumps the oxygenated blood out through the aorta to all parts of the body. The heart actually functions as two separate pumps: the right side receives deoxygenated blood and pumps it to the lungs, and the left side receives the oxygenated blood from the lungs and pumps it throughout the body.

Heart valves. Located within the heart are four **valves** that keep the blood moving forward and prevent backflow. The heart has two **atrioventricular** (AV) **valves.** They are located between the atria and ventricles. The right AV valve is located between the right atrium and right ventricle. It is called the *tricuspid* valve because it contains three flaps, or cusps. The left AV valve is composed of two cusps (bicuspid) and is commonly called the *mitral* valve. It is located between the left atrium and the left ventricle. Both the bicuspid and tricuspid valves open to allow blood to flow from the atria to the ventricles and then close rapidly to prevent backflow. Small, cordlike structures, chordae tendineae, connect the AV valves to the walls of the heart and work with papillary muscles located in the walls of the ventricles to make a tight seal to prevent backflow when the ventricles contract.

The two remaining valves, **semilunar valves,** are located at the points where the blood exits the ventricles. The pulmonary semilunar valve is located between the right ventricle and the pulmonary artery. Blood is pushed out of the right ventricle and travels to the lung via the pulmonary artery. The aortic semilunar valve is located

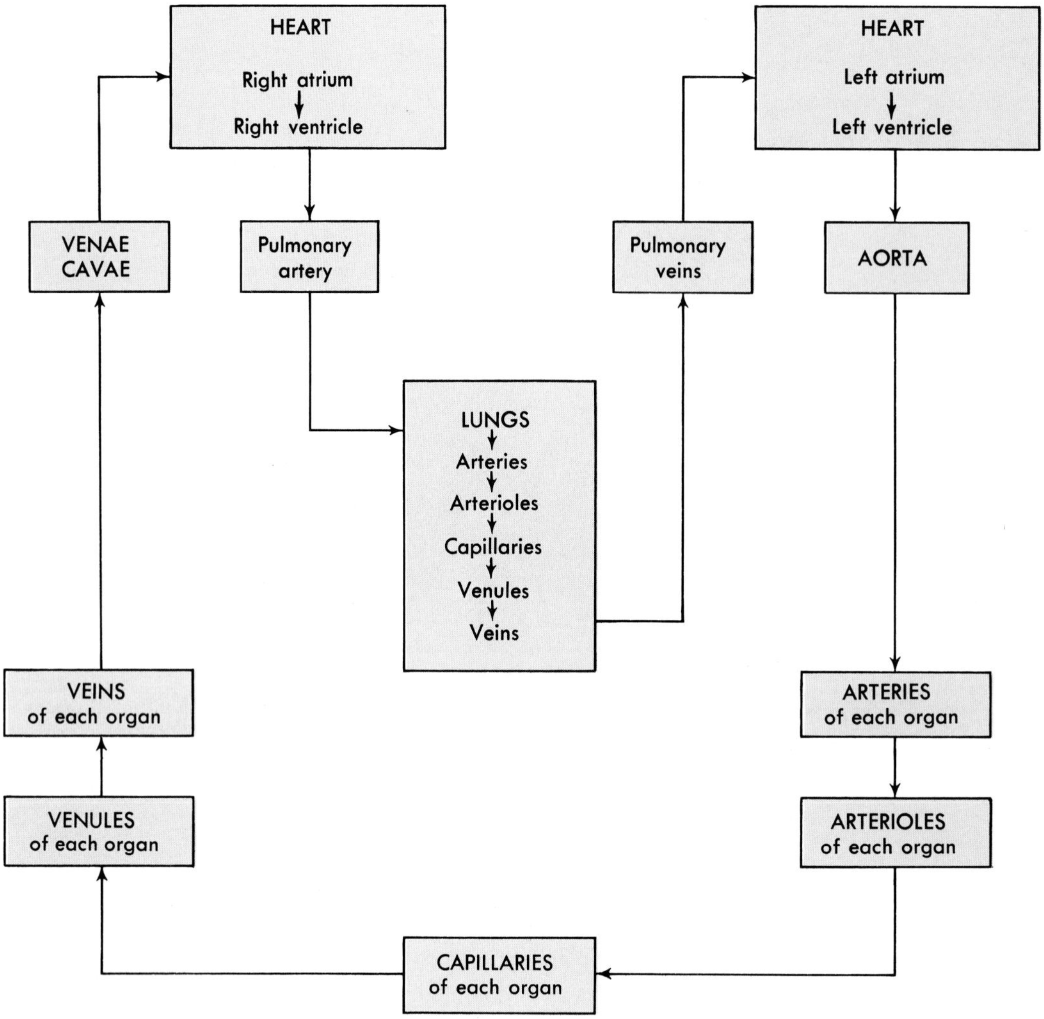

FIG. 32-7 Route of circulating blood.

between the left ventricle and the aorta. When the left ventricle contracts, the blood is forced into the aorta and the semilunar valve closes. Both of the semilunar valves are composed of three cusps that resemble a half moon, hence the name *semilunar*.

Blood Circulation Through the System

Coronary blood supply. The heart is responsible for pulmonary circulation (blood to and from the lungs) and systemic circulation (the entire body) (Fig. 32-7), but it is composed of muscle tissue and needs a blood supply of its own (coronary circulation) to stay healthy. The word *coronary* means resembling or being a crown. The coronary arteries form a crown around the myocardium (see Fig. 32-5, *B*). There are two branches immediately off the aorta that supply the myocardium with oxygen. They are the right and left coronary arteries. They bring oxygen and nutrition to the myocardium. Once the circulation is completed and the carbon dioxide and waste products have been collected, the blood flows into a large coronary vein, and finally into the coronary sinus, which empties into the right atrium. These two main arteries have many tiny branches that serve the heart. If an artery becomes occluded, these branches provide collateral circulation (alternate routes) to nourish the heart muscle. If the occlusion is severe, surgery and other procedures may be done. These treatments will be discussed later.

Electrical conduction system. Heart muscle tissue contains an inherent ability to contract in a rhythmic pattern. This ability is called *automaticity*. If heart muscle cells were removed and placed under a microscope, they would continue to beat. In addition, they have the ability to respond to a stimulus the same as nerve cells. This unique property is called *irritability*. Automaticity and irritability are two characteristics that affect the functions of the conduction system. Hormones, ion concentration, and changes in body temperature also affect the functions. These functions are the following:

- Conduction of messages around the heart
- Initiation of heartbeat
- Coordination of beating patterns between the atria and the ventricles

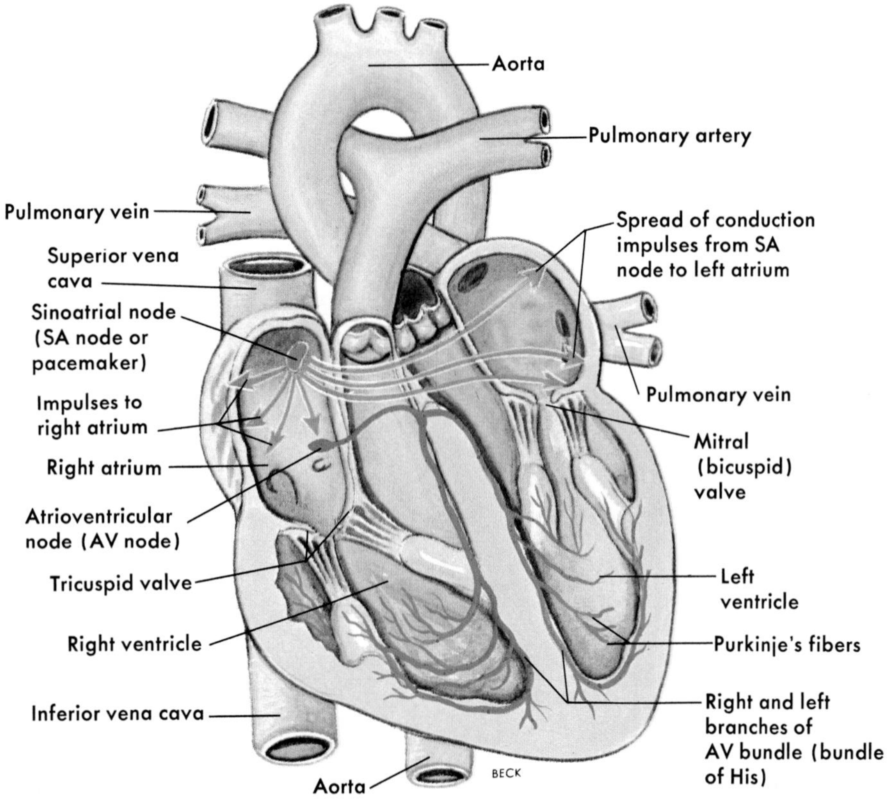

FIG. 32-8 The conduction system of the heart. The sinoatrial node in the wall of the right atrium sets the basic pace of the heart's rhythm, so it is called the "pacemaker."

The heartbeat is initiated in the sinoatrial (SA) node, which is located on the upper part of the right atrium just below the opening of the superior vena cava (Fig. 32-8). Because it regulates the beat of the heart, it is known as the *pacemaker,* and it causes contraction of the atria. Impulses are passed to the atrioventricular (AV) node, which is located in the base of the right atrium. The impulses are slowed by the AV node to allow the atria to complete contraction and to allow the ventricles to fill. The impulse then passes to a group of conduction fibers called the *bundle of His (AV bundle)* and break into right and left branches to travel to smaller branches called the *Purkinje fibers,* which surround the ventricles. The message travels very rapidly through the ventricles and causes contraction. This causes emptying of the ventricles.

Brief description of the impulse pattern:
SA node . . . AV node . . . bundle of His . . . right and left bundle branches . . . Purkinje fibers

Cardiac cycle. The cardiac cycle refers to a complete heartbeat. The two atria contract while the two ventricles are relaxed. When the ventricles contract, the two atria relax. The phase of contraction is called **systole,** and the phase of relaxation is called **diastole.** Complete diastole and systole of both atria and ventricles are a *cardiac cycle;* this takes an average of 0.8 second.

The heart sounds (*lubb* and *dubb*) are produced by closure of the valves. The first sound, lubb (long and low pitched) is heard when the AV valves close. The second sound, dubb (short, sharp sound) is heard when the semilunar valves close. Occasionally a murmur (swishing sound) can be heard. This can be a normal functional phenomenon produced by rapid filling of the ventricles or an abnormal condition produced by ineffective closure of the valves.

Electrocardiogram. As the heart goes through its cycle, tiny electrical currents are produced that can be measured and are of clinical value in diagnosing the condition of the heart. A normal tracing is shown in Fig. 32-9.

Each electrocardiogram (ECG) has three distinct waves, or deflections, called the *P wave,* the *QRS complex,* and the *T wave.* When the heart contracts, the electrical activity is called *depolarization. Repolarization* is the relaxation phase. The P wave represents the depolarization of the atria. The QRS complex represents the depolarization of the ventricles. The T wave represents the repolarization of the ventricles. Atrial repolarization is not represented but does occur; it is covered by the large QRS interval and cannot be seen on the ECG tracing.

Interpreting ECG tracings requires special knowledge.

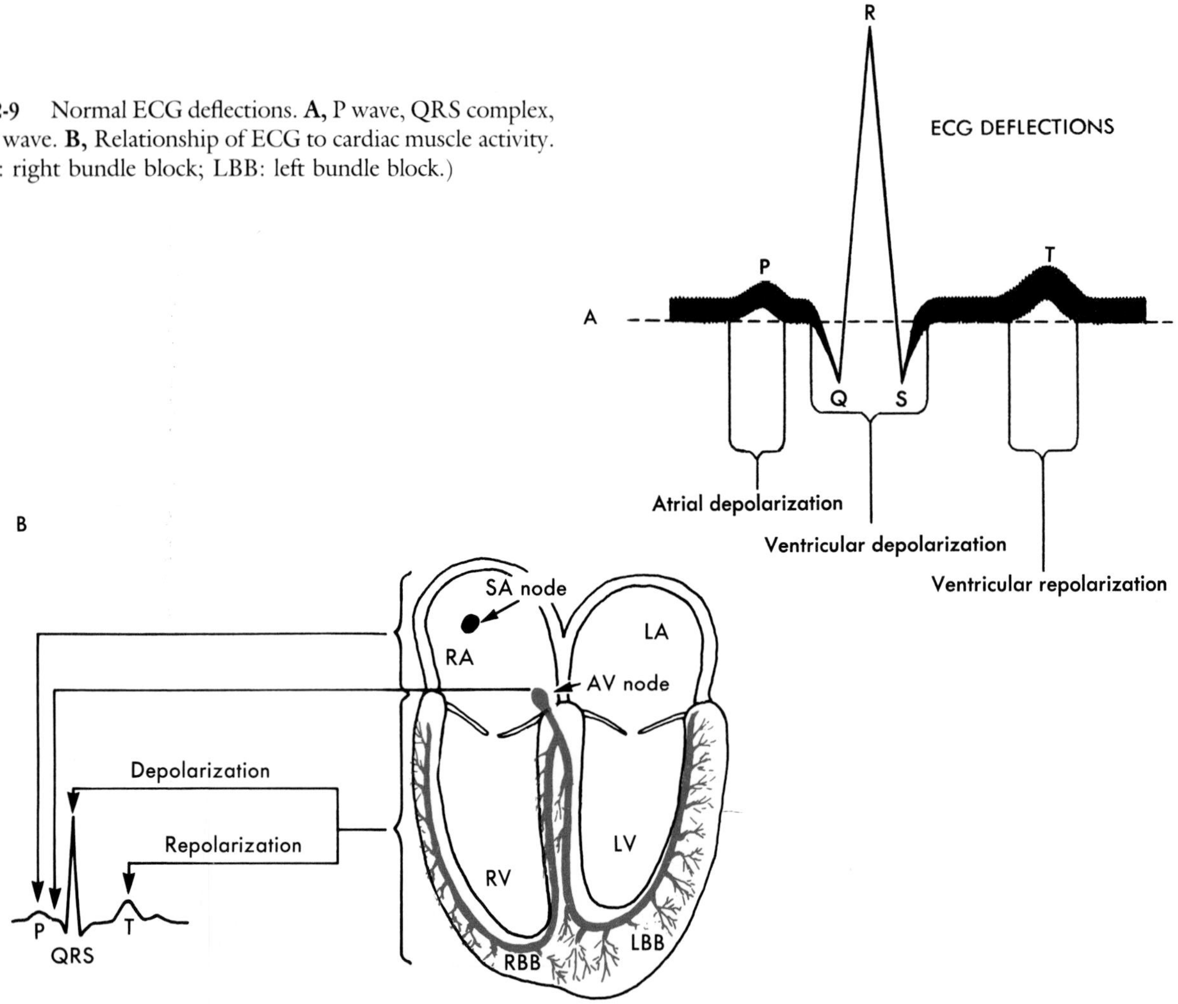

FIG. 32-9 Normal ECG deflections. **A,** P wave, QRS complex, and T wave. **B,** Relationship of ECG to cardiac muscle activity. (RBB: right bundle block; LBB: left bundle block.)

Interpretation is usually done by the physician, although many nurses have a basic understanding of ECGs. To interpret them, the reader considers the shapes of the waves and the time intervals between them. Many nurses, especially those working in critical care units, can identify changes in the tracing pattern.

Blood Vessels

There are three main types of blood vessels organized to carry blood to and from the heart. **Capillaries** connect the **arteries** to the **veins.** The veins return the blood to the heart. The heart delivers the blood to the arteries, which branch into tiny arteries called **arterioles,** which deliver the blood to the tissues. Within the various tissues, tiny microscopic vessels, capillaries, form an extensive network (50,000 miles), which allows for exchanges of products and by-products between the tissues and the blood. The capillaries then join with tiny veins, **venules,** which link with the larger veins and return to the heart.

A summary of the pattern:
Artery . . . arteriole . . . capillary . . . venule . . . vein

Structure of vessels. The walls of the vessels consist of three layers, or tunics: tunica externa, or adventitia (outermost); tunica media (middle); and tunica interna, or intima (innermost). The tunica externa is composed of connective tissue rich in elastic and collagen fibers. This layer is very thin in arteries but is the thickest layer of veins. The tunica media is composed of smooth (involuntary) muscle. It is the thickest layer of the large arteries. The interna is composed of flat epithelial cells, which allows the blood to flow freely.

Capillaries are microscopic and contain only the tunica interna. This allows for exchange of nutrients, oxygen, and carbon dioxide and other waste products as they pass among the cells in the tissues.

Circulation

Circulation refers to the movement of the blood throughout the body. Three major types of circulation will be discussed: systemic, pulmonary, and hepatic.

Systemic circulation. Systemic circulation occurs when blood is pumped from the left ventricle of the heart through all parts of the body and returns to the right atrium. When the oxygenated blood leaves the left ventricle, it enters the largest artery (2.5 cm, or 1 inch in diameter) of the body, the **aorta.** As the blood flows through the artery branches, the branches become smaller in diameter and are called *arterioles*. The blood continues to flow into microscopic structures called *capillaries*. The capillaries surround the cells, and the exchange of oxygen, nutrients, and carbon dioxide and other waste products occurs. The blood proceeds to tiny veins called *venules,* then to the larger structures called *veins,* and finally returns to the right atrium via the largest vein, the **vena cava.** The blood is now deoxygenated and needs to be replenished with oxygen. It is important to note that the upper portion of the vena cava (superior vena cava) returns blood from the head, neck, chest, and upper extremities. The inferior vena cava returns blood from the remaining distal portions of the body. To study the names and locations of the major arteries and veins of the body see Fig. 32-10.

Pulmonary circulation. The deoxygenated blood will now pass through pulmonary circulation to pick up the needed oxygen. Blood is pumped from the right atrium to the right ventricle, where it leaves the heart to travel via the pulmonary artery to the lungs. Once the blood reaches the lungs, it travels through arterioles to the capillaries. The microscopic capillaries surround the alveoli (air sacs), where oxygen diffuses into the bloodstream. The capillaries then connect with the venules and finally with the four pulmonary veins, which return the oxygenated blood to the left atrium of the heart. It is then pumped to the left ventricle, to the aorta, and systemic circulation is then repeated.

The blood circulation pattern is as follows:

1. Superior vena cava/inferior vena cava
2. Right atrium
3. Tricuspid valve
4. Right ventricle
5. Pulmonary semilunar valve
6. Pulmonary artery
7. Capillaries in the lungs
8. Pulmonary veins
9. Left atrium
10. Bicuspid valve
11. Left ventricle
12. Aortic semilunar valve
13. Aorta

See Fig. 32-7 for the blood circulation pattern through the body.

Hepatic portal circulation. Blood flowing through the liver takes a special route, and this is called *hepatic portal circulation*. Blood from the digestive organs does not empty into the inferior vena cava as from the other abdominal organs. Instead, it detours to the portal vein, which enters the liver. The blood travels through the liver capillaries. The liver cells remove excess glucose and store it as glycogen. They also remove and detoxify poisonous substances. The blood then empties into the hepatic veins, which empty into the inferior vena cava, which returns blood to the right atrium of the heart.

Lymphatic system. The lymphatic system is a subdivision of the cardiovascular system. It consists of the lymphatic vessels, the lymph fluid, and the lymph tissue. This system has three basic functions: (1) maintenance of fluid balance, (2) production of lymphocytes, and (3) absorption and transportation of lipids from the intestine to the blood stream.

Lymph. Lymph is a straw-colored fluid composed of water, lymphocytes, digested nutrients, oxygen, carbon dioxide, urea, and circulating hormones. Certain components of plasma from the blood diffuse into the area, surrounding and bathing the tissue cells. This fluid is called *interstitial fluid,* intercellular fluid, or tissue fluid. When this fluid moves into the lymphatic system, it is called *lymph*. This fluid differs from plasma because it contains less protein than plasma. It also contains leukocytes.

Lymphatic vessels. Lymphatic vessels are found throughout the body in vascular tissue. They are not found in the central nervous system, epidermis, the inner ear, the eyeball, or the spleen. The lymph vessels surrounding tissues are microscopic and are called *lymphatic capillaries*. These vessels join with larger vessels to form lymphatics. They form a meshlike network throughout the body and continue to unite until they join to form two large lymphatics, the thoracic duct and the right lymphatic duct.

All lymph flowing from the left side of the chest, head, neck, abdominal region, and lower legs flows through the thoracic duct. The thoracic duct then joins the left subclavian vein to empty into the superior vena cava and finally the right atrium of the heart. The right lymphatic duct receives lymph draining from the right arm, right side of the head, and upper trunk (Fig. 32-11). It travels to the right subclavian vein to the superior vena cava and finally to the right atrium of the heart. The lymph can travel in only one direction: from the organs toward the heart—never away from the heart.

Lymphatic tissue

Lymph nodes. Lymph nodes (glands) have two functions: (1) to filter impurities from the lymph—much like an oil filter in a car, and (2) to produce **lymphocytes** (WBCs). The body contains 500 to 600 lymph nodes. They are small, bean-shaped structures, usually appearing in groups. They range in size from 1 to 25 mm (0.04 to 1 in) in length. These groups are most numerous in the axillary, groin, abdomen, thorax, and cervical regions.

Tonsils. The tonsils are masses of lymphatic tissue embedded in the mucous membrane of the oral cavity and the pharynx. The pharyngeal tonsil (adenoid) is located in the posterior wall of the nasopharynx. The lingual

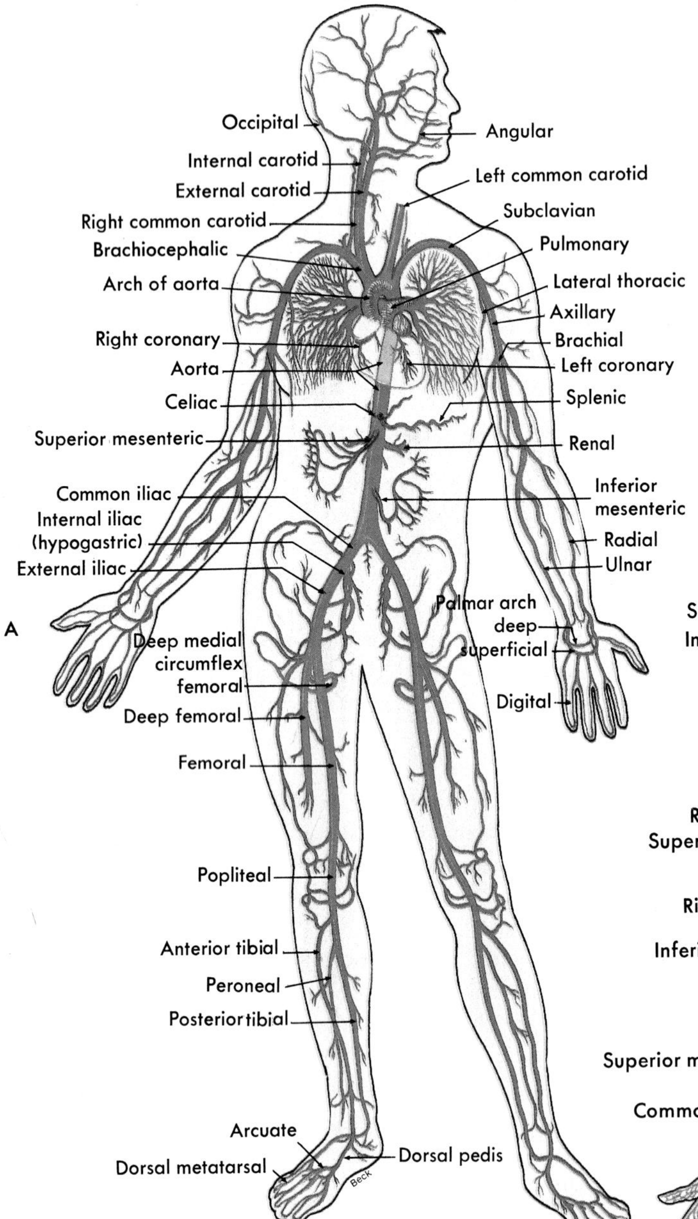

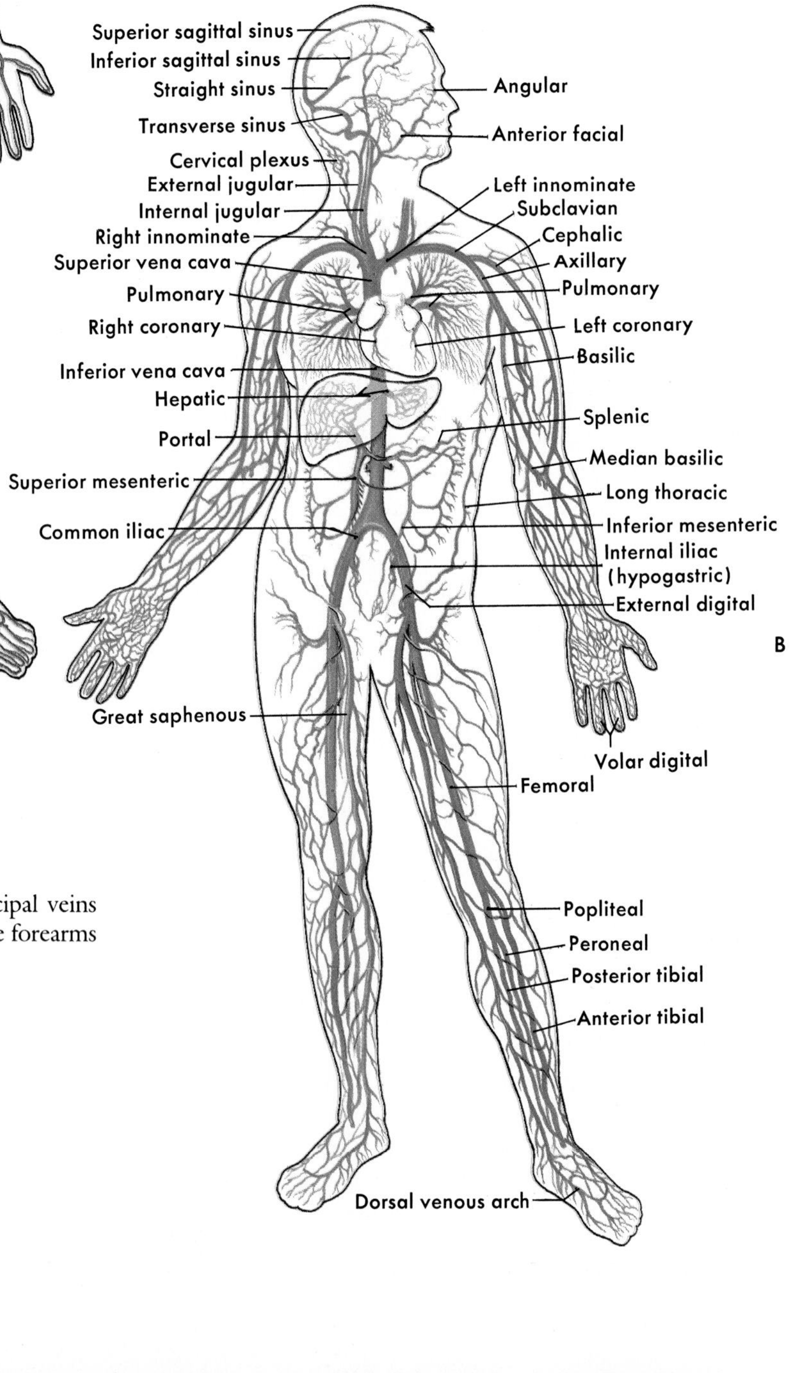

FIG. 32-10 **A,** Principal arteries of the body. **B,** Principal veins of the body. Only the superficial veins are shown on the forearms and hands.

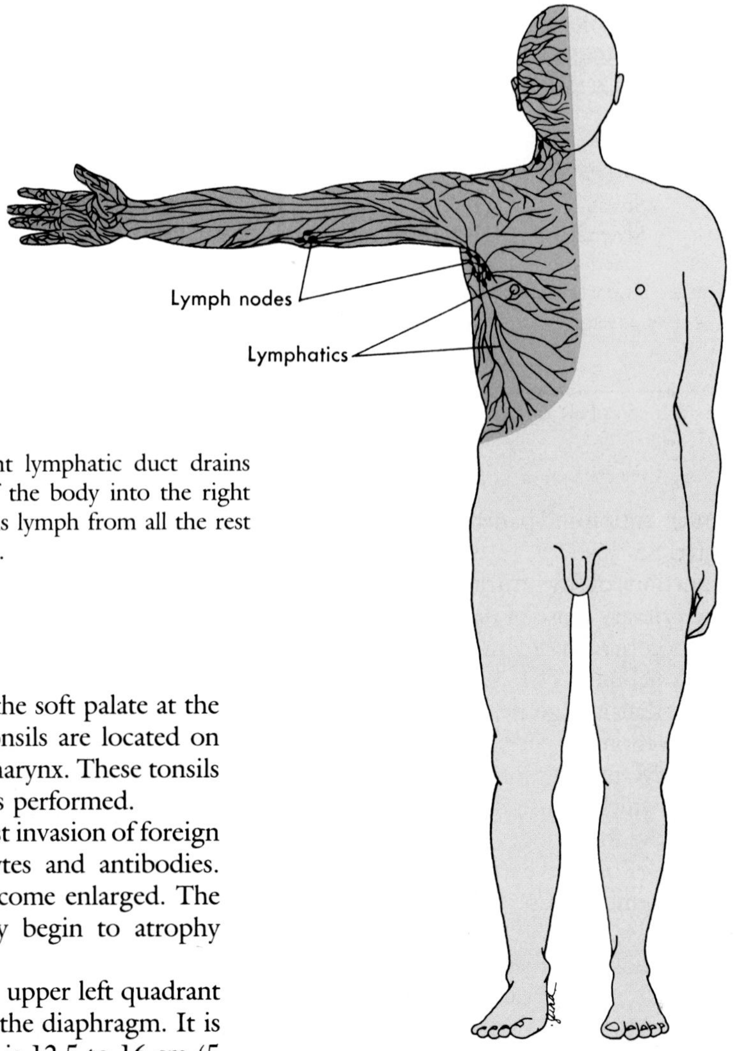

FIG. 32-11 Lymph drainage. The right lymphatic duct drains lymph from the upper right quarter of the body into the right subclavian vein. The thoracic duct drains lymph from all the rest of the body into the left subclavian vein.

tonsils are located on either side of the soft palate at the base of the tongue. The palatine tonsils are located on either side of the soft palate in the pharynx. These tonsils are removed when a tonsillectomy is performed.

The tonsils protect the body against invasion of foreign substances by producing lymphocytes and antibodies. They also trap bacteria and may become enlarged. The tonsils are larger in children. They begin to atrophy (shrink) at about age 7.

Spleen. The spleen is located in the upper left quadrant of the abdominal cavity, just below the diaphragm. It is protected by the lower three ribs. It is 12.5 to 16 cm (5 to 6 in) long and 5 to 7.5 cm (2 to 3 in) wide.

The spleen stores one pint of blood, which can be released in emergencies, such as hemorrhage. This large accumulation of blood gives it a unique deep purple color.

The main functions of the spleen are (1) to serve as a reservoir for blood, (2) to form lymphocytes, (3) to destroy worn-out red blood cells, and (4) to remove bacteria by phagocytosis (engulfing and digesting).

Thymus. The thymus is located in the upper thorax posterior to the sternum and between the lungs. The thymus gland functions in utero (before birth) and a few months after birth to develop the immune system. The thymus is responsible for the development of the T lymphocytes (discussed earlier). At puberty the thymus gland atrophies (shrinks) and eventually becomes replaced with fat and connective tissue.

Normal Aging Patterns of the Cardiovascular System

As the individual ages, the cardiovascular system undergoes certain normal changes. The heart muscle atrophies, and there are cellular changes in the blood vessel walls and valves. By the age of 65, the cardiac output has decreased by 30%.

The elderly are prone to dysrhythmias because of conduction defects of the electrical system. The valves of the heart have a tendency to calcify and become fibrotic.

All of these changes decrease the cardiovascular system's ability to function. The elderly need to be encouraged to exercise, to eat properly, and to get appropriate amounts of rest; this is good advice for any age group. With the advances in health care technologies, such as medications, surgical techniques, and diagnostic tests, such as cardiac catheterization, the elderly cardiac patient can live a better quality of life.

DISEASES AND DISORDERS OF THE CARDIOVASCULAR SYSTEM

The **cardiovascular** system supports the functioning of all other systems most efficiently when it is in optimal health. Achievement or maintenance of that status

BOX 32-1 RISK FACTORS ASSOCIATED WITH CARDIOVASCULAR DISEASE

UNCONTROLLABLE	CONTROLLABLE	HEALTH STATUS
Familial trait	Life-style	Diabetes mellitus
Age	Stress	Hyperlipidemia*
Sex	Sedentary activity	Hypertension*
Race		Obesity
	Tobacco usage*	Estrogen loss or oral contraceptive usage

* Denotes major factors that contribute to cardiovascular disease.

through nursing intervention and patient education is the focus of this chapter.

Although dysfunction of the cardiovascular system continues to be the primary cause of death in the United States, the public is becoming more informed in methods to avoid this health liability. The nurse in any health center will recognize that a large percent of that population will exhibit various aspects of heart disease. Achievement of effective nursing interventions relies on a knowledge base by which to use the nursing process. Components include the following:

- Skill in collection of objective and subjective data
- Understanding of the disease process and altered function
- Awareness of diagnostic test significance

The goal of data collection for cardiovascular nursing assessment will be to achieve an overview of signs and symptoms and related information to do the following:

- Establish a base for nursing intervention
- Correlate findings toward the participation in the development of nursing care plans

Collecting Data

Nursing data collection of the cardiovascular patient begins with a thorough health history, including symptoms, medications used, and dietary habits. Close attention to risk factors (Box 32-1), life-style, and psychosocial aspects gives insight into the individual and contributing factors in the condition. Physical findings further establish the data base. Considering these factors and the diagnostic study values will lead to a more thorough understanding of the disease manifestation and the needs or problems presented by the individual patient.

General Signs and Symptoms

The first aspects to be addressed in data collection are the signs and symptoms that may be presented by a patient with cardiovascular disease.

Pain, particularly chest pain, is the primary presenting symptom of heart disease. The patient may use the following terms to describe pain: dull, sharp, pressure, squeezing, crushing, viselike, grinding, and radiating. Location, duration, and intensity are determined. Precipitation of onset is noted. Pain originating from cardiac muscle ischemia is anxiety-producing. It may subsequently cause other symptoms, such as *nausea* and *vertigo* or *diaphoresis.* Chest pain is significant in forewarning heart damage.

On admission, careful attention to pain presentation can determine the need for analgesia for promotion of prompt relief. Relief of pain promotes cooperation and patient confidence in the nurse.

Dyspnea (shortness of breath or difficult breathing) is related to a heart condition and, on occasion, is accompanied by anxiety. The effect of exercise or exertion on the respiratory process is considered also when observing dyspnea. If the patient achieves comfort in breathing only through a sitting posture, the term **orthopnea** is applied.

Cough caused by fluid accumulation in the lungs is a body response that may be a source of discomfort to the patient. It may be accompanied by dyspnea. The patient may describe it as irritating, dry, productive, or spasmotic. The production of sputum with the cough is to be noted, especially if hemoptysis or frothy sputum is observed.

Fatigue may be expressed as "feeling tired all the time." This symptom relates to the decrease of blood flow and diminished oxygen supply to the tissues. It may be debilitating to the point of the patient being unable to perform the normal activities of daily living. *Depression* may accompany fatigue or result from it.

Edema, an abnormal retention of fluid in interstitial tissue spaces, is a common sign of heart disease and its complications. It is observed in heart failure, as well as renal dysfunction, venous obstruction, and inflammatory conditions. Edema is observed primarily in the ankles and feet. However, tightness of fingers and edema in the scrotal and sacral areas may occur.

Palpitation, a "pounding" or "racing" of the heart, is a symptom many patients become aware of when heart disease is diagnosed. Noticing the heartbeat, perhaps more frequently just before falling asleep, can be a frightening experience. Identified as a symptom of rhythmic disturbance, it can also be related to drug toxicity.

Syncope, or fainting, is a brief lapse in consciousness. Decreased blood flow to the brain relates it to the cardiovascular system. Vertigo may precede this symptom.

Careful attention to symptoms presented, as well as the patient reaction to the signs and symptoms, should be documented. The patient's perception of the problem and his ability to cope are important in establishing the plan of care. Family support and understanding are also noted. It may be helpful to use family aid in relating the health history or signs and symptoms.

Table 32-1 Medications Used in the Treatment of Various Cardiac Conditions

Classification	Drug	Action
Antibiotics	Penicillin Streptomycin Cephalosporin	Inhibit growth and eliminate infectious organisms.
Anticoagulants	Warfarin (Coumadin) Dicumarol Heparin Aspirin	Prevent blood from forming clots (emboli).
Antianginal agents/vasodilators	Isosorbide dinitrate (Isordil) Erythrityl tetranitrate (Cardilate) Dipyridamole (Persantine) Nitroglycerin preparations Pentaerythritol tetranitrate (Peritrate) Isosorbide dinitrate (Sorbitrate)	Reduce the workload of the heart by dilating blood vessel lumen, thus allowing increased blood flow.
Antihypertensives	Propranolol HCl (Inderal) Captopril (Capoten)	Control irregular heartbeat and elevated blood pressure.
Beta blockers	Propranolol (Inderal) Atenolol (Tenormin) Nadolol (Corgard)	Reduce myocardial oxygen demands, decrease heart rate, decrease contractility, decrease conduction, and decrease blood pressure.
Antidysrhythmics	Tocainide HCl (Tonocard) Quinidine sulfate Pronestyl Disopyramide (Norpace)	Treat and prevent cardiac dysrhythmias.
Cardiac glycosides	Digoxin Lanoxin	Control irregular heart rate and rhythm that occurs with CHF.
Calcium channel blockers	Verapamil HCl (Calan, Isoptin) Nifedipine (Procardia) Diltiazem HCl (Cardizem)	Treat spasms of coronary arteries that occur with exertional angina.
Diuretic agents	Furosemide (Lasix) Bumetanide (Bumex) Ethacrynic acid (Sodium Edecrin) Chlorothiazide (Diuril)	Remove excess fluid from tissues and blood stream.
Electrolyte replacement	K-Lor K-Lyte	Replace lost potassium caused by diuresis.

Medications

All medications the patient is taking must be noted, whether they are prescription or over-the-counter preparations. The nurse should consider the types or classifications of medications listed in Table 32-1.

Diet

Knowledge of the patient's diet helps the nurse understand his habits and plan for his discharge education. Caloric intake should focus on attaining and/or maintaining ideal weight. Sodium and fat restrictions are related to lowering blood levels of cholesterol and reducing fluid retention. Food-label-reading is emphasized for awareness of content. Baking, broiling, or steaming food is advised, as well as avoiding "fast foods." Relaxation at mealtime is stressed. This is an ongoing process and a point for education of the patient, because dietary habits are usually long established. The nurse should establish an understanding of the patient's diet knowledge to plan adequate care.

Initial Physical Observations

In noting signs and symptoms the nurse will realize that all body systems are affected by cardiovascular changes. Therefore all symptoms or signs, however remote, are noted. The general appearance is appraised first. Physical build is noted, with attention to any abnormalities. Posture may be relevant. Skin color is noted; cyanosis or pallor is observed. Texture, temperature and presence of edema are documented by proper description. Apical pulse is an accurate measure, with expected rate between 60 and 90 beats per minute. Activity may cause an increase of pulse rate. Blood pressure is accurately recorded, with attention to pulse pressure: the difference between the systolic and diastolic reading. A 30 to 40 point range is expected (e.g., BP: 128/90; pulse pressure:

36). Postural change may alter blood pressure. Usually the supine position is used. However, slight systolic elevation of 4 to 8 points may be shown if the patient is seated or standing. Rapid change of posture may produce a more radical change. The right and left arms may have different pressures, but these differences are slight and usually insignificant.

Diagnostic Evaluation

The nursing role is to physically prepare the patient for diagnostic procedures and to explain the examination to the patient. Cardiovascular function is evaluated through diagnostic examinations.

Radiological Examination

X-ray examination of the chest provides a film record of heart size, shape, and position and outline of shadows. Lung congestion is also shown, indicating heart failure, perhaps in the earliest stages.

Fluoroscopy, the action-picture x-ray, allows observation of movement. It is invaluable in pacemaker or intracardial catheter placement.

Angiogram is a series of x-rays taken after injection of radiopaque dye into an artery or vein. The circulatory process shows outlines of the heart and vessels. This procedure aids in diagnosis of vessel occlusion, pooling in various heart chambers, and congenital anomalies.

Arteriogram, or visualization of coronary arteries, is used to determine the extent of coronary occlusion by use of a radiopaque catheter threaded into areas suspect of occlusion.

Aortogram visualizes the abdominal aorta and the major leg arteries by use of dye injected through the femoral artery. X-ray visualization is employed. Aneurysms can be diagnosed, in addition to many other abnormalities. Contrast media to visualize the aortic arch and branches may also be employed.

Cardiac Catheterization

The passage of a catheter into the heart chambers through a peripheral vessel is used to measure (1) pressure within the heart and (2) blood volume relationship to cardiac competence. Valvular defects, occlusion, and congenital anomalies are determined. Blood samples are obtained. Contrast dye may be injected to allow better heart and vessel visualization (angiography). Because of the content of iodine in the contrast media, sensitivity is determined before injection to avoid allergic reaction, which could be a dangerous complication of this procedure. Cardiac catheterization is an invasive procedure, performed under sterile surgical conditions, and therefore must be preceded by a signed consent and standard preoperative testing. This procedure aids in diagnosis, prevents progression of cardiac conditions, and allows accuracy in evaluation and treatment of the critically ill patient.

Electrocardiography

The *electrocardiogram* (ECG/EKG) is a graphic study of the electrical activities of the myocardium to determine transmission of cardiac impulses through the muscles/conduction tissue. Rhythmic disturbance, myocardial damage, and hyperkalemia (elevated serum potassium) can be determined by the physician through ECG.

A standard ECG has 12 electrodes, or leads, which are placed on the chest in several positions and on both ankles and wrists. A conductive gel is used to enhance the contact and transmission. Straps attach the wrist and ankle leads, whereas rubber bulbs on metal suction cups are used on the chest leads. The patient is in a supine position. However, ambulatory ECG and exercise/stress test ECG require position variation. The machine, an electrocardiograph or galvanometer, records the energy wave of each heartbeat through a vibrating needle on graph paper, which feeds through the machine at a standard rate. This tracing—the ECG—is "read" or interpreted by a cardiac specialist (cardiologist). The reading can also be displayed on the fluorescent screen (oscilloscope) of a cardiac monitor. A graphic tracing may be printed out by the monitor.

Ambulatory ECG can be used to monitor heart rhythm over prolonged periods, usually 24 hours, and compared with various activities or patient symptoms. A Holter monitor (small portable recorder) is attached to the patient by one to four leads, with the recorder supported by a strap. It operates continuously to record the patterns and rhythms of the patient's heartbeat. In conjunction with the diary of activities and symptoms kept by the patient, the physician can note various events, times, and medication peaks that affect or precipitate dysrhythmias.

Exercise/stress ECG is another form of monitoring the heart's capability. It is accomplished in a laboratory setting during the performance of prescribed exertion by the patient. Tasks include use of treadmills, stair climbing, aerobic exercise, and other forms of exertion. Monitored carefully, the patient is coaxed to a limit of exertion to evaluate ischemia, dysrhythmia, and the extent of cardiac capability under extreme circumstances, thus setting the limit of exercise tolerance in cardiac disease.

Echocardiogram uses high-frequency ultrasound directed at the heart. The echo, or reflected sound, is graphically recorded. Size, shape, and position of cardiac structures are outlined. The focus of this diagnostic effort is to detect pericardial effusion, ventricular function, cardiac tumors, valvular function, and congenital heart disorder.

Phonocardiography involves the use of electrically recorded, amplified sounds. Special microphones attached to the patient's chest pick up cardiac sounds produced by pressure changes in the heart and great vessels. The sounds are graphically recorded on special phonograph paper so that a permanent record is available. Phonocardiography can be helpful in determining the exact timing and characteristics of murmurs and extra heart sounds.

Vectorcardiogram records heart action in three-dimensional loop—a variation of the standard 12-lead ECG.

Laboratory Examination

History and physical examination are supported by blood studies to aid the physician in diagnosing and monitoring the disease process. The nurse's responsibility is to prepare the patient by explaining the tests and the preparation required for each test. Common studies are addressed here; less common tests are noted with the presenting condition.

Blood cultures are crucial to the diagnosis of bacterial endocarditis.

Complete blood count (CBC) analyzes constituents of the blood. Low hemoglobin indicates oxygen supply interference and anemia; elevated white blood cell (leukocyte) count indicates infection or inflammation; and elevated red blood cell (erythrocyte) count indicates that the body is compensating for chronic hypoxia by increasing the manufacturing of red cells, such as in congestive heart failure.

Coagulation studies are useful in monitoring the patient receiving anticoagulant therapy, which is instituted in patients with myocardial infarction with congestive heart failure. These studies include *prothrombin time (PT)* and *partial thromboplastin time (PTT)*.

Erythrocyte sedimentation rate (ESR) is used to monitor or rule out inflammatory conditions of the heart. The sedimentation rate is elevated with MI and bacterial endocarditis and decreases when healing commences. The level of the ESR also indicates the extent of inflammation and infection in rheumatic fever.

Serum electrolytes focus on the body's balance of sodium, potassium, and calcium, necessary for myocardial muscle function. The physician compares serum levels with ECG changes.

Serum lipids are associated with vascular disease, particularly coronary artery disease (CAD). *Cholesterol* and *triglycerides* bound to plasma proteins are found in the blood as *lipoproteins*. Density levels vary according to the protein-fat ratio:

- VLDL (very-low-density lipoproteins) More fat than protein (primarily triglycerides)
- LDL (low-density lipoproteins) Equal fat and protein (50% cholesterol with moderate amounts of phospholipids)
- HDL (high-density lipoproteins) More protein than fat (approximately 50% protein—may serve a protective function, removing cholesterol from tissues)

Serum lipids are associated with risk of cardiovascular disease. A more elevated HDL is desired, whereas LDL or VLDL increases the risk for cardiovascular disease.

Arterial blood gases monitor oxygenation (PO_2; CO_2) and acid-base balance (pH). This test is useful in patients with unstable cardiac conditions to determine the blood oxygenation process and for physician evaluation of patients in cardiac failure.

DISEASES AND DISORDERS OF THE HEART

Coronary Atherosclerotic Heart Disease (CAHD)

The **coronary** arteries arise from the base of the aorta just below the semilunar valves (Fig. 32-12; see also Fig. 32-5, *B*). These arteries curve and angle in an attempt to adequately supply the heart muscle with oxygen and nutrients. These shapes, contours, and arrangements of the vessels allow for easy entrapment of substances that in-

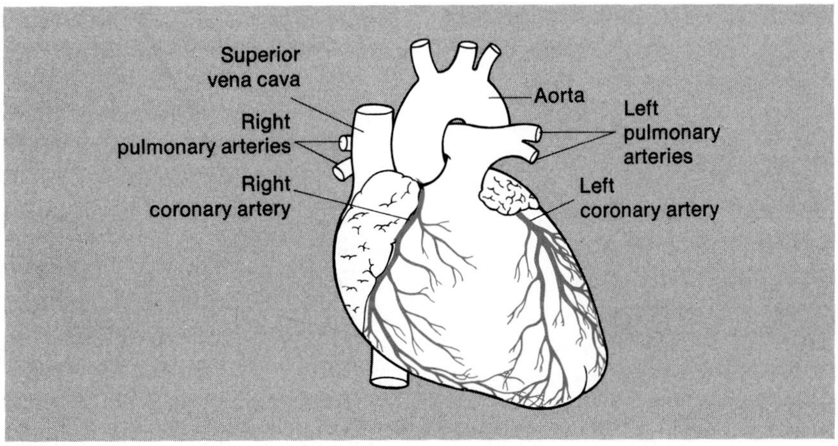

FIG. 32-12 Coronary arteries arise from aorta just above heart, one on left side and one on right side of aorta.

terfere with blood flow. In **anoxic** status (a condition of oxygen depletion) the heart cannot function to support the circulation process.

CAHD is a pathological condition affecting the coronary arteries, in which a narrowing of the artery lumen occurs, thereby preventing adequate blood supply. Etiology reveals an accumulated deposit of lipids, calcium, and fibrous tissue called **atheroma.** The resultant effect is myocardial **ischemia** (decreased blood supply), which, if it continues for any extended period, may lead to myocardial tissue necrosis (death of tissue).

Coronary Insufficiency

Etiology/pathophysiology. The main cause of coronary artery disease is **atherosclerosis,** a manifestation of **arteriosclerosis.** It usually involves larger arteries and their branches. Atherosclerosis is also called *arteriosclerotic heart disease, atherosclerotic coronary disease, coronary artery disease,* or *ischemic heart disease.* Abnormal accumulations of fatty deposits on the arterial walls (atheroma) characterize this condition. Arteriosclerosis, atrophy, and loss of elasticity of arterial walls contribute to the absence or decrease of myocardial blood supply.

Characterized by atheroma in the intima (the innermost layer, or membrane lining, of the vessel), this plaque formation constricts the **lumen,** (a channel or cavity within any organ), thickens the artery wall, and produces loss of elasticity. A chronic, mild inflammatory process sets up clotting within the vessel, producing a thrombuslike situation. Limited blood supply through constricted and narrowed vessels restricts normal blood flow. With progress of the condition, insufficient oxygen to myocardial tissue produces various degrees of disability. Resting behavior may be adopted to avoid ischemic symptoms. Many times the patient is not aware of self-imposed limitations until the disease symptoms progress considerably.

Clinical manifestations. Signs and symptoms will depend on the degree of occlusion (Fig. 32-13). The first sign of the condition may be angina (see pp. 722-725). Usually transient pain, especially on exertion, is noted. If discovered early in the disease process, CAHD can be treated before any extensive myocardial damage has occurred. Many times the patient remains asymptomatic, and it goes unrecognized while the collateral circulation (accessory or secondary vessel development) occurs. If CAHD is untreated, severe damage may result.

Assessment. Collection of *subjective data* includes noting the patient's description of pain relative to the onset, duration, and location. Intensity may be described as tightness, pressure, or squeezing pain in the substernal region, radiating to the upper chest, neck, shoulder, and inner arms. These symptoms may occur as a result of stress, exertion, or environment conditions: extreme cold, hot, or humid climates.

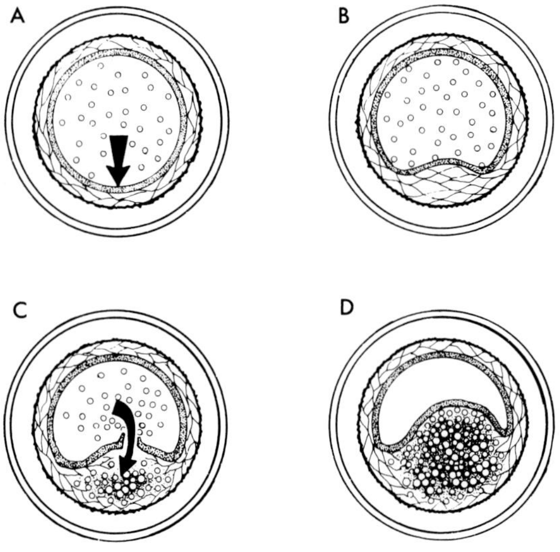

FIG. 32-13 Progressive development of coronary atherosclerosis. **A,** Injury to intimal wall. **B,** Lipoprotein invasion of smooth muscle cells. **C,** Development of fatty streak and fibrous plaque. **D,** Development of complicated lesion.

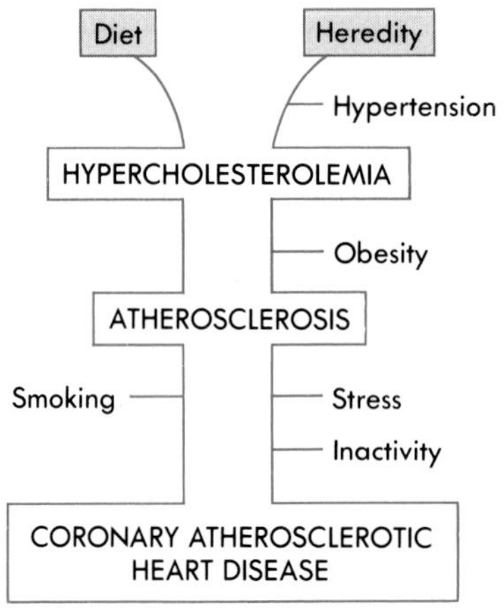

FIG. 32-14 Predisposing factors in the development of coronary atherosclerotic heart disease (CAHD).

Collection of *objective data* includes observing for vital sign alteration: elevation in blood pressure, pulse, and respiration and changes in cardiac rhythm are common. Outstanding risk factors for CAHD may be obvious (Fig. 32-14).

Diagnostic tests. The exercise stress test supports subjective data (exertional pain). ECG changes are often presented, but not always. Hyperlipidemia is found on blood examination. Hypertension may be noted when vital signs are observed.

Medical management. The medical approach may include any of three interventions for the patient with coronary artery disease: (1) medication, (2) percutaneous transluminal coronary angioplasty, and (3) bypass surgery. The intervention choice usually depends on the results of a coronary angiography—a procedure that aids in diagnosis of vessel occlusion and in determining whether surgery is advised. The purpose of treatment is to eliminate or reduce symptoms and decrease risk of disease progression to myocardial infarction (see pp. 725-729). In completely occluded arteries, the occurrence of myocardial infarction increases and damage is more severe.

Medication may be used alone or in conjunction with other therapies. The desired effect of medication is to improve efficiency of the heart and to reduce symptoms. It will not, however, eliminate blood vessel narrowing. Drugs commonly used are vasodilators, such as nitroglycerin and isosorbide (Sorbitrate); β-adrenergic blocking agents, such as propranolol (Inderal), metoprolol (Lopressor), and nadolol (Corgard); or calcium channel blockers, such as verapamil (Calan and Isoptin), nifedipine (Procardia), and diltiazem (Cardizem).

Percutaneous transluminary coronary angioplasty (PTCA) is an invasive procedure performed in the cardiac catheterization laboratory. The technique widens the narrowing in a coronary artery without surgery. *Percutaneous* denotes that the procedure is done through the skin; *transluminal* means that it is within the artery. Fluoroscopy is used to guide a catheter from the femoral or brachial artery to the coronary arteries to be treated. Inflation of a balloon in the catheter is achieved once it is positioned. The outward push of the balloon against the narrowing wall of the coronary artery reduces the constriction until it no longer interferes with blood flow to the heart muscle. Vessel patency is reestablished, thus *angioplasty* (vessel repair). This procedure may take 1 to 2 hours, with the patient usually awake but mildly sedated. Postprocedure nursing interventions are to continuously monitor the patient as with surgical recovery. Attention to the area of catheter insertion focuses on hemorrhage potential. Cardiac monitoring is effected.

Coronary artery bypass graft surgery (CABG) is a method of bypassing occluded vessels by grafting healthy vessels around the area of infarction or occlusion (Fig. 32-15). One end of the graft is sewn to the aorta and the other end to the coronary artery beyond the occlusion. Blood flow through the newly grafted vessel bypasses the occlusion, once again supplying the myocardium. The choice graft vessels are the saphenous vein from the leg or the internal mammary vein from the chest. The surgical procedure is performed under general anesthesia—sometimes after an ineffective PTCA. Recovery is usually monitored in the cardiac care unit for a few days before transfer to a medical-surgical unit.

Nursing interventions. The nursing approach is related to understanding and controlling factors that precipitate coronary insufficiency and to relieving activity intolerance. Pain on exertion can be controlled efficiently through medication intervention. Antianginals, such as Isordil and Cardilate, reduce the workload of the heart and restore adequate blood flow by means of vessel dilation. Thus the incidence of myocardial ischemia is lessened.

Although laser and surgical intervention may remove plaques and increase circulation, the nurse will focus patient education on prevention of disease progression. Medication intervention includes anticoagulant therapy, such as heparin or Coumadin, to decrease clotting complications, and antilipids to lower dangerous cholesterol levels.

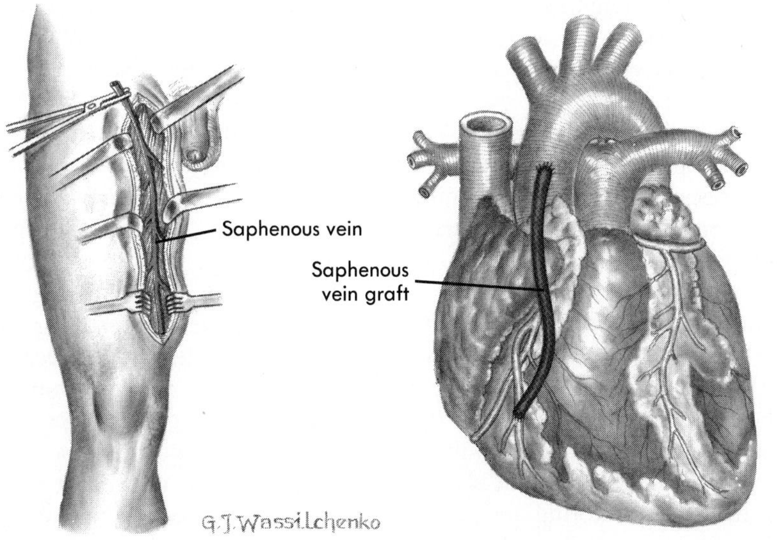

FIG. 32-15 Saphenous vein graft.

NURSING DIAGNOSES	NURSING INTERVENTIONS
Activity intolerance, related to hypoxic status	Advise patient to alter pace of life-style, avoiding pain-producing stress. Pace activity to decrease demand on circulatory system.
Pain, related to stress, exercise, or cold	Assess character of pain, relationship to activity, and patient tolerance. Teach medication approach to pain control with emphasis on administration by patient (after discharge).
Knowledge deficit, related to disease process and risk factors	Point out precipitating causes of pain and onset. Encourage avoiding cold exposure to lessen vasoconstriction. Discuss major risk factors and maintenance of high-level health status to avoid complications.

Patient teaching. Understanding the nature and progression of coronary artery disease is important in the education of the patient. The nurse will focus on precipitating causes and onset of pain, as well as citing risk factor control. The patient most at risk for coronary artery disease is the one with familial history of the disease. Early education may afford those at higher risk an opportunity to alter life-style.

Although the elderly are at greater risk because of the degenerative process, other factors also contribute to the condition. Men more frequently exhibit CAHD than women. However, women who use oral contraceptives or are of postmenopausal age are also vulnerable. Non-Caucasians exhibit symptoms more frequently than Caucasians. Although these factors cannot be changed, life-style can be adjusted to some degree. Cessation of smoking seems to result in the most obvious results and change. Avoiding stress or managing attitude adjustments is helpful. Because activity strengthens the circulatory system, advising the patient on exercise and physical maintenance as directed by the physician is desired.

Eating a diet low in fat and sodium and avoiding substances such as caffeine will improve health. The patient is encouraged to realize his responsibility for maintaining good health. Control of weight is an important factor when discussing the dietary aspects of this disease.

Patients should be taught (1) how to control the progression of diabetes mellitus, obesity, hyperlipidemia, and hypertension and (2) the proper health care management to offset the effects on the cardiovascular system.

It is important for the nurse to teach the patient the techniques of medication self-administration to reach the full therapeutic benefits. Patient education should stress the importance of medical monitoring and symptom reporting. Patient awareness of these interventions may reduce the progression of coronary artery disease.

Angina Pectoris

Etiology/pathophysiology. Anginal syndrome, or angina pectoris, is paroxysmal thoracic pain (a rapid onset of chest pain or pressure that begins and ends abruptly). This is a debilitating disorder caused by coronary atherosclerosis with myocardial anoxia. Blood supply to the myocardium is inadequate for its demand, thus causing myocardial ache. It is thought that sensory receptors that produce the pain are stimulated by lactic acid—a by-product of exertion. Certain factors precipitate the pain:

- Physical exertion
- Emotional excitement
- Extreme cold
- Heavy or irregular meals

Clinical manifestations. Pain is the outstanding characteristic of angina pectoris (Fig. 32-16). It has been described as sudden, dull to agonizing pain in the substernal chest region. It is known to progress to squeezing, viselike, crushing pain and thus is often confused with myocardial infarction symptoms. The pain often radiates down the left inner arm to the little finger and also upward to the shoulder and jaw. It is described as immobilizing.

The patient often has other symptoms, which include cold, clammy, ashen skin and diaphoresis. Anxiety and apprehension are noted. Diagnosis is often achieved at the primary level by the clinical manifestations. The location, onset, and duration of pain are usually explored first. If pain lasts more than 15 minutes in an acute attack, myocardial infarction is suspected. Environmental factors can contribute to angina, and it is often recognized by these factors. Any one of several factors may precipitate an anginal attack, including cold, emotional upset, unusually heavy meals, particularly at night, or any activity that increases the heart's workload or causes a decrease of blood flow to the myocardium.

Assessment. Collection of *subjective data* includes the nurse questioning the patient regarding location, intensity, radiation, and duration of pain. The patient may express a feeling that death is impending, especially if symptoms present at night. Night fear is then a reality. The patient may complain of suffocation or choking. Stress factors may precipitate symptoms.

Collection of *objective data* includes the nurse observing skin changes (pallor and perspiration); behavioral deviation; anxiety; posture to avoid movement that precipitates the pain; and vital sign changes (tachycardia and alternating weak and strong pulses).

Diagnostic tests. Electrocardiogram exhibits cardiac rhythm changes. Holter monitor correlation to activity pinpoints precipitating factors. The exercise stress test is valued in exhibiting these changes in a controlled atmosphere. It is imperative to note that the stress test is not administered during an anginal attack. Angiography or ventriculogram may be useful. The physician will often order cardiac enzymes studies to rule out a myocardial infarction.

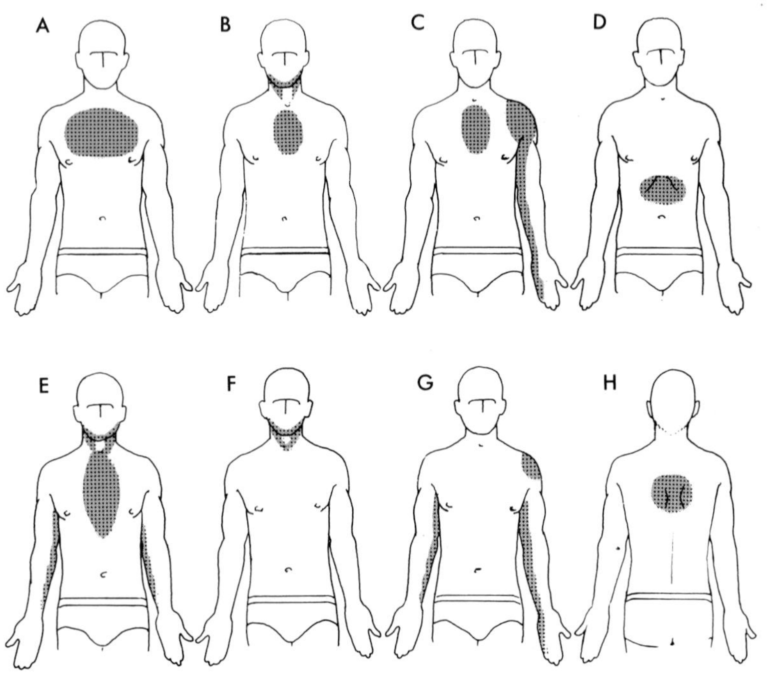

FIG. 32-16 Sites where ischemic myocardial pain may be referred. **A,** Upper chest. **B,** Beneath sternum radiating to neck and jaw. **C,** Beneath sternum radiating down left arm. **D,** Epigastric. **E,** Epigastric radiating to neck, jaw, and arms. **F,** Neck and jaw. **G,** Left shoulder, inner aspect of both arms. **H,** Intrascapular.

Table 32-2 Medication Management of Angina Pectoris

Classification	Agent	Action
Nitrates	Nitroglycerin (NTG); isosorbide	Dilates coronary arteries, collateral vessels, and peripheral vessels by relaxing smooth muscle walls. By reducing venous return, the workload of the heart is lessened. Blood is redistributed to ischemic myocardial areas. NTG administered sublingually is the method of choice for aborting the acute anginal attack; it relieves the anginal attack within 1 to 2 minutes. Long-acting nitrates are administered to prevent anginal attacks.
β-adrenergic blockers	Nadolol (Corgard); propranolol (Inderal)	Lowers myocardial O_2 demand, decreases heart rate, and lowers blood pressure by inhibiting circulating catecholamines on β-adrenergic receptors.
Calcium channel blockers	Diltiazem (Cardizem); nifedipine (Procardia)	Inhibits calcium influx across cell membrane, decreases workload of the heart, and improves O_2 supply by dilating coronary arteries.
Salicylates	Aspirin	Suppresses platelet coagulation by decreasing progression of CAHD.

Medical management. The primary goal of medical management is to accurately diagnose anginal pain, or syndrome, and to control the symptoms with medication or with behavioral change and alterations in life-style, which may be difficult and may require a long period for success. Some individuals may benefit from the support and structure provided by group activities (e.g., Weight Watchers, Smoke Enders, stress management workshops, and cardiac rehabilitation or exercise programs). The physician prescribes three major classes of medications in the treatment of angina: nitrates, β-adrenergic blockers, and calcium channel blockers (Table 32-2).

Percutaneous transluminal coronary angioplasty (PTCA) is used to dilate coronary arteries that are obstructed by atherosclerotic plaque. Coronary artery bypass graft (CABG) is a surgical revascularization procedure to increase coronary artery flow. Research is being conducted in the area of transluminal laser angioplasty to recanalize coronary arteries. Laser light has the ability to destroy atherosclerotic plaque.

Nursing interventions. The nursing interventions are centered on the following:

- Eliminating factors known to precipitate attack
- Relieving symptoms
- Preventing progression and complications of the condition
- Initiating medication therapy as ordered to control symptoms

Relief of anginal attacks or lessening the number of episodes is the primary goal of nursing intervention. Physical and psychological comfort measures should be carried out. Progress and goals should be discussed. The nurse should explain the purpose of diagnostic examinations and reinforce the physician's explanation of the results.

Dietary teaching includes reduction of cholesterol in the diet, control of caffeine usage (coffee and tea, which increase heart rate), and weight management coupled with moderate-size meals.

NURSING DIAGNOSES	NURSING INTERVENTIONS
Pain, related to myocardial ischemia	Maintain rest during episodes of pain. Record description of pain and activity before onset. Administer oxygen as indicated. Maintain diet as ordered; if chest pain occurs during eating, advise small feedings rather than two or three large meals.
Knowledge deficit, related to disease process	Discuss nature of angina pectoris: cause, risk factors involved, and importance of modification of controllable risk factors. Discuss management and nature of chest pain; assist in identifying precipitating factors. Avoid isometric activity: heavy lifting and pushing. Exercise regularly; encourage a regular home exercise program as ordered. Avoid sexual activities when fatigued; if chest pain occurs during sexual activity, stop and take nitrates if ordered. If pain persists or extreme fatigue occurs, report symptoms to physician.

Patient teaching. The focus of education is understanding the disease process and methods of control of anginal episodes, primarily through daily activity. Knowledge of the course of angina enables the patient to effectively cope with the condition. The patient is encouraged to decrease emotional tension and stress and to increase rest and relaxation to reduce the heart's workload. Readjustment of life-style may balance exertion and modify exercise. Avoiding tobacco reduces vasoconstriction. The nurse should stress the importance of complying with medication instructions. This will result in safety in self-administration and thus lower the patient's anxiety levels by more effective pain control.

THERAPEUTIC DIALOGUE

■ Mrs. Patterson, a patient with angina, has been admitted for further care, diagnosis, and treatment. After the initial nursing assessment, Nurse Chenier interviews the patient about the course of her anginal episodes. With the data she gathers, Nurse Chenier will be able to participate in the development of a program to educate Mrs. Patterson to minimize or control the attacks.

NURSE: I would like to ask you some questions, Mrs. Patterson, about the anginal pain that you are experiencing.

PATIENT: I already told Dr. Mark all about those attacks when I visited his office. His nurse Miss Gardner has all those records.

NURSE: Yes, I know. Your physician has asked us to help you plan a program for preventing or minimizing these attacks. With all of the information we gather, we can set goals for your care. We can also identify how angina relates to some of your activities.

PATIENT: OK, Miss Chenier, I would like to understand it better. Perhaps I would be less frightened when it happens. My friend Jeanette told me about her aunt who had angina—she died. That really worries me.

NURSE: We hope to decrease some of your fears, Mrs. Patterson, by helping you understand. First, when do your attacks usually occur?

PATIENT: Oh, mostly after a real busy day, you know—shopping, or after gardening or house cleaning. But a few times, I recall a spell after my sister-in-law Lisa visits. She and Tom—he's my husband—always seem to get into upsetting discussions. They never got along well. She upsets us both—prying and fussing.

NURSE: Have you noticed if a big meal is related to the anginal pain?

PATIENT: No, not really . . . Well, only when my sister-in-law is there. We hardly ever eat big meals any more, except when she comes. She expects to be fed well. Tom and I have cut down a lot. Big meals upset our systems—and then her—that harping on old problems and how she thinks we should run our lives! She upsets me so!

NURSE: Mrs. Patterson, I think we must talk more on how to handle stressful problems like Lisa. But first, could you describe the pain for me: Does it come on suddenly? How long does it last? What does it feel like?

PATIENT: Oh, no—not all of a sudden. It is just dull at times, like a stomach upset. But then, it travels up in my chest and gets really heavy—like a pressure. Sometimes, I declare, it makes my face and teeth hurt; and my arm, too—this one *(left)*—all the way down to my little fingers. If it's a really bad attack, I sometimes feel like I am going to vomit.

NURSE: Does your heart beat faster?

PATIENT: Oh, yes, and I just have to sit down and be quiet or I can't catch my breath. That's when I take the nitroglycerin. I carry it with me all the time now—in this special little container.

NURSE: I see. And how long does it take for the pain to stop after you take the medicine?

PATIENT: I use to think it took forever, but Tom—he times it for me—says it lasts about 15 to 20 minutes. I relax a little, and it passes.

NURSE: What about the weather, Mrs. Patterson? Have you noticed that it affects your attacks in any way?

PATIENT: I don't know if it is all those clothes or the weather, but I get more pains if I get out in all of that cold.

NURSE: Do you or your husband smoke?

PATIENT: Not any more. I gave up cigarettes when this angina started on me. I noticed the difference, too. Now, I can't even get in a room if people are smoking. I also cut down on the coffee when I retired. Dr. Mark said that the caffeine isn't good for the angina. All of the good things, they have to go when you get old!

NURSE: Maybe with some understanding of how certain activities and influences affect your condition, you can find new "good things" for you to enjoy just as much. Soon we will talk again. There are some effective coping methods to decrease your stress when Lisa visits that we can explore.

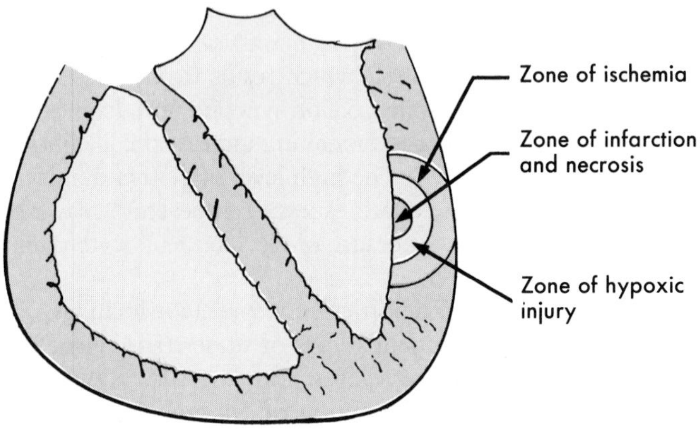

FIG. 32-17 The three zones of myocardial infarction.

BOX 32-2 **SIGNS AND SYMPTOMS OF MYOCARDIAL INFARCTION**

SUBJECTIVE SYMPTOMS	OBJECTIVE SIGNS
Pain	Pallor
Anxiety	Erratic behavior
Dyspnea	Hypotension, shock
Weakness, faintness	Cardiac rhythm changes
Nausea	Vomiting
	Fever
	Presence of risk factors

Coronary Occlusion

With the progression of atherosclerotic heart disease, any one of the coronary arteries may become obstructed. Atheroma and fibrous plaques, which occlude the coronary artery lumen, reduce blood flow and predispose to thrombus and embolus. This condition leads to infarction. An **infarct** is an area of tissue necrosis in a vessel, organ or a part, resulting from an interruption of blood supply to the affected area.

Myocardial Infarction (MI)

Etiology/pathophysiology. Myocardial infarction is an occlusion of a major coronary artery or one of its branches. An obstruction by atherosclerotic process or an embolus may interrupt the blood supply. Arteriosclerotic arteries are easily occluded and then deliver an amount of blood that is less than the myocardial demand. The extent of the infarct depends on the ability of the vascular network to rapidly develop collateral circulation. When the pathway of circulation is occluded, the body often compensates by forming new pathways, i.e., collateral circulation.

Decrease of oxygen to the myocardium may cause tissue necrosis in the affected area (Fig. 32-17). Onset of MI is usually sudden. Commonly, vasoconstriction has occurred when a blood clot forms or enlarges on an atherosclerotic lesion. Hemorrhage into the clot interrupts the blood flow, thus occluding the coronary vessels and ultimately causing tissue death. The soft, necrotic area gradually is replaced by fibrous tissue as the healing process occurs. With the occurrence of collateral blood supply, deficit circulation is achieved.

Clinical manifestations. Assessment of myocardial infarction is directly related to signs and symptoms (Box 32-2). However, an asymptomatic manifestation, known as *silent MI,* may occur. In such an undetected MI, the diagnosis may be incidental—derived from abnormalities found on routine diagnostic testing for other signs and symptoms.

The nurse will observe that pain, the characteristic symptom of MI, is recognized because of its sudden, severe, life-threatening manifestation. Often interpreted as indigestion initially, it radiates from the substernal origin to the shoulder, and progresses to the throat, jaw, and down the arm (the left side being more prevalent). Pain is often described as viselike, grinding, crushing, and stamina draining. It is long lasting—more than 5 minutes without lessening—and is not relieved by nitroglycerin, rest, or position change. Because of duration and intensity, the pain differs from that of anginal pain. Stress and anxiety related to this symptom often bring a feeling of impending doom.

Vital sign alteration includes decreased blood pressure and rapid pulse with dysrhythmia, accompanied by weakness and signs of shock, which result from a decreased cardiac output. Dyspnea, pallor, syncope, and diaphoresis coupled with nausea and vomiting increase the likelihood of a diagnosis of MI. The high level of pain and anxiety may cause loss of consciousness. Temperature may rise later in the episode because of elevated leukocyte count and ESR.

Assessment. Collection of *subjective data* includes observation of the patient's level of understanding of the MI symptoms. If the level of consciousness allows, the patient's input and perception of symptoms are important. The onset, location, and quality of pain will be of greatest importance. Dyspnea, vertigo, and weakness may be expressed. These symptoms will relate to pain, stress, and anxiety. Medical history can be a prime factor in the initial diagnostic data-gathering procedure.

Collection of *objective data* includes the nurse noting the patient's behavior, the posture, its relationship to pain, and the skin color. Vital signs reveal hypotension, pulse abnormalities, and early temperature elevation. The patient's normal values will be compared if available. If not, current vital signs will represent the baseline.

Family members may be able to aid in the nursing data collection, especially if the patient is unable to cooperate because of excruciating pain.

Diagnostic tests. When patient behavior, symptoms, vital signs, and presence of risk factors point to MI, changes in cardiac rhythm with elevation of cardiac enzyme levels (Fig. 32-18) strongly support the diagnosis. ECG deviations from normal cardiac rhythm are shown. Several ECG readings are used to follow and monitor cardiac distress. Dysrhythmias are noted by the physician and treated rapidly to prevent complication. The location of the infarct may be accomplished by Q wave abnormalities.

Significant laboratory value abnormalities will be present. Intracellular enzymes released into the blood stream

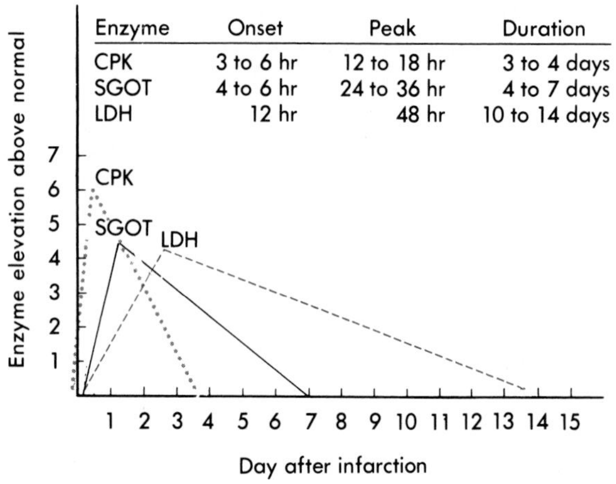

FIG. 32-18 Patterns of serum enzyme levels after myocardial infarction.

indicate tissue damage. WBC elevation (12,000 to 15,000/mm^3) is associated with severe infarcts. Leukocyte increase is a common result of necrotic tissue damage. Erythrocyte count and sedimentation rate elevation occurs in 24 to 48 hours. Nuclear scans aid in diagnosis by visualizing areas of the heart suffering inadequate perfusion. Pulmonary artery catheterization may be used to assess left or right ventricular function (denotes severity and location of infarct).

Medical management. The first goal of medical management is to stabilize the patient. Arrest of pain and prevention of cardiac arrest plus attainment of adequate tissue perfusion precede transfer to the nursing unit (see Table 32-3 for medications commonly prescribed). Attention to fluid overload and respiratory difficulties is also a priority of the physician. Complications and life-threatening occurrences of primary concern are as follows:

- Ventricular fibrillation and dysrhythmia
- Cardiac arrest
- Cardiogenic shock (Box 32-3)
- Pulmonary edema

ECGs and cardiac monitoring are performed, with careful observation to detect dysrhythmia. One fourth to one half of all deaths after hospital entry for MI result from heart failure. Control of this complication is vital. Cardiogenic shock is detected by ongoing monitoring of vital signs. Severe hypotension, tachycardia, mental confusion, and cold and clammy skin are signs of cardiogenic shock. Monitoring of cardiac enzyme studies is closely linked to physician management of patient activity and rehabilitative planning. Oxygen therapy is administered by nasal cannula for the first 24 to 48 hours and longer if pain, hypotension, dyspnea, or dysrhythmias persist.

Cardiac enzyme studies. Cell membrane damage or necrosis causes release of certain enzymes into the blood. Amounts found in the blood content are commonly elevated with incidence of myocardial infarction, defibrillation, trauma, and drug therapy (steroids, morphine, and antibiotics). Specific enzymes and elevation values follow.

Creatine phosphokinase (CPK or CK) is a muscle enzyme found in the brain, skeletal muscle, and myocardium. Isoenzymes of CK relate to the specific tissue and differentiate the sources.

- CK isoenzyme I (BB) originates from brain tissue.
- CK isoenzyme II (MB) originates from myocardial tissue.
- CK isoenzyme III (MM) originates in skeletal muscle.

CK MB

Normal range: 75 U/L; MI range: 10-25 times normal
Onset: 2-6 hours; Peak: 12-18 hours; Duration: 3-5 days
(See Fig. 32-18.)

Lactic dehydrogenase (LDH) is comprised of five isoenzyme components. Subunit LDH is found in cardiac muscle.

Table 32-3 Medications for Myocardial Infarction

Classification	Agent	Action
Vasopressors	Dopamine (Intropin)	Raise systemic arterial pressure and cardiac output.
Anticoagulants	Heparin; Warfarin (Coumadin)	Reduce incidence of clotting.
Analgesics	Morphine	Control pain.
Tranquilizers	Diazepam (Valium)	Decrease anxiety and restlessness.
Thrombolytic agents	Streptokinase	Use of thrombolytic (pertaining to dissolution of blood clots) agents when acute MI symptoms are less than 6 hours duration; these agents restore blood flow and salvage injured myocardium in certain patients.
Nitrates	Nitroglycerin; isosorbide	Dilate blood vessels, increase coronary artery blood supply, and decrease oxygen demands.
β-adrenergic blockers	Propranolol (Inderal); metoprolol (Lopressor)	Blocks β-adrenergic stimulation, and decrease myocardial oxygen demands.
Calcium channel blockers	Nifedipine (Procardia); diltiazem (Cardizem)	Dilate blood vessels, increase coronary artery blood supply, and decrease myocardial oxygen demands.
Salicylates	Aspirin	Decrease platelet adhesion and thus decrease thrombosis formation.
Antidysrhythmics	Lidocaine (Xylocaine) I.V.	Treat ventricular dysrhythmias.
Stool softeners	Surfak; Colace	Reduce straining at stool, prevent constipation produced by decreased mobility and use of constipating narcotics.
Diuretics	Furosemide (Lasix)	Control edema.
Electrolyte replacement	Slow-K	May be necessary when diuretics are used.

BOX 32-3 **CARDIOGENIC SHOCK**

An acute and serious complication of myocardial infarction and congestive heart failure is *cardiogenic shock*. It is characterized by low cardiac output and peripheral vascular system collapse. Left ventricular function is severely decreased, resulting in an inadequate blood supply to the vital organs. Immediate detection and treatment are necessary to prevent irreversible shock and death. Incidence of this complication proves fatal in 80% of the cases.

CLINICAL MANIFESTATIONS	SIGNS AND SYMPTOMS
Decreased cardiac output	
Myocardial ischemia	Dysrhythmias, chest pain
Cerebral hypoxia	Agitation, restlessness, confusion
Impaired tissue perfusion	
- Renal circulation decreased	Urinary output diminished or absent
- Anaerobic metabolism with lactic acidosis	Lactic acid accumulation in blood
Peripheral vascular system collapse	
Shock	Decreased blood pressure Narrowed pulse pressure Cyanosis, cold and clammy skin, tachycardia, and oliguria

MEDICAL MANAGEMENT

Recognition and control of life-threatening symptoms
- Oxygenation promotes tissue perfusion.
- Parenteral fluid acts as a volume expander.
- Drug therapy
  - Vasopressors: Raise arterial blood pressure.
  - Inotropics and cardiac glycosides: Increase cardiac contraction strength, and correct dysrhythmias.
  - Sodium bicarbonate: Combats lactic acidosis.

Normal range: 150-325 U/L; MI range: 2-4 times normal
Onset: 8-12 hours; Peak: 24-48 hours; Duration: 7-14 days

Serum-glutamic-oxaloacetic transaminase (SGOT) is found in heart tissue cells plus many other organ tissues of high metabolic activity. It is also indicative of dysrhythmia and angina.

Normal range: 12-40 U; MI range: 200 U (4-10 times normal)
Onset: 4-6 hours; Peak: 24-48 hours; Duration: 4-7 days

Assessment of enzyme level alterations supports other diagnostic data confirming myocardial infarction. The extent of damage can be determined by repeated monitoring. The physician's management of patient activity resumption is often based on cessation of cell breakdown.

Nursing interventions. By the time the patient arrives at the hospital, damage has usually occurred. Nursing interventions are divided into emergency care, intensive care, and the rehabilitative phase. Individualized care is indicated, with emergency problems being the first focus. Lifesaving measures, such as CPR and cardiac pacemaking and/or defibrillation, may be started immediately.

After a degree of stabilization in the emergency department, the patient may be transferred to the intensive care unit, where a specific regimen is individualized for his recuperation and rehabilitation (Box 32-4).

Nursing interventions on the medical-surgical unit may begin when intensive care is no longer necessary. This signifies progress to the patient and his family and is considered a psychological boost to care.

Initial vital signs and cardiac observation are carried out hourly with progression to 2-hour intervals until complete stabilization is reached. Promoting healing of the myocardium is a main objective of care; therefore rest—usually complete bed rest—is advised. After the second day, minimum effort is allowed. Progress to sitting in a chair for 10 to 15 minutes or on a bedside commode may be the activity allowed.

BOX 32-4 COURSE OF DISEASE AND HEALING PROCESS

Onset to 72 hours	Tissue degeneration, necrosis. Dysrhythmias—must be treated immediately.
72 hours to Week 1	Infarct softens. Aneurysm and cardiac rupture are prevalent complications.
Week 2	Capillary formation around necrotic area develops as collateral circulation begins (functional: 2 to 6 weeks).
Weeks 3 and 4	Scar forming occurs.
Weeks 8 to 12	Scar strengthens.

Maximum understanding of plans and procedures is necessary for low stress and anxiety levels of the patient. Visitors are limited to the immediate family and significant others, all of whom may be included in the plan for progress. A gradual increase in activity is permitted, with passive close observation to reactions and ongoing monitoring of cardiac change.

Control of pain is maintained. Exercise of muscles to prevent atrophy and stasis of blood supply begins with passive range-of-motion exercise, progressing to patient-initiated movement.

Diet is usually withheld until initial stabilization. When resumed, it will be one that will not increase the workload of the heart. Effort to conserve energy is important. Cardiac arrest and aspiration are complications to be considered. Liquid diet is progressed as tolerated to regular diet with restrictions. A low-carbohydrate, low-fat, easily digested, and calorie-controlled diet is desirable. Pulse-stimulating caffeine is withheld.

Prevention of complications is a primary objective. Antiembolic stockings are used. Ongoing assessment of cardiac status, dyspneic condition, and pulse change (rate, rhythm, and volume) is made and reported. Observation of patient response and mental status is used to plan the level of care and rehabilitation. Infusion of parenteral solutions or a Hep Lock remains in place to keep veins patent for any emergency treatment. Observation for signs of decreased cardiac output is ongoing (Box 32-5).

NURSING DIAGNOSES	NURSING INTERVENTIONS
Activity intolerance, related to ventricular dysfunction and fatigue	Maintain bed rest. Promote sleep patterns. Avoid sudden exertion. Apply antiembolic stockings to reduce complications. Use range-of-motion exercise when physician approves. Provide diversional outlet, e.g., reading or TV. Retrain elimination patterns to conserve energy.

BOX 32-5 SYMPTOMS AND SIGNS OF DECREASED CARDIAC OUTPUT

Hypotension
Tachycardia, dysrhythmias
Cool, clammy skin
Pallor, cyanosis
Weakness, fatigue
Mental changes
Decreased urinary output (oliguria)

NURSING DIAGNOSES	NURSING INTERVENTIONS
Pain, related to myocardial ischemia	Maintain bed rest and reduced activity. Administer O_2 as necessary and as ordered. Medicate with analgesia to decrease pain. Record response to nursing interventions. Teach relaxation techniques. Control environment for rest and minimal stress.
Ineffective breathing pattern, related to fluid volume excess	Assess respiratory function and abnormal breathing patterns. Regulate activity to O_2 balance. Adhere to low-sodium diet, thus reducing fluid volume. Encourage relaxation, and provide diversion.
Altered cardiopulmonary tissue perfusion, related to decreased cardiac output	Reduce cardiac workload—bed rest, relaxation. Maintain stability of blood force and flow. Monitor ECG for complications or regression. Monitor for complications: shock or congestive heart failure.
Anxiety (patient/family), related to fear of death, pain, and hospitalization	Assess level of anxiety and coping mechanisms. Assess grieving process (health loss). Reassure through patient education, encouraging family support, and allowing self-expression. Administer antianxiety agents and sedation as indicated. Encourage goal setting, patient decisions in care, and rehabilitation plan. Develop a relationship of trust.
Knowledge deficit (patient/family), related to disease process and therapeutic interventions	Discuss disease process. Cite limitations of activity. Discuss risk factors. Explain necessity for stress and anxiety control. Plan dietary management and weight control. Review necessity to continue treatment.

Patient teaching. The education process includes family participation, is detailed and specific, and is affected by the optimistic attitude and approach of the educators. The nurse will determine the level of the patient's comprehension. Teaching must result in maximum understanding and retention of facts. An individualized program is essential. Care should be taken to avoid tiring the patient. Adequate time must be provided for reinforcement and questions.

The patient who has had a myocardial infarction must learn to recognize the relationship of risk factors to his future health status. Often, denial of the MI diagnosis occurs after hospitalization, and nonadherence to the prescribed regimen results. Therefore a thorough program of written instructions and rehabilitative objectives must be presented to the patient during hospitalization. Some areas of concern will have been addressed by the nurse while caring for the patient.

Desired effect, side effects, and the prescribed regimen of medications must be explained. The patient is encouraged to discuss concerns with the physician, as well as report any untoward effects. Dietary restrictions seem to be the most difficult to accept. The dietician should begin teaching the diet regimen, and if the nurse can cite the rationale, teaching may be more successful. A list of restricted foods and acceptable substitutes may be explored. Resumption of normal activities is a concern of the patient during recuperation. The effect of activity on the heart and precisely how the cardiac workload can be lessened is stressed. Discussion of resumption of sexual activity should be tailored to the individual. A Medic-Alert identification is advised.

The rehabilitative plan. Rehabilitation of the patient recovering from a myocardial infarction begins as soon as his condition is stable. Total care by the nurse or significant others progresses to self-care. Daily activities are monitored to ensure progress and success. Usually a 7- to 15-day plan is enacted. It is flexible to meet the need: whether a longer or a shorter framework is desired. The nurse stresses that any level of activity that precipitates pain, dyspnea, blood pressure alteration, or dysrhythmia should be stopped and the program reevaluated. The plan progresses from complete bed rest to self-care activities of daily living with exercise as tolerated.

The discharge plan includes instructions for the first 2 months after hospitalization through discharge by the physician. The patient should be given the follow-up physician appointment before he leaves the hospital, as well as medications and instructions for administration. The nurse should instruct the patient to go directly home and to rest as soon as possible after arrival. Visitors, family, and coworkers should not visit until the patient is settled, and then only for brief periods.

Congestive Heart Failure (CHF)

Etiology/pathophysiology. This condition, known as heart failure, cardiac decompensation, cardiac insufficiency, or CHF, occurs when the heart is inefficient in its pumping capacity. This results in a collection of fluid in tissues and organs—hence the term *congestion.*

Etiological factors are associated with congenital heart conditions, coronary occlusion (MI), valvular heart disease, and a pericardial inflammatory condition. CHF is also attributed to infection, stress, hypertension, hyperthyroidism, hemorrhage, anemia, or fluid replacement therapy.

Because the left ventricle is most often affected by coronary atherosclerosis and hypertension, heart failure usually begins there. If untreated, the condition progresses to right-sided failure. Right ventricular failure can occur separately from left ventricular failure, but its appearance is more often a consequence of left-sided failure. Blood returning to the left atrium pools in the lungs as a result of inadequate pumping mechanics of the left ventricle.

Clinical manifestations. Early signs and symptoms of CHF include fatigue and dyspnea—especially in the supine position. This in turn causes insomnia, cough, and possibly hemoptysis. The onset of CHF may be acute, but it often progresses over months or years, rendering the patient chronically debilitated. When left ventricular function suddenly deteriorates, acute clinical signs and symptoms associated with pulmonary congestion and pulmonary edema result.

Depending on the degree of dysfunction of the heart, the location, and the severity of the condition, acute CHF may produce shock, cardiac arrest, and sudden death. This is usually the result of low cardiac output after myocardial infarct. Chronic CHF develops gradually with milder symptoms. The depletion of oxygen and nutrients is caused by reduced blood supply to tissues and organs. Waste products accumulate. Pumping inability causes venous stasis, resulting in tissue and organ congestion. The long-term result of CHF is constriction of ventricles, ventricular overload, and direct damage to the cardiac muscle. Signs and symptoms progress, depending on the stage of congestion and its relationship to forward or backward effects of left- or right-sided heart failure.

Backward versus forward heart failure. Backward versus forward heart failure is perhaps the oldest method of classifying heart failure. Backward failure is said to be the result of damming up of blood in the vessels proximal to the heart. Conversely, forward heart failure is the result of the inability of the heart to maintain cardiac output. The heart is part of a closed system; forward failure and backward failure will always be associated with each other.

Left ventricular failure. Decreased cardiac output of the left ventricle causes blood to dam up in the left side of the heart because it cannot be pumped efficiently. Increasing left ventricular pressures are transmitted to the left atrium and the pulmonary vascular bed, and the lungs become congested with fluid. Pulmonary edema and pleural effusion occur. Signs and symptoms include dyspnea, orthopnea, hemoptysis, and cough. The decreased cardiac output causes a diminished flow of blood to the kidneys and reduces the glomerular filtration rate. With reduced renal blood flow, sodium and water are retained in the body and contribute to generalized edema (anasarca).

Right ventricular failure. The most common cause of right ventricular failure is left ventricular failure. In right ventricular failure the right ventricle compensates in response to an increase in pulmonary artery pressure. The heart becomes less effective and is unable to maintain adequate output against the resistance. This results in blood damming back into the systemic circulation. Because of increased venous pressure and stasis, fluid is pushed out of the capillaries and venules. The liver and other organs become congested, and fluid escapes into the abdominal cavity, which results in ascites, sometimes as much as 2000 to 3000 ml. Pitting peripheral edema also occurs. It is also known as *dependent edema* because it occurs in dependent parts of the body, such as the legs or sacrum. The edema progresses into the thighs and external genitalia. Neck vein distention as a result of increased venous pressure also occurs and usually is observed when the patient is sitting.

Assessment. Collection of *subjective data* involves noting the patient's complaints of dyspnea and cough, caused by edema and pulmonary congestion. Gastrointestinal signs and symptoms include nausea and vomiting. Loss of strength accompanies feelings of anxiety and mental inefficiency. Palpitations are common.

Collection of *objective data* includes observing alterations in vital signs: pulse rate and rhythm (irregularities) and volume (strength). Palpitations accompany abnormal heart sounds (gallop and murmurs). Peripheral edema is evident in ambulatory patients, whereas the patient on bed rest exhibits sacral and external genitalia edema as well. Blood flow to the kidneys is diminished, resulting in oliguria and followed by nocturia (night diuresis).

Liver capsule distention, caused by increased venous pressure, may result in epigastric pain and ascites. Oxygen deficit in tissues results in cyanosis and general debilitation.

Diagnostic tests. The most common diagnostic tests for the patient with CHF include a chest x-ray study, which reveals cardiomegaly, pulmonary vascular congestion, and pleural effusion, and an ECG and echocardiogram, which reveal rhythm and rate abnormalities, usually indicative of underlying cardiac disorders and the cause of CHF.

Medical management. The objectives of medical intervention include the following:

- To increase cardiac efficiency with digitalis and vasodilators for expanded output
- To lower the oxygen requirement of the body systems through bed rest
- To provide oxygen to the tissues through oxygen therapy
- To treat edema and pulmonary congestion with diuretics and a sodium-restricted diet

Once the workload of the heart is decreased and diuresis of engorged tissues and organs is achieved, the activity ability of the patient will increase. These objectives are achieved by medication therapy, bed rest, and drug therapy (Table 32-4).

Table 32-4 Medication Therapy in Congestive Heart Failure

Classification	Agent	Action	Nursing Interventions
Cardiac glycosides	Digitalis preparations, such as digoxin (Lanoxin)	Strengthens cardiac force and efficiency. Slows heart rate. Increases circulation, effecting diuresis.	Monitor apical pulse to ensure rate above 60; monitor for toxicity (nausea, vomiting, anorexia, dysrhythmia, bradycardia, tachycardia, headache, fatigue, and blurred or colored vision).
Diuretics	Thiazides, such as chlorothiazide (Diuril), hydrochlorothiazide (Esidrix and Hydrodiuril)	Increases renal secretion of sodium. Safe for long-term use. Blocks sodium and water reabsorption in kidney tubules.	Monitor electrolyte depletion; weigh daily to ascertain fluid loss.
	Sulfonamides (loop diuretic), such as furosemide (Lasix)	Acts rapidly for less responsive edema.	Administer in AM, to prevent nocturia. Monitor for electrolyte depletion. Consider sulfa allergy (furosemide).
	Aldosterone antagonist (potassium-sparing), such as spironolactone (Aldactone)	Relieves edema and ascites that do not respond to usual diuretics. Blocks sodium-retaining and potassium-excreting properties of aldosterone.	Monitor for gastrointestinal irritation and hyperkalemia.
Potassium supplements	Potassium (K-Lyte)	Restores electrolyte loss.	Monitor blood potassium levels.
Sedatives and analgesics		Promotes rest and comfort. Relieves chest and abdominal pain. Lessens dyspnea.	Monitor rest and sleep benefits.
Nitrates	Nitroglycerin (Cardabid)	Dilates arteries. Reduces blood pressure.	Monitor blood pressure.

Pulmonary edema is a life-threatening complication of congestive heart failure. Progression of left-sided heart failure to engorgement of the pulmonary vasculature results in extravascular fluid accumulation in the lung interstitial space and alveoli. Involvement of bronchioles and bronchi follows, causing "drowning" in the serous fluids.

Signs and symptoms of acute CHF are exaggerated when pulmonary edema develops. Respirations are shallow, rapid, and dyspneic with blood-tinged, frothy sputum. Rales and wheezing are common. The rapid pulse delivery ranges from bounding to weak and thready. Cyanosis indicates oxygen deficit. Vein engorgement in the neck is noted, as is peripheral vessel edema. Anxiety, apprehension, and diaphoresis support indication by the patient of feelings of helplessness and impending doom.

Treatment aim is to reduce pulmonary congestion, improve oxygenation, and decrease anxiety. Positioning (Fowler's) reduces venous return to the thoracic region, and oxygen relieves hypoxia and dyspnea. Morphine in small doses induces a more relaxed respiratory process and lessens apprehension. Because of the potential for morphine-related respiratory depression, constant observation of breathing pattern changes is necessary. Diuresis per drug therapy is monitored to avoid significant electrolyte loss, hypovolemia, or drop in blood pressure. Phlebotomy to decrease blood volume and engorgement of organs is an infrequently used method because hemoglobin loss may contribute to a hypoxic condition.

Rotating tourniquets may reduce cardiopulmonary overload by temporarily pooling blood in the extremities (Fig. 32-19). The tourniquets occlude venous return but are not tight enough to suppress arterial flow. Pulses in extremities are monitored, as are blood pressure, skin temperature and color, and patient tolerance. Constant observation is essential during this procedure. Cuffs are applied to three extremities after baseline blood pressure is established. Inflation to a pressure less than systolic pressure allows palpable arterial pulse. After 15 minutes, one cuff is released and the previously free extremity cuff is inflated. A clockwise rotation is the pattern used. When discontinuing tourniquets, one at a time is released at 15-minute intervals to prevent sudden circulatory increase and subsequent overload.

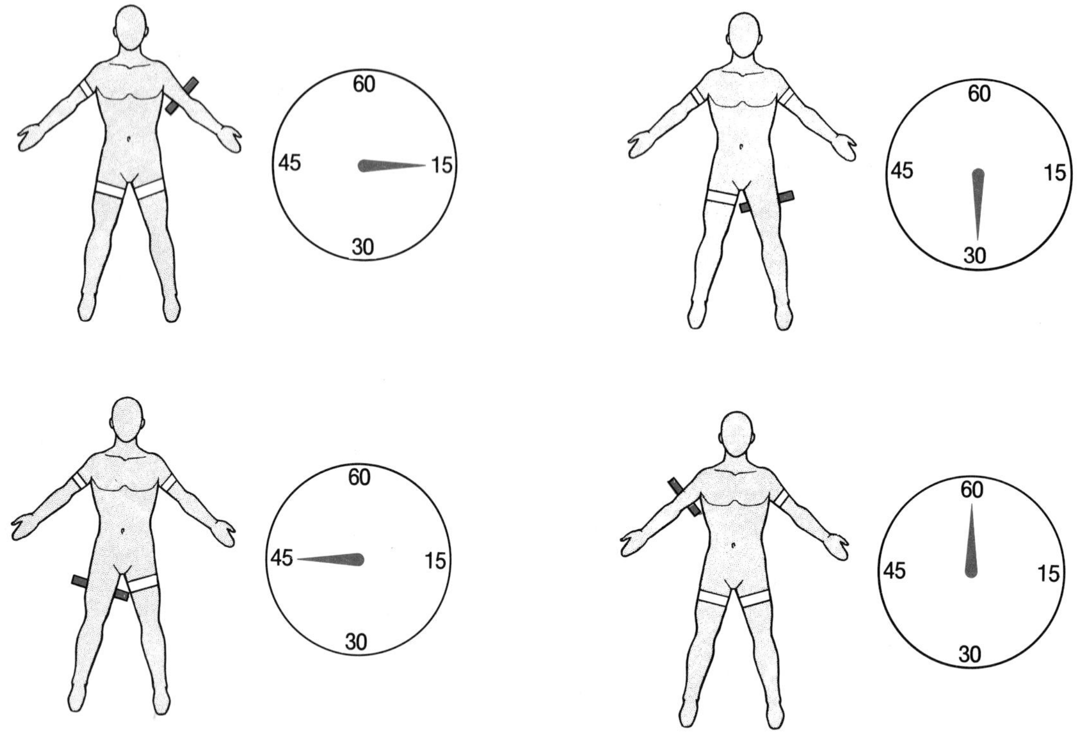

FIG. 32-19 Procedure for rotating tourniquets to reduce pulmonary edema. Note that tourniquets are rotated clockwise each 15 minutes and that one extremity remains free.

Nursing interventions. The nursing approach supports the objectives of medical treatment. Usually, bed rest, oxygen therapy, medication therapy, and diet control are the first interventions. Consideration of stress and anxiety is addressed through explanation and patient education along with nursing interventions.

In acute failure, administration of oxygen and medication should be of first concern. Decreasing oxygen requirements through complete bed rest will slow heart rate and increase cardiac and respiratory reserves. Anxiety produced from the effects of signs and symptoms and the fear of a life-threatening situation can be allayed by reassurance and explanation. Accurate interventions, observation, and reporting reduce the threat of such complications as embolus, thrombophlebitis, MI, and pulmonary edema.

In chronic failure or after the acute crisis, complete bed rest and freedom from stress should be maintained. This decreases cardiac workload. Fowler's position relieves pulmonary congestion by lowering venous return to the cardiopulmonary systems. Diaphragmatic pressure eases, and dyspnea becomes less prevalent. Relieving respiratory distress lessens oxygen requirements and aids in adequately supplying oxygen to tissues and organs.

The nursing interventions include measures to prevent disease progression and complications. Vital signs are monitored for changes. Signs of respiratory distress will be noted. The nurse will observe for signs of crisis and pulmonary edema. Symptoms of left-sided versus right-sided heart failure are carefully monitored. Urinary output is typically low, and edema is soft and pitting; legs are elevated to decrease edema.

The nurse should also note increase in abdominal girth and total body weight as indicators of the fluid retention common in heart failure. The nurse will auscultate lung fields to determine the presence of rales and rhonchi, coughing, and complaints of dyspnea. Restful sleep may be possible only in the sitting position or with the aid of extra pillows. Activity intolerance accompanied by extreme fatigue and anxiety is usually noted.

Cardiac Dysrhythmias

Etiology/pathophysiology. A **dysrhythmia** is a disturbance in the rate or rhythm of the heartbeat. It is an impulse conduction disorder and may be related to cardiac impulses originating outside the sinoatrial (SA) node.

The cause of the dysrhythmia may be organic, such as degenerative or inflammatory heart disease, or may originate in other systems, for example, vagal stimulation related to the central nervous system. Medication, electrolyte imbalance, or traumatic occurrences, such as surgical procedures, are also thought to effect dysrhythmias.

NURSING CARE PLAN: CARE OF THE PATIENT WITH CONGESTIVE HEART FAILURE

Mrs. Alicia Jons is a 55-year-old speech pathologist with a history of rheumatic heart disease and pericardial inflammatory constriction. She is self-employed in a stressful setting and reports episodes of essential hypertension. She complains of dyspnea, especially when lying flat. This has contributed to insomnia. In the past month she has had pedal edema several times and has noticed an enlargement of the abdomen, which prompted her to visit her physician Dr. Saltzenfeffer.

On admission Mrs. Jons' complaints include nausea, weakness, palpitations, and a sense of impending doom. She states that she was up all night going to the bathroom (excessive voiding). Nurse Beauxmer reported vital signs abnormalities, including pulse irregularity with bounding delivery. Auscultation of the heart and lungs reveals dysrhythmia, rales, and rhonchi. Abdominal inspection gives evidence of epigastric pain and abdominal enlargement. Digits are cyanotic and edematous. Pitting peripheral edema is demonstrated in the lower extremities.

ADMIT DIAGNOSIS: CHF (advanced)

MEDICAL ORDERS:
- Oxygen at 4 L/min per nasal cannula
- Bed rest with bedside commode
- I & O
- Weigh daily
- Diet: low sodium
- Medications: Lasix 40 mg BID; Slow-K tab ii TID; Lanoxin 0.125 mg QD; Maalox 30 ml QID
- Laboratory tests: Chest x-ray, echocardiogram, blood chemistry profile

Nursing diagnoses	Patient goals	Nursing interventions
Activity intolerance, related to dyspnea, weakness, and edema	Patient will adjust to and compensate for physical disabilities and will learn to conserve energy.	Reinforce importance of planning activities to conserve energy. Administer oxygen as prescribed. Elevate extremities, and observe dietary restrictions for edema control. Encourage gradually increasing activity within prescribed restrictions; monitor for intolerance. Assist with ADLs as necessary; encourage self-care as tolerated. Provide small, frequent feedings.
Decreased cardiac output, related to cardiac insufficiency	Patient's breathing will be easier; patient will be less dyspneic with activity.	Maintain bed rest and stress-free environment. Monitor vital signs, urinary output, and cardiac status frequently. Administer cardiac glycosides and diuretics accurately as ordered. Monitor serum electrolyte levels. Weigh daily to document fluid loss. Monitor accurate intake and output to assess renal output.

Continued.

NURSING CARE PLAN: CARE OF THE PATIENT WITH CONGESTIVE HEART FAILURE—cont'd

Nursing diagnoses	Patient goals	Nursing interventions
Anxiety and fear, related to knowledge deficit and health status change	Patient will express minimal anxiety; patient will state he feels more relaxed.	Give patient opportunities to explore feelings about effect of illness on life-style. Assist patient to identify personal strengths. Give medications to reduce anxiety, if prescribed. Encourage input and interaction from significant others.
Fluid volume excess, related to congestion of cardiovascular system	Patient will have a decrease of edema, weight, and abdominal girth. Patient will have no dyspnea with activity.	Weigh daily, record intake and output, and monitor laboratory reports. Measure abdominal girth daily. Administer medications: diuretic and potassium replacement, as prescribed. Maintain dietary restrictions: low sodium, fluid intake restrictions.

Each dysrhythmia affects the cardiovascular and related systems in a different and individual way. For example, increased cardiac workload may occur, or progression of coronary artery disease may result.

Clinical manifestations. Occasionally dysrhythmias may be asymptomatic. More often the following signs and symptoms are presented:

- Palpitation, headache, dyspnea, syncope, and chest pain are manifested in rapid rate dysrhythmias.
- Slow rate dysrhythmias exhibit syncope, dyspnea, and exertional fatigue.
- Hypotension is produced by blood force impairment, adding to the overall signs and symptoms that produce disability.
- Altered levels of consciousness and anxiety are also associated with dysrhythmias.

Diagnostic tests. Detection of dysrhythmia is accomplished by the physician's analysis of the ECG wave form or the Holter monitor. The ECG is normally represented graphically by a repetition of electrical impulses lettered *PQRST*. These waves occur at an established standard rate (60 to 100 times per minute), size, and shape. Medication therapy for dysrhythmias is shown in Table 32-5.

Common dysrhythmias. *Sinus bradycardia* occurs when the myocardium contracts steadily but at a rate of less than 60 contractions per minute. It may result from increased vagal tone (straining at stool), drug therapy (digitalis), or pathological conditions, such as myocardial infarct. Syncope and vertigo may be felt. Relief of the underlying cause and symptomatic treatment are the typical interventions.

Sinus tachycardia is characterized by rapid but regular heart rate, above 100 beats per minute. This condition increases the heart's workload, causing significant problems to patients with heart disease. Causes of tachycardia are emotion, exercise, physical stress, fever, shock, and excessive caffeine intake. Drug intoxication may be the cause. Signs and symptoms include fatigue and dyspnea. Treatment is aimed at correction of cause with a medication approach that includes propranolol (β-adrenergic blocker) and verapamil (calcium channel blocker).

Premature atrial contraction (PAC) is the result of atrial enlargement or ischemia, or may be caused by stress. The atrial beat occurs before the expected or normal sequence and is known as an *early P wave*. Usually this condition does not require treatment unless it threatens to develop into a more serious dysrhythmia. Signs and symptoms are palpitation, skipped beat or atrial flutter, vertigo, and anxiety. Quinidine is the drug of choice to treat and lower the number of ectopic beats. It is wise to restrict caffeine and nicotine.

Atrial flutter is a rapid, regular atrial contraction, which is sometimes asymptomatic or may produce dyspnea, palpitation, or tachypnea. Digoxin and quinidine are administered to slow and strengthen the heart rate.

Atrial fibrillation is a condition where a rapid atrial rate causes irregular ventricular beats. It is seen most frequently in rheumatic heart disease, mitral stenosis, and atrial infarction. Decreased cardiac output complicates the condition by stressing the cardiac workload. The signs and symptoms include palpitation, tachycardia, irregular pulse, and chest discomfort. Medication therapy includes

Table 32-5 Medication Therapy in Cardiac Dysrhythmias

Classification	Medication	Action	Action site
Cardiac depressants	Lidocaine; procainamide HCl; quinidine	Lowers heart rate	Myocardium
Antidysrhythmics; β-adrenergic blocking agents	Propranolol; isoproterenol	Increases rhythmicity	Myocardium
Cardiac glycosides	Digitalis preparations	Slows and strengthens heartbeat	Myocardium
Cholinergic blocking agents	Atropine	Increases heart rate	Autonomic nervous system

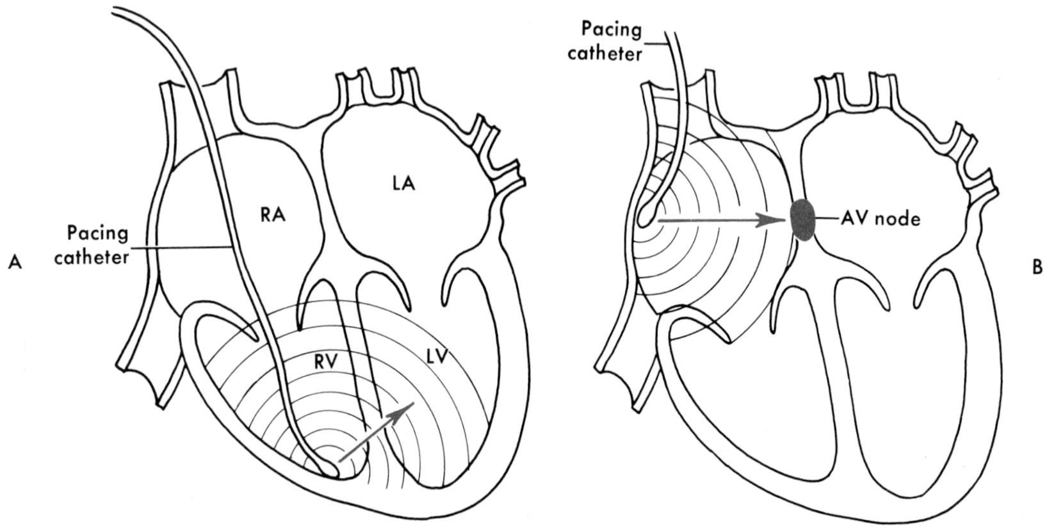

FIG. 32-20 **A,** Ventricular pacing. Impulses are initiated in ventricle. **B,** Atrial pacing. Impulses are initiated in atrium and travel to ventricles by normal conduction system.

digoxin and quinidine as explained above.

Premature ventricular contraction (PVC) is characterized by an early ventricular beat, which is seen in many forms of heart disease, especially myocardial infarction. It is also attributed to electrolyte imbalance, caffeine and alcohol stimulation, and excessive smoking (nicotine). The therapeutic approach is to treat the underlying cause and signs and symptoms: pain, palpitation, vertigo, and syncope. IV lidocaine is used to control PVC.

Ventricular fibrillation is marked by rapid and disorganized ventricle pulsation. There is no cardiac output. Marked hypotension occurs with immediate death if untreated. Cardiac arrest may occur. External defibrillation and ventilation are supported by parenteral lidocaine. Early signs and symptoms may include palpitation, dyspnea, nausea with vomiting, cyanosis, altered level of consciousness, and absent pulse.

Heart block is a conduction disorder whereby the AV node dysfunction blocks the SA node impulse relay to the ventricles. There are various degrees of heart block.

Heart block is associated with many heart conditions, such as myocardial infarction, myocarditis, and rheumatic heart disease. The toxic effects of digitalis, quinidine, or procainamide therapy can result in heart block.

In atrioventricular (AV) heart block, the contractions of the heart are weakened and therefore do not have enough force to send the blood from the atrium into the ventricle. The pulse rate is very slow (30 to 40 beats per minute).

In third-degree block, or complete heart block, none of the sinus impulses are conducted through the AV junction. The atrial rate is usually regular and of normal rate but faster than the ventricle rate. The ventricle rate is usually 30 to 45 beats per minute. Isoproterenol and temporary or permanent cardiac pacing (pacemaker) are used to treat third-degree block (Fig. 32-20).

NURSING DIAGNOSES	NURSING INTERVENTIONS
Pain, related to ischemia	Administer medication as ordered. Teach relaxation techniques. Institute position change, and support.

NURSING DIAGNOSES	NURSING INTERVENTIONS
Decreased cardiac output, related to cardiac insufficiency	Reduce cardiac workload by maintaining bed rest. Elevate head of bed 30 to 45 degrees for comfort. Restrict activities as ordered; plan care to avoid fatigue. Administer medication as ordered. Monitor for signs of drug toxicity.
Ineffective individual coping, related to fear and uncertainty of disease process	Assist patient with identifying strengths and coping skills. Supply emotional support. Teach relaxation techniques. Assess level of coping ability and family support level. Explain purpose of care as related to specific dysrhythmia. List symptoms to expect and to report to physician. Promote understanding of medication administration. Explain treatment goals. Explain importance of maintaining prescribed diet and fluid amounts. Explain importance of not smoking.

Defibrillation

Defibrillation is a synchronized cardioversion—an emergency procedure used to terminate ventricular fibrillation by delivery of a direct electric countershock to the patient, causing depolarization of the entire myocardium. The desired result is restoration of normal cardiac action through SA node control of cardiac impulse.

ECG verifies the diagnosis of ventricular fibrillation. Level of consciousness and vital signs are observed; parenteral support is maintained. An electrical charge of 200 to 400 watt seconds is delivered by the defibrillator through electrode paddles pressed flat against the chest wall. Additional shock may be required to accomplish normal cardiac rhythm.

After defibrillation, a comparison of the before and after rhythm pattern is made. Respiratory support is maintained. The patient is monitored continuously until stable. CPR may be required before or after this procedure.

Cardiac Arrest

The sudden cessation of cardiac output and circulatory process is termed *cardiac arrest*. Conditions effecting this circumstance are severe ventricular tachycardia, ventricular fibrillation, or ventricular asystole. Because of the manifestation of anaerobic tissue cell metabolism and respiratory and metabolic acidosis caused by absence of O_2-CO_2 exchange, immediate initiation of CPR is indicated to prevent major organ damage. Signs and symptoms of cardiac arrest include abrupt loss of consciousness with no response to stimuli, gasping respirations followed by apnea, absence of pulse (radial, carotid, femoral, and apical), absence of blood pressure, pupil dilation, and development of pallor and cyanosis.

Initiation of cardiopulmonary resuscitation is done by the first person to discover the condition. The aim is to reestablish heartbeat and ventilation. Prevention of severe damage to the brain, heart, liver, and kidneys as a result of anoxia is of primary concern. The **ABCs** of CPR should be remembered: **A**—open **A**irway; **B**—restore **B**reathing; and **C**—restore **C**irculation. (See Chapter 53.)

After successful CPR, the patient is on continuous ECG monitor. Chest x-ray examination and hemodynamic testing is done plus arterial blood gas and cardiac enzyme studies. Urinary output is monitored closely. Vital signs are taken every 15 minutes until stable. The ultimate medical intervention is to correct the underlying cause of the arrest.

The Pacemaker

A pacemaker is an electric apparatus used for maintaining a normal cardiac rhythm of myocardial contraction by electrically stimulating the heart muscle. It may be permanent, emitting the stimulus at a constant and fixed rate, or it may fire only on demand when the heart does not spontaneously contract at a minimum rate.

Catheter-like electrodes are placed within the area to be paced: atrium, ventricle, or both (Fig. 32-20). Indications for use include heart block or dysrhythmias, such as severe tachycardia or those dysrhythmias associated with myocardial infarction. After cardiac surgery, a temporary pacemaker may be necessary for a short period. This type is attached externally with an internal lead placed within the area to be paced (Fig. 32-21).

Nursing interventions. After placement of a pacemaker, the nurse closely monitors heart rate and rhythm by apical pulse and by ECG patterns. Vital signs and level of consciousness are checked frequently until stable. The insertion site is observed for erythema, edema, and tenderness, which could indicate the presence of infection.

Patient teaching. The patient should be informed of the necessity to continue medical management, and the nurse should advise that medical-alert identification should be carried, as well as pacemaker information. The nurse should emphasize the importance of reporting signs and symptoms of pacemaker failure: weakness, vertigo, chest pain, and pulse changes.

The patient should be taught potentially hazardous situations to avoid. Each pacemaker manufacturer can provide a list of devices that should be avoided by patients with pacemakers (e.g., older model microwave ovens). The patient should be taught to move away from any device that may be causing untoward symptoms, such as vertigo.

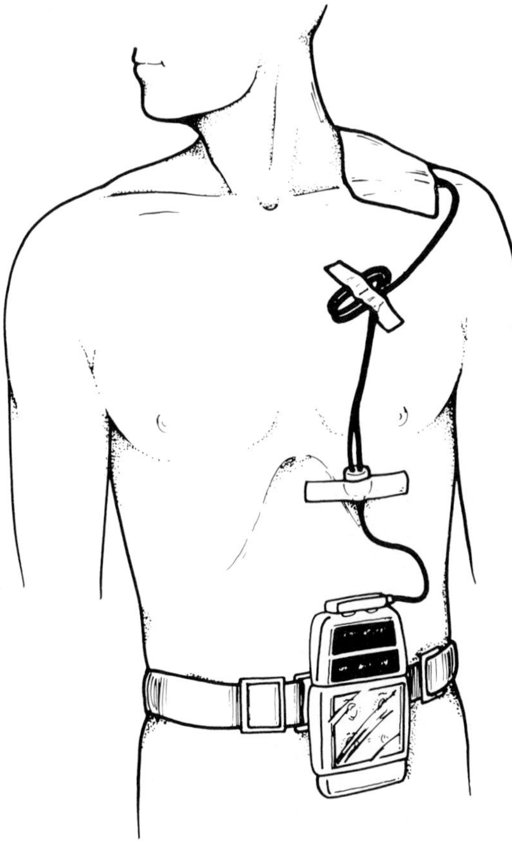

FIG. 32-21 Temporary external pacemaker.

The nurse teaches the patient how and when to take a radial pulse. The pulse should be taken at the same time each day and if symptoms of vertigo or weakness occur. The patient can expect to lead a reasonably normal life with full resumption of most activities as prescribed by the physician.

Inflammatory Diseases of the Heart

Inflammation is the response of tissues to injury or irritation, marked by erythema, heat, edema, and pain. Loss of function may result if the cause is not eliminated. The tissues of the heart are sensitive to bacterial, viral, and mycotic (fungal) infection, responding with inflammatory process and function loss.

Rheumatic heart disease

Etiology/pathophysiology. Rheumatic heart disease, a sequela of rheumatic fever, predominantly results from a childhood pharyngeal or upper respiratory tract infection (β-hemolytic streptococcus).

Ineffective treatment of infection results in delayed reaction and inflammation of the cardiac tissues (or the central nervous system, joints, skin, and subcutaneous tissues). Vegetation areas, called Aschoff bodies, develop in the myocardium and skin. Healing leaves scar tissue, which effects irreversible damage and subsequent disability of the area affected. Heart valves (most frequently mitral and aortic), when involved, fuse during healing, causing chronic valvular disorder. Rheumatic heart disease can be a recurrent condition with further damage occurring as each attack occurs.

Complications include mitral and aortic stenosis caused by thickened and fused valves. Heart failure and pulmonary edema occur with advanced disease. Surgical valvular replacement is often related to rheumatic condition or complication.

Clinical manifestations. Fever, increased pulse, anemia, joint involvement, and nodules on joints and subcutaneous tissue may be noted. Carditis can develop. When valvular involvement occurs, signs and symptoms are specific to each condition.

Assessment. Collection of *subjective data* may reveal joint pain (polyarthritis), as well as abdominal pain. There is also anorexia and fatigue.

Collection of *objective data* will include skin manifestations of small erythematous circles and wavy lines on the trunk and abdomen that appear and disappear rapidly (erythema marginatum). The nurse will observe involuntary, purposeless movement of the muscles if Sydenham's chorea (St. Vitus' dance), a disorder of the central nervous system, is present. An apical systolic murmur may be auscultated if carditis with valve involvement is present.

Diagnostic tests. Diagnosis is made through signs and symptom presentation and supported by laboratory study results. ECG shows cardiac dysrhythmia. Cardiac murmurs or friction rub can be heard. Sedimentation rate and leukocyte count will be elevated. Antibodies against the streptococci (measured by antistreptolysin O [ASO] titer) may be present.

Medical management. Intervention is more effective when approach is by preventive measures. Rapid treatment for pharyngeal infection, usually with prolonged antibiotic therapy, is desired. Bed rest is necessary in the acute phases. Symptomatic treatment and care is followed. Aspirin for joint pain and inflammation is accompanied by low heat application. A well-balanced diet, high in calories is supplemented by vitamins B and C and high volume fluid intake.

Nursing interventions. Bed rest during the initial attack is recommended, especially if carditis is present. After the acute stage, the child or young adult is treated at home. A schedule of daily events is reviewed with the patient and the parents.

Nursing interventions are carried out quickly and skillfully to minimize discomfort and prevent tiring the child.

Acquired valvular heart disease

Etiology/pathophysiology. The heart valves function to support forward blood flow through atria and ventricles into the pulmonary artery and aorta. Damage or impairment results from rheumatic heart disease, postinfarction insufficiency, or valve prolapse. Congestive heart failure will eventually occur if the stenosis or insufficiency worsens; valve replacement may be indicated.

Impairment of valvular function results in regurgitation or diminished force of blood flow. Stenosis, a thickening and contracture, can constrict and narrow the opening, thus obstructing blood flow. Infectious residuals of inflammatory heart conditions attribute to fusion and fibrosis of valves. Insufficiency or inadequacy means that imperfect closure allows blood regurgitation, backflow, or incompetence of the expected function.

Clinical manifestations. In valvular stenosis or valvular insufficiency the affected site cannot maintain a normal forward flow. Common sites and conditions are listed below in order of frequency of occurrence.

1. Mitral stenosis or insufficiency (most common)
2. Aortic stenosis or insufficiency
3. Tricuspid stenosis or insufficiency
4. Pulmonary stenosis or insufficiency (rare)

Assessment. Many of the signs and symptoms of valvular heart disease are related to decreased cardiac output. Therefore the data the nurse obtains are essentially the same for any person with valvular heart disease.

Collection of *subjective data* may include fatigue and weakness, dyspnea, angina, syncope, and heart palpitations.

Collection of *objective data* may reveal cyanosis, neck vein engorgement, diaphoresis, heart murmurs, adventitious lung sounds, rales, rhonchi, and presence of edema.

Diagnostic tests. ECG changes are noted; echocardiogram reveals a thickened valve and hypertrophy of affected atrium or ventricle. Chest x-ray study shows enlargement and calcification of valves. A cardiac catheterization is often performed, which demonstrates a valvular pathological condition.

Medical management. Treatment varies with the severity of the condition. Conservative treatment involves limitations of activity, reduction of sodium intake, and administration of digitalis and diuretics. If the patient becomes increasingly incapacitated when undergoing therapy, surgery may be necessary. Mitral stenosis can be treated surgically by a mitral commissurotomy, replacing the mitral valve. The surgeon makes an incision into the left atrium and inserts the finger, a knife, or a dilator through the valve and breaks apart the stenosed tissue. Aortic stenosis is treated by replacing the aortic valve. This is accomplished during open heart surgery using a perfusion pump.

Nursing interventions. Nursing interventions for the patient with valvular disease who is receiving medical therapy center primarily on continued monitoring. Fluid balance is monitored by daily weights and measuring and recording intake and output. Auscultation of heart and breath sounds is continued. The skin is observed for changes in appearance, capillary perfusion, and presence and extent of edema. The patient's activity tolerance is monitored, and evidence of dyspnea on exertion or fatigue should be noted.

Endocarditis

Etiology/pathophysiology. Endocarditis is an infection or inflammation of the inner membranous lining of the heart, particularly the heart valves. Classified on the basis of cause, it may result from invasion of an organism (bacterial endocarditis) or may be the result of injury to the lining. Endocarditis may develop after cardiac surgery, which in itself is traumatic.

Persons at risk include patients with rheumatic valvular disease, congestive heart disease, and degenerative heart disease. In some cases endocarditis is preceded by intrusive procedures, such as dental procedures, minor surgery, gynecological examinations, or indwelling urinary catheters. Other persons at high risk include those who "mainline" street drugs, because of the possibility of bacteremia from contaminated needles and syringes.

Bacteria, most commonly *Streptococcus viridans* or *Staphylococcus aureus, Staphylococcus epidermidis*, and enterococci, are deposited on the heart lining or valves. As the organism embeds into the tissue, a vegetative growth perforates the chambers or valve leaflets. Fibrin and calciferous growths of the vegetation may ulcerate and scar the valves or may break away, causing emboli, infection, or abscess in organs where they may lodge. The kidneys and spleen are often affected.

Clinical manifestations. Occurring in acute or subacute form, signs and symptoms progress either rapidly, in dangerous sequence during the acute phase, or gradually, with damage occurring over a long period.

Assessment. Collection of *subjective data* includes noting patient complaints of influenza-like symptoms with recurrent fever, undue fatigue, chest pain, headaches, and joint pain.

Collection of *objective data* may reveal the significant signs of petechia in the conjunctiva, mouth, and legs and anemia. Weight loss may occur. Pulse is rapid. Murmurs can be detected.

Diagnostic tests. ECG changes and chest x-ray examination denote evidence of CHF and heart enlargement. Laboratory findings indicate leukocytosis and increased sedimentation rate. Blood cultures determine causative organism, and sensitivity tests indicate the effective antibiotic needed for medical management.

Medical management. Management relies on bed rest to decrease the heart's workload. A massive dosage of antibiotics is administered—usually parenterally—to combat the organism for a prolonged time to eradicate all organisms. Before the use of antibiotics, patients with bacterial endocarditis could be expected to live about 1 year. Prompt treatment with intensive antibiotic therapy will now cure about 90% of patients with the disease.

Surgical repair of involved valves or valvular replacement necessitates postoperative nursing observation. Assessment for the occurrence of CHF—a complication of acute endocarditis—must be ongoing, to prevent valve destruction or patient death. Supporting the healing process, the diet recommended includes high-protein and high-caloric content with vitamin supplement.

Nursing interventions. The nursing interventions are based primarily on the signs and symptoms. Observation of the patient for petechiae, location of pain, vomiting, and fever is a nursing responsibility. If these signs and symptoms are observed, they should be reported at once. The patient needs encouragement to eat because of anorexia. It is vital that the nurse stresses the importance of maintaining bed rest.

Myocarditis. The inflammation of the myocardium may originate from rheumatic heart disease, an infectious process, or as a result of endocarditis or pericarditis. Symptoms will vary according to the site of manifestation. However, cardiac enlargement, murmur, gallop, and tachycardia are typically seen in myocarditis. Involvement and enlargement of the myocardium may result in dysrhythmia. Therapy is symptomatic and primarily follows the same approach as that of endocarditis: bed rest, antibiotics, and correction of dysrhythmias.

Pericarditis

Etiology/pathophysiology. Pericarditis is the inflammation of the membranous sac surrounding the heart. It may be manifested as an acute or a chronic condition. Trauma or bacterial, viral, or fungal infection is associated with acute pericarditis. It may occur as a complication of a systemic lupus erythematosus, scleroderma, azotemia, or myocardial infarction. Fibrosis of the pericardial sac develops in the chronic form.

Fibrous constriction and thickening of the pericardium occur gradually, causing compression severe enough to prevent normal filling during diastole. Surgical removal of the pericardium may be necessary to restore normal cardiac output.

Clinical manifestations. This condition differs clinically from other inflammatory conditions of the heart in that the presentation of debilitating pain—much like that of myocardial infarction—is common. Orthopneic positioning may promote relief. Dyspnea, fever, chills, diaphoresis, and leukocytosis are observed. Pericardial friction rub, grating, scratching, and leathery sounds are detected, as is dysrhythmia.

Decreased heart function to the level of cardiac failure can occur when the heart is compressed by excess fluid in the pericardial sac. Normally, a few drops of fluid is found in the pericardial sac, yet 150 to 200 ml may develop with incidence of pericarditis. When pericardial effusion restricts heart movement (cardiac tamponade), a pericardial tap (pericardiocentesis) may be performed to remove excess fluid and restore normal heart function.

Assessment. Collection of *subjective data* includes the patient's description of muscle aches, fatigue, and dyspnea. Excruciating chest pain is said to originate precordially and radiate to the neck and shoulders with severe and sudden onset.

Collection of *objective data* is noting expressed pain, obvious by orthopneic positioning and facial grimace on inspiration. Elevated temperature accompanies chills and may be followed by diaphoresis. Verbalizing anxiety, anticipation of danger, or uneasiness is common. Vital sign changes include pulse increase and rapid, shallow breathing. Pericardial friction rub and dysrhythmia may be noted by the physician assessment.

Diagnostic tests. ECG changes (dysrhythmia) will be noted. Echocardiogram will show the presence of pericardial effusion. Laboratory studies will show leukocytosis (10,000 to 20,000/mm^3 will be present) and the sedimentation rate will be elevated. Chest x-ray examination will show cardiac enlargement and pericardial effusion.

Medical management. Analgesia for comfort and relief of pain reassures the anxious patient. The physician prescribes salicylates for increased temperature, antibiotics for infection, and antiinflammatory agents (Indocin) and corticosteroids for a persistent inflammatory process. This requires nursing knowledge of untoward effects and nursing implications in the medication control of this condition. Surgical intervention—pericardial fenestration (pericardial window) or pericardiocentesis (pericardial tap)—may be performed to provide continuous drainage of pericardial fluid. Complications may include atelectasis and introduction of infectious agents.

Nursing interventions. The nurse will provide supportive measures and observe for complications in the patient with pericarditis. Bed rest is maintained to promote healing and decrease the cardiac workload. Nursing diagnoses and interventions for the patient with inflammatory heart conditions depend on the extent of the disease and complications.

NURSING DIAGNOSES	NURSING INTERVENTIONS
Decreased cardiac output, related to inflammatory process	Maintain bedrest with 30-degree head elevation. Assess vital signs q 2-4 hr as indicated by patient's condition. Administer medications as ordered. Monitor intake and output. Provide planned rest periods.
Altered nutrition: less than body requirements, related to loss of appetite	Assess for anorexia and weight loss; weigh daily; compare values. Encourage food intake high in protein and caloric value; provide supplemental feedings.
Pain, related to inflammatory process	Assess and record pain type and quality. Administer analgesia according to need, as ordered. Use comfort measures to provide physical support.

NURSING DIAGNOSES	NURSING INTERVENTIONS
Fluid volume deficit, related to ineffective myocardial action	Restrict sodium: monitor intake and output. Weigh daily; compare values. Administer diuretic therapy as ordered, monitoring electrolyte values. Observe respiration and pulse quality.
Knowledge deficit, related to disease process and home maintenance	Discuss disease process and symptoms to be reported. Discuss need for ongoing medical care. Explain necessity for rest, diversion, and program of structured exercise. Stress importance of avoiding potential for exposure to infections and seeking treatment if symptoms arise. Discuss medications, side effects, purpose, and administration techniques. Stress need for overall good heal maintenance, proper medical supervision, and dietary restrictions.

DISEASES AND DISORDERS OF THE VASCULAR SYSTEM

The blood supplies oxygenated, nutrient-rich components to body tissues and supports physical activity, removes metabolic by-products, and promotes healing. This circulatory function is accommodated by **patent**, unobstructed blood vessels that dilate and constrict, regulating volume according to varying need. The interruption of this process by vascular dysfunction can occur in any of the body parts or systems. Stasis of blood flow leads to ischemia and, ultimately, necrosis. Thrombus formation and accumulation of cellular waste further complicate and compromise tissue status.

Risk factors involved in vascular disease and disorder are inclusive of those presented earlier in this chapter. Education of the patient should be individualized to the specific risks presented, with emphasis on techniques to control the disease process and to strengthen health status for prevention of disease.

Diagnostic Procedures

Those previously presented diagnostic procedures are modified for vascular function diagnosis.

Angiography, arteriogram, and venography: Means of x-ray imagery of respective vessels injected with radiopaque contrast medium. Obstruction, constricture, neoplasm, or vessel route can be visualized.

Treadmill for intermittent claudication: Determines "cramping" related to physical exertion and the resultant rest relief. Rest pain, a burning sensation, may be identified after treadmill-induced symptoms.

Doppler ultrasonography: Used to measure blood flow by observation of reflected ultrasonic waves bounced off of moving structures (such as blood cells). Common placement sites include femoral, popliteal, and posterior tibial arteries. Valve patency is shown through the observations of the flow (see Fig. 13-6).

Nursing Assessment

The general physical assessment is enhanced by specific examination of the extremities, comparing bilateral similarities and differences. Information is compared with the history of general signs and symptoms and causes and with activity-rest relationship.

Clinical Manifestations of Peripheral Vascular Disease

Peripheral vascular diseases (PVD) are characteristically long-term conditions because of the slow healing process associated with circulatory impairment and nutritional deficiencies. The elderly are most commonly affected by this condition. Because of (1) inability to properly exercise, (2) poor nutritional status, and (3) knowledge deficit, PVD progression and complications are difficult to overcome. Related cardiovascular disease compounds the condition, resulting in medical management that is directed at multiple health problems.

Arterial Conditions and Disorders

Peripheral artery occlusion

Etiology/pathophysiology. Obstruction of peripheral arteries is linked to late-stage arteriosclerosis (arteritis obliterans) and atherosclerotic manifestation. Occlusive plaques, emboli, and damaged vessels are causative factors. Tobacco (nicotine) aggravates and potentiates the disorder.

This is a progressive disorder with symptoms paralleling Raynaud's and Buerger's diseases (discussed on pp. 741-742). Incidence is similar to that of arteriosclerotic heart disease and is prevalent in older men and patients with diabetes mellitus. Usually a disease of the lower extremities, it may also affect the great vessels. A buildup of agents causes circulatory impairment by progressively narrowing and obstructing vessels, thus preventing oxygen and nutrition to tissues.

Clinical manifestations. The patient with peripheral arterial occlusion will usually experience cold and pain in the affected extremities as the first and primary symptom. As the condition progresses, environmental temperature and activity will cause inability to function on a normal level. Noticing skin changes is common: coloration (ranges from cyanosis and pallor to erythema and rubor); edema; loss of hair; and inflammation. The nurse will assess pulse absence, asymmetry, and delayed healing caused by circulatory stasis. Numbness, rest pain, and cramping, which occurs because of ischemia, are found in the digits, legs, feet, or buttocks.

BOX 32-6 GENERAL SIGNS, SYMPTOMS, AND CAUSES OF VASCULAR DYSFUNCTION

SUBJECTIVE DATA

Pain **Intermittent claudication:** exertion initiates cramping pain that is relieved by rest.
Rest pain: burning sensation, intense enough to awaken patient.
General aches and pains accompanied by fatigue.

Cold Felt in extremities: moderate discomfort associated with inadequate circulation.

Fullness, tightness Noted in lower extremities: associated with edema and circulatory stasis.

Activity intolerance Associated with general circulatory inadequacy.

OBJECTIVE DATA

Muscular Changes

Flaccidity Noted on palpation: caused by decreased circulation and lactic acid accumulation.

Atrophy Results because of inactivity.

Skin Changes

Temperature Cool: cold to touch with decreased circulation.
Warmth over areas of inflammation: cellulitis, ulceration, thrombosis.

Color Cyanosis: inadequate oxygen-carrying hemoglobin, occlusion.
Rubor: prolonged vessel dilation causing bluish-red coloration.
Pallor: upon elevation of extremity, circulation is impaired.
with pressure application (pressing foot to floor), arterial vasodilation occurs.

Inflammatory process Ulceration, cellulitis, thrombophlebitis.
Inadequate perfusion of tissues to remove cellular wastes, potential tissue damage and slowing of healing process.

Pulse changes Absence/presence, symmetry, quality, and strength comparison.
Denotes circulatory embarrassment.

Healing ability Slowed.

Assessment. Box 32-6 represents the subjective and objective data for which the nurse should assess.

Diagnostic tests. Vascular examination, arteriography, and Doppler studies are used to obtain a diagnosis.

Medical management. Although prognosis is poor because of the general health and arterial status that usually accompanies this condition, care is aimed at relief of symptoms and preservation of the extremity(ies). Surgical procedures include bypass, grafting, endarterectomy (a surgical procedure that excises the tunica intima, or core, of an artery that has become thickened by atherosclerosis), and sympathectomy (a surgical intervention of part of the sympathetic nerve pathways, performed for the relief of chronic pain in vascular disease).

Nursing interventions/patient teaching. Information and instruction on the reduction of risk factors are the mainstays of intervention for the patient. For those patients who are obese, a reduction in weight will reduce the workload of the lower extremities. Many people find that losing weight is all that is needed to relieve the symptoms of claudication. Altering the diet to reduce the amount of fat in the blood may decrease the risk of further plaque development in the arterial system.

Smoking cessation is important; the nurse can inform the patient about the relationship between smoking and claudication, since this may be new information to the patient. The nurse can also provide written material or make a referral to a smoking cessation program.

It is important when teaching the patient about exercises to stress that the discomfort experienced with claudication is not harmful to the body. It is only a signal that there must be a pause to allow the arteries to rest and fill with blood. If individuals continue to be fearful of using the muscles and consequently do not use them to the point of claudication, there will be no stimulus for the development of collateral circulation. The patient must receive a medical clearance for exercise, and then a walking program should be developed that is consistent and fits into the patient's daily routine. The patient may be referred to a cardiac rehabilitation program.

Postoperative nursing intervention with emphasis on the specific procedure will be employed.

Raynaud's phenomenon

Etiology/pathophysiology. Intermittent attacks of ischemia of extremities—fingers, toes, ears, and nose—caused by exposure to cold or emotional stimuli is termed *Raynaud's phenomenon*. It is considered related to immunological disorders or occupational trauma (sometimes sustained by typists and jackhammer operators). The condition may be hereditary and usually affects women 16 to 35 years old. It is also noted more frequently in winter and in colder climates.

Arterial spasm and ischemic process occur, related to the thickening of the artery wall. Usually this affects one or two digits. If it affects the entire peripheral vascular system with bilateral, symmetrical manifestations, it is then termed *Raynaud's disease*.

Clinical manifestations. In cold conditions, pain and numbness of the fingers primarily are noted; this is accompanied by aching, throbbing, and burning. These symptoms are unrelieved by the usual attempt to warm the extremities and restore circulation. Vasoconstriction is present with pallor, characteristic color change from cyanotic to blanching, and finally reactive hyperemia with erythema. Fingertip ulceration may occur because of circulatory inadequacy and residual waste products.

Assessment. Box 32-6 lists the subjective and objective data that the nurse should observe.

Diagnostic tests. Doppler ultrasonography is used to study blood flow. A lumbar sympathetic block aids in evaluation of peripheral circulation. By blocking sympathetic nerves, vasodilation should occur. This examination should precede sympathectomy because it can determine its projected effectiveness. Laboratory immunological testing reveals abnormal antigen-antibody immune response.

Medical management. Management of Raynaud's condition is directed toward restoring normal sensation and avoiding precipitating factors: tempering exposure to cold with proper clothing and gloves and avoiding emotional stimuli that cause the vasoconstrictive reaction. Smoking and oral contraceptive drugs are not advised because they contribute to the condition. Injury to affected parts must be prevented. In situations of extreme manifestation, surgical intervention is considered. Medications include vasodilators, to decrease vasospasm while dilating vessels. Examples include cyclandelate (Cyclospasmol), phenoxybenzamine (Dibenzyline), and tolazoline (Priscoline).

Nursing interventions/patient teaching. After surgical intervention, the nurse will follow the usual postoperative intervention procedure. Reinforcing medical intervention includes patient teaching (Box 32-7) of risk factors and supportive approach. The nursing diagnoses and interventions are similar to those for arterial occlusive disease.

BOX 32-7 PATIENT TEACHING FOR RAYNAUD'S DISEASE

AVOID COLD

Use mittens (wool or cotton) in cold weather.
Use gloves to remove articles from the freezer.
Warm hands and feet by placing them next to another warm part of the body or placing them in warm (not hot) water; avoid hot water bottles or heating pads.

MANAGE STRESS

Anticipate stressful situations.
Examine present coping strategies, and determine whether new strategies are indicated.
Practice stress-reducing techniques.

STOP SMOKING

The nicotine in cigarette smoke stimulates constriction of the artery; "cutting down" will not improve the situation; complete smoking cessation is necessary.

Buerger's disease (thromboangiitis obliterans)

Etiology/pathophysiology. Buerger's disease, an occlusive vascular condition, begins in smaller vessels and progresses to larger vessels—arteries and veins alike. Although the cause is not fully understood, it is thought that smoking aggravates the condition.

Men of ages 20 to 40 years are primarily those affected by Buerger's disease. Inflammation affecting arteries, veins, and nerves of the lower extremities results in thrombus formation and vessel occlusion.

Clinical manifestations. Pain, as displayed by intermittent claudication, is accompanied by cold sensations of the feet. Weak peripheral pulse and cyanosis of the affected part indicate circulatory inadequacy. Phlebitis progressing to necrosis of toes and nailbeds may ultimately develop into gangrene. Inflammatory process is noted, especially if thrombus occurs.

Assessment. Box 32-6 presents the subjective and objective data that the nurse should observe.

Diagnostic tests. Arteriography visualizes vessels to pinpoint and differentiate the cause.

Medical management. Increasing circulation through exercise (which also develops collateral circulation) is a primary goal of care. Heat application is avoided, because of the resultant tissue need for increased oxygen. All factors that cause vasoconstriction or decreased blood supply to the extremity must be alleviated. Uncontrolled necrosis and gangrene may necessitate amputation; therefore these conditions are the focus of intervention. Sympathectomy may be performed in an attempt to relieve pain, but it is seldom successful.

Nursing interventions/patient teaching. Care of the extremities to prevent necrosis and gangrene includes hydration and cleanliness. Well-fitted shoes and socks alleviate pressure.

The most important single factor is teaching the patient the necessity for cessation of smoking. None of the palliative treatments are effective if the patient does not stop smoking. Nowhere is the cause and effect of smoking so dramatically presented as with Buerger's disease.

Nursing diagnoses and interventions are similar to those used for patients with arterial occlusive disease (see pp. 744-745).

Acute Arterial Occlusive Disorders

Certain arterial conditions develop as a result of the aging process or dietary and physical inadequacies or abuses. Insufficient blood flow occurs as a result of occlusive conditions or damaged vessels. Whereas some of these disorders are considered chronic disease processes, the **occlusion** onset may be sudden and threatening. The following brief presentations fall into this category. These disorders are diagnosed by Doppler ultrasonography, angiography, and through signs and symptoms manifested.

Embolus

Etiology/pathophysiology. An **embolus** is a foreign object circulating in the blood stream: air, gas, tumor, thrombus, or tissue. The danger of an embolus is the occurrence of lodging in and occluding a blood vessel.

Clinical manifestations. A sudden onset of pain is displayed in or around the affected area. If the embolus is in a peripheral artery, the skin temperature may become cool and the color may become pale, progressing to mottled, and finally, cyanotic, because of ensuing necrotic changes. Functional loss of the affected part is noted.

Diagnostic tests. Doppler ultrasonography and angiography are used to obtain a diagnosis.

Assessment. Collection of *subjective data* includes the nurse's awareness that occasionally pain is absent and the patient is not aware of the condition. Paralysis of the extremity, pallor, and coldness may be revealed.

Collection of *objective data* includes examination of the extremity, which may reveal asymmetry of pulses and cool-to-touch skin temperature with pallor to mottled appearance.

Medical management. Endarterectomy may be selected as the treatment of choice (Fig. 32-22). Balloon catheters are used to "ream" or excise tunica, intima, or the core of an artery affected by atherosclerosis. Removal of plaques and/or thrombi increases blood flow and lessens the danger of complication from emboli.

Embolectomy is another treatment available to suitable candidates. A longitudinal surgical incision into an artery for removal of a clot or embolus follows preoperative arteriogram that identifies the affected artery. Postoperatively, maintenance of a stable blood pressure is sought. This also reduces the predisposition of new clot formation.

Nursing interventions/patient teaching. The nursing interventions after both of these procedures include:

- checking peripheral pulses hourly for strength and quality
- recording vital signs, skin color, and temperature
- checking the incision for erythema, edema, and signs of infection

Prevention of these conditions is by far the most important intervention. The patient at risk is encouraged to adhere to activities that promote circulatory adequacy: exercise according to individual tolerance, proper diet, correct weight for size and age, and continued medical monitoring. Rest will reduce oxygen demand, and avoidance of injury may reduce severity or complication. In the acute stage, an embolus is life threatening and must be treated as an emergency situation. The nurse monitors

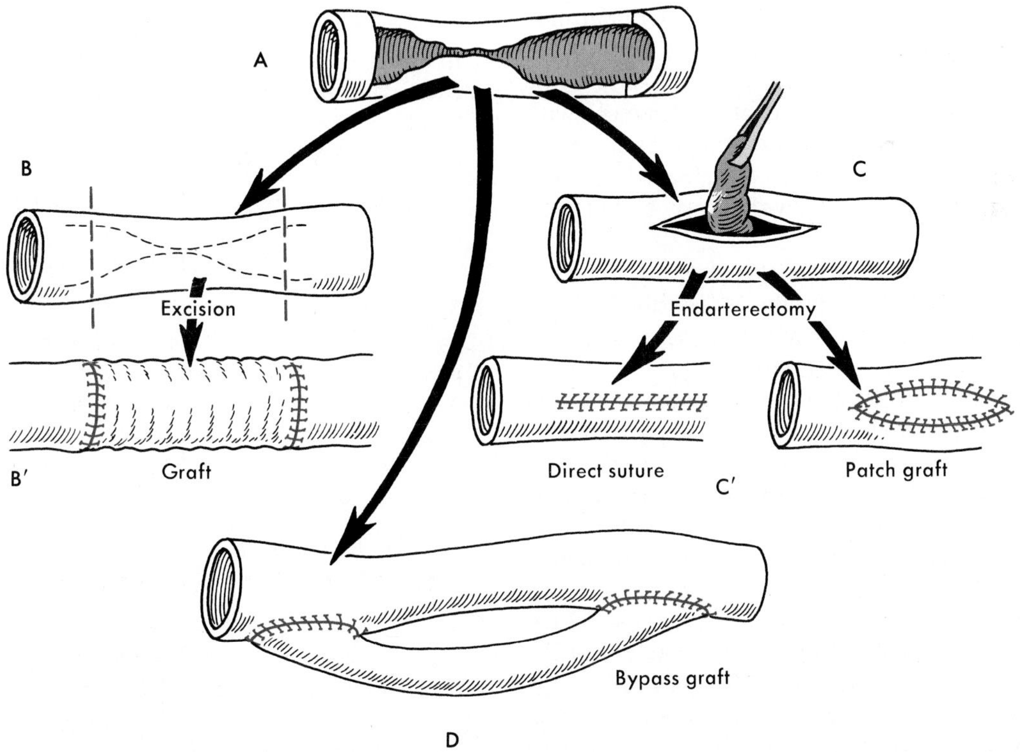

FIG. 32-22 **A,** Obstructed artery. Methods of restoring arterial blood flow include: **B,** excision; **B′,** graft; **C,** endarterectomy; **C′,** direct suture and patch graft reconstruction; and **D,** bypass graft. (Redrawn from Fairbairn JF and others: Peripheral vascular disease, Philadelphia, 1972, WB Saunders Co.)

BOX 32-8 PATIENT TEACHING FOR ARTERIAL OCCLUSIVE DISORDERS

- Avoid exposure to cold and chilling (causes vasoconstriction).
- Avoid constrictive clothing, rolled garters, socks with tight bands, girdles, and tight waistbands (impedes circulation).
- Adhere to medication regimen, and continue medical follow-up.

vital signs, bleeding into tissues, or signs of development of necrosis, which demands immediate medical attention. Administration of anticoagulant therapy must be careful and controlled with ongoing monitoring of prothrombin time. Surgical intervention requires preoperative preparation. Patient teaching strategies are listed in Box 32-8. Nursing diagnoses and interventions will be similar to those for arterial occlusive disease on pp. 744-745.

Thrombus

Etiology/pathophysiology. Platelets, clotting factors, fibrin, or cellular elements occlude arterial or venous vessels by attachment to the vessel wall. Blood vessel occlusion causes ischemic reaction—oxygen to tissues is diminished or absent. Development of an embolus is a threat.

Clinical manifestations. The occurrence of pain may be sudden, but usually this is a gradual development with increasing edema of the part. The skin is warm to the touch and may exhibit an indurated (hardened), painful area over the thrombosed vessel with display of rubescent discoloration.

Assessment. Collection of *subjective data* includes noting a gradual onset of symptoms as described by the patient, who identifies edema and changes in skin color and temperature. Pain may be reported.

Collection of *objective data* includes evaluation of blood supply to the extremities and gentle palpation of the affected part that reveals cyanosis or erythema of the area, accompanied by warmth and engorged tissue. Edema lessens if the extremity is elevated for any significant period. Pulses are palpable and more rapid than normal.

Medical management. The main objective of care in this condition is to reduce the risk of embolus (Table 32-6). Bed rest is ordered, with elevation of the part. Anticoagulant therapy is instituted (Box 32-9). Elastic stockings are used to prevent the condition from advancing and to protect the unaffected extremity. Analgesia is given as needed (Table 32-6). Reconstructive surgery or graft may be necessary (see Fig. 32-22).

Nursing interventions. The nurse should maintain the patient on bed rest during the acute phase and should perform range-of-motion exercises to the *unaffected* extremities. The extremity should be elevated to reduce edema and prevent venous **stasis**. An elastic stocking or bandage should be applied as ordered to increase blood flow and prevent venous stasis.

Table 32-6 Medication Administration for Peripheral Artery Disease

Classification	Agent	Action
Vasodilators	Isoxsuprine HCl (Vasodilan)	Lessens vasospasm
	Papaverine HCl (Pavabid)	Increases tissue perfusion
Anticoagulants	Heparin	Prolongs clotting time
	Warfarin (Coumadin)	Prevents thrombus formation
	Dicumarol	Prevents extension of clots
Fibrinolytics	Streptokinase (Streptase)	Dissolves necrotic tissue
	Fibrinolysin	Debrides necrotic tissue
Analgesics	Meperidine (Demerol)	Relieves pain
	Acetaminophen (Tylenol)	Relieves pain
Tranquilizers	Lorazepam (Ativan)	Manages anxiety Provides relaxation of stress reaction

NURSING DIAGNOSES	NURSING INTERVENTIONS
Activity intolerance, related to impaired physical mobility	Assess level of ability. Encourage controlled exercise, such as walking; provide passive ROM as ordered. Plan rest periods to conserve energy.
Pain, related to disease process	Assess pain level and coping ability. Teach relaxation measures and stress avoidance. Identify activity related to intermittent claudication; explain significance. Administer analgesics as needed.
Altered (peripheral) tissue perfusion, related to ischemia.	Assess pulses for quality, volume, and equality. Assess skin temperature and color for change. Maintain bed rest for decreased circulatory need. Position extremities for comfort and relief of edema. Use antiembolic stockings. Teach control of risk factors.
Knowledge deficit, related to disease process and home maintenance	Discuss symptoms and relation to condition and progression.

BOX 32-9 ANTICOAGULANT THERAPY

Aim	Medication therapy instituted to delay coagulation of the blood and prevent thrombus formation, especially in postoperative patients.	
Drugs	**Heparin**	**Warfarin (Coumadin)** **Dicumarol**
Route	Parenteral Infusion per pump Intermittent IV injection Intermittent subcutaneous injection	Oral
Dosage	20,000 to 30,000 units daily Continuous IV Divided doses	Coumadin 2 to 10 mg/day Dicumarol 25 to 200 mg/day
Laboratory tests	Prothrombin time (PT or pro time) determines clotting ability. Partial thromboplastin time (PTT) determines clotting ability. Platelet count checks for thrombocytopenia.	
Patient teaching	Wear medical alert identification bracelet or carry card with drug used and physician's name. Administer oral medication at same time (adhere to regular schedule). Avoid injury, e.g., bumping and razor cuts. Observe for complications and signs and symptoms to report to physician. Avoid alcohol (alters body response to therapy). Continue regimen without alteration (no catch-up doses). Consult physician before taking ANY medication.	

NURSING DIAGNOSES	NURSING INTERVENTIONS
	Explore importance of following regimen and therapeutic guidelines: medication, activity, and medical follow-up. Teach care of extremities and reporting of ulceration and delayed healing. Plan dietary guidelines: low calorie, low fat, low cholesterol, high protein, and vitamin supplements.

Patient teaching. To better recognize and cope with the presenting symptoms, the patient should understand the disease process. Risk factors must be identified, as should behaviors to exert a positive influence over their control. The nurse should make the patient aware of causative factors that initiate vasoconstriction: emotional stress, cold, humid environment, constrictive clothing, and smoking.

Taking prescribed medication to increase activity potential and tissue perfusion will decrease pain and discomfort. Understanding the medication use, action, and side effects is necessary, as is knowing the value of ongoing medical supervision. Exploring an exercise program tailored to the need and ability of the individual is essential for activity control.

Knowledge of skin integrity factors and protection of tissues against injury should be discussed with the patient to avoid infection and the progression of injuries. The nurse should explore with the patient the proper clothing for warmth in cold climates, skin care, and the value of exercise to increase collateral circulation. The nurse will teach the necessity for care of areas of necrosis and ulceration. The patient should be encouraged to see his physician as prescribed.

Dietary aspects to be taught include goals to promote healing, prevent advancement of the disease, and control weight to reduce pressure on extremities. A reduced-calorie, low-fat, low-cholesterol diet with increased vitamin and protein elements will be beneficial.

Aneurysm

Etiology/pathophysiology. Dilation of a weakened vessel wall, whether localized or diffuse, is termed *aneurysm.* Although more commonly the result of disease progression (infectious process or arteriosclerosis accentuated by hypertension), aneurysms are also caused by trauma or congenital defect. Because of greater pressure and blood flow force, aneurysms predominantly affect the thoracic and abdominal aorta. However, they are significant also in coronary and cerebral arteries. Peripheral vessels are affected also, especially the popliteal artery. The pathological effect of this condition is differentiated according to shape and site of presentation (Fig. 32-23).

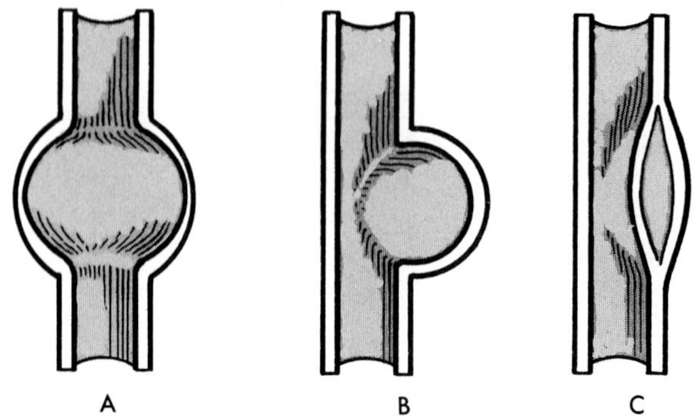

FIG. 32-23 Types of aneurysms. **A,** Fusiform. **B,** Saccular. **C,** Dissecting.

Fusiform aneurysm is a localized dilation of the entire circumference of the distended vessel. An elongated, tubular, or spindlelike enlargement occurs. *Saccular aneurysm* is a localized dilation of a small area of the involved vessel where the protrusion appears as a saclike enlargement. *Dissecting aneurysm* is a localized or diffuse dilation where artery wall layers tear with entry of blood into the separation. Longitudinal dissection of the vessel forms a cavity between the outer and middle vascular wall.

Pressure from the dilation interrupts circulatory function of adjacent organs or tissues. Functional loss or death as a result of hemorrhage after rupture is the outstanding threat of an aneurysm. Most common incidence is among men over age 60 and in smokers.

Clinical manifestations. The following are usual and common locations of aneurysms:

- Thoracic aortic aneurysm
- Abdominal aortic aneurysm
- Peripheral aneurysm

Assessment. Collection of *subjective data* involves awareness that most persons are asymptomatic but symptoms may occur, depending on how rapidly the aneurysm dilates and whether it is impinging on surrounding structures.

Collection of *objective data* includes observation of a pulsating enlargement that produces a blowing murmur on auscultation with a stethoscope. An aneurysm may rupture and cause hemorrhage, resulting in death without emergency surgical intervention.

Diagnostic tests. Fluoroscopy, chest x-ray studies, CT scan, ultrasound, and arteriography are means to diagnose the presence of an aneurysm.

Medical management. After diagnosis, aneurysms are monitored for complications—rupture, thrombosis, and ischemia with possible loss of the extremity because of gangrene. Control of hypertension is the first priority of care. Surgical intervention may be planned. A fusiform aneurysm can be removed and replaced with a graft of synthetic fiber, such as Dacron or Teflon, or with another vessel taken from another region of the patient's body. Saccular aneurysms can be removed and the vessel sutured, or a patch graft can be used to replace the deformity.

Postoperatively, kidney output is monitored, as is ECG for heart block complication. Medical management may be preferred over surgical intervention. In this circumstance, noting signs and symptoms with any changes will be significant. The prognosis is guarded.

Nursing interventions. Emotional support is important for the patient with an aneurysm. It is important to reinforce the physician's explanations of the complications. Emotional support for the patient's family should be given also. Accurate vital sign monitoring is of utmost importance, as is reporting any change or untoward signs or symptoms.

NURSING DIAGNOSES	NURSING INTERVENTIONS
Pain, related to pressure on surrounding structure	Assess level of pain and related symptoms. Administer analgesia as ordered. Assess source of pain, and report to physician.
Altered tissue perfusion, related to circulatory inadequacy	Assess circulation (especially extremities) by pedal pulse checks and capillary refill assessments. Examine skin for hematoma and abnormal pulsations. Be alert for complications.
Anxiety, related to feelings of impending death	Examine coping ability. Give emotional support to patient and family. Medicate as indicated: tranquilizers, analgesia. Maintain therapeutic environment.

Hypertension. Calculation of blood pressure measures cardiac output against peripheral vessel resistance: the pressure exerted on the walls of vessels by the blood force. Blood pressure persistently elevated above the normal range—higher than 140/90, or higher than 160 systolic in the elderly—is termed *hypertension*. This common disorder is characterized by abnormal elevations of systolic and/or diastolic pressures of small arterial vessels.

Etiology/pathophysiology. The cause of hypertension is related (1) to regulatory mechanisms that control arterial pressure through dilation and contraction of blood vessels and (2) to pathological factors in body function. Determination of cause is sometimes difficult, but it is important in medical management (Box 32-10).

The body reaction to hypertension is directly related to the cause: arterial walls become thickened, inelastic, and resistant to blood flow as a result of long-term hypertension. Hypertrophy and distention of the left ventricle may then develop, leading to congestive heart failure, angina, or myocardial infarction. The disease process precipitates severe complications and symptoms. Resistance of peripheral vessels and prolonged vascular pres-

BOX 32-10 FACTORS THAT CONTRIBUTE TO HYPERTENSION

Age: Adults—30 to 70 years
Sex: Females—Less frequent
Males— Higher occurrence for age group
Pain, emotion, stress
Activity: Exercise, diet
Disease process
Risks: Familial tendency
Race—More common (2:1) in African-Americans than in Caucasians
Health status—Obesity
—Elevated cholesterol level
Life-style—Alcohol excess
—Smoking
—Caffeine intake
—High sodium intake
Medication influence—Oral contraceptives
—Estrogen therapy

Table 32-7 Manifestations of Hypertension

Complications	Observations
CARDIOVASCULAR SYSTEM	
Left ventricular hypertrophy; failure	See specific disease condition for signs and symptoms.
MI; coronary vessel blowout	
Pulmonary edema	
CENTRAL NERVOUS SYSTEM	
Cerebrovascular accident	Abnormal neurological signs. Increased intracranial pressure. Transient ischemic attacks. Convulsive spasm.
EYE	
Retinal changes	Occipital headache.
Optic disc changes	Papilledema.
Hemorrhage	Photophobia. Capillary hemorrhage into conjunctival sac.
RENAL SYSTEM	
Kidney failure	Reduced urinary output.
Nephrosclerosis	Hematuria.

sure reduce blood supply to organs, resulting in system failure.

Clinical manifestations. Hypertension can be categorized into three classifications.

- *Primary/essential hypertension* is the most common presentation of this disorder. It develops without apparent cause and is not considered to be related to a pathological body process. In itself, the only significant finding is the elevated value of the blood pressure reading. Because of its asymptomatic quality, it is known as the "silent killer."
- *Secondary hypertension* is linked to pathological states: renal dysfunction, adrenal disease, thyrotoxicosis, toxic pregnancy, or cardiovascular disease. Autonomic nervous system regulatory factors are often the cause of this type of hypertension.
- *Accelerated/malignant hypertension* is a lethal form of the other two hypertensive classifications. It is a crisis blood pressure elevation that develops abruptly with severe manifestations. Rapid deterioration and serious organ damage occur without emergency treatment.

The patient with the most common type of hypertension (primary/essential) may be asymptomatic and remain undiagnosed until routine assessment presents the condition. Presenting signs and symptoms can be noted singly or in "like groups": vertigo, syncope, dyspnea, palpitations, anginal pain, and tinnitus (Table 32-7). A common complaint is that of awakening with an occipital headache. Eye hemorrhage is noted with very high, abrupt manifestation of hypertension. Papilledema and internal hemorrhage may be revealed. Epistaxis occurs, especially with altitude change. The more advanced hypertensive states show distended neck veins and associated carotid **bruit**. In late-stage hypertension, systems failure develops because of prolonged and intensified signs and symptoms; cardiac decompensation and hematuria can be present.

Assessment. Collection of *subjective data* includes questioning the patient about medical and familial history. Risk factors are identified. Complaints of memory lapse, headache, tinnitus, and cardiovascular signs and symptoms may be present. Although hematuria is not usually an early sign, attention to its occurrence is important. Family input can be valuable regarding observation of behavioral alteration and outward signs and symptoms such as capillary hemorrhage of the eye surface.

Collection of *objective data* includes proper determination of blood pressure readings. Hypertension is diagnosed when multiple measurements on subsequent visits or occasions reveal consistent elevation of diastolic pressure above 90 mm Hg (Box 32-11).

Diagnostic tests. Although the medical history and physical examination, including proper determination of blood pressure, are the main factors in hypertension diagnosis, other examinations are significant—especially in disease progression. On ECG studies, left ventricular hypertrophy as supported by x-ray examination is a significant finding. Chest x-ray examination will reveal cardiac size. Laboratory studies can target organ damage (hematocrit, BUN, urinalysis, serum potassium, renal function studies, IV pyelogram, and renogram).

BOX 32-11 **BLOOD PRESSURE RANGES**

ADULT

Systolic		**120**		**140**		**160**	
Diastolic	*Normal*	**84**	*High Normal*	**90**	*Moderate*	**100**	*Severe*

ELDERLY

Systolic		**140**		**160**		**180**	
Diastolic	*Normal*	**90**	*High Normal*	**100**	*Moderate*	**120**	*Severe*

Medical management. Hospitalization of patients specifically for hypertension is not common; most patients admitted to the hospital enter with problems unrelated to the condition. However, addressing the hypertensive condition is necessary to the holistic approach to patient care. Careful monitoring of medication interaction with hypertensive states, and relationship of other diagnoses to the condition is an important medical function. Blood pressure should be measured carefully to ensure accuracy. Daily weights are obtained when diuretic therapy is instituted. Rest is therapeutic. Bed rest is indicated if the accelerated type of hypertension is present. Stress reduction is encouraged. Medication therapy regimen to lower peripheral vessel resistance is followed (Table 32-8).

Nursing interventions. The nurse should be aware of the type of hypertension manifested in the patient and of the medical treatment goals. Signs and symptoms that produce discomfort should be assessed as to the source. A nonstressful environment should be maintained. Antihypertensive medications will be administered as ordered.

NURSING DIAGNOSIS	NURSING INTERVENTIONS
Knowledge deficit, related to disease progression and control	Determine level of understanding. Explain signs and symptoms and nature of disease. Review dietary controls. Discuss purpose of drug therapy. Emphasize necessity of adherence to medical regimen. Stress relaxation techniques.

Patient teaching. Awareness of the disease progression and the silent symptom aspect of hypertension is an essential element of patient teaching. The nurse should explain ill effects of medication management and side effects that should be reported to the physician.

Diet follows low-sodium and low-cholesterol intake with emphasis on weight management. Weight reduction is important if the patient is obese. Risk factors and contributing aspects must be reviewed, with emphasis on control of those that may increase the disease process—alcohol, caffeine, and smoking.

Table 32-8 Antihypertensive Medication Therapy

Classification	Agent	Action
Vasodilators	Hydralazine (Apresoline) Prazosin (Minipress)	Dilates peripheral vessels.
Adrenergic inhibitors (blocking agents)	Methyldopa (Aldomet) Reserpine (Serpasil) Propranolol (Inderal)	Displaces norepinephrine from storage sites. Lowers heart rate and thereby blood pressure.
Diuretics	Hydrochlorothiazide (Hydrodiuril) Furosemide (Lasix) Spironolactone (Aldactone)	Reduces fluid excesses in body tissues.
Sympathetic nervous system depressants and ganglion blocking agents	Captopril (Capoten)	Inhibits sympathetic activity.

Venous Disorders

The etiology, pathophysiology, clinical manifestations, and risk factors of common venous disorders are summarized in Table 32-9.

Assessment. Collection of *subjective data* includes a patient interview that focuses on leg pain and functional impairment manifestation. The patient may notice tenderness and taut skin. Calf site cramping and pain prevent activity.

Collection of *objective data* includes inspection of the extremity from the foot to the groin for asymmetry; this includes circumference measurement. Palpation reveals increased skin temperature with inflammatory process. Pulses are examined at femoral, popliteal, posttibial, and dorsalis pedis sites. Calf pain is initiated by foot dorsiflexion (Homans' sign). Observation is made for edema and vein enlargement or protrusion. Elevated temperature may be present.

Diagnostic tests. Doppler ultrasonography reveals diminished flow. Phlebogram views unfilled segments in affected vessel(s).

Table 32-9 Venous Disorders

Definition	Etiology	Pathophysiology	Clinical Manifestation	Risk Factors
THROMBUS				
Aggregation of platelets, fibrin, clotting factors, and cellular elements of blood attached to the vein wall	Stasis: immobilization, prolonged sitting or standing, or heart failure Hypercoagulability of blood Trauma to vessel wall, occlusion Infection, chemical irritation	Associated with cardiovascular disease: MI, CHF Blood dyscrasia Clot formation Lumen of vessel occluded Outflow inhibited	Variable, asymptomatic Muscle ache, calf pain Edema: extremity, ankle Erythematous site	Age: over 40, especially postoperative Smoking Health status Obesity Inactivity (bed rest) Trauma Previous venous insufficiency High emotional tension
DEEP VEIN THROMBOSIS				
Thrombus formation in the area below superficial vessels; deep vein location	Same as thrombus	Outflow severely limited Same as thrombus	Gradual onset Aching, cramplike pain Edema: extremity Skin temperature increased Color: cyanotic; rubescent Superficial veins: enlarged or normal, but prominent DANGER: dislodged clot (embolism)	Same
THROMBOPHLEBITIS				
Inflammation in the wall of a vein, often with clot formation	Trauma, occlusion most commonly Hemostasis Hypercoagulability	Vessel becomes thready, cordlike, sensitive to pressure Same as thrombus	Same as thrombus, except when inflammation is absent Pale, cool, edematous extremity	Same
PHLEBOTHROMBOSIS				
Clot formation without inflammation of vessel intima	Same as thrombophlebitis	Same as thrombophlebitis	Same as thrombophlebitis Absence of inflammation	Same

Medical management. Restoration of venous circulation to the fullest extent possible is the main objective of care. Prevention of complications is equally important: pulmonary embolism, myocardial infarction, cerebrovascular accident, ulceration, necrosis, or gangrene. Surgical intervention may include venous ligation or removal of a clot.

Nursing interventions. Identification of the risk of these conditions plus use of antiembolic stockings as ordered may aid in prevention of these conditions. If disease process is noted, positioning for comfort, bed rest with controlled exercise, and a medication regimen are the accepted interventions. The affected part is usually elevated, with moist heat application—except for deep vein thrombosis, where ice pack is more effective. Circulatory checks and monitoring of vital signs are ongoing, every 4 hours. After inflammation subsides, elastic stockings may be ordered.

NURSING DIAGNOSES	NURSING INTERVENTIONS
Pain, related to imflammation	Maintain bed rest: limit activity. Elevate and support affected extremity. Institute drug therapy for analgesia. Apply warm, moist heat; be aware that edematous sites burn easily.

NURSING DIAGNOSES	NURSING INTERVENTIONS
Impaired physical mobility, related to pain and edema	Reposition frequently: prevent pneumonia and other complications. Early ambulation is an objective; ROM exercise of unaffected extremity lessens muscle strength loss. Diversional activity provides emotional support.
Altered tissue perfusion, related to circulatory deficit	Confine to bed in acute phase. Check circulation frequently. Administer anticoagulant therapy as ordered. Be aware of laboratory values for coagulation. Implement graded exercise program as ordered. Teach significance of interventions.

Patient teaching. Knowledge of the cause, risk management, and manifestation of these conditions allows the patient to commit to choices and decisions regarding his health status. Awareness of occurrence of increased venous pressure with certain activities may result in avoiding their incidence: prolonged sitting or standing, along with excess body weight, straining related to heavy lifting or constipation, and constrictive clothing are examples.

Although elastic stockings are useful for ambulatory patients and after acute stage, their value in deep vein thrombosis is questioned. Proper measurement, application, and use is to be emphasized by the nurse. Warm clothing is recommended to offset chilling, which may result in vasoconstriction. It is common to rub an area where pain originates, yet any massage of extremities is *ill advised* because of danger of embolization of clots. The nurse should emphasize this point. All teaching procedures should be approached with a calm, reassuring attitude.

Chronic venous insufficiency

Etiology/pathophysiology. This condition is also referred to as *postphlebitic syndrome* because of its correlation to deep vein thrombosis. Small vessels dilate as a result of occlusion of return channels. The valves become incompetent, and backflow occurs. Prolonged increase of venous pressure results in thinning of vessel walls, which are less elastic and distend easily. Pressure in veins, especially in the ankles when the legs are in dependent positions, results in this vein congestion.

Clinical manifestation/assessment. Stasis of flow results in edema, discoloration, and pain in the lower legs. Venous congestion may eventually result in dermatitis, ulceration, and finally, cellulitis. Rupture of small vessels is evident on examination.

Diagnostic tests. Diagnosis is made on the basis of the signs and symptoms.

Nursing interventions. Prevention of chronic venous insufficiency is the most positive approach. Remembering that deep vein thrombosis is the forerunner of venous insufficiency, nurses should plan interventions with this complication in mind. Once the signs and symptoms manifest, palliative and symptomatic treatment is instituted.

Reduction of venous stasis may prevent ulceration. This may be accomplished by elevation of the lower extremities above the heart as frequently as possible. Sitting or standing for long periods increases the signs and symptoms and is ill advised. Antiembolic hose compress the superficial veins but must be well fitted and unrestricting rather than acting as a tourniquet. The affected extremities should be protected from trauma and be kept clean and dry. Careful washing and drying are accomplished before application of skin protection lotion.

Patient teaching. Wearing properly applied antiembolic stockings is emphasized, as well as leg elevation every 2 hours if possible. Avoidance of prolonged sitting or standing and proper weight management are encouraged. The previously mentioned skin care is recommended.

Stasis ulcers

Etiology/pathophysiology. As a result of vascular insufficiency and chronic venous congestion, necrotic, craterlike lesions of the skin develop on the lower legs. The elderly are more commonly affected. Obstruction, venous stasis, and varicose veins are forerunners of stasis ulcer. Congested vessels result in circulatory embarrassment and nutritional deficit to tissues usually supplied by these veins. Impaired skin integrity occurs, predisposing to an infectious process. Sloughing of tissue occurs, leaving craters and necrosis in the affected areas.

Clinical manifestations/assessment. Pain and tenderness accompany erythema and pruritus of tissues and skin. Edema may precede impaired skin integrity. Healing occurs slowly, if at all, leading to infection potential.

Diagnostic tests. Phlebography is used to confirm a diagnosis.

Nursing interventions. Cleanliness of ulcers and the entire affected area is accomplished by saline compresses or Burow's solution application or soaks. Necrotic tissue is debrided, and compression bandages are applied. Protection from trauma and infection is important.

NURSING DIAGNOSES	NURSING INTERVENTIONS
Altered peripheral tissue perfusion, related to ischemia	Maintain bed rest and elevation of extremities to reduce circulatory need. Prevent edema, trauma, and infection to enhance adequate healing. Address underlying cause to restore the circulatory process.
Dysfunctional grieving, related to the slow healing process and apparent gravity of the condition	Give emotional support and sufficient information to deal with care and management approach. Encourage self-expression.

Varicose veins

Etiology/pathophysiology. Varicosities are abnormally dilated, incompetent veins that, by their configuration, prevent valve cusps from meeting, thus effecting reflux of venous blood. Varicosities occur in the esophagus and the anal canal, but the saphenous veins of the lower extremities are the most commonly affected areas. Congenital defective valves, venous disorders, and prolonged strain on the vessels cause elongated, asymmetrical dilation. Poor posture and prolonged standing strains vessels and valves by adding pressure and interfering with venous return to the body trunk.

Weakened vessel walls are stretched, causing pooling with distended vessels. Refer to Chapter 31 for further discussion of hemorrhoids and esophageal varices.

Clinical manifestations. Although mild presentations of this condition may be asymptomatic, tortuous, disfigured veins cause leg fatigue, muscle cramping (especially nocturnal), and activity restraint. Edema and ulceration can precipitate pain. Complications include infection and ulceration.

Assessment. Collection of *subjective data* includes exploring the patient's history of vascular insufficiency, familial tendency, and initial occurrence. Occupational and risk factors are considered.

Collection of *objective data* includes examination of extremities, which allows comparison, pulse palpation, and skin assessment. Complications are noted, as well as observations of outstanding signs.

Diagnostic tests. Doppler ultrasonography records the circulatory process. Venography assesses the extent of dilation. The Trendelenburg test allows observation of venous filling: the patient is placed supine with legs raised until complete venous emptying occurs; tourniquet application above the knee before the patient stands allows venous filling to be observed; normal filling occurs from below the tourniquet, whereas varicosities with valve incompetence fill from reflux of upper legs and trunk.

Medical management. Correction of the underlying cause of varicosities is the primary approach of the physician, yet palliative care prevents aggravation of the condition: weight control and site injury avoidance. Mild signs and symptoms are controlled with elastic stockings, rest periods with leg elevation, and occupational choice that does not contribute to or worsen the signs and symptoms.

Surgical intervention may be necessary with recurrence or progression of varicosities, or if stasis ulcers develop. Cosmetic considerations are made also.

Vein ligation and stripping is the surgical procedure involving ligation of greater and/or lesser saphenous systems to divert peripheral circulation to deep veins. The patency of deeper vessels is established before surgery. The physician marks with ink the area before surgery because guidelines are difficult to establish when the patient is supine and tourniquet is in place.

Medial ankle and inguinal incisions are made. A plastic or metal stripping guidewire is inserted, threaded upward, and pulled out (upward), stripping the large, tortuous varicosities. Elastic compression bandage is applied, to be worn for at least 1 week. Increased peripheral circulation is expected.

Sclerosis injection is performed where isolated varicosities are noted. An irritating chemical solution, Sotradecol (3% sodium tetradecyl sulfate), is injected into the vein, producing intimal irritation, phlebitis, and fibrosis. This is not a curative therapy, but a palliative one.

Laser beam therapy is also used with some success on varicose veins.

Nursing interventions/patient teaching. The nurse should teach the patient to avoid venous stasis—no prolonged sitting, standing, leg crossing, or girdle use. Postoperatively, the nurse observes for hemorrhage and provides usual care. Legs are elevated, and early ambulation is encouraged even though it may be painful. Guarding against trauma is advised. No dangling is allowed, to prevent stasis. The nurse will educate the patient to expect site numbness, which disappears gradually.

NURSING DIAGNOSES	NURSING INTERVENTIONS
Pain, related to venous engorgement and fatigue	Assess level of discomfort, and educate to relieve with activity and analgesia. Control activity intolerance with rest, support stockings, and leg elevation.
Altered peripheral tissue perfusion, related to circulatory inadequacy	Correct posture to correct stasis. Limit activity to tolerance level. Administer drugs as ordered for circulatory increase. Prevent trauma, edema, and infection.
Body image disturbance, related to disfigurement	Advise use of supportive stockings for cosmetic value. Educate about preventive measures in accord with personal risk level. Discuss acceptance of limitations. Encourage self-expression.

Lymphatic Disorders

Lymphangitis

Etiology/pathophysiology. Inflammation of one or more lymphatic vessels or channels usually results from an acute streptococcal or staphylococcal infection in an extremity.

Clinical manifestations. Lymphangitis is characterized by fine, red streaks from the affected area to the groin or axilla. The infection is usually not localized, and edema is diffuse. Chills, fever, and local pain accompany headache and myalgia. Septicemia may occur; lymph nodes enlarge.

Medical management. Administration of penicillin or other antimicrobial drugs controls the infection. Hot, moist heat—soaks or packs—brings comfort.

Nursing interventions. Aseptic technique promotes healing. Rest and extremity elevation may relieve the pressure.

Lymphedema

Etiology/pathophysiology. This accumulation of lymph in soft tissue is caused by obstruction, an increase in the amount of lymph, or removal of the lymph channels and nodes. The condition may be hereditary.

If the lymphatic drainage function is disturbed, an inflammatory process may ensue.

Clinical manifestations. Massive edema and tightness cause pressure and pain in the affected extremities. It progresses toward the trunk and is aggravated by (1) standing, (2) pressure, as with pregnancy or premenstruation, (3) obesity, and (4) warm, humid environment.

Assessment. Collection of *subjective data* includes the nurse noting the patient's complaints of pain and pressure. Medical history of varicosities, pregnancy, or modified radical mastectomy is important.

Collection of *objective data* includes observation of the extremities for edema and palpation of pedal pulses.

Diagnostic test. Lymphography is used to differentiate from venous disorders.

Medical management. Diuretics and antimicrobials are administered as ordered. Mechanical management includes use of compression pumps and elastic sleeves or stockings on the affected limb. Diet restrictions include limiting sodium and avoiding spicy foods, which would precipitate thirst.

Nursing interventions. The primary goal of care is to increase lymphatic drainage and avoid trauma. Elevation of the extremities while asleep and periodically during the day will facilitate draining the tissues. Massage toward the trunk followed by active exercise (i.e., walking) decreases the edema. Avoidance of constrictive clothing, shoes, or stockings (except elastic stockings) is advisable. Meticulous skin care must be maintained, and every effort must be made to prevent infections.

An important nursing intervention is the provision of emotional support for the patient. Body image disturbance related to the appearance of the lymphedematous extremity should be addressed. Emphasizing that lymphedema need not prevent the individual from engaging in routine activity may increase self-esteem.

NURSING DIAGNOSIS	NURSING INTERVENTIONS
Impaired skin integrity, related to impaired lymphatic drainage	Protect engorged tissues. Consider physical therapy or passive exercise. Examine skin for impaired skin integrity. Gently handle affected parts. Apply skin-protecting moisturizers or emollients. Teach application of supportive stockings or elastic sleeves.

Patient teaching. The patient should be made aware of the progression of the condition and of the cause. If the disorder is long-term and ongoing, coping with its effects must be approached. Rationale behind nursing interventions must be explained to enhance the ongoing medical regimen. If unsightly results are permanent, the patient must consider acceptance rather than isolation.

DISEASES AND DISORDERS OF THE HEMATOLOGICAL SYSTEM

The hematological system includes the blood and the organs of blood production—the bone marrow and lymphatic tissue. The blood is the only organ in the body that exists in a fluid state. As such, it is the liaison between body organs and systems, carrying oxygen and nutrients, antibodies, hormones, and other substances related to body functions. The blood also transports cellular wastes and protects the body from infection.

Disorders of blood production, bone marrow, or lymphatic tissues will affect virtually all body systems. Disturbances in this delicate balance can produce life-threatening symptoms or occurrences, severe pain, and incapacitation.

Collecting Data

The nursing data collection is from diverse sources: patient and family observation, physical examination, and diagnostic evaluation results (Table 32-10).

Subjective data collection is vague and nonspecific at the disease process onset: malaise, fatigue, and weakness. History of illness, easy bruising, bleeding tendencies with petechiae, and ecchymosis may be related. Integumentary changes include pruritus, nonhealing cuts and bruises, draining lesions, jaundice, and palpable subcutaneous nodules. Edema and tenderness in lymph node regions may be accompanied by pain, sometimes severe. Gastrointestinal complaints are noted, as well as cardiovascular and respiratory changes. Neurological complaints may include headache, numbness, tingling, paresthesia, and behavioral alteration.

Objective data collection uses a system-by-system approach to confirm patient complaints. Manipulation of joints can reveal stiffness and hematoma and may produce pain. Oral cavity examination can reveal lesions, ulcers, signs of bleeding, or gingivitis. Cardiovascular and respiratory assessments include breath and heart sound variations and pain or dyspneic positioning. Anxiety is noted, as well as observation of diminished comprehensive ability. Listening and an unhurried interview may reveal many symptoms not previously mentioned.

Other Diagnostic Tests

Lymphangiography. This is a radiological examination used to detect lymph node metastatic involvement. Con-

Table 32-10 Diagnostic Blood Studies

Blood Test	Normal Values	Description	Associated Disease or Disorder
CBC with differential			
RBC	Males 4.8-5.5 million/mm^3 Females 4.4-5.0 million/mm^3	Actual cell count	Increased in polycythemia; decreased in anemia, leukemia, and posthemorrhage
Hgb	Males 13.5-18.0 g/dl Females 12-16 g/dl		Increased in polycythemia; decreased in anemias and after hemorrhage
Hct	Males 40%-54% Females 38%-47%		Same as above
WBC with differential			
WBC	5000-10,000/mm^3	Actual cell count	Increased with infectious process, leukemia; decreased with aplastic anemia, agranulocytosis, chemotherapy, and certain viral diseases
Neutrophils	60%-70%		
Eosinophils	1%-4%		
Basophils	0.5%-1%		
Lymphocytes	20%-40%		
Monocytes	2%-6%		
Erythrocyte sedimentation rate	0-20 mm/hr	Rate at which RBCs settle out of a tube of unclotted blood	Increased in tissue destruction; indicates infection when results are compared with elevation in WBC count
Reticulocyte count	0.5% to 2%	Number of reticuloctyes in whole blood	Low in hemolytic disease; increased in bone marrow hyperactivity and hemorrhage
Platelet count	200,000-300,000/mm^3	Actual cell count	Increased in granulocytic leukemia; decreased in thrombocytopenia or aplastic anemia
Prothrombin time	11-16 seconds	Rapidity of blood clotting	Detects plasma clotting defects, coagulation screening, and monitors Coumadin therapy
Partial thromboplastin time	60-85 seconds	Fibrin clot formation	Detects coagulation defects of the intrinsic system; deficiency of plasma clotting
Bleeding time	2-6 minutes	Amount of time for a small stab wound to stop bleeding	Prolonged in hemorrhagic disease; coagulation factor defect
Clotting time	3-9 minutes	Amount of time for blood in a tube to clot	Prolonged with deficiency in coagulation factors, vit. K; used to monitor anticoagulant therapy

trast medium is injected into a lymphatic vessel of the foot or hand, followed by radiological visualization of the lymphatic system.

Bone marrow aspiration or biopsy. This procedure is specific for establishing a diagnosis and for treatment response. Examination is made of cells: types, numbers, and maturation. The procedure is possible because normal bone marrow is soft and semifluid and can therefore be removed by aspiration through a needle. Bone marrow aspiration is most commonly performed in persons with marked anemia, neutropenia (decreased number of WBCs), acute leukemia, and thrombocytopenia (decreased number of platelets).

Special Procedures

Bone marrow transplant. This procedure is indicated in certain conditions and diseases such as immunodeficient states, cancer, leukemia, and recurrent aplastic anemia. A matched donor and recipient are essential to avoid rejection or complications. Specimens from twins, siblings, or self (autologous) while in remission are preferred.

After emotional and physical preparation, blood studies are done to set baselines and to assess the patient's status. A pathogen-free environment is established, with the patient placed on reverse isolation with monitoring for fever or infection. Medication therapy used in the preparation may include immunosuppressants, antibiotics, and antianxiety agents.

Bone marrow transplants are used increasingly in hematological malignancies after large doses of chemotherapy or radiation therapy. The amount of chemotherapy or radiation that can ordinarily be administered is limited because of its toxicity to the bone marrow. By transplanting bone marrow after these therapeutic modes, much larger therapeutic doses can be administered.

Bone marrow is obtained by multiple marrow aspirations under general or spinal anesthesia, usually yielding 500 to 800 ml of marrow. The marrow is cyropreserved (frozen) until used and then, after large particles are filtered out, administered intravenously to the recipient. The infused marrow repopulates the marrow of the patient after several weeks. There is great risk of toxicity to the patient, including infections, marrow rejection, and graft-versus-host disease. Medications supporting graft acceptance include cyclosporine (immunosuppressant) and chemotherapy (to prevent graft-versus-host complication).

Splenectomy. The surgical excision of the spleen may be performed to treat blood dyscrasias with incidence of splenomegaly; to treat trauma to the spleen; or to remove a diseased spleen. Preoperative assessment includes cardiovascular observation, respiratory function determination, and gastrointestinal evaluation. Postoperatively, these observations are compared with the baseline evaluations, and the patient is observed for infection or inflammation. Complication potential includes infection, hemorrhage, shock, and paralytic ileus. Parenteral therapy and nasogastric suction are maintained and observed. Management of postoperative pain is addressed. Movement and positioning to prevent infection or pneumonia is maintained.

Anemia

A disorder characterized by RBC, hemoglobin, and hematocrit levels below normal range, anemias also exhibit increased RBC destruction (hemolytic). Anemia causes delivery of insufficient amounts of O_2 to tissues and cells. Erythrocytes are classified according to size, shape, and color. Hemoglobin content is expressed as normochromic or hypochromic anemia, whereas RBC size is usually expressed as macro-, micro-, or normocytic.

Etiology/pathophysiology. Anemia can be caused by many factors. Hemorrhage or blood loss accounts for temporary anemia, whereas nutritional deficit can attribute to long-term iron-deficiency anemia. Marrow failure is linked to a disease process, toxic exposure, tumor, and unknown cause. A decrease in RBC production or RBC destruction results in a lower number of circulating red blood cells. Bone marrow hematopoietic function manifests the inability to produce the needed quantity.

Loss of the O_2-carrying element in the blood results in supply-demand imbalance in vital organs. Peripheral circulation compensates by shunting blood to vital organs, thus causing hypoxic status to other body parts. Rapid hematopoietic effort causes blood cell irregularities (immature RBCs) and inability to produce RBCs, with resultant decrease of RBC count.

Clinical manifestations. Although each manifestation has its specific signs and symptoms, some are also typical of all anemias. These signs and symptoms arise from decreased O_2 carrying capacity. The following are typical:

Fatigue	Confusion	Dyspnea
Exertional dyspnea	Palpitation	Pallor (mucous membranes and skin)
Dyspnea	Tachycardia	Vertigo
Headache	Cardiac dilation	Anorexia
Insomnia	Systolic murmur	Dyspepsia

Assessment. Collection of *subjective data* commonly includes expressions of weakness, dyspnea, fatigue, and vertigo. Anorexia and dyspepsia may accompany headache and insomnia, but the patient does not link these complaints to the condition unless questioning leads to this conclusion.

Collection of *objective data* includes observing signs of bleeding or shock (hypovolemic). Laboratory values show low red blood cell count, hematocrit, and hemoglobin. Pallor of skin and mucous membranes is present, and cardiac symptoms are noted and related to anemia. If anemia is a long-term presentation, the patient may have ulcerations of the extremities.

Diagnostic tests. Blood studies will show red blood cell count, hemoglobin, and hematocrit levels to be below normal. Serum iron, total iron-binding capacity, and serum ferritin levels are below normal. Reticulocyte count is increased because of immaturity of RBCs. Bone marrow study will show a deviation from normal findings. Peripheral blood smears enable identifications of abnormalities of shape and color of cells. A Schilling test reveals malabsorption of vitamin B_{12}.

Medical management. Intervention depends on the cause. Correction of the disease process may correct or lessen the anemic condition. Transfusion is appropriate for blood loss as is replacement of iron and vitamin B_{12} if these are deficient. Treatment is often specific to the particular anemia.

NURSING DIAGNOSES	NURSING INTERVENTIONS
Altered tissue perfusion, related to cardiovascular function	Observe vital signs and peripheral pulses for circulatory change. Monitor fluid and electrolyte status. Monitor cardiac and pulmonary status. Check skin and mucous membranes for hematoma, hemorrhage, and ecchymosis. Assess skin integrity.
Impaired gas exchange, related to RBC, hemoglobin, and hematocrit deficit	Evaluate ADL ability related to O_2 decrease. Assess activity response, dyspnea, and heart rate. Observe for cyanosis, hypoxia, and hypercapnia. Maintain bed rest as necessary and provide ROM exercise. Administer oxygen per route and flow as ordered. Explain activity-oxygen deficit relationship.
Activity intolerance, related to O_2 deficit secondary to decreased hemoglobin and hematocrit	Plan care to provide optimum rest. Assist in identifying factors causing intolerance. Assess ability to perform ADLs, ambulation, and exercise. Assess potential for injury caused by mobility impairment. Teach performing at own rate of ability, to reduce energy expenditure.

Patient teaching. Considerations for education will be tailored to the individual conditions and needs.

Types of Anemia

Hypovolemic anemia

Etiology/pathophysiology. Red blood cell and other component deficiency caused by an abnormally low circulating blood volume from hemorrhage is classified as *secondary anemia*. Blood loss of 1000 ml or more in an adult can be severe. It is usually related to internal or external hemorrhage caused by a surgical procedure, gastrointestinal bleeding, menorrhagia, trauma, or severe burns.

The loss of blood decreases the amount of circulating fluid and hemoglobin, and decreases the amount of oxygen carried to the tissues of the body. The tissues must have oxygen to survive. The degree of rapidity with which the blood loss occurs are related to the severity and number of signs and symptoms. RBC and Hct counts drop to half their normal range, resulting in hypovolemic shock.

Clinical manifestations. The following signs and symptoms are associated with hypovolemic shock.

- Physical collapse with prostration
- Circulatory dysfunction with inadequate tissue perfusion
- Decreased blood pressure and weak, thready, and rapid pulse
- Thirst
- Rapid respirations
- Cold, clammy skin
- Pallor
- Mental confusion
- Decreased urinary output
- **Without treatment, death will occur**

Diagnostic tests. RBC, hemoglobin, and hematocrit levels are severely decreased, often to half the normal values.

Medical management. In the case of massive hemorrhage, measures are taken to control the bleeding, treat for shock, and replace the volume of circulating fluid with blood transfusion, plasma, dextran (volume expander), or other intravenous therapy. Oxygen therapy is ordered to restore decreased available oxygen caused by decreased hemoglobin in the blood.

Nursing interventions. The nurse will monitor blood and fluid restoration and identify blood loss sites to control the bleeding. Patients should be kept flat and warm. Vital signs should be taken at frequent intervals. Care should be taken to prevent injury to a restless or confused patient. Intake and output is measured, with careful monitoring of urine output for oliguria caused by decreased renal perfusion.

Patient teaching. If the cause of the hemorrhage is a chronic problem, the patient should be taught to monitor bleeding amounts, occasion, and associated factors and to report to the physician immediately for treatment.

Pernicious anemia

Etiology/pathophysiology. This type of anemia is the result of a metabolic defect: the absence of an intrinsic factor secreted by the gastric mucosa. It is a progressive megaloblastic, macrocytic anemia affecting mainly older adults. The intrinsic factor is essential for absorption of vitamin B_{12} (cyanocobalamin).

Because the intrinsic factor is not available to combine with vitamin B_{12}, transport of this necessary vitamin to the ileum is prevented. Deficiency of the vitamin affects growth and maturity of all body cells. There is deficiency in the maturation of RBCs in the marrow. The erythrocyte membrane becomes fragile and ruptures easily. This vitamin is related to nerve myelination and, if absent, progressive demyelination and degeneration of nerves and white matter occur.

Clinical manifestations. Extreme weakness is noted with dyspnea, fever, and hypoxia. As the condition progresses, weight loss is apparent, as is slight icterus (jaundice) with pallor. The skin may appear a pale lemon-yellow color because of the excessive destruction of the red blood cells, which causes the bile pigments to increase in the blood serum. Edema of the legs occurs, as do intermittent constipation and diarrhea.

Assessment. Collection of *subjective data* will include noting the patient's complaints of palpitations, nausea, flatulence, and indigestion. There is soreness and burning of the tongue. Weakness and difficulty swallowing (dysphagia) may occur. Neurological symptoms may develop, including tingling of the hands and feet and loss of sense of body position.

Collection of *objective data* includes observing that the patient's tongue appears smooth and erythematous, with infection about the teeth and gums. Cerebral signs include mental confusion, personality changes, and behavior problems. Severe neurological impairments can result, which may include partial or total paralysis that results from destruction of the nerve fibers of the spinal cord.

Diagnostic tests. The Schilling test shows malabsorption of vitamin B_{12}. Bone marrow aspiration reveals abnormal RBC development.

Medical management. Cyanocobalamin injections (vitamin B_{12}), folic acid supplement, and iron replacement are ordered. If the anemia is severe, the patient may be transfused with packed red blood cells. Injections of vitamin B_{12} must be continued during the patient's lifetime. Treatment is individualized, but one injection every 2 months may keep the patient free of signs and symptoms. This condition, if untreated, can be considered terminal. Symptomatic approach in nursing intervention is appropriate.

Nursing interventions. The nursing interventions of the patient will depend to some extent on the stage of the disease. When the patient is confined to the hospital, vital signs should be checked every 4 hours. Special mouth care should be performed several times daily. The diet should be high in protein, vitamins, and minerals.

Patients with pernicious anemia are especially sensitive to cold, and extra lightweight, warm blankets may be needed. The goals of interventions are to conserve energy and prevent injury.

Patient teaching. Knowledge in regard to the disease process and the importance of following lifetime therapy is essential if the patient is to comply to treatment. Activity adjustment when signs and symptoms are present may lessen the patient's stress. The need for assistance for ADLs and for frequent rest periods should be impressed on the patient and significant persons involved in the care.

Aplastic anemia

Etiology/pathophysiology. Aplastic anemia (**aplasia**) is a condition that develops without known cause, but it is thought to be congenital. It is an immunological injury resulting in a decrease of bone marrow function. Secondary aplastic anemia is directly related to exposure to viral invasion, medications, chemicals, radiation, or chemotherapy, where the hematopoietic tissue is replaced by fatty marrow, causing a defect in RBC production.

Depression of erythrocyte production results in lowered hemoglobin and RBCs. Leukopenia and thrombocytopenia may develop.

Clinical manifestations. Repeated infections with high fevers may occur, along with fatigue, weakness, and general malaise. Dyspnea and palpitations occur. Mortality is high from complications of infection and hemorrhage. Bleeding tendencies are reported: petechiae, ecchymoses, bleeding gums, and epistaxis occurs, as well as gastrointestinal and genitourinary system bleeding.

Diagnostic tests. Bone marrow study (aspiration biopsy) shows hypoplastic or aplastic fatty deposits, a decrease in cellular elements, and depressed hematopoietic activity. Peripheral blood smears show that blood cells may be normocytic and normochromic.

Medical management. The cause of aplastic anemia must be identified promptly and removed or discontinued. Bone marrow suppression is expected with certain antineoplastic medications or radiation therapy, and frequent monitoring of laboratory values should be done to maintain control.

Blood transfusions are avoided if possible, to prevent iron overloading and the development of antibodies to tissue antigens. Platelet transfusions that are HLA (human lymphocyte antigen) matched are used to treat serious bleeding in the thrombocytopenic patient. Cautious use of blood transfusion is necessary to minimize the risk of rejection for the bone marrow transplant candidate.

A splenectomy may be required in patients with hypersplenism when that is the cause of destruction of normal platelets. Steroids and androgens are sometimes used to stimulate the bone marrow. Antithymocyte globulin has recently become an important therapy for patients who are not candidates for bone marrow transplantations.

Bone marrow transplantation is the treatment of choice

in patients under the age of 50 who have a compatible donor.

Nursing interventions. Proper observation and care after bone marrow study are essential. The object of care is to produce remission and prolong survival. Patients with aplastic anemia are highly susceptible to infection, and thus nursing interventions should be toward prevention. Strict aseptic techniques must be adhered to for dressing changes and intravenous site care. Meticulous care to prevent impaired skin and mucous membrane integrity includes avoiding intramuscular injections and administration of rectal medications or rectal temperatures. Protective devices, such as an Eggcrate mattress, are indicated. In the presence of thrombocytopenia, the nurse should observe carefully for any signs of bleeding and prevent even the slightest trauma. The patient's urine and stool should be monitored for occult or gross blood.

Patient teaching. All persons with aplastic anemia need to know how to protect themselves from infection and excessive bleeding.

Iron-deficiency anemia

Etiology/pathophysiology. If the total body iron level is below normal range and need, the synthesis of hemoglobin is impaired. Conditions that cause iron-deficiency anemia are bleeding disorders, ulcers, GI tumors, gastritis, and menorrhagia. Nutritional deficit, especially during time of increased need (pregnancy, rapid growth), may be the cause. Malabsorption of iron is the usual cause of this type of anemia.

Clinical manifestations. Pallor, fatigue, and weakness may accompany headache and vertigo. Exertional dyspnea occurs as does tinnitus. Paresthesia, or a "pins and needles" feeling in extremities, is often described. Pica (craving for unusual substances—mud, salt, starch) may be discovered by careful questioning of the patient. Many persons regard this practice as unusual and therefore fail to admit it.

Diagnostic tests. Blood studies show decreased hemoglobin, hematocrit, and serum iron and elevated serum iron-binding capacity. Serum ferritin shows low iron stores.

Medical management. The treatment of iron-deficiency anemia is to determine and correct the cause. Oral iron supplement is usually given in the form of ferrous sulfate. Because it may be irritating to the gastrointestinal tract, ferrous sulfate should be taken after meals. When the patient cannot tolerate oral preparations of iron, parenteral iron therapy is used. The Z-tract method of giving Imferon IM is preferable, to prevent skin staining.

Nursing interventions. Because the treatment course is directed toward diagnosis and alleviating the cause, the patient interview is important. Medication therapy for iron replacement is initiated as ordered.

Patient teaching. Education about nutritional needs relative to the condition may prevent this anemia. Foods high in iron include organ meats, white beans, leafy vegetables, raisins, molasses, dried fruit, and egg yolk.

Explanation of the side effects of iron therapy is essential to alleviate distress and to extend the therapy for the necessary time. Reporting signs and symptoms to the physician requires knowledge of those that are significant. Diarrhea or nausea is significant, but black, tarry stools are not (expected with iron therapy).

Sickle cell anemia

Etiology/pathophysiology. Sickle cell anemia is the most common genetic disorder in the United States. Sickle cell anemia occurs predominantly in the African-American population. A sickle cell is an abnormal, crescent-shaped red blood cell containing hemoglobin S—a defective hemoglobin molecule. This anemia is a severe, chronic, incurable condition that occurs in persons **homozygous** (having two identical genes) for hemoglobin S (Hgb-S). Sickle cell crisis is an episode of acute "sickling" of erythrocytes, which causes occlusion and ischemia in distal blood vessels. Sickling indicates a clumping or aggregation of these misshapen RBCs, which lodge in small vessels. *Sickle cell trait* is the **heterozygous** (having two different genes) form of sickle cell anemia whereby the individual has both hemoglobin S and hemoglobin A in the red blood cells. Signs and symptoms do not occur with this trait. However, the genetic implication is notable. Tissue hypoxia and ischemia occur, causing pain and edema as a result of inflammation. Fragile RBC destruction thus inhibits the oxygen-carrying function.

Clinical manifestations. Usually the patient is asymptomatic for the first year of life. However, periods of crisis then occur, accelerating the signs and symptoms. There are definite physical and probable emotional factors (stress) that precipitate a painful episode. Physical factors include events that cause dehydration or change the oxygen tension in the body, such as infection, overexertion, weather changes (cold), ingestion of alcohol, and smoking.[28] Loss of appetite and irritability with weakness follow minor infections. Abdominal enlargement with pooling of blood in the liver, spleen, and other organs may accompany jaundice. Joint and back pain are noted, as is edema of extremities. Complications include multisystems failure, infarctions, hemorrhage, and retinal damage leading to blindness.

Diagnostic tests. Hemoglobin electrophoresis is specific for detecting sickle cell crisis or anemia. A stained blood smear detects anemia only. Hematocrit and hemoglobin levels are below normal values. WBCs are increased with infection.

Medical management. Persons with mild sickle hemoglobin syndromes do not require treatment. In persons with high concentrations of sickle hemoglobin and frequent painful crises, treatment is required. Therapy includes rest, hydration, oxygen, analgesics for pain, and treatment for infections. Transfusion therapy may be given; the blood products generally used are packed red cells.

Nursing interventions. Supportive treatment follows symptom presentation: hydration and analgesia during crises and dilution of blood with increased fluid intake to reverse sickling. Monitoring the transfusion therapy for evidence of transfusion reaction is vital. Attention to fever and infection is important. Genetic counseling is indicated.

NURSING DIAGNOSES	NURSING INTERVENTIONS
Pain, related to thrombotic crisis	Place patient in proper anatomical alignment, and protect joint. Position by slow, gentle handling. Apply warmth with soaks or compresses to relieve discomfort. Give analgesics as ordered.
Knowledge deficit, related to disease process, complications, activity, and nutrition	Teach prevention of exacerbation by: ■ avoiding infection, dehydration, and O_2 deficiency ■ avoiding exertion beyond limitation ■ maintaining optimum health status ■ eating a high-caloric, high-protein, well-balanced diet and maintaining maximum fluid intake Instruct to report to physician: ■ joint or abdominal pain ■ fever or infection, hemorrhage, and hematuria Explain medication goals and importance of ongoing care. Identify disease process.

Polycythemia vera

Etiology/pathophysiology. This is a myeloproliferative (excessive bone marrow production) disorder with hyperplasia of bone marrow, which manifests with an increase in circulating erythrocytes, granulocytes, and platelets. It is a stem cell abnormality of unknown cause. Secondary to pulmonary and heart disease, polycythemia vera is also thought to be associated with prolonged high-altitude exposure. Bone marrow output of RBCs increases in response to hypoxic tissue conditions, causing viscosity of the blood, which impedes flow.

This multiorgan system disease is affected by hyperplasic bone marrow elements. Because of the increased erythrocyte mass, hypervolemic and hyperviscous (sticky) occurrence is 2 to 3 times normal. The sluggish circulatory process predisposes to infarctions of vital organs.

Clinical manifestations. This disorder is of gradual onset and has a progressive course of some length. It mainly affects men in middle age. As a result of venous distention and platelet dysfunction, the complications of esophageal varices, epistaxia, GI bleeding, and petechiae are seen.

Assessment. Collection of *subjective data* includes noting patient complaints of sensitivity to hot and cold and pruritus. Headaches, vertigo, tinnitus, and blurred vision are often present.

Collection of *objective data* includes noting eczema and dermatological changes. The skin may develop a reddened appearance. Elevated blood pressure accompanies left ventricular hypertrophy and angina.

Diagnostic tests. Arterial blood gases show O_2 concentration lower than normal. Plasma and red cell volume are increased. Hemoglobin, hematocrit, reticulocytes, and erythrocytes are increased. The basal metabolic rate (BMR) is increased without thyroid function alteration.

Medical management. Repeated phlebotomy decreases blood viscosity: removal of 500 to 2000 ml of blood until hematocrit maintains at 45%; the repeat of this procedure if hematocrit rises above 50%. If radiation or chemotherapy follows, patient stability is maintained.

NURSING DIAGNOSES	NURSING INTERVENTIONS
Altered cardiopulmonary, cerebral, gastrointestinal, and/or peripheral tissue perfusion, related to hyperviscosity of fluid and potential bleeding	Maintain position of comfort. When on bed rest, do not raise knee gatch. Provide active or passive ROM exercises q 2 to 4 hr. Check peripheral pulses and color and temperature of extremities q 4 to 6 hr. Report early signs or symptoms of thrombosis or bleeding to physician. If bleeding tendency, avoid invasive procedures when possible. Avoid trauma; provide soft-bristled toothbrush.
Activity intolerance, related to ischemia	Encourage adequate exercise and mobility to prevent stasis. Explain disease course and symptoms expected.

Nursing interventions/patient teaching. The nurse should alleviate knowledge deficit of this condition if it exists. The nurse should emphasize the importance of medical and nutritional regimen compliance. Diet teaching includes emphasis on avoiding foods that contain iron, while increasing calories and protein (because of BMR increase).

Signs and symptoms that need medical supervision include those of thrombosis (pain, edema, or erythema), and this must be stressed to the patient. Because this is a chronic illness, emotional support is imperative.

Agranulocytosis

Etiology/pathophysiology. This potentially fatal condition of the blood is characterized by a severe reduction in the number of granulocytes (basophils, eosinophils, and neutrophils). The white blood count is extremely low (leukopenia) as is a differential neutrophil count—less than 200/mm^3 (neutropenia).

Adverse medication reaction or toxicity is the primary cause of agranulocytosis. However, neoplastic disease and radiation therapy are often cited as causative. Viral and bacterial infections are possible causes of the condition. Heredity is also considered.

A suppression of the bone marrow by the causative agent reduces the number and production of white blood cells. Leukocytes, formed in the bone marrow, provide body protection against microorganisms. This protection is ineffective when bone marrow suppression has occurred.

Clinical manifestations. Fever, chills, headache, and fatigue are symptoms associated with infection and inflammatory process. Ulcerations of mucous membranes—mouth, nose, pharynx, vagina, and rectum—are found. Bronchial pneumonia and urinary tract infections are complications that occur in later stages.

Assessment. Collection of *subjective data* includes noting the common complaints of fever, extreme fatigue, and prostration. All medications taken, whether prescription or over-the-counter, are considered as possible causes of the condition.

Collection of *objective data* includes observing fever over 100.6° F. Erythema and pain from ulcerations may occur. Ulcerations are cultured for microorganisms. Lung and bronchial auscultation reveals rales and rhonchi because of trapped exudates.

AGRANULOCYTOSIS: CAUSATIVE CHEMICAL AGENTS

Antihistamines	Antibiotics (chloramphenicol)
Analgesics (Butazolidin)	Sulfonamides and derivatives
Antithyroid drugs	Phenothiazides (Thorazine, Prolixin, Sparine, Compazine)
	Diuretics

Diagnostic tests. Leukocytes and neutrophils will be below normal. A bone marrow study will show depression of activity.

Medical management. The main objective of treatment is to alleviate the responsible factors of bone marrow depression and to prevent or treat infection. Blood cultures may be done when fever is elevated, and cultures may be ordered if ulceration occurs. Transfusions are often ordered. Protective isolation may be instituted.

Nursing interventions. A patient with a compromised WBC system is highly susceptible to life-threatening infections. Nursing interventions are directed toward protecting the patient from potential sources of infection, and conscientious monitoring to detect the earliest signs of infection is necessary so that prompt therapy may be started. Meticulous washing of the hands by medical and nursing personnel and strict asepsis are mandatory.

Patient teaching. Patient and family members need frequent reminders to keep the environment meticulously clean and dustless. No person with any type of infection should come in contact with the patient. The patient should be taught to recognize the signs and symptoms of an infection and to notify the physician immediately if these occur.

NURSING DIAGNOSES	NURSING INTERVENTIONS
Potential for infection, related to depressed WBC (leukocytes) production	Maintain environment that is scrupulously clean. Be certain no person with any type of infection is allowed in contact with the patient. Observe for signs and symptoms of infection, such as elevated temperature and chills. Health care provider must wash hands meticulously and use strict asepsis for procedures.
Pain, related to ulceration or inflammatory process	Relieve pain through analgesia, ice collar, or warm saline gargles. Maintain bed rest for malaise and prostration. Support body parts in proper alignment.
Knowledge deficit, related to disease rarity	Teach causative agents. Inform of methods to reduce infection potential. Address diet for healing and comfort: high-vitamin (especially C), high-caloric, and soft or liquid diet as tolerated.

Bleeding Disorders

Etiology/pathophysiology. Release of blood from the vascular system results from trauma or vessel damage, vessel inadequacy, disturbance of function of platelets or clotting factors, or as a result of liver disease (impairment of clotting mechanisms).

The clotting mechanism is a hemostatic chain reaction. Vasoconstriction inhibits capillary leakage; hematoma compression provides pressure. Body reaction occurs: arterial blood pressure lowers. Any manifestation that alters this process predisposes to hemorrhage. The affected mechanism may be vascular, platelet dysfunction, or plasma coagulation factor alteration. The disorder may be congenital or acquired, possibly secondary to other disease or to medication toxicity.

Clinical manifestations. Skin and mucous membrane manifestations include petechiae and ecchymoses. Epistaxis and gingival bleeding are common. Circulatory hypovolemia is noted through hypotension, pallor, cool, clammy skin, and tachycardia. GI tract bleeding is common, with abdominal flank pain caused by internal bleeding. The central nervous system involvement includes altered response and malaise, to loss of consciousness or affected speech.

Assessment. Collection of *subjective data* includes noting a history of bleeding after surgical or dental procedures. The exposure to toxic or hazardous agents or to radiation may be revealed. Complaint of headache, extremity pain, easy bruising, oronasal bleeding, and numbness is noted. Medications taken may lead to suspicion of toxicity (aspirin).

Collection of *objective data* involves observation of pain upon pressure of abdomen, revealing liver and spleen tenderness, and perhaps enlargement. Examination of emesis and stool may show signs of bleeding. Joint examination exhibits motion pain.

Diagnostic tests. The platelet count will be low. The RBC count will be low with decreased hemoglobin. Coagulation time is altered. Bone marrow studies show abnormal cells.

Medical management. The underlying cause is assessed and corrected, and replacement transfusions may be ordered. Heparin therapy or medication toxicity is considered as a possible cause. Infections and complications are treated or prevented.

Nursing interventions. Many times medical intervention depends on accurate reporting and nursing observations. In bleeding disorders the nurse should monitor vital signs to note any signs of hypovolemic shock. Gentle movement of the patient is necessary to prevent trauma to the tissues. The nurse will monitor intravenous infusions and transfusions as ordered.

Specific Conditions

Vascular purpura. This blood disorder is characterized by hemorrhage into the tissues, particularly the skin and mucous membranes, producing ecchymoses and petechiae. Primarily caused by defective small vessels, spontaneous **extravasation** (seepage or escape of blood into tissues) occurs. This blood leakage into tissues is also related to such disease entities as diabetes mellitus or adrenocorticoid overproduction, vitamin C deficiency, and medication reaction. The effect ranges from minor to localized to a widespread hemorrhagic condition.

Platelet Disorders

Thrombocytopenia

Etiology/pathophysiology. A deficiency of the number of circulating platelets or change in the function of platelets alters the process of coagulation. Thrombocytopenia is an abnormal hematological condition in which the number of platelets is reduced. Decreased production occurs in aplastic anemia, leukemia, and tumors. Decreased survival occurs in the presence of antibody destruction, infection, or viral invasion. Increased platelet destruction is caused by disseminated intravascular coagulation. Splenomegaly results from entrapment of blood in the spleen.

The most common cause of increased destruction of platelets is thrombocytopenia purpura, which may be drug-induced or idiopathic (cause unknown, referred to as idiopathic thrombocytopenic purpura [ITP]). If the cause is medication-induced (Box 32-12), platelet counts usually return to normal 1 to 2 weeks after the medication is withdrawn. ITP occurs most commonly in the second and third decades of life and is caused by production of an autoantibody (IgG) directed against a platelet antigen.

Bleeding occurs from numerous small capillaries. This is the most common cause of bleeding disorders. It is related to bone marrow defect associated with neoplastic disease or immune response to drugs.

BOX 32-12 MEDICATIONS WITH THROMBOCYTOPENIC EFFECTS

Alcohol
Nonsteroidal antiinflammatory agents (azathioprine, D-penicillamine, phenylbutazone)
Oral hypoglycemics
Quinidine
Salicylates
Sulfonamides
Thiazides

Clinical manifestations. The major signs of thrombocytopenia observable by physical examination are petechiae and ecchymoses on the skin. Petechiae occur only in platelet disorders.

Assessment. Collection of *subjective data* includes questioning the patient about recent viral infections (they may produce a transient thrombocytopenia), medications in current use, and extent of alcohol ingestion.

Collection of *objective data* includes observing the patient for petechiae and ecchymoses throughout the skin. Epistaxis may be noted, as well as gingival bleeding.

Diagnostic tests. The tests include complete laboratory studies to ascertain the characteristics of all blood cells, which include platelet count, peripheral blood smear, and bleeding time. In addition, a bone marrow examination is performed to determine the presence of immature platelets. Examination also reveals presence or absence of primary bone marrow abnormalities, such as neoplastic invasion or aplastic anemia.

Medical management. The primary treatments are corticosteroid therapy and splenectomy. Other treatments may include gamma globulin or immunosuppressive drugs. Transfusions with platelet concentrates may be used in persons with thrombocytopenic bleeding.

Nursing interventions for bleeding disorders. The nurse will support the medical treatment regimen: specific intervention for specific disease cause. If medication toxicity is the cause, the medication is discontinued. Infections are prevented by meticulous asepsis and gentle handling of the patient. Plasma and platelet infusion and whole blood transfusions are monitored closely for reaction and effects on patients' conditions.

NURSING DIAGNOSES	NURSING INTERVENTIONS
Altered tissue perfusion, related to bleeding	Monitor vital signs and neurological status. Assess for bleeding and fluid imbalance. Check urine, stool, and emesis for blood.

NURSING DIAGNOSES	NURSING INTERVENTIONS
Altered tissue perfusion, related to bleeding—cont'd	Monitor invasive diagnostic procedure sites for bleeding. Maintain comfort measures and bed rest. Avoid trauma and infection. Observe patient receiving parenteral fluids and blood components carefully for untoward signs. Monitor potential sites of hemorrhage.
Pain, related to hemorrhage	Assess discomfort and pain level. Assess patient's ability to cope and his response to pain. Administer analgesia as ordered, and note patient response. Provide education.

Patient teaching. An understanding of the disease process and causative agents is necessary in forming a knowledge base for self-care and prevention of trauma or infection. Instructions of signs and symptoms, as well as preventive measures, must be approached: avoiding trauma and constipation and checking for presence of blood. The nurse should stress the importance of notifying the physician of signs and symptoms of bleeding.

Clotting Factor Defects

Hemophilia

Etiology/pathophysiology. This hereditary coagulation disorder is characterized by a disturbance of the clotting factors.

Hemophilia A, the more common type, lacks antihemophiliac factor VIII, which is needed to convert prothrombin to thrombin through thromboplastin component.

Hemophilia B (Christmas disease) exhibits a deficiency of factor IX with absence of plasma thromboplastin component (a plasma protein), resulting in nonformation of thromboplastin.

This is an X-linked hereditary trait that affects mainly males, but is manifested in females primarily as carriers. A decrease in the formation of prothrombin activators occurs as a result of the decrease in clotting factors.

The patient is at high risk for AIDS because of the need for cryoprecipitate concentrates and contamination with HIV virus. A small number of persons with hemophilia A have developed AIDS from transfusions of factor VIII concentrate. This problem should be eliminated in the future with the testing of all blood donors for evidence of HIV virus and, more recently, heat treatment of factor VIII concentrates that kills the AIDS virus.

Clinical manifestations. Internal or external hemorrhage occurs with large ecchymoses into tissue—especially muscles, which may show deformity, and joints, which become ankylosed. Small cuts can prove fatal; blood loss from simple dental procedures may be significant. Pain from the hemorrhage damage is significant.

Assessment. Collection of *subjective data* includes noting reports by patient and family of incidents of ecchymoses and hemorrhage from even the slightest trauma. Pain is associated with joint motion.

Collection of *objective data* includes noting the presence of blood in subcutaneous tissues, urine, or stool and noting edematous or immobile joints.

Diagnostic tests. Factors VIII and IX are absent or deficient. The prothrombin time may be prolonged, but often is normal. The partial thromboplastin time is prolonged. Laboratory personnel must be notified of the patients' disorder to alleviate further incident of trauma as a result of diagnostic procedures, e.g., venipuncture.

Medical management. Minimizing bleeding and relieving pain are the main directions of care. Transfusions and administration of factor VIII or IX concentrate may be prophylactic or used to stop the hemorrhage.

Nursing interventions. The nurse will control hemorrhages in emergency situations by pressure and cold application to the site. Support and reassurance are imperative. Education of the patient and entire family is significant because many persons may be involved in the patient care. The nurse will monitor transfusions of factor VIII concentrate.

NURSING DIAGNOSES	NURSING INTERVENTIONS
Altered tissue perfusion, related to blood loss from coagulation deficit	Assess for extent of hemorrhage. Prevent further hemorrhage or extension. Monitor vital signs and laboratory reports. Apply cold compresses to bleeding areas. Assess for anxiety, shock, confusion and decreased urinary output. Teach safety precautions to prevent trauma.
Pain, related to hemorrhage into tissues	Administer analgesia as ordered. Move patient gently and slowly, supporting joints. Prevent deformity through support, splints, and physical therapy. Administer warm soaks (avoid hot to alleviate extension of hematoma) as ordered.
Ineffective individual coping, related to long-term illness	Discuss disease process, altered life-style, and acceptance. Suggest genetic counseling. Encourage independence. Encourage compliance with medical regimen. Assess parental knowledge or guilt. Be an active listener.

Patient teaching. Avoiding injury and controlling bleeding are significant points. Physical activity within limits and avoiding trauma should be discussed by the nurse. Wearing of medical alert identification is encouraged. Supervision of young patients, as well as informing playmates, teachers and others, is important. Emergency care teaching includes immobilization of affected part, ice application, and consultation of physician. Diet to prevent obesity, which puts excess pressure on joints, is discussed. Regular dental care and preventive dental and medical measures are important aspects for the nurse to cover. Overprotection can sometimes be a factor to discuss. No aspirin or any other medication should be taken except with the physician's knowledge.

von Willebrand's disease

Etiology/pathophysiology. This inherited bleeding disorder is characterized by abnormally slow coagulation of blood and spontaneous episodes of GI bleeding, epistaxis, and gingival bleeding caused by a mild deficiency of factor VIII. It is common in postpartum periods, as menorrhagia, and after surgery or trauma. Although similar to hemophilia, it is not limited to occurring only in males.

Treatment includes administration of cryoprecipitate containing factor VIII, fibrinogen, or fresh plasma. Observation and nursing intervention for hemophilia can easily be adapted to this disorder.

Disseminated intravascular coagulation (DIC)

Etiology/pathophysiology. DIC is an acquired, hemorrhagic syndrome predisposed by septicemia, obstetrical complication, malignancies, tissue trauma, transfusion reaction, burns, or shock.

Plasma clotting factors are depleted during widespread clotting within small vessels. This in turn leads to a bleeding disorder and thrombosis.

Clinical manifestations. Bleeding is noted in mucous membranes, venipuncture or surgical sites, in GI and urinary tracts, and generally from all orifices, and ranges from occult to profuse. Dyspnea, hemoptysis, and diaphoresis with cold, mottled digits are observed.

Assessment. Collection of *subjective data* includes noting patient complaints of bone and joint pain. Visual changes occur.

Collection of *objective data* includes the nurse observing for occult or obvious bleeding. Skin and mucosa color and petechiae are noted. Abdominal tenderness may be shown.

Diagnostic studies. The coagulation profile shows prolonged clotting. The platelet count shows thrombocytopenia. Other tests show hypofibrinogenemia and factors V and VIII deficit.

Medical management. In keeping with medical therapeutic approach, the underlying cause is addressed and corrected and transfusion replacement and cryoprecipitate are ordered.

Nursing interventions. Protection from bleeding and trauma and pressure to sites of hemorrhage are essential nursing measures. Support and reassurance may aid in relieving high stress levels. Careful monitoring of vital signs and administration of transfusions and cryoprecipitate are necessary. (For patient teaching, see discussion on hemophilia on pp. 761-762.)

Neoplastic Disorders

Leukemia

Etiology/pathophysiology. Leukemia is a malignant disorder of the hematopoietic system, in which an excess of leukocytes accumulates in the bone marrow and lymph nodes. The cause, while unknown, is attributed to genetic origin, a virus, or exposure to radiation or chemotherapeutic agents that are toxic to bone marrow.

Bone marrow is replaced by rapidly developing white cells with abnormal numbers and forms of immature cells found in circulation and infiltrated into the lymph nodes, spleen, and liver. Organ enlargement occurs. Hematopoietic function is disturbed by incompetent bone marrow. Increased susceptibility to infection results.

Classification. Leukemia is classified according to the type of proliferating cells, the clinical course that occurs, and the duration of the disease. Examples include lymphocytic, granulocytic, or monocytic, and they are classified as to acute or chronic form.

Clinical manifestations. Signs and symptoms correlate with other disorders or conditions: anemia (pallor, fatigue, malaise, decreased activity tolerance), thrombocytopenia (petechiae, epistaxis, easy bruising, occult blood in stool or urine), and leukopenia (fever, upper respiratory and urinary infections). Enlarged lymph nodes may be the first sign of the disease in some persons.

Diagnostic tests. The white blood count is low, elevated, or excessively elevated. Bone marrow biopsy shows immature leukocytes. Chest x-ray examination shows mediastinal node and lung involvement and bone changes. Lymph node biopsy reveals excessive blasts (immature cells).

Assessment. Collection of *subjective data* includes noting patient complaints regarding symptoms that may seem unrelated at first. Pain in bones or joints as well as abnormalities of skin (petechiae, ecchymoses) and mucous membranes (bleeding) are often noticed. Fatigue, malaise, and irritability are usually present.

Collection of *objective data* includes noting those signs listed in clinical manifestations. Infections are common. Occult blood is shown in laboratory specimens of urine and stool.

Medical management. The object of treatment is to achieve remission or to control the symptoms. Chemotherapeutic agents, antibiotic therapy, and blood transfusion replacement are instituted by the physician (Box 32-13). Drug toxicity observation is noted.

Perhaps more dramatically than in any other malignant disorder, chemotherapy has improved the prognosis of children with acute lymphocytic leukemia (ALL). Untreated patients have a median survival time of 4 to 6 months. With current therapy of vincristine and prednisone, or mercaptopurine (6-MP), the medial survival rate is about 5 years, and approximately 50% of children with ALL can now be cured.

BOX 32-13 CHEMOTHERAPEUTIC AGENTS COMMONLY USED IN LEUKEMIA THERAPY

L-Asparaginase
Chlorambucil
Cyclophosphamide
Cytarabine
Daunorubicin
Doxorubicin
6-Mercaptopurine
Methotrexate
Prednisone
6-Thioguanine
Vincristine

Tremendous progress in the treatment of leukemia has been made during the past decade. This has come about with the use of a complex combination of medications and radiation therapy. Bone marrow transplantation may be selected as the treatment of choice in patients with suitable donors if the initial remission of the acute leukemia has been induced. Before the transplant the patient's bone marrow cells and leukemic cells must be killed by massive chemotherapy and total body irradiation. The patient may succumb to infection, hemorrhage, or graft-versus-host disease.

In chronic leukemia, which occurs almost entirely in adults and develops slowly, the desired objectives of treatment depend on the kind of cells that are involved. Medications commonly used include chlorambucil (Leukeran), hydroxyurea, corticosteroids, and cyclophosphamide (Cytoxan). Irradiation of lymph nodes is often used, and blood transfusion may be given if anemia is severe. Although medications are not curative in chronic leukemia, they help to prolong life. The median survival rate for chronic leukemia is 3½ to 5 years.

Nursing interventions. Prevention of infection by reverse isolation and teaching the avoidance of infectious agents is of utmost importance. Leukopenia can be fatal. The usual inflammatory process to control infection is decreased. Therefore frequent observation for signs and symptoms of infection is necessary. Thrombocytopenia-induced hemorrhage may be life threatening. Therefore prevention of this condition through safe, gentle care is a primary consideration. Pain may be controlled through analgesia as ordered and by comfort measures. Coping mechanisms may be strained because of pain, change of body image, or fear of death, and therefore support of patient and family is promoted through a positive nurse-patient-family relationship and referral to community support groups.

NURSING DIAGNOSES	NURSING INTERVENTIONS
Potential for infection related to disease process	Isolate from infectious agents. Teach self-protection. Provide support for emotional trauma related to isolation. Allow interaction in planning ADLs. Ensure rest, skin protection, and proper nutrition. Administer antibiotic therapy as ordered; maintain blood levels with therapeutic timed administration. Observe for infectious process.
Altered tissue perfusion, related to bleeding tendency	Assess for hemorrhage. Reduce trauma potential: gentle, safe care; nonrestrictive bedding or clothing. Avoid invasive procedures. Provide safe environment. Monitor parenteral fluids and transfusions carefully.
Pain, related to tissue infiltration	Administer analgesia when appropriate. Maintain stress-free environment: assess family impact and plan care and rest wisely. Provide diversional activities. Provide comfort and support in positioning.
Ineffective individual and family coping, related to diagnosis and disease process	Assess coping capabilities of patient and significant others. Discuss disease process and expectations. Alleviate knowledge deficit. Encourage questions and self-expression: listen actively, demonstrate compassion, reassure with touch and personal contact. Assess fear of threat of death: allow time for personal expression, and provide one-on-one discussion opportunity.

Patient teaching. Procedures, meaning of treatments, and care plan should be discussed by the nurse and the patient. The nature of the disease and previous information the patient has received should be discussed. Community resources for support and information are invaluable for education of the patient and family. Expectations of physical abilities, remission, and future plans should be examined. Continuation of medical regimen is encouraged, as is avoidance of situations where infection can be transmitted. Medication and diet information is important.

Malignant lymphoma

Etiology/pathophysiology. This tumor is a neoplastic disorder of lymphoid tissue. Cause is unknown, but a viral source is suspect. It is more common in males, Caucasians, and those of Jewish ancestry. This grouping includes non-Hodgkin's lymphomas and lymphosarcoma.

Tumors usually start in lymph nodes and spread to lymphoid tissue in the spleen, liver, GI tract, and bone marrow. Involvement of lymphoid tissue also results in malabsorption and bone lesions.

Clinical manifestations. Painless, enlarged lymph nodes are in the cervical area and fever, weight loss, anemia, pruritus, and susceptibility to infection develop. Pressure symptoms in the involved areas are noted. Pleural effusion, bone fractures, and paralysis are complications.

Assessment. Collection of *subjective data* includes observations of fatigue, malaise, and anorexia as frequent patient complaints. Fever and diaphoresis are noted also.

Collection of *objective data* includes examination of the abdomen, which suggests splenomegaly. Enlarged lymph nodes are also evident.

Diagnostic tests. A bone scan reveals fractures, lesions, and tumor infiltration. Blood studies show hypercalcemia. A Coombs' test is positive for antiglobulin. Biopsies of lymph nodes, liver, and bone marrow are done for specific evidence of a pathological condition.

Medical management. Once the diagnosis is made, the extent of the disease (staging) will be determined. Accurate staging is crucial to determine the treatment regimen. The therapeutic regimen for non-Hodgkin's lymphomas includes chemotherapy and radiation. Some chemotherapy agents used are cyclophosphamide (Cytoxan), vincristine (Oncovin), prednisone, doxorubicin (Adriamycin), bleomycin, and methotrexate. In general, radiotherapy is the initial treatment when the disease has a localized presentation. Chemotherapy is the mainstay of treatment of non-Hodgkin's lymphomas that are not localized.

Nursing interventions. Supportive care of the patient during radiation and chemotherapy is primary in nursing management. Observation for complications follows. Further intervention is similar to that for Hodgkin's disease.

Patient teaching. Explanations of the extensive workup in diagnosis and its importance for staging the disease for determining the treatment plan are an important focus of patient teaching in the diagnostic period.

Hodgkin's disease

Etiology/pathophysiology. Hodgkin's disease is a malignant disorder characterized by painless, progressive enlargement of lymphoid tissue. It affects males twice as frequently as females and the age incidence is from 15 to 35 years. Beginning as an inflammatory or infectious process, it develops into a neoplasm. Exact cause is unknown. Hodgkin's disease is thought to be an immune disorder (T cell disease).

Lymphoid tissue enlargement is first noticed in the cervical nodes and spleen and is characterized by abnormal or atypical cells. Sternberg-Reed cells (atypical histiocytes) increase in number, replacing normal cells.

Clinical manifestations. Anorexia, weight loss, and extreme pruritus are outstanding complaints associated with this condition. Low-grade fever and night sweats occur. Anemia and leukocytosis follow with development of complications of respiratory infections.

BOX 32-14 ANN ARBOR CLINICAL STAGING: CLASSIFICATION OF HODGKIN'S DISEASE

Stage I	Abnormal single lymph nodes Regional or single extralymphatic organ or site
Stage II	Two or more abnormal lymph nodes on the same side of the diaphragm Localized involvement of extralymphatic organs or sites
Stage III	Abnormal lymph node regions on both sides of diaphragm May be accompanied by spleen involvement May be accompanied by localized involvement of extralymphatic organs or sites
Stage IV	Diffuse and disseminated involvement of one or more extralymphatic tissues and/or organs—with or without lymph node involvement

Assessment. Collection of *subjective data* includes noting the common complaints of malaise and appetite loss. Pruritus is severe. Bone pain occurs later.

Collection of *objective data* includes palpating enlarged lymph nodes—cervical and supraclavicular. Splenomegaly, hepatomegaly, and abdominal tenderness are found. Excoriation of skin and evidence of scratching from pruritus are noted. Edema of the face and neck may be noticed. Weight and nutritional status is recorded.

Diagnostic tests. Treatment depends on diagnosis of the stage or extent of involvement. Blood studies show anemia (normocytic, normochromic), WBC increase, and an abnormal erythrocyte sedimentation rate. Chest x-ray examination shows a mediastinal mass. Lymphangiograms can detect retroperitoneal node involvement. Lymph node biopsy that includes laparoscopy for retroperitoneal nodes is done. CT scan and ultrasound can indicate an enlarged spleen or liver. The presence of Sternberg-Reed cells remains a hallmark for the presence of Hodgkin's disease.

Medical management. Treatment depends on the staging process (Box 32-14). The stage of the disease at the time of diagnosis affects the prognosis and the cure rate. For instance, 90% of Stage I patients may experience remission and cure; the percentage drops to 80% with Stage II. Lymphoid radiotherapy is effective with early stage Hodgkin's disease. For more advanced stages, chemotherapy is useful.

Combination chemotherapy is the treatment of choice for Stages IIIB and IV. Therapy of Stage IIIA is controversial and involves chemotherapy, radiation, or a combination of these therapies. The most commonly used combination is the MOPP regimen, which consists of mechlorethamine (nitrogen mustard), vincristine (Oncovin), procarbazine, and prednisone. Complete remissions are achieved in approximately 80% of these patients; long-term, disease-free remission and probable cure occur in 50% of this group. Long-term remission is often achieved with these two therapies.

Nursing interventions. The nurse will plan care according to the staging process level. Awareness of side effects of radiotherapy or chemotherapy is important in preparing the patient to deal effectively with the conditions. Comfort measures with focus on skin integrity are carried out. Soothing baths with antipruritic medication (as ordered) can be effective. Fever and perspiration may be controlled with medication and attention to increased fluid intake plus necessary linen changes to prevent further skin problems. Extensive tests must be explained to the patient because there is a tendency toward impatience and anxiety.

NURSING DIAGNOSES	NURSING INTERVENTIONS
Impaired skin integrity, related to pruritus and jaundice	Assess condition of skin and level of discomfort. Administer skin care by baths, medication, and keeping patient clean and dry. Monitor vital signs for fever; assess for perspiration and change linen, keeping it wrinkle free.
Pain, related to pruritus	Assess level and intensity of pain and ability of patient to cope. Administer medication for specific condition involved in discomfort. Use active and passive exercise, positioning for comfort. Teach relaxation techniques and diversional activity. Allow verbalization; be an active listener.
Potential for infection, related to immune system ineffectiveness	Protect the environment and teach the importance of possible reverse isolation. Use meticulous handwashing. Avoid contamination by infectious visitors. Maintain hygiene and cleanliness of area. Monitor vital signs, intake and output, respiratory status, and skin integrity.
Anxiety and fear, related to unknown outcome	Instruct patient on symptoms, disease progression, and treatment regimen. Encourage open communication and venting feelings. Encourage questions and problem solving.

Patient teaching. Understanding the disease is important to enable personal interaction in regard to self-care and retaining independence. The impact on the patient's life, as well as the effect on significant others, is a prime consideration of patient attitude and adjustment. Realistic approaches to the illness and therapies are imperative. Guidance toward counseling for stress management can be helpful. Special nutritional consideration for excess weight loss or undernourished condition is made.

REFERENCES AND SUGGESTED READINGS

1. Ames SW and Kneisl CR: Essentials of adult health nursing, Menlo Park, Calif, 1988, Addison-Wesley Publishing Co, Inc.
2. Anagnostakos NP and Tortora GJ: Principles of anatomy and physiology, ed 5, New York, 1987, Harper & Row, Publishers, Inc.
3. Baas L and Kretten C: Valvular heart disease, RN 50(11):30, 1987.
4. Bates BA: A guide to physical examination, ed 4, Philadelphia, 1987, JB Lippincott Co.
5. Beare PG and Myers JK: Principles and practice of adult health nursing, St Louis, 1990, The CV Mosby Co.
6. Brunner LS and Suddarth DS: Textbook of medical-surgical nursing, ed 6, Philadelphia, 1988, JB Lippincott Co.
7. Caldwell E and Hegner BR: Geriatrics: a study of maturity, ed 4, New York, 1986, Delmar Publishers, Inc.
8. Conover MB: Understanding electrocardiography: arrhythmias and the 12-lead ECG, ed 5, St Louis, 1988, The CV Mosby Co.
9. Dault LA, Nagy CS, and Collins JA: Reversing cardiac transplant rejection with orthoclone OKT3, Am J Nurs 89(7):953, 1989.
10. Douglas MK and Shinn JA: Advancement in cardiovascular nursing, Rockville, Md 1985, Aspen Publishers, Inc.
11. Doyle JE: Treatment modalities in peripheral vascular disease, Nurs Clin North Am 21:241, 1986.
12. Ellis K: When exercise can kill, RN 52(9):20, 1989.
13. Eyles MY: Mosby's comprehensive review of practical nursing, ed 10, St Louis, 1990, The CV Mosby Co.
14. Fong E, Ferris EB, and Skelley EG: Body structures and functions, ed 7, New York, 1989, Delmar Publishers, Inc.
15. Gaivlinski A: Saving the cardiogenic shock patient, Nurs '88, 18(12):34, 1988.
16. Hood G and Dincher J: Total patient care: foundations and practice, ed 7, St Louis, 1988, The CV Mosby Co.
17. Jarrett F and Hirsch SA: Vascular surgery of the lower extremity, St Louis, 1985, The CV Mosby Co.
18. Juleff G: Cracking open a blocked heart valve, Nurs '89 19(6):58, 1989.
19. Julian DG and Wenger NK: Management of heart failure, Boston, 1986, Butterworth Publishers.
20. Konradi D and Stockert P: A close-up look at leukemia, Nurs '89, 34, 1989.
21. Lamb IH: The angina that can kill, RN 48(8):28, 1985.
22. Long BC and Phipps WJ: Medical-surgical nursing: a nursing process approach, ed 2, St Louis, 1989, The CV Mosby Co.
23. Marieb EN: Essentials of human anatomy and physiology, Menlo Park, Calif, 1984, Addison-Wesley Publishing Co, Inc.
24. McCann ME: Sexual healing after heart attack, Am J Nurs 89(9):1143, 1989.
25. Memmler RL and Wood DL: Structure and function of the human body, ed 4, Philadelphia, 1987, WB Saunders Co.
26. Mosby's medical, nursing, and allied health dictionary, ed 3, St Louis, 1989, The CV Mosby Co.

27. Riegel B: Inpatient recovery following myocardial infarction and coronary artery bypass graft surgery, J Cardiovasc Nurs 2 (3):1, 1987.
28. Rozell MS, Hijazi M, and Pack B: The painful episode in sickle cell disease, Nurs Clin North Am 18(1):185, 1983.
29. Solomon EP and Phillips GA: Understanding human anatomy and physiology, Philadelphia, 1987, WB Saunders Co.
30. Strandness DE: Vascular disease: current research and clinical approach, Orlando, 1987, Grune & Stratton Inc.
31. Teplitz L: Clinical close-up on lidocaine, Nurs '89, 19(9):44, 1989.
32. Thibodeau GA and Anthony CP: Structure and function of the body, ed 8, St Louis, 1988, Times Mirror/Mosby College Publishing.
33. Tucker SM and others: Patient care standards: nursing process, diagnosis, and outcome, ed 4, St Louis, 1988, The CV Mosby Co.
34. Thrasher SB: What I didn't know really hurt me, RN 52(9): 49, 1989.

CHAPTER CHALLENGE

KEY POINTS

- The cardiovascular system is composed of the heart, blood vessels, and lymphatic structures.
- The functions of the cardiovascular system are to deliver oxygen and nutrients to the cells and to remove carbon dioxide and waste products from the cells.
- Blood is a thick, red fluid composed of plasma, red blood cells, white blood cells, and platelets.
- Type O-negative blood is the universal donor.
- The heart is a large pump (the size of a human fist) that propels blood through the circulatory system.
- The heart is composed of four chambers—two atria and two ventricles.
- There are two coronary arteries; they supply the heart with nutrition and oxygen.
- The electrical pattern of impulse starts with the sinoatrial node (SA node), which is the pacemaker of the heart; it initiates the heartbeat. This impulse travels to the atrioventricular node (AV node). From here the impulse travels to a bundle of fibers called the Bundle of His and finally to the Purkinje fibers.
- There are three kinds of blood vessels organized for carrying blood to and from the heart. They are the arteries, veins, and capillaries.
- Systemic circulation carries oxygen and nutrients to the body tissues.
- Pulmonary circulation sends deoxygenated blood from the right side of the heart to the lungs, picks up the oxygen, and returns the blood to the left side of the heart.
- Hepatic circulation diverts the blood from systemic circulation to the liver to store excess amounts of sugar and to detoxify any poisonous substances.
- The lymphatic system is a subdivision of the cardiovascular system. It consists of lymphatic vessels, lymph, and lymphatic tissue.
- The lymphatic system is responsible for the removal of impurities, the manufacture of lymphocytes (WBCs), and the production of antibodies.
- The tonsils are composed of lymphoid tissue and are responsible for the filtering of bacteria.
- The thymus gland is composed of lymphoid tissue in utero (before birth) and the early years of life. It aids in the development of the immune system.
- The spleen is also composed of lymphoid tissue and has many functions, such as filtering out old red blood cells, storing a liter of blood, producing antibodies, and phagocytosis of bacteria.
- The cardiovascular system supports the function of all other systems.
- Dysfunction of the cardiovascular system continues to be the primary cause of death in the United States.
- Control of risk factors through patient education may assist in decreasing the incidence of cardiovascular disease.
- Nurses' understanding and knowledge of diagnostic evaluation and normal expected outcomes are important to collection of data for assessment.

CHAPTER CHALLENGE—cont'd

KEY POINTS (cont'd)

- Arteriosclerotic heart disease and atherosclerosis are two of the most frequently diagnosed conditions, predisposing the patient to angina, infarction, and other disorders of the heart and blood vessels. It is therefore important for the nurse to focus patient education on prevention of these conditions.
- Dietary restrictions of fat, cholesterol, sodium, and caffeine are essential to health maintenance. Nursing responsibility includes conveying such information to patients.
- The nurse should be aware that enzymes released into the blood stream as a result of cell membrane damage or necrosis indicate recent myocardial infarction or trauma.
- Because myocardial anoxia from infarction and occlusion may result in necrosis and a nonfunctioning myocardium, restoration of oxygen through therapy ordered by the physician is an important nursing procedure.
- The nurse should understand the objective of anticoagulant therapy—that of prevention of thrombus formation in patients with a clotting tendency or prevention of postoperative thrombus.
- An awareness of the signs and symptoms of acute congestive heart failure—shock, cardiac arrest, and sudden death—is an essential part of the nurse's knowledge base to supplement collection of data for assessment.
- In assisting with care of the patient with a bone marrow transplant, it is important for the nurse to understand that the aim of the procedure is to provide the patient with functioning hematopoietic tissue until his own tissue is capable of physiologically healthy functioning.
- Understanding the cause of aplastic anemia—viral invasion, medications, radiation, and chemotherapy—enables the nurse to educate the patient regarding this immunological injury that manifests as bone marrow abnormalities.
- Nursing interventions for a patient with a pacemaker require knowledge of the objective: a pacemaker may be indicated for heart block, worn externally or implanted internally, and functions on an impulse only when patient pulse is absent or a fixed, continuous mode.
- Interventions by the nurse require knowledge that patent, unobstructed blood vessels carry oxygen and nutrients to body tissues and remove metabolic wastes.
- When monitoring the patient for an occlusive condition, the nurse should realize that a thrombus holds the threat of becoming an embolus; the danger of an embolus is occlusion of the circulatory process.
- Realizing that primary or essential hypertension—the most common type—develops without apparent cause and is sometimes undetected, the nurse should understand that it is therefore known as the "silent killer."

STUDY QUESTIONS

1. Another name for a red blood cell is:
   a. Leukocyte
   b. Monocyte
   c. Erythrocyte
   d. Platelet
2. Prothrombin is produced in the:
   a. Spleen
   b. Thymus
   c. Liver
   d. Stomach
3. The universal blood group donor is:
   a. O negative
   b. A positive
   c. O positive
   d. AB negative
4. The chamber of the heart responsible for pumping the oxygenated blood into the system is the:
   a. Right atrium
   b. Left atrium
   c. Left ventricle
   d. Right ventricle
5. The pacemaker of the heart is the:
   a. AV node
   b. SA node
   c. Bundle of His
   d. Purkinje fibers
6. The heart has the following number of chambers:
   a. 3
   b. 4
   c. 2
   d. Only 1
7. The largest organ of the lymphatic system is the:
   a. Thymus
   b. Spleen
   c. Tonsils
   d. Heart
8. The gland that plays a role in the development of the body's immune system is the:
   a. Tonsils
   b Thymus
   c. Spleen
   d. Liver
9. The nurse classifies the cause of angina pectoris as:
   a. Dysrhythmia triggered by stress
   b. Insufficient coronary blood flow
   c. Minute emboli discharged through the narrowed lumen of the coronary vessels
   d. Spasm of the vessel walls associated with excessive adrenalin secretion
10. Pain associated with myocardial infarction is all *except*:
    a. Relieved by rest and inactivity
    b. Substernal in location
    c. Sudden in onset, prolonged in duration
    d. Viselike and radiates to the shoulders and arms
11. Sudden loss of blood supply to a portion of the myocardium from an occluded coronary artery may lead to necrosis of that part of the myocardium. The necrosed tissue is termed:
    a. Coronary sclerosis
    b. Myocardial infarction
    c. Myocardial occlusion
    d. Coronary insufficiency
12. Endocarditis usually leads to:
    a. Inflammation of the chordae tendineae without permanent damage to the heart
    b. Permanent scarring and deformity of the heart valves, especially the mitral and aortic valves
    c. Scarring of the pulmonic valve
    d. Inflammation of the middle layer of the heart
13. The characteristic sign of pericarditis is:
    a. Friction rub
    b. Dyspnea
    c. Fever
    d. Hypoxia
14. The patient with CHF has physician orders for complete bed rest, meaning:
    a. He is encouraged to rest as much as possible
    b. While confined to bed, he may assume responsibility for his personal care
    c. He is confined to bed but is allowed to go to the bathroom as needed
    d. He must remain as quiet as possible, with any task requiring physical effort done for him
15. Congestive heart failure is best described as:
    a. An abnormality of the heart structure
    b. A decrease of blood flow through the heart and great vessels, resulting from failure of the heart to function effectively as a pump
    c. A result of a blood clot within one chamber of the heart
    d. A sudden spasm of the myocardium caused by a decreased blood supply

16. The sign of pitting edema in the lower extremities is indicative of:
    a. Left-sided failure (CHF)
    b. Right-sided failure (CHF)
    c. Pulmonary edema
    d. Aortic aneurysm
17. The patient with pitting edema has orders for daily weight check, to determine loss of:
    a. Body fat
    b. Appetite
    c. Tissue fluid
    d. Blood volume
18. Rotating tourniquets are useful to prevent pulmonary overload in CHF. The nurse will agree with all of the following statements *except*:
    a. No single extremity will be compressed for more than 45 minutes
    b. The amount of pressure in the cuff is of little importance
    c. One extremity is always free, while three of the four are compressed
    d. Discontinuation of the tourniquets involves releasing one at a time in 15-minute intervals
19. Anemia may be defined as:
    a. A decrease in the number of red blood cells and a deficiency of hemoglobin and hematocrit
    b. Iron deficiency
    c. Decrease in blood cells
    d. Loss of blood volume
20. Aplastic anemia is the term used to describe a condition in which:
    a. The activity of the bone marrow is depressed
    b. The bone marrow fails to produce lymphocytes
    c. The bone marrow fails to produce red blood cells
    d. Red cells are absent as a result of chronic blood loss
21. Treatment of polycythemia includes:
    a. Whole blood transfusions
    b. Platelet transfusion
    c. Phlebotomy with removal of 500 to 800 ml of blood
    d. Measures to stimulate the bone marrow to manufacture more red blood cells
22. Nursing assessment for a patient with leukemia includes observation for:
    a. Fever and infection
    b. Melena and hematuria
    c. Petechiae, ecchymoses
    d. All of these
23. Hemophilia is a hereditary bleeding disorder that:
    a. Has a higher incidence among males
    b. Is associated with joint bleeding, edema, and joint damage
    c. Is related to a genetic deficiency of a specific blood-clotting factor
    d. All of the above
24. The term *pacemaker* means:
    a. It stops the heartbeat on occasion for purposes of rest
    b. It initiates the heartbeat
    c. It causes an irregular heartbeat
    d. None of the above
25. The basis of electrocardiography is the fact that:
    a. The ventricles distribute oxygenated blood to the tissues
    b. The atria are the heart's receiving chambers
    c. An electrical charge is delivered to the heart
    d. Each contraction of the heart is accompanied by an electrical charge
26. The major complication that may arise from an angiogram is:
    a. Trauma of the vascular system
    b. Lack of patient cooperation
    c. Allergic reaction to the dye
    d. Infection after the procedure
27. Digoxin has many actions, but the chief action is that it:
    a. Decreases blood pressure
    b. Increases heart rate
    c. Prevents formation of blood clots
    d. Increases the force of myocardial contraction
28. Lasix 40 mg po daily may be considered:
    a. An effective cardiotonic
    b. A potent diuretic
    c. A useful drug for anemia treatment
    d. An antihypertensive
29. If the patient receives Lasix routinely, he should be observed for (electrolyte imbalance):
    a. Calcium excess
    b. Calcium deficit
    c. Potassium excess
    d. Potassium deficit
30. Angina is usually relieved by the following sublingually administered vasodilator:
    a. Reserpine
    b. Nitroglycerin
    c. Serpasil
    d. Digoxin

33

Care of the Patient with a Urinary Disorder

ALITA SELLERS
CAROLYN S. EDWARDS

LEARNING OBJECTIVES

After reading this chapter the student should be able to do the following:

- List the anatomical structures of the urinary system
- Discuss the nephron and its function
- Discuss the normal versus abnormal components of urine
- List the four processes involved in urine formation
- Discuss priorities for the special needs of the patient with urinary dysfunction
- Select nursing diagnoses specific for care of the patient with alteration in urinary function
- Describe the alterations in renal function associated with disorders of the urinary tract
- Identify the nurse's role in the care of the dialysis patient
- Appraise the changes in body image created when the patient experiences an alteration in urinary function
- Identify the effect of aging on urinary system function
- Identify teaching methods to meet the educational needs of the patient with urinary diversion
- Discuss the impact of renal disease on family function

RELATED TOPICS OF INTEREST

- Medical asepsis (Chapter 16)
- Specimen collection (Chapter 21)
- Diet therapy (Chapter 23)
- The surgical patient (Chapter 26)
- Fluids and electrolytes (Chapter 28)

KEY TERMS

Define the following:

- albuminuria
- anasarca
- anuria
- asthenia
- azotemia
- Bowman's capsule
- calyx
- cortex
- costovertebral angle
- creatinine
- cytological evaluation
- diuresis
- diuretics
- dysuria
- glycosuria
- hematuria
- hilus
- hydronephrosis
- ileal conduit
- ketosis
- medulla
- micturition
- nephron
- nephrotoxin
- nocturia
- oliguria
- pyuria
- residual urine
- retention
- ureters
- urolithiasis

ANATOMY AND PHYSIOLOGY

Daily, the cells throughout the body metabolize the ingested nutrients; this provides energy for the body, but also produces waste products. As protein breaks down, nitrogenous wastes—urea, ammonia, and **creatinine**—are produced. Excretion of these waste products is the primary function of the kidneys. The kidneys also assist in regulating the body's water, electrolytes, and acid-base balance. To perform this task the kidneys filter the blood much like an oil filter in a car removes the impurities from the oil.

The urinary system is composed of (1) two kidneys, which produce urine after filtering the wastes from the blood, (2) two ureters, which transport the urine from the kidneys to the bladder, (3) one bladder, which collects and stores the urine, and (4) one urethra, which transports the urine from the bladder to the outside of the body for elimination (Fig. 33-1).

This chapter will explore the filtering process, the composition of urine, and the pathway of urine removal from the body.

Kidneys

The kidneys are retroperitoneal (behind the peritoneum), just below the diaphragm. They are dark red, kidney bean–shaped organs 4 to 5 inches long and 2 to 3 inches wide. Because of the size and shape of the liver, the right kidney lies slightly lower in the abdominal cavity than the left kidney. They are surrounded by a layer of adipose tissue that anchors the kidneys in place. Near the center of the medial border is a notch or indentation called the **hilus** from which the ureter, blood, and lymph vessels enter and exit the kidney.

Gross anatomical structure. The outer covering of the kidney is composed of a strong layer of connective tissue called the *renal capsule.* Directly beneath the renal capsule is the renal **cortex,** which is soft and granular (Fig. 33-2). It contains 1.25 million renal tubules. These tubules are part of the microscopic filtration system. Immediately beneath the cortex is the medulla, which is a darker color. The **medulla** contains the triangular pyramids. Continuing inward, the narrow points of the pyramids (papillae) that empty into the calyces are seen. This innermost region is called the *renal pelvis,* and each pyramid empties into a **calyx** in this region. The renal pelvis is really an expansion of the upper end of the ureter; the ureter in turn drains the finished product, urine, into the bladder.

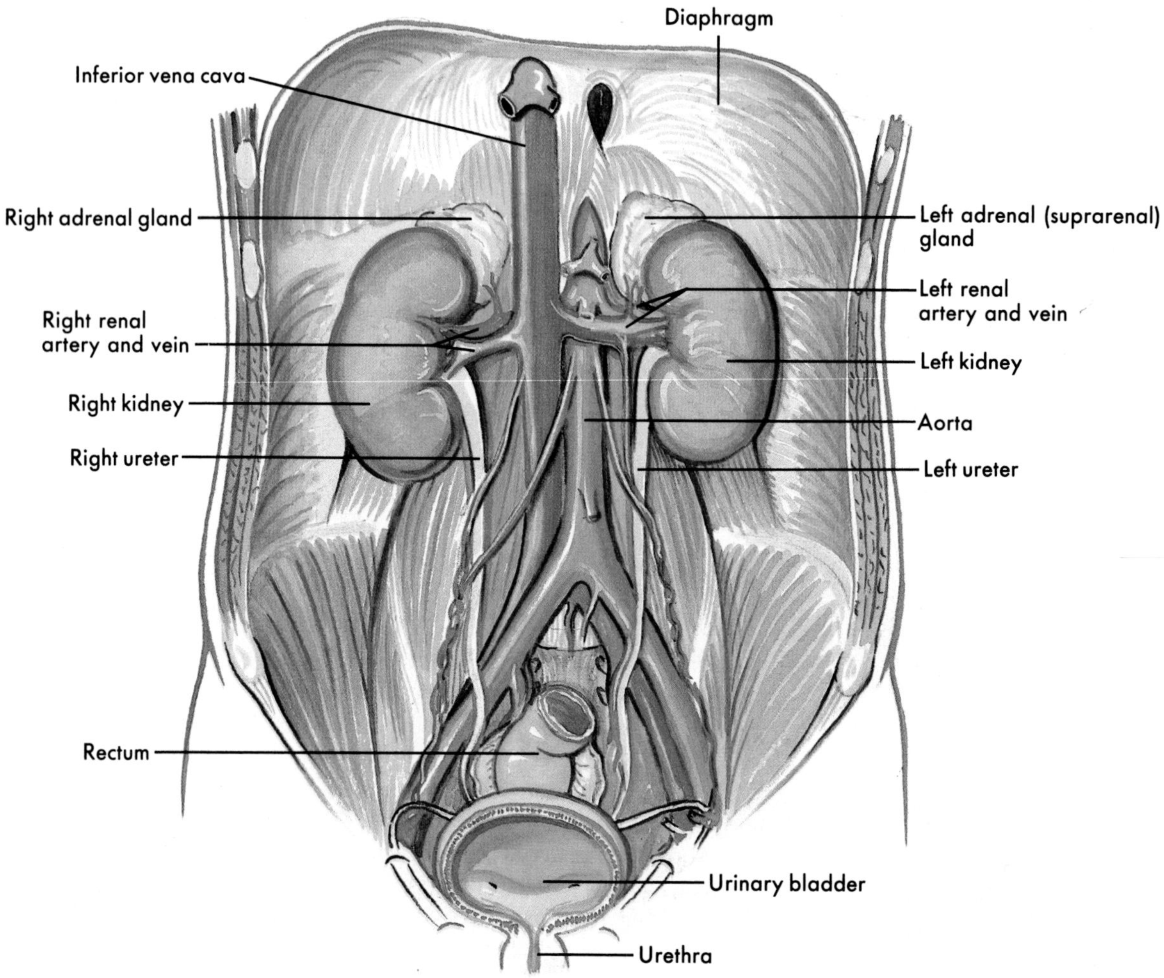

FIG. 33-1 Locations of urinary system organs.

FIG. 33-2 Coronal section through right kidney.

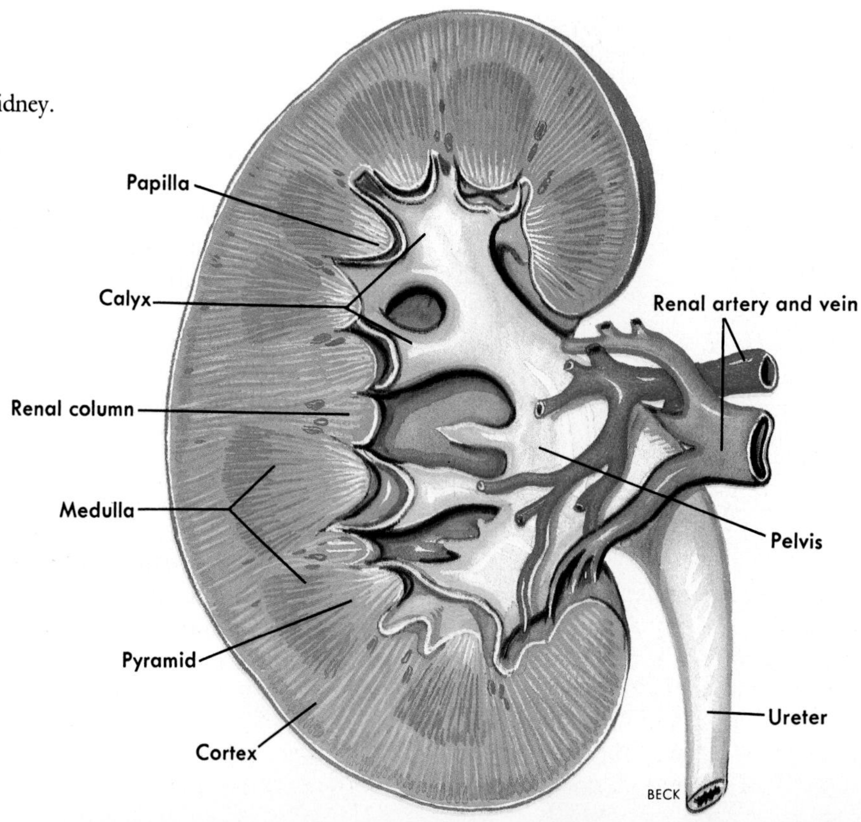

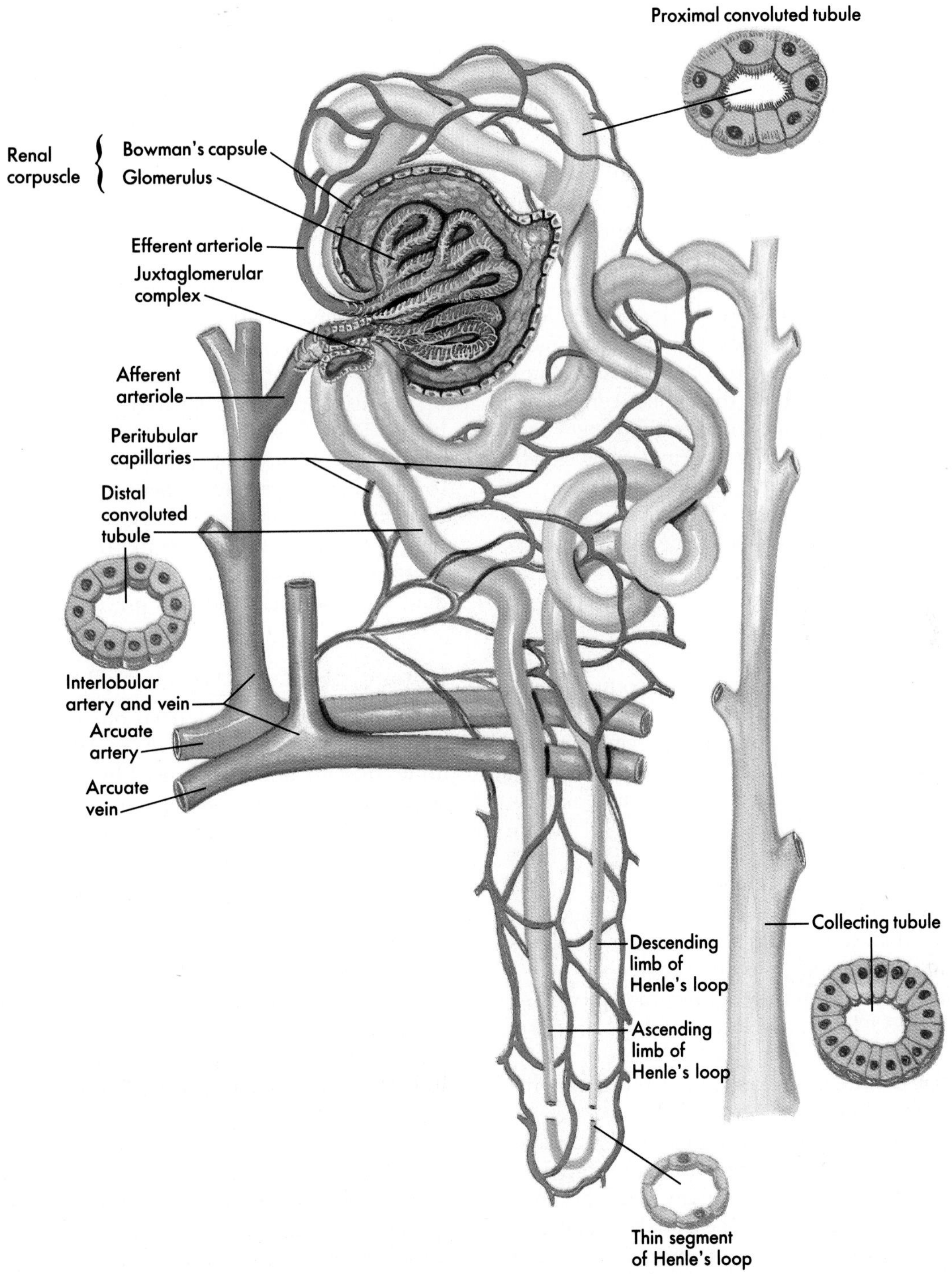

FIG. 33-3 The nephron unit. Cross sections from the four segments of the renal tubule are shown.

Microscopic structure

Nephron. Each kidney contains more than 1 million nephrons. The **nephron** is the functional unit of the kidney (Fig. 33-3). It is responsible for filtering the blood and processing the urine. It has three major functions: (1) it controls body fluid levels by selectively removing or retaining water; (2) it assists with the regulation of the pH of the blood; and (3) it removes toxic wastes from the blood. Approximately 60 times a day the body's entire volume of blood is filtered through the kidneys. Basically, the nephron consists of two main structures: the renal corpuscle and the renal tubule.

The renal corpuscle contains a tightly bound network of capillaries (glomerulus; pl. glomeruli) that are held inside a cuplike structure **(Bowman's capsule).** Blood is delivered to the glomerulus by the afferent arteriole; the blood leaves through the efferent arteriole. Fig. 33-3 shows that the afferent arteriole is much larger than the efferent arteriole. This blood flow pattern increases the pressure within the glomerular capillaries. This results in the first step of urine production—glomerular filtration. This filtrate contains blood plasma without the blood proteins and blood cells. The process continues as Bowman's capsule extends into the renal tubules. The efferent arterioles also connect to the peritubular capillaries that surround the renal tubules (see Fig. 33-3).

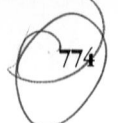

The second step of the process is reabsorption. As the filtrate leaves the Bowman's capsule, it enters a long, coiled, twisting tubule that descends in the center, much like a hairpin. The first segment of the tubule system is the proximal convoluted tubule; the second segment (the hairpin) is the loop of Henle; and the third segment is the distal convoluted tubule. The system is completed by the emptying of filtrate into the collecting tubules.

Reabsorption begins as soon as the filtrate reaches the tubule system. The filtrate contains important products needed by the body; water, glucose, and ions must be reabsorbed and returned to the blood for body use. In fact, 99% of the filtrate is returned to the blood.

The third and final step of the process is tubular secretion. In the second phase, tubular absorption dealt with reabsorption of materials from the filtrate into the blood. Tubular secretion is responsible for removing substances from the blood and adding it to the filtrate (urine). Some of the substances secreted are potassium and hydrogen ions, creatinine, urea, and ammonia. Certain drugs, such as penicillin, are also removed by tubular secretion. This third step, secretion, is responsible for ridding the body of certain remaining wastes and also controlling the blood pH. This secretion process occurs primarily in the distal and collecting tubules.

In summary, the three phases of urine formation (Fig. 33-4 and Table 33-1) and the location of the processes are as follows:

1. *Filtration* of water and blood products occurs in the glomerulus of Bowman's capsule.
2. *Reabsorption* of water, glucose, and important ions back into the blood occurs primarily in the proximal convoluted tubules, loop of Henle, and the distal convoluted tubules. The peritubular capillaries bring the blood supply to the area. This process reclaims important substances needed by the body.
3. *Secretion* of certain ions, nitrogen waste products, and drugs occurs primarily in the distal convoluted tubule. This process is the reverse of reabsorption; the substances move from the blood to the filtrate.

Hormonal influence on nephron function. When the body has suffered increased fluid loss through hemorrhage, diaphoresis, vomiting, diarrhea, or other means, the blood pressure drops, which decreases the amount of filtrate produced by the kidneys. The posterior pituitary releases antidiuretic hormone (ADH), which prevents excess water loss in the urine. ADH causes the cells of the distal convoluted tubules to increase their rate of water reabsorption. This returns water to the bloodstream, which increases the blood pressure to a more normal level and causes the urine to become very concentrated.

When there is decreased blood volume, decreased sodium ions, or increased potassium ions in the blood, the adrenal cortex releases the hormone aldosterone. This causes increased sodium retention, which results in increased potassium excretion. In addition, it causes increased water reabsorption by the tubules. This result produces homeostasis. If blood pressure is low, the cells of the juxtaglomerular apparatus release renin into the blood. There this hormone acts as an enzyme to activate a protein that causes blood vessels to constrict and thus to raise blood pressure. When the kidneys do not get enough oxygen, they release another hormone-like substance that acts as an enzyme to produce erythropoietin. Erythropoietin stimulates the red bone marrow to produce red blood cells and thus prevents anemia.

Urine Composition and Characteristics

The word *urine* comes from one of its components, uric acid. Daily the body urinates 1000 to 2000 ml of urine; this amount is influenced by several factors, such as mental and physical health, oral intake, and blood pressure. Urine is 95% water; the remainder is nitrogenous wastes and salts. It is usually a transparent yellow color with a characteristic odor. The normal urine is yellow because of urochrome, a pigment present in urine resulting from the body's destruction of hemoglobin. Urine is slightly acidic, with a pH of 4.6 to 8.0. Healthy urine is sterile, but at room temperature it rapidly decomposes and develops the odor of ammonia as a result of the breakdown of urea, one of the waste products.

Urine Abnormalities

A urinalysis, which studies the physical, chemical, and microscopic properties of urine, can give important diagnostic information. If the body's homeostasis has been compromised, certain substances may spill into the urine. Some of the more common substances include the following:

1. Albumin: The presence of albumin in the urine (**albuminuria**) indicates possible kidney disease, irritation of the kidney, increased blood pressure, or possibly irritation of the kidney cells from heavy metals.
2. Glucose: The presence of sugar in the urine (**glycosuria**) most often indicates a high blood glucose level. This condition is seen with diabetes mellitus,

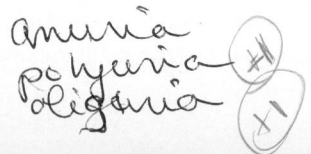

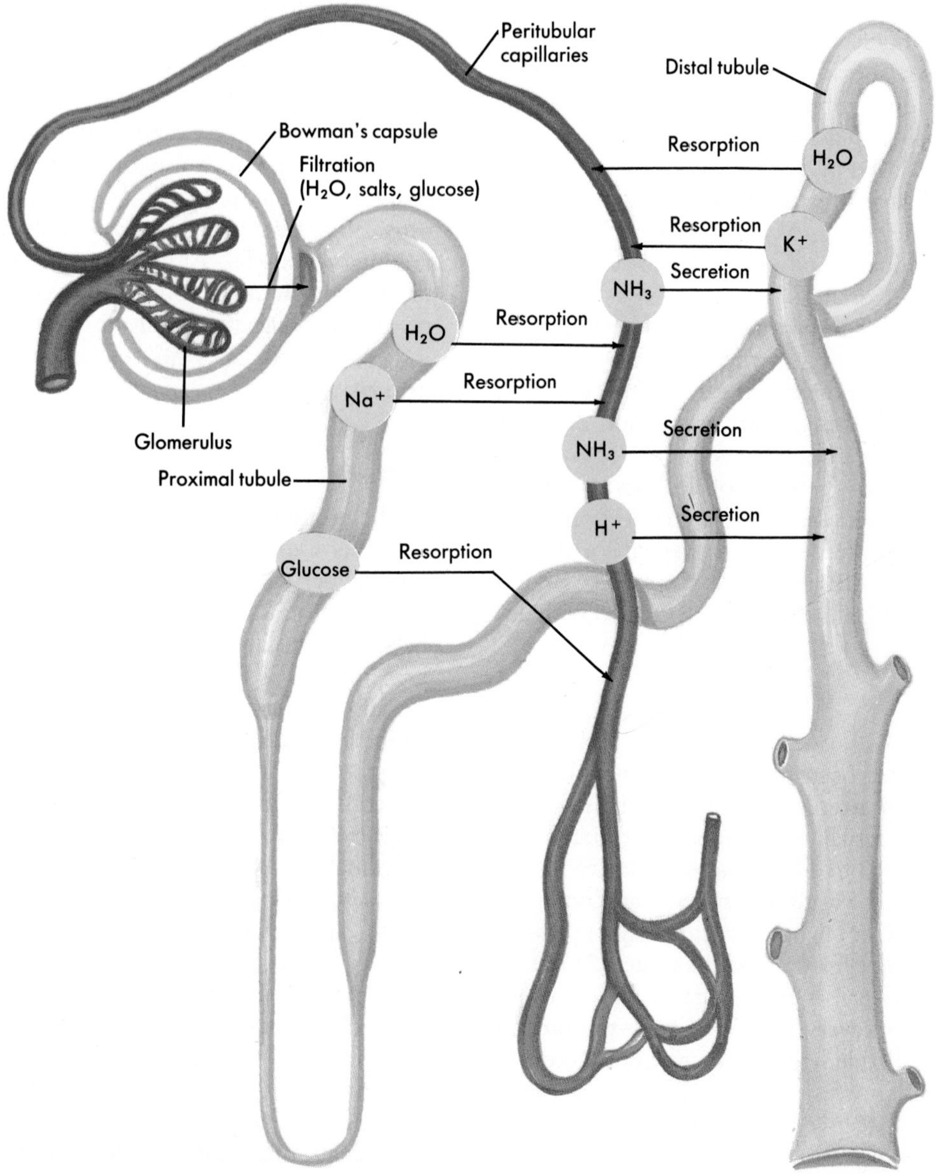

FIG. 33-4 Diagram of the steps in urine formation in successive parts of a nephron: filtration, resorption, and secretion.

Table 33-1 Functions of Parts of the Nephron in Urine Formation

Part of Nephron	Process in Urine Formation	Substances Moved and Direction of Movement
Glomerulus	Filtration	Water and solutes (e.g., sodium and other ions, nitrogen waste products, urea, uric acid, creatinine, glucose and other nutrients) filter out of glomeruli into Bowman's capsules
Proximal tubule	Resorption	Water and solutes
Loop of Henle	Resorption	Sodium and chloride ions
Distal and collecting tubules	Resorption	Water, sodium, and chloride ions
	Secretion	Ammonia, potassium ions, urea, uric acid, creatinine, hydrogen ions, and some drugs

because the pancreas is not producing enough insulin to metabolize the glucose. The blood glucose level increases above the renal threshold (point at which the kidney tubules can no longer reabsorb), and the glucose spills into the urine.
3. Erythrocytes: The presence of erythrocytes in the urine **(hematuria)** usually indicates infections, tumors, or kidney disease. Occasionally an individual may have a kidney stone and the irritation produces hematuria.
4. Ketone bodies: The presence of ketone bodies in the urine **(ketosis)** occurs when excessive quantities of fatty acids are oxidized in the liver. This condition is seen with diabetes mellitus, starvation diets, or diets too low in carbohydrates.
5. Leukocytes: The presence of leukocytes (white blood cells) occurs when there is an infection in the urinary tract. A sterile urine specimen for culture and sensitivity usually identifies the specific organism. The individual is then usually treated with antibiotics.

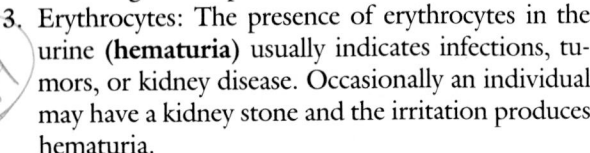

Ureters

Once the urine has been formed in the nephrons, it passes to the paired **ureters** through the hilus of the kidneys. Ureters are actually extensions of the kidney pelvis and they extend 10 to 12 inches to the lower part of the urinary bladder. The walls of the ureters are composed of three layers of tissue: (1) mucosa (inner layer) protects the lining of the ureter from the acidic urine; (2) muscle (middle layer), responsible for peristaltic waves, which produces contractions every 1 to 5 minutes—this propels the urine into the bladder (the more urine produced, the closer the peristaltic waves); and (3) fibrous coat (outer layer), which is a protective layer with fibrous extensions that anchor the ureters.

As the ureters leave the kidneys, they are retroperitoneal and pass under the urinary bladder before entering it. This anatomical position prevents backflow of urine, because pressure in the urinary bladder compresses the ureters.

Urinary Bladder

The urinary bladder (Fig. 33-5) is a temporary storage pouch for urine. It is composed of collapsible muscle and is located anterior to the small intestine and posterior to the symphysis pubis. As the bladder fills with urine, it elevates itself into the abdominal cavity and can actually be palpated. Under normal conditions the bladder can distend to hold 750 to 1000 ml of urine. When the bladder contains approximately 250 ml of urine, the individual has a conscious desire to urinate. This is because the stretch receptors become activated and a message is sent to the spinal cord. A moderately full bladder holds about 470 ml (1 pint) of urine.

Two sphincters, the internal and external, control the release of the urine. The internal sphincter is composed of involuntary muscle, and as the bladder becomes full, the stretch receptors cause contractions, pushing the urine past the internal sphincter. The urine then presses on the external sphincter, which is composed of skeletal or voluntary muscle. Although an individual feels the urge to void, it can be controlled. As the bladder continues to fill, the message will be sent at intervals, until it becomes necessary to respond to the message and urinate.

Urethra

The urethra is the terminal portion of the urinary system. It is a small tube that carries urine by peristalsis from the bladder to the outside of the body. In females it is embedded in the anterior wall of the vagina and exits between the clitoris and the vaginal opening. It is approximately ¼ inch in diameter and 1½ inches long. Because the urinary orifice (urinary meatus) is very close to the anus, it is fairly easy for *Escherichia coli (E. coli)* in the stool to enter the urinary meatus and cause a urinary infection. Young girls should be taught to cleanse anterior to posterior to decrease possible contamination.

In males the urethra is approximately 8 inches long. It leaves the urinary bladder, passes through the prostate gland, and extends the entire length of the penis. The urinary orifice is in the center of the distal area of the glans penis. In the male the urethra serves two functions: a passageway for urine and a passageway for semen.

In both sexes the mucous membrane that lines the urethra also lines the kidney pelves, ureters, and bladder. This anatomical feature is important, because infection can spread easily throughout the system.

Normal Aging Patterns

With aging the kidneys lose part of their normal functioning capacity; in fact, by the age of 70 the filtering mechanism is only 50% as efficient as at age 40. This occurs because of decreased blood supply and loss of nephrons.

In the aging female the bladder loses tone and the perineal muscles may relax; this can result in stress incontinence. In the aging male the prostate gland may become enlarged (this occurs in 75% of men by the age of 70) and leads to constriction of the urethra. Incomplete emptying of the bladder in both sexes increases the possibility of urinary infection. As always, assessing the amount, color, and odor of the urine may detect early symptoms.

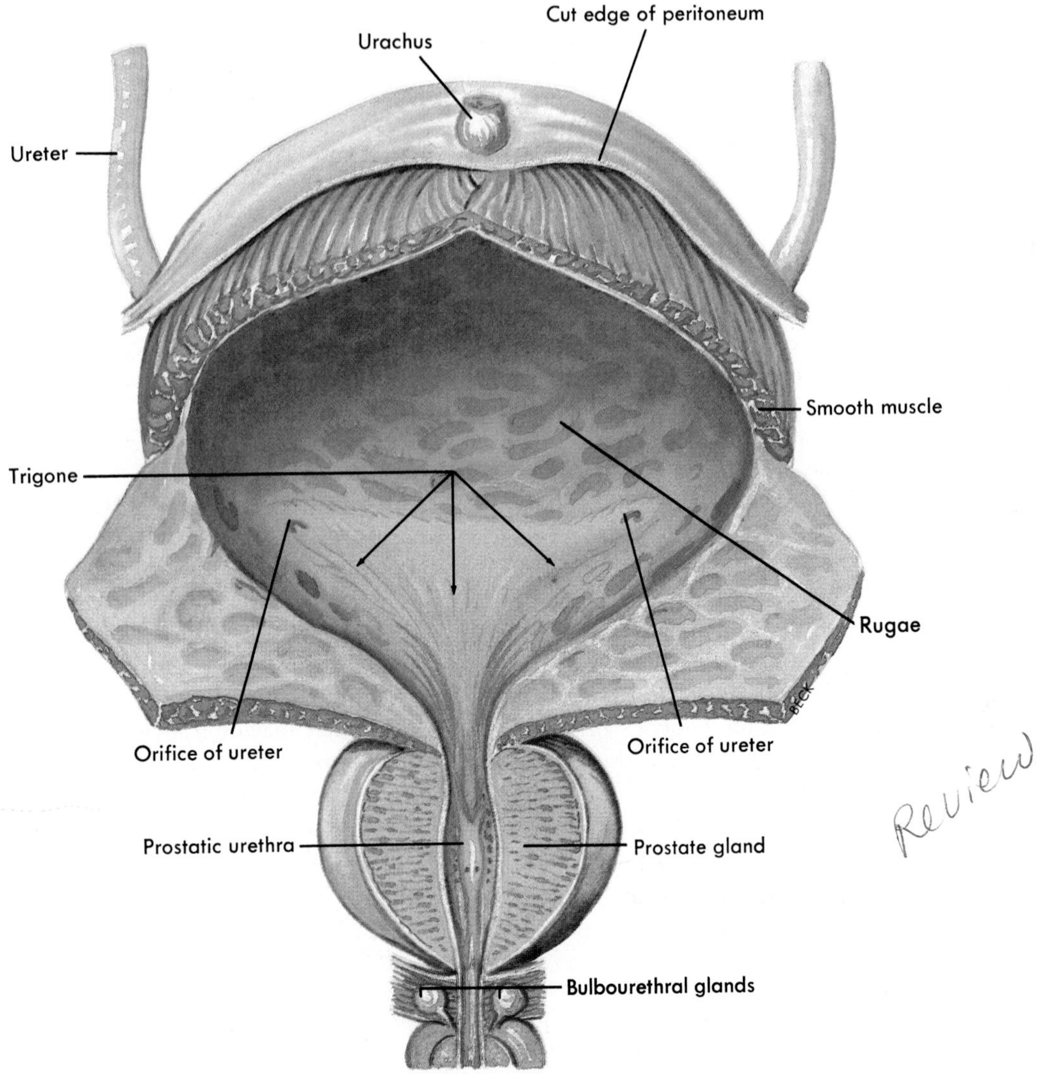

FIG. 33-5 The male urinary bladder, cut to show the interior. Note how the prostate gland surrounds the urethra as it exits the bladder.

CARE OF THE PATIENT WITH A URINARY DISORDER: GENERAL CONSIDERATIONS

Assessment of Urinary Function

Assessment of the urinary tract is included in baseline data for all patients. Assessment of the urinary tract is emphasized in special circumstances: (1) persons who may be at high risk for renal disease, such as individuals exposed to **nephrotoxins** (a substance with specific destructive properties for the kidneys) and those experiencing systemic changes from altered health states, such as pregnancy, diabetes mellitus, or hypertension; (2) conditions that may directly compromise renal function, including trauma, fluid depletion, or retention; and especially (3) patients with active or suspected renal disease.

The subject of urinary problems is a delicate one to approach, perhaps because the urinary system is closely associated with the reproductive system and cultural taboos surrounding sexuality. Often the patient's self-image and sexual performance are affected by altered urinary function. It is important for the nurse to be sensitive to the patient's feelings, guiding the interview to ensure accurate assessment while maintaining the patient's dignity.

The nursing assessment should include the patient's description of urine, urination patterns, sensation associated with urination, such as burning or pain, and difficulty starting or maintaining the urine stream. Advancing renal disease causes systemic changes, particularly in the respiratory and circulatory systems. The nurse assesses for signs and symptoms of fluid overload or depletion. The skin provides easily assessed clues about the patient's state of hydration. Dryness and pruritus occur from electrolyte imbalance and the buildup of waste products. Mucous membranes become dry if the patient fails to maintain adequate hydration. Uremic frost, the white sediment deposited on the skin from uremia, may be present, but this is seen less frequently because more effective management measures are now available.

Geriatric patients should be assessed for the effects of aging on renal functioning. Faulty renal circulation from generalized arteriosclerosis and a decrease in the number of functioning nephrons diminish the efficiency of the kidneys. Decreased bladder capacity, weakened musculature and sphincter tone, diminished innervation, and enlarged prostate in men interfere with sensation and bladder control. The role of the nurse in completing a physical assessment may vary widely in different care settings.

The nurse records the subjective and objective data findings for the nursing assessment. When possible, the patient's or family's own words should be recorded in quotation marks to describe the patient complaints; then objective assessment findings are documented, both normal and abnormal. The nurse selects NANDA-approved nursing diagnoses that describe the patient's problems. Suggested nursing diagnoses are included within the discussion of the urinary tract disorders and should be augmented with general medical/surgical principles where appropriate.

Diagnostic Tests

Diagnostic tests for urinary tract conditions include laboratory tests, radiological studies, and endoscopic procedures. Nursing responsibilities vary according to the studies performed. Nurses need to be aware of specific patient variables that may influence test results: state of hydration, nutritional status, or trauma.

Urinalysis. The most common urinary diagnostic study is the urinalysis. Table 33-2 provides a description of normal and abnormal constituents in the urine and possible factors that will influence test results. A urinalysis may be done in relation to conditions of other body systems because of the role of the kidneys in maintaining homeostasis. Urinalysis is completed on a clean-catch or catheterized specimen. A clean-catch urine specimen is obtained after cleansing the area surrounding the urinary meatus with an antiseptic solution. The patient voids a small amount into a nonsterile container, discards it, and continues to void into the sterile specimen container. The inside of the sterile specimen container and the lid must not be touched, because contamination alters test results. If it is necessary to obtain a catheterized specimen, aseptic technique must be maintained. If an indwelling catheter is in place, aseptic technique is used to obtain a urine sample through the port on the drainage tubing. A urine specimen for culture may be obtained using these same procedures (see Chapter 21).

There are various reagent strips available to test urine for abnormal substances. This is a quick reference that can be used in a clinic setting or at home. Easy-to-follow instructions accompany the specific reagent strips.

The nurse may be responsible for collecting a 24-hour urine sample. The first voiding is discarded and the time noted at the beginning of the 24-hour urine collection. For the next 24 hours all urine is collected and placed in a special laboratory container. Depending on the test ordered, the specimen container may contain special chemicals (preservatives) and/or the urine may need to be kept cold. The nurse should follow the institutional procedure manual.

Blood urea nitrogen. Blood urea nitrogen (BUN) is a laboratory test used to determine the kidney's ability to rid the blood of the nonprotein nitrogen (NPN) waste, urea, which results from protein breakdown (catabolism). The acceptable serum range for BUN is 8 to 23 mg/dl. For a more accurate test result, the patient should receive

Table 33-2 Urinalysis

Constituent	Normal Range	Variation Factors
Color	Pale yellow to amber	Diabetes insipidus, biliary obstruction, medications, foods
Turbidity	Clear to slightly cloudy	Phosphates, WBCs, bacteria
Odor	Mildly aromatic	Medication, bacteria
pH	4.6 to 8	Stale specimen, food intake
Specific gravity	1.003 to 1.030	State of hydration, diabetes insipidus
Glucose	Negative	Diabetes mellitus, medications, food intake
Protein	Negative	Renal damage that allows protein to escape through the glomeruli, muscle exertion
Bilirubin	Negative	Liver disease with obstruction or damage
Hemoglobin	Negative	Trauma, renal disease
Ketones	Negative	Diabetes mellitus, diet, febrile disease
Red blood cells	2 to 3/HPF	Blood dyscrasias, renal disease, bladder disease (cystitis, cancer), anticoagulant drugs, trauma
White blood cells	4 to 5/HPF	Renal disease, lower urinary tract disease
Casts	Rare	Alkaline urine, stasis

nothing by mouth (NPO) for 8 hours before blood sampling. If the BUN is elevated, preventive nursing measures should be instituted to protect the patient from possible disorientation or convulsions.

Creatinine clearance. Creatinine, a nonprotein nitrogen (NPN) substance, is present in blood and urine. Creatinine, a source of muscle energy, is utilized during muscle contraction and is then excreted by glomerular filtration. Levels are directly related to muscle mass and are usually measured for a 24-hour period. During the testing period, excessive physical activity should be avoided. A fasting blood sample is drawn at the onset of testing and another at the conclusion. All urine in the 24-hour period is collected, since any deviation will alter test results. An elevation in serum levels with a decline in urine levels indicates renal disease. Normal ranges are: serum—0.7 to 1.5 mg/dl; urine—110 to 150 ml/min (male), 100 to 130 ml/min (female).

Phenolsulfonphthalein. Secretory ability of the renal tubules is assessed by the phenolsulfonphthalein (PSP) test. The PSP test provides much the same data as the creatinine clearance test and is now being performed less often. The red dye, PSP, is injected intravenously, and at intervals urine samples are obtained. Normally 60% to 75% of the dye is excreted in the urine after 2 hours.

Concentration and dilution. A noninvasive examination to assess the kidney's ability to concentrate and dilute urine is done by withholding fluids and then giving the patient large amounts of fluids. Urine samples are taken during the test to check the specific gravity. Specific gravity will decrease with increased hydration in normal kidney function. With kidney damage the specific gravity does not change regardless of the fluid intake.

Assessment of osmolality, which measures the weight of the solute compared with its own weight, may be preferred over specific gravity. Regardless of the measurement used, the same testing procedure is followed. Plasma osmolality may be done in conjunction with the urine sampling when pituitary disorders are suspected.

Urine uric acid analysis. A urine uric acid analysis is a 24-hour urine collection to measure the body's production and consequent excretion of uric acid. The test determines the effectiveness of medication or the need for medication changes for patients who repeatedly form uric acid **urolithiasis** (calculi). There are no pretest preparations other than explaining the procedure for a 24-hour urine collection. Although dietary intake is not usually restricted during the test, it may influence the test results. The normal uric acid serum range is 2.7 to 7.7 mg/dl. The normal uric acid urine range is 250 to 750 mg/24 hours. The uric acid level may be altered in the presence of conditions such as multiple myeloma, chronic glomerulonephritis, gout, and polycythemia vera.

Kidney-ureter-bladder radiography (KUB). A KUB assesses the general status of the abdomen and evaluates the size, structure, and position of the urinary tract structures. No special preparation is necessary. The nurse should explain that the procedure involves changing position on the x-ray table, which may be uncomfortably firm. Abnormal findings related to the urinary system may indicate tumors, stones, glomerulonephritis, cysts, and other conditions.

Excretory urography or intravenous urography (IVU). IVU evaluates structures of the urinary tract and filling of the renal pelvis with urine. Many institutions use the term *intravenous pyelogram IVP* when referring to IVU. It is vital that the nurse determine whether the patient has an allergy to iodine, because it is the base of the radiopaque dye that will be injected into a vein. If the patient has previously had an allergic reaction, the physician may order a corticosteroid or an antihistamine to be administered before testing or, as an alternative, may order ultrasonography.

Because kidneys and ureters are positioned in the retroperitoneal space, gas and stool in the intestines interfere with radiographic visualization. Preparation usually includes a light supper, a non-gas-forming laxative, and nothing by mouth 8 hours before testing. In planning the testing regimen, the nurse should schedule urography before barium-based studies. When the dye is injected, the patient will experience a warm, flushing sensation and a metallic taste. During the procedure vital signs will be monitored frequently. X-ray films will be taken at various intervals to monitor movement of the dye. Abnormal findings may indicate structural deviations, hydronephrosis, calculi within the urinary tract, polycystic kidney disease, and other conditions.

Retrograde pyelography. Retrograde pyelography involves examination of the lower urinary tract with a cystoscope under aseptic conditions. The urologist injects radiopaque dye directly into the ureters to visualize the upper urinary tract. Urine samples can be obtained directly from the renal pelvis. Additional retrograde studies include the following:

Retrograde cystography: Radiopaque dye is injected through an indwelling catheter into the urinary bladder for visualization of the urinary bladder to evaluate its structure or to determine the cause of recurrent infections.

Retrograde urethrography: A catheter is inserted and dye injected as with the cystography to assess the status of the urethral structure.

Voiding cystourethrography. Voiding cystourethrography is used in conjunction with other diagnostic studies to detect abnormalities of the urinary bladder and urethra. Preparation includes an enema before testing. An indwelling catheter is inserted into the urinary bladder, and dye is injected to outline the lower urinary tract. X-ray films are taken, and the catheter is then removed. The nurse explains to the patient that he will be asked to void while x-ray films are being taken. Some patients may experience embarrassment or anxiety related to the procedure and should be given the opportunity to express their feelings. Structural abnormalities, diverticula, and reflux into the ureter may be detected.

Endoscopic procedures: cystoscopy. Endoscopic procedures are visual examinations of hollow organs using an instrument with a scope and light source. Because of the invasive nature of the procedure, an informed consent is necessary, and because the procedure is most often performed in the surgical suite, preoperative preparation is indicated. The urologist performs the procedure.

Cystoscopy is a visual examination to inspect, treat, or diagnose disorders of the urinary bladder and proximal structures. Patient preparation includes a description of the procedure. Usually the procedure is carried out using a local anesthetic after the patient has been sedated. Patient safety is paramount when he is sedated.

The patient will be placed in lithotomy position for the procedure, which may evoke embarrassment and anxiety. The thought of a scope being passed while he is awake may intensify these feelings. The nurse should provide an opportunity for the patient to verbalize his feelings.

The scope is passed under aseptic conditions after a local anesthetic, such as procaine, is instilled into the urethra (Fig. 33-6). The patient will experience a feeling of pressure as the scope is passed. Continuous fluid irrigation of the bladder is necessary to facilitate visualization. Care after the procedure includes hydration to dilute the urine. The first voiding after the procedure should be monitored, assessing time, amount, color, and any **dysuria** (painful urination).

Renal angiography. Renal angiography aids in evaluation of blood supply to the kidneys, evaluates masses, and detects possible complications after kidney transplantation. The patient should have oral intake withheld the night before the procedure. Because the procedure requires the passing of a small catheter into an artery to provide a port for the injection of radiopaque dye, when the patient returns from the x-ray department he will need to lie flat in bed for several hours to minimize the risk of bleeding. The puncture site should be assessed for bleeding or hematoma formation, and the pressure dressing at the site should be maintained. Circulatory status of the involved extremity will be assessed every 15 minutes for 1 hour, then every 2 hours for 24 hours.

Renal biopsy. The kidney can be biopsied by an open procedure similar to other surgical procedures on the kidney or by the less invasive method of needle biopsy, also called a *percutaneous biopsy.*

Precautions after the procedures include close monitoring of vital signs, maintenance of a pressure dressing at the puncture site, observation for bleeding, maintaining the patient in a supine position, and keeping the patient quiet for 4 hours, with limited activity for 24 hours. Normal diet with increased fluids will be instituted after the procedure. The patient should expect to see a small amount of blood in his urine, which should subside within 8 hours.

Computed tomography. Computed tomography (CT scan) differentiates masses of the kidney. Images are obtained by a computer-controlled scanner after the intravenous injection of a radiopaque dye. The nurse informs the patient that the table on which he is placed and the machine "taking pictures" will move at intervals and that it is very important to lie still. The CT body-scanning unit will take multiple cross-section pictures at several different sites, creating a three-dimensional "map" of the kidney structure.

Magnetic resonance imaging. Magnetic resonance imaging (MRI) uses nuclear magnetic resonance as its source of energy to obtain a visual assessment of body tissues. There is no special preparation of the patient for

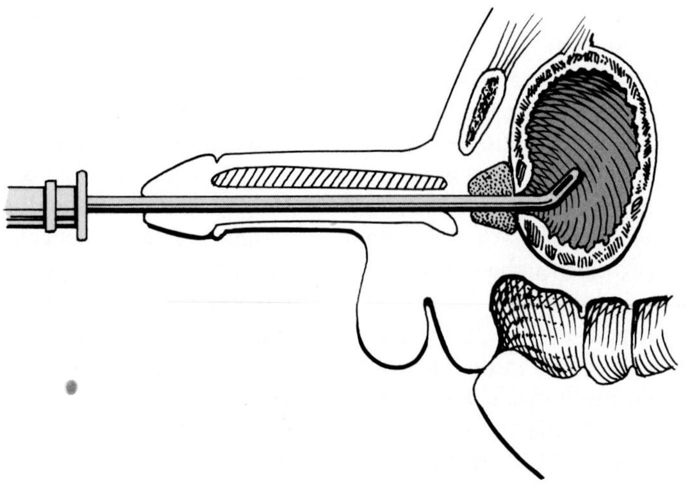

FIG. 33-6 Cystoscope inserted for examination of bladder.

MRI. It should be emphasized that the examination area will be confining and that a repetitive "pounding" sound will be heard (somewhat like the sound of a muffled jackhammer). MRI can be used for various diagnoses of pathological conditions of the renal system.

Ultrasonography. Ultrasonography is a diagnostic tool that uses the reflection of sound waves to produce images of deep body structures. The nurse should inform the patient that to carry out the procedure, a water-soluble jelly will be applied to the skin over the area to be studied to improve the transmission of sound waves. The sound waves are of a very high frequency that is inaudible to the human ear and will be converted into electrical impulses that will be photographed for study.

Ultrasonography of the kidney will visualize size, shape, and position of the kidney and delineate any irregularities in structure. Deviations from normal findings may indicate tumor, congenital anomalies, cysts, or obstructions. No special preparations are necessary.

Medication Considerations in Patient Care

The kidneys filter a wide range of water-soluble products from the blood, including medications. The kidney's effectiveness in removing certain medications from the blood may be affected by various conditions, such as renal disease, changes in the pH of urine, and age. Patients with renal disease will be administered reduced doses of medications to minimize further damage or drug toxicity. Alteration in urinary pH increases or decreases the absorption rate of certain medications. Elderly patients may have decreased physiological functioning, diminishing the kidneys' capacity for excretion of drugs. Diminished kidney function interferes with the filtration of water-soluble medications. The medications included in this discussion are not inclusive but are intended to be representative of those medications used in the management of renal and urinary disorders.

Medications that enhance urinary output (diuretics). Diuretics are administered to enhance urinary output. This action is achieved by increasing the kidney's filtration of sodium, chloride, and water at different sites in the kidney. Diuretics are used in the management of a variety of disorders, such as congestive heart failure and hypertension. Diuretics are classified by chemical form, as well as the site and type of action on the kidney. Box 33-1 lists generic or selected trade name diuretics.

The most widely used diuretics are the thiazide diuretics. Acting on the distal tubule, thiazide diuretics interfere with the reabsorption of chloride, sodium, and water. Thiazides have a rapid onset and extended action, with few side effects. This group of medications is used primarily to treat hypertension and edema associated with a variety of disorders, including renal problems such as end-stage renal disease. Adverse actions of these medications result largely from the changes in electrolytes that occur with **diuresis.** Particular care must be taken to compensate for the loss of potassium. Potassium chloride and dietary supplements are frequently prescribed with these medications.

Carbonic anhydrase inhibitors are weak diuretics and are not widely used. Acetazolamide (Diamox) is the most commonly used of the group.

Loop diuretics act by inhibiting the absorption of sodium and chloride in the loop of Henle. Furosemide (Lasix) and bumetanide (Bumex), frequently prescribed loop diuretics, cause significant diuresis. This group contains the strongest diuretic agents; they are used in a variety of disorders, including nephrotic syndrome, congestive heart failure, and pulmonary edema. The side effects of loop diuretics are the signs and symptoms associated with rapid fluid loss: vertigo, hypotension, and possible circulatory collapse, as well as decrease in serum potassium (hypokalemia).

Osmotic diuretics, such as mannitol, promote excretion of water by raising osmotic pressure of fluid in renal tubules; reabsorption of water increases and urinary output decreases. Osmotic diuretics are used to manage edema, promote systemic diuresis in cerebral edema, decrease intraocular pressure, and improve renal function in acute renal failure. In acute renal failure osmotics are used to attempt to prevent irreversible failure, but they are contraindicated in advanced stages of renal failure.

Potassium-sparing diuretics are weak and consequently are used in combination with other diuretics. Although the action of each of these medications is different, they all conserve potassium that is usually lost with sodium in diuresis. Spironolactone (Aldactone) is perhaps the most commonly prescribed of this group.

Patients receiving diuretics often have disease conditions such as congestive heart failure and pulmonary edema. Therefore nursing interventions include monitoring for signs and symptoms of fluid overload: changes in pulse rate, respirations, cardiac sounds, and lung fields. Daily morning weights should be recorded for the patient receiving diuretics. Accurate intake and output records

BOX 33-1 GENERIC (SELECTED TRADE) NAME DIURETICS

Loop diuretics
- Furosemide (Lasix), bumetanide (Bumex)

Osmotic diuretics
- Mannitol (Osmitrol)

Potassium-sparing diuretics
- Spironolactone (Aldactone)

Thiazides
- Chlorothiazide (Diuril)
- Hydrochlorprothiazide (HydroDIURIL)

Thiazide-related products
- Chlorthalidone (Hygroton)

should be kept, and blood pressure, pulse, and respirations should be documented 4 times a day until the medication is regulated and the vital signs remain stable. BUN, serum electrolytes, and urine are assessed as ordered. Diet instruction for the patient and family is important to avoid overuse of salt in cooking or as a table additive. A number of salt substitutes are currently on the market; however, the long-term effects of those potassium preparations are not known and could further complicate the renal patient's condition. The use of most diuretics, with the exception of the potassium-sparing diuretics, requires adding daily potassium sources (e.g., baked potatoes, raw bananas, apricots, or navel oranges). In some cases it is necessary for the physician to order potassium supplements to be taken in combination with the diuretic.

Medications that act on the bladder. Few medications are used specifically for treatment of conditions of the urinary tract. Oxybutynin chloride (Ditropan), an antispasmodic, is used for the treatment of bladder spasms by reducing the frequency of the bladder contractions. It is also used for the patient with a neurogenic bladder to inhibit the initial sensation to void.

Bethanechol chloride (Urecholine), a parasympathetic nerve stimulant, is used for urinary retention by contracting the detrusor muscle of the bladder. Side effects are of parasympathetic nerve stimulation: increased gastric motility with nausea, vomiting, and diarrhea, skin flushing, perspiration, and headache.

Phenazopyridine hydrochloride (Pyridium) is a urinary analgesic. It anesthetizes the mucous lining of the ureters and bladder as the medication is excreted from the body. It is used for the relief of discomforts associated with a urinary tract infection, such as burning, frequency, and urgency. It does cause the urine to become reddish-orange. The patient should be informed that this will happen but that it does not represent a problem. If the scleras of the patient's eyes become yellow, the medication should be discontinued and the physician notified.

Medications that are used for urinary tract infections. Certain antimicrobial agents are administered primarily for the treatment of infections within the urinary tract. These medications are selected according to Gram-stain sensitivity of the organism causing the infection. Cinoxacin (Cinobac) is used for recurrent urinary tract infections caused by these organisms: *Escherichia coli, Proteus mirabilis,* and other gram-negative microbes. Side effects include gastrointestinal irritation with loss of appetite, nausea, vomiting, abdominal cramping, and diarrhea. Allergic symptoms are skin rash, urticaria, and perineal burning. Methenamine mandelate (Mandelamine) is used for patients with chronic, recurrent urinary tract infections as a preventive measure after the use of antibiotics that clear the infection. Although side effects are rare, they include nausea, vomiting, skin rash, and urticaria (hives). Nalidixic acid (NegGram) is a urinary antiseptic that is used to treat gram-negative microbes, such as *E. coli* and *P. mirabilis*. The common side effects are drowsiness, vertigo, weakness, nausea, and vomiting. Nitrofurantoin (Furadantin, Macrodantin) is effective against both gram-positive and gram-negative microbes (e.g., *Streptococcus faecalis, E. coli,* and *Proteus*) in the urinary tract only. Common side effects are loss of appetite, nausea, and vomiting. Norfloxacin (Noroxin) is a broad-spectrum antibiotic effective against gram-positive and gram-negative organisms: *E. coli, P. mirabilis, Pseudomonas, Staphylococcus aureus, Staphylococcus epidermidis,* and others. Because of expense, however, its use is typically reserved for the treatment of organisms that are resistant to other agents. The most common side effects are vertigo, headache, and nausea.

Nursing interventions. Precautions should be taken in the nursing interventions of patients receiving antibiotics for urinary tract infections. The nurse should (1) report use of any other medications, since a number of medications are contraindicated because of negative drug interactions; (2) administer medications with food or milk to lessen gastrointestinal upset; (3) use Clinistix or TesTape, not Clinitest, since many of the medications cause false-positive results; (4) hydrate the patient to produce daily urinary output of 2000 ml, unless contraindicated; (5) instruct the patient to take all of the medication, even though the symptoms may subside quickly; (6) soothe skin irritation with cornstarch or a bath of bicarbonate of soda or very diluted vinegar; (7) observe the patient receiving NegGram for visual disturbances and offer appropriate assistance for ambulation or transfer; (8) monitor the patient receiving Furadantin or Macrodantin for signs of allergic response (e.g., erythema, chills, fever, and dyspnea)—if these symptoms develop, medication should be discontinued and the physician notified; and (9) report continuing signs of infection.

Nutritional Considerations in Patient Care

The nutritional needs of the patient with a urinary tract disorder vary with each disease process. Unique nutritional problems of the patient with a urinary tract disorder will be discussed later in the chapter. The presence of other systemic disease, such as diabetes mellitus, complicates the therapeutic diet of the patient with a urinary tract disorder. Some general guidelines include the following: (1) provide foods from each of the basic four food groups; (2) provide adequate hydration, with modifications according to physician order; unless the patient is on fluid restriction, daily fluid intake is 2000 ml to aid in flushing the urinary tract (some physicians prefer that the fluid be water only); (3) acid or alkaline foods may be restricted for patients who are prone to stone formation (see discussion on urinary calculi, pp. 801-803); and (4) restrict the amount of salt consumed in the diet. The patient receiving renal dialysis is on a special diet with many restrictions specific to his individual needs.

Maintaining Adequate Urinary Drainage

Urine clears the body of waste materials and aids in the balance of electrolytes. Conditions that interfere with urinary drainage may therefore create a health crisis. It is important to reestablish urine flow as soon as possible to prevent the buildup of toxins in the bloodstream. Patients who may be at risk to develop difficulty with urine elimination include patients who have undergone surgical procedures of the bladder, prostate, or vagina; patients with primary urological problems, such as urethral stricture; and those who are critically ill.

Urinary catheters are used to maintain urine flow, to divert urine flow to facilitate healing postoperatively, to introduce medications by irrigation, and to dilate or prevent narrowing of some portions of the urinary tract. Catheters may be used for intermittent or continuous urinary drainage. Urinary catheters may be introduced into the bladder, ureter, or kidney. The type and size of urinary catheter used are determined by the location and cause of the urinary tract problem. Catheters are measured by the French (F) system. Urethral catheters range in size from 14 to 24 F for adult patients. Ureteral catheters are usually 4 to 6 F. The physician always inserts ureteral catheters. The nurse is usually responsible for the insertion of indwelling catheters.

Types of catheters. Different types of catheters are used for different purposes. The coudé catheter with a tapered tip is selected for ease of insertion when enlargement of the prostate gland is suspected. The curved stylet is used to assist the physician in the insertion of a urethral catheter in a male patient. The Foley catheter is designed with a balloon near its tip so the balloon may be inflated after insertion, holding the catheter in the urinary bladder for continuous drainage. The Malecot and Pezzer or mushroom catheters are used to drain urine from the renal pelvis of the kidney. The Robinson catheter has multiple openings in its tip to facilitate intermittent drainage. Ureteral catheters are long and slender to pass into the ureters. The whistle-tip catheter has a slanted, larger orifice at its tip to be used if there is blood in the urine. The cystostomy, vesicostomy, or suprapubic catheter is introduced through the abdominal wall above the symphysis pubis. This catheter is used to divert urine flow from the urethra as needed to treat injury to the bony pelvis, urinary tract, or surrounding organs; strictures; or obstruction. The catheter is inserted via surgical incision or puncture of the abdominal and bladder walls with a trocar cannula. The catheter is connected to a sterile closed drainage system and secured to avoid pulling it out; the wound is covered with a sterile dressing. When the lower urinary tract has healed, the patient's ability to void is tested by clamping the catheter so the patient can try to void naturally. When the measured residual urine is consistently less than 50 ml, the catheter is usually removed and a sterile dressing is placed over the wound.

An external (Texas or condom) catheter is not a catheter but a drainage system connected to the external male genitalia. This noninvasive appliance is used for the incontinent male to minimize skin irritation from urine. The appliance is removed daily for cleansing and inspection of the skin. Use of the external catheter allows for a more normal life-style for the patient.

Nursing interventions. Nursing interventions for the patient with a urinary drainage system include employing a number of principles to prevent and detect infection and trauma (Skills 33-1 to 33-4):

1. Follow aseptic technique to avoid introduction of microorganisms from the environment. Never rest the collecting bag on the floor.
2. Record intake and output. For precision monitoring, such as hourly urine output, add a urometer to the drainage system. If urine output falls to less than 50 ml per hour, first check the drainage system for proper placement and so on.
3. Adequately hydrate the patient to flush the urinary tract.
4. Do not open the drainage system after it is in place except to irrigate the catheter, and then only with a specific order from the physician. It is important to maintain a closed system to prevent urinary infections.
5. Perform catheter care twice daily and as needed, using universal precautions. Each institution has a specific protocol for catheter care. Cleanse perineum with mild soap and warm water, rinse well, and pat dry. At times an antiseptic solution or ointment may be ordered to use at the catheter insertion site. Betadine ointment is often the agent of choice to place at the meatus and around the catheter to prevent infection.
6. Check the drainage system for leaks daily.
7. Avoid placement of the urinary drainage bag above the level of the catheter insertion, which would cause urine to reenter the drainage system and contaminate the urinary tract.
8. Prevent tension on the system or backflow of urine while transferring the patient.
9. Ambulate the patient if possible to facilitate urine flow. If the patient's activity must be restricted, turn and reposition every 2 hours.
10. Avoid kinks or compression of the drainage tube that may cause pooling of the urine within the urinary tract. Gently coil excess tubing, secure with a clamp or pin to avoid dislodging the catheter, and release the tubing before transferring or repositioning the patient.
11. Gently inspect the entry site of the catheter for blood or exudate that may indicate trauma or in-

Text continued on p. 791.

SKILL 33-1

CATHETERIZATION: MALE OR FEMALE

1. Wash hands.
2. Introduce self.
3. Identify patient by checking identification band.
4. Explain procedure to patient.
5. Close door and draw curtains to provide privacy.
6. Place waterproof absborent pad under patient's buttocks.
7. Position patient.
   a. Male: supine position with thighs slightly abducted allows relaxation of muscles and easy access to urinary meatus.
   b. Female: dorsal recumbent position with knees flexed and feet about 2 feet apart allows relaxation of muscles and easy access to urinary meatus.
8. Drape patient with bath blanket, covering upper body and shaping over both knees and legs, leaving genital area exposed.
9. Provide good light.
10. Arrange supplies and equipment on bedside table.
11. Put on disposable gloves.
12. Wash perineal area with warm soapy water and wash cloth.
13. Rinse and dry area.
14. Remove disposable gloves and place in paper bag.
15. Wash hands.
16. Open packaging using sterile technique.
17. Put on sterile gloves.
18. If indwelling catheter is used, test balloon by injecting normal saline or sterile water into balloon lumen until balloon is inflated, then aspirate saline or sterile water.
19. Open lubricant container; add antiseptic to cotton balls.
20. Wrap sterile towel around gloved hands. Place towel under edge of patient's buttocks. Nurse wraps edges of sterile towel around gloved hands to protect them from contamination while placing towel under edge of patient's buttocks.

STEP 22

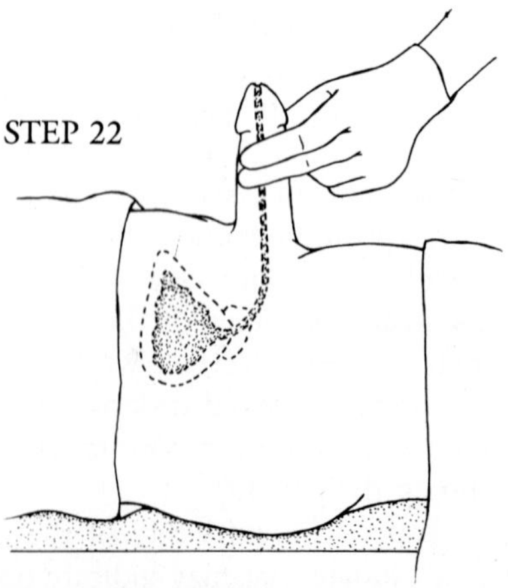

21. Lubricate catheter used for female for about 3.5 to 5 cm (1½ to 2 in). For a male, lubricate about 15 to 18 cm (6 to 7 in).
22. Cleanse perineal area using forceps to hold cotton balls soaked in antiseptic solution.
    a. Male
       (1) Grasp penis at shaft below glans with one hand; continue to hold throughout insertion of catheter.
       (2) With other hand, use forceps to hold cotton balls soaked in antiseptic solution.
       (3) Cleanse meatus in circular motion to decrease introduction of organisms into bladder.
       (4) Repeat cleansing two more times using sterile cotton balls each time.
    b. Female
       (1) Spread labia minora with thumb and index finger of nondominant hand to expose meatus; continue to hold throughout insertion of catheter.
       (2) With other hand, use forceps to hold cotton balls soaked in antiseptic solution.
       (3) Cleanse area from clitoris toward anus, using a different sterile cotton ball each time—first to the right of the meatus, then to the left of meatus, then down the center over meatus, using all cotton balls.
23. Pick up catheter with free sterile-gloved hand, near the tip; hold remaining part of catheter coiled in hand; place distal end in basin.

STEP 23

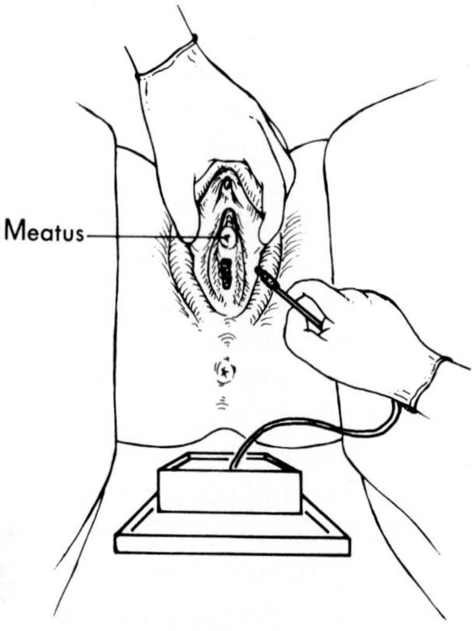

CATHETERIZATION: MALE OR FEMALE—cont'd

24. Insert catheter gently; urine flow begins quickly. Male urethra is longer (about 8 inches in length); urine flow may take a few seconds longer. Female urethra is short (about 1½ inches in length).
25. Collect urine specimen, if needed, by placing open lumen end of catheter into specimen container.
26. Type of catheter
    a. Indwelling catheter:
        (1) Inflate balloon with required amount of normal saline or sterile water.
        (2) Pull gently to feel resistance.
        (3) Attach end of catheter to collecting tube of drainage system, holding drainage bag below the level of bladder (many catheters are presealed to the collecting tube of the drainage system).
        (4) Attach collection bag to side of bed.
        (5) Secure catheter to patient to minimize tension and trauma to urethral opening.
            (a) Male
            Tape catheter to top of thigh or apply leg strap; allow slack for body movement.
            (b) Female
            Tape catheter to inner thigh or apply leg strap; allow slack for body movement.
        (6) Clip drainage tubing to bed linen; allow slack for body movement.
    b. Straight catheter:
        (1) Hold coiled catheter in hand with opening over basin.
        (2) Fully empty bladder (approximately 700 to 1,000 ml) unless institution policy differs.
        (3) Withdraw catheter slowly.
27. Dry perineal area.
28. Remove gloves; dispose of equipment, linen, and used materials.
29. Label urine specimen with patient's name, date, physician's name, and other pertinent information.
30. Reposition patient, remove drape, and cover patient.
31. Wash hands.
32. Check flow of urine and drainage tubing setup.
33. Open door or drapes.
34. Check patient for comfort level, catheter tubing placement, and whether patient has any questions.
35. Send urine specimen, if obtained, to laboratory.
36. Document procedure.
37. Report any unusual findings immediately.

STEP 26 a(1)

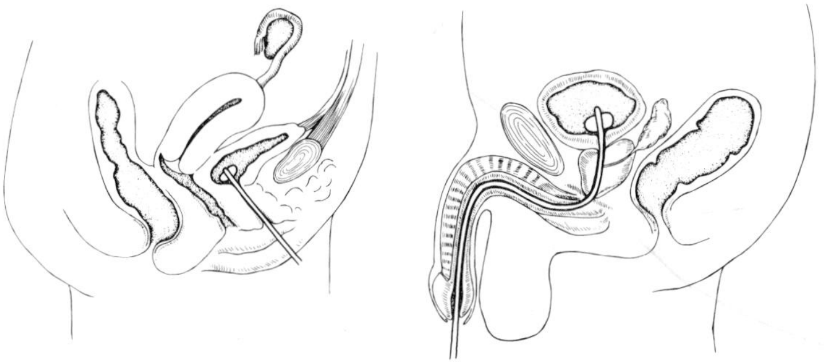

STEP 26 a(4)

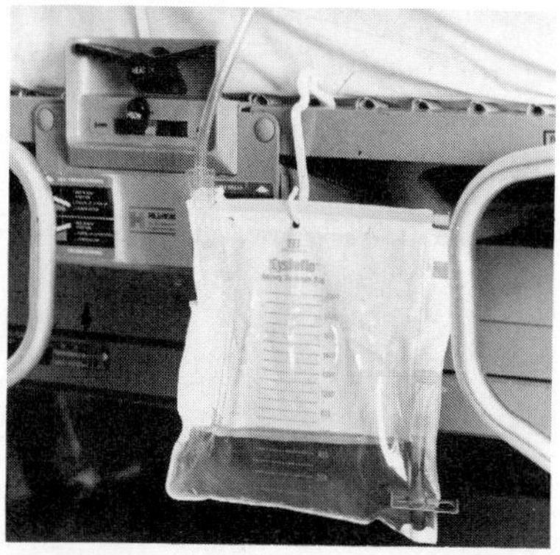

Continued.

SKILL 33-1

CATHETERIZATION: MALE OR FEMALE—cont'd

DOCUMENTATION

Sample charting

DATE	TIME	NOTES
8/28/90	8:45	Patient catheterized with #16 Foley catheter with 6 ml balloon inflated. Catheter taped to right thigh. Urine flow continuous without resistance. 300 ml of clear, amber urine obtained on insertion. Constant drainage bag attached and secured to bed frame. Urine specimen sent to laboratory. Patient tolerated procedure well. Side effects outlined for patient.

____
(nurse's signature)

SPECIAL CONCERNS

The following should be considered when caring for a patient with a catheter:

- Position patient for continuing flow of urine.
- Position constant drainage system to ensure flow of urine.
- Keep accurate output.
- Never disconnect the catheter except to irrigate; irrigate only with physician's order.
- Closed drainage system prevents contamination.
- Never elevate drainage bag above level of the patient's bladder or cavity being drained; teach the patient to carry the drainage bag at arm's length while ambulating.
- Attach drainage bag to bed frame; do not attach to side rails.
- Never allow drainage tubing or bag to touch floor.
- Check tubing for kinks or occlusions.
- Check drainage system for leaks or holes in plastic.
- Be sensitive to patient's feelings regarding catheter and constant drainage system.
- Determine level of understanding for need of catheter and limitation of movement with catheter.

PATIENT TEACHING

The catheterized patient should be instructed on the following:

- Caution patient not to lie on drainage tubing.
- Explain the side effects of a nonfunctioning catheter.
- Explain the importance of holding the catheter bag at arm's length while ambulating.
- Teach the need to report untoward signs and symptoms, such as a burning sensation, pressure in the bladder, elevated temperature, and chills.

SKILL 33-2 CATHETER CARE

1. Introduce self.
2. Identify patient by checking identification band.
3. Explain procedure to the patient.
4. Close door and draw curtains to provide privacy.
5. Wash hands.
6. Place waterproof disposable pad under patient's buttocks and to the side from which catheter care will be given.
7. Position patient
   a. Male: supine position
   b. Female: dorsal recumbent position
8. Drape patient with bath blanket exposing perineal area.
9. Open sterile supplies, using sterile technique, and arrange on bedside table.
10. Put on sterile gloves.
11. Place sterile drape over patient's perineum.
12. Hold cotton balls over container and pour antiseptic solution over them. Place in sterile basin or container.
13. With one hand expose urethral meatus:
    a. Male: retract foreskin; then hold penis erect.
    b. Female: gently retract labia minora away from urinary meatus, and hold in position.
14. Observe meatus, catheter, and surrounding tissue to assess normal or abnormal condition; determine presence or absence of inflammation, edema, malodorous exudate, color of tissue, burning sensation.
15. Wash the area at the meatus and around catheter with cotton balls:
    a. Male:
       (1) With one cotton ball cleanse around meatus and catheter in a circular motion.
       (2) Repeat two more times, using different cotton balls each time.
    b. Female:
       (1) With one cotton ball swab to one side of labia minora from anterior to posterior of anal area.
       (2) Repeat with second cotton ball on opposite side.
       (3) Repeat with third cotton ball down middle over meatus and around catheter; do not bring cotton ball up once descent has begun.
16. Discard soiled cotton balls in other basin in container.
17. With forceps, pick up cotton ball soaked in antiseptic solution and cleanse around catheter from urethral opening to approximately 10 cm (4 inches) to clean catheter of exudate.
18. Apply antibiotic ointment per physician's protocol to meatus and along catheter for 2.5 cm (1 inch).
19. Collect soiled material from bedside table and waterproof absorbent pad; discard into paper bag.
20. Remove drape; place in laundry hamper.
21. Remove gloves, and discard into plastic bag.
22. Retape or strap catheter to thigh to prevent trauma and pain from tension and pulling.
23. Reposition patient.
24. Check flow of urine through tubing.
25. Answer patient's questions about procedure.
26. Dispose of plastic bag.
27. Wash hands.
28. Document procedure.
29. Report any unusual findings immediately.

DOCUMENTATION
Sample charting

DATE	TIME	NOTES
12/6/90	10:00	Catheter care given. Large amount of dried, yellow exudate around catheter at meatus. Repeated cleansing of area with antiseptic solution until clean. Tissue area erythematous and edematous. Catheter draining clear amber urine. T 99.2 po, P 88, R 22. Reported to D. McClellan, RN.

____
(nurse's signature)

SPECIAL CONCERNS

The following should be considered when caring for the patient with a catheter:

- Provide intake for patient.
- Maintain intake and output record.
- Check patient's temperature every 4 hours for 24 hours if odor or exudate is present.

PATIENT TEACHING

The catheterized patient should be instructed on the following:

- Explain the need for the patient to drink fluids.
- Explain the need for meticulous catheter care.

SKILL 33-3

CATHETER IRRIGATION: OPEN, INTERMITTENT, CONTINUOUS

1. Introduce self.
2. Identify patient by checking identification band.
3. Explain procedure to patient.
4. Close door and draw curtains to provide privacy.
5. Wash hands.
6. Place waterproof absorbent pad under patient's buttocks and to the side from which bladder irrigation will be done.
7. Position patient
   a. Male: supine position
   b. Female: dorsal recumbent position
8. Drape patient with bath blanket, exposing perineal area.
9. Open sterile supplies using sterile technique, and arrange on bedside table.
10. Open method
    a. Pour sterile irrigating solution (sterile normal saline is used as an irrigating solution unless otherwise specified) into sterile graduated container, and recap solution bottle.
    b. Don sterile gloves.
    c. Place sterile basin between patient's legs, close to perineal area.
    d. Disconnect catheter from drainage system, and plug drainage tubing with sterile plug.
    e. Draw up 30 ml of sterile solution into syringe.
    f. Cleanse end of catheter with antiseptic swab.
    g. Place tip of syringe into end of catheter and gently inject solution.
    h. Withdraw plunger, and allow solution to drain into basin by gravity.
    i. If solution does not return, turn patient on side facing nurse.
    j. Repeat injection of solution until amount ordered is injected and returned.
    k. Remove plug from drainage tubing, and connect tubing to catheter.
    l. Measure solution to determine amount returned and amount of urine expelled.
11. Intermittent method (repeat steps 1 through 8 as described)
    a. Pour sterile irrigating solution (sterile normal saline is used as an irrigating solution unless otherwise specified) into graduated container.
    b. Draw up sterile solution into syringe.
    c. Clamp catheter below injection port.
    d. Cleanse port with antiseptic swab.
    e. Insert needle of syringe into port.
    f. Slowly inject solution into catheter to avoid bladder spasm and to dislodge clots, sediment, or other material.
    g. Remove syringe and clamp.
12. Continuous method
    a. Set up irrigating solution by attaching tubing to bag.
    b. Clamp off tubing so no solution flows through.
    c. Hang bag on IV pole.
    d. Open clamp, and allow solution to flow through tubing.
    e. Cleanse irrigating lumen on end of triple-lumen catheter.
    f. Connect irrigating solution tubing to catheter lumen.
    g. Restore flow as ordered; calculate drip.
    h. Deduct solution from urine in drainage bag when emptying.
13. Collect soiled material and waterproof absorbent pad; discard into plastic bag.
14. Remove bath blanket; place in laundry hamper.
15. Remove gloves, and discard into plastic bag.
16. Reposition patient.
17. Check flow of urine through drainage tubing.
18. Wash hands.
19. Record urine output on intake and output record.
20. Answer patient's questions about procedure.
21. Document procedure.
22. Report any unusual findings immediately.

SKILL 33-3

CATHETER IRRIGATION: OPEN, INTERMITTENT, CONTINUOUS—cont'd

DOCUMENTATION

Sample charting

DATE	TIME	NOTES
12/6/90	8:30	Continuous catheter irrigation started with 1000 ml normal saline at 20 gtt per min. Urine return light pink; layered in the tubing, had several small, dark, red clots. Urine flow is slow and constant. Patient tolerating procedure well. Encouraged patient to drink fluids.

____

(nurse's signature)

SPECIAL CONCERNS

The following should be considered when caring for the patient with a catheter:

- Provide intake for patient.
- Maintain intake and output record.
- Inject solution slowly into bladder, and allow to drain by gravity so as not to cause trauma or collapse bladder.

PATIENT TEACHING

The catheterized patient should be instructed on the following:

- Explain the need for the patient to drink fluids.
- Identify the side effects that may occur, and explain the need to report them immediately.

SKILL 33-4 DISCONTINUING A FOLEY CATHETER

1. Introduce self.
2. Identify patient by checking identification band.
3. Explain the procedure to the patient.
4. Close door and draw curtains.
5. Wash hands.
6. Place waterproof absorbent pad under patient's buttocks and to the side in which catheter will be removed.
7. Arrange supplies on bedside table.
8. Don sterile gloves.
9. Wash meatus and around catheter with sterile cotton balls soaked in antiseptic solution as per Skill 33-2.
10. Collect urine specimen, if ordered. Clamp off drainage between catheter and drainage tubing for about 15 minutes before collecting specimen. Leave drainage tubing intact and clamp tubing with rubber band. This allows adequate amount of urine (about 5 to 10 ml) for specimen collection. Cleanse port with antiseptic solution. Insert 22-gauge needle attached to 10 ml syringe into port of catheter. Urine will return in syringe when nurse pulls back on plunger. Place urine into correctly labeled sterile specimen container.
11. Deflate balloon by:
    a. Cleansing valve outlet with antiseptic solution on a swab.
    b. Inserting the barrel of a syringe into the tube extension used for inflating the catheter.
    c. Aspirating the fluid used to inflate the balloon.
    d. Being sure amount of fluid removed is same as amount inserted.
    e. Second method used by some institutions:
       (1) The balloon is emptied by cutting the tube extension used for inflating the catheter.
       (2) The liquid from the balloon is drained into an emesis basin or medication cup.
12. Place syringe in emesis basin; dispose of properly.
13. Carefully withdraw catheter out of meatus.
14. Inspect the catheter to be certain no remnants have remained in bladder; report promptly to charge nurse if this has occurred.
15. Untape catheter from patient's thigh.
16. Observe color of urine, condition of meatus. Check for abnormalities, infection, or other unusual effects.
17. Place catheter, urinary drainage tubing, and urinary drainage bag in plastic disposable bag.
18. Wash meatus with cotton balls soaked in antiseptic solution.
19. Remove urine from urinary drainage bag, and record amount of urine on intake and output sheet.
20. Remove and discard waterproof pad, gloves, urinary drainage system, catheter, and cotton balls into plastic disposable bag.
21. Discard syringe in special container.
22. Label urine specimen with patient's name, date, and other pertinent information, and send to the laboratory.
23. Explain to the patient the effects of catheter removal and need to drink fluids. Explain the need for the nurse to measure the voided urine. Check to see if the patient has questions.
24. Document procedure.
25. Report any unusual findings immediately.

DOCUMENTATION

Sample charting

DATE	TIME	NOTES
12/10/90	10:00	Urine specimen obtained from catheter port and sent to laboratory. Urine clear, amber color. 6 ml of solution aspirated from balloon valve. A #16 Foley catheter with a 6 ml deflated bag removed intact. Patient c/o slight burning sensation. 350 ml clear, amber urine in drainage bag. Encouraged patient to drink fluids and to be certain urine output is measured. Side effects outlined for the patient.

(nurse's signature)

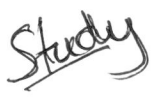

SKILL 33-4 DISCONTINUING A FOLEY CATHETER—cont'd

SPECIAL CONCERNS

The following should be considered when discontinuing the catheter:

- Provide fluid intake for patient.
- Provide easy access to bedpan, urinal, bedside commode, or bathroom with urine collection device.
- If bed patient, provide nurse call signal within reach.
- Maintain intake and output record.
- Check patient's temperature every 4 hours for 24 hours.
- When patient voids, check time, amount, color, and consistency.

PATIENT TEACHING

The patient should be instructed on the following when the Foley catheter has been removed:

- Explain to patient that it will take time for the urinary bladder to reestablish voluntary control of urine.
- Describe how to collect and measure urine output and the need for same.
- Explain the need for the patient to drink fluids.
- Tell the patient that it is common to feel some burning or discomfort in the meatal area when first voiding.
- Identify the side effects that may occur, and explain the need to report them immediately.

– Know Double Voided Specimen +1

fection. Observe the color and composition of the urine to note any blood or sediment. During drainage of the collection bag note the presence of malodor.

12. Collect specimens from the catheter by cleansing the drainage port with alcohol, then withdrawing the urine by using a sterile needle and a sterile 10 ml syringe using universal precautions. Send the urine specimen immediately to the laboratory.

After the urinary catheter is removed the patient may experience difficulty voiding until bladder tone and sensation return. If the patient complains of urinary retention, the nurse should institute the following measures:

1. If necessary, urination may be stimulated by running water, placing the patient's hands in water, or pouring water over the perineum. If the last method is attempted, the amount of water used should be subtracted in calculating the correct amount voided.
2. If the patient's condition permits, it is preferable, if female, to sit on a bathroom stool or commode, or if male, to stand to void.

The patient may experience some dribbling of urine after voiding as a result of dilation of the sphincter from the catheter. The time, amount, and color of the urine output should be recorded.

NURSING DIAGNOSES	NURSING INTERVENTIONS
Potential for trauma, related to insertion and maintenance of the catheter	Lubricate catheter. Secure catheter to leg. Move drainage bag when transferring patient. Provide adequate fluids. Administer urinary analgesic as ordered.

NURSING DIAGNOSES	NURSING INTERVENTIONS
Potential for infection, related to invasive use of catheter	Use aseptic technique. Complete meticulous catheter care. Administer antimicrobials as ordered. Keep urinary drainage system closed and patent. Avoid reflux of urine.

Patient education. The patient should be instructed about proper transfer from bed, chair, or stretcher and taught the principles of catheter care. Fluid intake should be encouraged to flush the urinary system.

Self-catheterization. Self-catheterization may be the intervention of choice for the patient who experiences spinal cord injury or other neurological disorders that interfere with urinary elimination. Intermittent self-catheterization promotes more independent function for the patient. At home there is less risk of cross-contamination than in the hospital, so the catheterization procedure can be safely modified as a clean technique, although the nurse will instruct the patient using strict surgical asepsis in the hospital because of the risk of infection there. The need for the patient to be alert for signs of infection and to have periodic evaluation by the physician should be emphasized. Institutional guidelines for catheter insertion technique should be followed.

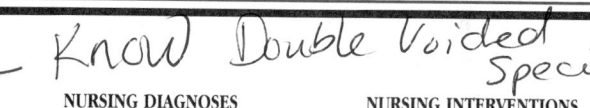

Bladder training. Bladder training involves developing the use of the muscles of the perineum to improve voluntary control over voiding; bladder training may be modified for different problems. In preparation for the removal of a urethral catheter, the physician may order a clamp/unclamp routine to improve bladder tone. For the patient with stress incontinence, the muscles of the perineum are exercised to assist in stopping urine flow. The nurse instructs the patient to perform Kegel or pubococcygeal exercises by tightening the muscles of the perineal floor. The patient can perhaps develop awareness of the appropriate muscle group by trying to stop the flow of urine during voiding. Having identified the correct muscles and the feeling of their contraction, the patient can be directed to tighten the muscles of the perineum, holding that tension for 10 seconds, then relaxing for 10 seconds. The exercises should be done initially in groups of 10, building to groups of 20, four times a day. Because muscle control develops gradually, it may take 4 to 6 weeks to develop measurable control of urine leakage.

For habit training, a voiding schedule is established. The nurse monitors the patient's voiding for a few days to identify patterns, or schedules voiding times to correlate with the patient's activities. Typical voiding times are on arising, before each meal, and at bedtime. The patient is assisted to void as scheduled. After a few days, the scheduled voiding pattern is evaluated by identifying its effectiveness in keeping the patient continent. The schedule is modified until continence is established. Fluid intake and medications may influence voiding patterns (that is, the patient may need to void 30 minutes after the ingestion of coffee or furosemide [Lasix] in response to the diuretic effect). Reduction of fluid intake during the hours preceding bedtime may aid in keeping the patient dry during sleep.

Alterations in Voiding Patterns

Urinary retention

Etiology/pathophysiology. Urinary **retention** is the inability to void even in the presence of an urge to void. The condition may be acute or chronic. With urinary retention the patient may not be able to empty the bladder, creating urinary stasis and increasing the possibility of infection.

Urinary retention may occur from a variety of causes: secondarily in response to stress; interference with the sphincter muscles during surgery to the perineum; occlusion of the urethra by calculi, infection, or tumor; medication side effects; or perineal trauma secondary to vaginal delivery. With chronic urinary retention the bladder capacity may be exceeded and the urine may overflow the bladder, causing incontinence.

Clinical manifestations. The signs and symptoms of urinary retention are sometimes vague and easily overlooked. The bladder becomes increasingly distended and may be palpated above the symphysis pubis. Urinary retention may cause the patient considerable discomfort and anxiety.

Assessment. Collection of *subjective data* includes noting patient complaints of frequency with or without symptoms of burning, urgency, and nocturia, and occasionally acute discomfort. Initial symptoms may not seem to be directly associated with urinary retention. Patients with diminished sensorium, as from spinal cord injury or organic brain disorder, may show signs of restlessness and irritability without direct complaints about difficulty voiding.

Collection of *objective data* includes assessing urinary bladder distention: palpable ovoid (egg-shaped) bladder, arising suprapubically, voiding frequently, voiding small amounts, and episodes of incontinence.

Medical management. Mechanical methods, such as the use of urinary catheters or surgical release of obstructions, may be necessary for the treatment of urinary retention. Urinary analgesics and antispasmodics are administered as prescribed to enhance relaxation.

Nursing interventions. The primary goal of nursing intervention is the reinstitution of normal voiding patterns. Regardless of the pathological findings and medical intervention, the nurse can greatly aid in the reinstitution of adequate voiding by supporting the patient's efforts with a private, relaxed environment. Bladder training approaches may assist the patient to empty his bladder. Warm showers or sitz baths may promote relaxation of the abdominal, gluteal, and sphincter muscles. Warm beverages may help the patient relax. If possible, the patient should be permitted to position himself in the most typical position for voiding: for the female sitting on a commode or bathroom stool is best; for the male standing may be more natural.

When continence is established, the patient may be catheterized intermittently to determine whether the bladder is emptying. The patient should void, and the amount should be measured. Immediately after the voiding the patient should be catheterized and the amount measured. The amount retained in the bladder is **residual urine** and should be less than 50 ml. If the underlying pathological condition remains unchanged, this patient may still be at risk for again developing retention; it is therefore important to teach the patient and/or primary caretaker to be observant for signs and symptoms of urinary retention and to notify the physician immediately if they return.

NURSING DIAGNOSES	NURSING INTERVENTIONS
Altered patterns of urinary elimination, related to sensory/motor impairment, neuromuscular impairment, or mechanical trauma	Establish urinary drainage. Develop voiding schedule. Teach Kegel exercises. Assist with skin care. Use protective clothing. Engage patient in social activities.

Urinary incontinence

Etiology/pathophysiology. Urinary incontinence is the involuntary loss of urine from the bladder. The patient may be totally incontinent, have dribbling, or experience leakage while lifting or sneezing (stress incontinence).

Incontinence may arise as a complication of many disorders, such as infection within the urinary tract, loss of sphincter control, or sudden change in the pressure within the abdomen. Incontinence may be permanent, as with spinal cord trauma, or temporary, as with pregnancy. Women with weakened structures of the pelvic floor are prone to stress incontinence. Although incontinence may occur in patients of any age, loss of control of urination is a particular problem for the elderly.

Clinical manifestations. The cardinal symptom of urinary incontinence is the involuntary loss of urine, which may or may not be the primary reason the patient seeks treatment.

Assessment. Collection of *subjective data* includes noting the patient's inability to control his urine. A woman may complain of urine leaking when she coughs, sneezes, or lifts heavy objects.

Collection of *objective data* includes the nurse being alert for clues that the patient is experiencing difficulty controlling the flow of urine. The assessment guidelines should be followed to clarify the patient's complaints.

Medical management. The management of incontinence depends on the underlying cause. If the problem arises from a disorder within the neck of the bladder, surgical repair may be necessary. The patient may require temporary or permanent urinary diversion or management with an indwelling catheter.

Nursing interventions. Bladder training exercises should be taught to improve the tone of the perineal muscles. Use of protective undergarments may help keep the patient and his clothing dry.

Neurogenic bladder

Etiology/pathophysiology. Neurogenic bladder means the loss of voluntary voiding control, resulting in urinary retention or incontinence. Neurogenic bladder is caused by a lesion of the nervous system that interferes with normal nerve conduction to the urinary bladder. The lesion may be caused by a congenital anomaly, such as spina bifida, a neurological disease, such as multiple sclerosis, or trauma, as in spinal cord injury. The two types of neurogenic bladder are *spastic* and *flaccid*.

Spastic (reflex or automatic) bladder is caused by a lesion above the voiding reflex arc (upper motor neuron) that results in a loss of sensation to void and a loss of motor control. The bladder wall then atrophies, decreasing bladder capacity. Release of the urine occurs on reflex, with little or no conscious control.

A flaccid (atonic, nonreflex) bladder, caused by a lesion of a lower motor neuron, continues to fill and distend, with pooling of urine and incomplete emptying. Because of the accompanying loss of sensation, the patient may not even experience discomfort that would indicate retention.

Clinical manifestations. Identification of the disease process is the first step in assessing the potential problem of neurogenic bladder. Prevention of complications is a major concern; infection occurs from urinary stasis and repeated catheterization. Retention of urine may lead to backup of urine (reflux) into the upper urinary tract and to the distention of the structures of the urinary tract. Renal failure is the leading cause of death in patients with neurogenic bladder.

Assessment. Collection of *subjective data* includes noting patient complaints consistent with the pathophysiology of the neurogenic bladder. The patient with a spastic bladder will experience urinary incontinence, whereas the patient with a flaccid bladder will describe infrequent voiding. Signs and symptoms of the presence of an infection may not be evident because of the patient's decreased nerve sensation.

Collection of *objective data* involves investigating the urinary status of the patient at risk for neurogenic bladder; this includes patients with a congenital anomaly, a neurological disease, or a spinal cord injury.

Diagnostic tests. Diagnostic testing is completed to assess the type and extent of damage to the urinary tract; chemistry studies monitor change in BUN and creatinine levels. X-ray studies outline structural changes that occur.

Medical management. Identification of patients at high risk for neurogenic bladder should be closely monitored. Assessment of urinary function should be started early in the course of treatment and antibiotics should be given to treat signs of infection. The patient is aided by the use of parasympathomimetic medication (for example, bethanechol chloride [Urecholine]) to increase the contractility of the bladder. It may be necessary for the patient to use intermittent self-catheterization or a urinary collection system if continence is not achieved.

Nursing interventions. The goal for management of the patient with neurogenic bladder is to establish urinary elimination and prevent complications. Because of the disturbance of neurological function, it may not be possible to reinstate normal voiding function. The patient with a spastic bladder may be placed on a bladder training program, with self-stimulation used every 2 hours to empty the bladder: the patient tries to initiate voiding by compressing the bladder by applying pressure to the abdomen suprapubically or by digital stimulation of the anal sphincter. Residual urine is then measured by catheterization. As the patient becomes more proficient in emptying the bladder, the times between the catheterizations are increased until voiding is achieved independently.

It is important to educate the patient to be alert for signs of the bladder becoming distended.

Management of the patient with a flaccid bladder is similar. The patient may be placed on a 2-hour voiding schedule for bladder training. Issues of self-esteem are crucial for this patient to remain in social settings. The nurse should provide a supportive, sensitive environment for the patient to discuss ways he can adapt to an altered self-image.

Surgical Procedures for Urinary Dysfunction

If damage to the urinary system cannot be corrected by medical management, surgical intervention may be necessary for temporary or permanent resection of the affected organ, such as when kidney function is lost. Dialysis is a viable management alternative, but a kidney transplant is preferable. It may become necessary for the patient to have a live or cadaver kidney replace the damaged kidney. Common surgical interventions and nursing intervention priorities are listed in Table 33-3. Preoperative and intraoperative management measures are the same as for major abdominal surgery and general anesthesia (see Chapter 26). Suggested nursing diagnoses include those for abdominal surgery.

Nephrectomy. Nephrectomy is the surgical removal of the kidney. Postoperative management for surgical removal of the kidney is based on the prevention and detection of hemorrhage by monitoring vital signs, especially pulse and blood pressure; observation for restlessness, gastrointestinal complications of nausea, vomiting, and abdominal distention; and establishment of adequate urinary drainage. Intake and output are recorded. If the thoracic cavity is opened during surgery, the patient will have chest tubes. Pain may compromise respiratory efficiency. Analgesics are administered as ordered to facilitate lung expansion and the patient's activity level. The patient is repositioned every 2 hours and ambulated as ordered. Dressings are changed according to the physician's order, and the amount and color of exudate are recorded.

Patient teaching. This includes instructing the patient to avoid heavy lifting, maintain hydration of 2000 ml each day unless contraindicated, monitor output, avoid use of alcohol, and avoid respiratory infections and hazardous activities that may cause assault to the remaining kidney.

Nephrostomy. Nephrostomy is an incision to drain the pelvis of the kidney. Catheters are used to drain the wound. Care must be given to prevent obstruction of the catheters with blood clots postoperatively. The amount of drainage from the catheters is measured and recorded, and dressings are changed frequently, keeping the skin clean using surgical asepsis. The patient is turned and positioned to the affected side when ordered to facilitate drainage and assist in respiratory ventilation. Irrigation of a nephrostomy catheter is a physician's procedure.

Kidney transplantation. There are special considerations for nursing interventions for a kidney transplantation recipient. Preoperative nursing intervention is complicated by the patient's fear and anxiety about transplantation and about possible rejection of the implanted organ. The patient is dialyzed until surgery can be satisfactorily completed. In surgery the nonfunctioning kidney remains in place and the donor kidney is positioned in the iliac fossa anterior to the crest of the ileum. The ureter is anastomosed into either the patient's ureter or bladder (Fig. 33-7).

Postoperatively the patient is assessed for signs of rejection and infection: apprehension, generalized edema, fever, increased blood pressure, **oliguria,** edema, and/or tenderness over the graft site. An immunosuppressive therapeutic agent, such as cyclosporine (Sandimmune), is used alone or in conjunction with steroids. Cyclosporine is considered the most effective drug to date in suppressing the immune system's efforts to reject tissue while leaving the recipient sufficient immune activity to combat infection. Immunosuppressive therapy increases the risk for infection and possible steroid-induced bleeding.

Patient teaching. Home follow-up becomes a life pattern for the transplantation patient. Patient education is

Table 33-3 Surgical Interventions and Nursing Intervention Priorities

Surgical Intervention	Nursing Intervention Priorities
Nephrostomy—surgical procedure in which an incision is made on the flank of patient so a catheter can be inserted into the kidney pelvis for drainage	Meticulous skin care, assessment for hemorrhage, accurate intake/output
Nephrectomy—surgical removal of kidney	Assessment for hemorrhage, promote respiratory effort, accurate intake/output
Cystectomy—surgical removal of bladder	Promote urinary drainage via ileoconduit, intake/output
Ureterosigmoidostomy—surgical procedure in which a ureter is implanted in the sigmoid colon of the intestinal tract	Meticulous skin care, monitor electrolyte imbalance, assess for signs and symptoms of infection
Cutaneous ureterostomy—surgical implantation of the terminal ends of the ureter under the skin	Meticulous skin care, assess for urinary obstruction, accurate intake/output

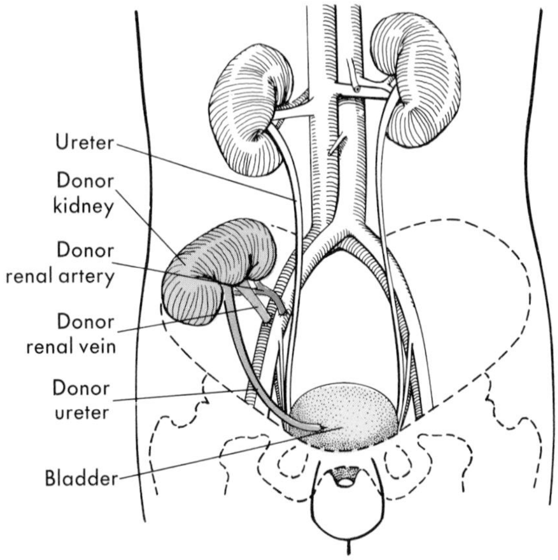

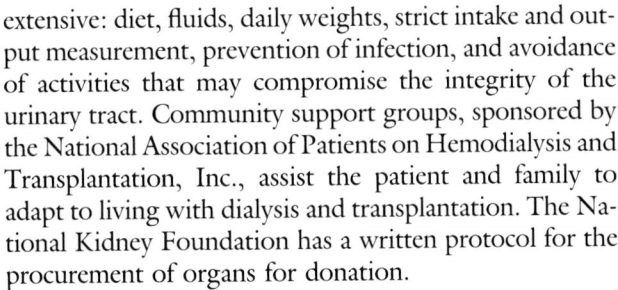

FIG. 33-7 Location of transplanted kidney showing anastomosis of renal artery, renal vein, and ureter.

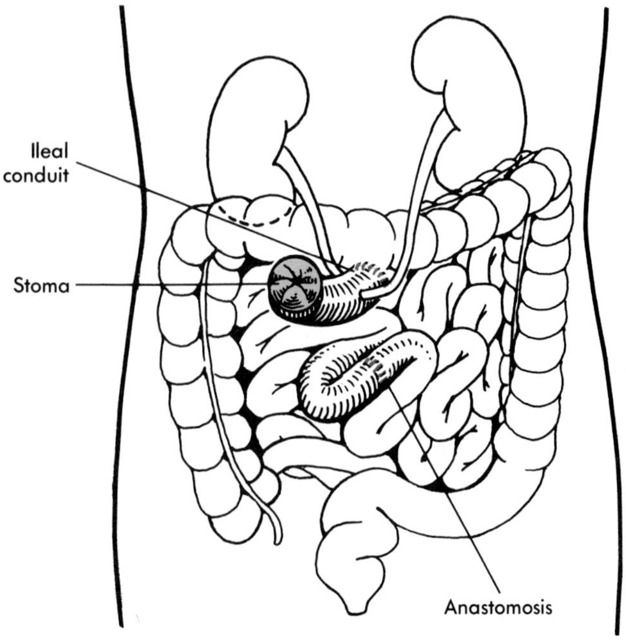

FIG. 33-8 Ileal conduit or ileal loop.

extensive: diet, fluids, daily weights, strict intake and output measurement, prevention of infection, and avoidance of activities that may compromise the integrity of the urinary tract. Community support groups, sponsored by the National Association of Patients on Hemodialysis and Transplantation, Inc., assist the patient and family to adapt to living with dialysis and transplantation. The National Kidney Foundation has a written protocol for the procurement of organs for donation.

Urinary diversion. Several types of procedures are used to divert the flow of urine when required for treatment of bladder cancer, invasive cancer of the cervix, neurogenic bladder, and congenital anomalies. Often a cystectomy is done to surgically remove the bladder.

The cystectomy patient presents a unique challenge because of the need to create an artificial port for urine elimination. The most common urinary diversion procedure is the *ileal conduit* (Bricker's procedure or ileal loop). In an ileal conduit procedure the ureters are implanted into a loop of the ileum that is isolated and brought to the surface of the abdominal wall (Fig. 33-8). Occasionally a segment of the sigmoid colon is isolated and used instead of the ileum (sigmoid conduit). The integrity of bowel function is maintained with the anastomosis of the remaining intestine. A drainage bag (urostomy bag or appliance) is fitted over the stoma to contain the constant drainage of urine. Continual urine drainage prevents increased pressure within the conduit that would cause backflow to the kidneys, compromise the circulatory integrity of the conduit, or rupture the surgical anastomosis. Decreased urine output and low abdominal pain may signal the onset of such problems. Complications of this procedure are wound infection or dehiscence, urinary leakage, ureteral obstruction, small bowel obstruction, stomal gangrene, contraction of the stoma, pyelonephritis, renal calculi, and/or a compromised respiratory state resulting from pain from the flank incision.

Postoperatively, urine flow is measured hourly. Output below 30 ml per hour should be reported to the physician immediately. A healthy stoma will appear moist and pink and may even bleed slightly. The skin around the stoma should be inspected daily for signs of bleeding, excoriation, and infection. Any odor of urine about the patient may indicate an infection or leak of urine from the drainage bag. Large quantities of water should be ingested to flush the ileal conduit. There will be mucus present in the urine from the intestinal secretions.

Care of the patient with an ileal conduit is a nursing challenge because of the continual leakage of urine through the stoma.

To change the urostomy bag, the urostomy bag is drained and removed. The skin is cleansed with water, and the new appliance is applied as outlined in the institution's standards of care. (See Chapter 31 for a discussion on stomal care.) When the stoma is healed, the bag is emptied at 2- to 3-hour intervals and a straight drainage tube connected to a drainage bag is used at night. A permanent urostomy bag can be left in place 4 to 7 days if it remains sealed. The nurse should recommend that the patient have two bags so one can be worn while the other is washed. Odor is controlled by using deodorant drops or tablets in the urostomy bag, avoiding

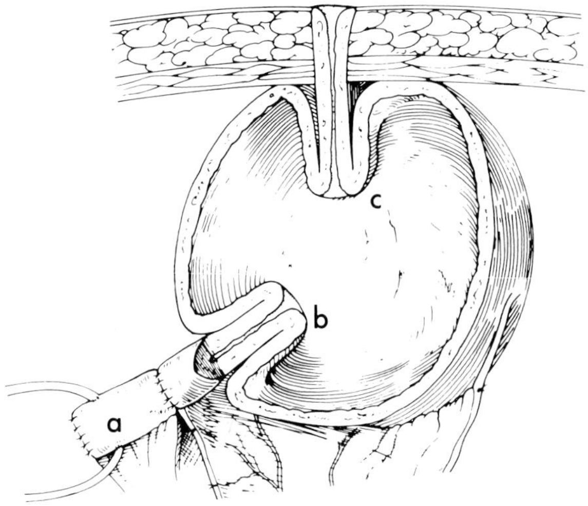

FIG. 33-9 Kock continent ileal reservoir: *a,* original ileal conduit with implanted ureters; *b,* reflux-preventing nipple valve; *c,* continence-maintaining nipple valve. (From Gerber A: J Enterostom Ther 12:15, 1985.)

odor-producing foods, such as beans, onions, cabbage, asparagus, high-fiber wheat, simple sugars, and milk in the lactose-intolerant patient, and cleansing the urostomy bag with a vinegar and water rinse and thoroughly drying.

Patient teaching. Patient teaching centers on the task of life-style adaptation: care of the stoma, nutrition, fluid intake, maintaining self-esteem in light of altered body image, modifying sexual activities, and early detection of complications. Patient teaching begins with appliance selection, sizing the stoma, and changing the appliance. The home health nurse can assist the patient in modifying his care to his home environment and by providing support during this stressful adjustment period.

The continent ileal urinary reservoir, or Kock pouch, is the implantation of the ureters into a segment of the small intestine that has been surgically removed from the rest of the bowel and anastomosed to the abdominal wall. Control of urine flow is achieved by the use of a nipplelike valve that prevents leakage of urine. To drain the urine from the reservoir, the patient inserts a catheter through the valve at regular intervals, thus minimizing the reabsorption of waste materials from the urine and reflux into the ureters (Fig. 33-9).

Urinary Tract Infections

Of nosocomial infections, 40% involve the urinary tract, with perhaps more than 75% of those associated with the use of urinary catheters. Urinary tract infection (UTI) is common in elderly patients, related to bladder obstruction or improper hygiene, and as a complication of acute and chronic illnesses. Immobility and sensory and multiple organ impairment may increase the probability of infection in the elderly. UTIs are second in frequency only to respiratory infections in children. Females are susceptible to UTIs because the urethra is short and proximal to the vagina and rectum.

Etiology/pathophysiology. UTIs are caused by pathogens that enter the urinary tract, with or without the presence of symptoms. Normally the flushing of the urinary tract with urine is sufficient to keep pathogens washed away. However, some conditions interfere with this process; urinary obstruction, ureterovesical or urethrovesical reflux, sexual intercourse, and catheterization may introduce bacteria into the urinary system. Many chronic health states predispose the patient to a UTI: diabetes mellitus, multiple sclerosis, hypertension, and diseases of the kidney.

Changes in urinary tract homeostasis allow the concentration of bacteria and increase the risk of infection. Risk of infection also increases with age, sexual activity, and impaired innervation. Infections of the lower urinary tract increase the risk of infection of the upper urinary tract.

Gram-negative microorganisms, such as *Escherichia coli, Klebsiella, Proteus,* or *Pseudomonas,* that commonly infect the urinary tract are usually from the gastrointestinal tract and ascend through the urinary meatus. Normally the body's defenses keep infections in check and clear them from the system before symptoms appear. If there is incomplete emptying of the bladder or reflux of urine, the retained urine supports growth of bacteria.

Clinical manifestations. The common symptoms associated with UTI are urgency, frequency, burning on urination, and microscopic to gross (visible without aid of microscope) hematuria. Infections of the urinary tract are identified by the location of the infection: urethritis (urethra), cystitis (urinary bladder), and pyelonephritis (kidney). Infections of the bladder are said to be *lower urinary tract infections*, whereas infections of the kidneys are *upper urinary tract infections*.

Assessment. Collection of *subjective data* includes noting patient complaints of pain or burning on urination, urgency, frequency, and excessive urination at night **(nocturia).** The patient may also relate a general feeling of tiredness and listlessness **(asthenia).** Abdominal discomfort, perineal pain, or back pain may be present, depending on the extent of the disease process and site of infection.

Collection of *objective data* involves palpation of the lower abdomen, which may produce discomfort over the urinary bladder. Urine may appear cloudy or blood tinged.

Diagnostic tests. Urine culture and bacteriology tests confirm the diagnosis. For patients with repeated UTIs or systemic disease, more detailed urological studies, such as an IVU and a voiding cystogram, are completed to assess the extent of involvement and damage to the structures of the urinary tract. Microscopic inspection of the urine often reveals bacteria, hematuria (blood in the urine), and pus **(pyuria).** Prostatitis is confirmed by patient history and culture of prostatic fluid or tissue.

Medical management. The goal of medical management is to eliminate bacteria from the urinary tract, thereby relieving symptoms, preventing damage to renal structures, and preventing spread of infection to other body systems. Antimicrobial medications are prescribed in either oral or parenteral single or multiple doses, depending on the severity of the infection, microbial sensitivity, cost, and the medications the patient can tolerate. Urinary antiseptics, such as methenamine mandelate or hippurate, may be used prophylactically in recurrent infections. Some of these medications are instilled directly into the bladder (Skill 33-5). If the infection is complicated by obstruction, that obstruction should be removed. If the patient experiences neurogenic bladder or other retention, the use of intermittent catheterization would permit urinary drainage.

Nursing interventions. Nursing intervention should be supportive, with patient education for adequate hydration and hygiene. Because there is a strong tendency for these infections to recur by either reinfection or persistent infection, patient education must include early detection. Comfort measures include a regime of antimicrobial agents, urinary analgesics, such as phenazopyridine HCl (Pyridium), adequate fluid intake, and perineal care. If treatment is effective, the patient should receive relief quickly.

Urethritis

Etiology/pathophysiology. Urethritis, inflammation of the urethra, is classified by the presence or absence of gonorrhea. Nongonorrheal urethritis is called *nonspecific urethritis* (NSU). NSU may be caused by monilial or trichomonal infections in women. Bacteria are present normally in the urethra but do not cause problems unless the integrity of the mucous membrane or tissues is interrupted, as when a catheter is in place or trauma has occurred.

Clinical manifestations. The clinical manifestations include inflammation of the urethra with pus formation in the mucus-forming glands within the lining of the urethra. Gonorrheal urethritis is evidenced by acute infection of the mucous membrane of the urethra that causes a purulent exudate from the meatus; the patient feels discomfort and burning on urination.

Assessment. Collection of *subjective data* should be done with an awareness that the patient may be asymptomatic or may complain of dysuria, urethral pruritus, and urethral discharge. Women may present with vaginal discharge or vulvar irritation.

Collection of *objective data* includes inspecting the urethra for purulent exudate or inflammation.

Diagnostic tests. These are usually limited to a Gram stain of the exudate to identify the pathogen.

Medical management. The first step in medical management is prevention of injury to the uretha during catheterization or sexual intercourse. Comfort measures include a regimen of antibiotics, adequate fluid intake to flush the system, and special care of the perineum using clean technique.

Nursing interventions. These should focus on patient education: avoid sexual activity until the infection clears; take all medications, especially antibiotics, to ensure the infection is resolved; use condoms for some protection from reinfection; and instruct sexual partners to be evaluated for urethritis to prevent continuing infections.

Cystitis

Etiology/pathophysiology. Cystitis is an inflammation of the wall of the urinary bladder, usually caused by urethrovesical reflux, introduction of a catheter or similar instrument, or perhaps by contamination from feces.

Cystitis is most common in women; the most common microorganism causing acute cystitis is *E. coli.* Conflicting data exist about the role of bubble baths, clothing, and hygiene in increasing the risk of cystitis in women. Cystitis in men usually occurs secondary to another infection, such as prostatitis or epididymitis.

Clinical manifestations. The common signs and symptoms associated with cystitis are dysuria, urinary frequency, and pyuria.

Assessment. Collection of *subjective data* includes assessment of the lower abdomen, which may detect discomfort over the urinary bladder. Patient complaints include burning on urination, dysuria, frequency, urgency, and nocturia.

Collection of *objective data* includes a clean-catch or

SKILL 33-5 BLADDER INSTILLATION

1. Introduce self.
2. Identify patient by checking identification band.
3. Explain procedure to the patient.
4. Close door and draw curtains to provide privacy.
5. Wash hands.
6. Place waterproof absorbent pad under patient's buttocks and to the side from which bladder instillation will be done.
7. Position patient
   a. Male: supine position
   b. Female: dorsal recumbent position
8. Drape patient with bath blanket, exposing perineal area.
9. Open sterile supplies using sterile technique, and arrange on bedside table.
10. Pour sterile prescribed medication or solution into sterile graduated container.
11. Don sterile gloves.
12. Place sterile basin between patient's legs, close to perineal area.
13. Disconnect catheter from drainage system, and plug drainage tubing with sterile plug to prevent infection.
14. Draw up prescribed amount of medication or solution into syringe.
15. Cleanse end of catheter with antiseptic swab.
16. Place tip of syringe into end of catheter, and inject solution slowly.
17. Clamp off end of catheter with sterile plug for period of time ordered to allow medication or solution to be absorbed by bladder.
18. Unclamp end of catheter, and allow remaining medication or solution to drain out by gravity.
19. Remove plug from drainage tubing, and connect tubing to catheter.
20. Measure solution to determine amount returned and amount of urine expelled.
21. Collect soiled material and waterproof absorbent pad, and discard into plastic bag.
22. Remove bath blanket; place in laundry hamper.
23. Remove gloves, and discard into plastic bag.
24. Reposition patient.
25. Check flow of urine through drainage tubing.
26. Record urine ouput on intake and output record.
27. Answer patient's questions about procedure.
28. Wash hands
29. Document procedure.
30. Report any unusual findings immediately.

DOCUMENTATION

Sample charting

DATE	TIME	NOTES
12/14/90		
	6:30	Penicillin 500 mg in 25 ml sterile water at room temperature instilled into the urinary bladder for 10 minutes. 20 ml returned. Solution returned clear. Flow was slow. Patient tolerated procedure well. Encouraged patient to drink fluids.

____
(nurse's signature)

SPECIAL CONCERNS

The following should be considered when preparing to perform a bladder instillation:

- Provide intake for patient.
- Maintain intake and output record.
- Triple-lumen catheter does not require disconnecting catheter from drainage tubing.
- Inject solution slowly into bladder, and allow to drain by gravity so as not to cause trauma or collapse bladder.

PATIENT TEACHING

The patient receiving a bladder instillation should be instructed on the following:

- Explain the need for the patient to drink fluids.
- Identify the side effects that may occur, and explain the need to report them immediately.

catheterized urinalysis with culture and sensitivity to aid in confirming the diagnosis and in determining the appropriate treatment.

Diagnostic tests. Microscopic inspection of the urine often reveals bacteria, hematuria, and pus. A voiding cystogram may be used to identify reflux of urine into the bladder. Diagnosis is confirmed by a clean-catch, midstream urinalysis that reveals a bacterial count greater than 100,000 organisms/ml. The most commonly found organism is *Staphylococcus* or *Candida*.

Medical management. For cystitis without the complications of obstruction or other underlying pathological conditions, medical management consists of single-dose or short-term therapy with an antimicrobial agent. If the treatment is effective, the patient should receive relief quickly. A repeat urinalysis 1 to 3 days after the initiation of the medication confirms the effectiveness of the intervention.

Nursing interventions. This should focus on teaching because there is a strong tendency for these infections to recur by either reinfection or persistent infection. The patient should be encouraged to drink 2000 ml of fluid per day. Accurate intake and output should be recorded.

Patient teaching. Teaching must include early detection. Long-term prophylaxis with low doses of medication may be necessary. Currently available is a simple urine test, Chem Strip LN, which allows the patient to test his own urine at the first sign of infection and to call the physician for a prescription.

Prostatitis

Etiology/pathophysiology. Prostatitis, inflammation of the prostate gland, occurs from infectious organisms such as bacteria or fungi traveling up the urethra, or from a variety of other reasons related to occlusion of the urethra (e.g., enlargement of the prostate gland).

Clinical manifestations. The patient experiences a burning sensation, discomfort in the perineum, dysuria, frequency, and urgency. Edema of the prostate gland may serve as an obstruction, causing urinary retention as a complication to the prostatitis. Pooling of urine may also foster stone formation. Other possible complications include epididymitis, pyelonephritis, or septicemia. Although the patient may be asymptomatic, the symptoms of acute bacterial prostatitis are usually those of a UTI with pain in the low back, perineum, or rectum. Because of the potential for relapse, the condition may become chronic.

Diagnostic tests. Diagnosis is confirmed by patient history and culture of prostatic fluid or tissue.

Assessment. Collection of *subjective data* includes noting complaints of fever, chills, and low back and perineal pain. Chronic bacterial prostatitis causes dysuria, urgency, frequency, nocturia, and pain in the lower abdomen or back, perineum, or genitalia.

Collection of *objective data* involves palpation of the prostate gland by the physician by rectal examination, which may reveal the prostate to be firm, edematous, and tender.

Medical management. If the condition is infectious, management focuses on control of the infection and prevention of the complications of abscess formation or septicemia. Broad-spectrum antimicrobial therapy is administered for 7 to 10 days. Intravenous antibiotic administration may be necessary to achieve sufficiently high medication levels in the blood and tissues.

Nursing interventions. Regardless of the pathological basis, comfort measures used are analgesics, sitz baths, and stool softeners to reduce pain, edema, spasm, and straining pressure in the pelvis.

Patient teaching. Teaching includes the medication regimen and avoiding alcohol, caffeine, and spicy foods. Sexual arousal and intercourse should be avoided in acute prostatitis; however, intercourse may be beneficial in the treatment of chronic prostatitis. Follow-up with the physician is crucial because of the likelihood that the disorder will become chronic.

Pyelonephritis

Etiology/pathophysiology. Pyelonephritis is an inflammation of the structures of the kidney—the renal pelvis, renal tubules, and interstitial tissue. Pyelonephritis is almost always caused by *E. coli*.

Pyelonephritis is usually seen in association with pregnancy; chronic health problems, such as diabetes mellitus or polycystic or hypertensive kidney disease; insult to the urinary tract from catheterization; or infection, obstruction, or trauma. Careful management of these disorders is important to prevent pyelonephritis.

The kidney becomes edematous and inflamed, and the blood vessels are congested. The urine may be cloudy and contain pus (pyuria), mucus, and blood. Small abscesses may form in the kidney.

Clinical manifestations. Either or both kidneys may be involved in acute pyelonephritis, causing chills, fever, and flank pain. Repeated episodes of pyelonephritis lead to a chronic disease pattern with atrophy of the kidney as the nephrons are destroyed. **Azotemia** (the retention in the blood of excessive amounts of nitrogenous compounds) develops if enough nephrons are nonfunctional.

Assessment. Collection of *subjective data* includes noting that in acute pyelonephritis the patient will become acutely ill, with malaise, chills, elevated temperature, and costovertebral angle pain. In the chronic phase, the patient may show unremarkable symptoms, such as a low-grade fever, nausea, and general malaise.

Collection of *objective data* includes assessing the patient for signs of infection: elevated temperature, pain over the affected kidney, costovertebral angle pain, and pus in the urine. Systemic signs occur as a result of the chronic disease: elevated blood pressure and gastrointestinal irritation.

Diagnostic tests. Diagnosis is confirmed by bacteria and pus in the urine and leukocytosis. A clean-catch or catheterized urinalysis with culture and sensitivity identifies the pathogen and determines appropriate antimicrobial therapy. An IVU will identify the presence of obstruction or degenerative changes caused by the infectious process. Assessment of BUN and creatinine levels of the blood and urine may be used to monitor kidney function.

Nursing interventions. The following nursing diagnosis and interventions are appropriate for the patient with pyelonephritis:

NURSING DIAGNOSIS	NURSING INTERVENTIONS
Altered patterns of urinary elimination, related to infection, and fluid volume excess, secondary to (2°) fluid retention and electrolyte imbalance	Monitor body temperature. Observe urine for cloudy appearance, high specific gravity, and hematuria. Assess for flank pain and tenderness over affected kidney. (The **costovertebral angle** [CVA] is one of two angles that outline a space over the kidneys.) Weigh daily. Institute strict intake and output monitoring. Observe for changes in fluid and electrolytes as evidenced by alteration in mental status, cardiac dysrhythmias, increase in blood pressure, thirst, and fluid retention. Administer urinary analgesics as ordered. Enhance patient comfort with a warm shower, back rubs, and a warm, soothing environment. Antimicrobial agents are used singly or in combination to control bacterial growth.

Patient teaching. The patient should be taught to identify the signs and symptoms of infection—elevated temperature, flank pain, chills, fever, nausea and vomiting, urgency, fatigue, and general malaise. He should also be taught indications, dose, length of course, and side effects of the medications. The nurse should emphasize the importance of follow-up care with the physician on a routine basis and when signs of infection arise.

Obstructive Disorders of the Urinary Tract

Etiology/pathophysiology. Obstruction at any point within the urinary tract can adversely affect function and alter structure. Causes of obstruction include strictures, kinks, cysts, tumors, stones, and prostatic hypertrophy. Obstruction may lead to alterations in blood chemistry and infection as a result of urine stasis, which provides a perfect medium for bacteria to thrive.

Clinical manifestations. The patient may be unaware of any problems initially if the obstruction is partial, allowing urine to drain and kidney function to remain within normal limits. With prostatic hypertrophy the obstructive process may be so gradual that the patient ignores the vague symptom of dull flank pain and seeks medical attention only when urination becomes acutely difficult. Acute pain occurs as the musculature is stretched by increasing pressure from urine accumulation and as muscular contractions increase in an attempt to move urine past the obstruction. This classic symptom is found with renal calculi and is called *renal colic.*

Assessment. Collection of *subjective data* includes noting the initial complaint of the continued need to void, although the patient may be able to void small amounts. Pain may range from dull flank pain to acute, incapacitating pain. Nausea and vomiting often accompany acute pain.

Collection of *objective data* includes noting on physical assessment, if the obstruction is in the bladder, the bladder will be palpable suprapubically because of urine retention. Retention with overflow occurs when the patient is unable to completely empty his urinary bladder and it quickly refills, causing the urge to void again. The nurse should assess time and amount of voidings and the degree of pain.

Diagnostic tests. As a quick evaluation the physician may order a KUB. Other diagnostic tests may include visual examinations with the aid of endoscopy, blood chemistry profile, and other x-ray studies as needed.

Medical management. Initial intervention will be to establish urine drainage and relieve discomfort. Conservative measures include insertion of an indwelling catheter, pain medication (usually narcotic), and an anticholinergic agent to decrease smooth muscle motility. It may be necessary to establish urine drainage surgically by inserting a catheter directly into the bladder through the abdominal wall (suprapubic cystostomy), into a ureter (ureterostomy), or into the kidney (nephrostomy).

Nursing interventions. These procedures require observation for hemorrhage, maintaining aseptic care of the surgical site, and providing a safe environment to prevent injury and infection. Box 33-2 provides general guidelines for the nursing interventions of the patient with urinary obstruction.

Hydronephrosis

Etiology/pathophysiology. **Hydronephrosis** (the dilation of the renal pelvis and calyces) may occur either unilaterally or bilaterally. Hydronephrosis is caused by obstructions of the urinary tract. These obstructions may be located in the lower urinary tract, in the ureters, or in the kidneys. The location of the obstruction will determine whether one or both kidneys are affected.

Obstructions generate pressure from accumulated urine that cannot flow past the obstruction. This pressure may cause functional and anatomical damage to the renal system. The renal pelvis and ureters dilate and hypertro-

BOX 33-2 NURSING INTERVENTION GUIDELINES FOR URINARY OBSTRUCTION

FLUID AND ELECTROLYTE BALANCE

Assess hydration status.
Monitor prescribed fluid replacement.
Monitor serum electrolytes.
Reinforce teaching of prescribed diet.
Maintain accurate intake and output measurements.

PREVENT COMPLICATIONS

Maintain urinary drainage.
Assess character of urine.
Assist with mobility.
Assess knowledge of treatment.

PROMOTE COMFORT

Provide quiet environment.
Alter care plan to meet needs.
Encourage self-care.
Administer medications.

PATIENT TEACHING

Special diet limitations, fluids.
Home medications (dosage, purpose, side effects).
Care of special equipment (catheter, drains).
Follow-up care.

phy. This pressure, if prolonged, causes fibrosis and loss of function in affected nephrons. If the condition is left untreated, the kidney may be destroyed.

Clinical manifestations. Hydronephrosis can occur without any symptoms as long as kidney function is adequate and urine can drain. The amount of pain is proportional to the rate of stretching. Slowly developing hydronephrosis may cause only a dull flank pain, whereas a sudden occlusion of the ureter, such as may occur from a stone, causes a severe stabbing (colicky) pain in the flank of the abdomen. Nausea and vomiting, which often accompany hydronephrosis, are caused by a reflex reaction to the pain and will usually be relieved as soon as the pain is controlled.

Assessment. Collection of *subjective data* involves questioning the patient about the presence of pain, including location, intensity, and character, and about the presence of nausea. The patient's voiding pattern should be discussed: frequency, hematuria, difficulty starting a stream of urine, dribbling at the end of **micturition** (voiding), nocturia, and burning on urination. Any history of obstructive disorders should be noted.

Collection of *objective data* includes assessing patients suspected of having hydronephrosis for vomiting, hematuria, urinary output, dyspnea, edema, a palpable mass in the abdomen, bladder distention on palpation, and tenderness over the kidneys or bladder.

Diagnostic tests. A urinalysis and serum renal function studies are obtained. X-ray examinations may include cystoscopy, retrograde pyelogram, IVU, KUB, CT scan, and ultrasound evaluation. Sometimes a renal biopsy is performed.

Medical management. Management is usually conservative if the condition is not severe. Surgical intervention is used to relieve the obstruction and preserve renal function. If the kidney is severely damaged, a nephrectomy may be necessary. If infection is present, antiinfective medications are administered. Antiinfectives, such as the penicillins, may be administered intravenously or intramuscularly. Penicillin may also be administered orally, as well as the sulfonamides (Gantrisin). Other medications used are the sulfamethoxazoles (Septra, Bactrim). Narcotics, such as morphine and meperidine, in combination with antispasmodic drugs, such as propantheline (Pro-Banthine) and belladonna preparations, are usually necessary to relieve severe, colicky pain.

Nursing interventions. Nursing interventions for the patient with hydronephrosis will include administering medications as ordered, monitoring intake (intravenous and oral) and output, observing for signs and symptoms of infection, and monitoring vital signs. The nurse will need to encourage the patient to take fluids and will also assess the patient for pain. Any drainage tubes will need to be kept open and anchored to avoid inadvertent displacement. If a catheter is present, regular catheter care will be necessary. If surgery has been performed, the dressing must be observed, because drainage of urine may continue for some time. The area should be kept clean and dry to avoid excoriation of the skin. Careful handwashing is important. All procedures should be explained to the patient and family.

Patient teaching. Patient teaching should include an explanation of the abnormality, along with the signs and symptoms of infection or obstruction. Measures to prevent infection should be explained, such as adequate fluid intake, good perineal hygiene, and regular emptying of the bladder.

Urolithiasis. Urolithiasis (urinary stones) can form in any area of the urinary tract (Fig. 33-10). Urolithiasis is a general term that encompasses all urinary stones, but they are also named specifically to indicate where they are located or formed: nephrolithiasis (stones in the kidney), ureterolithiasis (stones in the ureter), and cystolithiasis (stones in the bladder). Other descriptive terms are *calculi* (stones) and *lithiasis,* which means the formation of stones.

Etiology/pathophysiology. Urolithiasis results from minerals that have precipitated out of solution and adhere, forming stones that vary in size and shape. The event that initiates stone formation remains elusive, but some individuals are known to be predisposed: persons who are immobile, hyperparathyroid, or who have recurrent urinary tract infections.

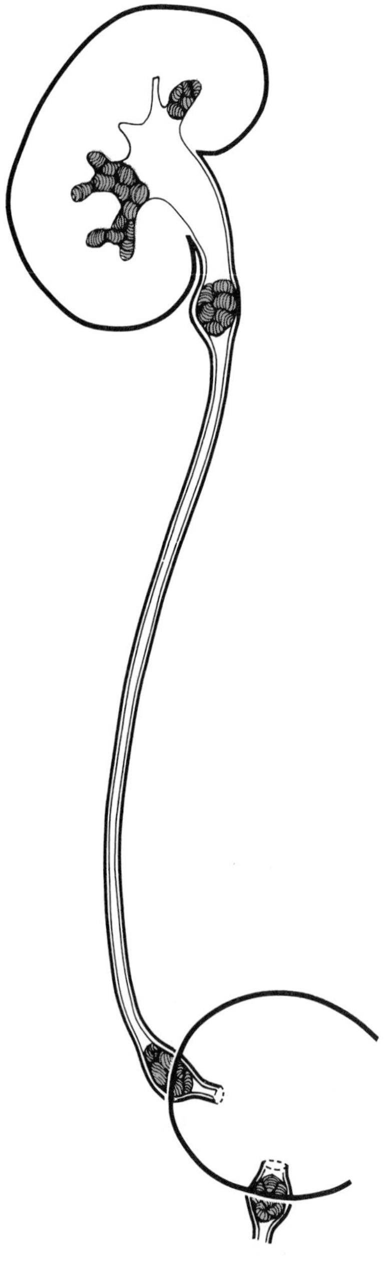

FIG. 33-10 Most common locations of renal calculus formation.

Clinical manifestations. Size and degree of mobility of the stone influence symptomatology. The patient with renal colic will seek care immediately, whereas a person with a less mobile stone may not seek assistance until signs of infection or hydronephrosis occur.

Assessment. Collection of *subjective data* may include the patient with mobile calculi complaining of intractable pain, usually accompanied by nausea and vomiting. The patient describes the pain as starting in the flank, and radiating into the groin, the genitalia, and the inner thigh. The patient with a less mobile stone will have symptoms associated with urinary infection or hydronephrosis.

Collection of *objective data* includes the nurse assessing for the presence of hematuria (gross or microscopic) on urinalysis, vomiting, and pain.

Diagnostic tests. Diagnostic tests include KUB, IVU, ultrasound, cystoscopy, and urinalysis. Other tests may be ordered to determine stone content, presence of infection, and alterations in blood chemistry that may influence stone formation. Twenty-four-hour urine examination may be done to detect abnormal excretion of calcium oxalate, phosphorus, and uric acid.

Medical management. Antimicrobial agents may be administered in the presence of infection or prophylactically. If stones are not passed, invasive techniques may be indicated. Stones in the lower tract can be removed by cystoscopy with stone manipulation or by surgical incision (Fig. 33-11). Terminology describes the location: ureterolithotomy, pyelolithotomy, and nephrolithotomy. Chemolytic agents may be instilled to dissolve stones. Extracorporeal shock-wave lithotripsy is an alternative to surgery. The patient is submerged in a special tank of water and ultrasonic shock waves are used to pulverize the stone. Urine must still be strained, even if a catheter is in place. Renal colic may still occur as the patient passes the stone fragments. Long-term manage-

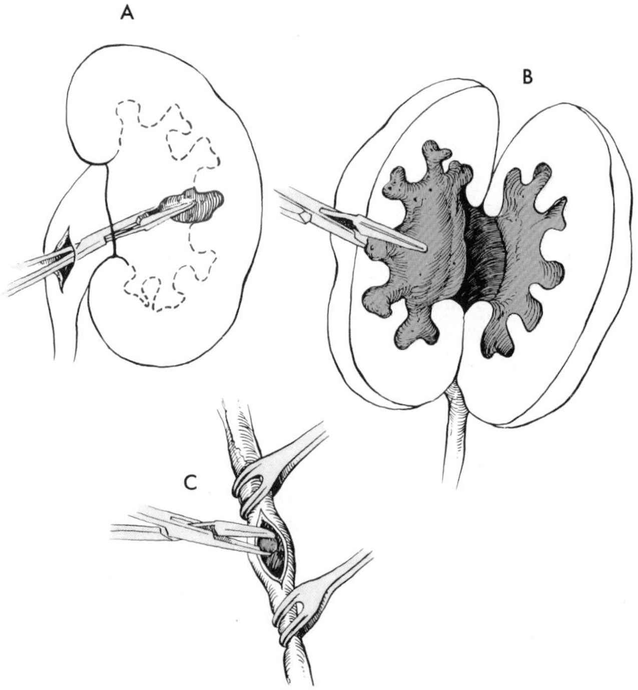

FIG. 33-11 Location and methods of removing renal calculi from upper urinary tract. **A,** Pyelolithotomy, removal of stone through renal pelvis. **B,** Nephrolithotomy, removal of staghorn calculus from renal parenchyma (kidney split). **C,** Ureterolithotomy, removal of stone from ureter.

ment may include dietary adjustments to influence the urine pH or to decrease availability of certain substances to discourage stone formation.

Nursing interventions. Stones are more likely to be passed if the person remains active and increases fluid intake. If pain is so severe as to require narcotic medication, the nurse must exercise discretion in allowing the patient out of bed. If nausea inhibits oral intake, the physician may order supplemental intravenous fluids. All urine will be strained. Because stones may be any size, even the smallest "speck" must be saved for assessment. The nurse should encourage fluids and administer analgesics as ordered. Pain should be monitored for passage of stone. Urine should be assessed for possible hematuria. BUN and creatinine should be monitored for indication of continuing urinary obstruction.

NURSING DIAGNOSES	NURSING INTERVENTIONS
Pain, acute, related to mobility of calculi	Develop pain management plan. Provide comfort measures. Provide diversional activities. Assess nature, intensity, location, duration, and alleviating factors of pain. Assess for nonverbal signs of pain (restlessness, wrinkled brow, clenched fists, elevated BP, and tachycardia. Monitor urine for flow, color, and amount. Provide nonpharmological comfort measures: a. Assist patient with assuming a comfortable position. b. Teach relaxation techniques. c. Provide diversional activity. d. Provide a restful environment. e. Encourage forcing fluids to dilute urine and flush stones. f. Assist patient with ambulation, if tolerated, to promote movement of stones. Administer antispasmodics and analgesics as ordered. Monitor and document pain relief and side effects of medications.
Potential for infection, related to obstruction	Monitor signs of infection. Provide nutrition/fluids. Discuss life-style factors that predispose to infection. Monitor for and report signs and symptoms of infection (elevated temperature, chills, flushed). Check temperature q 4 hr and report if above 101° F (38.5° C).

NURSING DIAGNOSES	NURSING INTERVENTIONS
Potential for infection, related to obstruction—cont'd	Note character of urine: report if cloudy and malodorous. Use good handwashing technique: teach and encourage patient to do the same. Instruct patient to avoid persons with infections.

Patient teaching. The nurse should instruct the patient about measures to prevent stone formation, obstruction, and infection. Prescribed diet, including fluid intake, should be discussed, as well as home medications (their purpose, dose, refills, and side effects). The patient should avoid inactivity by walking frequently. The need for follow-up with the physician should be emphasized, including keeping scheduled appointments and reporting difficulty of urination.

Although opinions vary greatly as to benefits of dietary restrictions, the nurse may be responsible for clarifying diet instructions. Fluid intake should be encouraged to at least 3000 ml of fluid in 24 hours unless contraindicated. Persons who are calcium stone formers may need to curtail their intake of dietary calcium (dairy products, antacids, and so on) to within minimum RDA guidelines. Persons who form oxalate stones should limit oxalate-containing foods (beans, deep-green leafy vegetables, cocoa, and so on).

Renal tumors

Etiology/pathophysiology. More common in men than in women, renal tumors are primarily adenocarcinomas that develop unilaterally and are often quite large when first detected. Renal cell carcinoma as a primary malignant tumor appears to arise from cells of the proximal convoluted tubules. Risk factors include pipe and cigar smoking, familial incidence, and preexisting renal disorders, such as adult polycystic kidney disease and renal cystic disease secondary to renal failure. Transitional cell tumors of the renal pelvis cause hematuria and can be confirmed by cytological study.

Clinical manifestations. The most common signs and symptoms are intermittent, painless hematuria, misleading the patient to defer seeking medical attention. Other symptoms appear after the malignant process has advanced: weight loss, dull flank pain, and a palpable mass in the flank area. Metastatic-related symptoms include respiratory distress and bone pain.

Assessment. Collection of *subjective data* includes a patient history of blood in the urine, which "comes and goes." When the bleeding occurs, there is usually no associated pain. In advanced stages of the illness, the patient will experience weight loss and dull flank pain.

Collection of *objective data* involves a physical assessment that reveals a mass in the flank area in advanced stages of the illness. Hematuria may be obvious, as well as symptoms related to systemic metastasis.

Diagnostic tests. Urinalysis will reveal hematuria in most patients. IVU will detect a renal mass, and ultrasonography will define composition of the mass in most instances. If indicated, other tests will be used to evaluate the status of other body systems; these include scans and MRI.

Medical management. Patients with localized disease usually respond well to radical nephrectomy. Radiation therapy and chemotherapy have proved to be of only minimal benefit.

Nursing interventions. Care of the patient with surgery of the urinary tract was addressed on pp. 794 and 795.

NURSING DIAGNOSES	NURSING INTERVENTIONS
Ineffective individual coping, related to powerlessness	Encourage patients to express feelings of frustration, anger, fear, and uncertainty. Actively listen. Observe for behavioral and emotional signs of grieving (denial, anger, crying, withdrawal, dependency). Support realistic hope: answer questions honestly. Provide assistance from other professionals to help patient with emotional changes (social worker, clergy, pyschologist, psychiatrist). Assist patient with identifying strengths and coping skills. Inquire as to how patient usually decreases tension and anxiety.
Knowledge deficit, related to limited information	Assess level of knowledge regarding care. Involve significant others in teaching process. Instruct patient on name of medications, dosage, schedule, purpose, and side effects. Teach patient to drink fluids generously unless contraindicated. Instruct patient to maintain mobility as tolerated. Instruct patients to avoid persons with infections.

Patient teaching. The patient should be instructed about community resources, support groups, and home health care. The nurse should emphasize the importance of follow-up care, including following discharge instructions and keeping return appointments.

Renal cysts

Etiology/pathophysiology. A single renal cyst may occur without clinical significance, but multiple cysts interfere with kidney function. The most clinically significant problems arise with polycystic kidney disease, which may be acquired or inherited. A patient with long-standing renal insufficiency or a dialysis patient may develop polycystic disease. Kidney function is compromised by the pressure of the cysts on kidney structures, secondary infections, and tissue scarring caused by rupturing of the cysts. The patient may progress to end-stage renal disease (ESRD).

Clinical manifestations. Symptoms are influenced by the degree of kidney structure involvement. The most common site is the collecting ducts, which fill with urine and/or blood. With extension of the disease process, fewer nephrons are available to maintain normal kidney function.

Assessment. Collection of *subjective data* includes noting the most common symptoms of abdominal and flank pain, followed by headache, gastrointestinal complaints, and voiding disturbances.

Collection of *objective data* involves an initial assessment that includes observation for systemic changes. The nurse should closely monitor blood pressure, which is usually elevated, and hematuria, and document the degree of patient complaints and response to intervention.

Diagnostic tests. Diagnosis is established by family history, physical examination, excretory urography, and imaging of cysts on x-ray examination or sonography. Blood chemistry results, such as urea and creatinine levels, are used to monitor the level of kidney function.

Medical management. There is no specific treatment for polycystic kidney disease. Medical treatment is aimed at relief of pain and symptoms of the disease. Heat and analgesics may relieve some of the discomfort caused by the enlarging kidneys. If the patient bleeds, heat should be discontinued and the patient should be placed on bed rest. Hypertension is treated vigorously with antihypertensive agents, diuretics, and fluid and dietary modifications. Because infections are common, antibiotics are often prescribed. As the disease progresses, dialysis or transplantation may be required.

Nursing interventions. Individual complaints and the severity of the disease process will influence nursing interventions. Patients and family members need to be given information about the availability of genetic counseling. The nurse should emphasize the need to report any changes in health status to the physician.

Tumors of the urinary bladder

Etiology/pathophysiology. Tumors of the urinary bladder range from benign papillomas to invasive carcinomas. The bladder is the most common site of cancer in the urinary tract, occurring more often in men than in women. Papillomas have the potential to become cancerous and are removed when detected.

Clinical manifestations. The patient may delay seeking medical attention, because the primary sign of bladder cancer is painless, intermittent hematuria.

Assessment. Collection of *subjective data* may include symptoms such as changes in voiding patterns, signs of urine obstruction, or renal failure, depending on the extent of the disease process.

Collection of *objective data* includes assessing the patient's understanding of his current health status, which will aid the nurse in planning teaching interventions. Accurate documentation of the time and amount of voiding, including the urine character, is indicated.

Diagnostic tests. Diagnostic tests include cystoscopy to obtain tissue samples for **cytological evaluation** (study of cells). Kidney function tests will assist in evaluation of overall renal status.

Medical management. The patient with local disease may be treated by removing the tissue by burning with an electric spark (fulguration), laser, instillation of chemotherapy agents, or radiation therapy. A partial or total cystectomy may be performed to remove invasive lesions. With complete removal of the urinary bladder, urinary diversion is necessary. (See pp. 795 and 796 for a discussion of ileal conduit or sigmoid conduit.)

Nursing interventions. The importance of follow-up care for the patient with papilloma must be emphasized. Care of the patient with bladder cancer will be influenced by the extent of the disease process, medical treatment, coincidental illness, and the patient's response to treatment. Observation of voiding patterns and urine character are necessary to monitor response to these therapies.

Patient teaching. Patient teaching is indicated so that the patient can return to optimum performance of activities of daily living. Suggested nursing interventions are addressed under surgical interventions, pp. 794-796.

Conditions Affecting the Prostate Gland

Benign prostatic hypertrophy

Etiology/pathophysiology. The prostate gland encircles the male urethra at the base of the urinary bladder. Its function is secretion of an alkaline fluid that helps neutralize seminal fluid and increases sperm motility. Enlargement of the prostate gland, benign hypertrophy (BPH), is a common occurrence in men older than 50 years. The precise cause of BPH remains unclear. Prostatic hypertrophy requires two conditions: aging and functioning testes.

Clinical manifestations. The patient will present with symptoms of urinary obstruction associated with inward pressure on the urethra by the enlargement of the prostate. Other clinical manifestations include complications of urinary obstruction, such as urinary tract infection, hematuria, oliguria, and signs of renal insufficiency.

Assessment. Collection of *subjective data* includes the patient describing the urine stream as difficult to start, slow, and painful, with complaints of frequency and nocturia (awakened by urgency to void two or more times).

Collection of *objective data* involves the nurse eliciting information to aid in determining the severity of the obstruction, in particular voiding patterns.

Diagnostic tests. On rectal examination, the physician may palpate the enlarged prostate gland, which has an elastic consistency. The hypertrophied prostate is symmetrically enlarged with a uniform, boggy presentation. Severity of the process can be determined through detecting alterations in blood chemistry, measuring residual urine, or by cystoscopy and/or IVU. Cytological evaluation will determine whether the process is benign or malignant.

Nursing interventions. Initial management is aimed at relieving the obstruction, usually by insertion of a Foley catheter. Care must be taken to avoid rapid decompression of the bladder to prevent rupture of mucosal blood vessels. Usually no more than 1000 ml of urine should be removed from a distended bladder initially. Physician's orders should be followed for the individual patient.

Prostatectomy (removal of the prostate gland) is indicated to relieve and/or prevent further obstruction of the urethra. The physician will choose the surgical approach for the prostatectomy after thorough appraisal of the patient. Preoperatively the physician may order an enema to reduce the possibility of the patient's straining to defecate after surgery, which could cause bleeding. Other preoperative preparations are standard, as noted in Chapter 26. There are four surgical techniques by which a prostatectomy may be done; they are presented in Box 33-3. They are (1) transurethral prostatectomy (TURP), (2) suprapubic prostatectomy, (3) perineal prostatectomy, and (4) retropubic prostatectomy (Fig. 33-12).

With BPH, a transurethral resection of the prostate (TURP) is less invasive and less stressful for the patient,

BOX 33-3 FOUR PROSTATECTOMY TECHNIQUES

1. Transurethral prostatectomy is done by approaching the gland through the penis and bladder using a resectoscope, a surgical instrument with an electric cutting wire for resection and cautery, to resect the lobes away from the capsule.
2. Suprapubic prostatectomy is accomplished by an incision through the abdomen; the bladder is opened, and the gland is removed from above with the finger.
3. Perineal prostatectomy requires an incision through the perineum between the scrotum and the rectum.
4. Retropubic prostatectomy is the method in which a low abdominal incision is made, but the bladder is not opened. The gland is removed by making an incision into the capsule encasing the gland.

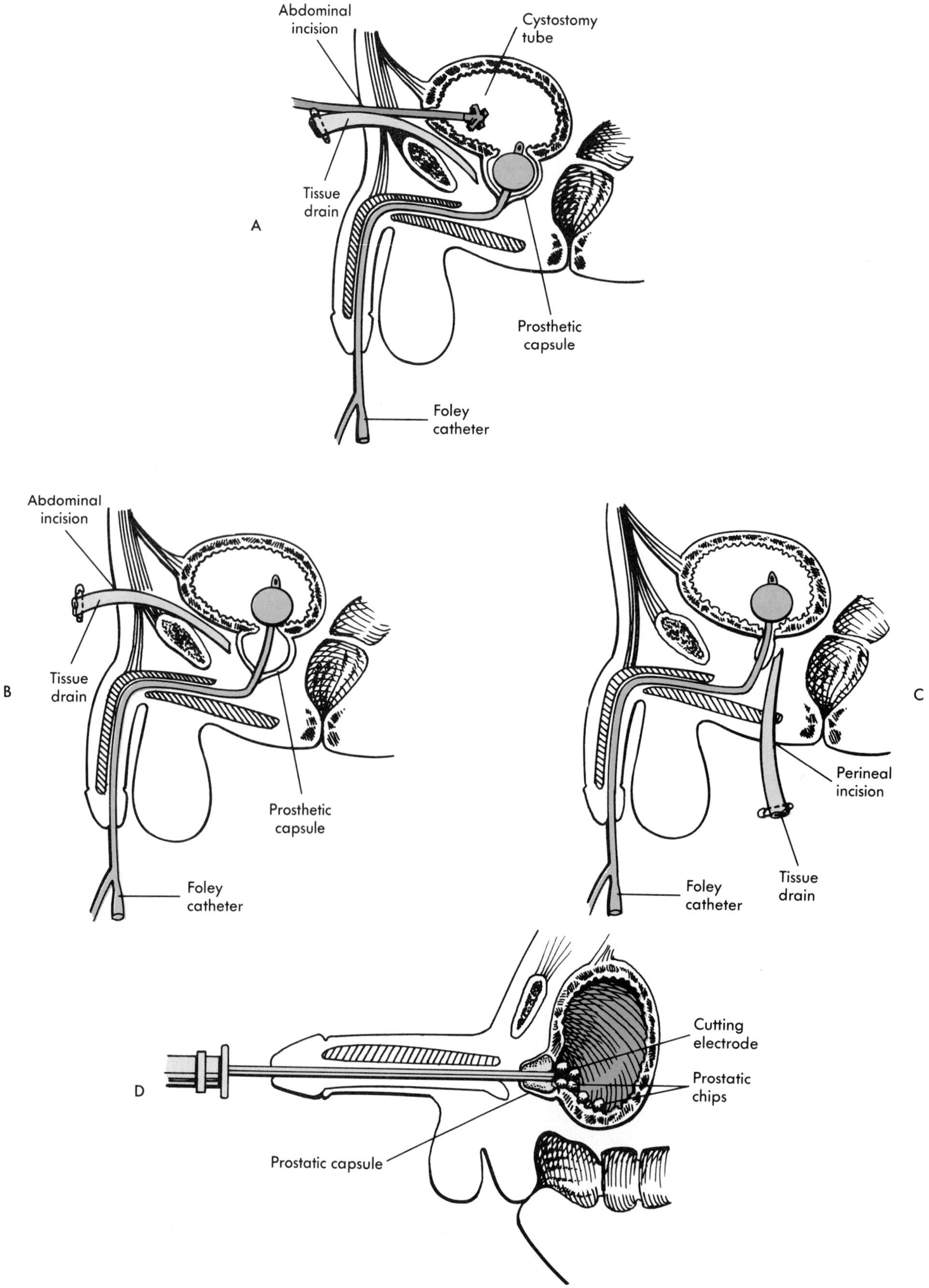

FIG. 33-12 Four types of prostatectomies. **A,** Suprapubic; note placement of inflated Foley catheter in prostatic fossa. **B,** Retropubic. **C,** Radical perineal; note tissue drain placed in incision between scrotum and rectum. **D,** Transuretheral resection of prostate gland by means of resectoscope. Note enlarged prostate gland surrounding urethra and tiny pieces of prostatic tissue that have been cut away.

especially the elderly patient or the patient with coincidental illness. Removal of the tissue is done through the urethra. With this procedure the outer capsule of the prostate gland is left in place, maintaining the continuity between the bladder and the lower urethra. Care of this patient is centered on observation of urine character and maintaining patency of the Foley catheter.

The patient who has a TURP may have continuous closed bladder irrigation or intermittent irrigation to prevent occlusion of the catheter with blood clots, which would cause bladder spasms. The patient and family need to know that hematuria is expected after prostatic surgery. Vital signs and urine color will be monitored every 2 hours for the first 24 hours to detect early signs of complications. With continuous bladder irrigation (CBI) the urine will be light red to pink, and with intermittent irrigation the urine will be a clear, cherry red color. Continuous irrigation is achieved by using a three-way catheter (one lumen for irrigation fluid, one for urine drainage, and one to the retention balloon) or by using two catheters (Foley and suprapubic—one for irrigation fluid and one for urine drainage). The irrigation solution is usually normal saline. To determine urine output, the nurse will subtract the amount of irrigation fluid used from the Foley catheter output to obtain actual urine. This is reported as "actual urine output." Catheter drainage tubes should be checked frequently for kinks that would occlude urine flow and cause bladder spasms. The patient should be advised not to try to void around the catheter, since this will contribute to bladder spasms. Hemorrhage is always a possibility. Belladonna and opium (B&O) suppositories are helpful to relieve bladder spasms.

Routine postoperative care is instituted. Prolonged sitting is to be avoided, because the resulting increased intraabdominal pressure may cause the operative site to bleed. The catheter will be removed when the urine becomes clear. The patient is informed that he may experience frequency, voiding small amounts with some dribbling initially. He should be instructed to void with the first urge to prevent increased bladder pressure against the operative site.

Some physicians may request that samples of the most recent voidings be saved for assessment. When the patient voids, the nurse records the time, amount, and color of each voiding.

A suprapubic or abdominal approach will require dressing observations and changes. When a suprapubic catheter is present, it will be cared for in the same manner as the Foley catheter. A perineal approach may also be used in the presence of malignancy. This patient will need emotional support related to the cancer and the impotence caused by surgery.

When the capsule of the prostate gland is removed, as with the perineal approach, there is no longer a connection between the bladder and the lower urethra. The area where these two structures are reconnected is usually supported by placement of the Foley catheter. Extreme care must be taken not to cause tension on the catheter, which would disturb the surgical area.

A care plan for the person with BPH is presented on pp. 808 and 809.

Cancer of the prostate

Etiology/pathophysiology. Prostatic cancer is most common in men older than 50 years. This insidious cancer usually starts as a nodule on the posterior portion of the prostate; therefore symptoms are not present initially. When the tumor causes urinary symptoms, the cancer is in advanced stages. At this point metastasis is common, with the most frequent sites being the pelvic lymph nodes and bone. Regular rectal examinations to detect any abnormalities of the prostate gland will led to early treatment and an increased survival rate.

Clinical manifestations. The patient will have symptoms related to urinary obstruction. Other symptoms will be determined by the presence and/or degree of metastasis.

Assessment. Collection of *subjective data* involves understanding that the patient with prostatic cancer may have no symptoms until the disease is advanced. The patient may seek medical intervention for BPH, which often accompanies prostate cancer, or when he experiences back pain or sciatica that occurs from metastatic changes in the bony pelvis.

Collection of *objective data* includes noting that if the tumor is of sufficient size, the patient may experience symptoms of obstruction such as dysuria, frequency, and nocturia. Metastatic changes may be seen in the lymph glands of the pelvis and in the bones of the lower spine, pelvis, and hips with associated signs and symptoms.

Diagnostic tests. On rectal examination by the physician, the involved area of the prostate gland will feel firm and fixed with hardened nodules typically in the posterior lobe of the gland. Definitive diagnosis is made by cytological examination. Serum acid phosphatase will be elevated when the disease process extends beyond the prostatic capsule. Other tests, such as a bone scan and serum alkaline phosphatase will be performed to assess the degree of metastasis.

Medical management. The stage of the disease process will influence the choice of treatment. A perineal approach for the removal of the prostate and surrounding structures may be used. This patient will need emotional support related to the cancer and the impotence caused by the surgery. Preoperative teaching should include an opportunity for the patient and his partner to discuss optional treatments and mortality rate. With removal of the prostatic capsule, there is no longer a connection between the urinary bladder and the lower urethra. The area where these two structures are reconnected is usually supported by placement of a Foley catheter. The catheter will remain indwelling for several postoperative days.

NURSING CARE PLAN: THE PATIENT WITH TRANSURETHRAL RESECTION PROSTATECTOMY FOR BENIGN PROSTATIC HYPERTROPHY

Mr. Smith is a 72-year-old retired automobile mechanic. He had been in his usual state of good health until about 4 months ago when he started to develop nocturia. Several weeks later he noted difficulty initiating voiding. He also noted mild dribbling after voiding. On physical examination his physician noted moderate enlargement of his prostate. He is being admitted for cystoscopy and possible TURP. His vital signs are stable. He is married and states that his wife is supportive. He lives in a two-story, single-family home.

Nursing diagnoses	Patient goals	Nursing interventions
Urinary retention, related to obstruction secondary to TURP	Patient will not experience retention of urine.	Monitor urinary output and characteristics. Maintain constant bladder irrigation as prescribed during first 24 hours. Maintain patency of indwelling urinary catheter by irrigating with CBI. Monitor intake and output. Encourage high fluid intake (2500 to 3000 ml/day). After catheter is removed, continue to monitor for signs of retention.
Pain, related to bladder spasm	Patient will state feeling more comfortable.	Teach patient not to try to void around catheter. Monitor patient at regular intervals for 48 hours to identify early signs of bladder spasm. Give prescribed medications (analgesics, antispasmodics). Tell patient spasms will decrease in intensity and frequency within 24 to 48 hours.
Potential for injury: hemorrhage or infection, related to surgery	Patient will experience minimized bleeding and will not manifest evidence of infection.	Monitor vital signs; report signs of shock or fever. Monitor appearance of urine for persistent bright red color rather than expected dark red beyond first few hours postoperatively. Teach patient to avoid Valsalva maneuver. Avoid use of rectal thermometers, rectal examinations, or enemas for at least 1 week. Maintain strict asepsis of urinary drainage system: hand irrigate *only* when necessary. Encourage high fluid intake.
Stress or urge incontinence, related to catheter removal after surgery	Patient will achieve urinary control.	Assess patient for dribbling after catheter is removed. If dribbling occurs: a. Tell patient this is common occurrence and continence will return. b. Teach perineal exercises.
Sexual dysfunction: potential, related to TURP	Patient will maintain sexual function	Give patient opportunity to discuss feelings about effects of prostatectomy on sexual intercourse. Provide information as necessary: a. Probable return of previous level of functioning. b. Occurrence of retrograde ejaculation (urine may have a milky appearance). Avoid sexual intercourse for 3 to 4 weeks after surgery

NURSING CARE PLAN: THE PATIENT WITH TRANSURETHRAL RESECTION PROSTATECTOMY FOR BENIGN PROSTATIC HYPERTROPHY—cont'd

Nursing diagnoses	Patient goals	Nursing interventions
Knowledge deficit, related to TURP	Patient will describe activity restrictions and need for medical follow-up.	Teach patient: a. Avoidance of heavy activities for 3 to 4 weeks (check with physician regarding resumption of long walks). b. Avoidance of straining at stool for 4 to 6 weeks; use of stool softeners or laxatives as necessary. c. Fluid maintenance of at least 2500 ml to 3000 ml/day d. Instructions for medical follow-up

In cases of advanced cancer, estrogen therapy may be used in attempt to alter the tumor growth. The patient may receive relief from such symptoms as pain or obstruction, but may, however, experience side effects of secondary sex characteristics and gastrointestinal complications. Radiation therapy may be used in advanced stages of the illness as primary or palliative treatment.

Because cure for cancer of the prostate is possible only when the tumor is discovered early, it is important to teach all male patients over the age of 50 to have annual or biannual rectal examination.

Nursing interventions. Postoperative nursing management is similar to that for perineal surgery, with special attention to maintenance of bowel and bladder function while keeping the surgical wound clean and avoiding pressure on the perineum and wound. Adequate fluid intake, modification of dietary selections, and perineal exercises may be used to promote regulation of bowel and bladder function. Extreme care must be taken to avoid trauma to the perineum to avoid possible perforation of the perineum, causing a fistula. Rectal temperature-taking, enemas, and use of rectal tubes are therefore forbidden. Extreme care must be taken not to cause tension on the Foley catheter, which would disturb the surgical area. The nurse observes the color of the urine for signs of bleeding. The patient will also have a tissue drain inserted during surgery to promote drainage from the wound in the perineum. Initially, there may be some small amount of urine from the drain, but this should stop in 1 or 2 days. Surgical asepsis should be followed during dressing changes. Irrigation of the perineum may be ordered to cleanse the wound and promote patient comfort. Analgesics should be administered as ordered for pain control in lower back, pelvis, upper thighs, and operative site.

Another possible complication of the surgery is urinary incontinence. The nurse should teach the patient how to keep himself clean. He may need an opportunity to discuss feelings of depression about his altered body function. Modification of life-style and maintenance of confidence are important for his return to preillness function.

Urethral Strictures

Etiology/pathophysiology. A urethral stricture is a narrowing of the lumen of the urethra that interferes with urine flow. Narrowing may be congenital or acquired. Acquired strictures may be caused by chronic infection, trauma, or tumor or as a complication of radiation treatment of the pelvis.

Clinical manifestations. Symptoms include dysuria, weak stream, splaying (spreading out) of the urine stream, nocturia, and increasing pain with bladder distention. In the presence of infection, fever and malaise may be apparent.

Assessment. Collection of *subjective data* includes noting a patient complaint of difficulty initiating the urine stream and the stream seeming to spray more than usual or even seeming to "fork."

Collection of *objective data* includes assessing for signs that may indicate an infectious process and gather information to describe the extent of the stricture and possible presence of an obstruction.

Diagnostic tests. Diagnosis can be confirmed by a voiding cystourethrogram, which demonstrates stricture. Additional diagnostic studies help evaluate damage caused by the obstruction.

Medical management. Correction of the stricture may be achieved by dilation or surgical release (internal urethrotomy).

Nursing interventions. Care includes adequate hydration to decrease discomfort when voiding and monitoring of urine output. Mild analgesics should be sufficient to relieve discomfort. Sitz baths may relieve discomfort and encourage voiding. Reconstruction (urethroplasty) of the urethra may require temporary urinary diversion (see care guidelines, p. 783). After the procedure a splinting catheter will support the suture line. Care must be taken not to cause tension on the catheter.

Urinary Tract Trauma

Etiology/pathophysiology. Any patient with a history of traumatic injury should be assessed for involvement of the urinary tract. Such injuries may include contusions or rupture of the urinary structures. A patient who has undergone abdominal surgery should also be observed for incidental injury sustained during the operation. Traumatic invasion of the urinary tract may be evident in open wounds to the lower abdomen, such as with gunshot or stab wounds. Contusion or laceration of the urethra may lead to urethral stricture and possible impotence in males secondary to soft tissue, blood vessel, and nerve damage.

Clinical manifestations. Urine output should be monitored hourly for amount and color, and any evidence of hematuria should be reported. The patient is assessed for abdominal pain and tenderness, which may indicate internal hemorrhage, peritonitis, or seepage of urine into the tissues.

Assessment. Collection of *subjective data* involves understanding that the trauma patient may be unable to relate any symptoms that would aid in the assessment of urinary tract involvement. If he is able to, any reference to the symptoms of hematuria is extremely important.

Collection of *objective data* includes a comprehensive assessment of the trauma patient reviewing all body systems. Assessment related to the urinary tract includes hourly measurement of intake and output, observation of urine character or difficulty voiding, evaluation of complaints of abdominal, flank, or referred shoulder pain, and evaluation of abdominal distention and girth.

Diagnostic tests. Diagnosis of traumatic involvement of the urinary tract may be aided by KUB, IVU, urinalysis, excretory urogram, and cystoscopy.

Medical management. Surgical intervention will be necessary for correction of tears or rupture of the integrity of the urinary tract, to reinstate urine flow. If damage to the structures is severe, removal of the kidney or bladder may be necessary, with the creation of urinary diversion as discussed earlier in this chapter.

Management of possible hemorrhage and prevention of infection are necessary preoperatively and postoperatively.

Nursing interventions. Nursing responsibility centers on identifying individuals at risk and detecting variations in assessment findings that indicate trauma to the urinary tract. The nurse should document and report all findings.

Noninfectious Disorders of the Urinary System

Nephrotic Syndrome

Etiology/pathophysiology. Nephrotic syndrome (nephrosis) is a group of symptoms characterized by marked proteinuria, hypoalbuminemia, and edema. Several events may precipitate the symptoms of nephrotic syndrome; the primary form of nephrosis occurs in the absence of glomerulonephritis or systemic disease, with the inciting event being an upper respiratory infection or allergic reaction.

Physiological changes in the glomeruli interfere with selective permeability. Blood protein is allowed to pass into the urine (proteinuria), causing a loss of serum protein (hypoalbuminemia). This decreases serum osmotic pressure, thus allowing fluid to seep into interstitial spaces, and edema occurs.

Clinical manifestations. The patient has severe generalized edema **(anasarca),** anorexia, fatigue, and altered renal function.

Assessment. Collection of *subjective data* includes noting patient complaints of loss of interest in eating, a constant feeling of being tired, and decreased urine output (oliguria). The patient may also relate problems with "swelling" of his face, hands, and feet.

Collection of *objective data* includes the nurse assessing the degree of fluid retention by monitoring daily weight, intake and output, respiratory effort, and level of consciousness. Skin integrity is assessed to determine special needs.

Diagnostic tests. Blood chemistry findings include hyperalbuminuria, hypoalbuminemia, and hyperlipidemia. Renal biopsy provides identification of the type and extent of tissue change. Other diagnostic testing will be performed to identify any underlying cause.

Medical management. Medical management depends on the extent of tissue involvement and may include the use of (1) corticosteroids to control symptoms, (2) potassium-sparing antihypertensives, such as spironolactone (Aldactone), or (3) antineoplastic agents (used for immunosuppressive effect). Diuretics are used to relieve edema. Hypoproteinemia may be treated with normal serum albumin and protein diet supplements, such as Meritene.

Nursing interventions. Nursing intervention includes monitoring of fluid balance (weight, measuring abdominal girth, intake and output), bed rest in the presence of extreme edema, and assessing for electrolyte imbalance. Skin care is very important, as is a gradual increase in activity as the edema is resolved.

Diet includes protein replacement using foods that provide high biological value (meat, fish, poultry, cheese, eggs) and restriction of sodium to decrease edema. Blood pressure is often elevated and should be monitored closely for changes.

Nephritis

Formerly called *Bright's disease,* nephritis encompasses a number of kidney disorders characterized by inflammation and abnormal function. Included in this group of disorders are acute and chronic glomerulonephritis.

Acute glomerulonephritis

Etiology/pathophysiology. Health history reveals that the onset of acute poststreptococcal glomerulonephritis symptoms was preceded by a throat or skin infection caused by streptococcus 2 to 3 weeks earlier. The organism is not present in the kidney. In some individuals streptococcal infections initiate an immune response, resulting in inflammation of glomeruli that allows excretion of red blood cells and protein in the urine. The condition is common in children and young adults. Recovery is usually achieved without residual damage, but it may progress to a chronic form in some individuals (usually adults).

Clinical manifestations. It is not unusual for family members to first note that the individual has "swelling" of the face, especially around the eyes, and a pale coloring. Some patients may be acutely ill with a multitude of symptoms, while others may be diagnosed on routine examination with only vague symptoms.

Assessment. Collection of *subjective data* includes noting the patient relating symptoms indicative of anorexia, nocturia, malaise, and exertional dyspnea.

Collection of *objective data* includes the nurses assessment of skin integrity and the degree of edema and observe urine for amount and color. Hematuria may be reflected in the urinalysis, or urine color may vary from smoky to frankly sanguineous (bloody) in appearance. Vital signs and the general condition of skin should be monitored.

Diagnostic tests. Diagnostic tests will reveal an elevated BUN, serum creatinine, potassium, erythrocyte sedimentation rate (ESR), and antistreptolysin-O titer (ASO titer). Urinalysis will show red blood cells and protein.

Medical management. Medical management includes treatment of primary symptoms while preventing complications to cerebral and cardiac function. Serum electrolyte levels (sodium and potassium) may indicate a need to adjust dietary intake of sodium and potassium. Level of consciousness should be monitored when the BUN is elevated.

A prophylactic antimicrobial agent, such as penicillin, may be administered for several months after the acute phase of the illness to protect against recurrence. Diuretics may be prescribed to control fluid retention and antihypertensives to reduce blood pressure.

Nursing interventions. Nursing intervention will be guided by individual patient needs, focusing on relief of symptoms and prevention of complications. Dietary intake will include protein restrictions, with carbohydrates providing a source of energy.

Nursing interventions include monitoring intake, output, and vital signs. Level of activity will be determined by the degree of edema and/or hypertension.

Chronic glomerulonephritis

Etiology/pathophysiology. With chronic glomerulonephritis there is usually no indication of an inciting event. Occasionally a patient with the acute variety will progress to a chronic phase. Most patients will not seek medical attention until renal function is compromised. Chronic disease is characterized by slow, progressive destruction of glomeruli with related loss of function. The kidney will actually decrease in size (atrophy).

Clinical manifestations. Symptoms may include malaise, morning headaches, dyspnea with exertion, visual and digestive disturbances, edema, weight loss, and fatigue. Physical findings include hypertension, anemia, proteinuria, anasarca, and cardiac and cerebral manifestations.

Assessment. Collection of *subjective data* includes the patient complaints of fatigue and a decreased ability to perform activities of daily living as a result of dyspnea. Morning headaches may also be noted. With this complaint it is important to obtain specific information about the location, pattern, and character of the headache. Questions should also elicit the presence of any visual disturbances.

Collection of *objective data* includes the nurse clarifying outward manifestations of headache and respiratory effort that may interfere with daily task performance. Careful assessment of the degree of edema will be documented, noting specific location and response to pressure by pressing the fingers into the edematous area and observing for pitting. The nurse observes urine for color and amount and monitors vital signs.

Diagnostic tests. Early disease shows albumin and RBCs in the urine, although renal function test results are within normal limits. With advanced destruction of nephrons the specific gravity becomes fixed and blood levels of nonprotein nitrogen wastes (creatinine and urea) increase.

Medical management. Medical management includes control of secondary side effects as discussed with acute glomerulonephritis, with the use of renal dialysis and

BOX 33-4

NURSING INTERVENTION GUIDELINES FOR NEPHRITIS

ACTIVITY

Bed rest until edema and blood pressure are reduced
Encourage quiet diversional activities
Ambulate gradually with assistance
Space activity to lessen fatigue

FLUID BALANCE MAINTENANCE

Implement dietary restrictions
Monitor intake and output
Document reactions to medication

DIET THERAPY

Protein restrictions to decrease nitrogenous wastes
Sodium restrictions to prevent further fluid retention
Increase calories for energy source

DRUG THERAPY

Prophylactic antibiotics
Antihypertensives
Diuretics
Drug interactions, side effects to expect and report

HEALTH MAINTENANCE

Recovery may be extended
Urine will be monitored for albumin and RBCs by physician
Teach early signs of fluid retention
Symptoms may resolve and then become worse
Normal activities may be resumed after urine is clear for a month, though the patient is not considered cured until the urine is free of albumin and RBCs for 6 months

possible kidney transplantation to provide elimination of wastes from the body.

Nursing interventions. Changes in vital signs and diagnostic tests are monitored to aid in choosing proper nursing interventions. Interventions parallel those noted with nephrotic syndrome and acute glomerulonephritis. Chronic glomerulonephritis may progress to end-stage renal disease (ESRD), necessitating related nursing interventions. Interventions are listed in Box 33-4.

NURSING DIAGNOSIS	NURSING INTERVENTIONS
Fluid volume excess, related to decreased urine output secondary to renal dysfunction	Assess understanding of therapeutic interventions. Monitor for and report signs and symptoms of fluid excess (hypertension, CHF, weight gain, edema). Measure and document intake and output q hr. Note amount and character of urine: report decreased urine output to physician.
Fluid volume excess, related to decreased urine output secondary to renal dysfunction—cont'd	Weigh patient daily at the same time with the same clothing and same scale. Restrict sodium as ordered. Replace fluids according to fluid loss as ordered. Provide ice chips to control thirst. Administer diuretics as ordered. Monitor electrolytes and report abnormal laboratory values, and signs and symptoms of electrolyte imbalances.

Patient teaching. Patient teaching includes emphasizing a health-promoting life-style, with prevention and early treatment of infections.

Renal Failure

An acute or chronic state, renal failure is characterized by the inability of the kidneys to excrete wastes, concentrate urine, and conserve or eliminate electrolytes.

Acute renal failure

Etiology/pathophysiology. Kidney function may be altered by interference with the kidney's ability to be selective in filtering blood or by an actual decrease in blood flow to the kidneys. A number of medical conditions can lead to acute renal failure, such as hemorrhage, trauma, infection, and decreased cardiac output. The course of acute renal failure (ARF) is divided into phases. In the *oliguric phase,* BUN and serum creatinine levels rise while urine output decreases; in the *diuretic phase,* blood chemistry levels begin to return to normal and urine output increases. Return to normal or near normal function occurs in the *recovery phase.*

Clinical manifestations. The patient with ARF may experience anorexia, nausea, vomiting, edema, and associated signs and symptoms of diminished renal function.

Assessment. Collection of *subjective data* includes the patient report of experiencing loss of appetite, nausea, and headache.

Collection of *objective data* involves physical findings that will depend on the state of the disease process. The nurse assesses for dry mucous membranes, poor skin turgor, urine output of less than 400 ml/24 hr, vomiting, and anasarca (generalized edema).

Diagnostic tests. Physical assessment, history, and elevated blood chemistry results to such tests as BUN and creatinine (azotemia) will confirm diagnosis. After the patient is stabilized, further studies may be done to assess for residual damage.

Medical management. Measures include administration of fluids and osmotic preparations to prevent decreased renal perfusion, manage fluid volume, and treat electrolyte imbalances. Renal dialysis may be necessary to manage systemic fluid shifts, especially cardiac and respiratory, and may be effective in removing some nephrotoxins.

Nursing interventions. Accurate documentation of urine output is necessary to identify the level of renal function. Azotemia may be revealed by blood chemistry studies. The patient with azotemia must be observed for changes in level of consciousness. Fluid status, vital signs, and response to therapies must be closely monitored. Frequent skin care with tepid water to remove urea crystals will be comforting. Diet should be protein sparing, high in carbohydrate, and low in potassium. Dialysis presents special nursing challenges (see p. 815).

Chronic renal failure (end-stage renal disease)

Etiology/pathophysiology. Chronic renal failure or end-stage renal disease (ESRD) exists when the kidneys are unable to regain normal function. As many as 80% of nephrons may be severely impaired before loss of renal function is detected. The most common causes of ESRD are pyelonephritis, chronic glomerulonephritis, glomerulosclerosis, chronic urinary obstruction, severe hypertension, diabetes mellitus, gout, and polycystic kidney disease.

ESRD represents a significant health problem worldwide, resulting in the death of thousands, and financial crisis for the patients and their families. The government does actively help defray costs through the Medicare program. ESRD develops slowly over an extended period as a result of kidney disease or other disease processes that compromise renal blood perfusion.

Clinical manifestations. The onset of symptoms may be so gradual and the symptoms so vague that the patient is unable to identify when the problems started. When questioned, he may be able to relate occurrences that seemed insignificant at the time. The clinical picture is usually unique to the individual patient. Common symptoms are headache, lethargy, asthenia (decreased strength or energy), anorexia, pruritus, elimination changes, **anuria** (urinary output less than 100 to 250 ml/day), muscle cramps or twitching, impotence, characteristic dusky, yellow-tan, or gray skin color from retained urochrome pigments, and symptoms characteristic of central nervous system involvement, such as confusion and mental lapses.

Other associated conditions are responsible for many of the symptoms the patient exhibits. Azotemia develops as excessive amounts of nitrogenous compounds build in the blood. Anemia occurs when the production of renal erythropoietin is decreased as a result of loss of kidney function. Acidosis, hypertension, and glucose intolerance may be present as a result of the insult to homeostasis.

Assessment. Collection of *subjective data* will include noting patient complaints of joint pain and edema, severe headaches, nausea, anorexia, intermittent chest pain, weakness, and in particular, fatigue.

Collection of *objective data* involves a nursing assessment that may yield unremarkable results, except for signs and symptoms that support the patient complaints. Uremic encephalopathy affects the central nervous system. Usually the first sign is a reduction in alertness and awareness.

Diagnostic tests. Diagnosis of ESRD is confirmed by elevated BUN and serum creatinine levels, electrolyte imbalance, and other indicators. Renal function studies assess the degree of damage and/or level of renal function.

Medical management. Medical management is instituted to delay the onset of end-stage renal disease as long as possible. Renal dialysis is initiated when necessary, and the patient may be prepared for renal transplantation. Medications are used, as with acute renal failure, to control systemic changes resulting from a shift in fluid and electrolyte balance, acidosis, possible hyperkalemia, possible seizure activity, hypertension, and infection.

Nursing interventions. Nursing interventions focus on restoring homeostasis. Measures to control fluid and electrolyte balance vary greatly, according to unique needs of the individual patient. Nutritional therapy is aimed at reserving protein stores and preventing production of additional protein waste products that the kidney would have to clear. The diet is high in calories from carbohydrates and fats—at least 2,500 to 3,000 calories daily. Other dietary restrictions are related to the patient's degree of acidosis. Potassium is retained; therefore foods high in potassium are restricted. Sodium is controlled at a level sufficient to replace sodium loss without causing fluid retention.

Nursing interventions for acute renal failure are also instituted for the chronic form. Emphasis is placed on emotional support for the patient who faces role changes and invasive treatments such as dialysis and/or transplantation. Box 33-5 offers guidelines for supporting the patient with renal failure. Fluid balance is of prime importance. The patient may have fluid equal to the amount excreted in the urine plus about 300 to 600 ml to compensate for insensible fluid loss (fluid lost through the lungs, perspiration, feces, and so on). Salt substitutes are not advised, because most contain potassium.

NURSING DIAGNOSES	NURSING INTERVENTIONS
Activity intolerance, related to weakness secondary to anemia, azotemia, and inadequate nutrition	Assess and document level of tolerance to activities. Encourage requesting of medications to promote comfort. Assess patient's present daily schedule. Identify factors that reduce patient's activity tolerance. Adjust patient's schedule to provide rest periods between activities and adequate nocturnal sleep.

BOX 33-5 NURSING INTERVENTION GUIDELINES FOR THE PATIENT WITH RENAL FAILURE

MONITOR FLUID AND ELECTROLYTE BALANCE

Assess intake and output (hourly may be indicated)
Weigh daily (same time, same clothing, same scale)
Assess overt (open to view) signs of hydration status (edema, turgor)
Assess covert (hidden) signs of hydration status (breath sounds, laboratory studies, and so on)

NUTRITION

Provide prescribed diet
Guide patient food selection
Plan fluid intake per shift within prescribed limits and according to patient preference
Reinforce diet instructions as indicated

PROMOTE COMFORT AND SAFETY

Provide quiet environment (sound and lighting)
Space nursing care to conserve patient energy
Medicate as needed for comfort
Skin care to alleviate discomfort resulting from pruritus
Mouth care as needed
Maintain asepsis during procedures
Prevent exposure to pathogens

PROMOTE COPING BEHAVIORS

Listen (patient and significant other)
Refer to pastoral care or religious support group
Provide private times with significant others
Offer interview with social services

DOCUMENTATION AND REPORTING

Document all relevant findings
Maintain open communications with supervisory staff
Adjust nursing care plan as indicated to meet changing patient needs

NURSING DIAGNOSES	NURSING INTERVENTIONS
Activity intolerance, related to weakness secondary to anemia, azotemia, and inadequate nutrition—cont'd	Limit visitors or length of stay as necessary. Allow patient to set daily activity goals. Encourage self-care activities and assist as needed. Maintain adequate nutrition. Praise attempts to increase activity.
Altered nutrition: less than body requirements, related to anorexia, nausea, vomiting, dietary restrictions	Monitor laboratory values and intake/output balance. Administer antiemetics before meals and prn. Assess nutritional status. Monitor patient's weight daily.
Altered nutrition: less than body requirements, related to anorexia, nausea, vomiting, dietary restrictions—cont'd	Consult with dietician to plan menus incorporating dietary restrictions, calorie requirements, and patient preference. Encourage patient to express feelings about dietary restrictions. Provide good oral hygiene before and after meals and prn. Provide smaller, more frequent meals if patient is nauseated or experiences early satiety. Administer vitamin supplements and iron as ordered.

Patient teaching. Patient teaching should emphasize food exchanges and fluid intake within restrictions.

Care of the patient requiring dialysis. Dialysis mimics kidney function, helping to restore balance when normal kidney function is interrupted temporarily or permanently. Dialysis involves either diffusion of wastes, drugs, or excess of electrolytes or osmosis of water across a semipermeable membrane into a dialysate fluid that is prescribed specific to individual patient needs. Dialysis is achieved by the process of extracorporeal hemodialysis or peritoneal dialysis.

Extracorporeal hemodialysis. Extracorporeal hemodialysis requires an access to the patient's circulatory system to route blood through the artificial kidney (dialyzer) for removal of wastes, fluids, and electrolytes, then return it to the patient's body. Temporary methods include subclavian or femoral catheters or an external shunt placed in the nondominant forearm. In ESRD, access can be achieved by constructing a direct or a graft arteriovenous fistula (Fig. 33-13). Hemodialysis is usually scheduled three times per week for 3 to 6 hours. Patients can be maintained on dialysis therapy and their lives prolonged pending the possibility of a kidney transplant.

Nursing interventions. Nursing intervention is dictated by individual patient conditions. The patient receiving renal dialysis may have other acute or chronic problems. Most patients are dialyzed on an outpatient basis. General nursing care guidelines are noted in Box 33-6.

Peritoneal dialysis. Peritoneal dialysis can be performed with a minimum of equipment and by the patient who is ambulatory. The time required for the peritoneal procedure is much longer, since the rate of exchange is slower. The principle of osmosis and diffusion through a semipermeable membrane is the same as in extracorporeal hemodialysis, but the peritoneum is used as the semipermeable membrane instead of the artificial kidney.

The physician places a catheter into the peritoneal space under aseptic conditions (Fig. 33-14). The dialyzing fluid is then instilled for a predetermined period and then drained. The ESRD patient may be maintained on peritoneal dialysis, continuous ambulatory peritoneal dialysis

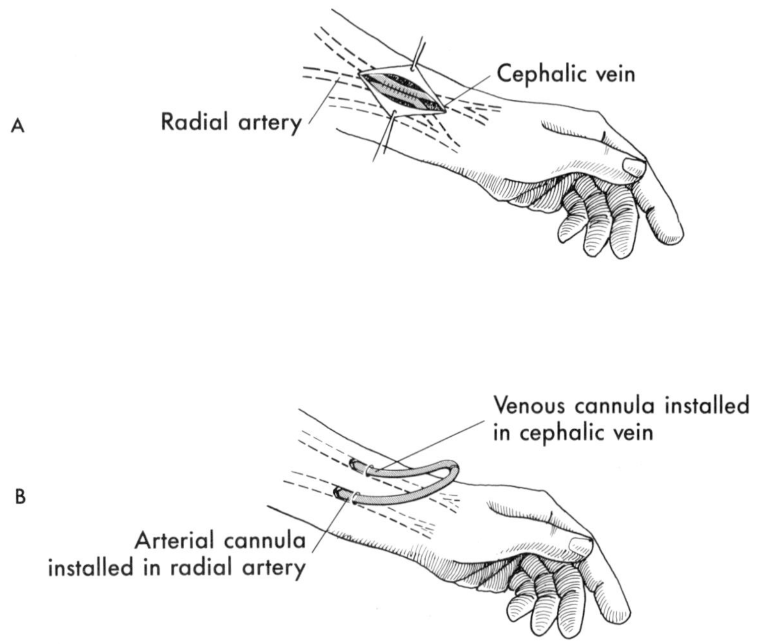

FIG. 33-13 Frequently used means for gaining vascular access for hemodialysis include, **A,** arteriovenous fistula, and **B,** external arteriovenous shunt.

BOX 33-6 NURSING INTERVENTION GUIDELINES FOR THE PATIENT UNDERGOING HEMODIALYSIS

PATIENT TEACHING

Reinforce explanation of dialysis procedure
Inform of community resources
Explain dietary restrictions
Self-care, general

MONITORING DURING DIALYSIS

Weigh before and after treatment
Vital signs every 30-60 minutes (B/P in arm without fistula)
Maintain orientation (thought processes may be altered)
Hemorrhage resulting from heparin use during dialysis
Equipment (interruption of procedure)

ACTIVITY

Diversions (reading, television, sleep)
Comfort (reclining, sitting, lying)
Dietary intake (may be hungry or nauseated)

CARE AFTER DIALYSIS OR BETWEEN TREATMENTS

Schedule fluid intake within restrictions
Monitor signs of fluid and electrolyte imbalance
Assess the access site for signs of infection
Post signs regarding location of access site; do not take blood pressure or perform a venipuncture on arm with access site
Assess, document, and report changes in general status
Skin care (bathe with tepid water to remove urea deposit)

(CAPD), or continuous cycle peritoneal dialysis (CCPD). The patient is taught to dialyze himself, which allows for much more freedom. Although hemodialysis can also be done at home, it is much more expensive and confining than CAPD.

Nursing interventions. Common complications associated with peritoneal dialysis guide nursing interventions. Hypotension may occur with excessive sodium and fluid removal. Peritonitis may arise from sepsis. Pain and/or hemorrhage may accompany instillation of the dialysate. Box 33-7 lists nursing intervention guidelines for peritoneal dialysis. Following are suggested nursing diagnoses for the patient receiving dialysis.

NURSING DIAGNOSES	NURSING INTERVENTIONS
Altered role performance, related to chronic illness, treatment side effects	Encourage verbalization of self-concept. Assist in identifying personal strengths. Assist patient and family with clarifying expected roles and those that must be relinquished or altered. Support grief work if lost role has occurred.

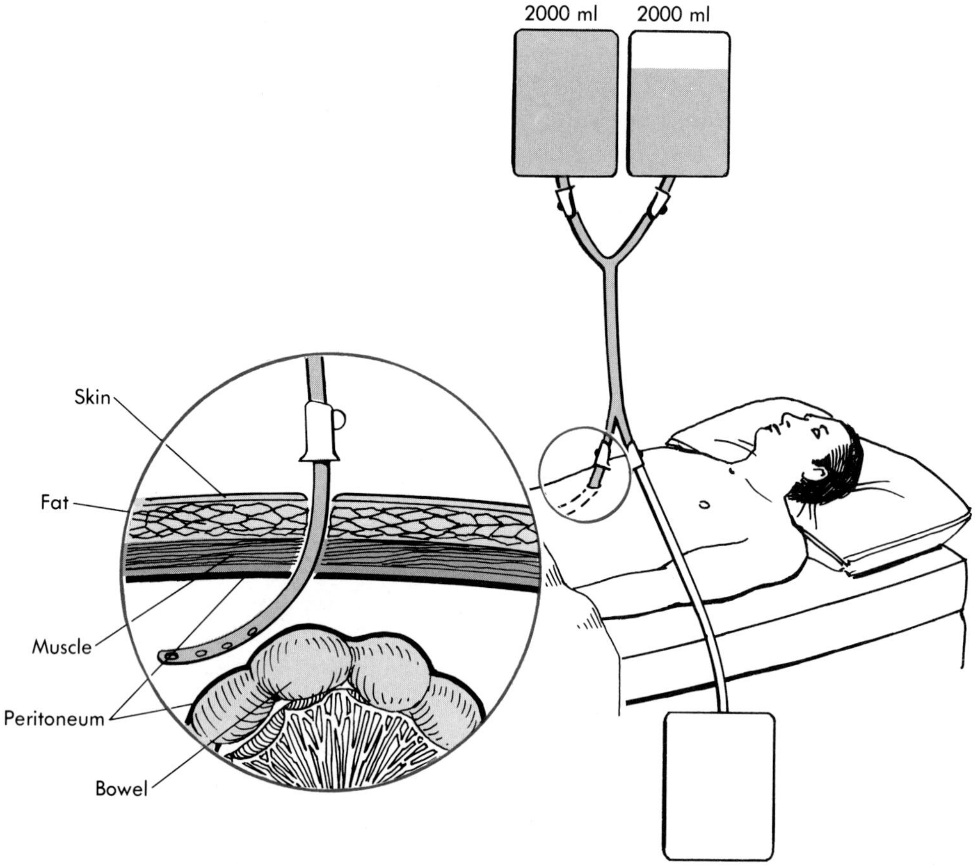

FIG. 33-14 Patient receiving peritoneal dialysis. Dialysis fluid is being inserted into peritoneal cavity.

NURSING DIAGNOSES	NURSING INTERVENTIONS
Altered sexuality patterns, related to altered body function	Encourage verbalization of sexual concerns. Inform physician of patient concerns.
Potential for infection, related to invasive techniques	Identify sources of potential infection. List signs of infection.
Fluid volume deficit, related to dialysis or inadequate fluid intake; fluid volume excess, related to retention or noncompliance with fluid restriction	Weigh every morning. Assess skin turgor. Monitor vital signs and laboratory studies. Measure intake/output. Restrict fluid intake

BOX 33-7 **NURSING INTERVENTION GUIDELINES FOR THE PATIENT UNDERGOING PERITONEAL DIALYSIS**

PATIENT TEACHING

Explanation of procedure
Signs of complications
Diet and/or fluid restrictions
Medication (schedule in relation to dialysis time)
Dialysate should be body temperature to lessen discomfort

MONITORING DURING DIALYSIS

Weigh before and after procedure
Hemorrhage (smoky, pink, or red-tinged dialysate)
Type of dialysate (tailored to patient needs)
Amount and timing of dialysate instillation
Vital signs

CARE BETWEEN DIALYSIS

Signs of peritonitis (pain, fever, cloudy fluid)
Strict aseptic care of catheter site
Weigh daily

REFERENCES AND SUGGESTED READINGS

1. Andressen GP: A fresh look at assessing the elderly, RN 52(6):28, 1989.
2. Ballinger PW: Merrill's atlas of radiographic positions and radiologic procedures, ed 6, St Louis, 1986, The CV Mosby Co.
3. Brunner LS, Suddarth DS, and Bare BG: Textbook of medical-surgical nursing, ed 6, Philadelphia, 1988, JB Lippincott Co.
4. Carpenito LJ: Nursing diagnosis: application to clinical practice, Philadelphia, 1988, JB Lippincott Co.
5. Cataldo CB, Nyenhui JR, and Whitney EN: Nutrition and diet therapy, St Paul, 1989, West Publishing Co.
6. Clayton BD: Basic pharmacology for nurses, ed 9, St Louis, 1989, The CV Mosby Co.
7. Dontas AS: Management of urinary-tract infections in the geriatric patient, Geriatr Med Today 6(61):41, 1987.
8. Eliopoulos C: Gerontological nursing, ed 2, Philadelphia, 1987, JB Lippincott Co.
9. Gasser TC, Larse EH, and Madsen PO: Prevention of indwelling catheter associated UTI, Infections in Medicine, Feb 1988, p 103.
10. Gerald MC and O'Bannon FV: Nursing pharmacology and therapeutics, ed 2, Norwalk, Conn, 1988, Appleton & Lange.
11. Glanze WD, editor: Mosby's medical and nursing dictionary, ed 2, St Louis, 1989, The CV Mosby Co.
12. Greenwood S: No more UTI misery, Women's Health, Jan/Feb 1989, p 18.
13. Griffith HW: Medical tests and diagnostic procedures, Philadelphia, 1989, Lea & Febiger.
14. Gruendemann BJ and Meeker MR: Alexander's care of the patient in surgery, ed 9, St Louis, 1991, The CV Mosby Co.
15. Gurklis JA and Menke EM: Identification of stressors and use of coping methods in chronic hemodialysis patients, Nurs Res 37(4):236, 1988.
16. Hamilton B: The seven ages of man, Nursing Times 85(15):68, 1989.
17. Hamilton PM: Basic pediatric nursing, ed 6, St Louis, 1990, The CV Mosby Co.
18. Heldrich FJ: Pinning down the diagnosis of UTI, Contemp Pediatr, April 1988, 52-78.
19. Henderson JS: Intermittent clean self-catheterization in clients with neurogenic bladder resulting from multiple sclerosis, J Neurosci Nurs 21(3):160, 1989.
20. Hoffmann SA: UTI's: everything you need to know about urinary tract woes, American Health, p 72, April 1989.
21. Hood GH and Dincher JR: Total patient care: foundations and practice, ed 7, St Louis, 1988, The CV Mosby Co.
22. Jaffe MS and Melson KA: Laboratory and diagnostic cards, St Louis, 1988, The CV Mosby Co.
23. Kim M, McFarland GK, and McLane AM: Pocket guide to nursing diagnoses, ed 3, St Louis, 1989, The CV Mosby Co.
24. Lederer JR et al: Care planning pocket guide, ed 3, Redwood City, Calif, 1990, Addison-Wesley Publishing Co.
25. Luckmann J and Sorensen KC: Medical-surgical nursing, ed 3, Philadelphia, 1987, WB Saunders Co.
26. Maher J, editor: Replacement of renal function by dialysis, ed 3, Dordrecht, Holland, 1989, Kluwer Academic Publisher.
27. Molavi A: Fluoroquinolones, AFP 37:5 279, 1988.
28. Moore MC: Pocket guide to nutrition and diet therapy, St Louis, 1988, The CV Mosby Co.
29. Neuman DK and Smith DAJ: Incontinence in elderly homebound patients, Holistic Nurs Pract 4(2):52, 1989.
30. Nissenson AR and Fine RN, editors: Dialysis therapy, Philadelphia, 1986, Hanley & Belfus, Inc./St Louis: The CV Mosby Co.
31. Nordstrom G: Urostomy patients: a strategy for care, Nurs Times 85(18):32, 1985.
32. Norris MK: Dialysis disequilibrium syndrome, Nurs 89 19:4, 1989.
33. Parsons CL: Do you think . . ., Postgrad Med 83(5):306, 1988.
34. Phipps WJ, Long BC, and Woods NF: Medical-surgical nursing, ed 4, St Louis, 1991, Mosby–Year Book, Inc.
35. Pieper B, et al: Inventing urine incontinence devices for women, Image 21(4):205, 1989.
36. Preshlock K: Detecting the hidden UTI, RN 52(1):65, 1989.
37. Richard CJ: Comprehensive nephrology nursing, Boston, 1986, Little, Brown & Co.
38. Roberts A: Systems of life No 170: Senior Systems-35, Nurs Times 85(12):55, 1989.
39. Roberts A: Systems of life No 171: Senior Systems-36, Nurs Times 85(19):61, 1989.
40. Sawyer DL: Potential for infections: a nursing diagnosis for the patient with an indwelling catheter, Focus Crit Care 16(1):46, 1989.
41. Scherer JC: Introductory medical-surgical nursing, ed 4, Philadelphia, 1986, JB Lippincott Co.
42. Schrier RW and Gottschalk CW, editors: Diseases of the kidney, ed 4, Boston, 1988, Little, Brown & Co.
43. Skidmore-Roth L: Mosby's 1991 Nursing drug reference, St Louis, 1991, The CV Mosby Co.
44. Stranghio L: Peritoneal dialysis made easy, Nurs 88 18(1), 1988.
45. Thompson JM and others: Mosby's manual of clinical nursing, ed 2, St Louis, 1989, The CV Mosby Co.
46. Tucker SM and others: Patient care standards, ed 4, St Louis, 1988, The CV Mosby Co.
47. Tulloch GJ: The incontinency taboo, Geriatr Nurs 10(1):19, 1989.
48. Turner SL: As women age: perspective on urinary incontinence, Rehabil Nurs 13(3):132, 1988.
49. Ulrich BT: Nephrology nursing: concepts and strategies, Norwalk, Conn, 1989, Appleton & Lange.
50. Way LW: Current surgical diagnosis and treatment, ed 8, Norwalk, Conn, 1988, Appleton & Lange.

CHAPTER CHALLENGE

KEY POINTS

- The kidneys lie retroperitoneally, just below the diaphragm.
- The filtering unit of the kidney is the nephron.
- Each nephron contains a glomerulus surrounded by a Bowman's capsule.
- The kidneys rid the body of wastes, maintain water and electrolyte balance, and maintain acid-base balance.
- Normal urine is transparent and yellow and contains waste products filtered by the kidneys.
- Assessment of the urinary tract is included in baseline data for all patients.
- The subject of urinary problems is an embarrassing topic for many patients; the nurse must be sensitive to the patient's feelings and be supportive.
- Aging may have a negative influence on urinary function, but many problems can be corrected.
- The kidneys filter a wide range of water-soluble products from the blood, such as medications, electrolytes, and metabolites.
- Dietary and medication modifications may be necessary for the patient with urinary dysfunction.
- Hydration status is monitored by daily weights, intake and output, laboratory studies, inspection of the skin and mucous membranes, and level of consciousness.
- Forty percent of nosocomial infections involve the urinary tract.
- Proper care of urinary catheters will decrease the chance of infections.
- Surgical intervention may be indicated for urinary dysfunction that cannot be corrected by medical management.
- Dialysis, which mimics kidney function, may be done temporarily or as a long-term therapy.

STUDY QUESTIONS

1. The filtering unit of the kidney is the:
   a. Medulla
   b. Cortex
   c. Nephron
   d. None of the above
2. Under normal circumstances, urine contains:
   a. Urea
   b. Glucose
   c. Albumin
   d. Leukocytes

Situation: Mr. Parker, 62 years old and retired, is admitted with a diagnosis of benign prostatic hypertrophy. He is scheduled for a transurethral resection of the prostate in the morning.

3. During Mr. Parker's preoperative teaching it is important to emphasize that after surgery he should expect:
   a. Red drainage from the catheter
   b. Limited intake of fluids
   c. A sodium-restricted diet
   d. Incisional drainage
4. Several hours postoperatively, Mr. Parker complains of a severe lower abdominal "spasmlike" pain. The first nursing intervention would be to:
   a. Inform the unit supervisor
   b. Increase the flow of the continuous bladder irrigation
   c. Administer the prescribed analgesic
   d. Check for kinks in the catheter and drainage system
5. The physician orders the removal of the indwelling catheter. Mr. Parker should be instructed that he should now anticipate:
   a. Fluid intake restrictions
   b. Normal voiding patterns
   c. Dribbling of urine
   d. No urine output for 6 to 8 hours

STUDY QUESTIONS (cont'd)

Situation: Ms. Wade, a 20-year-old college student, arrives at the clinic with lower pelvic pain and urinary frequency with burning and urgency.

6. The physician orders a urinalysis and urine culture to confirm the preliminary diagnosis of cystitis. To obtain the urine specimen, the nurse would first instruct Ms. Wade about:
   a. The catheterization procedure
   b. Obtaining a midstream clean-catch specimen
   c. Bringing in an early morning first-voiding specimen
   d. Limiting fluid intake for 8 hours to concentrate the urine
7. Diagnostic studies confirm the diagnosis of cystitis. Medications prescribed to treat cystitis include:

1. Bactrim DS	a. 1, 2
2. Meperidine	b. 2, 3, 4
3. Pyridium	c. 1, 3
4. Furosemide	d. 1, 2, 3, 4

Situation: Mr. Lemley, a 42-year-old construction worker, is admitted via the emergency room with a diagnosis of recurrent urolithiasis. He has been medicated with Demerol 100 mg and Phenergan 50 mg IM, 30 minutes ago. An IV of D_5W is being infused into his left forearm at 20 gtts/min.

8. Mr. Lemley is very restless and wants to walk. The nurse's main priority at this time is:
   a. Encouraging fluid intake
   b. Monitoring the IV
   c. Obtaining an assessment and history
   d. Maintaining a safe environment
9. The physician orders an intravenous urography. In preparation for the diagnostic study the nurse would first:
   a. Schedule the test with the x-ray department
   b. Order a light supper
   c. Explain the test procedure
   d. Administer a laxative
10. Mr. Lemley voids 360 ml of smoky-colored urine into the urinal. Using universal precautions, the nurse would:
    a. Strain the urine
    b. Discard the urine
    c. Save the urine for physician assessment
    d. Add the urine to a 24-hour collector
11. In teaching Mr. Lemley how to decrease the chance of further problems with urolithiasis, the nurse would encourage him to:

1. Increase water consumption	a. 1, 2
2. Avoid inactivity	b. 1, 3, 4
3. Adhere to dietary restrictions	c. 2, 3
4. Take medications as prescribed	d. 1, 2, 3, 4

Situation: Mr. Redman, a 49-year-old rural mailman, is admitted from outpatient surgery following a diagnostic cystoscopy with biopsy. He is accompanied by his wife and brother.

12. During interview Mr. Redman begins to cry when relating the reason for his admission. The nurse should:
    a. Continue the interview
    b. Tell him not to worry
    c. Wait quietly until he can continue
    d. Leave so he can be alone

34

Care of the Patient with a Respiratory Disorder

CONNIE M. WALLACE

LEARNING OBJECTIVES

After reading this chapter, the student should be able to do the following:

- Define the key terms.
- List and define the parts of the upper and lower respiratory tract.
- Describe the purpose of the respiratory system.
- Differentiate between external and internal respiration.
- List the ways in which oxygen and carbon dioxide are transported in the blood.
- List five nursing interventions to assist patients with retained pulmonary secretions.
- Identify those signs and symptoms that indicate a patient is experiencing hypoxia.
- Identify four strategies the nurse can teach patients to decrease risk of infection.
- List three medications commonly prescribed for the patient with tuberculosis.
- Compare/contrast nursing observations and interventions for the patient with chronic obstructive pulmonary disease (COPD) and the patient with pneumonia.
- List three nursing observations/interventions pertaining to the care of the patient with closed chest drainage.
- Discuss nursing interventions for the patient with a laryngectomy.
- State three possible nursing diagnoses for the patient with altered respiratory function.
- Identify nursing interventions relevant to psychosocial concerns of the patient with altered respiratory function.
- Discuss three risk factors associated with pulmonary emboli.

RELATED TOPICS OF INTEREST

- Signs, symptoms, and physical assessment (Chapter 13)
- Specimin collection (Chapter 21)
- The surgical patient (Chapter 26)
- Care of the patient with a cardiovascular or blood disorder (Chapter 32)
- Cardiopulmonary resuscitation (Chapter 53)

KEY TERMS

Define the following:

- adventitious
- alveolus
- apneic
- asthma
- atelectasis
- bronchiole
- bronchitis
- bronchoscopy
- chronic obstructive pulmonary disease (COPD)
- cilia
- cor pulmonale
- cyanosis
- dyspnea
- emphysema
- empyema
- epistaxis
- exacerbation
- extrinsic
- hemoglobin
- hemoptysis
- hilum (hilus)
- hypercapnia
- hypoventilation
- hypoxia
- intrinsic
- larynx
- orthopnea
- pharynx
- pleural effusion
- stertorous
- surface tension
- surfactant
- tachypnea
- thoracentesis
- trachea
- tracheostomy

ANATOMY AND PHYSIOLOGY

If an individual has experienced choking or has had to struggle for breath, the sensation of panic is a reminder that one cannot live without oxygen. For the millions of cells throughout the body to carry out their specialized activities, it is mandatory that they have a continuous supply of oxygen. External respiration, or breathing, allows this exchange of oxygen and carbon dioxide between the lungs and the environment. As air is inhaled, it is warmed, moistened, and filtered to prepare it for use by the body. The respiratory system works with the cardiovascular system to deliver the oxygen to the cells, where it is used to provide the cells with energy to carry out metabolism. Internal respiration refers to the exchange of oxygen and carbon dioxide at the cellular level. Oxygen enters the cells while carbon dioxide leaves the cells. These gases diffuse across the cell membranes into the bloodstream. The cardiovascular system plays the role of transporter. Failure of the respiratory or cardiovascular systems has the same result: rapid death of the cells from oxygen starvation. Fig. 34-1 shows the structural plan of the respiratory organs.

Upper Respiratory Tract

Nose. Air enters the respiratory tract through the nose. The air is filtered, moistened, and warmed as it enters the two nasal openings (nares) and travels to the nasal cavity. The nasal septum separates the nares. This entire area is lined with mucous membrane, which is vascular. This provides the warmth and moisture necessary. Normally a liter of moisture is secreted by this membrane every day.

Lateral to the nasal cavities are the three scroll-like bones called *turbinates* or *conchae* (Fig. 34-2), which cause the air to move over a larger surface area. This increase in surface area allows the air more time for warming and moisturizing. Lining the nasal cavities are tiny hairs, which trap dust and other foreign particles and prevent them from entering the lower respiratory tract.

Communicating with the nasal structures are the paranasal sinuses (Fig. 34-3). They are called the *frontal, maxillary, sphenoid,* and *ethmoid cavities.* They are hollow areas, which makes the skull lighter. It is believed they give resonance to the voice. They also are lined with mucous membrane that is continuous with the nasal cavity. Because of this, nasal infections can cause sinusitis, which is uncomfortable and difficult to treat.

The receptors for the sense of smell are located in the mucosa of the nasal cavities. They are the nerve endings of the olfactory nerve, the first cranial nerve. The nasolacrimal ducts, or tear ducts, communicate with the upper

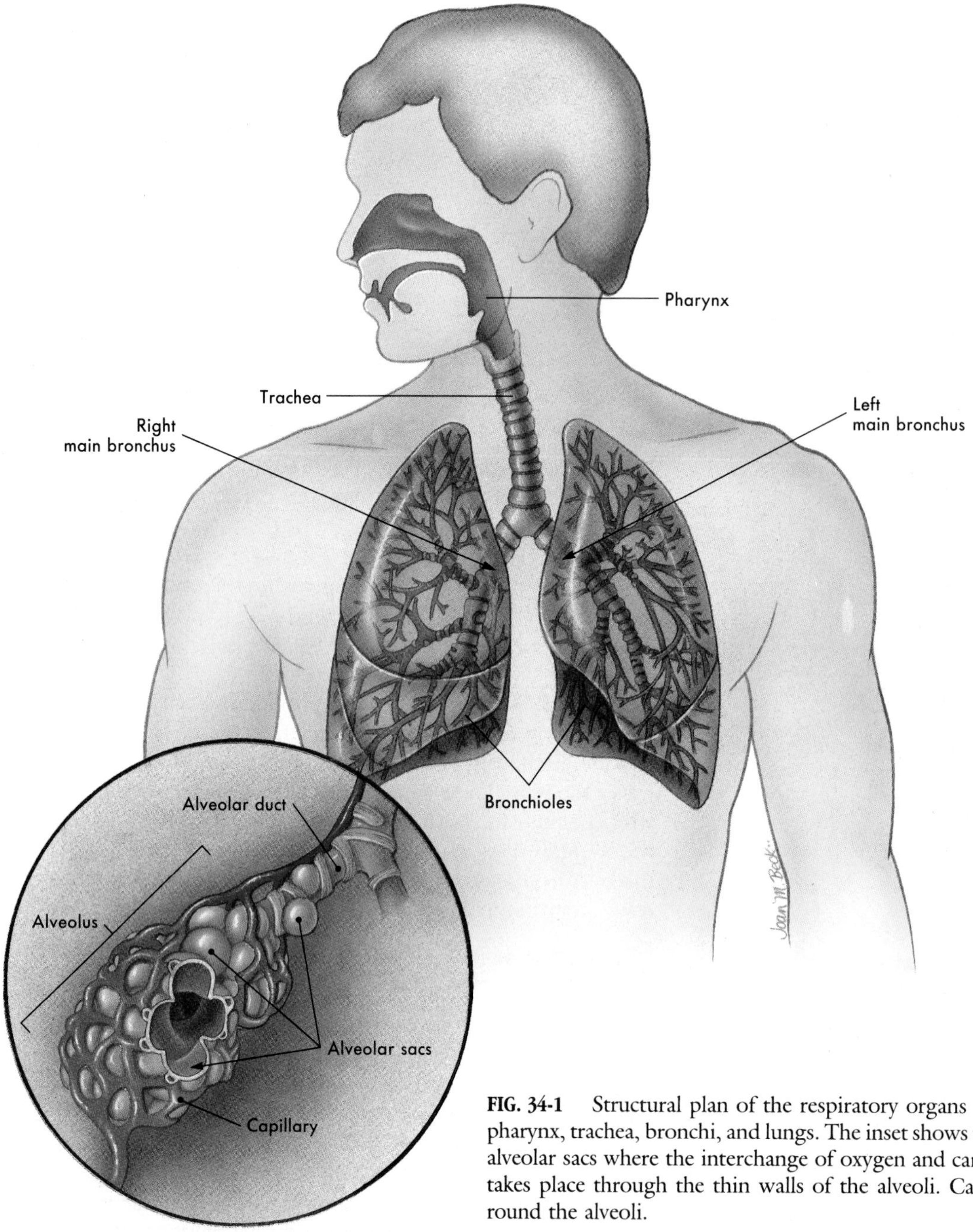

FIG. 34-1 Structural plan of the respiratory organs showing the pharynx, trachea, bronchi, and lungs. The inset shows the grapelike alveolar sacs where the interchange of oxygen and carbon dioxide takes place through the thin walls of the alveoli. Capillaries surround the alveoli.

nasal chamber. Hence when an individual cries, he has copious nasal secretions.

Pharynx. The **pharynx,** or throat, is approximately 5 inches long and is the passageway for both air and food. At the distal end of the pharynx, food passes to the esophagus. The pharynx is divided into three subdivisions: (1) nasopharynx (most superior portion); (2) oropharynx (posterior to mouth); and (3) laryngopharynx (directly superior to larynx).

The eustachian tubes enter either side of the nasopharynx, connecting it to the middle ear. Because the inner linings of the pharynx and the eustachian tubes are continuous, an infection of the pharynx can spread easily to the middle ear. This is very common in children.

In the mucous membrane of the pharynx are masses of lymphatic tissue called the tonsils. The adenoids (pharyngeal tonsils) are in the nasopharynx, whereas the palatine tonsils are in the oropharynx. Inflammation of these structures is referred to as *tonsillitis,* also very common in children. Physicians now recognize the importance of tonsils because of their lymphatic properties and thus their role in body defense mechanisms. Fewer tonsillectomy procedures are being performed.

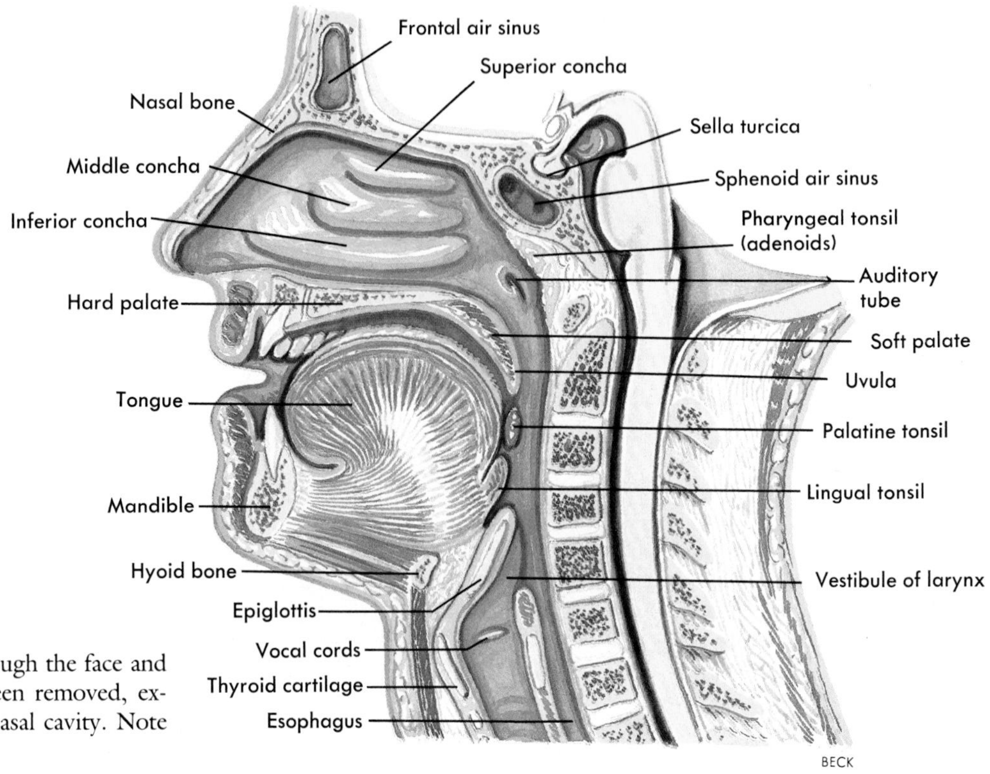

FIG. 34-2 Sagittal section through the face and neck. The nasal septum has been removed, exposing the lateral wall of the nasal cavity. Note the position of the conchae.

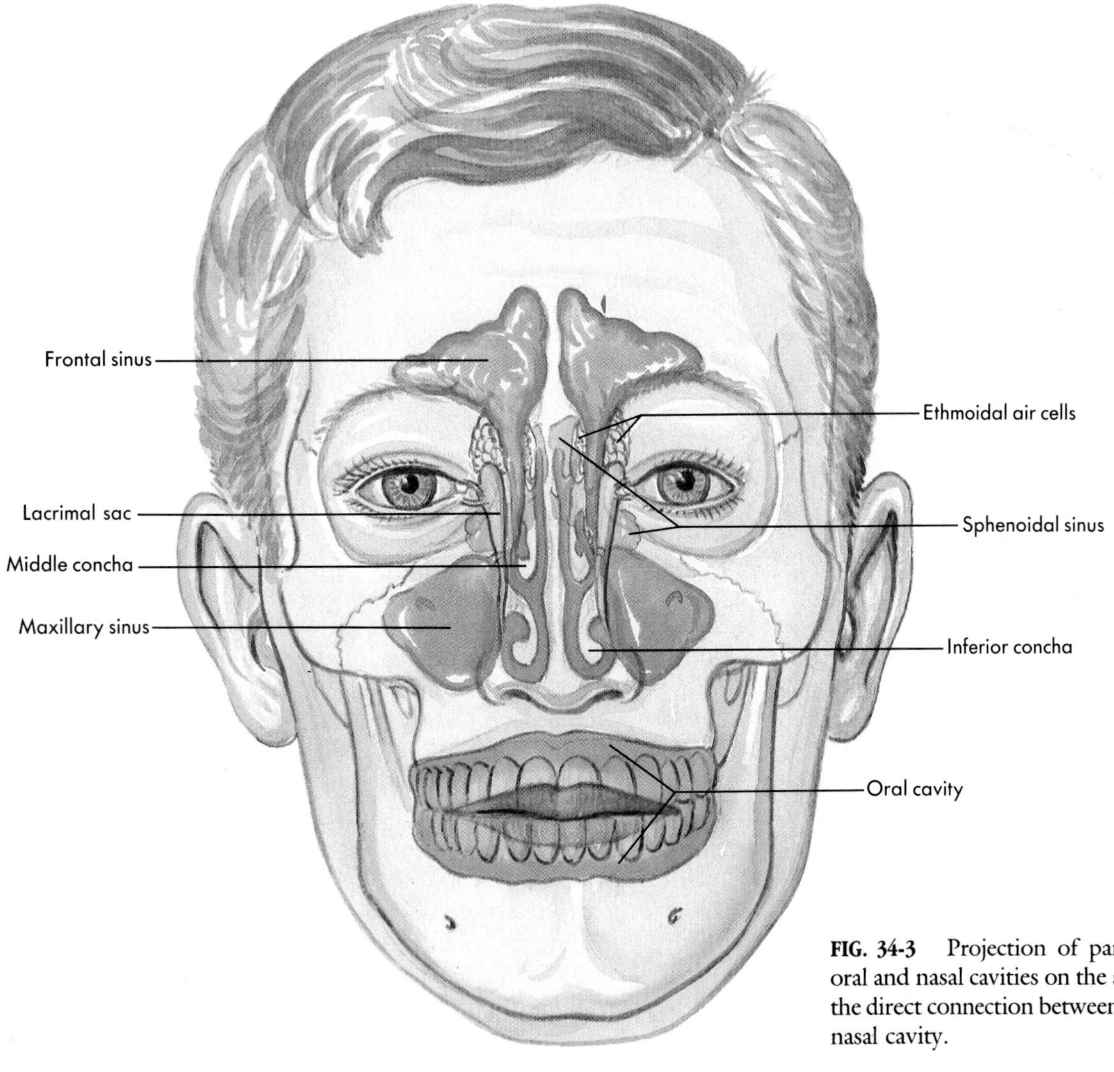

FIG. 34-3 Projection of paranasal sinuses and oral and nasal cavities on the skull and face. Note the direct connection between the sinuses and the nasal cavity.

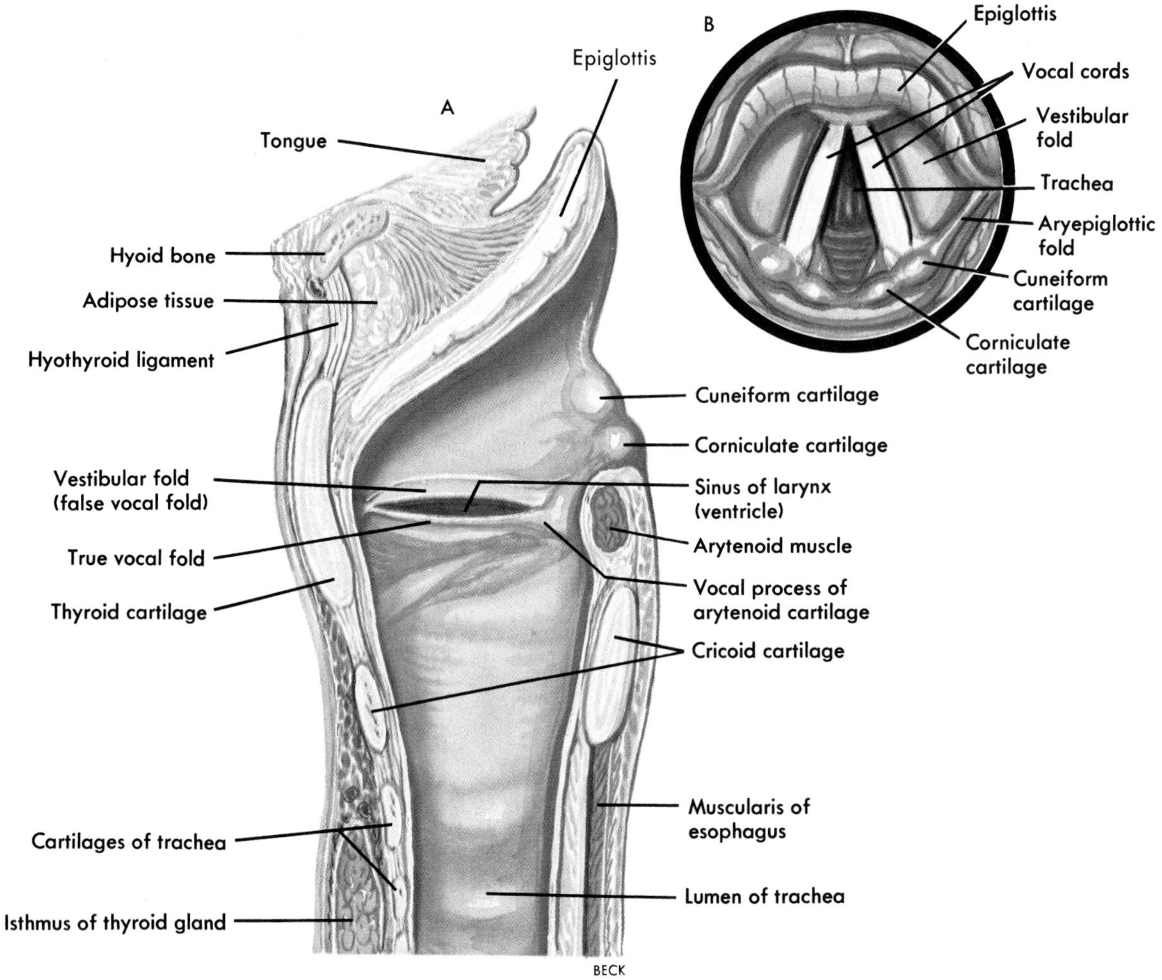

FIG. 34-4 **A,** Sagittal section through the larynx. **B,** Larynx and vocal cords as viewed from above through a laryngeal mirror.

Larynx (Fig. 34-4). The **larnyx,** or voice box, is supported by nine areas of cartilage and connects the pharynx with the trachea. The largest area of cartilage is composed of two fused plates and is called the *thyroid cartilage* or *Adam's apple*. It is smaller in females than in males. The epiglottis, a large, leaf-shaped area of cartilage, protects the larynx when swallowing. It covers the larynx tightly to prevent food entering the trachea and directs the food to the esophagus.

The larynx contains the vocal cords, which are muscular folds of tissue that extend from the lateral walls. During expiration air rushes over the vocal cords, which causes them to vibrate. This enables speech to occur. The opening between the vocal cords is called the glottis. The size of the vocal cords varies among individuals, which accounts for differences in pitch. Because the male usually has larger vocal cords, his voice is deeper than the female's.

Trachea. The **trachea,** or windpipe, is a tubelike structure that extends approximately 5 inches to the midchest, where it divides into the right and left bronchi. It lies anterior to the esophagus and connects the larynx with the bronchi. It contains C-shaped cartilaginous rings that keep it from collapsing. The open part of the C-shape lies posterior to the column, anterior to the esophagus. This allows for expansion of the esophagus during swallowing while still maintaining patency of the trachea. This is necessary for uninterrupted breathing. The entire structure is lined with mucous membrane with tiny **cilia** that sweep dust or debris upward toward the nasal cavity. Any large particles initiate the cough reflex, which is a protective mechanism that aids in the evacuation of foreign material. Sometimes, because of an airway obstruction, it becomes necessary to perform a **tracheostomy** (a surgical opening into the trachea). Once this procedure is completed, the individual breathes through the tracheal opening rather than the nose. The opening is below the larynx, so the air cannot pass over the vocal cords. The vocal cords cannot vibrate, and speech becomes physiologically impossible.

Lower Respiratory Tract

Bronchial tree. As the trachea enters the lungs, it divides into the right and left bronchi. The right bronchus enters into the right lung. It is larger in diameter and more vertical in descent. The left bronchus enters the left lung. It is smaller in diameter and slightly horizontal in position. Because of this design, foreign objects that are aspirated generally enter the right bronchus.

The large bronchi continue to divide into smaller structures called **bronchioles.** These structures continue to divide into smaller, tubelike structures called *terminal bronchioles* or *alveolar ducts*. All of these structures are lined with ciliated mucous membrane, as is the trachea.

The end structures of the bronchial tree are called *alveoli*. These saclike structures resemble a bunch of grapes. A single grapelike structure is called an **alveolus** (see Fig. 34-1). It is in this terminal structure of the bronchial tree that gas exchange takes place. Each alveolus is surrounded by a blood capillary, and diffusion of carbon dioxide and oxygen occurs.

Main bronchi and bronchioles. As stated, the lungs contain a right primary bronchus and a left primary bronchus. They consist of three layers of tissue. The outer layer is composed of fibrous tissue reinforced with cartilage. The middle layer is composed of smooth muscle. The innermost layer is mucous membrane coated with cilia. The bronchi connect the trachea to the smaller tubules, the bronchioles.

As the bronchi divide into the smaller structures, bronchioles, they lose the outer cartilage and fibrous tissue. Their walls are thinner and contain elastic tissue. It has been estimated that there are more than a million bronchioles in each lung. This branching and continual division of tubules make these structures resemble a tree with its branches—hence the name *bronchial tree*.

Alveoli. The terminal structure of the bronchial tree is the alveolus, a small, grapelike structure. Alveoli are contained in small sacs called the *alveolar sacs*. The walls of the individual alveoli are composed of a single layer of cells with elastic fibers intertwined. This enables them to contract and relax with breathing. In addition, each alveolus is coated with a thin covering of **surfactant.** This is a lipoprotein that reduces the **surface tension** of the alveolus and prevents it from collapsing between each breath. There are millions of alveoli in the lungs; they give shape and form to the lungs. They are filled with air, and lung tissue would float if submerged in water.

This tiny, grapelike structure is the most important feature of the respiratory system. It is here the oxygen diffuses into the cardiovascular system.

In the cardiovascular system the vessels get smaller and smaller until they reach the smallest structure, called a *capillary*, which is microscopic. In the lungs these capillaries surround the alveoli. Because the walls of the capillaries are thin and the walls of the alveoli are also thin, diffusion allows the oxygen to pass from the alveoli into the capillaries (Fig. 34-5). Once the oxygen enters the capillaries, it attaches itself to the red blood cells, more specifically, the hemoglobin portion of the red blood cells.

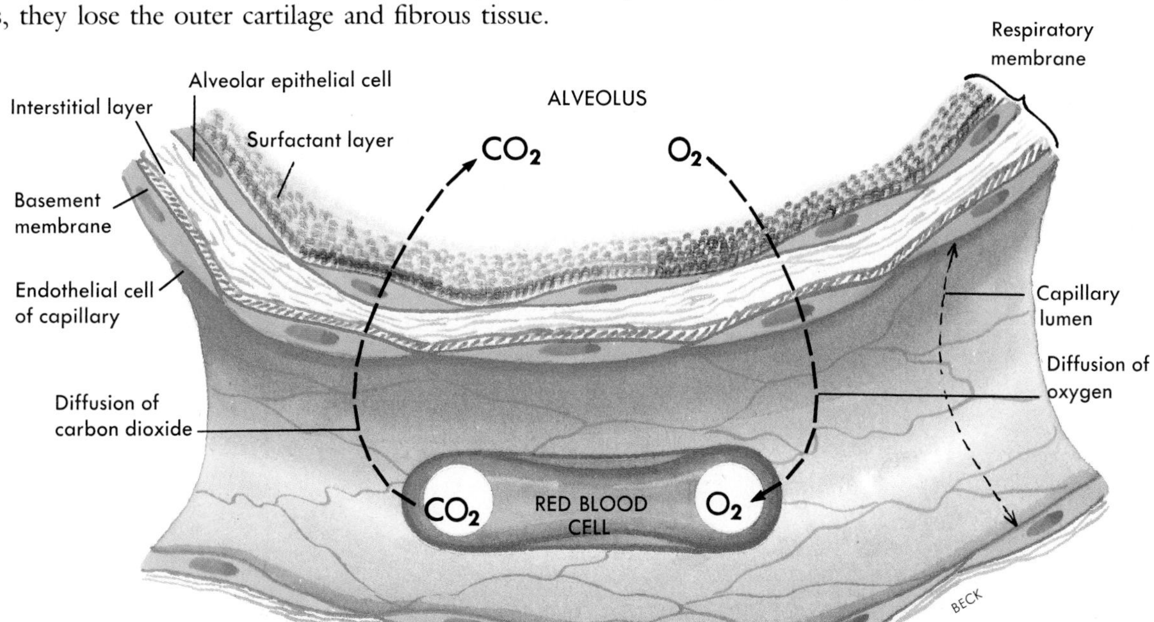

FIG. 34-5 A small portion of the respiratory membrane greatly magnified. An extremely thin interstitial layer of tissue separates the endothelial cell and basement membrane on the capillary side from the epithelial cell and surfactant layer on the alveolar side of the respiratory membrane. The total thickness of the respiratory membrane is less than 1/5000 of an inch.

The oxygen then continues in the bloodstream to the heart to be transported to the cells throughout the body.

Mechanics of Breathing

Thoracic cavity. The lungs occupy almost all of the thoracic cavity except the centermost area, the mediastinum, which contains the heart and great vessels. This cavity is enclosed by the sternum, ribs, and thoracic vertebrae. It is referred to as the *interpleural space.*

Lungs. The lungs are large, paired, spongy, cone-shaped organs (Fig. 34-6). They weigh approximately 2½ pounds. The right lung contains three lobes; the left lung contains only two lobes. Located approximately 1 inch above the first rib is the narrow part, the apex, or upper part, of each lung. The broad, lower part, the base of the lungs, lies on the diaphragm. The **hilum** is the medial portion and contains the pulmonary artery, pulmonary vein, main bronchus, and lymph nodes.

The lungs receive their blood supply through the pulmonary veins and pulmonary arteries, which come directly from the heart. The pulmonary artery comes from the right ventricle of the heart and brings deoxygenated blood to the lungs. It then flows through the thousands of tiny lung capillaries that are near to the air-filled alveoli. External respirations or the exchange of gases between the blood and alveolar air occurs by diffusion.

Diffusion is a passive process that results in movement down a concentration gradient; that is, substances move from an area of high concentration to an area of low concentration of the diffusing substance. Blood flowing through lung capillaries is low in oxygen. Oxygen is continually removed from the blood and used by the cells of the body. By the time it enters the lung capillaries, it is "low" in oxygen content. Because alveolar air is rich in oxygen, diffusion will cause movement of oxygen from the area of high O_2 concentration (capillary blood).

Diffusion of carbon dioxide also occurs between blood in lung capillaries and alveolar air. Blood flowing through the lung capillaries is high in carbon dioxide. As body

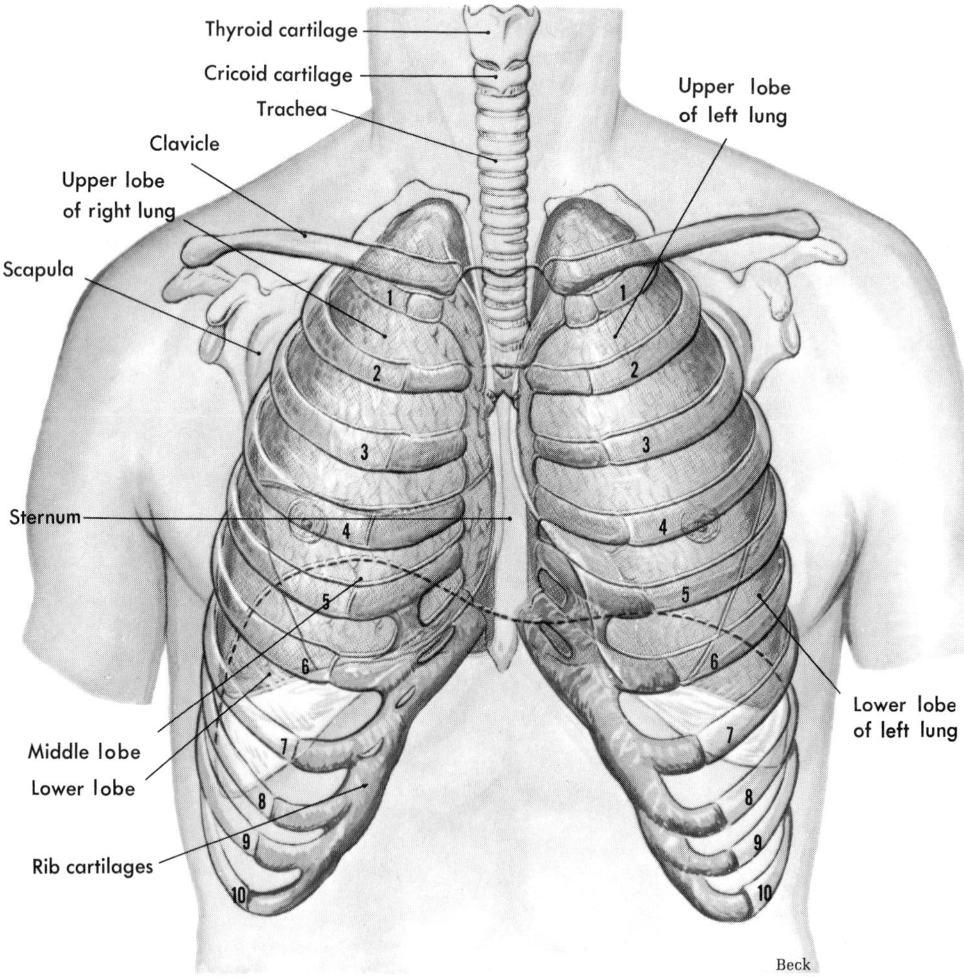

FIG. 34-6 Projection of the lungs and trachea in relation to rib cage and clavicles. Dotted line shows location of dome-shaped diaphragm at the end of expiration and before inspiration. Note that apex of each lung projects above the clavicle. Ribs 11 and 12 are not visible in this view.

cells remove oxygen from circulating blood, they add the waste product carbon dioxide to it. As a result, the blood in pulmonary capillaries eventually becomes low in oxygen and high in carbon dioxide. Diffusion of carbon dioxide results in its movement from an area of high concentration in the pulmonary capillaries to an area of low concentration in alveolar air. Then from the alveoli, carbon dioxide leaves the body in the expired air (see Fig. 34-5).

The capillaries surround the alveoli. The blood becomes rich with oxygen, goes to the pulmonary veins, returns to the left atrium, and continues to the left ventricle. It is then transported throughout the body.

The surface of each lung is covered with a thin, moist, serous membrane composed of tough endothelial cells. It is called the *visceral pleura.* The walls of the thoracic cavity are also covered with the same type of membrane, called the *parietal pleura.* The pleural cavity around the lungs is an airtight vacuum that contains negative pressure. The pressure within the lungs is atmospheric and is higher than in the pleural cavity. The negative pressure assists in keeping the lungs inflated. The visceral and parietal pleura produce a serous secretion, which allows the lungs to slide over the walls of the thorax during breathing. Usually the body produces the exact amount needed. If too much serous secretion is produced, it results in an accumulation of fluid in the pleural space called **pleural effusion.** This causes the pleural space to become distended and puts pressure on the lungs, making it difficult for the patient to breathe. The physician may decide to remove this fluid. A thoracentesis will be performed. A needlelike instrument is inserted into the pleural space, and the fluid is removed.

Another condition that could result is *pleurisy.* In this condition the pleura becomes inflamed and produces too little fluid. With each breath the patient experiences sharp chest pain.

Pressure changes. For breathing to occur, changes of pressure within the thoracic cavity must take place. Immediately preceding inspiration the air pressure inside the lungs is equal to the atmospheric pressure. For inspiration to occur, the lungs must have less pressure than the atmosphere. To achieve this, the volume of the lungs must be increased. The lungs need to expand for inspiration. This expansion causes an increase in lung volume and decreases the pressure in the lungs. To accomplish this (1) the external intercostal muscles contract and lift the ribs upward and outward; (2) the diaphragm contracts, which flattens and lowers its dome; and (3) the sternum is pushed forward, increasing the anteroposterior diameter. All of these activities occur simultaneously. They result in increased lung volume and decreased atmospheric pressure. As a result, the outside air rushes into the lungs (inspiration).

For expiration to take place, all structures relax; it is a passive process. The sternum drops back, the ribs move down, and the diaphragm moves up. These movements decrease the diameter of the thoracic cavity and return it to its resting state.

Respiratory movements/ranges. The rhythmic movements of the chest walls, ribs, and associated muscles when air is inhaled and exhaled make up the respiratory movements. The combination of one inspiration and one expiration makes one respiration, or respiratory movement. At rest the normal inspiration lasts about 2 seconds and expiration about 3 seconds.

Room air when inhaled contains about 21% oxygen; exhaled air contains 16% oxygen and 3.5% carbon dioxide. This represents the actual amount of oxygen used from a single breath.

When air enters the respiratory system, it must travel through the bronchial tree. As the tubes become smaller, the air moves slower until it reaches the alveoli, where it moves only by diffusion. Because the walls of the alveoli are thin and moist, the exchange of oxygen and carbon dioxide occurs readily.

The normal range of respirations for an adult at rest is about 14 to 20 breaths per minute. This rate can be affected by many variables: age, sex, activity, disease, and body temperature. For example, the respiratory rate for a newborn is 40 to 60 breaths per minute; early school age, 24 to 26 breaths; teenagers, 20 to 22 breaths; adults, 14 to 20 breaths. The normal range for females is usually slightly higher than for males.

Members of the health care team should assess all factors influencing the patient's respirations and should count the respirations without patient awareness to prevent alterations in the breathing pattern.

Regulation of respiration

Nervous control. The medulla oblongata and pons of the brain are responsible for the basic rhythm and depth of respirations. This rhythm can be modified according to the demands of the body. Other parts of the nervous system help to coordinate the transfer from inspiration to expiration. These areas are the pneumotaxic area, in the upper pons, and the apneustic area, in the lower pons.

Because the respiratory center can relay messages to the cerebal cortex, there is also some voluntary control, which allows alteration of breathing patterns. Breath can be held for a short period, but as the carbon dioxide level in the blood increases, the inspiratory area of the brain is stimulated, messages are sent to the inspiratory muscles, and breathing resumes on an involuntary basis. This mechanism makes it impossible to kill oneself by holding the breath.

Stretch receptors located in the walls of the bronchioles and alveoli respond to overinflation, as well as extreme deflation. Impulses alerting the status of inflation travel along the vagus nerve, and appropriate action is taken to prevent injury to the lung tissues.

Chemical stimuli. Carbon dioxide is considered the chemical stimulant for regulation of respiration, but it is actually the hydrogen ions that maintain the control. In the blood stream carbon dioxide combines with water to form carbonic acid, which immediately converts to hydrogen ions and bicarbonate ions. It should be remembered that the more hydrogen ions a solution contains, the more acidic it becomes. Therefore the more carbon dioxide in the blood, the more acidic the blood becomes. After exhalation the blood becomes more alkaline. The normal pH of blood is 7.35 to 7.45—a narrow range. Deviation from this range causes the patient to develop either alkalosis or acidosis.

Most of the oxygen transported to the cells is bound to the **hemoglobin** portion of the red blood cells. Normally this is a weak bond and is easily broken at the cellular level. Once the cells use the oxygen, carbon dioxide is given off and must return to the lungs. For carbon dioxide to reach the lungs it must travel on the bicarbonate ion. After reaching the lungs it is exhaled with expiration.

Respiratory measurements. A device called a *spirometer* is used to provide diagnostic information about the respiratory capacity of the lungs. The patient breathes into the device, and a tracing is made of the breathing ability (see Chapter 26).

Tidal volume refers to the amount of air inhaled and exhaled at rest. This is about 500 ml, or 1 pint. *Vital capacity* refers to a maximum inhalation followed by a maximum exhalation. This is 4500 to 5000 ml in an adult with healthy lung tissue. Total lung capacity refers to the total volume of air contained in the lungs after maximum inspiration. On the average this is about 6000 ml. Residual volume is the amount of air that remains in the lungs after maximum exhalation.

Modified respiratory movements. Such emotions as laughing, crying, sobbing, yawning, and sighing can be expressed. Respirations can also remove foreign matter from the respiratory tract by sneezing and coughing. Most of these responses are involuntary, but some of these movements can be initiated voluntarily. The most common movements are listed as follows:

- Cough: A deep breath is taken and the glottis closes. This results in a strong expiration, which forces the glottis open. In turn, air passes through the upper respiratory passageways with significant force.
- Sneeze: Air is forced through the nasal cavities instead of the oral cavity. The uvula closes the oral cavity, which aids in redirecting the forced air. A sneeze can clear the upper respiratory passageways.
- Sigh: A deep inspiration is followed with a short, forceful expiration.
- Yawn: A deep breath is taken with the mouth wide open, causing all the alveoli to ventilate, which does not happen with normal breathing.
- Sob: A series of convulsive inspirations are taken, immediately followed by a single, prolonged expiration. The glottis closes earlier than normal, and only a little air can reach the lungs.
- Cry: Normal inhalation is followed by exhalation with many short, convulsive movements. Facial grimaces are also present.
- Laugh: Same movements occur as with crying, distinguished only by the individual's facial expression.
- Singultus (hiccups): A sharp inspiratory sound is caused by stimulation or irritation of the phrenic nerve (which serves the diaphragm) when the diaphragm contracts, and the glottis closes.

ASSESSMENT OF RESPIRATORY FUNCTION

The function of the respiratory system is gas exchange (oxygen and carbon dioxide) at the alveolar/capillary level. This function depends on the lungs' capability for contraction and expansion, which in turn is influenced by musculoskeletal and neurological functions.

The respiratory system is always included in a physical assessment of the patient's general health. Certain types of patients require more extensive assessments. Included are those with acute or chronic respiratory or cardiac conditions, those with a history of respiratory impairment related to trauma or allergic reaction, or those who have recently undergone surgery or anesthesia. Because there is often a potential for physical and emotional responses to be correlated, the nurse should also inquire about any accompanying anxiety or stress. This information should be obtained in an unhurried, matter-of-fact manner.

The respiratory assessment will include collection of *subjective* data. During the interview the patient should be encouraged to describe any symptoms, such as shortness of breath, dyspnea on exertion, or cough. Data should include onset, duration, precipitating factors, and relief measures, such as position and use of over-the-counter or prescribed medications. If the patient has reported a cough, the nurse will ask him to describe the cough: productive or nonproductive; harsh, dry, or hacking; and color and amount of mucus expectorated. This information should be recorded as direct quotes from the patient when possible.

The nurse will then gather *objective data.* Initial observation will yield information on the patient's skin color and turgor. The nurse will note any obvious respiratory distress—dyspnea, wheezes, or **orthopnea.** To continue this assessment, the nurse will auscultate all lung fields anteriorly and posteriorly, noting the presence of adventitious lung sounds (see Fig. 13-5).

Diagnostic Tests

There are a variety of tests used to identify respiratory conditions. They include radiology studies, laboratory work, and more invasive measures. The nurse should be familiar with these tests so she can adequately prepare the patient.

Chest roentgenogram. Usually referred to as chest x-ray, this test gives information on alterations in size and location of the pulmonary structures and blood flow, as well as identifies the presence of lesions, foreign bodies, or fluid. The chest x-ray examination can be performed at different angles for greater clarification. The nurse should have the patient wear a hospital gown tied in back. Pins must not be used. Any article of clothing, such as a bra with metal hooks, must be removed, since the metal will produce a shadow on the film.

CT scan of lung. Computerized tomography (CT) scans take pictures of small layers of pulmonary tissue, usually to identify a pulmonary lesion. These views can be diagonal or cross-sectional, with a scanner rotating at various angles. Although this test is painless, noninvasive, and results in little radiation exposure, patient teaching is necessary before the procedure to offer explanations and allay anxiety.

Pulmonary function testing (PFT). Pulmonary function testing is composed of various procedures to obtain information on lung volume, ventilation, pulmonary spirometry, and gas exchange. Lung volume tests refer to the volume of air that can be completely and slowly exhaled after a maximum inhalation (vital capacity [VC]). Inspiratory capacity (IC) is the largest amount of air that can be inhaled in one breath from the resting expiratory level. Total lung capacity (TLC) is calculated to determine the volume of air in the lung after a maximal inhalation. Ventilation tests refer to the volume of air inhaled or exhaled in each respiratory cycle. Pulmonary spirometry tests refer to the amount of air that can be forcefully exhaled after maximum inhalation. These tests require the use of a spirometer.

One of the most important tools for diagnosing respiratory diseases is gas exchange, which refers to the capacity for carbon dioxide to be diffused. This component of the PFT determines the degree of function in the pulmonary capillary beds in contact with functioning alveoli.

Mediastinoscopy. A mediastinoscopy is a surgical endoscopic procedure in which an incision is created in the suprasternal notch, allowing the endoscope to be passed into the upper mediastinum. This is performed to gather a sample of lymph nodes for biopsy for tumor diagnosis. Because these lymph nodes receive lymphatic drainage from the lungs, they are of diagnostic value for carcinoma. This procedure is performed in the operating room, and the patient usually receives a general anesthetic agent.

Laryngoscopy. Laryngoscopy can be performed for either direct or indirect visualization of the larynx. Indirect laryngoscopy is probably the most common procedure for assessment of respiratory difficulties; this entails the use of a laryngeal mirror in the awake patient's mouth

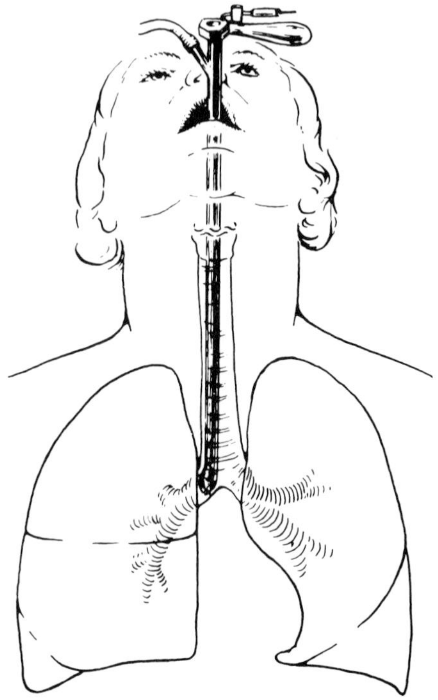

FIG. 34-7 Bronchoscope inserted through trachea into bronchus.

for visualization. This procedure can be used for biopsy or polyp excision.

Direct laryngoscopy requires local or general anesthesia and exposes the vocal chords with a laryngoscope passed down over the tongue.

Bronchoscopy. A **bronchoscopy** is performed by passing a bronchoscope into the trachea and bronchi. By use of either a rigid bronchoscope or a flexible, fiberoptic bronchoscope, the larynx, trachea, and bronchi can be visualized (Fig. 34-7). Diagnostic bronchoscopic examination includes observation of the tracheobronchial tree for (1) abnormalities, (2) tissue biopsy, and (3) aspiration of sputum for testing. A local anesthetic agent may be used, but an intravenous general anesthetic agent is usually given. The patient is treated as a surgical patient. Nursing interventions for patients after bronchoscopy are as follows:

1. Patient is on NPO status until gag reflex returns.
2. Patient is in semi-Fowler's position and turns on either side to facilitate removal of secretions, unless physician specifies another position.
3. Patient is monitored for signs of laryngeal edema or laryngospasms, such as stridor or increasing dyspnea.
4. If lung tissue biopsy is taken, sputum is monitored for signs of hemorrhage. NOTE: Blood-streaked sputum can be expected for a few days after biopsy.

Sputum specimen. Sputum samples frequently are obtained for microscopic evaluation, such as Gram stain and culture and sensitivity (Box 34-1). Sputum can be ob-

BOX 34-1 RANGE OF SPUTUM CHARACTERISTICS

COLOR	ODOR
Clear	None
White	Malodorous
Yellow	
Green	**BLOOD**
Brown	All the time
Red	Occasionally
Streaked with blood	Early morning

CONSISTENCY

Frothy
Watery
Tenacious

tained directly: the patient voluntarily expectorates sputum, which is collected in a sterile container. Usually early morning samples are collected on 3 consecutive days. If the patient cannot expectorate sputum (not saliva) spontaneously, sputum production may be induced by using a warm nebulizer mist of sodium chloride solution. The specimen should be properly labeled and sent immediately to the laboratory.

Sputum samples can also be obtained indirectly, such as with nasotracheal suctioning with a catheter or transtracheal aspiration. Care must be taken to ensure that the suction catheters remain sterile.

Cytology studies. Cytology tests can be performed on any body secretion, such as sputum or pleural fluid, to detect the presence of abnormal or malignant cells.

Thoracentesis. Thoracentesis involves the insertion of a needle into the pleural space. Indications for a thoracentesis include the following:

1. Removal of fluid for diagnostic purposes
   a. The pleural fluid can be examined for specific gravity, white blood cell count, red blood cell count, protein, and glucose
   b. The fluid can be cultured for pathogens and checked for the presence of abnormal or malignant cells
   c. The gross appearance of the fluid, the quantity obtained, and the location of the site of the thoracentesis should be recorded
2. Biopsy of the pleura
3. Removal of fluid when it is a threat to patient safety or comfort
4. Instillation of medication into the pleural space

Nursing interventions for the patient undergoing thoracentesis include the following:

1. Explain the procedure; every means should be used to relieve the patient's anxiety.
2. The procedure is usually carried out in the patient's room. The patient sits on the edge of the bed with his head and arms resting on a pillow placed on an overbed table. Patients who cannot sit up should be turned to the unaffected side with the head of the bed elevated 30 degrees.
3. Vital signs, general appearance, and respiratory status should be monitored throughout the procedure. Usually no more than 1300 ml of pleural fluid should be removed within a 30-minute period because of the risk of intravascular fluid shift with resultant pulmonary edema.
4. After thoracentesis, the patient is positioned on the unaffected side.

The specimen should be labeled and sent immediately to the laboratory as per physician's orders.

Arterial blood gases. This test yields definitive information on the patient's respiratory status and metabolic balance. The procedure is performed at the bedside. A heparinized syringe and needle are used to withdraw 3 to 5 ml of arterial blood, usually from the radial artery. Other possible sites include femoral or brachial arteries. After the sample is obtained, the nurse must place direct pressure on the puncture site for a minimum of 5 minutes to prevent hematoma formation and blood loss.

The blood gas values (Box 34-2) assess the patient's metabolic (acid-base) status by measuring the pH. Car-

BOX 34-2 GUIDELINES FOR INTERPRETING ABGs

1. Examine each value by itself.

NORMAL ABGs

pH	7.35-7.44
$Paco_2$	36-44 mm Hg
Pao_2	80-100 mm Hg
HCO_3	22-26 mEq/L
O_2 Saturation	≥95%

2. Determine whether the pH reflects acidity or alkalinity.
   pH of 7.35 and lower = acidity.
   pH of 7.45 and greater = alkalinity.
3. Which other value corresponds with that condition.
   NOTE: $Paco_2$ reflects respiratory factors; HCO_3 reflects metabolic factors.
   CO_2 is a potential acid, so CO_2 of greater than 45 = more acidity.
   HCO_3 is a basic (alkaline) substance, so HCO_3 of greater than 45 = more alkalinity.

EXAMPLE: A patient with acute exacerbation of COPD has the following ABGs:

pH	7.42
$Paco_2$	49 mm Hg
Pao_2	50 mm Hg
HCO_3	31 mEq/L
O_2 Saturation	84%

Because the pH is within a normal range, this is a compensated respiratory problem. The kidneys have increased the amount of bicarbonate they put into the blood to bring the pH to a normal level.

Table 34-1 Characteristics of Normal Breath Sounds

Sound	Characteristics	Findings
Vesicular	Heard over most of lung fields; low pitch; soft and short expirations	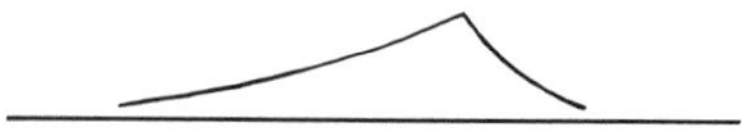
Bronchovesicular	Heard over main bronchus area and over upper right posterior lung field; medium pitch; expiration equals inspiration	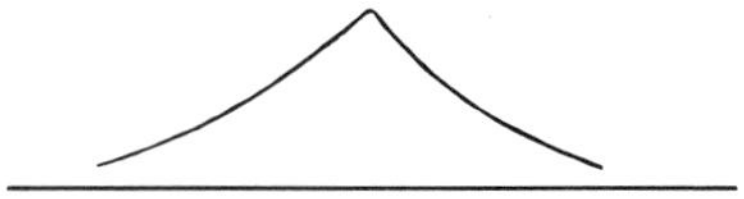
Bronchial	Heard only over trachea; high pitch; loud and long expirations	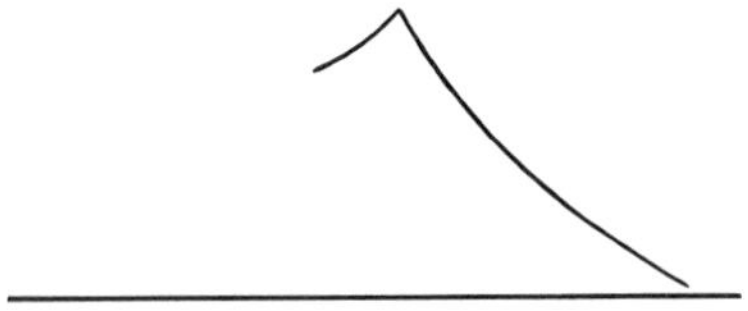

BOX 34-3 SIGNS AND SYMPTOMS OF HYPOXIA

- Apprehension, anxiety, restlessness
- Decreased ability to concentrate
- Decreased level of consciousness
- Increased fatigue
- Vertigo
- Behavioral changes
- Increased pulse rate; as hypoxia advances, bradycardia results
- Increased rate and depth of respiration; as hypoxia progresses, shallow, slow respirations develop
- Elevated blood pressure; if O_2 deficiency is not corrected, blood pressure will decrease
- Cardiac dysrhythmias
- Pallor
- Cyanosis
- Clubbing
- Dyspnea

bon dioxide tension is measured by $PaCO_2$ and will assess the patient's ventilation. The metabolic evaluation is assessed by measuring the bicarbonate (HCO_3). Oxygen saturation (PaO_2 and O_2) is also measured.

One aspect of nursing assessment important in the diagnosis of respiratory conditions is breath sounds heard on auscultation. Breath sounds will be difficult to hear if fluid is in the pleural space or if the patient is breathing shallowly. Abnormal breath sounds are called **adventitious** breath sounds.

See Table 34-1 for characteristics of normal breath sounds.

Another important aspect in collecting objective data in the nursing assessment is to be alert for signs and symptoms of hypoxia (Box 34-3).

DISORDERS OF THE UPPER AIRWAY

Epistaxis

Etiology/pathophysiology. The underlying cause of **epistaxis** is congestion of the nasal membranes, leading to capillary rupture. This condition is frequently caused by injury and occurs more frequently in men.

Epistaxis can be either a primary disorder or secondary to other conditions. It can be related to menstrual flow in women, as well as hypertension. Other causes include local irritation of nasal mucosa, such as dryness, chronic infection, or trauma (i.e., injury, vigorous nose blowing, or nose picking). A prime consideration of epistaxis is the many capillaries in the nasal passages.

Clinical manifestations. The primary observation is the presence of bright red blood draining from one or both nostrils. With a severe nasal hemorrhage adults can lose as much as 1 liter of blood per hour, but this loss is not prolonged.

Assessment. Collection of *subjective data* includes interviewing the patient and asking the patient to relate the duration and severity of bleeding and identification of precipitating factors, if possible.

Collection of *objective data* involves the nurse assessing the presence of bleeding from one or both nostrils. She will also need to determine whether the bleeding is occurring in the anterior or posterior portion of the nasal passageway. The nurse will assess the patient's blood pressure, TPR, and any evidence of hypovolemic shock.

Diagnostic tests. A hemoglobin and hematocrit determination will aid in establishing an estimate of the blood loss. PT and PTT will assist in identifying contributing factors, such as a bleeding tendency and clotting abnormalities. A rhinoscopy may be performed to locate the bleeding site as well as possible causes and treatment. This procedure involves inserting a lighted nasal speculum into the nasal cavity.

Medical management. There are many possible treatments for epistaxis, including nasal packing with cotton saturated with 1:1000 epinephrine to promote local vasoconstriction. Cautery can be either electrical (in which the bleeding vessel is burned [cauterized]) or chemical (a silver nitrate stick is applied to the site of the bleeding). Also, some physicians will prescribe antibiotics (penicillin) after the bleeding is controlled to minimize risk of infection.

Nursing interventions. Nursing interventions include applying pressure on the bridge of the nose to decrease blood flow to the area.

NURSING DIAGNOSES	NURSING INTERVENTIONS
Altered cerebral and/or cardiopulmonary tissue perfusion, related to blood loss	Assess vital signs and level of consciousness q 15 min and report any changes. Document estimated blood loss.
Potential for aspiration, related to bleeding	Elevate head of bed; place patient in Fowler's position with the head forward; patient should be encouraged to let the blood drain from the nose. Pinch nostrils; apply ice to head/neck; assist patient to clear secretions. Maintain airway patency. Instruct patient to expectorate any blood or clots rather than swallow them, which could cause nausea and vomiting.
Fear, related to perceived blood loss and difficulty swallowing	Instruct patient to mouth breathe to promote optimal air exchange, because anxiety will be increased when patient feels unable to breathe. Decrease sense of fear by staying with patient and offering reassurance in a calm manner. Promote patient's dignity by providing privacy.

Patient teaching. The patient (and his family, if possible) should be instructed not to pick, scratch, or otherwise irritate the nares. The patient/family should be instructed regarding the risks of foreign objects inserted in the nose (this is especially important in pediatric patients). The use of a vaporizer to keep nasal mucous membranes moist should be encouraged.

Deviated Septum and Nasal Polyps

Etiology/pathophysiology. Common conditions that cause nasal obstruction include nasal polyps or deviated septum caused by congenital abnormality or, more likely, injury.

The septum deviates from the midline and can cause a partial obstruction of the nasal passageway. Nasal polyps are tissue growths on the nasal tissues that are frequently caused by prolonged sinus inflammation.

Clinical manifestations. The major manifestations of nasal septal deviations and polyps are stertorous respirations, dyspnea, and sometimes postnasal drip.

Assessment. Collection of *subjective data* includes establishing the presence of previous injuries or infections, as well as sinus congestion. The patient will offer complaints of dyspnea.

Collection of *objective data* involves the nurse attempting to identify the condition and its location. The rate and character of the patient's respirations must be noted.

Diagnostic tests. Sinus x-ray studies will depict the presence of shadowy sinuses when nasal polyps are present, and a shift of the nasal septum will be evident with a septal defect. A deviated septum may also be present on visual examination.

Medical management. These conditions frequently require surgical correction, such as a submucous resection in which obstructive portions of cartilage or bone are removed from the nasal septum. Nasoseptoplasty may be done to reconstruct the nasal septum, or nasal polypectomy may be done to remove the polyps. Actions include nasal packing to control bleeding, if present, and maintaining nasal mucosa hydration with nasal irrigation of saline or application of a light layer of petroleum to the external nares to prevent drying. Medications include (1) corticosteroids (Prednisone), which will cause polyps to decrease or disappear; and (2) antihistamines for allergy signs and symptoms, to decrease congestion in both septal deviations and polyps. Antibiotic agents (penicillin) may be used in both conditions to prevent infection. Analgesics (acetaminophen [Tylenol]) may be given to relieve the headache that occurs with septal deviation.

Nursing interventions. Nursing interventions are generally aimed at maintaining airway patency and preventing infection. Postoperative intervention for nasal surgery will include monitoring closely for infection or hemorrhage and maintaining patient comfort.

NURSING DIAGNOSES	NURSING INTERVENTIONS
Ineffective airway clearance, related to nasal exudate	Document patient's ability to clear secretions, and note respiratory status. Elevate head of bed, and apply ice packs to face to decrease edema and bleeding. Change nasal drip pad as needed, documenting color, consistency, and amount of exudate.
Potential for injury, related to trauma to bleeding site associated with vigorous nose blowing	Assess and report exudate (as stated above). Instruct patient against blowing nose in immediate postoperative period, because this could increase edema and ecchymosis.

Patient teaching. The patient should be instructed to contact his physician if bleeding or infection develops.

The patient should be instructed to use nasal sprays and drops judiciously because of the possible rebound effect on nasal mucous membranes. He should be reminded to avoid nose blowing, vigorous coughing, or Valsalva maneuver (technique in which the patient holds his breath and bears down as if straining during a bowel movement) for 2 days postoperatively. The nurse should assure the patient that facial ecchymosis and edema may persist for several days after surgery.

Upper Airway Obstruction

Etiology/pathophysiology. Upper airway obstruction is precipitated by a recent respiratory event, such as traumatic injury to the airway or surrounding tissues. Common airway obstructions include dentures, aspiration of vomitus or secretions, and the most common airway obstruction in an unconscious person, the tongue.

Altered physiology includes any condition that could produce airway obstruction, such as laryngeal spasm caused by tetany resulting from hypocalcemia. Another cause may be laryngeal edema caused by injury.

Clinical manifestations. The main signs are **stertorous** (noisy) respirations, altered respiratory rate and character, and **apneic** periods.

Assessment. Collection of *subjective data* is limited because a patient is unable to talk when his airway is obstructed. The nurse therefore must make a prompt and accurate assessment of objective data.

Collection of *objective data* includes the nurse promptly assessing for signs of **hypoxia, cyanosis,** stertorous respirations, and wheezing or stridor (harsh, high-pitched sounds during respiration, caused by obstruction). As hypoxia progresses, the respiratory centers in the brain are depressed, resulting in bradycardia and shallow, slow respirations.

Diagnostic tests. Because this is a medical emergency, no diagnostic tests are needed. This condition is diagnosed by a prompt and accurate assessment.

Medical management. The patient may require an emergency tracheostomy to remove the obstruction. Depending on the cause of the obstruction, an artificial airway may need to be inserted to maintain patency. Examples of artificial airways include pharyngeal, endotracheal, and tracheal.

Nursing interventions. The most immediate nursing intervention will be that of opening the airway and restoring patency. This may be accomplished by properly repositioning the patient's head and neck, or it may require further maneuvers. The head-tilt/chin-lift practice is recommended by the American Heart Association because this technique minimizes further damage in the presence of a suspected cervical neck fracture. With a foreign body airway obstruction, the Heimlich maneuver is used (see Chapter 54).

NURSING DIAGNOSES	NURSING INTERVENTIONS
Ineffective airway clearance, related to obstruction in airway	Maintain secure airway. Administer oxygen as ordered. Suction as needed, and assess patient's ability to mobilize secretions. Monitor vital signs and breath sounds closely.
Potential for aspiration, related to partial airway obstruction	Monitor respiratory rate, rhythm, and effort. Assess and document breath sounds. Facilitate optimal airway and *functional* swallowing by elevating head of bed. Note amount, color, and characteristics of secretions. Suction as needed.

Patient teaching. The best goal of education is prevention. The patient and family should be taught how to assess for airway patency. Appropriate use of the Heimlich maneuver should be provided. Rationale for all treatments and procedures should be explained.

Cancer of the Larynx

Etiology/pathophysiology. Occurring most often in people over age 60, this condition is 5 times more common in men than in women. It appears to be correlated to heavy smoking and alcohol use, chronic laryngitis, vocal abuse, and family history. Because of the increase in the number of women who are heavy smokers, the incidence of carcinoma of the larynx is increasing.

Laryngeal cancer limited to the true vocal cords is slow growing; however, elsewhere in the larynx there is an abundance of lymph tissue, and cancer in these tissues spreads rapidly and metastasizes early to the deep lymph nodes of the neck.

Clinical manifestations. Progressive or persistent hoarseness is an early sign. Any person who is hoarse longer than 2 weeks should seek medical treatment. Signs of metastasis to other areas include pain in the larynx radiating to the ear, difficulty swallowing (dysphagia), a feeling of a lump in the throat, and enlarged cervical lymph nodes.

Assessment. Collection of *subjective data* includes assessing the onset and duration of symptoms. A complaint of referred pain to the ear (otalgia), as well as difficulty breathing **(dyspnea)** or swallowing, should be noted.

Collection of *objective data* includes examining sputum for the presence of blood **(hemoptysis).**

Diagnostic tests. Visual examination of the larynx with indirect laryngoscopy is done to determine the presence of laryngeal cancer. A health history will be helpful in making the diagnosis, and a biopsy and microscopic study of the lesion will be definitive.

Medical management. Treatment will be determined by

the extent of tumor growth. Radiation therapy or surgery is often performed. Surgery may include either a total or partial laryngectomy or a radical neck dissection. A partial laryngectomy is done to remove the diseased vocal cord and possibly a portion of thyroid cartilage, requiring the placement of a temporary tracheostomy (Skill 34-1), which will be closed when the edema has decreased. A total laryngectomy requires the placement of a permanent tracheostomy. Because the patient can no longer breathe through the nose, the sense of smell is absent. The voice is also absent, because the larynx is removed. There is no connection between the patient's mouth and his trachea.

A radical neck dissection to remove cervical lymph nodes is often done in conjunction with a total laryngectomy. This surgery entails removal of the sternocleidomastoid muscle, spinal accessory nerve, and the internal jugular vein, which results in one-sided shoulder droop.

SKILL 34-1 TRACHEOSTOMY CARE AND SUCTIONING

1. Check physician's orders.
2. Assess patient's tracheostomy for sanguineous exudate, edema, and respiratory obstruction.
3. Obtain supplies and equipment, and take to bedside.
4. Explain procedure.
5. Wash hands.
6. Pull curtain around bed and close door to room.
7. Position patient in semi-Fowler's position.
8. Provide paper and pencil for patient; because patient cannot speak, this offers means of communication for patient.
9. Position self at head of bed facing patient. Always face patient while cleaning a tracheostomy. Observe for respiratory difficulty and coughing, which might expel cannula.
10. Place towel or prepackaged drape under tracheostomy and across chest.
11. Prepare equipment and supplies on over-bed table.
    a. Open suction catheter, leaving it in its wrapper to maintain sterility and attach to suction machine.
    b. Pour cleansing solution in one basin and rinsing solution in another basin. The first basin should have hydrogen peroxide to cleanse mucus and secretions from inner cannula. The second basin should contain normal saline to rinse cannula. If basins are prepackaged and under sterile gloves, use one-glove technique to remove basins and pour solution with ungloved hand.
    c. Turn on suction machine.
    d. Apply other sterile glove.
12. Unlock and remove inner cannula, and place in hydrogen peroxide cleansing solution. Placing fingers on tabs of outer cannula prevents movement that may irritate surrounding tissue and cause pain and coughing. NEVER remove outer cannula. If it is expelled by patient, use hemostat to hold tracheostomy open and call for assistance.
13. Suction inner aspect of outer cannula.
    a. Withdraw sterile rinsing solution through catheter by placing thumb over suction control to moisten catheter.
    b. Ask patient to take several deep breaths or if patient is receiving oxygen, remove oxygen immediately before suctioning.
    c. Remove thumb from suction control or pinch catheter with gloved thumb and index finger; insert catheter 5 to 6 inches or as ordered. Depth of catheter should be length of outer cannula and extend approximately 1 to 2 inches beyond distal end.
    d. Apply intermittent suction by placing thumb on and off suction control, and gently rotate catheter as it is withdrawn.
    e. Suction for at least 10 to 15 seconds. (Do not suction longer than 15 seconds.) Holding your own breath until uncomfortable may provide same effect of not breathing that patient experiences.
    f. If mucus is tenacious, 4 to 5 ml sterile normal saline may be instilled into tracheostomy.
    g. Allow patient to rest between each episode of suctioning. If patient was previously receiving oxygen, it may be reapplied at the prescribed rate or as instructed. Suctioning can be exhausting and frightening for patient. Resting helps to regain depleted oxygen and renew strength.
    h. Rinse catheter with sterile solution, and repeat suction if needed.
    i. Turn off suction, and dispose of catheter.

SKILL 34-1

TRACHEOSTOMY CARE AND SUCTIONING—cont'd

14. Apply second sterile glove, if one-gloved technique is used, or apply new pair of sterile gloves.
15. Clean inner cannula:
    a. Use pipe cleaners and brush to clean inside and outside of inner cannula.
    b. Place inner cannula in sterile normal saline solution.
    c. Inspect inner and outer areas of inner cannula.
    d. Insert inner cannula and lock in place.
16. Clean skin around tracheostomy and tabs of outer cannula with hydrogen peroxide.
17. Thoroughly rinse cleansing solution from skin; place dry, sterile dressing around tracheostomy face plate.
18. Change cotton tapes (always do this last to prevent risk of cannula being expelled); attaching clean tape is done only when needed:
    a. Untie one side of cotton tape from outer cannula, and replace with clean one.
    b. Bring clean tape under back of neck. Securely hold tracheostomy tube in place to prevent movement of cannula that could stimulate coughing and expel cannula.
    c. Untie other side from outer cannula and replace with clean tape.
    d. Tie ends of two clean cotton tapes together and position knot at side of neck. Avoid placing knot at back of neck, which can cause pressure and discomfort to cervical vertebrae.
19. Provide mouth care.
20. Remove gloves.
21. Adjust top linens, and position patient in comfortable position as ordered.
22. Place call light, paper, and pencil within easy reach.
23. Dispose of soiled supplies in appropriate area.
24. Wash hands.
25. Reassess patient's tracheostomy for signs of bleeding, edema, and respiratory obstruction.
26. Record in nurse's notes: tracheostomy care performed, patient's response, respiratory assessment, suction performed, any adverse reactions, and condition of tracheal stoma. If oxygen is administered, note flow and method used.

Care of patient with cuffed tracheostomy tube

1. Follow steps 1 to 11.
2. Suction patient.
3. Connect syringe to pilot balloon valve.
4. Position stethoscope in sternal notch or above tracheostomy tube, and listen for minimal amount of air leak at end of inspiration.
5. Remove all air from cuff if no air leak is auscultated; this releases excessive air pressure.
6. While listening with stethoscope, slowly inflate cuff with 0.5 to 1 ml of air at a time. When no air leak is heard, stop injecting air and slowly withdraw up to 0.5 ml of air until air leak is auscultated with stethoscope.
7. If excessive air leak is heard, slowly add air as in step 6.
8. Remove stethoscope and cleanse diaphragm with alcohol swab.
9. Do not leave syringe attached to pilot balloon valve; remove syringe and either discard in proper container or store per agency's policy.
10. Reposition patient.
11. Wash hands.
12. Document as in Step 26.

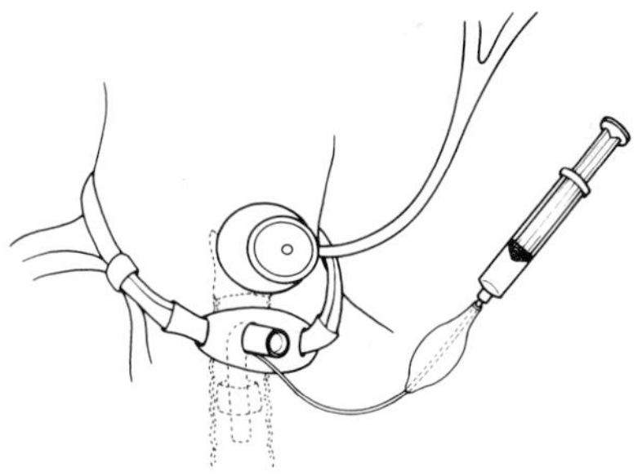

STEP 4

SKILL 34-2

CLEARING THE AIRWAY

1. Check physician's order.
2. Assess need for suctioning.
3. Explain procedure to patient.
4. Assemble equipment.
5. Wash hands.
6. Provide privacy.
7. Position patient.
   a. If patient is alert and conscious, place in semi-Fowler's position with head to one side; placing head to one side promotes drainage of secretions and facilitates insertion of the suction catheter.
   b. If patient is unconscious, place in side-lying position facing nurse.
8. Place towel lengthwise under patient's chin and over pillow.
9. Pour sterile normal saline solution into sterile container.
10. Don sterile gloves on dominant hand.
11. Turn on suction machine, and select appropriate suction pressure. Never suction with any more vacuum pressure than needed to remove the secretions, and use the smallest catheter that will remove the secretions well.

COMMON VACUUM SETTINGS

Children	60 to 80 mm Hg
Adults	80 to 100 mm Hg

COMMON CATHETER SIZES

Children	5 to 8 French (14 French for oral suctioning)
Adults	12 to 14 French (16 French for oral suctioning)

12. Aspirate solution through catheter by placing thumb over open end of connector or over vent to (1) check patency of suction catheter and suction pressure and (2) moisten catheter for ease of insertion.
13. Remove thumb from Y-connector opening or pinch catheter with thumb and index finger; if using suction catheter with vent, remove thumb from vent opening. This prevents injury to mucous membrane while catheter is being inserted.
14. Insert catheter.

    Oropharyngeal suctioning
    a. Gently insert catheter into one side of mouth.
    b. Glide catheter toward oropharynx without suction.

    Nasopharyngeal suctioning
    a. Holding catheter with thumb and index finger, place nasal catheter near patient's earlobe to tip of nose. Do not touch side of face, nose, or earlobe. This marks catheter for correct length of insertion at that point. From earlobe to tip of nose approximates depth of insertion.
    b. Lubricate catheter with water-soluble jelly. Water-soluble lubricant dissolves and thus buildup that may hinder airway is prevented.
    c. Hold catheter to observe its natural curvature and gently insert catheter into one side of nasal passage.

    Endotracheal suctioning
    a. Holding catheter with thumb and index finger, place endotracheal catheter near earlobe to tip of nose and extend to trachea to measure for correct length of insertion. Do not touch side of face, nose, or earlobe; maintain sterility.
    b. Lubricate catheter with a water-soluble jelly. This facilitates gliding catheter past nasal turbinates.
    c. Ask patient if either side of nose is obstructed and use unobstructed side. Hold catheter to observe its natural curvature, and gently insert catheter into one side of nasal passage.
    d. Stimulate coughing reflex, or ask patient to cough to guide catheter into trachea. If no cough reflex is present or if patient cannot assist, insert catheter when patient inhales; this avoids displacement of catheter into esophagus.
15. Apply suction by placing thumb over suction opening; rotate catheter gently as catheter is withdrawn.
16. Observe patient closely, and limit suction to 10 to 15 seconds.
17. Repeat suctioning if needed.
18. Allow 1 to 2 minutes' rest between suctioning if procedure must be repeated. If oxygen is administered by nasal cannula, mask, or other means, reapply oxygen during rest period. This provides rest and comfort and allows patient to regain oxygen supply. Time allowed for patient to rest between suctioning can vary from 1 to 2 minutes to 20 to 30 seconds, depending on patient's ability to tolerate procedure.

SKILL 34-2 CLEARING THE AIRWAY—cont'd

19. When suctioning is complete, suction between cheeks and gum line and under tongue; suction mouth last to prevent contaminating catheter.
20. If patient is alert and can cooperate, request patient to deep breathe and cough.
21. Place catheter in solution, and supply suction, which flushes secretions from catheter and tubing to maintain patency if procedure needs to be repeated.
22. Discard catheter: wrap catheter around gloved hand; pull glove off hand and over catheter. This reduces the spread of microorganisms and prevents direct contact with equipment and secretions.
23. Wash hands.
24. Place sterile, unopened catheter at patient's bedside to provide quick access to suction equipment if patient needs suctioning immediately.
25. Provide mouth care.
26. Observe patient's breathing patterns. Observe for decrease in anxiety, fatigue, and vital signs, and level of consciousness and color.
27. Document in nurses' notes: date, time, and method of suctioning, and color, odor, amount, and consistency of secretions. Include respiratory assessment after suctioning, and patient's response.

Nursing interventions. Airway maintenance through proper suctioning techniques is important (Skill 34-2). Skin integrity surrounding the tracheal opening should be assessed, being alert for signs of infection.

The nurse should monitor intake/output balance and assist with tube feedings as ordered. The nurse should explain to the patient that the tube feedings are a temporary measure and that when healing occurs in a few weeks, he may begin to eat normally again. The nurse should weigh the patient daily and assess hydration status for need for additional fluids; note skin turgor and observe for diarrhea.

Because of neck and facial disfigurement and loss of voice, a thorough psychosocial assessment and resultant interventions will be beneficial. The nurse should encourage communication through writing and facial and hand gestures.

Care of the tracheostomy. The term *tracheostomy* means an artificial opening made by a surgical incision into the trachea. After the surgical procedure is performed, the physician inserts a tracheostomy tube into the opening and secures it in place by cotton tapes around the patient's neck. This procedure is performed to provide the patient with a patent airway. Sterile gauze is placed around the opening under the flange of the outer tube for skin protection. The primary nursing responsibilities are to maintain a patent airway, keep the inner cannula clean, prevent impairment of surrounding tissue, and provide a means of communication for the patient.

The tubes used to maintain this artificial airway are commonly referred to as tracheostomy tubes. The tracheostomy tube is usually made of metal or plastic. Previously, the more common tracheostomy tube had three parts: outer cannula, inner cannula, and obturator. The obturator was placed within the outer cannula, with the round, blunt end protruding through the distal end of the cannula. This provided a smooth, rounded edge and made insertion less traumatic to the tissues and trachea. Once the outer cannula was in place, the obturator was removed and the inner cannula was inserted within the outer cannula and locked in place (Fig. 34-8).

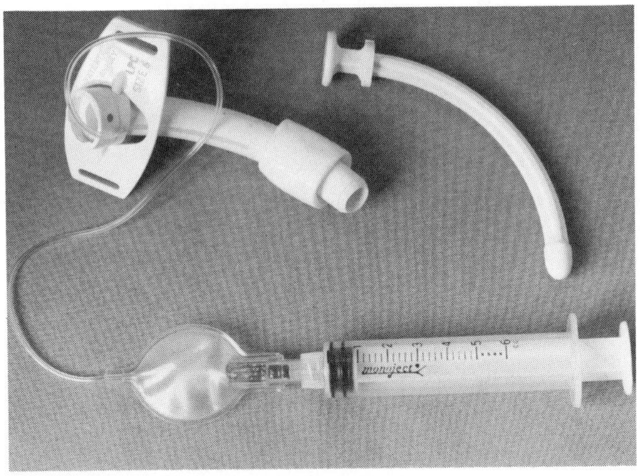

FIG. 34-8 Tracheostomy tube and inner cannula.

With today's knowledge and new materials, a single cannula tracheostomy is more commonly used. This type of tracheostomy is referred to as the *cuffed tracheostomy tube* (Fig. 34-9). It is made of plastic and has an inflatable cuff around the middle of the distal portion of the tube. The physician may order a cuffed tracheostomy tube to be used initially until the healing process of the tracheal stoma is complete. The cuffed tube (Fig. 34-10) is commonly used for temporary use, to hold the tube in place during special treatments, such as ventilation or IPPB, and to prevent aspiration during such activities as eating or taking medications.

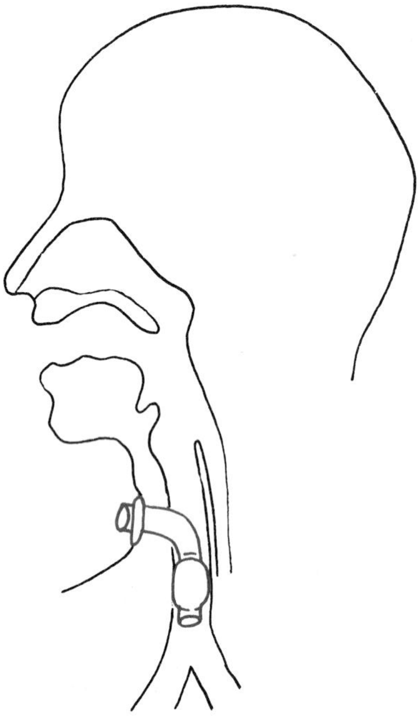

FIG. 34-9 Position of tracheostomy tube.

NURSING DIAGNOSES	NURSING INTERVENTIONS
Ineffective airway clearance, related to secretions or other obstruction	Suction secretions as needed. Provide tracheostomy care according to protocol; ensure the availability of emergency equipment (oxygen and tracheostomy tray). Offer small, frequent feedings, and give liquid or pureed food as tolerated to prevent choking. Teach patient stoma protection. Assess respiratory rate and characteristics q 1 to 2 hr. Maintain head of bed elevated at 30 degrees or higher. Turn, cough, and encourage deep breathing q 2 to 4 hr. Auscultate lung sounds. Provide constant humidity. Suction laryngectomy tube PRN, using aseptic technique; instruct patient to inhale as catheter is advanced. Clean inner cannula of laryngectomy tube q 2 to 4 hr and prn, using a solution of normal saline and hydrogen peroxide. Lavage laryngectomy tube before suctioning with 3 to 5 ml of a solution of normal saline q 2 to 4 hr.
Anxiety, related to inability to speak, isolation, mutilating surgery, diagnosis of cancer, and drooling	Keep call light within easy reach at all times. Locate patient close to nurses' station. Answer call light/bell as quickly as possible. Check patient frequently.

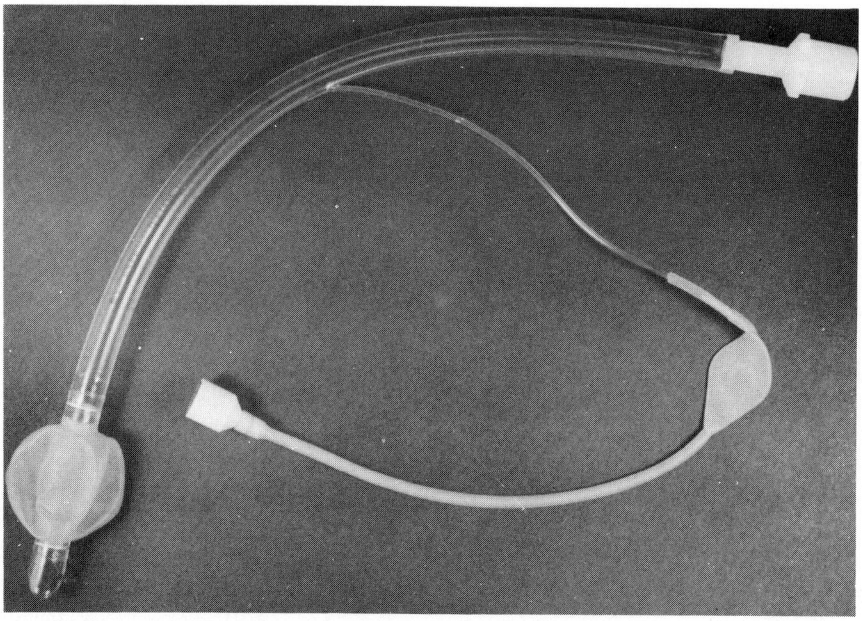

FIG. 34-10 Forregar high-volume, low-pressure cuffed endotracheal tube. Cuff shown here is not inflated. Low-pressure cuff is preferred because it is less likely to cause tracheal damage.

NURSING DIAGNOSES	NURSING INTERVENTIONS
Anxiety, related to inability to speak, isolation, mutilating surgery, diagnosis of cancer, and drooling—cont'd	Keep oral suction catheter beside patient to suction oral cavity. Encourage significant other to support patient. Provide information about alternative methods of communication.
Impaired verbal communication, related to removal of larynx	Provide patient with alternate implements for communication, including pencil, paper, Magic Slate, picture books, or electronic voice device. Keep call light/bell by patient's hand at all times. Ask patient questions that require a *yes* or *no* response, if possible, to avoid fatigue and frustration. Refer patient to local support groups, (e.g., Lost Chord Club) and the local chapter of the American Cancer Society. Assist with speech rehabilitation.
Self-esteem disturbance, related to disfiguring surgery	Assist patient to identify past strengths and coping mechanisms. Assess patient's body image concept, and note nonverbal responses to changes that have taken place. Provide patient with tissues to absorb oral secretions. Provide oral care, including mouthwash or half-strength hydrogen peroxide q 2 hr.

Patient teaching. Techniques of airway maintenance, such as oxygen usage, deep breathing, and coughing should be explained. The importance of dietary management in relationship to airway maintenance should be discussed. Optimal communication should be encouraged through speech rehabilitation and community support groups.

Respiratory Infections

Common cold (acute coryza)

Etiology/pathophysiology. The common cold is usually caused by one or more viruses; however it may become complicated by a bacterial infection. Signs and symptoms usually are evident within 24 to 48 hours after exposure. Sinus congestion causes increased sinus drainage leading to postnasal drip. The postnasal drip causes throat irritation, headache, and earache.

Clinical manifestations. An increased amount of thin, serous, nasal exudate and a productive cough are two of the most common signs. A sore throat and fever are often present. If the infection remains uncomplicated, it generally subsides in 1 week.

Assessment. Collection of *subjective data* includes the patient's complaints of sore throat, dyspnea, and congestion of varying duration.

Collection of *objective data* includes noting the color and consistency of the nasal exudate. A visual exam of the throat may reveal erythema, edema, and local irritation. The nurse will also document the presence and duration of fever.

Diagnostic tests. Throat and sputum cultures will indicate the presence and nature of microorganisms, which will then indicate the type of antibiotic agent to be prescribed.

Medical management. Medical management is aimed at accurate diagnosis and prevention of complications. Among the medications used are (1) aspirin or acetaminophen for analgesia and reduction of temperature (aspirin is not used in infants, children, and adolescents because of the danger of developing Reye's Syndrome); (2) a cough suppressant for a dry nonproductive cough; or (3) an expectorant for a productive cough. If the presence of a bacterial infection is confirmed, an antibiotic agent (such as erythromycin) will be prescribed.

Nursing interventions. Nursing interventions are aimed at promoting comfort. Such measures include encouraging fluids and applying warm, moist packs to sinuses.

NURSING DIAGNOSES	NURSING INTERVENTIONS
Ineffective airway clearance, related to nasal exudate	Encourage fluids to liquify secretions and aid in their expectoration. Use vaporizer to moisten mucous membranes and prevent further irritation.
Potential for infection, related to retained pulmonary secretions	Check temperature q 2 to 4 hr. Promote rest and comfort. Encourage coughing and deep breathing q 2 hr.
Health-seeking behaviors: illness prevention, related to preventing exacerbation or spread of infection	Remind patient and family of health maintenance behaviors to decrease risk of illness, such as adequate fluid and nutritional management and sufficient rest. Teach importance of hygiene measures to decrease spread of infection.

Patient teaching. The patient should be taught correct hand washing technique and proper disposal of tissues used for nasal secretions. The nurse should instruct the patient to limit his exposure to others during the first 48 hours and to check his temperature every 4 hours.

Tonsillitis

Etiology/pathophysiology. Tonsillitis can be an acute or chronic condition. It is the result of an air- or food-borne bacterial infection, often *Streptococcus*. It can also be viral, but this occurs less often. It appears to be most common in school-age children. Signs and symptoms of tonsillitis include sore throat, fever, chills, and anorexia. The tonsils become enlarged and often contain purulent exudate.

Clinical manifestations. Tonsillitis manifests itself clinically with enlarged, tender, cervical lymph nodes. Fever may be present with chills, general muscle aching, and malaise. Laboratory data reveal an elevated white blood cell count.

Assessment. Collection of *subjective data* includes monitoring the severity of throat pain and the possibility of referred pain to the ears. Headache or joint pain should be noted.

Collection of *objective data* includes a visual examination that shows increased throat secretions and enlarged, erythematous tonsils.

Diagnostic tests. Throat cultures will identify the causative microorganism, most commonly β-hemolytic streptococci. A complete blood count will be done to determine if the white blood count is elevated. It is not uncommon for the white blood count to be 10,000 to 20,000 per cubic millimeter.

Medical management. If antibiotics to which the offending organism is sensitive are administered early, infection subsides. Until recently tonsillectomy/adenoidectomy was the surgical intervention of choice. With this procedure the tonsils and adenoids are surgically excised because of chronic infection. Either general or local anesthesia is used. When a tonsillectomy/adenoidectomy is performed, hemostasis is of utmost importance, because the patient can lose a large amount of blood through hemorrhage without demonstrating any outward signs of bleeding. An important postoperative nursing intervention is to observe and report if the patient exhibits frequent swallowing, because this is often a subtle but reliable indication of excessive bleeding. The physician may be able to control minor postoperative bleeding by applying a sponge soaked in a solution of epinephrine to the site. The person who is bleeding excessively often is returned to the operating room for surgical treatment to stop hemorrhage.

Medications used in tonsillitis include analgesics and antipyretics, such as acetaminophen, and antibiotic agents, such as penicillin. Warm saline gargles are also beneficial.

Nursing interventions. One of the primary nursing goals for acute tonsillitis is to provide meticulous oral care, which will promote comfort and assist in combating infection.

Postoperative care for tonsillectomy includes maintaining intravenous fluids until the nausea subsides, at which time the patient may begin drinking ice cold liquids. The diet will be advanced to custard and ice cream and then to a normal diet as soon as possible. An ice collar should be applied to the neck for comfort and to reduce bleeding by vasoconstriction. Vital signs must be monitored to assess for hemorrhage, postoperative fever, or other complications. This surgery appears to be less common today because the role of lymphoid tissue in the body's immune mechanism has been determined.

NURSING DIAGNOSES	NURSING INTERVENTIONS
Pain, related to inflammation/irritation of throat	Assess degree of pain and need for pain medication. Document effectiveness of medication, and offer pain medication as ordered. Maintain bed rest, and promote rest. Offer warm saline gargles, ice chips, and ice collar as needed.
Potential fluid volume deficit, related to inability to maintain usual oral intake because of painful swallowing	Assess hydration status by noting mucous membranes, skin turgor, and urine output. Encourage increased oral intake: cold liquids, sherbet, and ice cream will be best tolerated; carbonated drinks may be taken if patient tolerates; avoid offering fruit juices, because they may burn throat.

Patient teaching. The patient or his family should be instructed that the patient should complete the entire course of the prescribed antibiotic. If he has had surgery (tonsillectomy and adenoidectomy [T&A]), dietary instruction should be offered regarding appropriate foods and liquids. The nurse should teach the patient to avoid attempting to clear the throat immediately after surgery (may initiate bleeding) and to avoid coughing, sneezing, or vigorous nose blowing for 1 to 2 weeks. The nurse should remind the patient to avoid overexertion and should ascertain that the patient and family know how to reach the physician in case of increased pain, fever, or bleeding.

Laryngitis

Etiology/pathophysiology. Laryngitis often occurs secondary to other respiratory infections. Laryngeal inflammation is a common disorder that can be either chronic or acute.

Acute laryngitis often accompanies viral or bacterial infections. Other causes include excessive use of the voice or inhalation of irritating fumes. Chronic laryngitis is usually associated with inflammation of laryngeal mucosa or edematous vocal cords.

Clinical manifestations. Clinical manifestation include hoarseness of varying degrees or even complete voice loss. The throat will feel scratchy and irritated, and the patient may have a persistent cough.

Assessment. Collection of *subjective data* includes the patient reporting progressive hoarseness and a cough that may be productive or may be dry and nonproductive. The nurse should attempt to identify any precipitating factors such as excessive voice use or increased exposure to inhaled irritants.

Collection of *objective data* includes the nurse evaluating and recording the characteristics (color, consistency, and amount) of sputum produced.

Diagnostic tests. Laryngoscopy will reveal abnormalities (edema, drainage) of vocal cords and erythematous laryngeal mucosa.

Medical management. Medications include antibiotics (such as erythromycin), analgesics/antipyretics for comfort, antitussives to relieve cough (such as Phenergan with codeine), and throat lozenges to promote comfort and decrease irritation.

Nursing interventions. General interventions include use of warm or cool mist inhalation via vaporizer. The patient should be encouraged to rest the voice by limiting verbal communication.

NURSING DIAGNOSES	NURSING INTERVENTIONS
Pain, related to throat irritation	Assess level of pain, and offer medications to promote comfort. Use steam inhalation as ordered.
Impaired verbal communication, related to edematous vocal cords	Instruct patient on the importance of resting the voice. Provide other means for communication (written word, gestures). Anticipate patient's needs whenever possible.

Patient teaching. If the patient receives antibiotic agents, the nurse should instruct him to finish the entire prescribed course. The patient should be reminded of the need to limit use of the voice. Patients who smoke should be encouraged to quit and also to limit exposure to irritating fumes.

Pharyngitis

Etiology/pathophysiology. Pharyngitis may be chronic or acute. It is the most common throat inflammation and frequently accompanies the common cold. Pharyngitis is usually viral in origin but can be caused by hemolytic streptococci, staphylococci, or other bacteria. There is increased evidence of gonococcal pharyngitis caused by the Gram-negative diplococcus *Neisseria gonorrhoeae*. A severe form of acute pharyngitis often is referred to as *strep throat*, because the streptococcus organism is commonly the cause. This disorder is contagious for 2 or 3 days after the onset of signs and symptoms and will usually resolve in 4 to 6 days unless secondary complications develop.

Clinical manifestations. Pharyngitis manifests itself clinically by a dry cough, tender tonsils, and enlarged cervical lymph glands. The throat appears erythematous, and soreness may range from slight scratchiness to severe pain with difficulty swallowing.

Assessment. Collection of *subjective data* includes any reported pharyngeal discomfort, presence of fever, or any difficulty swallowing.

Collection of *objective data* includes palpating for enlarged, edematous glands and associated tenderness and noting elevated temperature.

Diagnostic studies. Throat cultures will be done to document presence or absence of a bacterial infection.

Medical management. Commonly ordered medications include antibiotics, such as penicillin or erythromycin, to (1) treat severe infections or (2) prevent superimposed infections, particularly in persons who have a history of rheumatic fever or bacterial endocarditis. Analgesics/antipyretics, such as acetaminophen (Tylenol), are used to promote comfort.

Nursing interventions. The nurse should offer throat rinses/gargles and encourage oral intake. The importance of adequate rest and use of a vaporizer to increase humidity should be emphasized.

NURSING DIAGNOSES	NURSING INTERVENTIONS
Altered oral mucous membrane, related to edema	Provide warm saline gargles to promote comfort. Assess level of pain, and offer medications as ordered. Encourage oral intake of fluids. Offer frequent oral care.
Potential fluid volume deficit, related to decreased oral intake as a result of painful swallowing.	Observe and record patient's hydration status. Monitor intake, output, and patient's temperature. Maintain IV therapy if indicated.

Patient teaching. The nurse should perform and document medication teaching: the importance of completing the entire prescribed course of antibiotics and any side effects of medications. The patient should be instructed to avoid exposure to inhaled irritants and to use preventive measures, such as vaporizer and adequate fluid intake.

Sinusitis

Etiology/pathophysiology. Sinusitis can be chronic or acute, involving any sinus area, such as maxillary or frontal. This infection can be either viral or bacterial in origin and often is a complication of pneumonia or nasal polyps.

The underlying pathophysiology begins with an upper respiratory infection that leads to a sinus infection. If untreated, the sinus infection (sinusitis) may lead to meningitis, osteomyelitis, or septicemia.

Clinical manifestations. The patient with sinusitis often complains of a constant, severe headache with pain and tenderness in the particular sinus region. Frequently there is a purulent exudate.

Assessment. Collection of *subjective data* includes the patient reporting a decreased appetite or nausea. He may also complain of generalized malaise, headache, and pain in the sinus region.

Collection of *objective data* involves the nurse assessing vital signs, particularly temperature, and also assessing the character and amount of drainage.

Diagnostic tests. Sinus X-ray studies are frequently done to depict cloudy or fluid-filled sinus cavities. A simple way to diagnose sinusitis is with transillumination. This procedure involves shining a light in the patient's mouth with the lips closed around it; infected sinuses will look dark, and normal sinuses will transilluminate.

Medical management. Nasal windows or other surgical incisions can be created to allow better drainage and removal of diseased mucosal tissue. One of the most common surgical procedures to relieve chronic maxillary sinusitis is the Caldwell-Luc operation, which is a radical antrum operation involving the creation of an incision under the lip to remove diseased mucosal and bone tissue.

Medications used to treat sinusitis include antibiotic agents (penicillin), analgesics to relieve headache acetaminophen ([Tylenol], possibly with codeine), antihistamines (azatadine [Optimine]) to reduce congestion and secretions, and vasoconstrictors in the form of nasal sprays (Afrin) to reduce local vascular congestion.

Nursing interventions. Steam inhalation and warm, moist packs will facilitate drainage and promote comfort.

NURSING DIAGNOSES	NURSING INTERVENTIONS
Ineffective breathing pattern, related to nasal congestion	Assess respiratory status frequently, noting any changes; mouth breathing may be necessary because of nasal airway/sinus discomfort.
Pain, related to sinus congestion	Document comfort level. Assess need for pain medication, and document patient response. Elevate head of bed to promote drainage of secretions. Apply warm, moist packs four times/day to promote secretion drainage and provide relief.

Patient teaching. The aim of patient education is to prevent reoccurrence or complications of sinus infection. The patient should be instructed to be alert to signs and symptoms of sinusitis so early treatment can be obtained.

DISORDERS OF THE LOWER AIRWAY

Acute Bronchitis

Etiology/pathophysiology. Usually acute bronchitis is secondary to an upper respiratory infection, but it can be related to exposure to inhaled irritants. Inflammation of the trachea and bronchial tree causes congestion of the mucous membranes, which results in retention of tenacious secretions. These secretions can become a culture medium for bacterial growth.

Clinical manifestations. Acute bronchitis manifests itself by a productive cough, diffuse rhonchi/wheezes, dyspnea, chest pain, and low grade temperature. Generalized malaise and headache are also common symptoms.

Assessment. Collection of *subjective data* includes the patient's complaints of feeling poorly and experiencing headache and aching tightness in the chest.

Collection of *objective data* involves a nursing assessment that includes monitoring vital signs frequently, checking breath sounds, and noting the presence of rhonchi or basilar rales.

Diagnostic tests. The usual diagnostic aids include a chest X-ray examination to ensure clear lung fields and sputum specimen to determine the presence of associated bacterial infections.

Medical management. The medical management will promote a quick recovery by preventing further infectious complications. The physician may order sputum cultures periodically to ascertain that there is no secondary infection.

Medications that are frequently prescribed are cough suppressants (codeine), antitussives (dextromethorphan [Pertussin]), antipyretics (Tylenol), and bronchodilators (terbutaline [Brethine]). Antibiotics, such as ampicillin, may be ordered to combat an infectious process or to prevent its occurrence.

Nursing interventions. The goal of nursing interventions for acute bronchitis is to facilitate recovery and prevent secondary infections. Such actions include placing the patient on bed rest to conserve energy, using a vaporizer to add humidity to inhaled air, and increasing fluid intake.

NURSING DIAGNOSES	NURSING INTERVENTIONS
Potential for infection, related to retained pulmonary secretions	Assess for signs/symptoms of infection: fever, dyspnea, color and characteristics of sputum production. Administer antipyretics and antibiotics as ordered.
Ineffective airway clearance, related to tenacious pulmonary secretions	Assess patient's ability to move secretions; also note an increase in retained pulmonary secretions. Facilitate airway clearance by elevating head of bed and liquefying secretions by use of humidifier and adequate fluid intake (3000 to 4000 ml/day). Suction as needed. When offering fluids, avoid dairy products, which tend to produce more tenacious secretions.
Fatigue, related to prolonged coughing periods	Encourage rest periods between activities. Assess support systems and available resources; refer as necessary.

Patient teaching. The patient should be instructed on measures that will prevent exacerbation or reoccurrence of infection. Such measures include stressing the importance of increasing oral fluid intake, incorporating rest periods between activities, and teaching the patient the signs that may indicate worsening infection (purulent sputum and increased dyspnea). Medication teaching would involve emphasizing the importance of adhering to prescribed medication regimen and using analgesics and antipyretics to reduce fever and malaise. The nurse should teach the patient to limit his exposure to others, who may spread infection and to avoid smoking or other irritating fumes.

Legionnaires' Disease

Etiology/pathophysiology. The causative microorganism of this disease is *Legionella pneumophila,* first identified in 1977 when it caused a pneumonia outbreak at a convention of the American Legion. This organism thrives in water reservoirs, such as in air conditioners and humidifiers, and is transmitted through airborne routes. The *Legionella* microbe can progress in two different forms—influenza or Legionnaires' disease, which is characteristically lobar pneumonia. This causes lung consolidation and alveolar necrosis. The disease progresses rapidly (less than 1 week) and can result in respiratory failure, renal failure, bacteremic shock, and ultimately, death. The mortality has been 15% to 20% in a few localized epidemics.

Clinical manifestations. Clinical manifestations of Legionnaires' disease include markedly elevated temperature, headache, nonproductive cough, diarrhea, and general malaise.

Assessment. Collection of *subjective data* includes noting the patient's complaints of dyspnea, headache, and chest pain on inspiration.

Collection of *objective data* includes many significant signs associated with this infectious process. A markedly elevated temperature (102° F to 105° F) bears close watching and immediate interventions. Another sign the patient will exhibit is a nonproductive cough with difficult and rapid breathing. Auscultation of lungs will reveal rales or rhonchi. Because of the high fever and extreme respiratory effort, tachycardia and symptoms of shock may be present. Hematuria may develop, indicative of resulting renal impairment.

Diagnostic tests. Diagnostic tests to confirm *Legionella pneumophila* infection are cultures of blood, sputum, and pulmonary tissue or fluid. Chest X-ray studies will show patchy infiltrates and small pleural effusions.

Medical management. The physician may need to place the patient on assisted ventilation, which requires intubating the patient through an oral or nasal airway or directly via the trachea. Close observation for disease progression is required.

The patient may also require temporary renal dialysis because of acute kidney failure.

Medical management. To control and compensate for impaired/ineffective respiratory function, the patient will require oxygen therapy, possibly even mechanical ventilation. The patient will need adequate IV fluid therapy to maintain hydration and electrolyte status.

Antibiotic agents (erythromycin) will be given to treat the infection, and antipyretics will be administered to reduce the patient's temperature. The patient may also require vasopressors (dopamine or dobutamine) and analgesics to treat shock symptoms and promote comfort.

Nursing interventions. The patient will be maintained on bed rest, and intake and output will be monitored.

NURSING DIAGNOSES	NURSING INTERVENTIONS
Altered cardiopulmonary or renal tissue perfusion, related to lack of oxygen	Monitor and report signs and symptoms of impending shock (decreased blood pressure and increased pulse). Administer vasopressor drugs as ordered. Maintain hydration status and urinary output. Assess changes in level of consciousness. Assist with acute hemodialysis if indicated.
Ineffective breathing pattern, related to respiratory failure	Assess signs and symptoms of respiratory failure. Note respiratory rate, rhythm, and effort. Be alert to cyanosis and dyspnea. Assist with oxygen therapy or mechanical ventilation as ordered. Facilitate optimal ventilation—patient in semi-Fowler's position if condition tolerates; suction as needed. Have patient cough and deep breathe q 2 hr if able. Identify associated factors, such as ineffective airway clearance, pain, and altered level of consciousness.
Potential fluid volume deficit, related to hypovolemic shock	Administer prescribed IV solution. Monitor intake and output. Be alert to signs of impending renal failure—decreased urinary output and hematuria.

Patient teaching. Because of the many alarming actions necessary to treat this disease and its complications, patient and family education is important. The nurse should instruct the patient and family on the purpose of respiratory support—oxygen therapy or ventilator assistance—and how to use these procedures for the greatest benefit. Explanations should be provided of all procedures before their implementation. The purpose of hemodialysis and why it is required should be explained. The nurse should stress the importance of controlling the patient's temperature and fluid and electrolyte status. Emotional support should be offered to the patient and family as needed.

Tuberculosis

Etiology/pathophysiology. Tuberculosis is an infectious disease caused by the microorganism *Mycobacterium tuberculosis*. The population at risk includes those whose skin tests have recently converted, the elderly, anyone with chronic illness, such as diabetes, renal failure, or malignancy, or anyone who has been previously infected. Once the *Mycobacterium* bacilli have been inhaled by a susceptible host, they multiply on the alveolar surfaces, resulting in new tissue masses (infectious granulomas).

Clinical manifestation. The clinical manifestations are insidious. Generally there is fever, weight loss, weakness, and a productive cough. Later in the disease daily recurring fever with chills, night sweats, and hemoptysis are seen.

Assessment. Collection of *subjective data* includes the patient reporting loss of muscle strength and weight loss.

Collection of *objective data* includes evaluating and recording the amount, color, and characteristics of sputum produced.

Diagnostic tests. The most common diagnostic tool is the Mantoux test, in which the tubercle bacillus extract is injected intradermally on the inner aspect of the patient's forearm. The injection site is assessed 48 to 72 hours later. A positive reading (skin reaction) indicates that the patient has been exposed to *Mycobacterium tuberculosis,* but does not necessarily have the disease. A sputum test is also done to determine the presence of acid-fast bacilli (AFB). It is preferable to obtain the sputum specimen early in the morning, because secretions pool overnight and are less likely to be contaminated. A chest x-ray is obtained and characteristically will show patchy infiltrates on the lungs.

Medical management. The goals of managing pulmonary tuberculosis are to relieve the symptoms by eliminating all viable bacilli, restore the patient to optimal functioning, and prevent infection transmission.

Sometimes surgery is required for abscess drainage or treatment of spontaneous pneumothorax. However, the need for surgical intervention has greatly decreased since the advent of antimicrobial therapy. Primary antiinfective medications include isoniazid (INH), ethambutol (Myambutol), rifampin (Rifamycin), and streptomycin. These are generally prescribed in combination with a secondary drug such as pyrazinamide (Aldinamide) or paraaminosalicylate (P.A.S.) or kanamycin (Kantrex). The treatment regimen is usually 9 months or longer, with secondary medications prescribed for an additional 18 to 24 months.

Nursing interventions. Nursing interventions are focused on preventing complications and illness transmission. When the patient is hospitalized with active TB, isolation procedures must be followed. In order to assist the patient's compliance to the prescribed medication regimen, the nurse must develop a supportive relationship with him.

NURSING DIAGNOSES	NURSING INTERVENTIONS
Ineffective breathing pattern, related to pulmonary inflammation	Monitor breathing for evidence of dyspnea or symptoms of pneumothorax. Evaluate degree of respiratory effort, and assist as needed. Assess expectorated sputum for hemoptysis.
Potential for infection, related to patient contact	Use AFB isolation for patients who have positive sputum tests. Initiate antimicrobial medications as ordered. Implement secretion precautions for patients with external lesions. Instruct the patient to cough and sneeze into tissue and properly dispose to prevent organism transmission.
Altered nutrition: less than body requirements, related to infection	Offer high-protein, high-carbohydrate diet to provide adequate calorie intake to meet increased nutritional needs during infection. Encourage adequate intake by offering small, frequent feedings in a pleasant atmosphere.

Patient teaching. The nurse should teach the patient techniques of proper disposal and handwashing related to coughing and sneezing. These measures will decrease the spread of infection. The nurse should explain the importance of adhering to the medication regimen as ordered and the need for prolonged treatment. The patient should be instructed on medication, dosage, frequency, and possible side effects. The nurse should emphasize the need to report hemoptysis, dyspnea, vertigo, or chest pain. The patient should be reminded to maintain adequate fluid and nutritional requirements.

Pneumonia

Etiology/pathophysiology. Pneumonia may be bacterial *(Streptococcus, Staphylococcus,* or *S. pneumoniae,* also known as pneumococcus), viral, or atypical in origin *(Mycoplasma)*. It can also be caused by oversedation, inadequate ventilation, or aspiration. Pneumonia is most commonly seen in the winter and occurs most often in those over 60 years of age. Mycoplasmal pneumonia, however, is most common in children of school age and often spreads among family members.

The pathophysiology is determined by the causative agent; however, the basic underlying physiological changes remain the same: inflammation of pulmonary tissue in varying anatomical sites. Bacterial pneumonia may be either lobar, in which a whole lung lobe is consolidated, or bronchial, where the infectious process involves the bronchi. Mycoplasmal and viral pneumonia cause inflammation of the interstitial layers, and there are alveolar infiltrates. Aspiration pneumonia is nonbacterial in origin, resulting from foreign body aspiration, most commonly occurring when a patient has a decreased consciousness level because of drug overdose or seizure. It can also occur when there are invasive tubes altering the body's normal integrity, such as nasogastric and tracheostomy tubes. It can be a postoperative complication resulting from inadequate lung expansion during ineffective coughing and deep breathing.

An overview of the pathophysiology is as follows: (1) pulmonary cilia cannot remove accumulating secretions from the respiratory tract; (2) these retained secretions then become infected; (3) inflammation of some part of the respiratory tract develops, leading to a localized edema; (4) this causes decreased oxygen/carbon dioxide exchange. As stated, this process can begin in the bronchi or in the lobe of one lung, and it can become more extensive.

Clinical manifestations. There are many significant signs and symptoms seen in pneumonia. A productive cough is very common; color and consistency of sputum will vary depending on the type of pneumonia present. Severe chills, elevated temperature, and increased heart and respiratory rates accompany the painful, productive cough. Wheezing and dyspnea are associated with bronchopneumonia. Viral pneumonia is evidenced by a widely fluctuating fever, diaphoresis, and mucopurulent sputum.

Assessment. Collection of *subjective data* includes obtaining the patient's description of the history, onset, and duration of cough. He may complain of fever and night sweats.

Collection of *objective data* involves nursing assessment measures, including checking the level of consciousness and vital signs, especially temperature and respirations, every 2 hours or as ordered. The color, consistency, and amount of sputum produced should be noted. The nurse should inspect the thorax to determine the patient's use of accessory muscles in respiratory effort and note any cyanosis or dyspnea. The nurse will observe and document if the patient needs to use abdominal muscles or intercostal muscles to adequately breathe. On auscultation, the nurse will hear rales on inspiration and possibly a pleural effusion.

Diagnostic tests. Blood and sputum cultures will help in identification of organisms. Sputum for culture and sensitivity should be collected before initiation of antibiotic therapy, to identify the causative agent. Chest x-ray studies will reveal lobular changes in density. White blood cell count will be normal or even low in viral or mycoplasmal pneumonia, whereas it will be elevated in bacterial pneumonia. Pulmonary function tests may be done to determine whether lung volume is decreased, and arterial blood gas (ABG) values will be determined to identify altered gas exchange.

Medical management. If an accumulation of pus in the pleural space (empyema) occurs, the physician will insert a chest tube for drainage. The physician will also prescribe oxygen therapy and physiotherapy—chest percussion and postural drainage.

Commonly prescribed medications include antibiotics (penicillin), analgesics and antipyretics (Tylenol or aspirin), expectorants, and bronchodilators.

Nursing interventions. Nursing strategies are aimed at assisting the patient to conserve his energy. The nurse should allow rest periods and should facilitate optimal air exchange by placing the patient in high Fowler's position. Also, the patient should be positioned so that he lies on his affected lung side to promote optimal expansion of the functioning lung. Oral intake of fluids should be encouraged.

NURSING DIAGNOSES	NURSING INTERVENTIONS
Ineffective airway clearance, related to inability to mobilize secretions	Assess the patient's ability to clear secretions; assistive measures include encouraging oral liquids to liquefy secretions, elevating the head of the bed, suctioning as needed, and assisting with effective coughing techniques. Administer bronchodilator or expectorants as ordered. Assess respiratory rate, rhythm, and effort, noting any adventitious breath sounds.
Anxiety, related fear of inability to breathe effectively	Assess patient's present anxiety level and previous coping skills. Identify with patient's previous hospitalization experiences and response to same. Remember that much of the patient's anxiety may be exacerbated by air hunger. Deliver nursing interventions in a calm, proficient manner.

Patient teaching. The nurse should teach the patient and family necessary hygiene practices, such as (1) hand washing to limit the spread of infection, (2) proper handling of secretions, (3) covering the nose and mouth with a tissue when coughing or sneezing, and (4) expectorating into the container provided. Also the patient and family should be instructed to limit exposure to visitors. Medication teaching should stress following the prescribed regimen and understanding use and possible side effects. The nurse should remind the patient to drink large amounts of liquids. The patient should be taught effective coughing techniques and should be informed of the availability of pneumococcal vaccine.

Pleurisy

Etiology/pathophysiology. Pleurisy can be either a bacterial or viral infection. The underlying physiological change is an inflammation of any portion of the pleura. It may occur spontaneously but more frequently results as a complication of pneumonia.

Clinical manifestations. One of the first symptoms of pleurisy may be a sharp inspiratory pain, often radiating to the shoulder or abdomen of the affected side. Other signs and symptoms include dyspnea, cough, and elevated temperature.

Assessment. Collection of *subjective data* is awareness of a patient's complaint of chest pain on inspiration. He may also report an elevated temperature.

Collection of *objective data* includes the nurse's assessment of the nature of inspiratory pain, noting its radiation points. The nurse should monitor vital signs, especially temperature, every 2 or 4 hours. Respiratory rate and rhythm should be monitored and documented, noting dyspnea. On auscultation of the lungs the nurse will hear a friction rub.

Diagnostic tests. The presence of a friction rub may be considered to be diagnostic. Chest x-ray examination will depict inflammation, as well as the presence of a pleural effusion if fluid accumulates.

Medical management. The physician may inject an anesthetic block around the vertebra to block the intercostal nerves, thus relieving pain. Prescribed medications include antibiotics (penicillin) to combat the infection, analgesics (Demerol) to reduce discomfort, and antipyretics (Tylenol) for fever. Oxygen may be administered.

Nursing interventions. The patient should be positioned comfortably on the affected side, and heat may be applied to the area.

NURSING DIAGNOSES	NURSING INTERVENTIONS
Pain, related to stretching of the pulmonary pleura as a result of fluid accumulation	Assess patient's pain level and need for pain medication; administer as needed, documenting effectiveness. Assist with splinting affected side when patient coughs and deep breathes. Instruct patient to lie on affected side.
Impaired gas exchange, related to inability to deep breathe	Assess patient's level of consciousness, noting an increase in restlessness or confusion, which may indicate ineffective breathing. Reposition patient q 2 hr to prevent pooling of secretions and to promote optimal lung expansion. Elevate head of bed to facilitate optimal ventilation.

Patient teaching. The patient should be instructed to be alert to signs and symptoms of exacerbation—purulent sputum production, further increase in temperature, and increased pain. The nurse should teach the patient to effectively cough every 2 hours and to splint the affected side.

Pleural Effusion/Empyema

Etiology/pathophysiology. Once the pleural lining is inflamed (as in pleurisy), fluid can accumulate in the pleural space. This accumulation of fluid is known as pleural effusion. If the fluid becomes infected, it is called **empyema.**

The pathophysiology of pleural effusion lies in the alteration of pressure gradients or surface characteristics of capillaries. Empyema may be acute or can become chronic. In acute empyema there is inflammation of the affected area with a thin layer of fluid. If this goes untreated, the fluid thickens and the pleura becomes scarred and fibrosed, losing its elasticity.

Clinical manifestations. Pleural effusion is generally associated with other infectious processes or carcinoma involving altered capillary permeability. Empyema is usually seen after recent thoracic or upper abdominal surgery or blunt chest trauma. The patient may have a persistent fever in spite of receiving antibiotics.

Assessment. Collection of *subjective data* includes the patient verbalizing complaints of dyspnea and air hunger. He may also disclose feelings of fear and anxiety related to decreased levels of oxygen.

Collection of *objective data* in both pleural effusion and empyema includes the nurse's assessment of signs and symptoms of respiratory distress, such as nasal flaring, tachypnea, dyspnea, and decreased breath sounds. Breath sounds and vital signs, especially temperature, should be assessed frequently.

Diagnostic tests. Effusions or pleural fluid will be evident on chest x-ray examination. Often a thoracentesis (needle inserted into pleural space to aspirate excess fluid) will be done not only to obtain a specimen for culture to identify the causative agent, but to relieve the pressure and discomfort.

Medical management. Usually this condition requires a thoracentesis to remove fluid from the pleural space. A possible danger resulting from this procedure is removing fluid too rapidly; less than 1300 to 1500 ml at one time is recommended.

A chest tube may be inserted for continuous drainage and medication instillation. This tube will be sutured into place and covered with a sterile dressing.

The patient may have a thoracic drainage system in use. To prevent the lung from collapsing a closed system is usually used, which maintains the lung cavity's normal negative pressure. With this procedure one or, more commonly, two thoracotomy tubes are inserted into the pleural space and are attached to a closed-system, water-seal drainage. One catheter is inserted through a stab wound in the anterior chest wall; this is referred to as the *anterior tube*. It is used to remove air from the pleural space. The second tube is inserted through a stab wound in the posterior chest and is referred to as the *posterior tube*. It is primarily for the drainage of serosanguineous fluid or purulent exudate. The posterior (lower) tube may be larger in diameter than the anterior (upper) tube to prevent it from becoming occluded with exudate or clots (Fig. 34-11).

When chest tube drainage is initiated, a 2-liter clear glass bottle may be used, although other commercial devices, such as the Pleur-evac system (Fig. 34-12), are available. Approximately 300 ml of sterile water, or enough to fill the bottle 1 to 2 cm from the bottom, is added so the end of the glass rod is under water to maintain water-seal drainage and prevent air from entering the pleural cavity (Fig. 34-13).

Nursing interventions. General nursing measures include placing the patient on bed rest. The patient may be receiving oxygen therapy; if so, frequent oral care will help prevent drying of mucous membranes. Also, the nurse should encourage effective coughing and deep breathing techniques and respiratory treatments. If the patient has had a thoracentesis, a large sterile dressing

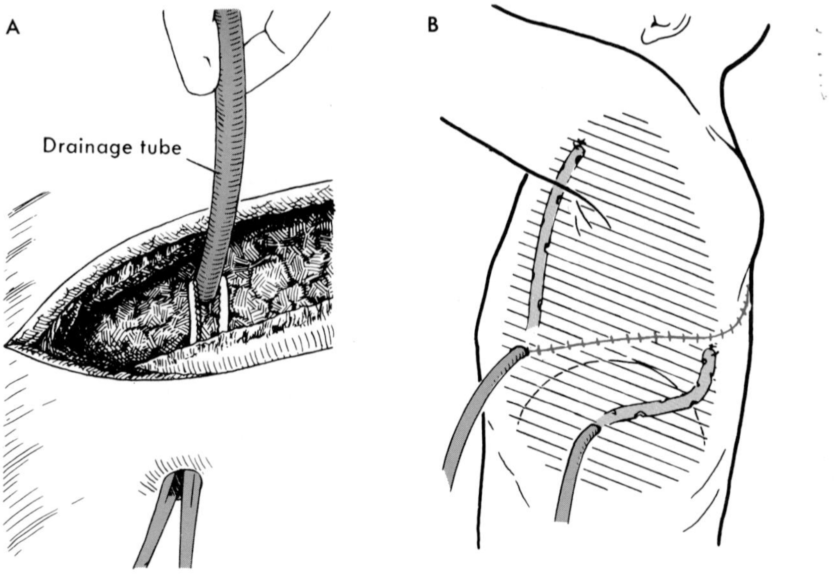

FIG. 34-11 **A,** Drainage tube inserted into pleural space. **B,** Note that upper and lower tubes are placed well into pleural space (From Johnson J, MacVaugh H, III, and Waldhausen JA: Surgery of the chest, a handbook of operative surgery, ed 4, Copyright © 1970 by Year Book Medical Publishers, Inc., Chicago. Used by permission.)

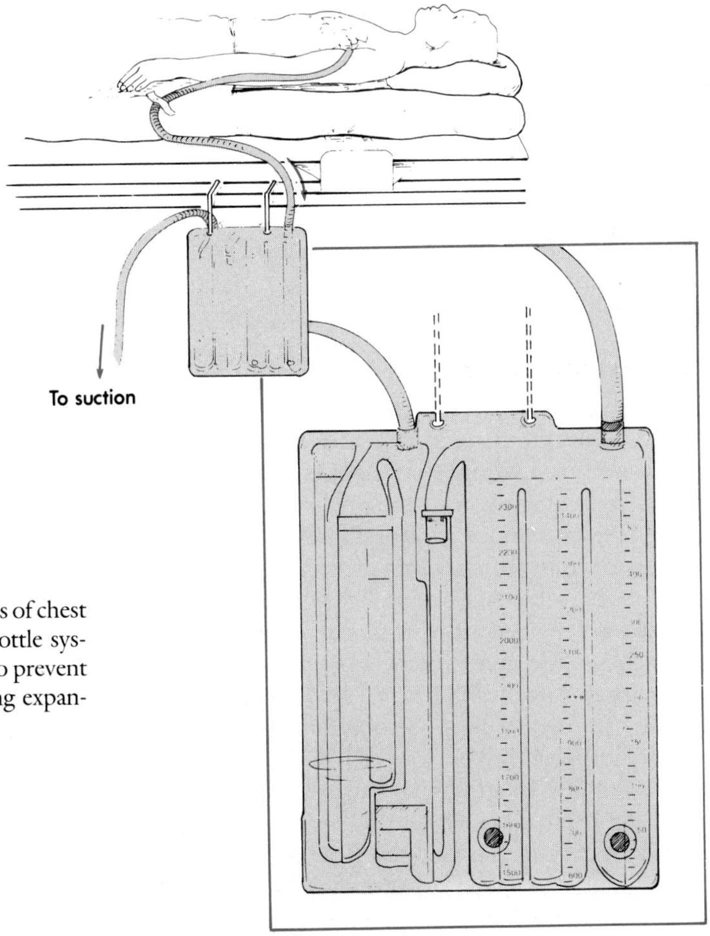

FIG. 34-12 Pleur-evac—one of several available brands of chest drainage systems. The system functions like a three-bottle system in that the unit collects drainage, maintains a seal to prevent air from entering the pleural cavity, and maintains lung expansion.

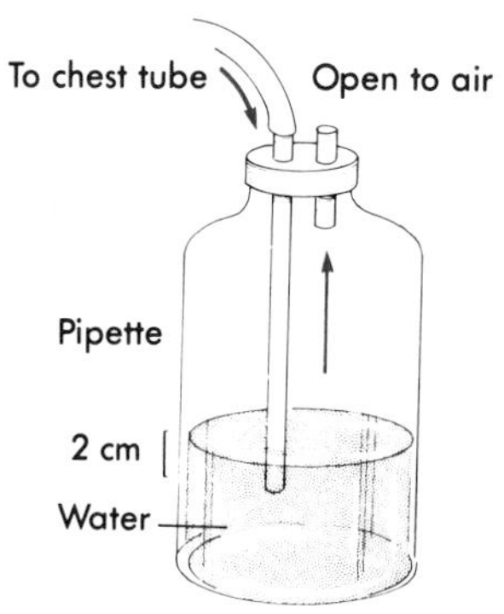

FIG. 34-13 Water-sealed closed chest drainage showing tip of tube under water.

will be applied, and the nurse will assess the dressing for drainage, noting color and amount.

The nurse must assure that patency of the chest tube system is maintained so that it can drain fluid adequately. Areas of concern include the following:

1. Proper system function: ensuring that the water in the water-seal chamber fluctuates when suction is applied; there should not be any bubbling in the water seal, because this indicates an air leak.
2. Potential atelectasis resulting from hypoventilation: assessing for increased dyspnea; checking chest X-ray studies frequently to compare degree of lung consolidation.
3. Increased air in the pleural space: noting any air leaks in the system; ensuring tubing is secure and remains patent.
4. Complication of infection; noting an increase in white blood cells, elevated temperature, and presence of purulent drainage.

While the chest tube is in place, the nurse will usually position the patient on the unaffected side to keep the tube from becoming kinked; however, the patient may assume any position of comfort in bed. There is no contraindication to ambulation with a chest tube in place, as long as the water-seal bottle remains below the level of the chest. The nurse must facilitate coughing and deep breathing procedures at least every 2 hours and auscultate breath sounds frequently. The nurse will document the amount and characteristics of pleural fluid drainage.

A key concern of the nurse is to determine what action to take if the chest drainage system becomes accidentally disconnected. In the distant past, nurses were taught to clamp the chest tube immediately. That placed patients with a persistent pneumothorax or copious mediastinal drainage at risk for a tension pneumothorax or cardiac tamponade (stoppage of the flow of blood to an organ or part of the body by pressure). Current practice is to not clamp the chest tube. The small amount of air that enters the pleural or mediastinal space can easily be evacuated by syringe or suction. As quickly as possible, the end of the chest tube should be placed in a container of sterile water or saline, such as the bottle of water used to fill the suction central chamber, until the drainage system can be replaced.

If the pleural chest tube is accidentally pulled out, in most cases the nurse should apply an occlusive dressing and notify the physician. If the patient develops respiratory distress, the dressing must be loosened or removed to allow air to escape.[5] The nurse can usually prevent a chest tube from being accidentally removed by careful attention to securing connections and positioning drainage tubings.

The patient will receive antibiotic agents and the nurse should administer them as ordered.

NURSING DIAGNOSES	NURSING INTERVENTIONS
Impaired gas exchange, related to ineffective breathing pattern	Assess for changes in level of consciousness, such as confusion, restlessness, or irritability, because these may indicate increasing hypoxia as a result of ineffective breathing. Monitor arterial blood gases. Encourage coughing and deep breathing to rid secretions and facilitate lung expansion. Reposition patient q 2 hr to prevent pooling of secretions. Assess for atelectasis.
Self-care deficit, related to mobility restriction	Assess patient's ability to care for self, and assist when needed. Encourage increasing activity level when fever is reduced and chest tubes are removed.

Patient teaching. The nurse should explain all procedures before their implementation. The patient should be prepared emotionally for chest tube insertion. The patient and family should be taught about his condition and the healing process. The nurse should instruct the patient on effective coughing and deep breathing techniques.

Atelectasis

Etiology/pathophysiology. Atelectasis occurs from occlusion of air (blockage) to a portion of the lung. Atelectasis is a common postoperative complication resulting from shallow breathing. All or part of the lung collapses, usually as a result of **hypoventilation**, which then leads to bronchial obstruction caused by mucus accumulation. A foreign body or a tenacious plug of mucus may completely occlude a bronchus, closing off all air to a portion of the lung. Atelectasis can also be the result of compression of lung tissue caused by emphysema, pneumothorax, or tumor.

The altered physiology depends on the site and degree of occlusion. If the main stem bronchus is obstructed, there will be severe ventilatory compromise. When a small bronchiole becomes obstructed, as with secretion accumulation, there are fewer signs and symptoms because the respiratory system will try to compensate. However, in either case atelectasis can lead to infection and lung damage.

Clinical manifestations. The patient will display dyspnea, **tachypnea**, pleural friction rub, restlessness, hypertension, and elevated temperature.

Assessment. Collection of *subjective data* includes the patient complaining of severe shortness of breath (**dyspnea**) requiring much effort, which results in fatigue. He may also verbalize a feeling of air hunger and resulting anxiety.

Collection of *objective data* includes the nurse noting decreased breath sounds and rales on auscultation. The nurse should assess vital signs frequently because hypertension will be present at first, followed by hypotension. Respiration rate and amount of effort required for breathing should be noted. The patient may exhibit altered levels of consciousness caused by hypoxia.

Diagnostic tests. Serial chest x-ray studies (frequently repeated x-ray examinations of same area done for comparison) will demonstrate atelectatic changes. Arterial blood gases will reveal a Pa_{O_2} of less than 80 mm Hg initially; this generally improves within the first 24 hours. Pa_{CO_2} will be normal or low, because of hypoventilation. A bronchoscopy may reveal a bronchial obstruction.

Medical management. Atelectasis frequently requires chest tube insertion as an attempt to reexpand the lung. Ventilation maintenance through intubation is frequently required.

Nursing interventions. Postoperatively, patients should be reminded to cough, deep breathe, and change positions every 2 hours. Early ambulation is encouraged. Incentive spirometry (Skill 34-3) and respiratory treatments with intermittent positive-pressure breathing (IPPB) may be ordered, as well as oxygen therapy. Chest physiotherapy with postural drainage will be administered (Skill 34-4). The patient may require suctioning; saline lavage often helps loosen secretions for easier removal. Prescribed medications may include bronchodilators (Bronkosol) to dilate the bronchioles and facilitate secretion removal, antibiotics to prevent infection, and mucolytic agents (acetylcysteine) to reduce the viscosity of the secretions.

NURSING DIAGNOSES	NURSING INTERVENTIONS
Ineffective airway clearance, related to inability to clear secretions	Assess patient's ability to move secretions, and assist if needed. Such measures are: reposition patient q 2 hr; encourage coughing and deep breathing, and suction as needed; liquify secretions using IPPB with nebulizer as ordered. Position patient as much as possible on unaffected side to promote maximum ventilation to affected side. Encourage adequate hydration to liquify secretions. Auscultate breath sounds frequently, documenting and reporting any changes. Assess color, consistency, and amount of secretions removed either via coughing or suction.
Ineffective individual coping, related to invasive medical regimen	Assess the patient's ability to comply with the prescribed regimen and to cooperate with nursing staff. Identify patient's emotional support systems.

SKILL 34-3 THE USE OF SPIROMETRY

Spirometry, referred to as *incentive spirometry*, is a procedure in which a device (spirometer) is used at the bedside at regular intervals to encourage the patient to deep breathe. Inspired measurement can be seen and used to encourage the patient to attain the established goal.

There are two general types of incentive spirometers:

1. *Flow-oriented inspiratory spirometer* This type of incentive spirometer is inexpensive and measures inspiration but not volume. It contains one or more clear plastic cylinder chambers that contain freely movable, colored, light-weight plastic balls. The patient is instructed to place the mouthpiece in the mouth and inhale slowly and deeply, which raises the balls in the cylinders. The patient is encouraged to keep the colored balls floating as long as possible. The cylinders are marked to measure the degree of elevation so that the degree of elevation and the length of time the patient can maintain elevation can be recorded (Fig. 26-4).
2. *Volume-oriented spirometer* This form of incentive spirometer maintains a known volume of inspiration. The patient is encouraged to breathe with normal inspired capacity. There are three primary purposes for the use of the incentive spirometer: to prevent or treat atelectasis, to improve lung expansion, and to improve oxygenation.

Continued.

SKILL 34-3 THE USE OF SPIROMETRY—cont'd

1. Check the physician's orders.
2. Assess patient's respiratory status and lung sounds. Indications for spirometry are (1) asymmetrical chest wall movement, (2) increased respiratory rate, (3) increased production of sputum, and (4) diminished lung expansion postoperatively.
3. Explain procedure, and instruct patient in the correct use of the spirometer. Frequently this is accomplished by the respiratory therapist. However, it may be the nurse's responsibility to follow up and promote proper technique.
4. Obtain supplies and equipment.
5. Wash hands.
6. Place prescribed incentive spirometer at the bedside.
7. Place patient in semi-Fowler's or high Fowler's position.
8. Place tissues and emesis basin within easy reach.
9. Instruct patient to completely cover mouthpiece with lips.
10. Instruct patient to (1) inhale slowly until maximum inspiration is reached, (2) hold breath 2 or 3 seconds, and (3) slowly exhale.
11. Instruct patient to relax and breathe normally for a short time. This prevents patient from hyperventilating and provides a resting period to prevent fatigue.
12. Instruct and encourage the patient to gradually increase depth of inspiration.
13. Offer mouthwash after spirometry is completed.
14. Store spirometer in an appropriate place, such as the bedside table, until next scheduled time.
15. Position patient as desired or as ordered.
16. Place call light within easy reach.
17. Wash hands.
18. Assess respiratory status, and evaluate patient's response to spirometry.
19. Document in nurses' notes: patient's respiratory status before and after incentive spirometry, type of spirometry, and any adverse effects from the procedure.

SKILL 34-4 PERFORMING PULMONARY PHYSIOTHERAPY (POSTURAL DRAINAGE)

1. Check physician's orders.
2. Assess respiratory status and lung sounds. This determines location of secretions before postural drainage and provides a baseline to note effectiveness of procedure.
3. Explain the procedure.
4. Obtain supplies and equipment.
5. Wash hands; don gloves.
6. Provide privacy.
7. Position patient according to the lung area to be drained (Fig. 34-21): provides gravitational drainage of secretions. Placing pillows for support will help provide comfort for the patient.
8. Place paper tissues and emesis basin within easy reach to collect secretions expectorated by patient.
9. Encourage deep breathing and coughing at intervals: facilitates bringing secretions toward the oropharynx where they can be expectorated or suctioned.
10. Cover patient with a light-weight blanket to prevent chilling.
11. Offer assistance with oral hygiene to provide comfort and reduce nausea if present.
12. Measure secretions if ordered; note color, amount, and consistency.
13. Position patient as desired or ordered after procedure.
14. Dispose of secretions and soiled tissues in appropriate area.
15. Remove gloves; wash hands.
16. Assess respiratory status, and evaluate patient's response.
17. Document in nurses' notes: patient's respiratory status before and after postural drainage; any secretions expectorated, including amount, color, and other characteristics; any adverse effect; and the patient's response to the treatment.

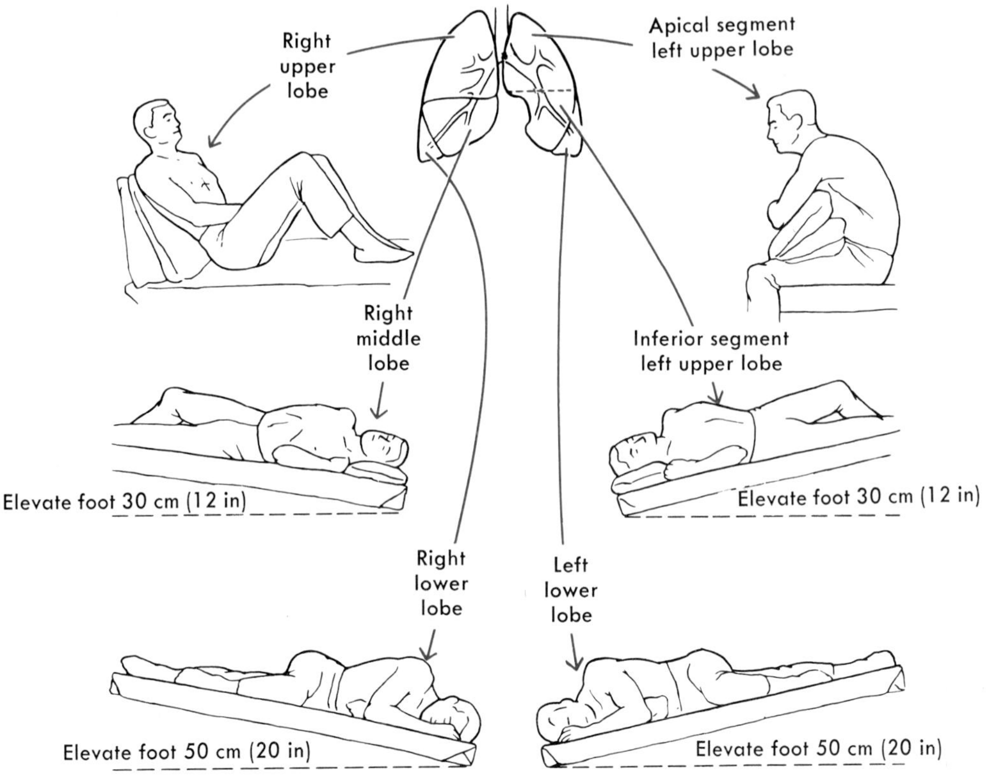

FIG. 34-14 Postural drainage requires that patient assume various positions to facilitate flow of secretions from various portions of lung into bronchi, trachea, and pharynx so that they can be raised and expectorated more easily. Drawing shows correct positions to drain various portions of lung.

Patient teaching. The nurse should instruct the patient on proper techniques for effective coughing and deep breathing, as well as other measures to facilitate optimal air exchange, such as increasing movement and changing position. Medication teaching should address rationale for prescribed medications, as well as side effects.

Pneumothorax

Etiology/pathophysiology. Pneumothorax occurs when the lung collapses because of air filling the pleural space. It can be secondary to a ruptured bleb on the lung surface (as in emphysema) or a severe coughing episode. It can be caused by a penetrating chest injury where the pleural lining is punctured, or a spontaneous pneumothorax can occur suddenly without an injury (Fig. 34-15).

When the pleural space is penetrated, air enters, thus decreasing the normal negative pressure. Consequently the lung cannot remain fully inflated.

Clinical manifestations. The patient may present with a recent chest injury. There will be decreased breath sounds on the affected side and a sudden, sharp chest pain with dyspnea. The patient may be diaphoretic and exhibit an increased heart rate and dyspnea. With a pneumothorax resulting from penetrating injury, there will be a sucking sound heard on inspiration.

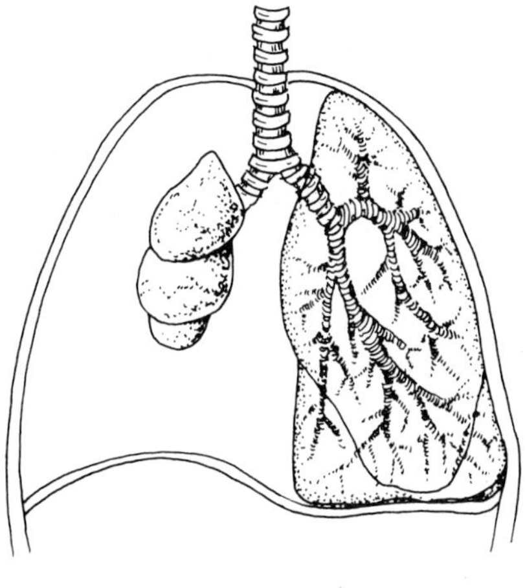

FIG. 34-15 Complete collapse of the right lung as a result of air in the pleural cavity (pneumothorax).

As positive pressure increases in the pleural space, the lung collapses. Because the lung tissue is no longer expanded, the mediastinum may shift to the unaffected side (mediastinal shift), placing increased pressure on the large vessels and resulting in decreased venous return.

Assessment. Collection of *subjective data* may include reporting a recent penetrating chest injury. He may also complain of shortness of breath of sudden onset and may indicate feelings of anxiety associated with air hunger.

Collection of *objective data* involves a nursing assessment that includes frequent vital signs, noting any change in respiratory and cardiac rate and rhythm. On auscultation the nurse will note bilateral unequal breath sounds, diminished on the affected side. Color, characteristics, and amount of sputum should be noted.

Diagnostic tests. Important findings to aid in diagnosis will come from the patient's history. For example, the patient may report a recent chest injury or a precipitating respiratory condition, such as **chronic obstructive pulmonary disease (COPD)**. Chest x-ray examination will reveal decreased lung expansion. Arterial blood gases will show a decrease in pH and PaO_2, with an increased $PaCO_2$.

Medical management. Surgery may be done to insert a chest tube (thoracotomy). The chest tube is inserted in the fifth and sixth intercostal space at the midaxillary line.

Nursing interventions. General measures include maintaining airway patency and providing adequate oxygenation. The nurse will need to assess and document patency of the chest tube system, keeping it free from kinks. If a chest tube is inserted, the nurse must note the color and amount of drainage and assess integrity of the dressing. The nurse will monitor blood pressure and place patient in high Fowler's position to promote airway clearance and lung expansion.

NURSING DIAGNOSES	NURSING INTERVENTIONS
Ineffective breathing pattern, related to nonfunctioning lung	Assess respiratory rate and rhythm, and note any signs of respiratory distress, such as dyspnea, use of accessory muscles, nasal flaring, and anxiety. Provide chest tube care, maintaining secure placement. Facilitate ventilation by elevating head of bed, and administer oxygen as ordered. Suction as needed to remove secretions. Encourage adaptive breathing techniques to decrease respiratory effort. Encourage rest periods interspersed with activities.
Impaired gas exchange, related to inability to breathe deeply	Assess for signs of hypoxia, i.e., restlessness, confusion, and irritability. Monitor arterial blood gases. Monitor fluid and electrolyte status and intake and output, being alert to changes caused by altered oxygenation.
Fear, related to feeling of air hunger	Assess patient's feelings of fear related to health concerns and feeling of air hunger. Identify positive coping methods, and support their use. Determine support systems available to patient.

Patient teaching. The nurse should explain the rationale for treatments—oxygen therapy and chest tube drainage—before their implementation. Effective breathing techniques and the need for ongoing medical care should be reinforced. The nurse should instruct the patient to limit exposure to people who may have infections, such as upper respiratory infection or influenza.

Lung Cancer

Etiology/pathophysiology. The incidence of lung cancer has been steadily increasing during the past 50 years in both men and women. In 1986 cancer of the lung surpassed breast cancer to become the number one cancer killer of women. Thus lung cancer is now the leading cause of death from cancer in both men and women. Tumors may result from metastasis anywhere in the body or may appear as primary tumors. Metastasis from the colon and kidney is common. Metastasis to the lung may be discovered before the primary lesion is known, and sometimes the location of the primary lesion is not determined during the person's life. It has been linked primarily with cigarette smoking. A history of smoking, especially for 20 years or more, is considered to be a prime risk factor. Occupational exposures, such as asbestos or chrome, are also risk factors. It is suspected that air pollutants may increase risk.

The mortality of persons with lung cancer depends primarily on the specific type of cancer and the size of the tumor when detected. Squamous cell carcinoma is the most common, followed by adenocarcinoma; undifferentiated small cell (oat cell) carcinoma is the least common. Most people who develop the disease are over 50 years of age.

Only 13% of lung cancer patients live 5 years or longer after diagnosis. The survival rate is 40% for cases detected in a localized stage; only 20% of lung cancers are discovered that early. Survival rates have improved only slightly over the past 10 years.[1]

Clinical manifestations. If the lesion is located peripherally, there are few symptoms and it may not be discovered until visualized on a routine chest x-ray examination. If the peripheral lesion perforates the pleural space, a pleural effusion will result and severe pain will occur. Central lesions originate from a larger branch of the bronchial tree. These lesions cause obstruction and erosion of the bronchus. Symptoms are hemoptysis, dyspnea, fever, and chills. Auscultation may reveal wheezing on the affected side as well.

As the disease progresses, metastasis may occur, along with weight loss. Primary lung tumors usually metastasize to the liver or to nearby structures, such as the esophagus, heart pericardium, or skeletal bone.

Assessment. Collection of *subjective data* includes the patient's complaints of a chronic cough and hoarsensss. He may also report weight loss and extreme fatigue. The nurse should interview the patient regarding his family history—especially a history of cigarette smoking and history of exposure to occupational irritants.

Collection of *objective data* includes assessing the cough, noting color (especially blood streaked) and consistency of sputum, as well as frequency, duration, and precipitating factors. Also the nurse should assess the characteristics of the cough (moist, dry, hacking) and effect of body position and should identify with the patient how he attempts to relieve his cough. The lungs should be auscultated to determine if unilateral wheezing is present.

Diagnostic tests. Chest x-ray studies and CAT scan of the lungs are used to identify the location and size of the tumor. Bronchoscopy with biopsy or brushings and sputum for cytology will indicate the presence of malignant cells. A mediastinoscopy may be done to determine whether spread of the tumor to the lymph nodes has occurred. Scalene lymph node biopsy is also done to determine metastasis. This biopsy is performed in the supraclavicular area.

Medical management. The treatment of lung cancer depends on the type and stage of lung cancer. Unfortunately, most patients are not diagnosed early enough for curative surgical intervention. It is estimated that one third of the patients are inoperable when first seen, and one third are found to be inoperable on exploratory thoracotomy. Of the third who are operable, the surgical mortality is 10% for pneumonectomy and 2% to 3% for lobectomy. A pneumonectomy is the most common surgical treatment. This consists of removing the entire lung. Because there is no lung left to require reexpansion, drainage tubes usually are not necessary. The fluid remaining in that area will consolidate eventually, which will help prevent a mediastinal shift. A lobectomy is performed when one lobe is involved rather than the entire lung. If only a portion of a lobe of a lung is involved, a segmental resection is done. Both a lobectomy and segmental resection require chest tube insertion to facilitate lung reexpansion. (See p. 848 for water-seal drainage [Fig. 34-13].) Radiation therapy and chemotherapy are often done in conjunction with surgery to enhance recovery. In small oat cell cancer of the lung, chemotherapy alone or combined with radiation has largely replaced surgery as a treatment of choice. A large percentage of these patients experience remission; in some cases the remission has been long lasting.[1] Presently about one third of the patients who have surgery experience tumor spread.

Nursing interventions. Nursing intervention is often directed at postsurgical interventions, including facilitating recovery and preventing complications by promoting effective airway clearance through frequent repositioning and coughing and deep breathing. The nurse will assess vital signs frequently, auscultating breath sounds. After routine postoperative vital signs check, the patient will be checked every 2 hours to ascertain stability; as the patient progresses, he will be checked every 4 hours.

Prescribed medications are primarily antineoplastic agents to prevent or reduce tumor growth. Medications will be given also for symptomatic relief: narcotic analgesics for pain control, antipyretics for fever, and antiemetics for nausea.

NURSING DIAGNOSES	NURSING INTERVENTIONS
Ineffective airway clearance, related to lung surgery	Facilitate optimal breathing by placing patient in a sitting position. Assist with position changes frequently. Promote coughing and deep breathing, providing necessary splinting. Encourage early ambulation to mobilize secretions.
Altered nutrition: less than body requirements	Encourage patient to eat by serving meal in calm, unhurried manner, offering assistance as needed. Provide pleasant environment for meals. Determine dietary preferences, and encourage family to bring special favorites. Offer small, frequent meals and nutritious snacks. Administer antiemetics before meals to prevent nausea. Monitor intake, output, and patient's weight to determine nutritional status and needs.
Impaired physical mobility	Assess patient's ability to ambulate, and assist as needed. Encourage range-of-motion exercises to maintain muscle strength. Encourage conservation of energy, and assess for signs of fatigue.

Patient teaching. The nurse should teach the patient effective coughing techniques. The patient and family should be instructed regarding nutritional needs and importance of maintaining physical mobility. If the patient smokes, he should be encouraged to quit. The nurse should also instruct the patient and family regarding signs and symptoms that could indicate recurrence or metastasis, such as central nervous system changes and arm or shoulder pain.

Pulmonary Edema

Etiology/pathophysiology. Pulmonary edema is an accumulation of serous fluid in interstitial lung tissue resulting from (1) left ventricular failure from too rapid infusion of crystalloid or colloid solutions or (2) barbiturate overdose.

With left ventricular heart failure, fluid leaves the vascular space and collects in interstitial fluid of the lung, leading to increased hydrostatic pressure. The two stages in the development of pulmonary edema are as follows:

1. **Engorgement**. Areas surrounding the vascular and bronchial structures become engorged as a result of interstitial edema. To compensate for this, pulmonary lymph flow increases, causing fluid reabsorption.

2. **Alveolar edema**. Blood plasma enters alveoli faster than coughing or compensatory mechanisms can accommodate. This leads to acute pulmonary edema, altered tissue perfusion, hypoxia, and eventually respiratory failure.

Clinical manifestations. The primary symptoms of pulmonary edema are dyspnea and related breathing disturbances. Labored respirations, tachypnea, tachycardia, **cyanosis**, and especially pink (or blood-tinged), frothy sputum are the most obvious signs. On examination, distention of the jugular neck veins is noted. The patient may also exhibit restlessness or agitation because of the resulting hypoxia.

Assessment. Collection of *subjective data* includes noting the patient's complaints of edematous ankles, fluid retention, and/or severe dyspnea.

Collection of *objective data* involves the nurse assessing for signs of respiratory distress. Such signs include nasal flaring and sternal retractions with inspiration, as well as rapid, stertorous respirations, restlessness, and confusion. On auscultation the nurse will most likely hear wheezing and rales. The patient may appear restless, confused, and apprehensive. On physical examination the nurse will often note a sudden weight gain caused by fluid retention, pitting edema in the feet or ankles, decreased urinary output as a result of retained fluid in the pulmonary vasculature, and a productive cough of frothy, pink sputum.

Diagnostic tests. Chest X-ray examination will reveal fluid infiltrates, indicating alveolar edema, increased pleural space fluid (pleural effusion), and enlarged heart (cardiomegaly). Arterial blood gases will be altered, with varying PaO_2 and $PaCO_2$ levels. There may be respiratory alkalosis or respiratory acidosis. Sputum cultures will be done periodically to rule out the presence of a bronchopulmonary infection.

Medical management. The physician will order oxygen therapy and may intubate the patient for adequate ventilation support. Medications will include diuretics to reduce alveolar and systemic edema by increasing urinary output (furosemide [Lasix]) and a narcotic analgesic, such as morphine sulfate, to decrease respiratory rate and lower the patient's anxiety level. Bronchodilators (aminophylline or theophylline) will be given to increase ventilation, and medications such as cardioglycosides (digoxin [Lanoxin]), will be used to treat underlying causative conditions.

Nursing interventions. One of the most important nursing measures is accurate assessment and documentation to identify any changes in the patient's condition. This will include assessment of respiratory status and frequent monitoring of intake and output, vital signs, arterial blood gases, and electrolyte values. The nurse will maintain oxygenation therapy as ordered—commonly delivered by Venturi mask at 40% to 70% concentration. Mechanical ventilation may be required, in which case the intubated patient will need oral care and tracheostomy care according to established protocol. Optimal air exchange must be facilitated by maintaining the patient in high Fowler's position. A patent IV line must be maintained, usually at a very slow rate to keep the vein open for medication administration (i.e., 30 ml/hr). This will prevent adding even more fluid to the overloaded patient. The patient will require extremely close monitoring of cardiac status and accurate measuring and recording of intake and output.

NURSING DIAGNOSES	NURSING INTERVENTIONS
Impaired gas exchange, related to excess fluid interfering with oxygen diffusion	Be alert to any signs indicating altered ventilation, such as restlessness, irritability, confusion, or apprehension. Monitor arterial blood gases, and RN to notify physician of any change. Monitor vital signs frequently, including cardiac rhythm. Administer oxygen therapy as ordered, and document patient response. Administer bronchodilators, cardiotonic glycosides, and other medications as ordered.
Fluid volume excess, related to altered tissue permeability	Assess indicators of patient's fluid volume status, such as breath sounds, skin turgor, and pedal/sacral/periorbital edema. Monitor intake and output accurately. Monitor electrolyte values closely, and RN to notify physician of alterations. Administer diuretics as ordered, and note patient response. Weigh patient daily on same scale at same time of day with same amount of bed linen and patient clothing. Provide low sodium diet to prevent excess fluid retention.
Fatigue, related to increased respiratory effort	Allow adequate rest periods interspersed with nursing interventions. Relate level of fatigue to patient activity, and modify accordingly. Encourage energy conservation; limit visitors as needed. Identify and promote patient's support systems.

Patient teaching. The patient should be taught effective breathing techniques. Medication teaching regarding actions, side effects, and dosage of prescribed medications should be given to the patient and family. The patient and family should be instructed on a low sodium diet and referred to the dietician for follow-up. The nurse should emphasize to the patient and family the signs and symptoms to observe that would indicate alteration in health, such as productive cough (noting the color and characteristics of sputum), activity intolerance, or the presence of edema.

Pulmonary Embolus

Etiology/pathophysiology. Pulmonary embolus usually occurs in patients identified to be at risk, such as the following:

- Those with prior thrombophlebitis
- Those who have recently had surgery, been pregnant, or given birth
- Women who are taking contraceptives on a long-term basis
- Those with a history of congestive heart failure, obesity, or immobilization from fracture; immobilization appears to be a key consideration

The basic alteration in this condition is the occlusion of a pulmonary artery caused by thrombus, air or fat embolus, or tumor. This occlusion results in obstructed blood supply to the lung tissue. Venous stasis, venous wall injury, and increased coagulability of blood cause the formation of a venous thrombus. The thrombus (usually in the deep veins of the lower extremities) dislodges and travels to the pulmonary artery where it becomes lodged. At the site of the embolus, lung tissue is ventilated but perfusion is inadequate because of the occlusion. As a result of this, arterial hypoxia develops.

Clinical manifestations. A pulmonary embolus manifests itself by a sudden, sharp abdominal or thoracic pain associated with dyspnea and hemoptysis. The respiratory rate will be rapid. In small areas of infarction, presenting signs and symptoms are a small amount of hemoptysis, pleuritic chest pain, elevated temperature, and increased white blood cell count. In large areas of infarction, symptoms include hypoxia, hypotension, and tachypnea. Lung sounds will be diminished, and rales may be present.

Assessment. Collection of *subjective data* includes noting the patient's report of presence and degree of dyspnea and chest pain. Nursing assessment will also include identifying the presence of associated risk factors.

Collection of *objective data* involves the nurse assessing for pleuritic pain and noting the nature of the patient's cough. Further assessment includes breath sounds, vital signs, and being alert for tachycardia and tachypnea. On auscultation the nurse will note any dullness in lung sounds and the presence of a pleural friction rub. In assessing the psychological response of the patient, the nurse will document the presence and degree of anxiety, which is often correlated to air hunger.

Diagnostic tests. Arterial blood gases will be significantly altered, depicting hypoxia and respiratory alkalosis. Chest x-ray examination shows an enlarged main pulmonary artery and generally many unilateral changes. CT scans of the lung may be helpful unless the patient has a history of congestive heart failure or chronic obstructive pulmonary disease, in which case an evaluation of the ventilation/perfusion ratio will be more definitive.

Medical management. Occasionally surgical intervention is the treatment of choice. When there are multiple pulmonary emboli present, an umbrella filter may be placed in the inferior vena cava to retain the emboli, preventing their migration to other parts of the body.

The physician will prescribe anticoagulant therapy to prevent clot formation. Initially heparin will be administered intravenously, either by way of continuous infusion on a pump or intermittent boluses. In the event of overheparinization resulting in profound bleeding, the treatment is intravenous administration of protamine sulfate. Heparin therapy is gradually tapered (it may take several days) while oral anticoagulation (Coumadin) is initiated. Effectiveness of Coumadin therapy is determined by monitoring prothrombin time (PT) values.

Some physicians prefer to use fibrinolytic agents, such as urokinase or streptokinase.

Nursing interventions. General nursing interventions include applying TED hose and elevating the lower extremities. The nurse should check peripheral pulses and frequently measure bilateral calf circumference to check for occlusion caused by a clot. The head of the bed may be slightly elevated, and oxygen will be administered by mask or nasal cannula to facilitate optimal gas exchange. The patient will promote lung expansion by coughing and deep breathing.

A major nursing intervention pertinent to heparin therapy is monitoring partial thromboplastin time (PTT), which should be maintained at 1½ to 2 times the control (or normal) values. Related nursing interventions will include assessing for signs of bleeding—epistaxis, hemoptysis, bleeding from gums or rectum, and ecchymosis.

Other general nursing interventions will include placing the patient on bed rest for the first few days and gradually increasing activity.

NURSING DIAGNOSES	NURSING INTERVENTIONS
Impaired gas exchange, related to alteration in pulmonary vasculature	Assess sensorium and vital signs q 2 hr or as needed, noting any changes indicative of altered oxygenation/ventilation. Monitor arterial blood gases frequently, reporting any increase or decrease of $PaCO_2$ and PaO_2 of more than 10 mm Hg. Be alert to any dysrhythmias.
Impaired physical mobility, related to fatigue associated with dyspnea	Encourage the patient to reduce the effort of breathing by using effective breathing techniques. Place TED hose on patient for continuous wear; remove at least q 8 hr. Deliver passive range of motion, and assist with position changes q 2 hr.

Patient teaching. Medication teaching is a major nursing concern. Often oral anticoagulation becomes a lifelong regimen that bears close monitoring, so the nurse must assess the patient's present knowledge base and expand on it. Preventive measures are also important, especially in the postoperative period. The nurse should teach the patient techniques to reduce venous pooling (which could precipitate thrombophlebitis), such as position changes and wearing nonrestrictive clothing. The patient must be told to avoid crossing the legs while in a sitting or lying position and also to avoid standing in one place for a prolonged period, because these activities increase venous pooling. The patient and family should be instructed on signs and symptoms to report to the physician, such as chest pain, dyspnea, and blood-tinged sputum or urine, which could result from anticoagulant therapy.

Adult Respiratory Distress Syndrome (ARDS)

Etiology/pathophysiology. There are many causes of ARDS, which results from either a direct or indirect pulmonary injury. Possible causes include viral or bacterial pneumonia, chest trauma, aspiration, or any type of shock. Drug overdoses, renal failure, and pancreatitis are also known to be causative factors.

Regardless of the cause of ARDS, there is a certain sequela of events in the body's response that remains the same. The surface of the alveolar capillary membrane becomes altered, causing increased permeability, which then allows fluid to leak into the interstitial spaces and alveoli. This creates pulmonary edema and hypoxia. The alveoli lose their elasticity and collapse, which causes the blood to be shunted through the impaired alveoli, hence interfering with oxygen transport. The damaged capillaries allow plasma and red blood cells to leak out, resulting in hemorrhage.

Clinical manifestations. ARDS manifests itself in 12 to 24 hours postinjury, resulting in lung tissue damage or hypovolemic shock, and 5 to 10 days after sepsis development, the patient will experience respiratory distress with altered breath sounds. There may be altered sensorium as a result of an elevated $Paco_2$ and decreased Pao_2. Additional symptoms will be cardiovascular in nature: tachycardia, hypotension, and decreased urinary output.

Assessment. Collection of *subjective data* involves a nursing assessment that will include background information and a history of the present illness (obtained from family members, because the patient is usually too ill to give details).

Collection of *objective data* involves the nurse being an astute observer of any change in the patient's condition, no matter how small or gradual. The nurse must make an accurate and thorough initial assessment so such changes will be quickly recognized. Initial assessment includes identifying and documenting respiratory rate, rhythm, and effort. Signs of dyspnea should be noted, such as nasal flaring, sternal retractions, or cyanosis. The nurse should auscultate the lungs and document the presence of rales, rhonchi, or wheezing and should maintain close observation of vital signs. Frequent assessment of the level of consciousness, with particular attention to increased restlessness or lethargy, is necessary.

Diagnostic tests. Pulmonary function tests will be done to determine the ease or difficulty of oxygen in crossing the alveolar capillary membrane. Arterial blood gases will show definitive changes: the Pao_2 will be decreased (less than 70 mm Hg), the $Paco_2$ will be increased (greater than 35 mm Hg), and the bicarbonate ion will be decreased (less than 22 mEq/L). Initially, HCO_3 increases in an attempt to buffer the elevated $Paco_2$ level, thereby maintaining pH in the normal range. The pH will be elevated initially but will steadily decrease as the patient's condition deteriorates. A chest X-ray examination will depict thickened bronchial margins and possibly diffuse infiltrates.

Medical management. The medical plan focuses on supportive treatment by maintaining adequate oxygenation and treating the cause—drug overdose, infections, or inhaled toxins. Medications commonly used to treat associated conditions include corticosteroids to treat pulmonary edema, aiding in restoring lung tissues to their normal structure and function. Morphine sulfate is commonly given to sedate restless patients and decrease respiratory rate. When the patient is intubated and ventilator dependent, a neurological blocking agent, such as Pavulon, may be administered to suppress the patient's own respiratory effort, relying on the controlled ventilator assistance.

Other medications may include cardiotonic glycosides (digoxin [Lanoxin]) to enhance cardiac function and antibiotic agents to prevent the further complication of infection.

Nursing interventions. The goal of nursing interventions is to provide adequate oxygenation and ventilation and to treat the multisystem responses caused by ARDS. Nursing intervention includes knowledge of mechanical ventilator settings and effects. Nursing intervention correlated to this is care pertinent to intubated patients, such as suctioning, providing oral care, and assessing for signs of inadequate ventilation. Arterial blood gases should be monitored closely and any changes reported.

Also, an accurate, ongoing assessment of cardiac function is important. The nurse should be alert for and document any rate or rhythm changes. The RN will notify the physician of any changes.

The nurse should assess vital signs and identify the presence of an elevated temperature so that cultures can be obtained to treat infections.

NURSING DIAGNOSES	NURSING INTERVENTIONS
Impaired gas exchange, related to tachypnea	Monitor arterial blood gases, and report any increase or decrease of $Paco_2$ and Pao_2 of more than 10 to 15 mm Hg. Address any factors that would contribute to restlessness and anxiety, because they increase the body's oxygen demand and will exacerbate the patient's already serious condition. Administer oxygen per order, assessing and recording patient response. Monitor electrocardiogram changes. Report any changes in vital signs and any change in patient's level of response, no matter how small or gradual.
Ineffective breathing pattern, related to respiratory distress	Assess respiratory rate, rhythm, and effort, being alert to signs of dyspnea, such as cyanosis and dyspnea. Facilitate optimal ventilation by proper positioning. Maintain airway patency by encouraging frequent coughing and deep breathing if able, or suctioning as needed.

Patient teaching. The nurse should teach the patient effective breathing techniques, emphasizing the importance of frequent position changes and coughing and deep breathing. If the patient is intubated, the nurse should explain all procedures before their implementation and should explain the importance of working *with* the ventilator and not trying to breathe independently. The patient should be reassured that the ventilator will breathe for him and that those breaths will be more effective than his own. The nurse should explain to the patient and family the importance of using rest and activity appropriately. Explanations of the purpose and side effects of all medications should be offered.

OXYGEN THERAPY

The element *oxygen* is a colorless, odorless, and tasteless gas that will not burn or explode. However, if combined with other factors, such as an electrical spark or fire, oxygen will support combustion and ignite. Nurses should follow all of the following safety precautions:

1. Place "No Smoking" and "Oxygen in Use" signs in conspicuous locations.
2. Instruct patient, family, and visitors that smoking is not permitted, because oxygen supports combustion.
3. Avoid the use of electrical appliances, such as razors, blankets, heating pads, and call signals; a nonelectrical signal, such as a hand bell, may be used in place of the electric call light.
4. Secure portable oxygen delivery systems, such as cylinders, to prevent falling or accidentally being tipped over.
5. Avoid placing oxygen cylinders near sources of heat, such as lamps or radiators.
6. Avoid clothing that is non–fire resistant.
7. Ensure that all electrical equipment is functioning appropriately and is well grounded. Avoid frayed, tangled, or cluttered cords, and do not overload circuits with too many appliances.
8. Know the institution's fire procedure and location of fire extinguishers.
9. Administer oxygen as ordered by a physician; the physician determines the method of administration and the flow rate of oxygen.

Oxygen therapy is frequently initiated by a respiratory therapist, who is a health care professional licensed to deliver treatment that will improve a patient's ventilation and oxygenation needs. Among the treatments often performed by a respiratory therapist is the intermittent positive-pressure breathing (IPPB) therapy. This is delivered by a mechanical device that hyperinflates a patient's lungs by applying positive pressure to the airways.

SKILL 34-5 OXYGEN ADMINISTRATION

1. Check physician's order.
2. Assess patient for signs of hypoxia and respiratory distress.
3. Assess patient's airway, and suction any secretions obstructing airway (see Skill 34-2).
4. Obtain supplies and equipment.
5. Explain procedure and necessity of precautions to take during oxygen therapy.
6. Place "No Smoking/Oxygen in Use" signs in conspicuous places.
7. Wash hands.
8. Provide privacy.
9. Position patient in Fowler's or semi-Fowler's position unless otherwise ordered, to allow for appropriate lung expansion.
10. Fill humidifier container to designated level, if used; use sterile, distilled water or as prescribed; this provides moisture in oxygen to prevent drying of the nasooropharyngeal mucosa.

Continued.

SKILL 34-5 OXYGEN ADMINISTRATION—cont'd

11. Attach flow meter to humidifer, and insert in proper oxygen source; most institutions have a central source of oxygen with a specially designed outlet. Flow meter must be properly secured to oxygen source.
12. Administer oxygen therapy:
    Nasal cannula: A simple two-prong plastic device that is used to deliver low concentration of oxygen. Nasal cannula allows patient to eat and talk normally and is appropriate for all age groups. Caution should be observed in proper placement of prongs to prevent oxygen coming in direct contact with nasal mucosa. Oxygen has drying effect on mucosa and interferes with moistening and warming air inhaled through nasal passage, making breathing uncomfortable for patient. It is nurse's responsibility to maintain method, flow rate, comfort, and safety of a patient receiving oxygen therapy.
    a. Attach nasal cannula to oxygen tubing (if it is not preattached), and then attach to flow meter.
    b. Place prongs in cup of water. Adjust flow meter to 6 to 10 L to flush tubing and prongs with oxygen. This determines patency and removes any microscopic particles that may be in the tubing. If water bubbles, tubing and prongs are patent.
    c. Adjust flow rate to the prescribed amount.
    d. Place a nasal prong into each naris of the patient. Adjust liter flow per physician's order; usually 2 L/min is prescribed.

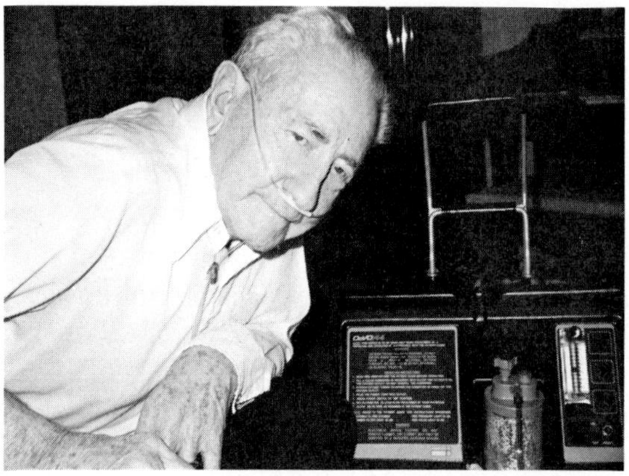

The nasal cannula can be used at home, as well as in the hospital.

    e. Adjust straps of the cannula over the ears and tighten under the chin. The fit should be snug and comfortable to prevent displacement of prongs.
    f. Place padding between strap and ears. Lamb's wool, gauze, or cotton balls may be used to prevent irritation.
    g. Provide slack of tubing, and secure to patient's garment to reduce risk of prongs causing pressure on the nares and displacement as patient moves or is repositioned.
    h. Maintain regular assessment.
       - Check cannula q 8 hr for possible obstruction.
       - Observe external nasal area and nares for skin impairment q 6 to 8 hr.
       - Check nares and prongs, and cleanse with cotton-tipped applicator as needed.
       - Check physician's orders for prescribed flow rate q 8 hr.
       - Maintain solution in humidifer container, if used, at appropriate level at all times.

    Nasal catheter: Administration of oxygen through a nasal catheter. This is less preferred than the use of the nasal cannula because it can traumatize the nasal mucosa on insertion, causing discomfort to patient.
    a. Attach nasal catheter to oxygen tubing, and then attach tubing to flow meter.
    b. Place catheter in cup of water, and turn on flow meter to 6 to 10 L to flush tubing.
    c. Adjust flow rate to prescribed amount; usually 2 L/min is ordered.
    d. Determine depth of insertion by using nasal catheter to measure from patient's earlobe to tip of nose. Marking place on catheter will assure nurse of proper length of insertion.
    e. Cover tip of catheter with water-soluble lubricant to reduce friction and trauma to nasal mucosa as catheter is inserted. Vaseline is never used because of danger of lipid pneumonia.
    f. Hold catheter to observe its natural curvature, and gently insert catheter into one side of nasal passage.
    g. Inspect mouth to visualize tip of catheter.
    h. Withdraw catheter approximately 1 cm (½ in), or until it is no longer visible.
    i. Tape catheter in place—may be taped to bridge of nose or side of cheek.

SKILL 34-5 OXYGEN ADMINISTRATION—cont'd

j. Provide slack of tubing, and secure to patient's garment.
k. Maintain regular assessments.
   - Alternate placement of catheter by using opposite nasal passage q 8 hr.
   - Observe external nasal area and nares for skin impairment q 6-8 hr.
   - Check nares, and cleanse with cotton-tipped applicator.
   - Check physician's orders for prescribed flow rate q 8 hr.
   - Maintain solution in humidifier container at proper level at all times.

Face mask. Administration of oxygen through face mask. Depending on patient's respiratory condition, physician may prescribe oxygen to be administered by oxygen mask. Mask is designed to fit snugly over patient's nose and mouth. There are different types of masks that may be used to meet patient's needs, such as Ventimask, nonrebreathing mask, and aerosol mask.

a. Adjust flow rate of oxygen per physician's order. Usually 6 to 10 L/min, which is measured in percentages, is prescribed. Respiratory therapist is usually responsible for maintaining proper flow. Observe for fine mist or bubbling in humidifier.
b. Allow patient to hold mask, and place your hand over patient's hand if possible. Placing mask over patient's face may cause feeling of suffocation and apprehension. This action allows patient to become accustomed to mask and to have some control of placing it on face.
c. Place mask over bridge of nose; then cover mouth.
d. Adjust straps around patient's head and over ears. Place cotton ball or gauze over ears under elastic straps.
e. Observe reservoir bag if one is attached to mask. This ensures mask is fitting appropriately by expanding and collapsing with patient's breathing. Complete collapse indicates oxygen flow should be increased.
f. Maintain regular assessments:
   - Remove mask and clean skin and dry q 1-2 hr.
   - Check physician's orders for prescribed flow rate q 8 hr.
   - Maintain solution in humidifier container, if used, at appropriate level at all times.

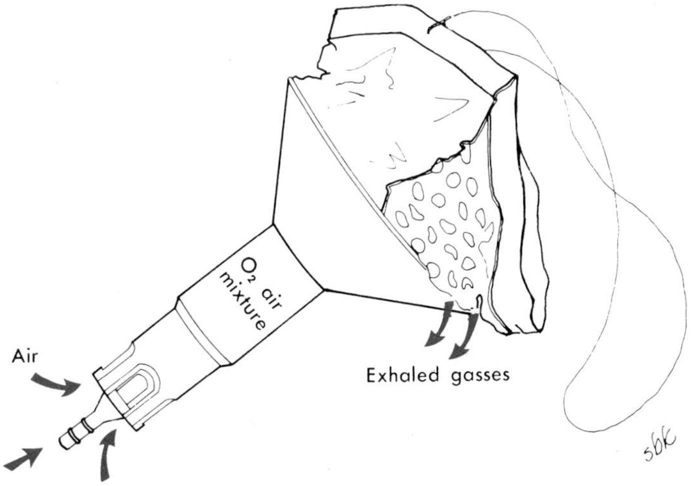

Ventimask allows air to be mixed with oxygen to provide diluted oxygen to patient.

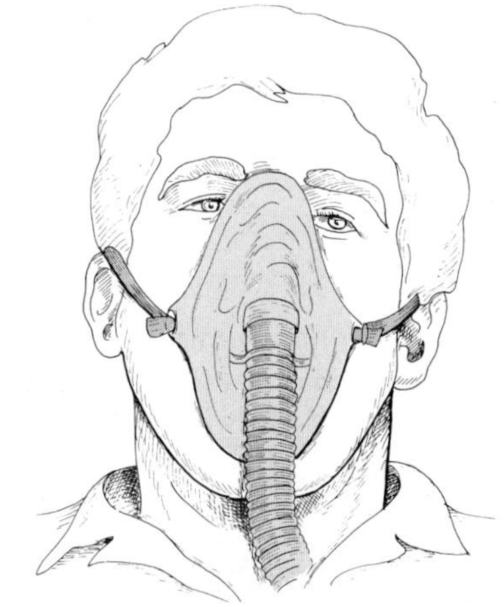

Simple face mask.

Continued.

SKILL 34-5

OXYGEN ADMINISTRATION—cont'd

Oxygen tent. Tent that provides fine mist, constant temperature, and high concentration and flow rate of oxygen. Mist is produced by humidification of oxygen confined within clear plastic canopy. Canopy encloses upper torso of patient. Psychological effect of covering patient's head may increase anxiety and therefore increase feeling of suffocation. Reassurance must be provided to relieve anxiety before placing patient in oxygen tent. Because canopy is clear, it allows patient to have visual contact with nursing staff and visitors. Some visual distortion of persons and objects can be expected when patient looks through canopy, and this should be explained. Because moisture accumulation frequently occurs from humidification of oxygen, primary responsibility of nurse is to keep patient warm and dry to prevent chilling. Clothing and bed linens may need to be changed more frequently. Tent also provides constant temperature, which is usually 70° F. Temperature may be adjusted for comfort of patient but should not exceed 10° over recommended temperature.

a. Place oxygen machine at head of bed for ease of draping canopy over head of bed and patient and to place humidifier where mist will be inhaled by patient.
b. Fan fold top sheet to patient's waist; may be used to secure front edge of canopy or to cover patient later if needed.
c. Set temperature to 70°, recommended setting unless ordered otherwise.
d. Turn machine on, and adjust flow rate to 10 to 12 L/min. Leave machine on until it registers appropriate temperature and oxygen concentration.
e. Placement of canopy:
   - Lift canopy over patient, and tuck back of canopy under head of mattress.
   - Tuck sides of canopy under sides of mattress at head of bed.
   - Place folded bath blanket lengthwise across patient's thighs.
   - Place lower, front edge of canopy to conform to shape of patient's thighs; place this edge of canopy within folded bath blanket.
   - Tuck folded bath blanket and canopy under sides of mattress to secure it and prevent leakage of oxygen.
f. Use zipper openings to provide care and administer medications: prevents large amounts of oxygen escaping and maintains control of temperature and humidity.
g. Maintain regular assessments
   - Check temperature, flow rate, and humidity at least q 4 hr.
   - Assess patient's response.
   - Check patient's clothing frequently, and change bed linens as needed.

12. Wash hands.
13. Document in nurses' notes: date, time, flow rate, method of oxygen delivery, temperature being maintained (if tent is used), respiratory assessment, patient's response, any changes in physician's orders, and any adverse reactions or side effects.

The signs and symptoms manifested by patients who might require oxygen will vary according to the degree of oxygen deficiency (see Box 34-3). See Skill 34-5 for O_2 administration.

Transtracheal Oxygen Delivery

Unlike a tracheostomy tube, a transtracheal cathether (Fig. 34-16) does not interfere with drinking, eating, or talking. The nasal cannula delivers oxygen only during inhalation, but the transtracheal oxygen delivery system delivers oxygen throughout the respiratory cycle. This allows the flow rate to be decreased for some patients. The low flow rates enable patients to use portable oxygen delivery systems longer between refills. It is recommended for those patients with congestive heart failure (CHF) and chronic obstructive pulmonary disease (COPD).

This method is especially adapted for home use. It allows the individual to be active. It may even be concealed under a shirt and tie. The transtracheal tract open-

SKILL 34-6 CARING FOR A TRACHEOSTOMY COLLAR OR T-PIECE

1. Wash hands.
2. Position the patient for comfort, usually in a semi-Fowler's position.
3. Inspect the rate of flow and the solution level for humidification often during the course of the patient's oxygen therapy.
4. Provide nose and mouth care to keep the mucosa lubricated, moist, clean, and fresh during the course of the patient's therapy.
5. Secure the collar or T-piece at the neck over the tracheostomy.
6. Adjust the oxygen flow rate according to the physician's order.
7. Adjust the temperature of the humidified oxygen.
8. Use large-lumen tubing from the oxygen source to the patient.
9. Condensation occurs within the tracheostomy collar or T-piece, so observe frequently.
10. The collar or T-piece and tubing should be removed frequently to be drained and cleaned to prevent the patient from aspirating the moisture.
11. As moisture collects, suction the tracheostomy and provide tracheostomy care as often as necessary.

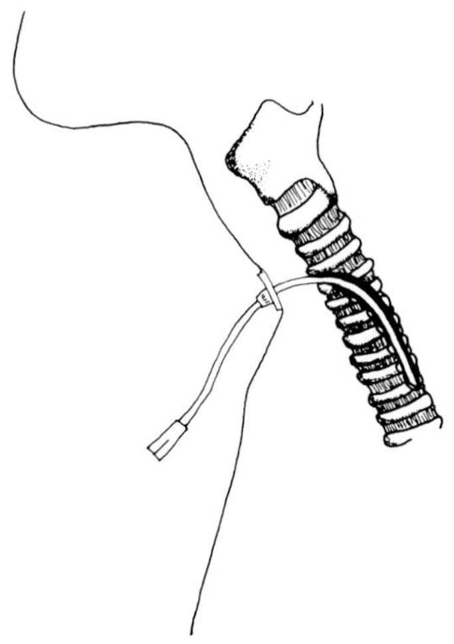

FIG. 34-16 A transtracheal catheter may be inserted into the trachea between the second and third tracheal cartilages.

ing should be inspected regularly for erythema, edema, or excessive exudate. (Small amounts of clear exudate are expected.) The area is cleaned twice daily with a cotton-tipped applicator. To remove dried exudate, hydrogen peroxide may be used to wash the neck. The transtracheal tract (like a tracheostomy) never truly heals as long as it is kept open for oxygen delivery.

A small oxygen tube is inserted through the transtracheal tract opening. Oxygen (O_2) is administered through the small oxygen tube. The tube is removed for cleaning. Oxygen is then administered through the nose. Clean technique is used. The transtracheal oxygen catheter may need cleaning several times a day. An extra transtracheal oxygen catheter is kept at the bedside. Usually the oxygen catheter is scrubbed with soap and water and rinsed. Skill 34-6 describes how to care for a tracheostomy or T-piece. The T-piece is the large plastic tubing fastened over the tracheostomy.

CHRONIC RESPIRATORY CONDITIONS

Chronic Obstructive Pulmonary Disease

Chronic obstructive pulmonary disease (COPD) includes emphysema, chronic bronchitis, asthma, and bronchiectasis.

Emphysema

Etiology/pathophysiology. **Emphysema** symptoms usually develop when the patient is in his 40s, with disability increasing by age 50 to 60. This condition is characterized by changes in the alveolar walls and capillaries.

A component of pulmonary connective tissue, lung elastin, is destroyed by an enzyme, which then causes decreased pulmonary surface area available for gas exchange. The bronchi, bronchioles, and alveoli become inflamed as a result of chronic irritation. Because of bronchiole lumen narrowing, air becomes trapped in the alveoli during expiration, causing alveolar distention (Fig. 34-17). The alveoli then rupture and scar, losing their elasticity. Oxygen in the arterial blood decreases, and CO_2 increases. This process is worsened by cigarette smoking and other inhaled irritants. Emphysema or other obstructive lung diseases can lead to **cor pulmonale,** in which the heart's right ventricle dilates and hypertrophies and may lead to right-sided congestive heart failure.

Clinical manifestations. The primary symptom of emphysema is dyspnea on exertion. Initially there is little

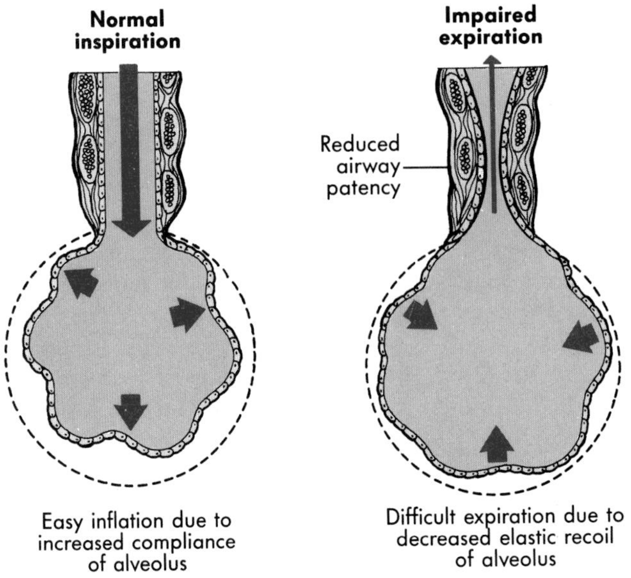

FIG. 34-17 Mechanisms of air trapping in emphysema. Damaged or destroyed alveolar walls no longer support and hold open the airways, and alveoli lose their property of passive elastic recoil. Both of these factors contribute to collapse during expiration.

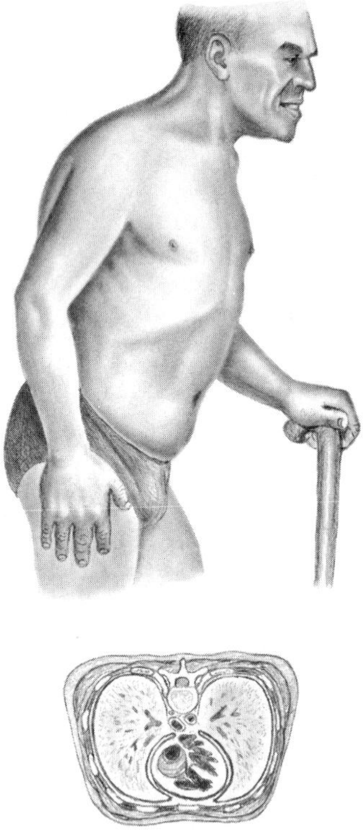

FIG. 34-18 Barrel chest. Note increase in AP diameter.

sputum production, but later it becomes copious. The patient will eventually appear barrel chested (an increased anteroposterior diameter caused by overinflation) and begin using accessory muscles for breathing (Fig. 34-18). He will exhibit spontaneous pursed-lip breathing and chronic weight loss.

Assessment. Collection of *subjective data* includes a nursing assessment that details a history of onset of symptoms. The nurse should note duration and intensity of dyspnea, cough, and sputum production (documenting color and amount). Also the patient's reported history of smoking and exposure to inhalants, and family history of respiratory disorders should be determined.

Collection of *objective data* includes assessment of presenting symptoms, such as tachycardia, tachypnea, peripheral cyanosis, and clubbing of fingers.

Diagnostic tests. Pulmonary function tests will be done to measure total lung capacity, which will be decreased with COPD. Residual volume is increased, as are compliance and airway resistance. Ventilatory response is decreased.

Arterial blood gases will reveal a decreased PaO_2, and $PaCO_2$ will often be increased. A chest X-ray examination will show widened intercostal spaces and flattened diaphragm with increased anteroposterior diameter (associated with barrel chest). Hematology studies should be done to determine if a positive alpha$_1$-antitrypsin assay exists (an enzyme deficiency causing airway abnormalities resulting in emphysema). Complete blood count will reveal elevated hemoglobin and hematocrit levels and polycythemia, caused by chronic hypoxia.

Medical management. The medical plan will include long-term management with home oxygen therapy and chest physiotherapy as needed. In an acute exacerbation the patient may require mechanical ventilation.

Prescribed medications will include bronchodilators (theophylline or aminophylline, isoproterenol [Isuprel], terbutaline [Brethine], metaproterenol [Alupent], and isoetharine [Bronkosol]) to enlarge the bronchioles for greater oxygenation and ease of secretion clearance, and corticosteroids to decrease pulmonary inflammation and obstruction. Antibiotics are frequently ordered to reduce the risk of infection related to retained pulmonary secretions. Diuretics will assist with fluid removal.

Nursing interventions. Nursing intervention will be directed at attempting to decrease the patient's anxiety and promote optimal air exchange. Such measures include elevating the head of the bed and administering *low flow* (1 to 2 L by nasal cannula) oxygen as ordered (see Skill 34-5). (This is extremely important for COPD patients, because a higher flow of oxygen delivery can be dangerous, since it diminishes the brain's respiratory (regulatory) center and can cause respiratory failure). The nurse should assist with chest physiotherapy and postural drainage (see Skill 34-4). Increasing oral intake of fluids will liquify secretions, thus aiding in their removal. Additionally, the use of a humidifier will enhance this process. Frequent oral care will promote comfort. The nurse should allow sufficient rest periods and should assist the patient in activities of daily living to prevent decrease in oxygen saturation levels.

NURSING DIAGNOSES	NURSING INTERVENTIONS
Ineffective airway clearance, related to narrowed bronchioles	Assess patient's ability to mobilize secretions, intervening as needed. Encourage coughing and deep breathing, frequent position changes, and increased oral intake (up to 2000 ml/day). Elevate head of bed; suction as needed. Assist with respiratory treatments. Auscultate lungs, reporting any changes in lung sounds.
Anxiety, related to feeling of dyspnea	Promote optimal air exchange to decrease anxiety. Assess patient's anxiety level, noting ability to cooperate with treatment regimen. Explain all procedures before their implementation. Encourage effective breathing techniques. Assess support systems available to patient, and mobilize resources.
Potential for infection, related to retained pulmonary secretions	Assess for indications of infection—sputum color, amount, and odor—as well as vital signs. Emphasize importance of reducing risk for secondary infection by decreasing exposure to others.

Patient teaching. The nurse should instruct the patient and family (1) on the importance of not smoking and of reducing exposure to other inhaled irritants and (2) effective breathing techniques (i.e., pursed-lip breathing) and relaxation exercises for anxiety control. Also, the nurse should teach the patient and family (1) how to prevent infection and (2) symptoms that should be reported to the physician. See the therapeutic dialogue and the patient care plan for the patient with emphysema.

THERAPEUTIC DIALOGUE: THE PATIENT WITH EMPHYSEMA

- Charles Oden, an 87-year-old man, lives at home with Annetta, his wife of 34 years. He was admitted to the hospital with acute **exacerbation** of emphysema. Mr. Oden has a 20-year history of emphysema, with progression of signs and symptoms. Signs and symptoms that he manifests are exertional dyspnea, expectoration of copious amounts of tenacious mucus, and fear of suffocation.

MR. ODEN: Will it always be like this? I am so short of air.

NURSE: Are you frightened?

MR. ODEN: I am not afraid of dying, but I worry about having to fight for my air.

NURSE: *(Gently touches Mr. Oden's arm)* Try taking slow, deep breaths, and concentrate on remaining calm.

MR. ODEN: Sometimes I can't even get to the bathroom and do my business—much less help Annetta with the dishes or even fill the bird feeder.

NURSE: Do you feel you are becoming a burden?

MR. ODEN: I have to be good to Annetta. I want to have something left to give her.

NURSE: I notice you are breathing more easily. I will be back to check on you, and perhaps we can continue this conversation.

Chronic bronchitis

Etiology/pathophysiology. Chronic **bronchitis** is characterized by a recurrent or chronic productive cough for a minimum of 3 months a year for at least 2 years. It is caused by physical or chemical irritants or an infection of bacterial or viral origin.

The underlying process is an impairment of cilia, so they can no longer move secretions. Mucous gland hypertrophy causes hypersecretion, altering cilia function. There is an increased susceptibility to infection. Chronic infection causes airway scarring, which causes obstruction. This increased airway resistance leads to bronchospasm. There is an altered oxygen-carbon dioxide exchange—**hypercapnia** and **hypoxia.**

Clinical manifestations. Primary signs include a productive cough, most pronounced in the mornings (this is often overlooked by cigarette smokers). There is also increased dyspnea and use of accessory muscles.

Assessment. Collection of *subjective data* includes obtaining a detailed history of smoking or exposure to ir-

NURSING CARE PLAN: THE PATIENT WITH EMPHYSEMA

Mr. Oden is an 87-year-old patient admitted with an exacerbation of COPD. His respirations are 32 and labored. He has nasal flaring and his nail beds are cyanotic. He presents with a barrel chest and digital clubbing. He states he has a productive cough. It is noted he expectorates tenacious yellow mucus. He appears anxious during the assessment.

Nursing diagnoses	Patient goals	Nursing interventions
Ineffective airway clearance, related to tenacious secretions	Patient will maintain patent airway as evidenced by decreased rhonchi, wheezes, tachypnea, dyspnea, and arterial blood gases within limits (for this patient).	Assess lung sounds q 2-4 hr. Encourage turning, coughing, and deep breathing q 2-4 hr. Suction PRN. Explain all medications used in inhalation therapy, and assist with treatment. Monitor effectiveness.
Potential for infection, related to retained tenacious secretions	Patient will be free from infection as evidenced by normal temperature and WBC, and sputum will be clear in color and decreased in amount.	Record TPR q 4 hr and more often if needed. Administer antipyretic PRN. Change position q 4 hr. Encourage fluids, and record intake and output every shift.
Anxiety, related to dyspnea and inability to verbalize	Patient will experience decreased anxiety as evidenced by verbalization of needs and concerns and statements of preference for more therapeutic coping methods.	Assess level of anxiety, and attempt to reduce by using calm, therapeutic interactions. Teach anxiety reduction techniques: pursed-lip breathing and controlled respirations. Assess family interactions; monitor as needed.

ritants, as well as family history of respiratory disorders. Also, the patient's current medication and treatment regimen should be determined.

Collection of *objective data* includes assessing the patient's productive cough, noting characteristics and amount of sputum. The nurse should assess the severity of dyspnea and presence of wheezing and should note the patient's level of restlessness. Also, when vital signs are checked, special attention should be paid to tachycardia, tachypnea, and elevated temperature.

Diagnostic tests. A CBC will show increased hemoglobin, hematocrit, and white blood cell count. Arterial blood gases will reveal respiratory acidosis and hypoxia. There will be an alteration in pulmonary function studies (increased airway resistance and residual volume) and often electrolyte abnormalities. Oximetry levels should be monitored on all patients with hypoxia.

Medical management. The medical plan is aimed at minimizing the disease progression and facilitating optimal air exchange by reducing spasms and secretions.

Prescribed medications will include bronchodilators (theophylline or aminophylline, isoproterenol [Isuprel], terbutaline [Brethine], metaproterenol [Alupent], and isoetharine [Bronkosol]) and mucolytics to enhance airway patency. Antibiotic agents (erythromycin) are commonly ordered.

Nursing interventions. The nurse should provide adequate hydration to liquify secretions and aid in their removal. The patient must be suctioned as needed and maintained on low-flow oxygen. The nurse should offer frequent oral hygiene and provide rest periods.

NURSING DIAGNOSES	NURSING INTERVENTIONS
Ineffective breathing pattern, related to retained pulmonary secretions	Assess degree of dyspnea, noting nasal flaring, sternal retractions, and pursed-lip breathing.

NURSING DIAGNOSES	NURSING INTERVENTIONS
	Instruct on effective breathing techniques. Suction as needed.
Fatigue, related to increased respiratory effort	Assess degree of fatigue, and with patient, use problem-solving techniques to explore techniques for decreasing fatigue. Provide treatments in calm, unhurried manner. Identify support systems, and refer if needed. Encourage adequate periods of rest.

Patient teaching. The nurse should teach the patient effective breathing techniques and instruct the patient and family on avoidance of infection exposure. Medication teaching should be provided, including action, rationale, and side effects. The nurse should stress the importance of increasing fluid intake. The patient and family should be encouraged not to smoke and to avoid using powders and aerosols.

Asthma

Etiology/pathophysiology. **Asthma** is a syndrome rather than a disease. It involves episodic increased tracheal/bronchial responsiveness to various stimuli, resulting in widespread narrowing of the airways, which usually improves either spontaneously or with treatment. It is classified as extrinsic or intrinsic. **Extrinsic** is caused by external factors; **intrinsic** is from internal causes, often triggered by respiratory infection.

Asthma can result from an altered immune response or increased airway resistance and altered air exchange. There are three mechanisms involved: (1) constriction of smooth muscles in airways leading to bronchospasm; (2) increased capillary permeability resulting in edema of mucous membranes with increased narrowing of airways; and (3) increased mucus secretion.

Clinical manifestations. Mild asthma is manifested by dyspnea on exertion and wheezing and is usually controlled by medications. An acute asthma attack usually occurs at night and will include tachypnea, use of accessory muscles, and nasal flaring. There will also be increased anxiety and diaphoresis. The patient will exhibit a productive cough of copious, thick mucus. Asthma can be triggered by external factors, such as dust, mold, or lint, or precipitated intrinsically by a respiratory infection or exercise.

Status asthmaticus is a severe, unrelenting attack that fails to respond to usual treatment. Symptoms of an acute attack are present, and the trapped air leads to exhaustion and respiratory failure.

Assessment. Collection of *subjective data* includes noting that the patient may report asthma-related factors: medications, self-care regimen, precipitating factors, and anxiety.

Collection of *objective data* includes the nurse assessing the presence of cyanosis, the amount of respiratory effort, and vital signs. The nurse should auscultate the lungs for wheezing and/or rhonchi.

Diagnostic tests. To diagnose asthma the physician will order arterial blood gases and pulmonary function tests. The chest X-ray examination is usually normal. However, there may be some hyperinflation related to trapped air. A sputum culture should be obtained to rule out secondary infection. A CBC will reveal increased hematocrit caused by hypoxia. If the patient reports he has been taking theophylline, a theophylline level should be drawn to determine whether the prescribed dose is maintaining a therapeutic level. This will also reduce the risk of complications as a result of toxicity.

Medical management. Once the acute event is over, the medical plan includes identification of precipitating factors and promoting optimal health.

Medications will include bronchodilators (epinephrine). IV aminophylline in a loading dose, subcutaneous terbutaline, or both may be given simultaneously and then in a maintenance dose for 48 to 72 hours; aminophylline blood levels should be monitored. Steroids (prednisone or Deltasone) are prescribed to decrease pulmonary inflammation and enhance airway patency. Aerosol therapy includes 1 to 2 inhalations of 0.5 ml isoetharine (Bronkosol) in 2.5 ml of saline. Antibiotic agents (ampicillin) are commonly administered prophylactically.

Nursing interventions. Nursing intervention includes ensuring adequate fluid intake and optimal ventilation. Measures to facilitate these goals include incorporating rest periods into activities and interventions, elevating the head of the bed, teaching effective breathing techniques, such as pursed-lip breathing, and providing oxygen therapy as ordered. The nurse should monitor vital signs and electrolytes.

NURSING DIAGNOSES	NURSING INTERVENTIONS
Ineffective breathing pattern, related to narrowed airway	Assess ventilation, and be alert for signs of increasing dyspnea, such as using accessory muscles, nasal flaring, dyspnea, pursed-lip breathing, or prolonged expiration. Maintain position to facilitate ventilation, such as elevated head of bed or leaning on overbed table. Assist with administration of respiratory treatments. Provide care in calm, unhurried manner. Attempt to minimize exposure to dust and other irritants by maintaining clean environment and use of humidifier.
Altered health maintenance, related to possible allergens in the home	Implement mutual problem-solving to explore with patient and family what stimulants may be in home environment, such as allergens.

NURSING DIAGNOSES	NURSING INTERVENTIONS
Altered health maintenance, related to possible allergens in the home—cont'd	Facilitate allergy testing if needed. Teach patient and family importance of avoiding exposure to known irritants.

Patient teaching. The nurse should educate the patient and family to identify signs and symptoms and precipitating factors, to avoid recurrent attacks. The patient should be instructed on relaxation techniques to use to manage anxiety. The importance of health maintenance measures, such as adequate fluid intake and effective breathing techniques, should be stressed.

Bronchiectasis

Etiology/pathophysiology. Bronchiectasis is a gradual, irreversible process which involves chronic dilation of bronchi and which eventually destroys bronchial elastic and muscular elements. This pulmonary muscle tone is gradually lost after one or, as is generally the case, repeated pulmonary infections in children and adults.

This condition is usually secondary to failure of normal lung tissue defenses (such as cystic fibrosis, foreign body, or tumor). It occurs as a complication of recurrence of an inflammation/infection process that gradually alters the pulmonary structures.

Clinical manifestations. Signs and symptoms occur after a respiratory infection. The signs and symptoms usually seen are dyspnea, cyanosis, and clubbing of fingers. There are paroxysms of coughing upon arising in the morning and when lying down. The severe coughing produces copious amounts of foul-smelling sputum. Fatigue, weakness, and loss of appetite are noted.

Assessment. Collection of *subjective data* includes noting the patient's report of difficulty breathing, weight loss, and fever.

Collection of *objective data* includes the nurse hearing fine rales and coarse rhonchi in the lower lobes on auscultation. The patient will exhibit a prolonged expiratory phase and increased dyspnea. Hemoptysis is seen in 50% of the patients.

Diagnostic tests. Chest X-ray examination will be essentially normal, but inflammation and mediastinal shift may be the result of overinflation of specific lobes. Sputum cultures can rule out the presence of a bacterial infection. CBC may show the presence of polycythemia, caused by pulmonary insufficiency (hypoxia). Pulmonary function tests will show a decreased forced expiratory volume.

Medical management. Oxygen will be ordered at low flow volume. The patient may require surgery if he does not respond to more conservative measures, such as medications, chest physiotherapy, and adequate hydration. Surgical removal of a portion of the lung is the only cure. If surgery is needed, the affected area will be removed (lobectomy).

Medications include mucolytic agents (acetylcysteine [Mucomyst]), as well as antibiotics and bronchodilators (theophylline or aminophylline).

Nursing interventions. General nursing interventions include using a cool mist vaporizer to provide humidity and increasing oral intake of fluids to aid in secretion removal. The nurse should assess vital signs and lung sounds every 2 to 4 hours. The patient should be suctioned as needed and assisted to turn, cough, and deep breathe every 2 hours. The nurse should assist with chest physiotherapy.

NURSING DIAGNOSES	NURSING INTERVENTIONS
Ineffective airway clearance, related to retained pulmonary secretions	Assess patient's ability to mobilize secretions, assisting as needed. Encourage postural drainage and coughing; suction if needed. Encourage frequent position changes to facilitate secretion mobility/removal. Maintain adequate hydration. Administer mucolytic agents as ordered, and note patient response.
Impaired physical mobility, related to decreased exercise tolerance	Assess patient's activity tolerance, and promote adaptive techniques, such as incorporating rest periods into activities. Promote a gradual increase of activity, noting patient tolerance. Problem solve with patient and family to identify methods of energy conservation and ways to implement them into life-style.

Patient teaching. The nurse should teach the patient and family environmental awareness (avoidance of smoke, fumes, and irritating inhalants). Smoking should be discouraged and appropriate rest/exercise practices should be taught. The nurse should perform medication teaching, including dosage, rationale, and side effects. The patient and family should be instructed on signs and symptoms of a secondary infection. The nurse should ensure that the patient knows how to reach the physician after discharge.

Cystic fibrosis

Etiology/pathophysiology. Cystic fibrosis is a genetic disorder of the exocrine glands that causes production of excessively thick mucus. It is thought to be related to an enzyme deficiency and is a multisystem disease affecting the respiratory system, pancreas, and sweat glands. The most common cause of death is progressive respiratory infections.

Bronchial obstruction occurs because of tenacious mucus, resulting in atelectasis and hyperinflation. This progresses to hypoxia, hypercapnia, and acidosis. The occurrence of mucostasis leads to pulmonary infection.

Clinical manifestations. The patient will present with respiratory distress: congestion, tachypnea, and dyspnea.

Rales and rhonchi will be heard on auscultation. The patient with cystic fibrosis will have a barrel chest and clubbing of fingers and toes. He will demonstrate a productive cough, cyanosis, and possibly headache or altered sensorium or level of consciousness.

Assessment. Collection of *subjective data* involves the nurse obtaining the patient's history and noting his present medication regimen, need for life-style alterations, and previous treatments or surgery. The nurse should determine the effectiveness of the patient's support systems and determine if intervention is needed.

Collection of *objective data* involves the nurse assessing the patient's respiratory status and effort, vital signs, appetite, and evidence of malnutrition.

Diagnostic tests. The diagnosis of cystic fibrosis is made by a sweat chloride level greater than 60 mEq/L (normal amount is 1 to 60 mEq/L) and is commonly diagnosed during childhood. Other diagnostic tests include chest x-ray studies (which may reveal disseminated infiltrates), pulmonary function tests, and sputum examination. Some physicians will also order arterial blood gases. Decrease or absence of pancreatic enzymes can also confirm cystic fibrosis.

Medical management. The goal of the medical plan is to decrease the occlusion of the bronchi by mucus. The patient may require surgery, such as a resection of blebs, or a tracheostomy to permit airway clearance and mechanical ventilation.

Prescribed medications include mucolytic agents, to combat the tenacious secretions, and expectorants (potassium iodide), to assist with their clearance. Bronchodilators, such as theophylline, are commonly ordered to facilitate airway patency. Antibiotic agents are frequently ordered (1) to treat infection or (2) prophylactically. A multivitamin supplement should be given.

Nursing interventions. Because cystic fibrosis is a multisystem disease, the nursing interventions are broad and address many systems. Interventions pertinent to respiratory symptoms will be addressed here. The nurse will determine that the patient's immunizations are current or, if needed, update as ordered. The nurse will assist with aerosol treatments and administer oxygen as ordered. A thorough dietary review must be completed, and the nurse can assist in planning a diet with increased calories and protein and decreased fat content. The nurse will also assist with the development of a network for psychosocial support.

NURSING DIAGNOSES	NURSING INTERVENTIONS
Ineffective airway clearance, related to tenacious pulmonary secretions	Determine patient's ability to mobilize secretions and assist as needed with chest physiotherapy. Administer medications as ordered, noting effectiveness. Provide adequate hydration to liquify secretions. Auscultate breath sounds frequently and report any changes. Assess productive cough, noting color, amount, and characteristics.
Altered nutrition: less than body requirements, related to altered digestion of fat, protein, and carbohydrates	Accurately weigh patient daily. Monitor intake and output, skin turgor and tone. Offer small, frequent, high-caloric, high-protein, low-fat feedings. Administer prescribed pancreatic enzyme at mealtime. Be alert to signs of malnutrition.
Family coping: potential for growth, related to chronic illness of family member	Assess and support patient/family's knowledge of disease and treatments. Explain all procedures. Identify coping skills, and support their use. Assist with contacting support systems as needed.

Patient teaching. The nurse should teach the patient effective breathing techniques and adaptive exercise/rest practices. The importance of up-to-date immunizations and the necessity of adhering to the prescribed medical/dietary regimen should be stressed.

REFERENCES AND SUGGESTED READINGS

1. American Cancer Society: Cancer facts and figures, New York, 1985, The Society.
2. Anagnostakos NP and Tortora GJ: Principles of anatomy and physiology, ed 5, New York, 1987, Harper & Row Publishers, Inc.
3. Asperheim M: Pharmacologic basis of patient care, ed 5, Philadelphia, 1985, WB Saunders Co.
4. Baer C and Williams B: Clinical pharmacology and nursing, Springhouse, Pa, 1988, Springhouse Corp.
5. Beare P and Myers J: Principles and practice of adult health nursing, St Louis, 1990, Mosby–Year Book.
6. Brunner L and Suddarth D: Textbook of medical-surgical nursing, ed 6, Philadelphia, 1988, JB Lippincott Co.
7. Doeschner S: Action stat! Pulmonary embolism, Nurs '88 18(9):33, 1988.
8. Erickson R: Mastering the ins and outs of chest drainage, Part I, Nurs '89 19(5):37, 1989.
9. Erickson R: Mastering the ins and outs of chest drainage, Part II, Nurs '89 19(6):46, 1989.
10. Fishbach F: A manual of laboratory diagnostic tests, ed 3, Philadelphia, 1988, JB Lippincott Co.
11. Fong E, Ferris EB, and Skelley EG: Body structures and functions, ed 7, Albany, NY, 1989, Delmar Publishers, Inc.
12. Harvey M: Controlling nasal hemorrhage, Nursing Times 83:48, 1987.
13. Hood G and Dincher J: Total patient care: foundations and practice, ed 7, St Louis, 1988, The CV Mosby Co.
14. Kersten L: Comprehensive respiratory nursing, Philadelphia, 1989, WB Saunders Co.
15. King K and O'Sullivan M: A respiratory resource program designed today for tomorrow, Nurs Manage 19(3):62, 70, 1988.
16. Lambert V and Lambert C: Psychosocial care of the physically ill: what every nurse should know, ed 2, Englewood Cliffs, NJ, 1985, Prentice-Hall, Inc.

17. Lockhart J and Griffin C: Action stat! Epistaxis, Nurs '86 16(11):343, 1986.
18. Long B and Phipps W: Medical-surgical nursing: a nursing process approach, ed 2, St Louis, 1989, The CV Mosby Co.
19. Luckman J and Sorenson K: Medical-surgical nursing: a psycho-physiologic approach, ed 3, Philadelphia, 1987, WB Saunders Co.
20. Marieb EN: Essentials of human anatomy and physiology, Reading, Mass, 1984, Addison-Wesley Publishing Co, Inc.
21. Memmler RL and Wood DL: Structure and function of the human body, ed 4, Philadelphia, 1987, JB Lippincott Co.
22. Phipps W and others: Medical-surgical nursing: concepts and clinical practice, ed 4, St Louis, 1991, The CV Mosby Co.
23. Potter P and Perry A: Basic nursing: theory and practice, St Louis, 1987, The CV Mosby Co.
24. Romanski S: Interpreting ABGs in four easy steps, Nurs '86 16(9):58, 1986.
25. Sarsony S: Respiratory distress, RN 51(4):47, 1988.
26. Seidel H and others: Mosby's guide to physical examination, St Louis, 1987, The CV Mosby Co.
27. Sexton D: Nursing care of the respiratory patient, East Norwalk, Conn, 1990, Appleton & Lange.
28. Solomon EP and Phillips GA: Understanding human anatomy and physiology, Philadelphia, 1987, WB Saunders Co.
29. Spearing C and Cornell D: Incentive spirometry: inspiring your patient to breathe deeply, Nurs '87 17(9):50, 1987.
30. Stevens S and Becker K: How to perform picture-perfect respiratory assessment, Nurs '88 18(1):57, 1988.
31. Thibodeau GA and Anthony CP: Structure and function of the body, ed 8, St Louis, 1988, Times Mirror/Mosby College Publishing.
32. Thompson J and others: Mosby's manual of clinical nursing, ed 2, St Louis, 1989, The CV Mosby Co.
33. Tucker and others: Patient care standards: nursing process, diagnosis and outcome, ed 4, St Louis, 1988, The CV Mosby Co.
34. Vasbinder-Dillon D: Understanding mechanical ventilation, Crit Care Nurse 8(7):42, 1988.
35. Winters C: Monitoring ventilator patients for complications, Nurs '88, pp. 38-41, June, 1988.

CHAPTER CHALLENGE

KEY POINTS

- When air is inhaled, it is warmed, moistened, and filtered to prepare it for use by the body.
- The most important structure of the respiratory system is the alveolus; it is here that actual air exchange occurs.
- For breathing to occur, pressure changes must occur within the thoracic cavity.
- The combination of one inspiration plus one expiration equals one respiration, or one respiratory movement.
- The primary function of the respiratory system is to exchange oxygen and carbon dioxide at the alveolar-capillary level.
- The ability of the lungs to expand and contract depends on musculoskeletal and neurological functions, as well as physiological conditions affecting the respiratory system.
- When obtaining a nursing history, the nurse will assess onset and duration of present signs and symptoms, previous respiratory conditions, current medications, family history, and exposure to irritants.
- Activity tolerance is frequently altered as a result of decreased oxygenation/ventilation.
- Anxiety can exacerbate pulmonary disorders, increasing the body's need for oxygen.
- Breathing exercises can improve ventilation.
- Effective breathing techniques include elevating the head and chest to maintain airway patency; deep breathing and coughing exercises to facilitate lung expansion; and pursed-lip breathing to decrease the effort of breathing.
- Adequate fluid intake and humidity help moisten secretions, thus aiding in their clearance.
- A thorough psychosocial assessment and resultant interventions are necessary for the patient with a laryngectomy, because of loss of voice and neck and facial disfigurement.
- Chest drainage serves a twofold purpose: it (1) drains air, blood, or fluid from the pleural space and (2) restores negative pressure. It requires a water seal to prevent air from reentering the pleural space.
- Techniques used in chest physiotherapy include percussion, vibration, and postural drainage.
- Nursing interventions after thoracic surgery that assist in preventing complications by promoting effective airway clearance are (1) frequent repositioning, (2) coughing, and (3) deep breathing.
- *Low flow* oxygen therapy is required for patients with COPD, because higher oxygen concentrations depress the body's own respiratory regulatory centers.
- Patients with respiratory disorders must reduce exposure to infection, because infection will further increase the body's oxygen demands.
- The definitive diagnostic test to confirm cystic fibrosis is a sweat chloride test.
- Chronic obstructive pulmonary disease includes emphysema, chronic bronchitis, asthma, and bronchiectasis.

STUDY QUESTIONS

1. The terminal structure of the bronchial tree is the:
   a. Alveolus
   b. Pulmonary vein
   c. Bronchioles
   d. Right bronchus
2. The volume of air inhaled and exhaled at rest is called:
   a. Total lung capacity
   b. Vital capacity
   c. Tidal volume
   d. Residual volume
3. The patient with respiratory acidosis will demonstrate all of the following *except:*
   a. Confusion
   b. pH of less than 7.36
   c. pH of more than 7.44
   d. Tachycardia
4. Sinusitis is an infection that may result in the following major complication if left untreated:
   a. Epistaxis
   b. Meningitis
   c. Pneumonia
   d. Acute coryza
5. The major complication of acute bronchitis is:
   a. It could become chronic bronchitis
   b. It could lead to meningitis
   c. It could lead to epistaxis
   d. It could lead to pneumothorax
6. Pleural effusion and empyema are similar except that empyema includes:
   a. The presence of fluid in the pleural space
   b. The presence of purulent fluid in the pleural space
   c. The presence of blood in the pleural space
   d. The presence of air in the pleural space
7. Pulmonary edema results from any of the following *except:*
   a. Damage to capillary walls
   b. Damage to pulmonary cilia
   c. Increased hydrostatic pressure within the capillaries
   d. Decreased osmotic pressure within the capillaries
8. Emphysema is characterized by:
   a. Changes in alveolar walls and capillaries
   b. Changes in bronchioles and bronchi
   c. Purulent drainage in the pleural space
   d. Sanguineous drainage in the pleural space
9. COPD is best treated by:
   a. Mechanical circulation
   b. High flow oxygen therapy
   c. Low flow oxygen therapy
   d. Mechanical ventilation
10. Asthma can be caused by extrinsic or intrinsic factors. Intrinsic factors include:
    a. Genetic predisposition
    b. Allergens in the environment
    c. Inhaled irritants
    d. Injury to trachea
11. Bronchiectasis often results from:
    a. Blood in pleural space
    b. Injury to trachea
    c. Repeated respiratory infections
    d. Tuberculosis
12. The diagnostic test for cystic fibrosis is:
    a. Decreased serum calcium level
    b. Elevated serum chloride level
    c. Decreased sweat chloride level
    d. Elevated sweat chloride level
13. The diet for patients with cystic fibrosis includes:
    a. High protein, high fat
    b. Low protein, low fat
    c. High protein, low fat
    d. Low protein, high fat

STUDY QUESTIONS (cont'd)

14. Patient teaching for those with respiratory conditions includes all *except:*
    a. Relaxation techniques
    b. Limiting exposure to irritants
    c. Use of humidifier to moisten secretions
    d. Encouraging dry air to prevent infections
15. The most common cause of airway obstruction in the adult is:
    a. Tongue
    b. Alcohol
    c. Sedatives
    d. Food
16. All of the following are signs and symptoms in hypoxia in the patient except:
    a. Restlessness
    b. Cyanosis
    c. Tachypnea
    d. Malaise
17. Which of the following is accurate in regards to ambulation of a patient with a chest tube in place:
    a. Patient is on bed rest
    b. Patient may dangle only
    c. Patient may ambulate with assistance
    d. Patient may stand but not walk
18. It is vitally important that the nurse does not allow an intravenous feeding to infuse too rapidly in a patient with compromised cardiac output, because of the complication of:
    a. Pulmonary edema
    b. Myocardial infarction
    c. Diuresis
    d. Decreased sensorium
19. A patient with COPD receives oxygen at a low flow rate of from 1 to 2 L because:
    a. Only slight dyspnea exists
    b. Hypercapnia is present
    c. The alveoli could become overdistended
    d. Respiratory arrest could occur

35

Care of the Patient with an Endocrine Disorder

SYLVIA LONG BALDWIN

LEARNING OBJECTIVES

After reading this chapter, the student should be able to do the following:

- Define the key terms.
- List and describe the endocrine glands and their hormones.
- Explain the action of the hormones on their target organs.
- Define the negative feedback system.
- List four clinical manifestations of diabetes insipidus.
- List three tests used in the diagnosis of hyperthyroidism.
- Give the clinical manifestations for patients with acromegaly, gigantism, pheochromocytoma, hyperparathyroidism, and hypoparathyroidism.
- Explain how to test for Chvostek's sign and Trousseau's sign.
- List two significant complications that may occur after thyroidectomy.
- Differentiate between the clinical manifestations of Cushing's syndrome and those of Addison's disease.
- Explain the interrelationship of diet, exercise, and medication in the control of diabetes mellitus.
- Describe the proper way to draw up and administer insulin.
- Differentiate between the signs and symptoms of diabetic ketoacidosis (DKA) and hypoglycemic reaction.
- List four nursing interventions that foster self-care in the diabetic patient's activities of daily living.

RELATED TOPICS OF INTEREST

- Diet therapy (Chapter 23)
- Principles and practice of medication administration (Chapter 25)
- Care of the patient with a reproductive disorder (Chapter 36)
- Normal pregnancy (Chapter 42)

KEY TERMS

Define the following:

- acetone
- adrenal glands
- adrenalin
- adrenocorticotropic hormone (ACTH)
- amenorrhea
- antagonist
- antidiuretic hormone (ADH)
- calcitonin
- Chvostek's sign
- cortisol
- dysphagia
- dyspnea
- endocrine glands
- endocrinologist
- estrogen
- exocrine glands
- follicle-stimulating hormone (FSH)
- glucagon
- glycosuria
- graafian follicle
- growth hormone
- hirsutism
- hormones
- hypercalcemia
- hyperglycemia
- hypocalcemia
- hypoglycemic
- hypokalemia
- idiopathic hyperplasia
- insulin
- insulin reaction
- irradiation
- ketoacidosis
- ketone bodies
- luteinizing hormone (LH)
- negative feedback
- neuropathy
- nodule
- oxytocin
- parathyroid glands
- parathyroid hormone
- pituitary gland
- polydipsia
- polyphagia
- polyuria
- progesterone
- prolactin
- somatotropin
- tetany
- thymus gland
- thyroid gland
- thyroid-stimulating hormone (TSH)
- Trousseau's sign
- turgor
- type I diabetes mellitus
- type II diabetes mellitus

There are two broad categories of glands: exocrine and endocrine. **Exocrine glands** have ducts that open onto the surface of the skin; examples are the sebaceous and sudoriferous glands. Their secretions usually serve protective or functional purposes. **Endocrine glands** are ductless; that is, they release their secretions directly into the bloodstream. These secretions have a regulatory function.

The endocrine system is composed of a series of ductless glands whose work is closely related to the nervous system. Both systems control homeostasis through communications within the systems. The nervous system exerts its control very rapidly through miles of nerve fibers. The endocrine system communicates more slowly through the use of **hormones,** which are chemical messengers that travel through the bloodstream to their target organ. When the hormone reaches its target, a metabolic change occurs.

The total weight of all the endocrine glands is less than half a pound, yet they exert a very powerful influence. The slightest change in hormonal levels can upset the metabolic balance of the entire body. Hormones can increase or decrease a normal body process by exerting an effect on its target organ. Too much or too little of a given hormone can interfere with the action of the other hormones, and for this reason they are somewhat interrelated. The endocrine glands (Fig. 35-1) have a generalized effect on metabolism, growth and development, reproduction, and many other body activities.

The amount of hormonal release is controlled by a **negative feedback** system. Information is constantly being exchanged between the target organ and the pituitary gland via the bloodstream regarding the impact of the hormone on the target organ. For example, after food is ingested the blood sugar (glucose) level increases. In response, the pancreas releases insulin into the blood to metabolize the glucose. As the blood glucose level drops, further release of insulin is inhibited. Because these responses are opposite to the stimulus, this mechanism is called negative feedback.

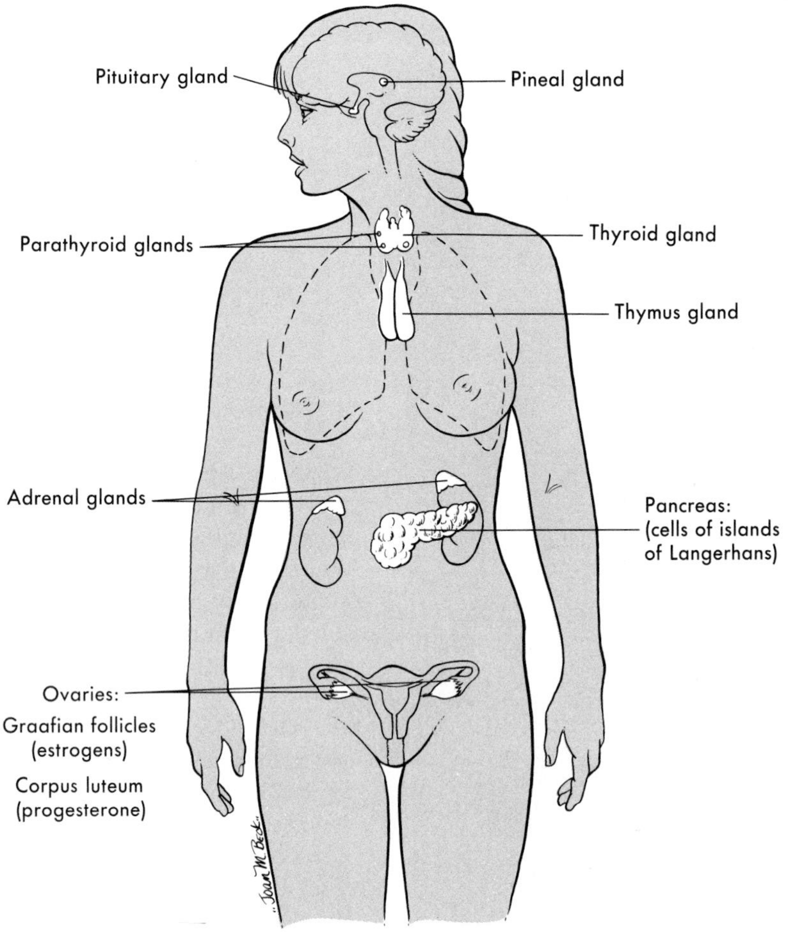

FIG. 35-1 Location of the endocrine glands in the female. Thymus gland is shown at maximal size at puberty.

Hormones are composed of protein or steroids. Protein hormones attach themselves to the cell walls of the target organ and cause a change within the cell as a result of their outside influence. Steroid hormones pass through the cell wall and combine with receptors within the cytoplasm, causing the nucleus to respond with change. Therefore protein hormones indirectly cause change within the target organ cells, whereas steroid hormones impart a direct change within the cell by actually entering the cell itself.

PROSTAGLANDINS

Prostaglandins, discovered in the early 1930s, are a group of hormone substances with one distinct difference: they are produced throughout the body by various tissues and localize their effect on that particular tissue. Most other hormones are produced by a specific organ and travel through the bloodstream to their target tissue. Prostaglandins also exert their effect on hormones that have travelled to the target tissue; they can increase or decrease the effect of these hormones.

ENDOCRINE GLANDS AND HORMONES

Pituitary Gland

The **pituitary gland** (hypophysis), the size of a small pea, is one of the most powerful glands in the body. It has been called the "master gland," because through the negative feedback system it exerts its control over the other endocrine glands. It is important to remember, however, that it works closely with the hypothalmus of the brain.

The pituitary is located in the cranial cavity in a small saddlelike depression in the sphenoid bone (the sella turcica). It is divided into two segments, each with specialized hormones. The first segment is called the *anterior pituitary* (adenohypophysis); the second is called the *posterior pituitary* (neurohypophysis). The gland is connected to the hypothalamus by a stalklike projection called the *infundibulum*. The hypothalamus actually produces the hormones of the posterior pituitary and releases them for storage in the posterior pituitary gland; they are in turn released from the posterior pituitary as a result of nerve impulses received from the hypothalamus.

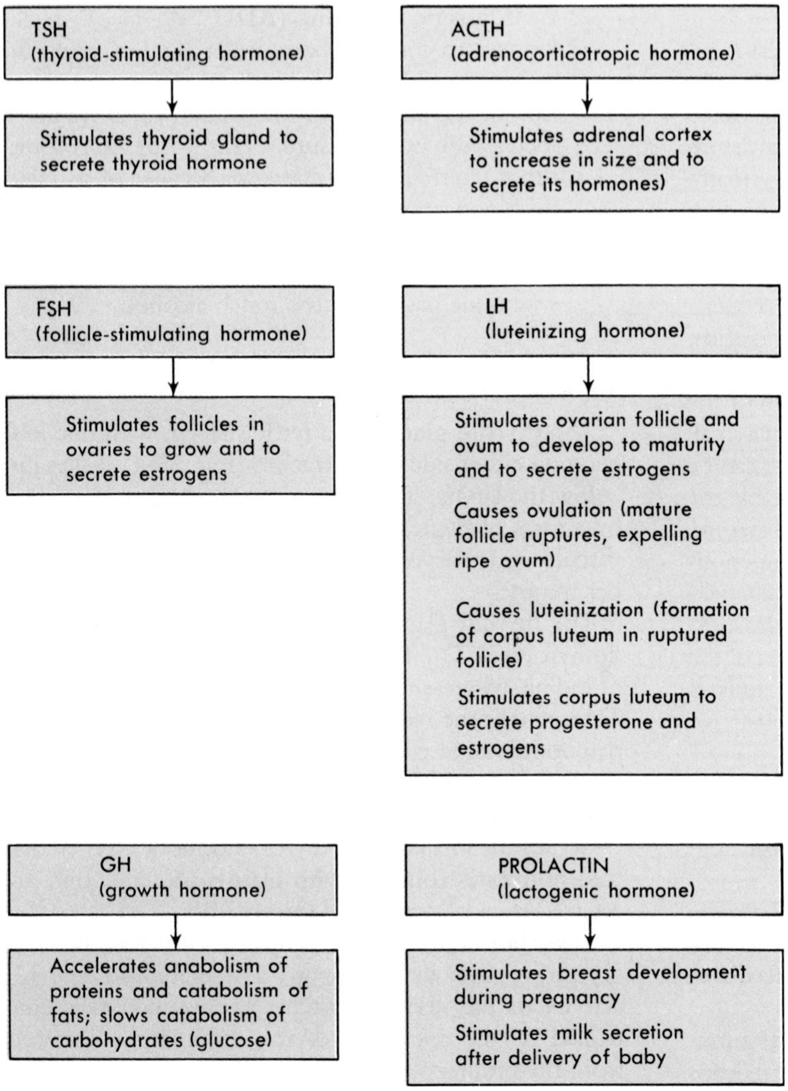

TSH
(thyroid-stimulating hormone)
Stimulates thyroid gland to secrete thyroid hormone
ACTH
(adrenocorticotropic hormone)
Stimulates adrenal cortex to increase in size and to secrete its hormones)
FSH
(follicle-stimulating hormone)
Stimulates follicles in ovaries to grow and to secrete estrogens
LH
(luteinizing hormone)
Stimulates ovarian follicle and ovum to develop to maturity and to secrete estrogens
Causes ovulation (mature follicle ruptures, expelling ripe ovum)
Causes luteinization (formation of corpus luteum in ruptured follicle)
Stimulates corpus luteum to secrete progesterone and estrogens
GH
(growth hormone)
Accelerates anabolism of proteins and catabolism of fats; slows catabolism of carbohydrates (glucose)
PROLACTIN
(lactogenic hormone)
Stimulates breast development during pregnancy
Stimulates milk secretion after delivery of baby

FIG. 35-2 Names and functions of anterior pituitary hormones.

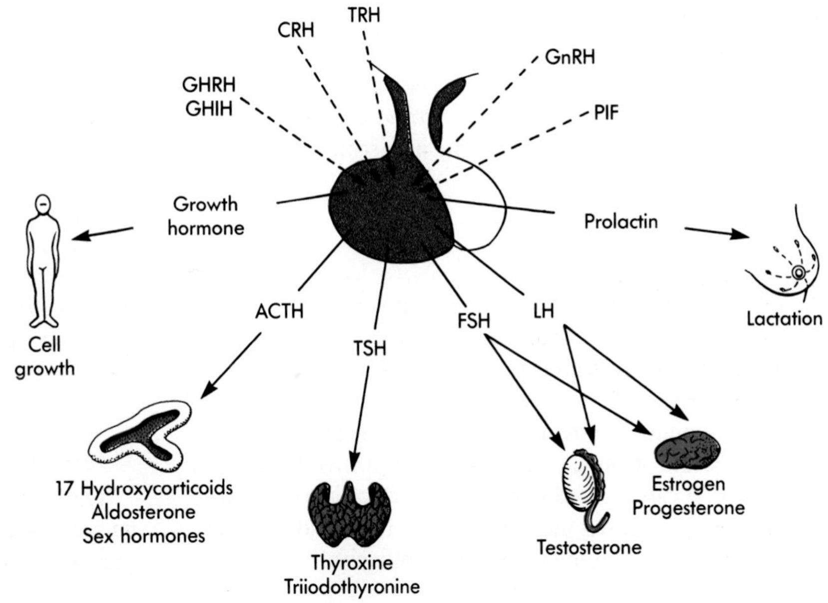

FIG. 35-3 Relationships between hormones of the hypothalamus, anterior pituitary gland, and target tissues are depicted. Only five released or inhibitory hormones have been chemically identified: growth hormone–releasing hormone *(GHRH)*; growth hormone–inhibitory hormone (*GHIH,* somatostatin); thyrotropin-releasing hormone *(TRH)*; corticotropin-releasing hormone *(CRH)*; and gonadotropin-releasing hormone *(GRH)*. Dopamine is thought to be a prolactin-inhibiting factor *(PIF)*. Each anterior pituitary hormone is shown with its respective target tissues: body cells *(GH)*; adrenal cortex *(ACTH)*; thyroid *(TSH)*; testes and ovaries (*FSH* and *LH*); and breasts *(prolactin)*.

Anterior Pituitary Gland

Six major hormones are secreted by the anterior pituitary gland. It constitutes about 75% of the total weight of the pituitary gland. Five of the hormones are called *tropic* hormones because they are responsible for the stimulation of other endocrine glands. Prolactin, the remaining hormone, causes the mammary glands to produce milk. These hormones and their functions are shown in Figs. 35-2 and 35-3 and are discussed below.

1. ***Somatotropin**—human growth hormone (HGH).* HGH speeds up the cells' anabolism of amino acids, which results in the formation of tissue proteins. This process stimulates the systemic growth of the body. A deficiency of this hormone results in a small but proportioned individual. This hormone can be administered in controlled situations to enable the individual to reach a more normal physical stature.
2. ***Prolactin**—lactogenic hormone.* Prolactin functions in the pregnant woman to develop the mammary glands for milk production. After delivery, the suckling of the infant stimulates the continuation of the production of milk. The actual release of milk is controlled by oxytocin, a hormone in the posterior lobe.
3. ***Adrenocorticotropic hormone (ACTH).*** ACTH stimulates the endocrine activity of the cortex portion of the adrenal glands. It operates on the negative feedback system.
4. ***Thyroid-stimulating hormone (TSH).*** TSH acts on the thyroid gland to increase thyroid hormone secretion; it also operates on the negative feedback system.
5. ***Follicle-stimulating hormone (FSH).*** FSH stimulates the growth of the graafian follicle that leads to ovulation in the female. In the male it leads to the development of sperm cells.
6. ***Luteinizing hormone (LH).*** LH initiates ovulation and release of the egg, followed by the formation of the corpus luteum (yellow body), which in turn produces the hormones estrogen and progesterone. In the male LH is called *interstitial cell–stimulating hormone (ICSH);* it causes the interstitial cells of the testes to produce sperm.

Posterior Pituitary Gland

Two hormones are released by the posterior pituitary; however, these were originally produced in the hypothalamus. They are stored in the posterior pituitary until needed by the body.

1. **Oxytocin.** Oxytocin promotes the release of breast milk and stimulates uterine contractions during labor. It can be used clinically to induce labor; it may also be used to increase uterine tone and prevent hemorrhage immediately after delivery.
2. **Antidiuretic hormone (ADH).** ADH causes the kidneys to conserve body water by decreasing the amount of urine produced. It also causes constriction of the arterioles in the body, which results in increased blood pressure. (This hormone is sometimes referred to as *vasopressin* because of its effect on blood pressure.) Alcohol consumption inhibits the secretion of ADH, which results in increased urinary output. This is possibly the reason for thirst when one has drunk too much alcohol.

Thyroid Gland

The **thyroid gland** is butterfly shaped, with one lobe lying on either side of the trachea (Fig. 35-4). It lies just below the larynx. The lobes are connected in the center by a mass of tissue called the *isthmus.* The gland is very vascular and receives approximately 80 to 120 ml of blood per minute.

The thyroid gland secretes thyroxine (T_4) and triiodothyronine (T_3). Thyroxine molecules contain 4 atoms of iodine, whereas triiodothyronine molecules contain 3. Thyroxine is the most abundant of these hormones, and triiodothyronine converts to thyroxine when it reaches the liver and the lungs; therefore these hormones will be discussed together. Adequate oral intake of iodine is necessary for the formation of thyroid hormones. When thyroid hormones combine with plasma proteins, they are referred to as *protein-bound iodine* (PBI).

These hormones have three main regulatory functions: (1) growth and development, (2) metabolism, and (3) activity of the nervous system. Their function is controlled by the release of thyroid-stimulating hormone from the pituitary gland.

Calcitonin is a hormone also released by the thyroid gland. This hormone works as an **antagonist** of the parathyroid hormone. It decreases blood calcium levels by causing calcium to be stored in the bones. It prevents **hypercalcemia,** a condition in which there is too much calcium in the blood. Administration of calcitonin has been used in conjunction with calcium intake to treat postmenopausal osteoporosis.

Laboratory tests are performed to monitor the function of the thyroid gland. Blood tests called T_3 and T_4 thyroid function tests are performed by mechanically tracing radioactive thyroxine in the body and observing the speed at which it enters the thyroid gland. Another frequently used test, the protein-bound iodine (PBI) test, estimates the amount of circulating iodine in the blood.

Parathyroid Glands

The **parathyroid glands** are located on the posterior surface of the thyroid gland (Fig. 35-4). Usually there are four of them, but sometimes there are as many as 10.

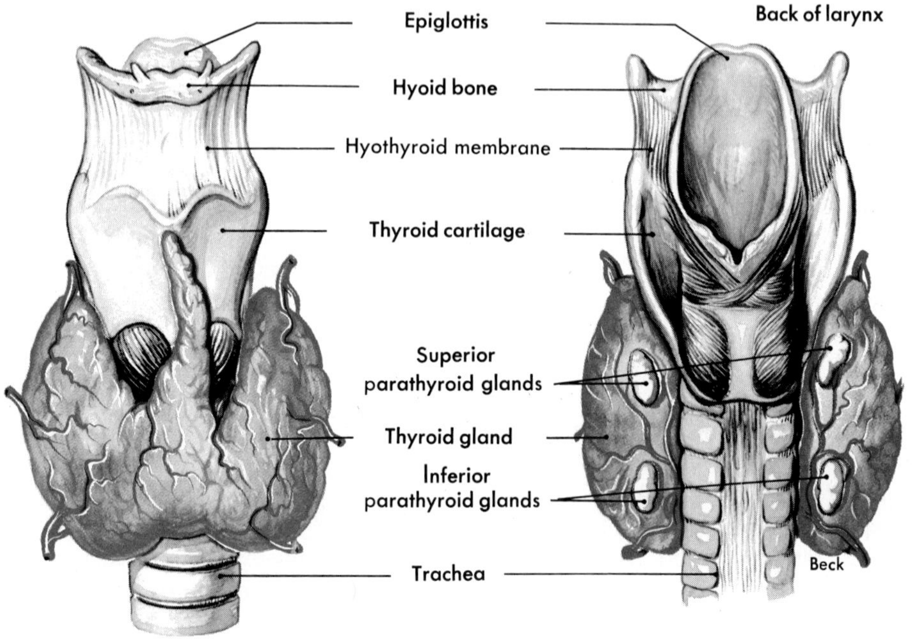

FIG. 35-4 Thyroid and parathyroid glands. Note their relations to each other and to the larynx and trachea.

These glands secrete **parathyroid** hormone (parathormone).

As an antagonist to calcitonin from the thyroid, parathyroid hormone tends to increase the concentration of calcium in the blood. It also regulates the amount of phosphorus in the blood. Under its influence, two changes occur in the kidneys: it increases the removal of calcium and magnesium from the urine that is being produced and accelerates the elimination of phosphorus in the urine.

The delicate balance of blood calcium is extremely important for normal body function. When blood calcium levels are low, the nerve cells become excited and stimulate the muscles with too many impulses, resulting in spasms **(tetany)**. When the blood calcium levels are abnormally high, heart function becomes impaired and can result in cardiac arrest.

Adrenal Glands

The **adrenal glands** (suprarenal glands) are small, yellow masses that lie directly atop the kidneys. The adrenal glands have two separate parts, much the same as the pituitary gland. Each part functions independently of the other. Both glands contain an outer section, the adrenal cortex, and a small inner section, called the *adrenal medulla*. Each gland is covered by a thin, fibrous capsule; directly beneath the capsule is a thick layer of fatty connective tissue.

Adrenal Cortex

The adrenal cortex (outer layer) is divided into three separate layers or zones. Each zone is composed of a certain type of cells and secretes a particular hormone. All three of the hormones secreted by the adrenal cortex are steroids. They are (1) mineralocorticoids, (2) glucocorticoids, and (3) sex hormones (androgens). Fifteen percent of the cortical volume lies directly beneath the connective tissue and is called the *zona glomerulosa*. It secretes a group of hormones called *mineralocorticoids*. As their name suggests, they are primarily involved in water and electrolye balance and indirectly in the management of blood pressure. Aldosterone, the principal mineralocorticoid, regulates sodium and potassium levels by exerting its effects on the kidney tubules. It decreases the level of potassium and increases the level of sodium in the bloodstream. The retention of sodium causes retention of water, which leads to an increase in blood volume and blood pressure.

The second group of hormones (glucocorticoids) are secreted by the middle layer, the *zona fasciculata*. The most important hormone of this group is **cortisol,** responsible for about 95% of glucocorticoid activity. It is involved in glucose metabolism and provides extra reserves of energy in times of stress. The secretion of glucocorticoids is regulated by the hormone ACTH, which is released by the pituitary. In times of stress large amounts of cortisol are released, initiating the process of *gluconeogenesis* in which amino acids are converted to glucose. This takes place in the liver, and the newly formed glucose is released in the bloodstream. The glucocorticoids exhibit antiinflammatory properties and many times are administered for such conditions as rheumatoid arthritis.

The inner zone, called the *zona reticularis,* releases the sex hormones. Small amounts of androgens (male sex hormones) and **estrogens** (female sex hormones) are secreted by this layer. In the adult the release of these hormones from the adrenals is a relatively small amount, and their impact on the system is insignificant.

Adrenal Medulla

The cells composing the adrenal medulla arise from the same type of cells as those of the sympathetic nervous system. Two hormones are released by the medulla during times of stress. Epinephrine (adrenalin) and norepinephrine can cause the heart rate and blood pressure to increase, the blood vessels to constrict, and the liver to release glucose reserves for immediate energy. This is a systemic preparation of the body for "the flight or fight" response that is needed in times of crisis. This whole process happens very quickly, because the messages are sent via the sympathetic nerve fibers. Once the message is received, the medulla pours epinephrine and norepinephrine into the bloodstream.

Pancreas

The pancreas is an elongated gland that lies posterior to the stomach. It is a very active organ in that it is composed of both endocrine and exocrine tissue. The exocrine activity involves production of digestive enzymes, which are transported through ducts to the small intestine. The islets of Langerhans, responsible for the endocrine activity of the pancreas, are tiny clusters of cells capable of producing hormones. These clusters number over a million and are microscopic. They secrete two major hormones, insulin and glucagon. The majority of the islet cells are *beta cells,* and they secrete insulin. The remaining islet cells are called *alpha cells,* and they secrete the hormone glucagon. Both hormones have an impact on the amount of glucose circulating in the blood but are antagonists (have the opposite effect).

Many hormones, such as glucagon, epinephrine, and the glucocorticoids, cause an increase in the blood glucose levels. Insulin is the only hormone that causes a decrease in blood glucose levels. When the proper amount of insulin is released, blood glucose levels remain between 65 and 120 mg/dl of blood. If the pancreas is unable to produce an adequate amount of insulin, the blood glucose level rises dramatically and may even spill into the urine. The circulating glucose cannot be metabolized, and the body begins to rely on fats and proteins for energy. At this point the body becomes dysfunctional, with serious complications.

On the other hand, when glucose levels are too low, the alpha cells of the islets release the hormone glucagon. Its target organ is the liver. The liver has stored glycogen as a reserve form of glucose. Glucagon stimulates the liver to break down the stored glycogen to glucose, which is released into the bloodstream. It also promotes an increase in the fatty acid levels in the blood by releasing fat stores from adipose tissue. This provides nutrients for glucose production.

These two hormones, glycogen and insulin, though antagonists, work together to keep glucose levels within normal ranges. When glucose ranges fall below normal, glucagon acts to raise it; when glucose ranges are too high, insulin is released to lower it.

Female Sex Glands

Deep in the lower abdominal region, lying to the upper right and left of the uterus, lie the almond-shaped ovaries, the two major sex glands of the female. The ovaries begin their production of hormones at puberty. At this time, the gonadotropin hormones stimulate the ovaries to release estrogen and progesterone in a rhythmic pattern—the menstrual cycle. The **graafian follicle** (a sac in which the egg matures) secretes the hormone estrogen. **Estrogen** is responsible for the development of the secondary sex characteristics: the appearance of axillary and pubic hair and the maturation of the reproductive organs. It also prepares the uterus monthly for the possibility of pregnancy. When the egg that has matured in the graafian follicle has been released at the midpoint of the menstrual cycle, a structure called the *corpus luteum* (yellow body) forms and releases progestrone. **Progesterone** maintains the preparation of the reproductive organs that was initiated by estrogen. If pregnancy occurs, progesterone levels remain high. If no pregnancy occurs, progesterone and estrogen levels fall, initiating the menstrual flow.

The placenta is a temporary endocrine gland that forms and functions during pregnancy. During this time the ovaries become inactive and the placenta releases the estrogen and progesterone needed to maintain the pregnancy.

A more in-depth discussion of these hormones can be found in Chapters 36 and 42.

Male Sex Glands

Suspended outside the body in a saclike structure, the scrotum, lie the two oval sex glands called the *testes*. The interstitial cells of the testes produce the hormone testosterone. It is responsible for the development of the secondary sex characteristics, including the appearance of axillary and pubic hair and the maturation of the reproductive organs. In addition, testosterone is responsible for the deepening of the voice, the appearance of a beard, and the development of muscle and bone mass. Unlike the female, whose eggs are present at birth, the male must continually produce sperm to remain fertile. Testosterone is necessary for sperm formation. If the levels of this hormone fall below normal ranges, sterility results.

Thymus Gland

The **thymus gland** lies in the upper thorax, posterior to the sternum. It produces the hormone thymosin, which plays an active role in the immune system. T lymphocytes (a type of white blood cell) are stimulated to carry out immune reactions to certain types of antigens. The thymus gland programs this information into the T lymphocytes in utero and during the first few months of life.

Pineal Gland

The pineal gland is a small, cone-shaped gland located in the roof of the third ventricle of the brain. It secretes the hormone melatonin, which seems to inhibit reproductive activities by inhibiting the gonadotropic hormones. This is particularly important in preventing sexual maturation until the child's body has reached adult size. After adulthood has been reached it possibly has an impact on the rhythm of the menstrual cycle. The pineal gland may also stimulate the adrenal cortex to secrete aldosterone.

DISORDERS OF THE PITUITARY GLAND (HYPOPHYSIS)

Acromegaly

Etiology/pathophysiology. An overproduction of somatropin (**growth hormone,** GH) in the adult causes acromegaly, a condition that afflicts an estimated 250 persons in the United States each year. The cause either may be **idiopathic hyperplasia** of the anterior lobe of the pituitary gland or may be attributed to tumor growth. Unfortunately, growth changes that occur in acromegaly are irreversible, even with adequate medical or surgical intervention.

Clinical manifestations. The subsequent overabundance of growth hormone produces many changes throughout the patient's body, including enlargement of the cranium and lower jaw, with separation and malocclusion of the teeth, bulging forehead, a bulbous nose, thick lips, enlarged tongue, and generalized coarsening of the facial features. The hands and feet become enlarged (Fig. 35-5), as do the heart, liver, and spleen; muscle weakness usually develops. Joints may hypertrophy and become painful and stiff. Male patients may become impotent, and female patients may develop a deepened voice, increased facial hair growth, and **amenorrhea**. If a tumor is present, pressure on the optic nerve may cause partial or complete blindness. Severe headaches commonly occur.

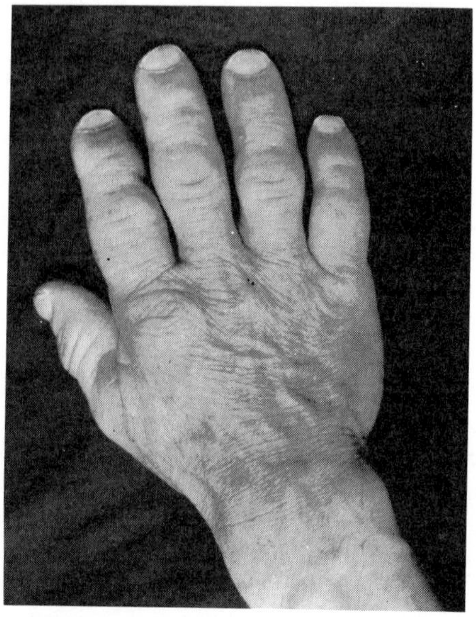

FIG. 35-5 Hand showing characteristics of acromegalic condition.

Assessment. Collection of *subjective data* includes determining the presence of headache and/or visual disturbances and any precipitating factors. Muscle weakness and its effect on the patient's ability to perform activities should be evaluated. Patients should be encouraged to verbalize emotional responses to sexual problems (such as impotence in males and masculinization in females).

Collection of *objective data* includes ongoing assessment of bone enlargement and joint involvement, evidenced by gait changes and increasing inability to perform other activities. The interval between doses of pain medication should be evaluated. Changes in the vital signs that may herald the onset of early congestive heart failure include dyspnea, tachycardia, weak pulse, and hypotension.

Diagnostic tests. Diagnosis of acromegaly is based on the patient's history and the clinical manifestations, as well as computed tomography (CT) scan and cranial x-ray evaluation. Laboratory tests confirm the presence of elevated serum GH levels. The patient's oral intake is restricted for 8 hours before this test.

Medical management. In the past, estrogens were administered to these patients. Newer medical treatments include bromocriptine mesylate (Parlodel) and somatostatin analogs, especially in patients who are not candidates for surgery or radiation therapy. These drugs are used in an attempt to suppress growth hormone secretion. Surgical treatment may include either cryosurgery (the use of subfreezing temperatures to destroy tissue) or transsphenoidal removal of tumor tissue. New **irradiation** procedures employing proton beam therapy have been used to destroy growth hormone–secreting tumors. Proton beam treatment uses very low doses of radiation, and therefore is much less destructive to adjacent tissues, such as the hypothalamus and temporal lobes, than conventional radiation therapy.

Nursing interventions. Nursing interventions are mainly supportive. If there is muscle weakness, joint pain, or stiffness, patients should be assessed for ability to perform activities of daily living. The presence of headache may impair the patient's ability to socialize and may also impede education. Worsening headache may indicate tumor progression. The diet should be soft and easy to chew, since jaw muscles and the temporomandibular joint may be involved. The patient should be encouraged to chew thoroughly, and the nurse should allow adequate time during meals, assisting when necessary. Fluids should be encouraged often. Nonnarcotic analgesics may be given for pain relief. Visual impairment may increase the risk of injury for these patients, so care should be taken to prevent stumbling into furniture or dropping objects.

As the body undergoes change, the patient may develop problems with self-esteem and may feel physically unattractive. There may be difficulties in communicating with significant others, and this may lead to disturbances in individual or family coping methods. Other complications of acromegaly are related to the enlargement of the liver, spleen, and heart. Cardiac dysrhythmias may develop, and the patient may experience heart failure. Abdominal girth may increase as a result of weight gain and inactivity, and respiratory difficulty may occur.

NURSING DIAGNOSES	NURSING INTERVENTIONS
Self-esteem disturbance	Convey respect and nonjudgmental acceptance of the patient as a person. Help the patient set achievable short-term goals.
Activity intolerance	Assess patient's current activity level and priorities for activity performance. Discuss with patient alternate ways of performing activities.
Potential for trauma	Assist patient to identify hazards in the environment. Help patient develop a plan to increase ambulation, asking for assistance as needed.

Patient teaching. The patient should remain under the supervision of a physician so that any complications can be diagnosed promptly and treated adequately. The patient should be taught exercises that can be performed at home, such as active range of motion of joints of the extremities and of the neck, to help prevent muscle atrophy and loss of movement.

Gigantism

Etiology/pathophysiology. Gigantism usually results from an oversecretion of GH as a result of hyperplasia of the anterior pituitary, and this hyperplastic tissue may develop into a tumor. Another possible cause is a defect in the hypothalamus, which directs the anterior pituitary to release excess amounts of GH.

Clinical manifestations. When this overproduction occurs in a child before closure of the epiphyses, there is an overgrowth of the long bones, which results in the attainment of great height, accompanied by increased muscle and visceral development. There is also an increase in weight, but body proportions are usually normal. Other kinds of gigantism may be caused by certain genetic disorders or by disturbances in sex hormone production. Once identified, these children should be referred for further medical evaluation and follow-up.

Assessment. Collection of *subjective data* includes assessment of the patient's understanding of the disease process, as well as the ability to verbalize emotional responses.

Collection of *objective data* requires frequent measurement of height. The patient's use of adaptive coping measures should be assessed, as well as family interactions.

Medical management. Medical management of children with gigantism may include surgical removal of tumor tissue or irradiation of the anterior pituitary gland, with a subsequent replacement of pituitary hormones as indicated. The physician will then observe the child for development of related complications, such as hypertension, heart failure, osteoporosis, thickened bones, and delayed sexual development.

Nursing interventions. Nursing interventions primarily include early identification of children who are experiencing increased growth rates compared with other children in their age-group. There are potential problems with self-image, especially if the child is a preteen who is a great deal taller than peers. Girls usually suffer more emotional trauma in this situation than boys do. The nurse must be understanding and compassionate and accentuate the positive aspects of being tall.

NURSING DIAGNOSES	NURSING INTERVENTIONS
Self-esteem disturbance: chronic low self-esteem	Be genuinely interested in and concerned about the patient. Help patient to identify problems in relating to others.
Ineffective individual coping	Assess patient's coping behaviors, stresses, and adaptive skills. Provide positive feedback.
Ineffective family coping	Provide adequate and correct information to patient and significant others. Help patient and family to identify strengths and weaknesses in interpersonal relationships.

Patient teaching. Early diagnosis of these patients is essential, because proper medical management can retard the height a child will reach. The importance of regular visits to the pediatrician or pediatric **endocrinologist** should be stressed to the parents.

Dwarfism

Etiology/pathophysiology. A condition in which there is a deficiency in growth hormone is called *hypopituitary dwarfism*. Most cases are idiopathic, but a small number can be attributed to an autosomal-recessive trait. In some cases there is also a lack of ACTH, TSH, and the gonadotropins.

Clinical manifestations. The most common clinical manifestation of dwarfism is that the child is shorter than his peers. These patients usually appear well proportioned and well nourished but appear younger than their chronological age. There may be problems with dentition as the permanent teeth erupt, because the jaws are underdeveloped. Sexual development is usually normal but delayed. Many dwarfs are able to reproduce normal offspring, unless there is an accompanying deficiency in gonadotropins. Because only a small number of children who experience short stature or delayed growth suffer from dwarfism, it is crucial that the diagnostic workup be thorough.

Assessment. Collection of *subjective data* includes assessment of the patient's understanding of the disease process, as well as emotional responses to it. A family history of dwarfism may reveal previously successful coping strategies. The patient should be encouraged to verbalize feelings. Normal intelligence is displayed by most of these children. The child's growth pattern should be compared with that of siblings and other relatives at comparable age periods. The child's history usually reveals a normal birth weight. It is important to determine when the child's growth retardation was first noted.

Collection of *objective data* includes regular measurement of height and weight to determine responses to GH and other hormones that may be administered. Current height and weight should be compared with standard growth charts.

Diagnostic tests. Diagnostic tests include x-ray evaluation of the wrist for bone age and a skull series to rule out a pituitary tumor. Definitive diagnosis is based on finding decreased plasma levels of growth hormone. The patient's oral intake should be restricted after midnight for this test.

Medical management. Medical treament involves replacement of GH by injection, as well as the addition of other specific hormones as needed to correct deficiencies. If a tumor is the cause of dwarfism, surgery is usually indicated.

Nursing interventions. Particular care should be exercised to identify children with growth problems. The physician will correlate the onset of growth retardation with symptoms of headache, visual disturbances, or behavior changes that might indicate tumor, so the nurse should be alert for these. The nurse should be careful not to make the parents feel guilty about any delay in seeking medical attention for their child.

NURSING DIAGNOSES	NURSING INTERVENTIONS
Body image disturbance	Encourage patient to verbalize feelings about body. Respect patient's need for privacy while performing personal hygiene.
Knowledge deficit: therapeutic regimen	Explain diagnostic and therapeutic measures, considering patient's level of understanding. Praise patient's efforts to cooperate with plan of treatment.

Patient teaching. The child should be encouraged to wear age-appropriate clothing and engage in activities with peers, because major problems with self-esteem can occur in dwarfism. The child's abilities and strengths should be emphasized, not physical size.

Diabetes Insipidus

Etiology/pathophysiology. Diabetes insipidus (*diabetes:* "sievelike, siphonlike"; *insipidus:* "tasteless") is a transient or permanent metabolic disorder of the posterior pituitary in which antidiuretic hormone (ADH) is deficient. The condition may be either primary or secondary to others, such as head injury, intracranial tumor, intracranial aneurysm, or infarct. Infections, such as encephalitis or meningitis, have been known to cause diabetes insipidus.

Clinical manifestations. Diabetes insipidus is characterized by marked polyuria and intense polydipsia. The urine is very dilute, looking much like water, with a low specific gravity (1.001 to 1.005), the normal being 1.005 to 1.03. Urinary output may exceed 10 L in a 24-hour period, whereas the average is 1.5 L in 24 hours. The patient craves cold or iced water and may drink 4 to 40 L of fluid daily, yet may become severely dehydrated and have increased levels of sodium in the blood. Even when unconscious after surgery or head trauma, these patients continue to produce copious quantities of urine.

Assessment. Collection of *subjective data* includes evaluation of the patient's understanding of the relationship of symptoms (such as thirst and polyuria) to the underlying cause. The patient should be able to verbalize the importance of *not* restricting oral fluids. The severity of thirst should be assessed. The patient may be very embarrassed about the constant need to drink and then empty the bladder and may voluntarily restrict social contacts and work activities. The patient is weak, tired, and lethargic.

Collection of *objective data* to be assessed includes skin **turgor**, color and specific gravity of the urine, and intake and output should be carefully monitored. The skin is dry, turgor is poor, and there is loss of body weight. Constipation may occur. The patient should be weighed daily in the early morning, before breakfast. The nurse should determine the presence of nocturia.

Diagnostic tests. Diagnosis is based on clinical manifestations, as well as urinary specific gravity and urinary ADH measurement. The fluid deprivation (water deprivation) test may be ordered to determine how well the pituitary is producing ADH and to help rule out other causes. A CT scan and x-ray evaluation of the sella turcica (the "Turkish saddle"–shaped depression in the sphenoid bone that houses the pituitary gland) may be done.

Medical management. Medical treatment involves administration of ADH preparations, either intramuscularly, subcutaneously, or by nasal spray. Coffee, tea, and other beverages containing caffeine are usually eliminated from the diet because of their possible diuretic effect.

Nursing interventions. Because of the potential for fluid volume deficit, the urinary output of pediatric and unconscious patients should be carefully monitored. Skin turgor should be assessed frequently, as should the condition of oral mucous membranes. The patient should be weighed daily. Oral fluids should not be limited in an effort to reduce urinary output.

NURSING DIAGNOSES	NURSING INTERVENTIONS
Fluid volume deficit (1)	Assess for signs and symptoms of dehydration (dry mouth, poor skin turgor, soft eyeballs, lowered BP, rapid pulse). Measure urinary output. Obtain daily weight.
Potential impaired skin integrity	Inspect skin for erythema, cyanosis, vesicles, and lesions. Prevent pressure on skin and skeletal prominences by turning and ambulating patient, use of sheepskin, Eggcrate mattress, or other measures. Increase fluid intake up to 2600 ml/day if possible. Encourage patient to eat food adequate in calories, protein, and vitamin C to promote healthy skin.

Patient teaching. The patient should be instructed to wear an alerting device, such as a necklace or bracelet, stating the diagnosis of diabetes insipidus. It is important that the patient remain under medical supervision for monitoring of the metabolic state, because the condition may worsen with time.

DISORDERS OF THE THYROID GLAND AND PARATHYROID GLANDS

Hyperthyroidism

Etiology/pathophysiology. Hyperthyroidism, also called Graves' disease, exophthalmic goiter, and thyrotoxicosis, is a condition in which there is increased activity of the thyroid gland, with overproduction of the thyroid hormones thyroxine (T_4) and triiodothyronine (T_3). As a result, all of the patient's metabolic processes are exaggerated. Although the exact cause of hyperthyroidism is unknown, it may result from extreme physical or emotional stress. It may occur during pregnancy, in adolescence, and in the presence of infection. There may be a genetic basis or autoimmune factors. The condition affects an estimated 0.4% of women but is seen much less often in men.

Clinical manifestations. Clinical manifestations are numerous and varied and may range from mild to severe. There is usually visible edema of the anterior portion of the neck as a result of enlargement of the thyroid. In severe cases, exophthalmos (bulging of the eyeballs) may occur, usually attributable to periorbital edema (Fig. 35-6).

Assessment. Collection of *subjective data* includes assessment of the ability to concentrate and the presence of memory loss. The patient may complain of dysphagia or may be hoarse. There is usually weight loss, even in the presence of a voracious appetite. The patient appears very nervous, jittery, excitable, and may experience insomnia. These patients are emotionally labile and may overreact to stressful situations.

Collection of *objective data* includes assessment of changes in the vital signs. The pulse is usually rapid, blood pressure elevated, and a bruit may be auscultated over the thyroid. The skin is warm and flushed, and the hair is fine and soft. Female patients may cease to menstruate. Elevated body temperature may be accompanied by intolerance to heat, with profuse diaphoresis. The presence of tremors of the hands should be noted. Behavior changes may include hyperactivity and clumsiness. Daily weighing usually shows weight loss.

Diagnostic tests. Diagnostic tests usually include those in Box 35-1.

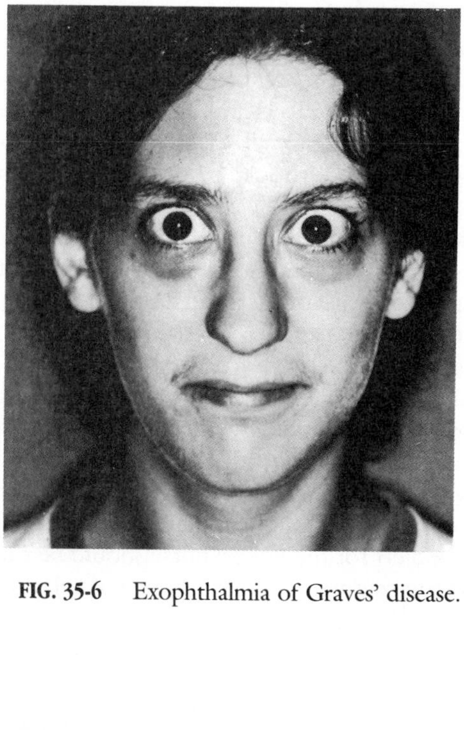

FIG. 35-6 Exophthalmia of Graves' disease.

BOX 35-1 **DIAGNOSTIC TESTS FOR HYPERTHYROIDISM**

PBI (protein-bound iodine). Reflects the level of circulating thyroid hormone. The patient should not have eaten large amounts of seafood for several weeks before the test. Substances containing iodine, such as dyes used for intravenous pyelogram (IVP), gallbladder studies, or bronchograms may cause incorrect test results. The normal PBI is 4 to 8 mg/dl. Elevated levels usually indicate hyperthyroidism.

T_3 (serum triiodothyronine). Measures the T_3 level in the blood serum. Normal is 70-190 μg/dl.

T_4 (serum thyroxine). Measures the T_4 level in the blood serum. Normal is 4.7 to 11 μg/dl. Some medications, such as oral contraceptives, steroids, estrogens, and sulfonamides, may be withheld for several hours before the T_3 and T_4 tests, but food and fluids are not withheld. Elevated levels of these tests usually indicate hyperthyroidism.

RAIU (radioactive iodine uptake test). Radioactive iodine, ^{131}I, is given by mouth to the fasting patient. After 2, 6, and 24 hours, a scintillator is held over the thyroid to measure how much of the isotope has been removed from the bloodstream. A hyperactive thyroid may remove up to 90% of the drug. This test may be affected by prior ingestion of iodine-containing substances or foods. It is necessary to obtain a signed consent form for this test. Also, any allergy to iodine should be noted on the request form, along with medications currently being taken. No radiation precautions are necessary.

Thyroid scan. ^{131}I is given to the patient either orally or intravenously. If an IV dose is given, the scan may be done in 30 to 60 minutes. A scintillation camera positioned over the patient's thyroid sends images that are received on an oscilloscope and may be printed out on special paper. A consent form must be signed for this test. No radiation precautions are necessary.

Table 35-1 Medications Commonly Used to Treat Hyperthyroidism and Hypothyroidism

Condition	Medication	Common Side Effects
Hyperthyroidism	Iodine or iodine products	Nausea, vomiting, diarrhea, abdominal pain
	Sodium iodide ^{131}I (Iodotope)	Sore throat, edema or pain in neck, temporary loss of taste, nausea, vomiting, painful salivary glands
	Methimazole (Tapazole), propylthiouracil (Propyl-Thyracil, PTU)	Rash or pruritus, vertigo, nausea, vomiting, loss of taste, paresthesias, abdominal pain
Hypothyroidism	Levothyroxine sodium (Levothroid, Synthroid, Eltroxin) Liothyronine sodium (Cytomel, Tertroxin) Liotrex (Euthroid, Thyrolar) Thyroglobulin (Proloid) Thyroid (Armour Thyroid, Thyro-Teric, Westthroid)	Nervousness, irritability, tremors, insomnia, tachycardia, hypertension, palpitations, cardiac dysrhythmias, vomiting, diarrhea, nausea, appetite changes, weight loss, menstrual irregularities, leg cramps, fever

Medical management. Medical treatment for hyperthyroidism may include administration of drugs that block the production of thyroid hormones, such as propylthiouracil or methimazole (Table 35-1). This may be followed after the acute stage by a therapeutic dose of sodium iodide (^{131}I; Iodotope), based on the patient's age, clinical manifestations, and estimated weight of the thyroid. This is done in an effort to destroy some of the hypertrophied thyroid tissue, and may need to be repeated once or perhaps twice in order to obtain the desired results. The patient will usually begin to notice a decrease in symptoms within 6 to 8 weeks after the first dose of the drug. An unfortunate sequela of this treatment in some patients is the development of hypothyroidism. For this reason, the patient must have adequate follow-up medical supervision. ^{131}I is not a radiation hazard to the nonpregnant patient but is absolutely contraindicated during pregnancy. Pregnant nurses should not care for this patient for several days.

Surgical treatment for hyperthyroidism is subtotal thyroidectomy, a procedure in which approximately five sixths of the thyroid is removed. Surgery is usually delayed, if possible, until the patient is in a normal-thyroid (euthyroid) state, because of the risk of excess bleeding during thyroidectomy, as well as postoperative thyroid crisis. Patients who have only mild hyperthyroidism will rarely be admitted to the acute care hospital. They will be followed by the physician in an office or clinic setting. However, the hospital nurse may come in contact with the patient because of admission for a different condition and will also care for these patients before and after thyroidectomy.

Nursing interventions. The hyperthyroid patient has a need for more nutrients because of increased metabolism, so diet therapy usually consists of food high in calories, vitamins (especially the B vitamins), minerals, and carbohydrates. Between-meal snacks are offered. Food should be soft and easily swallowed if there is **dysphagia**. Coffee, tea, and colas should be avoided because of their stimulant effect. Preoperative nursing interventions for the patient who is scheduled for a thyroidectomy should stress keeping the environment as stable as possible to prevent emotional strain. Visitors may have to be limited to ensure adequate time for the patient to rest. The room should be quiet and cool, not above 23° C (74° F). The nurse should encourage food and fluids to help replace electrolytes lost from perspiration. Attention should be paid to skin integrity for patients who are perspiring profusely. Keep the skin clean and dry, and change the patient's gown and bed linen as needed. Preoperative teaching is extremely important for this patient, and should include instructions on how to properly support the head while turning in bed or rising to a sitting or standing position. The nurse (or patient) should place both hands behind the head and maintain anatomical position while the rest of the body is being moved. The patient is also taught to deep breathe, but the physician will determine whether coughing is to be done postoperatively, since coughing puts a strain on the suture line. The nurse should inform the patient that a period of "voice rest" may be enforced for 48 hours postoperatively and that pencil and paper will be provided for writing notes instead of talking. Voice checks may be done every 2 to 4 hours, as ordered by the physician. The nurse asks the patient to say "ah" and checks for excessive hoarseness or voice change. Slight hoarseness is to be expected and should not be cause for alarm. Approximately 12.4% of thyroidectomy patients suffer some damage to the laryngeal nerve during surgery, but this is not always permanent.

Postoperative management of this patient includes keeping the bed in semi-Fowler's position, with pillows supporting the head and shoulders. The patient should be cautioned to avoid hyperextending the head to prevent excess tension on the incision, which is usually made in a naturally appearing horizontal crease in the anterior neck. There should be a suction apparatus and tracheotomy tray available for emergency use. A cool mist humidifer at the bedside may help soothe the throat and prevent coughing. Vital signs should be checked frequently, with special attention paid to the rate and depth of respirations and observation for any **dyspnea** related to edema in the operative site. Before any liquid is given orally, the nurse must be sure the swallowing and cough reflexes have returned. The nurse must be alert for signs of internal or external bleeding; early internal bleeding may be evidenced by restlessness, apprehension, an increased pulse rate, a decreased blood pressure, and a feeling of fullness in the neck. Later, cyanosis may develop, signaling an obstructed airway, and the surgeon must be notified immediately. The dressing on the neck should be inspected frequently for obvious external bleeding. The nurse should also check for bleeding at the sides and back of the neck and on top of the patient's shoulders, because oozing blood may pool there as a result of gravity. Most surgeons will allow a dressing to be reinforced as needed and loosened slightly if the patient complains that it is too tight.

Postoperatively, the diet initially will consist of clear, cool liquids, progressing to soft food as tolerated. This is followed by a regular diet as soon as possible in an effort to help the patient regain lost weight and correct any nutritional deficiencies.

In addition to hemorrhage, there are two significant postoperative complications after thyroidectomy for which the nurse must be ever watchful. The first is tetany. One possible cause of tetany is the inadvertent removal of one or more of the parathyroid glands during surgery. Another is edema in the operative area, which causes an occlusion of parathyroid release into the bloodstream, resulting in a low serum calcium level, the symptoms of which include numbness and tingling in the fingertips and toes and around the mouth. There may be carpal pedal spasms (muscle spasms in the hands and feet) and increased pulse, respirations, and blood pressure, accompanied by anxiety and agitation. Laryngeal spasm and stridor may occur. **Chvostek's sign** will be positive (an abnormal spasm of the facial muscles elicited by light taps on the facial nerve in patients who are hypocalcemic), and **Trousseau's sign** may also be positive (a test for latent tetany in which carpal spasm is induced by inflating a sphygmomanometer cuff on the upper arm to a pressure exceeding systolic blood pressure for 3 minutes—seen in hypocalcemia and hypomagnesemia). The condition may, if untreated, progress to convulsions or lethal cardiac dysrhythmias. Emergency treatment of tetany is the intravenous administration of calcium lactate, which should always be available postoperatively.

The other serious complication after thyroidectomy is thyroid crisis, or thyroid storm. Fortunately, it occurs rarely, and can usually be attributed to manipulation of the thyroid during surgery, which causes the release of large amounts of thyroid hormones into the bloodstream. If thyroid crisis occurs, it usually does so within the first

12 hours postoperatively. In thyroid crisis, all the signs and symptoms of hyperthyroidism are exaggerated. Additionally, the patient may develop nausea, vomiting, severe tachycardia, severe hypertension, and occasionally hyperthermia up to 41° C (106° F). Extreme restlessness, cardiac dysrhythmias, and delirium may also occur. The patient may develop congestive heart failure and may die. Emergency treatment of thyroid crisis includes intravenous administration of fluids, sodium iodide, and corticosteroids; antipyretics; and oxygen as needed. Prompt, adequate treatment usually results in dramatic improvement within 12 to 24 hours.

PREOPERATIVE NURSING DIAGNOSES	NURSING INTERVENTIONS
Potential hyperthermia	Assess body temperature at regular intervals. Regulate environment (room temperature, linens, clothing) to help keep patient comfortable.
Altered nutrition: less than body requirements	Encourage patient to eat prescribed diet, avoiding caffeine. Assess daily weight and food intake.
Altered thought processes	Explain procedures slowly; give a limited number of instructions and repeat if needed. Decrease external stimuli to minimize distractions and help patient concentrate.
Impaired skin integrity	Carefully assess skin daily. Keep linens dry and wrinkle free.

POSTOPERATIVE NURSING DIAGNOSES	NURSING INTERVENTIONS
Potential for aspiration	Ensure swallowing and cough reflexes present before oral intake. Encourage patient to drink slowly and chew food thoroughly.
Potential ineffective breathing pattern	Monitor rate and depth of respirations. Assess breath sounds and skin color. Encourage slow, deep breaths at least once an hour. Position to maximize respiratory effort.
Pain	Administer analgesics as ordered, and monitor relief. Use comfort measures (e.g., relaxation techniques, gentle backrub, distraction techniques).
Potential for infection	Use sterile technique when changing dressing on neck and during other invasive procedures. Assess body temperature every 4 hours, and report elevation to physician.

Patient teaching. Patient education after thyroidectomy includes stressing the importance of follow-up medical supervision. Thyroid function tests are done periodically to determine resolution of the hyperthyroid condition, as well as the possible development of hypothyroidism, a sequela that occurs in approximately 43% of surgical cases. Before leaving the hospital, the patient should be taught proper care of the incision site and symptoms that might indicate development of an infection, in which case the surgeon must be notified immediately.

Hypothyroidism

Etiology/pathophysiology. Hypothyroidism is the clinical state that occurs when the thyroid fails to secrete sufficient hormones, resulting in a slowing of all the body's metabolic processes. It may be caused by a condition of the thyroid itself or by a failure of the pituitary gland to furnish sufficient TSH for proper stimulation of thyroid secretion. It is sometimes an unfortunate sequela of the medical or surgical treatment of hyperthyroidism. It occurs most often in women aged 30 to 60 and is felt to be more common in the elderly than previously thought. Severe hypothyroidism in adults is called myxedema (Fig. 35-7). Congenital hypothyroidism is called cretinism (Fig. 35-8) and is estimated to occur in 1 of every 4000 to 5000 newborns.

Clinical manifestations. Clinical manifestations range from mild to severe and depend on the degree of thyroid hormone deficiency present. There is a slowing of all the body's metabolic processes, resulting in decreased production of body heat, intolerance to cold, and weight gain. Atherosclerotic changes may result in coronary artery disease.

Assessment. Collection of *subjective data* includes the patient's mental and emotional status, because he may display depression or paranoia, impaired memory, and general slowing of thought processes. There may be hearing and speech deficits. The patient is lethargic, forgetful, and irritable. Because of the body's slowed metabolism, anorexia and constipation may develop. Both sexes may

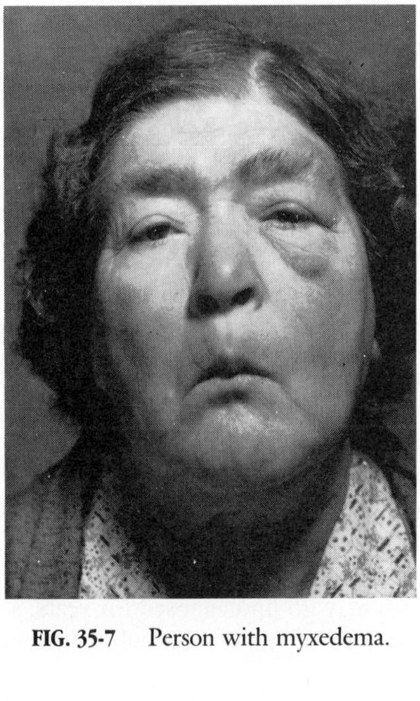

FIG. 35-7 Person with myxedema.

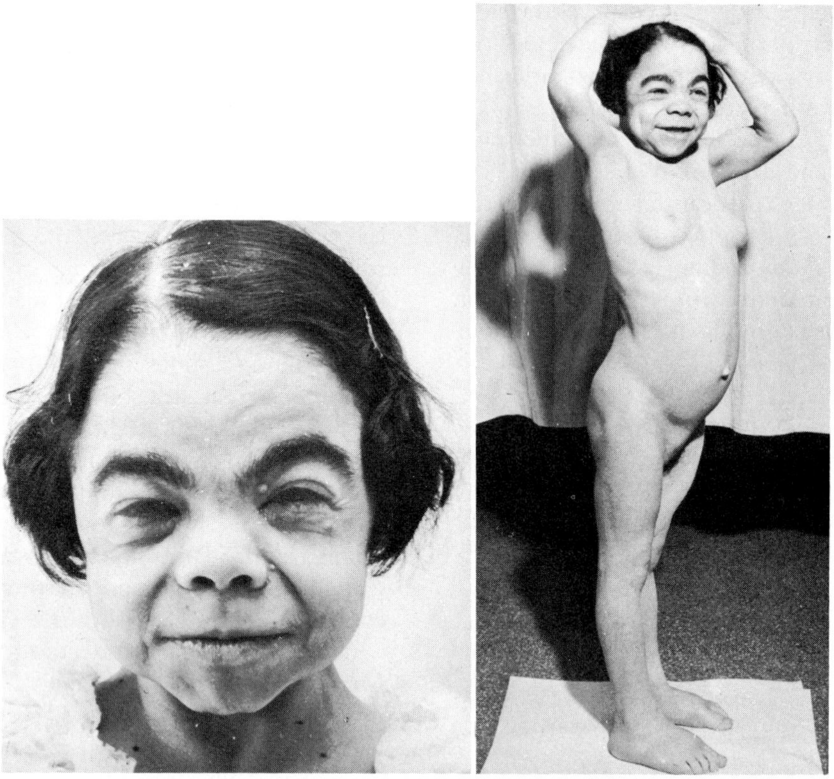

FIG. 35-8 Adult cretin (33 years old, untreated). Note characteristic cretinoid features, dwarfism (height 44 inches), absent axillary and scant pubic hair, poorly developed breasts, protruding abdomen, and small umbilical hernia.

experience decreased libido and reproductive difficulty. Female patients suffer from menstrual irregularities and may have difficulty conceiving or completing a pregnancy. Many experience spontaneous abortion, and this contributes to emotional distress and anxiety. The nurse should assess the patient's adaptive coping methods.

Collection of *objective data* includes assessment of the skin and hair. The hair thins and may fall out; the skin becomes thickened and dry. Facial features may enlarge to give the patient an edematous appearance. A masklike facial expression is common. The voice is characteristically low and hoarse. Decreased metabolism usually causes bradycardia, decreased blood pressure and respirations, and exercise intolerance. The patient's ability to perform activities may decrease because of weakness, clumsiness, and ataxia. The respiratory rate must be closely assessed after administration of any central nervous system depressant. The abdomen should be evaluated for distention, because *myxedema ileus* may occur.

Diagnostic tests. The diagnosis of hypothyroidism is based on the physical examination and history and on appropriate laboratory tests, such as the PBI, T_3, and T_4, which will show low levels of thyroid hormones. Subclinical cases may go undiagnosed for years, so the nurse should be aware of subtle clues while interviewing and caring for the patient. Recent research has suggested that mild hypothyroidism exists in approximately 5% of the population, more often in women. In children, when thyroxine replacement begins before epiphyseal fusion, the chance for normal growth is greatly improved.

Medical management. The treatment for hypothyroidism is replacement therapy, either with desiccated animal thyroid (Armour Thyroid), thyroglobulin (Proloid), or with synthetic products such as levothyroxine sodium (Levothroid) or liothyronine sodium (Cytomel) by mouth (Table 35-1). These drugs are usually given in the morning to enhance utilization of nutrients ingested during the daily meals. The patient will initially be given a low dose, with increases as necessary till the desired effect is achieved. A maintenance dose will then be established. The nurse should watch the patient for adverse effects of drug therapy, which mimic the signs and symptoms of hyperthyroidism. There is usually a dramatic change in the patient within a short time after replacement therapy begins.

Nursing interventions. Nursing interventions for the hospitalized severely hypothyroid patient center mainly on symptomatic relief. The room must be kept at least 20° to 23° C (68° to 74° F), and the patient should not be chilled during the bath or other procedures. Extra time should be allowed for physical care, so that the patient does not feel rushed. Accurate records of bowel elimination must be kept, since constipation may be severe. Stool softeners, bulk laxatives, or enemas may be ordered. A high-protein, high-fiber, low-calorie diet is given. Concentrated carbohydrates such as sweets should be avoided, to help prevent excess weight gain. The patient should be encouraged to take increased oral fluids. The nurse should watch for chest pain or dyspnea, accompanied by changes in the rate or rhythm of the heart, because this may indicate development of cardiac involvement. Since most hypothyroid patients are more susceptible to the effects of sedatives, hypnotics, and anesthetics, the nurse must be alert for possible adverse effects if these agents are given.

NURSING DIAGNOSES	NURSING INTERVENTIONS
Decreased cardiac output	Assess pulse, BP, skin color, and temperature. Schedule nursing activities around patient's activity cycle, with rest periods as needed to conserve energy.
Colonic constipation	Assess frequency and character of stools. Encourage oral fluid intake and high-fiber food intake.
Altered thought processes	Assess level of orientation to person, place, and time. Explain procedures slowly and simply, reinforcing them as necessary.

Patient teaching. Most hypothyroid patients do well with proper medical supervision, although they will probably have to take medication for the rest of their lives. Regular checkups are essential, because drug dosage may have to be adjusted from time to time. The patient should understand the desired effects of the medication and also the major adverse effects that might occur. The patient should be instructed to eat well-balanced meals of high-fiber foods, such as fruits, vegetables, and whole-grain cereals and breads; there should be adequate intake of iodine, in foods such as saltwater fish, milk, and eggs; fluids should be increased to help prevent constipation. The family should be told that mental and physical slowness may still be present but should improve with thyroid replacement therapy.

Simple (Colloid) Goiter

Etiology/pathophysiology. A simple, or colloid, goiter develops when the thyroid gland enlarges in response to low iodine levels in the bloodstream or when it is unable to utilize iodine properly. When the blood level of thyroxine is too low to signal the pituitary to decrease TSH secretion, the thyroid gland then responds by increasing the formation of thyroglobulin (colloid), which accumulates in the thyroid follicles and causes enlargement of the gland (Fig. 35-9). Most cases of simple goiter can be attributed to insufficient dietary intake of iodine, leading to this overgrowth of thyroid tissue.

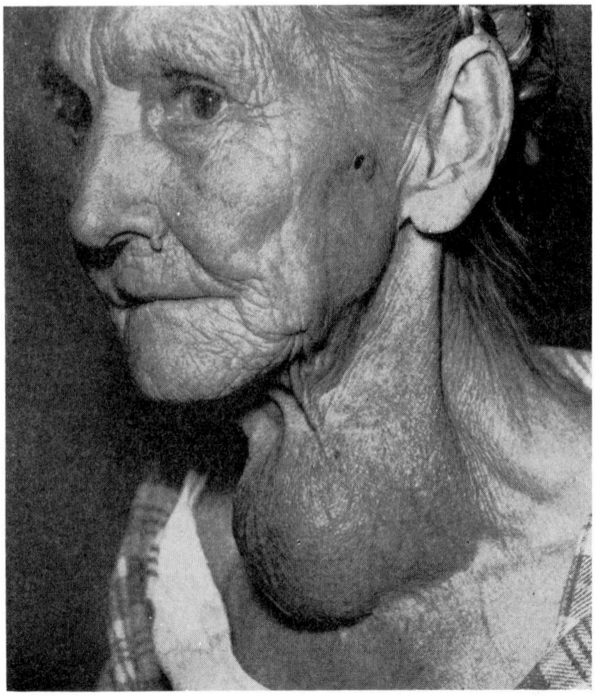

FIG. 35-9 Simple goiter.

Clinical manifestations. There are usually no manifestations of overt thyroid dysfunction, and the diagnosis is made essentially on the physical manifestations.

Medical management. Surgery may sometimes be performed for cosmetic effect, because this type of goiter can be very unsightly and damaging to the patient's self-image and self-esteem. If thyroidectomy is done, most of the gland is removed. Medical treatment consists of oral administration of potassium iodide, as well as foods high in iodine.

Assessment. Collection of *subjective data* focuses on assessing the patient's emotional response to the unsightly enlargement of the thyroid, and the patient should be encouraged to verbalize emotional reponses. The patient may only complain of symptoms of dysphagia, hoarseness, or dyspnea related to the pressure of the enlarged gland against the esophagus and trachea. Dysphagia may contribute to difficulty ingesting adequate food and fluids. The patient should be assessed for increasing dyspnea. The patient's understanding of the need for medication, diet therapy, and medical follow-up should be determined.

Collection of *objective data* includes assessment of increased goiter size, voice changes, and adequacy of food and fluid intake. The thyroid may be only slightly enlarged, or it may be so enlarged that surgery must be done to improve respiration or swallowing.

Nursing interventions. Nursing interventions after thyroidectomy (previously discussed) are aimed at prevention of complications such as bleeding, tetany, and thyroid crisis.

NURSING DIAGNOSES	NURSING INTERVENTIONS
Potential noncompliance: therapeutic regimen	Provide opportunities for patient to ventilate feelings about treatment plan. Correct misconceptions, and reinforce previous medical instructions. Stress importance of taking prescribed medications, having regular check-ups, and avoiding any identified goitrogenic foods.
Potential body image disturbance	Develop open and trusting relationship so patient will express feelings. Discuss ways to disguise thyroid enlargement (e.g., scarves, high collars, make-up).

Patient teaching. The nurse should stress the importance of adequate dietary intake of iodine. Medical supervision is recommended at regular intervals.

Cancer of the Thyroid

Etiology/pathophysiology. Cancer of the thyroid is a relatively rare malignancy, affecting approximately 25 of each 1 million people in the United States each year. However, more cases are expected, because between 1949 and 1960 many infants and children through adolescence were irradiated to shrink enlarged thymus tissue, tonsils, or adenoids and to treat severe cases of acne vulgaris. Cancer of the thyroid occurs more frequently in females, and more in Caucasians. The incidence rises as age increases. Most malignancies of the thyroid are papillary, well-differentiated adenocarcinoma, a type of cancer that grows slowly, is usually contained, and does not spread beyond the adjacent lymph nodes. Cure rates after thyroidectomy in these cases are excellent. Other cancers, follicular and anaplastic, though much more rare, have extremely low cure rates.

Clinical manifestations. The principal clinical manifestation of thyroid cancer is the presence of a firm, fixed mass or **nodule** that is felt on palpation of the gland. This nodule is painless. Only in rare instances have the symptoms of hyperthyroidism been seen.

Assessment. Collection of *subjective data* includes assessment of the patient's use of adaptive coping methods to deal with the diagnosis, as well as observation of the support system composed of the patient's significant others. The patient's understanding of the importance of medical follow-up should be assessed also.

Collection of *objective data* to be assessed includes progression of enlargement of the tumor area preoperatively, response to ^{131}I therapy, and skin involvement in the neck and torso after radiation therapy.

Diagnostic tests. Diagnosis of papillary thyroid cancer is suspected when a thyroid scan shows a "cold" nodule, indicating decreased uptake of ^{131}I. Benign adenomas and follicular cancers are usually visualized as "hot" nodules because of their increased uptake of the isotope. Thyroid function tests usually yield normal results. To confirm the diagnosis a thyroid needle biopsy may be done, but this should be attempted only by a skilled practitioner, since seeding of adjacent tissues may occur during the procedure. Metastasis can then result, with the prognosis becoming much more grave.

Medical management. Treatment of thyroid cancer is total thyroidectomy, with subsequent lifelong thyroid hormone replacement therapy. If metastasis is present at the time of the initial surgery, a radical neck dissection may be performed. In addition, radiation therapy, chemotherapy, and administration of ^{131}I may be done.

Nursing interventions. Nursing interventions for the patient after thyroidectomy (discussed previously) are instituted.

PREOPERATIVE NURSING DIAGNOSES	NURSING INTERVENTIONS
Anxiety	Encourage patient to discuss feelings about upcoming surgery. Monitor level of anxiety. Maintain a calm environment; try to decrease stressors.
Ineffective individual coping	Help patient identify previously successful coping methods. Teach new coping methods as needed.

Patient teaching. The patient should be aware of the importance of proper medical follow-ups to monitor thyroid hormone replacement therapy and to help ensure prompt diagnosis of any future metastatic lesions. Before discharge from the hospital, the patient should be taught proper care of the surgical incision.

Hyperparathyroidism

Etiology/pathophysiology. Hyperparathyroidism involves overactivity of the parathyroid glands, with increased production of parathormone. The cause of this condition may be a primary hypertrophy of one or more of the tiny parathyroid glands, usually in the form of an adenoma. It may also result from chronic renal failure, pyelonephritis, or glomerulonephritis. Parathyroid carcinoma is a rare condition, with rapid progress and a very grave prognosis. Hyperparathyroidism usually occurs in adults between 30 and 70 years of age, and twice as often in women.

Clinical manifestations. The primary clinical manifestation is **hypercalcemia.** This occurs as calcium leaves the bones and accumulates in the bloodstream. As a result, the bones become demineralized and may cause skeletal pain, pain on weight bearing, and pathological fractures (fractures that result from slight or no trauma to diseased bone). The high level of calcium in the blood may lead to the formation of kidney stones.

Assessment. Collection of *subjective data* includes assessment of the severity of skeletal pain, the degree of muscle weakness, and the effectiveness of analgesics. It is important to determine nursing measures that contribute to the patient's comfort and mobility. As neuromuscular function decreases, there is generalized fatigue, drowsiness, apathy, nausea, and anorexia; the degree of anorexia and nausea should be assessed. There may be constipation, personality changes, disorientation, and even paranoia. Symptoms that may indicate calculus formation are renal colic and dull back pain.

Collection of *objective data* includes careful observation for any skeletal deformity or abnormal movement of bone that might indicate a pathological fracture. The urine should be observed for quantity and the presence of hematuria and stones. There may be vomiting and weight loss. Hypertension and cardiac dysrhythmias may present significant problems. Changes in the serum calcium level may cause bradycardia and other cardiac irregularities (such as shortened Q-T interval). The level of consciousness may decrease, resulting in stupor or coma.

Diagnostic tests. X-ray examination may reveal skeletal decalcification. Blood parathyroid hormone (PTH) levels are increased, as are alkaline phosphate levels. The patient should receive nothing by mouth for 8 to 12 hours before these tests. The serum calcium level is elevated, while the serum phosphorus level is decreased. A differential diagnosis should be made to rule out multiple myeloma, Cushing's syndrome, vitamin D excess, and other causes of hypercalcemia.

Medical management. The treatment for hyperparathyroidism is surgical removal of an existing tumor, or removal of one or more parathyroid glands.

Nursing interventions. Preoperative nursing interventions include helping restore fluid and electrolyte balance by encouraging increased oral fluid intake, and by careful monitoring of the IV fluid therapy. The patient's intake and output should be monitored, because diuretics may be used. Furosemide (Lasix) is the diuretic of choice. Thiazide diuretics are not used, because they decrease renal excretion of calcium and thus increase the hypercalcemic state. Urine may be strained, since development of kidney calculi is not uncommon. Daily serum calcium levels may be ordered. The diet should be low in calcium, eliminating milk and other dairy products. Cranberry juice may be helpful in promoting acidic urine, thereby lessening the possibility of calculi formation. Some antacids are high in calcium and should not be used. The patient's pain should be accurately assessed and prescribed analgesics administered as needed. Postoperatively, the patient will be cared for in the same manner as after a thyroidectomy, with careful monitoring of intake and output. These patients commonly retain fluid in the tissues after surgery and will often have decreased urinary output. It is important to avoid overhydration at this point. The patient should be assessed frequently for signs of **hypocalcemia,** such as tetany, cardiac dysrhythmias, and carpopedal spasms. In the event that tetany does occur, calcium gluconate is usually administered intravenously.

NURSING DIAGNOSES	NURSING INTERVENTIONS
Activity intolerance	Assist patient to identify factors that increase or decrease activity tolerance and to eliminate or reduce painful, fatiguing activities. Encourage the patient to follow prescribed, individualized activity or exercise program.
Pain: skeletal, joint; renal colic	Assess factors that cause or worsen pain, and help patient adjust body mechanics or activity. Encourage adequate fluid intake, while assessing cardiac and renal output.
Potential for trauma	Assess for and eliminate potentially harmful factors in patient's environment. Instruct patient to use appropriate safety measures (e.g., walker, shower aids, siderails).

Patient teaching. The patient should be taught the principles of good body mechanics so that pathological fractures may be prevented during ambulation. The patient is reassured that bone pain should gradually decrease as electrolyte balance is restored and the condition is alleviated. The patient should be encouraged to participate in mild exercise as prescribed by the physician to regain muscle strength and a feeling of normal well-being. The nurse should teach the patient how to check the urine for the presence of stones or blood and how to monitor the pulse for any changes. The home environment should be evaluated and a plan developed for changes that may be necessary to prevent accidents.

Hypoparathyroidism

Etiology/pathophysiology. Hypoparathyroidism occurs when there is decreased **parathyroid hormone**, resulting in decreased levels of serum calcium. Idiopathic hypoparathyroidism is a rare condition, thought to be either autoimmune or familial in origin. Most commonly the cause is the inadvertent removal or destruction of one or more of the tiny parathyroid glands during thyroidectomy.

Clinical manifestations. Decreased parathyroid hormone levels in the bloodstream cause an increased serum phosphorus level and a decreased serum calcium level, resulting in neuromuscular hyperexcitability, involuntary and uncontrollable muscle spasms, and hypocalcemic tetany. Severe hypocalcemia may result in laryngeal spasm, stridor, cyanosis, and an increased possibility of asphyxia. In some patients, there is calcification of the basal ganglia in the brain, causing a parkinson-like syndrome with bizarre posturing and spastic movements.

Assessment. Collection of *subjective data* includes assessment of neuromuscular activity for symptoms such as dysphagia and numbness or tingling in areas of the skin. The patient may feel anxious, irritable, or depressed. The patient may experience headaches and nausea. Abdominal or flank pain may occur if a renal calculus attempts to pass down the ureter into the bladder. The effectiveness of narcotics used to relieve renal colic must be assessed.

Collection of *objective data* to be assessed includes the appearance of positive Chvostek's sign or Trousseau's sign. If laryngeal spasm and stridor should occur, cyanosis may appear. Cardiac output may decrease as a result of hypocalcemia, and the patient may develop dysrhythmias. Tetanic spasms of the extremities may be observed.

Diagnostic tests. Diagnostic laboratory studies confirm the presence of decreased serum calcium with increased urinary calcium, and increased serum phosphorus with decreased urinary phosphorus. Other possible causes of hypocalcemia, such as vitamin D deficiency, kidney failure, and acute pancreatitis, should be ruled out.

Medical management. The immediate treatment of hypoparathyroid tetany is intravenous administration of ionized calcium chloride (10%). This drug is very irritating to the vessel wall and should always be given very slowly, with a rate not to exceed 1 ml/min. The patient may complain of a hot feeling of the skin or tongue. If given too rapidly, intravenous calcium can precipitate cardiac arrest. Care should be taken that none of the drug escapes the vein and extravasates into the tissues, as sloughing may occur. After the initial IV dose, calcium may be continued in a slow IV infusion until tetany is controlled, then given orally. Vitamin D is usually also given orally to help increase the absorption and blood level of calcium.

Nursing interventions. Any patient receiving calcium, especially intravenously, must be monitored for signs of hypercalcemia. The most common clinical manifestations of this are vomiting, confusion, anorexia, abdominal pain, and weakness. The nurse should assess the patient for respiratory distress, renal involvement, and adverse reactions to calcium therapy, such as bradycardia, syncope, and hypotension. Calcium gluconate should be used cautiously in digitalized patients, because it may cause digitalis toxicity. Cimetidine (Tagamet) interferes with normal parathyroid functioning and should also be used carefully in these patients. The diet should contain foods high in calcium, such as dairy products, dark green vegetables, soybeans, and canned fish with the bones included. High-calcium snacks should be offered.

NURSING DIAGNOSES	NURSING INTERVENTIONS
Potential for injury	Assess for signs and symptoms of hypocalcemia (e.g., muscle spasms, laryngeal stridor, convulsion). Institute prescribed calcium therapy if need arises.
Potential fluid volume deficit	Assess intake and output, vital signs, and skin turgor. Encourage fluids as ordered.
Altered nutrition: less than body requirements	Give calcium replacement agents as scheduled. Monitor Chvostek's and Trousseau's signs. Arrange for dietitian to discuss dietary sources of calcium. Assess patient's intake of high-calcium foods.

Patient teaching. The patient should be taught the early symptoms of hypocalcemia and instructed to notify the nurse or physician if they occur. It is important that periodic blood levels of calcium and phosphorus be drawn while the patient is hospitalized. The patient should be taught to monitor the pulse for changes, as well as proper maintenance of fluid balance and the use of calcium supplements at home.

DISORDERS OF THE ADRENAL GLANDS

Hyperfunction (Cushing's Syndrome)

Etiology/pathophysiology. Cushing's syndrome (hypercortisolism) is a rare condition in which the plasma levels of adrenocortical hormones are increased. It occurs in only about 10 people in a million and is three times more common in women than in men. This syndrome may be caused by hyperplasia of adrenal tissue resulting from overstimulation by the pituitary hormone ACTH, by a tumor of the adrenal cortex, by ACTH-secreting neoplasms outside the pituitary (such as oat-cell carcinoma of the lung), and occasionally by overuse of corticosteroid drugs. The body's protective feedback mechanism fails, with resultant excess secretion of the adrenal hormones: glucocorticoids, mineralocorticoids, and sex hormones.

Clinical manifestations. This overabundance of hormones produces the signs and symptoms commonly associated with Cushing's syndrome, including moonface and buffalo hump. The arms and legs become thin as a result of muscle wasting. **Hypokalemia** is usually present. There is usually protein in the urine, as well as increased urinary calcium excretion, which may lead to the development of renal calculi. Osteoporosis results from abnormal calcium absorption, and kyphosis may develop. The patient is very susceptible to all kinds of infections, but the symptoms of these may be masked and not detected until the infection has progressed to a point that may be life threatening.

Assessment. Collection of *subjective data* includes assessment of the patient's ability to concentrate. Patients may feel irritable, and mental changes may develop. Some patients experience emotional instability, with severe mood swings, and occasionally a psychosis. Depression is very common, and the possibility of suicide is an ever-present concern for the nurse, who must be alert to subtle changes in the patient's affect, and must keep the environment free from objects with which the patient may inflict self-harm. Patients of both sexes may experience loss of libido and alterations in self-esteem; there may be concerns about sexual dysfunction. The patient should be encouraged to verbalize concerns about altered body image. Severe backache is often present and may signal a compression fracture of a vertebral body. The severity of back pain should be assessed, as well as nursing measures that contribute to the patient's comfort. Appetite usually increases, so the patient's understanding of special dietary restrictions should be assessed, as well as the understanding of the importance of medical follow-up.

Collection of *objective data* includes observation of the skin for the presence of ecchymoses and petechiae. The skin becomes thin and fragile and wound healing is delayed. There may be weight gain and abdominal enlargement, with development of striae, and this increased girth may contribute to difficulty with mobility. Weight should be monitored, because peripheral edema and associated hypertension are common. Impaired carbohydrate metabolism results in hyperglycemia. Women may experience **hirsutism,** menstrual irregularities, and deepening of the voice. Elevated body temperature may signal the presence of an undetected infection.

Diagnostic tests. Diagnosis is usually based on the clinical appearance of the patient and on the results of laboratory tests. Plasma cortisol levels are usually elevated. Plasma ACTH levels may be increased or decreased, depending on the location of a tumor. Skull x-ray evaluation may detect an erosion of the sella turcica in the presence of a pituitary tumor. Adrenal angiography will aid in diagnosing an adrenal tumor. Twenty-four-hour urine tests for 17-ketosteroids and 17-hydroxysteroids show increased levels present. Abdominal CT scan and ultrasound may help localize an abdominal tumor.

Medical management. Treatment is directed toward the causative factor. If an adrenal tumor is present, adrenalectomy is usually indicated for its removal. Pituitary tumors may be irradiated or removed surgically by transsphenoidal microsurgery. If the patient is unable to undergo surgery because of inoperable cancer elsewhere in the body or another preexisting serious condition, mitotane (Lysodren) therapy may be used. This cytotoxic agent is toxic to the adrenal glands and is given for at least 3 months, during which time the patient must be monitored for symptoms of hepatotoxicity, such as jaundice, gastrointestinal upsets, and pruritus. The diet should be lowered in sodium to help decrease edema. Reduced calories and carbohydrates will help control hyperglycemia, and foods high in potassium will help correct hypokalemia.

Nursing interventions. Important nursing interventions include gentle handling to prevent skin breakdown or excessive ecchymosis, as well as frequent assessment for areas of erythema, edema, or early signs of infection. The patient should be encouraged to turn frequently and ambulate as tolerated to eliminate undue pressure on bony prominences. Elbow and heel protectors and an Eggcrate mattress pad may help prevent decubiti in the bedridden patient. The patient should be encouraged to participate as fully as possible in normal ADLs, interspersing personal hygiene tasks with rest periods to prevent overtiring.

NURSING DIAGNOSES	NURSING INTERVENTIONS
Knowledge deficit: therapeutic regimen	Assess patient's understanding of prescribed medication and diet. Encourage patient to wear medical-alert devices and carry wallet identification cards.
Activity intolerance	Assess patient's current activity tolerance, and identify priorities for energy expenditures. Plan activity and rest periods with patient.
Fluid volume excess	Monitor daily weight, intake and output. Encourage compliance with salt restriction.
Self-esteem disturbance	Allow patient to verbalize negative feelings about body changes. Help patient set realistic goals based on physical tolerance.

Patient teaching. The patient's mental attitude is extremely important. The nurse should encourage verbalization of concerns and should also be watchful for the development of depression and the presence of suicidal thoughts. Patients should be helped to understand their prescribed medication, such as mitotane (Lysodren), as well as possible side effects. It is important to wear a medical alerting bracelet or necklace and to carry a wallet card stating the diagnosis of Cushing's syndrome. There may be a major life-style change to adjust to, and the aid of a social worker may be enlisted. Before adrenalectomy, the patient should be taught the importance of avoiding stress and avoiding infections. Postoperative teaching includes proper wound care and the symptoms of Addison's disease, which is sometimes an unavoidable sequela after this type of surgery.

Adrenal Hypofunction (Addison's Disease)

Etiology/pathophysiology. Adrenocortical insufficiency occurs when the adrenal glands do not secrete adequate amounts of glucocorticoids and mineralocorticoids. It

Table 35-2 Nursing Assessment of Patients with Cushing's Syndrome or Addison's Disease

Area of Assessment	Clinical Manifestations in Cushing's Syndrome	Clinical Manifestations in Addison's Disease
Cardiovascular	Mild to moderate hypertension	Postural hypotension, vertigo, syncope
Neurological	Impaired memory and concentration, insomnia, irritability	Lethargy, headache
Musculoskeletal	Muscle weakness, muscle wasting in extremities, back and rib pain, kyphosis	Muscle weakness, fatigue, muscle aches, muscle wasting
Integumentary	Skin thin; frequent petechiae and ecchymoses, hyperpigmentation, poor wound healing	Hyperpigmentation, decreased body hair
Self-care and hygiene	Tires easily	Tires easily; very susceptible to infections of all kinds
Nutrition/fluid balance	Increased appetite, moderate weight gain, edema, buffalo hump, moonface, obesity of trunk, hyperglycemia, need for decreased salt intake, reduced calories and carbohydrate, increased potassium intake	Nausea and vomiting, fluid and electrolyte imbalance, dehydration, weight loss, hypoglycemia, need for increased salt intake

may initially be seen as Addison's disease, a rather rare primary condition; it may result from adrenalectomy, pituitary hypofunction, or long-standing steroid therapy. Addison's disease can result from idiopathic adrenal atrophy, cancer of the adrenal cortex, or tuberculosis. Deficiencies in aldosterone and cortisol produce disturbances of the metabolism of carbohydrates, fats, and proteins, as well as sodium, potassium, and water. This results in electrolyte and fluid imbalance, dehydration, water loss, and hypovolemia.

Clinical manifestations. Clinical manifestations are directly related to imbalances in adrenal hormones, nutrients, and electrolytes.

Assessment. Collection of *subjective data* to be assessed includes the presence of nausea, anorexia, and craving for salt. Postural hypotension may be associated with lightheadedness, weakness, and syncope, resulting in reluctance to attempt normal activities. The patient may complain of severe headache, confusion, abdominal pain, or lower back pain, which could represent early symptoms of adrenal crisis. This patient tolerates stress poorly, feels anxious and apprehensive, and may thus suffer under emotional trauma more easily than a normal person would. It is important to assess emotional status and allow the patient to ventilate feelings about altered self-image. The nurse should also assess the patient's overall understanding of the disease process and the importance of medical treatment and follow-up.

Collection of *objective data* includes observation of changes in the color of the mucous membranes and the skin, with the appearance of darkly pigmented areas commonly observed. There is usually weight loss, which may be accompanied by vomiting and diarrhea. Hypoglycemia may contribute to the patient's fatigue; the nurse should assess the patient's ability to perform ADLs. An abnormally low or abnormally high body temperature, hyponatremia, and hypokalemia are signs of impending adrenal crisis.

See Table 35-2 for a nursing assessment comparison of patients with Cushing's syndrome and Addison's disease.

Diagnostic tests. Laboratory studies show decreased serum sodium, increased serum potassium, and decreased serum glucose. A 24-hour urine specimen shows decreased levels of 17-ketosteroids and 17-hydroxysteroids. Fasting plasma cortisol levels and aldosterone levels are low. A glucose tolerance test may yield abnormal results.

Medical management. Medical treatment involves the prompt restoration of fluid and electrolyte balance, as well as replacement of the deficient adrenal hormones. Fludrocortisone (Florinef) is usually the drug of choice. The diet should be high in sodium and low in potassium.

Nursing interventions. The nurse should carefully assess the circulatory status of the patient, keep accurate intake and output records, and record daily weight. Skin turgor should be checked and fluids offered frequently. Vital signs are monitored at regular intervals, with particular attention paid to the temperature and blood pressure. The patient is also monitored for response to prescribed steroid drugs and any adverse effects promptly reported to the physician. The environment must be kept as free from stressors as possible. Visitors and hospital personnel should be screened for the presence of infectious disease and excluded from the patient's room. This patient should be continually assessed for signs of developing adrenal (addisonian) crisis, in which there may be a sudden, severe drop in blood pressure, nausea and vomiting, an extremely high temperature, and cyanosis, progressing to vasomotor collapse and possibly to death. Emergency treatment is intravenous administration of corticosteroids in a solution of saline and glucose.

NURSING DIAGNOSES	NURSING INTERVENTIONS
Potential for infection	Assess environment for stressors. Screen visitors and personnel for contagious disease. Monitor temperature routinely. Stress importance of prescribed medications.
Altered peripheral tissue perfusion	Monitor vital signs and intake and output. Have patient make position changes slowly; monitor for vertigo, visual changes.
Sleep pattern disturbance	Decrease amount of external stimuli. Use comfort measures (e.g., backrub, dark room, relaxation techniques). Do not disturb patient when sleeping.
Fluid volume deficit (1)	Assess skin turgor for dehydration. Encourage compliance with increased dietary salt.

Patient teaching. Before discharge from the hospital, the patient must be taught the importance of adhering to the prescribed drug therapy, having regular medical checkups, and immediately reporting all illnesses, even a cold, to the physician. The patient should understand the importance of avoiding stress, one of the major precipitating factors in adrenal crisis, and should be encouraged to eliminate excess stressors. Other factors include overexertion, diarrhea, infection, decreased intake of salt, exposure to cold, and surgery. The nurse should teach the patient to wear a medical alerting bracelet or necklace and to carry a wallet card.

Pheochromocytoma

Etiology/pathophysiology. A pheochromocytoma is a chromaffin cell tumor, usually found in the adrenal medulla, that causes excessive secretion of epinephrine and norepinephrine. These tumors occur most often between the ages of 20 and 60 and are almost always benign; only about 10% are malignant.

Clinical manifestations. The principal manifestation of pheochromocytoma is hypertension, which may be intermittent but is usually persistent. Hypertensive crisis episodes may occur, during which the blood pressure may fluctuate widely, sometimes as high as 300/175. Signs and symptoms may be triggered by an identifiable factor, such as overexertion or emotional trauma, or they may occur for no apparent reason. Extreme hypertension may result in cerebrovascular accident, kidney damage, and retinopathy. Cardiac damage may occur, resulting in congestive heart failure.

Assessment. Collection of *subjective data* to be assessed during hypertensive crisis includes the presence of severe headache and palpitations. The patient may feel nervous, dizzy, and dyspneic and may experience paresthesias. There may be nausea and intolerance to heat. Anxiety is common, and the patient may have trouble sleeping. The nurse should question the patient about the occurrence of symptoms in relation to identifiable factors such as excess stress or overexertion and should assess the coping methods identified.

Collection of *objective data* includes frequent measurement of blood pressure and respiratory rate for increases and of pulse for tachycardia. There may be tremors, diaphoresis, dilated pupils, glycosuria, and hyperglycemia. The nurse should assess responses to prescribed medications.

Diagnostic tests. A 24-hour urine test (the VMA, or vanillylmandelic acid test) will be used to diagnose pheochromocytoma. VMA is the main urinary metabolite of epinephrine and norepinephrine. A test that may be used to confirm the results of the VMA is the total urine catecholamine test, which also requires a 24-hour specimen. Elevations of these metabolites will confirm the diagnosis. CT scan of the adrenal glands, along with IVP (intravenous pyelogram) may help in locating the tumor. Oral intake is restricted for 8 hours before IVP, and laxatives are usually administered the evening before the test.

Medical management. Treatment is usually surgical removal of the tumor, if possible, and sometimes removal of the adrenal gland as well. Preoperatively, the patient may be given alpha-adrenergic blocking agents such as phentolamine mesylate (Regitine) or phenoxybenzamine HCl (Dibenzyline) in an effort to control hypertension. Metyrosine (Demser) may be given to help inhibit catecholamine production, and the drug must be continued on a long-term basis if a tumor is inoperable.

Nursing interventions. Postoperative care is carried out in the same manner as for any major abdominal surgery, with the following special concerns. If the patient has undergone adrenalectomy, large amounts of hydrocortisone will be given. The patient must be watched carefully for fluctuations in blood pressure caused by adrenal manipulation during surgery, with subsequent release of epinephrine and norepinephrine. These fluctuations may be severe and life threatening if cardiovascular collapse occurs. The patient should avoid excess stress and must be allowed adequate time to rest; sedatives may be given to ensure this. A careful intake and output record should be kept and intravenous solutions administered exactly as ordered. Vasopressors and corticosteroids may be given. The diet should be free from stimulants, such as coffee, tea, and soft drinks containing caffeine.

NURSING DIAGNOSES	NURSING INTERVENTIONS
Altered tissue perfusion: cardiopulmonary, renal	Monitor BP and pulse and record intake and output. Eliminate smoking and caffeine-containing beverages.
Activity intolerance	Assist with gradual position changes from lying to sitting or standing. Limit activity as needed, to prevent increased hypertension.
Anxiety	Help patient identify stressors. Assess previous satisfactory coping methods with patient. Encourage patient to verbalize feelings of powerlessness and loss of control.

Patient teaching. Follow-up 24-hour urine tests (VMA, catecholamines) may be done to determine return to normal levels. When this goal is achieved, the patient is pronounced cured and may resume normal activities. If the tumor has proved inoperable, it is important that the patient remain under lifelong medical supervision, and the importance of compliance with prescribed treatment is stressed. Medical alert jewelry should be worn and a wallet card carried. The patient should be taught self-monitoring of blood pressure and instructed when to call the physician if elevation occurs.

DISORDERS OF THE PANCREAS

Diabetes Mellitus

Etiology. Diabetes mellitus, or DM (*mellitus:* "sweet or related to honey"), is a systemic metabolic disorder that involves improper metabolism of carbohydrates, fats, and proteins. This condition may be caused by a decrease or absolute lack of **insulin** production by the beta cells of the islets of Langerhans in the pancreas or by the decreased activity of the insulin that is secreted. There are several types of diabetes mellitus, but in each type, hyperglycemia is present as the principal clinical manifestation. Although the exact cause of DM is unknown, a number of factors have been demonstrated as contributing to its development: genetic predisposition, viruses (such as coxsackievirus B, rubella, and mumps), the aging process, diet and life-style, and ethnicity. Obesity is felt to be a major factor. Recent research has suggested that the T lymphocytes may play a role in the development of autoimmune destruction of the pancreatic insulin-producing cells.

Types of diabetes mellitus. There are two main types of diabetes mellitus: **type I** (insulin-dependent) **diabetes mellitus** (IDDM) and **type II** (non-insulin-dependent) **diabetes mellitus** (NIDDM). Type I was formerly called juvenile diabetes, or juvenile-onset diabetes. Type II was formerly called adult-onset diabetes, or maturity-onset diabetes. Other types of DM patients include those diagnosed with such conditions as pancreatitis, genetic syndromes, malnutrition, chemical- or drug-induced disease, and pregnancy. There are some distinct differences between type I and type II diabetes (Table 35-3). In type I (IDDM), destruction of beta cells in the pancreatic islets results in deficient insulin *production*, but the patient retains normal sensitivity to insulin action. In type II (NIDDM), the main problem seems to be an abnormal resistance to insulin *action*. Regardless of the type of DM, all of these patients have impaired glucose tolerance. Only 5% to 10% of all diabetics are type I, but since they do not produce adequate amounts of endogenous (produced by the body) insulin, they must take regular injections of exogenous (from outside the body) insulin or they will die. Type II diabetics are usually diagnosed after age 40, and 80% of these patients are overweight, with a familial

Table 35-3 Comparison of Diabetes Mellitus Type I (IDDM) and Diabetes Mellitus Type II (NIDDM)

	Type I	Type II
Age at onset	Usually 30 years or younger	Usually more than 40 years
Body weight	Normal or underweight	80% are overweight
Symptoms at onset	Sudden; polydipsia, polyuria, weight loss, weakness, fatigue; glycosuria, hyperglycemia; acidosis, progressing to DKA	Gradual; may be asymptomatic at onset; later, may develop signs and symptoms of type I; others include slow wound healing, blurred vision, pruritus, boils or other skin infections; vaginal infections in women
Treatment	Diet, exercise, and insulin	Diet and exercise *or* diet, exercise, and oral hypoglycemic agents, *or* diet, exercise, oral hypoglycemic agents, and insulin during times of illness
Incidence of complications	Frequent	Frequent
Psychosocial and sexual concerns	Irritability; altered body image; mood swings, depression; menstrual irregularities; hirsutism; decreased libido	Altered body image; amenorrhea; decreased libido; poor tolerance to stress

history of diabetes. They are usually able to secrete sufficient amounts of insulin, but their body tissues are unable to properly utilize it. These patients can usually achieve good control of their disease by diet and oral hypoglycemics, using insulin only when first diagnosed and during times of illness, surgery, or other periods when the body's insulin level is out of control.

Pathophysiology. In normal metabolism, the end-products of digestion (glucose, fatty acids and glycerol, and amino acids) are absorbed into the venous circulation and carried to the liver, where they may then be either used immediately or stored for later use. The liver can change glycerol and fatty acids into glucose, and glucose into triglycerides, as needed. Fatty acids may also be changed into **ketone bodies**, such as **acetone**, which serve as fuel for the muscles of the body and as an energy source for the brain. Glucose storage takes place in the form of glycogen in the liver. Free glucose in the bloodstream can always be used by the brain and kidney, since it is not necessary for insulin to be present to enable glucose molecules to enter the brain cells or the glomeruli. But insulin *must* be present for muscle cells and other body cells to be able to utilize glucose. Glycogen can be changed back into glucose as needed by the body for energy. In the diabetic patient, lack of proper amounts of insulin, or its inadequate utilization, impairs the use of glucose by the body. Thus the excess glucose accumulates in the bloodstream, and **hyperglycemia** exists. To rid the body of this abnormal amount of glucose, the kidneys will excrete it in the urine. This is called **glycosuria**, a condition that necessitates an extra amount of water for proper dilution of the urine. The patient then develops **polyuria**, producing large amounts of urine, and also experiences **polydipsia.** Often the patient is unable to drink enough fluid to compensate for polyuria and may become dehydrated. Even though there is excess glucose available in the bloodstream, it cannot be utilized by the body tissues without the help of insulin. So the cells are not properly nourished, and **polyphagia** develops. In spite of increased food intake, metabolism remains faulty, and the patient loses weight. Since carbohydrates cannot be utilized properly, proteins and fats are broken down and ketone bodies used excessively for heat and energy. Because ketone bodies are acid substances, the patient may develop acidosis. Diabetic **ketoacidosis** (DKA), formerly called diabetic coma, may develop, and the patient could die.

Clinical manifestations. The clinical manifestations of type I diabetes mellitus include the three classic "polys": polyuria, polydipsia, and polyphagia. As ketone bodies accumulate in the bloodstream, imbalances of sodium, potassium, and bicarbonate result. Type II diabetics, most of whom are older than age 40, experience very different signs and symptoms. In the early stages of the disease, the patient may be asymptomatic but later may complain of symptoms associated with type I, plus a number of others. These patients may not seek medical care until a severe complication such as kidney involvement, retinopathy, or gangrene occurs.

Assessment. Collection of *subjective data* to be assessed includes hunger, thirst, and nausea. In addition to frequent urination of large amounts, the patient may complain of nocturia, weakness, and fatigue. There may be blurred vision, seeing halos around lights, and headache. Symptoms such as cold extremities, cramping pain in the calves and feet during exercise or walking, decreased sensation to pain and temperature in the feet, and numbness and tingling of the lower extremities may occur. There may be pruritus. Male patients may become impotent. The patient may verbalize negative feelings about his or her body and the ability to cope with the illness. The nurse should assess coping methods, as well as the patient's knowledge about the disease process. Misunderstandings and lack of interest may result in inadequate skills necessary to manage the diabetic life-style, such as diet planning, injections, and exercise programs. The patient's understanding of the importance of compliance with prescribed medical treatment should be assessed, as well as the patient's willingness to obtain adequate follow-up.

Collection of *objective data* includes assessment of the skin, since slow wound healing, boils, carbuncles, and ulcerations are common. Women with diabetes mellitus may experience frequent vaginal infections, and vaginal discharge is often bothersome. In type I patients, weight loss and muscle wasting may be seen, but many type II patients remain obese. The skin on the lower extremities may appear shiny and thin, with less hair present. The legs and feet may feel cold to the touch, and there may be ulcerated areas. Gangrene of the toes is a dreaded sign. The nurse should assess the patient's ability to perform blood and/or urine testing and proper injection of insulin.

Diagnostic tests. Diagnosis of DM is made on the basis of clinical manifestations, plus the patient's history and laboratory findings. The patient with random blood glucose over 200 mg/dl should be further evaluated. Blood tests commonly done include those in Box 35-2.

Since 1982 the American Diabetes Association (ADA) has recommended SMBG instead of urine testing in any patient with IDDM. This is accomplished in a number of ways. Blood from a fingerstick may be placed on a reagent strip and compared with a color chart, or it may be placed into a reflectance meter. Another type of meter uses a glucose sensor instead of a meter, and test strips are not used; instead, a drop of blood is placed directly into the machine. Self-monitoring blood glucose (SMBG) is the monitoring tool of choice because it provides an accurate picture of current blood glucose levels. Its use in NIDDM patients is usually limited to stabili-

BOX 35-2 **DIAGNOSTIC TESTS FOR DIABETES MELLITUS**

Fasting blood sugar (FBS). After an 8-hour fast, blood is drawn. The normal is 60 to 110 mg/dl of venous blood.

Oral glucose tolerance test (OGTT). After an 8- to 12-hour fast, a venous blood specimen is drawn and a urine sample is collected and discarded. Then the patient is given a measured amount of carbohydrate solution orally. Blood and urine samples are obtained at 30 minutes, 1 hour, and 2 hours after ingestion of the solution. The test may continue for up to a total of 4 hours, as ordered by the physician. In nondiabetic patients, blood sugar returns to normal in about 2 hours. In diabetics this does not occur; values will remain higher than normal for a longer time. Blood samples are drawn by the laboratory technician and urine samples are collected by the nurse, if this test is done on a hospital inpatient. The patient may usually have water orally during the testing time to facilitate the collection of urine samples. The nurse must properly label each timed specimen.

Serum insulin. Absent in IDDM; normal to high in NIDDM.

Postprandial (after a meal) blood sugar (PPBS). A fasting patient is given a measured amount of carbohydrate solution orally. An alternate method is to have the patient eat a measured amount of foods containing carbohydrates, fats, and proteins. A blood sample will be drawn 2 hours after completion of the meal. Elevated plasma glucose over 160 mg/dl may indicate the presence of DM.

Patient self-monitoring of blood glucose (SMBG). A blood sample is obtained by the fingerstick method, by either the patient or the nurse, and tested using a dipstick or machine.

zation of glucose control after initial diagnosis and during periods of instability of control, such as infections. SMBG is more expensive than urine testing but is felt to result in fewer hospitalizations for the patient, so it is probably more cost effective on a long-term basis. If overall achievement of control is accomplished and complications reduced proportionally, the cost then becomes negligible.

Urine tests are not as reliable as blood tests but are still done in many hospitals, usually with dipsticks that measure the percentages of glucose and/or acetone in a urine sample. The patient may be instructed to test the urine at home. There are several methods of accomplishing this, but regardless of which is employed, a double-voided specimen should be tested each time. Urine that has accumulated in the bladder for several hours will be much less accurate in determining the true amounts of glucose and ketones than a fresh specimen will. In the older person with diabetes, the point at which glucose will be spilled into the urine is set higher than in the younger person. In other words, the "renal threshold" is set higher, and blood glucose may actually be very high, yet the urine will test negative for glucose. To obtain a specimen for testing, the patient should empty the bladder completely, then 30 to 60 minutes later, void again, and perform the test on this specimen. If the patient has an indwelling catheter, the tubing should be drained into the collection bag, then clamped for 30 minutes, after which a specimen is drawn from the port with a sterile syringe and needle to prevent contamination of the closed system. Some of the products used to test the urine for glucose only are Clinitest tablets (Ames), Chemstrip bG (Bio-Dynamics), Tes-tape (Lilly), and Diastix (Ames). Acetone testing products include Ketostix (Ames) and Acetest tablets. Ketodiastix (Ames) may be used to test for both glucose and acetone. The manufacturer's directions on all packages of these products and others must be followed exactly, because inaccurate results may occur otherwise. The results from glucose testing are usually recorded in percentage, ranging from 0% to 5%. The amount of acetone is represented by a color change, in shades of pink to purple, recorded as negative to large amounts. Testing for acetone should be done routinely when glucose in the urine is 1% or more and also during illness or during periods of high stress, because the presence of acetone in the urine indicates the possibility of impending ketoacidosis.

Medical management. Medical treatment for DM, no matter what type, consists mainly of *diet, exercise, and medication,* the major goal being to achieve control of the disease and prevent complications. It is hoped that the patient will assume a large part of the responsibility for self-care, with emphasis on optimal wellness instead of illness. Since 1921, when Drs. Charles Best and Frederick Banting first isolated insulin, medical science has made many dramatic strides in the care of the diabetic. But physicians depend on the valuable help obtained from other members of the health care team, especially nurses. Every newly diagnosed patient must undergo an intensive and extensive education program to learn proper diet, medication routines, home testing of blood and urine, and the role of exercise. The importance of the nurse as a teacher cannot be overemphasized.

Diet. Diet therapy for the diabetic is aimed at helping to achieve a normal blood glucose level and attaining or maintaining ideal body weight, while ensuring proper growth and/or body maintenance. The services of a dietitian should be enlisted for each newly diagnosed diabetic. The menu must be individualized, taking into consideration the patient's age, weight, activity level, lifestyle, ethnic background, and food preferences. The ability to choose and pay for groceries, prepare food, and properly store leftovers must be assessed. After discharge from the hospital, detailed dietary instructions will be of no use to the patient who does not have money, cooking skills, and appliances necessary to comply with them. If the patient is a member of a family, the person who will be planning and preparing the meals must be educated along with the patient, and this person should be taught how to fit the patient's dietary needs into the family menus. The physician and dietitian will decide the proper amounts of each nutrient in the dietary prescription. Diets are based on ADA recommendations, and patients may obtain additional information and menus from that organization at no cost.

Quantitative diabetic diets consist of measured amounts of food in the basic four food groups, with 50% to 55% of caloric intake from carbohydrates, 25% to 20% from proteins, and 25% or 30% from fats. Complex carbohydrates and polyunsaturated fats are best for these patients to use. Concentrated carbohydrates such as candy or other sweets should not be used by the diabetic for whom an ADA diet is prescribed.

The *qualitative* diet is unmeasured and more unstructured, stressing moderation when selecting food from the basic four food groups and reducing the use of simple carbohydrates, saturated fats, and alcohol. This diet may be used for the patient whose blood glucose levels are not extremely high, for the pediatric patient, or the patient who is noncompliant with the ADA diet.

Insulin-dependent patients are usually given midafternoon and bedtime snacks in addition to their regular three meals a day. It is important that food intake be evenly distributed throughout the day, taking insulin dosage and exercise into consideration. The patient who plans to engage in strenuous exercise may be able to eat more food, because exercise increases the absorption rate of insulin, thereby enabling muscles to utilize glucose more effectively. (For further information on diabetic diets, see Chapter 23.)

Diabetics should do a fingerstick blood glucose level test before each meal and at bedtime until their disease is under control. Thereafter, they usually only test once or twice a day, as directed by the physician, unless they become ill or their diabetes becomes uncontrolled. Urine testing may be done at home, instead of blood testing, but should be on a regular basis, such as before meals, using a double-voided specimen each time.

The patient may need follow-up visits with a dietitian as well as with the physician. Obese NIDDM patients are encouraged to lose weight, because many are then able to control their diabetes with only diet and exercise, eliminating the need for medication. The IDDM patient should try to attain and maintain ideal weight, because better control of the condition usually results. Good control of DM is desirable in helping prevent complications.

Exercise. The diabetic should exercise regularly. The physician will help determine the best type of exercise for each patient. Exercise is beneficial, not only because it aids in promoting proper utilization of glucose, but also because it is important to the overall functioning of the cardiovascular system and will increase the patient's feeling of well-being.

Medications. Insulin and oral hypoglycemics are the drugs of choice for diabetic patients (Table 35-4). Insulin administration is necessary for all type I patients and in type II patients who cannot be controlled on diet or oral hypoglycemics alone. Insulin may be obtained from the pancreatic tissue of pigs or cows and has recently been produced synthetically employing recombinant DNA techniques using *Escherichia coli* bacteria. Insulin is a hormone and is absorbed into the patient's bloodstream. There are many types and brands of insulin. A number of different chemicals can be added to insulins to potentiate their action, and these types cannot be administered intravenously. Only regular insulin can be given IV. Insulin is given subcutaneously, and in rare instances, such as in DKA, is given intramuscularly to some patients. When giving insulin, the nurse must be careful to inject into the *subcutaneous pocket* (space between the fat and muscle layers) only, avoiding depositing the medication directly into the fat or muscle (Fig. 35-10). Insulin is packaged in vials containing 40, 100, or 500 units/ml. Syringes are calibrated by units, and may be 30 units (0.3 ml), 50 units (0.5 ml), or 100 units (1 ml) size. Needles are very fine, usually 25- to 32-gauge, to be as atraumatic to the tissue as possible. Regardless of the units in a vial or on a syringe, the nurse *must* be sure that these match before drawing up a dose of insulin. Needles and syringes used now in the hospital are of the disposable type (Fig. 35-11). However, some older diabetics may still be using glass syringes and metal needles in the home, sterilizing them by boiling. A bottle of insulin that is open and currently in use does not have to be kept in the refrigerator. In fact, it is now felt that insulin should be administered at room temperature, not straight from the refrigerator, to help prevent lipodystrophy. However, any extra bottles on hand should be stored in the refrigerator.

Box 35-3 offers guidelines for preparation of a dose of insulin, one or two types at a time.

Patients who self-inject insulin at home may want to have a family member oversee the procedure. Nurses administering insulin injections should always have the dose drawn up in the syringe checked by another licensed person to prevent medication errors. The diabetic patient should ideally be taught self-injection technique before discharge from the hospital. However, some patients are unable to perform this because of physical problems or intellectual incapacity, visual disturbances, or age. In these cases, family members or others have to administer the injections. Before discharge, either the patient or the significant other, or both, must display the ability to correctly draw up and inject insulin. In a newly diagnosed patient, regular insulin may be injected before each meal. After reasonable control of hyperglycemia is achieved,

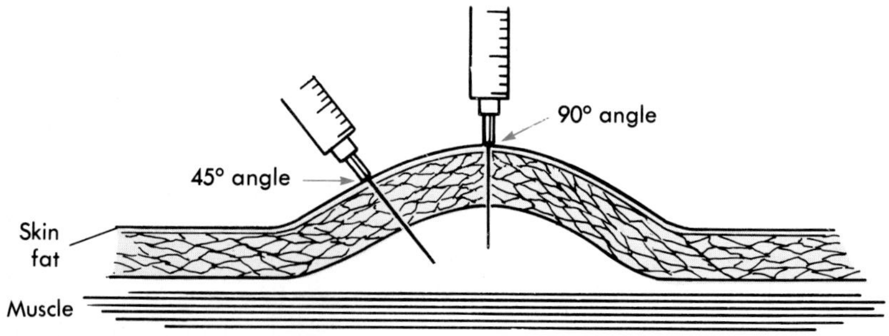

FIG. 35-10 Insulin is injected into the pocket between subcutaneous fat and muscle occurring when the skin is pinched up. The angle of injection may be 45 degrees or 90 degrees.

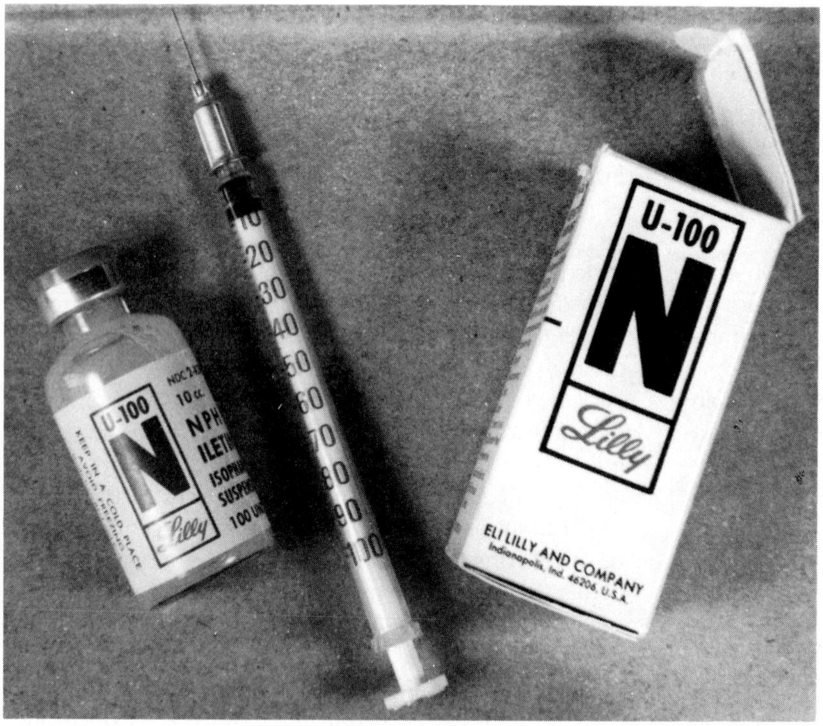

FIG. 35-11 U-100 insulin and disposable U-100 insulin syringe.

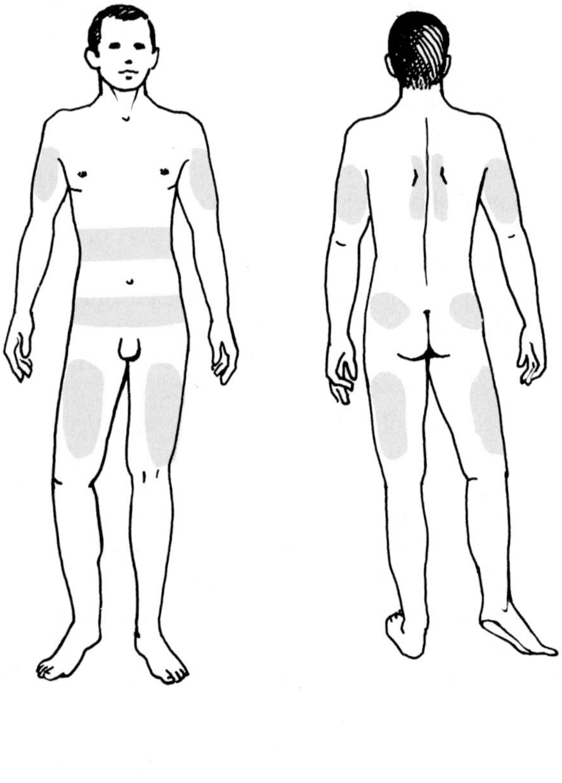

FIG. 35-12 Rotation of sites for insulin injections.

BOX 35-3 PREPARATION OF INSULIN

1. Thoroughly wash hands with warm water and soap.
2. Assemble all equipment needed, such as needle and syringe unit, prep sponge, and insulin.
3. Turn the insulin vial onto its side and gently rotate between the hands several times to be sure it is mixed. The precipitate should be evenly blended. This does not need to be done with regular insulin because it has no precipitate. Never shake insulin vigorously, because this creates air bubbles.
4. Clean the rubber stopper on the vial with a prep sponge.
5. Remove the needle cover and draw in the same amount of air as units of insulin to be injected.
6. Insert the needle into the rubber stopper of the vial and then inject air; invert the bottle with the syringe unit attached, making sure the tip of the needle is below the level of the insulin so air will not be drawn into the syringe.
7. Pull back slowly on the plunger, a few units past the desired dose of insulin.
8. Inspect for air bubbles in the syringe; if any are seen, gently tap the barrel until they rise to the top, then push back into the vial with plunger, to the level of the desired dose of insulin.
9. Holding onto the barrel and plunger, remove the syringe unit and put the needle cover back on. Check insulin dose with a second licensed nurse. Proceed with injection procedure.

TWO INSULINS

1. Follow steps 1 through 5 at left.
2. Insert the desired amount of air into the vial of the longer-acting insulin first.
3. Inject the desired amount of air into the shorter-acting insulin vial; leave the syringe unit in this vial, invert, and proceed through steps 6 through 9 but do not inject yet. *Set the vial of shorter-acting insulin out of reach to prevent accidental reuse.*
4. Insert the needle into the vial of longer-acting insulin, being careful to hold onto the plunger so none of the insulin in the syringe enters that vial.
5. Slowly pull the plunger to the level of the combined total of both types of insulin desired (e.g., regular 10 U, NPH 30 U, totalling 40 U). Do not pull extra units into the syringe! Take special care not to get any air bubbles into the syringe, because they will displace some of the insulin and make the dose incorrect. If this happens, you will have to discard the whole syringeful and start all over again. Check insulin dose with a second licensed nurse.
6. If the dose is correct, proceed with the injection procedure.

Table 35-4 Types of Insulin

Type	Onset of Action (hr)	Peak of Action (hr)	Duration of Action (hr)
RAPID-ACTING			
Regular	½-1	2-4	4-8
Crystalline zinc	<1	2-4	5-8
Semilente	<1	4-7	10-12
INTERMEDIATE-ACTING			
NPH or Humulin N	2-4	6-12	18-28
Globin zinc	2-4	6-10	12-18
Lente	1-4	8-12	18-24
Mixtard; Novolin 70/30	½	4-8	24
LONG-ACTING			
Protamine zinc (PZI)	4-8	14-24	36+
Ultralente	4-8	18-24	36+

the dosage schedule may be changed to once a day, in the morning before breakfast, with the type of insulin being intermediate- or long-acting. See Table 35-4 for types of insulin. Sometimes diabetic patients take two doses of insulin, in divided doses given before breakfast and before the evening meal. The nurse should be alert for signs of hypoglycemia at the peak of action of whatever type of insulin the patient is taking, and the patient should be instructed to notify a member of the nursing staff if any of the following signs of **hypoglycemic (insulin) reaction** occur: faintness, sudden weakness, excessive perspiration, irritability, hunger, palpitations, trembling, or drowsiness.

After appropriate blood or urine testing, the patient will choose an injection site. The subcutaneous pocket is the desired layer into which insulin should be injected. Insulin should *not* be injected into the muscle, because it enters the bloodstream too quickly and could cause hypoglycemia. Site selection is crucial, as is site rotation (Fig. 35-12). Because of differing anatomical absorption rates of insulin, it is currently recommended that injections should be given in all the available areas in a site, such as the thigh, before moving to another site. In this way the diabetic may take eight or more injections, spaced 1 to 1½ inches apart, thus allowing the tissues in other sites to recover more fully before being used again. This technique helps prevent lipodystrophy and lipoatrophy, conditions that can lead to unsightly lumps under the skin and inhibition of insulin absorption. If the patient engages in heavy exercise, an injection site may be chosen where movement will not be as great, because exercise of a body part may increase insulin absorption.

The technique for insulin injection is described in Box 35-4.

There are several new delivery systems now available to the diabetic who finds injections emotionally and/or physically uncomfortable. These include automatic injectors, the jet stream (needleless) injector, and the button infuser.

Oral hypoglycemics are compounds that stimulate the beta cells in the pancreatic islets to produce insulin. These drugs are *not* an oral form of insulin. The two groups of hypoglycemics are the biguanides (DBI) and the sulfonylureas (Table 35-5). Biguanides are rarely used now because of their toxicity. The sulfonylureas cannot be taken by persons who are allergic to sulfa drugs. The main side effect of oral hypoglycemics is hypoglycemic reaction.

Another drug that may be used in the treatment of diabetes mellitus is **glucagon**. Glucagon is a hormone normally secreted by the alpha cells of the pancreas. It stimulates the liver to change stored glycogen into glucose, which is then released into the bloodstream. Glucagon is available in a purified, crystallized form for reconstitution and subcutaneous, intramuscular, or intravenous administration in the event of loss of consciousness as a result of hypoglycemic reaction. The usual dose is 0.5 mg to 1.0 mg for adults, with smaller doses for children. Some form of oral carbohydrate, such as milk and crackers, should be given after the patient regains consciousness. A commercially prepared kit containing glucagon is carried by many diabetics, along with concentrated carbohydrate such as candy or glucose gel.

The surgical treatment of diabetes mellitus, type I (IDDM), is a new and largely experimental area. Two procedures are now available to selected patients. One is pancreas transplant, a procedure first performed at the University of Minnesota in 1966. The other is implantation of an insulin-infusion pump under the skin. Much research into these two surgical procedures is currently being conducted, as is pancreatic islet transplant between identical twins.

Nursing interventions. Persons with diabetes may be hospitalized as a direct result of their disease process, or they may have a different primary diagnosis. The main focus of nursing interventions must always be on the primary diagnosis, but the nurse must remember that the patient is also diabetic and is susceptible to a number of complications in addition to all those experienced by nondiabetic patients.

Daily routine for the diabetic patient includes accurate monitoring of blood glucose levels, either by fingerstick specimens or by laboratory testing. Urine testing, when done, should be on a second-voided specimen each time. Careful attention to diet is important, and the nurse should note the amount of food eaten at each meal and record it accurately. If the type I patient is not hungry, is nauseated, or cannot eat for any other reason, the next dose of insulin may be withheld and administered later, as determined by the physician. If the patient does not like the types of food on the meal tray, the dietitian should be consulted and a visit arranged.

Good skin care is essential for the diabetic, because poor circulation, so common in diabetes, can lead to the development of skin problems. Any abnormalities such as cuts, scratches, or lesions anywhere on the body should be reported to the physician and treated before infection develops. Special foot care is crucial for this patient, because poor circulation and decreased nerve sensation

BOX 35-4 TECHNIQUE FOR INSULIN INJECTION

1. Follow steps 1 through 9 or 1 through 6 from Box 35-3, as before, to prepare the insulin dose.
2. Don disposable gloves.
3. Clean the injection site with a prep swab, using a circular motion. Allow the alcohol to dry. Place the swab between the last two fingers of the hand not used to inject the insulin.
4. Pick up the syringe and remove the needle cover and lay it aside. Hold the syringe like a dart.
5. Using the other hand, gently pinch up at least a 2-inch fold of tissue (not just the skin!).
6. Quickly insert the needle into the top (apex) of the fold, entering the *subcutaneous pocket*. The "soft spot" technique is to insert the needle about 1 inch to the side of the apex of the fold, into softer tissue, entering the pocket. The needle should be inserted at a 90-degree angle unless the patient is very thin and has little subcutaneous tissue. In that case, the angle may be reduced by up to 45 degrees.
7. Release the skin fold and use that hand to steady the barrel of the syringe. Pull back on the plunger to check for blood. If any is seen, remove the syringe unit and start over with a second dose of insulin.
8. If no blood is seen, inject the insulin over a period of 3 to 5 seconds.
9. Place the alcohol swab against the needle hub, at the injection site, and pull the syringe unit straight out in one swift motion. Gently press on the injection site for a few seconds, but *do not massage the site.*
10. Carefully place the entire unit, uncapped, into the sharps container provided.
11. Record the injection site and insulin dose on a chart or other documentation sheet and store insulin and other supplies properly.

Table 35-5 Sulfonylureas

Generic and Brand Name	Usual Daily Dose	Onset of Action (hr)	Peak of Action (hr)	Duration of Action (hr)
Acetohexamide (Dymelor)	250-1500 mg	1	4-5	12-24
Chlorpropamide (Diabinese, Glucamide)	100-500 mg	1	3-6	24-48
Glipizide (Glucotrol)	5-40 mg	1	2-6	12-24
Glyburide (DiaBeta, Micronase)	2.5-20 mg	1	2-4	24
Tolazamide (Tolinase)	100-1000 mg	4-6	4-8	12-24
Tolbutamide (Orinase, Glucamide)	500-3000 mg	½-1	3-5	6-12

(neuropathy) increase the danger of ulcers or other abnormal lesions developing into gangrene. Many patients seek the services of a podiatrist for their foot care. The patient should thoroughly wash the feet with soap and water every day, dry them thoroughly, and inspect them carefully for cracks, blisters, or foreign objects, paying special attention to the area between the toes. Foot soaks or powders are not recommended. Clean socks should be worn daily, and tight garters should be avoided. The toenails should be clipped straight across so the edges do not become ingrown. The nurse should *never* trim the toenails of a diabetic patient without a physician's written order. No hot water bottles or heating pads should be put on the feet, because burns may occur and not be felt. Sturdy, properly fitting shoes should be worn, and the patient should not go barefoot at any time. The physician should be notified immediately of any injury to the toes or feet.

The diabetic who is receiving insulin should be watched very carefully for development of hypoglycemia, especially when the particular kind of insulin being injected is at its peak of action. Hypoglycemia is seen much less frequently in patients receiving oral hypoglycemics, but it can occur.

The emotional aspects of diabetes are numerous, and many patients experience a period of denial after the initial diagnosis. Some patients become very depressed. Since this disease affects all age groups, nursing interventions must be tailored to fit the needs of each patient. Diabetics must have help in working through their feelings, so the nurse must be a good listener and be supportive at all times. The patient who does not satisfactorily resolve any major problems in accepting the diagnosis of diabetes mellitus may be noncompliant with the treatment plan.

The nurse who supervises the diabetic in a home setting must encourage the patient to take the prescribed medication faithfully, eat the right kinds of food, test blood and/or urine correctly, and exercise regularly. If a family member is going to be responsible for the patient's care, the nurse must make sure that the caregiver is functioning adequately in this role. Some patients live alone and do very well caring for themselves, with occasional visits from a home health or public health nurse. Others who have visual disturbances, circulatory problems, or other conditions may need daily visits and more actual nursing intervention, such as help with hygiene, arrangements for meals, and administration of insulin injections. See the nursing care plan for the patient with diabetes mellitus on pp. 902 and 903.

Acute complications. One of the acute complications of DM is coma, which may be attributed to three different causes. The first type of coma is diabetic ketoacidosis (DKA), which results from inadequate amounts of insulin present or from inadequate insulin utilization. The second type, hyperglycemic hyperosmolar nonketotic coma (HHNC), involves no acidosis or ketonemia, but results from excess glucose presence, diuresis, and dehydration without adequate fluid replacement. The third type is hypoglycemic reaction, which results from an excess amount of insulin available, with an inadequate amount of glucose present. DKA and hypoglycemic reaction are compared and contrasted in Table 35-6. Emergency care of the patient experiencing DKA or hypoglycemia is found in the emergency boxes on p. 905.

Another acute complication diabetics face is the development of infections of any kind. The presence of hyperglycemia and ketonemia hinders the phagocytic action of leukocytes. An infection can therefore become more severe and last longer, with poor wound healing taking place. The possibility of DKA increases in the presence of infection, and diabetic control is harder to achieve. Diabetics are often hospitalized for treatment of infections that might be handled on an outpatient basis for the nondiabetic patient.

Long-term complications. Long-term complications of diabetics include blindness, cardiovascular problems, and renal failure. Diabetes causes more new cases of blindness in the United States than any other disease process. Diabetic retinopathy involves progressive changes in the microcirculation of the retina, resulting in hemorrhages, scar tissue formation, and various degrees of retinal detachment. New surgical techniques such as laser beam coagulation of retinal vessels may improve vision for selected patients with early diagnosis. Vascular changes in

Text continued on p. 906.

NURSING CARE PLAN: THE PATIENT WITH DIABETES MELLITUS

DATA: Mrs. Toren is an obese, 52-year-old married woman with NIDDM diagnosed 3 years ago. She was referred to a short-term ambulatory diabetes education program by her physician for instruction on insulin administration since blood glucose control had not been achieved with dietary measures.

The nurse history identified the following:

1. She saw referral as necessary but perceived it and inability to control weight and blood glucose as a personal failure.
2. She maintained inconsistent sleep/activity schedule. (Worked as an LPN 8 PM to 8 AM Saturday and Sunday with 2 to 4 hours sleep during day; arose at 8 AM and retired at 11 PM on other days.)
3. She had accurate knowledge about dietary modifications and had participated successfully in several weight reduction programs with 20- to 40-pound weight loss each time.
4. She does not exercise consistently.
5. She has monitored blood glucose on others and once or twice on self (self-monitoring of blood glucose [SMBG]).
6. She states that work is important to her; satisfactions were derived from work and group socialization, and it "keeps me busy."
7. She fears that her husband will die suddenly at home. Two years ago she had performed CPR when he had a cardiac arrest at home. Realizes that she maintains work schedule "to keep me from worrying about husband."

Objective data included blood glucose, 220 mg/dl; weight, 200 lb; BP 134/84; urine, glucose 2% with no ketones present.

Collaborative nursing actions include teaching Mrs. Toren those measures that would help her achieve control of blood glucose (insulin, diet, and exercise) and to detect, prevent, and treat hypoglycemic reactions. The nurse reported Mrs. Toren's work schedule to the physician and asked for insulin dosage alterations on weekends. The physician was unaware of her work schedule and stated that blood glucose control could not be optimum with this schedule.

Nursing diagnoses	Patient goals	Nursing interventions
Knowledge deficit: Self-injections, self-blood glucose monitoring, related to lack of exposure	Patient will independently administer to self.	Support patient as necessary to self-inject insulin.
	Patient will perform SMBG accurately.	Observe patient's skill in SMBG; correct as necessary.
	Patient will use measurements obtained by SMBG to achieve blood glucose below 140 mg/dl.	Review with patient the effect of activity, dietary intake, and insulin on blood glucose.
	Patient can detect and treat hypoglycemia.	Instruct patient on frequency and timing of SMBG.
		Review with patient signs and symptoms and treatment measures.
		Refer to dietician for modification of diet necessary with insulin and for verification of diet knowledge.
Altered health maintenance, related to ineffective coping skill	Patient will state at least one change that will improve blood glucose control.	Teach patient effects of stress, lack of exercise, and activity pattern on blood glucose.
		Explore with patient willingness and ability to change behaviors: sleep/activity, coping, and exercise.
		Engage patient in mutual problem solving; refrain from prescribing.
		Explore sources for long-term support in learning more effective coping skills; suggest support groups: 1. For spouses of patients with myocardial infarction 2. For weight loss and *maintenance* of weight loss 3. Available at work in health service program
		Suggest to patient that she seek a trial period on day shift on weekends

Table 35-6 Comparison of Diabetic Ketoacidosis and Hypoglycemic Reaction

Assessment	Ketoacidosis (DKA)	Hypoglycemic Reaction
Type of diabetes	Type I (IDDM)	Type I (IDDM) or type II (NIDDM)
Cause	Inadequate insulin present	Too much insulin or oral hypoglycemic agent present
Patient history	Omitted or insufficient dose of insulin; infection; stress; GI upsets; dietary noncompliance	Reduced food intake; delayed meal; too much exercise
Onset of symptoms	Hours to days	Minutes to hours
Previous diagnosis as diabetic	Almost always	Yes; on medication
Age of patient	Usually younger patient	Usually younger patient
Appearance of skin	Hot, dry	Cool, moist
Breath	Fruity (from acetone)	Normal
Mucous membranes	Dry	Moist
Respirations	Deep; may have Kussmaul respirations (air hunger) as a result of metabolic acidosis	Rapid, shallow
Neurosensory	Drowsiness, to coma	Impaired consciousness; personality changes; may lose consciousness
Blood pressure	Low	Normal
Glycosuria and ketonuria	Present	Absent
Polyuria and polydipsia	Present	Absent
Hunger	Absent; may have nausea, vomiting	Present; may be nauseated
Blood glucose level	Usually 300-800 mg/dl	Usually below 50 mg/dl
Emergency treatment	Insulin, usually regular	Glucose (oral or intravenous) or glucagon (subcutaneous, intramuscular, or intravenous)

DIABETIC KETOACIDOSIS (DKA)

USUAL TREATMENT DURING ACUTE STAGE

- Fluid replacement with normal saline intravenously: initially given rapidly using 18-gauge needle and pump controller
- Small dosages of regular insulin: given IV; regular insulin is only kind given IV
- IV replacement of potassium to help move insulin into cells
- Oxygen administration; insertion of nasogastric tube: connected to intermittent suction
- Cardiac monitoring; central venous pressure (CVP) and Swan-Ganz monitoring if available
- Foley catheter usually inserted with intake and output monitored hourly
- Vital signs and neurological status assessed frequently
- Hourly determination of blood glucose level (finger stick or venous sample)

NURSING INTERVENTIONS DURING AND AFTER DKA

- Keep airway patent.
- Maintain patent intravenous infusion at prescribed rate.
- Keep accurate intake and output record.
- Do accurate blood/urine testing for glucose/acetone.
- Monitor vital signs frequently, and assess cardiac status on monitor.
- Assess level of consciousness frequently, and perform neurological checks as ordered.
- Assess the causation of DKA.

HYPOGLYCEMIC REACTION

IMMEDIATE TREATMENT: If Conscious

Give patient 10 to 20 g of oral glucose in some form, such as 4 oz orange juice or regular soft drink (*not* diet drink), half of any kind of candy bar; commercially prepared concentrated dextrose tablets or glucose paste; 1 tube Cake Mate Icing gel (small); 2 tsp sugar or honey; 6 jelly beans or gumdrops; 5 or 6 Lifesavers or other roll candy; 4 animal crackers; 1 granola bar.

IMMEDIATE TREATMENT: If Unconscious

Squeeze one tube of glucagon gel between teeth and gums, in buccal space, or give glucagon 0.5 to 1.0 mg subcutaneously or intramuscularly; get patient to hospital.

Hospitalized patients may receive intravenous bolus of 20 ml of 50% glucose or 50 ml of 20% glucose; glucagon may be given intravenously. May need IV 10% or 20% glucose at 100 ml/hr to follow.

NURSING CARE DURING AND AFTER HYPOGLYCEMIC EPISODE

- Stay with the patient; check vital signs and do fingerstick blood glucose levels.
- Monitor for worsening of condition, or relief of symptoms.
- If patient becomes unconscious, administer glucagon buccal, subcutaneously, intramuscularly, or intravenously.
- Be sure patient ingests food such as milk, crackers with peanut butter (6), or 1 slice cheese and 6 crackers after symptoms terminate.
- Observe closely for 1 to 2 hours after cessation of symptoms.
- Notify physician about the hypoglycemic reaction.
- Assess reason the reaction may have occurred.

EMERGENCY

THERAPEUTIC DIALOGUE

■ Justin, age 15, has been a diabetic for the past 4 years. He is a ninth grader and today is visiting the school nurse, Mrs. Burnett, for a routine update of his records. The nurse senses that he is troubled about something, because he does not display his usual outgoing, friendly behavior.

NURSE: You seem a little down today, Justin. Is there something you'd like to discuss with me?

JUSTIN: No, it's nothing. I'm okay.

NURSE: I know it's hard to put your thoughts into words sometimes. I want you to feel free to tell me anything you'd like to. I'd really like to help.

JUSTIN: *(Silence for a few seconds.)* There's nothing anyone can do about it, anyway, so what's the use?

NURSE: If you'll tell me what's bothering you, I'll do my best to help, and if I can't, maybe I can find someone who can.

JUSTIN: It's just that some of the kids are spreading rumors about me telling everyone that I "shoot up" on drugs! They just don't understand that I *have* to take my insulin! I wish I was normal like all the other kids!

NURSE: It must be really hard for you, feeling different from the others. But a lot of *them* have physical problems, too, like asthma and acne. Very few people have perfect health, Justin. Do you think they're trying to be mean, or are they just uneducated about your particular problem?

JUSTIN: I don't know. I guess they just don't know any better, so they make fun of kids that are different. Some of the guys make fun of Joe because he has to wear glasses . . . *(Stops to think)*.

NURSE: Is there any way we could help them understand about diabetes and why you have to inject insulin? What about the Health Fair at the mall next week?

JUSTIN: My doctor said the American Diabetes Association will have a booth and volunteers will be doing blood glucose testing. Maybe I could work there a couple of hours, and maybe I could make a poster and put it up in our science lab so all the kids in my class could see it.

NURSE: That's a great idea! I know that volunteers of all ages are needed. Why don't we call the local ADA office and get your name on the list of workers?

JUSTIN: Okay—and I'll talk to Mr. Wilson, my science teacher, about putting up a poster. Thanks, Mrs. Burnett! Maybe if the kids understand more about diabetics they won't think I'm so weird. Well, 'bye now. I'll come back after my last class today to see what time I'm supposed to be at the mall!

diabetics, especially capillary changes, contribute to the development of renal sclerosis, often progressing to end-stage renal disease (ESRD). Many of these patients have to undergo either peritoneal dialysis or hemodialysis as a result. Diabetes contributes to accelerated atherosclerotic changes in the blood vessels, so many diabetics experience myocardial infarction, stroke, and the development of gangrene in the lower extremities. A great number of diabetics have to undergo amputation as a result of this. Additionally, nervous system manifestations (diabetic neuropathy) are commonly seen, which cause pain and decreased sensation in the extremities and contribute to the development of diabetic gangrene. Many diabetic men experience problems with impotence or premature ejaculation. Diabetics of either sex may have orthostatic hypotension and bladder or bowel dysfunction.

NURSING DIAGNOSES	NURSING INTERVENTIONS
Knowledge deficit: diabetes mellitus	Assess level of understanding of disease process. Institute diabetic teaching plan. Have patient participate in planning daily routine, anticipating discharge and home care.
Powerlessness	Provide opportunities for patient to express feelings about self and illness. Encourage patient's participation in all aspects of self-care. Provide positive reinforcement. Maintain calm, confident attitude.
Altered peripheral tissue perfusion	Assess peripheral pulses, skin color, temperature, capillary refill. Teach patient to avoid pressure against popliteal area and to avoid constricting hose and socks.
Potential fluid volume deficit	Assess skin turgor for dehydration. Encourage intake of noncaloric liquids.
Altered nutrition: potential for more than body requirements	Arrange consultation with dietitian and reinforce the dietary prescription. Allow patient to verbalize concerns about diet.
Potential impaired skin integrity	Assess feet daily for skin changes and pressure areas. Instruct patient regarding proper foot care. Encourage good hydration and nutritional status.
Ineffective individual coping	Assist patient to assess personal strengths and weaknesses, current stressors, and stress-management skills. Encourage maximal self-care. Assist patient in determining realistic goals. Refer patient to appropriate agencies and services (local support groups, American Diabetes Association).
Potential for injury	Instruct in proper self-injection of insulin; have patient perform return demonstration. Reinforce instructions regarding availability of glucose and glycogen sources. Remove potentially hazardous objects from environment.
Potential noncompliance: diabetic management	Establish therapeutic relationship so patient can express negative feelings. Correct misconceptions about treatment regimen. Assist patient in setting long-term goals for lifetime optimal disease management. Involve significant others whenever possible, and encourage communication between them and the patient.

Patient teaching. There are many important areas of education for the diabetic, including the importance of proper administration of insulin or oral hypoglycemics, as well as their side-effects (see Therapeutic Dialogue); the symptoms of hyperglycemia and hypoglycemia; methods of testing blood glucose levels and of urine testing for glucose and acetone; planning and preparing the prescribed diet; and personal hygiene, emphasizing skin and foot care. The nurse should stress the interrelationship between diet, medication, and exercise. The patient should be instructed to visit the dentist regularly and have an annual examination by an ophthalmologist. Because infections and illnesses of any kind could result in loss of diabetic control, the patient should be instructed to notify the physician at the first sign of any illness. Special plans for travel include providing extra insulin vials and syringes, carrying food and some form of concentrated carbohydrate, and arranging for SMBG or urine testing. Provisions for adequate rest time must be made, because exhaustion may lead to changes in the diabetic's overall condition.

Before discharge from the hospital, the patient should verbalize an understanding of how complications may be prevented and display an interest in maintaining optimal wellness. The nurse should stress the importance of regular medical checkups. The social aspects of diabetes mellitus cannot be ignored. Patients need to learn about lifestyle adjustment and should wear medical alert jewelry and carry medical information wallet cards at all times. Decisions such as whether to attempt pregnancy should be thoroughly explored by women with diabetes. Above all, the patient must accept the responsibility for self-care and recognize that making the right choices can affect life expectancy as well as the quality of life. A current trend is for hospitals to employ a diabetes nurse specialist to develop and implement patient and staff education.

Although the life expectancy for the diabetic is usually decreased, current research and recent advances have led to the hope of a much better prognosis. Early diagnosis and prompt, accurate treatment is essential in promoting longevity. The diabetic's quality of life has been enhanced by better ways to control hyperglycemia and by earlier recognition of developing complications.

REFERENCES AND SUGGESTED READINGS

1. Anagnostakos NP and Tortora GJ: Principles of anatomy and physiology, ed 5, New York, 1987, Harper & Row, Publishers, Inc.
2. Beall GN: Immunologic aspects of endocrine diseases, JAMA 258(20):2956, 1987.
3. Brenner ZR: Diagnostic tests and procedures: applying the nursing process, East Norwalk, Conn, 1987, Appleton & Lange.
4. Byrnes CA: What's new in the diabetic diet, Nurs '87 17(8):58, 1987.
5. Cooper DS: Subclinical hypothyroidism, JAMA 248(2):246, 1987.
6. Decker JL and Gorden P, editors: Understanding and managing diabetes, New York, 1987, Avon Books.
7. Fong E, Ferris EB, and Skelley EG: Body structures and functions, ed 7, Albany, NY, 1989, Delmar Publishers, Inc.
8. Galloway JA, Potvin JH, and Shuman ER, editors: Diabetes mellitus, ed 9, Indianapolis, 1988, Eli Lilly & Co.
9. Hood GH and Dincher JR: Total care, ed 7, St Louis, 1988, The CV Mosby Co.
10. Kim MJ, McFarland GK, and McLane AM: Pocket guide to nursing diagnoses, ed 3, St Louis, 1989, The CV Mosby Co.
11. Lockhart JS and Griffin CW: Tetany, Nurs '88 18(8):33, 1988.
12. Marieb EN: Essentials of human anatomy and physiology, California, 1984, Addison-Wesley Publishing Co.
13. McHenry LM and Salerno E: Mosby's pharmacology in nursing, ed 17, St Louis, 1989, The CV Mosby Co.
14. Memmler RL and Wood DL: Structure and function of the human body, ed 4, Philadelphia, 1987, JB Lippincott Co.
15. Mosby's medical and nursing dictionary, ed 3, St Louis, 1990, The CV Mosby Co.
16. O'Neil JR: Thyroid crisis, Nurs '87 17(11):33, 1987.
17. Phipps WJ, Long BC, and Woods NF: Medical-surgical nursing: concepts and clinical practice, ed 4, St Louis, 1991, The CV Mosby Co.
18. Point Study Group: One-year trial of a remote-controlled implantable insulin infusion system in Type I diabetic patients, Lancet II (8616):866, 1988.
19. Potter PA and Perry AG: Basic nursing theory and practice, ed 2, St Louis, 1991, The CV Mosby Co.
20. Raymond CA: Acromegaly said to respond to proton therapy, JAMA 259(6):788, 1988.
21. Raymond CA: Insulin-dependent diabetes mellitus called epidemiologist's dream, JAMA 259(11):1614, 1988.
22. Rivkees SA, Bode HH, and Crawford JD: Long-term growth in juvenile-acquired hypothyroidism: the failure to achieve normal adult stature, N Engl J Med 318(10):599, 1988.
23. Solomon EP and Phillips GA: Understanding human anatomy and physiology, Philadelphia, 1987, WB Saunders Co.
24. Tarn AC and others: Predicting insulin-dependent diabetes, Lancet I(8590):845, 1988.
25. Thatcher G: Insulin injections: the case against random rotation, Am J Nurs 85(6):690, 1985.
26. Thibodeau GA and Anthony CP: Structure and function of the body, ed 8, St Louis, 1988, Times Mirror/Mosby College Publishing.
27. Thomas V: Life sciences for nursing and health technologies, California, 1974, Technicourses, Inc.
28. Thompson JM and others: Mosby's clinical manual of nursing practice, ed 2, St Louis, 1989, The CV Mosby Co.
29. Treseler KM: Clinical laboratory and diagnostic tests, ed 2, East Norwalk, Conn, 1988, Appleton & Lange.
30. Tucker SM and others: Patient care standards, ed. 4, 1988, The CV Mosby Company.
31. Waldrop JW: The demographics of diabetes, American Demographics, pp 45-47, April, 1987.
32. Whaley LF and Wong DL: Essentials of pediatric nursing, ed 3, St Louis, 1989, The CV Mosby Co.
33. Whaley LF and Wong DL: Nursing care of infants and children, ed 4, St Louis, 1991, The CV Mosby Co.
34. Williams SR: Nutrition and diet therapy, ed 5, St Louis, 1988, The CV Mosby Co.

CHAPTER CHALLENGE

KEY POINTS

- Endocrine glands are ductless glands that release chemicals (hormones) into the bloodstream to regulate body activities.
- The pituitary gland located in the brain is the master gland of the endocrine system.
- Hormones have a generalized effect on metabolism, growth and development, and reproduction.
- The endocrine glands regulate themselves by a series of negative feedback messages.
- The hormones secreted by the endocrine glands affect tissues of the entire body, and an imbalance in their levels may contribute to pathological changes in many different systems.
- Acromegaly and gigantism, disorders of the pituitary gland, result in growth changes that may lead to negative effects on the patient's self-image and self-esteem.
- Diabetes insipidus is a disorder of the posterior pituitary and must not be confused with diabetes mellitus, a disorder of the pancreas.
- When caring for the hyperthyroid patient, the nurse must provide for adequate rest periods and be sure that fluid and food intake meet the patient's nutritional needs.
- The emotions of the hyperthyroid patient are very labile, so the nurse must try to eliminate sources of stress from the environment, to help prevent emotional trauma.
- ^{131}I should not be administered to a pregnant patient because of the risk of danger to the fetus; pregnant nurses should not care for these patients.
- Three postoperative complications may be life threatening to the thyroidectomy patient: hemorrhage, tetany, and thyroid crisis.
- The hypothyroid patient may experience sluggish mental and physical functioning, so the nurse must be patient and allow adequate time for nursing routines.
- The prognosis for papillary adenocarcinoma of the thyroid is excellent, because few of these tumors metastasize.
- When administering intravenous calcium chloride to any patient, the nurse must be careful that none of the drug extravasates, because tissue sloughing may result.
- The extreme hypertension often seen in patients with pheochromocytoma may result in CVA.
- Depression is very common in the patient who suffers from Cushing's syndrome; the nurse must be alert for suicidal thoughts and suicide attempts by this patient.
- The three main facets of medical treatment for the patient with diabetes mellitus are diet, exercise, and medication.
- IDDM is usually first diagnosed in persons under the age of 30; NIDDM is more commonly found after age 40, and the incidence increases with the aging process.
- The elderly diabetic may have a very high blood glucose level before excreting any into the urine because of an increased renal threshold for glucose.
- The diabetic diet must be individualized, taking many factors into consideration, such as age, life-style, food preferences, and the ability to cook and store food.
- The insulin-dependent diabetic must have access to a source of quick glucose at all times, in the event of a hypoglycemic reaction.
- The nurse must become familiar with the clinical manifestations of both DKA and hypoglycemic reaction to properly assess diabetic patients, as well as educate them in self-care.
- Patients on insulin therapy and oral hypoglycemics must be observed carefully during the time of peak action of the medication, and treatment must be initiated promptly if hypoglycemia develops.
- DKA can result in seizures, brain damage, or death for the diabetic patient.

STUDY QUESTIONS

1. The hormones responsible for "fight or flight" are:
   a. Estrogen and testosterone
   b. FSH and LH
   c. Epinephrine and norepinephrine
   d. Calcitonin and parathormone
2. The hormones responsible for blood calcium levels are:
   a. Calcitonin and parathormone
   b. Estrogen and progesterone
   c. Melatonin and FSH
   d. Thyroxine and parathormone
3. The main characteristics of diabetes insipidus are:
   a. Severe headache and visual disturbances
   b. Massive weight loss and poor skin turgor
   c. Decreased blood sodium level and oliguria
   d. Intense polydipsia and marked polyuria
4. Thyroidectomy should be postponed, if possible, until the patient is in a euthyroid state because of:
   a. The possibility of excess bleeding during the surgery
   b. The danger of thyroid crisis preoperatively
   c. The demands placed on the patient's physical reserves
   d. The danger of damage to the laryngeal nerve during surgery
5. After thyroidectomy, internal bleeding in the operative area may cause the following:
   a. Increased blood pressure, with decreased pulse rate
   b. Restlessness and a feeling of fullness in the neck
   c. Severe bouts of nonproductive coughing
   d. The appearance of bright red blood on the dressing
6. Emergency treatment of thyroid crisis includes administration of:
   a. Sodium calcium IV, slowly
   b. Sodium iodide and corticosteroids IV
   c. Large amounts of thyroid hormone orally
   d. Electrolyte solutions containing glucose, IV
7. Chvostek's sign and Trousseau's sign are tests to determine:
   a. Presence of low levels of blood calcium
   b. Presence of high levels of blood calcium
   c. Presence of low levels of blood sodium
   d. Presence of high levels of blood sodium
8. The main clinical manifestation of pheochromocytoma is:
   a. Hypotension
   b. Hypertension
   c. Hypercalcemia
   d. Hypoglycemia
9. The most common cause of diabetes mellitus is:
   a. Eating too many sweets
   b. A viral infection
   c. Genetic predisposition
   d. Not known fully at this time
10. The proper rotation of insulin injection sites is important primarily for the prevention of:
    a. Hypoglycemia
    b. Subcutaneous infections
    c. Lipoatrophy and lipodystrophy
    d. Malabsorption of insulin
11. If urine testing for glucose is done, the most accurate results will be obtained by:
    a. Testing of the first morning voided specimen
    b. Using a catheterized urine sample
    c. Use of the dipstick method
    d. Testing a double-voided specimen
12. The diabetic patient experiencing a hypoglycemic reaction will probably have which of the following signs and symptoms:
    a. Hot, dry, flushed skin; polyuria
    b. Moist, cool skin; hunger; weakness
    c. Blood glucose level of 300 mg/dl or higher
    d. Large amounts of ketones in the urine

36

Care of the Patient with a Reproductive Disorder

HAZEL WALKER

LEARNING OBJECTIVES

After reading this chapter, the student should be able to do the following:

- Define the key terms.
- List and describe the functions of the organs of the male reproductive tract.
- List and describe the functions of the organs of the female reproductive tract.
- Discuss menstruation and the hormones necessary for a complete cycle.
- Discuss the impact of illness on the patient's sexuality.
- List nursing interventions for patients with menstrual disturbances.
- Discuss nursing interventions for the patient undergoing diagnostic studies related to the reproductive system.
- Discuss the importance of the Papanicolaou smear test in early detection of cancer.
- Discuss four important points to be addressed in discharge planning for the patient with pelvic inflammatory disease (PID).
- List four nursing diagnoses pertinent to the patient with endometriosis.
- Identify the clinical manifestations seen in the patient with a vaginal fistula.
- Discuss the four major areas of postoperative concerns in the nursing interventions for a patient undergoing hysterectomy.
- Identify four nursing diagnoses pertinent to the patient with ovarian cancer.
- Describe six important points to emphasize in the teaching of breast self-examination.
- Compare five surgical approaches for the patient with cancer of the breast.
- Discuss nursing interventions for the patient after a mastectomy.
- List several discharge planning instructions for the mastectomy patient.
- Describe nursing interventions for the patient with prostatitis.
- Distinguish between hydrocele and varicocele.
- Discuss the importance of monthly testicular self-examination beginning at 15 years of age.
- Discuss patient education related to prevention of sexually transmitted diseases.

RELATED TOPICS OF INTEREST

- Care of the patient with AIDS (Chapter 40)
- Care of the patient with cancer (Chapter 41)
- Normal pregnancy (Chapter 42)
- Normal labor and delivery (Chapter 43)
- Care of the mother and newborn (Chapter 44)
- Care of the mother and newborn at risk (Chapter 45)

KEY TERMS

Define the following:

- amenorrhea
- areola
- Bartholin's gland
- candidiasis
- carcinoma in situ
- cervix
- chancre
- *Chlamydia trachomatis*
- circumcision
- climacteric
- coital
- colporrhaphy
- colposcopy
- Cowper's glands
- cryptorchidism
- culdoscopy
- curettage
- dysmenorrhea
- dyspareunia
- endometriosis
- epididymis
- epididymitis
- fallopian tubes
- fundus
- genitalia
- hymen
- hypermenorrhea
- hysterosalpingo-oophorectomy
- labia majora
- laparoscopy
- mammography
- menarche
- menorrhagia
- metrorrhagia
- Papanicolaou (Pap) smear test
- phimosis
- prepuce
- procedentia
- quadratectomy
- seminal vesicles
- spermatogenesis
- trichomoniasis
- tylectomy
- vagina
- zygote

Conception and birth are made possible through the dynamics of the normally functioning male and female reproductive systems. Reproduction of like individuals is necessary for the continuation of the species. The male and female sex glands (gonads) produce the gametes (sperm and ova) that unite to form a fertilized egg (zygote), the beginning of a new life. This chapter is dedicated to the understanding of the unique characteristics of both of these systems.

ANATOMY AND PHYSIOLOGY

Male Reproductive System

The organs of the male reproductive system include the testes, the penis, a ductal system, and the accessory glands (Fig. 36-1). These structures have various functions: producing and storing sperm, depositing sperm for fertilization, and developing the male secondary sex characteristics.

Testes (testicles). The two oval testes (gonads) are enclosed in a saclike structure, the scrotum, which lies suspended from the exterior abdominal wall. This keeps the temperature in the testes below the normal body core temperature, which is necessary for viable sperm production and storage.

Each testis is divided into lobules by a fibrous tissue called the *tunica albuginea.* Each lobule contains one to three coiled seminiferous tubules that produce the sperm cells. After puberty millions of sperm cells are produced daily. Small clusters of interstitial cells surround the seminiferous tubules throughout the testes. These cells (cells of Leydig) are responsible for the production of the male sex hormore *testosterone.* Testosterone is responsible for the development of male secondary sex characteristics.

Ductal system

Epididymis. Sperm produced in the seminiferous tubules immediately travel to a network of ducts called the

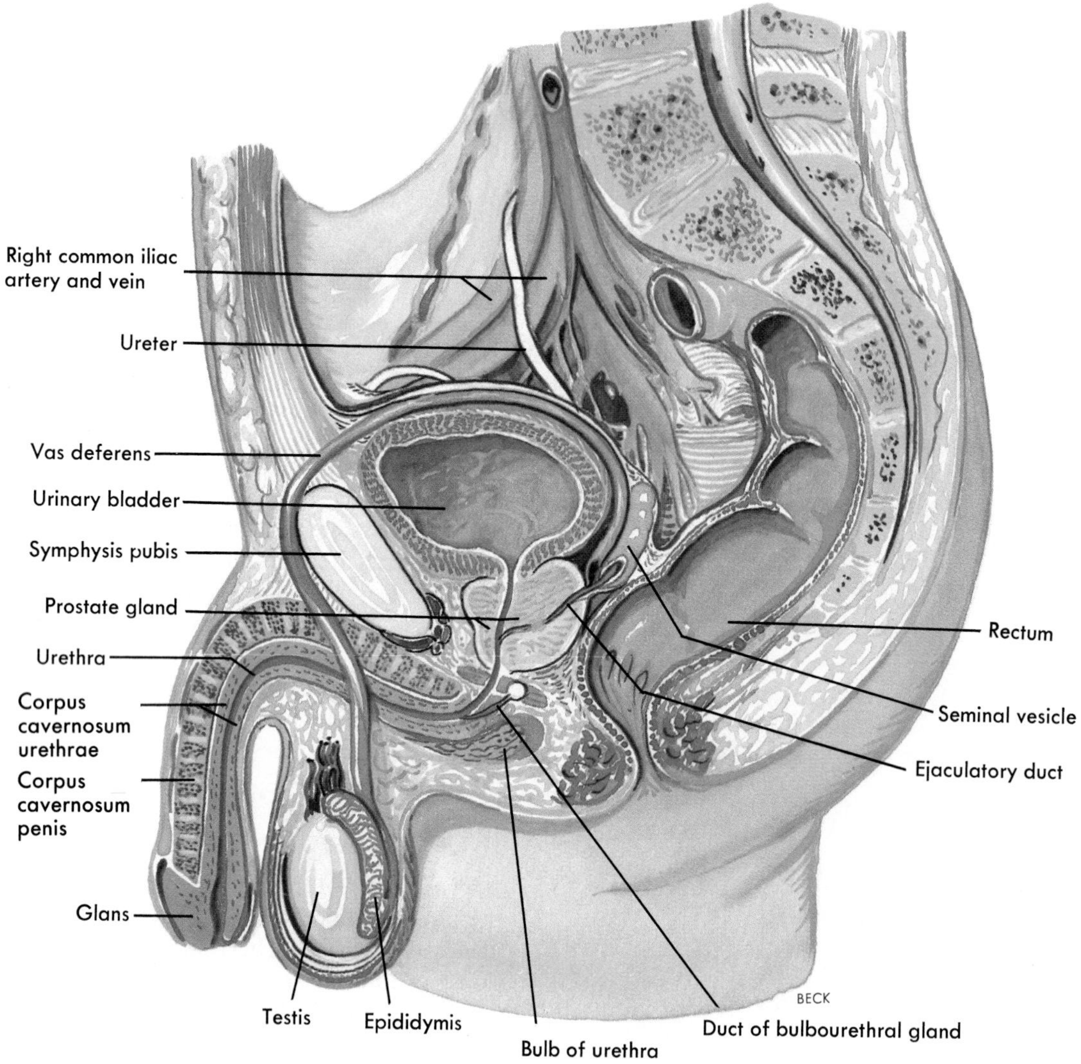

FIG. 36-1 Longitudinal section of the male pelvis showing the location of the male reproductive organs.

rete testis. These passageways contain cilia that sweep the sperm out of the testes into the **epididymis,** a tightly coiled tube structure that lies superior to the testes and extends posteriorly. The immature sperm are stored here to mature and gain strength to enable them to fertilize the ovum. This maturing process can last from a few hours to 10 days. If the sperm are not used after 4 weeks, they are reabsorbed into the body. With sexual stimulation the walls of the epididymis contract, forcing the sperm along the reproductive system.

Ductus deferens (vas deferens). The ductus deferens is approximately 18 inches long and rises along the posterior wall of the testes. As it moves upward it passes through the inguinal canal into the pelvic cavity and loops over the urinary bladder. The ductus deferens, nerves, and blood vessels are enclosed in a connective tissue sheath called the *spermatic cord*.

If a man elects to be sterilized for birth control management, it is a simple procedure to make small slits on either side of the scrotum and sever the ductus deferens. This procedure is called a *vasectomy*. It renders the man sterile because sperm can no longer be expelled.

Ejaculatory duct and urethra. Behind the urinary bladder, the ejaculatory duct connects with the ductus deferens. It is only 1 inch long. It unites with the urethra to pass through the prostate gland. The urethra extends the length of the penis, ending at the bulb of the penis with the urinary meatus. The urethra carries both sperm and urine, but because of the urethral sphincter it does not do so at the same time.

Accessory glands. The ductal system transports and stores sperm. The accessory glands, which produce the liquid portion, seminal fluid (semen), include the seminal vesicles, prostate gland, and the Cowper's glands. The thick, alkaline fluid makes up 60% of the volume of the semen. Alkalinity protects the sperm from the acid condition of the vagina and increases the motility of the sperm. With each ejaculation (2 to 5 ml), approximately 200 to 500 million sperm are released. Although it takes only one sperm to unite with one egg to cause fertilization, it takes many sperm to break down the outer coating of the egg (zona pellucida) to allow entry of the single sperm.

Seminal vesicles. The **seminal vesicles** are paired structures that lie at the base of the bladder and produce 60% of the volume of semen. In addition to its alkalinity, the fluid is high in fructose, a sugar that provides nourishment and energy for the sperm. The fluid is released into the ejaculatory duct to meet with the sperm.

Prostate gland. The single, doughnut-shaped prostate gland surrounds the neck of the bladder and urethra; it secretes 20% of the volume of the thick, alkaline semen. It is a firm structure about the size of a chestnut, composed of muscular and glandular tissue. The ejaculatory duct passes obliquely through the posterior part of the gland. With the aging process the prostate gland often hypertrophies, leading to difficulty in urination, because the gland surrounds the urethra.

Cowper's glands. The tiny, pea-sized **Cowper's glands** (bulbouretheral glands) secrete a clear mucus that drains into the urethra. This fluid contributes to the total volume of the semen and also provides lubrication during sexual intercourse.

The urethra and penis. The male urethra serves the twofold purpose of conveying urine from the bladder and carrying the reproductive cells and secretions to the outside. The cylindrical penis is the organ of copulation. The shaft of the penis ends with an enlarged tip called the *glans penis*. The skin covering the penis lies in folds around the glans; this tissue is called the **prepuce** or foreskin. This excess tissue is sometimes removed in a surgical procedure called *circumcision* to prevent **phimosis** (a tightness of the prepuce of the penis that prevents the retraction of the foreskin over the glans).

Three masses of erectile tissue containing many sinuses fill the shaft of the penis. With sexual stimulation the sinuses fill with blood, causing the penis to become erect. After the penis ejaculates the semen, it returns to its flaccid state.

Sperm. At puberty, sperm production **(spermatogenesis)** begins and continues throughout life. The mature sperm consists of three distinct parts: (1) the head, which contains the enzyme hyaluronidase, (2) the midpiece, which carries on metabolism to provide energy for locomotion, and (3) the tail or flagellum, which propels the sperm. Mature sperm, once deposited in the female reproductive system, live approximately 48 hours. If they come in contact with a mature egg, the enzyme on the head of the sperm bombards the egg in an attempt to break down the coating of the egg (zona pellucida) (Fig. 36-2). It takes thousands of sperm to break the coating, but only one sperm enters and causes fertilization, and the remaining sperm disintegrate.

Female Reproductive System

The organs of the female reproductive system include the ovaries, uterus, fallopian tubes, and vagina (Figs. 36-3 and 36-4). These organs, along with a few accessory structures, produce the ovum, house the fertilized egg, maintain the embryo, and nurture the newborn infant. The ability to conceive and nurture this new human being requires the intricate balance of many hormones and the menstrual cycle.

Ovaries. The paired ovaries (gonads) are the size and shape of almonds. They are covered with epithelium and are located bilateral to the uterus, immediately inferior to the fallopian fimbriae. They are supported by the ovarian and broad ligaments. At puberty they release the female sex hormones estrogen and progesterone and release a mature egg during the menstrual cycle. Each ovary contains 30,000 to 40,000 microscopic ovarian follicles.

At puberty, the female's body prepares for ovulation (Fig. 36-5) and the possibility of pregnancy each 21 to 45 days. The normal or usual cycle is 28 days. This series of preparations is called the menstrual cycle and will be discussed in detail later in the chapter.

The ovaries prepare an egg (ovum) in a pocket- or envelope-shaped structure called a *graafian follicle*. The cells of the follicle walls secrete estrogen. When an ovum has ripened, the follicle ruptures and releases the ovum from the surface of the ovary into the abdominal cavity. The fingerlike projections of the fallopian tubes, fimbriae, sweep the ovum into the fallopian tubes. Once this mature ovum has been expelled, the follicle is transformed into a solid glandular mass called the *corpus luteum,* which means "yellow body." This structure secretes both estrogen and progesterone. Normally the corpus luteum shrinks and is replaced by scar tissue called *corpus albicans*.

Fallopian tubes (oviducts). The **fallopian tubes** are connected to either side of the upper portion (fundus) of the uterus. They are approximately 12 cm (4 inches) long with fimbriae at the distal ends. The entire inner surfaces of the tubes are lined with cilia. They are composed of three layers of tissue: (1) mucosa, the inner layer, (2) muscle, the middle layer, and (3) serosa, the outer layer. When the graafian follicle of the ovary ruptures and releases the mature ovum, the fimbriae sweep the mature ovum into the fallopian tube. Fertilization takes place in the outer third of this tube, and the fertilized egg **(zygote)** is moved along the tube by the combination of muscular peristaltic movements and the sweeping action of the cilia. If the mature ovum is not fertilized, it disintegrates. In about one of every 250 pregnancies, the zygote imbeds

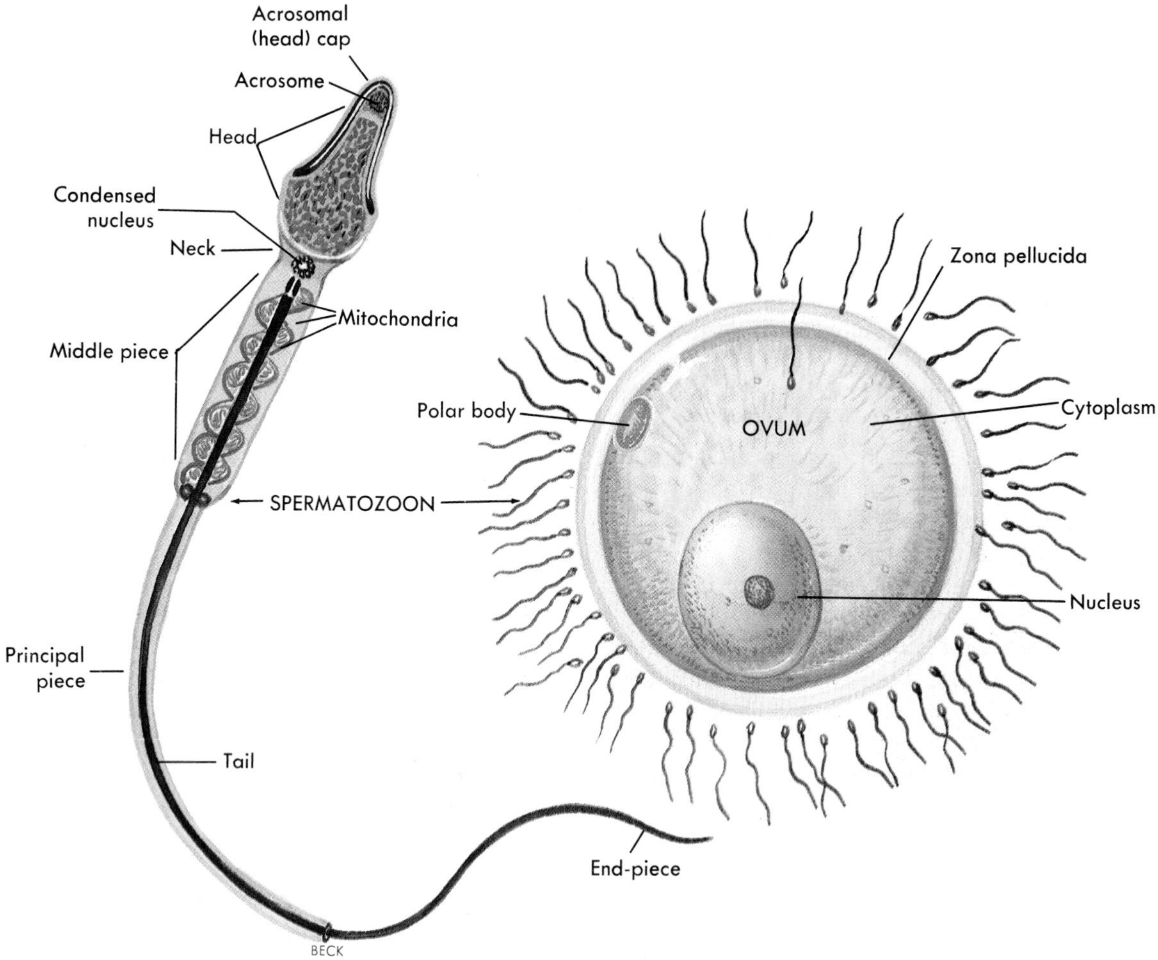

FIG. 36-2 Left, a sex cell (spermatozoon) greatly enlarged. Right, a female sex cell (ovum) surrounded by sperm at time of fertilization.

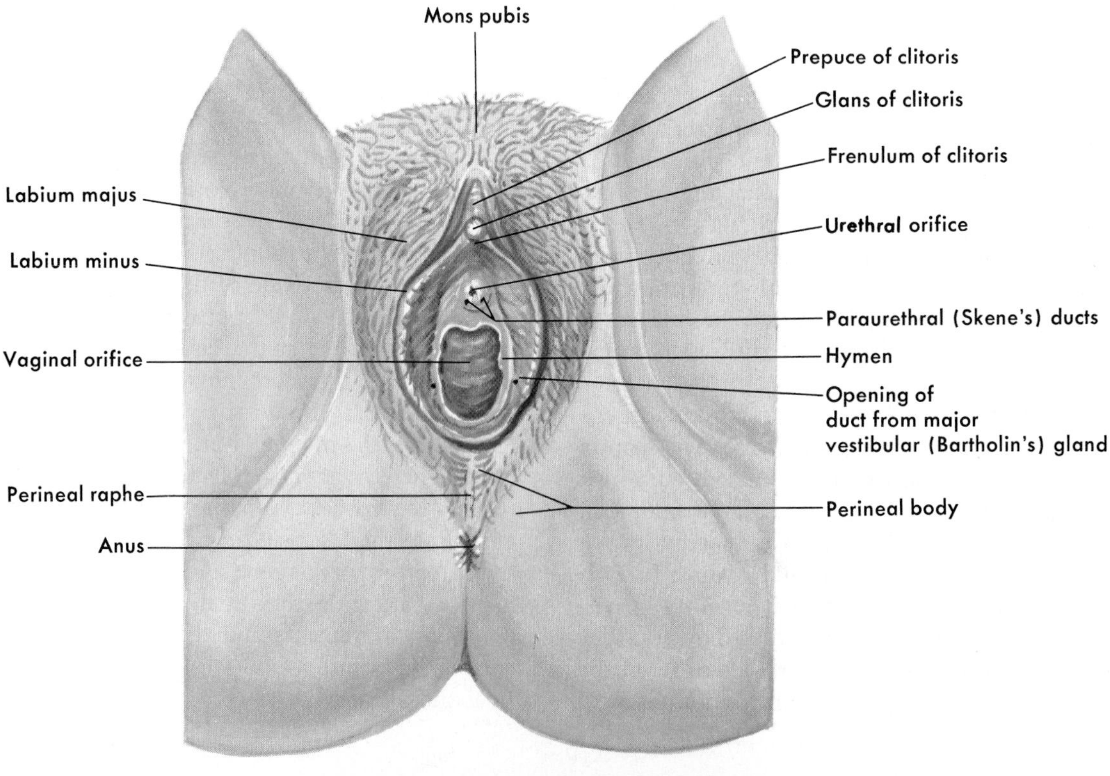

FIG. 36-3 External female genitals (the vulva).

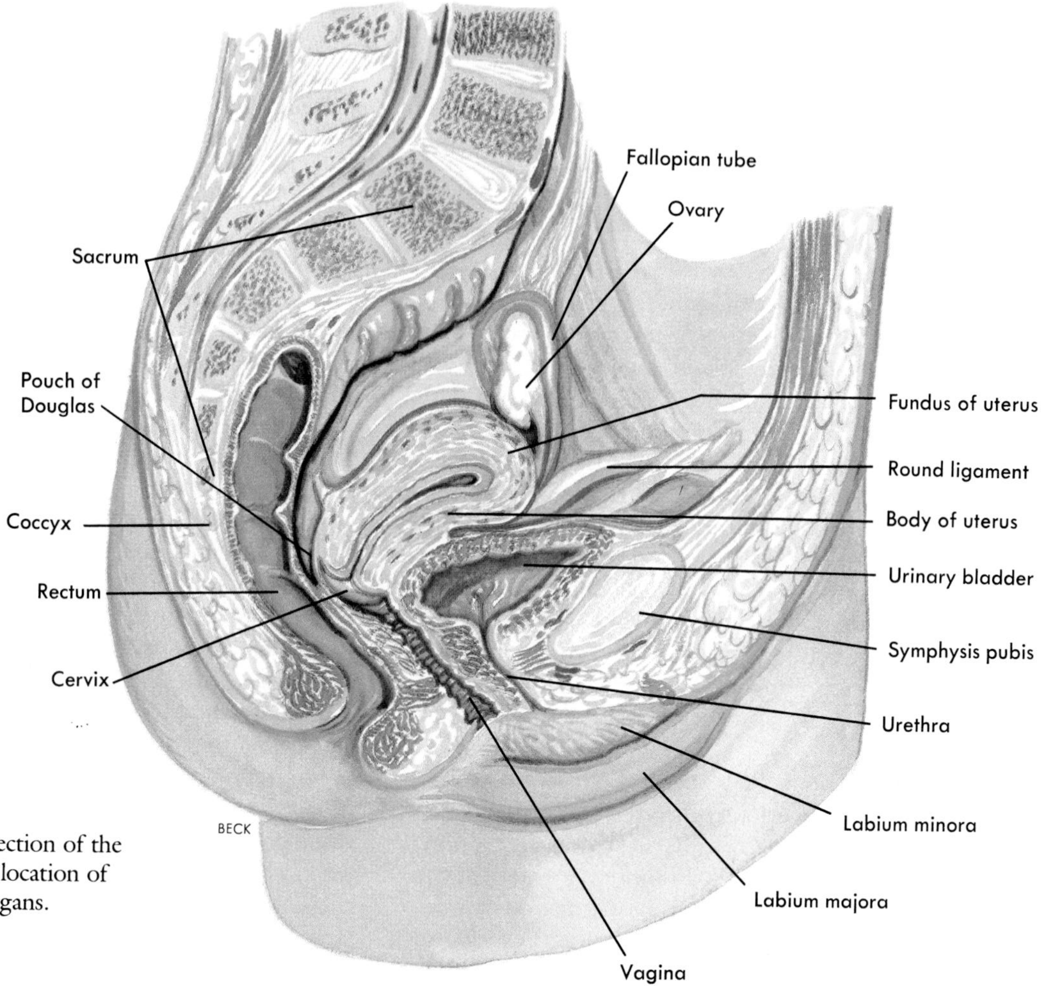

FIG. 36-4 Longitudinal section of the female pelvis showing the location of the female reproductive organs.

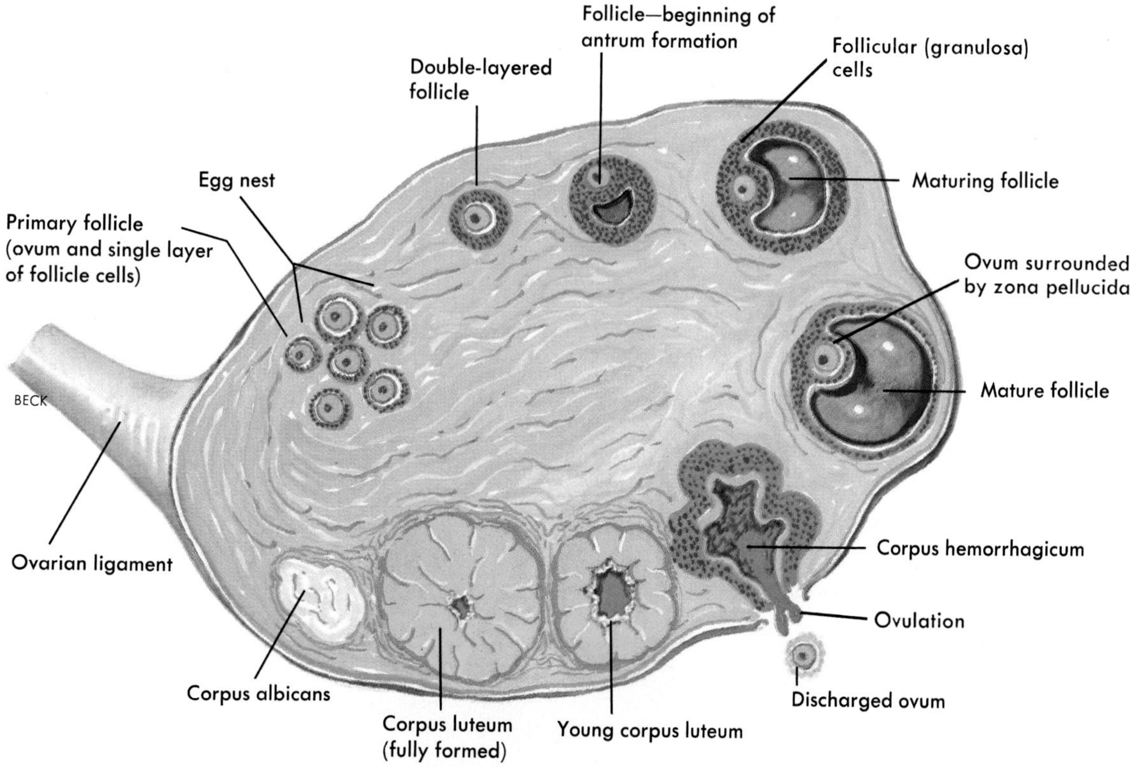

FIG. 36-5 Mammalian ovary showing successive stages of ovarian (graafian) follicle and ovum development. Begin with the first stage (egg nest) and follow around clockwise to the final stage (corpus albicans).

in the fallopian tube rather than sweeping along to the uterus. This condition is called *ectopic pregnancy* and results in the rupturing of the fallopian tube, a medical emergency.

Uterus. The uterus is shaped like an inverted pear and measures 3 inches (7.5 cm) by 2 inches (5 cm) by 1 inch (2.5 cm) in the nonpregnant state. It is situated between the urinary bladder and the rectum and is supported by the broad and round ligaments. It consists of three layers of tissue: (1) endometrium, the inner layer, composed of mucous membrane, (2) myometrium, the middle layer, composed of muscle tissue, and (3) perimetrium, the outer layer, composed of serous membrane.

The uterus is divided into three major portions (Fig. 36-6). The upper, rounded portion of the uterus, the **fundus,** is the insertion site of the fallopian tubes. The larger midsection is called the *corpus* or body. The smaller, narrower lower portion is called the **cervix.** Part of the cervix actually descends into the vaginal vault. During pregnancy the uterus is capable of enlarging up to 500 times its size.

The uterus is a remarkable organ. Each month it prepares for implantation of a fertilized ovum. If pregnancy does not occur, the lining sloughs off with menstruation. If pregnancy does occur, it allows for development of the fetus for 9 months. At the end of this period it goes through a series of contractions (labor) and expels the infant. To prevent hemorrhage after childbirth it contracts sharply. Because the muscle fibers run in all directions and the blood vessels are intertwined between them, this clamping action prevents bleeding.

Vagina. The **vagina** is a thin-walled, muscular, tubelike structure approximately 3 inches (7.5 cm) long. It is located between the urinary bladder and the rectum. The superior portion articulates to the cervix of the uterus; the inferior portion opens to the outside. The vagina is lined with mucous membrane, which is responsible for most of the lubrication during sexual activity. The walls of the vagina normally lie in folds called *rugae.* This enables the vagina to stretch to receive the penis during intercourse and to allow the passage of the infant during the birth process.

The external opening of the vagina is covered by a thin membrane called the **hymen.** For centuries the hymen was a symbol of virginity, but it is now realized that rigorous exercise or insertion of a tampon for menstrual flow may tear the hymen. If the hymen has remained intact, it is ruptured with coitus (intercourse).

External genitalia. The reproductive structures located outside the body are the external **genitalia** or vulva. Included are the mons pubis, labia majora, labia minora, clitoris, and vestibule.

Located superior to the symphysis pubis is a mound of fatty tissue, covered with coarse hair. This structure is the mons pubis. Extending from the mons pubis to the perineal floor are two large folds of tissue called the **labia majora** (large lips). These structures protect the inner structures and are also covered with pubic hair. In addition, the labia majora contain sensory nerve endings and an assortment of sebaceous (oil) and sudoriferous (sweat) glands. Directly beneath the labia majora lie the

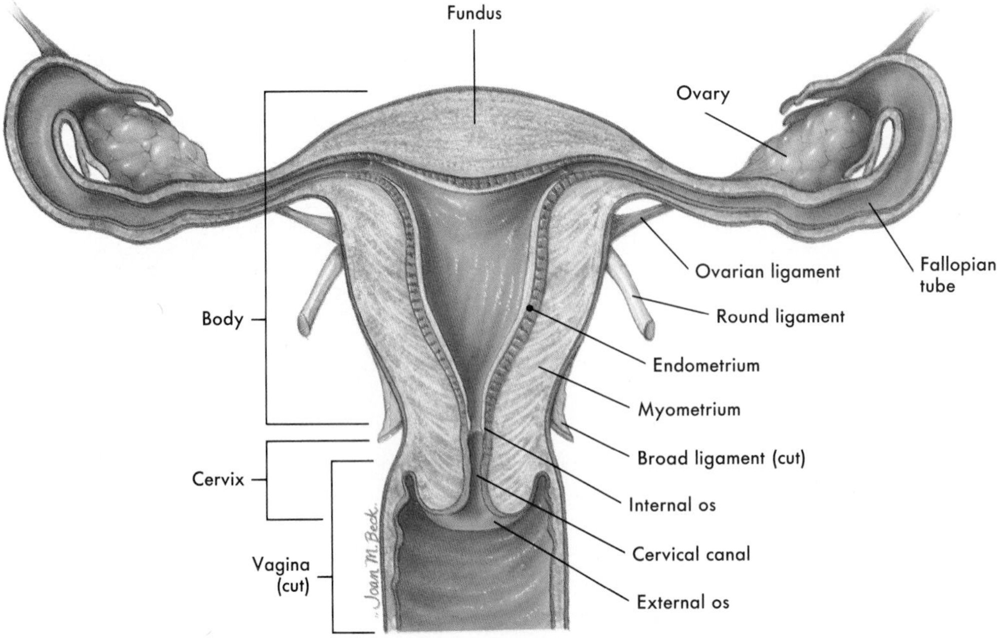

FIG. 36-6 Sectioned view of the uterus showing relationship to ovaries and vagina.

labia minora (small lips); these are smaller folds of tissue, devoid of any pubic hair, that merge anteriorly to form the prepuce of the clitoris.

The clitoris is comparable to the male penis. It too is composed of erectile tissue that becomes engorged with blood during sexual stimulation. It is the center of sexual excitement for the female.

The space enclosing the structures located beneath the labia minora is called the vestibule. It contains the clitoris, urinary meatus, hymen (if present), and the vaginal opening.

Accessory glands. Bilateral to the urinary meatus lie the paraurethral or Skene's glands. These glands are responsible for the secretion of mucus and are similar in function to the prostate gland in the male. Bilateral to the vaginal opening are the greater **Bartholin's** (vestibular) **glands.** These glands secrete a mucuslike secretion that lubricates the area for sexual intercourse. Their secretion is similar to the fluid released by the bulbourethral glands in the male.

Perineum. The area enclosed by the posterior end of the labia (forchette) and the anterior portion of the anus is called the *obstetrical perineum;* the area enclosing the region containing the reproductive structures is referred to as the *general perineum.* The perineum is diamond shaped and starts at the symphysis pubis and extends to the anus. Sometimes with childbirth, the physician clips the perineum extending from the forchette in a procedure called an *episiotomy* to prevent tearing of tissue with childbirth.

Mammary glands (breasts). The breasts are attached to the pectoral (chest) muscles by connective tissue and to the skin and deep fascia by ligaments of Cooper (suspensory ligaments) (Fig. 36-7). Breast tissue is identifiable in both sexes. During puberty several things occur to the female breasts that change the size, shape, and ability to function.

Each breast contains 15 to 20 lobes that are separated by adipose tissue. The amount of adipose tissue is responsible for the size of the breast. It is important to realize that size of the breast has no impact on the ability of the breast to function—to produce and eject milk. Within each lobe there are many lobules that contain milk-producing cells (alveoli or acini); these lobules lead directly to the lactiferous ducts that empty directly into the nipple.

The nipple is composed of smooth muscle that allows it to become erect. The dark pink tissue surrounding the nipple is called the **areola.** Small papillae on the aerola are called the *tubercles of Montgomery.* These structures are sebaceous glands that secrete oil to keep the nipple supple, to prevent it from drying and cracking.

Milk production does not start until the woman has given birth. At this time, under the influence of prolactin, the milk is formed. The hormone *oxytocin* allows the milk to be released. The amount of milk produced is directly related to the stimulus of the suckling infant. The more the infant nurses, the more milk is produced.

Menstrual cycle. At puberty, the female reproductive system, under the influence of hormones, prepares itself

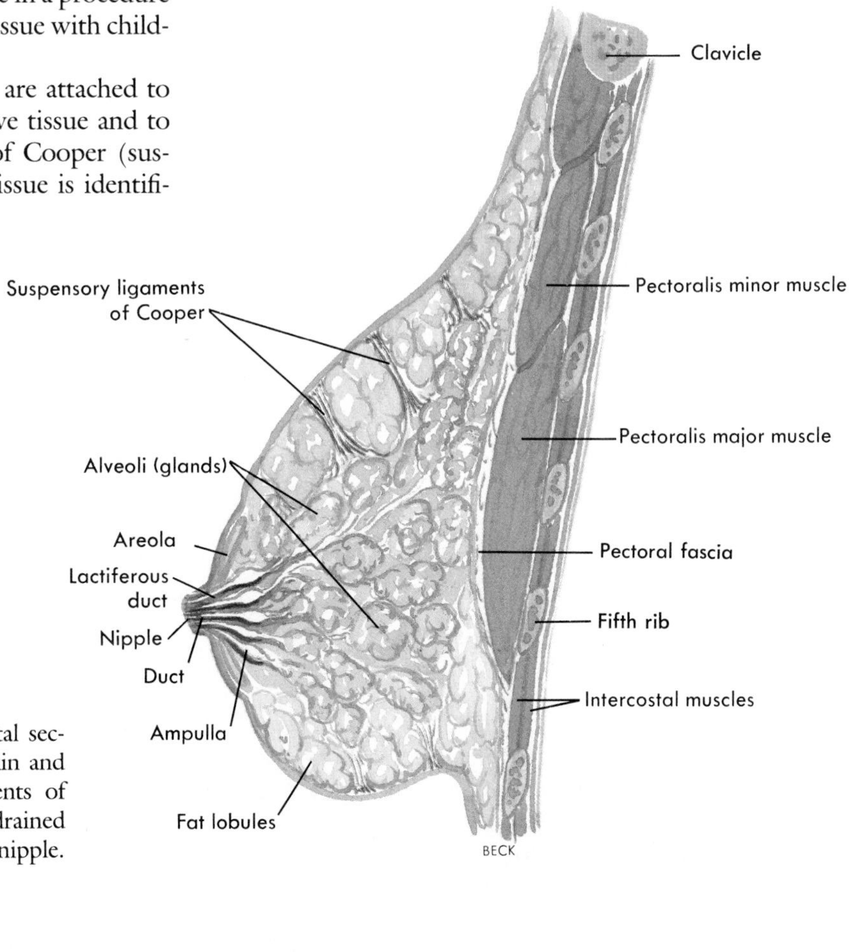

FIG. 36-7 Lateral view of the breast (sagittal section). The gland is fixed to the overlying skin and pectoral muscles by the suspensory ligaments of Cooper. Each lobule of secretory tissue is drained by a lactiferous duct that opens through the nipple.

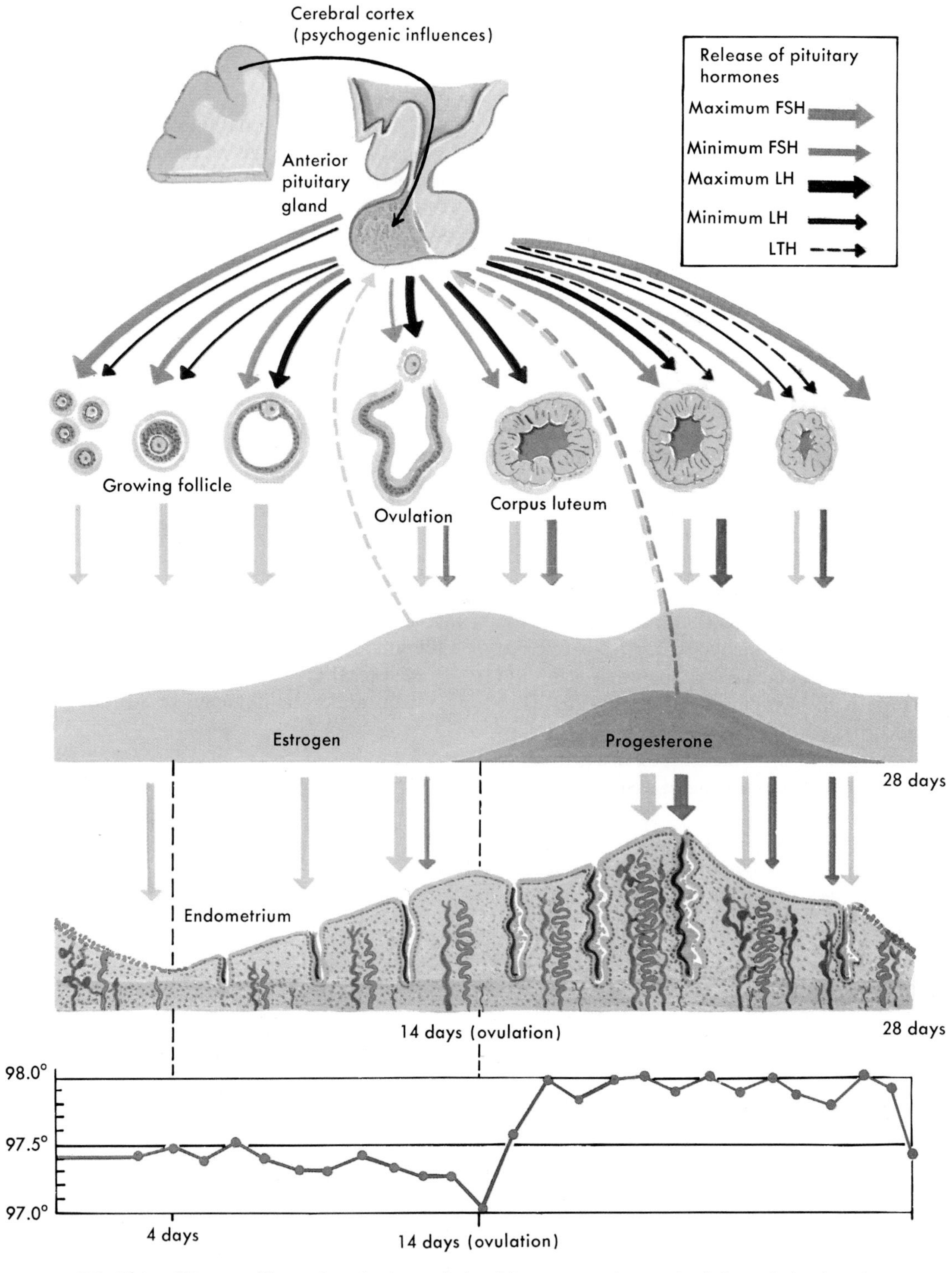

FIG. 36-8 Diagram illustrating the interrelationships among the cerebral, hypothalamic, pituitary, ovarian, and uterine functions throughout a usual 28-day menstrual cycle. The variations in basal body temperature are also illustrated.

for the possibility of pregnancy. The major changes occur within the uterus. The inner lining, the endometrium, is prepared to receive and nurture a fertilized ovum. It will nurture this egg, allowing it to grow through embryonic and fetal stages and finally to the birth of the infant.

Menarche, the first menstrual cycle, usually begins around the age of 12 years. Each month, for 30 to 40 years, an ovum matures and is released about 14 days before the next menstrual flow. This, on average, occurs every 28 days. If fertilization occurs, menstrual cycling subsides and the body adapts to the developing fetus (see Chapter 42).

Generally speaking, the menstrual cycle can be divided into three phases: menstrual, preovulatory, and postovulatory. For our discussion, we will use the 28-day cycle to explore what happens (Fig. 36-8). On days 1 through 5 of the cycle the endometrium sloughs and is accompanied by 1 to 2 ounces of blood loss. The anterior pituitary begins to release follicle-stimulating hormone (FSH); as the level of FSH increases the egg matures within the graafian follicle. From days 6 through 13 (preovulatory phase) estrogen is released from the maturing graafian follicle. This estrogen causes the vascularization and thickening of the uterine lining. On day 14 the anterior pituitary releases luteinizing hormone (LH), which causes the rupture of the graafian follicle and the release of the mature ovum. During days 15 through 28 (postovulatory phase) the developing corpus luteum releases estrogen and progesterone, which maintains the vascularization of the uterus if pregnancy does occur. If this is the case, the corpus luteum continues to release estrogen and progesterone to maintain the uterine lining until the placenta is formed, which then takes over the job of hormonal release. If pregnancy does not occur, the corpus luteum lasts for 8 days and then disintegrates. At this point the hormone level decreases over several days and menstruation starts again.

For a more detailed discussion of the menstrual cycle, problems of menstruation, see pp. 923-926.

Effects of Normal Aging Patterns on the Female Reproductive System

Menopause occurs in the normal female between the ages of 48 and 52 years. During this time the menstrual flow ceases and hormonal levels decrease. This is the period when a woman may experience "hot flashes" (a sudden warm feeling) that are caused by the decrease in estrogen production. Changes also occur in the reproductive organs. The vagina loses elasticity. The breasts and vulva lose some adipose tissue, which results in decreased tissue turgor. The bones may also become brittle and prone to osteoporosis.

In the male there is no menopausal period. Sperm production decreases but does not cease. In later years, testosterone production decreases, but not dramatically.

Basically, as long as the older individual is healthy, there is nothing in the aging process that prohibits normal sexual function.

HUMAN SEXUALITY

Sexuality is recognized as a function of the total personality but may be altered by interfering disorders of the reproductive system. Abnormalities may lie within the reproductive system itself or through the interaction with other body systems that may be malfunctioning.

In 1984, the Sex Information and Education Council (SIECUS) provided a position statement regarding sexual health care and mandated that providers of health services:

1. Recognize the importance of sexual health for people of all ages and life-styles
2. Understand how the variations in health, such as those resulting from pregnancy, illness, disease, surgery, diet, and medication, may affect an individual's sexuality
3. Assess the individual's sexual functioning and sexual concerns as integral parts of health care and make appropriate interventions and resources available

SIECUS advocates that education in sexual health concerns, needs, and therapies become a part of the professional training in all health care fields, at both entry and continuing education levels.

Sexual Health and Education

The goals of sex education are to promote sexual health and sexuality as a natural part of life. The sexuality concept includes touching, being touched, love, sex relationships, behaviors, and the manner in which men and women relate to each other and to others.

Human sexuality courses in medical and nursing schools are receiving more attention in the last decade. Courses are being offered for increasing self-acceptance of one's own sexual feelings, skills for communication, clarifying of sexual values, and recognition of sexual myths. There has been an increase in the number of textbooks and articles in professional publications and journals regarding sexuality.

The increased attention given to sex education has stirred an interest in and a demand for treatment of sexual problems. Patients were once ashamed, anxious, or embarrassed to acknowledge a sexual issue. Currently the demand for treatment has led to more openness. There are answers to questions concerning sexual functioning, practices, alternatives, inadequacies, and compatibility.

Illness and Sexuality

All patients are sexual, and their total health is affected by their emotions, behaviors, beliefs, attitudes, and knowledge of sexuality. Sexual health is a component, along with emotional and physical health, of the patient's total health-need picture. The nurse who is concerned with all components of the patient's health and welfare can demonstrate support as a part of care when the patient expresses sexual problems and concern at the time of illness.

Illness may cause changes in one's self-concept and an inability to function sexually. Medications, stress, fatigue, and depression also affect sexual functioning. Alcohol abuse can lead to a reduced sex drive and inadequate sexual functioning.

Disinterest or lack of desire for sexual activity generally occurs with patients at the time they are preoccupied with symptoms of illness. Most often these sexual symptoms disappear as patients recover from the acute phase of illness and sexual activity is resumed. However, some illnesses, such as diabetes mellitus, end-stage renal disease, spinal cord injuries, and heart disease, may cause patients some concerns or actual inabilities with sexual function.

Changes in the nervous system, circulatory system, or genital organs may lead to sexual health problems. The patient with spinal cord injuries can experience an interruption of the peripheral nerves and spinal cord reflexes that involve sexual responses. Spinal cord–injured men and women have reported orgasm in spite of complete denervation of all pelvic structures. They reported that the orgasm was satisfying and led to a comfortable resolution stage of sexual excitement for many of them.

Each type of body structure change that causes sexual health problems needs to be discussed with the patient. Because sexuality is a part of the total individual, sexual function needs to be openly discussed and alternatives recommended for optimal sexual health. The patient needs to investigate these recommendations and express results of being able or not being able to employ alternatives for sexual gratification.

Sexual dysfunction of the diabetic patient can occur when the disease is not well controlled. The dysfunction generally disappears when the lack of control is diagnosed and treated. Impotence is found in approximately half of the men who have diabetes and is generally related to poor control of the diabetes. Sexual counseling is important to (1) provide accurate information about the sexual aspects of the disorder, (2) dispel the patient's faulty assumptions and expectations, and (3) give advice designed to optimize the level of sexual self-esteem and dispel the guilt that is frequently found with both partners.

A mastectomy results in both physical and emotional trauma. The resultant disfigurement is only one of multiple problems that are being faced. Patients must grapple with these problems as well: (1) how to cope with cancer, (2) how the operation will affect the relationship with the spouse or significant other, (3) how can they relate to the strangeness of their own body, and (4) how their sexual life will be affected. Problems that arise with pelvic irradiation for cancer of the cervix are much harder to treat than those of mastectomy, because the entire physiology of the vagina is altered by the radiation and there is a true loss of function. With the mastectomy the function that is lost is the ability to nurse an infant. The goal for the patient and partner is to face the issue straightforwardly, so that both partners can acknowledge the diagnosis and true feelings can be acknowledged and discussed. If feelings are repressed—not verbalized or shared—both the patient and the significant other may suffer.

For the patient undergoing a mastectomy, her sexual self-concept and intimate physical interactions can and will be affected. Two variables that influence a woman's sexual function are (1) sufficient self-love and acceptance and (2) positive attitudes and feelings about sexuality. The male partner should be persuaded to face his own feelings so that he is able to offer support to his partner. Therapeutic counseling before surgery can aid the patient's and partner's acceptance and recovery after surgery.

HEALTH HISTORY

Health history data should be relevant to the developmental stage of the patient. Information about reproductive health and sexuality can form a large portion of the data collection. This history is as important as the physical and mental information as a basis for determining appropriate nursing diagnoses and interventions. Data collected about sexual health, sexual relations, birth control methods, sexually transmitted disease, and the use of chemical substances provide an opportunity to clarify any misconceptions, myths, and hearsay that may be revealed during history-taking.

Data Collection: Female

Data collection for adolescent and adult women focuses on the reproductive tract with the menstrual, gynecological, and obstetrical history.

The menstrual history includes the time of menarche (onset of menstrual flow) to the climacteric (cessation of menstrual cycle), as to: (1) age of onset, (2) date of last menstrual flow, (3) usual amount and volume of flow (number of pads used per day), (4) presence of **dysmenorrhea** (painful menstruation), **menorrhagia** (excessive flow), **amenorrhea** (absence of flow), or **metrorrhagia** (excessive spotting between cycles), and (5) other difficulties during menses.

The gynecological assessment includes data on (1) vaginal discharge (odor, color, frequency, and duration), (2) vaginal pruritus (itching), (3) vaginal irritation with coital activity, (4) date and results of the last Papanicolaou (Pap) test, (5) types of birth control methods or kinds of contraceptives used, and (6) family history of cancer of the reproductive system.

If the female has conceived, information should be collected as to the gravidity (number of pregnancies) and parity (number of births), abortions, miscarriages, and stillbirths. Assessment of the breast includes (1) tenderness of the breast areas, (2) pain, (3) masses in any specific areas, (4) presence of nipple discharge, (5) knowledge and frequency of breast self-examination, and (6) date of last mammogram, if applicable.

Data Collection: Male

The data collected from the male adolescent and the adult male include (1) urological history about voiding difficulties and/or any discharge from the penis, (2) characteristics of the urine (odor, color, amount, and frequency), (3) information on prostate and/or testicular problems, (4) masses or lesions on genitalia, (5) frequency of testicular self-examination, (6) frequency of professional testicular examination, (7) nature of measures to prevent infections, and (8) birth control measures. In addition, the nurse should note concerns about sexual health and the **climacteric** voiced by the patient.

DIAGNOSTIC TESTS FOR PROBLEMS OF THE REPRODUCTIVE SYSTEM

Diagnostic Tests for the Female

The pelvic examination is performed by a physician and is advantageous for visualization and palpation of the vulva, perineum, vagina, cervix, ovaries, and uterine surfaces. During the pelvic examination specimens are frequently obtained for diagnostic purposes. The pelvic examination progresses from the visualization and/or palpation of the external genital organs for edema and irritations to inspection for abnormalities of the internal organs. To visualize internal organs the physician inserts a vaginal speculum. The physician may do a rectovaginal examination to evaluate abnormalities or problems of the rectal area and the posterior internal organs.

Colposcopy provides direct visualization of cervix and vagina. The patient is prepared for a pelvic examination. The vaginal speculum is inserted, followed by the insertion of the colposcope for inspection of the area. The color of the tissue, presence of growths and lesions, and condition of the vascularity are observed and specimens obtained as necessary.

Culdoscopy is another diagnostic procedure that provides visualization of the uterus and adnexa (uterine appendages, ovaries, fallopian tubes) and small intestine. The patient is given a local, spinal, or general anesthetic. After the anesthetic is administered, the patient is assisted to a knee-chest position. The culdoscope is passed through the vaginal wall in back of the cervix. The area is examined for tumors, cysts, and endometriosis. During the procedure conization (removal of eroded or infected tissue) may be done. This procedure is generally done on an outpatient basis.

Laparoscopy provides direct visualization of the uterus and adnexa. Preparation of the patient includes insertion of a Foley catheter to maintain bladder decompression for an open view. The procedure is usually done with a general anesthetic. A small incision is made beneath the umbilicus. The cervix is grasped by forceps and a lighted laparoscope is inserted through the incision. Carbon dioxide may be introduced to distend the abdomen for easier visualization. If a biopsy is to be done or organs are to be manipulated, a second incision may be made in the lower abdomen to allow for instrument insertion. The ovaries and fallopian tubes may be observed for masses, ectopic pregnancy, adhesions, and pelvic inflammatory disease. Tubal ligations may be done using this procedure.

Papanicolaou (Pap) smear test is most widely known for its use in the early detection of cervical cancer. Scrapings of secretions and cells are taken from the cervix and spread on a glass slide. The slide is sprayed with a fixative and sent to the laboratory for analysis. It is important that slides be properly labeled. The label should give the date, time of the last menstrual period, and whether the woman is taking estrogens or birth control pills. Annual tests are advised for women who (1) are over 40 years of age, (2) are in high-risk categories for cervical cancer (3) have had previous positive reports, and (4) are sexually active women under 20 years of age. If a Pap test is positive or suggests a malignancy, a cervical biopsy is done to confirm the diagnosis.

Biopsies are procedures in which samples of tissues are taken for evaluation to confirm or locate a lesion. Tissue is aspirated by special needles or removed by forceps or through an incision.

A *cervical biopsy* is done to evaluate suspicious cervical lesions and to diagnose cervical cancer. The biopsy is generally done without anesthesia. For direct visualization the colposcope is inserted through the vaginal speculum and the cervical site is selected and cleansed and tissue is removed. The area is packed with gauze or a tampon to check the blood flow.

A *breast biopsy* is performed to differentiate benign or malignant tumors. Breast biopsy is indicated for patients with palpable masses, suspicious areas appearing from mammography, and persistent encrusted, purulent, inflamed, or sanguineous discharge from the nipples. The procedure is performed by needle biopsy, under local anesthetic, or by open biopsy with general or local anesthetic. In a needle biopsy, fluid is aspirated from the breast and is expelled into a specimen bottle. Pressure is placed on the site to stop bleeding. When bleeding has ceased, an adhesive bandage is applied. In an open biopsy, an incision is made in a portion of the breast to expose the mass; tissue portions are incised, or the whole mass may be incised. Specimens of selected tissue may be frozen and stained for rapid diagnosis. The wound is sutured and a bandage is applied. The incision site should be observed for bleeding, tenderness, and erythema.

An *endometrial biopsy* is performed to collect tissue for diagnosis of endometrial cancer and analysis for infertility studies. The procedure is generally performed at the time of menstruation when the cervix is dilated and cells are more easily obtained. The cervix is locally anesthetized, a curette is inserted, and tissue is obtained from selected sites of the endometrium.

Conization of the cervix is indicated when eroded or

infected tissue is to be removed or there is a need for confirmation of cervical cancer. A cone-shaped section is removed when the mass is confined to the epithelial tissue. After surgery the area is packed with gauze to control bleeding. The patient is observed for bleeding and is generally discharged from the hospital the same day.

Dilation and **curettage** is a procedure performed to obtain tissue for biopsy, to correct cervical stricture, and/or treat dysmenorrhea. The patient is prepared for general anesthesia. While the patient is anesthetized the cervix is dilated and the inside of the uterus scraped with a curette. A packing may be inserted for hemostasis and a perineal pad is applied for absorption of drainage.

Cultures and smears are collected to examine and identify infectious processes, presence of abnormal cells, and hormonal changes of the reproductive tissue. Specimens collected for smears are prepared by spreading the collected smear on a glass slide and covered with a second slide or sprayed with a fixative. Specimens should be handled with aseptic technique and caution should be observed to avoid transfer and spread of organisms. Cultures are taken from exudates of the breast, vagina, rectum, and/or urethra. Sexually transmitted diseases and mastitis are diagnosed by isolation of the causative organisms.

Schiller's iodine test is used for the early detection of cancer cells and to guide the physician in doing a biopsy. An iodine preparation, applied to the cervix, produces a brown stain for normal vaginal cells. Glycogen, which is present in normal cells, will stain brown when the iodine solution is applied. Abnormal or immature cells do not absorb the stain. This method of detection is valuable but is not entirely reliable, because normal cells sometimes lack glycogen, and malignant tissue at times will contain glycogen. After the procedure the patient should wear a perineal pad to avoid staining of the clothing.

Radiographic examinations are performed to detect abnormal tissue, locate abnormal structures, and observe patency of ducts.

Hysterograms and hysterosalpingograms are studies for visualizing the uterine cavity to confirm (1) tubal abnormalities (adhesions and occlusions), (2) presence of foreign bodies, (3) congenital malformations, and (4) traumatic injuries. The patient is placed in the lithotomy position. A speculum is inserted in the vagina, a cannula is inserted through the speculum into the cervical cavity, and a contrast medium is injected through the cannula. As the contrast medium progresses through the cavity, the uterus and fallopian tubes are viewed by the fluoroscope and films are taken.

Mammography is a radiographic technique used to detect breast cysts or tumors, especially those not palpable on physical examination. It is believed that the average breast tumor is present for 9 years before it is palpable. Mammography is helpful as a screening procedure for those with a family history of breast cancer. It is recommended by the American Cancer Society that baseline mammograms be performed on women between the ages of 35 and 39; every 1 to 2 years for women 40 to 49 years of age; and yearly for women 50 years of age and beyond.

At the time of scheduling of the procedure the nurse advises the patient to refrain from using body powders, deodorants, and ointments on the breast areas, because this could cause false-positive results. Before the procedure the patient is provided with a patient gown and asked to remove jewelry and upper garments. The patient is asked to sit or stand in an upright position and rest one breast on the x-ray table. A compressor is placed on the breast, and the patient is asked to hold her breath as an anterior view is taken. The machine is rotated and again the breast is compressed and a lateral view is taken. The procedure is repeated on the other breast. The patient may be asked to wait until the x-ray films are read. Xeromammography involves recording of the radiographic images on a selenium-coated plate and transferring the images to a special paper. This process enables enhancement of edges and sharpening of images.

Magnetic resonance imaging (MRI) provides excellent visualization of tissue without the use of a contrast medium or ionizing radiation. It is not as readily available or economical as other diagnostic methods.

In pelvic ultrasonography, high-frequency sound waves are passed into the area to be examined and images are formed on a screen—similar to an x-ray film. Ultrasound is useful in detecting foreign bodies (such as IUDs), distinguishing between cystic and solid tumor bodies, evaluating fetal growth and viability, detecting fetal abnormalities, and detecting ectopic pregnancy. Generally it is noninvasive, safe, and painless. Fluids are encouraged. The nurse should explain to the patient that a full bladder is essential to the accuracy of the test.

Tubal insufflation (Rubin test) involves transuterine insufflation of the fallopian tubes with carbon dioxide (Fig. 36-9). The procedure enables evaluation of the patency of the fallopian tubes and may be part of a fertility study. Tubal insufflation takes approximately 30 minutes and is usually performed on an outpatient basis.

All pregnancy tests, regardless of method, are based on detection of human chorionic gonadotropin (HCG), which is secreted after the fertilization of the ovum. Regardless of method, it is important to know that the tests do not indicate whether the pregnancy is normal. False positives may occur.

Diagnostic Tests for the Male

Testicular biopsy is a means to detect abnormal cells and the presence of sperm. The testing can be done by aspiration or through an incision. The anesthetic used de-

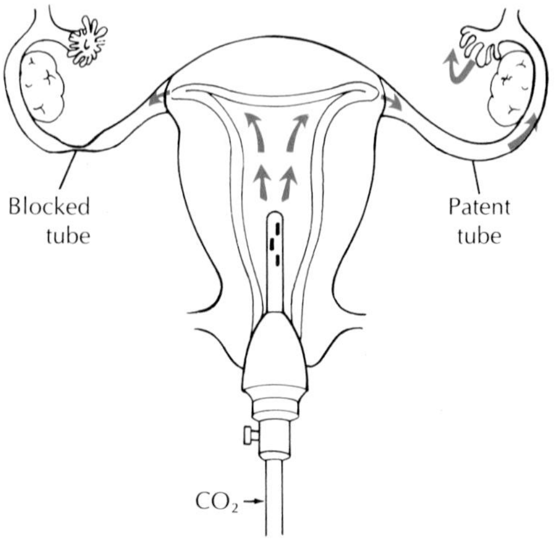

FIG. 36-9 Rubin test. Carbon dioxide escapes into abdominal cavity through patent left uterine tube.

pends on the choice of technique. Postbiopsy care consists of comfort measures with a scrotal support, ice pack, and analgesic medications. Warm sitz baths for edema may be helpful. The nurse should instruct the patient to call the physician if bleeding occurs.

Semen analysis can be performed to substantiate the effectiveness of a vasectomy, to detect semen on the body or clothing of a suspected rape victim, and to rule out paternity. The procedure is generally one of the first tests to be performed on the male patient to evaluate fertility. Collection of semen for evaluation of fertility may be by manual stimulation, coitus interruptus, or the use of a condom.

Prostatic smears are obtained to detect and identify microorganisms and tumor cells in the prostate. The physician massages the prostate by way of the rectum, and the patient voids into a sterile container prepared with additive preservative. The specimen is collected and a smear is prepared in the laboratory. It is possible to detect some cases of cancer and even tuberculosis of the prostate gland by this method.

In *cystoscopy*, the prostate and bladder of the male can be examined by passing a lighted cystoscope through the urethra to the bladder. The examination is usually performed without anesthesia, but a local anesthetic may be instilled into the bladder. This can be done for both men and women to detect bladder infections and tumors.

Other diagnostic studies for men include the prostatic-specific antigen (PSA), the alkaline phosphatase (ALP) test, and the acid phosphatase (ACP) test. These specific tests are useful in diagnosing benign prostatic hypertrophy, prostatic cancer, bone metastasis in prostatic cancer, as well as other disease conditions. See Box 36-1 for nursing interventions for patients undergoing diagnostic tests.

BOX 36-1 **NURSING INTERVENTIONS FOR THE PATIENT UNDERGOING DIAGNOSTIC STUDIES**

1. Explain the examination carefully.
2. Provide privacy.
3. Obtain a signed consent when necessary.
4. Prepare the skin for surgery.
5. Assess the patient for allergies.
6. As appropriate, request that the patient partially or completely disrobe and remove all jewelry. Provide gown and/or drape.
7. Give preexamination instructions; NPO status if indicated.
8. Encourage verbalization and discussion of fears.
9. Administer preexamination medication as ordered by physician.
10. Occasionally it will be necessary to advise patients to go without medications for 24 hours. A medication history should be obtained.
11. If the specimen is to be collected at home, stress the importance of handling all specimens precisely as directed.
12. It may be necessary to monitor vital signs.
13. Be attentive during examination; offer support as necessary.
14. Relay any immediate concerns to the physician as appropriate.
15. Guide patients to follow any postexamination instructions.
16. Inform the patient that some discomfort can be expected. Minor discomfort can be relieved by mild analgesics such as aspirin or Tylenol, but if pain becomes more intense the physician should be notified. Most discomfort is temporary.
17. When pertinent, tell patients to rest and to avoid any heavy lifting following the examination for 24 hours as directed by the physician.
18. When relevant, advise the patient to avoid douching or intercourse until the site is healed. Consult the physician.
19. Caution patients to report any bleeding from an incisional area.
20. Advise the patient to avoid the use of tampons as directed by the physician.
21. Inform the patient how test results may be obtained.

THE REPRODUCTIVE CYCLE

Menarche

Menarche, the beginning of menses, designates the first menstrual cycle. Menarche is the signal that sexual maturation of the young female has occurred and that the body is capable of supporting pregnancy.

The menarche occurs from 9 to 17 years of age, the average age being 12.5 years. The cycle length varies from

BOX 36-2 HEALTH TEACHING FOR MENSTRUATION

1. Knowledge of the physiological process
2. Factors that may alter the menstrual cycle: stress, fatigue, exercise, acute or chronic illness, changes in climate, or working hours and pregnancy
3. Personal hygiene
   a. Wear pads during early period of heavy flow
   b. Change tampons frequently to decrease risk of toxic shock syndrome
   c. Consult physician if tampons cause discomfort
   d. Take a daily shower for comfort (warm baths may relieve slight pelvic discomfort)
   e. Keep perineal area clean and dry; cleanse from anterior to posterior
   f. Cotton underwear preferred
      Nylon panty hose and tight-fitting slacks cause retention of moisture and should not be used for extended periods of time
   g. Feminine hygiene products, such as vaginal sprays and suppositories, may contribute to a feeling of cleanliness.
   h. A daily douche is not recommended, because it changes the protective bacterial flora of the vagina and predisposes the woman to infection
4. Exercise
   a. Exercise is not contraindicated and may help prevent discomfort
   b. Modify exercise if fatigue occurs
5. Diet
   a. Restrict salt intake if fluid retention is present
   b. Consult a physician if fluid retention persists after menstruation
6. Discomfort
   a. For mild discomfort take aspirin or acetaminophen (Tylenol), apply warmth, and rest
   b. For prolonged, severe discomfort, consult a physician

24 to 32 days, the average cycle lasting 29 days. The duration of the flow is from 1 to 8 days, the average being 3 to 5 days. The amount of flow is from 10 to 75 ml, the average being 35 ml per cycle.

The nurse should help patients promote reproductive and sexual health. Nurses may have the opportunity to instruct or counsel women about personal hygiene. Personal cleanliness is a health habit that should be promoted for all patients and implemented in each care plan. This is especially meaningful during menstruation. See Box 36-2 for health teaching for menstruation.

Disturbances of Menstruation

Because of the relationship between the menstrual cycle and the body's mechanisms of hormonal secretion, a decrease or increase in the activity of the hormonal glands can disturb menstruation. The most common disturbances include the following:

Amenorrhea: absence of menstrual flow
Dysmenorrhea: painful menstruation
Abnormal uterine bleeding
Hypermenorrhea/menorrhagia: excessive bleeding (amount and duration)
Metrorrhagia: bleeding between menstrual periods

Another disturbance of the menstrual cycle is premenstrual syndrome. This will be discussed later in the chapter.

Suggested nursing diagnoses are anxiety, ineffective coping, fear, pain, knowledge deficit, and low self-esteem. Nursing interventions are based on specific behaviors, symptoms, and treatments.

Amenorrhea. Amenorrhea (absence of menstrual flow) is normal before puberty, after menopause, during pregnancy, and sometimes during lactation. Menstrual flow may also be absent or suppressed as a result of hormonal abnormalities or surgical interventions such as a hysterectomy (surgical removal of the uterus).

Etiology/pathophysiology. Amenorrhea is classified as *primary* when menarche has not occurred by the age of 17 to 18 years. The cause may be a congenital defect. *Secondary* amenorrhea means that there has been an initial menarche but flow has ceased for at least 3 months or there has been an absence of vaginal fluid for 12 months, coupled with a history of irregular bleeding. Causes for secondary amenorrhea may be normal pregnancy; frequent, vigorous exercise, as in women athletes; or an emotional disorder such as depression, anorexia (lack of appetite), or bulimia (an insatiable craving for food, often resulting in episodes of continuous eating followed by purging).

Assessment. Early diagnosis and prompt management are necessary if more serious reproductive and genital problems are to be prevented. The nurse should urge the sexually active woman to see a physician as soon as a menstrual period is missed. Maintaining health during pregnancy is vital for both the mother and the fetus. Women who suspect their amenorrhea is caused by menopause can be examined by a physician to confirm this.

Obtaining a family history is important. Emotional factors (behaviors) that may influence the menstrual cycle should be assessed. A menstrual history should include (1) the number of periods missed and (2) whether amenorrhea was present previously. Recent use of medications and drugs needs to be determined.

Diagnostic tests. Beyond the preliminary workup and when pregnancy is not a possibility, the diagnostic study for primary and secondary amenorrhea is the same. This study includes the following:

Pelvic examination
Blood, urine, and hormonal analysis
Determination of existing tumors
Papanicolaou (Pap) smear

Medical management. Treatment is based on the underlying cause and must be determined on an individual basis. It may mean hormonal therapy, or, as in a majority of cases, surgical intervention may be necessary.

Nursing interventions. Nursing interventions for women with amenorrhea may include the following.

NURSING DIAGNOSIS	NURSING INTERVENTIONS
Ineffective individual coping, related to lack of menstrual flow	Acknowledge patient's feelings. Provide emotional support. Refer to counseling as necessary. Explain diagnostic procedures. Provide information, privacy, or consultation as indicated for sexual concerns.

Patient teaching. The nurse should encourage compliance with treatment and emphasize the importance of follow-up visits with the physician for treatment, therapy, and further evaluation of treatment efficacy.

Dysmenorrhea. Uterine pain with menstruation, commonly called "menstrual cramps," is dysmenorrhea. Primary dysmenorrhea that is not associated with pelvic disorders usually develops when ovulatory function is established (under 20 years of age), and there is no underlying organic disease. Often it will disappear or decline after pregnancy or by the late twenties. Secondary dysmenorrhea is painful menstruation caused by organic disease such as pelvic inflammatory disease (PID) or endometriosis and most often occurs in women over 20 years of age.

Studies in industry and schools have shown it to be the greatest single cause of absenteeism among women. It is one of the most common health problems for which women seek treatment.

Etiology/pathophysiology. The causes of dysmenorrhea can be related to endocrine imbalance, increase in prostaglandin secretions, or associated with chronic illnesses, fatigue, and anemia.

A recent theory proposes that hypercontractility of the uterus resulting from higher-than-normal levels of prostaglandins may be the cause of dysmenorrhea. Whatever the cause, the symptoms and pain are real. Conditions that cause general debilitation, such as inadequate diet and exercise, anemia, and fatigue, are often related to dysmenorrhea.

Assessment. Many women have systemic symptoms of breast tenderness, abdominal distention, nausea and vomiting, headache, vertigo, palpitations, and excessive perspiration.

The nurse should assess the woman for colicky and cyclic pain and, infrequently, dull pain in the lower pelvis that radiates toward the perineum and back. This pain may be experienced 24 to 48 hours before menses or at the onset of menses.

Family history is important, because dysmenorrhea has been reported to be significantly increased among mothers and sisters of women with dysmenorrhea.

Secondary dysmenorrhea is suspected if the symptom begins after 20 years of age. It has been described as a steady or cramping pain and may be specific to the site of pelvic disorder.

Diagnostic tests. Diagnostic studies to rule out organic causes for dysmenorrhea include pelvic examination, laparoscopy, dilation and curettage, and hystersalpingography.

Medical management. Treatment of secondary dysmenorrhea is aimed at the cause. Surgical and medication intervention may be appropriate, depending on the severity and type of pathological condition.

If no organic cause is found, the nurse should instruct the woman to exercise and eat nutritious foods, especially those high in fiber, and to avoid constipation (see Chapter 22).

Local applications of heat and mild analgesics are prescribed. Medications found effective for the treatment of dysmenorrhea include aspirin, which causes vasodilation of blood vessels, and prostaglandin inhibitors such as ibuprofen (Motrin) and naproxen sodium (Anaprox). Oral contraceptives have been used to suppress ovulation by inhibiting prostaglandin levels.

Nursing interventions. Nursing interventions for women with dysmenorrhea include the following.

NURSING DIAGNOSES	NURSING INTERVENTIONS
Knowledge deficit, related to lack of education concerning disease process and treatment	Present information on orientation to the hospital setting, disease process, procedures to be performed, medications, and treatments. Prepare for information; questions and answer sessions according to patient needs. Teach procedures patient must know how to perform. Obtain feedback. Be certain learning has taken place. (Reinforce teaching as needed.) Develop a trusting relationship. Involve patient in care.
Pain, related to biological agent	Assess nature of pain. Observe nonverbal cues. Encourage pain reduction techniques as appropriate. Explore best method for controlling pain (medication, positioning, comfort measures such as backrub or use of heat or cold, etc.). Monitor vital signs. Provide quiet environment, calm activities. Promote wellness; discuss with significant other(s) ways in which they can assist the patient.

Patient teaching. The nurse should instruct women to maintain good posture, to exercise, and to practice good nutrition, and encourage a positive attitude. Women who are unable to engage in activities because of dysmenorrhea should be urged to seek health care.

Abnormal uterine bleeding. Abnormal uterine bleeding may take many forms. Two of these will be discussed: hypermenorrhea and metrorrhagia.

Hypermenorrhea is excessive bleeding at the time of the regular menstrual flow. In younger women it may be attributable to endocrine disturbances but in older women it is usually indicative of inflammatory disturbances or uterine tumors. Emotional or psychological problems may also affect uterine bleeding. The severity of hypermenorrhea is usually estimated in terms of numbers of pads or tampons used in excess of those used for the regular menstrual flow.

Metrorrhagia is the appearance of uterine bleeding between the regular menstrual periods or after menopause. It merits early diagnosis and treatment, because it may be indicative of cancer or benign tumors of the uterus.

Diagnosis is made by a routine speculum and pelvic examination. Also used to diagnose gynecological causes of hypermenorrhea and metrorrhagia are the endometrial biopsy and dilation and curettage (D&C).

The nurse should (1) assess for bleeding, pain, vaginal secretions, and psychosocial concerns, (2) encourage the woman to express her feelings, (3) explain the importance of recording dates, type of flow, and number of sanitary pads or tampons used, (4) teach the patient pain-relieving techniques, and (5) explain the importance of sharing concerns with her partner.

Women of all ages need to be educated about the importance of follow-up care when abnormal uterine bleeding is initially detected.

Premenstrual syndrome (PMS). PMS occurs in 30% to 50% of females between the ages of 25 to 45 years. It differs from dysmenorrhea because it has no relation to ovulation.

Etiology/pathophysiology. It is believed that PMS is related to the neuroendocrine events occurring within the anterior pituitary. It is known that there is a loss of intravascular fluid into the body tissues, which causes water retention, bloating, and weight gain.

The syndrome occurs 7 to 10 days before the menstrual period and usually subsides within the first 3 days after the onset of the menstrual flow.

Intake of sodium and use of alcohol, tobacco, and caffeine should be evaluated as possible causes.

Clinical manifestations. Symptoms are multiple and vary among individuals and may be behavioral or physical. Behavorial symptoms include irritability, lethargy (inactivity), fatigue, sleep disturbances, and depressions. Headache, vertigo, backache, acne, paresthesia (burning, tingling) of hands and feet, and allergies, if present, may become worse. There are many symptoms that may appear alone or in combination with other symptoms. Some women accept the symptoms as being normal and only after the symptoms become severe do they seek medical help.

Assessment. Collection of *subjective data* needs to be specific as to the symptoms and combination of symptoms that occur with each woman. Each patient is asked to maintain a log for three consecutive menstrual cycles of symptoms and activities that relate to the menstrual period. The collected information can be analyzed and symptoms treated accordingly.

Collection of *objective data* pertinent to the syndrome, especially the inability to perform activities of daily living in the multiple roles as wife, mother, and career person, should be assessed by the nurse.

Diagnostic tests. Diagnostic tests include evaluation of estrogen and progesterone levels to rule out hormonal imbalances, and determination of glucose levels, which may be a factor leading to irritability. Dietary analysis may reveal the need for adjustments or alterations.

Medical management. PMS has no single treatment and no specific medication. Some physicians prescribe analgesics, diuretics, and progesterone. The patient's diet should be reviewed, and initially a high-protein, well-balanced diet is suggested (see Chapter 22).

Nursing interventions. Nursing interventions for the woman with premenstrual syndrome include the following.

NURSING DIAGNOSIS	NURSING INTERVENTIONS
Anxiety, related to PMS	Encourage verbalization of feelings. Acknowledge existence of the syndrome and its symptoms. Encourage the patient to keep a menstrual symptom calendar to document the cycle and nature of the symptoms. Encourage the patient to plan activities during the symptom-free part of her cycle. Administer supplements of vitamin B_6, calcium, and magnesium as prescribed. Encourage daily exercise and relaxation. Encourage self-help groups and the reading of self-help literature (group support tends to reduce stress). Provide emotional support with a nonjudgmental and caring manner. Assist in identifying possible sources of anxiety. Assist in identifying coping mechanisms.

Patient teaching. The patient should assume responsibility for following a dietary plan of eating small meals and eliminating or restricting sugar, alcohol, caffeine, and nicotine, which may minimize the symptoms of PMS.

Climacteric. The climacteric is the phase of the aging process of women and men who are making a transition from a reproductive phase to a nonreproductive stage of life. The phase occurs in middle adulthood and marks the onset of a decrease in hormone secretion, cessation of ovulation and menses, and physical changes.

Menopause. The female climacteric is called *menopause*. Female menopause is the normal cessation of the menstrual cycle, which appears on an infrequent cycle for a period of time that usually does not exceed 2 years. As long as the menstrual cycle occurs, no matter how infrequently, ovulation continues and the potential for conception exists.

Etiology/pathophysiology. Menopause is the normal decline of ovarian function resulting from the aging process. Menopause begins in most women between 40 and 55 years of age and is characterized by infrequent ovulation, decreased menstrual function, and eventually cessation of the menstrual flow. Surgical removal of the uterus and/or ovaries will cause cessation of the menstrual flow.

Decline in ovarian function produces a variety of symptoms, such as a decrease in the frequency, amount, and duration of the menstrual flow, spotting, amenorrhea, and polymenorrhea (increased number of menstrual periods). Symptoms can last from a few months to several years before menstruation ceases permanently. Menopause is not considered to be completed until 1 year after the last menstrual period.

Clinical manifestations. Physical changes that occur in the body systems do not generally develop until after permanent cessation of menstruation. Changes of the reproductive system include shrinkage of vulval structures, atrophic vulvitis, shortening of the vagina, and dryness of the vaginal wall. There is pelvic relaxation of supporting structures as a result of the decrease in estrogen. Cystitis, pyuria (pus in the urine), and urinary frequency and urgency may appear as changes of the urinary system. There is a loss of skin turgor and elasticity, increase in subcutaneous fat, decrease in breast tissue, and thinning of hair of the axilla, head, and pubis. About 25% of postmenopausal women develop osteoporosis.

Assessment. Collection of *subjective data* should include family history. The nurse should determine whether family members and/or significant others are aware of the transition and if they are supportive. Emotional illness, if present, should be noted. "Hot flashes" caused by glandular imbalances may become prominent. Other symptoms may include fatigue, vertigo, headache, nausea, dyspareunia, palpitations, and chest and neck pain. With some there is an emotional feeling of being unwanted and some may fear growing old. Both could cause depression.

Collection of *objective data* includes an awareness that some patients may display frequent crying spells and/or outbursts of anger. The use of contraceptives should be explored. Frequency, amount, and duration of the menstrual flow need to be assessed. Diaphoresis, weight gain, and vomiting, as well as tachycardia, may occur. The nurse is in a position to note many of these disturbances.

Diagnostic tests. Tests include analysis of hormonal levels. Other diagnostic testing may be indicated by symptoms. Some examinations are performed to rule out possible conditions such as cancer.

Medical management. Typically, estrogen therapy is administered cyclically, usually in the form of conjugated equine estrogens (Premarin) taken orally from days 1 to 25; from days 15 to 25 medroxyprogesterone acetate (Provera) is taken. Thereafter, this cycle is repeated. A transdermal estrogen system (Estraderm) in the form of skin patches is also currently being evaluated as a long-term modality for osteoporosis. Some physicians recommend calcium supplements, which are available in many forms, but the generic calcium carbonate products are the most cost effective.

Nursing interventions. Education regarding menopause should occur before its onset. Many women appreciate opportunities made by nurses to discuss menopause. An exercise program should be set up that includes both movement and weight-bearing. Walking is an excellent weight-bearing exercise. Other exercises include bicycling, stationary cycling, and aerobic dancing. Patients should be advised to avoid activities such as jogging that would add pressure to weight-bearing joints. Nursing interventions include the following.

NURSING DIAGNOSES	NURSING INTERVENTIONS
Self-esteem disturbance, related to concerns about femininity, sexuality, and aging	Encourage patient and/or significant others to verbalize concerns. Confirm accurate information. Correct information related to self-concept issues. Avoid value judgments. Refer patient to couple, family, and/or sex therapy as appropriate. Provide understanding and support as appropriate.
Knowledge deficit regarding patient's physiological and psychological changes, related to climacteric and menopause	Explain the process of climacteric and menopause, depending on the patient's ability to comprehend. Explain importance of keeping fit, eating a well-balanced diet, getting adequate rest and sleep, avoiding stress and fatigue, and continuing contraception until indicated by physician. If estrogen replacement therapy is ordered, inform patient about side effects. Instruct patient to report any vaginal bleeding occurring 6 months or more after last menstrual period. Inform patient of the availability of water-soluble lubricants if needed before coitus.

Patient teaching. The nurse should emphasize that the climacteric is normal and self-limiting, and menopause is not the end of the patient's sex life. A nutritious diet and weight control will improve physical condition, and an exercise program promotes vitality. Interest and participation in activities will help decrease anxiety and tension. Skin creams and lotions can be used to prevent drying,

BOX 36-3 KEGEL EXERCISES

Kegel exercises are performed to help strengthen and tighten muscles that support the pelvic organs. These muscles (pelvic floor) are used to stop the flow of urine. To perform Kegel exercises while standing or sitting, tighten the pelvic floor muscles as hard as you can. Hold for 5 seconds, then release. Repeat at least 10 times. This exercise can be done many times throughout the day. Practice while urinating: try to stop the flow of urine by tightening the pelvic muscles.

pruritus, and cracking skin. The nurse should encourage the woman to perform breast self-examination monthly and monitor calcium intake. Contraceptives should be used for 1 year after the last menstrual period. The patient can obtain a prescription for treatment of pruritus or burning of the vulva. Women can practice Kegel exercises daily (Box 36-3) to strengthen pelvic muscles. A water-soluble lubricant such as K-Y jelly can be used to prevent dyspareunia (painful intercourse). The side effects of any medications or hormonal therapy should be explained. The nurse should emphasize that an annual physical examination is important for maintaining good health.

Male climacteric. The climacteric is less pronounced in men and may not even be apparent in many men.

Etiology/pathophysiology. The appearance of the climacteric phase is gradual and occurs between the ages of 55 and 70. There is a gradual decrease of testosterone levels and seminal fluid production. The impact is largely psychological, possibly because of the recognition of some reduction of sexual activity and interests.

Clinical manifestations. Manifestations are mostly physiological changes. Erections require more time and are not as full or firm. The prostate gland enlarges, and secretions diminish; seminal fluid decreases. The physical changes occur as the man grows older, and the most noticeable signs are thinning and loss of hair from the head, chest, axilla, and pubis. There may be some flushing and chilling. Muscle tone is decreased.

Assessment. Collection of *subjective data* generally reveals that the man is at the peak of his career or possibly considering retirement. He interprets the decreased sexual needs as a loss of productivity and sexual power. Therefore the assessment should invite verbalization of emotions with coping mechanisms.

Collection of *objective data* includes assessment of behaviors that may be causing the man to be stressed and concerned. Changes that he has noted regarding his lifestyle and feelings of loss of self-worth should be expressed.

Diagnostic tests. Diagnostic tests include a complete physical examination to rule out abnormalities of structure and function.

Nursing interventions. Nursing interventions for men experiencing male climacteric include the following:

NURSING DIAGNOSIS	NURSING INTERVENTIONS
Ineffective individual coping, related to situational crisis (climacteric)	Show understanding and concern. Assist the patient in identifying how the problem affects his life and future, his family, and significant others. Encourage the patient to verbalize whether factors could be influencing the way he sees the problem. Assist the patient in identifying strengths and coping skills and the nature and strength of situational support. Collect data about current and potential sources of support. Assist the patient in planning alternative solutions. Give positive reinforcement.

PATIENT TEACHING. The patient should be informed that the climacteric is normal. The nurse should encourage patients to verbalize their fears and to seek counseling if stress increases.

Impotence. Impotence is the inability of an adult man to achieve penile erection. Several forms are recognized: functional impotence (psychological basis), anatomical impotence (results from a physical defect of genital structures), and atonic impotence (involves disturbed neuromuscular function). The nurse can best understand impotence by developing a broad understanding of the factors that contribute to the condition.

Medical management. Medical treatment is based on careful assessment of the causative factors. It is known that such medications as antihypertensive, antidepressive, and antianxiety agents, as well as some cardiac agents, may cause impotence. Illicit or abused substances such as alcohol, cocaine, and nicotine are also known to cause impotence. Such disease conditions as diabetes mellitus and end-stage renal disease may also be a causative factor in the diagnosis of impotence.

There are mechanical devices available for the patient with impotence. Surgical implantation of a penile prosthesis may be performed as a "day-stay" procedure or may require hospitalization for 5 or more days, depending on the patient and the type of device used (Fig. 36-10).

Nursing interventions. The nurse is responsible for teaching the patient to administer hormonal medication (testosterone) and to watch for side effects. The nurse should advise the patient to take oral hormonal replacement drugs with meals to prevent nausea.

The nurse should advise the patient about signs and symptoms of infection of the implant, including tenderness of the penis, fever, dysuria, and signs of urinary tract

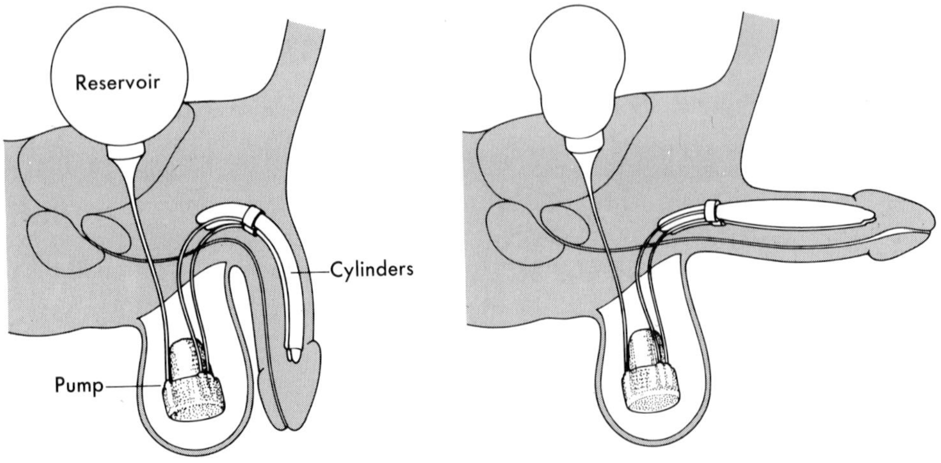

FIG. 36-10 The Scott inflatable prosthesis has both erect and flaccid positions designed to mimic normal erectile function.

infection. The nurse should educate the patient to seek medical attention promptly if infection occurs.

Infertility

Etiology/pathophysiology. Infertility is defined as the inability to conceive after 1 year of sexual intercourse without birth control measures. Primary infertility refers to couples who have never conceived. Secondary infertility refers to couples who have conceived but now are not able to do so.

The age of the woman has a significant bearing on her ability to conceive. The most fertile time of a woman's life is during the twentieth to twenty-ninth year. The most fertile time of a man's life is in his late teens and early twenties. A man's fertility does not decrease much as he grows older, but a woman's fertility drops dramatically as she ages.

Infertility may be caused by impaired sperm or ovum production or an occlusion within the reproductive system that prevents the sperm and ova from meeting. Infections of the reproductive tract, such as pelvic inflammatory disease, and sexually transmitted diseases, such as syphilis, are frequently associated with infertility. Because the man may be the infertile partner in one third of cases of infertility, the quality and quantity of the sperm may be questioned. The primary causes of female infertility are tubal insufficiency and ovarian and uterine conditions such as endometriosis or congenital defects.

Assessment. Collection of *subjective and objective data* includes physical examination and health histories for both partners, to make the infertility assessment and prepare a plan of treatment.

Diagnostic tests. Specific testing is necessary to rule out systemic diseases such as diabetes mellitus, neoplasms, hepatic and renal diseases, and viral conditions. Genetic defects and disorders of the testes are explored. Diagnostic testing can produce a great deal of anxiety and stress. This testing may continue for fairly long periods with or without favorable results. Male testing is somewhat simpler and most of the time is not as expensive. If there is reason to suspect infertility or sterility of the man, it is appropriate to test him first. Male infertility testing includes semen analysis, which measures the quantity and quality of semen, volume of sperm cells, sperm motility, and sperm density; and endocrine imbalance testing, which explores possible disruption of the pituitary gonadotropins and testosterone production.

Female testing focuses on the ovulation process and reliability of the reproductive organs. Female infertility testing includes (1) basal body temperature to assess ovulation, (2) endometrial biopsy, which confirms ovulation and endometrial cyclic changes, (3) endocrine studies to detect the nature of the functioning of the adrenal and thyroid glands with anovulation cycles, (4) Rubin's insufflation test, which determines tubal patency, and (5) hysterosalpingography and hysterography to assess the position and alignment of the reproductive organs.

Male and female interaction studies include the (1) Huhner test, which examines the cervical mucus for motile sperm cells after intercourse at midmenstrual cycle, (2) immunological or immunoglobin (antibody) testing for detection of spermicidal antibodies in the sera of the woman, and (3) testing both the man and woman for normalcy of their sex chromosomes.

Medical management. Medical treatment for any infertile couple depends on the cause of the infertility.

Medications causing dysfunctions can be discontinued and/or adjusted. Artificial creams, oils, and lubricants and douching can be discontinued. The man whose sperm production is low may need testosterone, vitamins, and nutritional counseling. He may need to avoid wearing jockey shorts and avoid hot tubs and saunas that may keep his testicles too warm. The woman who has endocrine deficiencies may be treated to gain the necessary balances. Surgery may be necessary to reconstruct anatomical defects.

Nursing interventions. Patients who are infertile experience guilt, disappointment, and alterations in self-esteem. Many also experience the inability to conceive as a loss and demonstrate typical grief reactions. The nurse must be sensitive to these feelings and help patients identify their reactions and coping strategies. During counseling the nurse also provides information about alternatives or options for parenting.

INFECTIONS OF THE FEMALE REPRODUCTIVE TRACT

Infections of the female reproductive tract are most commonly found in the vagina, cervix, fallopian tubes, and adjacent areas. The vagina is lubricated and protected by flora containing Döderlein's bacilli, an acid pH, and secretions from the vaginal and cervical cells.

Causative organisms of vaginal infections are multiple. The most common organisms that cause infection are *Escherichia coli, Candida albicans,* and *Trichomonas vaginalis.* Infections are more likely to occur when the flora and the acidity of the vagina are disturbed by administration of medication (birth control pills and antibiotics), stress, malnutrition, douching, aging, and disease. Yeast organisms grow best in an acid pH (−4.7), whereas *Trichomonas* and organisms causing nonspecific vaginitis flourish on a pH (5+), which is more alkaline.

Organisms are often introduced from external sources by way of unclean douche nozzles, poor hygiene, inadequate handwashing, neglected nail care, soiled clothing, and intercourse. Vaginal infections can be sexually transmitted and unless both partners are treated, the infection returns.

Simple Vaginitis

Etiology/pathophysiology. Vaginitis is a common vaginal infection. It is usually caused by *E. coli,* an organism found in feces and the rectum. It may be caused by staphylococcal and streptococcal organisms, *T. vaginalis* (a flagellated protozoan), *C. albicans* (a yeastlike fungus), and *Gardnerella* bacillus.

Vaginitis is an inflammation of the vagina. If the patient changes perineal pads and/or tampons infrequently an irritation of the vaginal tract and inner groin occurs. This creates a medium suitable for organism growth. Examination of the vaginal walls will show a profuse foamy (bubbly) exudate if the cause of the vaginitis is *T. vaginalis.* If *C. albicans* is the causative agent, a thick, cheese-like discharge results. Bacterial vaginitis produces a milk-like discharge with a foul odor.

Clinical manifestations. The exudate in vaginitis is yellow, white, or grayish white, curdlike, and generally accompanied by pruritus, burning, and edema of the surrounding tissue. Voiding and defecation generally intensify the symptoms.

Assessment. Collection of *subjective data* includes assessment of menstrual history, age at menarche, length of cycles, duration and nature of flow, any dysfunctions, birth control methods, medications taken, family history of diabetes mellitus, previous vaginal infections, and sexually transmitted diseases. Sexual practices and information about signs of infection in the sex partner should be elicited. Dysuria may occur as a consequence of local irritation of the urinary meatus.

Collection of *objective data* includes observation for excoriations of the skin caused by scratching, in which case secondary infection may result. The specific type of exudate is observed.

Diagnostic tests. Diagnostic tests include direct visual examination of the vagina, culture of the organism, and bimanual examination to assess for inflammation of the vagina and its surrounding tissues.

Medical management. Vaginal infection can be treated by a variety of methods. The major goals are to cure the infection, prevent reinfection, prevent complications, and prevent infection of the sexual partner or partners. Douching is frequently prescribed for treatment, as well as local applications of vaginal suppositories, ointments, and creams. (See Skill 36-1.)

Nursing interventions. The nurse should advise the patient of the importance of handwashing before and after vaginal application of medications. Applications of heat in the form of douches, perineal irrigations, or sitz baths may be administered.

NURSING DIAGNOSES	NURSING INTERVENTIONS
Pain, related to vaginal discharge	Flush vaginal flora with acid douche (15 ml white vinegar with 1000 ml water) as ordered. Antibiotic creams may be applied after douche as ordered. Sitz bath for edema.
Potential for infection, related to invasion of pathogenic organisms	Cleanse perineum with witch hazel cleansing pads after defecating and voiding as ordered.
Knowledge deficit, related to good personal body hygiene	Provide appropriate teaching.
Potential for infection, related to sexually transmitted disease	Administer medication and treatments as ordered. Teach preventive methods, such as use of condoms
Sexual dysfunction, related to discomfort and pain	Recommend that partner be checked for infection and treated as necessary to avoid reinfection.

Patient teaching. Most patients with vaginal infection are directed to abstain from sexual intercourse during the period of treatment. The male partner's use of a condom

SKILL 36-1 PERFORMING A VAGINAL IRRIGATION (DOUCHE)

1. Review physician's order.
2. Identify patient.
3. Explain procedure to patient.
4. Suggest elimination.
5. Obtain and prepare supplies:
   Douche kit (bag, tubing, and nozzle)
   1000 to 1500 ml of irrigating solution at 100.5° to 110° F (40.5° to 43.3° C)
   Bedpan
   Disposable gloves
6. Assist patient onto bedpan; head of bed may be raised slightly for patient's comfort. Inspect perineal area. If necessary, don gloves, and perform perineal care.
7. Don clean gloves.
8. Allow sufficient solution to run through tubing to expel air and to moisten nozzle; allow some solution to flow onto patient's perineal area to test degree of warmth of solution.
9. Separate labia while directing some solution to flow over outer area.
10. Insert nozzle downward and backward. *Gently* rotate nozzle within vagina during irrigation.
11. Position container of irrigation solution at height that will not allow the solution to instill too quickly (18 to 24 inches above patient's hips).
12. Instruct patient to tighten her perineal muscles as if to suppress urination, and then relax: repeat four or five times throughout irrigation.
13. When all solution has been instilled, remove nozzle, allowing the patient to expel remaining solution.
14. Dispose of equipment per agency's policy.
15. Dispose of gloves, and wash hands.
16. Perform any necessary comfort measures.
17. Document observations and patient's reaction.

until symptoms of infection disappear may be advised. The patient is also instructed that her sexual partner should be treated.

Senile Vaginitis or Atrophic Vaginitis

This condition occurs in women after menopause and upon aging. Low estrogen levels cause the vulva and vagina to atrophy and become susceptible to the invasion of bacteria. The exudate causes pruritus, edema, and skin irritations. Estrogen, vaginal suppositories, and ointments may be applied.

Cervicitis

Cervicitis, infection of the cervix, is one of the most common diseases of the reproductive system. The infection occurs from vaginal infection or sexually transmitted disease, such as *Chlamydia trachomatis* infection, gonorrhea, herpes II, or trichomoniasis. The infection often follows childbirth or abortion when lacerations occur. Therapy is specific to the causative organism. Symptoms are backaches, whitish exudate, and menstrual irregularities. If cervicitis remains untreated, the tissues are continually irritated and the infection may spread to other pelvic organs. Personal hygiene and frequent warm tub baths can minimize odor and discomfort. Local applications of vaginal suppositories, ointments, and creams are usually prescribed.

Pelvic Inflammatory Disease

Pelvic inflammatory disease (PID) is any acute, subacute, recurrent, or chronic infection of the cervix (cervicitis), uterus (edometritis), fallopian tubes (salpingitis), and ovaries (oophoritis) that has extended to the connective tissues lying between the broad ligaments.

Etiology/pathophysiology. The most common causative organisms are *Neisseria gonorrhoeae, Streptococcus, Staphylococcus, Chlamydia,* and tubercule bacilli. PID can follow the insertion of a biopsy curette or an irrigation catheter, abortion, pelvic surgery, sexual intercourse, or infection during pregnancy. The condition may occur with or without gonorrheal infection and may be mild or severe.

When conditions or procedures alter or destroy the cervical mucus, the bacteria present ascend into the uterine cavity. Pelvic examination and movement of the reproductive organs are painful. PID is very serious, because it may cause adhesions and produce sterility. Sexually active women with more than one partner are at higher risk for PID.

Clinical manifestations. The patient is usually hospitalized to isolate the organism and plan the treatment. The patient and those assisting with the care should be informed of all precautions that are necessary and be instructed in handwashing techniques, gowning and gloving, and disposition of soiled items. Symptoms are temperature elevation, chills, severe abdominal pain, malaise, nausea and vomiting, and malodorous purulent vaginal exudate.

Assessment. Collection of *subjective data* relates to the severity of the disorder, pain, time of onset, and frequency—primary infection or continuous reinfection. Sexual history, pelvic examinations, and pelvic procedures are important, because they may reveal the origin of the pathogen.

Collection of *objective data* invites assessment of the knowledge of the patient, level of discomfort, and coping mechanisms used. The patient should be assessed for fever and the amount and characteristics of vaginal discharge.

Diagnostic tests. Diagnostic tests include Gram stains of secretions from the endocervix, urethra, and rectum. Culture and sensitivity testing identifies organisms and is helpful in selection of antibiotics for treatment. Laparoscopy or ultrasonographic visualization of the pelvic inflammation may be necessary to confirm the extent of infection. Leukocyte count and erythrocyte sedimentation rate are also assessed to confirm an infection process.

Medical management. The goal of treatment is to control and eradicate the infection by preventing the infection from spreading to other body systems. Treatment includes systemic antibiotics administered intravenously and/or intramuscularly.

Nursing interventions. Nursing interventions include (1) following the medical plan of treatment, (2) monitoring vital signs and progress of treatment, (3) providing fluids to avoid dehydration, (4) performing palliative measures for comfort in bathing, changing of perineal pads, personal hygiene, and warm douches, (5) providing patient support with a positive, nonjudgmental attitude, (6) positioning the patient in Fowler's position to facilitate drainage, and (7) following isolation techniques related to gowning, gloving, and environment.

NURSING DIAGNOSES	NURSING INTERVENTIONS
Pain, related to infection process	Manage pain with analgesics as ordered; assess effectiveness of pain relief measures. Provide comfort measures.
Potential for fluid volume deficit, related to inadequate intake, fatigue, pain, and fluid losses caused by elevated temperature	Maintain parenteral fluids as ordered. Provide adequate oral intake of fluids as prescribed. Monitor intake and output.
Potential for ineffective individual coping, related to condition	Provide emotional support. Encourage verbalization of feelings. Provide therapeutic environment for the patient.
Potential for altered health maintenance, related to insufficient knowledge of condition and complication	Patient teaching includes understanding of the significance of pelvic inflammatory disease and the importance of complying with medication therapy.

Patient teaching. Discharge planning should include patient teaching and instructions for (1) contacting the physician if a low-grade fever persists or purulent vaginal discharge occurs, (2) understanding the significance of the pelvic inflammation condition, (3) understanding the importance of compliance with medication therapy, (4) handwashing technique and practices of body hygiene with bathing, avoidance of tampons, frequent changing of perineal pads, and clean clothing, (5) understanding of the importance for the sexual partner to be examined and treated to avoid recurrence of the PID, and (6) recognizing that intercourse is sometimes very painful after an occurrence of PID and that sexual activity should be avoided until advised by a physician.

Toxic Shock Syndrome

Etiology/pathophysiology. Toxic shock syndrome (TSS) was first identified in the 1970s. It is an acute bacterial infection caused by *Staphylococcus aureus* and usually occurs in women who are menstruating and using tampons (particularly superabsorbent tampons). Women at greatest risk are those who insert tampons with their fingers instead of with inserters, women with chronic vaginal infections, and women with genital herpes. TSS can also occur in nonmenstruating women.

Clinical manifestations. Often the woman will have flu-like symptoms for the first 24 hours. Between days 2 and 4 of the menstrual period the patient may have an elevated temperature (up to 102° F [39° C]), vomiting, diarrhea, myalgia, hypotension, and signs suggesting the onset of septic shock. Sore throat, headache, and a red macular palmar or diffuse rash followed by desquamation of the skin, hands, and feet may develop, urinary output is decreased, and the urea nitrogen level is elevated. Disorientation may occur from dehydration and release of toxins. Pulmonary edema and inflammation of mucous membranes may occur.

Assessment. Collection of *subjective data* includes determining whether the patient has recently used tampons, and how long she used a single tampon before changing it. Information should be obtained about myalgia, sore throat, headache, and fatigue.

Collection of *objective data* includes assessing for edema. The palms and soles should be assessed for the presence of an erythematous rash. Desquamation and sloughing occur within 1 to 2 weeks after the rash. The patient's level of consciousness should be noted. The presence of hypotension is a sign of TSS. Nonpurulent inflammation of the conjunctiva and hyperemia of the oropharynx and vagina are also signs of TSS.

Diagnostic tests. Blood tests will demonstrate leukocytosis, thrombocytopenia, and elevated levels of bilirubin, urea nitrogen, creatinine, SGOT (AST), SGPT (ALT), and CPK. Blood and urine cultures should be taken along with throat cultures when appropriate, and vaginal and genital specimens should be evaluated.

Medical management. Treatment of TSS varies because of the range in types of and severity of symptoms. Antibotic therapy is given according to the results of the culture and sensitivity tests performed. Parenteral therapy is given to maintain proper fluid balance. Laboratory data are evaluated for electrolyte imbalance caused by vomiting and diarrhea, elevated BUN suggesting renal involvement, and elevated enzymes suggesting liver dysfunction.

Nursing interventions. When the patient is hospitalized, bed rest is prescribed and antibiotics are administered. Close monitoring of vital signs and fluid status is important. If there is respiratory distress, oxygen therapy is instituted.

NURSING DIAGNOSES	NURSING INTERVENTIONS
Anxiety, related to TSS	Encourage patient to verbalize fears. Provide quiet, therapeutic environment. Provide support and understanding.
Potential for fluid volume deficit, related to vomiting and diarrhea	Monitor amount, frequency, and characteristics of vomitus and diarrhea. Assess tissue turgor for evidence of dehydration. Assess patient for dry mucous membranes, and monitor parenteral fluids with electrolytes as ordered. Monitor intake and output.
Pain, related to myalgia	Provide comfort measures. Administer analgesics as ordered.

Patient teaching. Since the use of tampons during menstruation has been linked to TSS, it is recommended that superabsorbent tampons not be used. If tampons are used, they should be alternated with the use of pads. Tampons should be changed frequently (every 4 hours) and should be inserted carefully to avoid abrasions. Patients who have had TSS should not use tampons. The patient should be taught to wash hands thoroughly before inserting a tampon. Women who are menstruating and develop a sudden high fever accompanied by vomiting and diarrhea should be counseled by the nurse to seek immediate medical attention. If the woman is wearing a tampon, she should remove it immediately.

DISORDERS OF THE FEMALE REPRODUCTIVE SYSTEM

Endometriosis

Endometriosis is a condition in which endometrial tissue appears outside the uterus.

Etiology/pathophysiology. The tissue can be found on the ovaries, fallopian tubes, and uterus, within the abdominal cavity, and in the vagina (Fig. 36-11). The spread of the tissue is believed to be through the lymphatic circulation, or by menstrual backflow to the fallopian tubes and pelvic cavity, or through congenital displacement of the endometrial cells.

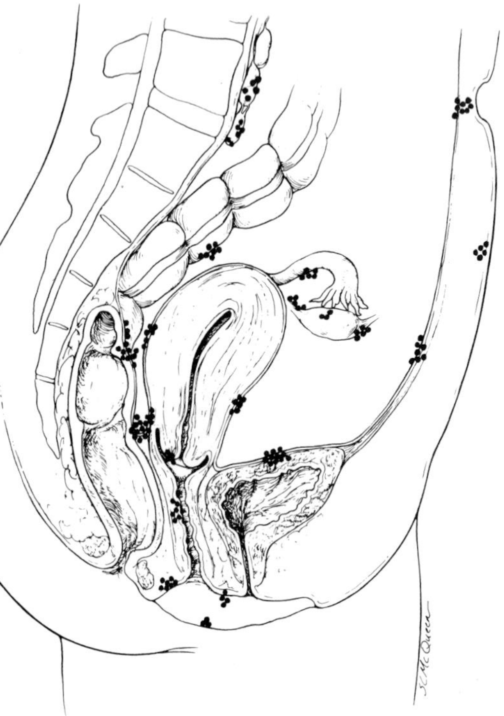

FIG. 36-11 Common sites of endometriosis.

The tissue responds to the normal stimulation of the ovaries, bleeds each month, and forms an endometrial crust, which causes an endometrial cyst. The endometrial cyst may rupture and cause further reproduction of tissue.

Clinical manifestations. Symptoms are lower abdominal and pelvic pain with or without pain in the rectum. It may be unilateral or bilateral and may radiate to the lower back, legs, and groin. Symptoms are more acute during menstruation and subside after menstruation. Endometriosis occurs with women over the age of 30. Women who have not conceived or lactated are at greater risk. Pregnancy is encouraged, because it is believed that an interruption of the menstrual cycle will slow the progress of the disorder. Pregnancy is also advised for women who want children, because a complication of endometriosis is infertility.

Assessment. Collection of *subjective data* includes obtaining a history of the patient's symptoms, including pelvic pain with menstruation, aching, cramping, a bearing-down sensation in the pelvis, or lower back dyspareunia (sexual intercourse is accompanied by pain). The type of pain may indicate the presence of ripe cysts that are about to rupture or may indicate the formation of infected tissue. The patient may reveal a history of menstrual irregularities such as amenorrhea.

Collection of *objective data* involves noting signs, which generally appear 5 to 7 days before menses and last 2 to 3 days. Signs may include abnormal uterine bleeding.

Diagnostic tests. Laparoscopy with a biopsy of the lesions may confirm the diagnosis. Regular pelvic examinations are recommended to monitor the progression of endometriosis.

Medical management. Medical treatment consists of high-dose antiovulatory medications to inhibit ovulation and induce a state physiologically similar to pregnancy and therefore suppress menstruation. Synthetic androgens such as danazol may be prescribed to arrest proliferation of the endometrium and to prevent ovulation, and thus to produce atrophy of the displaced endometrium. Occasionally women will have spontaneous disappearance of endometriosis. Some women who become pregnant remain asymptomatic after pregnancy. When the involvement is severe, surgery may be necessary. A laparoscopy may be performed to remove endometrial implants and to remove adhesions. Lasers may be used to vaporize the small implants of endometrial tissue. A total hysterectomy, oophorectomy, and salpingectomy may also be done.

Nursing interventions. The nurse should reinforce the physician's explanation of the expected results of treatment, instruct the patient regarding the dosage, frequency, and side effects of prescibed medications, and emphasize the importance of regular check-ups and of reporting abnormal vaginal bleeding. The nurse should also encourage the patient to verbalize her concerns. The nurse should assist the patient with comfort measures and help her with adaptive reponses to self-concept.

NURSING DIAGNOSES	NURSING INTERVENTIONS
Pain, related to displaced endometrial tissue	Institute comfort measures to cope with pain, such as medications and warm compresses to abdomen. Maintain bed rest when pain is most severe.
Anxiety, related to unpredictable nature of the illness	Provide emotional support during symptoms by encouraging verbalization of concerns, making correct responses, and referral to appropriate resources. Assist to develop effective coping mechanisms.
Sexual dysfunction, related to painful intercourse or infertility	Relate importance of communicating fears and concerns, which lead to anxiety.
Altered health maintenance, related to insufficient knowledge of condition and medication therapy	Instruct patient to take medications as prescribed and rationale for same.

Patient teaching. The nurse caring for a patient who has endometriosis should reinforce the physician's explanation of the expected results of treatment, teach the patient pain-relieving techniques, instruct the patient regarding the dosage and frequency and possible side effects of prescribed medication, and emphasize the importance of regular checkups and the importance of reporting any abnormal vaginal bleeding.

Vaginal Fistula

A fistula is defined as an abnormal opening between two organs.

Etiology/pathophysiology. Vaginal fistulas are caused by an ulcerating process resulting from cancer, radiation, weakening of tissue by pregnancies, and surgical interventions.

Vaginal fistulas are named for the organs involved (Fig. 36-12):

- Urethrovaginal fistula: opening between the urethra and vagina
- Vesicovaginal fistula: opening between the bladder and vagina
- Rectovaginal fistula: opening between the rectum and vagina

Clinical manifestations. Fistulas are recognized by their exudate, which has a distinct odor of urine or feces. Generally a bladder infection is present. The vesicovaginal fistula causes a constant trickling of urine into the vagina; a rectovaginal fistula allows feces and flatus to enter the vagina.

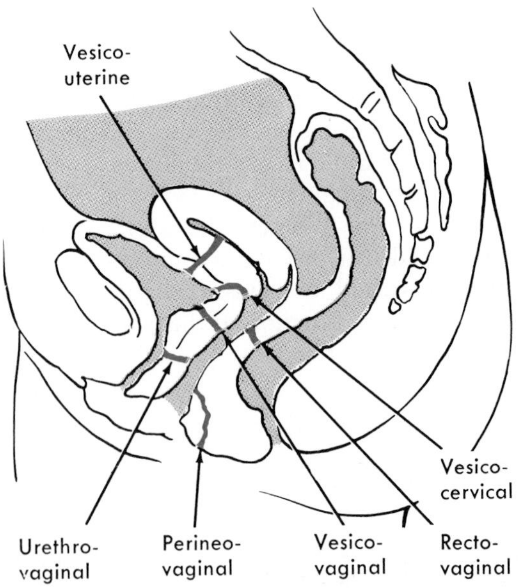

FIG. 36-12 Types of fistulas that may develop in vagina and uterus.

Assessment. Collection of *subjective data* includes the patient's understanding of the exudate that occurs as well as of any causative factors. The patient will report the presence of urine or feces from the vagina.

Collection of *objective data* that should be assessed includes any behaviors that indicate stress, anxiety, and pain. The patient may express feelings of disturbance in self-esteem because of the condition. The nurse should observe for urine or feces on the perineal pad.

Diagnostic tests. Diagnostic testing includes methylene blue instillation in bladder, and an intravenous pyelogram and/or cystoscopy to assist in the location of the fistula. Pelvic examination is performed.

Medical management. In some cases fistulas will heal spontaneously. Healing is promoted by an increase in vitamin C and protein in the diet. If inflammation is present, the treatment is delayed to allow inflammation to subside. The patient is given oral or parenteral antibiotics. If the organ tissue is healthy, a surgical approach is recommended. The surgical approach may be similar to anterior or posterior colporrhaphy, which will be discussed later in the chapter. Fistulas that are difficult to repair or very large may require urinary or fecal diversion.

Nursing interventions. Soiling from leakage of urine or stool into the vagina is disturbing for the patient. Sitz baths, deodorizing douches, perineal pads, and protective undergarments will be necessary. If the fistula is repaired surgically, a Foley catheter will be inserted postoperatively to prevent strain on the suture line caused by a full bladder. Nursing diagnoses and interventions include the following.

NURSING DIAGNOSES	NURSING INTERVENTIONS
Impaired skin integrity, related to exudate and irritation	Teach and assist in caring for the skin with douches, creams, and Sitz baths.
Sexual dysfunction, related to pain during sexual activity	Offer support and understanding of distress toward sexual activities and self-esteem.
Ineffective individual coping, related to abnormal vaginal exudate	Actively listen. Teach patient douche cleansing and meticulous care of perineal area. Encourage adaptive coping behaviors.
Fear, related to concern about outcome of surgical therapy or medical treatment	Encourage verbalization of fears. Answer questions honestly.

Relaxed Pelvic Muscles

The most common problems resulting from relaxed pelvic muscles are displaced uterus with prolapse and or procidentia, cystocele, urethrocele, rectocele, enterocele, and malpositions of the uterus.

Displaced uterus. Normally the uterus lies with the cervix at a right angle to the long axis of the vagina, and the body of the uterus is inclined slightly forward. A displaced uterus is usually congenital, but may be caused by childbirth. Backward displacement may be retroversion or retroflexion. Retroversion position places the cervix at the normal axis, but the body of the uterus is directed toward the sacrum. In retroflexion the angle of the body of the uterus is on the cervix. The patient has backache, muscle strain, leukorrheal discharge, and heaviness in the pelvic area and tires easily. Treatment consists of a pessary and possible uterine suspension.

Uterine prolapse and procidentia

Etiology/pathophysiology. Uterine prolapse is a herniation of the uterus into the vagina and at times beyond the vulva **(procidentia)** (Fig. 36-13). When the uterus loses its support, the organ descends and prolapses into the vaginal canal. In uterine procidentia there is a protrusion of the uterus, vaginal wall, rectum, and bladder.

Obstetrical trauma, overstretching of the uterine muscle support system, coughing, straining, and lifting heavy objects contribute to uterine prolapse and procidentia.

Clinical manifestations. The woman with uterine prolapse or procidentia may complain of urinary incontinence, retention, constipation, backache, and vaginal exudate from the increased pressure exerted by the prolapsed uterus. The symptoms may increase with coughing or prolonged standing.

Medical management. A vaginal pessary may be of some help, but the surgical correction is generally a vaginal hysterectomy with anterior and posterior repair. It is also called an anteroposterior colporrhaphy.

Cystocele and rectocele

Etiology/pathophysiology and clinical manifestations. When the tissue, muscles, and ligaments that support the uterus and perineum have been stretched and weakened by childbearing, multiple births, and/or cervical tears, the organs gradually move into other positions. The relaxation of the tissues, muscles, and ligaments of the bladder causes a displacement of the bladder into the vagina. This is referred to as a *cystocele* (Fig. 36-14). Clinical symptoms are urinary urgency, frequency, and/or incontinence, fatigue, and pelvic pressure. A large cystocele prevents complete emptying of the bladder, which leads to bacterial growth and infection.

The relaxation of the supporting tissues to the rectum causes the rectum to move toward the posterior vaginal wall and form a rectocele (Fig. 36-15). The rectocele causes constipation, rectal pressure, heaviness, and hemorrhoids.

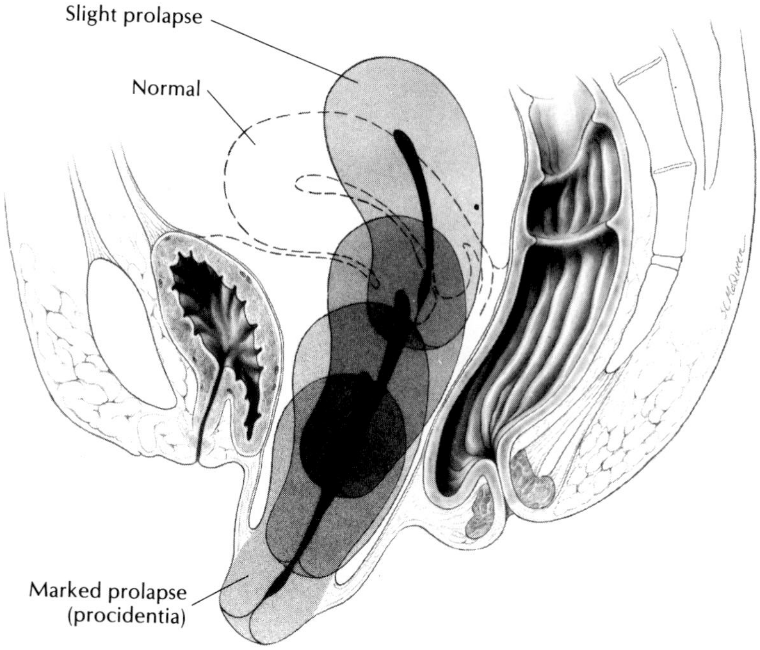

FIG. 36-13 Prolapse of the uterus. (Redrawn from Symmonds RE: Relaxation of pelvic supports. In Benson RC, editor: Current obstetric and gynecologic diagnosis and treatment, ed 5, Los Altos, Calif, 1984, Lange Medical Publications.)

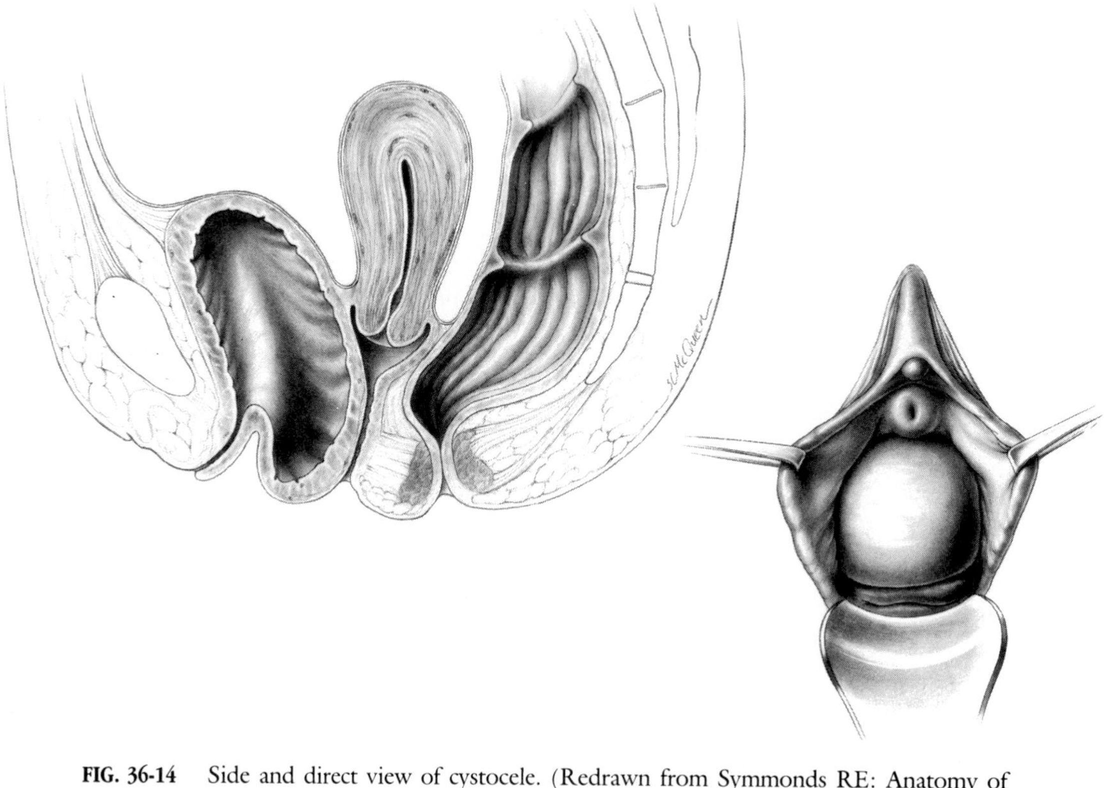

FIG. 36-14 Side and direct view of cystocele. (Redrawn from Symmonds RE: Anatomy of the female reproductive system. In Benson RC, editor: Current obstetric and gynecologic diagnosis and treatment, ed 5, Los Altos, Calif, 1984, Lange Medical Publications.)

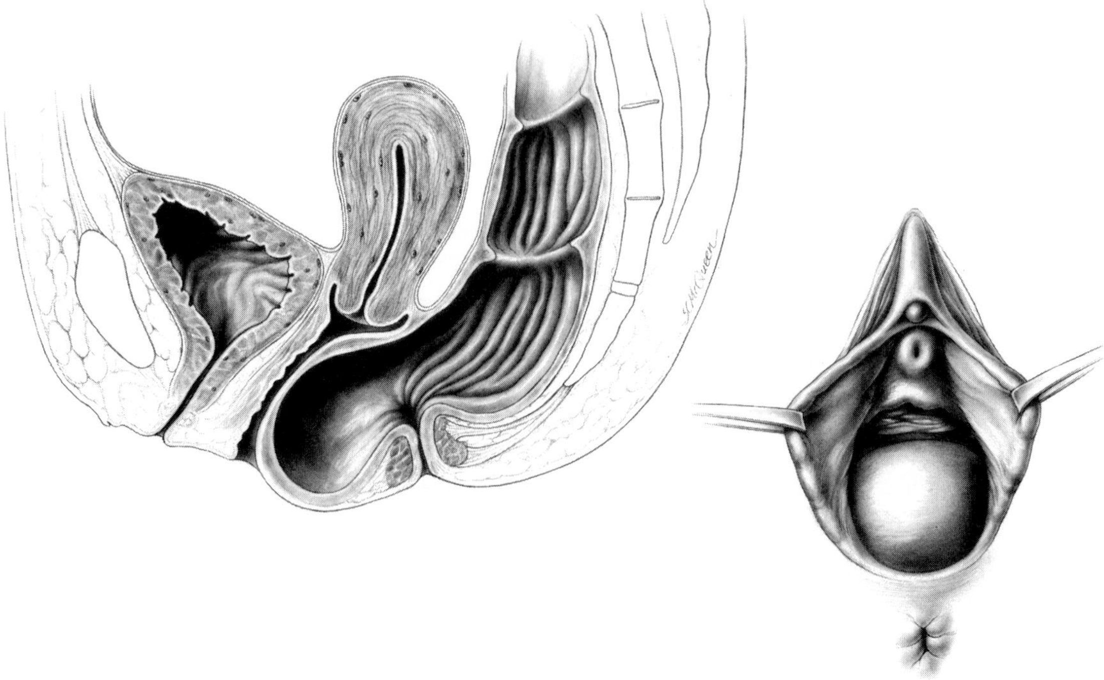

FIG. 36-15 Side and direct views of rectocele. (Redrawn from Symmonds RE: Relaxations of pelvic supports. In Benson RC, editor: Current obstetric and gynecologic diagnosis and treatment, ed 5, Los Altos, Calif, 1985, Lange Medical Publications.)

Medical management. Correction of cystocele and rectocele is by surgical repair, involving shortening the muscles that support the bladder and repair of the rectocele. This is known as anterior-posterior or anteroposterior **colporrhaphy.** It is sometimes referred to as an A&P repair.

Nursing interventions. Preoperative and postoperative nursing interventions include the following. Preoperative care for colporrhaphy is especially important in ensuring as clean an operative area as possible. Patients may be given a cathartic followed by enemas to be sure the bowel is completely empty. A liquid diet for 48 hours before surgery will help keep the bowel empty. A cleansing vaginal douche is given the evening before and the morning of surgery. Postoperative care includes checking vital signs and observing for hemorrhage. A retention catheter is usually inserted into the bladder to keep it empty and prevent pressure on sutures. It is important to keep the fecal residue as soft as possible; some physicians order only liquids for several days, or they may order mineral oil to be given every night. An oil retention enema may be ordered, but cleansing enemas are not given. The perineal area is cleansed carefully using surgical asepsis. Early ambulation is encouraged.

Patient teaching. The patient should be advised against standing for long periods or lifting heavy objects. Coitus must be avoided until healing occurs, usually about 6 weeks.

Benign Tumors of the Uterus

Etiology/pathophysiology. Fibroid tumors or leiomyomas are benign tumors arising from the muscle tissue of the uterus. It has been estimated that 20% to 25% of women over 30 years of age develop uterine fibroid tumors (myomas). Because their growth is stimulated by ovarian hormones, uterine fibroids tend to disappear with menopause. They rarely become malignant.

The size and number of myomas vary. Most are found in the body of the uterus, but some occur in the cervix or may involve the broad ligaments.

Clinical manifestations. The symptoms are primarily pressure from an enlarging pelvic mass, pain (including dysmenorrhea), abnormal uterine bleeding, and abnormally long or heavy bleeding **(menorrhagia)** with menstrual periods. If the fibroid tumor becomes large enough to cause pressure on other structures, there may be backache, constipation, and urinary symptoms.

Assessment. Collection of *subjective data* includes asking the patient about the presence of pain with menstruation or abnormally heavy flow. The patient is asked to describe her symptoms, which may include pelvic fullness or heaviness, constipation, urinary frequency or urgency, and menorrhagia.

Collection of *objective data* includes assessing the patient for excessive heavy discharge of blood by observing the number and saturation of perineal pads.

Diagnostic tests. Diagnostic studies may include a pregnancy test, dilation and curettage (D&C), laparoscopy, and ultrasonography.

Medical management. The treatment of fibroid tumors depends on the symptoms and the age of the patient, whether more children are desired, and how near to menopause the woman is. If there is severe bleeding or obstruction, a hysterectomy may be necessary.

Nursing interventions and patient teaching. For preoperative and postoperative nursing interventions for the patient who has a hysterectomy, see pp. 938-940 and Chapter 26. The nurse caring for a patient with fibroid tumors should reinforce the physician's explanation of the treatment plan—either a total hysterectomy or pelvic examination at regular intervals to monitor the status of the fibroid tumor. The nurse instructs the patient about the dosage and frequency of prescribed medications and possible side effects. The patient with menorrhagia should be taught to include adequate iron in her diet to prevent iron deficiency anemia from the extra blood loss. The importance of regular checkups to monitor the status of the fibroid tumor should be emphasized, and the nurse can encourage the patient to express her feelings and assist her with appropriate coping mechanisms.

NURSING DIAGNOSES	NURSING INTERVENTIONS
Pain, related to fibroid tumors	Assess pain location, onset, and duration. Administer analgesics as ordered. Provide comfort measures as needed.
Self-esteem disturbance, related to the presence of fibroid tumors	Encourage verbalization of concerns. Be an active listener.

Ovarian Cysts

Etiology/pathophysiology. Ovarian cysts are benign tumors that arise from dermoid cells of the ovary or from a cystic corpus luteum or graafian follicle.

Clinical manifestations. Ovarian cysts enlarge and are palpable on examination. They may cause no symptoms, or they may result in a disturbance of menstruation, a feeling of heaviness, and slight vaginal bleeding.

Medical management. The cysts are usually removed before they become malignant or obstruct blood supply to the ovaries.

Nursing interventions. Nursing interventions are similar to those for the patient having an abdominal hysterectomy (see pp. 938-940).

Hysterectomy

A hysterectomy involves the removal of the uterus, including the cervix. This procedure may be done for many conditions, such as dysfunctional uterine bleeding, endometriosis, malignant and nonmalignant tumors of the uterus and cervix, and disorders of pelvic relaxation and uterine prolapse.

Various terms are used to describe the removal of the uterus. A total hysterectomy is the removal of the entire uterus. The vagina remains intact and intercourse is possible even though childbearing is not. Estrogens are still released. Menopause will occur naturally because the ovaries are still present. A total abdominal hysterectomy with bilateral salpingooophorectomy (TAH-BSO) is the removal of the uterus, fallopian tubes, and ovaries. It is sometimes called panhysterosalpingooophorectomy. A radical hysterectomy also includes the removal of the pelvic lymph nodes. If the ovaries are removed with these surgeries, there is a surgically induced menopause.

Vaginal hysterectomy. A vaginal hysterectomy may be done for a prolapsed uterus. It is not used nearly as often as the abdominal approach. The vaginal approach is selected for the patient who cannot tolerate abdominal surgery or prolonged anesthesia. There is no abdominal incision. The uterus is removed through the vagina. Advantages of the vaginal entrance are that there is no wound dehiscence, there is less pain, complications are less likely, hospitalization is shorter, and there is no abdominal scar. The most important disadvantage is that there is a limited view of the operative field for visualizing intrapelvic and intraabdominal organs. Other disadvantages are risk of bleeding and postoperative infection.

Abdominal hysterectomy. An abdominal hysterectomy is preferred when there is a need to explore the pelvic cavity and if the fallopian tubes and ovaries are to be removed. There are three procedures for an abdominal hysterectomy, named according to the extent of the surgery performed. *Subtotal hysterectomy* refers to the removal of the corpus (the larger upper portion or body) of the uterus and leaves the cervical stump in place. *Total hysterectomy* is the removal of the entire uterus, including the cervix, but leaving the fallopian tubes and ovaries in place. *Total hysterectomy with bilateral salpingooophorectomy* or **hysterosalpingooophorectomy** involves the removal of the entire uterus plus the fallopian tubes and the ovaries.

Nursing interventions for the hysterectomy patient

Preoperative interventions. When the physician has explained the surgery to the patient, the nurse can reinforce the explanation and answer questions the patient might have. The nurse should encourage verbalization of fears. Additional preoperative instructions are given to help the woman prepare for recovery postoperatively. The nurse should instruct the patient how to turn, cough, and deep breathe.

Before a vaginal or abdominal hysterectomy, the colon is emptied to prevent postoperative distention. The patient may be on a low-residue diet for several days preoperatively. Enemas may be given the evening before surgery.

The bladder may be decompressed to prevent pressure on the suture site and to protect it from accidental trauma during surgery. The indwelling catheter will generally remain in place for 1 or 2 days after surgery.

An antiseptic vaginal douche may be ordered to decrease microbial invasion of the surgical site.

If the surgeon anticipates excessive manipulation of the intestines, a nasogastric tube may be inserted to prevent abdominal distention. The patient should be instructed about the purpose of the tube and that it will be kept in place for a few days after surgery.

Surgical preparation of the skin includes the surgical prepping of the abdomen, pelvis, and perineum. The patient will sign a consent form and oral intake will be restricted from midnight on.

Postoperative interventions. Postoperative nursing interventions focus on monitoring vital signs and preventing urinary retention, intestinal distention, and venous thrombosis. If a retention catheter was inserted, it should be kept patent and connected to closed drainage. Meticulous catheter care is performed to prevent bladder infection. If no retention catheter is in place, the patient must be checked frequently for bladder distention; an accurate urine output is recorded. The incidence of urinary retention is greater after a hysterectomy than after any other type of surgery, because some trauma to the bladder unavoidably occurs. If the patient does not have a catheter and is unable to void, catheterization every 8 hours may be necessary. Occasionally the patient will have residual urine. The physician often orders catheterization of the patient to check for residual urine; 60 ml or less is within the normal range.

A nasogastric tube may be inserted. A small up-and-down flush enema may be ordered to help relieve distention. Early ambulation is very helpful to return the bowel to normal function. When bowel sounds have returned and flatus is being expelled, the patient is allowed liquids by mouth and a gradual increase in return to solid foods.

Patients undergoing pelvic surgery are more susceptible to venous stasis and thrombophlebitis because of trauma to blood vessels. The patient is usually permitted to be out of bed on the first postoperative day, but the nurse should encourage the patient to dangle her legs and to sit on the side of the bed before standing and walking to prevent the effects of postural hypotension. Antiembolic stockings may be used to prevent thrombus or embolus formation, and legs should be exercised frequently when the patient is in bed. The patient should avoid bending her knees and gatching the bed or placing pillows under her knees. These activities could cause pooling of blood in the pelvic cavity, resulting in stasis in the lower extremities. The patient at risk for thromboembolic disease may receive low-dose heparin to prevent thrombus formation.

Analgesics such as meperidine (Demerol) may be ordered for relief of pain. Slight vaginal drainage may occur for 1 or 2 days, but any unusual bleeding should be reported to the physician.

The nurse will observe the abdominal dressing on the patient with an abdominal hysterectomy for evidence of hemorrhage. Surgical asepsis is carried out for the dressing change. The patient usually receives intravenous feedings for several days postoperatively. The rate of flow and the condition of the IV site are carefully monitored.

NURSING DIAGNOSES	NURSING INTERVENTIONS
Knowledge deficit, related to preoperative and postoperative period	Obtain feedback of patient's knowledge of surgery and preoperative and postoperative procedures. Clarify any misconceptions related to outcome of the surgical procedure, such as fear of sexual dysfunction, mood swings, and loss of femininity. Provide education related to surgical menopause. Provide emotional support to patient and her partner.
Altered patterns of urinary elimination, related to postsurgical sensorimotor impairment	Connect indwelling catheter to closed gravity drainage. Give meticulous catheter care as indicated. Record color and amount of urinary output. Promote micturition at regular intervals when catheter is removed. Catheterize for residual urine as ordered.
Potential for self-esteem disturbance, related to body image change and value of reproductive organs	Encourage verbalization with significant others. Relate importance of communicating anything that causes anxiety. Reinforce correct information and provide factual information to correct any misconceptions.
Pain, related to abdominal incision	Assess postoperative pain. Administer analgesics as ordered. Assist patient in splinting abdominal incision while coughing and ambulating.
Altered peripheral tissue perfusion, related to pelvic surgery, thrombophlebitis	Do not elevate the bed in the knee gatch position. Assess proper placement of antiembolic stockings every 4 hours as ordered. Assist in passive and active leg exercises every shift.

NURSING DIAGNOSES	NURSING INTERVENTIONS
Altered peripheral tissue perfusion, related to pelvic surgery, thrombophlebitis—cont'd	Encourage ambulation. Assess legs for erythema, increased tenderness, severe cramping, positive Homans' sign every shift.

Patient teaching. Before the patient's discharge, the physician will explain to the woman and her partner that there should be no sexual intercourse for 4 to 6 weeks after surgery. If there has been an abdominal incision, there may be further restrictions on heavy lifting (nothing over 10 pounds), walking up and down stairs, and prolonged riding in the car. Riding in the car may cause pelvic pooling and development of a thrombus in the legs.

The patient should know that vaginal drainage is normal for about 2 to 4 weeks after an abdominal hysterectomy.

The patient should avoid wearing any tight clothing such as a girdle or knee-high hose, which might constrict circulation to the surgical site and cause venous stasis.

There are several signs and symptoms of infections that should be reported by the patient to the physician if they occur: (1) erythema, edema, exudate, or increased tenderness along surgical incision, (2) increased malodorous vaginal exudate, (3) a temperature of 101° F (38.3° C) or more, and (4) any problems with urinating, such as difficulty starting to void, voiding too often, voiding small amounts, or a burning sensation while urinating (indicative of a bladder infection).

CANCER OF THE FEMALE REPRODUCTIVE TRACT

Cancer is the second most common cause of death in women, and malignant tumors of the reproductive tract represent a significant portion of the total number of deaths from cancer.

Ovarian cancer is the fifth most frequently occurring cancer in women. Uterine cancer, principally arising in the cervix, is the sixth most common cancer of women, ranking behind cancer of the (1) breast, (2) colon and rectum, (3) endometrium, (4) lung, and (5) ovary. Cervical cancer often affects women in their reproductive years and with the diagnostic Pap smear the cancer can be detected in its early stages. Unfortunately, only 10% to 15% of women in the United States obtain a Pap smear each year.

Endometrial cancer is primarily a disease of women over 50 years of age, but the incidence among younger women is increasing. Most cases of ovarian cancer occur in women over 50, but malignant neoplasms of the ovaries may occur at all ages.

Cancer of the Cervix

Cancer of the cervix is usually a squamous cell carcinoma. Unless treated in its early stages, the tumor invades the vagina, pelvic wall, bladder, rectum, and regional lymph nodes.

Etiology/pathophysiology. Women who become sexually active in their teens are at a higher risk for cancer of the cervix, as are those who have had multiple sexual partners, those who have multiple births, and those of lower socioeconomic status. There is an increased incidence of cervical carcinoma in young women whose mothers took diethylstilbestrol (DES) during pregnancy as treatment to prevent spontaneous abortion.

Viral and chronic infections and erosions of the cervix are most likely significant in the development of cancer. **Carcinoma in situ** is a preinvasive, asymptomatic carcinoma that can only be diagnosed by microscopic examination of cervical cells. Once it is diagnosed, it can be treated early without radical surgery. Carcinoma in situ of the cervix is essentially 100% curable.

Clinical manifestations. Most cervical cancer is silent in the early stages and offers few symptoms. The two chief symptoms are leukorrhea and irregular vaginal bleeding or spotting between menses. Bleeding often occurs after coitus or after menopause. Bleeding at first appears as very slight, but as the disease progresses, the bleeding increases in amount. The vaginal exudate becomes watery and then increases as a dark, bloody exudate that has an offensive odor caused by necrosis and infection of the tumor mass. As the cancer progresses, the bleeding may become constant and increasing in amount. With advanced stages there is severe pain in the back and upper thighs and legs.

Assessment. Collection of *subjective data* includes the nurse urging women to have regular health appraisals and pelvic examinations, so that cancer of the cervix can be detected in its earliest stages. The patient will present no symptoms in the early stages of cancer of the cervix. If the tumor becomes more invasive, the patient will experience back and leg pain, weight loss, and malaise.

Collection of *objective data* includes assessing the patient for abnormal vaginal discharge by observing the sanitary pads. The vaginal exudate may be watery to dark red and malodorous. The number and saturation of the perineal pads should be noted. If the tumor becomes more invasive, the patient will be assessed for anemia, fever, and the presence of lymphedema.

Diagnostic tests. The following tests are performed to determine the presence of cervical cancer: (1) Pap smear, (2) Schiller's test, (3) physical examination, (4) cervical biopsy, and (5) additional diagnostic studies, such as chest x-ray evaluation, intravenous pyelogram, cystoscopy, sigmoidoscopy, or liver function studies to determine the extent of invasion.

Medical management. Carcinoma in situ is treated by

removal of the affected area. This removal can be accomplished by a variety of techniques, including electrocautery, laser, conization, and hysterectomy. Conization is the removal of a cone-shaped section of the cervix. This surgery is particularly useful to preserve childbearing function.

Early carcinoma of the cervix can be treated with a hysterectomy or intracavitary radiation (see Chapter 41).

A radical hysterectomy with pelvic lymph node dissection may be required for more extensive lesions. The treatment plan is tailored to each patient based on the extent of the disease.

Nursing interventions. Nursing interventions should include verbal reassurance. In advanced cancer of the cervix, the nurse should position the patient comfortably, change her position slowly, maintain the patient's body alignment, provide pain relief measures, change the patient's dressings and sanitary pads frequently, and assess color, odor, and amount of drainage. The skin is assessed for impairment. (See pp. 938-940 regarding nursing interventions for the patient having a hysterectomy.)

NURSING DIAGNOSES	NURSING INTERVENTIONS
Fear, related to diagnosis of cancer	Assist patient with recognizing and clarifying fears and with developing coping strategies for those fears. Be an active listener.
Impaired skin integrity, related to drainage	Assist and teach patient to perform perineal care every 3 to 4 hours. Keep skin dry. Change sanitary pads every 3 to 4 hours or more frequently if needed.
Self-esteem disturbance, related to body image change and value of reproductive organs	Encourage patient's comments and questions about condition. Encourage verbalization with significant others. Provide factual information to correct any misconceptions.
Pain, related to complication of metastasis	Assist patient in assuming a position of comfort. Administer analgesics as ordered. Keep patient pain free.

Patient teaching. The nurse can both educate and encourage patients to assume responsibility for their health by having a yearly Pap smear. The nurse should encourage patients to seek prompt medical assistance for any abnormal vaginal exudate.

Cancer of the Endometrium

Etiology/pathophysiology. Cancer of the endometrium (uterine cancer) usually affects postmenopausal women. Endometrial cancer is usually an adenocarcinoma. The tumor is more likely to be localized, but may spread to the cervix, bladder, rectum, and surrounding lymph nodes. It is the most common malignancy of the female genital tract. Those in high-risk groups are women with a history of irregular menstruation, difficulties during menopause, obesity, hypertension, diabetes mellitus, those who have not had children, and those with a family history of cancer of the uterus. Women who have used high-level estrogen birth control pills and estrogen replacement therapy to treat menopausal symptoms have a greater likelihood of developing endometrial cancer.

The tumor in situ is slow growing. Invasion and metastasis occur later, with spread to the cervix and myometrium and ultimately to the vagina, pelvis, and lungs.

Clinical manifestations. About 50% of patients with postmenopausal bleeding have cancer of the uterus. Its progress is slow, metastasis occurs late, and the symptom of irregular vaginal bleeding often appears early enough to allow for cure of the disease. In premenstrual or postmenopausal women, any abnormal bleeding or spotting should be reported.

Assessment. Collection of *subjective data* includes the nurse assisting the patient in identifying and reporting changes in reproductive or sexual health. The patient may report abdominal pressure and pelvic fullness. The patient will have a history of postmenopausal bleeding and leukorrhea. Pelvic and back pain and postcoital bleeding are late signs and symptoms.

Collection of *objective data* includes the nurse observing the patient for color and amount of vaginal exudate on perineal pads. The nurse will assess the patient for complaints of pain and enlarged lymph nodes.

Diagnostic tests. Pelvic and rectal examination and D&C are used to diagnose cancer of the endometrium.

Medical management. Treatment of cancer of the endometrium depends on the stage of the tumor and the woman's health. Surgery, radiation, or chemotherapy may be used to remove the tumor and/or treat metastasis. For early cancer of the endometrium, a total abdominal hysterectomy and bilateral salpingo-oophorectomy are done. Intracavitary radiation followed by a hysterectomy and bilateral salpingo-oophorectomy may be done for the early stage of endometrial cancer (stage I). Patients with stage II disease may receive pelvic irradiation to cause shrinkage and help prevent spread. Afterward the patient will undergo a hysterectomy. Patients with stage III and IV disease are uncommon, and treatment is tailored for each patient based on extent of disease.

Nursing interventions. See pp. 938-940 concerning care of the patient undergoing a hysterectomy; also see Chapter 41 for care of the patient with intracavitary radiation.

Patient teaching. Health teaching and follow-up after discharge should emphasize the need for regular physical examination by the physician and the importance of compliance with the prescribed treatment plan.

Cancer of the Ovary

Etiology/pathophysiology. Ovarian cancer, the fifth most common cause of cancer death in women, is the leading cause of gynecological death in the United States. There is no known method for detecting ovarian cancer at an early stage. Women between the ages of 50 and 59 have the greatest number of cases of ovarian cancer, but it can occur at any age. In the early stages the tumors are asymptomatic and when detected usually have spread to other pelvic organs. Females at high risk are those who are infertile, anovulatory, nulliparous, and habitual aborters. Ovarian cancer commonly spreads by peritoneal seeding of the cancer cells. Common sites of metastasis are the peritoneum, omentum, and bowel surfaces.

Clinical manifestations. In the early stages the symptoms may cause vague abdominal discomfort, flatulence, and mild gastric disturbances. As the tumor progresses, abdominal girth enlarges from the presence of ascites, and there is flatulence with distention. Other symptoms that can be present are urinary frequency, nausea, vomiting, constipation, and weight loss.

Assessment. Collection of *subjective data* includes awareness that cancer of the ovary is difficult to detect. The patient will report symptoms of abdominal discomfort, gastric disturbances (such as nausea and constipation), and urinary frequency.

Collection of *objective data* includes the nurse observing any increase in the abdominal girth. The patient may void at frequent intervals because of pressure on the bladder. The patient may be dyspneic related to ascites and pressure on the diaphragm.

Diagnostic tests. Ovarian cancer is diagnosed by palpation of a pelvic mass and aspiration of ascitic fluid and detection of cancer cells in the fluid. A laparotomy is performed to determine the stage of the cancer.

Medical management. Ovarian cancer treatment often involves surgery alone or with radiation or chemotherapy. Surgical intervention may be a total abdominal hysterectomy with bilateral salpingo-oophorectomy and omentectomy (excision of portions of the peritoneal folds).

Nursing interventions. Nursing interventions for any patient with ovarian cancer include management similar to that for patients undergoing abdominal hysterectomy and receiving chemotherapy and external radiation. (See pp. 938-940 and Chapter 41.)

Because ovarian cancer is generally at an advanced stage at the time of diagnosis, despite the woman's feeling well, support and encouragement to comply with the treatment regimen is an important nursing intervention. As the disease progresses, the nurse will become involved in activities to increase the patient's comfort.

NURSING DIAGNOSES	NURSING INTERVENTIONS
Pain, related to metastatic process	Establish trusting relationship with patient.
Pain, related to metastatic process—cont'd	Monitor and document pain characteristics. Administer prescribed analgesics every 3 to 4 hours to control pain. Provide environment conducive to comfort and rest.
Ineffective breathing pattern, related to ascites and pressure on diaphragm	Maintain patient in semi-Fowler's position. Observe for respiratory distress. Administer oxygen as prescribed. Assist the patient to turn, cough, and deep breathe every 2 to 4 hours. Monitor vital signs.
Fluid volume excess, related to ascites	Monitor intravenous fluids. Maintain accurate intake and output. Weigh patient daily. Observe for signs of edema. Measure abdominal girth daily.
Ineffective patient and family coping: compromised, related to poor prognosis	Assess present coping abilities. Encourage and allow time for verbalization of feelings. Support patient's coping strengths, and discuss alternative coping measures. Involve patient and significant others in nursing interventions and procedures.

PROBLEMS OF THE FEMALE BREAST

Fibrocystic Breast Condition

Etiology/pathophysiology. Fibrocystic breast condition involves benign tumors of the breasts, usually occurs in women 30 to 50 years of age, and is rare in postmenopausal women. This suggests that the occurrence is related to ovarian activity.

The cysts are characterized by numerous cellular changes, with an abnormal amount of epithelial hyperplasia and cystic formation within the mammary ducts. The cysts rarely become malignant, but the risk of breast cancer does increase for women who have fibrocystic breast condition; therefore the cysts are observed with great caution.

Clinical manifestations. Cystic lesions are often bilateral and multiple. The cysts are soft, well differentiated, tender to touch, and freely movable. The lumpiness and tenderness are more apparent before menses.

Diagnostic tests. The disorder is diagnosed by mammography or ultrasound and confirmed by biopsy. As a therapeutic measure, the cyst is aspirated by needle and syringe to empty the secretions, and the fluid is sent to the laboratory for cytological examination. Aspiration produces a turbid, nonhemorrhagic yellow, greenish, or brownish fluid.

Medical management. When cysts recur in the same area and repeated aspirations are ineffective, surgical excision of the cyst may be done.

Conservative treatment is the usual approach to fibrocystic breast condition. The usefulness of eliminating methylxanthines from the diet (coffee, tea, cola) is still controversial, but it is the least expensive therapy. Many women have reported a lessening of symptoms after altering their diet, even though findings by palpation and mammogram were not significantly changed. Danocrine (danazol) may be prescribed to inhibit FSH and LH production, thereby decreasing ovarian production of estrogen. Danocrine may cause weight gain, hot flashes, menstrual irregularities, hirsutism, and deepening of the voice. Vitamin E may also be prescribed, but its efficacy has not been proved.

Patient teaching. The nurse should instruct the patient to perform breast self-examination 1 week after menses and be able to recognize the presence of cysts and note any changes.

Acute Mastitis

Acute mastitis is an acute bacterial infection usually caused by *Staphylococcus aureus* or streptococci. It is most often observed during lactation and late pregnancy. The infection may result from inadequate cleanliness of the breasts, a nipple fissure, or infection in the infant. The breasts are tender, inflamed, and engorged, causing the milk flow to be obstructed.

Treatment is application of warm packs, support to the area by a well-fitting brassiere (which also supplies comfort), and systemic treatment with antibiotics.

Chronic Mastitis

Chronic mastitis tends to develop in women between 30 and 50 years of age and is more common in those who have had children, have had difficulty with inverted and cracked nipples, and have had problems with nursing their infants. A traumatic blow to the breasts allows the fat to necrose in the area and form abscesses. There is an increased fibrosis of the tissue, which causes cysts to form. The cysts are tender, painful, and palpable on examination. The disorder is generally unilateral and benign and most frequently occurs in obese women. Treatment is the same as for acute mastitis.

Breast Cancer

Breast cancer is the most common malignancy affecting women in the United States. The incidence of breast cancer in men is rare—less than 1%. Statistics of 1989, estimating cancer incidences by site and sex, reveal that breast cancer incidence is the highest, at 28%, of all sites. It is estimated that breast cancer will occur in 1 of every 10 women in the United States. The 5- to 10-year survival rate has improved from 65% in 1970 to 82% in 1982.[7] This is probably related to early detection and improved treatment therapies. Vital to the process of detection are monthly breast self-examination, breast imaging with mammography and other diagnostic studies to detect small tumors before they can be palpated, and periodic breast examinations by a physician.

BOX 36-4 PREDISPOSING FACTORS FOR FEMALES AT HIGH RISK FOR BREAST CANCER

1. Sex: being a female introduces a high risk
2. Age: higher incidence occurs with women over age 40 and in the postmenopausal phase of life
3. Race: Caucasian in the middle or upper socioeconomic class
4. Genetics: women whose mother and sisters have developed cancer
5. Menarche: occurred before the age of 12
6. Parity (total number of pregnancies): decreased for women if birth is before 18 years; increased for unmarried women and infertile women, women who become pregnant after the age of 35
7. Menopause: late menopause after the age of 55
8. Other cancer: had other cancer such as endometrial, ovarian, and colon; if cancer has appeared in one breast, it is more likely to occur in the other breast

Etiology/pathophysiology. The cause of breast cancer is unknown. The high incidence occurring in women implies hormonal cause. Predisposing factors for women at high risk are shown in Box 36-4.

Other possible risks that influence cancer formation are exposure to heavy radiation, immunodeficiency (reduced protection against disease), estrogen therapy, high dietary fat intake, and fibrocystic breast condition.

Breast cancer is usually an adenocarcinoma, arises from the epithelium and develops in the lactiferous ducts, and infiltrates the parenchyma (the tissue of an organ other than the supporting or connective tissue). The cancer occurs most often in the upper outer quadrants of the breasts of women who have not given birth or breast-fed a child. A slow-growing breast cancer may take up to 8 or 9 years to become palpable or to have reached the size of a small pea. Metastasis is by the lymphatic system and bloodstream. The most common sites for metastasis are bone, lungs, pleura, breast site, central nervous system, and liver, in that order. When referring to estimated growth rate of breast cancer, the term "doubling time" indicates the time it takes malignant cells to double in number. Assuming that the doubling is constant and that the neoplasm originates in one cell, a carcinoma with a doubling time of 100 days may not reach clinically detectable size, 1 cm, for 8 years. Rapid growing cancers have a much shorter preclinical course and a greater tendency to metastasize to regional nodes or more distant sites by the time a breast mass is discovered.[9]

Clinical manifestations. Breast tumors are usually small, movable, and isolated with defined edges. There may be a change in skin color, tenderness present, puckering and/or dimpling (peau d'orange—appearance of an orange skin) of tissue, nipple discharge, and/or retraction of the nipple and axillary tenderness.

More than 70% of breast cancers are detected by the patient. Breast self-examinations should be performed at monthly intervals, preferably on an established routine examination 1 week after menses. Breast examination for the postmenopausal woman should be done on the same day of each month (Fig. 36-16). If on the monthly examination there are questionable findings, the patient should not hesitate to immediately contact her physician. The points emphasized in Box 36-5 should be used in teaching breast self-examination.

Diagnostic tests. Diagnosis of tumors is generally made by physical examination combined with mammography or ultrasound, and if necessary, confirmed by biopsy. If the screening mammogram indicates a problem or if the woman has a breast mass, a xeromammogram may be done. The xeromammogram provides a uniform image of the breast, giving a wide exposure.

A biopsy is an incisional procedure done in the operating room. The patient may be scheduled for removal of the breast if the biopsied tissue confirms malignancy. This type of scheduling reduces performing surgery twice and may be the choice of many women. Frequently patients prefer to have a discussion with physician and family regarding the biopsy report and to discuss alternative modes of treatment before a mastectomy is performed. Radiographic studies may be obtained before or after the biopsy to detect possible metastasis (Fig. 36-17) to the brain, chest, liver, and bones. Further confirmation may be needed to determine the status of lymph nodes of the axillary and the supraclavicular areas.

Medical management. The intervention for treatment of breast cancer depends on the stage of the tumor, the age and health status of the patient, the hormonal status, and the presence of estrogen receptors in the tumor. Radiation, chemotherapy, and surgery alone or in combination are the most common modes of treatment of cancer of the breasts (see Chapter 41).

Staging. After breast surgery and axillary dissection, the staging process is completed. The universal staging and classification system for breast cancer agreed on in 1987 is the tumor, node, metastasis (TNM) system (Box 36-6).[11] Staging depends on size of the tumor, size and presence or absence of nodal malignancy, and presence or

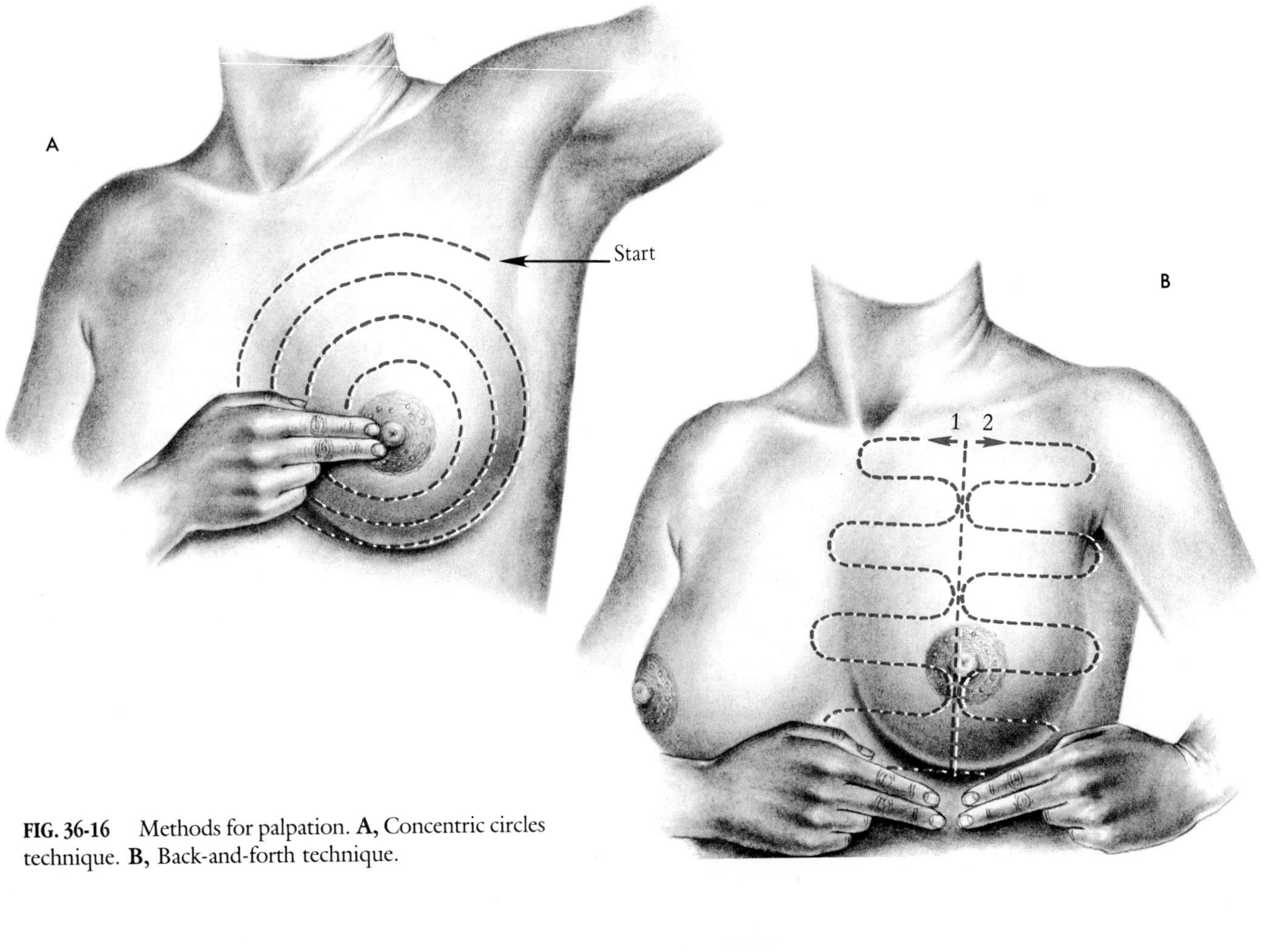

FIG. 36-16 Methods for palpation. **A,** Concentric circles technique. **B,** Back-and-forth technique.

BOX 36-5 **TEACHING BREAST SELF-EXAMINATION**

1. The majority of breast lumps are not cancer.
2. Most cancerous breast lesions are curable.
3. Breasts should be examined each month between the fourth and seventh day of the menstrual cycle, when they are least congested, and on the same day of each month for postmenopausal women.
4. Visual inspection and palpation should be done.
5. Visual inspection should be done when the woman is stripped to the waist and looking in a mirror, using the following arm positions: arms at rest at sides, hands on hips and pressed into hips, contracting chest muscles; hands over the head (torso in upright position); hands over head (torso leaning forward).
6. Palpation may be done in the shower when the soap and water assist the hands to glide over the skin. However, the examination of large breasts and axillae is better done in a supine position rather than a standing position.
7. The entire breast should be examined in a systematic way, moving clockwise, with a circular motion.
8. Specific examination of the nipple, through compression for discharge, and the areola, through palpation, should not be forgotten.
9. Any breast change should be reported to the physician.

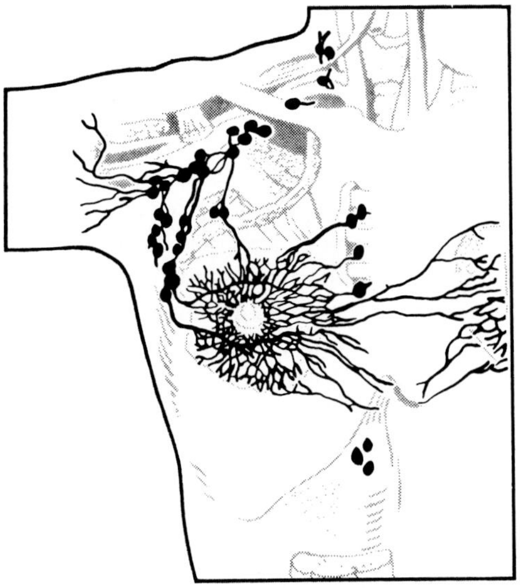

FIG. 36-17 Lymphatic spread of breast cancer. (From A cancer source book for nurses, rev ed, New York, 1981, American Cancer Society, Inc.)

absence of distant metastasis. Tumors are classified from stage 0 to stage IV.

Surgical interventions. Surgery plays a vital role in the management of breast cancer. Tissue biopsy, inspection

BOX 36-6 **TNM STAGING**

Stage 0: tumor in situ that has no nodal or metastatic involvement and is noninvasive

Stage I: tumor is 1 to 2 cm or smaller, with no nodal or metastatic involvement

Stage II: tumors 2 to 5 cm, with or without nodal involvement and no metastasis

Stage III: tumors 5 to 10 cm, usually with lymph node involvement and no metastasis

Stage IV: denotes any size tumor, with or without nodal involvement with distant metastasis

and biopsy of lymph nodes in the axillary areas, radiological examinations, and laboratory reports are aids in making the decision that surgery should be performed. Several surgical approaches may be selected for the removal of the breast carcinoma (Fig. 36-18). Types of approaches include the following:

1. A lumpectomy (**tylectomy,** tumorectomy) is the removal of a circumscribed area that includes the tumor. This type of surgery is usually done when the tumor is small and is on the peripheral area of the breast. The breast contour and muscle support are preserved if possible. The patient and physician may decide to use local irradiation of the breast to destroy potentially microscopic cancer cells in the area.
2. A partial mastectomy **(quadratectomy)** is the removal of the tumor plus a wedge of normal tissue that surrounds the tumor and possibly a portion of overlying and underlying fascia that covers the breast and chest muscle. Augmental surgery may be required at a later time, because this surgery can be disfiguring.
3. A subcutaneous mastectomy is the removal of malignant breast tissue, leaving the breast skin surface and nipple in place. At this time a prosthesis can be implanted if surgical conditions are considered appropriate.
4. A simple mastectomy is the removal of the entire breast. The skin flap is retained to cover the incised area. Both pectoralis major and pectoralis minor muscles are left intact.
5. A modified radical mastectomy is performed when the tumor is 4 cm or larger, if it is invasive, or if the patient and physician decide this procedure is in the patient's best interest. In this operation all breast tissue, overlying skin, nipple, and pectoralis minor muscle are removed, as are samples of lymph nodes from all surrounding positions; at times all adjunct lymph nodes are also removed.
6. A radical mastectomy involves removal of the breast, major and minor pectoral muscles, all lymph

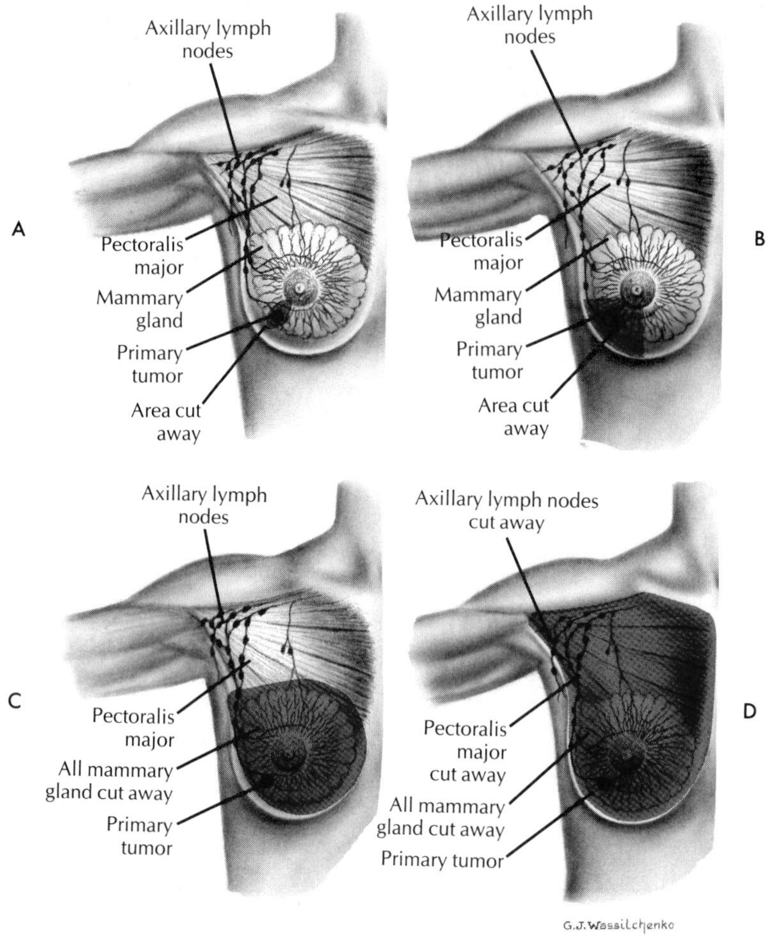

FIG. 36-18 Four ways to deal surgically with cancer of the breast. **A,** Lumpectomy (tylectomy). **B,** Quadrectomy (segmental resection). **C,** Total (simple) mastectomy. **D,** Radical mastectomy.

nodes, fat, and fascia. A skin graft may be used to cover the incised area. This type of surgery is seldom done in the United States, because refined techniques of pathological evaluations, radiation therapy, and chemotherapy have made it unnecessary in most cases.

Nursing interventions. The physician will discuss with the patient and family the rationale for mastectomy and the manner of coping with the cosmetic effects of and psychological response to the operation. Patients often have questions about possible alternatives to standard or modified mastectomy.

The patient may be confused with so many options of therapy and surgical interventions. During this time the nurse plays an active role as listener and reinforcer of information provided by the physician and providing responses that can encourage and assist the patient to verbalize her concerns and recognize her feelings about the surgery. The emotional preparation of the patient may be more important than the physical preparation. Often there is grieving for the lost body part.

Preoperative preparation enlists the participation of patient, support group, and nursing staff so that progressive care can continue, beginning at admission through surgery, recovery, and the postoperative period. The essential admission assessment provides data that are helpful in planning care by the nurse and patient. Nursing diagnoses can be developed and a plan of care individualized for the patient according to her needs. (See the Nursing Care Plan on pp. 947-948.)

It is important for the nurse to assess and identify the members of the patient's support system to know their strengths and concerns about the pending treatment and interventions. Support does not always need to come from the immediate family and close circle of friends. Outside support and resources can come from coworkers, religious groups, oncology clinicians, psychologists, and Reach To Recovery support groups. It is important to openly discuss the patient's fears, and this is often done by the nurse who has established a therapeutic relationship with the patient and family.

Reach To Recovery volunteers have been a source of information, encouragement, and support for the female with breast cancer. The organization is based on the premise that rehabilitation for a woman with breast can-

NURSING CARE PLAN: THE PATIENT UNDERGOING MASTECTOMY

Nursing diagnoses	Patient goals	Nursing interventions
Fear, related to the extent of the disease and surgical intervention	Patient will be able to state fears. Patient will be able to state a positive improvement in coping. Patient can describe type of surgical procedures. Patient can recite postoperative interventions that will occur.	Encourage expression of feelings. Provide a calm, supportive environment. Provide information on coping mechanisms. Encourage consultation with resource persons, e.g., psychologist, clergy, nurse specialist, and Reach to Recovery. Use support of family/significant others. Encourage patient's comments and questions about surgery and postoperative care.
Potential for infection, related to surgical incision	Skin will remain free of signs and symptoms of infection. Vital signs and WBC values will be maintained within normal limits.	Assess skin integrity. Instruct on signs and symptoms of infection. Assess and report abnormal vital signs and elevated WBC; skin changes and comfort level. Observe and record amount of exudate. Check drainage tubing for patency.
Body image disturbance, related to surgical procedure	Patient will verbalize acceptance of altered body image as evidenced by absence of weeping, irritability, verbalization of discomfort with present body, and attempting difficult physical or mental tasks despite limitations.	Encourage patient's comments and questions about surgery, progress, and prognosis. Reinforce correct information, and provide factual information to correct any misconceptions. Relate importance of communicating anything that causes anxiety. Encourage patient to verbalize and explore feelings regarding impact missing body part might have on patient's functioning as a sexual partner and in activities of daily living. Encourage patient to look at and touch the changed body part when she demonstrates readiness. Encourage use of rehabilitation services (e.g., Reach for Recovery, Wellness Community). Check drainage tubing for patency.
Pain, related to incision	Patient will verbalize site and nature of pain; will relate comfort increase. Patient will demonstrate willingness to participate in self-care activities. Patient will interact positively with staff and significant others. Patient will demonstrate relaxed facial expression and body movements.	Assess attitude toward pain; record verbal and nonverbal cues. Explore methods for controlling pain, e.g., medications, visual imagery, controlled breathing, and diversionary activities; monitor effectiveness. Position patient on back or unaffected side in semi-Fowler's position.

NURSING CARE PLAN: THE PATIENT UNDERGOING MASTECTOMY—cont'd

Nursing diagnoses	Patient goals	Nursing interventions
Impaired physical mobility, related to surgery, pain, and discomfort	Patient's mobility will be restored to optimum level. Patient will willingly participate in exercise program. Patient will verbalize comfort levels. Patient will regain ROM of affected arm.	Assist in activity progression from sitting to ambulating. Encourage participation in exercise program for affected arm. Turn and reposition every 2 hours or as needed; position for body alignment. Encourage bilateral use of arms in activities, such as personal hygiene.
Knowledge deficit, related to home care management	Patient and/or significant other will demonstrate understanding of home care and follow-up instructions through interactive discussion and actual return demonstration.	Assess current level of learning and determine needs.
	Patient will exhibit increased interest in exercise program as shown by verbal and nonverbal cues and will demonstrate correct method of postoperative arm exercises.	Explain importance of exercise to tolerance; instruct patient to stop at point of pain.
	Patient will verbalize the necessity of healing to occur before a permanent prosthesis is worn.	Discuss types of prosthesis available and instruct on not wearing permanent prostheses until incision is completely healed.
	Patient will verbalize/demonstrate how to change dressing on her incision.	Teach care of incision.
	Patient will identify and recite signs/symptoms of infection.	Discuss signs and symptoms to report to physician: erythema, pain, edema, drainage, elevated temperature. Emphasize need to gradually resume activities of daily living. Explain that incision and/or chest wall may feel numb.
	Patient will verbalize/demonstrate procedure for breast self-examination.	Instruct patient to examine remaining breast once a month.
	Patient will verbalize specific precautions to prevent infection and lymphedema in affected arm.	Caution patient to avoid allowing blood to be drawn from or IV to be started in affected arm. Caution patient to avoid injections, vaccinations, and taking of BP in affected area. Emphasize importance of follow-up outpatient care.

cer should include communication with, and support from, another who has shared a similar situation and who has learned to cope and resume her normal activities.

Nursing interventions for patients who undergo surgery of the breast include monitoring vital signs and observing for symptoms of shock or hemorrhage, since many large blood vessels are involved in the procedure. Drains such as a Davol or Hemovac may be placed in the axilla to facilitate drainage and prevent formation of a hematoma. Postoperative dressings are usually constrictive and bulky and may tend to embarrass respiratory effort as well as cause pain and discomfort. When the vital signs are stable, the patient is placed in a 45-degree Fowler's position to promote drainage. The position should be changed frequently, and deep breathing and coughing are encouraged.

Some patients may experience incisional pain for several days after surgery and when doing arm exercises. There may be complaints of numbness and referred pain in the arm of the operative area. The pain radiates to the shoulder and the back because of severance of peripheral nerves. Most of the nerves regenerate, but there are cases of residual numbness. Pain medication may be given as the patient feels she needs it. Care must be exercised to prevent oversedation. It is important for the patient to deep breathe and cough to prevent postoperative atelectasis.

Physicians differ in opinion about the best positioning of the affected arm. Some physicians place the affected arm in the dressing and place it in a sling for a couple of days postoperatively. If the arm is not restricted by dressings, it may be elevated on a pillow with the hand and wrist higher than the elbow and the elbow higher than the shoulder joint. This will facilitate the flow of fluids by the lymph and venous routes and prevent lymphedema.

Usually the patient is allowed to ambulate on the first postoperative day. Assistance to move out of bed will be needed to have the patient learn to maintain balance because of breast removal and bulky dressings. If a modified or radical mastectomy has been the surgical intervention, the defense mechanisms are lessened by the removal of lymph nodes.

Patients should be taught not to have any procedures involving the arm on the affected side—blood pressure readings, injections, intravenous infusion of fluids, or blood drawing, which may cause edema or infection, and to guard against infections from burns, needle pricks (sewing), and gardening injuries. Removing lymph nodes and channels increases the risk of developing lymphedema, even years after surgery. Referral to physical therapy may be indicated to control lymphedema if it develops. The patient should be instructed to avoid sleeping on the involved arm. Clothing on the affecting arm should be nonconstricting. Bracelets and watches should be worn on the unaffected arm (Box 36-7).

The longer the edema persists the more difficult it is to manage. Diuretics and low-sodium diets are often prescribed. If the edema persists, elastic stockinette is measured for precise fit to avoid venous flow constriction. The sleeve is applied from the wrist to the shoulder and worn when the patient is out of bed. When the patient is sleeping, the arm is positioned to aid venous flow. If the lymphedema is severe, the physician may order Jobst extremity therapy. There is an automatic inflation and deflation of a pneumomassage sleeve that can be placed on the arm. The compression pump is strictly contraindicated when there is evidence of acute phlebitis, perivascular lymphangitis, or cellulitis.

Isometric exercises are helpful for increasing the circulation and development of the collateral lymph system. Opening and clenching fingers and squeezing a rubber ball can be started in the first few postoperative days. This activity provides extension and flexion of the wrist and elbow. The activity is equivalent to sewing, knitting, typing, and playing piano when at home.

Preventing muscle contractures. Specific exercises may be ordered to restore the muscle strength and full range of motion of the affected area. The nurse or the therapist should instruct the patient and encourage the continuation of the exercises on discharge. Many of the exercises may be incorporated into activities of daily living as normal daily tasks are assumed (Fig. 36-19).

Exercising can be painful but can be accepted as a challenge by the patient with the support group encouraging her. The challenge can be met and the results of

BOX 36-7 HAND AND ARM CARE AFTER BREAST SURGERY

1. Prevention of infection
   a. Wear gloves when cleaning with harsh detergent.
   b. Wear gloves when gardening.
   c. Avoid injections, vaccinations, and venipuncture in involved arm.
   d. Use cuticle remover in preference to cutting cuticles.
   e. Sew with a thimble.
   f. Avoid chapped hands; use lanolin cream daily.
   g. Take care when using equipment that might cut, scrape, or abrade.
   h. Shave underarms with an electric razor.
   i. Avoid insect bites; use insect repellent.
2. Prevention of constricting circulation
   a. Do not take blood pressure in involved arm.
   b. Wear loose clothing; avoid tight bra straps or tight sleeves.
   c. Wear watch or jewelry on uninvolved arm.
   d. Carry purse on uninvolved arm or shoulder.
3. Prevention of burns
   a. Wear padded mitts to reach in oven; use potholders.
   b. Prevent sunburn; use sunscreens with SPF of 15; cover arms during prolonged exposure.
4. Prevention of drag or pull
   a. Carry heavy packages on uninvolved arm.
   b. Avoid motions that increase centrifugal force.
5. Immediately report any signs of erythema, edema, warmth, or pain.

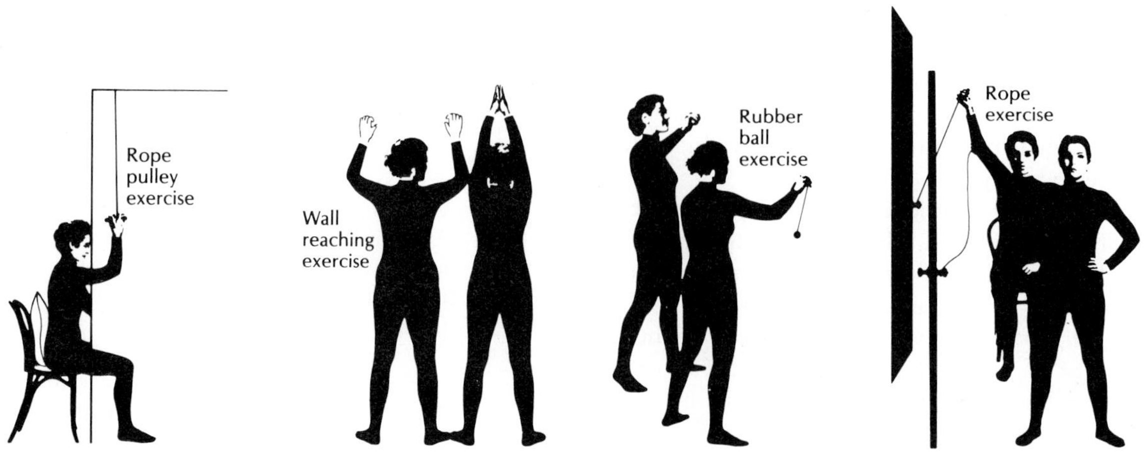

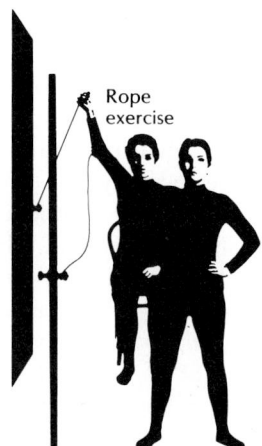

FIG. 36-19 Exercises after mastectomy.

muscular strengthening achieved. The patient should be encouraged to continue the exercises after discharge.

Body image acceptance. After losing a breast, many patients experience grief over the loss of a body part. This acute grief is like a crisis and may last 4 to 6 weeks. Grief makes the fact of loss real. The process of grieving is essential for personal adaptation to the loss. The nurse can assist the patient to find helpful coping mechanisms. When deep breathing exercises are started immediately after surgery and the patient has been able to splint the area, and while exercising her arm, the woman will recognize the absence of the breast through touch. Dressing changes and incision cleansing with patient involvement make the absence real. Being involved and responsible for the dressing and incision allows a more personal approach to the patient. At this time support by the nurse is very important. The nurse can provide a mirror or seat the patient in front of the mirror so that the patient can see the operative site being cleansed and dressed. The nurse must be very sensitive to the patient and be alert for signs of readiness by the patient to become involved in care and accepting of the loss of the body part. The incisional area may be erythematous and edematous, but the discoloration will gradually lessen and the site will become more comfortable. The patient should be encouraged to apply and massage cocoa butter or a cream to make the incisional line softer. The patient should be counseled that it takes time to accept the loss and heal emotionally as well as physically.

Prosthesis. A breast prosthesis should not be worn unless authorized by the physician. There are many breast forms available. Forms are made of gels and molded silicone. Most forms are covered with soft fabric and are light in weight and feel like breast tissue. In selecting a breast form there is a shape for each type of breast, because each woman's body is different and each woman's surgery is different. Forms have been developed that can be fitted for a right or left breast, slanted for the breast that was slanted or a full breast with an outer curve that simulates the extension of the breast under the axilla and upward on the chest. It is advisable to have a skilled fitter from a reliable company to fit the prosthesis.

A well-fitted brassiere is essential before choosing the shape form. If the woman is very active and desires a pocket or restraining cup, the brassiere needs to be equipped for it. Brassieres can be purchased with these adaptions. Some available forms can be worn against the skin with no underpadding or bra cups. Most forms can be washed with water and mild detergent to keep the form clean and supple. Many prostheses are waterproof and can be worn swimming; when wet they do not "weigh down" the wearer with heaviness.

When the patient is being fitted with a prosthesis, the best assurance that the fit is right is when:

1. The brassiere fits snugly around the rib cage
2. The prosthesis fills the bottom of the bra cup
3. The prosthesis projects the same as the remaining breast, with form bulk and nipples in position
4. The breasts are separated when the bra is centered
5. The top of the bra cup is filled and appears like the other breast

Breast reconstruction. The patient whose disease is limited to the breast may benefit from reconstructive surgery. Some patients have reconstructive surgery done at the time of the original surgery; others wait until they have completed adjuvant chemotherapy or radiation to be sure that the area is disease free. Breast reconstruction can produce psychological benefits and for many women provide them with a renewed sense of wholeness and a return to a normal state. The most important indicators for reconstruction are the patient's motivation and desire for the procedure.[13] The prime determinant for the procedure is the clinical status of the patient. Goals for reconstruction are to select the simplest type that meets the patient's needs and expectations to match the opposite breast in size, shape, and contour.

Nipple reconstruction is usually performed as a separate procedure after the breast reconstruction has been completed. Nipple construction is generally from available tissue at the site or harvested tissue from the opposite breast. New techniques allow the nipple to be done from tissue and subcutaneous tissue of the breast mound. Areola reconstruction is provided by obtaining pigmented skin from the upper thigh or by using skin from the lateral chest area.

INFLAMMATORY DISORDERS OF THE MALE REPRODUCTIVE SYSTEM

Prostatitis

Etiology/pathophysiology. Prostatitis is an acute or chronic infection of the prostate gland. It is commonly a result of bacterial invasion from the urethra. The causative organisms include *Escherichia coli, Klebsiella, Proteus, Pseudomonas, Streptococcus,* and *Staphylococcus.*

Bacterial invasion originates in the bloodstream and/or from a descending infection from the kidneys.

Clinical manifestations. Symptoms include sudden onset of chills and fever. There is urgency and frequency of urination, dysuria (pain on urination), cloudy urine, perineal fullness, low back pain, arthralgia (pain in the joints), and myalgia (pain in the muscles). When the gland is palpated, there is tenderness, edema, and firmness. In chronic prostatitis, many patients may appear to be asymptomatic, but generally the same symptoms exist as in the acute phase with a lesser degree of intensity.

Diagnostic tests. Diagnostic testing includes culture and sensitivity tests of the urethra, prostatic fluid, and urine for organism identification and appropriate antibiotic therapy. Prostatic fluid is collected by prostate massage and expression of fluid. The pH of the fluid is generally elevated. A rectal examination done by the physician reveals gland tenderness and edema.

Medical management. Medical management includes antibiotic therapy and periodic digital massages of the prostate by the physician to increase the flow of infected prostatic secretions.

Nursing interventions. Nursing interventions primarily focus on symptoms and include (1) a full explanation of antibiotic therapy and the need for compliance with treatment, (2) supportive care such as bed rest to relieve strain and pain of the perineum and suprapubic area, sitz baths to promote muscle relaxation, and stool softeners to prevent straining on defecation, (3) monitoring intake and output, and (4) encouraging follow-up care for evaluation of the inflammation.

NURSING DIAGNOSES	NURSING INTERVENTIONS
Pain, related to disease process	Assess type and location of pain; provide analgesics as ordered. Bedrest to promote comfort.
Pain, related to disease process—cont'd	Provide nonpharmacological comfort measures: 1. Assist patient with assuming comfortable position. 2. Provide diversional activity. 3. Provide a restful environment.
Potential for self-esteem disturbance, related to fear of impotence	Encourage patient to express feelings. Actively listen. Encourage adaptive coping behaviors.
Knowledge deficit, related to illness and outcome	Instruct patient in necessity to comply with taking prescribed medication and to follow orders for activity level.

Epididymitis

Etiology/pathophysiology. Epididymitis is an infection of the cordlike excretory duct of the testicles. It is one of the common infections of the male reproductive tract. The causative organisms are *Staphylococcus aureus, E. coli,* and *Streptococcus* and *Gonococcus* species. The inflammation is associated with urethral strictures, cystitis, and prostatitis.

Symptoms can occur after trauma to the genital area, after instrumentation of the urethra and cystocopy, and after physical exertion or prolonged sexual activity. Abscesses can form and cause desquamation (flaking) of tissues. The infection can be bilateral and may recur. With repeated infections sterility can occur.

Clinical manifestations. Severe pain appears suddenly in the scrotum and radiates along the spermatic tube. Edema appears and the patient develops a "duck walk" or "waddling gait" because of the sensitivity and pain that walking stimulates. The scrotal area becomes tender. Pyuria (pus in urine) is present. Chills and fever are noted.

Diagnostic tests. Diagnostic testing includes examining the first daily flow of urine and sending a midstream specimen to the laboratory to check for pyuria. The epididymis is massaged by the physician and a fluid expression specimen is sent to the laboratory. Physical examination of the scrotum is performed. The WBC is monitored for leukocytosis.

Medical management. Medical management includes a regimen of bed rest and support of the scrotum. Heat or cold may be applied, and the appropriate antibiotic is administered. If abscess formation occurs, incision and drainage (I&D) of the scrotum may be required.

Nursing interventions. Nursing interventions for patients with epididymitis include (1) bed rest during the acute phase of illness, (2) support of the testicular area, with scrotal support during bed rest and athletic support when ambulatory, (3) ice compresses to the area in the initial phase and sitz baths in later stages to hasten recovery, and (4) explaining the need for compliance with antibiotic therapy until all signs of inflammation have disappeared.

DISORDERS OF MALE GENITAL ORGANS

Phimosis

Etiology/pathophysiology. Phimosis is a condition in which the prepuce is too small to allow retraction of the foreskin over the glans. Phimosis is often congenital but may be acquired as a result of local inflammation or disease. The condition is rarely severe enough to obstruct the flow of urine but may contribute to local infection because it does not permit adequate cleansing treatment.

Medical management. A surgical procedure **(circumcision)** may be performed in which a part of the foreskin is removed, leaving the glans penis uncovered.

Nursing interventions. After a circumcision a sterile petrolatum gauze dressing is applied and changed after each voiding. The nurse should always observe the patient for unusual bleeding.

Hydrocele

Etiology/pathophysiology. A hydrocele is an accumulation of fluid between the membranes covering the testicle and the membrane enclosing the testicle. The scrotum slowly enlarges as the fluid accumulates. Pain occurs if the hydrocele develops suddenly. Most hydroceles occur in males over the age of 21. The actual cause is not known, but it may develop as a result of trauma of the area, orchitis (inflammation of the testes), or epididymitis.

Medical management. Treatment includes aspiration of fluid from the sac or surgical removal of the sac to avoid constriction of the circulation of the testicles. After aspiration the pain is relieved and the scrotum can be examined more easily.

Nursing interventions. Nursing interventions consist of maintaining bed rest, scrotal support with elevation, ice to edematous areas, and frequent changes of dressings to avoid skin irritation.

Varicocele

Varicocele occurs when the veins within the scrotum become dilated. Obstruction and malfunctioning of the veins cause engorgement and elongation, which does not allow adequate drainage of the blood. The symptoms are a pulling sensation that causes a dull aching and pain accompanied by edema of the scrotal area. The treatment is surgical removal of the obstruction. Nursing interventions include bed rest with scrotal support, ice to the incisional site, and medication for discomfort as ordered.

CANCER OF THE MALE REPRODUCTIVE TRACT

The more common tumors of the male reproductive tract involve the testes, prostate gland, and penis. Most tumors of the male reproductive system are malignant.

Men should be taught to do testicular self-examination. The examination takes 3 minutes and should be done monthly. The best time to do a testicular self-examination is after the man has had a warm shower and the scrotal skin is relaxed. Each testicle should be rolled gently between the thumb and fingers of both hands, examining for lumps or nodules. If any lumps or nodules are found, a physician should be consulted promptly.

Cancer of the Testes

Etiology/pathophysiology. Cancer of the testes is the second most common malignancy in men 25 to 35 years of age and is the most common cause of death in this age-group. The causes are unknown. The incidence of this cancer is higher in men with **cryptorchidism** (failure of testes to descend into the scrotum). Other associated factors are testicular atrophy and scrotal trauma.

Clinical manifestations. The symptoms of early disease include an enlarged scrotum, and a firm, painless, smooth mass in the testicular area is noted. At times the patient may speak of a feeling of heaviness. Diagnosis is generally revealed when the patient complains of the presence of the mass or at the time of a routine physical examination.

Medical management. Orchiectomy (removal of the testes) is the principal procedure for removing a testicular tumor. Surgery is generally followed by radiation and/or chemotherapy. Often a retroperitoneal lymph node dissection is performed to remove affected nodes and to assist in determining the stage of the tumor. Staging a testicular tumor helps determine the treatment. The prognosis is often not favorable, and death may occur within months or a few years.

Nursing interventions/patient teaching. The first priority for nursing in the care of patients who have or are at risk for a tumor of the testes is early detection of cancer by testicular self-examination. Young men should be taught to perform self-examination monthly beginning at 15 years of age.

Cancer of the Penis

Etiology/pathophysiology. Cancer of the penis is rare. It generally appears in men over 50 years of age. Men who have not been circumcised, have not maintained good personal hygiene, or have had sexually transmitted diseases are at risk.

Clinical manifestations. The tumor is painless, and a wartlike growth or ulceration on the gland under the prepuce is present. It is common for mestastasis to occur to the inguinal nodes and adjacent organs.

Diagnostic tests. Biopsy confirms the diagnosis.

Medical management. Surgical intervention requires removal of as little tissue as possible, but it may be necessary to do a partial or total amputation of the penis as well as remove the adjacent tissue and inguinal lymph nodes. When mestastasis involves the bladder and rectum, more radical surgery may be needed, and outlets for urinary or fecal elimination are provided by creating an ileoconduit and a colostomy. The surgeon may place a suprapubic catheter into the bladder as a means of draining the urine from the bladder.

Nursing interventions. Nursing interventions include providing emotional support. If amputation of the penis is required, the patient faces the psychological trauma associated with loss of sexuality and loss of ability to urinate through the penis. Nursing interventions include monitoring urine output by suprapubic catheter or if an ileoconduit was performed, monitoring urine in the urostomy bag. Elevation of the scrotum controls edema. The nurse will provide comfort measures to control pain. See Chapter 33 for a discussion of cancer of the prostate.

SEXUALLY TRANSMITTED DISEASES

Today, despite sweeping advances in the diagnosis and treatment of communicable diseases, the incidence of infections transmitted through intimate or sexual activities continues to increase worldwide.

Sexually transmitted diseases (STDs), previously called *venereal diseases*, are infections that are usually transmitted during intimate sexual contact. They may have other routes of transmission (e.g., an infected mother to her newborn), occur with or without symptoms, and have long periods of asymptomatic infectivity.

Any sexually active person may be at risk for a sexually transmitted disease. Persons who have frequent sexual contact with multiple partners are at very high risk. Common characteristics of these individuals are young, single, urban, poor, male, and homosexual. Because some STDs persist and are infectious for long periods (herpes genitalis or AIDS), even persons in mutually monogamous sexual relationships are at some risk. The proliferation of acquired immunodeficiency syndrome (AIDS) since the late 1970s has produced an urgent reason to educate sexually active individuals to the risk of unprotected sexual contact.

As of December 1988, the Centers for Disease Control (CDC) reported 82,764 cumulative cases of AIDS in the United States and estimated that another 102 million people were infected with human immunodeficiency virus (HIV), the causative organism of AIDS. These are sobering statistics indeed. The number of people contracting the traditionally defined STDs (e.g., syphilis, gonorrhea) is even greater. Gonorrhea is estimated to infect 250 million people worldwide and nearly 3 million in the United States each year. Annual syphilis incidence is about 50 million cases worldwide and 25,000 in the United States. No reliable statistics exist for the "new generation" STDs, such as trichomoniasis, herpes simplex virus (HSV), venereal warts, scabies, and others; these are probably even more prevalent. In addition, bowel pathogens such as *Salmonella*, amoeba, hepatitis A and B, and the herpes viruses may be sexually transmitted.

Despite the physical and emotional discomfort, the possibility of long-term disability (infertility, chronic infectivity), and advances in diagnosis and treatment that sharply decrease the period of infectivity, STDs continue to be among the world's most common communicable diseases. Three main factors are responsible: (1) unprotected sex, (2) antibiotic resistance, and (3) treatment delay. The following is a discussion of some of the more commonly diagnosed sexually transmitted diseases.

Herpes Genitalis

Etiology/pathophysiology. Herpes genitalis or herpes simplex virus (HSV) is a treatable, but not curable, infectious viral disease, characterized by recurrent episodes of acute, painful, erythematous, vesicular eruptions (blisters) on or in the genitalia or rectum.

The two closely related forms are designated types I and II. Most persons are infected in infancy with type I during feeding or kissing by adults. There are infrequent recurrences around the lips. A prior infection with HSV I confers relative immunity to HSV II. This immunity may enable persons infected with HSV I to be completely resistant or have a less dramatic HSV II infection.

HSV II is usually acquired sexually after puberty in the genital or anal regions.

Clinical manifestations. Symptoms appear as fluid-filled vesicles after the incubation period and in women usually occur on the cervix, which is considered the primary site, but may also be seen on the labia, rectum, vulva, vagina, and skin and on the glans penis, foreskin, and penile shaft of men. Other lesions may appear on the mouth and anus. Vesicles may rupture and develop into shallow, painful ulcers; they are erythematous with marked edema and tenderness. Lymph nodes may become involved. Initial lesions last from 3 to 10 days and recurrent lesions have a duration of 7 to 10 days. The infection may be accompanied by fever, malaise, dysuria, and in women, leukorrhea. Sites are painful in the presence of fever, stress, or emotional upset or when exposed to intense heat. Complications are rare.

Medical management. Diagnosis is based on the physical examination and the patient history. The diagnosis is confirmed by appearance of the virus on tissue cultures. There is no known cure for HSV. Ointments such as acyclovir inhibit the virus. Antibacterial agents combat secondary infections.

Nursing interventions/patient teaching. The nurse should advise the patient that genital lesions should be kept clean and dry. Hands should be washed thoroughly after touching a lesion. Loose, absorbent underclothing is usually more comfortable than close-fitting clothing. Sitz baths decrease lesional discomfort and enhance urinary and bowel elimination. The patient should be taught that sexual intercourse during the active lesion phase increases the risk of transmission and may also be painful. Future sexual partners and health care providers should be advised of recurring or latent infections. The nurse should teach the role of stress, poor nutrition, and insufficient rest related to recurrences of symptoms. Women patients need a yearly Pap test and should inform their physician in the event of future pregnancies so that the course of the disease can be monitored closely; there is a possibility of spontaneous abortion. The nurse should provide the patient with nonjudgmental support and with the contact number of the local herpes support group if one exists.

Syphilis

Etiology/pathophysiology. The coiled spirochete *Treponema pallidum* causes syphilis. Congenital syphilis occurs in about 1 in 10,000 pregnancies, generally in the minority population. The age-group of the highest incidence is 20 to 40 years. Transmission occurs primarily through sexual contact during the primary, secondary, and latent stages of the disease. Prenatal infection from the mother to the fetus is possible. The organism thrives in the warm parts of the body and can be destroyed by soap and water. The spirochete penetrates intact skin as well as openings in the mucous membrane of the genital organs, rectum, and mouth.

Clinical manifestations. Each stage of syphilis has its peculiar symptoms: primary, secondary, latent, and tertiary syphilis. The signs and symptoms of syphilis range from the clean-based, painless **chancre** of primary syphilis to the skin rashes of secondary syphilis. Moist, raised, gray to pink lesions of the genital or perirectal skin, enlarged lymph nodes, fever, fatigue, or infections of the eyes, bones, liver, or meninges may occur. In the late stages of syphilis dementia, pain or loss of sensation in the legs and destruction of the aorta occur. Destructive inflammatory masses can appear in any organ.

Diagnostic tests. Diagnostic tests that are available include the Venereal Disease Research Laboratory (VDRL) slide test and rapid plasma reagin (RPR) test.

Medical management. Penicillin is the drug of choice of syphilis, but the treatment regimen varies according to the stage of the disease. When the patient is allergic to penicillin, erythromycin or tetracycline is used.

Nursing interventions. Nursing interventions, other than the routine implications for patients with STDs, include monitoring for drug reaction to penicillin, stressing good handwashing technique with the patient, encouraging follow-up visits with the physician, and informing the patient that he or she should absolutely not engage in sexual intercourse until cured.

Gonorrhea

Etiology/pathophysiology. Gonorrhea is caused by *Neisseria gonorrhoeae*, a gram-negative diplococcoid bacterium, and almost exclusively follows sexual contact. It is the most commonly reported communicable disease in the United States. It is estimated that at least 2 million unreported cases occur each year. The disease is most common in the 20 to 24 age-group, closely followed by the 15 to 19 age-group. Those who are at risk are sexually active individuals and women who use birth control pills or are otherwise susceptible to infections. Gonorrhea is not limited to the genital organs; it can infest the mouth and the throat through oral sex with an infected partner. It may also infect the eyes. Three times as many males are infected as females. The incubation period of gonorrhea is 3 to 5 days.

Clinical manifestations. Some infected males may be asymptomatic after the incubation period but in a short time develop symptoms of urethritis, dysuria, infection with a purulent discharge, and edema of the affected area. Most females remain asymptomatic but may show a greenish-yellow discharge from the cervix. Other female symptoms, which may vary depending on the infected site, are urinary frequency, purulent discharge from the urethra, pruritus, burning and pain of the vulva, vaginal engorgement and erythema, abdominal pain and distention, muscular rigidity, and tenderness. As the infection spreads, nausea, vomiting, fever, and tachycardia may develop. Other symptoms that appear may include pharyngitis, tonsillitis, rectal burning, pruritus, and purulent rectal discharge.

Diagnostic tests. Diagnosis is determined by cultures from the site of infection. Cultures isolate the organism and establish an identification. An important concern in treatment for gonorrhea is coexisting chlamydial infection (see pp. 955-956). This infection has been documented in up to 45% of gonorrhea cases when adequate chlamydial cultures are performed.

Medical management. Medications recommended are oral amoxicillin or penicillin G procaine intramuscular. For proven or suspected penicillin-resistant strains of gonorrhea, spectinomycin or ceftriaxone intramuscular is the medication of choice. Tetracycline is contraindicated with pregnancy because of potential adverse effects for the fetus. With adequate treatment, the prognosis is excellent, but recurrence is common.

Nursing interventions/patient teaching. The nurse should advise patients that loose, absorbent underclothes, changed frequently after perineal/penile cleansing, will enhance comfort. Sitz baths decrease lower abdominal discomfort and dysuria. The patient should avoid infecting sexual partners. The patient should also be taught that sterility may occur as a result of gonorrhea.

The nurse should obtain laboratory specimens as ordered. Alternative methods of birth control can be discussed as appropriate. The nurse encourages notification of present and past sexual partners of the diagnosis and the need for them to promptly seek medical care.

Trichomoniasis

Etiology/pathophysiology. Trichomoniasis is a sexually transmitted disease caused by the protozoan *Trichomonas vaginalis*, which affects about 15% of sexually active females and 10% of sexually active males. The incubation period is 4 to 28 days. Trichomoniasis is usually transmitted by sexual intercourse, and at times by dirty douche nozzles and douche containers and moist washcloths. Occasionally the newborn develops an infection from an infected mother. *T. vaginalis* thrives when the vaginal mucosa is more alkaline than normal. Frequent douching and use of oral contraceptives and antibiotics raise the normal pH of the vagina.

Clinical manifestations. Most males and females are asymptomatic. The male symptoms are mild to severe transient urethritis, dysuria, frequency of urination, pruritus, and purulent exudate. Approximately 70% of infected females are asymptomatic; symptoms when present include profuse, frothy gray, green, or yellow malodorous discharge, pruritus, edema, tenderness of vagina, dysuria, frequency of urination, spotting, menorrhagia, and/or dysmenorrhea. Symptoms may persist for a week to several months. Symptoms may be more pronounced after menstruation and/or during pregnancy.

Diagnostic tests/medical management. Diagnosis is based on the microscopic examination of the vaginal discharge that identifies *T. vaginalis*. Treatment for both males and females is oral metronidazole (Flagyl) in small doses for 7 days or one large single dose. The patient should avoid alcoholic beverages, because alcohol can cause a reaction with signs and symptoms of confusion, headache, cramps, vomiting, and possible convulsions. Metronidazole can cause the urine to turn dark brown.

Nursing interventions. The nurse should counsel the patient to avoid alcohol during treatment, inform patients that their urine may turn dark orange or brown, and counsel patients to avoid douches, sprays, and powders. The patient should be taught how to disinfect douche nozzles, applicators, diaphragms, and the toilet area. The nurse encourages the patient to wear loose-fitting clothing and cotton underwear, encourages follow-up visits with the physician, and discusses the need to contact sex partners to encourage their treatment.

Candidiasis

Etiology/pathophysiology. Candidiasis (candidosis, moniliasis) is a mild fungal infection that appears in men and women. Candidal infections are usually caused by *Candida albicans* and *Candida tropicalis*. The fungi are a part of the normal flora of the gastrointestinal tract, mouth, vagina, and skin. The infection often occurs when the glucose level rises from diabetes mellitus or when resistance is lowered from diseases such as carcinoma. Radiation, immunosuppressant drugs, hyperalimentation, antibiotic therapy, and oral contraceptives may predispose individuals to candidiasis. The male and female display symptoms of scaly skin, erythematous rash, and at time exudates that appear under the breasts, between the fingers, and in the axillae, groin, and umbilicus.

Clinical manifestations. If the mother is infected, a newborn can contract oral *thrush* during delivery. The infant may display a diaper rash. Nails become edematous and have a darkened, erythematous nail base from which there is purulent exudate. Thrush may appear on the mucous membranes of the mouth and cause edema and engorgement. The infant may have a edematous tongue that can cause respiratory distress. The female patient may have a cheesy, tenacious white discharge accompanied with pruritus, and an inflamed vulva and vagina. The male presents symptoms of an infected penis with purulent exudate. Systemic infections are represented by chills, fevers, and general malaise.

Diagnostic tests/medical management. Diagnosis is based on evidence of the *Candida* species on a Gram stain of collected specimens from scraping of the vagina and penis, from pus, and from sputum from the mouth. Treatment consists of treating and improving any underlying condition, such as controlling diabetes mellitus, discontinuing antibiotics and oral contraceptives, and catheter therapy. Nystatin (Mycostatin) is effective for superficial candidiasis; topical amphotericin B is effective for skin and nail infections.

Nursing interventions. The nurse should emphasize the use of prescribed ointments, sprays, and creams as indicated for each part of the body affected. Teaching includes the method for insertion of vaginal suppositories (to be inserted high into the vagina when in a dorsal recumbent position) and to remain on back for 30 minutes to allow suppository absorption. Sexual partner(s) should be encouraged to have examination and treatment. Good handwashing techniques should be taught to avoid reinfection or the transfer of the fungi. The nurse encourages pregnant women to accept treatment to prevent infection of the newborn at the time of delivery.

Chlamydia

Etiology/pathophysiology. *Chlamydia trachomatis,* a Gram-negative, intracellular bacterium, causes several commonly sexually transmitted diseases. Cervicitis and urethritis are most common, but like the gonococcus, *Chlamydia* also causes epididymitis in men and salpingitis in women. Chlamydial infections may be the most commonly occurring sexually transmitted disease in the United States. Although both men and women may have asymptomatic infection, women are more likely to be asymptomatic carriers despite deep pelvic infections, such as infection of the fallopian tubes and pelvic inflammatory disease (PID).

Clinical manifestations. In men symptoms may include a scanty white or clear exudate, burning or pruritus around the urethral meatus, urinary frequency, and mild dysuria. Symptoms of cervicitis in women may include one or more of the following: vaginal pruritus or burning, dull pelvic pain, low-grade fever, vaginal discharge, and irregular bleeding.

Diagnostic tests. A recently developed test, the fluorescein-labeled monoclonal antibody test, provides a ready basis for diagnosis. Treatment can be initiated promptly based on a confirmed diagnosis.

Medical management. The drug of choice for treatment of chlamydial infection is tetracycline. Pregnant patients or patients who are allergic to tetracycline can be treated with erythromycin. Penicillin, the drug of choice to treat gonorrhea, may temporarily suppress the multiplication of chlamydia, but usually does not provide a cure.

Nursing interventions. Patients' physical symptoms are commonly complicated by their emotional responses to STDs. Complaints of depression, anger, fear, and guilt are common and need to be addressed if education and treatment are to be effective. Outcome is also influenced by educational and income level, primary language, health insurance coverage, and support network. The focus of patient education is on prevention (Box 36-8).

BOX 36-8 PREVENTION OF SEXUALLY TRANSMITTED DISEASES

- Individuals should reduce the number of partners they have sex with—preferably to one person.
- Avoid contact with individuals known to be infected or who are at high risk of infection.
- Avoid contact with the genital area if signs and symptoms develop.
- Hands and the genital-rectal area should be washed before and immediately after having intercourse.
- Special attention must be given to washing the foreskin.
- A mouthwash or gargle with hydrogen peroxide (1 part to 3 parts of water) or Listerine antiseptic may slightly reduce the risk of oropharyngeal STD infection.
- Use barrier (condom) contraceptives with new partners.
- Use a water-based lubricant.
- Void after intercourse.
- Avoid excess douching.
- If an STD infection is suspected, seek medical help immediately.
- Individuals with multiple sex partners should seek an STD examination twice a year or more if needed.

Acquired Immunodeficiency Syndrome

Acquired immunodeficiency syndrome (AIDS) is the ultimately fatal, advanced stage of a chronic retroviral infection that gradually destroys the cell-mediated immune system. For a more detailed discussion on this sexually transmitted disease, see Chapter 40.

FAMILY PLANNING

Methods of Contraception

Advances in drug therapy and family planning technology have made available a range of options for individuals wishing to prevent or plan conception. Birth control planning involves moral, religious, cultural, and personal values, and the nurse should be sensitive to these factors when discussing birth control with patients.

There are several types of birth control procedures or devices that can be employed. The selection of the particular method should be based on the health of the individual, effectiveness of the method, cost, ease of use, and age and parity (total number of pregnancies) of the patient. Willingness of the patient to comply with use and preference of the couple are two additional factors taken into consideration when selecting a method of contraception. The nurse can help by reinforcing information given by the physician and encouraging patients to seek more information, directing them to the source.

Contraceptive methods and products can be categorized as surgical, hormonal, barrier, and behavioral. Surgical and hormonal methods will be addressed here.

Surgical methods. Sterilization is a permanent, effective method of birth control that can be performed for men or women. Many states have laws regulating this method of birth control; in some states the husband and wife must both sign a release for the operative procedure. Persons who have not had children are often advised against sterilization.

Vasectomy is the operation performed on a man to terminate the passage of sperm through the vas deferens (Fig. 36-20). There are several ways to perform this procedure, and it can generally be done in the physician's office, in same-day surgery centers, or in ambulatory surgical units.

Although the procedure is intended to be permanent, the patient may wish to reverse the procedure because of remarriage or death of a child. This procedure is known as *vasovasotomy*. Research is being considered to develop a device that permits a reversible vasectomy.

Sperm counts will be required for 6 weeks or until semen is tested free of sperm. The nurse should advise

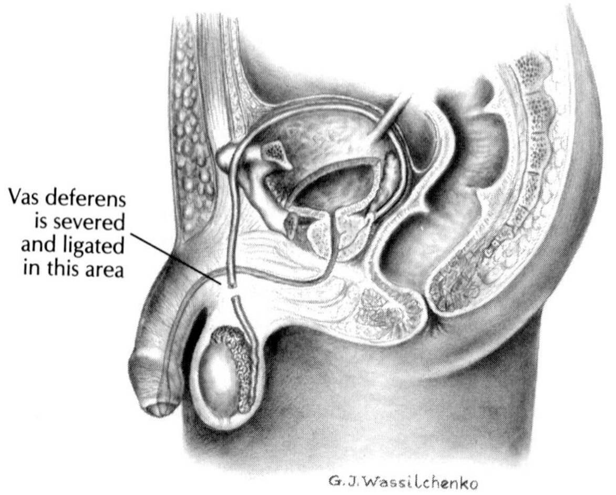

FIG. 36-20 Vasectomy. Sperm duct severed (and ligated).

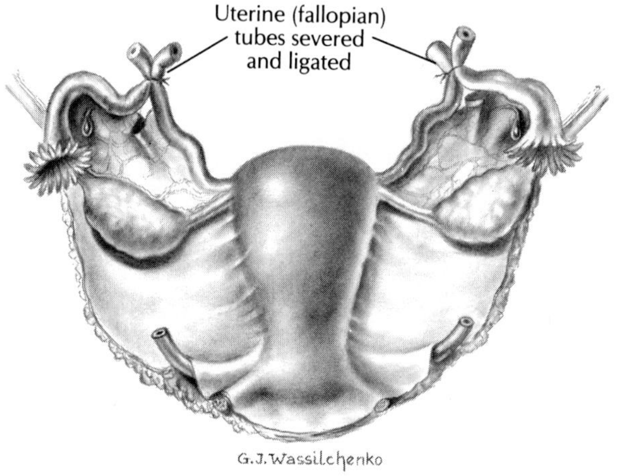

FIG. 36-21 Tubal ligation. Oviduct ligated and severed.

the patient that until the semen tests free of sperm, the ability to impregnate exists.

Tubal ligation (Fig. 36-21) is the surgical sterilization approach for women. There are various approaches used to accomplish this procedure, some of which are ligation, clips, bands or rings, and coagulation. This intervention can be performed through the abdomen or through the vagina. Regardless of method, only a short hospitalization is required. After surgery, ova will not pass through the fallopian tubes. The menstrual cycle, however, will remain normal because the ovaries continue to produce estrogen. Reconstruction of the tubes is possible, with a 50% success rate. A tubal ligation may be performed at the same time other abdominal surgeries are done. The abdominal approach to the tubal ligation is often called *Band-Aid surgery* because a very small incision requiring only a Band-Aid is necessary.

The nurse should advise the patient that she will be allowed up after recovery from anesthesia. She may even be discharged the same day. Postoperative discomfort is minor. There may be abdominal cramping and perhaps a transitory headache. The patient should avoid strenuous exercises and lifting. If there is a vaginal discharge or if spotting appears, the patient should wear a perineal pad.

Hysterectomy (removal of the uterus) and oophorectomy (removal of the ovaries) are other surgical procedures that will cause the woman to be sterile. These were discussed on pp. 938-940 and 942.

Hormonal contraceptives. Oral contraceptives (birth control pills) are hormonal contraceptives taken orally. Birth control pills are a popular and easy form of contraception that is close to 100% effective. The pill, which is taken by the woman, inhibits release of follicle-stimulating hormone (FSH), and subsequently the menstrual cycles are anovulatory (the ovaries do not release ova).

Birth control pills have the advantage of being easy to take, not requiring use of a contraceptive device before intercourse, and being highly effective. They are prescribed by the physician, and the woman should have a yearly physical examination while taking birth control pills. The woman must remember to take the pill daily. If she forgets to take one, she is usually advised to take two the next day. If she misses more than two pills she should stop taking the pills for that cycle, wait 7 days, and then restart the regimen. It is advisable to use another form of contraception for that cycle. The pills should be stored carefully. The pills are affected by high humidity and should be kept in a dry place; extreme heat should be avoided because heat can decrease potency of the pills.

Some women experience various side effects when using the pills, particularly during the first few months. The signs and symptoms are usually similar to those during the first trimester of pregnancy: nausea, vomiting, weight gain, and breast swelling. The nurse advises patients to take the pills after a meal to lessen the nausea. It will be helpful to take the pills at the same time each day. Women taking birth control pills are more susceptible to vaginal infections.

Oral contraceptives have been demonstrated to have a relationship to certain cardiovascular disorders; consequently women with hypertension, thromboembolic diseases, or a history of circulatory disease, varicosities, or diabetes mellitus should be discouraged from using birth control pills. Smoking increases the risk of cardiovascular complication in women taking birth control pills.

Other side effects are often related to birth control use. As research findings are published, more information is available to use in considering birth control pills as a method for contraception. The nurse is in a position to assist the patient to interpret the information for her individual needs.

Some research has been conducted in the use of male

contraceptives. Under investigation in the United States and elsewhere are antispermatogenic agents that create temporary infertility by interfering either with spermatogenesis or with the sperm's ability to fertilize ova. These agents can be given by injection or taken orally.[19]

REFERENCES AND SUGGESTED READINGS

1. Anagnostakos NP and Tortora GJ: Principles of anatomy and physiology, ed. 5, New York, 1987, Harper & Row, Publishers, Inc.
2. Beare PG and Myers JD: Principles and practice of adult health nursing, St Louis, 1990, The CV Mosby Co.
3. Billings D and Stokes LG: Medical-surgical nursing, ed 2, St Louis, 1987, The CV Mosby Co.
4. Bobak IM, Jensen MD and Zalar MK: Maternity and gynecologic care, ed 4, St Louis, 1989, The CV Mosby Co.
5. Bostwick J: Breast construction following mastectomy, CA-A J Clin 39(1):40, 1989.
6. Bowen LW et al: Toxic shock syndrome following carbon dioxide, Am J Obstet Gynecol 154(1):145, 1986.
7. Brunner LS and Suddarth DS: The Lippincott manual of nursing practice, ed 4, Philadelphia, 1990, JB Lippincott Co.
8. Caldwell E and Hegner BR: Geriatrics: a study of maturity, ed 4, New York, 1986, Delmar Publishers, Inc.
9. D'Agostino NS: Managing nutrition problems in advanced cancer, Am J Nurs 89(1):50, 1989.
10. Fong E, Ferris EB, and Skelley EG: Body structures and functions, ed 7, New York, 1989, Delmar Publishers, Inc.
10a. Gray G et al: A clinical data base for advanced cancer patients: implications to nursing, Cancer Nurs 11:47, 1988.
10b. Hatchor RA et al: Contraceptive technology, ed 13, New York, 1986, Irvington Publishers.
11. Hood GH and Dincher JR: Total patient care, ed 7, St Louis, 1988, The CV Mosby Co.
12. Long BC and Phipps WJ: Medical-surgical nursing, ed 2, St Louis, 1989, The CV Mosby Co.
13. Malasanos L et al: Health assessment, St Louis, 1990, The CV Mosby Co.
14. Marieb EN: Essentials of human anatomy and physiology, Menlo Park, Calif, 1984, Addison-Wesley Publishing Co, Inc.
15. Memmler RL and Wood DL: Structure and function of the human body, ed 4, Philadelphia, 1987, WB Saunders Co.
16. Monier M and Laird M: Contraceptives: a look at the future, Am J Nurs 89(1):496, 1989.
17. Moorhouse MF and Doenges ME: Nursing diagnosis, care planning, and documentation, Philadelphia, 1990, FA Davis Co.
18. Phipps WJ, Long BC and Woods NF: Medical-surgical nursing, ed 4, St Louis, 1991, The CV Mosby Co.
19. Rosenthal T and Nuttall K: Premenstrual syndrome (PMS), J Pract Nurs 37(4), 1987.
20. Seidel HM et al: Mosby's guide to physical examination, ed 2, St Louis, 1991, The CV Mosby Co.
21. SIECUS Report: SIECUS position statement on sexual health care, 13(2):5, 1990, SIECUS, Inc.
22. Silverbery E and Luber J: Estimated cancer incidence by site and sex, CA-A J Clin 39(1):3, 1989.
23. Solomon EP and Phillips GA: Understanding human anatomy and physiology, Philadelphia, 1987, WB Saunders Co.
24. Thibodeau GA and Anthony CP: Structure and function of the body, ed 8, St Louis, 1988, The CV Mosby Co.
25. Tucker S et al: Patient care standards, ed 4, St Louis, 1988, The CV Mosby Co.
26. Van Tyle JH and Sagranes R: Premenstrual syndrome: diagnoses, etiologies, therapy, J Pract Nurs 3(4):19, 1988.
27. When patients with genital herpes turn to you for answers, Am J Nurs 19(8), 1989.
28. Williams ND, editor: Contraceptive technology 1986-1987, ed 13, New York, 1986, Irvington Publishers.
29. Zatuchni GL et al: Male contraception: advances and future prospects, Philadelphia, 1986, JB Lippincott Co.

CHAPTER CHALLENGE

KEY POINTS

- All patients are sexual, and their total health is affected by their emotions, behaviors, beliefs, attitudes, and knowledge of sexuality.
- Sperm are produced in the seminiferous tubules and stored in the epididymis.
- Testosterone, the male sex hormone, is responsible for male secondary sex characteristics.
- Seminal fluid is produced in the seminal vesicles, prostate gland, and Cowper's glands.
- In the female, each month an egg matures in the graafian follicle, which is located in the ovary.
- The acini cells in the mammary glands produce milk after the birth of a child.
- The menstrual cycle prepares the uterus and causes ovulation to occur each month.
- Because of the relationship between the menstrual cycle and the body's mechanisms of hormonal secretion, a decrease or increase in the activity of the hormonal glands can disturb menstruation.
- Early diagnosis and prompt management are necessary if reproductive and genital problems of a more serious nature are to be prevented.
- Health teaching for patients with menstrual disturbances includes a knowledge of the physiological process, factors that alter menstruation, personal hygiene, exercise, diet, and pain management.
- Discharge planning is vital to prevent reinfection after pelvic inflammatory disease.
- Pregnancy is encouraged in the patient with endometriosis, because it will slow the progress of the disorder; infertility is a complication as the condition continues.
- Postoperative nursing interventions for the patient having a hysterectomy include monitoring vital signs and prevention of urinary retention, intestinal distention, and venous thrombosis.
- It is important to educate women in the necessity of having a yearly Papanicolaou smear examination of the cervix as a method of early detection of cervical cancer.
- It is a nursing responsibility to teach breast and testicular self-examination.
- Several surgical approaches may be selected for the removal of breast carcinoma: lumpectomy, partial mastectomy, simple mastectomy, modified radical mastectomy, and radical mastectomy.
- Discussion of hand and arm care, prevention of muscle contractions, body image acceptance, and fitting for a prosthesis are all areas to be addressed in discharge planning for a patient after a mastectomy.
- Nursing interventions for a patient with prostatitis include the need for compliance with treatment, supportive care such as bed rest and sitz baths, and monitoring intake and output.
- A hydrocele is an accumulation of fluid between the membranes covering the testicle and the membrane enclosing the testicle, whereas a varicocele occurs when the veins within the scrotum become dilated.
- Young men should be taught to perform testicular self-examination beginning at 15 years of age.
- Any sexually active person may be at risk for a sexually transmitted disease.
- The focus of patient education related to sexually transmitted diseases is on prevention.

STUDY QUESTIONS

1. The hormone responsible for ovulation is:
   a. FSH
   b. LH
   c. Estrogen
   d. Progesterone
2. The male gonads are the:
   a. Seminiferous tubules
   b. Scrotum
   c. Epididymis
   d. Testes
3. Sexuality and total health are affected by all of the following except:
   a. Socioeconomic factors
   b. Myths, beliefs, and attitudes
   c. Knowledge of sexuality
   d. Sexual behaviors
4. Illness may cause changes in one's self-concept and inability to function sexually:
   a. False
   b. True
5. Which of the following are disturbances of menstruation:
   a. Menarche and climacteric
   b. Toxic shock syndrome and candidiasis
   c. Amenorrhea, dysmenorrhea
   d. Leukorrhea
6. Which of the following statements is not true of infertility:
   a. Infertility may cause sperm and ovum production
   b. Infertility is caused by infections of the reproductive tract
   c. Infertility is caused by occlusion of fallopian tubes
   d. Infertility is caused by chronic mastitis
7. All of the following are true of patient education related to the climacteric except:
   a. It is normal and self-limiting
   b. An exercise program promotes vitality
   c. Contraceptives should be used for 1 year after the last menstrual period
   d. It marks the end of the patient's sex life
8. Pelvic inflammatory disease is any acute, subacute, recurrent, or chronic infection of the:
   a. Vagina, cervix, uterus
   b. Cervix, uterus, fallopian tubes, ovaries, and connective tissue lying between the broad ligaments
   c. Uterus, fallopian tubes, ovaries
   d. None of the above
9. All of the following correctly describe endometriosis *except:*
   a. Endometrial tissue appears outside of the uterus
   b. Rupture of an endometrial cyst causes reproduction of endometrial tissue
   c. Symptoms are more acute after menstruation
   d. Pregnancy is encouraged to slow the progress of the tissue reproduction
10. Correction of cystocele and rectocele is by surgical repair known as:
    a. Anteroposterior colporrhaphy
    b. Laparoscopy
    c. Dilation and curettage
    d. Total hysterectomy
11. Postoperative nursing interventions for a patient having a hysterectomy include all of the following except:
    a. Monitoring vital signs
    b. Prevention of urinary retention
    c. Observation for intestinal obstruction
    d. Assessment for lymphedema

STUDY QUESTIONS (cont'd)

12. An increase in abdominal girth and dyspnea resulting from pressure on the diaphragm are two clinical manifestations noted in cancer of the ovaries caused by:
    a. Development of ascites
    b. Metastasis to the bowel
    c. Dilation of the alveoli
    d. Bladder distention
13. Which of the following best describes when a self-breast-examination should be performed by a premenopausal female:
    a. During menstruation
    b. Between fourth and seventh day of the menstrual cycle
    c. The same day of each month
    d. None of the above
14. A lumpectomy, also called tylectomy or tumorectomy, is usually performed when:
    a. The tumor is 4 cm or larger
    b. The tumor is invasive
    c. The tumor is small and is on the peripheral area of the breast
    d. The tumor plus a wedge of normal tissue and fascia is to be removed
15. After a modified radical mastectomy, drains such as a Davol or Hemovac may be placed in the axillae to:
    a. Facilitate drainage and prevent formation of a hematoma
    b. Control numbness and referred pain
    c. Decrease the postoperative complications of atelectasis
    d. Prevent postoperative phlebitis in the affected arm
16. The following are often causative organisms of epididymitis *except:*
    a. *Staphylococcus aureus*
    b. *Escherichia coli*
    c. Gonococcus
    d. Pneumococcus
17. An accumulation of fluid between the membranes covering the testicle and the membrane enclosing the testicle describes:
    a. Varicocele
    b. Prostatitis
    c. Hydrocele
    d. Epididymitis
18. The prognosis for testicular cancer is usually:
    a. Unfavorable
    b. Favorable
19. All of the following are sexually transmitted diseases *except:*
    a. Herpes genitalis
    b. Amenorrhea
    c. Trichomoniasis
    d. Gonorrhea
20. Which of the following statements is true concerning the patient with a sexually transmitted disease:
    a. Female patients need a Pap test at least every 2 years
    b. During treatment the patient is unable to transmit the STD
    c. The patient should use an oil-based lubricant if vaginal dryness occurs
    d. The patient should wear loose, absorbent underclothing, change frequently, and frequently cleanse perineal area

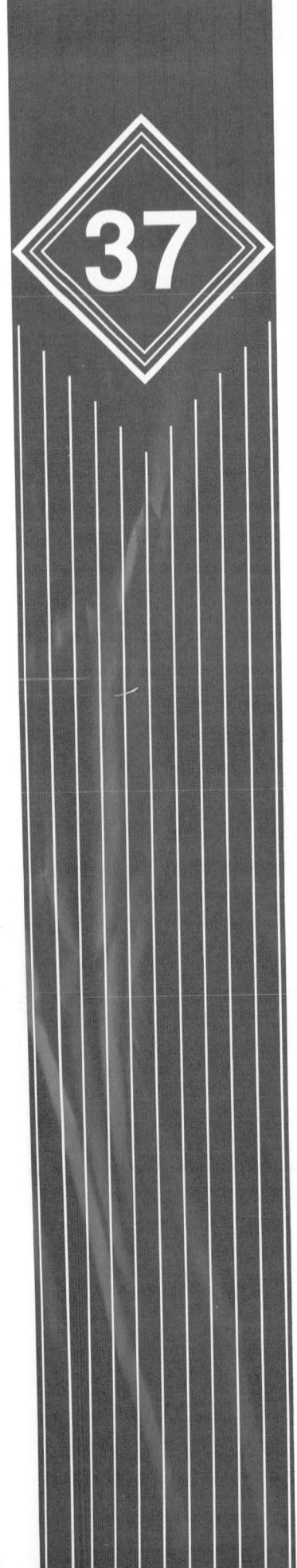

37

Care of the Patient with an Eye or Ear Disorder

PATRICIA HELMER OLES
KAREN H. RICHARDSON

LEARNING OBJECTIVES

After reading this chapter, the student should be able to do the following:

- Define the key terms.
- List the major sense organs, and discuss their anatomical position.
- List the parts of the eye, and define the function of each part.
- Compare and contrast the function of the rods and cones.
- List the three parts of the ear, and discuss the function of each.
- Discuss the effects of noise pollution on the internal structures of the ear.
- Describe two changes in the sensory system that occur as a result of the normal aging process.
- Identify factors influencing assessment of the eye and ear.
- Describe the techniques used in assessment of the eye and ear.
- Identify the purposes and procedures of diagnostic tests of the eye and ear.
- Describe signs and symptoms of various disorders of the eye and ear.
- Record significant normal and abnormal data in the patient's chart.
- Identify the nursing intervention associated with medical-surgical interventions of the eye and ear.
- List communication tips for hearing and sight impaired persons.
- Give patient instructions regarding care of the eye and ear in accordance with written protocol.
- Use an agency nursing care plan in the delivery of patient care.

RELATED TOPICS OF INTEREST

- Diet therapy (Chapter 23)
- Principles and practice of medication administration (Chapter 25)
- The surgical patient (Chapter 26)
- Care of the aging (Chapter 48)

KEY TERMS

Define the following:

- accommodation
- astigmatism
- aqueous humor
- audiometry
- canal of Schlemm
- cataract
- cerumen
- choroid
- color blindness
- conjunctiva
- conjunctivitis
- constriction
- convergence
- cornea
- cryosurgery
- diabetic retinopathy
- enucleation
- eustachian tube
- exophthalmos
- glaucoma
- incus
- iridectomy
- iris
- keratoplasty
- labyrinthitis
- lens
- malleus
- mastoiditis
- mydriatic
- myopia
- myringotomy
- ossicles
- otitis
- pinna
- proprioceptors
- punctum
- pupil
- refraction
- sclera
- semicircular canals
- Snellen
- stapedectomy
- stapes
- strabismus
- tinnitus
- tympanic membrane
- tympanoplasty
- vertigo
- vitreous humor

The sensory system constantly gathers information through millions of receptors scattered throughout the body and delivers it to the brain for interpretation. This process allows humans to survive safely by allowing appropriate responses to external stimuli. The five major senses are taste, touch, smell, sight, and hearing. The sense of balance (equilibrium) is linked with hearing, because the sensors are located within the ear.

ANATOMY OF THE EYE

The eye is a marvelous spherical structure, only 1 inch in diameter. Seventy percent of the sensory structures of the body are in the eye. The optic tracts contain more than 1 million nerve fibers that carry messages from the eye to the brain, where they are interpreted. Only a small portion of the eye is visible externally; the remainder is enclosed in the skeletal bones of the face and cushioned by layers of fat.

Accessory Structures of the Eye

The accessory structures of the eye—the eyebrows, eyelids, eyelashes, and lacrimal apparatus—function mainly as protective devices. In addition, six external eye muscles control gross eye movement and allow the eyes to focus on any object in the visual field. Superior to the eyes are the eyebrows, which are composed of coarse hair; they protect the eyes from perspiration and foreign objects and shade the eyes from direct rays of the sun.

The upper and lower eyelids protect the anterior portion of the eye. As a reflex in response to danger, they close automatically. They close with sleep to keep the eye moist. Blinking spreads lubricating secretions over the eye when an individual is awake. Lashes protrude from both the upper and lower lids to shade the eye and prevent debris from entering it.

The structures of the lacrimal apparatus (Fig. 37-1) manufacture and drain tears to keep the eyeball moist and sweep away debris that might enter the eye.

Tears are composed of a watery secretion that contains

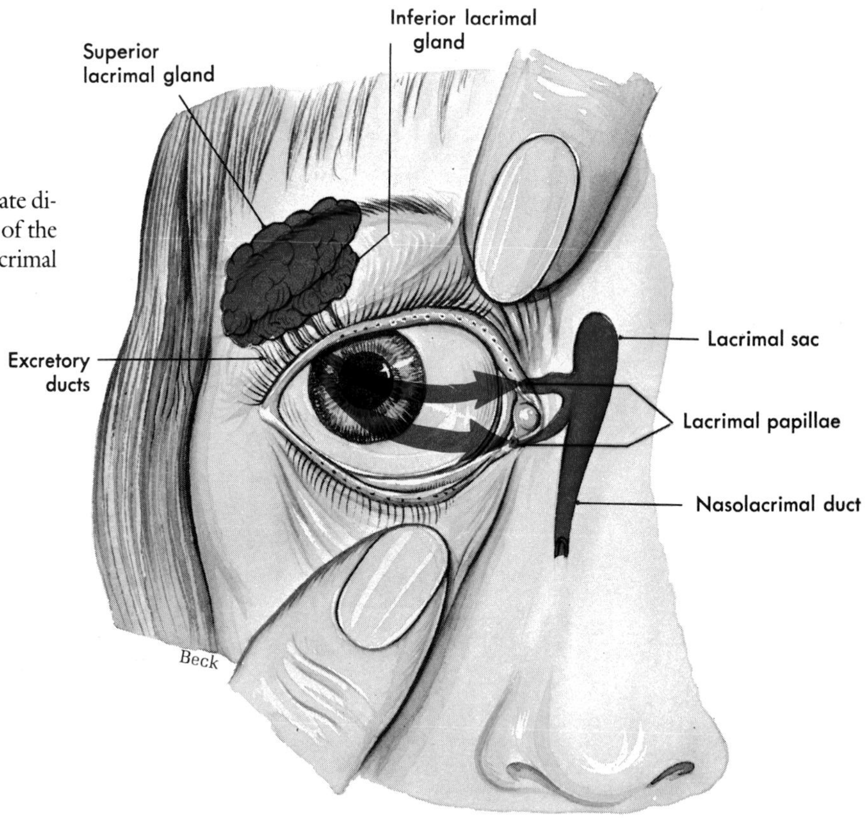

FIG. 37-1 Lacrimal apparatus. Arrows indicate direction of drainage from the excretory ducts of the lacrimal glands across the eye to the nasolacrimal duct.

salts, mucus, and a bactericidal enzyme called *lysozyme*. The lacrimal glands are located superior and lateral to each eye. Blinking causes tears to flow medially to the lacrimal ducts, which empty into the lacrimal sacs. The lacrimal sacs in turn empty into the nasolacrimal ducts and drain into the nasal cavity.

The six external eye muscles are controlled by the third, fourth, and sixth cranial nerves. They are attached to the sclera or white part of the eye. The eyes are able to move laterally, medially, superiorly, and inferiorly. Occasionally, children develop a condition commonly called *lazy eye*, which involves a weak or elongated eye muscle and is characterized by visual disturbances. It is usually easily corrected with eye exercises or surgical shortening of the muscle.

The conjunctiva (Fig. 37-2) is a thin mucous membrane that lines the inner aspect of the eyelids and the anterior surface of the eyeball to the edges of the cornea. Sometimes the blood vessels of the conjunctiva become dilated because of irritation or congestion, and the individual is said to have "bloodshot" eyes.

Structure of the Eyeball

The eyeball (Fig. 37-3) is composed of three layers or tunics. The outermost layer is the fibrous tunic, composed of thick, white connective tissue called the **sclera** or white of the eye. The sclera gives shape to the eyeball and because of its toughness protects the inner eye structures. The central anterior portion of the sclera, the **cornea,** is transparent and covers the colored portion of the eye, the iris. The cornea is the eye's window to the world, allowing light rays to enter the inner portion of the eye. Located at the border or junction of the sclera and cornea is a special structure called the **canal of Schlemm.** It is a venous sinus that aids in controlling intraocular pressure (the pressure within the eyeball).

The middle layer is the vascular tunic. It contains the choroid, the ciliary body, and the iris. The posterior portion of the middle layer is called the **choroid,** a thin, dark brown membrane that lines most of the internal area of the sclera. It is highly vascular and supplies nutrients to the retina. The choroid contains a large amount of pigment, which absorbs light rays and prevents them from reflecting outside the eye. The anterior portion of the vascular tunic forms the ciliary body, a muscular ring that holds the lens in place and changes the shape of the lens for near or far vision. The ciliary body also attaches to the **iris,** a pigmented muscular ring that resembles a doughnut. A black hole in the center of the iris is called the **pupil.** The color of the iris varies from shades of blue to brown; this is determined by the amount of pigment the iris contains and is an inherited characteristic. The iris lies between the cornea and the lens and regulates the amount of light entering the eye, much like a camera lens. Two sets of smooth muscles control the iris, which in turn affects the pupil. In bright light the circular muscle fibers of the iris contract and the pupil contracts; in dim light the radial muscle fibers of the iris contract and the pupil dilates.

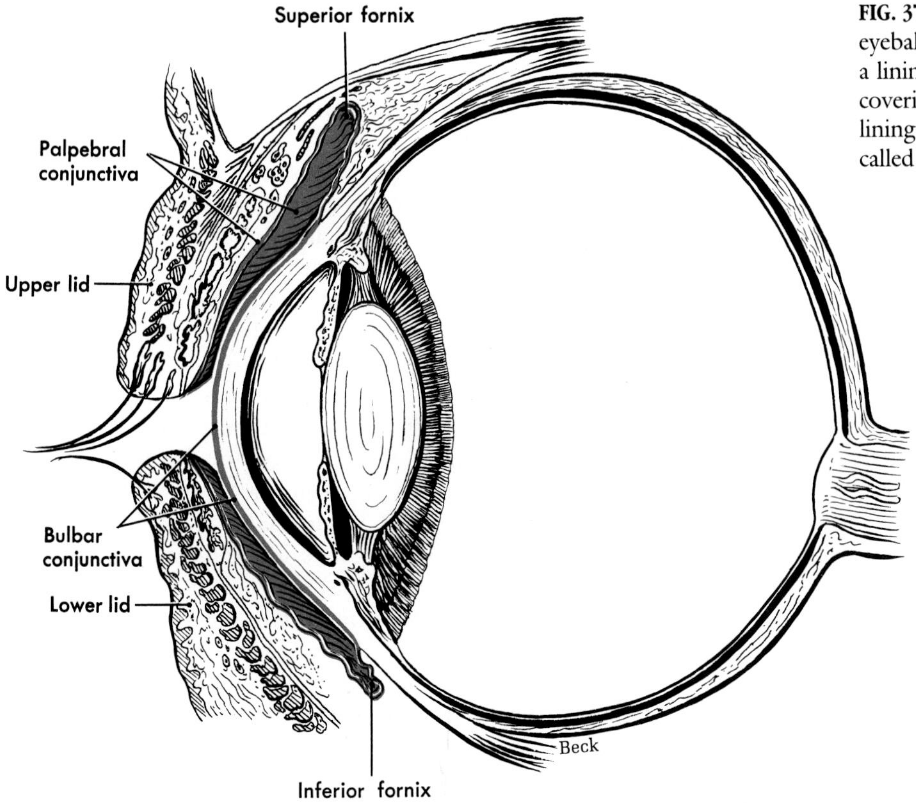

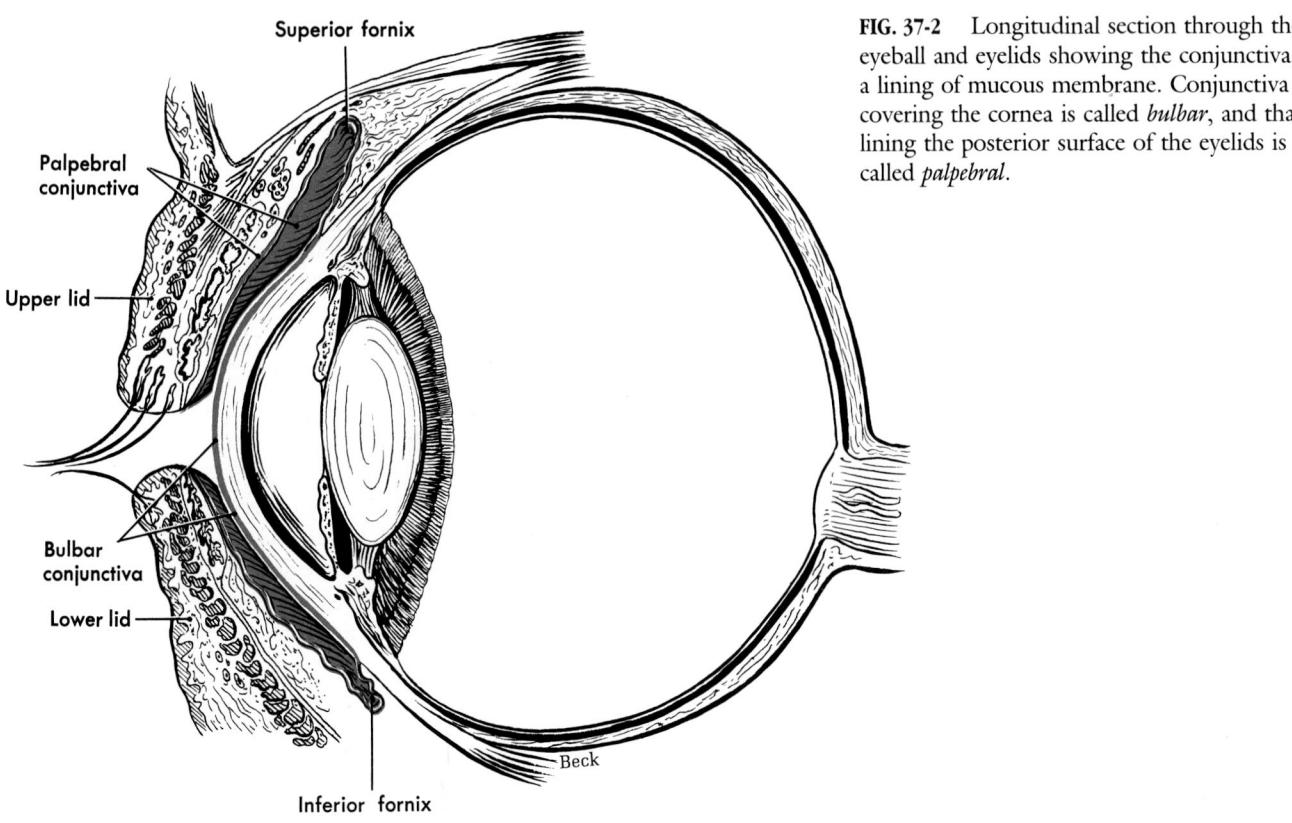

FIG. 37-2 Longitudinal section through the eyeball and eyelids showing the conjunctiva, a lining of mucous membrane. Conjunctiva covering the cornea is called *bulbar*, and that lining the posterior surface of the eyelids is called *palpebral*.

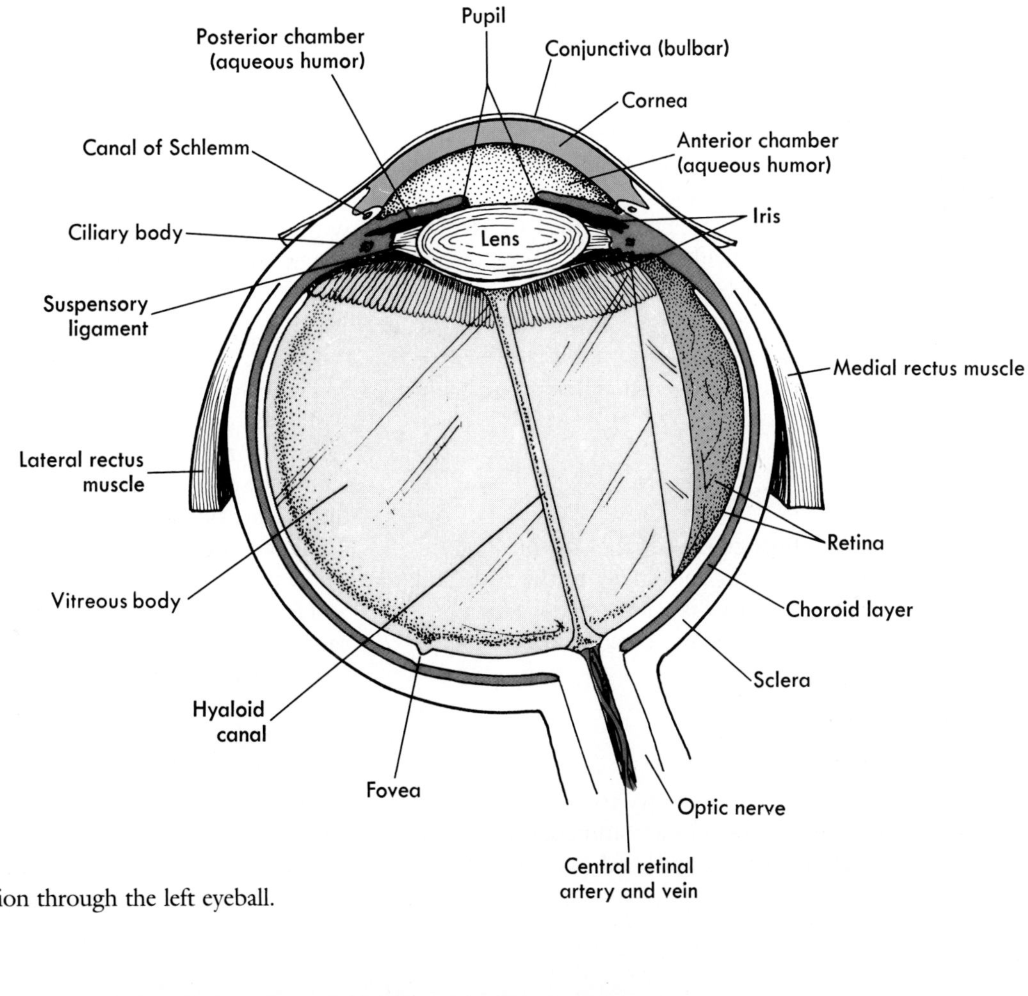

FIG. 37-3 Horizontal section through the left eyeball.

The innermost tunic of the eye is the retina, which lies only in the posterior portion of the eyeball. Located within the retina are specialized sensory cells called *rods* and *cones* (photoreceptors). They are responsible for the conversion of light to nerve impulses, which are transported through the optic nerve to the brain, where an image is formed. The rods and cones are scattered throughout the retina, except where the optic nerve exits the eye. This area is called the *optic disc* or blind spot. Rods control vision in dim light and allow sight in shades of gray; they are also responsible for peripheral vision. Cones allow vision in bright light and in color. They are concentrated in the fovea centralis, the area of most acute vision. This is a small, depressed area in the posterior portion of the retina. Color pigments that are sensitive to light allow the rods and cones to function. Vitamin A is responsible for the production of these pigments. There are three types of cones sensitive to three distinct colors: red, green, and blue. The absence of any of these three types causes **color blindness.** The most common type of color blindness is red-green blindness. Color blindness is an inherited condition occurring primarily in males.

Chambers of the Eye

The eye is divided into two chambers by the lens. Anterior to the lens is the aqueous chamber (anterior chamber). It is filled with a clear, watery fluid **(aqueous humor)** similar to blood plasma. It is continually secreted by the ciliary bodies of the choroid. To maintain normal intraocular pressure it drains through the canal of Schlemm into the bloodstream. Aqueous humor helps maintain the shape of the eyeball, keeps the retina attached to the choroid, and refracts light.

The posterior chamber, located behind the lens, is filled with **vitreous humor,** a jellylike substance. Vitreous humor gives shape to the eyeball, keeps the retina attached to the choroid, and also refracts light. It differs from the aqueous humor not only in composition but also in production. It is formed during embryonic development and is not continually replaced.

PHYSIOLOGY OF VISION

Light must travel through the cornea, aqueous humor, pupil, lens, vitreous humor, and finally to the rods and cones of the retina. The image is transported via the optic nerve to the visual center of the cerebral cortex of the brain.

Image Formation of the Retina

Four basic processes are necessary to form an image: (1) refraction of light rays, (2) accommodation of the lens, (3) constriction of the pupil, and (4) convergence of the eyes.

Refraction. Refraction is the bending of light rays. Light is bent as it passes through the colorless structures of the eye, allowing light from the environment to focus on the retina. The light from a large area can be focused on a small area.

Accommodation. The process of **accommodation** is the focusing for near objects (less than 20 feet away). For near vision to occur, the ciliary muscle must contract, which pulls the choroid toward the lens, thus causing the lens to shorten and thicken and giving it a convex appearance. This allows the lens to bend light rays toward the fovea centralis.

Constriction. To assist with accommodation, **constriction** of the diameter of the pupil must occur to prevent light from entering the periphery of the lens. If light entered the periphery, it would not focus on the retina and the image would be blurred.

Convergence. Convergence is the movement of both eyes medially to allow light rays from an object to hit the same points on both retinas. The extrinsic eye muscles control this movement. As the object becomes closer, the eyes turn toward the nose; this allows binocular vision (seeing the same object with both eyes).

ANATOMY AND PHYSIOLOGY OF THE EAR

The external ear (pinna or auricle) reveals only a portion of the complex organ of hearing. Within the ear lie many structures that allow hearing and interpretation of sound and assist in maintaining equilibrium (balance). Anatomically, when examining the ear from the external structures to the internal structures, one finds three distinct parts: the external ear, middle ear, and inner ear (Fig. 37-4). The external and middle ear deal exclusively with sound waves, while the inner ear deals with sound waves and equilibrium.

External Ear

The external ear is composed of **pinna** (outer flap of tissue and cartilage), the external auditory canal, and the **tympanic membrane** (eardrum). It is designed to collect sound waves and channel them to the middle ear. The upper part of the pinna is composed of elastic cartilage, while the lower part, the lobe, is mainly soft fleshy tissue. The whole structure is attached to the head by ligaments and muscles. The center opens into the external auditory canal.

The external auditory canal, or meatus, is a tube 2.5 cm, or 1 inch, long that terminates at the tympanic membrane. The walls of the canal are composed of bone lined with cartilage; this cartilage is continuous with the cartilage of the pinna. The epithelium (skin) covering the canal is thin and very sensitive. It contains cilia (tiny hairs) and specialized sebaceous (oil) glands called *ceruminous glands*. They secrete **cerumen** (ear wax), which protects

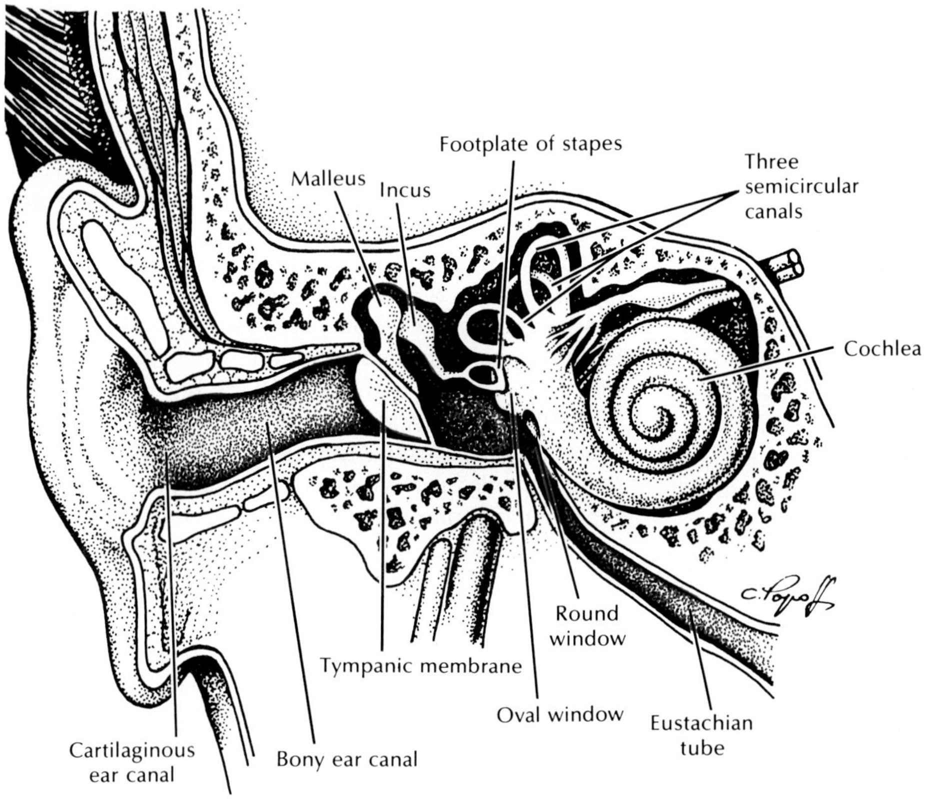

FIG. 37-4 External auditory canal, middle ear, and inner ear.

the lining from infection. The cilia, in combination with the cerumen, also prevent foreign objects from entering the ear. Because the canal is composed of epithelium, it is subject to the same irritations and infections as the skin covering the body. Foreign objects must not be inserted into the canal, because the skin is delicate and the tympanic membrane could be ruptured.

As sound waves travel through the external auditory canal, they hit the tympanic membrane, causing it to vibrate. The vibration transmits the sound waves to the middle ear.

Middle Ear

The middle ear, or tympanic cavity, is a small air-filled chamber located within the temporal bone. The **eustachian** (auditory) **tube** connects the middle ear to the nasopharynx. This tube equalizes the air pressure on either side of the tympanic membrane. When one swallows or yawns, the tube allows air to enter the middle ear, which equalizes the middle-ear and external-ear pressure. Because the pharynx, eustachian tube, and middle ear are all covered with a continuous mucous membrane, infection can travel very easily from the throat to the middle ear. This is often seen in young children. The posterior wall of the middle ear opens into the mastoid process, an area filled with air spaces, which also aids in equalization of air pressure. Infection of the middle ear, if untreated, can spread to the mastoid process.

Extending along the middle ear chamber are three small bones **(ossicles)** that carry sound waves from the external ear to the inner ear. These three small bones are named according to their shape: the **malleus** (hammer), **incus** (anvil), and **stapes** (stirrup). The internal surface of the tympanic membrane is connected to the first of these three bones, the malleus. The malleus transfers sound waves to the incus, which in turn transfers it to the stapes. The stapes pushes against the oval window, a small membrane that marks the beginning of the inner ear. This pressure of the stapes against the oval window results in vibration and sets the fluid of the internal ear into motion.

Internal Ear

The most important portion of the ear, the inner ear or labyrinth, is a series of canals. Structurally, it contains the bony labyrinth, which is lined with the membranous labyrinth. The bony labyrinth is filled with a fluid called *perilymph* and contains three subdivisions called the cochlea, vestibule, and **semicircular canals.** The membranous labyrinth is a series of sacs and tubes that contain a thicker fluid called *endolymph*. The endolymph and perilymph have different chemical compositions, but they are both fluids and both conduct sound waves through the inner ear system.

The cochlea resembles a snail's shell and contains the

organ of Corti, the organ of hearing. It contains many hearing receptors or hair cells. These cells respond to sound waves by stimulating the cochlear nerve (a branch of the eighth cranial nerve—the vestibulocochlear nerve), which transmits the message to the brain. These hair cells may become damaged from *noise pollution* (i.e., high-intensity sounds such as those produced by jet engines, factory equipment, and rock and roll bands). Once these cells are damaged or destroyed, hearing becomes permanently damaged.

Deeper in the inner ear, past the cochlea, is the vestibule or the oval central portion of the bony labyrinth. The vestibule contains receptors that respond to gravity. They provide information on which way is up and which way is down, allowing an individual to remain in an upright position. Extending upward from the vestibule are three semicircular canals responsible for maintaining balance and equilibrium. They contain sensory hair cells and endolymph. The motion of the endolymph stimulates the hair cells, which stimulates the receptors; then the message is sent to the brain for interpretation.

OTHER SPECIAL SENSES

Taste and Smell

On the tongue of the average adult there are approximately 10,000 taste buds; some are also located on the inner aspect of the cheeks. Taste buds are the receptors for four basic sensations. They respond only to substances in solution; otherwise, they are not activated. The four taste sensations and the locations of the taste buds that detect them are as follows:

Sweet—located in the tip of the tongue, they respond to sugar and other sweet substances.

Sour—located on the sides of the tongue, they respond to acid content of foods.

Salty—located on the tip of the tongue, they respond to metal ions contained in foods.

Bitter—located on the posterior portion of the tongue, they respond to alkaline or basic ions contained in foods.

The taste receptors send their messages to the taste center of the cerebral cortex of the brain. It is important to note that the sense of taste works very closely with the sense of smell for the identification of various foods. The senses of touch and sight are also involved.

The receptors for the sense of smell (olfactory receptors) are located in the roof or upper part of the nasal cavity. The olfactory receptors, embedded in the epithelium, each send cilia into the nasal chamber. On inhalation, an odor comes in contact with the olfactory receptors, and the message is then sent to the brain. Memory for certain odors is long-standing; certain odors stimulate certain memories (e.g., pine scent, Christmas; talcum powder, infants). All persons have special memories that come to mind when certain odors are smelled. The body is not able to regenerate olfactory cells; once they are damaged, the sense of smell is impaired.

Touch

The receptors for touch (tactile receptors) are located throughout the integumentary system. They respond to touch, pressure, and vibration. The most abundant receptors are the Meissner's corpuscles and pacinian corpuscles. Meissner's corpuscles, found in the fingertips, interpret fine touch and vibration. The pacinian corpuscles are located throughout the body but particularly in the joints, mammary glands, and external genitalia of both sexes. They are sensitive to pressure and vibration. Other receptors called *free nerve endings* are located throughout the body and interpret painful stimuli and temperature.

Position/Movement

Proprioception (sense of position) maintains the proper position of the body. **Proprioceptors,** located in the muscles, tendons, and joints, work in conjunction with the semicircular canals of the inner ear to maintain proper coordination. They orchestrate the body for running, walking, dancing, and many other activities. Once they receive information from the environment, they send it to the cerebellum for interpretation.

NORMAL AGING PATTERN OF THE SENSORY SYSTEM

As an individual ages, the lens of the eye hardens and becomes too large for the eye muscles, thus causing a loss of accommodation. It loses some of its transparency and becomes more opaque, and glare begins to become a problem. Concurrently the pupil becomes smaller and decreases the amount of light that reaches the retina, and one needs brighter lighting to read.

The aging ear loses the ability to hear high frequencies, probably as a result of deterioration of the nerve fibers and breakdown of the cells in the organ of Corti.

The remaining senses undergo slight changes that decrease their reaction or threshold time, which results in slower response or diminished sensation.

CARE OF THE PATIENT WITH AN EYE DISORDER

Specific Nursing Considerations for the Patient with an Eye Disorder

An initial consideration in caring for the patient with an eye disorder would include review of the following:

Eye pain, pruritus, excessive tearing, floaters, light flashes, discharge, visual changes, or blind spots

Table 37-1 Normal Findings of the Adult Eye

Area Examined	Findings
Eyelids	Blink reflex to light or touch intact. Lid margins just above corneal borders.
Eyeball	Eyeball does not protrude beyond supraorbital bridge of frontal bone. Eyeball is usually moist; moisture may be diminished in the older adult.
Conjunctivae	Palpebral (eyelid): Pink, uniform blood vessels without discharge. Bulbar: Clear, tiny red vessels; in the older adult, the bulbar conjunctiva may lose luster.
Sclera	Generally white. May have yellow-tan dots in a dark-skinned individual.
Cornea	Transparent, smooth, convex. In the older adult, a gray ring around cornea (arcus senilis) may be present as a result of lipid deposits.
Iris	Round, intact, bilateral coloration. In the older adult, color may be paler and shape less regular.
Pupil	Equal, round, reactive to light and accommodation. Response to light is equal bilaterally. In the older adult constriction response may be slower.
Internal eye (including retina, vessels, and optic disk)	Retina is intact. Vessel structure is intact and bilaterally similar in pattern. Optic disk has well-defined border.
Visual acuity	
Distant vision	20/20 (able to read line 20 of eye chart at a distance of 20 feet).
Near vision	Able to read newspaper print at 14 inches.
Peripheral vision	Side vision is 90 degrees from central visual axis. Upward 50 degrees; downward 70 degrees.
Eye movement	Coordinated eye movement bilaterally.
Color perception	Able to properly identify eye colors of major groups: red, blue, and green.

Current medication for the eye disorder
Side effects of medications, if any
Use of glasses or contact lenses
Adequacy of current eyewear prescription
Personal habits related to care of eyewear

Once the information has been gathered and communicated, the nurse assists with the eye examination. The results of the initial examination are compared with normal findings (Table 37-1).

Diagnostic Testing

Once the initial eye examination is completed, the patient may require additional diagnostic testing. The major diagnostic eye tests are explained in Table 37-2.

Additional eye tests may be required to assist in the diagnosis. The Amsler grid is used to detect a defect of the macular area of the retina. The tangent screen evaluates central and peripheral fields of vision. The Goldmann perimetry test detects and evaluates the progression of **glaucoma,** which affects peripheral vision. Exophthalmometry measures the degree of forward placement of the eye, known as **exophthalmos** (protrusion of the eyeball). Slit-lamp examination is done to examine the conjunctiva, **lens,** vitreous humor, iris, and cornea. The Schirmer test evaluates the function of the major lacrimal glands. Fluorescein angiography is used to examine the microvascular structures of the eye and assess patency of the lacrimal system.

DISORDERS OF THE EYE

Blindness and Near Blindness

Etiology/pathophysiology. Blindness is a loss of visual acuity that ranges from partial to total loss of sight. It may be congenital or acquired.

The World Health Organization (WHO) has determined that in the United States there are approximately 1 million people who are legally blind. Legal blindness refers to individuals with a maximal visual acuity of 20/200 with corrective eyewear and/or visual field sight capacity reduced to 20 degrees. (The normal visual field range is 180 degrees.)

Categories have been established to help determine the exact extent of the vision loss and what assistance measures are appropriate for the individual. These categories range from low vision loss (20/70 to 20/200) to three categories of blindness (20/400, 20/1200, and no light perception).

Congenital blindness results from various birth defects. Acquired blindness in adults occurs as a result of such disorders as diabetic retinopathy, glaucoma, cataracts, and retinal degeneration; acute trauma is also a common cause.

Clinical manifestations. The degree of vision loss will depend on the extent of trauma or disease. Symptoms may include diplopia, pain, presence of floaters and flashes of light, and pruritus or burning of eyes. Additional physical manifestations of the visually impaired patient include loss of peripheral vision, halos (colored

Table 37-2 Major Diagnostic Eye Tests

Test	Purpose	Equipment	Procedure	Patient Teaching
Snellen test (Eye chart test for visual acuity: letters, numbers, or symbols are arranged on the chart in decreasing size from top to bottom)	Assessment of visual acuity; used as screening test	Snellen chart; eye patch/cover	1. Patient stands 20 ft from chart. 2. Covers one eye. 3. Asked to read above or below the 20/20 line. 4. Repeats step 3 using the other eye. 5. Findings are documented.	1. Explain test. 2. If findings are abnormal (i.e., other than 20 ft required to read the chart line), encourage patient to seek further eye testing.
Color vision	Prerequisite for driver's license	Color chart or machine	1. Color dots are reflected on a background of mixed colors. 2. Patient identifies color patterns on the test field. 3. Finding are documented.	1. Explain procedure. 2. Encourage patient to seek further testing when results indicate inaccurate recognition of color patterns.
Refraction	Measurement of visual acuity to determine refractory errors such as: **myopia** (nearsightedness), hyperopia (farsightedness), presbyopia (inability to focus on close objects), and astigmatism (blurred vision)	Retinoscope or sample lenses	1. Ophthalmologist/optometrist asks patient to indicate clear/blurred vision with each lens change in the retinoscope.	1. Explain procedure. 2. Examiner discusses results with patient and encourages appropriate corrective measures.
Ophthalmoscopy	Evaluation of underlying structures of the eye; routine screening	Ophthalmoscope; **mydriatic** drops to dilate the pupil	1. Mydriatic drops applied. Mydriatic drops are contraindicated in patients with narrow-angle glaucoma. 2. As pupil dilation occurs, the room is darkened. 3. Patient is instructed to remain still and focus on a stationary object. 4. Examiner uses ophthalmoscope to view internal eye structure. 5. Findings are documented.	1. Explain procedure. 2. Instruct patient that effects of the drops will last no longer than 1 hour. 3. Sunglasses are required when outside or in brightly lit room until pupils return to normal size. 4. Examiner discusses results with patient and encourages corrective measures.
Tonometry	Measurement of intraocular pressure to detect tumors and glaucoma	Tonometer Topical anesthetic may be used	1. Examiner places tonometer on cornea. 2. Pressure readings are obtained. 3. Findings are documented.	1. Explain procedure. 2. Encourage patient to relax to avoid false high readings. 3. Eyes are not to be rubbed for approximately 30 minutes to avoid corneal irritation. 4. Contact lenses may be reinserted 2 hours after completion of test.

circles around the cornea), a sense of orbital pressure, bulging of the eye(s), and any difference in the appearance of an eye structure, such as the pupil.

The wide variety of emotional symptoms associated with blindness may range from fear, anxiety, disorientation, depression, helplessness, and hopelessness to acceptance.

Assessment. Collection of *subjective data* may include noting the patient complaint of blurred vision as an early symptom of an eye disorder. It is important to determine the onset, severity, and duration of the symptoms, as well as any factors that relieve symptoms.

Collection of *objective data* may include observing squinting and rubbing of the eyes. It is important to note the patient's compensation measures, such as use of a magnifying glass. The use and effectiveness of assistive eyewear are also determined.

Emotionally the patient may experience poor interpersonal communication skills and coping mechanisms. Because self-care skills may be impaired, a blind individual may isolate himself or herself, causing additional physical and emotional difficulties.

Diagnostic tests. The initial examination begins with an ophthalmoscopic examination. Other tests may include color and light vision tests and peripheral vision tests.

Medical management. Corrective eyewear (contact lenses and glasses) is the first method of medical management for a partially sighted individual. If the visual defect results from an inflammatory disorder, medication is prescribed, appropriate to the causative agent.

Additional assistive devices for a visually impaired patient include canes, Seeing Eye dogs, magnifying systems, and telescopic lenses. The patient should be evaluated by an eye specialist to determine which devices are best suited. Some of the more technologically complex devices are expensive and may not be covered by insurance.

Canes are the most frequently used device for the partially or totally blind person. They are lightweight and portable and allow the patient simple maneuvering. The drawback to their use is that overhead objects are not usually detected. The newer laser canes provide more information about objects in front and at head and foot levels, but these are not readily available and are expensive. Seeing Eye dogs allow the blind person mobility that would otherwise be difficult. Trained dogs steer the patient away from obstacles, both aerial and stationary.

Surgical correction of the visual defect may provide eyesight. New laser surgeries provide excellent results in selected cases.

Nursing interventions. The nurse might falsely assume that patients should be in the acceptance phase if the blindness has been present for years. This is not necessarily the case. Complications of long-term blindness may result in physical and emotional problems. Physically, the patient may be malnourished from diminished self-care cooking skills. The patient may also have secondary infections related to poor hygiene practices. Assistance with activities of daily living is a primary focus of patient care. Adequate time should be provided to allow the patient to assist in self-care. Emotional aspects of nursing care include appropriate communication (Box 37-1).

BOX 37-1 GUIDELINES FOR COMMUNICATING WITH BLIND PERSONS

1. Talk in a normal tone of voice.
2. Do not try to avoid common phrases in speech, such as "See what I mean?"
3. Introduce yourself with each contact (unless well known to the person).
4. Explain any activity occurring in the room.
5. Announce when you are leaving the room so the blind person is not put in the position of talking to someone who is no longer there.

The impact of vision loss affects not only the patient, but also family, friends, and the community. Coping mechanisms differ among individuals. It is a nursing responsibility to educate, assist, counsel, and prevent complications. A comprehensive approach to patient care is essential with blind individuals. Use of government and community resources is absolutely necessary; individuals should be encouraged to contact the Department of Health and Human Services for resources and assistance. When a total approach is taken, the patient's successful adjustment to home, work, and society is possible. Blind individuals are capable of leading a full and active life and need to be treated as such.

NURSING DIAGNOSES	NURSING INTERVENTIONS
Fear	Determine the patient's level of fear. Orient the patient to use persons and the environment. Use therapeutic touch. Avoid loud sounds that may startle the patient.
Potential for injury	Use protective devices, such as side rails and canes. Alter surroundings to afford safety—clear passageways, nonslip rugs, and so on.
Feeding self-care deficit	Describe the meal tray contents; arrange foods by texture and temperature; describe the location of the foods by the clock method (e.g., orange juice at 11:00 position, spoon at 9:00).

Patient teaching. The patient will require instruction on ambulatory safety. Aspects to include in the instructions are walking slowly, using verbal clues from the walking companion, and encouraging the patient to touch objects or borders.

Table 37-3 Common Refractory Errors

Condition	Description	Etiology/Pathophysiology	Clinical Manifestations	Assessment
Astigmatism	Defect in the curvature of the eyeball surface	May be hereditary or a muscular deficit Occurs when the light rays cannot be focused clearly in a point on the retina because the spherical curve of the cornea is not equal in all meridians	Blurring of vision	*Collection of subjective data:* Complaints of eye discomfort, difficulty in focusing
Strabismus	Eyes unable to focus in the same direction; commonly called "cross-eyed" Esotropia: eye turns in the direction of the nose Exotropia: eye turns outward	May result from neurological or muscular dysfunction or may be inherited Only one eye can fix on an object, since the optic axes do not focus simultaneously	Eyeball position is not symmetrical	*Collection of subjective data:* States difficulty following objects *Collection of objective data:* One eye focuses or follows an object rather than both eyes

SKILL 37-1 REMOVAL OF CONTACT LENSES

Rigid lens

Method 1

a. Place finger at outer canthus of eye.
b. Pull skin obliquely upward, then straight down.
c. Lens will appear on lower lashes as the upper lid moves downward.
d. If lens moves off center, reposition it by gentle pressure on lid or lens itself.

Method 2

a. Place finger or thumb of each hand at base of eyelashes (upper and lower).
b. Bring eyelids together, trapping the lens (the lens will eject).
c. If lens moves off center, reposition it by gentle pressure on lid or lens itself.

Method 3

a. Using eye irrigation set, gently flush eye with sterile normal saline solution.
b. Retrieve lens in curved basin.

Method 4

a. Use small suction device shaped like a miniature "plumber's helper."
b. Place over center of lens and pull lens off gently.

Soft lens

a. Pull upper lid up with one thumb.
b. Be sure lens is in place before attempting removal.
c. Move lens over conjunctiva before grasping it, if possible. If lens does not move freely, put several drops of sterile saline solution in eye, close lid, and wait 1 minute before trying again.
d. Grasp lens with thumb and forefinger or other hand and pinch the soft lens (it will pop off).

The walking companion should precede the patient by about 1 foot and have the patient's hand on the companion's elbow to provide security. For both short-term and long-term blindness, if total vision is affected, a description of the surroundings is appropriate.

Refractory Errors

Astigmatism and strabismus

Etiology/pathophysiology. Common refractory errors are included in Table 37-3.

Clinical manifestations. Refer to Table 37-3.

Assessment. Refer to Table 37-3.

Diagnostic tests. Common tests used in the diagnosis of refractory errors include ophthalmoscopy, retinoscopy, visual acuity tests, and refraction tests.

Medical management. Many refractory errors are treated with the use of corrective eyewear. Although corrective eyewear is the more common treatment, the preferred treatment is surgical correction.

Nursing interventions. The hospitalized patient wearing corrective eyewear requires daily assistance in cleansing and maintenance. If eyeglasses are worn, the lenses are washed daily with a mild or diluted glass cleaner and rinsed before drying with a soft cloth. Screw fittings should be checked to make sure they are secure. Contact lenses are cared for based on the manufacturer's directions. Removal for cleaning is described in Skill 37-1. Safety should be maintained when corrective eyewear is not worn.

NURSING DIAGNOSIS	NURSING INTERVENTIONS
Fear and/or anxiety	Explain all procedures and diagnostic tests. Orient patient to the environment, offer reassurance and understanding, and identify anyone entering the room to prevent startling the patient.

Patient teaching. The patient should be encouraged to see an optometrist or ophthalmologist yearly to keep the eyewear prescription current. The patient should be instructed on the use and care of eyewear; complications may result if the patient does not follow use and care instructions.

Inflammatory and Infectious Disorders of the Lid

Hordeolum, chalazion, and blepharitis. The most commonly seen infection and inflammatory disorders of the lid are listed in Table 37-4.

Clinical manifestations. Refer to Table 37-4.

Assessment. Refer to Table 37-4.

Diagnostic tests. The eyelid margin is examined. Culture and sensitivity tests of any drainage may be ordered. Visual disturbances are also noted.

Medical management. Antiinfective agents are prescribed. Localized incision and drainage of a cyst or stye may be performed under local anesthesia. Warm normal saline compresses are ordered for 10 to 20 minutes two to four times a day.

Nursing interventions. A primary objective of nursing care for the patient with an infectious or inflammatory process of the lids is prevention of the spread of infection. Care should be taken when applying compresses (Skill 37-2). Handwashing is essential before contact with the eye.

Patient teaching. Instructions should be provided on the use of prescribed drops or ointments (see Skill 25-6). The patient is taught the use of warm compresses and informed about specific hygiene practices, such as keeping hands clean and away from the eyes and replacing mascara after 3 to 6 months, since the oils decompose and may harbor bacteria. The patient is cautioned to avoid irritating fumes or smoke, which may cause the patient to rub the eyes, leading to further infection. The use of eye makeup is discouraged until all inflammation subsides.

Conjunctivitis

Etiology/pathophysiology. **Conjunctivitis** is an inflammation of the **conjunctiva** resulting from bacterial or viral infection, allergy, or environmental factors. It is commonly called *pink eye*.

Acute bacterial conjunctivitis is usually transmitted by direct contact with a contaminated object. Pneumococcal, staphylococcal, streptococcal, and gonococcal organisms are the major causative agents. The hands are the most common transmitter of bacteria from the contaminated object to the eye. The eye, because of its warmth, moisture, and extensive vascularization, provides the bacteria with an excellent medium for multiplication. Conjunctivitis represents about two thirds of the 1 million cases per year of eye inflammation and infection. The disease is usually self-limiting, leaving no permanent impairment.

Viruses of the respiratory or intestinal tract may result in a secondary infection of the eye. The two more common viral agents are *Chlamydia trachomatis* and type 1 herpes simplex. Trachoma, a highly contagious form of conjunctivitis, is caused by a strain of the *C. trachomatis* virus. Transmission is by direct contact with an ocular discharge. It is rare in the United States but is a major cause of blindness in the Far East and Mediterranean countries.

Clinical manifestations. The inflammatory process that results from the contamination produces erythema of the conjunctiva, edema of the lid, and a crusting discharge on the lids and cornea. This infection, if untreated, leaves the eyelid scarred with granulations that invade the cornea, resulting in loss of vision.

Assessment. Collection of *subjective data* includes an awareness that during allergy seasons and because of exposure to environmental irritants, the patient may report pruritus, burning, and excessive tearing.

Table 37-4 Common Infections/Inflammatory Disorders of the Lid

Condition	Description	Etiology/Pathophysiology	Clinical Manifestations	Assessment
Hordeolum (Stye)	Acute infection of eyelid margin or sebaceous glands of the eyelashes	Frequently caused by the staphylococcus organism One or more pustules may form	Abscess localized to base of eyelashes, with edema of lid	*Collection of subjective data:* Localized tenderness and pain resulting from edema; pain diminished after pustule ruptures *Collection of objective data:* Raised, erythematous area on eyelid Pustule drainage
Chalazion	Inflammatory cyst on the meibomian gland at the eyelid margin; may require weeks to develop into a cyst	May be caused by infection; associated with diabetes mellitus, gout, and anemia	Discomfort, mass on eyelid, edema, visual disturbance	*Collection of subjective data:* Pressure felt as eyelid closes over cornea Patient may describe vision changes *Collection of objective data:* Cyst formation Eyelid edema
Blepharitis	Inflammation of eyelid margins	Ulcerative: caused by bacterial infection, usually staphylococcal organisms Nonulcerative: caused by psoriasis, seborrhea, or allergic response	Pruritus, erythema of eyelid, eyelid pain, photophobia Excessive tearing may occur in nonulcerative type	*Collection of subjective data:* Eye pruritus Lids adhere together after sleep *Collection of objective data:* Eyes erythematous Patient rubs eyes Sensitivity to light Tear spillage

SKILL 37-2

APPLICATION OF WARM MOIST EYE COMPRESSES

1. Use sterile technique when infection or ulceration is present; clean technique may be used for allergic reactions.
2. Use separate equipment for bilateral eye infections.
3. Wash hands before treating each eye.
4. Temperature of compresses should not exceed 49° C (120° F).
5. Change compresses frequently over 10 to 20 minutes.
6. Do not exert pressure on eyeball.
7. Sterile petrolatum may be used on skin *around* eyes, if desired, to protect skin.
8. If sterility is not necessary, moist heat may be applied by means of a clean washcloth.

Collection of *objective data* includes observing eyes that are erythematous, with edema of the lid. A dried exudate may be noted.

Diagnostic tests. The conjunctiva is scraped for bacteria and stained for microscopic examination.

Medical management. Medical treatment is similar to that for blepharitis.

Nursing interventions. The lid and lashes are cleansed of exudate with normal saline. Warm compresses are applied two to four times a day. When allergies are present, cold saline compresses may be ordered for control of edema and pruritus. Eye irrigations with normal saline or lactated Ringer's solution may be prescribed to remove secretions. Topical antibiotics and adrenocortical steroid medications are administered. Eyepads are contraindicated, because they enhance bacterial growth.

NURSING DIAGNOSES	NURSING INTERVENTIONS
Pain: pruritus	Apply warm or cold compresses. Administer prescribed eye medications; ensure proper installation of eyedrops and ointments; administer eye irrigation as prescribed. Administer analgesics as ordered.
Actual or potential sensory/perceptual alterations (visual)	Assess patient's limitations in visual sensory perception. Implement safety measures as appropriate.

Patient teaching. The patient and family should be instructed to avoid contact with the eyes or soiled materials when an infection is present. Individual washcloths and towels are to be used. The patient is instructed to wash hands if contact is made with the eyes and before any treatments and is also taught to perform and describe treatments such as irrigations, compresses, and medication administration. The patient should avoid noxious fumes or smoke and should not wear contact lenses during the suppuration period.

Inflammatory and Infectious Disorders of the Cornea and Sclera

Keratitis

Etiology/pathophysiology. Keratitis, an inflammation of the cornea, may result from injury, irritants, allergies, viral infection, or diseases such as congenital syphilis, smallpox, and some nervous disorders. It may be superficial and involve the epithelial layer only or invade the subepithelial layer and the endothelial membrane. The layers of the eye are innervated, and thus when inflammation is present pain will be acute. Ulcers may form in the eye membrane layers, resulting in scattered scarring of the corneal surface.

Pneumococcus, Staphylococcus, Streptococcus, and Pseudomonas are the most common types of bacterial causes of keratitis. The viral agent most often responsible for corneal inflammation is the herpes simplex virus. Keratitis can be triggered by stress, illness, and exposure to ultraviolet light. The condition may be associated with the use of ophthalmological steroid medications. Overuse or abuse of topical steroids may injure epithelial cells.

Another form of keratitis is acanthamoebic keratitis. The *Acanthamoeba* organism is found in the soil, airborne dust, fresh water, and the noses and throats of healthy humans. This organism is often found to be resistant to antimicrobial agents. Contact lens wearers are more susceptible, because traditional cleaning agents for lenses include rinsing with clean or distilled water. People who swim frequently are at greater risk, because the amoeba is not killed by usual methods of disinfection, such as chlorine.

Clinical manifestations. Severe eye pain is the most common symptom that differentiates this disease from other eye inflammatory diseases. If uncontrolled, keratitis may result in blepharospasms and vision loss. Other symptoms include photophobia, tearing, edema, and visual disturbances.

Assessment. Collection of *subjective data* includes noting the severity and duration of the pain, the extent of light sensitivity, and any vision loss.

Collection of *objective data* includes assessing the patient for facial grimacing, lacrimation, and photophobia.

Diagnostic tests. Depending on the causative agent, a variety of diagnostic tests may be ordered, including culture and sensitivity tests, fluorescein staining, and Gram staining. Ophthalmoscopic examination is also performed.

Medical management. Medical management includes topical antibiotic therapy. Systemic antibiotics may be prescribed for severe cases. Cycloplegic-mydriatic drugs may be ordered, which paralyze the ocular muscles of accommodation and dilate the pupil. Analgesics are used to control pain associated with acute inflammation. Pressure dressings may be ordered to relax the eye muscle and decrease discomfort. These dressings are often applied to both eyes, since the eyes move together. Warm or cold compresses two to four times daily are prescribed for symptomatic relief. Epithelial debridement of loose tissue may be performed. Surgical management involves a corneal transplant, known as **keratoplasty.**

Nursing interventions. The focus of nursing interventions for keratitis includes control of pain, safety, and prevention of complications.

NURSING DIAGNOSES	NURSING INTERVENTIONS
Potential for infection	Assess eye drainage to determine whether isolation is required. Administer eye and systemic medications to control and prevent the spread of infection.
Pain	Administer topical anesthetics if ordered to reduce spasms. Apply pressure dressing to the eye(s) to rest the muscle activity. Apply warm or cold eye compresses (as ordered) two to four times daily to control pain.
Potential for injury	Install topical anesthetic medications for pain reduction. Ensure safety measures, such as moving needed objects close to the patient, orienting the patient to the environment, and using side rails if the patient is hospitalized. Assist patient in ambulation as indicated.

Patient teaching. The nurse should provide information on self-care of a corneal abrasion. The patient must also learn to wash the hands before instilling medication and to prevent infection by not rubbing the eyes. The patient

Table 37-5 Noninfectious Disorders of the Lacrimal Gland

Condition	Description	Etiology/Pathophysiology	Clinical Manifestations	Assessment
Dry eye	Inadequate tear production from the lacrimal gland	Lacrimal dysfunction Congenital: conditions such as trigeminal nerve Acquired: conditions such as arthritis, systemic lupus erythematosus, leukemia, lymphomas, or infectious disorders Medication therapy (e.g., atropine, antihistamines, β-adrenergic blockers that reduce tear production)	Stinging, burning, pain, lacrimation, and insufficient mucus production to the eyeball surface	*Collection of subjective data:* Includes the degree of pain (which may vary), the feeling of a foreign substance in the eye, complaints of environmental irritations, and determination of contact lens wear
Excessive tearing	Overproduction of tears	Eye infection Presence of a foreign body in the eye Tear spillage resulting from an occlusion in the drainage system Environmental stimulants/injuries Medications, such as cholinergic drugs	Blurred vision, erythema, edematous puncta or conjunctiva	*Collection of objective data:* Includes observing the patient for eye rubbing, tear spillage, and facial grimacing

is instructed to note any change in discharge or increase in pain and to notify the physician immediately.

Noninfectious disorders of the lacrimal gland. Table 37-5 discusses conditions of the lacrimal gland.

Diagnostic tests. The definitive test for dry eye is the Schirmer test. Normal results should indicate 10 to 15 mm of wet paper.

Medical managment. Medical management for dry eye includes artificial tear replacement. Many nonprescription products are available for this purpose.

Estrogen therapy may be prescribed for postmenopausal women. Medications that may cause dry eye as a side effect are limited, if possible. If an infection accompanies the dry eye syndrome, antibiotic therapy will be prescribed.

As many environmental irritants as possible are eliminated. If contact lenses cause local irritation and dry eye, a change in the prescription or type of lens is advised.

Results of the fluorescein staining test for excessive tear disorder are considered normal if the dye disappears from the lacrimal cul-de-sac within 1 minute.

When excessive tearing results from environmental irritants, the patient is encouraged to eliminate the noxious element. Filtering machines are available to control pollen and dust levels in the environment.

Surgical repair of an injured punctal sac by correctly aligning the eyelid margin or by probing an obstructed **punctum** (opening to the tear duct) to allow for tear reabsorption is the advised method of treatment.

Nursing interventions. Nursing interventions for patients with dry eye and excessive tearing include patient safety and education, as discussed below.

NURSING DIAGNOSIS	NURSING INTERVENTIONS
Potential for injury	Note lubrication of eye surfaces. Document level of discomfort. Instill medications as ordered.

Patient teaching. The patient should be instructed on instilling eye medications, and appropriate hygiene practices should be reinforced. Instructions are given on avoiding irritants.

Noninfectious Disorders of the Lid

Ectropion and entropion

Etiology/pathophysiology. Two noninfectious conditions cause an abnormal turning of the eyelid margins: ectropion and entropion.

Ectropion is the outward turning of the eyelid margin. There are two types—atonic and cicatricial. In the elderly patient, it is common for the orbicularis oculi muscle to be relaxed. This condition is atonic ectropian.

Cicatricial ectropian involves either eyelid margin. The most common causes are eyelid laceration and burns of the conjunctival tissue.

Entropion is an inward turning of the eyelid. The lower eyelid margin is the most frequently involved. The conjunctival membrane lining the eyelid and part of the eyeball are exposed. Entropion is caused by atrophy of the eyelid tissue, spasms of the oculi muscle, or scarring of the tarsal plate (dense connective tissue that stiffens the eyelid) resulting from congenital origin or trauma. Varying degrees of atonia exist in the elderly; this is considered common.

Clinical manifestations. Ectropion and entropion are

Clinical manifestations. Ectropion and entropion are characterized by abnormal direction of the eyelid, with tear spillage and corneal dryness.

Assessment. Collection of *subjective data* includes noting the degree of vision loss and determination of tear loss and/or dryness of the cornea.

Collection of *objective data* includes observing the extent to which the patient can perform ADLs and the presence of any eyelid margin inflammation.

Diagnostic tests. The physician determines these conditions through a visual and ophthamological examination.

Medical management. Medical intervention consists of topical medications to reduce conjunctival and corneal inflammation or drying. Surgery is the preferred method of treatment. A resection of the tarsal plate, removal of the scarred tissue, or tightening of the oculi muscle is the choice to permanently repair these conditions.

Nursing interventions. Interventions for ectropion and entropion involve monitoring the medical treatment and reporting its progress. If the eyelid is surgically repaired, the patient should be monitored for safety considerations.

NURSING DIAGNOSIS	NURSING INTERVENTIONS
Sensory/perceptual alterations (visual)	Caution the patient regarding loss of depth perception and peripheral vision. Assist the patient with self-care activities. Observe the intactness of the eye patches. Provide safety through the use of side rails. Note any eyelid margin inflammation. Change dressings as ordered. Instill medications as prescribed.

Injury and infection are complications of unsuccessful postoperative therapy. Successful therapy involves minimal visual disturbances.

Noninfectious Disorders of the Lens

Cataracts

Etiology/pathophysiology. A **cataract** is an opacity, or clouding, of the lens. The lens is normally clear and transparent. As one ages, there is a gradual opacification of the lens. When a cataract develops, the lens becomes foggy and prevents vision. If a large enough portion of the lens becomes opaque, light cannot reach the retina. Cataracts are not contagious, as some individuals believe. People often feel that cataracts cause blindness or result from cancer. This is false information and the patient needs to be educated about the pathophysiology of the condition.

Cataracts may be congenital or acquired from systemic disease, trauma, toxins, intraocular inflammation, and aging. Senile cataracts, associated with the elderly, are the most common type.

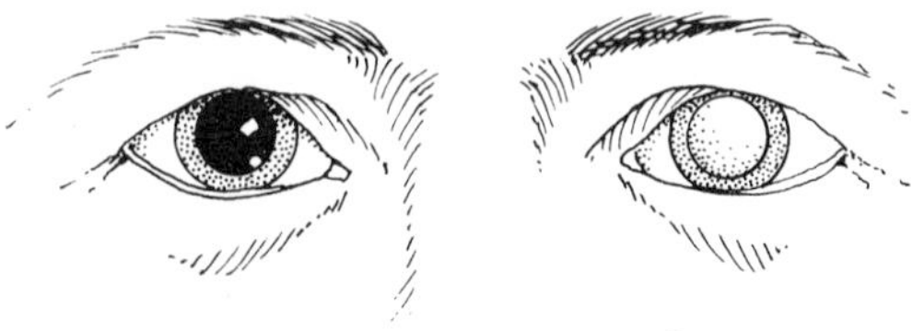

FIG. 37-5 Cataract, visible in the left eye as white opacity of the lens, is seen through the pupil.

Clinical manifestations. Symptoms of a cataract include blurring of vision, diplopia, photosensitivity, and difficulty in driving at night; no pain is associated with cataract formation. There is an opacity in the center portion of the lens (Fig. 37-5).

Assessment. Collection of *subjective data* includes noting blurring of vision as often the first symptom to be expressed by the patient. The nurse should note any subjective complaints, such as "hazy" or "fuzzy" vision.

Collection of *objective data* involves observing the patient for difficulty in reading, noting whether the patient brings newsprint close to the eyes. Sensitivity to light should also be noted.

Diagnostic tests. Ophthalmoscopic examination is the primary evaluative method.

Medical management. Medical intervention involves monitoring the patient for changes in vision associated with an increasing size of the cataract. Surgery is the only definitive method of treatment and can be performed at any age. It may be done using local or general anesthesia. There are two methods of surgery: intracapsular and extracapsular extraction.

Intracapsular surgery involves removing the lens and its entire capsule. The extracapsular method, the most common form of treatment, removes the lens and anterior capsule without removing the posterior capsule. Healing is rapid with this method.

During surgery, the physician may implant an intraocular lens (Fig. 37-6) in the anterior or posterior chamber. When intraocular lenses are not implanted, the physician will prescribe external lenses or glasses. Special contact lenses for cataracts provide the patient many options for comfort.

Nursing interventions. Preoperative and postoperative nursing care is a primary nursing responsibility (see the nursing care plan, p. 978, for nursing diagnoses and intervention).

Cataract symptoms usually develop slowly and can easily be detected. Annual examinations, especially for persons 40 and older, should be encouraged. If a cataract is treated early, blindness is usually prevented. Surgery provides about a 90% success rate of acceptable levels of vision.

NURSING CARE PLAN: THE PATIENT WITH AN EYE DISORDER

Nursing diagnoses	Patient goals	Nursing interventions
Potential for injury, related to altered visual acuity	Patient will not have any evidence of injury	Preoperative Instill eye drops as prescribed Administer preoperative medications or sedatives as ordered. Explain postoperative procedures to expect, such as patches and eye drops. Postoperative Instill hydriatic/cycloplegic and corticosteroid eyedrops as prescribed. Instruct patient to avoid sudden head movement, heavy lifting, coughing, sneezing, vomiting, or straining with elimination which causes increased intraocular pressure. Maintain prescribed eye patch/shield in position during specified hours. Remove environmental barriers to ensure safety. Keep side rails up at all times. Plan all care with patient: explain routines of what will happen and when. Visit frequently and announce yourself on entering room. Assist with and teach deep breathing exercises. Check with physician for any special positioning and/or precautions. (If turned, position patient on the unaffected side.) Elevate head of bed 30 degrees as ordered. Assist with and teach active and passive range-of-motion exercises every 4 hours. Increase activities and ambulation as ordered; assist as needed. Teach self care activities and assist as needed.
Sensory/perceptual alteration (visual), related to trauma/disease of the eye	Patient will attain maximum functioning within limits of visual impairment.	Determine nature of visual symptoms, such as degree of vision loss or pain. Note eye and/or lid imflammation, edema, or appearance changes. Determine the patient's visual limitations. Provide self-care assistance and unit orientation. Reinforce discharge instructions for the patient and family regarding home care follow-up. Maintain safety precautions regarding physical environment. Encourage the patient to wear prescribed glasses during activity. Reinforce that limitations in vision will be present during the healing phase, especially with peripheral and depth perception.
Knowledge deficit, related to unfamiliarity with the eye disorder	Patient and/or family will obtain adequate knowledge related to care of the eye.	Reinforce preoperative/postoperative instructions on eye care. Reinforce correct technique regarding medication administration. Demonstrate and request return demonstration on eye patch dressing changes. Observe the patient's knowledge of contact lens use and care. Reinforce safety precautions that should be observed as a result of vision loss. Encourage the patient to report any sudden symptoms of severe pain, sudden vision loss, or signs of infection. Encourage the patient to carry identification regarding date of recent eye surgery.
Anxiety/fear, related to visual impairment	Patient will experience less anxiety/fear.	Observe level of patient/family anxiety. Note patient's coping mechanism related to vision loss. Encourage ventilation of feelings and concerns. Support patient/family's positive actions toward adapting to visual limitations.

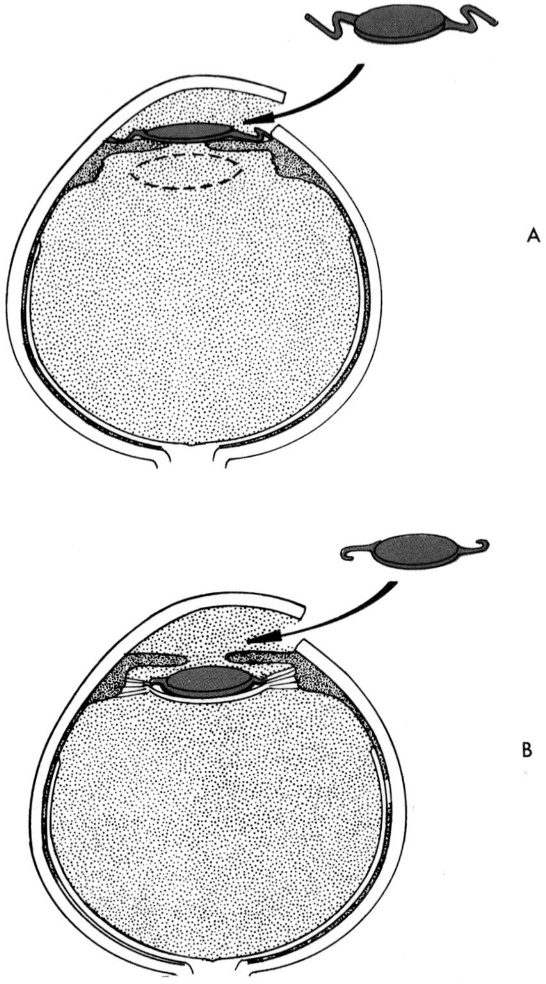

FIG. 37-6 Intraocular lens. **A,** Anterior lens implant in front of iris. **B,** Posterior lens implant behind iris.

THERAPEUTIC DIALOGUE

■ Mary, age 71, has been experiencing decreased vision for the past 5 years. She seeks medical attention and is told that surgery will be required to correct her condition. While talking to the patient, the nurse senses her reluctance to comply with postoperative treatment.

PATIENT: I'm too old to go through all the routines that the doctor wants me to. It involves too much.

NURSE: I know that surgery is a concern for you. You must have many emotions that you are feeling right now. It's understandable that you have concerns about your recovery.

PATIENT: There's so much to think about and remember.

NURSE: The doctor and our staff are here to help make your recovery as easy as possible for you. Tell me what bothers you the most.

PATIENT: What if I go home and fall? I could reinjure my eye or break something, like my hip.

NURSE: There are several things that you and your family can do to prevent any injury to yourself. The doctor and staff will explain these things very carefully to you.

PATIENT: I'm afraid I'm too old to learn.

NURSE: (*Touching the patient*) The staff will provide as much time and support as you need to help you learn. I have a feeling that you will surprise yourself at how well you do!

PATIENT: My doctor thinks I'll have no problems. *(After a few seconds)* Maybe the doctor and you are right.

NURSE: I suggest you talk to the doctor about your feelings. Together, we'll help you in any way we can.

PATIENT: I guess anything's possible! Thanks for your understanding. Being old isn't easy. Yet, as my husband used to say: "You're never too old to learn!"

BOX 37-2 **TEACHING THE PATIENT AFTER EYE SURGERY**

1. Sleep on unaffected side for the prescribed time (3 to 4 weeks) to prevent pressure on operated eye.
2. Wash hands before instilling eyedrops or changing eyepad.
3. If an eyepad is required:
   a. Use two oval eyepads, to provide snug but gentle pressure to prevent blinking against resistance.
   b. Apply tape (paper or silk) diagonally from above nose to lower cheek.
4. Apply metal eye shield at night to protect eye.
5. Use glasses indoors and sunglasses with side sections outdoors to protect eyes from foreign substances and ultraviolet light until healing occurs.
6. Avoid rubbing or pressing on the eye (creates pressure and may dislodge sutures).
7. Avoid showers and shampooing hair (soap may irritate eye) for specified period as instructed; the time period differs from 1 day to up to 2 weeks.
8. Avoid bending at the waist or lifting heavy objects for a least 1 month to prevent increased intraocular pressure (IOP) or adhesions of the iris.
   a. To pick up objects from floor, kneel while keeping head erect.
   b. To put on stocking or to tie shoes, sit and raise foot to reach hand while keeping head erect.
   c. Long pick-up "forceps" can facilitate picking up small objects from the floor without having to bend over.
9. Avoid straining with bowel movements or with other activities and avoid violent coughing (increases IOP).
10. Limit reading (back and forth movement may loosen stitches); television is usually permitted.
11. Report signs of edema, discharge, or pain to physician (may indicate infection or hemorrhage).

Patient teaching. The nurse should reinforce postoperative instructions and observe the patient's correct use of eye medications and eye patches before discharge. The nurse should assess the patient's knowledge of contact lens use and care. Safety measures appropriate to vision alterations should be discussed, and the patient should be encouraged to notify the physician of any complications such as pain, erythema, drainage, or sudden visual changes. If sudden pain occurs, the nurse should call the physician. See Therapeutic Dialogue, p. 979, and see Box 37-2 for postoperative eye surgery teaching.

Disorders of the Retina

Diabetic retinopathy

Etiology/pathophysiology. **Diabetic retinopathy** is a disorder of retinal blood vessels characterized by capillary microaneurysms, hemorrhage, exudates, and the formation of new vessels and connective tissue.

Diabetic retinopathy usually appears 10 years after onset of diabetes mellitus. The incidence increases in relationship to the length of time the patient has had the disease. The disorder occurs more frequently in patients with long-standing, poorly controlled diabetes mellitus.

The initial stage of diabetic retinopathy may last for several years. The blood vessels in the retina begin to widen and become tortuous. Microaneurysms then develop at the periphery and small hemorrhages develop. These may disappear but leave in their place scars that can decrease vision. Increased capillary permeability causes protein exudate.

As the disease progresses, new blood vessels form on the retina and into the vitreous. These new vessels rupture, causing decreased vision. Absorption of some of the blood can occur, which will improve vision until another hemorrhage occurs. Significant vision loss will eventually occur as these hemorrhages continue. Vitreous contraction and full detachment can occur as the vessels and surrounding tissue become fibrous.

Clinical manifestations. Symptoms include microaneurysms, which can only be identified by ophthalmoscopy in the initial stage. In the advanced stages, the patient will have progressive vision loss and the presence of "floaters," which are minute products of the hemorrhage.

Assessment. Collection of *subjective data* must include assessing the length and control of diabetes mellitus. The patient will have varying degrees of vision loss, from decreased vision to blindness. The patient's knowledge of therapy should be assessed.

Collection of *objective data* involves noting that in the early stages there are no symptoms; as the disease progresses, vision is diminished.

Diagnostic tests. Indirect ophthalmoscopy shows dilated and tortuous vessels and narrowing or obliteration of the arteries. Opacities, hemorrhages, and microaneurysms can be seen.

Slit-lamp examination provides magnification of the lesions.

Medical management. Surgical intervention includes photocoagulation and/or vitrectomy. Photocoagulation destroys new blood vessels, seals leaking vessels, and helps to prevent retinal edema by use of a laser beam. (See the discussion of photocoagulation on p. 987). A vitrectomy may be performed when photocoagulation is not possible.

NURSING DIAGNOSES	NURSING INTERVENTIONS
Fear	Determine patient's knowledge of purpose and procedure of photocoagulation.
Anxiety	Assure the patient that the procedure is painless and takes approximately 15 to 20 minutes. A family member or friend must be available to drive the patient home.

Patient teaching. The patient should follow the same instructions at home as for the patient undergoing eye surgery (see Box 37-2).

Macular degeneration

Etiology/pathophysiology. Macular degeneration is a condition of the aging retina characterized by slow, progressive loss of central and near vision. There are two types of macular degeneration. The first, called wet type, has new vessel growth in the macular region that occurs suddenly. The macula becomes displaced, and scarring occurs.

The second, known as the dry type, is the more common. Degenerative changes are the cause: lipid deposits occur, followed by slow atrophy of the macular region, including the retina.

Clinical manifestations. The main symptom of macular degeneration is gradual and variable bilateral loss of central vision. One eye may have a greater loss than the other eye. Color perception may also be affected.

Assessment. Collection of *subjective data* includes noting that the patient may have difficulty distinguishing colors correctly. The nurse should assess for visual disturbances and coping mechanisms for the loss.

Collection of *objective data* includes the nurse noting the degree to which the patient can centrally view objects.

Diagnostic tests. Indirect ophthalmoscopy is used to detect opacity, hemorrhage, and new blood vessel formation. In addition, retinal detachment or other abnormalities can be seen.

Medical management. Photocoagulation may be used, but only if the areas of new vessels have not grown into the macula. This procedure may be useful in the wet type if treatment is begun within the first few days after onset of symptoms. There is no treatment for the dry type.

Nursing interventions. The patient needs patience and understanding in order to cope with the continuing loss of sight. The nurse needs to assist the patient through the process of acceptance of loss of sight. Maintaining safety is important because only peripheral vision exists.

NURSING DIAGNOSIS	NURSING INTERVENTIONS
Sensory/perceptual alterations (visual)	Note the extent of visual loss and the level of difficulty with ADLs; assist the patient to develop ways of performing these activities. Determine the patient's support systems and elicit help, if available.

Patient teaching. The nurse instructs the patient about the disease process, stressing that peripheral vision will be maintained. The patient is provided ways to maintain as much independence as possible, and family and friends can learn the areas in which to assist the patient.

Retinal detachment

Etiology/pathophysiology. Retinal detachment is a separation of the retina from the choroid in the posterior area of the eye (Fig. 37-7). This usually results from a hole in the retina that allows vitreous humor to leak between the choroid and the retina.

The immediate cause may be severe trauma to the eye, such as a contusion or penetrating wound. In most cases, however, retinal detachment is the result of internal changes related to aging and sometimes inflammation of the eye. Retinal detachment may also occur in debilitated patients when there is sudden severe physical exertion.

As the detachment progresses there is an interruption in the transmission of visual images from the retina to the optic nerve. The result is a progressive loss of vision to complete blindness.

Clinical manifestations. Symptoms include a sudden or gradual development of flashes of light, followed by floating spots and progressive loss of vision.

Assessment. Collection of *subjective data* includes noting patient complaints of flashing lights unilaterally and floaters. There is a progressive vision restriction in one area. If the tear is acute and extensive, the patient will describe a sensation of a "curtain being drawn" across the eye.

Collection of *objective data* includes observing the patient for the ability to perform ADLs. The level of anxiety associated with coping is also assessed.

Diagnostic tests. Indirect ophthalmoscopy is used to detect pallor of the retina as well as the detachment. Three-mirror gonioscopy provides a magnified view of any retinal lesions. Slit-lamp examination magnifies the lesions.

Medical management. The treatment of choice is early surgical intervention. One of four surgical procedures may be performed.

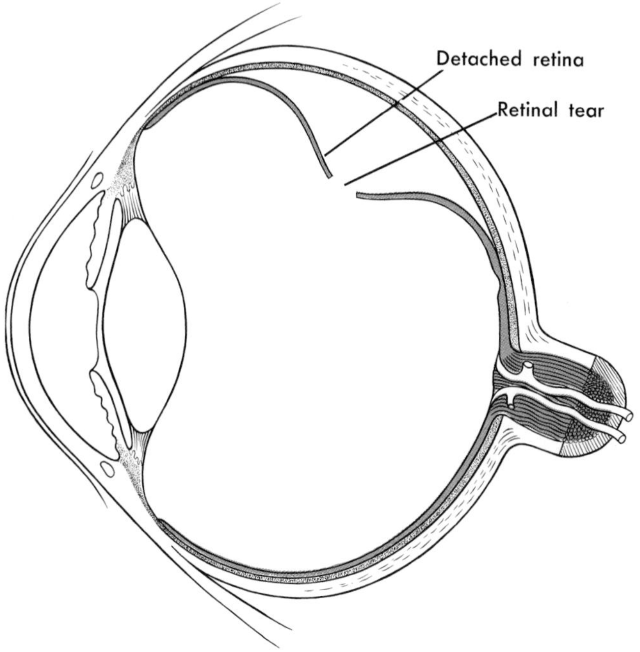

FIG. 37-7 Retinal detachment.

Photocoagulation is used to burn localized tears or breaks that may have occurred in the posterior portion of the eyeball. This causes an eventual sealing of the tear or break.

Cryosurgery is used to "freeze" the borders of a retinal hole with a frozen-tipped probe. The probe is applied to the scleral surface directly over the retinal hole area. The hole seals when the resultant inflammatory process produces scarring.

Diathermy is used to burn a retina break using an ultrasonic probe. The probe is applied to the scleral surface directly over the retinal break. Sealing occurs from the resultant inflammatory and scarring process.

Scleral buckle is used to hold the retina and choroid together. Scarring can then occur and permanently seal the tear or hole.

Nursing interventions. Postoperative management includes cycloplegic-mydriatic and antiinfective eye drops. Eye patches are applied over only the operative eye or both eyes, providing the required rest of the eye for 1 to 2 days. Safety measures are essential, since the eyes are patched.

Depending on the procedures, the position of the head postoperatively may vary. If air is injected into the vitreous, the head will be positioned with the unaffected eye upward with the patient on the abdomen or sitting forward for 4 to 5 days.

Dark glasses are prescribed to decrease the discomfort of photophobia.

NURSING DIAGNOSIS	NURSING INTERVENTIONS
Anxiety	Allow the patient the opportunity to discuss feelings and fears about the possible loss of vision. Answer questions honestly and correct any misunderstandings. Explain the reasons for restrictions of activities and procedures.

Patient teaching. Temporary restrictions of reaching, work, and activity should be discussed with the patient (see Box 37-3).

BOX 37-3

TEACHING THE PATIENT WITH RETINAL DETACHMENT

- Return to sedentary activity in 2 weeks; no heavy lifting or active physical activity for 6 weeks, or as instructed by physician.
- Check with physician concerning shampooing of hair.
- Limit reading for 3 weeks (or as instructed by physician).
- Use correct technique for administration of eye medications.
- Report to ophthalmologist any signs of further detachment (flashes of light, increase in "floaters," blurred vision).
- Report for medical follow-up visits as instructed.

Disorders of Intraocular Pressure

Glaucoma

Etiology/pathophysiology. Glaucoma is an abnormal condition of elevated pressure within an eye because of obstruction of the outflow of aqueous humor. It is associated with a progressive loss of peripheral vision.

Glaucoma is found in persons who are middle-aged and older. Approximately 12% to 15% of all blindness in the United States results from glaucoma. It is seldom seen in persons under 35 years of age but may occur in infancy.

Glaucoma occurs when there is an obstruction of the aqueous humor drainage that increases the intraocular pressure (Fig. 37-8). Damage to the optic nerve results.

Open-angle glaucoma, also known as chronic simple glaucoma, is a common form of the disease. The course of the disease is slowly progressive and results from degenerative changes. It is often bilateral.

Closed-angle glaucoma, also known as acute glaucoma, occurs if there is an abrupt angle change of the iris, causing rapid vision loss and dramatic symptoms.

Clinical manifestations. In open-angle glaucoma, the patient has no signs or symptoms during the early stages of the disease. As the symptoms become apparent, they include tunnel vision, eye pain, difficulty adjusting to darkness, halos around lights, and inability to detect colors. Intraocular pressures will be elevated.

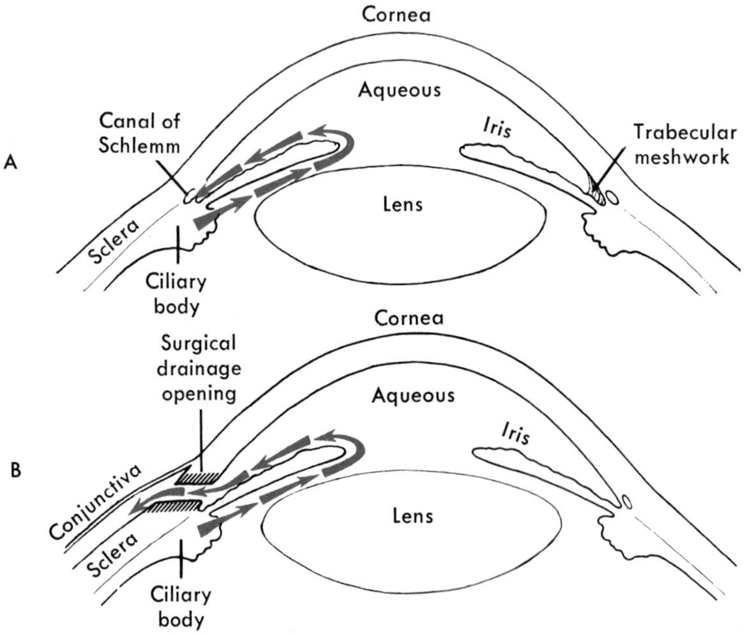

FIG. 37-8 **A,** Originating from ciliary processes, aqueous humor flows through the pupil into the anterior chamber and normally leaves the eye by way of the canal of Schlemm. **B,** In glaucoma, normal aqueous outflow is occluded. Purpose of glaucoma surgery is to create a new channel through which aqueous can leave the eye.

Closed-angle (acute) glaucoma produces severe pain, decreased vision, and nausea and vomiting. The sclera is erythematous, and the pupil is enlarged and fixed. The patient sees colored halos around lights. There is an acute increase in the intraocular pressure.

Assessment. Collection of *subjective data* includes noting the time of day when the eye pain occurs. Frequency, intensity, and duration of the pain are also assessed. Complaints of peripheral vision loss, maladaptation to darkness, and halos seen around lights are noted. Severity of headaches and presence of nausea and vomiting are determined.

Collection of *objective data* includes noting that the patient will have a need for frequent eyeglass prescription changes. Elevated intraocular pressures are also present.

Diagnostic tests. Tonometry is used to test for intraocular pressure (Fig. 37-9). A patient with glaucoma would test above the normal range of 10 to 22 mm Hg. Visual field studies will show a decline in the patient's peripheral vision.

Medical management. Open-angle glaucoma is medically treated by the use of beta-blockers, miotics, and carbonic anhydrase inhibitors. A beta-blocker, such as Betoptic, will reduce intraocular pressure. Miotics, such as pilocarpine, constrict the pupil and allow aqueous humor to drain out of the canal of Schlemm. Carbonic anhydrase inhibitors, such as Diamox, decrease the production of aqueous humor. The result is a lowering of intraocular pressure. Surgery is done when medications do not control the pressure and consists of a trabeculectomy or laser trabeculoplasty. Trabeculectomy is the removal of corneoscleral tissue, usually the canal of Schlemm and trabecular meshwork. This produces an increase in the outflow of aqueous humor. Laser trabeculoplasty produces openings in the trabecular meshwork.

Closed-angle glaucoma is medically treated with osmotic diuretics, such as mannitol, carbonic anhydrase inhibitors, and miotics. Surgical treatment includes a peripheral iridectomy or an iridotomy. A peripheral **iridectomy** is the removal of part of the iris. The procedure is performed with the patient under general anesthesia; this often restores drainage of the aqueous humor. Postoperatively the patient is observed for signs and symptoms of local hemorrhage or excessive pain. An iridotomy is an incision into the iris of the eye to create an opening for aqueous flow. A local or general anesthetic may be used. Postoperatively the dressing is observed for signs of drainage.

Nursing interventions. Nursing interventions involve protecting the patient's safety, monitoring compliance to therapy, and reinforcement of discharge instructions (see the nursing care plan, p. 978).

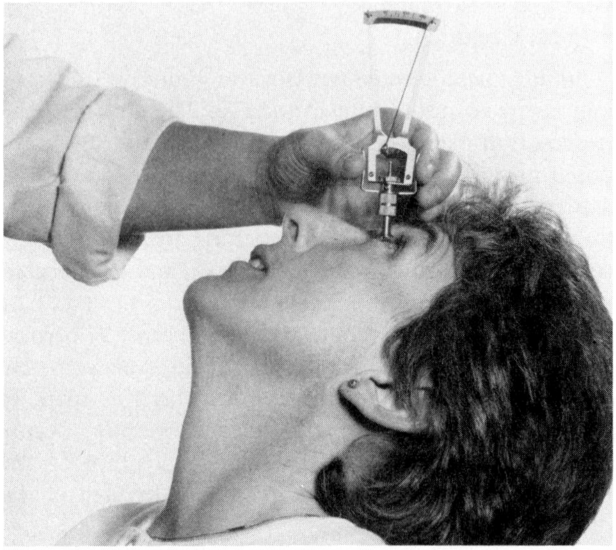

FIG. 37-9 Measurement of intraocular pressure with the Schiötz tonometer.

BOX 37-4 **TEACHING THE PATIENT WITH GLAUCOMA**

1. Medical supervision will be required for the rest of life.
2. Eye drops *must* be continued as long as prescribed, even in the absence of symptoms.
   a. Blurred vision decreases with prolonged use.
   b. Avoid driving for 1 to 2 hours after administration of miotics.
3. To prevent complications:
   a. Press lacrimal duct for 1 minute after eyedrop insertion to prevent rapid systemic absorption.
   b. Have reserve bottle of eyedrops at home.
   c. Carry eyedrops when away from home.
   d. Carry card identifying glaucoma and the eyedrops solution prescribed.
4. Bright lights and darkness are not harmful.
5. There is no apparent relationship between vascular hypertension and ocular hypertension.
6. Report any reappearance of symptoms immediately to ophthalmologist.
7. If admitted to hospital for a different medical condition, alert the staff of continued need for prescribed eyedrops.
8. Avoid the use of mydriatic or cycloplegic drugs (e.g., atropine) that dilate the pupils.

Today's method of medical and surgical management provides the patient with an excellent prognosis for a full recovery. Complications are few if care is early in the course of the condition. When glaucoma is ignored or noncompliance to therapy is noted, blindness may occur.

Patient teaching. The areas of education are covered in Box 37-4.

Injuries to the Eye

Corneal injuries

Etiology/pathophysiology. Corneal injuries result from injuries to corneal layers of the eye. The cornea is the convex, transparent outermost layer of the eye. It is composed of five layers of tissue and is uniform in nature. The cornea is nonvascular; therefore no bleeding occurs from injury unless subcorneal structures are involved. The cornea is kept moist by tear production and is protected from daily insult by the eyelid.

Foreign bodies are the most common cause of corneal injury. Dust particles, propellants, and eyelashes may lodge in the conjunctiva or cornea. The eyes blink in response to the irritant, and further irritation occurs from the upper lid closing frequently, thus moving the foreign body into deeper layers or a wider area of the cornea.

Burns often occur in the home and workplace. When burns affect the eye, it is considered a medical emergency. Depending on the chemical causing the burn, the damage may be superficial or deep. Chemical irritants such as acids and alkalines and metal flashes from acetylene blowtorches cause significant pain, depending on the depth of chemical erosion.

Abrasions and lacerations are usually superficial scratches that occur from injuries to the eye, such as fingernails or clothing. They may be painful, depending on the depth of the abrasion.

Penetrating wounds are the most serious corneal injuries. Eye structures may be injured permanently, resulting in total blindness. Infection may result from the introduction of microorganisms on the penetrating object.

Clinical manifestations

- Foreign bodies—produce pain on movement of the eyeball or when the eyelid moves over the eyeball during blinking. Excessive tearing, erythema of the conjunctiva, and pruritus may occur also.
- Burns—acute pain and burning are the primary symptoms with any topical burn to the eye.
- Abrasions and lacerations—produce mild to severe pain, depending on the depth of corneal involvement. The pain may be transitory and slight, or spasmotic and deep.
- Penetrating wounds—result in varying degrees of pain. If underlying structures are involved, pain may be absent because the nerves have been severed.

Assessment

Foreign bodies. Collection of *subjective data* includes noting the time and type of injury. The patient is assessed for the degree and severity of eye pain and vision loss. The patient should be asked about any first-aid treatment provided.

Collection of *objective data* includes observation of the foreign body and extent of damage. When the intracapsular area has been penetrated, fluid will be leaking from the eye.

Burns. Collection of *subjective data* includes determining the degree of pain. It is important to assess the substance causing the burn and any first-aid treatment that has been provided. Vision loss is determined by the physician.

Collection of *objective data* includes noting the extent of the burn in and around the eye, including eyelashes and eyebrows, and assessing the condition of the eyeball.

Abrasions and lacerations. Collection of *subjective data* includes assessing the patient for the degree of pain following the incident and how the injury occurred. Treatments used at the time of injury are noted.

Collection of *objective data* includes assessing the degree of damage of the eyeball and surrounding structures, and any vision loss is noted.

Penetrating wounds. Collection of *subjective data* includes noting the time and causative factors related to the injury. Presence and severity of pain are assessed. Determine any first-aid treatment rendered.

Collection of *objective data* includes determining the type and size of the penetrating object. Fluid leakage from the eye is noted. The damage of surrounding structures is assessed.

Diagnostic tests. Tests include visual and ophthalmoscopic examination, fluorescein staining, peripheral vision tests, and slit-lamp examination.

Medical management. Foreign bodies are medically treated with a flush of normal saline when the object is near the sclera and conjunctiva; it can then be removed by a clean swab or tissue. Cotton is not to be used, because it may scratch the cornea. If the object is not easily flushed away, the individual must see an ophthalmologist to have the object removed. Antibiotic topical eye ointments are ordered.

Burns are medically treated with a prolonged, 15- to 20-minutes or longer tap water flush immediately after burn exposure. This will help prevent scar formation. The eyelids are separated during the flush procedure. The patient is then treated in a local emergency department or physician's office for follow-up care. Home remedy first-aid treatment should not be done. Topical antiinfective agents are ordered for the eye. Abrasions and lacerations of the eye are medically cleaned with a normal saline solution. Antibiotic therapy, usually topical, is prescribed.

See Box 37-5 for eye safety measures and Table 37-6 for first-aid for eye injuries.

Immediately after a penetrating wound injury, both the eyes should be covered while transporting the patient to the hospital because both eyes work in synchrony.

BOX 37-5 EYE SAFETY MEASURES

1. Avoid frequent rinsing of eyes with unprescribed solutions.
2. Discard any ophthalmic solution that is cloudy, discolored, has been open for ≥3 months, or contains particles.
3. Avoid self-treatment of an eye inflammation with a medication prescribed for a previous eye disorder.
4. To avoid eye strain:
   a. Use a good light for reading or doing work that requires careful visual focus.
   b. When reading or focusing eyes for long periods, look at distant objects for a few minutes at repeated intervals to rest eyes.
5. Avoid rubbing eyes.
6. Wash hands before touching eyes.
7. Wear safety glasses when engaging in activities that could injure the eyes.
8. Wear dark glasses for prolonged exposure to very bright light (such as sunlight or snow or water).
9. Flush eyes with copious amount of water when any irritating substances are accidentally introduced.
10. Do not attempt to remove foreign bodies from the cornea; cover eye and seek medical attention.
11. If a speck of dust blows in eye, pull upper lid over lower lid and let the tears wash the speck to the inner canthus or lower lid, where it may be safely removed.

Covering the eyes prevents the eye from involuntarily moving with the other eye. A shield reduces further injury but must not touch the foreign object. A Styrofoam cup provides adequate coverage and is readily available. The foreign object should not be removed except by a trained physician.

Nursing interventions

Foreign bodies—the nurse will assist with the required irrigation of the eye (Skill 37-3).

Burns—the nurse will assist with the flushing process and providing eye medications as ordered.

Abrasions and lacerations—the nurse will assist with cleaning the eye as ordered and providing general first-aid (see Table 37-6).

Penetrating wounds—the nurse should note whether the pupil on the affected side becomes irregular. This results when the iris of the affected eye moves to occlude the wound area. Infection potential is high; therefore topical and systemic antibiotics are ordered. If the wound is small, self-healing occurs. If the wound is large or deep, enucleation of the eye may be performed.

Table 37-6 First-Aid for Eye Injuries

Injury	Interventions
Burns: chemical, flame	Flush eye immediately for 15 to 20 minutes or longer with cool water or any available nontoxic liquid; seek medical assistance.
Loose substance on conjunctiva: dirt, insects	Lift upper lid over lower lid to dislodge substance, produce tearing; irrigate eye with water if necessary; do not rub eye; obtain medical assistance if above interventions fail.
Contact injury: contusion, ecchymosis, laceration	Apply cold compresses if no laceration present; cover eye if laceration present; seek medical assistance.
Penetrating objects	Do not remove object; place protective shield over eye (e.g., paper cup); cover uninjured eye to prevent excess movement of injured eye; seek medical assistance.

Effective and immediate therapy is crucial for any injury to the eye. If treatment is interrupted, ineffective, or not sustained, permanent eye damage will occur. The most frequent complications include infection, vision disturbances, and blindness.

NURSING DIAGNOSIS	NURSING INTERVENTIONS
Pain	Note the level of pain, using a grade of 1 to 10. Administer ordered local and/or systemic analgesics; administer antiinfective topical agents, and apply warm or cool compresses as ordered.

Patient teaching. The nurse should ensure that the patient can apply ointments and dressings, if ordered. The patient is instructed in the use of other therapy devices, such as warm or cool compresses. Proper handwashing techniques are taught. Dark sunglasses are to be worn by the patient if cycloplegic or mydriatric eye drops are used. Instruct the patient to avoid future episodes of chemical or environmental hazards. The patient should understand discharge instructions, including the need for follow-up physician visits and symptoms to report. The nurse should determine the patient's knowledge about the progress of therapy.

Surgeries of the Eye

Enucleation. Eye **enucleation** is the surgical removal of the eyeball. It is often necessary after severe eye trauma but may be done for other reasons, such as malignant

SKILL 37-3

EYE IRRIGATION

1. Place patient lying toward side to be irrigated to prevent fluid from flowing into other eye.
2. A plastic squeeze bottle is used unless very large amounts of fluid are needed.
3. Direct the irrigating fluid along the conjunctiva from the *inner* to the outer canthus.
4. Avoid directing a forceful stream onto the eyeball.
5. Avoid touching any eye structures with irrigation equipment.
6. A piece of gauze may be wrapped around the gloved index finger to raise upper lid for better cleaning if heavy discharge is present.
7. Place an emesis basin at side of face to collect irrigating fluid.

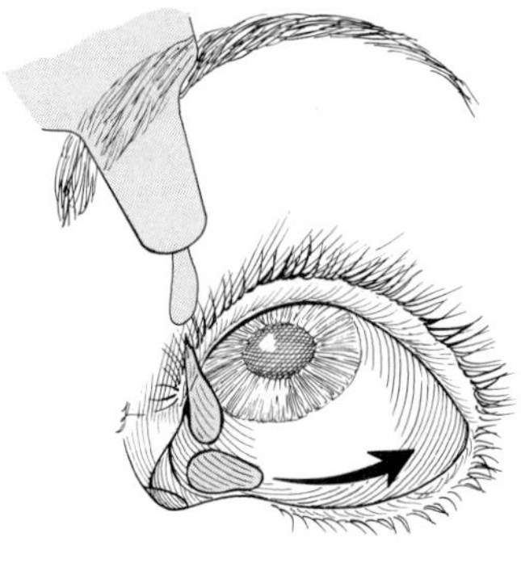

STEP 3

tumors. Surgical methods vary from removal of the entire eyeball or the eyeball contents to removal of the eyeball and all underlying structures.

Nursing interventions. Preoperative care includes determining the patient's feelings about the surgical intervention. It may be a welcome relief from pain and pressure of a malignancy. For other patients it is a disfiguring surgery that leads to a drastic change in life-style. Other nursing responsibilities include therapeutic dialogue between the physician and patient regarding the exact nature of the surgery. If a prosthesis (commonly called "glass eye") is used, the nurse should ensure that the patient understands its care.

Postoperatively a pressure dressing is applied over the socket of the eye to control hemorrhage. The nurse observes the dressing at least every hour for the first 24 hours. The patient is questioned about any pain on the affected side of the head or any headache, which might indicate hemorrhage or infection. These findings should be reported to the physician immediately. Routine postoperative procedures of coughing and turning on the affected side are discouraged to prevent sutures from dislodging. A prosthetic eye may be worn once healing occurs, usually in 4 to 6 weeks.

Keratoplasty (corneal transplant). Keratoplasty is the excision of the corneal tissue, followed by surgical implantation of a cornea from another human donor. It is done to replace damaged cornea resulting from trauma, ulceration, or congenital deformities of the cornea. The surgery can be successful if the area of implantation is small. The possibility of donor rejection is high when large amounts of tissue replacement are required. Rejection normally begins about 3 weeks after surgery. Medications to suppress rejection (e.g., cyclosporine) may be ordered. If the cornea is perforated from ulcer formation or from surgical implantation, vision will be destroyed.

Corneal grafts are taken usually within 5 hours after death from a donor who is ideally between 25 and 35 years old. An appropriate donor is an individual who died of injury or acute disease. The corneas of persons with chronic or communicable diseases, such as hepatitis, AIDS, or cancer, are not appropriate for transplantation. The donor eye should have normal light perception and projection. The donor tissue is best used within 48 hours after removal. The nurse is often the individual most accessible to the family when questions of organ donation occur. Responsibilities would include notification of appropriate supervisory personnel.

Keratoplasty is performed with the patient under local or general anesthesia. The transplanted tissue is sutured into place to maintain graft alignment and a watertight wound.

Nursing interventions. Preoperatively the nurse encourages the patient to express fears related to surgery and gives instructions in the use of protective eyeglasses if eye medication is used, causing dilation. The nurse maintains safety in the environment by use of safety devices and orienting the patient to each new environment.

The surgical areas are cleansed and prepared as ordered, usually with an antiseptic solution. Preoperative teaching includes deep breathing and turning to reduce any complications associated with surgery. Coughing is discouraged, because sutures may break. Dietary restrictions, if ordered, should be maintained; a light breakfast may be allowed if the surgery is done with the patient under a local anesthesia. Prescribed medications are administered.

Postoperatively the nurse ensures that correct postoperative positioning is maintained; the patient is usually positioned on the back or nonoperated side until the physician allows turning to the operated side. Activity restrictions as ordered are reinforced to prevent injury to the eye. Safety measures are employed until the patient is able to ambulate safely. Anyone coming into the room should announce his or her presence. The patient should avoid bending, lifting, and straining for approximately 1 month to prevent intraocular pressure or suture tension.

Progressive activity should be prescribed by the physician. Regular postoperative visits with the eye surgeon should be encouraged. The nurse should report any severe or progessive pain to the surgeon immediately, as well as any complaints of erythema, loss of vision, or photophobia that would occur with corneal rejection. Systemic and ophthalmic medications are administered. Strict surgical asepsis must be maintained during dressing changes. Staff, the patient, and the family must wash hands thoroughly before any contact with the eye area. The patient should be instructed to avoid the use of such irritants as powder, perfume, and propellants, which might cause sneezing and displacement of sutures. The patient should not rub the eye area, or contamination of the site or suture displacement may result. The patient's diversional activities should be assessed; television is usually permitted, but reading is limited because of the side-to-side movement of the eyes. The lateral motion of the eye may cause loosening of sutures. If an eye patch or a metal eyecup shield is ordered, the nurse can demonstrate care. The eye patch is applied snugly to inhibit the blink reflex and allow the eye to rest. The metal eyecup shield is used during the night to protect the eye from trauma. Discharge instructions should be obtained from the physician regarding use of eyewear.

Photocoagulation. Using a laser, a small, intense beam of light is directed into a small spot on the retina. Conversion into heat energy occurs and coagulation of tissue protein occurs, which is called *photocoagulation*.

Photocoagulation is a nonsurgical procedure usually performed on an outpatient basis. Without surgical intervention, the structures of the eye remain undisturbed and only the sealing of leakage and offending tissue destruction occurs.

Photocoagulation is useful in diabetic retinopathy to cauterize hemorrhaging vessels. It cannot increase visual acuity but can prevent further loss. Usually no hospitalization or postoperative medical management is required.

Nursing interventions. Postoperative assessment for patients who have undergone photocoagulation therapy includes assessment of vision. There may be a constriction of peripheral fields, and central vision may temporarily be decreased. A decrease in night vision and a headache resulting from the laser's bright light may also occur.

Vitrectomy. A vitrectomy is the removal of excess vitreous fluid caused by hemorrhage and replacing it with normal saline. Any scar tissue may also be removed.

Postoperative management includes the prescription of topical eye medication for 4 to 6 weeks. Acetaminophen or acetaminophen with codeine is prescribed for pain management.

A pressure patch to the operative eye is placed immediately after surgery. Ice packs to reduce inflammation are ordered.

Nursing interventions. The patient is required to maintain a position on the abdomen or sitting forward resting the nonoperated side of the head on a table to allow air that is in the eye to float against the retina. These positions are maintained for 4 to 5 days. This is not required if oil has been injected into the eye during the vitrectomy instead of normal saline.

Dark glasses are prescribed postoperatively to decrease the discomfort of photophobia.

Postoperative assessment includes assessment of the eye patch, ice packs, and abnormal vital signs, especially fever. The dressing should be assessed for bleeding.

Patient teaching. The aspects of patient education are detailed in Box 37-2.

CARE OF THE PATIENT WITH AN EAR DISORDER

Specific Nursing Considerations for the Patient with an Ear Disorder

Once the history and general assessment have been done, the nurse should focus on aspects related to the ear. Additional information would include the following:

- Occurrence of ear drainage, tinnitus, vertigo, wax build up, pressures, pain, and pruritus
- Behavioral indications of hearing loss (see Box 37-7)
- History of medications used for ear disorders, specifically those known to be ototoxic, such as those listed in Box 37-6
- Current medications for the ear disorder
- Side effects of medication, if any
- Associated speech pattern abnormalities
- Use of assistive hearing devices
- Home remedies that cause ear trauma

The nurse communicates the gathered data to the ap-

BOX 37-6 SELECTED OTOTOXIC DRUGS

ANTIBIOTICS

Streptomycin
Dihydrostreptomycin
Gentamicin (Garamycin)
Neomycin
Kanamycin
Vancomycin
Polymyxin B/Colistin
Chloramphenicol (Chloromycetin)
Capreomycin

DIURETICS

Ethacrynic acid (Edecrin)
Furosemide (Lasix)
Acetazolamide (Diamox)

SALICYLATES

Acetylsalicylic acid (aspirin)

OTHER DRUGS

Quinine
Chloroquine
Nitrogen mustard
Bleomycin
Quinidine

propriate personnel and documents the findings in the patient record. The next step in the assessment process is to prepare the patient for the initial otoscopic diagnostic evaluation.

Diagnostic testing

Otoscopy. With an otoscope the examiner can visualize the external auditory canal and the eardrum, or tympanic membrane. Normally, the tympanic membrane is disk shaped and pearl gray or pale pink in color. This is the initial examination of the ear, performed before other testing. One responsibility of the nurse is to explain to the patient the purpose and procedure of otoscopy. The patient should be reassured that this is a painless test requiring only about 5 minutes, with slight pulling of the ear upward and backward during the procedure.

Tuning fork tests. The two most common tests using tuning forks are the Weber and Rinne tests. These tests are used to determine hearing loss as well as data related to the type of loss.

The Weber test evaluates the lateralization of sound. A vibrated tuning fork is placed on the patient's forehead or on the maxillary incisors. If hearing is normal, the loudness of sound will be equal in both ears.

The Rinne test is used to compare air conduction with bone conduction. The base of a vibrating tuning fork is placed on the patient's mastoid process; this tests bone conduction. When the tone is no longer heard, the vibrating prongs are then placed ½ inch from the external auditory meatus of the ear until the sound is no longer heard; this tests air conduction. The difference is noted. A patient with normal hearing perceives the sound for a longer period when conduction is by air than by bone.

Nursing responsibility in both the Weber and Rinne tests includes explanation of the purpose and procedure of the tests. The nurse should stress that the patient will need to concentrate and indicate through the use of hand signals in which ear or ears the sound is heard in the Weber test and when no longer heard in the Rinne test. In addition, the nurse should assure the patient that the test is painless and requires only a few minutes.

Audiometric testing. **Audiometry** is the testing of the acuity of the sense of hearing. Various audiometric tests determine the lowest intensity of sound at which an individual can perceive an auditory stimulus (hearing threshold), hear different frequencies, and distinguish different speech tones.

Nursing responsibilities include providing the patient with the purpose and procedure of each test. Any required responses by the patient should be reviewed.

Vestibular tests. Vestibular testing measures balance and equilibrium. The Romberg and past-point tests are used for patients complaining of dizziness or disequilibrium.

The Romberg test measures the patient's ability to perform specific tasks with eyes open and then with eyes closed. The normal response is maintaining balance throughout the entire test.

Past-point testing measures the patient's ability to touch the examiner's finger with eyes closed.

The nurse's responsibility is to explain the purpose and procedure of each test. Safety measures are taken to prevent patient injury during the Romberg test if the patient cannot maintain balance.

DISORDERS OF THE EAR

Loss of hearing (deafness). Deafness is characterized by a partial or complete loss of hearing. Any ear disorder can cause interference with hearing to some degree. Interference with sound wave transmission can be caused by fluid accumulation and inflammations, fixation of the ossicles, and inner ear disorders that interfere with sound vibrations (Fig. 37-10).

More than 6 million people in the United States have some degree of bilateral hearing loss. More than 50% of these people are over 65 years of age. Recognition, diagnosis, and early treatment may help to prevent further impairment and damage.

The implications of hearing loss are great. Hearing is needed to develop speech and conceptual ability; thus

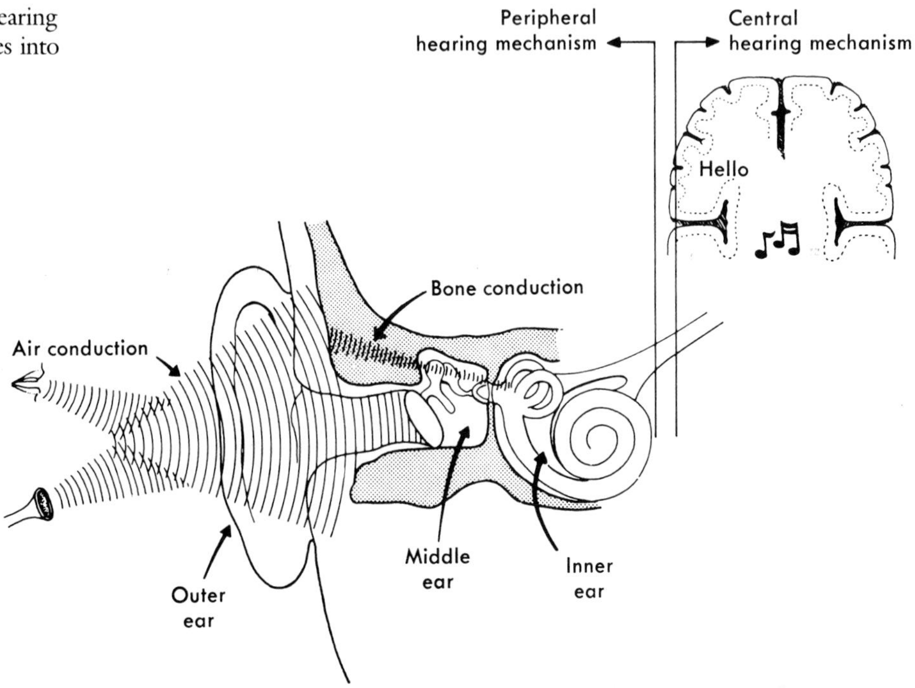

FIG. 37-10 Schema of functions of hearing mechanism as it translates sound waves into meaningful sensations.

hearing loss may well affect personality development and intelligence test responses when the hearing impairment is severe and congenital. This may have implications for the person's education and socialization. As the loss of hearing increases, the person may socially withdraw because of the inability to understand and be understood; this could lead to isolation and depression.

Types of hearing loss. There are six types of hearing loss: conductive, sensorineural, mixed, congenital, simulated, and central.

In conductive hearing loss, sound is inadequately conducted through the external or middle ear to the sensorineural apparatus of the inner ear. Sensitivity to sound is diminished, but clarity or interpretation of the sound is not changed. When increased volume compensates for the loss, then hearing is normal; therefore a hearing aid can be helpful.

In sensorineural hearing loss sound is conducted through the external and middle ear in a normal way, but a defect in the inner ear results in its distortion, making discrimination difficult. This type of hearing loss is usually caused by trauma, infectious processes, presbycusis (hearing loss caused by aging), or exposure to ototoxic drugs. Destruction of cochlear hair by intense noise may also cause sensorineural loss. Amplifying sound, such as with a hearing aid, will help some people with this type of loss. Many people have an intolerance to loud noise and would not be helped by a hearing aid.

Mixed hearing loss is a combined conductive and sensorineural hearing loss.

Congenital hearing loss is present from birth or early infancy. Anoxia or trauma during delivery may be causes. Rh incompatibility may also be a cause. The mother's exposure during pregnancy to syphilis or rubella and the use of ototoxic drugs during pregnancy may also be causes.

Simulated hearing loss is a loss of hearing in which there is no organic cause. It is also known as functional psychogenic or nonorganic hearing loss.

Central hearing loss occurs when the brain's auditory pathways are damaged, as in cerebrovascular accident.

Clinical manifestations. Clinical manifestations may vary, depending on the degree of deafness. Symptoms may range from such subtle clues as requests for repeating information to more obvious signs of nonresponse.

Assessment. Collection of *subjective data* includes noting the onset and progression of the condition, deficit in one or both ears, family history, history of head trauma, exposure to noise, current medications, visual or speech disorders, and any other ear symptoms.

Collection of *objective data* must include an assessment of behavioral clues that indicate a hearing difficulty. (See Box 37-7 for behavioral clues indicating difficulty hearing.)

Diagnostic tests. Conductive hearing loss produces lateralization of sound to the deaf ear in the Weber test. Results of the Rinne test show that sounds transmitted through bone conduction are heard longer than or equal to sounds transmitted through air conduction.

Sensorineural hearing loss produces lateralization of sound to the better ear in the Weber test. Results of the

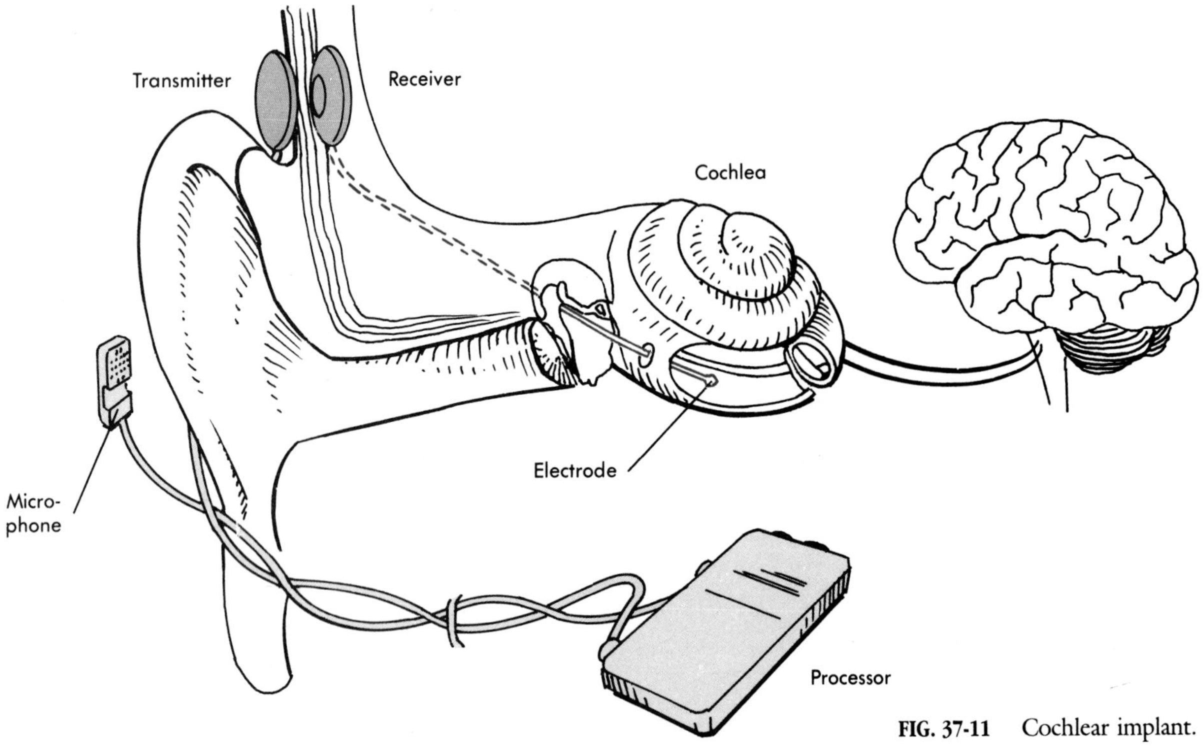

FIG. 37-11 Cochlear implant.

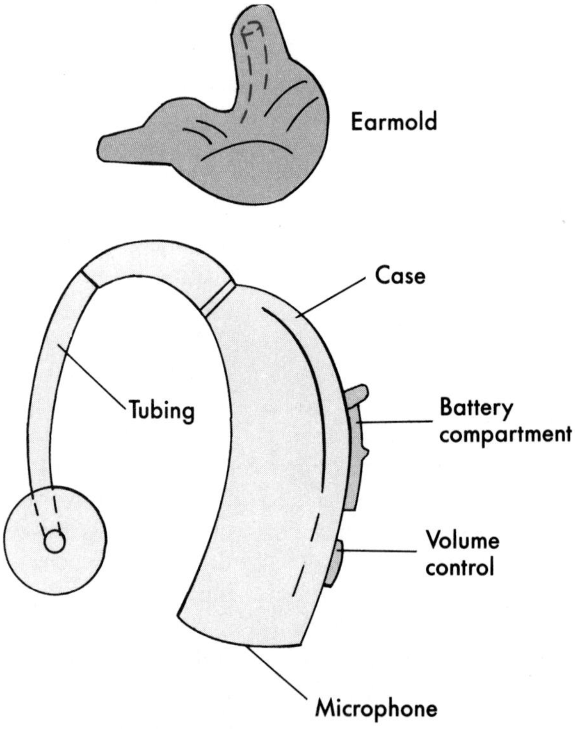

FIG. 37-12 Parts of a hearing aid.

BOX 37-7 BEHAVIORAL CLUES INDICATING DIFFICULT HEARING

Any adult who
- Is irritable, hostile, hypersensitive in interpersonal relations
- Has difficulty in hearing upper frequency consonants
- Complains about people mumbling
- Turns up volume on television
- Asks for frequent repetition and answers questions inappropriately
- Loses sense of humor; becomes grim
- Leans forward to hear better; face serious and strained
- Shuns large- and small-group audience situations
- May appear aloof and "stuck-up"
- Complains of ringing in the ears
- Has an unusually soft or loud voice
- Repeatedly asks, "What did you say?"

BOX 37-8 CARE OF HEARING AID

1. Wash earmold or plug daily in mild soap and water using a pipe cleaner to cleanse the cannula.
2. Dry earmold or plug thoroughly before reconnecting it to the receiver.
3. Keep an extra battery and cord available at all times.
4. When hearing aid is not in use, turn aid off and open battery compartment.
5. If hearing aid whistles, reinsert earmold.
6. If hearing aid fails to work:
   a. Check the on-off switch
   b. Inspect earmold for cleanliness
   c. Examine battery for tightness of fit
   d. Examine cord plug for tightness of insertion
   e. Examine cord for breaks
   f. Replace battery and/or cord

BOX 37-9 FACILITATING COMMUNICATION FOR PERSONS WITH IMPAIRED HEARING

1. Get the person's attention by raising an arm or hand.
2. Start with the light on your face; this will help the person speech read.
3. Face the person when speaking.
4. Speak clearly, but do not overaccentuate words.
5. Speak in a normal tone; do not shout. Shouting overemploys normal speaking movements and may cause distortion and be too loud for the person with sensorineural damage. If the person has conductive loss only, sometimes making the voice louder without shouting is helpful.
6. If the person does not seem to understand what is said, express it differently. Some words are difficult to "see" in speech reading, such as *white* or *red*.
7. Move closer to the person and toward the better ear if the person does not hear you.
8. Write out proper names or any statement that you are not sure was understood.
9. Do not chew gum or cover the mouth when talking to a person with limited hearing.
10. Observe for inattention that may indicate tiredness or lack of understanding.
11. Use phrases to convey meaning rather than one-word answers. State the major topic of the discussion first and then give details.
12. Do not show annoyance by careless facial expression. Persons who are hard of hearing depend more on visual clues for acceptance.
13. Encourage the use of a hearing aid if the person has one; allow the person to adjust it before speaking.
14. If in a group, repeat important statements and avoid asides to others in the group.
15. Avoid the use of the intercommunication system as this may distort sound and cause poor communication.
16. Do not avoid conversation with a person who has hearing loss.

Adapted from Conover M and Cober J: Nurs Clin North Am 5:497, 1970.

Rinne test show that air-conducted sounds are heard longer than bone-conducted sounds, but not twice as long.

Audiometric testing determines the type of hearing loss and the degree of impairment.

Medical management. Medical management depends on the type of impairment. Surgical procedures may be required. Hearing aids or cochlear implants may be used when appropriate. A cochlear implant (Fig. 37-11) is used for people with complete hearing loss. A small computer changes the spoken words into electrical impulses that are transmitted to an implanted cochlear coil.

Nursing interventions. Patients with partial hearing loss may benefit from a hearing aid (Fig. 37-12). The patient is assisted in caring for the hearing aid as detailed in Box 37-8.

NURSING DIAGNOSIS	NURSING INTERVENTIONS
Sensory/perceptual alterations (auditory)	Facilitate communication with the patient by following the interventions provided in Box 37-9.

Patient teaching. The nurse assists the patient in learning to care for a hearing aid, if prescribed. The patient can be instructed to request that others speak slowly or more clearly and repeat if necessary.

Inflammatory and Infectious Disorders of the Ear

External otitis

Etiology/pathophysiology. External **otitis** or otitis externa is an inflammation or infection of the external canal or the auricle of the external ear and is sometimes called *swimmer's ear.* External otitis may be acute or chronic.

External otitis can be caused by allergy, bacteria, fungi, viruses, and trauma. Allergic reaction can stem from nickel or chromium in earrings. In addition, chemicals in hair sprays, cosmetics, hearing aids, and medications, especially sulfonamides and neomycin, are common sources of allergy. Common bacterial agents are *Staphylococcus aureus, Pseudomonas aeruginosa,* and *Streptococcus pyogenes.* Frequently the viruses herpes simplex and herpes zoster are implicated. The external ear may also be affected by eczema, psoriasis, and seborrheic dermatitis. Fungi such as *Aspergillus* and *Candida* may also be causes. External otitis is more prevalent during hot, humid weather.

Trauma from cleaning or scratching the ear canal with a foreign object, such as a cotton swab, bobby pin, or finger, may result in irritation and possible introduction of infectious organisms. Certain activities allow moisture to become trapped in the ear, creating medium for infection; these include use of earphones, hearing aids, earplugs, earmuffs, and stethoscopes. Excessive swimming may wash out the protective cerumen, remove skin lipids, and lead to secondary infection.

Malignant external otitis is a rare, lethal form caused by *Pseudomonas* and occurring mostly in patients with diabetes. It is a bone-destroying infection that quickly involves all surrounding ear structures. Mortality of 50% to 75% occurs unless the condition is treated early.

Clinical manifestations. The acute inflammatory process produces pain with movement of the auricle or chewing and often the entire side of the head aches. Erythema, scaling, pruritus, edema, watery discharge, and crusting of the external ear may occur.

With chronic external otitis there is usually pruritus, but no pain with movement of the auricle. A discharge is also present.

Assessment. Collection of *subjective data* includes determining the onset, duration, and severity of pain, which is crucial to the assessment of inflammatory disease of the ear. The patient should be questioned about any home remedies used to treat infections. Knowledge of preventive measures is also assessed.

Collection of *objective data* includes noting a discharge, which may be watery or yellow and tenacious with a fetid odor. The discharge will be black if from a fungal infection. There may be a partial loss of hearing or the feeling that the ear is occluded if the ear canal is edematous or is obstructed by adenoids. Palpation of the external ear may produce pain.

Diagnostic tests. A culture of the discharge is obtained to identify bacterial, viral, or fungal organisms.

Medical management. Oral analgesics such as codeine may be used if the pain is severe. Corticosteriods (1% hydrocortisone) may be used to reduce edema and to allow antibiotics to penetrate. A wick is inserted into the ear canal to prevent loss of medication from the canal and maintain continuous absorption of the medicine. The physician orders frequency of the wick change. Antimicrobial agents such as antibiotic or antifungal eardrops may be used. The most commonly used contain 0.5% neomycin or 10,000 U/ml of polymyxin B. Systemic antibiotics may be used if the infection is severe. The specific antibiotic used will be based on the results of the culture.

Nursing interventions. The ear canal is carefully cleansed (Skill 37-4). Heat may be applied to the external ear for pain relief. An adequate method of communication is implemented. Eardrops are instilled (See Skill 25-7).

Acute external otitis may become a chronic problem. If the infection remains untreated and enters the brain, death can occur.

NURSING DIAGNOSIS	NURSING INTERVENTIONS
Pain	Apply warm compresses as ordered. Administer prescribed analgesics, and instill ordered ear medications.

Patient teaching. The nurse ensures that the patient has the knowledge to prevent further infection and can care for the infected ear.

Otitis media

Etiology/pathophysiology. Otitis media, an inflammation or infection of the middle ear, is the most common disorder of the middle ear. Acute otitis media is most often caused by *Haemophilus influenzae* or *Streptococcus pneumoniae.* Chronic otitis media is usually caused by Gram-negative bacteria, such as *Proteus, Klebsiella,* and *Pseudomonas.* In addition, allergy, mycoplasma, and several viruses may be factors.

Otitis media occurs more frequently in children, especially at 6 to 36 months of age, in the winter and early spring. Children's shorter and straighter eustachian tubes provide easier access of the organisms for the nasopharynx to travel to the middle ear.

The patient usually has had a recent upper respiratory infection. The infection ascends via the eustachian tube and involves the lining of the entire middle ear. Usually only one ear is affected.

Viral infections frequently cause a serious otitis media. Retraction of the tympanic membrane occurs with a buildup of sterile serous exudate. If there is a secondary bacterial infection, purulent exudate collects behind the tympanic membrane, causing it to bulge. This is called *purulent otitis media.*

SKILL 37-4 EAR IRRIGATION

1. Wash hands.
2. Explain steps of procedure and advise patient about sensations that might be experienced.
3. Assist patient to either a side-lying or a sitting position with head tilted toward affected ear. Position emesis basin under ear. (Patient may help hold basin.)
4. Place towel over patient's shoulder just under ear and emesis basin.
5. Inspect auditory canal for any accumulation of cerumen or debris. Remove with cotton applicator and solution.
6. **Check irrigating solution for proper temperature.**
   Fill bulb syringe with appropriate volume.
7. Straighten auditory canal for introduction of solution. In infants, pull auricle (or pinna) down and back. In adults, pull auricle up and back.
8. With tip of syringe just above canal, irrigate gently by creating steady flow of solution against roof of canal.

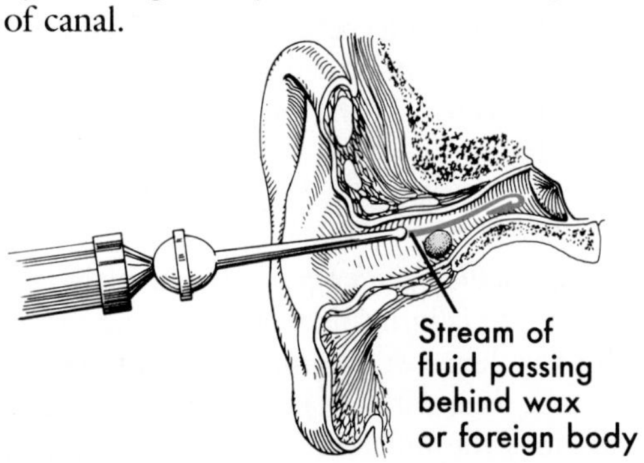

STEP 8

9. Continue irrigation until all debris has been removed or all solution has been used.
10. Assess patient for onset of dizziness or nausea. Onset of symptoms may require temporary cessation of procedure.
11. Dry off auricle and apply cotton ball to auditory meatus.
12. Position patient on side of affected ear for 10 minutes.
13. Remove equipment and wash hands.
14. Return to patient to assess character and amount of drainage and determine patient's level of comfort.
15. Record in nurse's notes patient's response to irrigation and note type, temperature, and volume of solution used and character of drainage.
16. Return to patient after 10 minutes to remove cotton ball and reassess drainage. Patient may resume normal level of activity.

Clinical manifestations. The patient will experience a sense of fullness in the ear and also have severe, deep throbbing pain behind the tympanic membrane. This severe pain may disappear if the tympanic membrane ruptures. Hearing loss, **tinnitus,** and fever may also be present.

Assessment. For information on collection of *subjective data,* refer to the discussion of external otitis, p. 992.

Collection of *objective data* is the same as for external otitis, with the exception of noting pain on palpation of the external ear.

Diagnostic tests. A culture of the purulent drainage is obtained to identify the causative organisms.

Medical management. Antibiotic therapy is based on results of the culture. Analgesics such as codeine are prescribed for severe pain. Sedatives are prescribed for children to provide rest and pain relief. Local heat is used and nasal decongestants are ordered.

Needle aspiration of secretions collected behind the tympanic membrane may be necessary. **Myringotomy**—a surgical incision of the eardrum to relieve pressure and release purulent exudate from the middle ear—may be required.

Nursing interventions. Inner ear pressure may cause discomfort, requiring pain medication to be prescribed. Sedatives may be ordered for young children.

Hearing loss may also occur. Effective communication is essential. Parents of young patients should be alerted to the fact and their help enlisted in monitoring the level of loss.

Chronic otitis media caused by repeated attacks of acute otitis media may result in a permanent perforation of the tympanic membrane. The result is a slight to moderate conductive hearing loss.

A growth called *cholesteatoma* occurs when a tympanic membrane perforation allows squamous epithelium of the external auditory canal to enter and grow in the middle ear. Enlargement is slow, but the mass can expand into the mastoid antrum and destroy adjacent structures.

Mastoiditis, which is an infection of one of the mastoid bones, may develop. It is usually an extension of a middle ear infection that was untreated or inadequately treated. Signs of mastoiditis should be reported immediately, including earache, fever, headache, malaise, and large amounts of purulent drainage.

NURSING DIAGNOSIS	NURSING INTERVENTIONS
Impaired skin integrity	Note and report any outer ear purulent drainage. Keep ear clean and dry; sterile cotton may be used if ordered to absorb drainage. Monitor temperature, and report changes.

BOX 37-10 TEACHING FOR THE PATIENT WITH AN EAR INFECTION

PREVENTION OF FURTHER INFECTION

1. Protect ear canal during showers (cotton with petrolatum in external canal; use a shower cap over ears).
2. Avoid swimming during infection or following a perforated eardrum; avoid swimming in contaminated water when infection is healed.
3. Continue antibiotic therapy for prescribed number of days, even when symptoms disappear.
4. Get adequate and early treatment of upper respiratory tract infections and allergic conditions.

CARE OF INFECTED EAR

1. Use correct eardrops insertion or ear irrigations, as prescribed.
2. Wash hands before and after changing cotton plugs to prevent secondary infection.
3. Keep external ear clean and dry to protect skin from drainage.

SIGNS REQUIRING MEDICAL ATTENTION

Fever
Return of ear pain or drainage

Patient teaching. The nurse should ensure that the patient and parents are aware of the necessity to complete the entire course of antibiotic therapy. Children are to be fed upright to prevent nasopharyngeal flora from entering the eustachian tube. The patient is instructed to blow the nose gently and not forcefully. If a myringotomy has been performed, the patient and parents are instructed to change the cotton in the outer ear at least twice a day (Box 37-10).

Labyrinthitis

Etiology/pathophysiology. **Labyrinthitis** is an inflammation of the labyrinthine canals of the inner ear. Labyrinthitis is the most common cause of **vertigo.** A common cause is a viral upper respiratory infection that spreads into the inner ear; other causes include certain drugs and foods. The vestibular portion of the inner ear may be destroyed by streptomycin. Tobacco, and alcohol may also be causative factors. A rarer form of labyrinthitis is caused by bacteria. It is usually associated with middle ear and mastoid infections.

Clinical manifestations. Severe and sudden vertigo are the most common symptoms of labyrinthitis. Also present are nausea and vomiting, nystagmus, photophobia, headache, and ataxic gait.

Assessment. Collection of *subjective data* should include noting the frequency and duration of the vertigo, as well as any safety measures taken by the patient during an attack. Other symptoms, such as hearing ability, ringing in the ears, and vomiting, are assessed. Because fear is associated with the attacks, the patient's feelings should be explored.

Collection of *objective data* includes noting any jerking movement of the eyeballs, unilaterally or bilaterally. Color and moisture of skin are assessed to determine the extent of autonomic response.

Diagnostic tests. Electronystagmography may show a diminished or absent nystagmus with stimulation. Audiometeric testing shows a low-tone sensorineural hearing loss.

Medical management. There is no specific treatment for labyrinthitis. Usually antibiotics and dimenhydrinate (Dramamine) or meclizine HCl (Antivert) for vertigo are prescribed. If nausea and vomiting persist, parenteral fluids are administered.

Nursing interventions. It is important to note the frequency and degree of vertigo. Antibiotics and medications for vertigo are administered. Fluid intake is assessed to ensure dehydration does not occur. Labyrinthitis usually resolves itself with little or no hearing impairment.

NURSING DIAGNOSIS	NURSING INTERVENTIONS
Potential for injury	Keep side rails up. Note presence of vertigo before patient ambulates. Supervise ambulation. Caution the patient not to attempt ambulation alone and to call for help.

Patient teaching. The nurse instructs the patient concerning vertigo using the information in Box 37-11.

BOX 37-11 TEACHING FOR THE PATIENT WITH VERTIGO

1. Nature of the disorder
   a. Physiological basis for the vertigo
   b. Avoidance of any known precipitating factors
   c. Rationale for a low-salt diet
2. Actions to take during an attack
   a. Lie down immediately and call for help if necessary at the first signs of an attack
   b. If driving when an attack occurs, pull over immediately to the curb
   c. Lie immobile and hold head in one position until vertigo lessens
3. Ask for assistance when ambulating if dizzy
4. Take prescribed medications as instructed even if no recent attacks have occurred; check with physician before discontinuing any medication
5. Symptoms requiring medical attention: changes in symptoms or nature of attacks

Obstructions of the ear

Etiology/pathophysiology. Ear canal obstruction is usually caused by impaction or excessive secretion of cerumen or by foreign bodies, including insects. Children often place beans, beads, pebbles, and small toys in their ears. Usually these objects are found on routine examination.

Obstruction by cerumen can be caused when excessive amounts are produced by overactive glands, or from impaction of cerumen in narrow or tortuous ear canals.

Clinical manifestations. The obstruction may cause the ear to feel occluded. There may be presence of **tinnitus** or "buzzing," pain in the ear, and slight hearing loss.

Assessment. Collection of *subjective data* includes interviewing the patient about any possible foreign bodies being introduced into the ear and any home remedies used to remove the object. If the patient is a child, determination is made of risk factors causing ear obstructions, such as beads or nuts.

Collection of *objective data* involves the nurse noting any presence of a foreign body in the external ear canal. Children are observed for tugging of the pinna.

Diagnostic tests. Otoscopic examination provides visualization of the cause of the obstruction.

Medical management. Medical management includes removal of cerumen by irrigation or cerumen spoon. Foreign objects are removed with forceps, if possible. Insects are smothered with drops of an oily substance and removed with forceps. Medications, such as carbamide peroxide 6.5%, may be used to soften cerumen. Surgical removal of the foreign object may be necessary.

Nursing interventions. The nurse assists with the irrigation of the ear (see Skill 37-4). Medications are instilled into the ear as ordered.

NURSING DIAGNOSIS	NURSING INTERVENTIONS
Sensory/perceptual alterations (auditory)	Note the presence and amount of hearing impairment and/or tinnitus. Assure the patient or parents that once the obstruction is removed, any hearing loss or tinnitus should disappear.

Patient teaching. The nurse informs the patient and parents about the danger of placing objects in the ears. The nurse also reinforces the method for preventing cerumen obstruction through the instilling of 1 to 2 drops of an oily substance at night. This is followed by hydrogen peroxide in the morning and cleaning with a soft cotton wick.

Noninfectious Disorders of the Ear

Otosclerosis

Etiology/pathophysiology. Otosclerosis is a condition in which irregular ossification in the bony labryinth of the inner ear (especially of the stapes) occurs, causing tinnitus, then deafness.

The cause is unknown, although about half of the patients with the disease have a family history of the disease. Women are affected twice as often as men. Frequently pregnancy triggers a rapid onset of this condition. Previous ear infections are not believed to be related to otosclerosis.

Gradual replacement of normal bone, in the otic capsula, by highly vascular otosclerotic bone occurs. This replacement bone is described as spongy. Calcification of the area follows, and conductive hearing loss is then produced.

Clinical manifestations. The patient with otosclerosis will experience a slowly progressive conductive hearing loss and will describe a low- to medium-pitched tinnitus. The deafness is usually first noted between the ages of 11 and 20.

Assessment. Collection of *subjective data* includes noting the degree and progression of hearing loss or tinnitus. Family history for the disease is assessed.

Collection of *objective data* includes assessment of behavioral clues related to hearing loss as outlined in Box 37-7.

Diagnostic tests. Otoscopy will reveal a normal eardrum. A pink blush called *Schwartz's sign* may be seen through the ear; this is indicative of a high degree of vascularity in active otosclerotic bone. The result of the Rinne test shows sounds transmitted by bone conduction lasting longer than by air conduction in the affected ear. The Weber test results are the reverse from normal hearing. Audiometric testing shows a lateralization of sound more to the affected ear. The Weber test in otosclerosis would result in a lateralization of sound to the affected ear. Audiometric testing may show minimal to total hearing loss. Hearing loss ranges from mild in the early stages to total loss in the later stages.

Medical management. Otosclerosis is usually treated with a stapedectomy to restore hearing (see stapedectomy, p. 997). When a stapedectomy is not indicated, an air conduction hearing aid may be prescribed.

Nursing interventions. Nursing diagnoses and interventions of otosclerosis are specific to poststapedectomy care. (See the discussion of stapedectomy, p. 997.)

Patient teaching. Refer to the discussion on ear surgery, p. 999.

Ménière's disease

Etiology/pathophysiology. Ménière's disease is a chronic disease of the inner ear characterized by recurrent episodes of vertigo, progressive unilateral nerve deafness, and tinnitus.

Ménière's disease is most common in women between the ages of 50 and 60 years. The cause is unknown, although occasionally the condition follows middle ear infection or trauma to the head. There are usually several yearly attacks until the disease either resolves itself or progresses to complete deafness in the affected ear.

There is an increase in endolymph fluid, either from increased production or decreased absorption. This causes increased pressure in the inner ear labyrinth. Attacks of severe vertigo, tinnitus, and progressive deafness result from this increased pressure. Usually one ear only is involved.

Clinical manifestations. The patient experiences recurrent episodes of vertigo with associated nausea and tinnitus, and hearing loss may be present. During an attack, vomiting, diaphoresis, and nystagmus may occur. These attacks last from a few minutes to several hours. Sudden movements often aggravate the symptoms.

Assessment. Collection of *subjective data* includes noting the frequency and severity of the vertigo attack. History and knowledge of the disorder and circumstances that precipitate an attack are noted. Assessment is made of actions taken by the patient during an attack and the degree of relief those actions provide.

Collection of *objective data* includes determining unilateral or bilateral hearing loss. The nurse observes the patient for associated symptoms during an attack.

Diagnostic tests. Audiologic tuning fork tests show a sensorineural deficit. Vestibular testing shows lack of balance.

Medical management. There is no specific therapy for Ménière's disease. Fluid restriction, diuretics, and a low-salt diet are prescribed in an attempt to decrease fluid pressure.

Dimenhydrinate (Dramamine), meclizine HCl (Antivert), and diphenhydramine (Benadryl) are prescribed for use between attacks. In acute attacks the medications may be given intravenously. Atropine is also given for its anticholinergic effect during these acute attacks.

For preservation of hearing, surgical procedures may be performed. Approximately 5% to 10% of the patients with Ménière's disease require surgery. These surgeries and subsequent nursing care are discussed in Table 37-7.

Nursing interventions. The nurse should maintain the prescribed low-salt diet and administer diuretics as ordered. The patient may have some auditory deficit, which will require alternate methods of communication. If the patient's tinnitus becomes distressing, an increase in background noise, such as music, may provide some relief.

Table 37-7 Surgery for Ménière's Disease

Type	Description	Residual	Postoperative Care
Surgical destruction of labyrinth	Extraction of membranous labyrinth by suction; access to inner ear through external canal (stapes and incus removed)	Destroys remaining hearing	Bed rest and NPO until vertigo subsides in 1 to 3 days Avoid sudden movement of head for 1 to 2 weeks Take action to prevent falls from unsteadiness for 1 to 3 weeks
Endolymphatic subarachnoid shunt	Insertion of drain tube from endolymphatic sac into subarachnoid space; access through mastoid	Preserves hearing in 60% to 70% of patients	Monitor for dizziness (rare)
Cryosurgery	Application of intense cold to lateral semicircular canals to decrease sensitivity or to create an otic-periotic shunt; access through mastoid	Preserves hearing in 80% of patients	Monitor for dizziness for 2 days Take action to prevent falls from unsteadiness for 2 to 3 weeks
Vestibular nerve section	Dissection of cranial nerve VIII (vestibular portion); access through mastoid or through cranial drilling over roof of internal auditory canal	Preserves hearing in 90% of patients	Same as for surgical destruction of labyrinth

NURSING DIAGNOSIS	NURSING INTERVENTIONS
Potential for injury	Keep side rails up. Assist with ambulation, and instruct the patient to call for assistance before attempting to ambulate. Have the patient sit or lie down when vertigo occurs. Have the patient move slowly and avoid turning the head suddenly. Administer medications, as prescribed. Position patient on unaffected side. Stand in front of patient, and prevent head turning. Avoid bright or glaring lights around patient. Place all needed supplies so that patient does not have to turn head.

Patient teaching. The nurse provides information about a low-salt diet and taking diuretics. The patient should be warned to avoid reading when vertigo or tinnitus is present. The patient is instructed to avoid smoking to prevent vasoconstriction. The patient should learn to identify precipitating factors and the proper actions to take when an attack occurs: (1) sit or lie down immediately, (2) stop the car and pull over to the side of the road, and (3) keep medication available at all times. See nursing care plan for patient with Ménière's disease, p. 998.

SURGERIES OF THE EAR

Stapedectomy

Stapedectomy is the removal of the stapes of the middle ear and insertion of a graft and prosthesis. The stapes that has become fixed is replaced so that vibrations can again transmit sound waves through the oval window to the fluid of the inner ear.

Using a local anesthetic, the surgeon removes the stapes, and the opening into the inner ear is covered with a graft of body tissue. One end of a small plastic tube or piece of stainless steel wire is attached to the graft, while the other end is attached to the two remaining bones of the middle ear.

Nursing interventions. Postoperative management consists of an external ear packing to ensure healing; the packing is left in place 5 or 6 days. The patient should remain in bed for approximately 24 hours, depending on physician preference. Gradual activity, when allowed, is provided. The patient is kept flat with the operative side facing upward to maintain the position of the prosthesis and graft; therefore the nurse makes certain that the patient is not turned.

Possible complications of the stapedectomy include infection of the outer, middle, or inner ear. Displacement or rejection of the prosthesis or graft may occur, or perilymph fluid may leak around the prosthesis into the middle ear, causing ringing in the ears and vertigo.

Nursing diagnoses and interventions are provided on p. 999.

Tympanoplasty

Tympanoplasty is any of several operative procedures on the eardrum or ossicles of the middle ear designed to restore or improve hearing in patients with conductive hearing loss. These operations may be used to repair a

NURSING CARE PLAN: THE PATIENT WITH MÉNIÈRE'S DISEASE

Nursing diagnoses	Patient goals	Nursing interventions
Anxiety, related to effects of disorder	Patient will experience decreased signs of anxiety.	Encourage patient to explore concerns about decreased hearing and effects of vertigo attacks and to take action in relation to the concerns. Explore patient's knowledge of the disorder and correct misunderstandings. Encourage realistic hope about expected hearing ability as described by physician. Refer patient to necessary support services, such as social worker or audiologist.
Sensory/perceptual alterations: vestibular, auditory	Patient will describe actions to avoid vertigo. Patient will interact with others accurately.	Help patient identify avoidable actions that precipitate vertigo attacks. Encourage patient to move slowly and not turn head suddenly when vertigo is present. If tinnitus is distressing, increase background noises such as music. If hearing is decreased: a. Use measures to facilitate communication with hearing impaired. b. Refer patient to audiologist, if appropriate.
Potential for injury and trauma, related to vertigo	Patient will not sustain injury.	Keep side rails up when patient with dizziness is in bed. Assist with ambulation as needed. Encourage patient to sit or lie down and to remain immobile if signs of dizziness occur. Teach patient to stop car at side of road immediately at first signs of dizziness while driving.
Bathing/hygiene, dressing/grooming, feeding, toileting, self-care deficit, potential	ADL needs will be met. Patient will function as independently as condition permits.	Provide desired foods and fluids if nausea is present. Assist with hygiene as needed while encouraging independence; place hygiene supplies so that patient does not have to turn head. Provide sufficient time for ADL so patient can move slowly.
Ineffective coping, individual	Patient will identify coping pattern and resultant effects. Patient will describe alternative coping behaviors.	Make decisions regarding safety of patient and others when patient is unable to do so. Assist patient to identify usual coping behaviors and the consequences of the behaviors. Assist patient to identify personal strengths. Teach patient alternative coping behaviors (see Chapter 49).
Knowledge deficit	Patient will describe nature of disorder, therapy, and safety measures.	Teach patient about the disorder, therapy, and need for medical follow-up. Teach patient ways to protect self from injury and to prevent vertigo attacks when possible.

BOX 37-12 **TEACHING FOR THE PATIENT AFTER EAR SURGERY**

1. Change cotton in ear daily as prescribed
2. Open mouth when sneezing or coughing and blow nose gently one side at a time for 1 week (to prevent increased ear pressure and infection)
3. Keep ear dry for 6 weeks (to prevent infection)
   a. Do not wash hair for 1 week
   b. Protect ear when outdoors using two pieces of cotton (use petrolatum jelly on outer ball)
   c. Protect ear with shower cap when bathing
4. Wear ear protectors as necessary for exposure to loud noises
5. Follow activity guidelines
   a. No physical activity for 1 week
   b. No exercises or active sports for 3 weeks
   c. Return to work in 1 week (3 weeks for strenuous work)
6. Avoid exposure to persons with upper respiratory tract infections
7. Avoid airplane flights for at least 1 week (to prevent effects of pressure changes)

perforated eardrum, for otosclerosis, or for dislocation or necrosis of one of the small bones of the middle ear.

Nursing interventions. Postoperative management consists of bed rest until the next morning. The head of the bed is to be elevated 40 degrees and the patient's operative side facing upward. Medications include narcotic analgesics; tetracycline HCl (Achromycin) as an antiinfective agent; and meclizine HCl (Antivert) for vertigo.

Postoperatively the presence of bleeding, the amount, color, and consistency of drainage, and temperature must be noted and reported. Complaints of vertigo when the patient is getting out of bed should be noted; with sudden movements, nausea and vertigo may occur. Keep the head of the patient's bed elevated 40 degrees. Possible complications include infection and displacement of the graft.

Nursing diagnoses and interventions are provided in the discussion of myringotomy, which follows.

Myringotomy

Myringotomy is a surgical incision of the eardrum. It is performed to relieve pressure and release purulent exudate from the middle ear. The procedure is done under either local or general anesthetic.

A myringotomy may be performed in one of two ways. Using a myringotomy knife, the surgeon makes a curved incision in the drumhead. In the second procedure, a heated wire loop is touched for about 1 second to the drumhead, producing a 2 mm hole.

Nursing interventions. Pus and fluid may drain immediately, requiring suctioning. Cotton placed in the ear is used to absorb the drainage, which may continue for several days.

The incision usually heals quickly with little scarring. Disruption of hearing does not usually occur.

Postoperative management includes cotton in the ear for absorption of drainage. Cotton should be changed frequently to avoid recontamination of the surgical area. Medications commonly used are tetracycline (Achromycin) and polmyxin B (Neosporin) eardrops as antiinfective agents. Tylenol with codeine may be used for pain.

Postoperatively the nurse monitors for signs of drainage and bleeding and reports any occurrence. Incisional pain or hearing impairment should be noted.

NURSING DIAGNOSES	NURSING INTERVENTIONS
Impaired physical mobility	Note patient's ability to comply with bed rest order. Keep the patient's operative side up; do not allow the patient to be turned.
Activity intolerance	Keep side rails up. When movement is allowed, begin gradually. Administer prescribed medications for pain and vertigo as needed.
Potential for injury	Note and report any drainage or bleeding. Assist with ambulation when it is allowed.

Patient teaching. Provide the information outlined in Box 37-12 to patients or parents and ensure their understanding.

REFERENCES AND SUGGESTED READINGS

1. Anagnostakos NP and Tortora GJ: Principles of anatomy and physiology, ed 5, New York, 1987, Harper & Row, Publishers.
2. Bajart AM: Common eye problems in the older woman—dry eye syndrome, cataracts, glaucoma and macular degeneration, Women's Health 10(2/3):85, 1985.
3. Brunner LS and Suddarth DS: Textbook of medical-surgical nursing, ed 6, Philadelphia, 1988, JB Lippincott Co.
4. Caldwell E and Hegner R: Geriatrics: a study of maturity, ed 4, New York, 1986, Delmar Publishers, Inc.
5. Diagnostics—the nurses' reference library, Nursing 86 Books, Springhouse, Pa, 1986, Intermed Communications, Inc.
6. Fong E, Ferris EB, and Skelley EG: Body structures and functions, ed 7, 1989, Delmar Publishers, Inc.
7. Goldman R: For your eyes only: eye injuries (Pictorial), Emergency 19(12):27, 1987.
8. Goldstein J: Pharmacology of ophthalmic drugs: anesthetics, mydriatics and cycloplegics and ocular hypotensives, J Ophthalm Nurs Technol 6(4):146, 1987.
9. Gottsch JD and others: Cataracts: diagnosis and treatment, Hosp Med (Suppl) 23(4):21, 1987.
10. Graber RF: Removing a foreign body from the eye (Pictorial), Patient Care 19(21):96, 1985.
11. Havener WH and others: Nursing care in eye, ear, nose, and throat disorders, ed 5, St Louis, 1986, The CV Mosby Co.
12. Hearing loss: basic anatomy of the ear (Pictorial), Hosp Med 22(7):160, 1986.
13. Hood GH and Dincher JR: Total patient care: foundations and practice, ed 7, St Louis, 1988, The CV Mosby Co.
14. Hughes GB: Textbook of clinical otology, New York, 1985, Thieme-Stratton, Inc.
15. Lent-Wunderlich L and others: Helping your patient through eye surgery, RN 49:6, 1986.
16. Levene B: Sorry nurse, I can hear you but I can't understand you, Nurs 85 (Oxford) 2(41):1221, 1985.
17. Long B and Phipps WJ: Medical-surgical nursing: a nursing process approach, ed 2, St Louis, 1989, The CV Mosby Co.
18. Luckman J and Sorensen KC: Medical-surgical nursing: a psychophysiologic approach, ed 3, Philadelphia, 1987, WB Saunders Co.
19. Malamed M: The injured eye, Emerg Med 20(17):86, 1988.
20. Marieb EN:Essentials of human anatomy and physiology, Calif, 1984, Addison-Wesley Publishing Co., Inc.
21. Memmler RL and Wood DL: Structure and function of the human body, ed 4, Philadelphia, 1987, WB Saunders Co.
22. Pagana KD and Pagana TJ: Diagnostic testing anad nursing implications, ed 2, St Louis, 1986, The CV Mosby Co.
23. Pappas JJ and others: Hearing loss: new techniques to correct defects and enhance sounds, Consultant 26(9):129, 1986.
24. Petrowski DD: Care of an artificial eye after enucleation, J Ophthalm Nurs Technol 5(4):135, 1986.
25. Phipps WJ, Long B, and Woods NF: Clinical handbook of medical-surgical nursing, ed 1, St Louis, 1987, The CV Mosby Co.
26. Phipps WJ, Long B, and Woods NF: Medical-surgical nursing: concepts and clinical practice, ed 3, St Louis, 1987, The CV Mosby Co.
27. Potter PA and Perry AG: Fundamentals of nursing: concepts, process, and practice, ed 2, St Louis, 1989, The CV Mosby Co.
28. Riley MA: Nursing care of the client with ear, nose, and throat disorders, New York, 1987, Springer Publishing Co.
29. Schremp PS: Discharge instructions: providing continuity of care for ophthalmic patients—what does the departing surgical patient need to know? J Ophthalm Nurs Technol 4(2):30, 1985.
30. Seidel HM and others: Mosby's guide to physical examination, St Louis, 1987, The CV Mosby Co.
31. Soll DB and others: Drugs and glaucoma, Am Fam Phys 34(1): 181, 1987.
32. Solomon EP and Phillips GA: Understanding human anatomy and physiology, Philadelphia, 1987, WB Saunders Co.
33. Thibodeau GA and Anthony CP: Structure and function of the body, ed 8, St Louis, 1988, Times Mirror/Mosby College Publishing.
34. Thompson JM and others: Mosby's manual of clinical nursing, ed 2, St Louis, 1989, The CV Mosby Co.
35. Tucker SM and others: Patient care standards, ed 4, St Louis, 1988, The CV Mosby Co.
36. Vader L: End-stage glaucoma and enucleation: an ophthalmic nursing challenge (case study), Ophthalm Nurs Forum 3(4):1, 1989.
37. West R: ABC's of cataract surgery preparation: assessment, briefing and counseling, J Ophthalm Nurs Technol 6:156, 1987.

CHAPTER CHALLENGE

KEY POINTS

- The five major senses are taste, touch, smell, sight, and hearing/balance.
- Seventy percent of the sensory structures of the body are located in the eye.
- The accessory structures of the eye are the eyebrows, eyelids, eyelashes, and the lacrimal apparatus.
- The three tunics of the eyeball are the fibrous tunic (sclera), the vascular tunic (choroid), and the retina.
- The two chambers of the eye are the aqueous chamber (which contains aqueous humor) and the posterior chamber (which contains vitreous humor).
- Image formation at the retina requires four basic processes: refraction, accommodation, constriction, and convergence.
- The photoreceptors of the retina are the rods and cones. The rods control vision in dim light and the cones control vision in bright light. The cones are also responsible for color vision.
- Light entering the eye must travel through the cornea, aqueous humor, pupil, lens, vitreous humor, and finally, the retina.
- The ear is divided into three distinct parts: the external ear, middle ear, and inner ear.
- The external ear flap is called the pinna (auricle); it extends into the external ear canal.
- The middle ear contains the ossicles and the entrance of the eustachian tube and ends with the tympanic membrane.
- The internal ear contains the vestibule, cochlea, and semicircular canals.
- The organ of Corti is the organ of hearing; it is located within the cochlea.
- The semicircular canals are responsible for the sense of balance and equilibrium.
- The tastebuds differentiate four basic tastes: sweet, sour, salty, and bitter. Food must be in solution for interpretation, because it is a chemical reaction that occurs.
- Normal aging causes decreased hearing and sight as a result of normal physiological changes of the structures.
- Individuals with chronic disease or who are over the age of 40 should be examined yearly to detect eye abnormalities or so that changes in current therapy may be prescribed.
- Refractory errors include conditions referred to as hyperopia (farsightedness), presbyopia (farsightedness related to the aging process), and astigmatism (objects waver).
- Ranges of 20/20 to 20/40 vision are considered normal, whereas 20/200 is defined as legal blindness.
- Cataracts are an opacity of the lens and may be surgically removed by intracapsular or extracapsular extraction.
- Glaucoma is a slow, progressive disorder involving increased intraocular pressure. It is related to occlusion of aqueous humor drainage.
- Loss of hearing may result from infection, trauma, or use of ototoxic drugs, or may be a congenital condition.
- Conductive hearing loss is a decrease in amplification, whereas sensorineural hearing loss is interference within the inner ear.
- Prevention of serious complications of ear disorders, such as infections, mastoiditis, and brain abscess, requires early detection and treatment.
- Potential for injury is the primary nursing diagnosis for the patient experiencing vertigo, which occurs in labyrinthitis and Ménière's disease.
- An essential communication tip for speaking to the hearing impaired is to face the patient and to speak clearly without shouting.

STUDY QUESTIONS

1. Another name for the incus, malleus, and stapes is:
   a. Tympanic membrane
   b. Ossicles
   c. Pinna
   d. Major structures
2. The organ of hearing is the:
   a. Semicircular canals
   b. Organ of Corti
   c. Tympanic membrane
   d. Oval window
3. The structure responsible for maintaining balance is the:
   a. Organ of Corti
   b. Oval window
   c. Semicircular canals
   d. Tympanic membrane
4. Another name for the tympanic membrane is:
   a. Pinna
   b. Eardrum
   c. Oval window
   d. Cerumen
5. The innermost tunic or covering of the eyeball is the:
   a. Retina
   b. Sclera
   c. Cornea
   d. None of the above
6. The structures responsible for color vision are the:
   a. Rods
   b. Cones
   c. Iris
   d. Lens
7. What structure is the eye's window to the world:
   a. Iris
   b. Cornea
   c. Sclera
   d. Lens
8. All the following are diagnostic eye tests except:
   a. Amsler grid test
   b. Tangent screen test
   c. Goldman perimetry test
   d. Rinne test
9. A primary objective of nursing care for the patient with an infectious/inflammatory process of the eyelid is:
   a. Administering antibiotics
   b. Flushing of the eye with sterile ophthalmic solution
   c. Prevention of further infection
   d. Maintaining bed rest
10. When assisting a blind person to ambulate, the nurse should:
    a. Precede the patient with the patient's hand on the nurse's elbow
    b. Follow the patient with the nurse's hand on the patient's elbow
11. The first symptom to be expressed by a person developing a cataract is often:
    a. Pain in the eyes
    b. Blurring of vision
    c. Loss of peripheral vision
    d. Dry eyes
12. After cataract surgery, the correct posture for the patient to assume while picking up an object from the floor is to:
    a. Kneel while keeping head erect
    b. Bend at the waist
13. Nursing interventions for the blind patient that are beneficial in the nursing diagnosis of Self-care deficit: feeding are all of the following except:
    a. Feeding the patient
    b. Describing the meal tray content
    c. Arranging foods by texture and temperature
    d. Describing the location of foods by the clock method

STUDY QUESTIONS (cont'd)

14. A surgical procedure for correction of the pathophysiology in diabetic retinopathy is:
    a. Enucleation
    b. Scleral buckle
    c. Photocoagulation
    d. Trabeculoplasty
15. Tunnel vision, eye pain, difficulty in adjusting to darkness, halos seen around lights, and failure to detect colors are all symptoms seen in:
    a. Cataracts
    b. Detached retina
    c. Entropion
    d. Chronic glaucoma
16. In first-aid treatment for eye injuries where a chemical burn has occurred, the correct immediate intervention would be:
    a. Applying sterile eyepads; seeking medical attention
    b. Flushing eyes immediately for 15 minutes with cool water or an available nontoxic liquid; seeking medical assistance
17. The two most common tests using tuning forks for auditory testing are:
    a. Slit-lamp and Schirmer tests
    b. Tonometry and fluorescein tests
    c. Weber and Rinne tests
    d. Snellen and Goldmann tests
18. Conductive hearing loss results when:
    a. Sound is delivered through the external and middle ear but a defect in the inner ear results in distortion
    b. Sound is inadequately delivered through the external or middle ear to the inner ear
    c. There is no organic cause but a functional problem exists
    d. The brain's auditory pathways are damaged
19. Which of the following is helpful in facilitating communication for persons with impaired hearing:
    a. Facing the person when speaking
    b. Overaccentuating words
    c. Shouting
    d. Using one-word answers
20. Otitis media is more frequent in children 6 to 36 months of age because their eustachian tubes are:
    a. Shorter and wider for easier access of organisms from nasopharynx to middle ear
    b. Longer and wider for easier access of organisms from nasopharynx to middle ear
    c. Shorter and straighter for easier access of organisms from nasopharynx to middle ear
21. The primary symptom of inflammation of the labyrinthine canals of the inner ear is:
    a. Severe pain
    b. Vertigo
    c. Headache
    d. Malaise
22. The surgical procedure for treatment of otosclerosis is:
    a. Surgical destruction of the labyrinth
    b. Dissection of cranial nerve VII (vestibular portion)
    c. Myringotomy
    d. Stapedectomy
23. Postoperative teaching for the patient after ear surgery should include:
    a. Changing cotton from ear canal hourly
    b. Blowing nose gently both sides at a time
    c. Teaching patient to open mouth when sneezing or coughing
    d. Limiting activities for 3 weeks

38

Care of the Patient with a Neurological Disorder

ELIZABETH SCHENK

LEARNING OBJECTIVES

After reading this chapter, the student should be able to do the following:

- Define the key terms.
- Name the two structural divisions of the nervous system.
- List the three parts of the neuron and describe the function of each part.
- Describe the "all or none" law and its impact on the nervous system.
- Discuss the difference between the motor neuron and the sensory neuron.
- List the main parts of the brain.
- List the coverings of the brain.
- Describe the difference between gray matter and white matter.
- Discuss the parts of the peripheral nervous system.
- Describe how the peripheral nervous system works in conjunction with the central nervous system.
- Name the 12 cranial nerves and list the areas they serve.
- List three physiological changes that occur in the nervous system with aging.
- Explain three parts of the neurological assessment.
- Explain the importance of prevention in problems of the nervous system and give at least one example of prevention.
- Explain the mechanism that occurs with increased intracranial pressure.
- List five signs and symptoms of increased intracranial pressure.
- List five nursing interventions that decrease intracranial pressure.
- Give examples of two degenerative neurological diseases and two diseases related to infection of the nervous system and explain the pathophysiology involved.
- Define the following terms: cerebrovascular accident, cerebral thrombosis, cerebral embolism, transient ischemic attack, and cerebral hemorrhage.
- State two complications of brain surgery and the signs and symptoms seen with each complication.

RELATED TOPICS OF INTEREST

- Care of the patient with an eye or ear disorder (Chapter 37)
- Care of the patient with AIDS (Chapter 40)
- Care of the patient with cancer (Chapter 41)
- Care of the aging (Chapter 48)
- Mental health concepts (Chapter 49)
- Rehabilitation nursing (Chapter 52)

KEY TERMS

Define the following:

- acetylcholine
- acceleration-deceleration injury
- agnosia
- aneurysm
- anomia
- aphasia
- apraxia
- aura
- autonomic dysreflexia
- axon
- bradykinesia
- brainstem
- cerebellum
- cerebrospinal fluid
- cerebrovascular accident
- cerebrum
- clonus
- concussion
- contracture
- contusion
- craniectomy
- craniotomy
- decerebrate rigidity
- decorticate rigidity
- degenerative diseases
- demyelination
- dendrite
- diabetes insipidus
- diencephalon
- diplopia
- dopamine
- dura mater
- dysarthria
- dysphagia
- endorphins
- fasciculation
- flaccid
- Glasgow Coma Scale
- global cognitive dysfunction
- gray matter
- gyri
- hemianopsia
- hemiplegia
- hyperreflexia
- medulla oblongata
- meninges
- motor (efferent) neurons
- neurilemma
- neuromuscular junction
- neurotransmitter
- norepinephrine
- nystagmus
- paralysis
- parasympathetic nervous system
- percutaneous cordotomy
- peripheral nervous system
- plaques
- pons
- postictal period
- prodromal
- proprioception
- receptor
- reflex
- rhizotomy
- sensory (afferent) neurons
- serotonin
- status epilepticus
- sympathetic nervous system
- tonic-clonic movements
- transient ischemic attack
- unilateral neglect
- ventricle
- white matter

The nervous system is responsible for communication and control within the body. It interprets or processes the information received and sends information to the appropriate area of the brain or spinal cord, from which a response is generated. The nervous system is the body's link with the environment. It works in conjunction with the endocrine system to maintain the body's homeostasis. The nervous system reacts in split-seconds, whereas the hormones secreted by the endocrine glands work more slowly in initiating a response.

ANATOMY AND PHYSIOLOGY

Structural Divisions

There are two main structural divisions of the nervous system (Fig. 38-1). The first division, the central nervous system (CNS), is composed of the brain and the spinal cord. It occupies a central or medial position in the body and is responsible for interpreting incoming sensory information and issuing instructions based on past experiences. The second component is the peripheral nervous system, which lies outside the central nervous system. It is composed of 12 pairs of cranial nerves and 31 pairs of spinal nerves. The cranial nerves carry impulses to and from the brain, whereas the spinal nerves carry impulses to and from the spinal cord. Sensory neurons (nerve cells) throughout the body send messages to the CNS, and motor neurons carry the message from the CNS to the appropriate muscle, gland, or structure.

The peripheral nervous system contains two main divisions: the somatic nervous system and the autonomic nervous system. The somatic nervous system sends messages from the CNS to the skeletal muscles (voluntary muscles). The autonomic system transmits messages from the CNS to smooth muscle, cardiac muscle, and certain glands. The autonomic system is sometimes called the *involuntary nervous system*, because its action takes place without conscious control.

Cells of the nervous system. There are two broad categories of cells within the nervous system. The first category, the neurons, are the transmitter cells. They carry

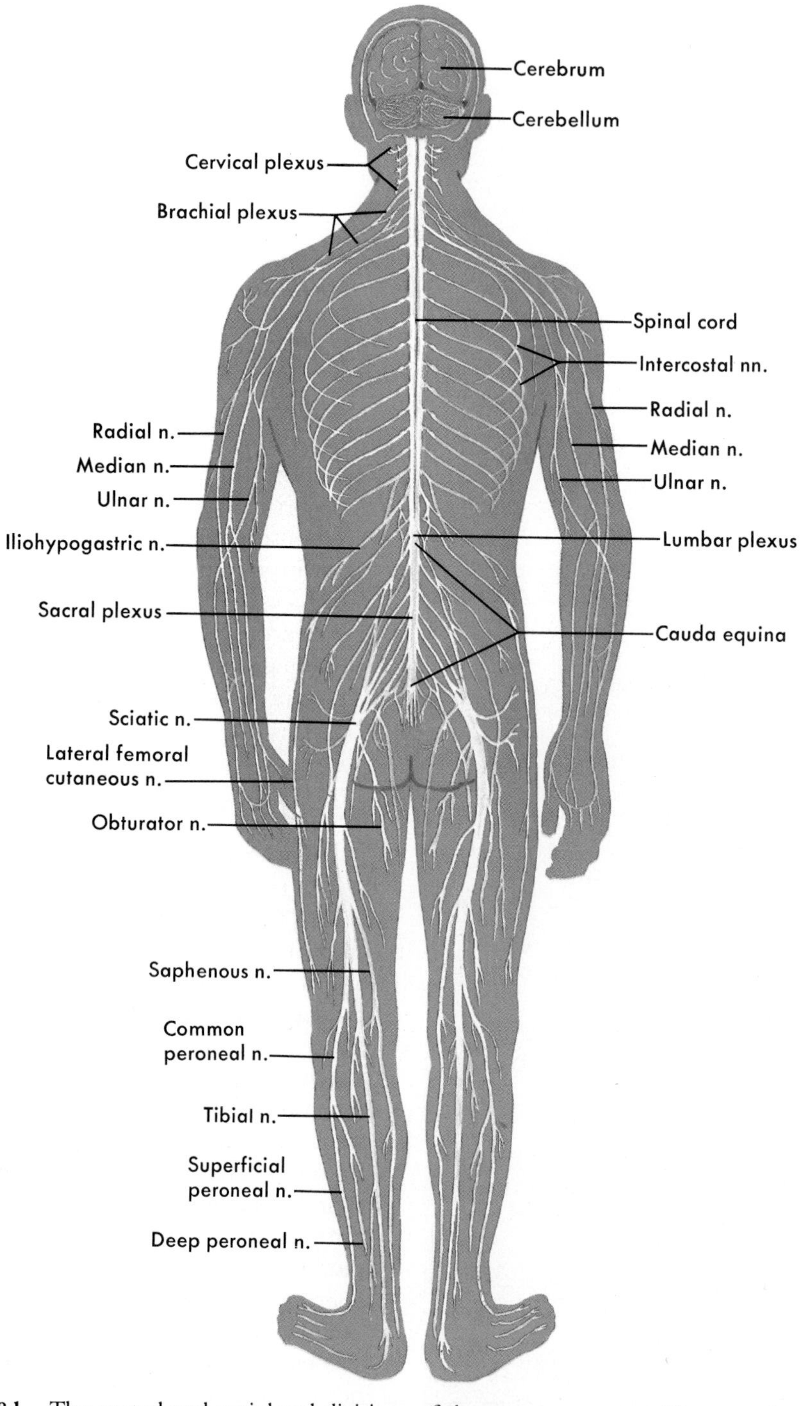

FIG. 38-1 The central and peripheral divisions of the nervous systems. The central nervous system (CNS) consists of the brain and spinal cord. The peripheral nervous system is composed of the cranial and spinal nerves.

the messages to and from the brain and spinal cord. The second category, the neuroglia or glial cells, are the support cells to the neurons. They support and protect the neurons while producing cerebrospinal fluid, which bathes the structures of the CNS.

Neuron structure. A neuron (nerve cell) is a separate unit and is composed of three main structures: the cell body, the axon, and the dendrites (Fig. 38-2). The cell body contains a nucleus surrounded by cytoplasm. The **axon** is a single projection extending away from the cell body; it transmits impulses away from the cell body. The **dendrites** are branching structures that extend from the cell body and receive impulses. Between each neuron is a gap (space) called the *synapse*.

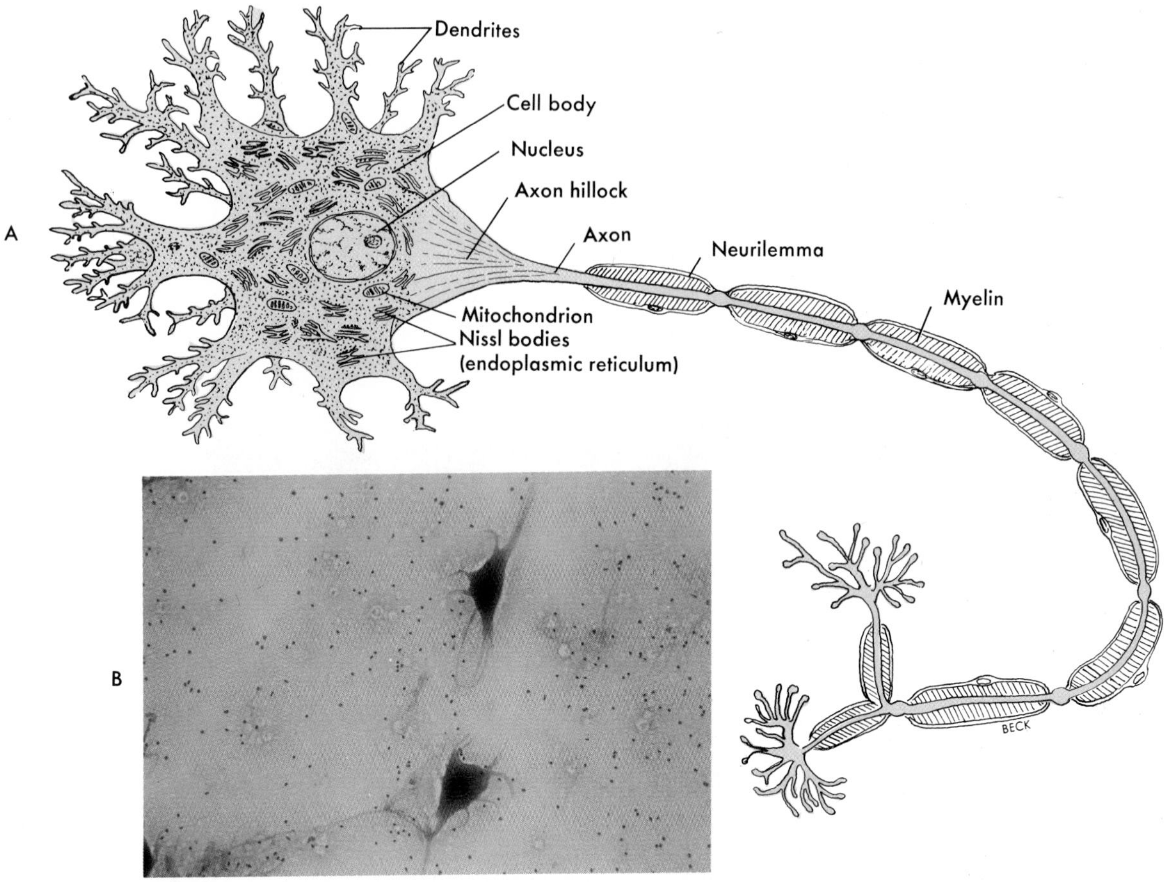

FIG. 38-2 **A,** Diagram of a typical neuron showing dendrites, cell body, and axon. **B,** Photomicrograph of neurons.

All neurons are governed by the "all or none law," which means there is never a partial transmission of a message—the impulse is either strong enough to elicit a response or too weak to generate the message.

Neurotransmitters. Special chemicals called **neurotransmitters** have been identified and have many different properties. The most well-known neurotransmitters are acetylcholine, norepinephrine, dopamine, and serotonin.

Acetylcholine plays a role in nerve impulse transmission; it spills into the synapse area and speeds the transmission of the impulse. The enzyme *cholinesterase* is then released to deactivate the acetycholine once the message or impulse has been sent. This happens very rapidly and continuously as each impulse needs to be relayed.

Norepinephrine has an impact on maintaining arousal (awakening from a deep sleep), dreaming, and regulation of mood (e.g., happiness, sadness).

Dopamine primarily effects motor function; it is involved in gross subconscious movements of the skeletal muscles. It also plays a role in emotional responses. In Parkinson's disease there is a decrease in dopamine levels, and the individual suffers from tremors, or involuntary, trembling muscle movements. (This will be discussed in detail later in the chapter.)

Serotonin, another neurotransmitter, induces sleep, affects sensory perception, controls temperature, and has a role in control of mood.

In the past few years another group of chemical messengers has been discovered; they are known as *neuropeptides*. Some of these messengers function as neurotransmitters, but generally they increase or decrease the response of the other neurotransmitters. In 1975 enkephalins were discovered; they are the body's natural pain relievers. Enkephalins are thought to inhibit the pain impulses and bind with the same receptors in the brain that chemicals such as morphine and other narcotics bind with.

Chemical **endorphins** have been isolated in the pituitary and have several functions. They suppress pain and are linked with memory and learning, sexual activity, and many more functions.

Neuron coverings. Many neuron fibers (axons and dendrites) are covered with a white, waxy, fatty material called *myelin* (Fig. 38-3). Myelin increases the rate of transmission of impulses and protects and insulates the fibers. Axons leaving the CNS are wrapped in layers of myelin with indentations called nodes of Ranvier. These

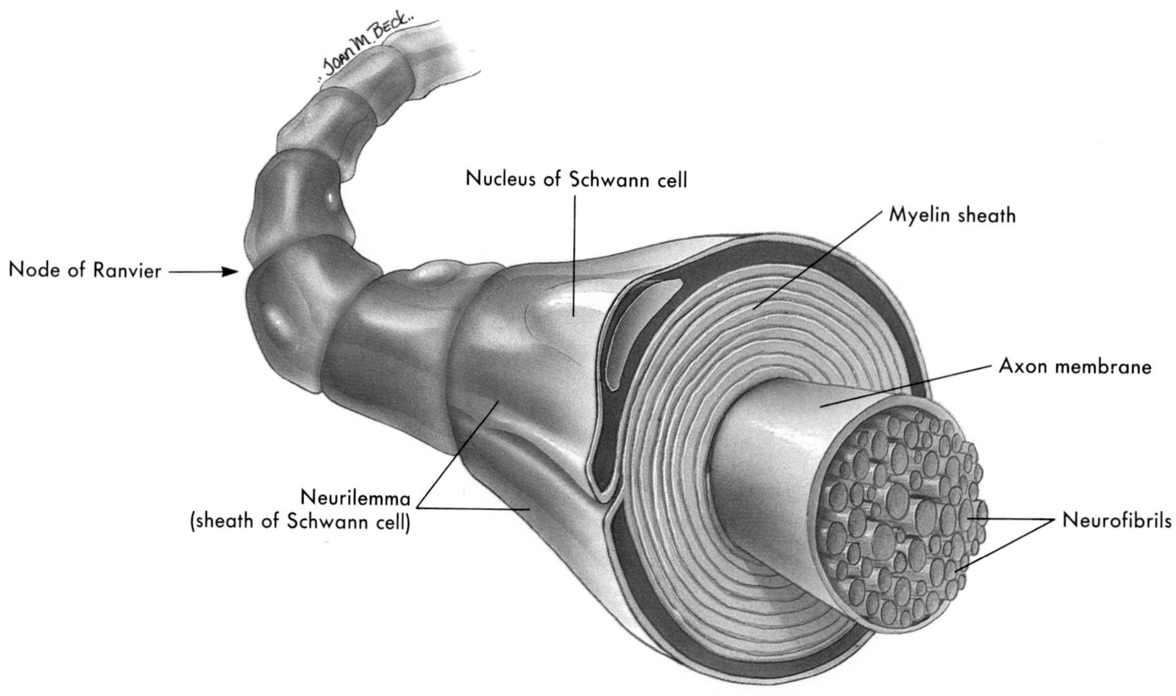

FIG. 38-3 Diagram of a nerve fiber and its coverings. This myelinated axon is located outside the central nervous system. Myelin is produced by the concentric layers of the Schwann cell. The neurilemma is the outer sheath of the Schwann cell and is indented by successive nodes of Ranvier.

nodes further increase the rate of transmission, because the impulse can jump from node to node.

In the peripheral nervous system, the myelin is produced by Schwann cells. The outer membrane of the Schwann cells gives rise to another layer called the **neurilemma**. The neurilemma is a very important layer, because it helps to regenerate injured axons. Thus regeneration of nerve cells occurs only in the peripheral nervous system. Cells damaged in the CNS result in permanent damage (paralysis), because they do not have neurilemma and are not able to regenerate.

Neuron classification. Neurons are classified according to the direction of the message they transmit. **Sensory (afferent) neurons** transmit messages to the brain and spinal cord. **Motor (efferent) neurons** transmit messages away from the brain and spinal cord. The sensory neurons carry information for interpretation; the motor neurons carry information for response to the interpreted information.

Nerve fibers. Groups or bundles of nerve fibers wrapped in connective tissue and lying outside the CNS are called *nerves*. Groups of nerve cell bodies that lie outside the CNS are called *ganglia*.

Inside the CNS the terminology changes. The bundles of nerve fibers are called *tracts* and the cell bodies are called *nuclei*.

Nerve impulses. A nerve cell impulse is the ability of the cell to change the electrical charge on the cell membrane and transmit the electrical current along the cell membrane. Because of positive and negative ions concentrated on either side of the membrane, the inside of the membrane at rest is negative as compared with the outside. A nerve impulse is a local reversal in the charge on the cell membrane that then spreads along the membrane like an electrical current.[30] The neuron has the ability to respond to a stimulus and convert it into a nerve impulse; this is called *irritability*. The nerve cell also has the ability to transmit the impulse to other neurons; this is called *conductivity*.

Nerve cell impulses are stimulated by pressure, temperature, or chemical changes and are governed by the "all or none" law.

Transmission of nerve impulses. In the resting phase the cell membrane of the nerve cell is negatively charged. During this period, the predominant extracellular ion is sodium and the predominant intracellular ion is potassium. An impulse brings about a sudden shift in the sodium and potassium across the cell membrane and reverses the electrical charge. This sudden change is called an *action potential*. Once the impulse has been transmitted, the cell membrane returns very rapidly to its former state.

The Central Nervous System

The central nervous system, composed of the brain and spinal cord, functions somewhat like a computer but is much more complex. The cranium protects the brain and the vertebral column protects the spinal cord.

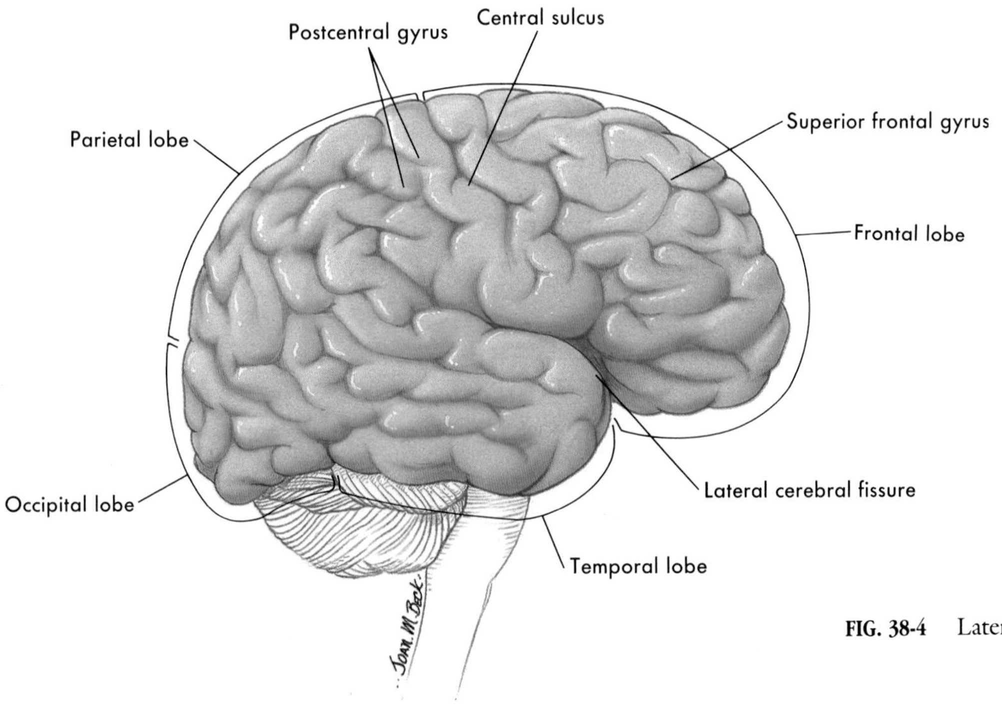

FIG. 38-4 Lateral view of the brain.

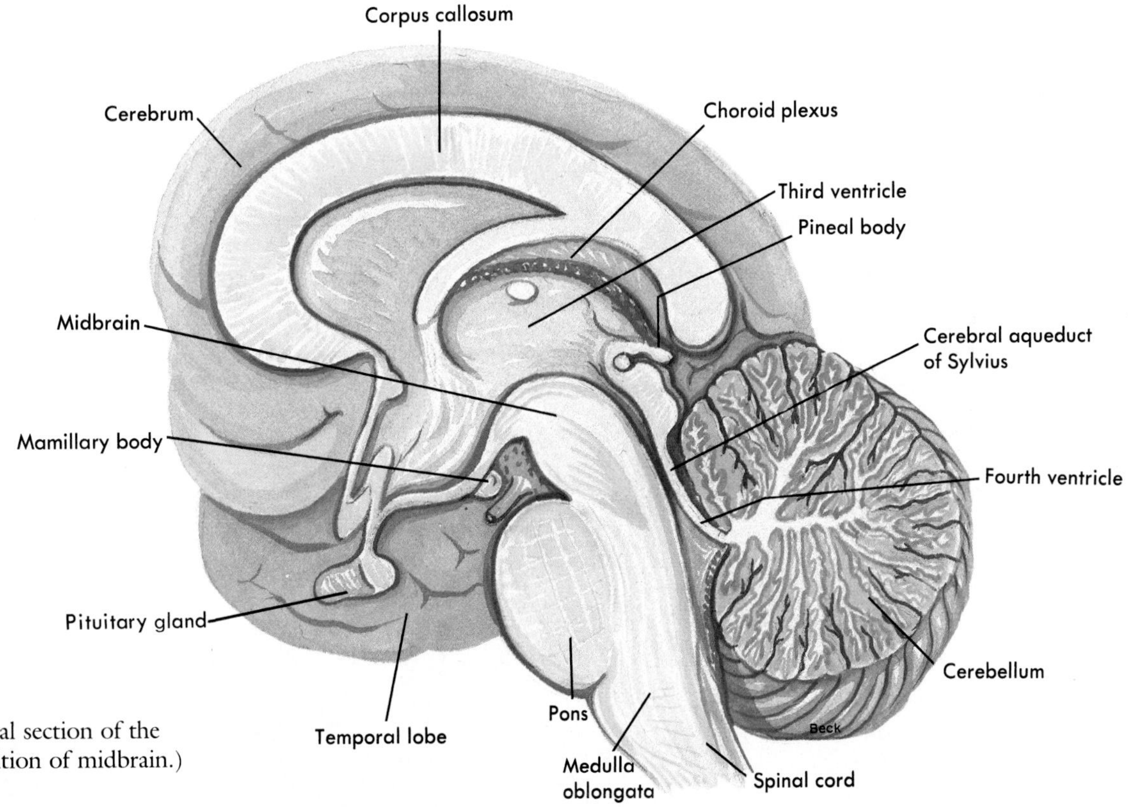

FIG. 38-5 Sagittal section of the brain. (Note position of midbrain.)

Brain. Specialized cells in the brain's mass of convoluted, soft, gray or white tissue coordinate and regulate the functions of the central nervous system. The brain is one of the largest organs, weighing approximately 3 lb (6.6 kg). It is divided into four principal parts: the cerebrum, the diencephalon, the cerebellum, and the brainstem (Figs. 38-4 and 38-5).

Cerebrum. The **cerebrum** is the largest part of the brain. It is divided into the right and left hemispheres. The outer portion of the cerebrum is composed of **gray matter** and is called the *cerebral cortex*. It is arranged in folds that are called **gyri** (convolutions); the grooves are called *sulci* (fissures). A deep fissure divides the right and left hemispheres; it is called the *longitudinal fissure*. A

BOX 38-1 CEREBRUM FUNCTIONS

FRONTAL LOBE

Written speech (ability to write)

Motor speech (ability to speak)

Motor ability—directs movements of body; the left side of the brain controls the right side of the body, and the right side of the brain controls the left side of the body

Intellectualization—the ability to form concepts, to think

Judgment formation

PARIETAL LOBE

Contains the sensory area; the impulses from the skin, such as touch, pain, and temperature, are interpreted

Ability to recognize body parts

Ability to determine left from right

Determination of shapes, sizes, and distances takes place here

TEMPORAL LOBE

Memory storage

Integration of auditory stimuli; this lobe receives and interprets impulses from the ear

OCCIPITAL LOBE

Contains the visual area for interpreting impulses from the retina of the eye

Understanding of the written word

bridge or connecting structure, the corpus callosum, links the two hemispheres. Other fissures divide the hemispheres into four lobes that are named for the bones lying over them: the frontal lobe, the parietal lobe, the temporal lobe, and the occipital lobe (see Chapter 30 for the location of cranial bones). The interior of the cerebrum is composed of **white matter** consisting of bundles of nerve fibers (tracts). Throughout the white matter are small islands of gray matter called *basal ganglia*. The basal ganglia play an important role in body movement and posture. The functions of the four lobes of the cerebrum are described in Box 38-1. See Fig. 38-6 for localization of function in the cerebral cortex.

Diencephalon. The **diencephalon** is often called the *innerbrain*: it lies directly beneath the cerebrum. It contains the thalamus and the hypothalamus. The thalamus, an oval structure with two lobes, is approximately 1 inch (3 cm) in diameter; it composes four fifths of the diencephalon. The thalamus serves as a relay station for some sensory impulses while interpreting other sensory messages, such as pain, light touch, and pressure.

The hypothalamus, which lies below the thalamus, plays a vital role in the control of body temperature, fluid balance, appetite, and certain emotions, such as fear, pleasure, and pain. Both the sympathetic and parasympathetic divisions of the autonomic system are under control of the hypothalamus, as is the pituitary gland. Thus the hypothalamus influences the heartbeat, the contraction and relaxation of the walls of the blood vessels, hormone secretion, and other vital body functions.

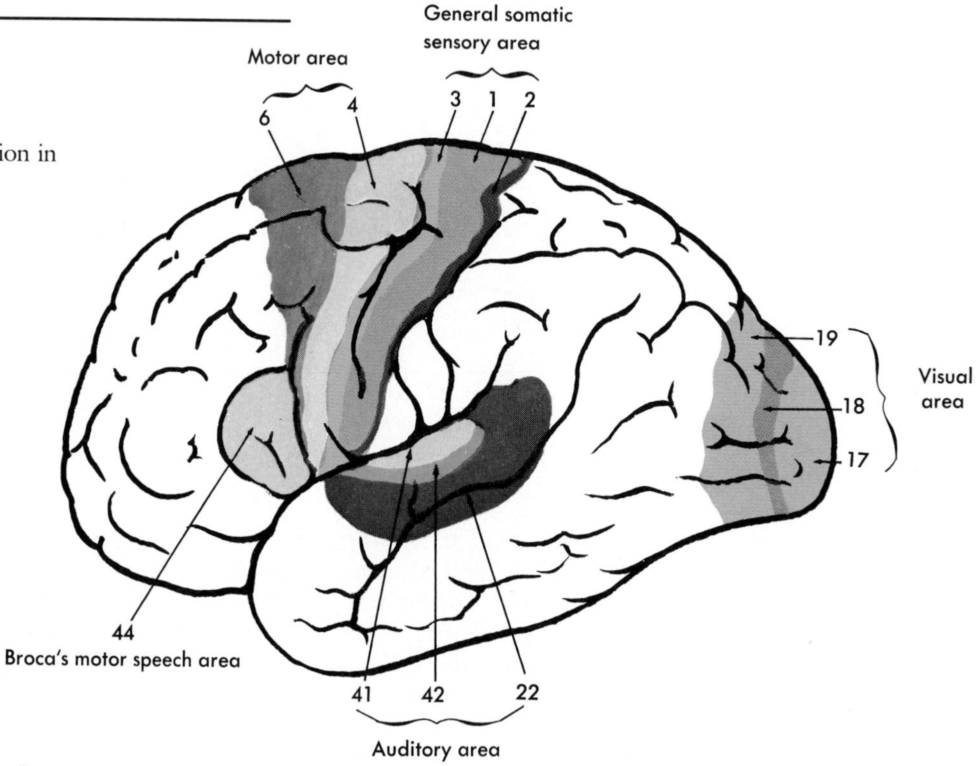

FIG. 38-6 Localization of function in the cerebral cortex.

Cerebellum. The **cerebellum** lies posterior and inferior to the cerebrum. It is the second largest portion of the brain. The cerebellum contains two hemispheres with a convoluted surface much like the cerebrum. Structurally it resembles a small head of cauliflower.

The cerebellum is mainly responsible for coordination of skeletal muscles and maintenance of balance, equilibrium, and muscle tone. Sensory messages from the semicircular canals in the inner ear send their messages to the cerebellum.

Brainstem. The **brainstem** is located at the base of the brain and contains the midbrain, pons, and medulla oblongata. These structures serve to connect the spinal cord and the cerebrum (Box 38-2). The brainstem carries all nerve fibers between the spinal cord and the cerebrum.

Midbrain. The midbrain forms the superior portion of the brainstem. It is responsible for motor movement, the relay of impulses, and auditory and visual reflexes. It is the origin of cranial nerves III and IV.

Pons. The **pons** connects the midbrain to the medulla oblongata. The word *pons* means "bridge." It is the origin of cranial nerves V through VIII. The pons is composed of myelinated nerve fibers and is responsible for sending impulses to the structures inferior and superior to it. It also contains a respiratory center that complements respiratory centers located in the medulla.

Medulla oblongata. The **medulla oblongata** is the distal portion of the brainstem. It is the origin of cranial nerves IX through XII. The medulla contains the cardiac center that regulates the heartbeat and force of the contraction. It also contains the respiratory center that controls the rhythm of breathing. A vasomotor center regulates the diameter of the blood vessels, which aids in control of the blood pressure. The medulla also controls the coordination of swallowing, coughing, sneezing, vomiting, and hiccuping (singultus).

Coverings of the brain and spinal cord. The brain and spinal cord are surrounded by three protective coverings (membranes) called the **meninges** (Fig. 38-7). The outermost covering, the **dura mater**, is a tough, fibrous membrane that adheres to the skull. The middle layer, the arachnoid membrane, resembles a spiderweb with **cerebrospinal fluid (CSF)** filling its spaces. The innermost layer, the pia mater, is a thin, vascular layer with many blood vessels that provides oxygen and nourishment to the nervous tissue. These three layers protect the brain and spinal cord and also bathe it in cerebrospinal fluid.

Ventricles. The ventricles (four in all) are spaces or cavities located in the brain (Fig. 38-8). Each hemisphere of the cerebrum has a lateral ventricle. These connect to the third ventricle in the diencephalon. The fourth ventricle is dorsal to the pons. CSF is formed continuously

BOX 38-2 BRAINSTEM FUNCTIONS

DIENCEPHALON (THALAMUS AND HYPOTHALAMUS)

Receives sensory impulses (pain, temperature, and touch)

Acts as relay station

Controls pain threshold

Acts in synthesis of vasopressor and oxytocin

Helps maintain wakeful state

Controls temperature

Generates emotional response

PONS

Pneumotaxic center (rhythmicity of respirations)

Connection between medulla, midbrain, and cerebellum

Origin of cranial nerves V, VI, VII, and VIII

MIDBRAIN

Motor movement

Relay of impulses

Postural reflex patterns

Auditory reflexes

Righting reflex

Some control of vision

Origin of cranial nerves III and IV

MEDULLA OBLONGATA

Cardiac, vasomotor, and respiratory center

Center for cough, swallowing, and singultus

Role in reticular activating system

Origin of cranial nerves IX, X, XI, and XII

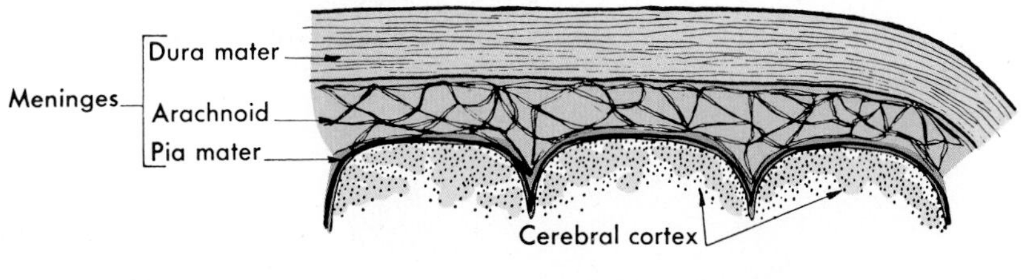

FIG. 38-7 Schematic drawing showing the structure of the meninges around the brain.

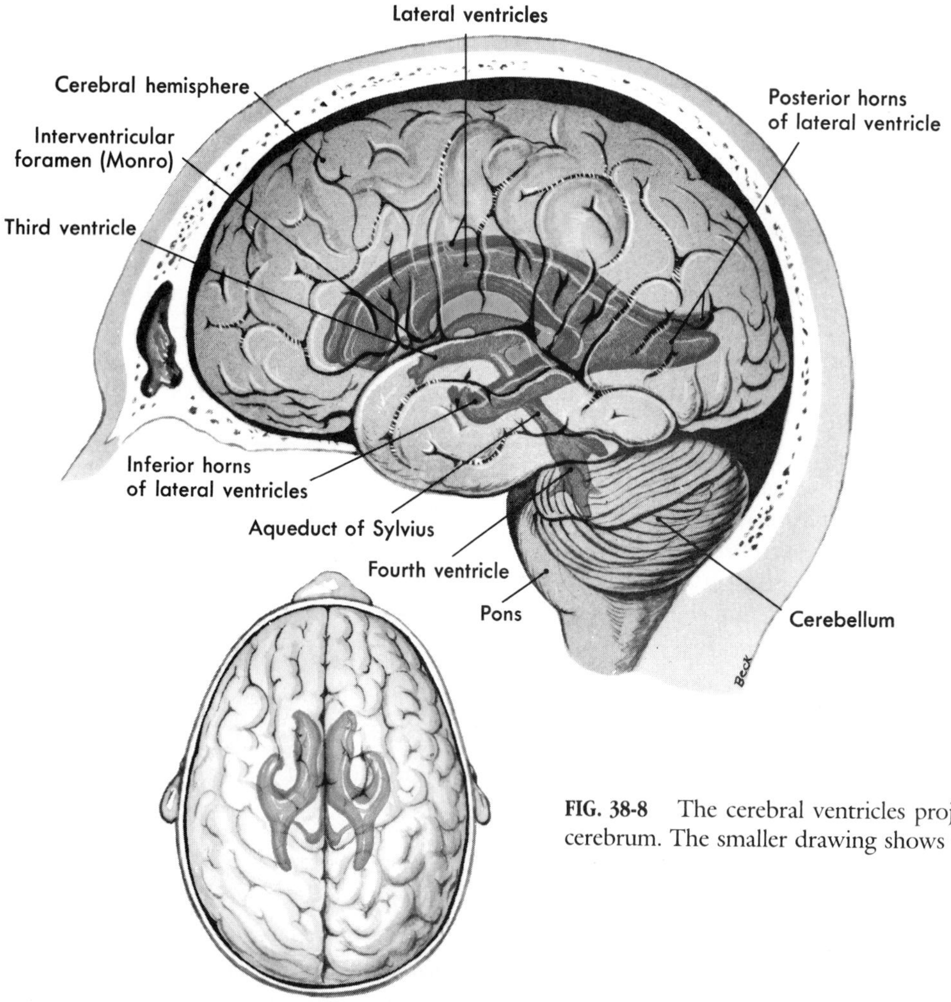

FIG. 38-8 The cerebral ventricles projected on the lateral surface of the cerebrum. The smaller drawing shows the ventricles from above.

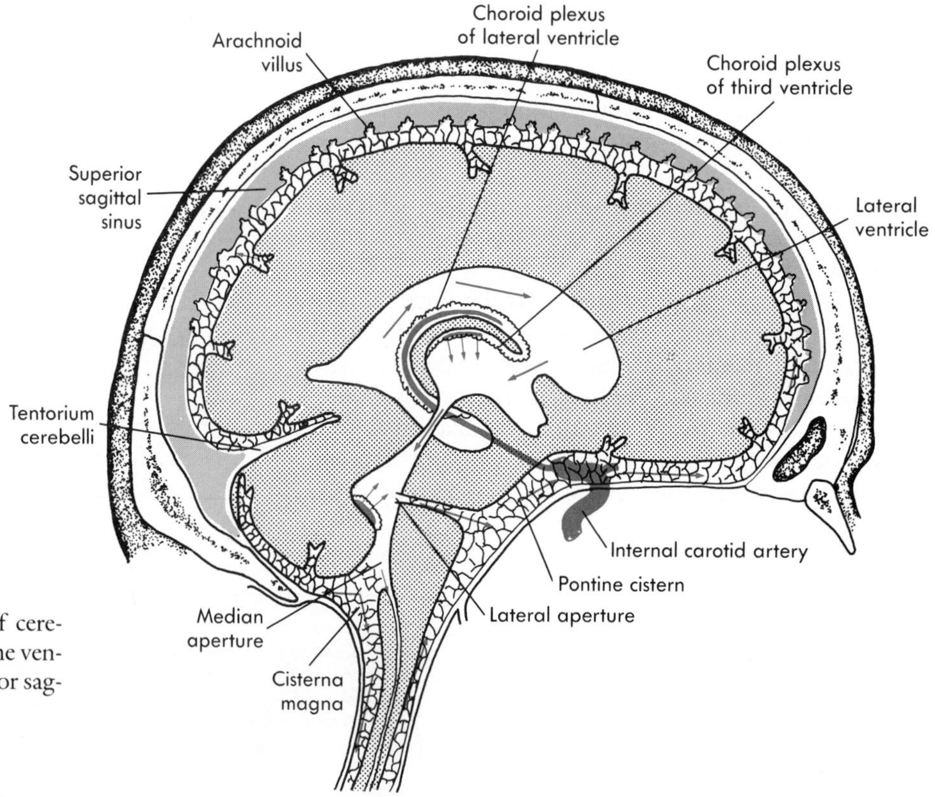

FIG. 38-9 Pathway of circulation of cerebrospinal fluid from its formation in the ventricles to its absorption into the superior sagittal sinus.

from fluid filtering out of the blood in a network of capillaries called the *choroid plexus* (Fig. 38-9). The choroid plexus lines the roofs of the ventricles. The cerebrospinal fluid flows from the lateral ventricles down through the interventricular foramen (Monro) into the third ventricle; it continues down the aqueduct of Sylvius into the fourth ventricle. Openings in the roof of the fourth ventricle allow the fluids to flow into the subarachnoid spaces around the brain and the spinal cord. The flow of fluid is from the blood in the choroid plexuses, through the ventricles, the central canal, the subarachnoid spaces, up into arachnoid granulations projecting up into venous sinuses, and returning to the venous circulation.

The cerebrospinal fluid is clear and resembles plasma. It contains proteins, glucose, urea, and salts; it also contains certain substances that form a protective barrier that prevents some (but not all) harmful substances from entering the brain and spinal cord. This fluid cushions the brain and spinal cord, protecting them from trauma.

In a 24-hour period, the choroid plexus secretes about 500 to 570 ml of CSF. Only about 125 to 150 ml is circulating at any given time. It delivers nutritive substances and removes waste and toxic substances from the cells of the CNS.

Spinal cord. The spinal cord is a 17- to 18-inch (45 to 48 cm) cord that extends from the brainstem to the second lumbar vertebra (at the level of the lower edge of the ribcage). It has two main functions: it conducts impulses to and from the brain, and it serves as a center for reflex actions. The center of the spinal cord forms the letter H. This area is composed of **gray matter** (dendrites and cell bodies of neurons), while the outer portion is composed of **white matter** (myelinated nerve fibers).

The white matter contains the spinal tracts (groups of axons that carry the messages). The ascending tracts carry the messages to the brain, and the descending tracts carry the messages away from the brain.

The spinal cord is responsible for certain **reflex** activities (e.g., knee jerk) (Fig. 38-10). A sensory neuron sends the information to the cord, a central neuron (located in the cord) interprets the impulse, and a motor neuron sends the message back to the muscle or organ involved. Thus a message is sent, interpreted, and acted upon without traveling to the brain.

The Peripheral Nervous System

The **peripheral nervous system** is composed of 31 pairs of spinal nerves, 12 pairs of cranial nerves, and the autonomic nervous system.

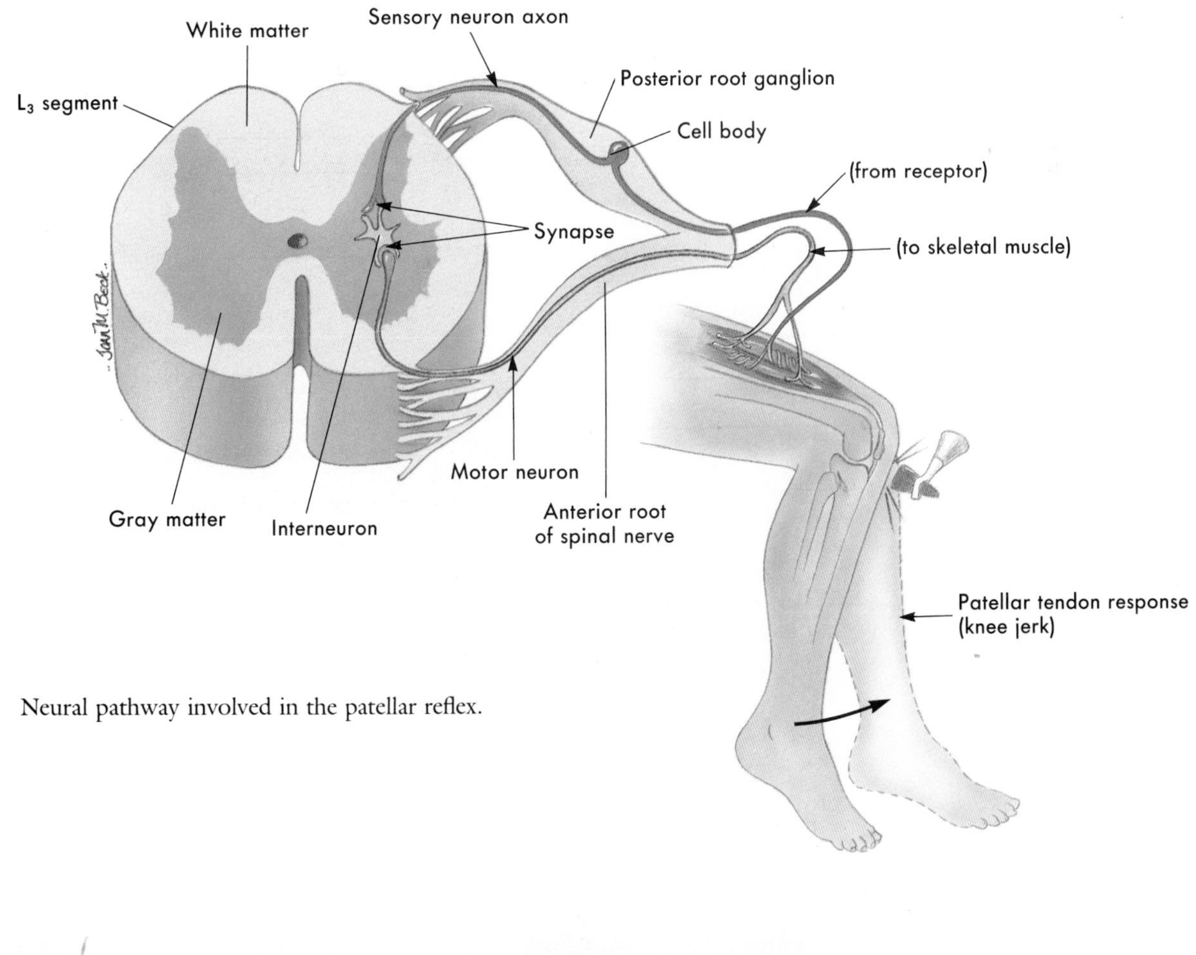

FIG. 38-10 Neural pathway involved in the patellar reflex.

Spinal nerves. The 31 pairs of spinal nerves are all mixed nerves. This means they transmit sensory information to the spinal cord through afferent neurons and motor information from the CNS to the various areas of the body through efferent neurons. The spinal nerves are named according to the corresponding vertebra (e.g., C1, C2). Each spinal nerve has two attachments to the spinal cord. The dorsal root attaches posteriorly and consists of afferent fibers (sensory), while the ventral root attaches anteriorly and consists of efferent fibers (motor). Each dorsal root has an enlarged area composed of gray matter (dorsal root ganglion), which consists of the cell bodies of the sensory neurons.

As the spinal nerves leave the spinal cord they develop several branches (plexuses). The most important plexuses are as follows:

1. Cervical plexus, which serves the shoulders, neck, and diaphragm
2. Brachial plexus, which serves the arms, wrists, and hands
3. Lumbar plexus, which serves the lower abdomen, buttocks, and anterior thighs and legs
4. Sacral plexus, which serves the lower trunk and posterior surface of the thighs and legs

Cranial nerves. There are 12 pairs of cranial nerves, which attach to the posterior surface of the brain, mainly the brainstem (Fig. 38-11). The cranial nerves are always written in Roman numerals (e.g., I, II, III). All 12 pairs conduct impulses between the head, neck, and brain, excluding the vagus nerve (X), which also serves organs in the thoracic and abdominal cavities. Table 38-1 lists the names of the cranial nerves, where the impulses are conducted, and their functions.

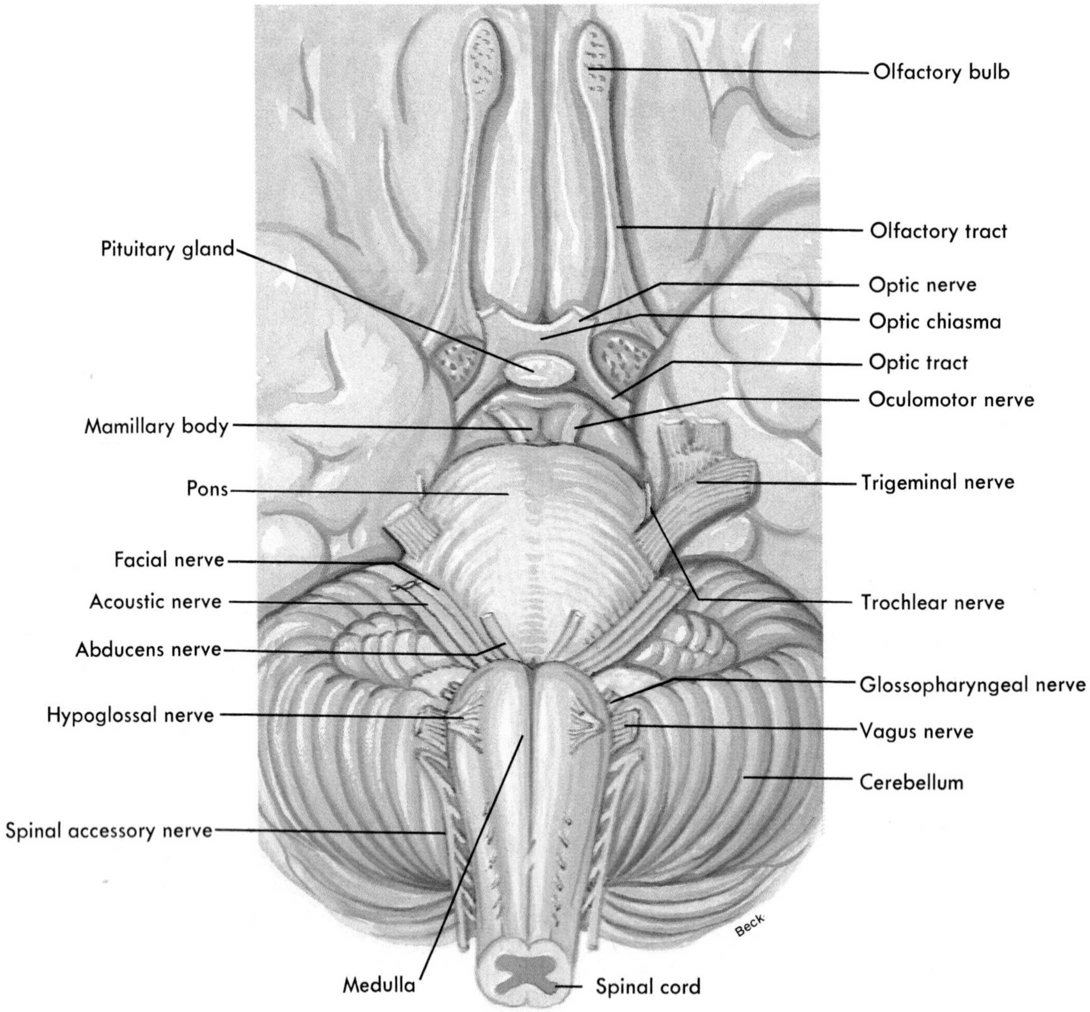

FIG. 38-11 Undersurface of the brain showing attachments of the cranial nerves.

Table 38-1 Cranial Nerves

Nerve*	Conducts Impulses	Functions
I Olfactory	From nose to brain	Sense of smell
II Optic	From eye to brain	Vision
III Oculomotor	From brain to eye muscles	Eye movements
IV Trochlear	From brain to external eye muscles	Eye movements
V Trigeminal (or trifacial)	From skin and mucous membrane of head and from teeth to brain; also from brain to chewing muscles	Sensations of face, scalp, and teeth, chewing movements
VI Abducens	From brain to external eye muscles	Turning eyes outward
VII Facial	From taste buds of tongue to brain; from brain to face muscles	Sense of taste; contraction of muscles of facial expression
VIII Acoustic	From ear to brain	Hearing; sense of balance
IX Glossopharyngeal	From throat and taste buds of tongue to brain; also from brain to throat muscles and salivary glands	Sensations of throat, taste, swallowing movements, secretion of saliva
X Vagus	From throat, larynx, and organs in thoracic and abdominal cavities to brain; also from brain to muscles of throat and to organs in thoracic and abdominal cavities	Sensations of throat, larynx, and of thoracic and abdominal organs; swallowing, voice production, slowing of heartbeat, acceleration of peristalsis
XI Spinal accessory	From brain to certain shoulder and neck muscles	Shoulder movements; turning movements of head
XII Hypoglossal	From brain to muscles of tongue	Tongue movements

*The first letter of the words of the following sentence are the first letters of the names of cranial nerves: "On Old Olympus' Tiny Tops A Finn And German Viewed Some Hops." Many generations of students have used this or a similar sentence to help them remember the names of cranial nerves.

The Autonomic Nervous System

This portion of the nervous system controls the activities of the smooth muscle, cardiac muscle, and all of the glands. The autonomic nervous system is not a separate nervous system but a subdivision of the peripheral nervous system.

It is misleading to think of this system as the "automatic" system, although most of its activity is performed on an unconscious level. Its primary function is to maintain internal homeostasis; for example, it strives to maintain a normal heartbeat, a constant body temperature, and a normal respiratory pattern.

To maintain this homeostasis, the autonomic system has two divisions: the **sympathetic nervous system** and the **parasympathetic nervous system**. These two divisions are antagonistic—one slows an action, while the other accelerates the action. For example, the sympathetic system increases the heartbeat, while the parasympathetic system decreases the heartbeat.

Table 38-2 lists the antagonistic functions of the sympathetic and parasympathetic nervous systems. It is important to note that both these systems function simultaneously, but they have the ability to dominate each other as the need arises. In times of stress, the sympathetic system takes over to prepare the body for "flight or fight." The heartbeat increases, the blood pressure increases, and the adrenal glands increase their secretions. To calm the body after the crisis, the parasympathetic system becomes dominant, slowing the heartbeat and decreasing the blood pressure and adrenal hormone output.

CARE OF THE PATIENT WITH A NEUROLOGICAL DISORDER

The clinical picture for the patient with neurological problems is often complex. Understanding these conditions requires knowledge of the anatomy and physiology of the nervous system (see pp. 1005-1015). The nervous system coordinates and controls all activities of the body by acting as an electrical conductance system. It performs four basic functions, including the receiving of information (stimuli) over sensory (afferent) pathways, the communicating of information between distal parts of the body, the processing of information received at conscious and reflex levels to determine responses, and the transmitting of information over motor (efferent) pathways to body organs. This is done via the neuron, which is the basic unit of the nervous system.

Changes in the Nervous System with Aging

The effects of aging on the nervous system are variable. The changes that occur include a loss of brain weight and a substantial loss of neurons (1% a year after age 50), with the cortex losing cells faster than the brainstem. The remaining cells undergo structural changes. There is also

Table 38-2 Autonomic Functions

Visceral Effectors	Parasympathetic Control	Sympathetic Control
HEART MUSCLE		
	Slows heartbeat	Accelerates heartbeat
SMOOTH MUSCLE		
Of most blood vessels	None	Constricts blood vessels
Of blood vessels in skeletal muscles	None	Dilates blood vessels
Of digestive tract	Increase peristalsis	Decrease peristalsis; inhibits defecation
Of anal sphincter	Inhibits—opens sphincter for defecation	Stimulates—closes sphincter
Of urinary bladder	Stimulates—contracts bladder	Inhibits—relaxes bladder
Of urinary sphincters	Inhibits—opens sphincter for urination	Stimulates—closes sphincter
Of eye		
Iris	Stimulates circular fibers—constriction of pupil	Stimulates radial fibers—dilation of pupil
Ciliary	Stimulates—accommodation for near vision (bulging of lens)	Inhibits—accommodation for far vision (flattening of lens)
Of hairs (pilomotor muscles)	No parasympathetic fibers	Stimulates—"goose pimples"
GLANDS		
Adrenal medulla	None	Increases epinephrine secretion
Sweat glands	None	Increases sweat secretion
Digestive glands	Increases secretion of digestive juices	Decreases secretion of digestive juices

a general decline in interconnections of **dendrites**, a reduction in cerebral blood flow, and a decrease in brain metabolism and oxygen utilization. The neurons may contain senile **plaques**, neurofibrillary tangles, and the age pigment lipofuscin. There is often an altered sleep/wakefulness ratio, a decrease in the ability to regulate body temperature, and a decrease in the velocity of nerve impulses. The blood supply to the spinal cord is decreased, resulting in decreased reflexes.[7]

Normal changes in the nervous system associated with aging are *not* the same as senility, organic brain disease, or Alzheimer's disease. Many older persons reach old age with no functional deterioration of the nervous system.

Prevention of Neurological Problems

Many conditions of the nervous system have no known cause. Other neurological problems can be prevented or their effects reduced by modifying life-style factors. Neurovascular diseases occur in part as a result of defined risk factors. These are the same factors that also increase the risk of cardiac disease and include high blood pressure, high blood cholesterol levels, cigarette smoking, obesity, stress, and lack of exercise.

The avoidance of cigarette smoking has been found to decrease the incidence of lung cancer. This is significant for the nervous system, because cancer of the lung often metastasizes to the brain.

Prevention of neurological problems resulting from trauma is a major challenge. These injuries include the fairly common diagnoses of spinal cord injury and head injury, which occur frequently in young persons. Patient teaching regarding avoiding such injuries should include the following:

- Avoidance of drug and alcohol use
- Safe use of motor vehicles—use of automobile seat belts, helmets with motorcycles and snowmobiles
- Safe swimming practices—avoidance of diving in shallow water
- Safe handling and storage of firearms
- Use of hardhats in dangerous construction areas
- Use of protective padding as needed for sports

Neurological diseases, such as meningitis or a brain abscess, that occur as a result of infection can sometimes be prevented by prompt treatment of ear and sinus infections. The practice of safe and responsible sex is important, because some neurologically related diseases, such as syphilis and AIDS, are spread by sexual contact. Safe practices include abstinence, monogamy, and the use of condoms. Treatment for drug abuse, especially intravenous use, is important, as in the prevention of AIDS.

Neurological Assessment

History. A comprehensive history is essential to the diagnosis of neurological disease. This includes specifics about symptoms experienced, as well as the patient's understanding and perception of what is happening. Obtaining information from family members and/or significant others may also be extremely helpful. The same format should be followed routinely to make sure information is complete.

For patients with suspected neurological conditions, the presence of many symptoms or subjective data may be significant. These include the following[25]:

- Headaches, especially ones that first occur after middle age, or ones that change in character; headaches that are worse in the morning or awaken a person from sleep are especially significant
- Clumsiness or loss of function in an extremity
- Change in visual acuity
- Any new or worsened seizure activity
- Numbness or tingling in one or more extremities
- Pain in an extremity or other part of the body
- Personality changes or mood swings
- Extreme fatigue or tiredness

Mental status. Assessment of the neurological patient's mental status is important. An examination of mental status generally includes orientation (person, place, and time), mood and behavior, general knowledge (such as the names of the presidents of the United States), and short-term and long-term memory. The patient's attention span and ability to concentrate may also be assessed.

It is important to document mental status in terms that are specific. For instance, it is better to document "oriented to name, date, and hospital" than to document "oriented."

Level of consciousness. A decreasing level of consciousness is the earliest symptom of increased intracranial pressure. Restlessness, disorientation, and lethargy may be seen first. Observations are recorded in terms of behavior and signs—not labels such as "confused."[15] One way of classifying level of consciousness is found in Box 38-3.

Glasgow Coma Scale. A way to standardize observations of patients in terms of neurological function is the **Glasgow Coma Scale** (Fig. 38-12). It was developed in 1974

BOX 38-3 LEVELS OF CONSCIOUSNESS

Alert	Responds appropriately to auditory, tactile, and visual stimuli
Confusion	Disoriented, unable to follow simple commands, thinking slowed, inattentive
Stupor	Responds to verbal commands with moaning or groaning, if at all
Semicomatose	Unable to cooperate, responds only to pain—response may range from purposeful to decerebrate to decorticate
Comatose	Unable to respond to any external stimuli; loss of brain functions

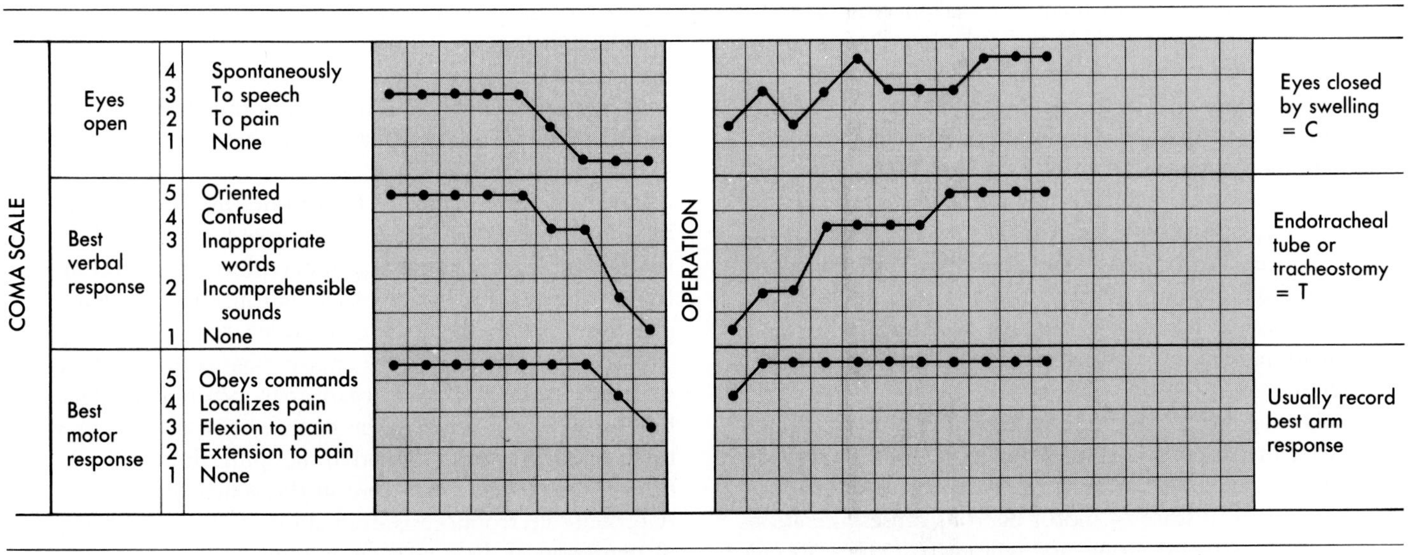

FIG. 38-12 Glasgow Coma Scale, demonstrating measurement of level of consciousness. Record "C" if eyes are closed by edema; record "T" if endotracheal tube or tracheostomy tube is in place. Notice change in patient's condition just before and after surgery.

and consists of assessment of three parts of the neurological assessment: eye opening, best motor response, and best verbal response.

The stronger the stimulus needed to obtain a response, the lower the patient's score. The number value assigned to each part of the scale is added to yield an objective score. The score for a patient who is not neurologically impaired is 14 to 16, depending on the system used. The lowest possible score is 3. Generally, any score of 7 or less is commonly accepted as a definition of coma. The scale has a high degree of consistency even when used by staff of varied experience.

Language and speech. It is important to assess the language and speech capability of the neurological patient. Speech is a function of the dominant hemisphere, which is on the left side of the brain for all right-handed people and most left-handed people. **Aphasia** is a disorder of language caused by damage to the speech-controlling areas of the brain (Broca's area in the frontal lobe and Wernicke's area in the posterior part of the temporal lobe). It includes all areas of language, including speech, reading, writing, and understanding. Aphasia has been subdivided as follows:

1. Sensory aphasia or receptive aphasia—inability to comprehend the spoken word or written word
2. Motor aphasia—inability to use symbols of speech (also called expressive aphasia)
3. Global aphasia—inability to understand the spoken word, as well as to speak

Anomia is a form of aphasia characterized by the inability to name objects. **Dysarthria** is defined as difficult, poorly articulated speech that usually results from interference in the control over the muscles of speech. The general cause is damage to a central or peripheral nerve.

Cranial nerves. Assessment of cranial nerve function is another important part of the neurological assessment. The 12 pairs of nerves emerge from the cranial cavity through openings in the skull. (See Table 38-1 for specifics of cranial nerve classification and assessment.)

Motor function. Evaluation of motor status of the neurological patient will detect abnormalities in the normal functioning of nerves and muscles. Motor function disturbances are the most commonly encountered neurological symptom. In general, the parts of the motor status examination include gait and stance, muscle tone, coordination, involuntary movements, and the muscle stretch reflexes.

Damage to the nervous system often causes a serious problem in mobility. A loss of function is called **paralysis**; a lesser degree of movement deficit is called *paresis*.

Injury or disease of motor neurons causes alterations of muscle strength, tone, and reflex activity. The specific signs and symptoms seen vary according to whether the lesion involves an upper motor neuron or a lower motor neuron. Muscles may be **flaccid**, with absent deep tendon reflexes, or they may be spastic, with increased reflexes. With some muscle problems, the affected muscle shows small, localized, spontaneous and involuntary contractions called **fasciculations**. With other problems, **clonus** (a forced series of alternating contractions and partial relaxation of a muscle) may occur.

Sensory and perceptual status. The sensory examination is the most difficult part of the neurological evaluation. Specific alterations in sensation that should be assessed include pain, touch, temperature, **proprioception** (the ability to know the position of the body without looking at it), and the ability to "know" objects by the sense of touch.

In clinical settings it is usually not feasible or necessary to complete the total neurological examination during shift-to-shift assessments of the patient. In many settings, however, such as intensive care units, the neurological checks may be done as frequently as every hour. Factors that are the most important include orientation, level of consciousness, muscle strength, ability to speak, involuntary movements, and any abnormal posturing.

Laboratory Tests

Blood and urine tests. Assessment of the neurologically impaired patient includes a variety of blood and urine tests. A culture of the urine may rule out infection involving the urinary tract. Other urine testing may indicate the presence of **diabetes insipidus**. Urine drug screens may be done to rule out drug use as a cause of lethargy or to identify specific drugs ingested.

Arterial blood gas values may be an important diagnostic tool in monitoring the oxygen content of the blood. The gases may be altered with neurological diseases such as Guillain-Barré syndrome, in which breathing patterns may be altered. Blood tests that are routinely done may help narrow the diagnosis of neurological disorder.

Cerebrospinal fluid. Examination of the **cerebrospinal fluid** (CSF) can yield information about many neurological conditions.

Normally there are up to 10 lymphocytes per milliliter of spinal fluid. An increase in the number of cells may indicate an infection, such as tuberculosis or a viral infection. Bacterial infections such as tuberculous meningitis often lower the CSF glucose level, as well as the chloride levels. A culture or smear examination is done to determine the causative organism in meningitis. Spinal fluid protein is elevated when degenerative diseases or a brain tumor is present. Blood in the spinal fluid indicates hemorrhage from somewhere in the ventricular system. A protein electrophoresis evaluation may give evidence of neurological diseases such as multiple sclerosis (Box 38-4).

Other tests. Plain skull x-ray films of the head and vertebral column are useful in ruling out fractures of the skull and cervical vertebrae. Since the development of the

BOX 38-4 **NORMAL CHARACTERISTICS OF CEREBROSPINAL FLUID (CSF)**

Specific gravity	1.007
pH	7.35 to 7.45
Chloride	120 to 130 mEq/L
Glucose	50 to 80 mg/dl
Pressure	80 to 200 mm/water
Total volume	80 to 200 ml (15 ml in ventricles)
Total protein	15 to 45 mg/dl (lumbar) 10 to 25 mg/dl (cisternal) 5 to 15 mg/dl (ventricular)
Gamma globulin	6% to 13% of total protein
Cell count	
RBC	None
WBC	0-5 0-10 cells (all lymphocytes and monocytes)

CT scan, skull x-ray films are not used as extensively as before.

Computed tomography (CT) scan. The purpose of the CT scan, also called the *CAT scan*, is to detect pathological conditions of the cerebrum and spinal cord using a technique of scanning without radioisotopes. There is no special physical preparation of the patient for the test. The CT scan takes 20 to 30 minutes if done without contrast medium and about 60 minutes if the scan is also done with contrast. The procedure is painless, except for the slight discomfort that occurs when an intravenous line is started for the injection of the contrast dye. There is also some discomfort in lying still, and possible feelings of claustrophobia as a result of the head being positioned in the head holder. If contrast medium is used, it is important for the nurse to document and report to the physician any history of allergy to iodine and seafood, because iodine is present in the contrast medium.

During the procedure, the patient lies supine with the head positioned within a rubber head holder to prevent air gaps between the machine and the scalp. The head is scanned in two planes simultaneously and at various angles. Each image that appears is a specific layer of brain tissue. The computer displays a printout that indicates areas of increased densities (e.g. tumors or thrombi).

Brain scan. Like the CT scan, the brain scan's purpose is the detection of pathological conditions of the cerebrum. It uses radioactive isotopes and a scanner. There is no special physical preparation of the patient. The procedure takes approximately 45 minutes for the actual scan. The patient is injected with a radioisotope (mercury or sodium pertechnetate [Tc 99m]). While the patient lies still, a scanner is passed over the brain area. Concentrated areas of uptake are reflected. There are generally no adverse effects from the procedure and only minimal discomfort associated with the intravenous administration of the radioactive isotopes. If mercury is used as the isotope indicator, a mercurial diuretic (meralluride [Mercuhydrin]) is administered several hours before the procedure to allow a greater concentration of the mercury to be circulated to brain tissue, since meralluride minimizes the uptake of mercury by the kidneys.

MRI scan. The magnetic resonance imaging (MRI) scan uses magnetic forces to image body structures. It has relevance in the nervous system as a way to detect pathological conditions of the cerebrum and spinal cord. Because the scan involves a magnetic force, the patient should be cautioned to remove watches, credit cards, and other metal from the clothing before entering the scanning room. The patient should also be questioned about the presence of any metal in the body that would preclude the use of the scan, such as orthopedic appliances, aneurysm clips, and pacemakers.

During the procedure the patient lies supine with the head positioned in a head holder. The test takes 45 to 60 minutes. The procedure is painless, except for discomfort in lying still and possible feelings of claustrophobia. The patient should be warned that the machine makes different and somewhat loud noises during the scanning procedure.

PET scan. Another evaluative measure that is similar to the CT scan and MRI scan is the positron emission tomography (PET) scan. In this procedure the patient receives an injection of deoxyglucose with radioactive fluorine. The area in question is scanned and a color composite picture is obtained. Shades of color give an indication of the level of glucose metabolism; this then can be translated into indications of a pathological state. As with the CT scan, discomfort is minimal. The patient should be aware of the need to lie still for the duration of the scan, usually about 45 minutes.[39]

Lumbar puncture. A lumbar puncture is often performed as part of the diagnostic workup of the patient who may have a neurological problem. It is contraindicated in patients who might have increased intracranial pressure, because the withdrawal of fluid may cause the medulla oblongata to herniate downward into the foramen magnum.

The purpose of the lumbar puncture is to obtain CSF for examination or relief of pressure or to allow the introduction of dye or medication. It is a common procedure, usually done in the patient's room. The procedure takes 10 to 15 minutes. Slight pain and pressure may be felt as the dura is entered. A sharp, shooting pain down one leg may occur, caused by the needle coming close to a nerve.

The patient is usually positioned on the side with the knee and head flexed at an acute angle. This allows for maximal lumbar flexion and separation of the interspinous spaces. After anesthetizing the area with a local anesthetic, the physician inserts the needle below the level of the spinal cord, at the L4-L5 or L5-S1 interspace. The inner needle is removed to allow for drainage and measurement of spinal fluid. The level-of-fluid column in the manometer is used to measure the pressure. Fluid may be collected for various tests or to relieve pressure. The first specimen of spinal fluid may contain blood from slight bleeding at the site of the puncture. This specimen should not be sent for cell count.

After the procedure, the patient lies flat in bed for several hours. The site of the puncture should be assessed for any leakage, as evidenced by moisture on the bandage or around the puncture site. Headache is fairly common and is thought to be caused by the loss of spinal fluid through the dura mater. If a headache develops, bed rest, analgesics, and ice to the head may help.

Electroencephalogram. The electroencephalogram (EEG) is used to provide evidence of focal or generalized disturbances of brain function by measuring the electrical activity of the brain. There is no special preparation for this test, but the patient is encouraged to be quiet and rest before the procedure, unless it is to be a sleep-deprived EEG. With this, the patient is kept awake the night before the test, and the EEG is usually done first thing in the morning. The EEG usually takes about 1 hour to complete. The hair and scalp of the patient should be clean. The electrodes are placed on the scalp with collodion in a set pattern to cover all scalp areas. There is no pain associated with the EEG.

The basic resting rhythm of the electroencephalogram is affected by opening the eyes or altering attention. Recordings are sometimes made while the patient is asleep or sleep deprived, when the seizure threshold may be lowered. Comparisons are made of different patterns of the recordings (Fig. 38-13). After the test the patient should be allowed to rest. The patient should be assisted if necessary in washing the hair and removing the collodion from the scalp.

Myelogram. The myelogram is commonly used to identify lesions in the intradural or extradural compartments of the spinal canal by observing the flow of radiopaque dye through the subarachnoid space. The two types of dyes most commonly used are metrizamide and iophendylate (Pantopaque) dye. Before the procedure the patient's baselines of lower extremity strength and sensation are assessed and documented. The patient is informed that the procedure takes about 2 hours. The patient should also be told that there may be slight discomfort as the dura is entered and that he may be asked to assume a variety of positions during the procedure.

If the patient is scheduled for a metrizamide myelogram, he should not take some drugs for 24 to 48 hours before the scan because they lower the seizure threshold, one of the side effects of the dye. These drugs include

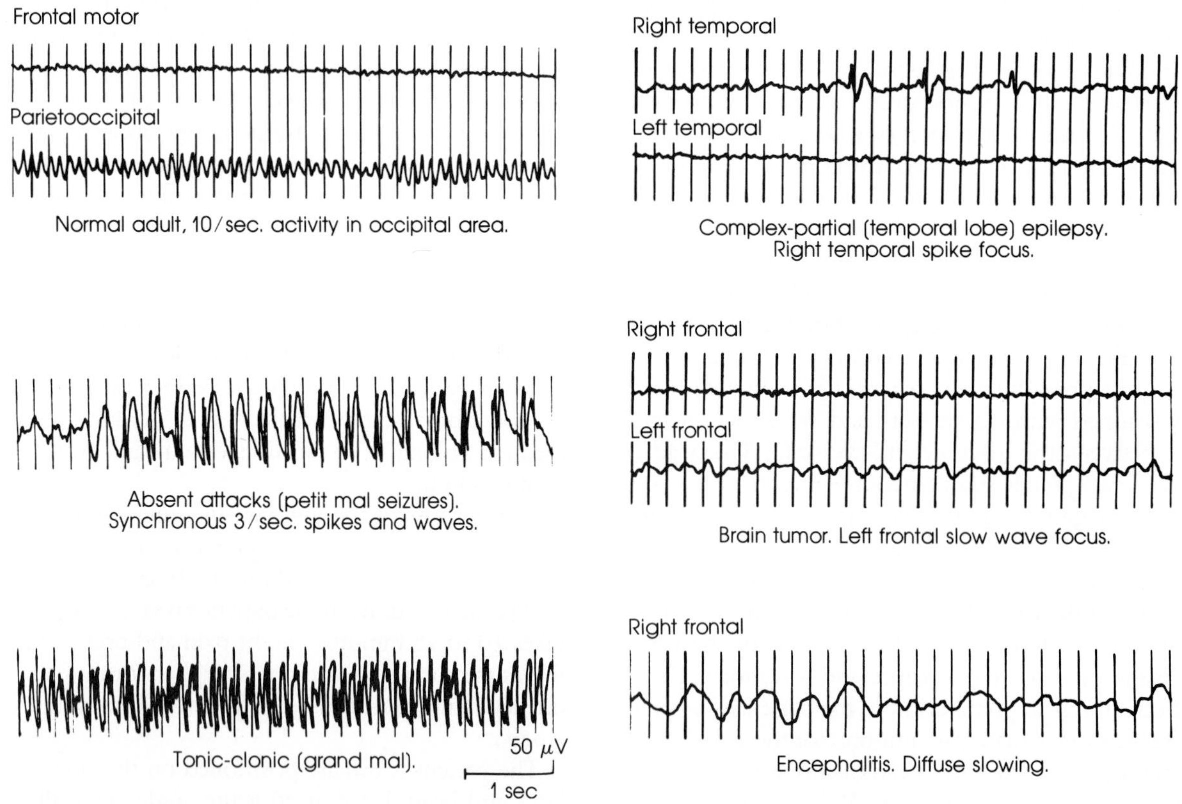

FIG. 38-13 Tracings of electroencephalogram. The normal tracing is demonstrated, as are several pathological states.

the phenothiazines, tricyclic antidepressants, CNS stimulants, and amphetamines.

The patient is usually positioned on his side with both knees and the head flexed at an acute angle to allow maximal flexion of the lumbar area for ease in performing the lumbar puncture. After the puncture is performed, the inner needle is removed to allow drainage of CSF, measurement of pressure, and collection of specimens. The dye is instilled and the needle is removed. The patient is then turned to various positions so the spinal cord can be visualized while fluoroscopic and radiopaque films are taken. After the procedure is completed, Pantopaque dye must be removed via another lumbar puncture to prevent serious irritation of the meninges. Metrizamide dye does not have to be removed. The patient usually undergoes a CT scan 4 to 6 hours after a metrizamide myelogram.

Care after the procedure varies, depending on the dye used. With a Pantopaque myelogram, the patient lies flat in bed overnight. No pillow is used, and the head of the bed is not elevated. The site of the puncture should be observed for any leakage of CSF, and the strength and sensation of the lower extremities should be assessed. Headache is fairly common after the procedure.

If the patient has had a myelogram using metrizamide dye, his head and thorax must remain elevated to at least 30 to 50 degrees for at least 8 hours and then elevated to at least 30 degrees for another 24 hours. Fluid intake is encouraged to assist in absorption of the dye. Common side effects with this dye include nausea, vomiting, and seizures, as well as nonspecific behavior changes. The peak risk for these side effects is 4 to 6 hours after completion of the procedure. The site of the puncture and strength and sensation of the lower extremities are assessed. The patient must avoid the use of the same drugs that were restricted before the procedure for 24 to 48 hours, because they lower the seizure threshold. Despite the side effects, the advantages of the metrizamide myelogram are many. The dye is less viscous and allows better visualization of smaller areas than that obtained with a myelogram using Pantopaque dye.

Angiogram. The angiogram (cerebral arteriography) is a fairly common procedure used to visualize the cerebral arterial system by injecting radiopaque material. It allows the detection of arterial aneurysms, vessel anomalies, ruptured vessels, and displacements of vessels by tumors or masses.

Before the procedure the patient is usually given clear liquids, although in some institutions all oral intake is restricted. The patient must be assessed for any allergy to iodine because the dye contains iodine. If the femoral approach is to be used, it is helpful to assess and mark the locations of the bilateral pedal pulses. If the carotid artery is used, the neck circumference is measured as part of the baseline data. Immediately before the procedure, baseline vital signs and pulses are measured, and a neurological check is performed and recorded.

The test takes approximately 2 to 3 hours. The patient may experience discomfort in lying still for that period of time. When the dye is injected, most patients complain of feeling extremely hot and seeing flashes of light.

The patient is positioned supine on the x-ray table. A local anesthetic agent is used to anesthetize the area of the puncture site. The catheter is introduced percutaneously and introduced into the relevant vessels. At times, the catheter may be inserted directly into the carotid or vertebral arteries. After all the injections are done, the catheter is withdrawn and pressure is applied to the puncture site for at least 15 minutes.

After the procedure, bed rest is ordered for a specified time, usually 4 to 6 hours. Vital signs are checked frequently (at times as often as every 15 minutes), and a neurological check is performed with every vital sign check. The site of the puncture is assessed frequently for the presence of a hematoma. With a femoral stick, the pulses distal to the site are checked for evidence of arterial occlusion. With a carotid stick, the patient is assessed for any difficulty breathing or swallowing or an increase in the girth of the neck.

The patient undergoing this procedure is at risk for cerebral vascular accident, as well as an increase in intracranial pressure. Any change in level of consciousness or other parts of the neurological assessment should be promptly reported.

Digital subtraction angiography. In digital subtraction angiography (DSA), abnormalities of the cerebrovascular system are identified using a process that removes overlying structures from the image, so that clinically significant details can be displayed in an enhanced way. Often the same vessels used for an angiogram are used with the DSA. Care of the patient before and after the procedure is the same as that for the patient undergoing angiography.

Electromyogram. An electromyogram (EMG) is used to measure the contraction of a muscle in response to electrical stimulation. It provides evidence of lower motor neuron disease, primary muscle disease, and defects in the transmission of electrical impulses at the **neuromuscular junction**, such as in myasthenia gravis. There is no special preparation for the test. The test takes approximately 45 minutes for one muscle study. The patient needs to know that there will be discomfort when the electrode is inserted into the muscle and when the electrical current is used. The muscle may ache for a short time after the procedure.

During the test, an electrode is inserted into selected skeletal muscles. An electric current is passed through the electrode, and the machine graphs the variations of muscle potentials (voltage). After the procedure it is important to assess the patient for signs of bleeding at the site of the electrode insertion. The patient may need an analgesic for discomfort and a rest period.

Echoencephalogram. An echoencephalogram uses ultrasound to depict the intracranial structures of the brain. It is especially helpful in detecting ventricular dilation and a major shift of midline structures in the brain as a result of an expanding lesion. The preparation of the patient, the actual procedure, and aftercare are similar to those of the brain scan.

Other tests. Several other tests are used to detect neurological problems of the ventricles and cisternal system. These include the **ventriculogram** and the **pneumoencephalogram**. Both tests use air as a contrast; it is inserted into the ventricular system. The ventriculogram is usually performed in the operating room under general or intravenous anesthesia. The pneumoencephalogram is done rarely since the advent of less-invasive procedures such as the CT scan. After either procedure the patient is often quite uncomfortable, with a headache and nausea. Side effects are common until the air is absorbed, usually in 24 to 48 hours.

Common Neurological Problems

Headaches

Etiology/pathophysiology. Headache is a common neurological complaint; its significance is variable and it can result from many different causes. The source of recurring headache should be determined through careful physical examination with appropriate neurological assessment. Some tumors may produce no symptoms except for headache for a long period.

The exact mechanism of head pain is not known. Although the skull and brain tissues are not able to feel sensory pain, pain arises from the scalp and its blood vessels and muscles and from the dura mater and its venous sinuses. Pain also arises from the blood vessels at the base of the brain and from cervical cranial nerves. Blood vessels may dilate and become congested with blood. Headaches can be classified as vascular, tension, and traction-inflammatory. Vascular headaches include migraine, cluster, and hypertensive headaches. Tension headaches may arise from psychological problems of tension or stress or from medical problems such as cervical arthritis. Traction-inflammatory headaches include those caused by infection, intracranial or extracranial causes, by occlusive vascular structures, and by temporal arteritis.

Clinical manifestations. Headache pain may be made worse by stress or tension. Knowledge of the patient's perception of the effect of stress on the headache pain is important in planning effective interventions.

Migraine headaches are unusual in that there are **prodromal** (early signs and symptoms of a developing condition or disease) signs and symptoms that occur before the acute attack. These may include any of the following: visual field defects, experiencing unusual smells or sounds, confusion, paresthesias, and paralysis of a part of the body (in rare cases). During a migraine headache, signs and symptoms may include nausea, vomiting, sensitivity to light, chilliness, fatigue, irritability, diaphoresis, edema, and other signs of autonomic dysfunction.

Assessment. Collection of *subjective data* includes the patient's understanding of the headache, possible causes, and any precipitating factors. It is important to determine what measures relieve the symptoms, as well as the location, frequency, pattern, and character of the pain. This includes the site of return of the headache, time of day, and intervals between the headaches. The initial onset of the headache, presence of any symptoms that occur before the headache or associated symptoms, the presence of allergies, and any family history of similar headache patterns are also important to assess.

Collection of *objective data* includes any behaviors indicating stress, anxiety, or pain. Changes in the ability to carry out activities of daily living, an abnormally raised body temperature, and the presence of sinus drainage may be important. Abnormalities noted during the physical examination portion of the neurological assessment should also be documented. (See therapeutic dialogue below.)

Diagnostic tests. It is important to evaluate headaches that are not transient. Usual testing includes a neurolog-

THERAPEUTIC DIALOGUE

NURSE: Can you describe your problem to me?
PATIENT: It's a pain in my head.
NURSE: When did this pain start?
PATIENT: About a month ago.
NURSE: Did anything else happen at that same time?
PATIENT: My daughter left home for college.
NURSE: How did you feel about that?
PATIENT: I was really upset. She was my baby. I can't believe that she's gone.
NURSE: Was there anything else that you noticed at the same time? Like an increased temperature or nasal drainage?
PATIENT: No, I don't think so.
NURSE: What made the headache worse?
PATIENT: Thinking about my loneliness.
NURSE: What made the headache better?
PATIENT: Sleeping or taking a Valium.
NURSE: Have you had trouble sleeping or noticed that your appetite was worse?
PATIENT: I wake up early in the morning. I don't feel much like eating.
NURSE: Have you lost weight?
PATIENT: About 10 pounds in the last month.
NURSE: Can you tell me what the pain feels like?
PATIENT: It's a pain that goes through my whole head. It throbs and gets worse in the evening.
NURSE: What do you think is the cause of the headache?
PATIENT: I guess maybe I'm upset that my daughter left.

ical examination, a CT scan (MRI or PET scan may also be done), a brain scan, skull x-ray films, and a lumbar puncture. A lumbar puncture is not done, however, if there is evidence of increased intracranial pressure or if a brain tumor is suspected, because quick reduction of pressure produced by removal of the spinal fluid may cause brain herniation. In these situations, a CT scan is done first.

Medical management

Dietary counseling. Some foods may cause or worsen headaches. These include foods containing tyramine, nitrates, or glutamates. One example of this is monosodium glutamate (MSG), often used in the preparation of Chinese foods. Other substances that may provoke headaches include vinegar, chocolate, yogurt, alcohol, fermented or marinated foods, ripened cheese, cured sandwich meat, caffeine, and pork.

Psychotherapy. Patients with headaches may respond to psychotherapy. This is not to say that the headache pain is not physiological in nature, but counseling can help the patient to develop awareness of stress factors and to deal with the pain. The patient may need help in expressing feelings about intractable headache pain.

Medications. Medications are often used to treat headache. These will be described in terms of their use for migraine, cluster, and tension headaches.

MIGRAINE HEADACHES. Acetylsalicylic acid (aspirin) may be helpful after a migraine headache has developed. Ergotamine tartrate preparations taken early in the attack may prevent progression of the headache. These drugs are usually successful in treating migraines. Ergotamine tartrate preparations act by constricting cerebral blood vessel walls and reducing cerebral blood flow. They can be given orally, sublingually, rectally, or by injection. These preparations are also available in combinations with other drugs, such as caffeine, phenobarbital, and belladonna. Side effects of ergot preparations include nausea, vomiting, numbness and tingling, muscle pain, and changes in heart rate. They cannot be taken by pregnant women, because they stimulate contractions of the uterine smooth muscle.

Other drugs that may be used include nonnarcotic analgesics, such as phenacetin, acetaminophen, or propoxyphene (Darvon). Codeine may be prescribed. Propranolol hydrochloride (Inderal) has been used in the prophylactic treatment of migraine and other vascular headaches.

CLUSTER HEADACHES. Because the pain associated with vascular cluster headaches is often extremely severe, narcotic analgesics, sometimes given intramuscularly, are used. Patients with cluster headaches usually feel fine between attacks, so no analgesic is needed during these times.

TENSION HEADACHES. Nonnarcotic analgesics are often used to treat tension headaches. These include acetaminophen, propoxyphene, phenacetin, and acetylsalicylic acid (aspirin). Narcotic analgesics such as codeine may be prescribed, along with a medication such as diazepam (Valium) for relief of tension. However, because these drugs are often subject to abuse, it is much better to counsel patients to develop other ways to relieve headaches.

Nursing interventions. Since stress and emotional upsets may precipitate some headaches and worsen others, relaxation and rest should be facilitated. This includes relaxation techniques, planned sleeping hours, and regular rest periods. The patient may need the nurse to help him do this. Alcohol should not be used to relieve tension, because it may become addicting and has been found to be a significant cause of cluster headaches. Regular physical exercise may also help to prevent headaches, especially ones caused by tension.

If a patient is suffering from a severe headache, the nurse should plan nursing interventions so that only essential activities take place. Interventions should be grouped so that the patient has adequate time to rest.

Comfort measures. Other treatments that may be helpful for a patient with a headache include cold packs applied to the forehead or base of the skull. Pressure applied to the temporal arteries may be helpful. Persons with migraine headaches, especially, are usually most comfortable lying in a dark room with minimal auditory stimulation.

Identifying triggering factors. Triggering factors associated with severe and recurring headaches may include fatigue, alcohol, stress, seasonal climate changes, hunger, allergies, and menstruation. The nurse may need to help the patient identify these factors. They can be assessed through ongoing observation of the patient's personality, habits, and activities of daily living, as well as career plans, work habits, family relationships, coping mechanisms, and relaxation activities. A diary or journal kept by the patient may be helpful in determining these factors.

NURSING DIAGNOSES. Nursing diagnoses and interventions for the patient with headache include, but are not limited to, the following.

NURSING DIAGNOSES	NURSING INTERVENTIONS
Anxiety, related to pain	Provide quiet environment. Encourage verbalization of concerns. Provide diversional activities.
Pain, acute or chronic, related to disease process	Administer analgesics as ordered. Provide comfort measures. Maintain nonstressful environment. Encourage pain reduction techniques as appropriate: rocking movements, external warmth, breathing patterns.

Patient teaching. Teaching is an important part of the nursing intervention of the patient with headaches. Topics include (1) avoidance of factors that trigger headaches, (2) relaxation techniques including biofeedback, (3) importance of maintaining regular sleep patterns, (4) medications to be used (including dose, actions, and side effects), and (5) the importance of follow-up care.

Neurological pain

Etiology/pathophysiology and clinical manifestations. Neurological pain, other than headache, is common. The transmission of pain is not fully understood, but patients may experience disabling pain either caused by a disorder within the nervous system or caused peripherally at a distant part of the body.

The transmission of pain impulses is not fully understood. Neurological pain may arise from lesions involving the peripheral cutaneous nerves, the sensory nerve roots, the thalamus, and the central pain tract (lateral spinothalamic) at some level. Each produces characteristic pain. Pain receptors are not adaptable, and pain impulses continue at the same rate as long as the stimulus is present. They are specific for pain only. Pain receptors can be activated by cellular damage; certain chemicals such as histamine; heat; ischemia; muscle spasm; and sensations of cold and pruritus that go beyond a specific level of intensity.

Pain that is described as unbearable and does not respond to treatment is classified as *intractable*. It is chronic and often debilitating, and may prevent the patient from functioning in activities of daily living.

Assessment. The perception of pain is highly subjective. Collection of *subjective data* includes the patient's understanding of the pain, any precipitating factors, and measures that relieve stress, including medication. The site, frequency, and nature of the pain are important, as well as the usual coping patterns of the patient when under stress. The presence of associated symptoms and measures that make the pain worse are important subjective data.

The quality of pain and its distribution are important factors to assess. Pain may vary from mild to excruciating. Some terms that are important include the following[25]:

Paresthesia—abnormal sensation
Hyperalgesia—increased pain sensation
Hypoalgesia—decreased pain sensation
Analgesia—blocked pain sensation
Dysesthesia—pain sensation caused by a stimulus that normally would not be painful
Referred pain—pain that occurs in a site other than its origin
Causalgia—intense, continuous, burning pain
Local pain—occurring as a result of direct stimulation of pain receptors

Collection of *objective data* may be limited when assessing neurological pain. Objective factors that should be assessed are any behavioral signs indicating pain or stress, a change in the ability to carry out activities of daily living, any muscle weakness or wasting, vasomotor responses (such as flushing), abnormalities of spinal reflexes, and abnormalities noted during the sensory examination.

Diagnostic tests. Diagnostic tests for the patient in pain may include electrical stimulation used to define the pain to a greater degree. Psychological testing may be part of the workup. If back or neck pain is present, a myelogram is usually performed.

Medical management

Nonsurgical methods of pain control. Neurological pain sometimes responds to other methods of pain control. These include transcutaneous electrical nerve stimulation (TENS) and spinal cord stimulation. Both techniques use electrodes applied near the site of pain or on or around the spine. The stimulator is used to modify the sensory input by blocking or changing the painful sensation with a stimulus that is perceived to be less painful or nonpainful. Acupuncture has also been used to treat patients with neurological pain.

NERVE BLOCK. A nerve block is used to control intractable pain. It involves the injection of a local anesthetic, alcohol, or phenol close enough to a nerve to block the conduction of impulses. Sources of pain often treated with a nerve block include trigeminal neuralgia, cancer, or peripheral vascular disease. The duration of effect is from several months to several years.

MEDICATIONS. Medications are often used to treat patients with neurological pain. These often include nonnarcotic analgesics such as acetaminophen, propoxyphene (Darvon), phenacetin, and acetylsalicylic acid. Narcotics may be prescribed, as well as muscle relaxants, but these drugs may lead to abuse.[42] The emphasis should be on helping the patient learn other measures to control the pain.[41]

Surgery. In cases of intractable pain that does not respond to more conservative measures, surgery may be necessary to reduce or abolish pain. Neurosurgical procedures that may be done include neurectomy, **rhizotomy**, cordotomy, and **percutaneous cordotomy**.[31]

These procedures all have potential complications that need to be considered before the decision is made to perform surgery. For example, a patient who undergoes a cordotomy may be expected to have difficulties with postural hypotension, ability to feel hot or cold, and possibly motor and bowel function. Temporary edema of the cord from the procedure may lead to temporary paralysis or leg weakness.

Nursing interventions

Comfort measures. A patient with neurological pain may be very uncomfortable and should be assisted to assume a position of comfort. For example, the patient with back pain should avoid movements that cause direct or indirect movement of the spinal cord. The patient may find lying in a supine position uncomfortable. The nurse should help the patient find a comfortable position and may need to actively assist the patient in turning or moving. Straining when having a stool can intensify pain, and a stool softener may be needed. The nurse should offer prune juice and a high-fiber diet and encourage up to 2000 ml a day or more of fluids.

Promotion of rest and relaxation. As with headache, stress and emotional upsets may precipitate or exacerbate neurological pain. Rest and relaxation should be facilitated, with planned sleeping hours and rest periods as needed.

Some patients with pain, especially intractable pain, may respond well to psychotherapy. This does not mean that the pain does not have a physiological basis, but counseling can help the patient develop awareness of what makes the pain worse and how to cope with the discomfort.

NURSING DIAGNOSES. Nursing diagnoses and interventions for neurological pain are the same as those listed previously for headache, with the addition of the following.

NURSING DIAGNOSES	NURSING INTERVENTIONS
Potential for disuse syndrome, related to lack of use of a body part as a result of pain	Explain need for regular exercise program to maintain joint mobility: ROM exercises to all body joints q2h to 4h. Be positive and reassuring in approach.
Feeding, bathing/hygiene, dressing/grooming, self-care deficit, related to pain	Provide basic ADL needs as necessary, but encourage patient to begin to participate at ability level. Provide sufficient time for ADLs. Facilitate use of self-help devices as needed. Provide for total hygiene as indicated.

Patient teaching. Teaching is an important part of the nursing interventions of the patient with neurological pain. Teaching should include at least the factors that are taught to the patient with headache. Also important is the awareness of physical methods such as positioning the body to increase comfort and the structuring of the home and work setting to keep stressors at a minimum.

Increased intracranial pressure

Etiology/pathophysiology and clinical manifestations. Increased intracranial pressure is a complex grouping of events that occurs because of multiple neurological conditions. It often occurs suddenly, can progress rapidly, and often requires surgical intervention. It is a potential complication in many neurological conditions and can rapidly lead to death if not arrested and reversed.

Specific causes of increased intracranial pressure include space-occupying lesions that increase tissue volume, cerebrospinal problems, and cerebral edema. An increase in any one of the contents of the cranium is usually accompanied by a reciprocal change in the volume of one of the others. This is because the cranial vault is rigid and nonexpandable. The buildup of pressure may occur slowly over weeks or rapidly, depending on the cause. Usually one side of the brain will be more involved, but both sides of the brain will eventually be involved.

As the pressure increases within the cranial cavity, it is first compensated for by venous compression and cerebrospinal displacement. As the pressure continues to rise, the cerebral blood flow decreases and inadequate perfusion of the brain occurs. This inadequate perfusion starts a vicious cycle that causes the PCO_2 to increase and the PO_2 and the pH to fall. These changes cause vasodilation and cerebral edema. This edema leads to further increased intracranial pressure, which causes increased compression of neural tissue and an even greater increase in intracranial pressure.

When the pressure buildup is greater than the brain's ability to compensate, pressure is exerted on surrounding structures where the pressure is lower. This movement of pressure is called *supratentorial shift* and can result in herniation.

As a result of herniation of the brain, the brainstem is compressed at various levels, which in turn compresses the vasomotor center, the posterior cerebral artery, the oculomotor nerve, the corticospinal nerve pathway, and the fibers of the ascending reticular activating system. The life-sustaining mechanisms of consciousness, blood pressure, pulse, respiration, and temperature regulation are all impaired.

Assessment. The detection of increased intracranial pressure must occur early while it is still reversible. The ability to make accurate observations, interpret observations intelligently, and record observations carefully is most important for the nurse working with patients with increased intracranial pressure.[21]

Collection of *subjective data* for a diagnosis of increased intracranial pressure includes the patient's understanding of the condition, presence of any visual changes (**diplopia** or blurred vision), and a change in the ability to think. The diplopia usually results from paralysis or weakness of one of the muscles that controls the eye movement. It often occurs fairly early in the process of increased intracranial pressure. The presence of nausea or pain, especially headache, is also important. The headache is thought to result from venous congestion and the tension in the intracranial blood vessels as the cerebral pressure rises. Headache that occurs with increased intracranial pressure usually increases in intensity with coughing, straining at stool, or stooping. It is usually present in the early morning and may awaken the patient from sleep.

Collection of *objective data* includes a change in the level of consciousness.[22] A decreasing level of consciousness is an early sign of increased intracranial pressure. This may include disorientation, restlessness, or lethargy. Observations are recorded in terms of behaviors and symptoms, not in terms of labels. It is important to chart what is seen, not what is inferred.

Pupillary signs may also change with increased intra-

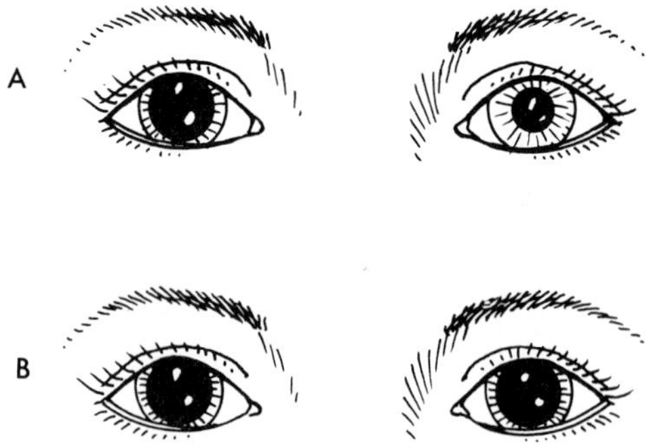

FIG. 38-14 A, Unequal pupils, also called anisocoria. B, Dilated and fixed pupils, indicative of severe neurological deficit.

cranial pressure. Pupillary responses are controlled by cranial nerve III (oculomotor nerve). As the brain herniates, the nerve is compressed with the top part of the nerve being affected first. The ipsilateral pupil (when the lesion is in one hemisphere) remains dilated and is incapable of constricting. The pupil appears larger than that of the affected side and does not react to light. As the intracranial pressure increases and both halves of the brain become affected, bilateral pupil dilation and fixation occurs. Dilating pupils that respond slowly to light are a sign of impending herniation. A pupil that is fixed and dilated is sometimes called a "blown pupil" and is an ominous sign that *must* be reported to the physician immediately[32] (Fig. 38-14).

Changes in the blood pressure and pulse are seen with increasing intracranial pressure. Herniation causes ischemia of the vasomotor center, which excites the vasoconstrictor fibers, causing the systolic blood pressure to rise. If the intracranial pressure continues to increase, diastolic blood pressure may fall, resulting in a widening pulse pressure.

Pressure in the vasomotor center also increases the transmission of parasympathetic impulses through the vagus nerve to the heart, causing a slowing of the pulse. A widened pulse pressure, increased systolic blood pressure, and bradycardia are together called *Cushing's response*. It is considered an important diagnostic sign of late-stage increased intracranial pressure.

Brain herniation produces respiratory problems that are variable and related to the level of the brainstem compression or failure. The breathing pattern may be deep and stertorous (snorelike) or periodic (Cheyne-Stokes) respirations. Ataxic breathing may also occur; this is an irregular and unpredictable breathing pattern with random, shallow, and deep breaths and occasional pauses. It is seen in patient with medulla oblongata damage. As intracranial pressure increases to fatal levels, respiratory paralysis occurs.

Failure of the thermoregulatory center because of compression occurs later with increased intracranial pressure. It results in high, uncontrolled temperatures. This hyperthermia increases the metabolism of brain tissue.

Compression of the upper motor neuron pathway (corticospinal tract) interrupts transmission of impulses to the lower motor neuron, and progressive muscle weakness occurs. The presence of the Babinski sign, hyperreflexia, and ridigity are additional signs of decreased motor function. Seizures may occur. Herniation of the upper part of the brainstem produces **decerebrate rigidity** (fixed posture with arms, legs, and trunk extended and with flexion of the palms and plantar joints) or **decorticate rigidity** (fixed posture with flexion of the arm, wrist, and fingers with adduction of the arms and extensors and internal rotation of the legs). The worsening of motor problems is significant, because it means that the intracranial pressure is continuing to increase[19] (Fig. 38-15).

Vomiting and singultus are two objective signs that may be seen with increased intracranial pressure. The vomiting is often projectile in nature. Singultus is caused by compression of the vagus nerve (cranial nerve X) that occurs as brainstem herniation occurs.

One last objective sign is papilledema, which is detected with the use of an ophthalmoscope (usually a physician function). As intracranial pressure increases, the pressure is transmitted to the eyes through the cerebrospinal fluid and to the optic disc. As the optic disc becomes edematous, the retina is also compressed. The damaged retina cannot detect light rays. Visual acuity is lessened as the blind spot enlarges. Papilledema is also called a *choked disc*.

Diagnostic tests. The diagnosis of increased intracranial pressure is usually made with a computed tomography or magnetic resonance scan, which can show actual structural hernation and shifting of the brain. Most of the time, however, acute increased intracranial pressure is a medical emergency and there is little time for diagnostic tests. The diagnosis must be made on the basis of frequent and careful observation and neurological testing. *The presence of even subtle changes can be very significant.*

In some postoperative or critically ill patients, internal measuring devices are used to diagnose increased intracranial pressure. One of the most common requires the placement of a hollow screw through the skull into the subarachnoid space. The device is connected to a transducer and oscilloscope for continuous monitoring. Waveforms are produced that indicate the intracranial pressure.

Medical management. The prevention of increased intracranial pressure may not be possible, but prevention of further increases in pressure with resulting damage to the brain is crucial. The medical treatment of the patient with increased intracranial pressure depends on the cause of the pressure. For example, surgery may be done to remove a tumor. If surgery is not possible, efforts are made to reduce the pressure through the use of drug therapy or other measures.

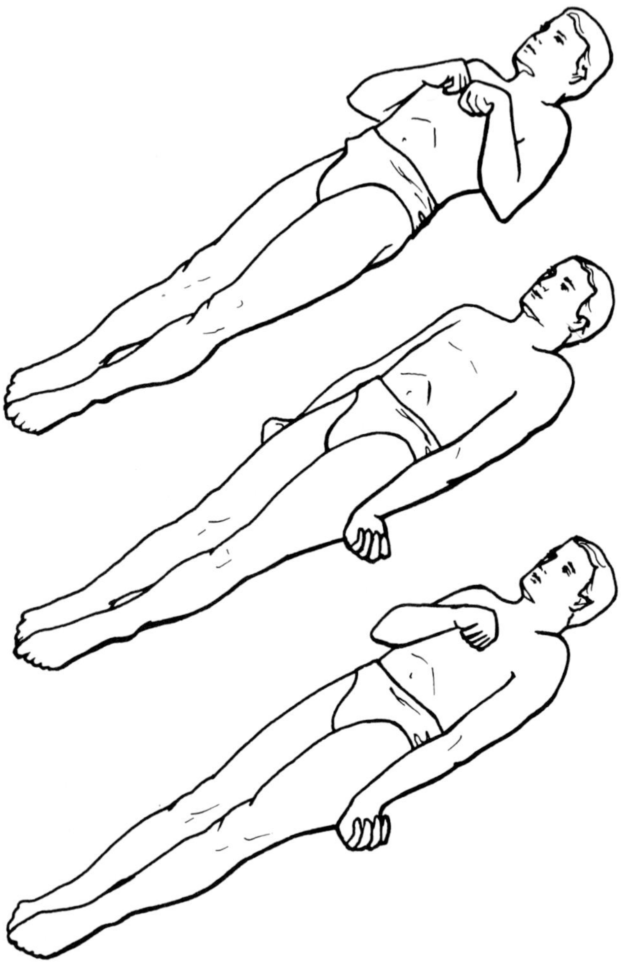

FIG. 38-15 **A,** Decorticate posturing: flexion of arms, wrists, and fingers with adduction in upper extremities. Extension, internal rotation, and plantar flexion in lower extremities. **B,** Decerebrate posturing: all four extremities in rigid extension, with hyperpronation of forearms and plantar extension of feet. **C,** Flexion of arm, wrist, and fingers on right side of body. Rigid extension with hyperpronation of left forearm. Plantar extension of feet.

Mechanical decompression. Rapidly rising intracranial pressure can be relieved by mechanical decompression. This may include a **craniotomy**, in which a bone flap is removed and then replaced, or a **craniectomy**, in which the bone flap is removed and not replaced. The craniectomy is often done when pressure is high. Other means of decompression may include drainage of the ventricles or any subdural hematoma.

Endotracheal intubation may be necessary. With the use of controlled ventilation, the P_{CO_2} can be lowered to below normal, which causes a slightly alkalotic pH. The decrease in the P_{CO_2} and the increase in pH will decrease vasodilation and decrease intracranial pressure.

Medications. Three types of medications are usually administered to patients with increased intracranial pressure: osmotic diuretics, corticosteroids, and anticonvulsants. Osmotic diuretics are also called hyperosmolar drugs. They draw water from the edematous brain tissue. An example of this type of medication is mannitol. It begins to reduce increased intracranial pressure within 15 minutes, and its effects last for 4 to 6 hours. Glycerol is another osmotic diuretic that is sometimes used.

The corticosteroid that is usually given is dexamethasone. With this drug, monitoring of blood glucose levels is important because steroids can affect carbohydrate metabolism and glucose utilization.

Anticonvulsants are given to prevent seizures. Phenytoin (Dilantin) is the most commonly given drug. It can be given intravenously but is usually not given intramuscularly because of poor absorption. Narcotics and other drugs that cause respiratory depression are avoided.

Nursing interventions

Conservative measures. Conservative measures to reduce venous volume may be implemented.[25] These include the following[44]:

1. Elevate head of the bed to 30 to 45 degrees to promote venous return
2. Place neck in neutral position (not flexed or extended)

3. Position patient to avoid flexion of the hips, waist, and neck as well as rotation of the head, especially to the right
4. Instruct patient to avoid isometric or resistive exercises
5. Restrict fluid intake
6. Implement measures to help patient avoid Valsalva maneuver (any forced expiratory effort against a closed airway, such as straining to have a stool)
7. Have a Foley catheter in place if the patient is not alert because of the large amount of urine that is produced
8. Perform suctioning only as necessary and only oropharyngeal
9. Administer oxygen via mask or cannula to improve cerebral perfusion
10. Use hypothermia blanket to control body temperature (increased body temperature increases brain damage)

NURSING DIAGNOSES. Nursing diagnoses and interventions for the patient with increased intracranial pressure may include, but are not limited to, the following.

NURSING DIAGNOSES	NURSING INTERVENTIONS
Ineffective breathing pattern, related to neuromuscular impairment	Maintain patent airway; avoid flexion of neck. Administer oxygen and humidification as ordered. Provide oral nasopharyngeal airway as indicated for managing secretions; suction oropharynx prn.
Sensory/perceptual alteration: visual, tactile, related to altered cerebrovascular perfusion	Maintain method of communication. Maintain safe environment. Anticipate needs of patient.
Potential for injury, related to physiological effects of sustained elevations in intracranial pressure	Elevate head of bed 30 degrees. Maintain body position: avoid semiprone or prone position. Avoid compression of neck veins. Check blood pressure, pulse, and respiration q 30 min. Perform neurological check q 30 min using Glasgow Coma Scale; report any findings below 8 to physician.

Patient teaching. The patient with increased intracranial pressure is often unresponsive. However, information about procedures that are being done should be shared with the patient and the family. This may help both be as cooperative as possible.

Alterations in muscle tone and motor function

Etiology/pathophysiology. Motor function disturbances are the most commonly encountered neurological symptoms. Damage to the nervous system often causes serious problems in mobility.

Clinical manifestations. Injury or disease of motor neurons results in alterations of muscle strength, tone, and reflex activity. The specific clinical manifestations differ according to the location of the neurological lesion.

Assessment. Collection of *subjective data* for patients with motor problems includes the patient's understanding of the problem and possible causes. The initial onset of the symptoms, measures that improve symptoms, and the presence of clumsiness or incoordination or abnormal sensation are important to assess. If the lesion occurs suddenly, as in spinal cord injury from trauma, subjective symptoms may be minimal. If the motor deficit develops slowly, subjective symptoms may be so subtle that they are at first ignored.[26]

Collection of *objective data* includes coordination, muscle strength, muscle tone, and the presence of any muscle atrophy. Reflexes are often checked, as well as the presence of clonus or fasciculations and the ability to move muscles. Any abnormal gait is significant, as well as a change in the ability to carry out ADLs.

Diagnostic tests. One of the most common procedures for detecting pathological conditions of muscle is the electromyogram. It detects the various types of electrical activity and abnormal patterns that may appear in resting muscle in the presence of pathology.

Medical management. Patients with motor problems may have problems with spasticity. Muscle relaxants may be used to decrease tone and involuntary movements. Some commonly prescribed medications include baclofen (Lioresal), dantrolene sodium (Dantrium), and diazepam (Valium). Common side effects of these drugs include drowsiness and vertigo. These side effects are increased by the use of alcohol or other depressants.

Some patients may have severe swallowing difficulty (**dysphagia**) and require prefeeding and feeding exercises. In patients at severe risk for aspiration, a video fluoroscopy with barium may be done to rule out aspiration. The procedure requires the patient to swallow a small amount of liquid or semisolid barium while a fluoroscopic examination is being done.

For patients with paralysis, the eye on the affected side of the body may need to be protected if the lid remains open and there is no blink reflex. The patient is at high risk for corneal scratches or irritation. Irrigation with a physiologic solution of sodium chloride may be used, followed by eye drops. An eye pad may be used to keep the eye closed, although eye shields are preferable.

Nursing interventions

Safety needs. Patients with paralysis have significant safety needs. This includes protection from falling, including the use of side rails when the patient is in bed and a chair restraint when the patient is in a chair, especially if balance cannot be maintained. If the patient also has a sensory problem, which often accompanies paralysis, the danger to a part of the body may not be realized. An example is the patient with a CVA who is not aware that a hemiplegic arm is hanging over the side of the wheelchair arm.

The eye on the affected side of the body should be cleaned and assessed for signs of infection on a regular basis, usually at least three times a day. The patient must also learn to inspect affected body parts for injury.

Skin over bony prominences needs to be inspected regularly for signs of pressure. Paralyzed persons are at risk for skin impairment and should be taught to turn themselves in bed and to reposition themselves in the bed or chair independently, if possible. If the patient is unable to turn independently, the nurse carries out this function. Usually the patient is turned from one side to another or from one side to the back to the other side. Repositioning also includes weight shifts, done by the patient or by staff. These weight shifts may include controlled leaning from one side to another or push-ups done by the patient. If the patient is not able to do the activity, he is taught to take the responsibility to remind the staff when it is time to do the weight shift.

Paralyzed or weakened areas should be inspected at least daily for any signs of skin impairment. A mirror is often used to assist in the assessment of skin by the patient. With this, the patient is able to visualize all skin areas and is not as dependent on staff or family.

Activity needs. The extremities of a person who has an acute motor problem may be flaccid at first. Spasticity of muscles develops gradually. The joints then become flexed and fixed in useless, deformed positions unless preventive measures are taken.

The nurse should carefully place the extremities in a normal anatomical position to prevent deformity. Counterpositioning may be helpful. In **hemiplegia**, for example, the affected upper extremity is pulled inward at the shoulder joint and the wrist drops; in the lower extremity the knee flexes and the foot drops. In counterpositioning the nurse positions the patient so that the shoulder and upper arm are in abduction, the elbow is flexed, the wrist is dorsiflexed, the knee is in neutral position, and the foot is dorsiflexed. If the person is supine, a pillow can be placed between the upper arm and body to hold the arm in abduction. Physical therapists and occupational therapists can provide splints and braces that can aid in positioning.

In positioning, footboards may be used to prevent footdrop, although some feel that these contribute to increased spasticity and should not be used routinely for patients who have muscle spasms. High-topped tennis shoes can help prevent footdrop, if initiated early, or other devices, such as splints or braces. In some hospitals, casts are applied to patients' lower extremities to prevent footdrop. A sling or hook hemi-harness may be useful to support the affected arm to prevent shoulder subluxation.

The prone position is excellent for patients who are able to tolerate it. Not only is the chance of skin impairment decreased with this position, but it also causes extension of the hip and knee joints, and the ankles by means of gravity. A pillow placed under the chest may help patients comfortably assume this position.

Positioning of the paralyzed person is extremely important. Complications such as footdrop and flexion contractures of the knee seriously limit mobility. As a result, the level of self-care and independence is diminished. Most joint deformities in a paralyzed person are preventable with early and continuing nursing interventions.

In addition to positioning, interventions for the person with paralysis include range of motion (ROM) exercises to all joints. These may be passive (carried out by the nurse) or active (carried out by the patient). Passive range of motion is indicated at least three times daily for all joints that the patient cannot voluntarily move.

Nutritional needs. Patience and persistence are often necessary in giving food and fluids to the patient with hemiplegia. Important nursing measures include avoiding foods that cause choking, checking the affected side of the mouth for accumulation of food and resultant poor hygiene, not mixing liquids and solid foods, and encouraging the patient to take small bites. If the patient has dentures they should be worn. The patient should sit at a 90-degree angle with the head up and chin slightly tucked. The head should not be extended and the patient should be encouraged to tip the head toward the unaffected side while swallowing.[9,20] Assistive devices for feeding include utensils with universal cuffs, covered plastic cups, scoop dishes, plate guards, and Asepto syringes. (See Fig. 48-1.) These enable the patient to assist himself to a greater degree and be less dependent on the staff. These devices are usually available through therapists in most hospitals.

Activities of daily living. During the acute rehabilitative phases of a motor problem, patients with paralysis are taught how to carry out daily activities to the extent that they are able. A variety of devices are available to assist with dressing and grooming. The occupational therapist becomes involved in many of these activities, including homemaking. It is important to stress the concept of the rehabilitative team in managing these patients. The patient is taught to compensate for weakness or paralysis. It is important for the nurse to give the patient the time to do activities on his own if he is able. It is often easier and faster to do things for the patient, but this defeats the purpose of rehabilitation.

Psychological adjustments. The person with paralysis may need assistance in adjusting to the change in his body. The loss of the ability to function independently is traumatic, and the patient may have fears of rejection, as well as loss of self-esteem and concerns about the future.[16] A grief reaction similar to that described in the stages of dying and death may occur. At times, the patient may relate to the paralyzed part of the body as though it were not a part of him and may have nicknames for the body part. Nursing interventions are essential in helping the patient cope with the loss of function and change in body image. This includes praising the patient for achievements, encouraging him to talk about his fears and grief, and helping him see that there is life after disability. It might be helpful to have the patient visited by someone with the same disability who has been successfully rehabilitated.

NURSING DIAGNOSES. Nursing diagnoses and interventions for the patient with alterations in muscle tone and motor function include, but are not limited to, the following.

NURSING DIAGNOSES	NURSING INTERVENTIONS
Impaired physical mobility, related to neuromuscular impairment	Perform active or passive ROM exercises q4h to all extremities, neck, hands, fingers, wrists, elbows, knees. Provide physical therapy as ordered: massage and stretching exercises. Maintain planned rest periods. Encourage ambulation to tolerance. Arrange for necessary assistive devices for home care needs.
Anticipatory grieving, related to perceived or actual loss of body function	Provide emotional support; actively listen to patient's concerns about body image changes. Encourage communication with family and/or significant other. Deal with feelings of frustration, helplessness, and powerlessness associated with loss of motor function.
Potential for disuse syndrome, related to impaired functioning of body part	Perform hand, finger, foot exercises; assist in active and passive ROM exercises q2h to 4h. Assist patient with using supportive devices as indicated: overhead trapeze, braces, walker, cane. Encourage use of involved side when possible. Instruct patient to use unaffected extremity to support weaker side (e.g., lift involved left leg with right leg or lift involved left arm with right arm).
Impaired or potential impaired skin integrity, related to pressure on bony prominences	Administer skin care q4h; keep skin meticulously clean, dry, lotioned, and massaged. Use Eggcrate mattress. Assess skin for erythema or excoriation q2h. Turn q2h. Encourage nutritional diet and adequate fluid intake.

Patient teaching. Teaching is an extremely important part of caring for the person with motor problems. Appropriate teaching activities include the following: safety needs, skin care, activity needs (range of motion and positioning), medications (dosage, action, times, and side effects), the importance of good nutrition, activities of daily living, bowel and bladder care, and the importance of follow-up care. Written instructions are helpful to reinforce teaching and for the patient to refer to when he returns home. Family members should be taught, to prepare them for when they will need to assume some of the care for the patient.

Alterations in sensory and perceptual function

Etiology/pathophysiology. The presence of a lesion anywhere within the sensory system pathway, from the **receptor** to the sensory cortex, alters the transmission or perception of sensory information. The parietal cortex is of major importance in interpretation of sensation. Loss, decrease, or increase in sensation of pain, temperature, touch, and proprioception results in difficulty in daily functioning. Any alteration lessens the patient's ability to be completely protected from inadvertent injury.

One specific loss is proprioception, or the ability to know the position of the body and its parts without directly looking at the part. **Agnosia** is a total or partial loss of the ability to recognize familiar objects or persons through sensory stimuli.

Assessment. Collection of *subjective data* includes the patient's understanding of the sensory disturbance, measures that relieve symptoms (including medications), and the presence of symptoms that occur with the sensory problem. An example is the person who experiences weakness of a hand at the same time that he feels numbness and tingling. The onset of the sensory problem and the specific site in the body are important information to collect.

Collection of *objective data* includes noting the patient's ability to perform purposeful movements or to recognize familiar objects.

Medical management. Refer to medical management on pp. 1028-1029.

Nursing interventions. The most important nursing intervention for the patient with sensory dysfunction is teaching the patient protective measures in relation to the sensory deficit or alteration. This includes helping him learn to inspect parts of the body that have no feeling or protecting sensitive body parts from the discomfort of linen rubbing over them. If a patient has a deficit in one sense, he should be taught to compensate with another (e.g., the patient who learns to lip read because of a hearing deficit; the patient with **hemianopsia** who is taught to scan the printed page).

NURSING DIAGNOSES. Nursing diagnoses and interventions for the patient with a sensory or perceptual problem are the same as those for the patient with a motor problem with the addition of the following.

NURSING DIAGNOSIS	NURSING INTERVENTIONS
Potential for injury, related to sensory/perceptual alteration	Maintain safe environment. Teach patient to protect body parts that have decreased sensation. Teach patient to inspect body parts for possible injury. Protect patient from sustaining injury from hot liquid or heating pads.

Patient teaching. The teaching for a patient with a sensory deficit is essentially the same as that for the patient with a motor deficit (See p. 1030).

Specific Neurological Disorders

Functioning of the neurological system can be interrupted for a variety of reasons. These include conduction abnormalities, degenerative changes, vascular diseases, infection, trauma, and tumors. Selected disorders in each area will be discussed.

Conduction abnormalities

Epilepsy or seizures

Etiology/pathophysiology. The incidence of epilepsy has been recorded throughout history. Seizures occur in all races and affect men and women equally. There is no apparent geographic distribution. In many the onset of seizures is before the age of 20, but it can begin at any age. The incidence is about 1 in every 200 to 300 persons.

Clinical manifestations. Seizures can be classified according to the varied features of the attack. This includes grand mal (major or generalized), petit mal, psychomotor, Jacksonian or focal, and miscellaneous (myoclonic and akinetic) seizures. See Table 38-3 for a description of seizures.

Epilepsy can be defined as a transitory disturbance in consciousness or in motor, sensory, or autonomic function with or without a loss of consciousness. It is associated with sudden, excessive, and disorderly discharges in the neurons of the brain that result in the sudden, violent, involuntary contraction of a group of muscles. The patterns or forms of seizures vary and depend on the area of the brain from which the seizure arises. Seizures occur for a variety of reasons, including hypoglycemia, infection, and electrolyte inbalance.

The excessive neuronal discharges may result in a tonic convulsion, with alternate contraction and relaxation of opposing muscle groups. This gives the characteristic **tonic-clonic** jerking movements of the body. Seizures are

Table 38-3 Characteristics of Seizures

Type of Seizure	Incidence	Characteristics	Clinical Signs	Aura	Postictal Period
Grand mal	Most common	Generalized, characterized by loss of consciousness for several minutes	Aura Cry Loss of consciousness Fall Tonic-clonic movements Incontinence	Yes Flashing lights Smells Spots before eyes (Scotomas) Vertigo	Yes Need for sleep 1 to 2 hrs Headache common
Petit mal	Usually occur during childhood and adolescence Frequency decreases as child gets older	Sudden impairment in or loss of consciousness with little or no tonic-clonic movement Occurs without warning Has tendency to appear a few hours after arising or when person is quiet	Sudden vacant facial expression with eyes focused straight ahead All motor activity ceases except perhaps for slight symmetric twitching about eyelids Possible loss of muscle tone Consciousness returns	No	No
Psychomotor	Occur at any age	Sudden change in awareness associated with complex distortion of feeling and thinking and partially coordinated motor activity	Behaves as if partially conscious Often appears intoxicated May do antisocial things such as exposing self or carrying out violent acts	Yes Complex hallucinations or illusions	Yes Confusion Amnesia Need for sleep

Continued.

Table 38-3 Characteristics of Seizures—cont'd

Type of Seizure	Incidence	Characteristics	Clinical Signs	Aura	Postictal Period
Psychomotor—cont'd		Longer than petit mal	Autonomic complaints, such as shivering, may occur Urinary incontinence		
Jacksonian-focal	Occur almost entirely in patients with structural brain disease	Depends on site of focus May or may not be progressive	Commonly begin in hand, foot, or face May end in grand mal seizure	Yes Numbness Tingling Crawling feeling	Yes
Myoclonic	May antedate grand mal by months or years	May be very mild or may have rapid, forceful movements	Sudden involuntary contraction of muscle group, usually in extremities or trunk No loss of consciousness	No	No
Akinetic	Not common	Peculiar generalized tonelessness	Person falls in flaccid state Unconscious for minute or two	Rarely	No

followed by a rest period of variable length, called the **postictal period**. During this period the patient usually feels groggy and acts confused. Complaints of headache and muscle aches are common. Usually the patient sleeps after a seizure and may experience amnesia for the event.

When recurrent, generalized seizure activity occurs at such frequency that full consciousness is not regained between seizures, it is called **status epilepticus**. This is a medical emergency and requires medical and nursing interventions to prevent death from brain damage resulting from prolonged hypoxia and exhaustion. The nursing interventions always involve ensuring that there is a patent airway and that the patient is protected from injury. Medications used to stop the seizure activity may be of such volume that he is rendered unconscious. The nurse must then assume total care of the patient's needs. A Foley catheter will usually be inserted and the patient will have an intravenous line. The patient may be intubated and receiving ventilatory support. The skin should be protected from injury. Care should be used with restraints if the patient is awake and active so that they do not cause injury if he begins to have a seizure.[12]

Assessment. Collection of *subjective data* includes the patient's awareness of the disorder and any precipitating factors. The presence of an **aura** preceding a seizure is important to consider. An aura occurs in about 50% of all patients with grand mal seizures. The exact character of the aura varies from person to person and is specific to the individual. Awareness of an aura allows the person to be aware of the impending seizure and seek safety and privacy.

Collection of *objective data* includes the number of seizures occurring within a specific time, the character of the seizure, and any behaviors noted and injuries suffered. The character of the seizure should be described as completely as possible, including duration, the nature of the patient's movements, whether the patient was incontinent, any cries or sounds that were made, and the level of alertness.

Diagnostic tests. The most common test used to evaluate seizures is the electroencephalogram (EEG). It allows a specific diagnosis of the nature of the seizure. This test was described earlier in the chapter. (See Fig. 38-13.)

Medical management

MEDICATIONS. Treatment of patients with a seizure disorder almost always includes the use of one or more of the anticonvulsant drugs (Table 38-4). The choice of medication depends on the type of seizure. Failure to take the prescribed medication or to take an adequate dose is often the cause of failure in treatment. Blood levels

Table 38-4 Anticonvulsants used to prevent and control seizures

Drug	Use Related to Seizure Type	Toxic Effects
Phenytoin sodium (Dilantin)	Grand mal, focal, psychomotor	Ataxia, vomiting, nystagmus, drowsiness, rash, fever, gum hypertrophy, lymphadenopathy
Phenobarbital (Luminal)	Grand mal, focal, psychomotor	Drowsiness, rash
Primidone (Mysoline)	Grand mal, focal, psychomotor	Drowsiness, ataxia
Ethosuximide (Zarontin)	Petit mal, psychomotor, myoclonic, akinetic	Drowsiness, nausea, agranulocytosis
Trimethadione (Tridione)	Petit mal	Rash, photophobia, agranulocytosis, nephrosis
Diazepam (Valium)	Grand mal and status epilepticus, mixed	Drowsiness, ataxia
Carbamazepine (Tegretol)	Grand mal, psychomotor	Rash, drowsiness, ataxia
Valproic acid (Depakene)	Petit mal, absent seizures	Nausea, vomiting, indigestion, sedation, emotional disturbance, weakness, altered blood coagulation
Clonazepam (Clonopin)	Petit mal, akinetic, myoclonic Grand mal seizures	Drowsiness, ataxia, hypotension, respiratory depression

may be checked to provide an accurate check on the therapeutic level of the medications taken. If medication is not effective, surgical removal of the brain tissue where the seizure occurs may be done.[41]

Activities of daily living. The majority of patients with seizures are able to control the seizures with medications and so can lead a very normal life. Until seizures are controlled, activities such as driving a car, operating machinery, or swimming should be avoided. Maintaining adequate rest and good nutrition are also important. Alcohol use should be avoided. If the patient is receiving long-term phenytoin (Dilantin) therapy, good hygiene practices for the mouth and teeth are important because of the side effect of edematous and enlarged gums (gingival hyperplasia). The patient should wear a medical alert bracelet or tag.[12]

Nursing interventions

CARE DURING A SEIZURE. The primary goals of the nurse and the family caring for a patient having a seizure are protection from aspiration and injury and observation and recording of the seizure activity. The patient should never be left alone. If the patient is sitting or standing, he should be lowered to the floor in an area away from furniture and equipment. If there is time, clothing may be loosened around the neck. No effort should be made to restrain the patient during the seizure. The nurse should not try to pry open the jaw to place a padded tongue blade. The tongue blade may be inserted between the back teeth early in the seizure if it can be accomplished before the tonic-clonic movements begin. Padded side rails may be used, especially if seizures often occur during sleep.[13]

NURSING DIAGNOSES. Nursing diagnoses and interventions for the patient with seizures may include, but are not limited to, the following.

NURSING DIAGNOSES	NURSING INTERVENTIONS
Ineffective airway clearance, related to mucus accumulation in oropharyngeal area during seizure.	Place patient in side-lying position to prevent aspiration and ensure airway patency. Suction secretions prn.
Anxiety, related to threat to self-concept, powerlessness	Instruct in and encourage use of relaxation exercises, deep breathing techniques. Encourage verbalization of fears. Provide restful environment. Provide emotional support.
Potential for injury, related to rapid onset of altered state of consciousness and seizure activity	Pad side rails. If patient is out of bed during seizure activity, assist him to floor and remove objects that may harm him. Place padded tongue blade at bedside; use if able to insert before tonic-clonic movements begin. Maintain patent airway. Inform patient of seizure and reorient if necessary.

PATIENT TEACHING. Teaching for the patient with a seizure disorder usually includes the use of medications, including dose, action, and side effects, as well as the importance of avoiding alcohol. Safety measures to avoid injury, good oral hygiene, the importance of adequate rest and diet, and the importance of taking medications even if the patient is seizure free should be emphasized. Any restrictions on activities, the importance of follow-up care, and how to access community resources are taught. The patient should be encouraged to avoid excessive stress and to wear a medical alert tag or bracelet.

Degenerative diseases. The term **degenerative diseases** is used to refer to neurological disorders in which there is a premature aging of nerve cells, which is caused by suspected metabolic disturbance or the cause is unknown. Three diseases will be discussed: multiple sclerosis, Parkinson's disease, and Alzheimer's disease.

Multiple sclerosis

Etiology/pathophysiology. Multiple sclerosis (MS) is a common degenerative neurological disease that affects many people. The cause is unknown, although genetics have been implicated, because there is a higher rate of the disease among relatives. Persons living in temperate climates have an increased risk of the disease. Viral and immunological causes for the disease have also been suggested.

The onset of symptoms is usally between the ages of 20 and 40. The course of the disease is estimated to be 12 to 25 years. The highest number of persons with MS live in the Great Lakes area, the Pacific Northwest, and the north Atlantic states.

Multiple foci of **demyelination** are distributed randomly in the white matter of the brainstem, spinal cord, optic nerves, and cerebrum. During the demyelination process, the myelin sheath and the sheath cells are destroyed, causing an interruption or distortion of the impulse so that it is slowed or blocked. There is evidence of partial healing in areas of degeneration, which explains the transitory nature of early symptoms.

Clinical manifestations. Because of the wide distribution of areas of degeneration, the variety of signs and symptoms in multiple sclerosis is greater than in other neurological diseases. These include visual problems, urinary incontinence, fatigue, weakness or incoordination of an extremity, sexual problems such as impotence in men, or swallowing difficulties. The majority of persons have early remissions that may last for a year or more. Exacerbations may be aggravated or precipitated by fatigue, chilling, or emotional disturbances.

Assessment. Collection of *subjective data* includes the patient's understanding of the disease. The presence of eye problems such as diplopia, scotomas (spots before the eyes), and blindness is important. The patient may also talk about weakness or numbness of a part of the body, fatigue, emotional instability, bowel and bladder problems, vertigo, or loss of joint sensation. In men, the presence of impotence is significant. Pain is not a common symptom.

Collection of *objective data* includes documented abnormalities in neurological testing that may include **nystagmus**, muscle weakness and spasms, changes in coordination, or a spastic, ataxic gait. There may be evidence of behavior changes such as euphoria, emotional lability, or mild depression. Urinary incontinence, difficulty in swallowing, and intention tremors of the upper extremities may be present.

Diagnostic tests. Examination of the cerebrospinal fluid in patients with multiple sclerosis usually shows elevated gamma globulin and an increased WBC. A CT scan may show enlargement of the ventricles. The MRI scan has been found very helpful in the diagnosis of multiple sclerosis.[29]

Medical management

MEDICATIONS. There is no specific treatment for multiple sclerosis, although many different remedies have been tried. Favorable results often occur with the use of adrenocorticotropic hormone (ACTH) and the corticosteroids such as prednisone or dexamethasone (Decadron). These may be given orally, intramuscularly, or intravenously. The effects of ACTH and the steroids on the demyelinating process are unknown. If steroids are used in high doses at the start of an exacerbation, the episode seems to resolve more rapidly.

ELIMINATION. Urinary frequency and urgency may respond to propantheline bromide (Pro-Banthine). Cholinergic drugs such as bethanechol chloride (Urecholine) can sometimes help the patient with a neurogenic bladder by exerting a direct antispasmodic effect on smooth muscles. Because urinary tract infections are a major problem in MS, some patients are given prophylactic doses of medications such as trimethoprim and sulfamethoxazole (Bactrim, Septra) or nitrofurantoin (Macrodantin). Cystometric studies can be helpful in defining the specific bladder problem.

The patient should be encouraged to drink adequate fluids (at least 2000 ml a day). If the patient suffers from constipation, a stool softener such as docusate sodium (Colace) may be used, as well as prune juice. If spasticity is a problem, drugs such as diazepam (Valium), dantrolene sodium (Dantrium), and baclofen (Lioresal) may be helpful in preventing or decreasing the spasms.

Nursing interventions

NUTRITION. A well-balanced diet with high-fiber foods and adequate fluids is important. Obesity will make it more difficult for the patient to meet daily needs and maintain mobility. The patient who is obese should be referred to the dietitian and be placed on a calorie-restricted diet that will help the patient lose weight slowly, while receiving adequate nutrition.

SKIN CARE. It is important to teach the patient with multiple sclerosis and/or the caregiver to turn the patient frequently to avoid skin impairment. Devices to relieve pressure, such as Eggcrate or air mattresses, may be helpful. Because of sensory involvement, the patient may not feel discomfort that signals the need to change position.

ACTIVITY. Patients with multiple sclerosis are encouraged to exercise regularly, but not to the point of fatigue. Daily rest periods may be helpful. During an acute exacerbation, patients are often kept as quiet as possible; this includes bed rest.

One side of the body is often more affected than the other. The patient must learn to stabilize the gait by leaning toward the less-involved side. If the foot slaps forward when he is walking, the patient should be taught to put the foot down in a pronounced fashion and rolling the weight forward on the side of the foot.

CONTROL OF ENVIRONMENT. Hot baths should be avoided, because they often increase weakness. Traveling in hot weather should be planned to prevent travel during the warmest part of the day. If at all possible the patient should be in air-conditioned surroundings during the summer.

Persons with multiple sclerosis do best in a peaceful and relaxed environment. They may have slowness of speech and slowness in the ability to respond, as well as sudden explosive emotional outbursts of crying or laughing. The patient and family will need support in terms of this behavior.

NURSING DIAGNOSES. Nursing diagnoses and interventions for the patient with multiple sclerosis may include, but are not limited to, the following.

NURSING DIAGNOSES	NURSING INTERVENTIONS
Potential for powerlessness, related to physical limitations imposed by progressive physical deterioration, loss of body control, and/or threat to physical integrity	Provide emotional support, thorough explanations, and reassurance. Be alert to emotional changes and mood swings. Encourage patient's participation and expression of needs and feelings. Maintain planned rest periods. Encourage self-care as indicated. Provide physical care as indicated.
Altered nutrition: less than body requirements	Maintain high-calorie, high-vitamin, high-protein diet. Assist patient in selection of beneficial foods. Serve meals attractively and maintain pleasant surroundings. Promote small, frequent meals. Report alterations in eating and drinking patterns to physician. Administer oral hygiene before meals.
Bathing/hygiene, dressing/grooming, feeding, toileting self-care deficit, related to limitations in physical mobility imposed by disease process	Assist with or provide physical hygiene as indicated by physical ability. Maintain appropriate bathing temperatures. Administer oral hygiene q4h and prn. Catheterize intermittently as indicated; teach self-catheterization when possible. Plan bladder dysfunction program as appropriate for spasticity or flaccidity. Institute bowel control program. (establish regular bowel routine, avoid constipation). Assist in dressing/grooming as indicated. Provide nutritious, attractive meals.
Body-image disturbance, related to neurophysiological deficits resulting from disease process	Be supportive of patient's emotional needs relating to changes in body image. Acknowledge concerns about body image. Encourage participation in MS support groups. Emphasize need for diversional activities, such as reading, watching television, hobbies, and games.
Knowledge deficit regarding disease process	Explain nature of disease, emphasizing that this is not a hereditary condition. Explain that warm weather and hot baths may increase weakness. Emphasize importance of avoiding fatigue and becoming overworked or emotionally stressed, since these may be precipitating factors in exacerbation. Explain importance of exercising regularly and the need to maintain rest periods. Discuss need for patient support when ambulating with walker, cane, or braces as indicated. Explain importance of maintaining skin integrity. Explain importance of avoiding persons with infections. Encourage independence and self-care to point of tolerance.

PATIENT TEACHING. Teaching is important for both the patient with multiple sclerosis and significant others. In late stages of the disease the care functions usually have to be assumed by someone other than the patient. Important points include those for the patient with motor and sensory problems (see p. 1030.) In addition, it is important to teach about the importance of spacing activities and avoiding temperature extremes, and the potential for emotional lability. The nurse should make sure that the patient and/or family has the address of the nearest multiple sclerosis society or support group.

Parkinson's disease

Etiology/pathophysiology. Parkinson's disease (parkinsonism) is one of the more common diseases of the nervous system. It may also be referred to as *idiopathic Parkinson's* or *spasmus agitans*. It was first described by James Parkinson in 1817. The mean age of onset is 60 years, and the prevalence increases with age. The incidence is about 130 per 100,000 population. It affects both sexes equally, as well as all races.

Etiological factors in Parkinson's disease include viral, toxic, vascular, and genetic causes. Some believe that arteriosclerosis may be a causative factor. Drug-induced parkinsonian syndromes occur with drugs that interfere with the synthesis or storage of dopamine or interfere with the striatal dopamine receptors. These drugs include reserpine (Serpasil), phenothiazines, butyrophenones (haloperidol), and cocaine.

Clinical manifestations. In Parkinson's disease, there is no true paralysis and no loss of sensation. It has some characteristics of upper motor neuron involvement. It is characterized by muscular tremors and rigidity. Defects in judgment and emotional instability may occur, but intelligence is not impaired. A decrease in blinking is seen. All signs and symptoms increase with fatigue.

Assessment. Parkinson's disease starts with subtle symptoms and progresses slowly. Collection of *subjective data* includes symptoms of fatigue, presence of incoordination, judgment defects, emotional instability, and heat intolerance. The patient's understanding of the disease should be assessed.

Collection of *objective data* includes the presence of tremor, which is the outstanding sign of the disease. This has been described as a pill-rolling motion of the fingers or a resting tremor. **Bradykinesia** (an abnormal condition characterized by slowness of voluntary movements and speech) is present with rigidity and loss of postural reflexes. Muscle rigidity leads to a masklike appearance of the face and slowed, monotonous speech; drooling; moist and oily skin; and a shuffling, propulsive gait that the patient may not be able to stop until he meets an obstruction. Swallowing may be abnormal, and the patient may be constipated. He may have a scaly, erythematous rash, particularly near the ears and eyebrows and in the scalp and nasolabial folds.

Diagnostic tests. There is no diagnostic test for Parkinson's disease. The clinical examination and history and the patient's response to medication confirm the diagnosis. If there is a history of chronic dementia, the CT scan may show cerebral atrophy. The EEG may show minimal slowing, and the upper GI evaluation may show decreased motility.

Medical management

MEDICATIONS. Treatment for Parkinson's disease is based on easing of the symptoms of the disease. There are several different drugs that may be used that have had a dramatic effect on the course of the disease:

Trihexyphenidyl hydrochloride (Artane)
Benztropine mesylate (Cogentin)
Procyclidine hydrochloride (Kemadrin)
Biperiden lactate (Akineton Lactate; injection)
Levodopa (Dopar)
Amantadine hydrochloride (Symmetrol)
Carbidopa-levodopa (Sinemet)

After prolonged treatment with some of the drugs, side effects may increase, and the effectiveness of the medication may decrease. It may be helpful to admit the patient to the hospital, during which all drugs are withdrawn for a time. The medications are then restarted, and often much smaller doses will produce favorable results. Complications such as aspiration can occur during this time, because withdrawal of the drugs causes immobility and rigidity.

SURGERY. Surgery that involves destroying portions of the brain that control the rigidity or tremor has been found helpful with some patients. Newer experimental surgery includes transplanting part of the adrenal gland into the brain. Medications are discontinued several days preoperatively so that symptoms will be at their maximum at the time of surgery.

Nursing interventions

ACTIVITY NEEDS. Special attention should be paid to posture. Lying on a firm bed without a pillow may help prevent the spine from bending forward. Holding the hands folded behind the back when walking may help to keep the spine erect and prevent the arms from falling stiffly at the sides. The patient cannot be hurried, because it will make the bradykinesia worse.

FEEDING. When the disease is advanced, aspiration is a real concern. Care should be taken during feeding. Unless the disease is well controlled by medication, drooling can be a problem and increases with general excitement. When patients are dressed, garments with generous pockets for an ample supply of tissues will help them to be less conspicuous.

ELIMINATION. The patient with Parkinson's disease may feel urgency and hesitancy in voiding. Measures appropriate for the patient with multiple sclerosis also apply to these patients.

Chronic constipation may be a real concern. The patient should be on a diet high in fiber and roughage for bulk. The nurse should encourage oral fluid intake, and stool softeners, suppositories, and prune juice are often helpful. Mild cathartics such as milk of magnesia are used if required.

NURSING DIAGNOSES. Nursing diagnoses and interventions for the patient with Parkinson's disease are the same as for multiple sclerosis, with the addition of the following.

NURSING DIAGNOSIS	NURSING INTERVENTIONS
Constipation, related to decreased intestinal motility	Encourage fluids to 3000 ml daily unless contraindicated. Encourage diet high in fiber and roughage. Stool softeners and suppositories are helpful. Enemas are discouraged, because they further decrease motility. Prune juice is offered.

NURSING DIAGNOSIS	NURSING INTERVENTIONS
Potential for aspiration, related to disease process	Ensure that when patient is eating, he sits at 90-degree angle with head up and chin slightly tucked, avoiding extending the head. Do not mix liquids and solid foods. Encourage patient to take small bites of food.

PATIENT TEACHING. Education for the patient with Parkinson's disease should include the importance of taking medications on the prescribed time schedule. The importance of good skin care must be stressed, as well as the importance of keeping active so that the patient remains as mobile as possible. Proper positioning should be demonstrated to the patient and family if they will be taking care of the patient. Proper feeding techniques to reduce the risk of aspiration should be taught to the family and patient. (See interventions for Potential for Aspiration.)

Altzheimer's disease

Etiology/pathophysiology. Alzheimer's disease is a degenerative disorder that affects the cells of the brain and causes impaired intellectual functioning. It is a common cause of dementia in the older person and affects men and women in equal numbers. One person in 20 will develop Alzheimer's disease by age 65; 1 in 10 will have it by age 75; and 1 in 3 will have it by age 90. Alzheimer's may strike persons in their forties and fifties. The cause is unknown. The changes in the brain of patients with Alzheimer's disease include the presence of plaques in the brain. These changes were first discovered in 1907 by the German neurologist Alois Alzheimer.

Clinical manifestations. The progression of Alzheimer's disease is commonly divided into four stages. In the early stage a person with Alzheimer's has relatively mild memory lapses and may have difficulty in using the correct word. His attention span is decreased, and he may be disinterested in his surroundings. In the second stage the person has more obvious memory lapses, especially with short-term memory, and usually may be disoriented to time. Loss of personal belongings is common, as is confabulating (making up stories) to explain the loss of memory. By the time a person reaches the third stage, he is totally disoriented to person, place, and time, and motor problems such as **apraxia** (an impairment in the ability to perform purposeful acts) interfere with the ability to carry out daily functions. Wandering is common. In the terminal, or fourth stage, severe mental and physical deterioration is present. Total incontinence is common.

There may be some variations in these stages. However, all persons with Alzheimer's disease experience a steady deterioration in their physical and mental status, usually lasting 7 to 15 years until death occurs.

Assessment. Memory loss is the first symptom usually noticed in Alzheimer's disease, combined with the inability to carry out normal activities. Other evidence may be the presence of agitation and/or restlessness. It is important to rule out other conditions such as pernicious anemia, drug reactions, depression, or hormonal imbalances.[15]

Diagnostic tests. There is no diagnostic test specific for Alzheimer's disease. A CT scan may be used to rule out other pathological conditions. A family history of Alzheimer's disease is significant. At times the diagnosis can only be confirmed at the time of autopsy.

Medical management. The case of the patient with Alzheimer's disease can be frustrating for the physician, because the treatment options are so limited. Often medications make the condition worse. Drugs such as lorazepam (Activan) or haloperidol (Haldol) in small doses may be necessary to lessen agitation and unpredictable behavior.

Nursing interventions. Nursing interventions are directed toward maintaining adequate nutrition. This can be a challenge, because often the patient will not sit still long enough to eat. Finger foods may be helpful, as well as letting the patient eat while walking. Frequent feedings with high nutritive value are important. Encouraging fluids up to at least 2000 ml a day is also helpful.

Safety demands a special mention. Because of memory problems, patients with this disease often do dangerous things, such as walking outside while not dressed, turning on stoves, wandering away, and setting fires. Measures that the family can take include removing burner controls from the stove at night, double-locking all doors and windows, and keeping the person under constant supervision. One very frustrating part of the disease is that many patients sleep for only short periods and are awake most of the night.[4]

PATIENT TEACHING. Most of the time education is directed at the family, because by the time the patient is diagnosed there is serious mental impairment. The family should be helped to set a realistic schedule that also allows them time for rest and relaxation. If necessary, the family may need to consider placing the patient in a long-term care facility. The family should be put in touch with the local support group for Alzheimer's disease.[14,46]

Vascular problems. Interference with function because of vascular conditions is a common cause of neurological impairment. Two conditions will be discussed in this section: cerebrovascular accident and intracerebral hemorrhage.

Cerebrovascular accident

Etiology/pathophysiology. **Cerebrovascular accident** (CVA or stroke) is the most common disease of the nervous system and is ranked as the third leading cause of death in the United States, with about 200,000 deaths

NURSING CARE PLAN: THE PATIENT WITH ALZHEIMER'S DISEASE

Mrs. Akers is a 65-year-old widow who had been a seamstress. She has a progressive history of memory loss, paranoia, confusion, and agitation. She was diagnosed as having Alzheimer's disease 2 years ago. Her family kept her at home until 6 months ago, when she was admitted to a long-term care instituion.

The nursing history and data obtained indicated the following:

1. She is incontinent of urine about 50% of the time.
2. She usually sleeps for about 3 to 4 hours a night.
3. She is incontinent of stool.
4. She tends to wander if not observed.
5. She is confused as to time and place and her environment; she often thinks the nurses are her children.
6. Her health is good except for the Alzheimer's disease.
7. Her verbal expression is good.
8. Her weight is in the 90th percentile for her height.

Nursing diagnoses	Patient goals	Nursing interventions
Anxiety, related to cognitive impairments	Patient will express minimal anxiety.	Assess cause of anxiety. Use calm, undemanding, unhurried approach. Encourage exercise. Keep nursing interventions consistent and simple. Minimize patient's choices in care. Teach relaxation techniques.
Impaired verbal communication, related to motor or cognitive deficits	Patient will be able to express needs.	Maintain calm atmosphere; avoid rushing. Listen carefully to patient's verbalization. Speak slowly and distinctly. Try to anticipate patient's needs. Encourage speech therapy.
Functional incontinence, related to condition and cognitive impairment	Patient will be continent.	Take patient to bathroom at regular intervals. Encourage adequate fluid intake (at least 2000 m/day.) Determine patient's preference for fluid. Place sign on door indicating "Toilet" or "Bathroom." If patient has urgency, ensure proximity to bathroom. Simplify closures on clothing. Avoid fluids before bedtime. Use adult diapers prn.

NURSING CARE PLAN: THE PATIENT WITH ALZHEIMER'S DISEASE—cont'd

Nursing diagnoses	Patient goals	Nursing interventions
Altered nutrition: less than body requirements resulting from agitation	Patient will maintain weight.	Provide properly balanced diet. Administer diet as ordered; present one course at a time (e.g., salad first, then entree). Assist patient in cutting food as needed. Provide finger food when possible. Offer frequent snacks. Attempt to redirect to eating. Weigh at least monthly. Consult with dietitian.
Potential for injury, related to cognitive problems	Patient will remain free of injury.	Provide constant supervision. Remove safety hazards from environment. Have patient wear well-fitting tie shoes. Use restraints only when necessary. Introduce all caregivers by name each time; repeat on regular basis. Give single, simple instructions. Use exercise to tire patient. Use medication only as needed.
Sleep pattern disturbance, related to agitation	Patient will sleep 6 hr per night.	Avoid use of caffeine. Control environmental disturbances, noise. Maintain quiet environment: close doors; pull drapes and dividers; decrease stimuli. Provide night lights, soft music. Coordinate nursing functions to allow for rest periods and fewer interruptions at night. Maintain balance of daytime activity and rest. Increase activity to tolerance. Limit sleep during daytime. Provide comfort measures. Use medication only as necessary. Wear colored uniforms if white causes patient agitation.
Feeding, dressing/grooming, bathing/hygiene self-care deficit, related to cognitive deficit	Patient will have minimal deficit in self-care.	Use nonverbal cues or demonstration as adjunct to verbal cues. Provide few choices (e.g., in choosing clothes). Do not hurry patient. Assist as needed.
Potential for ineffective family coping: compromised, related to long-term deteriorating effects of disease process	Family and/or significant others will demonstrate ability to cope with disease process.	Provide emotional support. Refer family to support groups. Refer to social services for financial concerns and potential placement. Refer to home care services for potential in-home assistance for home maintenance management problems. Ensure that family and/or significant others are informed about disease process and physician's instructions for supportive care.

annually. Strokes affect persons in all age groups, but the greatest number of persons are between 75 and 85 years of age. Strokes leave many persons with residual effects.

CVAs are caused by a number of pathological processes; these include thrombosis, embolism, and hemorrhage. Many underlying factors are also contributing causes: atherosclerosis, heart disease, hypertension, kidney disease, peripheral vascular disease, and diabetes mellitus. Other risk factors include obesity, high serum cholesterol, cigarette smoking, stress, and a sedentary lifestyle. Oral contraceptives also increases the risk of stroke.

Clinical manifestations. Permanent damage can result from a CVA because of anoxia of the brain. The type of permanent deficits will depend on the area of the brain that is affected. The area of the brain affected depends on which cerebral vessels are involved.[16,49] The vessel most commonly affected is the middle cerebral artery. Frequently, the patient is unconscious and may experience convulsions. Both unconsciousness and convulsions result from generalized ischemia and the brain's response to abrupt hypoxia.

Cerebral thrombosis. Thrombosis is the most common cause of CVA, and the most common cause of cerebral thrombosis is atherosclerosis. Additional disease processes that cause thrombosis are hypotension and other types of vascular injury such as arteritis. CVA resulting from thrombosis is seen most often in the 60- to 90-year-old age group. Thrombi usually occur in larger vessels and are associated with damage to the vessel wall. The internal carotid arteries are a common source of thrombi.

Symptoms of this type of CVA tend to occur during sleep or soon after arising. This is thought to result partly from the fact that recumbency causes a lowering of blood pressure, which can lead to brain ischemia. Postural hypotension may also be a factor. Neurological signs and symptoms frequently worsen for the first few hours after a **CVA**.

Cerebral embolism. Embolism is the second most common cause of CVA. Persons who have CVAs resulting from embolism are usually younger. The emboli most commonly originate from a thrombus in the heart, often caused by rheumatic heart disease with mitral stenosis and atrial fibrillation or myocardial infarction.

Emboli usually affect small vessels and are commonly found at points of bifurcation in blood vessels. They most frequently occur in the midcerebral artery.

Cerebral hemorrhage. Intracerebral or intracranial hemorrhages include bleeding into the brain itself or bleeding into the subarachnoid space. The bleed causes damage by destroying and replacing brain tissue. Intracranial hemorrhages are the third most common cause of CVAs. The peak incidence of aneurysms occurs in persons who are 35 to 60 years of age. Women are more frequently affected than men.

An **aneurysm** is often the cause of hemorrhage. An aneurysm is a weakening of the wall of a blood vessel. It ruptures as a result of a small hole that occurs in a part of the aneurysm. The hemorrhage spreads rapidly, producing localized changes and irritation to the cerebral vessels. The bleeding usually stops when a plug is formed consisting of fibrin platelets. The hemorrhage begins to absorb within 3 weeks. Recurrent rupture is a serious risk 7 to 10 days after the initial hemorrhage.[11]

Transient ischemic attack. The term **transient ischemic attack** (TIA) refers to transient ischemia with temporary episodes of neurological dysfunction that vary in severity. The most common deficit is contralateral weakness of the lower face, hands, arms, and legs; transient dysphasia; and some sensory impairment. Between attacks the neurological status is normal.

The major importance of TIAs is that they warn the patient of the existence of an underlying pathological condition. At least one third of patients who experience TIAs will have a CVA in 2 to 5 years.

Assessment. Collection of *subjective data* that is important with a patient experiencing a CVA includes the description of the onset of symptoms, the presence of headache, any sensory deficit, such as numbness or tingling, the ability to think clearly, and the presence of visual problems. In the case of a hemorrhage the headache may be described as sudden and explosive. The patient's ability to understand the condition should be assessed.

Collection of *objective data* includes the presence of hemiparesis or hemiplegia, any change in the level of consciousness, signs of increased intracranial pressure, respiratory status, and the presence of aphasia. The exact clinical picture varies, depending on the area of the brain affected. When the midcerebral artery is affected, as is most common, the symptoms seen include contralateral paralysis or paresis, contralateral sensory loss, dysphasia or aphasia if the dominant hemisphere is involved, spatial-perceptual problems, changes in judgment and behavior if the nondominant hemisphere is involved, and contralateral (homonymous) hemianopsia.[15]

Diagnostic tests. A lumbar puncture is often performed; blood in the spinal fluid will indicate a hemorrhage. A CT scan may show an area of decreased density, and a brain scan will show an area of diminished perfusion. Following TIAs, a cerebral angiogram or digital subtraction angiogram (DSA) may be done.

Medical management. If the patient has had a stroke as a result of an aneurysm, surgery may be necessary to prevent a rebleed. The surgery consists of a craniotomy and tying off or clipping of the aneurysm. If the base of the aneurysm is too large for these procedures to be done, it may be coated with a liquid, adherent, plastic substance that hardens to form a firm support for the weakened vessel wall.

After a TIA, a carotid endarterectomy may be performed. This includes cleaning out the occluded carotid artery. It may be useful in preventing a stroke.

In an attempt to prevent further thrombosis or emboli,

the physician may prescribe dicumerol and heparin if it is certain that the cause is cerebral thrombosis. The use of anticoagulants is controversial. Some patients may be treated with various types of vasodilating agents, although the effectiveness of this type of therapy is not well established. Drugs to reduce intracranial pressure, such as dexamethasone (Decadron), may be given. Suppositories such as bisacodyl (Dulcolax) are generally prescribed to be given daily or every other day. However, some physicians order stool softeners, laxatives, or enemas.

Fluids may be restricted for the first few days after a CVA in an effort to prevent edema of the brain. The patient will be fed intravenous fluids, or a nasogastric tube may be inserted and tube feedings begun.

The length of time the patient remains in bed depends entirely on the type of CVA suffered and the judgment of the physician in regard to early mobilization. Some physicians prescribe fairly long periods of rest after CVAs, whereas others believe in early mobilization that begins a day or two after the accident has occurred.

Nursing interventions. Goals in the initial phase are directed toward survival needs of the patient and prevention of further complications. Neurological assessment is done at regular intervals but at least every shift to detect changes in status and any complications such as worsening stroke. Some patients may be unconscious as a result of increased intracranial pressure and will need total care (see pp. 1025-1028).

Because nutrition is a concern and the patient may have great difficulty in swallowing at first, tube feedings may be necessary, as well as intravenous fluids unless the patient is more alert. (See the section on motor and sensory problems for a discussion of techniques to assist in feeding the patient with dysphagia.[9,20])

If the patient is responsive after the onset of the stroke, the nurse needs to help the patient assume as much self-care as possible. This includes assisting with teaching the patient one-handed dressing techniques and ways of feeding himself with one hand. It is important to reinforce teaching by other members of the health team.

The patient with a CVA may be incontinent at first. It is important to remove the urinary catheter (if there is one) as soon as possible to prevent urinary tract infection. The patient should be put on a bladder training program to assist in regaining continence. This usually includes taking the patient to the bathroom every few hours and encouraging fluids (at least 2000 ml per day). The patient's normal bowel pattern before the stroke needs to be assessed and included in the nursing care plan if possible. If the patient has difficulty with communication, the use of a picture of a bathroom or toilet can be useful.

Return of motor impulses and movement in involved extremities occurs in stages, lasting from hours to months. Recovery may also halt at a specific stage and progress no further. Return of function is significant for functional use of extremities but also increases the possibility of **contractures.** Appropriate nursing interventions to prevent contractures include passive exercise, active exercise, strength-building of the unaffected side, and early ambulation to promote the return of muscle function. (See the discussion of motor problems, pp. 1028-1030.)

Patients may experience a loss of proprioception with a stroke. This may include **apraxia** and **agnosia** (a total or partial loss of the ability to recognize familiar objects or persons). The nurse can assist the patient with activities by repeating directions and demonstrating care. If the patient has hemianopsia, which is common, the patient should be approached from the nonparalyzed side for care. The patient should be taught to scan past midline to the side where there is the deficit. These patients may also fail to recognize that they have a paralyzed side. This is called *unilateral neglect.* This patient must be taught to inspect this side of the body for injury and to protect it from harm. These patients often show poor judgment and may move impulsively or unsafely. They need to be observed for this and safety precautions should be taken if needed until the patient can learn to compensate for this lack of judgment. Crying or emotional lability is common.

It is important to foster the patient's sense of self-esteem in the midst of his disability. The nurse must always treat the patient as an adult, not as a child. The patient's successful efforts and gains in self-care should be praised and reinforced.

COMMUNICATION PROBLEMS. Many CVA patients have speech problems, including dysarthria and aphasia. The patient may be frustrated and should be approached in a unhurried manner. Often, the patient does much better with communication when he does not feel pressured to speak. The nurse may find that giving the patient a communication board is helpful. The nurse should wait for the patient to communicate, rather than prompting him or finishing his sentence before he has a chance to find the appropriate word. Inability to articulate does not mean that the patient has decreased cognitive abilities.

NURSING DIAGNOSES. The nursing diagnoses and interventions for the patient with a CVA include, but are not limited to, the following.

NURSING DIAGNOSES	NURSING INTERVENTIONS
Ineffective airway clearance, related to inability to maintain secretions	Position body and head to avoid obstruction of airway and provide optimal secretion removal. Suction secretions prn. Provide oral or nasopharyngeal airway to maintain airway patency. Auscultate chest for breath sounds q2h to 4h. Administer oxygen/humidification as ordered. Monitor arterial blood gases and hemoglobin.

NURSING DIAGNOSES	NURSING INTERVENTIONS
Body image disturbance, related to neurophysical deficits	Determine patient's perception of change in body image and subsequent threat to self. Encourage verbalization (if able) such as anger, fear, frustration, and anxiety about altered functioning of body part. Encourage patient to look at and touch changed body part. Assist family in adapting to change by providing resources, encouraging verbalization, and including family members in care. Assess own attitudes and values related to one's physical appearance. Teach patient and family the stages of grief and importance of grief work.
Impaired verbal communication	Speak slowly and distinctly. Phrase questions that can be answered by yes or no (or by appropriate signals). Try to anticipate patient needs. Provide call signal within reach of unaffected hand. Begin speech therapy as soon as possible.
Altered cerebral tissue perfusion, related to ischemic injury	Maintain bed rest, with head of bed elevated 15 to 60 degrees. Check q15 to 30 min to assess alterations in circulatory status; immediately report any sudden changes in blood pressure or pupillary or neurological status. Check rectal temperature q2h to 4h; hypothermia or cooling measures may be needed. Maintain parenteral fluid as ordered.
Impaired home maintenance management, related to individual family member, lack of finances, or family organization	Refer patient and family to services of social worker. Involve patient (if possible) and family members in problem-solving solutions to individual needs. Arrange for necessary assistive devices through home health. Encourage expression of feelings and discuss concerns.
Total incontinence	Monitor urinary output and signs of retention or incontinence. Assure patient that urinary problems will probably improve. Provide catheter care if retention catheter is needed initially. Offer bedpan or urinal after meals and at regular intervals. Provide fluids to maximum amount prescribed; provide greater amounts before 4 PM. Use disposable adult diaper or external urinary system as indicated.
Potential for injury, related to changes in sensory-perceptual function	Maintain seizure precautions. Maintain safe environment. Use side rails with padding as indicated. Maintain quiet environment. Use soft restraints as indicated. Maintain bed in low position.
Knowledge deficit regarding disease process	Teach patient and family prescribed therapy to be carried out at home, plans for increased patient independence, professional and community resources necessary to achieve long-term goals, and plans for follow-up care.
Impaired physical mobility, related to neuromuscular impairment	Encourage active ROM and exercises of unaffected extremities. Encourage patient to move in bed as able. Teach patient how to sit up on side of bed and to transfer to chair when permitted. Support activities initiated by physical therapy staff. Encourage ambulation when possible and provide support. Provide shoe support for transfer and ambulation.
Altered nutrition: less than body requirements, related to impaired ability to swallow	Provide IV fluids and tube feedings as prescribed during initial period. Assess ability to swallow before initiating feedings. Position patient with head elevated and turned to unaffected side when feeding patient. Provide foods initially that are easier to swallow (soft or pureed foods except for mashed potatoes). Use training cup or feeding syringe for fluids as necessary. Inspect mouth for food trapped in cheek pockets. Be patient when feeding patient and provide directions for swallowing, as needed. Encourage patient to feed self as soon as possible; provide self-help devices as necessary.
Bathing/hygiene self-care deficit, related to impaired physical mobility and alteration in cognitive process	Administer skin care q4h. Use oil-based lotions. Inspect area over bony prominences q4h for any skin impairment. Maintain body alignment. Provide physical hygiene as indicated. Encourage patient to assist himself as able. Praise efforts at personal hygiene.

PATIENT TEACHING. The teaching for a patient with a CVA includes teaching the patient about techniques to compensate for the deficits suffered as a result of the stroke. In this the nurse functions as part of the rehabilitation team. This rehabilitation must start at the time of admission to the acute care facility. The patient will probably be attending occupational and physical therapy and may need speech therapy.

If the patient is receiving medication (e.g., for hypertension), it is important to teach the patient and/or family about side effects and the schedule for taking the medication. Plans for follow-up should be discussed. The patient and/or family may be referred to a stroke club for support.

The patient's family needs to be taught techniques to enhance safety and communication. If the patient has a problem with dysphagia, the family needs to be taught appropriate techniques. Instructions should be written out for the patient or family to refer to after discharge. Most rehabilitation centers will also include therapeutic leaves as a way to test the family's skills and knowledge. Each pass or leave has specific goals, and feedback is obtained from the family about additional teaching that may be needed. The family and patient should also be educated about the perceptual problems associated with stroke, along with techniques that compensate for these deficits (e.g., writing down instructions for the patient who has trouble carrying out an activity alone).

Infection/inflammation

Etiology/pathophysiology. Interference with function because of infection or inflammation is a common occurrence. Some specific conditions include meningitis, encephalitis, brain abscess, Guillain-Barré syndrome, herpes zoster, neurosyphilis, and AIDS. Only meningitis and AIDS will be discussed in this chapter.

The nervous system may be affected by a variety of organisms and may suffer from toxins of bacteria and viruses. These toxins reach the nervous system from a variety of sources, including adjacent bones, blood, or lymph. Meningitis can occur as a result of an invasive procedure such as surgery.

Assessment. Subjective and objective assessment are important in any patient who has infection of the nervous system. Collection of *subjective data* includes a history of infection, such as an upper respiratory infection, and the presence of discomfort that may include headache or stiff neck. The initial onset of symptoms, any difficulty in thinking, and the presence of weakness may be important. The patient's understanding of his condition should be assessed.

Collection of *objective data* includes behavioral signs indicating discomfort or disorientation, as well as an inability to carry out ADLs. The physical assessment part of the neurological assessment may reveal abnormalities; the presence of a fever, vomiting, abnormal CT results, seizures, altered respiratory patterns, tachycardia, and meningeal irritation is significant. The patient's level of consciousness and orientation should be assessed.

Diagnostic tests. Many of the infections of the nervous system can be diagnosed by examining the cerebrospinal fluid. A CT scan or an EEG may also be done.

NURSING DIAGNOSES. Nursing diagnoses and interventions for the patient with an infection/inflammation are the same as for cerebrovascular accident, with the addition of the following.

NURSING DIAGNOSES	NURSING INTERVENTIONS
Hyperthermia, related to inflammatory response to CNS infection	Assess temperature q2h and prn. Provide cooling measures prn; avoid cooling to point of shivering. Administer antipyretics as ordered. Administer antibiotics as ordered. Monitor parenteral fluids as ordered. Control exposure to extremes in temperature. Assess TPR q2h as indicated.
Altered thought processes, related to neurophysiological response to infection	Protect patient from self-injury. Provide soft restraints to prevent injury. Introduce self to patient and establish rapport to prevent agitation. Relate date, time of day, and recent activities. Speak in kind tone, using short, simple sentences. Maintain a therapeutic environment.

PATIENT TEACHING. Education for the patient with an infection includes teaching about the disease process, the treatments involved, and the expected outcomes. If the patient is seriously ill, the initial teaching focuses on the family. Other aspects of teaching for motor and sensory problems may also be relevant for the patient with an infection or inflammation, depending on the symptoms demonstrated.

Meningitis

Etiology/pathophysiology and clinical manifestations. Meningitis is an acute infection of the meninges. It is usually caused by one of several organisms, including pneumococci, meningococci, staphylococci, streptococci, *Haemophilus influenzae,* and viral aseptic agents. The effect of the bacteria in the subarachnoid space is an inflammatory reaction in the pia mater and arachnoid and in the CSF. Pus accumulates, and the bacteria may injure nervous tissue.

Meningitis can be classified as bacterial or aseptic. The incidence of bacterial meningitis is higher in fall and winter, when upper respiratory tract infections are common. Pathological changes that can occur include hyperemia of the meningeal vessels, edema of brain tissue, increased intracranial pressure, a generalized inflammatory reaction with exudation of white blood cells into the subarachnoid spaces, and associated hydrocephalus caused by exudate occluding the ventricles.

Two abnormal signs that occur with meningitis are Kernig's sign (inability to extend the legs completely without extreme pain) and Brudzinski's sign (flexion of the hip and knee when the neck is flexed). The onset of meningitis is usually sudden and is characterized by severe headache, stiffness of the neck, irritability, malaise, and restlessness. Nausea, vomiting, and delirium develop, as well as increased temperature, pulse rate, and respirations.

Diagnostic tests. Meningitis is diagnosed by examining the cerebrospinal fluid. A culture and sensitivity test is done to ascertain the pathogenic organism. A CT scan of the head and an EEG are also ordered.

Medical management. Treatment of meningitis consists of massive doses of antibiotics. Multiple antibiotics are often used. The medication is usually given intravenously or intrathecally (directly into the spinal canal). Hyperosmolar agents or steroids may be needed to decrease intracranial pressure. Anticonvulsants may be given to prevent seizures.

Nursing interventions. Respiratory isolation is required until the pathogen can no longer be cultured from the nasopharynx. This is usually accomplished after 24 hours of effective antibiotic therapy. Other nursing interventions include the general care given a critically ill patient who may be irritable, confused, and unable to take fluids. Dehydration is common and the patient almost always has an intravenous line. The room is kept darkened and noise is kept to a minimum, since any increase in sensory stimulation may cause a seizure. If the patient is disoriented, safety precautions need to be taken, including restraints if needed.

Acquired immunodeficiency syndrome

Etiology/pathophysiology. Acquired immunodeficiency syndrome (AIDS) is a disease that has serious implications for the nervous system, with more than 40% of AIDS patients having neurological symptoms. Patients develop neurological symptoms either as a result of infection with HIV itself or as a result of associated infections.[1,34] See Chapter 40 for a discussion of AIDS.

Clinical manifestations. Patients with AIDS may have ADC (AIDS dementia complex), which is known as subacute encephalitis. This may be manifested as difficulty in concentrating or a recent memory loss, which may progress to a **global cognitive dysfunction** (generalized impairment of intellect, awareness, and judgment). Patients may also experience opportunistic infections such as meningitis, herpes simplex, cytomegalovirus, toxoplasmosis, and cryptococcal meningitis. Primary malignant lymphomas of the CNS may also develop.

Diagnostic tests. The diagnostic tests used to determine whether a neurological problem is related to AIDS include serological studies, a lumbar puncture, and CT scan. At times, a cerebral biopsy may be necessary to make the differential diagnosis.

Medical management. Treatment of the patient with neurological problems related to AIDS depends on the nature of the infection. Various methods of treatment have included administration of antiviral, antifungal, and antibacterial agents. Radiation has been used on the affected part of the brain. Experimental therapies including iron dextran (Imferon) have been attempted. Mortality remains high despite aggressive therapy.

Nursing interventions. The patient is likely to be confused, and the nurse needs to reorient him frequently. Safety measures such as padded side rails may be necessary to prevent injury to the patient, who may have seizures.

The patient may experience pain and have difficulty sleeping. It is important to administer medications to the patient as needed and to structure activities to avoid waking him from sleep. The patient may also have visual problems associated with the disease, and the nurse must be careful to orient the patient to nursing interventions.

Most patients with AIDS experience depression and powerlessness about the nature of the disease. They may isolate themselves from others. Patients should be encouraged to talk about their fears and concerns, be assisted to find emotional support, and be referred to a support group. The nurse needs to maintain a nonjudgmental attitude.

The patient may be incontinent of bowel and bladder. It is important to encourage an active bowel and bladder program. If the patient is experiencing diarrhea, it is important to keep the rectal area as clean and dry as possible and administer antidiarrheals if ordered. The patient may also have difficulty with nausea. Foods that the patient likes should be offered in small, frequent meals. Tube feedings or hyperalimentation may be needed if the patient agrees.[35]

Trauma. Interference with neurological function can occur as a result of trauma. Parts of the nervous system commonly subjected to trauma include the craniocerebrum, the spinal cord, and peripheral nerves. Only the first two will be discussed in this chapter.

Craniocerebral trauma

Etiology/pathophysiology. Craniocerebral trauma, or head injury, causes death or serious disability in people of all ages. Head injury is the second most common cause of neurological injuries and the major cause of death between ages 1 and 35. Causes of head injury include motor vehicle accidents, falls, industrial accidents, assaults, and sports trauma.

Craniocerebral trauma may result in injury to the scalp, skull, and brain tissues. Injuries vary from minor scalp wounds to concussions and open fractures of the skull with severe damage to the brain. The amount of obvious damage is not indicative of the seriousness of the trouble. Effects of severe head injury include cerebral edema, sensory and motor deficits, and increased intracranial pressure.

Injuries to the brain can result from direct or indirect trauma to the head. Indirect trauma is caused by tension strains and shearing forces transmitted to the head by stretching of the neck. Direct trauma occurs when the head is directly injured. This results in an **acceleration-deceleration injury**, with rotation of the skull and its contents. Bruising or contusion of the occipital and frontal lobes and the brainstem and cerebellum may occur.

Clinical manifestations. Head injuries may be open or closed. Open head injuries result from skull fractures or penetrating wounds. The amount of injury with this type of wound is determined by the velocity, mass, shape, and direction of the impact. A skull fracture (linear, comminuted, depressed, or compound) may also occur. Fractures of the base of the skull are more serious because of their location, near the medulla.

Closed head injuries include **concussions** (a violent jarring of the brain against the skull), **contusions,** and lacerations. Lacerations of the scalp bleed profusely because of the large vascularity in the region. Hemorrhage resulting from craniocerebral trauma may occur in the following sites: scalp, epidural, subdural, intracerebral, and intraventricular. Epidural and subdural hematomas require careful and continuous observation by the nurse. Epidural hematomas form as blood collects rapidly between the dura and skull. If lethargy or unconsciousness develops after the patient regains consciousness, an epidural hematoma may be suspected and needs immediate treatment.

A subdural hematoma forms as venous blood collects below the dura. Because the bleeding is under venous pressure, the hematoma formation is relatively slow. The clot will cause pressure on the brain surface and will displace brain tissue. If a patient who has been conscious for several days after head injury loses consciousness or develops neurological symptoms, a subdural hematoma should be suspected. Subdural hematomas may be classified as acute, subacute, or chronic.

Assessment. Collection of *subjective data* includes the patient's understanding of the injury and the resulting pathological processes. Determining how the injury happened and whether the patient has headache, nausea, or vomiting is important. Abnormal sensations and a history of a loss of consciousness and of bleeding from any orifice should be noted.

Collection of *objective data* includes the status of the respiratory system, level of alertness and consciousness, and size and reactivity of the pupils; these should be checked frequently. The nurse also assesses the patient's orientation, motor status, vital signs, the presence of bleeding or vomiting, and abnormal speech patterns.

Medical management. Immediate care of the patient with a head injury is directed toward lifesaving measures and the maintenance of normal body function until recovery is ensured. It is extremely important to maintain a patent airway and ensure adequate oxygenation. Suctioning may be necessary (but never through the nose because of the possibility of a skull fracture), as well as the administration of oxygen. Arterial blood gas levels are checked.

Medications are used to reduce cerebral edema and increased ICP, which are common problems in patients with head injuries. Medications include mannitol and dexamethasone. Codeine or other analgesics that do not depress the respiratory system are used for pain control. Anticonvulsants may be given to prevent seizures. Measures to control elevated temperatures are taken because hyperthermia increases brain metabolism, resulting in brain damage.

Nursing interventions

PREVENTION OF INFECTION. The patient's ears and nose are checked carefully for signs of blood and serous drainage, which indicate that the meninges are torn and spinal fluid is escaping. No attempt should be made to clean out the orifice. If there is evidence of drainage from the nose, the patient should not cough, sneeze, or blow the nose. If there is a question about whether drainage is CSF, a Tes-Tape will show a positive reaction for sugar. Meningitis is a possible complication when communication with the meninges and the nose or ears occurs.

EMOTIONAL SUPPORT. It is not uncommon that the patient with a head injury shows a loss of memory and loss of initiative. Behavioral problems associated with a lack of judgment and restlessness may also occur.[36,47] Restlessness in the head-injured patient may be caused by the need for a change of position, pain, or the need to empty the bladder. These patients need firm but gentle care, with specific guidelines for what behavior is allowed. It is not helpful to argue with the patient. It may be helpful to redirect his attention. Memory aids such as a log book or written schedule can be very useful in assisting him with orientation.

The length of convalescence will depend on the amount of brain damage and how rapid the recovery is. Many patients with head injury will recover physically but will have behavioral and psychological problems that make it difficult for them to function independently. (See Chapter 52.)

NURSING DIAGNOSES. Nursing diagnoses and interventions for the patient with a head injury are the same as for the patient with a CVA, with the addition of the following.

NURSING DIAGNOSIS	NURSING INTERVENTIONS
Impaired social interaction, related to cognitive and affective deficits from neurophysiological trauma	Encourage and support verbalization about feelings, medical conditions, and current treatment; listen nonjudgmentally. Build trust through consistency and keep promises. Involve patient in his own plan of care. Give full attention to patient during verbal interactions and recognize qualities to promote self-esteem.

PATIENT TEACHING. A patient with a head injury may be seen in the emergency room but not be admitted to the hospital. Such a patient needs to be taught about observations for complications. Teaching for patients with a head injury and who have residual deficits severe enough to require rehabilitation is similar to that needed for patients with motor or sensory problems.

Spinal cord trauma

Etiology/pathophysiology. Spinal cord injury from accidents is a common and increasing cause of serious disability and death. Approximately 10% of traumatic injuries to the nervous system involve the spinal cord. Most

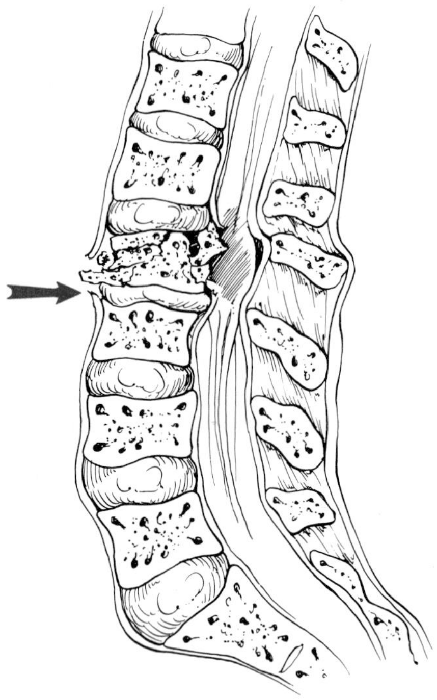

FIG. 38-16 Damage to spinal cord and distortion of adjacent structures that may occur in traumatic injuries to spine.

BOX 38-5 MUSCLE FUNCTION AFTER SPINAL CORD INJURY

SPINAL CORD INJURY	MUSCLE FUNCTION REMAINING	MUSCLE FUNCTION LOST
Above C4	None	All, including respiration
C5	Neck Scapular elevation	Arms Chest All below chest
C6-C7	Neck Some chest movement Some arm movement	Some arm, fingers Some chest All below chest
Thoracic	Neck Arms (full) Some chest	Trunk All below chest
Lumbosacral	Neck Arms Chest Trunk	Legs

persons involved with spinal cord injuries are males between the ages of 18 and 25. Automobile, motorcycle, diving, surfing, and other athletic accidents and gunshot wounds are major causes of spinal cord injury.

The soft tissue of the spinal cord is protected by the vertebral column. Injuries that occur to this column include a simple fracture, compressed or wedged fracture, comminuted or burst fractures, or dislocation of the vertebrae (Fig. 38-16). As a result the cord is often damaged. Severe traumatic lesions of the spinal cord may result in total transection of the spinal cord or a tearing of the cord from side to side at a particular level, with a complete loss of spinal cord functions. This total transection is also called a *complete cord injury*. With this type of injury, all voluntary movement below the level of the trauma is lost. A partial transection or *incomplete injury* involves a partial transection or injury of the cord. Quadriplegics are patients who sustain injuries to one of the cervical segments of the spinal cord. Paraplegics are those whose lesions are confined to the thoracic, lumbar, or sacral segments of the spinal cord. The symptoms of an incomplete injury are variable (Box 38-5).

Clinical manifestations

SPINAL SHOCK. Initially, in most spinal cord injuries, there is a period of flaccid paralysis and a complete loss of reflexes below the trauma. Sensory and autonomic functions are also lost. This is called *areflexia* or spinal shock and is temporary. During this time the patient may need temporary respiratory support.[24,39]

AUTONOMIC DYSREFLEXIA. One complication of spinal cord injury that is extremely important to understand is **autonomic dysreflexia** or **hyperreflexia**. It occurs in patients with cord injuries above the sixth thoracic vertebra and most commonly in patients with cervical injuries. Autonomic dysreflexia occurs as a result of abnormal cardiovascular response to stimulation of the sympathetic division of the autonomic nervous system. The clinical signs include bradycardia, hypertension, diaphoresis, "goose flesh," severe headache, and nasal stuffiness. Patients tend to develop individual symptoms of this condition and are soon able to recognize them.[35]

The most common cause of this condition includes a distended bladder or a fecal impaction. It is a medical emergency that requires immediate treatment to prevent a CVA, blindness, or death. (See emergency box, p. 1047.)

SEXUAL FUNCTION. In most cases men experience impotence, decreased sensation, and difficulties with ejaculation. Impairment of fertility is common. The experience of orgasm is described as different than before the injury. Women with spinal cord injury are able to continue to perform sexually, although perception of sexual pleasure is usually altered.

Assessment. Collection of *subjective data* includes information about the nature of the injury, presence of any

AUTONOMIC DYSREFLEXIA

EMERGENCY

- Place patient in sitting position to decrease blood pressure.
- Check patency of catheter for kinking. If catheter is occluded, insert new catheter immediately.
- Check rectum for impaction.
- If it is necessary to remove impaction, an anesthetic ointment should be used.
- Administer ganglionic blocking agent such as hexamethonium or a vasodilator such as nitroprusside (Nipride) as ordered if conservative measures are not effective.
- Continue monitoring blood pressure.
- Send urine for culture if no other cause is found; urinary infection can lead to symptoms of autonomic dysreflexia.

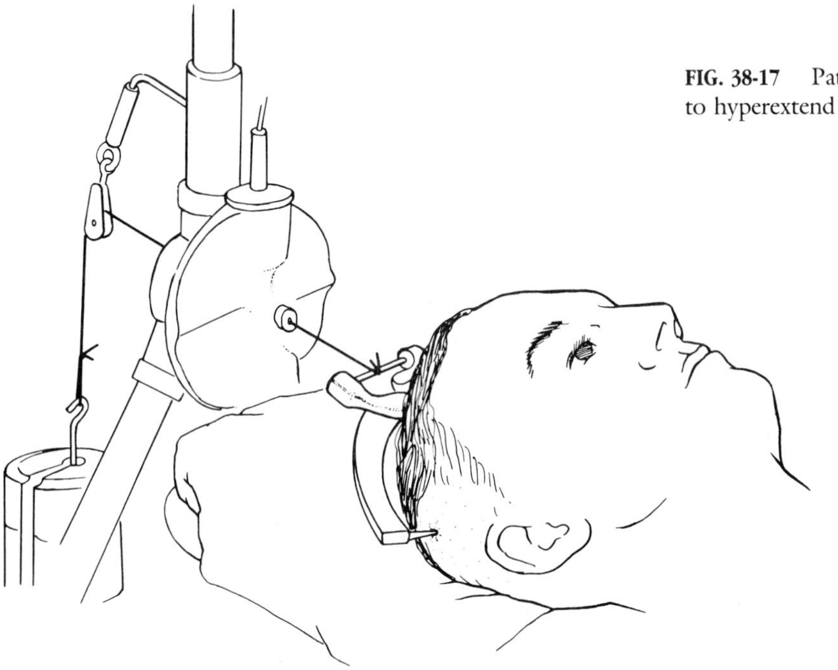

FIG. 38-17 Patient with Crutchfield tongs inserted into skull to hyperextend head and neck.

dyspnea, and unusual sensations. The presence of pain, any loss of consciousness, and the absence of sensation on sensory examination are important to assess.

Collection of *objective data* includes the level of alertness and consciousness, orientation, pupil size and reactivity, motor strength, skin integrity, and bowel and bladder status, including distention. It is important to assess for other injuries, such as fractured bones or head injury.

Diagnostic tests. X-ray films are often taken first to detect any cervical vertebra fracture or displacement. A spinal tap or myelogram may also be done to detect occlusion. A CT scan and MRI scan may be helpful to rule out spinal cord injury.

Medical management. Immediate care after spinal cord injury is directed toward realignment of the bony column in the presence of fractures or dislocations. The measures involved may include simple immobilization, skeletal traction, or surgery for spinal decompression. Skeletal traction may include Crutchfield tongs (Fig. 38-17), halo traction (see Fig. 30-24), or a Stryker or Foster frame. Bracing may be used for thoracic or lumbar injuries. Often a surgical decompression is not performed until after a period of skeletal traction if the injury involves the cervical region.

Nursing interventions

MOBILITY. Throughout all stages of hospitalization of the patient with a spinal cord injury, nursing and medical interventions are directed toward restoration of structural or body integrity. All efforts are taken to ensure that the skin is intact, that contractures do not develop, and that range of motion is maintained. Early mobilization is important. When patients, especially quadriplegics, begin to sit up, it may be necessary to wrap the legs with elastic wraps to encourage venous return. Slowly increasing the angle of sitting up is essential to prevent hypotension. A recliner wheelchair is usually necessary.

URINARY FUNCTION. Usually a Foley catheter is inserted initially; later bladder training is started (see Chapter 33). Intermittent catheterization is often used. Fluid intake that exceeds 2000 ml per day is encouraged.

BOWEL FUNCTION. Patients are usually started on a bowel program early in their hospital stay. At first bisacodyl (Dulcolax) suppositories are given at regular intervals—usually every other night. This is followed by digital stimulation to further stimulate peristalsis. The goal is to eliminate the need for suppositories. Other aids to bowel programs are the use of adequate fluids (usually at least 2000 ml per day), stool softeners, and prune juice.

NURSING DIAGNOSES. Nursing diagnoses and interventions for the patient with a spinal cord injury are the same as those for the patient with a motor or sensory problem, with the addition of the following.

NURSING DIAGNOSES	NURSING INTERVENTIONS
Ineffective breathing pattern, related to neurogenic or traumatic injury	Maintain patent airway. Auscultate breath sounds. Be cognizant of assisted ventilation and oxygenation being ordered, as well as measurement of vital capacity to ensure adequate ventilation. Be aware that tracheostomy may be indicated. Maintain nasal and oropharyngeal airway and suction as needed.
Dysreflexia, related to neurophysiological trauma to spinal cord above sixth thoracic vertebra	See emergency box on p. 1047 for emergency interventions.
Knowledge deficit regarding diagnosis and potential home management	Ensure that patient and significant other are informed about disease and prognosis. Prepare for chronicity and duration of rehabilitative process. Discuss medications: name, dosage, route, side effects, and purpose. Refer to appropriate rehabilitative and counseling resources.
Powerlessness, related to actual or perceived body image changes	Encourage communication between patient and family or significant others. Encourage independence when possible; be aware of limitations. Involve patient in decision-making process when formulating care plan. Help patient set small, realistic goals. Give positive reinforcement for independent functioning. Assist patient in identifying areas over which he has control. Support all verbalization of feelings, especially anger.
Altered patterns of urinary elimination, related to sensory-motor impairment	Check carefully for voiding and for distention of the bladder. Teach patient intermittent self-catheterization if indicated. Teach patient Credé's maneuver as indicated (See Chapter 33.) Foley if indicated; administer meticulous aseptic technique in changing catheters. Teach patients signs of infection. Encourage patient to have a genitourinary checkup at least yearly. Maintain fluid intake of 3 to 4 L daily unless contraindicated. Adult diapers may be necessary.

PATIENT TEACHING. Teaching of the patient with a spinal cord injury includes education about autonomic dysreflexia and about sexual functioning after spinal cord injury. Other teaching points are found in the sections of this chapter dealing with the patient with motor or sensory problems (see p. 1030).

Tumors

Intracranial tumors

Etiology/pathophysiology and clinical manifestations. Intracranial tumors include both benign and metastatic lesions. All areas and structures of the brain can be affected. Primary intracranial tumors, or *neoplasms*, arise from the cells of brain tissue and the pituitary and pineal glands. These include gliomas, meningiomas, pituitary tumors, and neuromas. Metastatic tumors also occur frequently in the brain. Brain tumors are named from the tissues from which they arise. (See Chapter 41.)

Assessment. Collection of *subjective data* includes the patient's understanding of the diagnosis, as well as changes in personality or judgment and the presence of abnormal sensations or visual problems. Complaints of unusual odors may be present with tumors of the temporal lobe. Headache, hearing loss, or the inability to carry out daily activities is also important to assess.

Collection of *objective data* includes motor strengths, gait, the level of alertness and consciousness, and orientation. The pupils are assessed for response and equality. The presence of seizures in an adult is significant. Speech abnormalities, cranial nerve abnormalities, and symptoms of increased intracranial pressure are also significant.

Diagnostic tests. No one procedure is entirely diagnostic of brain tumors, but a CT scan is often the basis for the diagnosis. Other tests that may be performed include the brain scan, MRI, PET scans, and the EEG. Arteriography may also be done.

Medical management. The general method of treatment for intracranial tumors includes surgical removal when feasible, radiation, and chemotherapy. The choice of therapy is determined by the tumor type and site. A combination of methods is often used.

SURGERY. A surgical opening through the skull is called a *craniotomy*. Following removal of the bone, an incision is made into the meninges, and the tumor is removed. The removed bone is carefully preserved and may be replaced at the end of surgery if there is no indication of infection or increased intracranial pressure (IICP). The removal of part of the skull without replacement is called *craniectomy*.

Nursing interventions. Preoperative preparation of both the patient and the family is important. Specific fears may be related to a permanent change in appearance, dependency, and possible death. A baseline neurological assessment is important. Treatments and procedures, including the shaving of hair, are explained. Usually hair is shaved in the operating room. It is then given to the patient who may choose to have it made into a wig. The family needs to be prepared for the appearance of the patient after surgery.

Postoperative care is determined by the patient's condition. Most patients spend 1 or 2 nights in an intensive care unit, under close nursing observations, with frequent neurological checks. The patient should be assessed carefully for indications of increased ICP. The patient may have residual motor or sensory problems as a result of the tumor or surgery. (The interventions needed were previously described in this chapter.)

NURSING DIAGNOSES. Nursing diagnoses and interventions for the patient with a brain tumor are the same as those for CVA, with the addition of the following.

NURSING DIAGNOSES	NURSING INTERVENTIONS
Anxiety, related to unknown outcome of disease process	Observe for signs of increasing anxiety. Assist in identifying successful coping skills. Maintain a calm, unhurried manner. Teach relaxation exercises and techniques. Administer tranquilizers and sedatives as ordered. Allow for verbal expression of anger. Use touch, reassurance, and positive body language.
Pain, related to pressure on brain	Assess type and location of pain. Administer analgesics as ordered and assess effectiveness of pain relief measures; narcotics such as morphine, which depress respirations, are not used. Turn and change position q2 to 4h. Provide back rubs and skin care. Maintain planned rest periods. Assist patient with alternate comfort measures.
Sensory/perceptual alterations: visual, auditory, kinesthetic, tactile, related to compression/displacement of brain tissue	Maintain method of communication. Provide for social interaction. Maintain safe environment. Provide orientation and appropriate level of stimuli.
Altered thought processes, related to altered circulation and/or destruction of brain tissue	Protect patient from self-injury. Provide soft restraints as indicated. Assist patient in self-care activities. Speak in kind tone using short, simple sentences. Give one direction at a time. Relate date, time of day, and recent activities. Maintain a therapeutic environment. Keep equipment and personal possessions in same place. Encourage socialization.

REFERENCES AND SUGGESTED READINGS

1. Ake J and Perlstein L: AIDS: impact on neuroscience nursing practice, J Neurosci Nurs 19:300, 1987.
2. Anagnostakos NP and Tortora GJ: Principles of anatomy and physiology, ed 5, New York, 1987, Harper & Row, Publishers, Inc.
3. Barker E and Higgins R: Managing a suspected spinal cord injury, Nurs 88 19(4):52, 1988.
4. Beck C and Heacock P: Nursing interventions for patients with Alzheimer's disease, Nurs Clin North Am 23(1):95, 1988.
5. Burns E and Buckwalter K: Pathophysiology and etiology of Alzheimer's disease, Nurs Clin North Am 23(1):11, 1988.
6. Caldwell E and Hegner BR: Geriatrics, a study of maturity, ed 4, New York, 1986, Delmar Publishers, Inc.
7. Christ M and Holboch F: Gerontologic nursing, Springhouse, Pa, 1988, Springhouse Publishing.
8. Colling J: Educating nurses to care for the incontinent patient, Nurs Clin North Am 23(1):279, 1989.
9. DiIorio C and Price M: Swallowing: an assessment and practice guide, Am J Nurs 90:38, 1990.
10. Findley L: Altered consciousness, Nurs 84 2:663, 666, 1984.
11. Fode N: Subarachnoid hemorrhage from ruptured intracranial aneurysm, Am J Nurs 88:5, 1988.
12. Fong E, Ferris EB, and Skelly EG: Body structures and functions, ed 7, New York, 1989, Delmar Publishers, Inc.
13. Friedman D: Taking the scare out of caring for seizure patients, Nurs 88 18(2):52, 1988.
14. Given C, Collins C, and Given B: Source of stress among families caring for relatives with Alzheimer's disease, Nurs Clin North Am 23(1):69, 1989.
15. Gray-Vickrey P: Evaluating Alzheimer's patients—the importance of being thorough, Nurs '89 18(2):34, 1988.
16. Hahn K: Left vs. right: what a difference the side makes in stroke, Nurs 87 17:4, 1987.
17. Hendrickson S: Psychological care of the patient with neurological dysfunction, J Neurosurg Nurs 16:202, 1984.
18. Hinkle J and others: Restoring social competence in minor head-injured patients, J Neurosci Nurs 18:268, 1986.
19. Hood GH and Dincher JR: Total patient care, ed 7, 1988, The CV Mosby Co.
20. Hufler D: Helping your dysphagic patient eat? RN 50:9, 36, 1987.
21. Jess L: Assessing your patient for increased intracranial pressure, Nurs 87 17:6, 1987.
22. Jess L: Investigating impaired mental status: an assessment guide you can use, Nurs 88 18:6, 1988.
23. Johnson S, Omery A, and Nikas D: Effects of conversation on intracranial pressure in comatose patients, Heart Lung 18:1, 1989.
24. Kirby N: The individual with high quadriplegia, Nurs Clin North Am 24(1):179, 1989.
25. Kirk E and Bradford L: Effects of alcohol on the CNS: implications for the neuroscience nurse, J Neurosci Nurs 19:326, 1987.

26. Konikow N: Alterations in movement: nursing assessment and implications, J Neurosurg Nurs 17:61, 1985.
27. Long BC and Phipps WJ: Medical-surgical nursing, ed 2, St Louis, 1989, The CV Mosby Co.
28. Mauser G: Neuromuscular respiratory failure—what the nurse knows makes a difference, J Neurosci Nurs 20110:117, 1988.
29. McBride E and DiStefano K: Explaining diagnostic tests for MS, Nurs 88 18(2):68, 1988.
30. Memmler RL and Wood DL: Structure and function of the human body, ed 4, Philadelphia, 1987, WB Saunders Co.
31. Mosby's medical and nursing dictionary, ed 2, St Louis, 1986, The CV Mosby Co.
32. Norman S: The pupil check, Am J Nurs 82:588, 1982.
33. Palmer M: Incontinence: the magnitude of the problem, Nurs Clin North Am 24:1, 1989.
34. Perlstein L and Ake J: AIDS: an overview for the neuroscience nurse, J Neurosci Nurs 19:296, 1987.
35. Peterson T: Action stat: autonomic dysreflexia, Nurs 87 17:33, 1987.
36. Plylar P: Management of the agitated and aggressive head-injured patient in an acute care setting, J Neurosci Nurs 21:353, 1989.
37. Price M and DeVroom H: A quick and easy guide to neurological assessment, J Neurosurg Nurs 17:313, 1985.
38. Reimer M: Head-injured patients, Nurs 89 19:3, 1989.
39. Romeo J: The critical minutes after spinal cord injury, RN 41:4, 61, 1988.
40. Rudy E: Advanced neurological and neurosurgical nursing, St Louis, 1985, The CV Mosby Co.
41. Santilli N and Sierzant T: Advances in the treatment of epilepsy, J Neurosci Nurs 19:144, 1987.
42. Schaefer S: Relieving pain—an analgesic guide, Am J Nurs 88:815, 1988.
43. Solomon EP and Phillips GA: Understanding human anatomy and physiology, Philadelphia, 1987, WB Saunders Co.
44. Stevens S and Becker K: A simple, step-by-step approach to neurological assessment, Part 1, Nurs 88 18:9, 1988.
45. Stevens S and Becker K: A simple, step-by-step approach to neurological assessment, Part 2, Nurs 88 18:10, 1988.
46. Stevenson J: Family stress related to home care of Alzheimer disease patients and implications for support, J Neurosci Nurs 22:179, 1990.
47. Thibodeau GA and Anthony CP: Structure and function of the body, ed 8, St Louis, 1988, Times Mirror/Mosby College Publishing.
48. Tucker SA and others: Patient care standards, ed 4, St Louis, 1988, The CV Mosby Co.
49. Whitney F: Relationship of laterality of stroke and emotional and functional outcome, J Neurosci Nurs 19:158, 1987.

CHAPTER CHALLENGE

KEY POINTS

- The nervous system is the body's link with the environment. It allows the interpretation of information and appropriate action to occur.
- The two main structural divisions of the nervous system are the central nervous system and the peripheral nervous system.
- The central nervous system is composed of the brain and the spinal cord.
- The peripheral nervous system is composed of the nerve cells lying outside of the central nervous system. It is composed of the somatic nervous system and the autonomic nervous system.
- A nerve cell is composed of three parts: the dendrite, the cell body, and the axon. The space between each nerve cell is called the synapse.
- All neurons are governed by the "all or none" law, which means there is never a partial transmission of a message. The impulse must be strong enough to elicit a response, or the impulse is not transmitted.
- Myelin is a white, waxy, fatty material that covers neuron fibers. It increases the rate of transmission of impulses and protects and insulates the fibers.
- Another material that covers neuron fibers is found only in the peripheral nervous system. It is called neurilemma, and it helps to regenerate injured axons.
- The brain and spinal cord are protected by the bony coverings (skull and vertebral column), the cerebrospinal fluid, and the three meninges (pia mater, arachnoid, and dura mater).
- The cerebrum is the largest part of the brain and contains five major areas: motor, sensory, visual, speech, and auditory. The cerebrum governs the ability to reason and make judgments.
- The diencephalon lies beneath the cerebrum and contains the thalamus and hypothalamus. The thalamus serves as a relay station, while the hypothalamus has several roles, such as temperature control, water balance, and appetite.

CHAPTER CHALLENGE—cont'd

KEY POINTS (cont'd)

- The cerebellum is the second largest portion of the brain and is responsible for coordination of skeletal muscles and maintenance of balance and equilibrium.
- The peripheral nervous system is composed of the cranial nerves, the spinal nerves, and the autonomic nervous system.
- The autonomic nervous system contains two subdivisions: the sympathetic nervous system and the parasympathetic nervous system. The sympathetic nervous system "speeds" things up and the parasympathetic nervous system "slows" things down.
- Normal changes of aging are not the same as senility, Alzheimer's disease, or organic brain damage.
- The source of any headache should be determined through neurological testing, because it may be a symptom of a serious pathological condition.
- A lumbar puncture should not be done if there is evidence of increased intracranial pressure because of the danger of brain herniation.
- Any increase in the volume of one of the contents of the cranium (brain, blood vessels, and cerebrospinal fluid) results in increased intracranial pressure, because the cranial vault is rigid and does not expand.
- Classic signs of increased intracranial pressure include restlessness, disorientation, headache, contralateral hemiparesis, an ipsilaterally dilated pupil, and visual changes that include blurring and diplopia.
- Nursing intervention measures can significantly influence intracranial pressure.
- Epilepsy is a transitory disturbance in consciousness or in motor, sensory, or autonomic functions with or without loss of consciousness, caused by sudden, excessive, and disorderly electrical discharges of the brain.
- Early symptoms of multiple sclerosis are usually transitory.
- Cerebrovascular accident (CVA) is the most common disease of the nervous system and can be caused by thrombus, embolus, or hemorrhage.
- Approximately 40% of patients with AIDS have neurological symptoms that result from infection from HIV itself or from associated complications of AIDS.
- Many patients with head injury may recover physically, but they will have behavioral and psychological problems that make it difficult for them to function independently.
- The signs and symptoms of intracranial tumors result from both local and general effects of the tumor.
- Autonomic dysreflexia in the patient with spinal cord injury is a medical emergency that demands quick nursing interventions.
- The first sign of increased intracranial pressure may be a lessening of the state of consciousness.
- It is important to document patients' behaviors in terms of what is seen, not what is inferred.

STUDY QUESTIONS

1. The central nervous system works with what system to maintain homeostasis in the body:
   a. Endocrine
   b. Integumentary
   c. Musculoskeletal
   d. None of the above
2. Special chemicals that assist in the transmission of a message are called:
   a. Dendrites
   b. Axons
   c. Neurotransmitters
   d. Cell bodies
3. The neuron has special structures that receive impulses and transmit them to the cell body. They are called:
   a. Axons
   b. Dendrites
   c. Cell bodies
   d. Neurotransmitters
4. The nodes of Ranvier:
   a. Increase the speed of message transmission
   b. Decrease the speed of message transmission
   c. Increase regeneration of the nerve cell
   d. Decrease regeneration of the nerve cell
5. Another name for the "innerbrain," which contains the hypothalamus and thalamus, is the:
   a. Cerebrum
   b. Cerebellum
   c. Diencephalon
   d. Brainstem
6. Which part of the brain is mainly involved in coordination of skeletal muscles, maintenance of balance, and control of muscle tone:
   a. Cerebrum
   b. Cerebellum
   c. Diencephalon
   d. Brainstem
7. Which part of the brain contains the respiratory center:
   a. Medulla
   b. Thalamus
   c. Hypothalamus
   d. Cerebrum
8. This covering of nerve tissue allows regeneration:
   a. Myelin
   b. Nodes of Ranvier
   c. Neurilemma
   d. Pia mater
9. A total or partial loss of the ability to recognize familiar objects or persons through sensory stimulation is which of the following:
   a. Apraxia
   b. Agnosia
   c. Aphasia
   d. Dysphagia
10. How much cerebrospinal fluid circulates in the ventricular system at any one time:
    a. 50-100 ml
    b. 125-150 ml
    c. 175-200 ml
    d. 500-570 ml
11. Which is not a normal aging change of the neurological system:
    a. Altered sleep/wakefulness ratio
    b. Senile changes of mental ability
    c. Reduction in cerebral blood flow
    d. Decrease in brain weight
12. What is the most significant symptom of increased intracranial pressure:
    a. Pupil changes
    b. Ipsilateral paralysis
    c. Vomiting
    d. Decreasing level of consciousness
13. Which test should not be done if there is an indication of increased intracranial pressure:
    a. CT scan
    b. MRI scan
    c. Lumbar puncture
    d. Electroencephalogram
14. What nursing intervention is contraindicated in the presence of a head injury:
    a. Suctioning through the nose
    b. Suctioning through the mouth
    c. Turning from side to side
    d. Range of motion exercises
15. What may be the first sign of increased intracranial pressure:
    a. Unequal pupils
    b. Decorticate posturing
    c. Change in the level of consciousness
    d. Projectile vomiting
16. When a patient has a motor neurological problem, flexion contractures may occur. Which are characteristic of contractures:
    a. Abduction and extension
    b. Extension and adduction
    c. Abduction and flexion
    d. Flexion and adduction

STUDY QUESTIONS (cont'd)

17. Which of the following is not a cause of autonomic dysreflexia:
    a. Kinked catheter
    b. Bowel impaction
    c. Infection
    d. Low temperature
18. What is the first nursing intervention that is necessary if a patient has autonomic dysreflexia:
    a. Sit the patient upright
    b. Check for bowel impaction
    c. Give medication as ordered
    d. Place the patient in supine position
19. What nursing intervention is appropriate for the patient with AIDS:
    a. Isolating the patient so that others are not exposed
    b. Keeping the patient active so that he does not have a chance to worry about the diagnosis
    c. Encouraging the patient to talk about fears and concerns
    d. Providing three large meals a day
20. A patient is not able to tell the position of the body without looking at it. What is this called:
    a. Agnosia
    b. Apraxia
    c. Proprioception
    d. Sensory loss
21. Which nursing intervention would be helpful in reducing increased intracranial pressure:
    a. Spacing nursing interventions to allow for rest
    b. Suctioning hourly to keep the airway patent
    c. Adding extra blankets to keep the patient warm
    d. Turning the patient frequently to prevent skin impairment
22. Which nursing intervention would not be appropriate for the patient with multiple sclerosis:
    a. Taking the patient to the bathroom frequently
    b. Giving a hot bath to ensure cleanliness
    c. Encouraging fluids to prevent urinary infection
    d. Using a suppository to help evacuate the bowel
23. If a patient who has been conscious for several days after a head injury becomes less responsive, what should be suspected:
    a. Epidural hematoma
    b. Ruptured aneurysm
    c. Skull fracture
    d. Subdural hematoma
24. What nursing intervention is not helpful for the patient with a swallowing problem (dysphagia):
    a. Encouraging the patient to hyperextend the neck
    b. Encouraging the patient to take small bites
    c. Not mixing solids and liquids together
    d. Encouraging a relaxed environment for eating
25. Patients with a seizure often experience a warning feeling before a seizure. What is this called:
    a. Postictal period
    b. Tonic sign
    c. Aura
    d. Convulsions
26. The appropriate intervention for the nurse to take during a grand mal seizure include all of the following except:
    a. Turning head or body to one side to aid with airway
    b. Prying open jaws to place padded tongue blade
    c. Remaining in attendance with patient
    d. Loosening constrictive clothing, especially around neck
27. In a patient with a cerebrovascular accident who has hemianopsia, which is the best side for the nurse to approach:
    a. Nonparalyzed side
    b. Paralyzed side
28. Which of the following signs and symptoms are not indicative of autonomic dysreflexia:
    a. Bradycardia
    b. Hypotension
    c. Diaphoresis
    d. Severe headache
29. Which of the following is often a problem in advanced Parkinson's disease:
    a. Paralysis
    b. Dementia
    c. Aspiration pneumonia
    d. Sjögren's syndrome

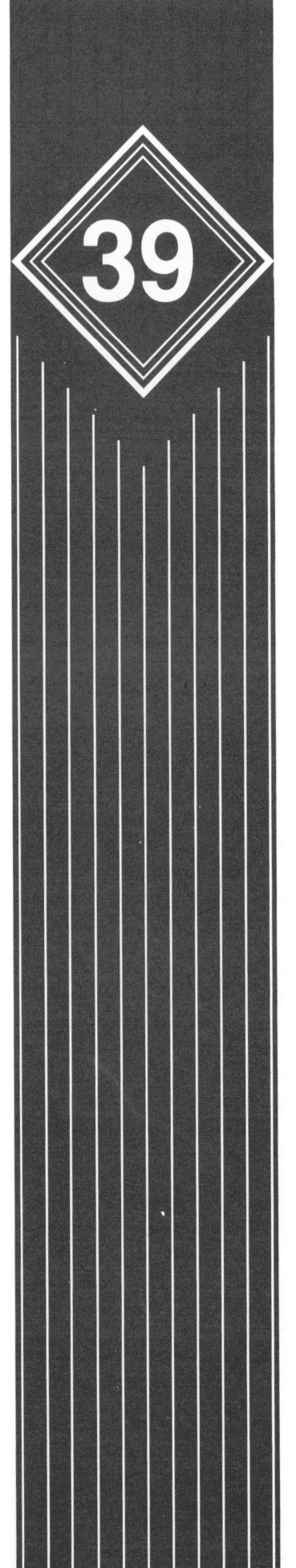

39

Care of the Patient with an Immune Disorder

IVA L. MUELLER

LEARNING OBJECTIVES

After reading this chapter, the student should be able to do the following:

- Define the key terms.
- Describe the two major types of immunity: innate and adaptive.
- Review the mechanisms of immune response.
- Explain the terms *immunocompetent, immunodeficient,* and *autoimmunity*.
- Discuss the hypersensitivity diseases.
- Outline the immediate aggressive treatment in anaphylaxis.
- Describe the nursing care plan for a patient with systemic lupus erythematosus.
- Explain an immunodeficiency disease.

RELATED TOPICS OF INTEREST

- Cells, tissues, and membranes (Chapter 27)
- Care of the patient with an integumentary disorder (Chapter 29)
- Care of the patient with a respiratory disorder (Chapter 34)
- Care of the patient with AIDS (Chapter 40)
- Care of the patient with cancer (Chapter 41)

KEY TERMS

Define the following:

- adaptive immunity
- allergen
- antigen
- attenuated
- autoimmune
- autologous
- cellular immunity
- humoral immunity
- hypersensitivity
- immune serum
- immunity
- immunization
- immunocompetent
- immunodeficiency
- immunogen
- immunoglobulin
- immunology
- immunosuppressive
- immunotherapy
- innate immunity
- lymphokine
- nonspecific immunity
- perennial
- proliferation
- specific immunity

NATURE OF IMMUNITY

The role of the immune system is to protect the body from disease. Resistance to disease is referred to as **immunity.** There are two major subclassifications of immunity: innate (natural) and adaptive (acquired) immunity (Fig. 39-1). Innate immunity is nonspecific, whereas adaptive immunity is specific. The study of the immune system is **immunology.**

Innate or Natural Immunity

The body's first line of defense against disease **(innate immunity)** protects locally against the external environment. The innate system is composed of the skin and mucous membranes, cilia, stomach acid, tears, saliva, sebaceous glands, and secretions and flora of the intestine and vagina. These organs, tissues, and secretions provide biochemical and physical barriers to disease. The first line of defense provides **nonspecific immunity** to the individual.

Adaptive or Acquired Immunity

The body's second line of defense against disease **(adaptive immunity)** protects the internal environment. The systemic immune system is composed of highly specialized cells and tissues, including the thymus, spleen, bone marrow, blood, and lymph (Fig. 39-2). Adaptive or acquired immunity includes both humoral and cell-mediated immunity. The characteristics of an adaptive immune system are specificity (specific) and memory. This **specific immunity** results from the production of antibodies in the cells. Antibodies develop naturally after infection or artificially after vaccinations. Another function of the immune system is to maintain homeostasis by removing damaged elements from the system. The third function is to provide the body with a surveillance network to guard against development, growth, and dissemination of tumor cells.

The cells of the immune system are the macrophages and the lymphocytes. When organisms pass the epithelial barriers, phagocytes become activated. Phagocytes also have the ability to migrate through the bloodstream to the tissues for the body's second line of defense against disease. Phagocytes engulf and destroy microorganisms that pass the skin and mucous membrane barriers. These cells also assist in the immune response by carrying antigens to the lymphocytes.

Lymphocytes include the T cells and B cells (Fig. 39-3) and the large, granular lymphocytes also known as NK or natural killer cells. Approximately 80% of the lymphocytes are T cell lymphocytes.

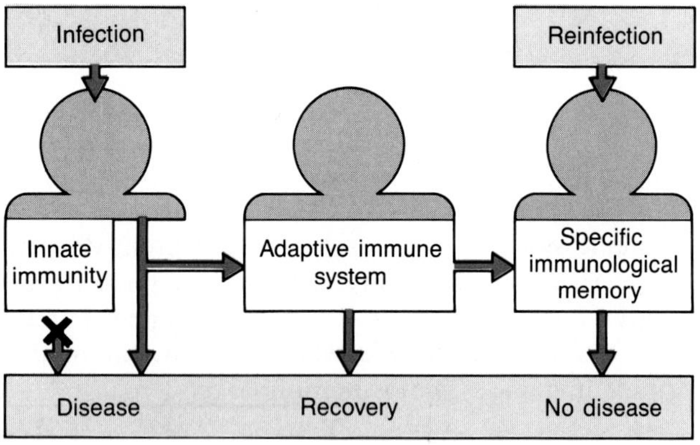

FIG. 39-1 When an infectious agent enters the body, it first encounters elements of the innate immune system. These may be sufficient to prevent disease, but if not, a disease will result and the adaptive immune system is activated. The adaptive immune system produces recovery from the disease and establishes a specific immunological memory, so that after reinfection with the same agent, no disease results. The individual has acquired immunity to the infectious agent.

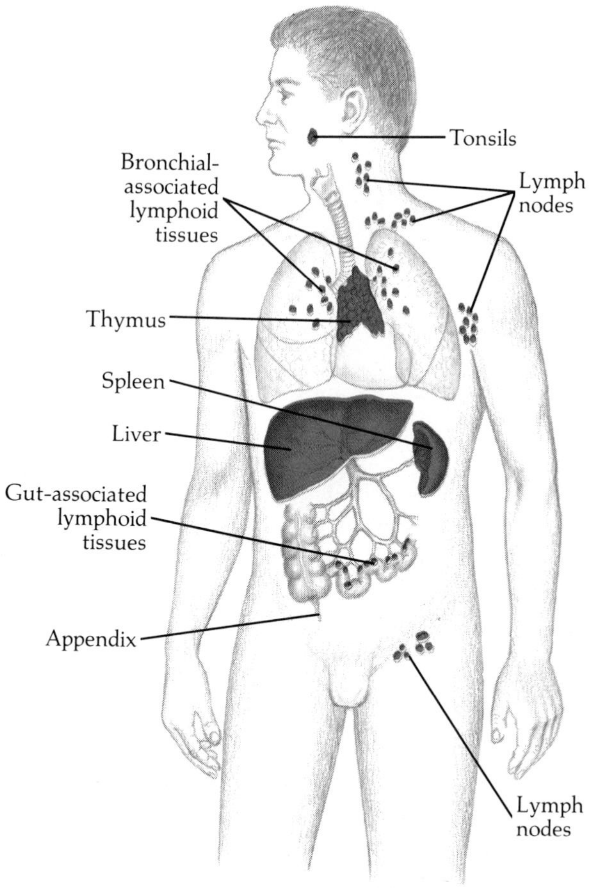

FIG. 39-2 Organization of the immune system.

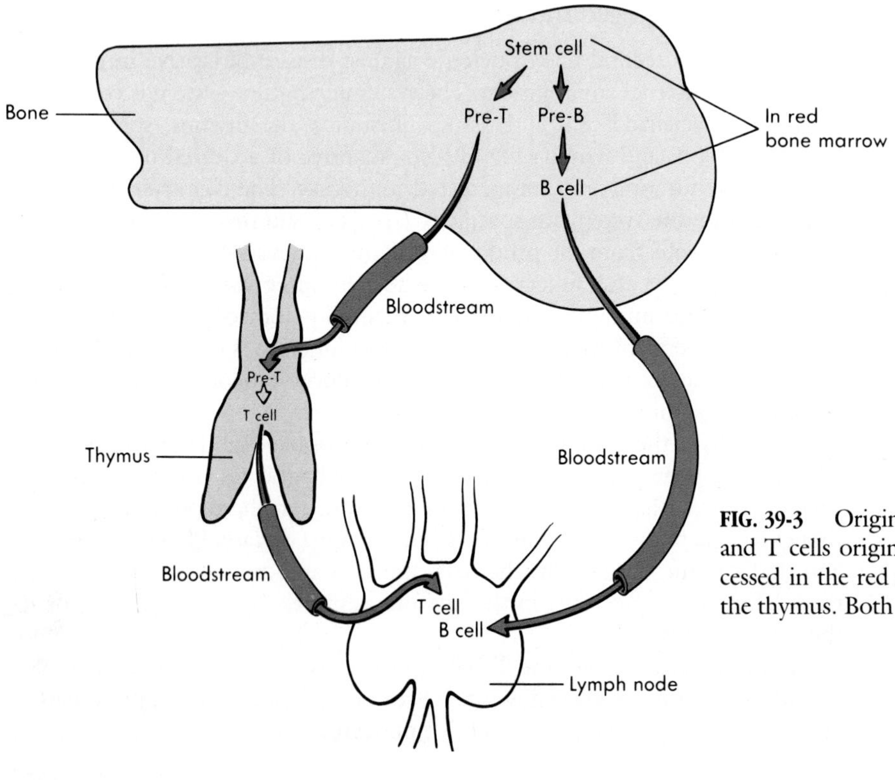

FIG. 39-3 Origin and processing of B and T cells. Both B and T cells originate in red bone marrow. B cells are processed in the red marrow, whereas T cells are processed in the thymus. Both cell types circulate to other lymph tissues.

When activated, T cells release a substance called **lymphokine,** which has a profound effect on other T cells and attracts macrophages to the area. In addition to these functions, in the antigen-antibody reaction, T cells cooperate with the B cells to produce antibodies but do not produce antibodies themselves. T cells are responsible for cell-mediated immunity and provide the body with protection against viruses, fungi, and parasites. T cells also provide protection in allograft (transfer of tissue between two genetically dissimilar individuals of the same species) and against malignant cells.

B cells comprise approximately 20% of the lymphocyte population. B cells cause the production of antibodies and proliferate (increase in number) in response to a particular **antigen.** B cells migrate to the peripheral circulation and tissues and eventually are filtered from the lymph and stored in the lymphoid tissue of the body.

It is significant to note that the initial formation of B cells does not require antigen stimulation or any other environmental stimuli. However, B cell **proliferation,** reproduction, or multiplication depends on antigen stimulation. B cells are responsible for humoral immunity. B cells produce antibodies and provide protection against bacteria, viruses, and soluble antigens.

Humoral Immunity

Humoral immunity is mediated by the B cells. B cells produce antibodies in response to antigenic challenge. On first exposure to a given antigen, a primary humoral response is initiated. This response is generally slow compared with subsequent antigen exposures. Memory B cells cause antibody proliferation at a much more rapid rate once the body has experienced a primary antigen exposure. It does not matter if primary exposure is caused by antigen or **immunization** agent; the memory response is more rapid and more sustained after initial exposure.

Antigen is presented to the T cell helper population by the macrophage. Most are then taken to the B cells, and the B cell initiates production of antibody assisted by helper T cells. Suppressor T cells maintain the humoral response at a level appropriate for the stimulus.

Antibodies produced by one's own body are said to provide active immunity. Antibodies formed by another in response to a specific antigen and administered to an individual will provide only temporary or passive immunity.

Even though humoral immunity is mediated by the B cell population, helper T cells and suppressor T cells have a function and are vital to the **immunocompetent** person. Both the number and functions of the helper and suppressor T cells help determine the strength and persistence of an immune response. The normal ratio of helper T cells to suppressor T cells is 2:1 in the body. When this ratio is disrupted, autoimmune and immunodeficient diseases occur.

Exposure to antigen and response with antibody may activate either (1) the humoral complement system, which results in breakdown of the bacteria and release of lysosomes to destroy bacteria or (2) the antigen/antibody reaction, which results in degranulation of most cells and release of histamine, which produces the symptoms of allergy. Antigen is referred to as **allergen** when symptoms of allergy occur. Antigen is referred to as **immunogen** when immunity results.

THE COMPLEMENT SYSTEM

The complement system is a system of approximately 20 serum proteins that interact with each other and with other components of the innate (natural) and adaptive (acquired) immune systems. Normally, complement enzymes are inactive in plasma and body fluids. When an antigen and antibody interact, the complement system is activated. Complement functions in a "step by step" series much like the clotting mechanism, but with a different purpose. The complement system can destroy the cell membrane of many bacterial species, and this action attracts phagocytes to the area.

CELLULAR IMMUNITY

Cellular immunity results when T cells are activated by an antigen. Whole cells become sensitized in a process similar to that which stimulates the B cells to form antibodies. Once these T cells have been sensitized, they are released into the blood and body tissues where they remain indefinitely. On contact with the antigen to which they are sensitized, they will attach to the organism and destroy it. Cellular immunity is effective against fungi, viruses, and tumors and is the major reaction in the rejection of organ transplants.

Hypersensitivity reactions are cell-mediated responses of the body. For review, see Box 39-1.

GENETIC CONTROL OF IMMUNITY

More is being discovered about the genetic role in immunity. There is a genetic link to both well-developed immune systems and also poorly developed or compromised immune systems.

The immune system develops at different rates and at different times in fetal and early life. For humans, the bone marrow provides the continuous service of stem cells and all of the other cells involved in the immune response.

TOLERANCE

Immunological tolerance is the development of nonreactivity toward particular antigens and as such is the

BOX 39-1

REVIEW OF THE MECHANISMS OF IMMUNE RESPONSE

- The skin and mucous membranes are natural barriers to infectious agents. When these barriers are crossed, the immune response is begun in the immunocompetent host.
- The first time an antigen enters the body, the antigen is processed by macrophages and presented to lymphocytes. Responses of B cells to the antigen in humoral immunity require interaction with T helper cells, which assist B cells in responding to the antigen by proliferating, synthesizing, and secreting the appropriate antibody. Antigen are then neutralized by antibody or can form immune complexes or be phagocytosed by macrophages or neutrophils.
- Humoral immunity is not effective against intracellular organisms. Once the organisms have penetrated the host's cells, the antibody cannot function. Cellular immunity is the primary defense against intracellular organisms. In cellular immunity the antigen is processed by macrophages and recognized by T cells. T cells produce lymphokines, which further attract macrophages and neutrophils to the site for phagocytosis, or cytotoxic killer T cells can respond directly.
- Any B cell or T cell lineage could lead to immunodeficiency, as well as to defects in the complement or phagocytic systems.

reverse of immunity. Tolerance is enhanced by immunosuppressive drugs. The fundamental basis of the immune system is tolerance to "self" tissues and lack of tolerance to foreign tissue or antigen, marked by an appropriate immune response. Failure of the appropriate response may be marked by a failure to respond against foreign protein or a hypersensitivity reaction.

THE IMMUNE RESPONSE

There are two ways of assisting the body to develop immunity: immunization and immunotherapy. The theory behind immunization is to have controlled exposure to a disease-producing pathogen, developing antibody production while preventing disease. The first immunization is credited to Edward Jenner (1796), who observed that individuals who had had cowpox became immune to the disease. The idea of administering "attenuated [weakened] microbes" developed, and the scientific approach was applied by Louis Pasteur. Vaccines and toxoids are altered, **attenuated** in such a way as to reduce their degree of power without losing their ability to produce antibodies. In immunization, the immune system mounts a greater response to second encounter with antigen. The vaccine, or toxoid, stimulates humoral immunity, which provides protection from disease for months to years.

Immunotherapy consists of injecting a person with a very diluted antigen (allergen) to which the patient has a type I hypersensitivity. The strength of the dilution is increased over a long period, and weekly injections are given over a 1- to 3-year period. The theory behind immunotherapy is to assist the individual to build a tolerance to the allergen without developing fever or increased signs and symptoms. *Desensitization* is another term used for *immunotherapy*. It is indicated for patients with clinically significant disease in whom avoidance of the allergen or treatment with medication has proven to be inadequate. It is considered safe in properly selected patients but does present problems, which include a lengthy, expensive process and a potential for severe anaphylaxis.

Immunotherapy may be coseasonal, preseasonal, or **perennial.** Perennial therapy is most widely accepted, since it allows for a higher cumulative dose, which produces a better effect. Perennial therapy usually begins with 0.05 ml of a 1:10,000 dilution and increases to 0.5 ml in a 6-week period. The amount given again decreases to 0.05 ml while the dilution lessens to 1:1000 to begin the next series. The amount increases each week until a 0.5 ml dose is given. The next cycle begins with a 0.05 ml dose of 1:100 dilution. Over another 6-week period, the amount administered will increase to 0.5 ml. Perennial therapy is administered subcutaneously. The patient must always be observed for at least 20 minutes after administration, since hypersensitivity reaction or anaphylaxis may occur. The treatment protocol for anaphylaxis with immunotherapy is generally accepted to be 0.3 ml of 1:1000 adrenalin chloride subcutaneously every 15 minutes for 3 doses.

Most patients are begun on immunotherapy at the physician's office, and subsequent weekly injections are given until the maintenance level is reached. Home administration by the patient or a family member is acceptable once maintenance level is reached. Interrupted regimens because of illness may place the patient at risk for reaction. The physician should be consulted before administering a dose of diluted allergen if illness or interruption of time schedule has occurred while the patient is on maintenance immunotherapy.

Alterations in the Immune Response

Failure of the immune system occurs in several ways and expresses itself in mild to severe form. There are many points in which the system can malfunction while attempting to provide the body with protective defense.

It is thought that failures occur because of genetic factors, developmental defects, infection, malignancy, injury, drugs, or altered metabolic states.

Severity of altered immune response disorders ranges from mild to chronic to life threatening and is categorized as follows:

I **Hypersensitivity** disorder: involves allergic response and tissue rejection

II **Immunodeficiency** disease: involves altered and failed immune response

III **Autoimmune** disease: involves extensive tissue damage resulting from an immune system that seemingly reverses its function to one of self-destruction.

HYPERSENSITIVITY DISORDERS

Hypersensitivity disorders arise when harmless substances, such as pollens, danders, foods, and chemicals, are recognized as foreign. The body mounts an immune response in much the same way it does to any foreign protein. The result, however, differs. The host becomes sensitive after first exposure, and on subsequent exposure the allergic individual exhibits hypersensitivity reaction. Chronic exposure leads to chronic allergy response, which ranges from mild to incapacitating symptoms.

Hypersensitivity disorders are believed to be a genetic defect that allows increased production of IgE (**immunoglobulin** E—a humoral antibody). Exposure to antigen may occur by inhalation, ingestion, injection, or touch (contact). Symptoms occur as a result of histamine release and may be local (gastrointestinal, skin, respiratory, conjunctival) or systemic (anaphylaxis). The exact mechanism and pathway of these inflammatory responses are not clearly understood.

It is known that a combination of interrelated factors occurs with increased severity of symptoms. These factors include those found in Box 39-2.

BOX 39-2 **FACTORS INFLUENCING HYPERSENSITIVITY**

Host response to allergen. The more sensitive the individual, the greater the allergic response.

Exposure amount. Generally, the greater the amount of allergen the individual is exposed to, the greater the chance of severe reaction.

Nature of the allergen. Most allergy reactions are precipitated by complex, high molecular weight, protein substances.

Route of allergen entry. Most allergens enter the body via gastrointestinal and respiratory routes. Injections of venoms and medications hold a more severe threat of allergic response.

Repeated exposure. Generally, the more the individual is exposed, the greater the response.

Diagnostic Tests

Hypersensitivity illnesses are diagnosed largely through patient history and physical examination. Laboratory studies are supportive tools for diagnosis and therapy.

A thorough history is the most important diagnostic tool. A detailed history is taken, listing (1) onset, nature, and progression of symptoms, (2) aggravating and alleviating factors, and (3) frequency and duration of symptoms. Environmental, household, and occupational factors are assessed. Common offenders include pollens, spores, dusts, food, drugs, and insect venoms. Many but not all offenders are seasonal in nature. Symptoms generally vary from mild upper respiratory manifestations, such as sneezing and excessive nasal secretions, to watery, itching eyes. Skin symptoms are often eczema-like or urticarial. Diarrhea may be a gastrointestinal complaint in some individuals. More severe symptoms include those of the lower respiratory tract, such as coughing, wheezing, chest discomfort, breathing difficulties, and shock. Shock would soon be followed by cardiovascular collapse and respiratory arrest. The complete history will assist in accurate diagnosis.

The physical examination should include a thorough assessment of the skin, middle ear, conjunctiva, nasooropharynx, and chest.

Laboratory studies are usually not necessary unless allergic symptoms are severe and protracted. A complete blood count (CBC), skin testing, total serum IgE levels, and a specific IgE level for a particular allergen may be ordered. The latter test is called *RAST* (radioallergosorbent test).

Overview of Medical Management

Treatment of hypersensitivity disorders includes (1) symptom management with medications, (2) environmental control, and (3) immunotherapy. The most effective treatment is environmental control, which includes avoidance of the offending allergen.

Pollens are seasonal and can be avoided at season peaks or with air conditioning and limiting time spent outdoors. Mold spores can be reduced with dry conditions and air filters. House dust can be controlled with damp dusting, air filters, and decreased use of carpet and overstuffed furniture. Most other offending allergens can simply be avoided (food, drugs, chemicals, and stinging insects).

Medications are used to treat and alleviate symptoms. Antihistamines compete with histamine by attaching to the cell surface receptors and blocking histamine release. Antihistamines therefore must be initiated soon after exposure or taken on a regular basis. Drowsiness, mucous membrane dryness, and occasionally central nervous system excitation are side effects of the earlier antihistamines. Examples of these include pseudoephedrine (Actifed), diphenhydramine (Benadryl), chlorpheniramine (Chlor-Trimeton), and brompheniramine (Dimetapp). A more recent member, terfenadine (Seldane) does not cause the drowsiness and is therefore more desirable for those who experience drowsiness with antihistamine use.

Overview of Nursing Interventions

Assessment. Assessment should involve predominantly the integumentary, gastrointestinal, respiratory, and cardiovascular systems. The nurse should be aware of the seasonal nature of the complaints.

Collection of *subjective data* includes pruritus, nausea, and uneasiness.

Collection of *objective data* includes sneezing, excessive nasal secretions, lacrimation, inflamed nasal membranes, skin rash or areas of raised inflammation, diarrhea, cough, wheeze, impaired breathing, and hypotension.

Nursing diagnoses. Nursing diagnoses for patients with atopic illness include (1) potential for injury, related to exposure to allergen, (2) activity intolerance, related to malaise, and (3) potential for infection, related to inflammation of protective mucous membranes.

Patient teaching. Patient teaching should revolve around the specific diagnosis. The patient should be informed regarding seasonal avoidance of the offending allergens and should understand the therapeutic medication plan. The nurse will focus on health promotion and health teaching for self-care management.

Urticaria

Etiology and pathophysiology. Urticaria (hives) occurs as a local allergic response, generally to foods. Offending foods may include oranges, strawberries, nuts, tomatoes, and shellfish. Food coloring may precipitate symptoms in some individuals.

Clinical manifestations. The pruritic lesions are IgE-mediated tissue responses and are pale pink, raised wheals. The wheals are transient and may disappear and then recur elsewhere on the body. They may involve any part of the body, including skin, mouth, and larynx, and may occasionally cause respiratory and gastrointestinal tract symptoms.

Nursing interventions. Allergic urticaria is self-limiting, and treatment other than allergen avoidance may not be necessary. Local application of Caladryl or calamine lotion may be used. Antihistamines and epinephrine may be used to hasten relief of more extensive reactions.

Angioedema

Etiology and pathophysiology. Angioedema is a form of urticaria. It occurs in the subcutaneous tissue, whereas urticaria is a skin and mucous membrane lesion. Angioedema is caused by the same offenders that cause urticarial lesions.

Angioedema is characterized by local edema of an entire area, such as an eyelid, thumb, or lip. Seldom does more than a single edematous area appear at a time.

Medical management. Treatment to relieve angioedema may include the use of antihistamine drugs—epinephrine or corticosteroids.

Nursing interventions. A cold pack or cold compress may be used.

Allergic Rhinitis and Allergic Conjunctivitis (Hay Fever)

Etiology and pathophysiology. These atopic allergic conditions are a result of antigen/antibody reactions occurring in the nasal membranes, nasopharynx, and conjunctiva from inhaled or contact allergens. Many infants, children, and adults have this seasonal or perennial conditions, resulting in absences from school and work.

Rhinitis and conjunctivitis occur as the result of antigen/antibody reaction. Ciliary action slows, mucosal gland secretion increases, leukocyte (eosinophil) infiltration occurs, and because of increased capillary permeability and vasodilation, local tissue edema results.

Common allergens causing allergic rhinitis and conjunctivitis (hay fever) are tree, grass, and weed pollens, mold spores, fungi, house dusts, mites, and animal danders. Other allergens include some foods, drugs, and insect stings.

Clinical manifestations. Acute ocular manifestations include edema, photophobia, excessive tearing, blurring of vision, and pruritus.

Individuals with rhinitis complain of excessive secretions or inability to breathe through the nose because of congestion and/or edema.

Serious otitis media symptoms can occur if the eustachian tubes are occluded. These symptoms occur more in childhood, with the individual complaining of ear fullness, ear popping, or decreased hearing.

Assessment. The initial complaints of seasonal rhinitis and conjunctivitis include severe sneezing, congestion, pruritus, and lacrimation (watery eyes). Cough, epistaxis, and headache may also occur. More chronic symptoms include headache, severe nasal congestion, postnasal drip, and cough. If not treated, chronic sufferers eventually develop secondary infections, such as otitis media, bronchitis, sinusitis, and pneumonia.

Medical management. Treatment goals are to relieve symptoms and prevent infections and other complaints, such as malaise, extreme fatigue, and severe headaches. Avoiding the allergen is effective. Perennial use of antihistamines is recommended. Changing from one antihistamine to another seasonally may help to impede tolerance to any one medication.

BOX 39-3 CONTROL OF ENVIRONMENTAL ALLERGENS

1. Use air conditioner and air filters; change furnace filter monthly.
2. Use synthetic overstuffed furniture, pillows, and mattresses—no kapok or feathers.
3. Avoid wool clothing. Use garment bags to decrease dust.
4. Damp dust floors.
5. Avoid dried plants.
6. Avoid drying laundry outdoors during seasonal peaks of allergens.
7. Avoid outdoor exposure during seasonal peaks of offending pollens, especially on windy days.
8. Have no fur-bearing pets.
9. Avoid gardening, lawn mowing, and damp, musty places.

BOX 39-4 SELF-CARE MANAGEMENT AND COMFORT MEASURES TO RELIEVE SYMPTOMS

Congestion. Keep head of bed elevated 45 degrees to facilitate drainage. Humidify air. Use decongestant as directed.

Eye discomfort. Apply warm compress. Use synthetic "tears." Avoid sprays, makeup, or other irritating contactants.

Headaches. Administer analgesics. Apply hot pack over facial sinuses.

Fatigue. Plan rest periods. Be aware of potential interference to activity that may occur related to drug therapy.

Decongestants may be added and used intermittently for 3 to 5 days if congestion occurs. Common over-the-counter decongestants, such as phenylephrine, pseudoephedrine, chlorpheniramine, and phenylpropanolamine, are contained in familiar products, such as Actifed, Triaminic, and Robitussin.

Long-term, consistent use of topical or nasal corticosteroids is highly recommended. Included are beclomethasone (Vancenase, Beconase), dexamethasone (Decadron, Turbinaire), and flunisolide (Nasalide). Corticosteroids require a prescription.

Pressure headaches may require narcotic analgesics until symptoms are relieved. Hot packs over facial sinuses offer relief if headache is related to sinus congestion.

Nursing interventions. Because these atopic illnesses are self-limiting, the nurse will focus on health promotion and health maintenance teaching to provide for self-care management.

Patient teaching. The nurse's responsibilities in patient education are as follows:

1. Teach patient ways to avoid the allergen (Box 39-3).
2. Teach patient self-care management through symptom control (Box 39-4).
3. Teach medication action and usage; assess for medication effectiveness.

Atopic Dermatitis

Etiology and pathophysiology. Atopic dermatitis (eczema) is an inflammatory skin response to certain allergenic offenders. It is characterized by dry, erythematous, raised pruritic lesions, often occurring facially and at the antecubital and popliteal spaces.

Clinical manifestations. Atopic dermatitis occurs in individuals with a strong family history of allergy. Allergens may be contactant or ingested.

Assessment. Generally, in contact dermatitis the allergic manifestation occurs locally where the contact occurred, such as nettle rash on fingertips or on the leg that brushed the plant. Eczema occurs on the face and at the antecubital spaces. Both are manifestations of antigen/antibody reaction and are IgE mediated.

Medical management, nursing interventions, and patient teaching. Treatment modalities include hot moist packs, emollients, and topical steroid creams. The nursing diagnosis is impaired skin integrity. Intervention includes skin care and application of topical medication.

Patient education should include avoidance of the allergen, application of a thin layer of steroid cream after skin cleansing or hot moist packs, and prevention of skin breakdown through use of lotions and emollients and decreased use of soaps and dry heat.

Anaphylaxis

Etiology and pathophysiology. The most severe allergic reaction that is IgE-mediated is anaphylaxis, or systemic reaction to allergens. The antigens causing anaphylaxis include (1) venoms, (2) drugs, such as penicillin and aspirin, (3) contrast media dyes, (4) insect stings, and (5) some food.

Clinical manifestations. In anaphylaxis, the reaction occurs very rapidly after exposure, from seconds to a few minutes. If left untreated, the symptoms can lead to death in a relatively short time. Fatal reactions are associated with a fall in blood pressure, laryngeal edema, and bronchospasm, leading to cardiovascular collapse, myocardial infarction, and respiratory failure.

In anaphylaxis, massive release of mediators initiates

events in target organs throughout the body. Skin and gastrointestinal symptoms may occur, although respiratory and cardiovascular symptoms predominate. Anaphylactic reactions are classified as mild, moderate, and severe.

Assessment. Early recognition of symptoms and early treatment may prevent severe reactions and even death. Generally, the more rapid the onset, the more severe the outcome. Overall, the individual may have a feeling of uneasiness that increases to a sense of foreboding and leads to a fear of impending death. The skin may or may not be involved. Urticaria and pruritus may be present in mild and moderate anaphylaxis, whereas cyanosis and pallor may be seen in severe reactions. Upper respiratory symptoms range from congestion and sneezing to edema of the tongue and larynx with stridor and occlusion of the upper airways. Lower respiratory symptoms will follow, including bronchospasm, wheezing, and severe dyspnea. Gastrointestinal (GI) symptoms will increase from nausea, vomiting, and diarrhea to dysphagia and involuntary stools. The patient may have cardiovascular symptoms, such as tachycardia and hypotension. Symptoms may increase, and the patient may display coronary insufficiency, vascular collapse, dysrhythmias, shock, cardiac arrest, respiratory failure, and death.

Medical management. Immediate aggressive treatment is the goal in anaphylaxis. At the first sign, 0.5 ml of epinephrine (Adrenalin Chloride) 1:1000 is given subcutaneously. It may be repeated at 15-minute intervals as prescribed by the physician. Benadryl 50 to 100 mg may be given IM or IV as indicated for allergic symptoms. If moderate to severe symptoms occur, IV therapy may be initiated to prevent vascular collapse and the patient may be intubated to prevent airway obstructions. Oxygen may be administered by mask. Aminophylline may be given to relieve bronchospasm.

Nursing interventions. These measures include the following:

1. Assess vital signs continuously.
2. Assess intake and output.
3. Assess respiratory status, including dyspnea, wheezing, and decreased breath sounds.
4. Assess circulatory status, including dysrhythmias, tachycardia, and hypotension.
5. Assess mental status, including anxiety, malaise, confusion, and coma.
6. Assess skin status, including erythema, urticaria, cyanosis, and pallor.
7. Assess GI status, including nausea, vomiting, diarrhea, and incontinence.

The diagnosis is most often made by a history of signs and symptoms. Looking and listening to the anxious patient should be a leading clue to suspecting anaphylaxis.

An alert diagnostician will question the patient about recent exposure to known antigens that cause anaphylaxis (Table 39-1). Most laboratory studies would not be beneficial.

Table 39-1 Common Allergens Causing Anaphylaxis

Drugs	Venoms	Foods
Vaccines	Honeybees	Peanuts
Allergen extracts	Wasps	Brazil nuts
Enzymes	Hornets	Cashew nuts
Penicillins		Berries
Sulfonamides		Shellfish
Dextrans		Egg albumin
Hormones		
Contrast media		
Anesthetic agents		

NURSING DIAGNOSES	NURSING INTERVENTIONS
Potential for injury related to exposure to allergen	Maintain airway. Administer medications as ordered.
Ineffective breathing pattern related to edema, bronchospasm, and increased secretions	Administer oxygen if ordered. Monitor vital signs. Suction if necessary.
Decreased cardiac output related to increased capillary permeability and vascular dilation	Monitor IV fluid infusions as ordered. Monitor vital signs. Monitor intake and output. Obtain complete allergy history. Document symptoms, interventions, and response.

Patient teaching. The nurse's responsibilities in patient education are as follows:

1. Reassure patient during procedures.
2. Teach patient avoidance of allergen.
3. Teach patient the use of Medic-Alert identification.
4. Teach patient preparation and administration of epinephrine subcutaneously.

Transfusion Reactions

Transfusion reactions are a hypersensitivity disorder and are best illustrated by reactions that occur with mismatched blood.

Careful selection of blood donors is important in prevention of transfusion reaction, followed by careful type and cross-matching of blood from donor to recipient. Storage of blood and administration protocol are important in blood reaction prevention. Blood and blood components should be refrigerated at specific temperatures until ½ hour before administration. Blood must be administered within 4 hours after refrigeration; blood components within 6 hours after refrigeration. Donor and recipient numbers are specific and must be thoroughly checked and the patient identified with an armband. All blood and blood products are administered through microaggregate filters. The nurse should monitor for adverse effects.

Transfusion reactions are labeled mild, moderate, and severe. The most severe reactions occur within the first 30 minutes, moderate reactions within 30 to 90 minutes, and mild reactions may be delayed late in the transfusion or hours to several days after transfusion.

Mild transfusion reaction symptoms include dermatitis, diarrhea, fever, chills, urticaria, cough, and orthopnea. Treatment includes (1) stopping the transfusion and (2) administering saline, steroids, and diuretics. Transfusion may continue at a slower rate.

In moderate reactions, in which fever, chills, urticaria, and wheezing occur after the first 30 minutes of administration, the transfusion is stopped and saline is continued. Antihistamines and epinephrine may be given. The physician decides if the transfusion is to continue. With severe reaction, the transfusion is stopped and saline is given to provide venous access. It is recommended that the blood or blood product be returned to the laboratory for immediate testing if any type of reaction occurs.

The best method for prevention of transfusion reaction is autologous transfusion, or use of one's own blood, for replacement therapy. Weeks to months in advance of expected need, the patient donates blood to be frozen and stored for personal use.

DELAYED HYPERSENSITIVITY DISEASE

Delayed hypersensitivity reactions occurring 24 to 72 hours after exposure are mediated by T cells accompanied by release of lymphokines. Delayed reaction contact dermatitis, such as after contact with poison ivy, is one example. Tissue transplant rejection is another example. Only transplant rejection will be discussed.

Transplant Rejection

Transfer of healthy tissue or organs from a donor to recipient has been done for many years. The immune process that protects the body from foreign protein is the same process at work in tissue transplant rejection. Knowledge of the function of the immune system enabled medical experts to find a way to control the rejection process. It is now possible to prepare the body before tissue transplant for grafting to be successful.

Autograft, or transplantation of tissue from one site to another on an individual, is successful. It is used after trauma and in reconstructive surgery.

Isograft is transfer of tissue between genetically identical individuals, such as identical twins.

Allograft is a term applied to the transplantation of tissue between members of the same species. Because few humans are born with an identical twin, allograft is the most common form of tissue transplant.

Antigenic determinants on the cells lead to graft rejection via the immune process. Therefore before transplant, recipient tissue is as closely matched as possible to donor tissue antigenic determinants. Tissue matching leads to a better chance of success.

Tissue rejection does not occur immediately after transplantation. It takes several days for vascularization to occur. Seven to ten days after blood supply is adequately established, sensitized lymphocytes appear in sufficient numbers for sloughing to occur at the site.

Graft rejection is slowed through use of chemical agents that interfere with the immune response process. Included are corticosteroids, cyclosporine A, and azathioprine. This chemical therapy is referred to as **immunosuppressive** therapy.

Infection is a threat to the immunosuppressed patient. Meticulous aseptic technique is required when caring for these individuals. Prophylactic antibiotic therapy may be advisable, and good skin care is necessary. Visits to the bedside are limited in frequency for both staff and family. Persons with infection are not allowed at the bedside.

IMMUNODEFICIENCY DISEASES

The first evidence of immunodeficiency disease is an increased susceptibility to infection. The problem can manifest as recurrent infection or chronic infection. Unusually severe infection with complications or incomplete clearing of an infection may also indicate an underlying immunodeficiency.

Defects in genes leading to immunodeficiency provide a hereditary link to the diseases.

Agammaglobulinemia

Etiology and pathophysiology. Agammaglobulinemia is a primary immunodeficiency disease of B cell deficiency occurring in boys. This severe deficiency illness is characterized by severe, recurrent, pyogenic infections.

Most primary immunodeficiency diseases are believed to be caused by single genetic defects.

Secondary immunodeficiency disease is acquired. An example is AIDS (see Chapter 40 for further discussion).

Multiple Myeloma

Etiology and pathophysiology. Multiple myeloma, a neoplastic immunodeficiency disease, occurs most frequently after age 40 and affects twice as many men as women. Onset is gradual and insidious and often goes unrecognized for years while the individual experiences frequent, recurrent bacterial infections. This increased susceptibility to infection follows disturbances of antibody formation by abnormal plasma cells. Suppression of normal antibody levels is seen in this plasma cell tumor disease. Incidence of multiple myeloma has increased and now approaches that of Hodgkin's disease.

Clinical manifestations. The disease process will show a proliferation of malignant plasma cells and development of single or multiple bone marrow tumors. This is followed by bone destruction throughout the body with dissemination into lymph nodes, liver, spleen, and kidneys.

The skeletal system symptoms typically involve the ribs, spine, and pelvis. Individuals complain of bone pain that increases with movement. Some develop pathological fractures accompanied by severe pain.

In the individual with multiple myeloma, disruption of production of erythrocytes, platelets, and leukocytes occurs because of crowding of the marrow by the abnormal proliferation of plasma cells. This leads to increased infection, anemia, and increased potential for bleeding. Calcium and phosphorus drain from bones, leading to hypercalcemia and renal problems.

Assessment. Collection of *subjective data* includes assessment of the patient's complaints of pain, including location, intensity, and duration. The patient's understanding of the disease, verbalization of discouragement, hopelessness, and desires for emotional and spiritual support should be addressed.

Collection of *objective data* includes assessing the patients facial expression for signs of increased pain with movement, the ability to perform activities of daily living, increased body temperature, increased potential for bleeding, changes in urine characteristics, and effectiveness of medication administration.

Diagnostic tests. Diagnosis of multiple myeloma is made with x-ray studies, bone marrow biopsy, and laboratory examination of blood and urine.

X-ray examinations reveal widespread demineralization and osteoporosis. Bone marrow studies reveal large numbers of immature plasma cells, which normally account for only 5% of marrow population. Bence Jones protein appears in the urine.

Medical management. Treatment is symptomatic, since multiple myeloma is not curable.

Radiation and chemotherapy are initiated to both reduce tumor size and impede tumor growth. Radiation is used in small doses. The antineoplastic drugs of choice are the alkylating agents, such as melphalan (Alkeran) and cyclophosphamide (Cytoxan). Bone marrow depression occurs as a side effect, and therefore the CBC is monitored during treatment.

Hypercalcemia and pain also should be addressed. Hospitalization to administer corticosteroids and fluids may be required.

Nursing interventions. Care of the patient with multiple myeloma should focus on pain relief, prevention of infection and bone injury, and maintenance of hydration. Attention to the psychosocial, emotional, and spiritual needs is also indicated.

NURSING DIAGNOSES	NURSING INTERVENTIONS
Potential for injury, related to osteoporosis	Protect from bone injury; use log roll, turning sheet.
Pain, related to disease process	Administer analgesics as ordered. Assess contributing factors.
Fluid volume deficit: actual, related to impaired renal function	Increase fluid intake to 3000-4000 ml/day. Maintain intake and output record.
Potential for infection, related to stasis of body fluids and immunosuppression	Administer antibiotics as ordered. Maintain aseptic technique. Monitor vital signs.
Spiritual distress, related to intense suffering	Listen to patient complaints of anger, concern, alienation from God; refer to religious counselor or significant others who could provide support.

Patient teaching. The nurse's responsibilities in patient education are as follows:

1. Teach patient to avoid traumatic bone injury.
2. Teach patient pain control modality.
3. Teach patient importance of hydration.
4. Teach patient prevention of infection.
5. Assist patient to identify spiritual resources.

AUTOIMMUNE DISORDERS

Autoimmune disorders are failures of the tolerance to "self." Autoimmune disorders may be described as an immune attack on the self and result from the failure to distinguish "self" protein from "foreign" protein.

As a person ages, the probability of failure in any system occurs. It is not clearly understood what happens when autoimmune responses occur.

Whatever the cause, autoimmune disorders exist. There are many illnesses now believed to be in this classification. Included are pernicious anemia, Guillain-Barré syndrome, rheumatic fever, rheumatoid arthritis, ulcerative colitis, and male infertility. These conditions are discussed elsewhere in the text. The following are autoimmune diseases.

Myasthenia Gravis

Etiology and pathophysiology. Myasthenia gravis is an unpredictable autoimmune disorder occurring primarily in women in the 18- to 25-year age group and men in the 50- to 60-year age group. It is not considered hereditary, and the incidence is somewhere between 2 to 10 in every 100,000 population.

The defect is thought to be an alteration in neuromuscular transmission that causes muscular weakness. One theory is that acetylcholine is either blocked or deactivated at postsynaptic receptor sites because of acetylcholine antibodies. Myasthenia so limits muscle contraction that severe weakness occurs with increased activity.

Clinical manifestations. Myasthenia gravis occurs in both ocular (pertaining to the eye) and generalized forms. In ocular myasthenia gravis, the symptoms include ptosis (eyelid droops) and diplopia (double vision). The generalized variety may vary from mild to severe symptoms. The patient may complain initially of ptosis and diplopia. Skeletal weakness, dysarthria (difficult or inarticulate speech), and dysphagia (difficult swallowing) may follow. In more severe cases or as the disease progresses, the patient will complain of severe ocular, pharyngeal, and respiratory muscle weakness. Bowel and bladder sphincter weakness occurs with severe loss of muscle control.

There may be a tendency for the head to fall forward, and there may be weak, nasal-sounding speech. Upper extremity involvement is to be anticipated, and occasionally the lower extremities are weak. Muscle atrophy does not occur, reflexes are normal, and cerebral function remains intact. Dyspnea and severe respiratory weakness are very problematic. Periods of exacerbation and remission are expected.

Assessment. Collection of *subjective data* includes the complaints of weakness; double vision; eye, throat, and respiratory muscle weakness; dyspnea; swallowing difficulties; and urinary and bowel incontinence. The patient may or may not complain of upper and/or lower extremity weakness.

Collection of *objective data* includes ptosis, nasal-sounding speech, and loss of muscle control.

Complications with myasthenia gravis include respiratory distress, pneumonia, choking, and swallowing difficulties.

Diagnostic tests. A detailed history and physical examination may suggest an autoimmune disorder.

The IV anticholinesterase test is a reliable diagnostic tool. Edrophonium chloride (Tensilon) or neostigmine bromide (Prostigmin Bromide) is administered IV, and the patient response is carefully evaluated. Muscle function improves dramatically in a short time with patients who have the illness.

Actual diagnosis can be made partly on the basis of electromyography (EMG).

Medical management. Anticholinesterase drugs, such as neostigmine (Prostigmin) and pyridostigmine (Mestinon), may be administered. These medications allow acetylcholine to accumulate at synapses and promote nerve impulse transmission.

Corticosteroids may or may not be used as adjunct therapy.

Immunosuppressants, such as azathioprine (Imuran) and cyclophosphamide (Cytoxan), are also used.

Physical therapy, such as range-of-motion exercises, may be beneficial in muscle function. Braces, splints, walkers, and canes may assist the patient in achieving some independence.

Nursing interventions. Nursing interventions of the patient with myasthenia gravis include nursing diagnosis, interventions, and teaching related to muscle weakness and disturbance in self-esteem.

Nursing intervention is aimed at assessing respiratory status and minimizing complications.

NURSING DIAGNOSES	NURSING INTERVENTIONS
Impaired physical mobility, related to muscle weakness	Plan activities and rest to reduce fatigue. Assess functional ability.
Ineffective breathing pattern, related to muscle weakness	Elevate head of bed. Suction airway as indicated. Supervise use of durable medical equipment.
Bowel/urinary incontinence, related to decreased muscle control	Establish bowel program. Provide incontinence aids. Palpate bladder. Catheterize intermittently.
Potential for injury, related to trauma	Assess muscle strength, and gross and fine motor coordination.
Impaired verbal communication, related to muscle weakness	Provide slate board and picture board. Validate nonverbal communication.
Bathing/hygiene self-care deficit, related to spasticity or muscle weakness	Determine individual strengths and skills. Assist with necessary adaptations.
Self-esteem disturbance: situational low self-esteem, related to powerlessness	Assess patient interaction with significant others, encourage expression of feelings.
Impaired swallowing, related to muscular weakness, choking	Provide for food and fluids more easily swallowed; remain with patient during meals.

Patient teaching. The nurse's responsibilities in patient education are as follows:

1. Teach safety measures; teach use of assistive mobility devices, braces, and walkers.
2. Teach good posture and use of accessory muscles; assist patient with learning breathing exercises.
3. Instruct in use of laxatives or stool softeners; schedule social activities within time frame of bowel program.
4. Teach use of Credé maneuver, Valsalva maneuver to increase intraabdominal pressure; teach self-catheterization program; stress need for adequate fluid intake.
5. Identify need for safety devices; discuss need for and sources of supervision and available day care programs.
6. Teach alternate communication skills; refer to speech therapy.
7. Refer to occupational therapy and respite care.
8. Teach learning strategies for dealing with feelings and acceptance of strengths and weaknesses.
9. Consult with physician and/or dietary department regarding optimum diet plan.

Systemic Lupus Erythematosus

Etiology and pathophysiology. Systemic lupus erythematosus (SLE) is a systemic inflammatory disorder characterized by antibody formation directed against **autologous** (origin within self) tissues and serum protein factors.

The disease is chronic and incurable and is multicausal in origin. Immunological, hormonal, genetic, and possible viral factors contribute to onset of this disease, which is most prevalent in women of childbearing age. Nine times more women than men are affected by this disorder, and three times as many African-Americans as Caucasians are affected. About 10% of cases occur later in life. Survival rates have increased to longer than 15 years after diagnosis with this disorder. Earlier treatment modalities have contributed toward a better prognosis.

SLE is considered a serious illness despite advances in treatment. The cause remains unclear, and more than one factor is likely. Genetic predisposition seems apparent in most instances, coupled with an inciting agent or factor.

T suppressor cells are decreased in the person with SLE. In addition, T suppressor cells that are present function in a limited manner. Antibodies develop against other antigens.

Clinical manifestations. Clinical manifestations are nephritis, pericarditis, synovitis, organic brain syndromes, peripheral neuropathies, anemia, leukopenia, thrombocytopenia, coagulopathies, immunosuppression, and dermatitis.

Refer to Table 39-2 for pathogenic occurrences in body systems.

Diagnostic tests. Diagnostic tests for systemic lupus erythematosus can be seen in Box 39-5.

Many of these test results are positive in the presence of inflammatory disease. No single test is considered conclusive for diagnostic purposes. However, positive results of one or more diagnostic tests along with at least three other critieria may lead to the diagnosis of SLE. This would include the following criteria:

1. Butterfly rash
2. Photosensitivity
3. Oral ulcers
4. Arthritis of peripheral joints
5. Pleuritic pain, pleural effusion, or pericarditis
6. Renal disorders as evidenced by the presence of protein and/or cellular casts in the urine
7. Neurological signs, such as seizures of unknown cause
8. Hematological disorders, such as hemolytic anemia, leukopenia, lymphopenia, or thrombocytopenia, in absence of other diagnostic reasons
9. Immunological disorder identified with positive LE prep or antinuclear antibody (ANA) or double-stranded DNA (ds-DNA)
10. Positive ANA in absence of patient use of drugs known to cause drug-induced lupus erythematosus

Medical management. SLE is best treated symptomatically. Attempts to induce remission of the disease, to alleviate exacerbations early, and to prevent complications are goals of therapy.

Drug therapy includes use of nonsteroidal antiinflammatory agents, such as acetylsalicylic acid (ASA) and indomethacin (Indocin), and corticosteroids, such as prednisone, in low doses given several times a day. Methylprednisolone may be used intravenously in cases of exacerbation.

Peak amounts of steroids are given to achieve remission. Doses are then decreased slowly until a maintenance dose is reached.

Topical corticosteroid creams are used for the rash of SLE.

Antineoplastic drugs such as azathioprine (Imuran), cyclophosphamide (Cytoxan), or chlorambucil (Leukeran) may be used therapeutically to achieve remission or to control symptoms of the illness.

BOX 39-5 DIAGNOSTIC TESTS FOR SYSTEMIC LUPUS ERYTHEMATOSUS

Antinuclear antibody (ANA)	Rapid Plasma Reagin (RPR)
Complement	Skin or muscle biopsy
CBC	C-reactive protein (CRP)
Sedimentation rate	Coombs test
Coagulation profile	LE prep
Rheumatoid factor	Urinalysis

Table 39-2 Pathogenic Occurrences in Body Systems

Musculoskeletal	Inflammation of vessels, tendons, and muscle tissue occurs because of deposits of fibrin.
Gastrointestinal	Ulceration occurs on mucosal membranes because of degeneration of a collagen tissue.
Renal	Glomerular sclerosis and inflammation occur.
Hematological	Cells are destroyed, and interference with coagulation occurs because of circulating antibodies.
Cardiovascular Pulmonary Cutaneous Neurological	Inflammatory processes occur across these systems.

Antiinfective agents are used both to treat and to prevent infections in the patient with SLE.

Peritoneal dialysis or hemodialysis may be indicated in patients with moderate to severe renal involvement.

Analgesics and diuretics may be used to treat symptoms often found in SLE individuals.

Supportive therapy, such as balanced diet, a balance of rest and activity, and reduction of exposure to the sun, may also be indicated.

Nursing interventions. Because SLE is a multisymptom disease, a thorough assessment is indicated. The plan of care should be individually tailored to include (1) skin care, including teaching avoidance of direct sunlight and use of protective clothing and sunscreen, (2) balancing rest and activity, (3) assisting the patient to recognize changes in condition, (4) early recognition of symptoms of infection, (5) stress reduction, and (6) balanced nutrition and reduction of sodium intake. Because the disease is one of exacerbation and remissions, each exacerbation will intensify the patient's stress and subsequent ability to cope. The nurse should provide psychosocial, emotional, and spiritual support.

Patients with impaired immune system function must endure the consequences of chronic and/or incurable disease. A caring and gentle approach to patient care, as well as understanding, will help alleviate the burden and stress of these illnesses. See the nursing care plan for the patient with SLE.

NURSING CARE PLAN: THE PATIENT WITH SYSTEMIC LUPUS ERYTHEMATOSUS

Nursing diagnoses	Patient goals	Nursing interventions
Impaired skin integrity, related to skin rash (butterfly across face), hair loss, skin atrophy, discoid lesions involving other parts of the body	Patient will verbalize understanding of skin care regimen and positioning schedule. Patient will demonstrate behaviors to promote skin healing. Patient will experience improved wound/lesion healing.	Inspect skin and describe lesions' size, characteristics, and changes noted. Monitor for signs of infection. Assess nutritional status and areas at risk for pressure. Develop positioning schedule. Use appropriate devices, such as air mattress, Eggcrate mattress, sheepskin, or foam padding, where indicated. Provide optimum nutrition. Teach skin care maintenance.
Fear, related to separation from support system (hospitalization, treatments, and threat of death)	Patient will acknowledge fear. Patient will use effective coping measures. Patient will demonstrate problem solving and use resources effectively.	Assess signs of denial, depression. Listen to patient concerns. Allow patient to express feelings freely.
Self-esteem disturbance, related to baldness, dependence on others for care	Patient will verbalize understanding of altered body image. Patient will accept self with loss of self-esteem. Patient will perform self-care activities within level of own ability. Patient will identify personal community resources that can provide assistance.	Recognize behavior indicative of overconcern with body and its processes. Record emotional changes. Set limits on maladaptive behavior.
Bathing/hygiene self-care deficit, related to weakness and restricted activity	Patient will verbalize importance of personal hygiene.	Assist in ADLs.

REFERENCES AND SUGGESTED READINGS

1. Benjamini E and Lostowitz S: Immunology, a short course, New York, 1988, Alan R Liss, Inc.
2. Bergman HD: The treatment of systemic lupus erythematosus, Pract Nurs 39(1):50, 1989.
3. Butler S: Current trends in autologous transfusion, RN 52(11) November 1989.
4. Ciranowics MN and others: Immune disorders, Nurses' Clinical Library, Nursing 85 Books, Springhouse, Pennsylvania, 1985, Springhouse Corp.
5. Clark WR: The experimental foundations of modern immunology, ed 3, New York, 1986, John Wiley & Sons, Inc.
6. Gurevich I and Tafuro P: Nursing measures for the prevention of infection in the compromised host, Nurs Clin North Am 20 (1):257, 1985.
7. Hood GH and Dincher JR: Total patient care, St Louis, 1988, The CV Mosby Co.
8. Lee BA: Living with lupus, Pract Nurs 36(4):37, 1986.
9. Macmillan M: Community care of a patient with multiple sclerosis, Nurs 89 3(33):28, 1989.
10. Mosby's medical, nursing, and allied health dictionary, ed 3, St Louis, 1990, The CV Mosby Co.
11. Nass T: Helping the patient who has lupus, RN 50(10):69, 1987.
12. Phipps WJ and others: Medical-surgical nursing: concepts and clinical practice, ed 4, St Louis, 1991, The CV Mosby Co.
13. Rhynsburger J: How to fight myasthenia's fatigue, Am J Nurs 89(3) March 1989.
14. Roitt I, Brostoff J, and Male D: Immunology, ed 2, London, 1989, Gower Medical Publishing, Ltd.
15. Schmitt DM: Helping Gwen to keep going, Nursing 19(3):54, 1989.
16. Sherman SL: Community health nursing care plans, New York, 1985, John Wiley & Sons, Inc.
17. Snyder LA and Peter NK: How to manage organ donation, Am J Nurs 89(10), Oct 1989.
18. Thompson JM and others: Mosby's manual of clinical nursing, ed 2, St Louis, 1989, The CV Mosby Co.
19. Thompson RA: Recent advances in clinical immunology, No 4, New York, 1987, Churchill Livingstone, Inc.
20. Weir DM and others: Cellular immunology, ed 4, vol 2, Boston, 1986, Blackwell Scientific Publications, Inc.

CHAPTER CHALLENGE

KEY POINTS

- The two major forms of immunity are innate and acquired or adaptive.
- T lymphocytes, B lymphocytes, and macrophages are the three major cells active in acquired immunity.
- B lymphocytes produce antibodies.
- T lymphocytes do not produce antibodies, but assist the B cell.
- T lymphocytes release lymphokines.
- Macrophages trap, process, and present antigen to T lymphocytes.
- Supportive therapy, such as balanced diet, balance of rest and activity, and reduction of exposure to the sun, is indicated in chronic debilitating diseases, such as SLE.
- Muscular weakness that impairs respiratory function and bowel and bladder function and results in a potential for injury is a key factor in myasthenia gravis.
- Infection is a primary threat to the immunosuppressed patient. Aseptic technique is required when caring for these patients. Good skin care is necessary.
- Careful selection of blood donors and careful typing and cross-matching of blood are important in prevention of transfusion reaction.
- Early recognition of symptoms followed by early treatment may decrease the severity of allergic reaction.
- Avoidance of the offending allergen is an important teaching concept related to atopic allergy.

STUDY QUESTIONS

1. Innate or natural immunity is:
   a. The body's first line of defense against and protects locally against the external environment
   b. The body's second line of defense against disease and protects the internal environment
   c. Mediated by B cells to produce antibodies in response to antigenic challenge
   d. An immunity that is specific
2. Humoral immunity is mediated by:
   a. T cells
   b. B cells
3. Cellular immunity develops when which cells are activated by an antigen:
   a. T cells
   b. B cells
4. Desensitization is another term for:
   a. Autoimmune disorders
   b. Adaptive immunity
   c. Immunotherapy
   d. Immunodeficiency disease
5. Immune disorders that result from failures of the tolerance to "self" responding immunologically to one's own antigens are called:
   a. Immunodeficiency disorders
   b. Hypersensitivity disorders
   c. Desensitization disorders
   d. Autoimmune disorders
6. In caring for the patient with systemic lupus erythematosus, it is important to teach the patient:
   a. To avoid direct sunlight and to wear protective clothing, dark glasses, head coverings, etc.
   b. Alternate communication skills
   c. Self-catheterization
   d. Use of accessory muscles; assist with learning breathing exercises
7. While doing a nursing history, the nurse should recognize that the most common initial symptoms of systemic lupus erythematosus are:
   a. Petechiae in the skin, epistaxis, pallor
   b. Hematuria, increased blood pressure, and edema
   c. Tachycardia, tremors, and loss of weight
   d. Painful muscles and joints, stiffness, and inflammation of joints
8. Coseasonal, preseasonal, and perennial are terms related to:
   a. Cellular immunity
   b. Humoral immunity
   c. Immunocompetence
   d. Immunotherapy
9. Nursing assessment of the patient with hypersensitivity disease includes the following systems:
   a. Musculoskeletal system
   b. Genitourinary systems
   c. Skin and respiratory systems
   d. Gastrointestinal system
10. In allergic diseases, the most important teaching concept is:
    a. Immunotherapy regimen
    b. Avoidance of the allergen
    c. Antihistamine administration
    d. Adrenalin administration
11. Nursing care of the immunosuppressed patient should include:
    a. Prophylactic antibiotic therapy
    b. Meticulous aseptic technique
    c. Restriction of all visitors
12. In addition to prevention of infection and maintaining adequate hydration, the patient with multiple myeloma should be taught:
    a. Effective pain control
    b. Avoidance of sunlight
    c. Socialization technique

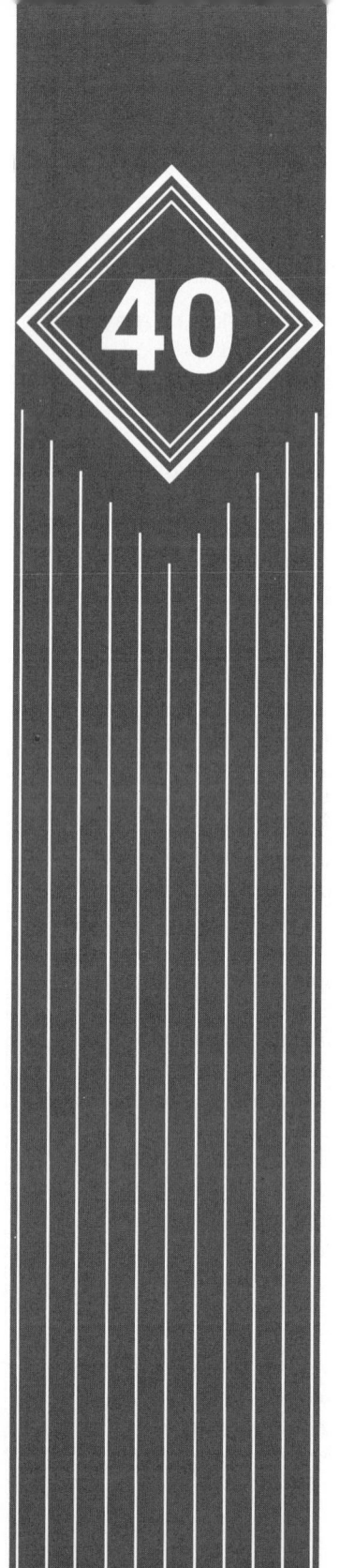

40

Care of the Patient with AIDS

IVA L. MUELLER

LEARNING OBJECTIVES

After reading this chapter, the student should be able to do the following:

- Define the key terms.
- Relate the clinical manifestations indicative of AIDS.
- List the modes of transmission of AIDS.
- Identify the causative agent of AIDS.
- List the "at risk" groups for AIDS.
- List diagnostic tests for AIDS.
- Describe the prevention of AIDS.
- Describe treatment modalities for AIDS.
- Identify opportunistic infections associated with AIDS.
- Implement a plan of care for the patient with AIDS.
- Identify support systems available to the patient, including presence of and relationship with friends and extended family.

RELATED TOPICS OF INTEREST

- Care of the patient with a reproductive disorder (Chapter 36)
- Care of the patient with an immune disorder (Chapter 39)

KEY TERMS

Define the following:

- acquired immunodeficiency syndrome (AIDS)
- AIDS-related complex (ARC)
- asymptomatic
- Centers for Disease Control (CDC)
- host
- human immunodeficiency virus (HIV)
- immunodeficiency
- immunotropic
- Kaposi's sarcoma (KS)
- lymphadenopathy
- myalgia
- neurotropic
- opportunistic infection
- persistent generalized lymphedema (PGL)
- persons with AIDS (PWA)
- *Pneumocystis carinii* pneumonia (PCP)
- retrovirus
- seroconversion
- T cell

AIDS is the acronym for **acquired immunodeficiency syndrome.** This disease is an epidemic phenomenon of the 1980s. After recognition of what were thought to be rare disease conditions in a few young gay men in California and New York, the **Centers for Disease Control (CDC)** was soon to learn of similar disease occurrences among intravenous drug users and persons with hemophilia. This led to what is now referred to as the AIDS epidemic.

The CDC defines AIDS as "a disease at least moderately predictive of a defect in cell-mediated immunity, occurring in persons with no known cause for diminished resistance to that disease."

AIDS weakens the immune system of the **host,** lowering the resistance to infectious diseases. These diseases, known as **opportunistic infections,** seize the opportunity to move into the person who has a damaged immune system.

STATISTICS

Statistics regarding AIDS change monthly. Since AIDS was first recognized in the early 1980s, nearly 100,000 confirmed cases have been recorded. An estimated 1 to 2 million people are believed to be infected with the virus but are not yet confirmed as having AIDS, since the disease AIDS is the end stage of the infection.

No group can be considered safe or at a lower risk than another. The percentage of growth by group is rapidly changing (Table 40-1). Estimates for number of cases in 1991, or 10 years after the first diagnosed case in the United States, are alarming. The figure ranges between 270,000 and 385,000 cases. It is further estimated that AIDS will be the leading cause of death in the 19- to 40-year-old age group in 1991.

New York and California lead in number of cases, presently accounting for 40% of all cases. Florida, Texas, New Jersey, Illinois, Pennsylvania, Georgia, Massachusetts, and the District of Columbia complete the list of leading states for reported AIDS cases.

ETIOLOGY

The virus causing AIDS is now globally known as **human immunodeficiency virus (HIV).** HIV is a **retrovirus** that is both **immunotropic** and **neurotropic,** attacking the immune and nervous systems. Retroviruses live within the host cell, replicate, and tend to endure for extended periods. Therefore HIV infection is considered to be lifelong. When the retrovirus HIV enters the body, it attacks primarily the T cell. Eventually this leads to a disturbance of the immune system.

Table 40-1 Cases of AIDS by Groups

	Fall 1988	Winter 1990
Homosexual/bisexual men	62%	60%
Intravenous drug users	19%	20%
Homosexual and intravenous drug users	7%	7%
Persons who have hemophilia/coagulation disorders	1%	1%
Recipients of transfusion/blood components	4%	2%
Heterosexual population	3%	5%
Others (includes health care workers, infants, and children)	3%	3%

Table 40-2 Transmission Modes

SEXUAL ACTIVITY

Homosexual males
Heterosexual
  Male to female
  Female to male
Homosexual females

PERINATAL

Mother to infant in utero
Breast milk to baby

BLOOD-BORNE

Intravenous drug users
Persons with hemophilia
Recipients of contaminated blood transfusion
Health care workers
  Needle sticks
  Nonintact skin

OTHER MODES

Organ transplant

BOX 40-1 BEHAVIORS RELATED TO AIDS TRANSMISSION

Not risk behaviors

- Living in the same house
- Eating food handled by the HIV infected person
- Using the same swimming pool
- Exposure to the cough or sneeze of the HIV-infected person
- Casual kissing

At-risk behaviors

- Unprotected vaginal and anal sexual intercourse
- Sharing of needles
- Transfusion of contaminated blood and blood products
- Organ transplants from an infected donor
- Artificial insemination from an infected donor
- Oral sex
- Intimate kissing

BOX 40-2 RISK-REDUCTION BEHAVIORS

1. Abstinence from sexual activity for the young
2. Monogamous sexual relationships for the adult
3. Promotion of safe sex or protected sex through use of an undamaged latex condom
4. Avoidance of oral/anal sex and other practices that mix blood or body fluids
5. Avoidance of drug abuse; no sharing of needles

TRANSMISSION/RISK

There are three major routes of transmission of AIDS: (1) sexual, (2) blood, and (3) transplacental/perinatal. Though HIV has been isolated in other fluids, such as saliva, tears, urine, brain/cerebrospinal fluid, and bone marrow, documentation of disease transmitted through these sources has not occurred.

However, infected breast milk has been known to transmit HIV from mother to infant. If the breast milk does not contain gross blood, it is not considered to be infectious to health care personnel.

When the retrovirus HIV enters the body, it begins to attack a specialized group of white blood cells called T-4 or helper **T cell** lymphocytes. As the virus reproduces, the T-4 lymphocyte is destroyed. Eventually so many T-4 helper cells are lost that the remaining cells cannot function. This ultimately leads to a disturbance of the immune system.

According to the CDC:

> All persons who are antibody positive for HIV, whether they are symptom free or ill, must be considered potentially infectious to others by sexual transmission, by sharing drug injection equipment, by childbearing, or by donation of blood, semen, or organs.
>
> Transmission of AIDS is directly related to behavior in the majority of cases (Box 40-1).

Transmission of AIDS and hepatitis B is similar. The virus is neither particularly contagious nor hardy. The mode of transmission is extremely limited, and the virus is susceptible to the most common antiseptic procedures (Table 40-2).

HIV is most often transmitted by HIV-infected persons who do not have AIDS. These so-called "healthy carriers" may be infected by the virus without knowing it and unwittingly transmit it to others.

Because AIDS is 100% preventable, yet once developed is not curable, it has clearly made health care professionals look to prevention of the disease.

Prevention is aimed at risk-reduction behaviors, education, and universal precautions (Box 40-2).

Clinical Manifestations

Despite what is now known about AIDS, much is unknown or not as yet discovered. It is known that not every individual infected with the HIV will develop AIDS. Some persons may feel well and simply be carriers. This could lead to their unknowingly infecting others, who will become ill with the disease.

Asymptomatic carriers may be symptom free for months to years although the virus is present in their body secretions, such as semen, vaginal secretions, tears, breast milk, saliva, and sweat. Also, in the first few weeks after infection with HIV, there is absence of symptoms. Therefore those who have just recently been infected and those who may be **asymptomatic** AIDS carriers contribute to potential transmission of HIV even before they are aware of the illness.

After a few weeks, influenza-like symptoms or a mononucleosis-like syndrome may occur with fever, chills, pruritic rash, headaches, **myalgia**, sore throat, vomiting, diarrhea, or swollen lymph nodes.

These symptoms usually occur within 2 to 6 weeks after exposure but may be unrecognized as HIV. **Seroconversion,** or the point at which the virus can be identified in the blood, may not occur until 8 to 12 weeks or longer after exposure. Individuals then may remain asymptomatic for months to years, during which time they may appear well and feel well.

Others, however, develop a variety of symptoms, often chronic in nature, that are not yet defined as AIDS symptoms. This group of individuals is classified as having **AIDS-related complex,** or **ARC.** ARC includes such manifestations as **lymphadenopathy,** chronic fatigue, unexplained weight loss, persistent fever, diarrhea, night sweats, and laboratory findings reflective of immune system dysfunction. Individuals with helper T cell counts above 800/ml have a relatively unimpaired immune system, whereas those with counts of less than 400/ml probably will progress to symptomatic illness. At least two clinical symptoms and two abnormal supporting laboratory test findings are generally required before a diagnosis of ARC is made. An individual may lack a diagnosis of opportunistic infection, yet once ARC develops, there is considerable immune system damage.

The incubation period for AIDS ranges from a few months to more than 5 years from time of infection to full-blown disease. There is a shorter incubation period in infants, the elderly, and persons with preexisting **immunodeficiency** disease. Some authorities believe that **persistent generalized lymphedema (PGL)** comes between the ARC and AIDS stages of illness.

The AIDS patient has a dysfunction of the immune system unrelated to recent transplant or another diagnosed immune system disease. A large percentage of patients with AIDS develop opportunistic infection. The organisms causing opportunistic infection in those patients do not cause infection in the noncompromised host. Frequently the opportunistic infection is ***Pneumocystis carinii*** **pneumonia (PCP)** or **Kaposi's sarcoma (KS).** Relapse may occur, and the infections are potentially life threatening (Table 40-3).

Table 40-3 Commonly Seen Opportunistic Infections and Malignant Neoplasms in the HIV Patient

Disease	Causative Organism	Signs and Symptoms	Diagnosis	Treatment
OPPORTUNISTIC INFECTIONS				
Pneumocytic Carinii (PCP)	Protozoan	Fever, productive or nonproductive cough, shortness of breath, tachypnea, weight loss, chills, cyanosis, intercostal retractions, decreased breath sounds, and tendency for recurrence is high.	Biopsy x-ray examination shows infiltrates with granular, butterfly pattern; irregular lobar consolidation; laboratory values that show decreased arterial blood gases and gallium scan, which shows pneumonia, infection—nonspecific for organism, are indicative but not diagnostic of PCP.	Antibiotic therapy of at least 21 days' duration. Pentamidine and a combination of sulfamethoxazole and trimethoprim have been useful. DFMO and dapsone have been tried experimentally.

Continued.

Table 40-3 Commonly Seen Opportunistic Infections and Malignant Neoplasms in the HIV Patient—cont'd

Disease	Causative Organism	Signs and Symptoms	Diagnosis	Treatment
VIRAL INFECTIONS				
Herpes simplex	Herpes simplex virus (HSV) type II	Oral or rectal lesions, or both, in cluster-like groupings; the lesions are painful, pressure sensitive, and highly contagious.	Cultures of lesions.	Topical medications, such as acyclovir.
Cytomegalovirus (CMV)	Cytomegalovirus	Retinitis with fever, fatigue, vision loss, blindness, or disseminated disease with fever, fatigue, weight loss, mononucleosis-like symptoms, pneumonitis, diarrhea, abdominal pain, ulceration of the esophagus and stomach, adrenalitis, or meningitis.	Laboratory examination of blood, urine, or semen.	No effective treatment for this disease that causes damage to lungs, kidneys, eyes, brain, and other organs; any treatment is considered experimental. DHPG may be used to control retinitis.
MALIGNANT NEOPLASMS				
Kaposi's sarcoma (KS)	A malignancy in which the cytomegalovirus and Epstein-Barr virus have been isolated; KS is believed to occur because of defect in cell-mediated immunity.	Early stage: pink-blue macule, which advances to a larger, deeper red-purple lesion of the face and mouth—painless. Mid-stage: dark red-brown or red-blue, tumor-like, painful lesions over the body. Advanced stage: oral or skin lesions, lymph nodes, and visceral involvement; edema of face, lymphedema of extremities, pulmonary edema, respiratory distress, gastrointestinal symptoms.	Biopsy of tissue.	Chemotherapy is considered the treatment of choice; drugs used include vincristine, vinblastine, etoposide (VP-16), doxorubicin, bleomycin, and methotrexate.

DIAGNOSTIC TESTS

Enzyme-linked immunosorbent assay (ELISA) is an AIDS virus antibody test that detects antibodies to the organism causing the disease. For most persons, this test could detect marker antibodies at about 10 to 12 weeks after exposure. Some persons may not experience seroconversion or detection for the marker antibodies for as long as 6 months after exposure.

Because the ELISA test is very sensitive and therefore positive for other antibodies, one positive test does not give a positive diagnosis for HIV seroconversion. False positive results may occur, especially in multiparous women. The cost of this test is approximately $15.

A positive ELISA test leads to confirmation by use of the Western blot test, a confirmatory test for presence of HIV antibodies. It is more specific than ELISA and eliminates false positives. The test however is not considered infallible. The cost is approximately $50.

Most blood samples are automatically tested through both ELISA and Western blot if a positive test result is obtained. The same sample is then screened twice more. After two positive results on ELISAs, a Western blot is done usually from the original sample.

Any person notified of positive test results has a further need for psychological and emotional support. Counseling is important, and the patient should have further medical evaluation to determine immune status. The patient should be told what to expect in the disease process, how to prevent further transmission, and what support systems are available.

ASSESSMENT

A comprehensive plan of care is established after a thorough assessment by a team of professionals, including physicians, nurses, clergy, dieticians, and social workers. A social history, including the patient's sexual activity, drug use, needle exposure, and travels, is done. A history of the patient's medications, illnesses, surgeries, childhood diseases, and sexually transmitted diseases is also included. Assessment is an ongoing process at the time of diagnosis, during treatment, when new signs and symptoms occur, at times of relapse, and at the terminal stage.

Collection of Subjective Data

Subjective data early in HIV infection include chills, myalgia, and increasing weakness. These relatively mild symptoms are often considered influenza-like symptoms to the patient. During the ARC stage, the patient may complain of chronic fatigue and anxiety. With a full-blown diagnosis of AIDS, assessment will also include the subjective symptoms of recurrent infections with chills, myalgia, and headache.

Collection of Objective Data

Objective data include frequent relapses into influenza-like syndromes, including persistent fever, vomiting, and diarrhea. The nurse will note the patient has increasing difficulties in carrying out activities of daily living. There is unexplained weight loss, a wasting appearance of the individual, unusual susceptibility to infection, body lesions, night sweats, and lymphadenopathy.

Social needs and conflicts occur throughout the illness. Social conflicts can be related to public exposure, AIDS laboratory testing, stigma, sexual activity, employment, insurance, social support limitation, and for some, separation from family.

After completing the assessment, the results of diagnostic tests are evaluated, and a plan of care for the patient is developed.

TREATMENT

AIDS is often referred to as a wasting illness. There is no cure for AIDS, and the mortality is high. Few live beyond 2 years after diagnosis. A vaccine in development since October 1987 may protect against HIV infection by creation of a preexisting immunity. This vaccine is yet unnamed and may not be available for decades. It offers no help to **persons with AIDS (PWAs).** Azidothymidine (AZT) is an antiviral agent being tested to determine its ability to halt the effects of HIV. The drug has shown some early positive results, but evaluation of its side effects, long-term effectiveness, and safety for various categories of AIDS patients continues.

NURSING INTERVENTIONS

Nursing interventions for the patient with AIDS ranges from simple, common nursing measures to complex care related to the multiple physical and psychosocial problems that are associated with the disease. Exacerbations of symptoms and increasing debilitation may affect the patient's ability to perform activities of daily living. In addition, the patient may have several AIDS-related diseases occurring simultaneously. The patient with AIDS suffers from chronic illness, and as the disease progresses, physical debilitation increases, respiratory illnesses intensify, and mental changes occur.

The nurse should deal with personal feelings surrounding the disease before attempting to care for the patient with AIDS. It is not uncommon for the nurse to have mixed feelings, even negative feelings toward the patient, the disease, or the behaviors involved in transmission of the illness. These feelings should be identified, expressed, and dealt with before approaching patient care. The nurse must see the patient as a human being with an urgent need to be loved and cared for with compassion, support, and dignity.

A nursing care plan for an AIDS patient is illustrated on pp. 1076-1077. Common nursing problems are included. The patient with AIDS is often weak as a result of nutritional problems and diarrhea. Many have impaired skin integrity because of lesions or infections. Repeated respiratory infections leave the patient unable to maintain a job and often impair ability to perform personal care, such as feeding, dressing, and toileting. A caring bedside nurse, a supportive family member, or a close friend is often the only one the patient with AIDS trusts and depends on.

The nurse may find it difficult to know what to say to the patient with AIDS. Words are one way to convey caring. Listening is another important tool. Also a nurse can develop a good therapeutic relationship with the patient by allowing the patient to assist and participate in the planning of care and decisions regarding care (see therapeutic dialogue, p. 1077).

Infection control guidelines for hospital and home care

NURSING CARE PLAN: THE PATIENT WITH AIDS

Nursing diagnoses	Patient goals	Nursing interventions
Diarrhea, related to inflammation, irritation, or malabsorption	Patient will verbalize understanding of causative factors. Patient will experience improved bowel function. Patient will tolerate increased variety of foods. Patient will maintain adequate hydration.	Assess onset and pattern of diarrhea: record frequency, amount, characteristics. Assess for fecal impaction. Promote relaxation and decreased stress. Limit caffeine, high-fiber foods, milk, and fruits. Increase fluid intake. Record intake and output if indicated. Apply skin barrier if needed to protect from skin breakdown. Give medications as ordered. Diaper patient if infected.
Social isolation, related to altered state of wellness, alternations in physical appearance, and inability to engage in satisfying personal relationships	Patient will express increased sense of self-worth. Patient will demonstrate a trust in the health care provider. Patient will participate in community support group.	Assess patient's feelings about self. Identify support systems available to the patient, including family, friends, and community support groups. Establish a therapeutic relationship; spend time with patient; listen carefully; encourage verbalization of feelings. Involve patient with others having similar circumstances.
Activity intolerance, related to weakness	Patient will report measurable increase in activity tolerance.	Identify activities that are too strenuous; plan care with rest periods. Provide for progressive activity as patient tolerates. Inform patient when evidence of progress occurs.
Altered nutrition: less than body requirements, related to inadequate food intake and related to abdominal cramping with food ingestion	Patient will experience increase in body weight and appetite. Patient will report a decrease in abdominal cramping with use of antispasmodics.	Assess ability to chew. Note food intolerances; provide diet modifications and dietary supplements. Encourage foods that appeal to the patient. Provide frequent oral care. Weigh weekly. Assess needs for parenteral nutrition.
Ineffective airway clearance, related to infection, secretions	Airway will be patent. Patient will verbalize preventative measures. Patient will experience improved vital signs and breathing.	Elevate head of bed; change position every 2 hours; encourage deep breathing, coughing, exercises. Give medications as ordered. Assess for increased signs of respiratory distress. Teach patient contributing causes and prevention.

NURSING CARE PLAN: THE PATIENT WITH AIDS—cont'd

Nursing diagnoses	Patient goals	Nursing interventions
Impaired skin integrity, related to disruption of skin surface, trauma	Patient will demonstrate behaviors to promote healing. Patient will experience improvement of wounds and lesions.	Inspect skin on a daily basis; describe lesions and changes observed; monitor for signs and symptoms of infections; keep area clean with mild soap and water. Perform and instruct in aseptic/clean technique for dressing changes and proper disposal of soiled dressings. Provide soaks if ordered; expose wound to air if indicated. Teach skin care.

THERAPEUTIC DIALOGUE

NURSE: I need to take a look at the abscess on your anus.

PATIENT: Do you have to? I take care of it myself, and I do a portable sitz bath after every stool. I keep it real clean.

NURSE: I'm sure it bothers you to have people look . . . *(Recognizes patient's sensitivity)*

PATIENT: Well, everybody wants to look. I've shown it so many times, I guess one more wouldn't hurt. I get so tired of it though. *(Does not look at nurse while speaking)*

NURSE: Have you had the abscess a long time? *(Gives patient space by verbalizing rather than going directly to the exam)*

PATIENT: Yeah, it's been draining for almost 2 months now, but it isn't as painful and it doesn't drain so much anymore.

NURSE: Well, if it's ok with you, I could look at it today, and then later on I would be able to tell you how much improvement is made. If not, I could wait and assess it on my next visit, whichever you'd rather. *(This allows the patient to help make the decision. Nurse looks directly at the patient to show she is not uncomfortable.)* Actually, I wouldn't have to assess it every visit. *(Allows patient some control over his plan of care)*

PATIENT: Well go ahead. Be sure you wear gloves because it's draining some. Be careful, it hurts if you press on it. Some nurses are rough. *(Patient shows concern for the caregiver while expressing own needs)*

NURSE: There are signs of improvement. No deep redness . . . there is still some deeper pink color around the open area. Obviously you are doing a good job with the sitz baths. *(Nurse shows concern and regard for the patient)*

can be found in Box 40-3. These universal guidelines may be used in any health care setting and for all patients, not only those with a diagnosis of AIDS.

Practical/vocational nurses are a vital part of the health care team for the AIDS patient. They function under the direction of the physician and professional nurse, along with social service workers, therapists, clergy, family, and volunteers.

PWAs have considerably more psychosocial problems than others with terminal illness. They face uncertainty, isolation, fear, and depression. The condition is fatal, it is contagious, it has no cure, and it has media attention. The disease affects support groups, intimacy, sexuality, role status, self-sufficiency, appearance, competency, and employment. The PWA faces many losses: physical, emotional, social, economic, psychological, and often spiritual. In addition, many of those diagnosed with AIDS, unlike others with fatal illness, must face family reactions. The PWA often must face "coming home," coping with stigma of social discrimination, and bereavement.

Parents with AIDS who have children with AIDS face even greater challenges. Who will care for their child? Most agencies are not prepared for this situation. These parents die not knowing how their child will be provided for. They cannot "get their house in order." Children with AIDS are the totally innocent. Approximately 80% contracted the illness in utero and the remaining 20% from blood and blood products/hemophilia. Who will love and care for them? These innocent victims often live out their lives in hospitals. They are often rejected for foster care and never know a real home life.

Time and age are additional factors. Once AIDS is

BOX 40-3 INFECTION CONTROL

Universal Precautions

Hospital recommendations include the following:

- Handwashing before and after patient contact in the patient room.
- Gloves worn only with direct contact with specimens, body fluids, soiled linens, soiled surfaces, and dressings.
- Gowns worn to protect clothing during direct patient care and removed and discarded in room.
- Masks and protective eye wear worn during procedures with aerosols or activity where splashes may occur; a mask worn when needed to protect the severely immunodepressed patient.
- Needles not recapped, discarded with other sharps in a rigid, puncture-proof container.
- Disposable paper wastes, used gloves, and dressings discarded in plastic bag in room; disposed with contaminated articles per hospital policy.
- Soiled linen bagged in room and double bagged as per protocol for handling contaminated material.
- Specimens bagged and labeled.
- Nondisposable items autoclaved, or washed with soap and water, or per hospital protocol.
- Usually there are no precautions with food trays unless the patient has copious oral or respiratory secretions; the use of disposable utensils, dishes, and trays should then be considered.
- Door to room need not be closed; a private room is recommended only, for example, if the patient cannot control secretions or cannot maintain scrupulous hygiene.
- Disposable Ambu bags and airways available in patient room at all times.

POSTMORTEM TECHNIQUE

Wear gown and gloves; double bag the body and label.

CMV (cytomegalovirus), HIV, and herpes virus are potentially dangerous to fetal development; pregnant women should be excused from care.

BOX 40-4 FUNDING SOURCES FOR CARE OF AIDS PATIENTS

Medicaid and SSI (Supplementary Security Income)	54%*
Private insurance	17%
Personal reserves	17%
Medicare	2%

*Approximated at time of writing.

diagnosed, 80% will die within 2 or 3 years. This most often occurs in the fourth decade of life, the peak death period for PWAs.

Economic Factors

Economic stress is severe for PWAs as it is with others who have slowly debilitating illnesses. Often financial problems occur between the time of being physically unable to work and the time of formal diagnosis of disability. The time lapse before financial aid becomes available is stressful emotionally, mentally, and economically (see Box 40-4 for funding sources). AIDS challenges the health care system like no other disease today.

Social Factors/Reactions

Social stigma and widespread discrimination were initial social reactions. Legal questions continue to arise regarding the patient's right to work, right to rental of homes and apartments, deliberate transmission of the disease, right to attend school, premarital screening, and anonymity. Fear of the illness and fear of the person with AIDS are the great social challenges.

Patient Education

The patient should be involved in the plan of care as much as possible. As new developments occur, the patient should be informed. At the time of diagnosis, it is important to teach the patient about the disease and its transmission modes. The patient who is HIV positive should be advised to alert his dentist and other health care providers about the diagnosis. Blood and organs should not be donated. The patient should be taught to modify sexual habits, that is, decrease the number of partners, use condoms, explore alternative sexual activity, avoid oral/anal sex, and avoid sharing needles. Patient teaching should be centered on health maintenance, balanced diet, balance of rest and activity, and health care follow-up. It may be beneficial to teach the patient methods of self-assessment for recurrent infections. The patient also should be taught all aspects of his care at home to maintain independence.

AIDS has taught health care workers to be more aware of the human condition so that they can deal with their own prejudices, judgments, and concerns. Health care workers are challenged by the AIDS patient, whose needs and sufferings require more than nursing skill, education, and technology. A spirit of compassion stemming from a genuine willingness to serve the needs of another is essential in caring for the patient with AIDS.

REFERENCES AND SUGGESTED READINGS

1. Advocacy for AIDS patients is helping all patients, RN, p 65, May 1989.
2. AIDS ethics and the truth, Am J Nurs 89(7):924, 1989.
3. AIDS: acquired immunodeficiency syndrome and other manifestations of HIV infection, Park Ridge, NJ, 1987, Noyes Publications (Edited by GP Wormser).
4. AIDS: the women, San Francisco, 1988, Cleis Press (Edited by I Rieder and P Ruppelt).
5. Bakerman S: Understanding AIDS, Greenville NC, 1988, Interpretive Laboratory Data Inc.
6. Beril MT and others: Living with AIDS, RN, pp 81, 87, March 1988.
7. Brown R: AIDS cancer and the medical establishment, New York, 1986, Robert Speller and Sons Publishers, Inc.
8. DeVita T, Jr, Hellman S, and Rosenburg S: AIDS etiology, diagnosis, treatment, and prevention, Philadelphia, 1985, JB Lippincott Co.
9. Doenges M and Moorhouse M: Nursing diagnosis with interventions, ed 2, Philadelphia, 1988, FA Davis Co.
10. Drugs that keep AIDS patients alive, RN, p 35, Feb 1989.
11. Farthing CF and others: A color atlas of AIDS, Chicago, 1986, Year Book Medical Publishers, Inc.
12. Flaskerud J: AIDS/HIV infection: a reference guide for nursing professionals, Philadelphia, 1989, WB Saunders Co
13. Hamilton D: Little things can mean a lot: living with AIDS, a nurse's story, Nurs '88 18(5):61, 1988.
14. Jager H: AIDS and AIDS risk patient care, New York, 1988, John Wiley & Sons, Inc.
15. Kubler-Ross E: AIDS: the ultimate challenge, New York, 1987, Macmillan Publishing Co.
16. Lechtenberg R and Hollenberg S: AIDS in the nervous system, New York, 1988, Churchill Livingstone, Inc.
17. Masters W, Johnson V, and Kolodny R: Crisis: heterosexual behavior in the age of AIDS, New York, 1988, Grove Press, Inc.
18. Matlock R, Forbes C, and Evatt B: Blood and blood products and AIDS, Baltimore, 1987, The John Hopkins University Press.
19. MMWR Morbidity and Mortality Weekly Report, vol 36, no 25, Aug 1987, Department of Health and Human Services Public Health Services, CDC, Atlanta.
20. Parentesis VP and others: AIDS: acquired immunodeficiency syndrome. I. J Pract Nurs 38(2):18, 1988.
21. Perdow S: Facts about AIDS: a guide for health care providers, Philadelphia, 1990, JB Lippincott Co.
22. Pratt RJ: AIDS: a strategy for nursing care, London, 1986, Arnold Edward Publishers, Ltd.
23. Schofferman J: Hospice care of the patient with AIDS, Hospice J 3(4):51, 1987.
24. Thompson J and others: Clinical nursing, ed 2, St Louis, 1989, The CV Mosby Co.
25. Ungvarski P: Coping with infections that AIDS patients develop, RN 51(11):53, 1988.
26. Wiley K and others: Care of AIDS patients: student attitudes, Nurs Outlook 36(5):244, 1988.

CHAPTER CHALLENGE

KEY POINTS

- AIDS is caused by the retrovirus HIV.
- AIDS is transmitted by three routes: (1) sexual, (2) blood, and (3) perinatal.
- AIDS transmission is directly related to behavior in approximately 90% of all cases.
- At-risk groups include (1) the sexually active, (2) intravenous drug users, and (3) in utero offspring of numbers 1 and 2.
- AIDS is 100% preventable but is incurable.
- AIDS is the end stage of HIV infection and is marked by opportunistic infections.
- It is safe to live with a person with AIDS and to attend school or work with these individuals. Universal blood and body fluid precautions must be used, as well as sexual abstinence and no shared needles.
- AIDS is not spread through casual contact.
- HIV-positive persons should not donate blood, sperm, or organs. These individuals should not share needles with others and should avoid oral/genital contact and exchange of body fluids through intimate kissing and sexual activity.
- Social stigma. Widespread discrimination and legal questions regarding rights to work, to attend school, and to rent homes were initial social reactions to AIDS.
- AIDS has taught the health care worker to be more aware of the human condition, and to deal with one's own prejudices, judgments, and concerns.
- The nursing diagnoses in AIDS patients include: diarrhea; social isolation; activity intolerance; altered nutrition: less than body requirements; ineffective airway clearance; and impaired skin integrity.

STUDY QUESTIONS

1. AIDS is a disease of the immune system caused by:
   a. Cytomegalovirus
   b. Herpes simplex virus
   c. *Pneumocystis carinii*
   d. Human immune deficiency virus
2. Patients infected with HIV generally die of: (1) AIDS, (2) recurrent infections, or (3) malignancies:
   a. 1 and 2
   b. 2 and 3
   c. 1 and 3
   d. 1 only
3. Behaviors not considered risks in the transmission of AIDS include: (1) abstinence, (2) sex with one person, (3) casual kissing, or (4) exposure to the cough of the HIV-infected person:
   a. All of these
   b. None of these
   c. 1 and 2
   d. 2, 3, and 4
   e. 1, 3, and 4
   f. 1, 2, and 3
4. In the transmission of AIDS, two of the following are considered risk behaviors: (1) intercourse, (2) donation of an organ for transplant, (3) sharing of needles, or (4) living with a person with AIDS:
   a. 1 and 2
   b. 2 and 3
   c. 1 and 3
   d. 1 and 4
   e. 2 and 4
5. To be diagnosed as having AIDS, the patient must have a compromised immune system without known immune system disease or recent transplant and:
   a. Present with opportunistic infection
   b. Present with a positive ELISA or Western blot test
   c. Present with weight loss, fever, and generalized lymphedema
6. Which of the following are considered risk-reduction behaviors in the transmission of AIDS: (1) monogamous sexual relationships in adults, (2) promotion of safe sex with use of a fresh condom, (3) avoidance of sex and other practices that mix blood or body fluids, or (4) avoidance of drug abuse—no shared needles:
   a. 1, 2, and 3
   b. 2, 3, and 4
   c. All of these
   d. Only 1
7. The virus that causes AIDS attacks primarily: (1) the blood and skin system, (2) the organs and brain, (3) the immune system, or (4) the respiratory system:
   a. 1 and 2
   b. 2 and 3
   c. 3 and 4
   d. only 3
8. One of the following is a true statement. Circle the true statement:
   a. Direct contact with the blood or body fluids of an HIV-positive person may transmit the disease AIDS
   b. To contract AIDS, one must be exposed to the blood or body fluids of a person with AIDS
9. One of the following statements regarding the disease AIDS is NOT true. Circle the correct response.
   a. HIV is found in blood, body fluids, semen, and breast milk
   b. The HIV organism is considered hardy and difficult to kill
   c. The HIV isolated in tears, saliva, breast milk, and urine has not been documented in the transmission of the disease

41

Care of the Patient with Cancer

JOYCE ELIZABETH MYERS

LEARNING OBJECTIVES

After reading this chapter, the student should be able to do the following:

- Define the key terms.
- List seven risk factors for the development of cancer.
- State seven warning signs of cancer.
- Indicate the incidence of cancer as one of the leading causes of death in the United States.
- Define terminology used to describe cellular changes, characteristics of malignant cells, and types of malignancies.
- Name the cytological examination that is used to identify the presence of cancer cells.
- Describe the process of metastasis.
- Explain common reasons for delay in seeking medical care when a diagnosis of cancer is suspected.
- List common diagnostic tests used to identify the presence of cancer.
- Explain why biopsy is essential in confirming a diagnosis of cancer.
- Define the systems of tumor classification: *grading* and *staging*.
- Describe the nursing interventions for the individual undergoing each: surgery, radiation therapy, chemotherapy, immunotherapy, and bone marrow transplantation.

RELATED TOPICS OF INTEREST

- Diet therapy (Chapter 23)
- The surgical patient (Chapter 26)
- Care of the patient with a reproductive disorder (Chapter 36)
- Care of the patient with an immune disorder (Chapter 39)
- Dying and death (Chapter 55)
- Hospice care (Chapter 56)

KEY TERMS

Define the following:
- alopecia
- anaplasia
- benign neoplasm
- biopsy
- cachexia
- carcinogen
- carcinoma
- differentiated
- dysplasia
- glioma
- hyperplasia
- leukemia
- leukopenia
- malignant neoplasm
- mammogram
- metastasize
- multiple myeloma
- neoplasia
- oncology
- Papanicolaou test
- sarcoma
- stomatitis

Oncology is the sum of knowledge regarding tumors; it is the branch of medicine that deals with the study of tumors. Oncology nursing is the care of people with cancer. Until the recognition of AIDS, probably no other medical diagnosis produced as much fear as cancer. The American Cancer Society indicates that in a lifetime, cancer will affect three of four families in the United States. Of every five deaths in the United States from all causes, one is from cancer. Cancer is the second leading cause of death.

Cancer affects people of all ages. Although cancer occurs more frequently in the aged than in other age groups, more children age 3 to 14 years die of cancer than of any other disease.

Cancer of the lung is the major site for new cases of cancer and the cause of the highest number of deaths from cancer for both men and women. The other primary sites where cancer originates in highest frequency are the colon, rectum, breast, uterus, ovary, prostate gland, and bladder. There has been a significant increase in the number of cases of skin cancer (Fig. 41-1).

DETECTION AND PREVENTION OF CANCER

Carcinogenesis and the Primary Prevention of Cancer

Carcinogenesis is the term used for the various factors that are possible origins of cancer. Primary prevention of cancer consists of changes in lifestyle habits to eliminate or reduce exposure to **carcinogens,** which are substances known to increase the risk for the development of cancer.

Risk factors include the following:

1. *Smoking* It is estimated about 83% of people who develop lung cancer are smokers. Twice as many smokers are diagnosed with bladder cancer than nonsmokers.
2. *Dietary habits* Diet plays a role in the development of cancer of the colon, rectum, and breast. A diet high in fiber and low in fat is recommended for prevention (Box 41-1). Obesity should be avoided.
3. *Exposure to radiation* Avoid midday exposure (11 AM to 3 PM) to ultraviolet rays in sunlight unless protected by an effective sunscreen or clothing. Sunlamps and tanning booths also emit ultraviolet rays and have the same risks as sunlight. In addition, the effects of radiation commonly used for medical diagnosis and treatment are also known to be carcinogenic. (Exposure should be limited and monitored.)
4. *Exposure to environmental and chemical carcinogens* Some of these include fumes from rubber and chlorine, dust from cotton and coal,

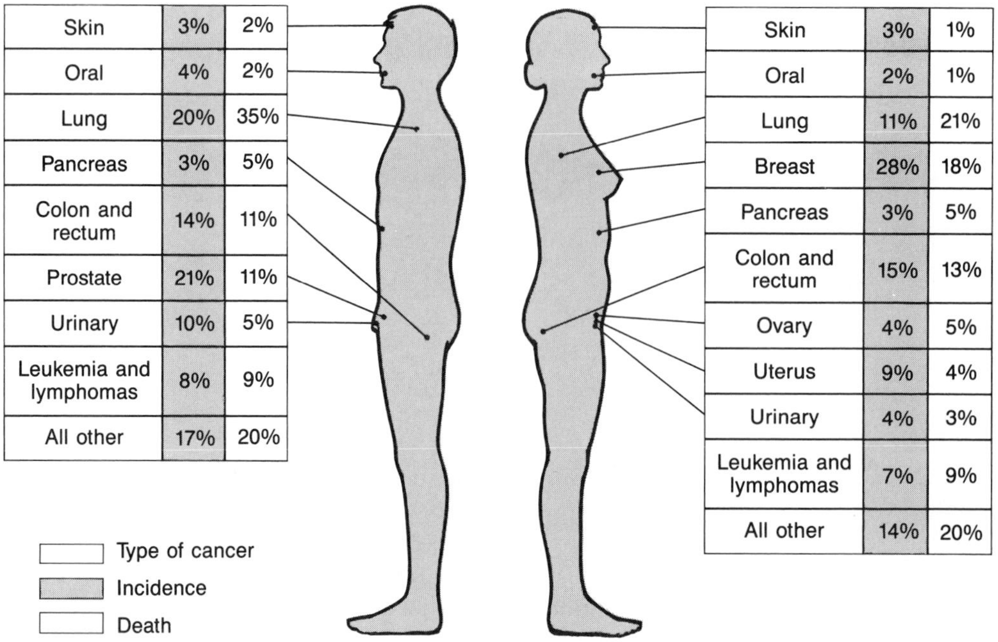

FIG. 41-1 Comparison of cancer incidence and deaths by site and sex (1989 estimates). (From American Cancer Society: Cancer facts and figures, New York, 1989, The Society.)

BOX 41-1 FOODS TO REDUCE CANCER RISK

- Vegetables from the cabbage family, such as:
  broccoli
  cauliflower
  brussels sprouts
  all types of cabbage and kale
- Vegetables high in β-carotene, such as:
  carrots squash
  peaches broccoli
  apricots
- Rich sources of vitamin C, such as:
  grapefruit red and green peppers
  oranges broccoli
  canteloupe tomatoes
  strawberries
- Lean meat, fish, skinned poultry
- Low-fat dairy products, including white cheese rather than yellow
- Avoid salt-cured, smoked, or nitrite-cured foods

include fumes from rubber and chlorine, dust from nickel, chromate, asbestos, and vinyl chloride. There is a greater incidence of bladder cancer among people who live in urban areas and among those who work with dyes, rubber, or leather.

5. *Smokeless tobacco* Use increases the risk of cancer of the mouth, larynx, throat, and esophagus.
6. *Frequent heavy consumption of alcohol* This may result in oral cancer and cancer of the larynx, throat, esophagus, and liver.

Secondary Prevention of Cancer

Secondary prevention of cancer includes the following measures:

1. Planned periodic examinations and the recognition of cancer's warning signals (Box 41-2), which enable the individual to obtain medical attention early. Early detection provides the time needed to diagnose and initiate treatment before cancer has reached an advanced stage.
2. Colorectal tests (men and women)
   a. Digital-rectal examination every year after age 40
   b. Hematest stool for blood every year after age 50
   c. Proctosigmoidoscopy every 3 to 5 years after age 50
3. Pelvic examination for women must include a Papanicolaou test: annually after 18 years of age.
4. Breast cancer detection
   a. Monthly self-examination (men and women)
   b. Part of physical examination (men and women)
   c. **Mammogram** baseline needed age 35 to 39; then every 1 or 2 years, based on findings; every year after age 50 (women only). Mammography can detect a mass before it can be felt.

It is reported that 4 of 10 patients (40%) who are diagnosed with cancer today will be alive 5 years after

BOX 41-2	CANCER'S SEVEN WARNING SIGNALS

If you have a warning signal, see your doctor.

1. Change in bowel or bladder habits
2. A sore that does not heal
3. Unusual bleeding or discharge
4. Thickening or lump in breast or elsewhere
5. Indigestion or difficulty in swallowing
6. Obvious change in wart or mole
7. Nagging cough or hoarseness

diagnosis. If other problems are not also present, such as heart disease, accidents, and old age, the expected survival rate may increase to 49%.

Beginning at high school years, all women should be taught to examine their breasts each month, 2 or 3 days after the menstrual period ends. After menopause, a woman should choose a day to help remind her, such as the first day of each month. A woman needs to become familiar with the appearance and feel of her breasts. This will help her identify any change from one month to the next. Any abnormality, such as a discharge from the nipples, puckering, dimpling, or scaling of the skin, is sig-

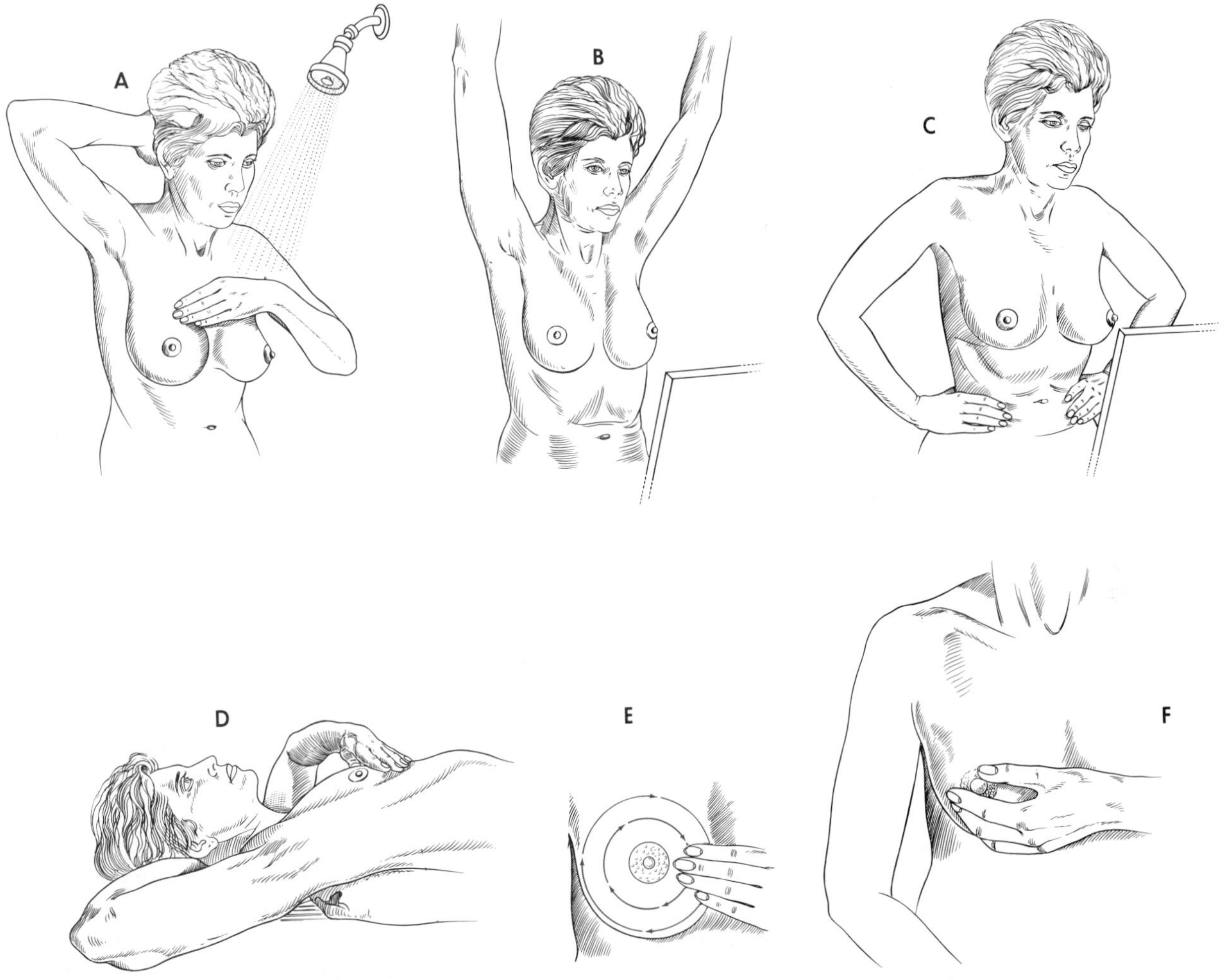

FIG. 41-2 Breast self-examination. **A,** Examine breasts during bath or shower, since flat fingers glide easily over wet skin. Use right hand to examine left breast and vice versa. **B,** Sit or stand before a mirror. Inspect breasts with hands at sides and then raised overhead. Look for changes in contour or dimpling of skin. **C,** Place hands on hips and press down firmly to flex chest muscles. **D,** Lie down with one hand under head and pillow or folded towel under that scapula. **E,** Palpate that breast with other hand, using concentric circle method. It usually takes three circles to cover all breast tissue. Include the tail of the breast and the axilla. Repeat with other breast. **F,** End in a sitting position. Palpate the areola areas of both breasts, and inspect and squeeze nipples to check for discharge.

nificant, as well as the palpation of any lump or thickness. The following is a guide in examining the breasts:

1. Inspect the breasts before a mirror; raise arms behind head and also place hands on hips with shoulders and elbows pulled forward; gently squeeze the nipples to determine if any discharge is present.
2. While bathing, when the breasts and hands are wet, slide the fingers over the skin to check each breast with the opposite hand; use the flat surface of two or three fingers; this is a good practice for men, as well as women.
3. In the lying-down position, place a towel or small pillow under the shoulder of the breast being examined to flatten the breast and make it easier to feel; use the flat surface of two or three fingers of the hand opposite the side being examined; gently palpate each breast, moving in at least three circles of different distances from the nipple at different points, such as 1 o'clock, 2 o'clock, 3 o'clock, and continuing to the 12 o'clock position.

The upper, outer tail of the breast that extends to the axilla and the entire axillary area must also be checked (Fig. 41-2).

Nurses should teach breast self-examination to all patients, emphasizing that any problem identified should be brought to the attention of a physician. Any delay is a waste of valuable time if cancer is present.

Men should be taught to check the scrotum for enlargement, thickening, or the presence of a lump felt in the testicles. This should be done monthly, after a warm bath or shower. It should be emphasized that a physician must be contacted to determine the significance in any changes from the normal, smooth consistency of the testes.

A common reason for delay in diagnosing cancer is because early malignant changes do not produce pain. Cancer is insidious in onset and may often be far advanced before the individual experiences any symptoms.

PATHOPHYSIOLOGY OF CANCER

Normal cells divide and make new cells that are like the parent cells. When malignant cells change, they become unlike parent cells. They are not differentiated or recognizable as being the same in size or shape as normal cells. Cancer cells can divide and multiply but not in a normal manner. Instead of limiting their growth to meet specific needs of the body, they continue to reproduce in a disorderly and unrestricted manner.

Neoplasia is the term for uncontrolled or abnormal growth of cells. **Neoplasms** may be **benign** or **malignant** (Box 41-3). The growths are also called *tumors*. They may be localized or invasive. The following types of cellular growth have been identified:

BOX 41-3 GENERAL CHARACTERISTICS OF NEOPLASMS

BENIGN TUMORS	MALIGNANT TUMORS
1. Slow, steady growth	1. Rate of growth varies—usually rapid
2. Remains localized	2. Metastasizes
3. Usually contained within a capsule	3. Rarely contained within a capsule
4. Smooth, well defined, moveable when palpated	4. Irregular; more immobile when palpated
5. Resembles parent tissue	5. Little resemblance to parent tissue
6. Crowds normal tissue	6. Invades normal tissue
7. Rarely recurs after removal	7. May recur after removal
8. Rarely fatal	8. Fatal without treatment

- **Hyperplasia**—increase in the number of cells of a tissue.
- **Metaplasia**—one type of mature cell is changed to another type, usually as a result of chronic irritation or inflammation, a vitamin deficiency, or chemical exposure; the changes may be reversible.
- **Dysplasia**—difference in size, shape, or arrangement of cells from other cells in the same tissue; these changes may also result from chronic irritation or inflammation, chemicals, or radiation; dysplasia may be reversible.
- **Anaplasia**—a characteristic of malignancy, where there is loss of differentiation that identifies cells by their origin and degree of maturity. Anaplastic cells lack normal cell characteristics and have large, irregularly shaped nuclei. These cells have undergone changes that identify them as different from the parent cells of their specific location. Mitosis (cell division) in cancer is more rapid and disorderly, resulting in atypical cells. Malignant neoplasms may progress and destroy surrounding tissues. They may also **metastasize** from the primary site of origin to distant sites by direct spread of tumor cells to body cavities or through circulation by way of the blood and lymphatic vessels and diffusion or seeding within a body cavity.

In addition to the carcinogenic factors that have been identified that may bring about malignant cellular changes, certain viruses have also been suspected. There is also strong evidence to suggest that there are genetic factors that result in the predisposition to the development of cancer.

The body's immune system is responsible for recognizing and destroying malignant cells. The immune system may be weakened by cancer-producing substances, tumor cells, and the aging process.

Description, Grading, and Staging of Tumors

Tumors are described according to the parent tissue of the specific location in the body. **Carcinoma** is the term used for malignant tumors composed of epithelial cells. **Sarcoma** refers to the malignant tumor of connective tissues, usually presenting as a painless swelling.

Tumors are classified grade 1 to grade 4 by the degree of malignancy. Grade 1 is the most differentiated tumor (most like the parent tissue) and the least malignant. Grade 4 is the least **differentiated** tumor (unlike parent tissue) and highly malignant.

The tumor, node, metastasis (TNM) system of staging cancer is used to indicate tumor size, spread to lymph nodes, and extent of metastasis (Box 41-4). This system is used to direct treatment, predict prognosis, and contribute to cancer research by ensuring reliable comparison of different patients.[14]

A tumor may be named for its location, for its cellular makeup, or for the person by whom it was first identified. (Table 41-1 lists different locations and types of tumors.)

Exfoliative cytology **(Papanicolaou** [Pap] smear **test)** is a means of studying cells that the body has shed during

BOX 41-4 TNM CANCER STAGING CLASSIFICATION SYSTEM

T* subclasses	T_x—tumor cannot be adequately assessed T_o—no evidence of primary tumor T_{is}—carcinoma in situ T_1, T_2, T_3, T_4—progressive increase in tumor size and involvement
N† subclasses	N_x—regional lymph nodes cannot be assessed clinically N_o—regional lymph nodes demonstrably abnormal N_1, N_2, N_3, N_4—increasing degrees of demonstrable abnormality of regional lymph nodes
M‡ subclasses	M_x—not assessed M_o—no (known) distant metastasis M_1—distant metastasis present, specify site(s)
Histopathology	G_1—well-differentiated grade G_2—moderately well-differentiated grade G_3, G_4—poorly to very poorly differentiated grade

From American Joint Committee for Cancer Staging and End Results Reporting: Manual for Staging of Cancer, Chicago, 1977, American Joint Committee.
*T—Primary tumor.
†N—Regional lymph nodes.
‡M—Distant metastasis.

Table 41-1 Classification of Neoplasms

Parent Tissue	Benign Tumor	Malignant Tumor
EPITHELIUM		
Skin and mucous membrane	Papilloma Polyp	Squamous cell carcinoma Basal cell carcinoma Transitional cell carcinoma
Glands	Adenoma Cystadenoma	Adenocarcinoma
ENDOTHELIUM		
Blood vessels	Hemangioma	Endothelioma Hemangioendothelioma Angiosarcoma
Lymph vessels	Lymphangioma	Lymphangiosarcoma Lymphangioendothelioma
Bone marrow		**Multiple myeloma** Ewing's sarcoma Leukemia
Lymphoid tissue		Lymphosarcoma Reticulum cell sarcoma (difficult to classify because of cell embryology) Lymphatic leukemia Hodgkin's disease Malignant lymphoma

Continued.

Table 41-1 Classification of Neoplasms—cont'd

Parent Tissue	Benign Tumor	Malignant Tumor
CONNECTIVE TISSUES		
Embryonic fibrous tissue	Myxoma	Myxosarcoma
Fibrous tissue	Fibroma	Fibrosarcoma
Adipose tissue	Lipoma	Liposarcoma
Cartilage	Chondroma	Chondrosarcoma
Bone	Osteoma	Osteogenic sarcoma
Synovial membrane	Synovioma	Synovial sarcoma
MUSCLE TISSUE	**MYOMA**	**MYOSARCOMA**
Smooth muscle	Leiomyoma	Leiomyosarcoma
Striated muscle	Rhabdomyoma	Rhabdomyosarcoma
NERVE TISSUE		
Nerve fibers and sheaths	Neuroma	Neurogenic sarcoma
	Neurinoma (neurilemoma)	
	Neurofibroma	Neurofibrosarcoma
Ganglion cells	Ganglioneuroma	Neuroblastoma
Glia cells	**Glioma**	Glioblastoma
		Spongioblastoma
Meninges	Meningioma	
PIGMENTED NEOPLASMS		
Melanoblasts	Pigmented nevus	Malignant melanoma
		Melanocarcinoma
MISCELLANEOUS		
Placenta	Hydatidiform mole	Chorion-epithelioma (choriocarcinoma)
	Dermoid cyst	Embryonal carcinoma
		Embryonal sarcoma
		Teratocarcinoma

the normal sequence of growth and replacement of body tissues. If cancer is present, cancer cells are also shed.

The results of the Pap test may be reported as:

Class 1 Absence of atypical or abnormal cells
Class 2 Atypical cytology but no evidence of malignancy (may indicate infection)
Class 3 Cytology suggestive of but not conclusive for malignancy
Class 4 Cytology strongly suggestive of malignancy
Class 5 Cytology conclusive for malignancy

Except for a *Class 5 report,* abnormal Pap test reports require additional examination of tissue to confirm a diagnosis.

DIAGNOSIS OF CANCER

Persons who show signs of cancer should undergo diagnostic testing to confirm or rule out the diagnosis. The only definite way to determine the presence of malignant cells is to obtain tissue **biopsy** for microscopic examination. This can sometimes be accomplished by the Papanicolaou test or by aspiration with a needle inserted directly into the tumor. Cells or tissue can also be obtained using an endoscope to directly visualize an internal structure through a body cavity or through a small incision. Endoscopes are rigid or flexible tubes containing a magnifying lens and a light. Endoscopes vary in diameter and length according to the structure being examined; that is, the bronchoscope is used to visualize the tracheobronchial tree; the sigmoidoscope is used to examine the sigmoid colon.

In addition to tissue examination, other diagnostic studies determine the depth of the specific lesion and identify other structures that may have been invaded. These include x-ray and scanning procedures. Commonly ordered x-ray studies are the chest x-ray, mammography, gastrointestinal series, barium enema, and intravenous pyelogram.

Tomography is the special technique of making multiple x-ray films at different depths of a specific area, organ, or structure. The details of each thin section can be clearly visualized.

Computed tomography (CT scan) uses x-rays and a computed scanning system to produce and record images of specific structures at different angles. The entire body can be scanned to detect the presence of any abnormal lesion. Computed tomography is especially helpful to detect small lesions that may not be seen by radiographs or tomography.

Radioisotope studies require the injection or ingestion of a radioactive substance. A scanning device is used to identify the distribution of the substance in different areas of the body. Concentration of the radioisotope in a specific organ, such as the thyroid or brain, identifies tumor in that location (may be primary or metastatic).

Ultrasound testing is a noninvasive procedure using high-frequency sound waves to examine internal structures of the body. As a transducer is moved over the area being studied, an ultrasound beam is directed through the tissues, which reflects back to the transducer where the sound waves are converted into electrical impulses, which produce an image on a display screen. Ultrasound can show the size, consistency, and shape of the structure being studied and is most helpful in distinguishing between cystic and solid tumors. Ultrasound is not used to examine bones or air-filled organs. The procedure is painless. Persons having ultrasonography will feel the transducer moving over their skin and may need to hold their breath for brief periods and to remain still while the procedure is being done.

Magnetic resonance imaging (MRI) is a painless diagnostic procedure that does not involve any exposure to radiation. As the person reclines on a narrow surface that moves into a cylindrical tunnel containing magnetic coils, radio frequency energy waves produce signals that are processed by a computer and displayed as images on a video monitor. The images can be recorded on film or magnetic tape for permanent storage. This test is currently used in the diagnosis of intracranial and spinal lesions and of cardiovascular and soft tissue abnormalities. The procedure also provides information about changes within cells of soft tissues, arteries, veins, the brain, and spinal column.

The person having MRI must not have any magnetic materials on his body during the test. (No jewelry may be worn.) MRI cannot be done if the person has any metallic implants in his body, such as a pacemaker, an orthopedic nail, or aneurysm screw.

The person having the test can talk to those performing the test by means of a microphone placed inside the scanner tunnel. He should be told that he will hear the sound waves thumping on the magnetic field. He must lie still while the test is being done, which may take longer than an hour to obtain the images needed.

Commonly used laboratory tests include the following:

1. *Measurement of acid phosphatase and alkaline phosphatase levels in the blood*

   Acid phosphatase is elevated if cancer is in the prostate gland. Alkaline phosphatase is elevated if there is metastasis to the bone or liver.

2. *Serum calcitonin level*

   Calcitonin is a hormone secreted by the thyroid gland in response to a rising serum calcium level. The level is increased in the blood of people who have cancer of the thyroid. It may be elevated with breast cancer and oat cell cancer of the lung. Calcitonin stimulation testing may be used in addition to the baseline level testing to confirm a diagnosis. It is essential that the person having this test does not eat or drink during the night before the test.

3. *Carcinoembryonic antigen (CEA) serum level*

   Normally, production of CEA stops before birth, but may begin again if a neoplasm develops. This test cannot be used as a general indicator of cancer because there are other reasons why the level may be elevated. The level is elevated in people who smoke. It is found in increased amounts in the blood of people with colorectal cancer. The test assists in the evaluation of cancer treatment where a rising CEA may indicate tumor recurrence or metastatic disease.

4. *Stool examination for blood*

   The cause of blood in the stool must be identified to rule out the possibility of cancer. The guaiac test is commonly used to detect occult (hidden) blood in the stools. Names of other commonly used tests for occult blood in the stool are Hematest, Occultest, and Hemoccult test. Early detection self-tests are available for home use. If blood is found, the person should seek immediate medical attention. For accurate test results for the presence of blood, it is essential that the person not have any of the following foods or medications for 4 days before the test:

   Red meat
   Turnips
   Melons
   Aspirin
   Vitamin C

The test must be performed on three consecutive bowel movements.

People need to be urged to follow through with additional diagnostic testing that may be recommended as a result of initial tests.

MANAGEMENT OF CANCER

Surgery

By the time it is decided that surgery is needed to remove a cancerous lesion, cancer cells may already be spread to other areas. The goal of surgery is to remove all malignant cells. This includes the removal of the tumor, surrounding tissue, and regional lymph nodes that may be present. It is believed that surgical intervention for cancer may release cells to metastasize throughout the body.[8] This has been reduced in laboratory animals by the use of anticoagulants. Surgery in conjunction with chemotherapy and/or radiation therapy may increase the destruction of cancer cells. The effects of cancer drugs and radiation treatments administered before, during, and after surgery are being investigated. A surgical cure may result from a well-isolated lesion removed in the very early stages, such as in cancer of the skin, testicle, or cervix. Surgery may be performed for many reasons—preventive, diagnostic, curative, and palliative.

Surgery may be performed to remove polyps in the colon before they undergo any malignant changes. Occasionally, prophylactic mastectomy is done to prevent breast cancer in those identified to be at very high risk because of family history or other factors.

If the cancerous lesion has already metastasized, surgery may provide palliation by relieving some of the associated problems, such as obstruction, ulceration, hemorrhage, or pain.

The pituitary, adrenals, ovaries, or testes may be surgically removed to help control the growth and spread of malignancies caused by hormonal stimulation.

Reconstructive surgery may be needed to improve body functions and appearance after some types of surgery, such as radical mastectomy. When this is anticipated, preoperative counseling by the surgeon and the nurse will help the patient consider the long-range outcome instead of the immediate, initial surgical procedure.

Nursing considerations. If the nurse is not present when the physician explains recommendations for care, she must ask the physician what has been told to the patient and his family. This is essential to reinforce the information given by the physician. Patients and families are usually frightened and may not remember all that the physician has explained to them.

The patient should have confidence and trust in those responsible for his care. Positive feelings and attitudes promote relaxation and help reduce anxiety and fear. The nurse should encourage the patient to ask his physician any questions he has regarding potential risks as a result of a given treatment (see therapeutic dialogue). A patient needs to feel that he has made the right decision to follow through with plans recommended by the physician.

The use of laser beams is increasing as an alternative for some surgical procedures. The laser beam vaporizes tissue with little bleeding and low risk of infection. Currently the major uses of laser surgery are in ophthalmology, gynecology, urology, neurosurgery, and otolaryngology. The chief discomfort while undergoing laser surgery is that the person must lie very still while the laser is in use.

Preparing the patient for a surgical procedure must include an explanation of what to expect postoperatively. Preoperative teaching is discussed in Chapter 26.

When surgery may result in a changed body image, such as mastectomy, laryngectomy, or formation of an ostomy, the patient may benefit from talking with another person who has had the same type of surgery. The American Cancer Society sponsors support groups. They also specially prepare volunteers to visit individuals who need these types of surgical procedures. *Reach to Recovery,* the *Lost Chord Club,* and the *Ostomy Club* are some of the special groups that are available in some local communities.

A patient's spouse or significant other should see the surgical site as soon as possible after surgery so that before discharge, the patient can talk about reactions and feelings and ask questions while professional staff are available to assist.

THERAPEUTIC DIALOGUE

■ Patient scheduled for modified radical mastectomy

NURSE: Good afternoon, Mrs. Smith. My name is Ms. Johnson. I'm your nurse this evening. How are you feeling?

PATIENT: I'm feeling all right now; it's tomorrow I'm dreading.

NURSE: Would you like to talk about it? What are you dreading?

PATIENT: The doctor told me he has to remove my whole left breast and even cut under my arm to remove any lymph nodes that may be there.

NURSE: You said you were dreading having this done.

PATIENT: I was hoping that the only thing he'd have to do is remove just the lumps. I dread the thought I will look so different.

NURSE: Do you know about some of the choices you have to help you maintain your appearance?

PATIENT: Yes, I've heard about special brassieres, but how about when I undress and my husband sees my chest.

NURSE: Have you talked to him about how you feel?

PATIENT: I've tried to. He tells me it won't make any difference.

NURSE: Do you feel it will make a difference because your physical appearance has changed?

PATIENT: I don't know. I will be the same person. Maybe I just can't accept what's happening to me. I'm afraid.

Radiation Therapy

Radiation therapy can be used to cure or control cancer that has spread to local lymph nodes or to treat tumors that cannot be removed.

Radiation may be used preoperatively to reduce the size of a tumor. Postoperative radiation may be indicated to destroy malignant cells not removed by surgery. Radiation may be used to slow the growth of malignant tumors.

Radiation may be delivered externally or internally.

External therapy may be directed toward superficial lesions or may be targeted to deeper structures within the body.

External radiation therapy. When external radiation is planned, the specific area on the body is marked to indicate the port for external radiation to be directed. These markings must not be washed off. If the area becomes wet while bathing, pat the area with an absorbent towel to dry the skin. Help the patient to understand the need to protect this area. Also instruct him to avoid the use of any ointments, lotions, or powder on this area. The physician may approve specific lotions or creams for drying skin. The patient should be told to protect the radiated area from direct sunlight and to avoid applications of heat or cold, since these would increase erythema, drying, and pruritus of the skin, which is common over an irradiated area.

A diet high in protein and calories and a fluid intake of 2 or 3 quarts of fluid per day must be encouraged. The person undergoing radiation therapy should be assured that lethargy and fatigue are not uncommon during treatment and that frequent rest periods are helpful.

Half of all people with cancer are treated with radiation therapy at some point. For many of these, radiation therapy is the only therapy needed to destroy the cancer.[12]

Internal radiation therapy. General principles to be followed when caring for the patient treated with internal radiation are the following:

1. Assemble materials and plan ahead to provide several nursing care measures at the same time when entering the patient's room.
2. Stand at the greatest distance away from the site where an internal radiation device is in the patient's body.
3. Limit the time needed for close contact near the site being irradiated. If direct, prolonged care is needed, nurses should wear a lead apron.

Unsealed internal radiation is administered intravenously or orally so that it is distributed throughout the patient's body. Special precautions must be taken to prevent exposure to radiation from direct contact with the patient or from contact with any of his body tissue or fluid (Box 41-5).

Radioactive implant (brachytherapy) is the insertion of sealed radioactive materials temporarily or permanently into hollow cavities, within body tissues, or on the body's surface. The radioactive source delivers a specific radiation dose continuously over hours or days. A highly concentrated radiation dose is delivered in or near a tumor. This technique is generally combined with a course of external radiation therapy to increase the dosage to a specific site. Certain organs, such as the uterus and vagina, are natural receptacles for the placement of an applicator that can be loaded with radioactive material. Radioactive needles, wires, seeds, beads, or catheters may be inserted directly into tumor tissue (Figs. 41-3 and 41-4).

BOX 41-5 PREVENTION OF RADIATION HAZARDS

Unsealed Internal Radiotherapy

1. Radioactive iodine
   a. Use special precautions for urine
      (1) Collect in lead-lined container, label
      (2) Take to radioisotope laboratory for disposal
      (3) Follow approved institution protocols for spilled urine
   b. Monitor linen and equipment for contamination, using a Geiger-Muller counter, before removal from room
   c. Label and store radioactive linen in lead containers or burn
   d. Use paper dishes and burn after use
   e. Wash skin and equipment with soap and water, if contaminated, then monitor
   f. Wear gloves when handling linen
   g. Air room for at least 24 hours or until monitoring shows radioactivity is negligible
2. Radioactive phosphorus
   a. Follow skin and equipment contamination procedures as for radioactive iodine
   b. Place vomitus and dressings in lead-lined container, label, and take to radioisotope laboratory for disposal
3. Radioactive gold
   a. Place contaminated linen in container, label, send to radioisotope laboratory
   b. Burn dressings and tissues or send to laboratory for disposal
   c. If the patient dies, place a conspicuous tag on body to warn the mortician

Children younger than 18 years and pregnant women should not be allowed to visit implant patients. Approved visitors should be advised regarding the recommended limit of time and safe distance to stay with the patient.[19]

When cancer of the cervix is treated with the use of an applicator containing a radioactive material, the applicator is placed in the vagina. The following special nursing measures are indicated[13]:

1. Place "Radiation in Use" sign on the patient's door.
2. Prevent dislodgment. Keep patient on strict bed rest. Instruct the patient not to turn from side to side or onto the abdomen. Do not raise the head of the bed more than 30 to 45 degrees.
3. Do not give a complete bed bath while the applicator is in place, and do not bathe the patient below the waist. Do not change bed linen unless necessary.

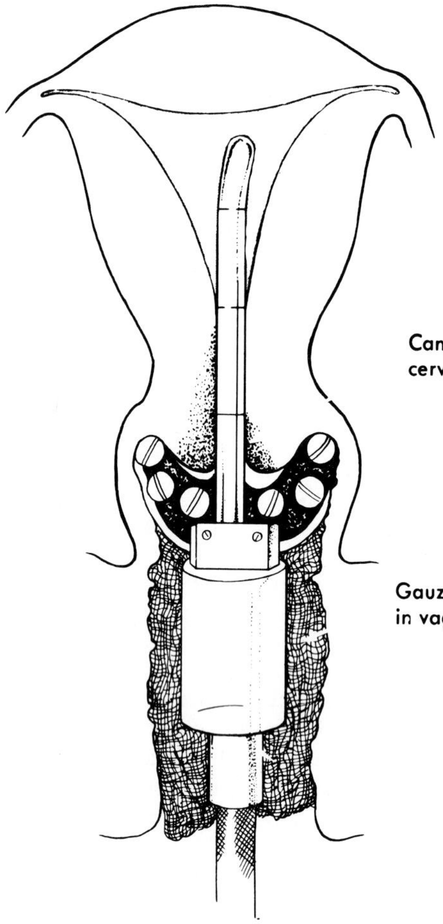

FIG. 41-3 Ernst applicator in place for treatment of cancer of the cervix. Note gauze packing in the vagina to help maintain applicator in position.

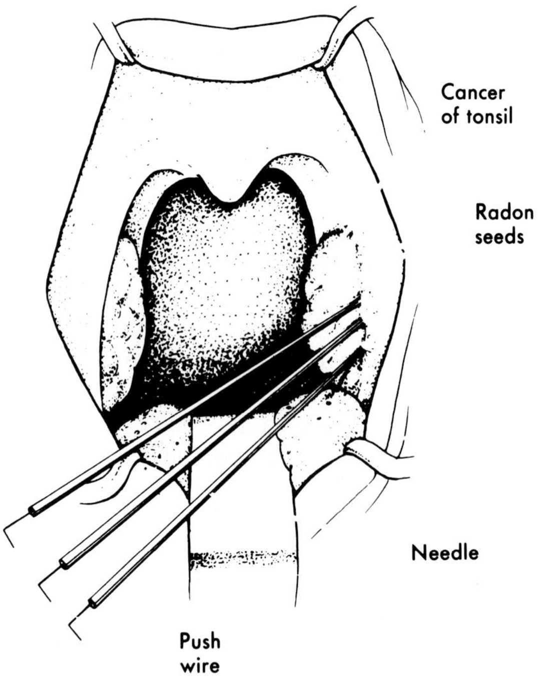

FIG. 41-4 Radium emanations may be sealed in tiny gold tubes (radon seeds) and left indefinitely within tissue into which they are inserted. Schema shows insertion into tonsil.

4. Encourage the patient to do active range-of-motion exercises with both arms and mild foot and leg exercises to minimize the hazards of immobility. Patient will wear antiembolism stockings (TED hose).
5. Monitor vital signs every 4 hours, observing for elevations in temperature, pulse, and respirations. Temperature above 100° F should be reported to the physician.
6. Observe for and report the development of any rash or skin eruption, excessive vaginal bleeding, or vaginal discharge.
7. Keep accurate intake and output record. Encourage a fluid intake of at least 3 L daily. An indwelling catheter is in place to reduce the size of the bladder and decrease effects of radiation on the bladder. Check to be sure it is draining well.
8. Serve diet as ordered—usually a low-residue diet to minimize peristalsis and bowel movement, which might lead to dislodgment of applicator.
9. Check position of applicator every 4 hours.
10. Keep long-handled forceps and a special lead container in the patient's room for use by the radiologist, should the implant become dislodged. *Never touch a dislodged applicator or any other materials that have fallen out of the patient. These may contain the radiative sources.* Any bed linens, dressings, or pads that have been changed for the patient must be checked with a radiation survey meter before removing them from the patient's room.
11. After the applicator is removed, the indwelling catheter is usually removed and a douche and enema are generally prescribed.
12. Precautions are no longer needed after removal. Encourage ambulation and gradual resumption of activities.
13. Sexual intercourse is usually delayed for 7 to 10 days.
14. Instruct the patient to notify the physician of nausea, vomiting, diarrhea, frequent or painful urination, or a temperature above 100° F.[13]

Chemotherapy

Chemotherapy drugs are used to reduce or slow the growth of metastatic cancer. A combination of chemotherapeutic agents may be more effective than a single drug. Chemotherapy drugs are often effective in preventing the multiplications of cancer cells or destroying them. Normal tissues are also affected. Tissues that multiply rapidly are affected the most, such as the hematopoietic system, hair follicles, and the gastrointestinal system, which may result in the side effects of **leukopenia**, anemia, thrombocytopenia, **alopecia, stomatitis,** nausea, vomiting, and diarrhea.

Many of the problems that may be experienced by people undergoing chemotherapy are the same as those that may result from radiation therapy (depending on the target site and amount of radiation). The nurse must help the patient realize that some of the problems are the result of therapy and not a sign that the cancer is increasing. Some of these are included below.

NURSING DIAGNOSES	NURSING INTERVENTIONS
Tissue integrity, impaired: oral mucous membrane, related to stomatitis (inflammation of the mouth); xerostomia (decreased salivation)	Assist with frequent, careful oral hygiene and hydration; use very soft toothbrush. Give soothing oral lozenges; use ice chips and frequent sips of ice water; avoid hot beverages; use lip balm for dryness.
Nutrition, altered: less than body requirements, related to anorexia (results from changes in taste and smell); nausea/vomiting; dysphagia (difficulty in swallowing); aspiration; diarrhea; malabsorption; cachexia	Provide adequate, easily digestible, soft, bland diet. Give small, frequent, highly nutritional foods to meet the extra demands created by energy used by malignant cells; allow extra time needed to eat.
Fatigue, related to anemia	Arrange rest periods before mealtimes and at frequent periods throughout day. Provide slow, individualized schedule for activities; wheelchair/walker may conserve energy.
Potential for infection, related to weakened immune system; leukopenia	Protect against infections—especially from other people. Observe and promptly report to physician any signs of inflammation at injection sites or insertion sites of any peripheral or central intravenous lines.
Potential for trauma, related to fatigue, increasing weakness, and thrombocytopenia	Protect from injuries that may result in bleeding; inspect for evidence of bleeding or bruising; use smallest needles for injections.
Self-esteem disturbance: situational low self-esteem, related to changes in appearance if cachexia is experienced as a result of advanced cancer	Encourage active participation in planning and care for self; assist with hair care to maintain attractive appearance.
Diversional activity deficit, related to decreased energy as a result of anemia	Provide time for viewing or listening to favorite TV or radio programs; encourage hobby or games with other people; encourage visitors and conversation regarding current events; assist to participate in selected activities, such as church, the theater, or shopping at selected stores (conserve energy); plan eating out in a favorite restaurant for special occasions; arrange short drives to favorite locations, such as beach, parks, lakes.
Pain, related to late-stage problems resulting from progressive cancer	Assist to develop and maintain trusting relationship with caregivers. Provide medications as ordered before pain intensifies. Provide comfort measures, such as good alignment and frequent position changes. Encourage relaxation by use of soft music and quiet environment.
Knowledge deficit, related to outcomes of problems and treatment for cancer	Be realistic and honest in discussions regarding the future. Assist to identify and fulfill planning for personal business and family matters with awareness of shortened life-expectancy if a poor prognosis has been established.
Anxiety/fear, related to the diagnosis of cancer	*Listen* with genuine interest and concern.
Impaired tissue integrity, related to damage to integumentary tissue: alopecia	Give reassurance that problem is usually not permanent. Assist to choose an attractive wig to have when needed.
Activity intolerance, related to fatigue, decreased mobility, and effects of debilitating disease	Change position frequently (at least every 2 hours). Provide range-of-motion exercises every 8 hours.
Impaired skin integrity, related to decreased mobility and altered nutritional status	Massage over bony prominences each time position is changed. Use Eggcrate foam mattress or alternating air pressure mattress. Keep sheet smooth (no wrinkles). Inspect carefully for potential development of decubitus.
Ineffective individual and family coping, related to feelings about diagnosis of cancer, change in body image, feelings of powerlessness/inability to control outcome of disease	Encourage communication/sharing of feelings among family members.

Chemotherapy has proven effective in treatment of many cancer patients. In 1980 more than 46,000 cancer patients were cured with the use of anticancer drugs, either alone or combined with radiation and/or surgery.[6]

Nurses must learn about each drug being administered

to anticipate the expected side effects and plan the nursing interventions needed.

There are safety guidelines for the preparation and administration of chemotherapeutic agents, since they may be absorbed into the skin or inhaled. The major types of chemotherapeutic agents used for the treatment of cancer include the following:

Alkylating agents — interfere with DNA replication; cell-cycle phase nonspecific
Nitrosoureas — inhibit DNA replication
Antimetabolites — inhibit enzymes of nucleic acid synthesis; generally cell-cycle phase specific
Vinca alkaloids — bind to microtubular proteins; necessary for cell division during mitosis; cell-cycle phase specific
Antitumor antibiotics — inhibit DNA and RNA synthesis; generally cell-cycle phase nonspecific
Hormones — affect the growth pattern of hormonally responsive tumors

Immunotherapy

When conventional treatment for cancer is not sufficient, immunotherapy may be recommended. This therapy is given to stimulate the body's natural immune system. The immune system has the ability to control cancer cells. Experiments have demonstrated the body does have a defense mechanism against cancer. Some of the agents that stimulate the body's natural immune system include Bacille Calmette-Guérin (BCG), interferons, interleukin-2, and specific malignant cell antibodies produced in the laboratory from actual tumor cells from a patient's body. When these agents are used, nurses must accurately observe and record patient responses and promptly report potential adverse reactions. New techniques for treating cancer are being developed, and many believe that the future holds new hope for otherwise terminally ill people.

Bone Marrow Transplantation

Bone marrow may be removed from an individual for his own use at a later time, or an individual may be given bone marrow removed from another person. Bone marrow aspirations are prepared so that they can be administered intravenously after large doses of chemotherapy or radiation therapy. Bone marrow transplantation is also used for treatment of people with acute **leukemia** or Hodgkin's disease. The infused bone marrow will stimulate production of healthy blood cells. Infection and rejection are possible risks.

There are many *unproven* methods for the treatment of cancer, and many cancer patients become victims of "false hope" practices.

Nurses should communicate genuine concern for cancer patients. This includes reinforcing information explained to patients by their physicians regarding the expectations of their specific treatments. Patients may become discouraged by toxic side effects and other problems they experience while undergoing conventional cancer therapies. Nurses should allow extra time to listen to patients with cancer express their feelings and to encourage them to follow the guidelines of conventional medical practice that offer the most hope.

The number of cancers that are being cured is rising daily. In 1980, 136,000 cancer patients were reported to be free of the disease for 5 years or more after having radiation treatments alone or combined with other therapies.[12]

ADVANCED CANCER

Pain Management for the Patient with Advanced Cancer

Pain may be experienced with advanced cancer as a result of compression on nerves. Pain is caused also by destruction of the spinal column and bone as a result of metastasis. Lymphatic or venous obstruction causes pain. Pain also results where there is inflammation, ulceration, infection, and tissue necrosis. Pain may result from the treatments for cancer, such as surgical procedures and the effects produced by chemotherapy or radiation therapy.

Because pain with advanced cancer is chronic, recurring, and increasing in intensity, it may be accompanied by depression. A combination of analgesics, antidepressant or antianxiety agents, or mood elevators may be used for pain management. Continuing relief is better provided by administering the medications on a regularly scheduled basis rather than only when needed. In addition to the oral, rectal, and parenteral routes for administering pain medications, intraspinal infusion or an infusion implant reservoir may be used to deliver narcotic analgesia slowly and continuously.

Adequate rest, sleep, diversion, and other meaningful activities will also help in the management of pain.

Fear and anxiety increase as a result of pain. Many cancer patients feel increased pain is a sign their condition is worsening and death is imminent. Pain increases their fear, and the cycle of pain continues.

The combination of (1) appropriate pain relief methods, (2) the opportunity to make personal and spiritual peace if there are unresolved conflicts in relationships with others, and (3) someone to listen and offer comfort is probably the most effective pain reliever known.[1] Nurses have a vital role in the assessment and management of pain by recording the type, duration, severity, and location, and measures that have relieved or not relieved the patient. The patient with cancer is often in a state of **cachexia,** and therefore positioning, meticulous skin care, offering nutritious fluids and foods, and other comfort measures to promote relaxation and rest will also help to reduce pain and severe fatigue.

Caring for the Patient with Advanced Cancer

The patient and his family may become irritable and angry with caregivers when suffering and progressive problems are experienced. Nurses should understand that these feelings are not directed toward them personally but have emerged from the circumstances associated with the patient's disease. Kind understanding and continued warm, responsive caring are the best approaches. The patient may not hear the explanations that have been given when feelings are at a high level. By listening and administering kind and gentle nursing care, the nurse may communicate more effectively than with words. Touch may also be appropriate to add the dimension of another human being's awareness of the emotional distress being experienced.

The Terminal Prognosis

Coping with the multiple problems experienced when one has advanced cancer can lead to a sense of helplessness and hopelessness in spite of all efforts. The patient and his family may look forward to death as a relief from unrelenting suffering.

Spiritual activities may provide mental and emotional strength in spite of physical deterioration. The patient may ask the nurse to read the Bible to him or to pray with or for him, or he may request that a minister, priest, or rabbi be called to visit him. Spiritual strength may help the patient and his family to cope with continuing problems encountered in the cancer experience.

The hospital social worker assists the patient/family in planning to meet the immediate needs for home care. Arrangements for any special supplies and equipment are made before discharge. The nurse plays a major role in teaching the patient and at least one family member (significant other) how to continue any special care needed at home, such as dressing changes, irrigations, the management of a feeding tube, or the care of a central venous line for administration of parenteral nutrition or medications.

Throughout the hospital stay, nurses must take advantage of time available to promote self-care to the extent possible. Assessment of readiness to learn and ability to assume active participation in caring for self is a major responsibility of nurses. Advanced clinical nursing specialists may need to be consulted to provide individualized guidelines for teaching patients. Plans for patient education must be written on the nursing care plan. Evidence of the patient's comprehension and ability to care for himself must be documented, and assistance needed from others must be planned and provided for accordingly. Continuity of care is the goal in discharge planning. Hospice services can be arranged in most communities for those who have advanced cancer. There are free-standing hospices, hospices within a hospital or skilled nursing facility, or at-home arrangements. The primary focus of hospice is enhancing the quality of life for the individual, not prolonging life. Efforts are directed toward relief from pain and other problems. Skilled professional care and voluntary support services are provided to assist the patient and family to live life to the fullest each day.[11] See Chapter 56 for a discussion about hospice care.

REFERENCES AND SUGGESTED READINGS

1. Advanced cancer: living each day, US Department of Health and Human Services, National Cancer Institute, 1985.
2. Brunner L and others: Textbook of medical-surgical nursing, ed 6, Philadelphia, 1988, JB Lippincott Co.
3. Byrne CJ and others: Laboratory tests: implications for nursing care, Menlo Park, Calif, 1986, Addison-Wesley Publishing Co, Inc.
4. Ca—a cancer journal for clinicians: American Cancer Society, Inc. 38(3):176, 1988.
5. Cancer facts and figures—1988, The American Cancer Society, Inc.
6. Chemotherapy and you, US Department of Health and Human Services, National Cancer Institute, 1987.
7. Dudas S and Carlson C: Cancer rehabilitation, Oncol Nurs Forum 15(2):183, 1988.
8. Hood G and Dincher J: Total patient care: foundations and practice, ed 7, St Louis, 1988, The CV Mosby Co.
9. Morra M: Choices: who's going to tell the patients what they need to know, Oncol Nurs Forum 15(4):421, 1988.
10. Mosby's medical, nursing, and allied health dictionary, ed 3, St Louis, 1990, The CV Mosby Co.
11. Phipps W and others: Medical surgical nursing: concepts and clinical practice, ed 3, St. Louis, 1987, The CV Mosby Co.
12. Radiation therapy and you, US Department of Health and Human Services, National Cancer Institute, 1986.
13. Snyder C: Oncology nursing, Boston, 1986, Little, Brown & Co, Inc.
14. Springhouse Corporation: Diagnostic tests handbook, Springhouse, Penn, 1987 Springhouse Corp.
15. St. Vincent's Medical Center: Lasers: the healing light, Involved: 14, Jacksonville, Fla, 1989.
16. Taptich B and others: Nursing diagnosis and care planning, Philadelphia, 1989, WB Sanders Co.
17. Thompson JM and others: Mosby's manual of clinical nursing, ed 2, St. Louis, 1989, The CV Mosby Co.
18. Thorne SE: Helpful and unhelpful communications in cancer care: the patient perspective, Oncol Nurs Forum 15(2):167, 1988.
19. Ziegfeld C: Core curriculum for oncology nursing, Philadelphia, 1987, WB Saunders Co.

CHAPTER CHALLENGE

KEY POINTS

- It is currently estimated that one of every five people in the United States will get cancer during his lifetime; and of the people who do, more than 50% may die from the disease within 5 years.
- There is strong evidence that what people eat or drink or their life-style habits predispose to the development of cancer.
- It is important to have periodic physical examinations and to seek medical attention promptly if one of the warning signs of cancer develops.
- A common reason for a delay in diagnosing cancer is because early malignant changes are not accompanied by pain.
- Seeking medical attention when any warning signs occur is also frequently delayed because people fear the possible diagnosis of cancer and hope the signs and symptoms will just go away.
- The diagnosis of cancer has a profound effect on family members, as well as the patient himself. Shock, disbelief, denial, anger, and fear are experienced. The feelings are accompanied by a high degree of anxiety and a sense of helplessness.
- The American Cancer Society sponsors organized support groups for individuals with the same types of cancer. Some of these are *Reach to Recovery*, the *Lost Chord Club*, and the *Ostomy Club*. Prepared volunteer visitors are available in most communities to visit a newly diagnosed patient on the approval of the responsible physician.
- Spiritual strength assists the patient and his family to cope with the problems experienced as a result of cancer. Based on the patient's preference, religious counsel may be helpful.
- The concepts of rehabilitation should be applied in planning care for the patient with cancer that will promote the highest level of functioning possible.

STUDY QUESTIONS

1. In the United States, death from cancer ranks:
   a. First
   b. Second
   c. Third
   d. Fourth
2. In which of the following sites does cancer result in the highest number of deaths:
   a. Bladder
   b. Breast
   c. Colon
   d. Lung
3. Which of the following is an example of primary prevention of cancer:
   a. Change in life-style habit, such as smoking cessation
   b. Planned, periodic physical examinations
   c. Recognition of one of cancer's warnings signs
   d. Breast self-examination
4. Which of the following tests can be used to make a definite diagnosis of cancer:
   a. Biopsy
   b. Mammography
   c. Tomography
   d. Ultrasound testing
5. Which of the following tests cannot be done if the patient has a metallic implant in his body:
   a. Computed tomography
   b. Magnetic resonance imaging (MRI)
   c. Radioisotope studies
   d. Ultrasonography
6. If an individual finds a small lump in one of the breasts, which action is best:
   a. Prompt examination by a physician is needed
   b. It is best to wait at least 1 month to be sure the lump remains
   c. Physical examination should be postponed until the lump enlarges
   d. Warm moist compresses should be applied at least 3 times a day to help reduce the size
7. For accurate test results for the presence of blood in the stool, which of the following foods must be avoided for 4 days before the test:
   a. Chicken, broccoli, or squash
   b. Fish, cabbage, or potatoes
   c. Milk or milk products
   d. Red meat, turnips, or melons
8. Which of the following medications must be avoided 4 days before testing for occult blood:
   a. Aspirin and vitamin C
   b. B complex vitamins
   c. Fat-soluble vitamins (A, D, E, or K)
   d. Antibiotics
9. It is necessary to perform tests for occult blood in the stool:
   a. One time only
   b. On at least 2 consecutive stools
   c. On at least 3 consecutive stools
   d. On at least 4 consecutive stools
10. Which of the following laboratory tests is elevated in people who smoke:
    a. Carcinoembryonic antigen (CEA) serum level
    b. Serum calcitonin
    c. Acid phosphatase
    d. Alkaline phosphatase
11. When caring for a patient who has an applicator with radioactive implants in his throat, the nurse should:
    a. Stand near the patient's head so that the patient can clearly see the nurse continuously while they are talking
    b. Remain outside the room to avoid any contact with the patient
    c. Stand near the foot of the patient's bed when talking, and limit the time close to the patient
    d. Not be concerned with the time or distance, but avoid touching the patient's body
12. Which of the following is an example of an agent that stimulates the body's natural immune system:
    a. Antimetabolites
    b. Antibiotics
    c. Interleukin
    d. Hormones
13. Chemotherapeutic drugs used for cancer:
    a. Cure malignant tumors
    b. Reduce or slow the growth of metastatic cancer
    c. Stop the process of metastasis
    d. Increase the body's resistance against cancer
14. The person with leukopenia has a special need for which of the following nursing interventions:
    a. Provision of adequate fluid intake
    b. Protection from falls
    c. Protection against infection, especially for other people
    d. Limitation of activities
15. The person with thrombocytopenia must be protected by which of the following nursing measures:
    a. Limitation of activities and socialization
    b. Provision of frequent oral hygiene with a firm toothbrush
    c. Encouragement to use a wheelchair to conserve energy
    d. Use of the smallest needles for injections

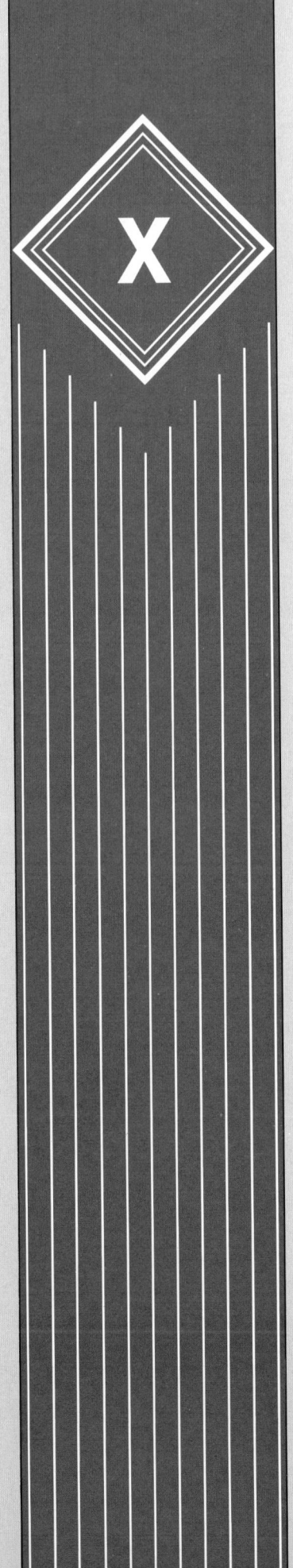

X

Maternal and Neonatal Nursing

Nursing gives me the opportunity to give of myself to someone else who has a need. Nursing is being there when a new life enters into this world and sharing the happiness it brings. It is sharing tears with the family that has lost a loved one. It is the way patients' faces light up when you tell them you are their nurse. My life has been touched and made richer by being a nurse. My hope is that I have given, as well as received.

STELLA NETHERTON
Student Nurse

42

Normal Pregnancy

GLORIA E. WOLD

LEARNING OBJECTIVES

After reading this chapter, the student should be able to do the following:

- Define the key terms.
- Explain the physiology of conception.
- Discuss the anatomical and physiological alterations that occur during pregnancy.
- Identify the components of antepartal assessment.
- Compare the presumptive, possible, and positive signs of pregnancy.
- Recognize the common discomforts of pregnancy.
- List the danger signs that might occur during pregnancy.
- Describe nutritional requirements during pregnancy.
- Identify nursing diagnoses relevant to care of the prenatal patient.

RELATED TOPICS OF INTEREST

- Basic nutrition (Chapter 22)
- Care of the patient with a reproductive disorder (Chapter 36)

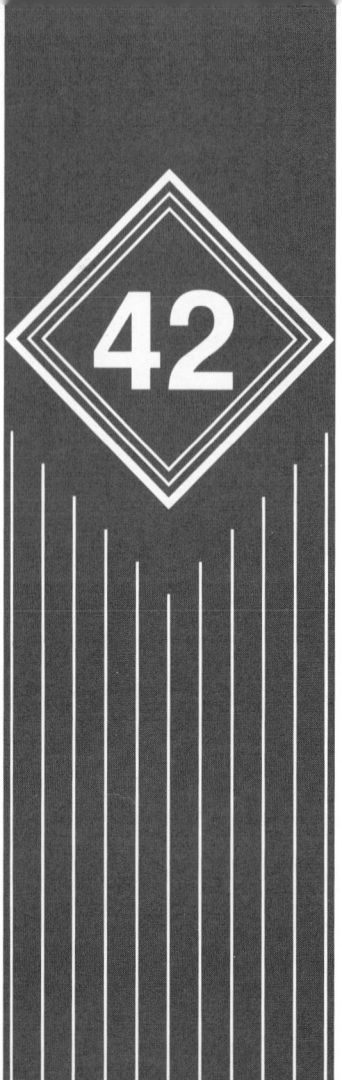

KEY TERMS

Define the following:

- blastocyst
- ectoderm
- ectopic
- endoderm
- flagellar
- gravida
- implantation
- lanugo
- mesoderm
- morula
- multigravida
- multipara
- nullipara
- nulligravida
- -para
- teratogenic
- viable
- zygote

Few experiences in life are as exciting and challenging as childbearing. The changes that occur in a relatively short time are profound and dramatic. Childbearing is a challenge to the new mother, to the newly developing or changing family unit, to society, and to the nurse who assists in the childbearing process.

THE PHYSIOLOGY OF PREGNANCY

To comprehend the physiological changes of pregnancy, the nurse must understand the normal anatomy and physiology of the male and female reproductive systems. It is particularly important to review the menstrual cycle and related hormonal activity. It is also important to recognize that specific cells, ova in the female and sperm in the male, carry genetic messages to their offspring. These cells, when united, result in a new individual with a unique genetic makeup, parts of which come from each parent.

Fertilization

During sexual intercourse sperm carried in the ejaculatory semen of the male enters the vagina of the female. By **flagellar** (whiplike) movement the sperm travel through the mucus of the cervical canal (if the mucus is receptive), enter the uterine chamber, and move into the ampulla—the outer third of the fallopian tube. If the timing is such that an ovum has been produced and is also within the ampulla of the tube, fertilization may occur. Fertilization takes place when the sperm joins or fuses with the ovum; this is also called *conception*. The fusion of the sperm into the ovum requires approximately 24 hours. Once fertilization has occurred, the new cell is referred to as a **zygote** or fertilized ovum. This cell carries 46 chromosomes (44 autosomes and 2 sex chromosomes). At the moment of fertilization the sex of the zygote and all other genetic characteristics are determined and do not change.

Implantation

The zygote moves through the uterine tube by ciliary action and some irregular peristaltic activity. It requires 3 to 4 days to enter the uterine cavity. During this time the zygote is in a phase of rapid cell division called *mitosis*. Further changes result in formation of a structure called the **morula**, which develops into the **blastocyst.** After the blastocyst is free in the uterine cavity for 1 to 2 days, the exposed cell walls of the blastocyst (called the *trophoblast*) secrete enzymes that are able to break down protein and penetrate cell membranes. These enzymes allow the blastocyte to enter the endometrium and implant. The action of the enzymes normally stops short of the myometrium but may cause slight bleeding in some individuals. This is called *implantation bleeding*. While this bleeding is rarely more than spotting, it may confuse some women who think that they had a very light and short menstrual cycle when they are really pregnant.

The condition of the uterine lining is critical if **implantation** of the zygote is to occur. The endometrium during the secretory phase of the menstrual cycle has an enriched vascular bed with enlarged blood vessels and an increased store of glycogen, which will support development of the embryo if implantation occurs. Implantation usually occurs in the fundus of the uterus on either the anterior or posterior surfaces. If uterine conditions are not suitable, it is unlikely that implantation will occur. If intrauterine vascular or hormonal conditions cannot sustain the implanted embryo, a spontaneous abortion will occur. Most spontaneous abortions occur during the first 8 weeks of pregnancy for these reasons. **Ectopic** pregnancy, where implantation occurs outside of the uterine cavity, also poses serious problems. These conditions will be discussed further in Chapter 45.

During the first few weeks after implantation, primary villi appear. These villi are able to use maternal blood vessels as a source of nourishment and oxygen for the developing embryo. This occurs during the stage of development, from the time of implantation, about 2 weeks after conception, until the seventh or eighth week. It is also during these first few weeks that the first stages of the chorionic villi occur. Chorionic villi secrete human chorionic gonadotropin (HCG), a hormone that stimulates the continued production of progesterone and estrogen by the corpus luteum. This is the reason that ovulation and menstruation cease during pregnancy. Primary villi also synthesize protein and glucose for approximately 12 weeks, until the fetus is adequately developed to meet its own needs. The chorionic villi become the fetal portion of the placenta.

Embryonic/Fetal Development

Until the time of implantation, the germinal phase, the cell mass is referred to as the **zygote**. During this period the fertilized ovum develops from the two original cells into a many-celled organism. The zygote develops two separate and distinct cavities, the amniotic cavity and the yolk sac. The amniotic cavity has walls lined with the **ectoderm** and a cavity filled with amniotic fluid. The yolk sac is lined with the **endoderm,** which supplies nourishment until implantation. A third layer of primary cells, the **mesoderm,** is located between the two cavities. The embryo develops at the point at which these three layers meet, called the trilaminar embryonic disk. Various structures and organs arise from each of these layers.

The embryonic stage begins with implantation and comprises approximately the first 8 weeks of pregnancy. During the embryonic stage, the three primary cell layers differentiate into tissue and layers, which form the placenta, embryonic membranes, and the embryo itself. During the embryonic stage, cell growth is rapid. A simple heart begins beating, and rudimentary forms of all the major organs and systems develop. By the end of this stage, the embryo has acquired a human appearance. Starting with the ninth week the embryo is referred to as the fetus, and the fetal stage begins.

Many structures are developing simultaneously in the embryo; therefore when an infant is born with one birth defect or abnormality, the physician will check for others that are likely to be present. During the early weeks of pregnancy, often before a woman even knows that she is pregnant, **teratogenic** agents, such as drugs, medication, radiation, and infectious agents, can cause serious harm. Rubella, which is usually a mild childhood disease, is serious if developed at this stage of pregnancy. This virus can affect all of the germ layers and cause serious anomalies, such as cardiac defects, deafness, and mental retardation.

The prenatal calendar, Table 42-1, describes fetal development and maternal changes throughout pregnancy.

Embryonic/Fetal Physiology

The placenta. The *placenta* (Greek, "flat plate"), is a disklike organ made up of about 20 sections called *cotyledons*. It is a unique structure, present only during pregnancy. From a few beginning cells this organ develops rapidly. At full term the placenta looks like a large red disk with a diameter of 15 to 20 cm (6 to 10 inches) and a thickness of 2 to 3 cm (1 inch). It normally weighs between 400 and 600 g (1 pound to 1 pound 5 ounces). The bulk of the placenta is fetal in origin. It appears dark red and has a rough surface; the cotyledons are apparent as distinct lobes with clefts or divisions between each lobe. The fetal side is smooth and shiny. It consists of the membranes of the amniotic sac that encases the fetus.

As already mentioned, the placenta functions as an endocrine gland secreting HCG (human chorionic gonadotropin) and the steroidal hormones estrogen and progesterone, which maintain the pregnancy. In addition, the placenta is the site of the exchange of nutrients, oxygen, and waste products between the fetus and the maternal circulation. While the placenta allows transfer of oxygen and nutrients through such processes as diffusion, active transport, and others, it also has the ability to block the transfer of certain substances. Some viruses are able to cross the placental barrier, but most bacteria are too large to cross. Some drugs do not cross the placenta, but most do cross and can cause serious harmful effects on the growing embryo/fetus. After delivery the placenta is of no further use and is expelled.

Table 42-1 Prenatal Calendar (Using Fertilization Age)

General Developmental Characteristics (Schematically Pictured)		Average Weight and Size	Possible Maternal Findings and Diagnostic Aids
GERMINAL STAGE (1 TO 10 DAYS)			
First week 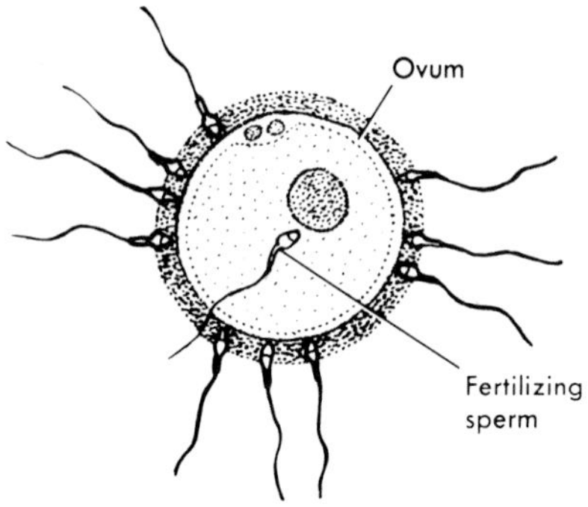	*Zygote* forms: ovum fertilized in fallopian tube undergoes cell divisions (cleavage) on way to uterus	Just visible to eye	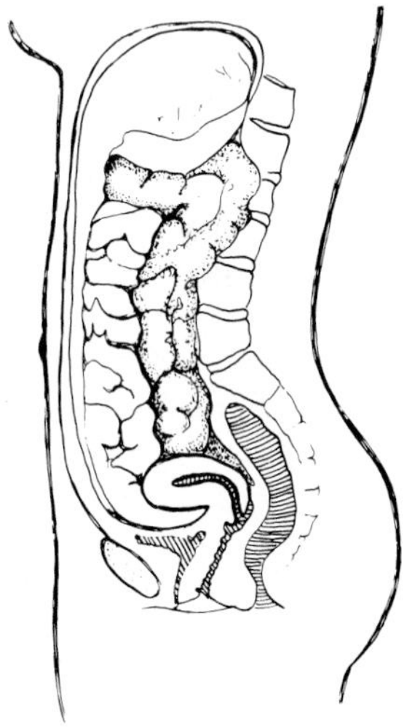 Normal female pelvis before implantation (sagittal section)
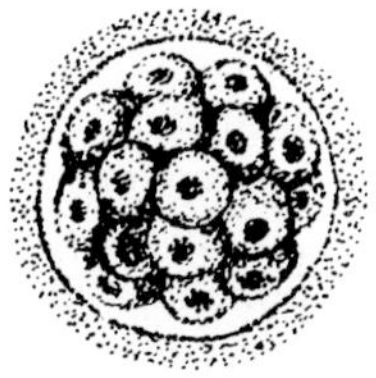	*Morula* forms: solid mass of about 16 microscopic cells resembling mulberry; enters uterus on third day		
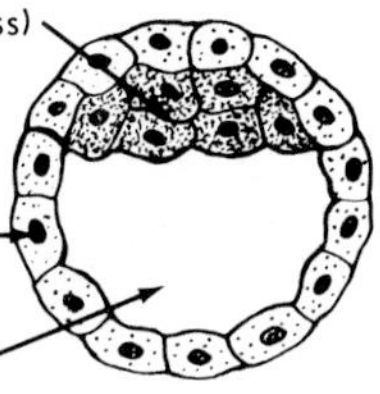	*Blastocyst:* morula develops fluid-filled cavity; *trophoblast:* outer wall of blastocyst; *embryoblast:* inner cell mass from which embryo eventually forms		
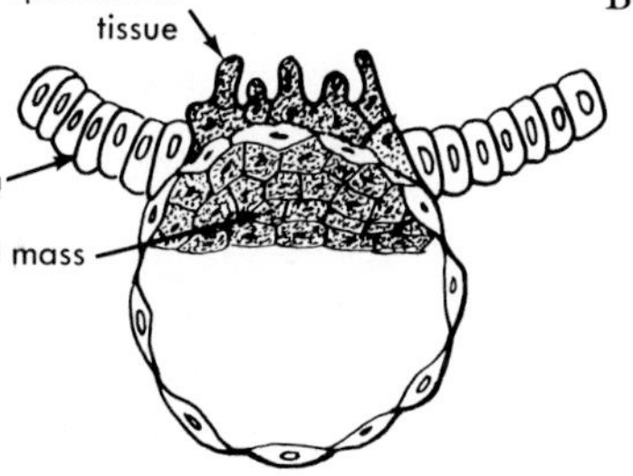	Beginning implantation of blastocyst in endometrium by invading trophoblastic tissue ±7 days		

Continued.

Table 42-1 Prenatal Calendar (Using Fertilization Age)—cont'd

General Developmental Characteristics (Schematically Pictured)		Average Weight and Size	Possible Maternal Findings and Diagnostic Aids
EMBRYONIC STAGE (10 DAYS TO 8 WEEKS)			
Second week 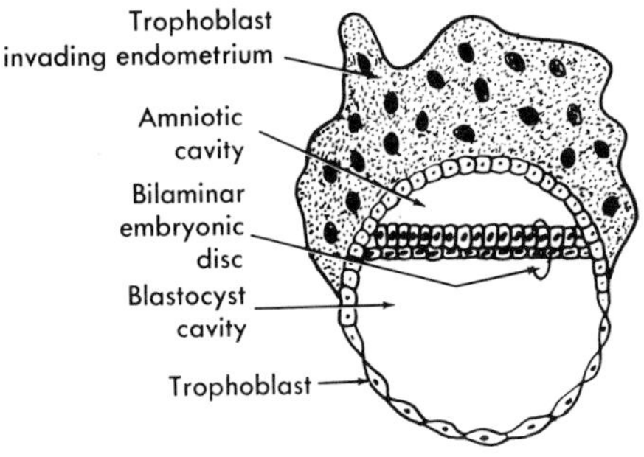 	Implantation deepens and is completed; primitive uteroplacental circulation originates from enlarging trophoblast and maternal endometrial tissues *Amniotic cavity* appears as opening between inner cell mass and invading trophoblast; a thin lining becomes amnion Two-layered (bilaminar) embryo called *embryonic disk* develops, formed by ectoderm and endoderm *Yolk sac* present		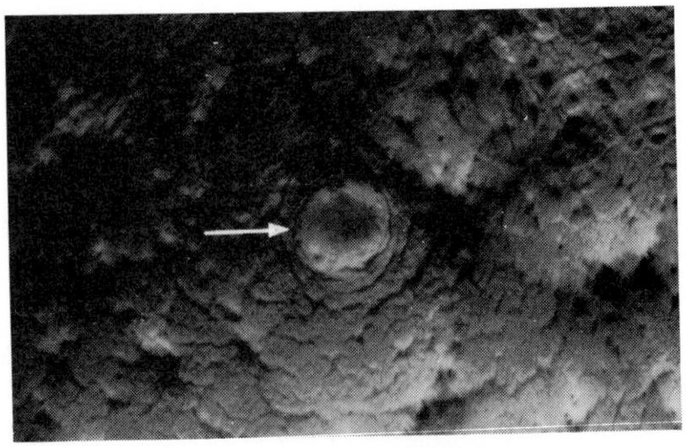 Implantation site of human embryo at about 12 days (*see arrow*) Endometrium covers blastocyst, producing elevation or wartlike bulge on uterine surface
Third week 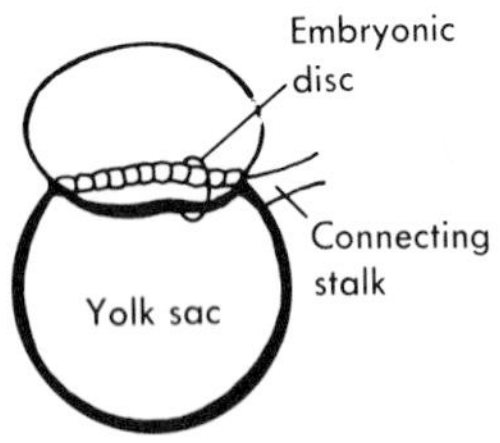 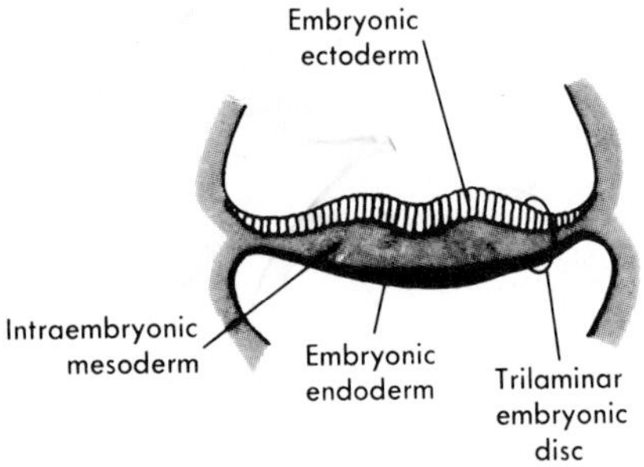 	Thickening in midline of ectoderm gives rise to *mesoderm,* a third layer between ectoderm and endoderm forming trilaminar embryo; basic embryological beginnings of body systems and organs Three basic embryonic layers: 1. *Endoderm:* forerunner of lining of gastrointestinal tract from pharynx to rectum; epithelial parts of trachea, bronchi, lungs, liver, pancreas, and urinary bladder 2. *Ectoderm:* forerunner of mucous membrane, tooth enamel, hair, nails, mammary glands, and nervous system 3. *Mesoderm:* forerunner of heart and blood vessels, spleen, blood and lymph cells, bones, and muscles Neural tube, beginning of central nervous system, forms in midline of cranial portion of ectoderm	2 to 3 mm (1/10 inch)	Amenorrhea Human chorionic gonadotropin (HCG) in urine beginning 10 days after conception, but tests not always sensitive Ultrasonogram may reveal pregnancy as early as 3 to 4 weeks postconception

General Developmental Characteristics (Schematically Pictured)		Average Weight and Size	Possible Maternal Findings and Diagnostic Aids
Fourth week 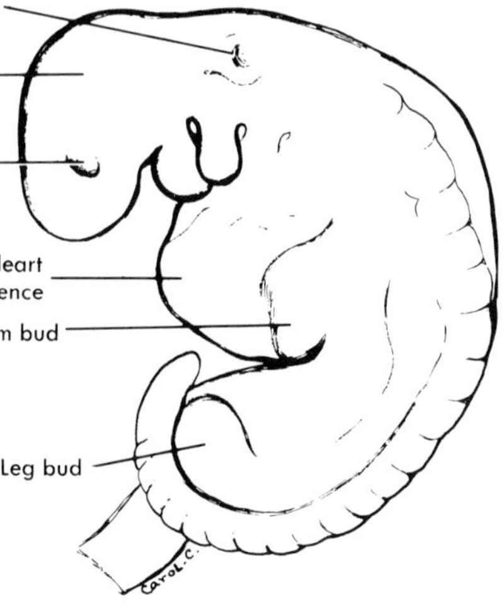	Cells group in mesoderm to form primitive blood vessels and blood cells; heart tube forms and contracts to circulate blood by end of third week; umbilical vessels pass through connecting stalk to placenta Flat, disklike embryo folds to form typical C-shaped cylinder Rapid development of forebrain portion of neural tube Heart prominence seen Arm and leg buds; forerunners of ears and eyes appear Primitive gut formed with incorporation of dorsal yolk sac	5 mm (1/16 in)	Nausea and vomiting Urinary frequency Breast tenderness, tingling, swelling Montgomery's tubercles visible Uterine enlargement Increased cervical secretion
Fifth through seventh weeks 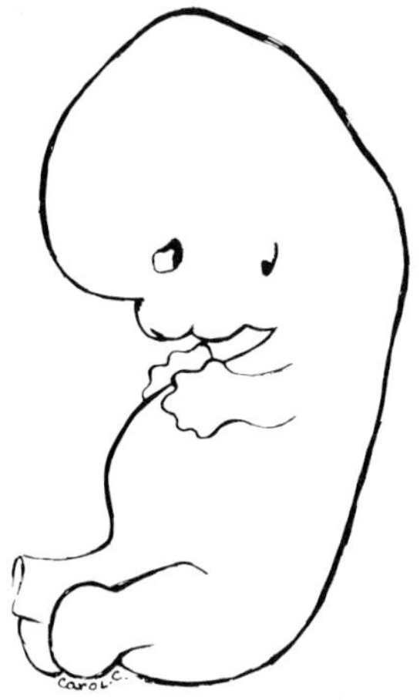 By end end of seventh week all essential systems present	Rudimentary lungs, kidneys Rapid brain development Retina of eye forms Heart becomes chambered Fingers, toes, and eyes are becoming visible Palate and upper lip forming Gastrointestinal tract develops; part of intestine still in umbilical cord Rapid formation of urogenital systems	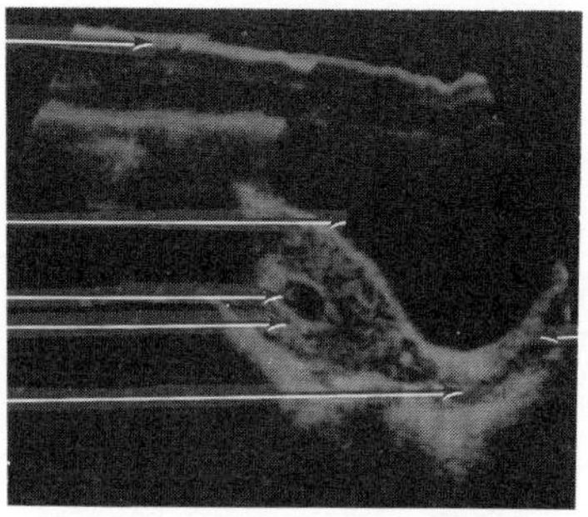	Softening of cervix (Goodell's sign) Softening of uterine isthmus (Hegar's sign) Violet coloration of cervix and vagina (Chadwick's sign)
FETAL STAGE (EIGHTH WEEK TO BIRTH)			
Eighth through tenth weeks 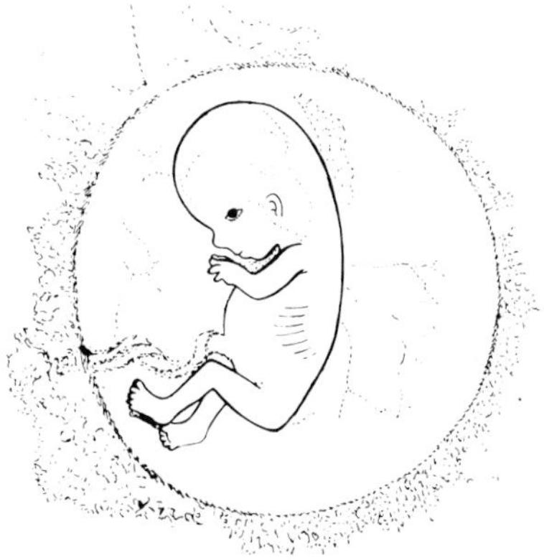	Development mainly involves growth and maturation of structures begun in embryo; fetus less vulnerable to effects of drugs, most infections, and radiation Head almost half fetal length at 8 weeks (illustration shows fetus within amniotic sac)	3 cm (1 1/8 in) 2 g (1/15 oz)	

Continued.

Table 42-1 Prenatal Calendar (Using Fertilization Age)—cont'd

General Developmental Characteristics (Schematically Pictured)		Average Weight and Size	Possible Maternal Findings and Diagnostic Aids
Eleventh through twelfth weeks 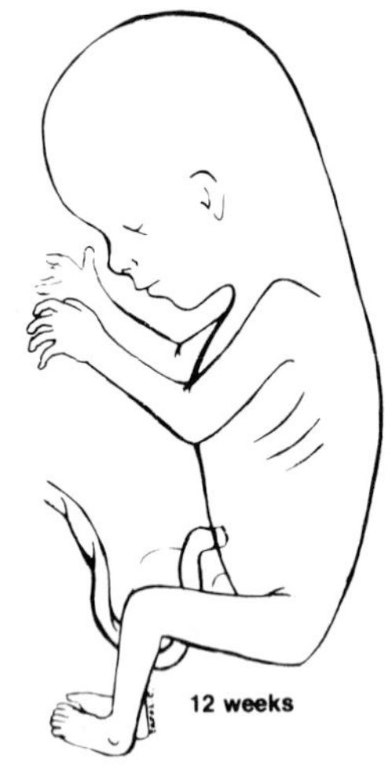 	Facial features forming Eyelids present and fused Intestine retracted from umbilical cord into abdomen Palate fusion complete External sex identification possible Well-defined neck Nail beds beginning Tooth buds forming	Crown-heel length: 11.5 cm (4½ in), 20g (⅔ oz)	Frequent urination and nausea have usually disappeared Fetal heart tone may be detected with Doppler techniques 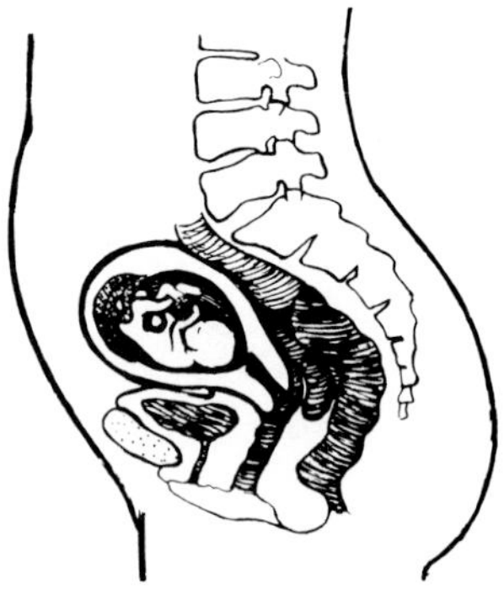 Fundus of uterus rises above pubic bone between 12 and 16 weeks
Thirteenth through sixteenth weeks 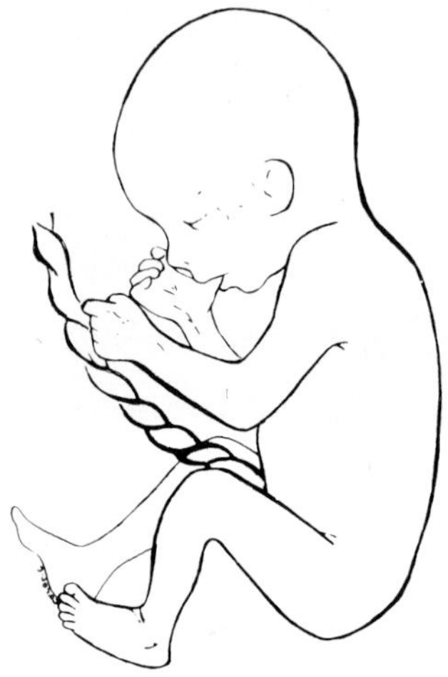	Rapid growth of limbs and trunk; head less prominent Active fetus Skeleton calcified on x-ray examination by sixteenth week Increasing respiratory movement detected by sonogram Approximately 150 to 280 ml amniotic fluid present Placenta distinct	19 cm (7½ in) 100 g (3⅓ oz)	Start of maternity clothing(?) Amniocentesis between fourteenth and sixteenth weeks Quickening felt at 16 weeks(?) 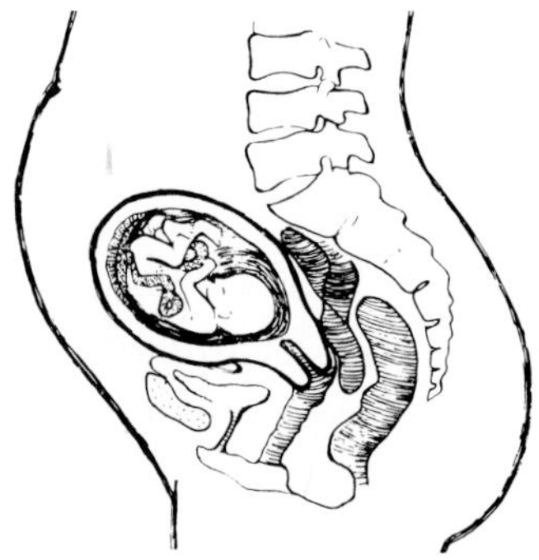 Fundus half distance between pubis and umbilicus at 16 weeks(?)

Table 42-1 Prenatal Calendar (Using Fertilization Age)—cont'd

General Developmental Characteristics (Schematically Pictured)		Average Weight and Size	Possible Maternal Findings and Diagnostic Aids
			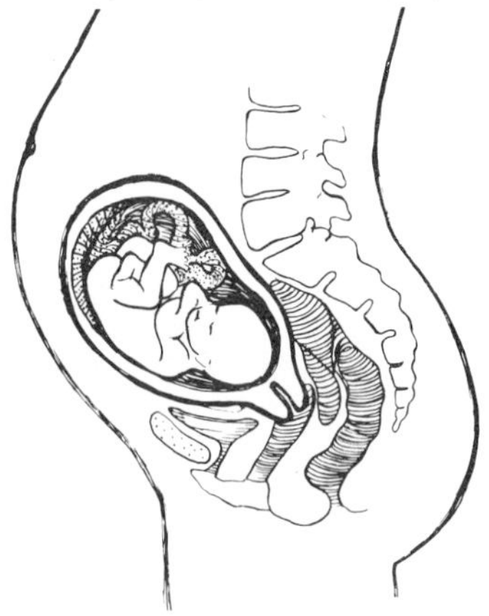
Seventeenth through twentieth weeks 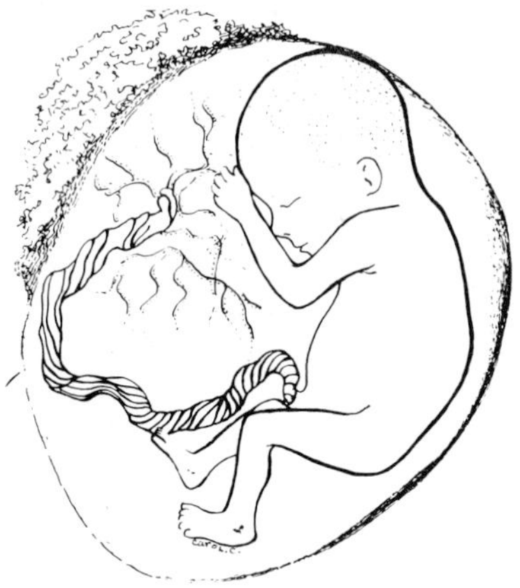	Eyebrows, lanugo, and vernix appear Nipples barely visible (illustration shows placental relationship) Scalp hair visible Fetus able to hear sounds within mother and in external world	22 cm (8¾ in) 300 g (10 oz)	Quickening at 16 to 18 weeks Fetal heart tone detected by standard fetoscope (18 to 20 weeks) Secondary areola prominent Fundus at umbilicus or slightly above
Twenty-fourth week Only rare survivals 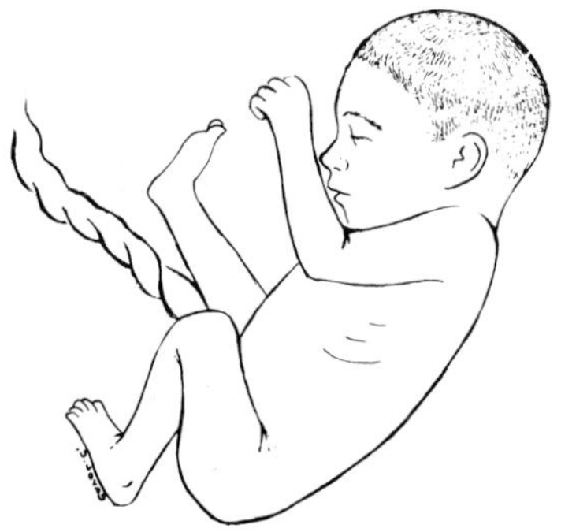	External ear soft, flat, shapeless Skin wrinkled, translucent, appears pink; blood in capillaries shows Lanugo covers body	32 cm (12½ in) 600 g (1¼ lb)	Chloasma (mask of pregnancy) Striae may develop 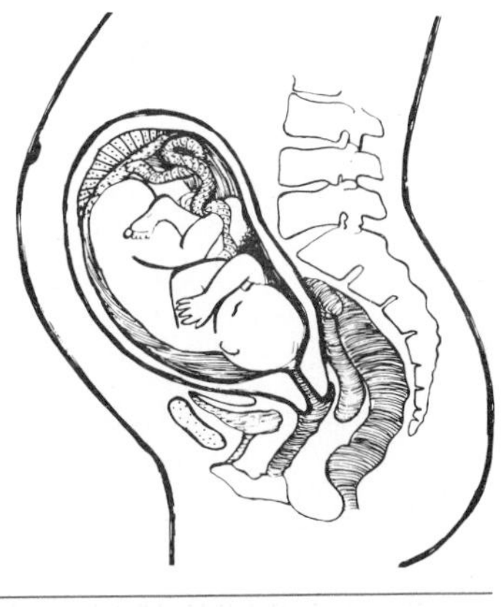

Continued.

Table 42-1 Prenatal Calendar (Using Fertilization Age)—cont'd

General Developmental Characteristics (Schematically Pictured)		Average Weight and Size	Possible Maternal Findings and Diagnostic Aids
Twenty-eighth week 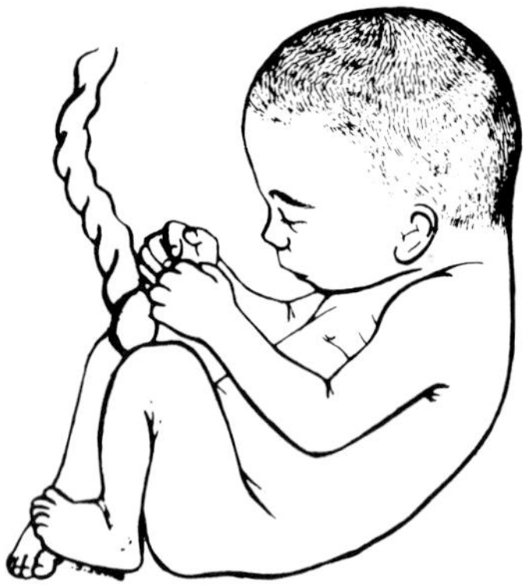	Subcutaneous fat appears, fingernails and toenails Testes at internal inguinal ring or below Eyes open Scalp hair well developed	36 cm (14 in) 1100 g (2¼ lb)	
Thirty-second week 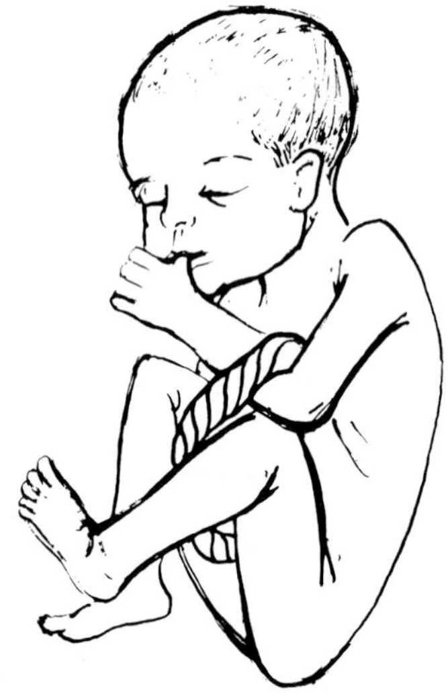	Hair fine and wooly Nails to fingertips Prominent clitoris; labia majora small and separated Skin pink and smooth 1 or 2 creases on anterior portion of soles Breast areolae visible but flat	41 cm (16 in) 1800 g (3¾ lb)	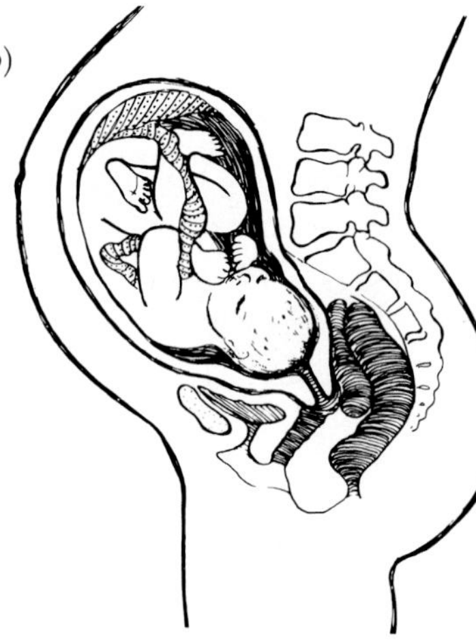

Table 42-1 Prenatal Calendar (Using Fertilization Age)—cont'd

General Developmental Characteristics (Schematically Pictured)		Average Weight and Size	Possible Maternal Findings and Diagnostic Aids
Thirty-sixth week 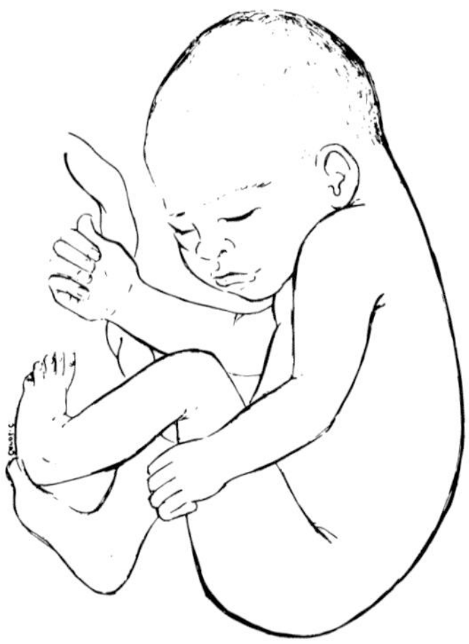	Body, limbs more rounded Skin thicker, whiter, lanugo disappearing Breast tissue develops under nipples Scrotal rugae few Testes in inguinal canal Sole creases involve anterior two thirds of sole	46 cm (18 in) 2200 g (4½ lb)	Dyspnea resulting from pressure on diaphragm Lightening in primigravidas about 38 weeks Urinary frequency returns Increasing prominence of Braxton Hicks contractions Milk may appear in breasts In primigravida, characteristic effacement may be noted by pelvic examination
FULL TERM			
Thirty-eighth through forty-second week 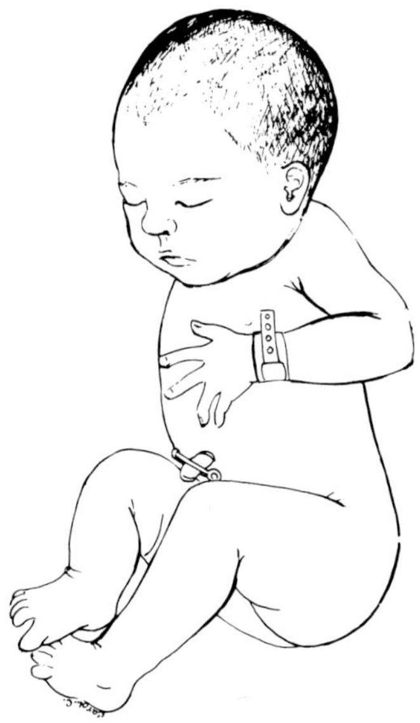	Skin whitish pink Lanugo gone from face Hair in single strands Vernix decreasing Areola 5 to 6 mm with 7 to 10 mm breast tissue Ear well defined by outer incurving to lobe, erect from head Testes in scrotum Labia majora meet in midline; cover labia minora and clitoris	51 cm (20 in) 3200+ g (6.6+ lb)	At term 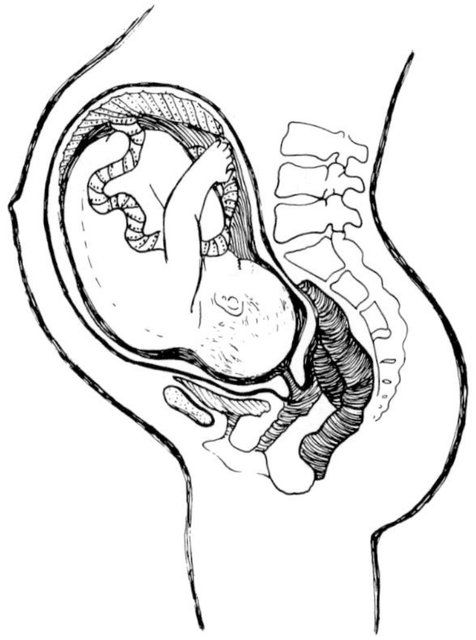

The Fetal Membranes

The amniotic sac is composed of two layers, both originating in the zygote. The outer layer, the chorion, attaches to the fetal portion of the placenta. The inner layer, the amnion, blends with the fetal umbilical cord. These membranes appear to be very fragile, but in fact are strong enough to contain the fetus and amniotic fluid even at full term.

The Umbilical Cord

The umbilical cord joins the embryo to the placenta. It originates in the fetal portion of the placenta and is normally attached near the center. The cord is normally 50 to 55 cm (20 to 22 inches) long and approximately 2 cm (less than 1 inch) in diameter at the time of delivery. Umbilical cords can vary widely in appearance. The major part of the cord is a pale white, gelatinous-mucoid substance called *Wharton's jelly.* This substance prevents compression of the blood vessels. Normally two arteries and one vein are apparent and may give a ropelike appearance to the cord. The vein carries oxygenated blood to the fetus; the arteries carry deoxygenated blood back to the placenta. The cord has no pain receptors, so cutting at the time of delivery does not cause pain.

Amniotic Fluid

Amniotic fluid acts as a cushion against mechanical injury, helps to regulate fetal temperature, and allows the developing embryo/fetus room for growth. The amount of fluid changes from about 30 ml (1 ounce) at 10 weeks

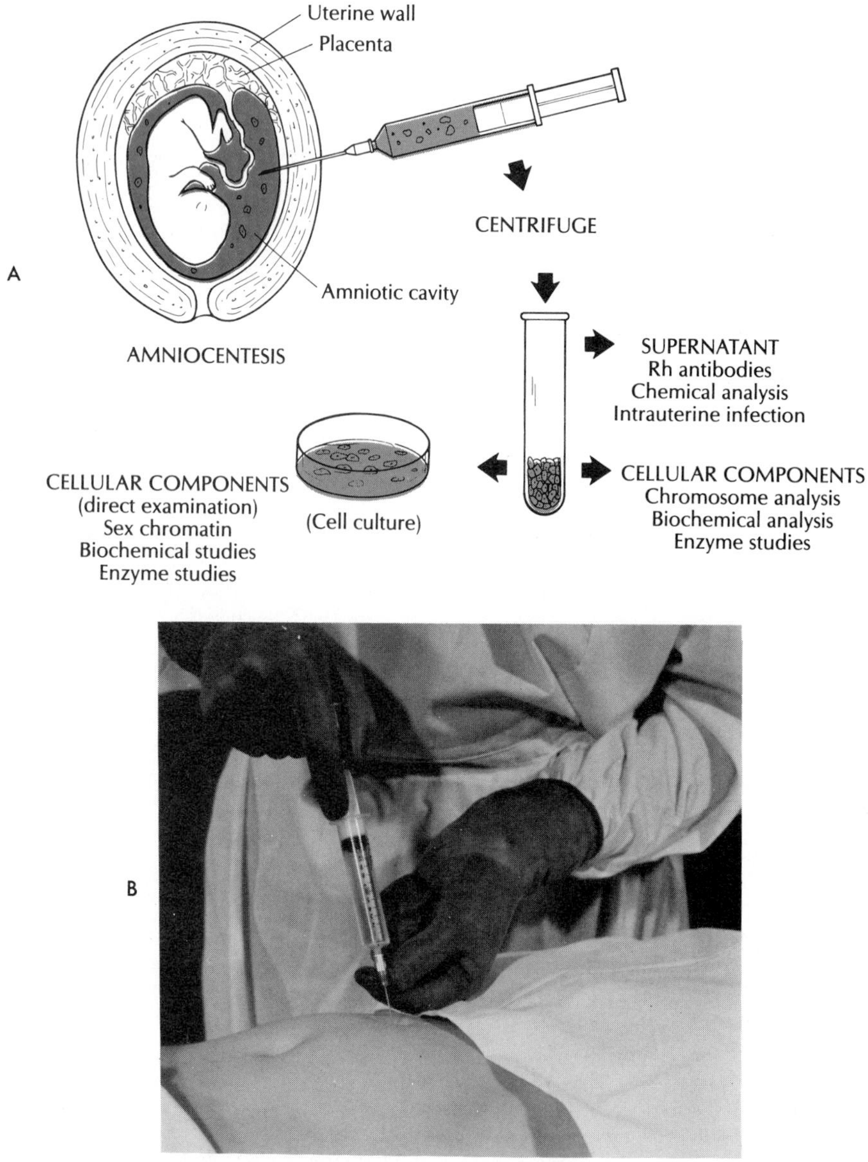

FIG. 42-1 **A,** Amniocentesis and laboratory use of amniotic fluid aspirant. **B,** Transabdominal amniocentesis, (**B,** Courtesy of March of Dimes.)

to as much as 1 L at delivery. This slightly alkaline fluid is changing continuously. Amniotic fluid contains albumin, urea, uric acid, creatinine, bilirubin, lecithin (phospholipids for fat metabolism), sphingomyelin (a compound consisting of lipids and sphingosine, found in high concentrations in the brain and other tissues of the nervous system), fructose, fat, leukocytes, proteins, epithelial cells, enzymes, and **lanugo** hair.

Amniocentesis can be done in the later stages of pregnancy. This procedure involves removal of amniotic fluid by passing a needle through the abdominal wall (Fig. 42-1). Examination of the fluid can reveal information on the development, maturity, health, and sex of the fetus. Amniocentesis is not without risks and is performed only to obtain necessary medical information.

MATERNAL PHYSIOLOGY

Hormonal changes

Estrogen and progesterone levels remain elevated for the first 8 to 10 weeks of pregnancy as a result of human chorionic gonadotropin, which supports the corpus luteum. After this time the placenta takes over production and maintains necessary levels. As long as these levels are high, FSH, LH, and ovulation are suppressed, as is menstruation.

Uterus

The uterus enlarges during pregnancy as a result of hormonal stimulus, increased vascularity, hyperplasia (new muscle fiber and tissue), and hypertrophy (enlargement of existing fiber and tissue). The nonpregnant uterus is pear shaped and weighs approximately 50 g (2 ounces). By the third trimester it is egg shaped and has increased in weight to 1000 g (2.2 pounds). At term it is capable of holding a fetus, placenta, and amniotic fluid totaling more than 4000 g (8.5 pounds).

The consistency of the tissue changes also. Changes in the cervix and fundus, along with an altered position in the pelvis, are early signs of pregnancy.

The uterus, which in a nonpregnant state is a pelvic organ, will rise to the base of the ribcage. The superior aspect of the uterus (the fundus) will be located at the level of the xiphoid process when the pregnancy reaches completion.

ANTEPARTAL ASSESSMENT

General Physical Assessment

When a woman suspects she is pregnant and visits the physician's office or clinic, assessment should begin. Ideally the woman has been receiving regular medical attention and is already known by the physician. Unfortunately, because of cost or frequent changes of residence, many people do not receive regular, routine health care. Many women also seek the attention of a specialist, an obstetrician, during pregnancy. This necessitates establishing a new doctor-patient relationship and a total review of the health history.

On the first visit demographic (study of the human population) data such as age, occupation, marital status, and insurance information are obtained. This basic information helps the physician and nurse identify potential areas of concern. For example, an adolescent woman who is 15, single, unemployed, a high school dropout, with no insurance presents a very different set of concerns from those of a 25-year-old, married, college graduate with comprehensive insurance.

A basic family and personal medical history is obtained. To anticipate any problems, the physician must be aware of any genetic diseases present in either the mother's or father's families. A family history that includes genetic diseases may increase the concerns of a pregnant woman until she is assured that her baby is normal. If serious genetic problems are known, many couples seek genetic counseling before they consider having children.

A personal medical history is taken and a review of systems is done. Information about such chronic diseases as cardiac problems, hypertension, diabetes mellitus, and infectious diseases (e.g., rubella, AIDS and other sexually transmitted diseases) is obtained, as any history of accidents or previous surgeries is documented. Significant findings in these areas may indicate the potential for problems and the need for early medical and nursing intervention. High-risk pregnancies involving these conditions will be discussed in Chapter 45.

Life-style patterns including recreational activities, nutrition, and eating habits, use of prescription medication or street drugs, alcohol, work exposure to hazardous conditions, and smoking are assessed. Early detection of problem situations and correction of these can reduce hazards to the woman and prevent detrimental effects on the growth and development of the fetus.

A basic physical examination, including measurement of height and weight and vital signs, assessment of heart, lungs, and reflexes, and a general physical inspection of skin and mobility, is normally done. Basic blood work includes (1) hemoglobin and hematocrit assessment, (2) serology tests for detection of infectious diseases such as syphilis, and possibly for AIDS and hepatitis, (3) blood typing and Rh factor determination, and (4) rubella titer. Routine urinalysis is done to test for glucose, protein, and ketones. Pregnancy tests may be ordered if the pregnancy has not already been confirmed. All of these tests increase the data available and enable the physician and nurse to plan comprehensive care.

Obstetrical Assessment

In addition to the general health history and physical examination, information about the woman's gynecological, menstrual, and obstetrical history is obtained. This includes the use of contraceptives and the regularity of the menstrual period, including frequency, duration, amount of flow, presence of pain, and any other significant comments. Any history of gynecological surgery, vaginal discharge, or herpes infection is reviewed. The physician may ask questions also regarding exposure to DES (diethylstilbestrol), since daughters of women who took DES during pregnancy have an increased risk of spontaneous abortion caused by incompetent cervix.

The woman's number of pregnancies and their outcomes are discussed. This includes the course of the pregnancy with special attention to any complications, the type of delivery (vaginal or cesarean), the presence of any complications during delivery, the use of forceps or other medical assistance, the type of anesthetic used, the condition of the newborn, and any complications of the postpartum period.

Gynecological Examination

The gynecological examination normally includes palpation and auscultation of the abdomen, visualization of the cervix and vagina, evaluation of the bony pelvis, palpation of the uterus externally or bimanually, depending on the situation, and an examination of the vulva, perineum, anus, and rectum. If a Papanicolaou, or Pap, smear is needed, this may be obtained at the beginning of the examination. The nurse is often called on to prepare the necessary equipment and assist in this examination. The nurse should also provide explanations and emotional support to the patient.

DETERMINATION OF PREGNANCY

Many times it is a suspicion of pregnancy that brings a woman to the doctor's office. After the entire history and physical examination have been done, the physician can determine with varying degrees of certainty that this is in fact true.

Presumptive Signs

The presumptive signs below are indicators that a woman may be pregnant, but these signs may also be indicators of other conditions not related to pregnancy. Box 42-1 summarizes the signs of pregnancy.

1. Amenorrhea: Absence of menstruation is frequently an early sign of pregnancy but can also be seen with other hormonal conditions, changes in environment, malnutrition, fatigue or stress, and in menopause.
2. Nausea and vomiting: The number of potential causes for nausea and vomiting is limitless and in and of itself is not indicative of pregnancy.
3. Frequent urination: As the uterus enlarges it is common for a woman to experience urinary frequency. However, many other conditions ranging from diabetes mellitus and cystitis to emotional stress can cause urinary frequency.
4. Breast changes: Swelling, tingling, and tenderness of the breasts are common during pregnancy, along with changes in pigmentation of the areola. Many women experience similar changes during the normal menstrual cycle.
5. Change in the shape of the abdomen: Abdominal enlargement is typically seen in the second trimester of pregnancy but can also be caused by tumors or organomegaly (enlargement of any organ).
6. Quickening: The subjective sensation of fetal movement first occurs at about 16 to 18 weeks' gestation. At times intestinal peristalsis or gas can be mistaken for fetal movement.
7. Skin changes: Pigment changes, such as darkening of some areas of the body such as the areola, may occur, possibly indicating pregnancy. These changes can also be caused by endocrine disturbances. During the pelvic examination the physician may note that the vagina, cervix, and sometimes the vulva will have a violet or purplish discoloration, which appears at about 6 to 10 weeks' gestation. This is called *Chadwick's sign*. In addition to pregnancy, this sign can be caused by any condition that causes pelvic congestion.

Probable Signs

The probable signs below indicate a high likelihood that the woman is pregnant. These signs are not, however, 100% reliable indicators. Box 42-1 summarizes the signs of pregnancy.

1. Changes in the reproductive organs: Enlargement of the uterus indicates a high probability of pregnancy, particularly if accompanied by changes in the consistency of the isthmus of the uterus (the segment between the fundus and the cervix). A softening of this segment is called *Hegar's sign* (Fig. 42-2). This change, and a softening or increased pliability of the cervix called *Goodell's sign*, are most commonly seen in pregnancy. Ballottement, which may be used at approximately 16 to 18 weeks' gestation, is a technique that involves palpating the uterus in such a way that the rebound of the floating fetus is felt by the examiner's finger (Fig. 42-3).
2. Positive pregnancy tests: Tests are administered using either blood or urine and function by measuring the level of HCG. Many of these tests are now available over the counter in drugstores; however, the reliability of these products is only as good as the technique used in collecting the urine specimen

and performing the test. Tests administered by the physician are generally between 95% and 99% accurate. Over-the-counter tests tend to yield either false positive readings, in which the woman is not pregnant but the test indicates she is, or false negative readings, in which the test indicates the woman is not pregnant when in fact she is. The greatest advantages of pregnancy tests are that they can be administered early in pregnancy and are reasonably inexpensive. If the test results are positive and other indicators such as uterine changes are abnormal, the physician may suspect complications such as an **ectopic** (outside the uterus) pregnancy or hydatidiform mole (abnormal growth of a fertilized ovum in which a large vascular mass, but no fetus, develops). Hydatidiform mole frequently results in a highly reactive pregnancy test, and the test may continue to indicate positive results even after surgical removal of the mole.

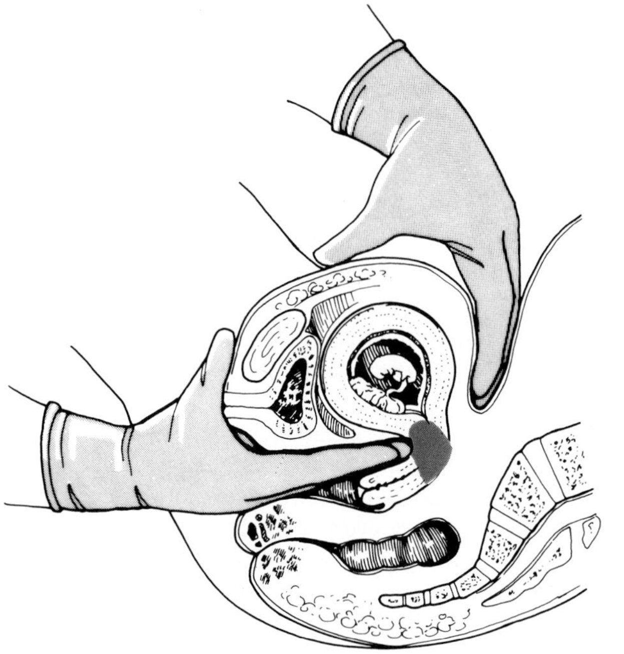

FIG. 42-2 Hegar's sign. Bimanual examination for assessing softening of isthmus while the cervix is still firm.

Positive Signs

Positive signs are those that occur only with pregnancy and are not present at any other time. Box 42-1 summarizes the signs of pregnancy.

1. Visualization: The fetal skeleton seen on x-ray examination is a positive sign of pregnancy, but use of radiation is generally limited during pregnancy because of possible danger to the fetus. Ultrasonic tracing of the fetus is also a positive indication of pregnancy.
2. Fetal movement: Fetal movement may be detected by a trained observer such as a physician or midwife.
3. Auscultation of fetal heart beat: At 10 to 12 weeks' gestation a Doppler or ultrasonic transmitter can be used to detect the fetal heart tone. After 18 weeks, traditional equipment such as a fetoscope can be used to ausculate the fetal heart rate.

BOX 42-1 SIGNS OF PREGNANCY

PRESUMPTIVE	PROBABLE	POSITIVE
Amenorrhea	Changes in the reproductive organs:	Radiographic visualization
Nausea and vomiting	Hegar's sign	Fetal motion detected by trained observer
Urinary frequency	Goodell's sign	Auscultation of fetal heart sounds
Breast changes	Ballottement	
Abdominal changes	Positive pregnancy tests	
Quickening		
Skin changes: Chadwick's sign		

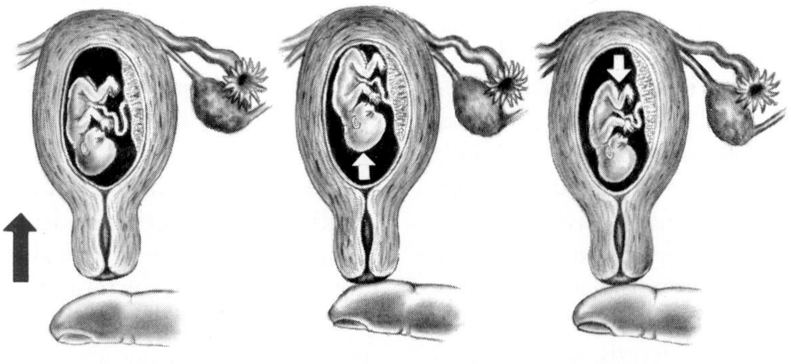

FIG. 42-3 Internal ballottement (18 weeks).

Determination of the Estimated Date of Confinement

Normal human pregnancy, counting from the first day of the last menstrual period, is about 280 days, 40 weeks, 10 lunar months (28 days each), or slightly more than 9 calendar months.

The estimated date of confinement (EDC), often known as the "due date," involves calculations based on the woman's menstrual cycle. The most common method is called *Nagele's rule.* Using this rule one would start with the *first day* of the woman's last menstrual period and add seven days, then count back 3 months. For example, if the first day of the last menstrual period was June 14, counting back three months to March 14 then adding 7 days would yield an EDC of March 21. Studies reveal that only a small percentage of infants are actually born on the date predicted; most deliveries, however, do occur within 1 to 10 days before or after the EDC.

If the woman does not keep a menstrual record, calculation of the EDC may be more difficult. The physician must then rely on observations such as quickening, estimation of fetal size by palpation, or ultrasonic tests, all of which can be unreliable. If it is imperative that the physician know the level of fetal maturity, specialized tests can be performed later in the pregnancy.

Obstetrical Terminology

Specific terms are used in obstetrics to describe the number of times a woman has been pregnant and has given birth. **Gravida** (fr. Latin root *gravidus*, "heavy") indicates a pregnant woman. To this term Latin numerical prefixes are added to indicate number of pregnancies, such as *primigravida* (one), **nulligravida** (none), and **multigravida** (multiple). Similarly, prefixes to the Latin root **-para** (to bring forth) denote the number of births, such as *primipara*, **nullipara, multipara.** A shorthand method of keeping track of a patient's obstetrical history is used in many facilities; for example, to record the gravida/para, "1/0" indicates the first pregnancy with no viable births.

A more detailed five-part description is sometimes used. The first digit represents the total number of pregnancies, including the present one; the second digit indicates the number of term deliveries; the third indicates the number of premature deliveries; and the fourth indicates the number of abortions. *Abortion* is a medical term indicating loss of a fetus before the age of viability; "miscarriage" is often the term used in everyday speech. The fifth indicates the number of children living. This is sometimes confusing, because it does not indicate how a child may have died. It also does not include the outcome of an ongoing pregnancy, because this cannot be known until after delivery. In other words, if all children died in an auto accident, the last number would be 0, even if all of the pregnancies and deliveries were normal. For example, a descriptive number such as 5-3-2-0-4 indicates that a woman has been pregnant 5 times, delivered 3 full-term infants, and 2 preterm infants, has had no abortions, and has 4 living children.

ANTEPARTAL CARE

Health Perception/Health Management

Most pregnant women want to learn more about pregnancy, childbirth, and motherhood (provided no serious problems in the area of role relationship, coping, or self-perception are occurring). Pregnancy is one time in life when most women see the importance of regular medical supervision and are more willing to make changes in their habits than any other time. It seems that most women are willing to think of their baby first and to do everything that is best for the infant.

Pregnancy is an excellent time to establish good general health practices if these have been lacking. Many women do not have regular physical examinations or Pap smears or do home screening tests such as self-breast examinations until they become pregnant. The high motivation level makes this a good time for the nurse to teach patients about health maintenance practices. (See Chapters 36 and 41 for a discussion of self-breast examination.)

Early in pregnancy the woman often begins to seek information and make choices regarding how and where she wishes to give birth. The nurse can help provide information regarding the options available in a particular community. These options are discussed further in Chapter 43.

Routine care during pregnancy begins with the initial examination and history, as previously described. Appointments are recommended once a month through the seventh month, once every 2 weeks for the next month, and then once every week until delivery. If any problems occur or the physician suspects anything unusual, such as a multiple pregnancy, the schedule of visits may be altered. Dental care should continue during pregnancy. Any major dental work, such as oral surgery or extractions, is usually delayed until after delivery.

Smoking during pregnancy can be dangerous to the developing fetus. Oxygen deprivation can lead to decreased intrauterine growth and low birth weight.

Drinking alcoholic beverages during pregnancy is also contraindicated, particularly during the first trimester. Fetal alcohol syndrome will be discussed in Chapter 45.

Taking any medication or drugs during pregnancy, including over-the-counter drugs, should be avoided. As mentioned, most drugs are able to cross the placenta and are transmitted to the fetus. Only medications prescribed by the physician should be taken. Street drugs such as marijuana and cocaine are very dangerous to both mother and fetus and must be avoided.

Today many women continue to work throughout

BOX 42-2 DANGER SIGNS DURING PREGNANCY

Visual disturbances—diplopia, blurring, or spots

Headaches—severe, sudden, or continuous

Edema—swelling of the face, presacral area, or fingers

Rapid weight gain—in excess of normal gain for gestation

Pain—severe abdominal or epigastric pain

Signs of infection—fever, chills, diarrhea, changes in vaginal drainage, pain or burning with urination

Vaginal bleeding—no matter how slight

Vaginal drainage—anything other than normal mucus

Persistent vomiting

Muscular irritability or convulsions

Absence or decrease in fetal movement once felt

pregnancy. It is important that the work environment be checked for chemicals and other hazards.

Danger Signs During Pregnancy

While there are many changes and normal discomforts during pregnancy, certain signals indicate the need for immediate medical attention. These danger signs are listed in Box 42-2. The pregnant woman should be taught these danger signs. The nurse must stress the importance of contacting the physician promptly if any of these signs are present.

Nutritional/Metabolic Health Pattern

Weight gain. Nutritional needs change substantially during pregnancy, since the mother must meet not only her own nutritional needs but also those of the developing fetus. This does not mean that the woman must "eat for two" by doubling her food intake; this will only lead to extra body weight, which adds to discomfort and increases the stress on all body systems. Weight gain is no longer tightly controlled, but most physicians recommend weight gain in the 21- to 35-pound range as most desirable. Only 2 to 4 pounds should be gained during the entire first trimester; a gain of about 1 pound per week for the remainder of the pregnancy is normal. Inadequate weight gain or sudden excessive weight gain may indicate problems with nutrition or complications.

Nutritional requirements

Caloric intake. Pregnancy places additional demands on the mother's metabolism. To meet her needs and those of the fetus, caloric needs increase about 300 calories per day on average—slightly less early in pregnancy, slightly more later in pregnancy. The woman's activity level must also be taken into account when determining desirable caloric intake. If problems are encountered in determining caloric needs, a dietician should be consulted.

The pregnancy diet is a modification of a normal diet based on the four food groups, with increases in those nutrients needed for fetal development. Protein, which supplies amino acids for tissue and blood production, is very important. Milk, which is rich in calcium, is an important nutrient for pregnant women. Fats are important as an energy source and carbohydrates are needed to meet total caloric needs. Inadequate carbohydrate intake can lead to abnormal metabolism of protein, decreasing the amount available for growth. (See Chapter 22.) Dietary recommendations are summarized in Tables 42-2 and 42-3.

Minerals and vitamins. Calcium and phosphorus are necessary for bone and tooth mineralization in the fetus. They also affect the acid-base balance of the body. Iron is essential to prevent anemia, which would decrease the oxygen-carrying ability of the blood. Oxygen transport is very important during pregnancy, because the mother must not only meet her own needs but also meet the needs of the developing fetus. A normal hematocrit level in nonpregnant women is 38% to 47%. During pregnancy this may drop as low as 34% as a result of a condition called *physiological anemia of pregnancy*. The total red blood cell volume normally increases during pregnancy; however, there is an even greater increase in plasma volume. This results in a decreased hematocrit level, even if nutrition and iron intake are adequate. If iron intake is inadequate, serious anemia may result. Vitamin intake should follow the recommended daily allowance for both water- and fat-soluble forms. Some that are of particular importance are vitamins C and D and folic acid. Vitamin C requirements are increased in pregnancy to aid in tissue formation; vitamin D is necessary for absorption and utilization of calcium. Folic acid is necessary for fetal growth and prevention of anemia. Vitamin and mineral supplements are frequently prescribed by the physician and should be taken as directed.

Pica. Pica is the craving and eating of substances that are not normally considered edible. The reason for this condition is not known, but it is more common in certain cultural groups and regions of the country. It may be seen in children and occasionally during pregnancy. Substances such as clay or laundry starch are commonly ingested. Although not toxic, both of these may interfere with iron absorption, resulting in anemia. Large amounts of clay may also result in fecal impaction.

Common discomforts. Many pregnant women experience some discomforts of the GI tract during pregnancy. Excessive salivation (ptyalism) is mentioned by some women; it is thought that this occurs in response to the high levels of estrogen during pregnancy. While it may be uncomfortable and awkward at times, it causes no

Table 42-2 Daily Food Plan for Pregnancy and Lactation

Food	Nonpregnant Woman	Pregnant Woman	Lactating Woman
Milk, cheese, ice cream, skimmed milk or buttermilk (food made with milk can supply part of requirement)	2 C	3-4 C	4-5 C
Meat (lean meat, fish, poultry, cheese, occasional dried beans or peas)	1 serving (3-4 oz)	2 servings (6-8 oz); include liver frequently	2½ servings (8 oz)
Eggs	1	1-2	1-2
Vegetable* (dark green or deep yellow)	1 serving	1 serving	1-2 servings
Vitamin C–rich food* Good source—citrus fruit, berries, cantaloupe Fair source—tomatoes, cabbage, greens, potatoes in skin	1 good source or 2 fair sources	1 good source and 1 fair source or 2 good sources	1 good source and 1 fair source or 2 good sources
Other vegetables and fruits	2 servings	4-6 servings	4-6 servings
Bread† and cereals (enriched or whole grain)	4 servings	4 servings	4 servings
Butter or fortified margarine	Moderate amount	Moderate amount	Moderate amount

*Use some raw daily.
†One slice of bread equals 1 serving.

Table 42-3 Sample Menus

	Nonpregnant Woman	Pregnant Woman	Lactating Woman
Breakfast	120 ml (4 oz) orange juice ½ C oatmeal 240 ml (8 oz) milk Coffee or tea*	120 ml (4 oz) orange juice ½ C oatmeal 240 ml (8 oz) milk Coffee or tea*	120 ml (4 oz) orange juice ½ C oatmeal 240 ml (8 oz) milk Coffee or tea*
Morning snack		Fruit and/or cheese†	Fruit and/or cheese†
Lunch	1 tuna fish sandwich made with: 2 slices whole wheat bread ½ C tuna fish Diced celery and onion to taste, mayonnaise,* lettuce* 1 medium apple 240 ml (8 oz) milk	1 tuna fish sandwich made with: 2 slices whole wheat bread ½ C tuna fish, 1 hard-boiled egg Diced celery and onion to taste,* mayonnaise,* lettuce* 1 medium apple 240 ml (8 oz) milk	1 tuna fish sandwich made with: 2 slices whole wheat bread ½ C tuna fish 1 hard-boiled egg Diced celery and onion to taste, mayonnaise,* lettuce* 1 medium apple 240 ml (8 oz) milk
Afternoon snack		½ C salted peanuts 120 ml (4 oz) milk	½ C salted peanuts 240 ml (8 oz) milk
Dinner	3 oz roast beef ½ C egg noodles* with sautéed poppy seeds* ¾ C cut asparagus Salad made with: 1 C torn spinach Sliced mushrooms and radishes to taste* Oil and vinegar* Coffee or tea	6 oz roast beef ½ C egg noodles* with sautéed poppy seeds,* 1 pat butter ¾ C cut asparagus Salad made with: 1 C torn spinach Sliced mushrooms and radishes to taste,* tomato Oil and vinegar* 240 ml (8 oz) milk Coffee or tea	6-9 oz roast beef ½ C egg noodles* with sautéed poppy seeds,* 1 pat butter ¾ C cut asparagus Salad made with: 1 C torn spinach Sliced mushrooms and radishes to taste,* tomato Oil and vinegar* 240 ml (8 oz) milk Coffee or tea
Evening snack		1-2 oatmeal raisin cookies* 120 ml (4 oz) milk	2 oatmeal raisin cookies* 240 ml (8 oz) milk

Adapted from Nutrition during pregnancy and lactation, Sacramento, 1975, Maternal and Child Health Branch, California Department of Health Services.
*This food is optional and is added to the basic diet.
†Serving size determined by caloric or dietary need.

serious problems and disappears either later in pregnancy or after delivery. Use of astringent mouthwash or chewing gum or sucking on hard candy may provide some relief.

Nausea in the early stages of pregnancy is a common complaint. This most typically occurs when the woman awakens in the morning; hence the name "morning sickness." It can, however, occur at any time of the day. This is thought to be caused by increased HCG levels and changes in carbohydrate metabolism. If the nausea is mild, it can usually be controlled by slowly eating a few soda crackers or dry toast before rising from bed. Smaller, more frequent meals are also suggested. Avoidance of spicy or greasy food helps in some cases. Morning sickness rarely lasts beyond the fourth month. If it lasts longer, is more severe, and particularly if it involves vomiting, the physician should be contacted. The most severe form is called *hyperemesis gravidarum*. The cause of this is not clear, but untreated, it can lead to dehydration, fluid and electrolyte imbalance, acid-base imbalance, and altered kidney and cardiac function. Fetal death may also result. Hospitalization with close medical supervision, including administration of IV feeding, may be required.

Heartburn from gastric reflux into the esophagus can be caused by the increasing size of the fetus in the abdominal cavity, which displaces the stomach. Increased progesterone level, which causes relaxation of the cardiac sphincter, and decreased gastric mobility, which delays the emptying time of the stomach, can also contribute to the problem. Smaller meals taken more often, decreased fat intake, low-sodium antacids, and avoiding lying down after meals often give relief.

Skin changes. Changes in pigmentation are often seen during pregnancy as a result of increased amounts of melanocyte-stimulating hormone. The changes occur primarily in areas that already have greater pigmentation, such as the areolas, nipples, vulva, perianal area, and linea alba (midline of the abdomen from pubis to umbilicus), which darkens and is called the *linea nigra*.

Chloasma, the mask of pregnancy, is an irregular darkening of the pigment of the cheeks, forehead, and nose. These changes are frequently more obvious in women with darker hair and skin and may be worsened by sun exposure. This generally disappears or fades significantly soon after delivery.

Striae gravidarum, or stretch marks, are reddish, wavy streaks that can appear on the thighs, abdomen, and breasts. These are more common with distention but may occur even in relatively thin women. They usually fade after delivery.

Spider nevi and palmar erythema (reddened palms) are sometimes seen. These are caused by increased blood flow resulting from high estrogen levels. Both usually disappear when the pregnancy ends.

Changes in hair growth and consistency, even significant loss of scalp hair, are noted by some women. This is usually temporary unless other physiological problems are active.

Occasionally, decreased emptying of the gallbladder may result in subclinical jaundice, which causes generalized pruritus.

Hygiene practices. Bathing or showering during pregnancy should continue as part of routine hygiene. Increased perspiration is common, and good personal hygiene is important to prevent body odor. Tub bathing may become difficult in the later months of pregnancy because of changes in mobility and balance. Some physicians restrict tub baths in the last month of pregnancy, since the cervix may have begun to dilate. Douching is not recommended, even though the woman may have increased vaginal discharge. If the vaginal drainage causes pruritus or other symptoms, this should be reported to the physician.

It is not essential for a woman to buy special clothing, but whatever garments are chosen should be comfortable and should not restrict movement. It is important to avoid circulation-restricting clothing such as garters. Larger bras may be necessary as breasts enlarge; too snug a bra may interfere with breathing.

Elimination

Gastrointestinal system. Slowing of intestinal peristalsis can result in abdominal distention, flatulence, and constipation. Constipation can also be related to the iron supplements that are being taken.

Hemorrhoids can result from straining as a result of constipation. They can also be caused by the enlarged uterus putting pressure on the pelvic blood vessels, slowing venous return from the lower extremities. Women with a history of cholelithiasis may experience problems with this as a result of an increased cholesterol level, which is common during pregnancy. Adequate fluid intake, dietary roughage, and exercise may help reduce problems related to constipation.

Urinary system. Frequency of urination is a common complaint of pregnancy. During pregnancy the mother must excrete not only her own waste products but also those of the fetus. Urinary output increases during pregnancy and the specific gravity decreases. Early in pregnancy the enlarging uterus irritates the bladder by putting pressure on it. This continues until the uterus rises into the abdominal cavity. Later in pregnancy, when the presenting part descends into the pelvis, the pressure and symptoms return. Kegel's exercises can be taught to help tone the muscles of the perineum and help prevent stress incontinency (see Chapter 36).

Dilation of the ureter and kidneys may occur, particularly on the right side, as a result of placental progesterone and pressure from the enlarging uterus. Restricted circulation in the pelvis as the uterus enlarges increases the risk of bladder trauma and urinary tract infection.

Activity/Exercise

Normal activity should continue throughout an uncomplicated pregnancy. If a woman regularly participates in a fitness program or sport, she probably can continue with most activities. This should be discussed with the physician if there are any doubts. High-risk activities or those that require a great deal of balance and coordination are discouraged. Common sense is the best guide.

Fatigue is a common complaint during pregnancy. The woman must pace herself and not overdo tiring activities.

Change in balance and posture occur as the fetus increases in size. To compensate for the shifting center of gravity, the lumbodorsal curve increases (lordosis). This may result in low backaches. Hormonal influence on pelvic bones, resulting in joint relaxation, can lead to a waddling gait. Footwear with low heels and the use of good body mechanics will help reduce discomfort.

Leg cramps are a common occurrence. These may relate to pressure on the pelvic blood vessels and nerves or altered calcium and phosphorus balance. Dorsiflexion of the foot may help reduce these cramps. Dependent edema and varicose veins can also result from increasing intraabdominal pressure. Many women wear support hose to reduce edema; resting with legs elevated is also helpful.

Round ligament pain or tenderness in the lower abdomen is a result of stretching of the ligaments by the enlarging uterus. There is no way to prevent this, but good body mechanics helps minimize discomforts.

Shortness of breath may be experienced as the uterus enlarges and pushes the diaphragm upward, reducing the size of the chest cavity. Avoiding large meals, which distend the stomach, and maintaining good posture will help reduce this problem. The exercises in Figs. 42-4 and 42-5 are often recommended to help reduce discomfort and to prepare for childbirth.

Rest/Sleep

Early in pregnancy few changes in sleep patterns are experienced. However, as the size of the abdomen increases it may become increasingly difficult for the woman to find a position of comfort, particularly for those women who prefer to sleep in the prone position. The supine position is not recommended as a woman approaches her due date, because this may cause excessive pressure on the aorta and vena cava as a result of the increased size of the uterus. The woman may experience syncope and vertigo. The supine position also may result in decreased circulation for the fetus. A side-lying position is recommended.

Placing pillows under the legs and abdomen will promote good body alignment and rest. Naps at intervals during the day can be helpful, but these are not always possible with busy life-styles.

Sexuality/Reproductive

Breast changes. Breast changes begin early in pregnancy. Many women complain of tingling and a feeling of fullness. Increased sensitivity is also common. Generally the breasts increase in size preparatory to lactation.

Sexual activity. Sexual desire and activity may change during pregnancy. Unless there are complications in the pregnancy or the bag of waters has ruptured, there is no **physiological** reason to limit sexual activity during pregnancy. Many factors will have a strong influence on the frequency and type of sexual activity. Both the woman and her partner may experience fears or concerns related to sexual activity during pregnancy. There are many cultural, religious, and psychological influences, and it is important for the partners to communicate their fears, concerns, and needs to each other. Many women experience a decrease in desire as a result of hormonal changes and the multiple discomforts that may be occurring. Change in body shape and body image may also cause concern. Discussion of various coital positions and sexual activity that does not include intercourse is appropriate. The physician or nurse may promote this discussion by introducing the topic during routine prenatal care.

Increased vaginal secretions are common during pregnancy. Leukorrhea, an increase in vaginal mucus, results from hormonal changes. If the discharge changes in color or odor, the physician should be informed.

Vaginal bleeding. Vaginal bleeding at any time during pregnancy should be reported to the physician. Sexual activity should cease until the cause of the bleeding is determined and should be resumed only when the physician determines that no danger exists.

Coping/Stress Tolerance

Pregnancy is a developmental landmark. Physiologically it marks the onset of adulthood, no matter what the actual age of the woman. As with other significant developmental changes, anxiety is normal. All of the physical and hormonal changes of pregnancy place additional stress on the woman. Fears are plentiful. Will the labor and delivery be painful? Will the baby be normal? Will she be able to provide proper care? Will there be enough money? Mood swings and ambivalence (conflicting emotions) are common as the woman works through her fears and comes to grips with the reality of pregnancy and how this pregnancy will affect her life.

Problem-solving skills and methods of coping that worked in the past are used in an attempt to adjust to this new situation. It is important to provide support as this problem solving occurs and to help the woman work through her unique situation. Explanation of the normal physiological changes and discomforts is important. Listening and allowing the woman adequate time to verbalize her fears can also help reduce anxieties.

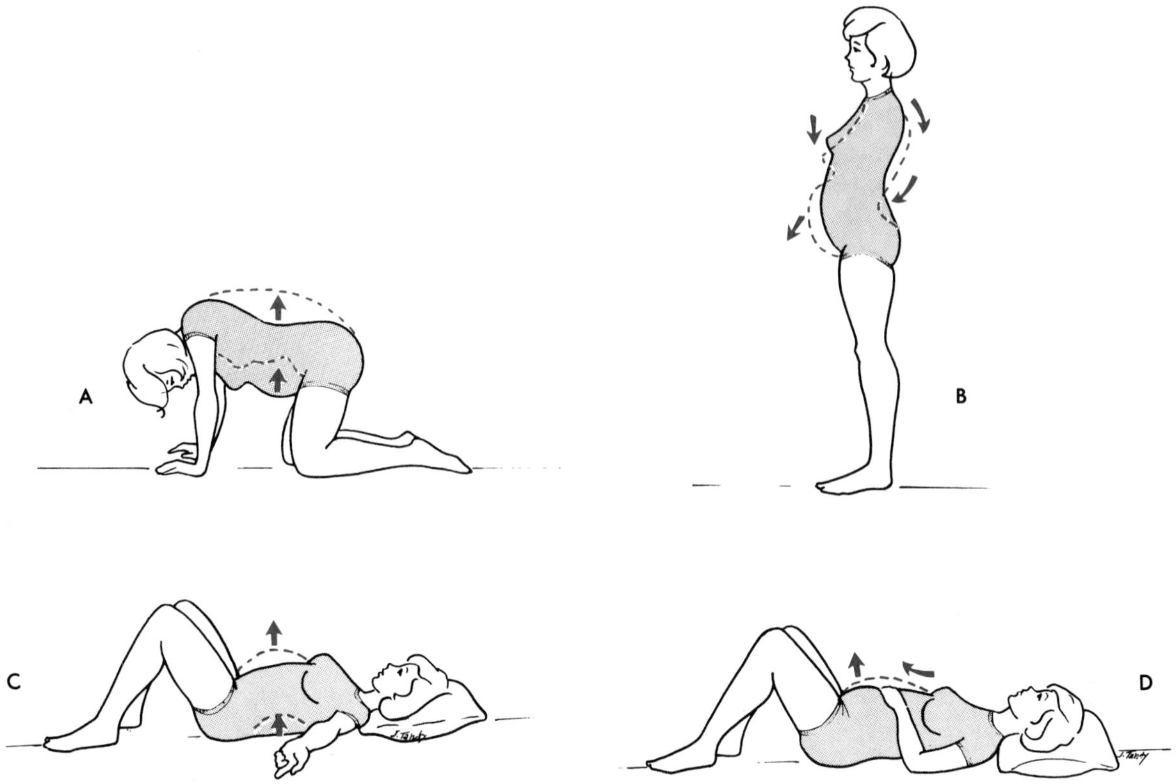

FIG. 42-4 Exercises. **A-C,** Pelvic rocking relieves low backache (excellent for relief of menstrual cramps as well). **D,** Abdominal breathing aids relaxation and lifts abdominal wall off uterus.

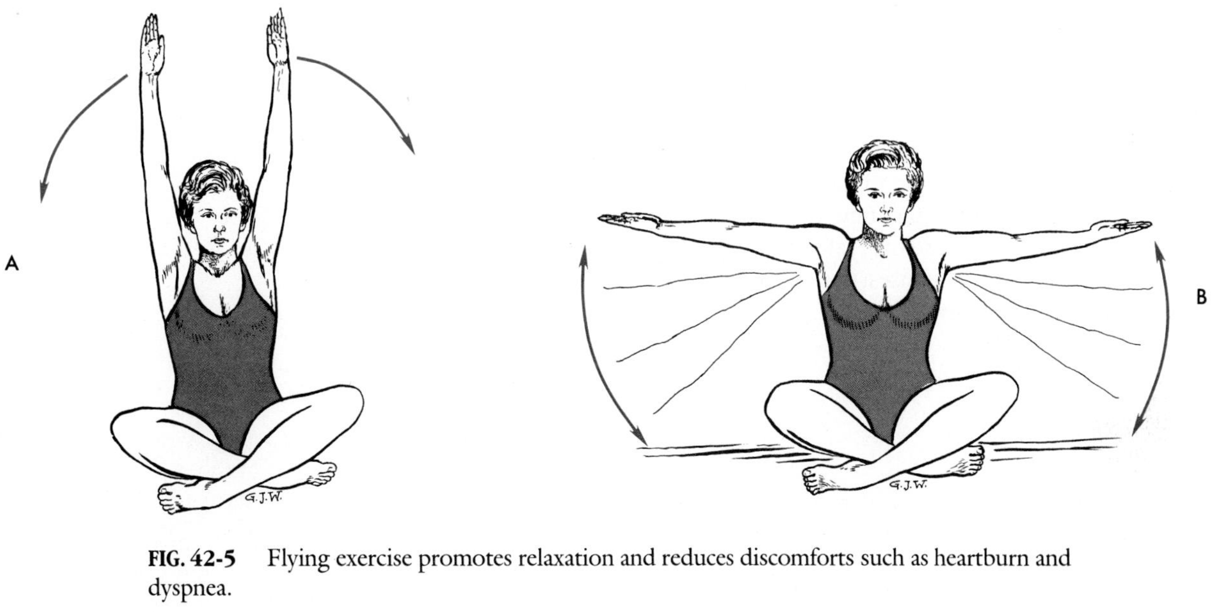

FIG. 42-5 Flying exercise promotes relaxation and reduces discomforts such as heartburn and dyspnea.

Role/Relationship

The expectant woman has generally held several roles in her life, such as child, student, employee, and wife. Pregnancy introduces a totally new role, that of mother. The woman often looks to her own life for persons to model and tends to seek guidance from family and friends. Culture will have much to do with how she will define her role.

There are also changes in the dynamics between the woman and the baby's father, particularly with the first pregnancy. She is no longer just a wife or girlfriend; she is a mother. While she is coping with the role change to mother, he is coping with a role change to father.

Self-Perception/Self-Concept

The rapid changes in body shape and size can lead to changes in self-image. Many women feel that they are not attractive when they are pregnant. They may also feel a loss of control related to the changes taking place. They are no longer free to do as they please, since anything that they do may affect the growing fetus.

Cognitive/Perceptual

Although sensory changes are uncommon with pregnancy, blurring or diplopia may indicate problems with pregnancy-induced hypertension. See Chapter 45 for further discussion.

Prenatal education is important. Most physicians give explanations during routine visits, but the time available is too brief to meet all of the average woman's needs. The nurse should play an important role in prenatal education. Many low-cost pamphlets are available and should be provided whenever possible. Libraries and bookstores also have many good books on prenatal care. Classes are held in many hospitals, clinics, public health agencies, and schools. Special classes that teach methods of prepared childbirth such as Lamaze and Dick-Read methods are also available. Information regarding classes is available through most clinics or physicians' offices.

Critical areas in prenatal teaching include discussion of the common discomforts of pregnancy, the danger signs of pregnancy, nutritional counseling, safety teaching, and a general hygiene review. Exercises that help prepare a woman for childbirth are also valuable.

Value/Belief

There are many cultural and religious influences on the pregnant woman. It is important not to generalize when giving care; not all members of a cultural group will behave in exactly the same way. It is always wise to discuss beliefs with each individual to determine her unique cultural practices, and if the practices do not cause harm, they should be included in planning care. An example of this would be inclusion of ethnic foods in the diet. If the practices are potentially harmful, such as starch-eating or refusal to take prescribed medication, the nurse should try to find a way of persuading the woman to accept safer practices. If unable to do this, the nurse must accept that the pregnant woman is not willing to change her beliefs and should find a way to work with her to minimize complications.

NURSING PROCESS SUMMARY

When performing a nursing assessment on a pregnant woman the various health patterns listed in Table 42-4 should be reviewed to help focus observations. The nurse is not limited to the questions indicated but may use these as a starting point. Any significant observations or responses will indicate the need for a more in-depth assessment. It is important to consult with a more experienced nurse or a physician if the significance of any data is in question.

Table 42-4 also suggests possible nursing diagnoses and nursing interventions that may be helpful in planning nursing care.

Table 42-4 Nursing Process and the Prenatal Patient

Pattern	Data Collection	Possible Nursing Diagnoses	Nursing Interventions
Health management	Does the patient keep appointments? Are medications taken as prescribed? Does the patient avoid alcohol, cigarettes, and other drugs? Does patient perform breast self-exam? Is patient aware of danger signs?	Noncompliance Knowledge deficit	Identify cause of noncompliance; provide emotional support; provide explanations; teach and provide literature on breast self-exam and danger signs
Nutritional/metabolic	Is diet adequate per recommended daily allowance? Is fluid intake adequate? How much weight has been gained/lost? How rapidly is the weight changing? Has she noticed any edema of feet or ankles?	Altered nutrition: less than body requirements; more than body requirements Fluid volume deficit Fluid volume excess	Initiate dietary consultation; review basic food groups; provide literature
Activity/exercise	What type of exercise is practiced? Does the woman complain of backache? Has the physician placed any limits on activity?	Potential for injury Activity intolerance Pain	Stress importance of pacing activities, wearing proper footwear, avoiding hazardous activity
Elimination	Has pattern of urine elimination changed? Has bowel elimination pattern changed? Is there any burning with urination? Pain with defecation? Constipation? Diarrhea?	Diarrhea Constipation Altered patterns of urinary elimination Potential for infection	Discuss dietary interventions to prevent constipation; teach Kegel's exercises; review signs of urinary tract infection
Rest/sleep	Has sleep pattern changed? Increased fatigue noticed? Does patient take naps or rest periods? Do any positions cause discomfort?	Sleep pattern disturbance Fatigue	Discuss positioning for comfort and possibility of naps
Cognitive/perceptual	Has the patient noticed any vision changes? Blurring? Headaches? Has she enrolled in any prenatal classes? Does she attend them?	Potential for injury Knowledge deficit	Provide information about prenatal classes; review danger signs of pregnancy
Role/relationship	Does she feel confused regarding her changing role? Have interpersonal dynamics with husband, boyfriend, mother, friends changed?	Altered role performance Altered family processes	Listen, involve significant others in teaching; possible social service contact if serious problems with dynamics observed
Coping/stress tolerance	What fears or anxieties are verbalized? How has her self-image changed?	Anxiety Fear Ineffective coping	Listen, provide explanations at patient's level of understanding; provide written materials
Value/belief	What is the patient's cultural background? What are her religious practices?	Spiritual distress	Incorporate cultural practices into care whenever possible; consult minister, priest, rabbi for specific information if needed

REFERENCES AND SUGGESTED READINGS

1. Aaronson LS and Macnee CL: Tobacco, alcohol and caffeine use during pregnancy, J Obstet Gynecol Neonatal Nurs 18:279, 1989.
2. Bernhardt JH: Potential workplace hazards to reproductive health, J Obstet Gynecol Neonatal Nurs 19:53, 1990.
3. Bobak IM and Jensen MD: Essentials of maternity nursing, St Louis, 1991, The CV Mosby Co.
4. Burroughs A: Bleir's maternity nursing, ed 5, Philadelphia, 1986, WB Saunders Co.
5. Doenges M and Moorhouse M: Nurse's pocket guide to nursing diagnosis with interventions, ed 2, Philadelphia, 1988, FA Davis Co.
6. Fischbach F: A manual of laboratory diagnostic tests, ed 3, Philadelphia, 1988, JB Lippincott Co.
7. Fishbein EG and Phillips M: How safe is exercise during pregnancy? J Obstet Gynecol Neonatal Nurs 19:45, 1990.
8. Ingalls AJ and Salerno MC: Maternal and child health nursing, ed 7, St Louis, 1990, The CV Mosby Co.
9. Jaffe MS and Melson KA: Maternal-infant health care plans, Springhouse, Pa, 1989, Springhouse Corp.
10. Ladewig PW, London ML, and Olds SB: Essentials of maternal-newborn nursing, ed 2, Redwood City, Calif, 1990, Addison-Wesley.
11. Ladewig PW, London ML, and Olds SB: Maternal newborn nursing: a family-centered approach, ed 3, Menlo Park, Calif, 1988, Addison-Wesley.
12. Pillitteri A: Maternal-newborn nursing; care of the growing family, ed 3, Boston, 1985, Little, Brown & Co.
13. Pritchard JA, MacDonald PC, and Gant GF: Williams' obstetrics, ed 17, New York, 1985, Appleton-Century-Crofts.

CHAPTER CHALLENGE

KEY POINTS

- Pregnancy is a normal process that involves many complex physiological changes in the mother.
- During a period of 280 days, two initial cells join and develop into a unique, viable human being.
- Unique structures such as the placenta, membranes, umbilical cord, and amniotic fluid protect and support the developing fetus. These structures are discarded when the pregnancy is completed and they are no longer necessary.
- All aspects of the mother's life-style can potentially affect her developing fetus.
- Many drugs and viruses can cross the placenta and present serious hazards to the developing embryo, particularly during the first trimester of pregnancy.
- While pregnancy is a normal process, regular and ongoing medical attention is important throughout pregnancy.
- Many signs and symptoms of pregnancy are similar to those manifested by other medical conditions. The positive signs of pregnancy are visualization of the fetus, fetal motion detected by a trained observer, and auscultation of fetal heart sounds.
- Every pregnant woman should be aware of the danger signs during pregnancy and contact her physician if any of these are present.
- Nutritional needs change during pregnancy. To support normal growth and development of the fetus, caloric needs increase, as well as mineral and vitamin requirements.
- Many discomforts may occur during pregnancy. The nurse should be aware of measures that can reduce these discomforts without causing harm to the mother or fetus.
- Pregnancy is a time of role adjustment for both the prospective mother and father. All family members are affected by the addition of a new member.
- Education-for-childbirth classes are widely available. It is highly recommended that prospective parents contact their physician or other health providers in their community and attend these classes.

STUDY QUESTIONS

1. A woman who has never been pregnant is referred to as a:
   a. Nulligravida
   b. Primipara
   c. Primigravida
   d. Multipara
2. Fertilization occurs in the:
   a. Ovary
   b. Fallopian tube
   c. Uterus
   d. Any of the above
3. Ovulation and menstruation cease during pregnancy because of:
   a. Low levels of both estrogen and progesterone
   b. Low level of estrogen and high level of progesterone
   c. High levels of both estrogen and progesterone
   d. High level of estrogen and low level of progesterone
4. Organ formation and discrimination occurs during:
   a. Fertilization
   b. The first trimester
   c. The second trimester
   d. The third trimester
5. Which of the following is involved in the oxygenation and nutrition of the fetus:
   a. Placenta
   b. Amniotic fluid
   c. Chorion
   d. Wharton's jelly
6. A *presumptive* sign of pregnancy is:
   a. A positive pregnancy test
   b. Nausea and vomiting
   c. Hearing fetal heart sounds
   d. Uterine enlargement
7. A *positive* sign of pregnancy is:
   a. Fetal heart tones
   b. A positive pregnancy test
   c. Feeling of fetal movement by the mother
   d. Positive Chadwick's sign
8. The expected date of confinement is calculated by:
   a. Counting back 7 days from the first day of the last menstrual period and adding 3 months
   b. Counting back 3 months from the first day of the last menstrual period and adding 7 days
   c. Counting back 3 months from the last day of the last menstrual period and adding 7 days
   d. Counting back 7 months from the first day of the last menstrual period and adding 9 days
9. A danger sign during pregnancy that should be reported promptly is:
   a. Urinary frequency
   b. Severe headaches
   c. Backache
   d. Edematous ankles
10. Preparation-for-childbirth classes are important to:
    a. Prepare the father to go into the delivery room
    b. Give the expectant mother a chance to socialize with other pregnant women
    c. Reduce fears by explaining the process of labor and delivery
    d. Teach the pregnant woman exercises for weight control

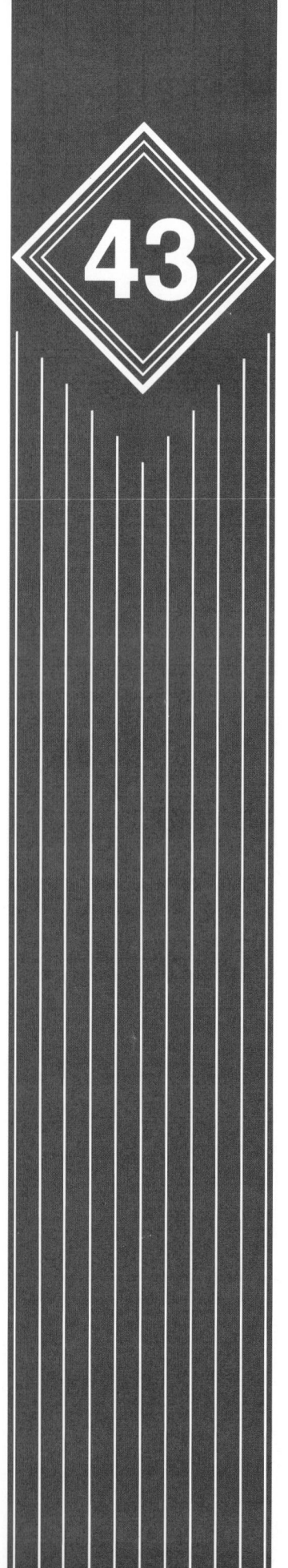

43

Normal Labor and Delivery

GLORIA E. WOLD

LEARNING OBJECTIVES

After reading this chapter, the student should be able to do the following:

- Define the key terms.
- Recognize the signs of impending labor.
- Distinguish between true and false labor.
- Describe fetopelvic disproportion.
- Discuss the "powers" involved in labor and delivery.
- Identify the mechanisms of labor.
- Describe the stages of labor.
- Explain the components of assessment during labor and delivery.
- Identify nursing diagnoses relevant to the woman in labor.
- Discuss medical interventions related to labor and delivery.
- Discuss nursing interventions related to labor and delivery.

RELATED TOPICS OF INTEREST

- Cultural aspects of nursing care (Chapter 12)
- Care of the patient with a reproductive disorder (Chapter 36)
- Care of the mother and newborn at risk (Chapter 45)

KEY TERMS

Define the following:

- amniotomy
- attitude
- Braxton Hicks contractions
- descent
- effacement
- engagement
- expulsion
- extension
- external rotation
- fetopelvic disproportion
- flexion
- internal rotation
- lie
- lightening
- oxytocic
- oligohydramnios
- position
- presentation
- restitution
- surfactant
- uterine inertia

NORMAL LABOR

Onset of Labor

In most pregnancies the fetus reaches maturity and the uterus begins the process of labor at exactly the right time. Although this process has been occurring throughout human history, researchers are still trying to discover the exact cause for the onset, or beginning, of labor.

Theories of Labor

Although there is no known cause for the onset of labor, there are several theories. These fall into two main categories—those based on mechanical changes and those based on hormonal changes.

One mechanical theory involves uterine stretching. It is based on the principle that once a hollow body organ reaches a certain state of distention, it will spontaneously contract and empty. For example, a full bladder will empty by incontinence and a distended stomach will empty by vomiting. It is hypothesized that when the uterus stretches to a certain size it will empty spontaneously. However, the wide variation of uterine size between different pregnancies in the same woman makes this a weak theory. For example, a woman may have one pregnancy in which she delivers a 6-pound baby at term. In her next pregnancy she may again reach term, but this time delivers twins each weighing 6 pounds.

There are several hormonal theories for the onset of labor based on either an increase or decrease in hormones. In some of the theories, the source of the hormones is the mother; in other theories, it is the fetus. Some suggest the production of increased amounts of hormones acts as a trigger to start labor; others hypothesize a decrease in hormone levels is the trigger. Some of the more common theories relating to hormones are (1) oxytocin stimulation, (2) progesterone withdrawal, (3) estrogen stimulation, and (4) fetal cortisol. These and others are possible but not proven.

Signs of Impending Labor

Although we do not know what causes labor, we can recognize when labor is about to begin by watching for certain signs.

As early as 2 weeks before the onset of labor the woman may notice that the fetus seems to have settled or "dropped" into the pelvis. This is called **lightening** and is seen most often in nulliparas. Once this has occurred the woman often notices that urinary frequency returns. She may be able to breathe more normally, since there is more space in the abdominal cavity. Multiparas may not experience this change until they are in active labor.

Occasionally a woman may experience a leakage or sudden outflow of fluid from the vagina. This may be urine, or it may be amniotic fluid, indicating a rupture of the amniotic sac. A simple test with nitrazine paper can distinguish between these. Without washing the area, the paper is moistened with the discharge. If the paper reacts (turns blue), the discharge is probably amniotic fluid. If the test is nonreactive, the membranes are probably intact. The amniotic sac generally ruptures after labor has begun. If it ruptures before labor starts, medical attention is essential. Rupture of the bag of waters (BOW) leads to increased risk of infection. If labor does not occur within 24 hours after rupture of the membranes, the physician will usually attempt to start labor by administering medication.

The amount of vaginal drainage typically increases as term approaches, and a blood-tinged mucus called the *bloody show* may be observed. This "show" is the mucus that occluded the opening of the cervix during pregnancy. Vaginal examination may reveal that the cervix has begun to change consistency. The cervix begins to soften, and in true labor it also begins to thin (efface) and open (dilate).

Backache and contractions of the uterus, called **Braxton Hicks contractions,** are common as the pregnancy approaches term. These contractions vary from mild to moderate in severity. They remain irregular and do not dilate the cervix.

Some women notice a slight loss of weight (1 to 3 pounds) a few days before labor, and others report a last-minute burst of energy.

True labor is marked by the onset of regular, rhythmic contractions that cause progressive dilation and **effacement** of the cervix.

Table 43-1 Comparison of True and False Labor

True Labor	False Labor
Contractions follow a regular pattern.	Contractions rarely follow a pattern.
Contractions come closer together, are stronger, and tend to last longer.	Contractions vary in length and intensity.
Contractions get stronger with ambulation.	Contractions frequently stop with ambulation or position change.
Contractions seem to start in the lower back and then travel to the lower abdomen.	Contractions may be felt in the back, but are most often noticed in the fundus.
Contractions are usually not stopped by controlled breathing, sedation, or other relaxation interventions.	Contractions eventually stop with relaxation interventions.
The cervix softens, effaces, and dilates.	The cervix may soften, but there is little or no change in effacement or dilation.
The fetus continues descent into the pelvis.	There is no significant change in the fetal position.

False Labor Versus True Labor

Because many women fear that they will go to the hospital at the wrong time, nurses should explain how true labor differs from false labor. These differences are described in Table 43-1. It is also important to stress that when there is any doubt, medical attention should be obtained. At times even experienced professionals find it difficult to differentiate the early stages of true labor from false labor.

LABOR AND DELIVERY

Alternative Labor and Delivery Sites

When the woman suspects that the onset of true labor has begun, she typically notifies her physician or nurse midwife and her significant others. A plan for delivery should have been established during the pregnancy. Delivery can be planned in a traditional hospital setting, a birthing room, or at home. A traditional labor and delivery setting tends to be very medically oriented and may seem physically and emotionally "sterile and cold" to many women. In this traditional method visitors to the woman in labor are strictly limited. Only the spouse or one significant other is allowed to be present during labor and delivery. Typically, many room changes occur: the mother is admitted to a labor room, then transferred to a delivery room, after delivery is moved to a recovery room, and finally to a postpartum room. Many women dislike this and find the restriction of visits with loved ones and the frequent moves disturbing. Despite these considerations, the traditional hospital is a safe setting. All of the personnel and equipment needed in case of emergency are readily available.

To avoid the negative aspects of the traditional system, some women want to give birth at home. This plan must be agreed on by the physician or nurse midwife. Home delivery is permitted only when an uncomplicated delivery is expected and the physician has reasonable confidence that no harm will come to either the mother or infant. An unplanned delivery at home could lead to serious problems. If an emergency occurs, precious time is lost transporting the mother or infant to the hospital where the necessary support is available.

Birthing centers are a fairly recent development. These centers are generally located within the hospital but are structured to be more homelike. The attitude of the staff is more open and welcoming to the spouse and significant others. The entire birthing process and often the entire stay at the facility will take place in one room. This eliminates many of the negative factors of the traditional hospital setting but provides the safety of having all necessary personnel and equipment available. For these reasons, alternative birthing centers are becoming increasingly popular.

The Process of Labor and Delivery

To understand the complex process of labor and delivery it is important to examine each of the factors involved. These factors are frequently called the four *P*'s:

passage	The pelvis and soft tissues
passenger	The fetus
powers	Contractions and voluntary effort
process	All parts working together

The Passage

The pelvis. The superior portion of the pelvis (iliac segment of the innominate bones) functions as a support for the uterus and fetus during the late months of pregnancy. These bones aid in directing the fetus into the inferior (lower) portion of the pelvis, which is called the *true pelvis*. The two sections are divided by an imaginary line called the *linea terminalis* or pelvic inlet.

The size and shape of the true pelvis are of more importance than those of the false pelvis, because the fetal head must be able to pass through this section of the pelvis for vaginal delivery to occur. Four different types of pelves are recognized. Each of these has a unique shape and characteristics, as shown in Table 43-2.

The true pelvis is further divided into three segments, the inlet, the cavity or midpelvis, and the outlet (Fig. 43-1). Several methods are available to the physician for evaluating the size of the true pelvis:

1. Palpation: Externally, the physician can use a pelvimeter to determine the distance between the ischial tuberosities. This helps the physician estimate the distance between the ischial spines, which can otherwise be obtained only by pelvic x-ray examination. Internally, the physician can palpate additional bony prominences to determine pelvic adequacy.
2. Pelvimetry: With x-ray films from different views the physician can accurately measure the bony prominences. However, this measurement is usually done at a time other than pregnancy if there has been an injury or known developmental problem, such as rickets. Pelvimetry is not routinely done during pregnancy, because the radiation may be harmful to the fetus.
3. Ultrasonography: Sound waves above the range of human hearing can also be used to estimate pelvic adequacy. Because ultrasound does not involve the use of radiation, it is generally regarded as safe for

Table 43-2 Comparison of Pelvic Types

	Gynecoid (50% of Women)	**Android (23% of Women)**	**Anthropoid (24% of Women)**	**Platypelloid (3% of Women)**
Brim	Slightly ovoid or transversely rounded	Heart shaped, angulated	Oval, wider anteroposteriorly	Flattened anteroposteriorly, wide transversely
	Round	Heart	Oval	Flat
Depth	Moderate	Deep	Deep	Shallow
Side walls	Straight	Convergent	Straight	Straight
Ischial spines	Blunt, somewhat widely separated	Prominent, narrow interspinous diameter	Prominent, often with narrow interspinous diameter	Blunted, widely separated
Sacrum	Deep, curved	Slightly curved, terminal portion often beaked	Slightly curved	Slightly curved
Subpubic arch	Wide	Narrow	Narrow	Wide
Usual mode of delivery	Vaginal Spontaneous Occiput anterior position	Cesarean Vaginal Difficult with forceps	Vaginal Forceps/spontaneous occiput posterior or occiput anterior position	Vaginal Spontaneous

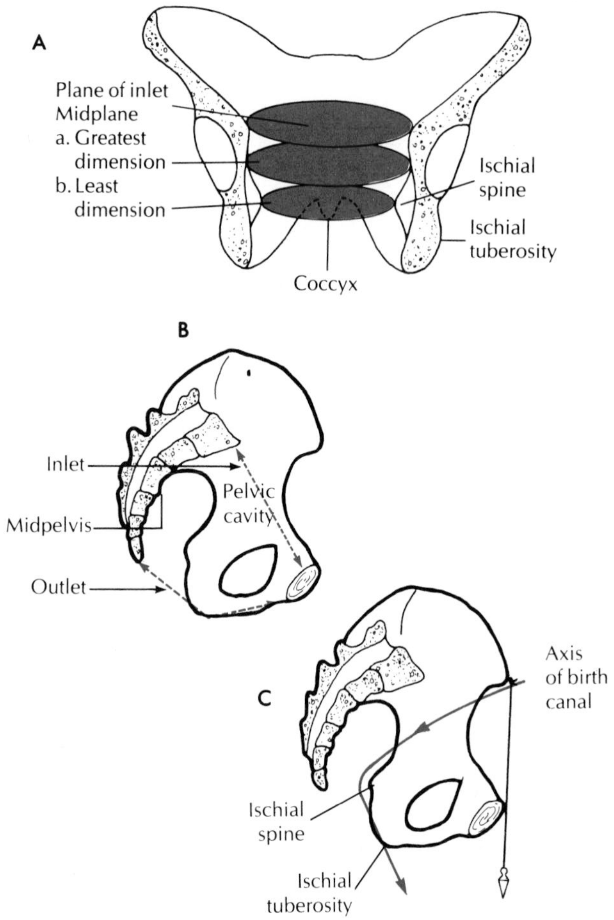

FIG. 43-1 Pelvic cavity. **A,** Inlet and midplane. (Outlet not shown.) **B,** Cavity of true pelvis. **C,** Note curve of sacrum and axis of birth canal.

the fetus. In more than 20 years of obstetrical use, no detrimental effects have been observed. Because ultrasound can visualize soft tissue, it is also helpful in gathering information regarding fetal growth, multiple pregnancy, placental location, and abnormal presentation that may complicate delivery.

It is important to understand that adequacy of the pelvis is relative. At the time of each delivery the physician must determine whether the pelvis is adequate to allow passage of this particular fetus. While there are certain measurements that are considered "normal," the size and position of the fetus make each situation unique.

The soft tissues. During labor the uterus, cervix, vagina, and muscles of the perineum change in consistency and shape to allow passage of the fetus in the following ways.

Uterine tissues. During labor the walls of the upper section of the uterus have a thickened musculature that provides the force during contractions. The muscle walls of the lower section become thinner and act as a passive tube. Located between the two sections is a band of tissue called the *physiological retraction ring* (Fig. 43-2).

Cervical tissues. As contractions of the muscular upper segment apply downward pressure, the uterine contents (fetal presenting part) efface and dilate the cervix.

The vagina. In response to hormonal changes during pregnancy, the vagina undergoes many changes. Increased blood supply (vascularity), increased thickness of the mucosa, loosening of the connective tissue, and enlargement (hypertrophy) of smooth muscle cells all make the vagina capable of stretching (dilating) to allow passage of the fetus.

The perineum. The muscles of the pelvic floor are stretched and thinned by the pressure of the presenting part. The anus may appear dilated and bulging.

The Passenger

To be born, the fetus must be able to exit through the bony passageway just described. This is a major challenge, since at term the fetus weighs approximately 7 pounds and is 20 to 21 inches long.

The fetal skull. Because the fetal skull is usually the largest part of the body, the delivery of the head poses

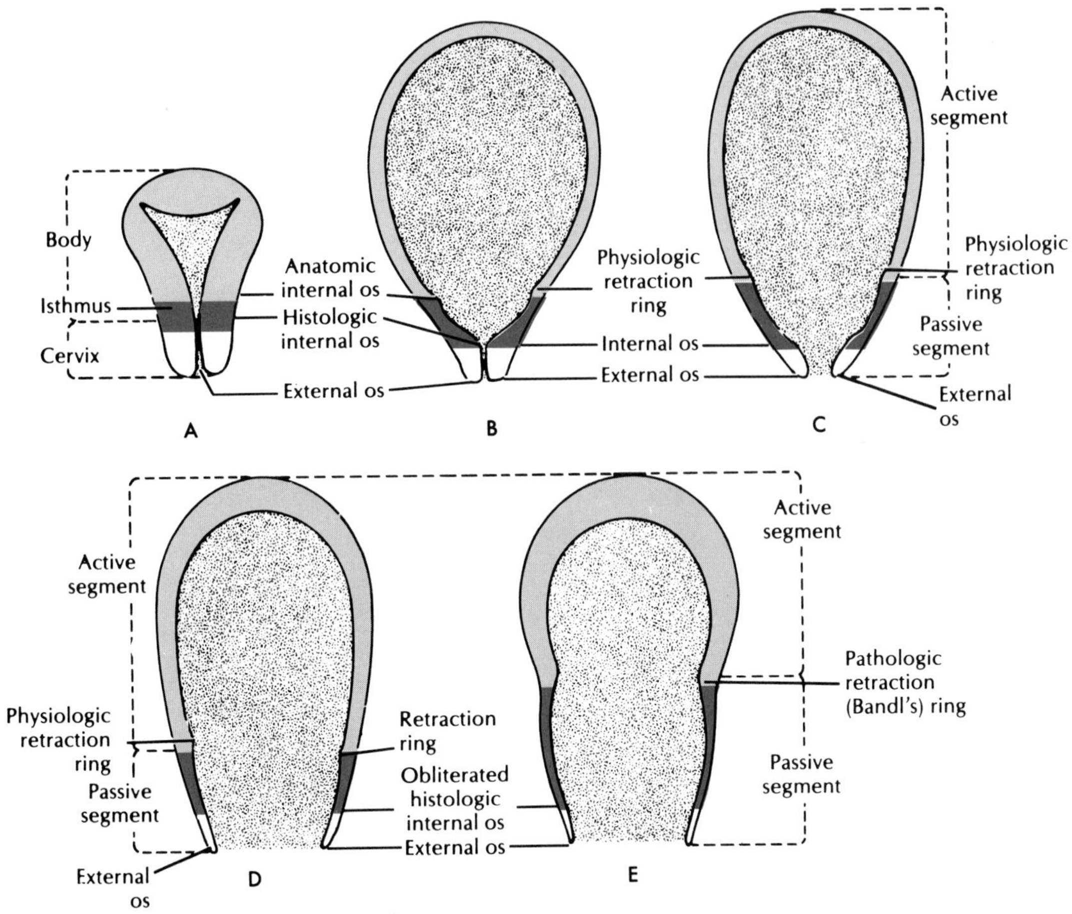

FIG. 43-2 Progressive development of segments and rings of uterus at term. Note comparison between **A,** nonpregnant uterus, **B,** uterus at term, and **C,** uterus in normal labor in early first stage, and **D,** second stage. Passive segment is derived from lower uterine segment (isthmus) and cervix, and physiological retraction ring is derived from anatomical internal os. **E,** Uterus in abnormal labor in second-stage dystocia. Pathological retraction (Bandl's) ring that forms under abnormal conditions develops from physiological ring.

the greatest concern. The shoulders and pelvis, which are more mobile, do not often cause problems.

The bones of the fetal skull are not rigidly joined (fused). This allows the bony plates to move and overlap as they progress through the maternal pelvis. This reshaping of the skull bones in response to pressure against the maternal pelvis is called molding.

The major bones of the skull are the two frontal bones, two parietal bones, two temporal bones, and the occiput.

These are joined by membranous spaces called the *sutures*. Where sutures meet, there are larger membranous areas called the *fontanels* (Fig. 43-3). The anterior fontanel (bregma) tends to be larger and diamond shaped, since it is formed by four bones. The posterior fontanel is smaller and triangular, since only three bones adjoin. Palpation of the sutures and fontanels through the cervix permits the physician or nurse to determine the presentation of the fetus during labor. The largest transverse diameter of the skull is the biparietal measurement. If this is too large, the skull may not be able to enter the mother's pelvis.

Fetal attitude. The relationship of body parts to one another is called **attitude.** At term, the ideal attitude for the fetal body is flexion. The back is bowed outward, the chin is touching the sternum, the arms are crossed on the chest, and the thighs are flexed on the abdomen. This is called the **fetal position.** This attitude is ideal, because it takes up minimal space and allows the best angle of approach to the pelvis. If there is insufficient room because of too little amniotic fluid **(oligohydramnios),** multiple pregnancies, or anatomical variations in the mother, the attitude may be altered, leading to complications of labor or delivery.

Fetal lie. Fetal **lie** is the relationship of the cephalocaudal (head-to-buttocks) axis of the fetus to the cephalocaudal axis of the mother. If the spine of the fetus is parallel to the spine of the mother, the lie is called *longitudinal*. This could be cephalic presentation (head

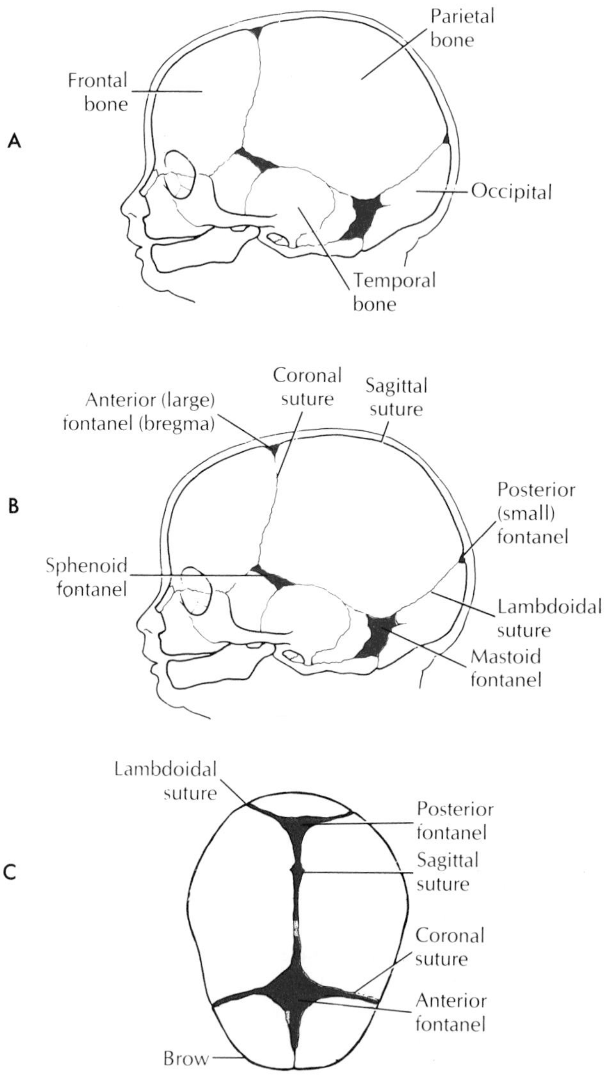

FIG. 43-3 Fetal head at term. **A,** Bones; **B,** fontanels; and **C,** sutures.

down) or breech presentation (buttocks down). The lie is longitudinal in 99% of deliveries. If the spine of the fetus is perpendicular to that of the mother, it is called *transverse* lie. Only 1% of deliveries involve a transverse lie. This is most common in women who have had many pregnancies (resulting in weakened abdominal walls), maternal pelvic contracture, or placenta previa, which will be discussed in Chapter 45. During pregnancy, while the fetus is small it changes lie frequently. By term the fetal lie seldom changes because the space available is limited.

Fetal presentation. Fetal **presentation** describes the part that will be in contact with the cervix. This is determined by both attitude and lie.

In about 96% of deliveries the presentation is cephalic. In cephalic presentation some part of the fetal head is in contact with the cervix. There are four types of cephalic presentation: vertex (region between the fontanels), brow, face, and mentum (chin).

In about 3% of deliveries the presentation is breech. In breech presentations either the buttocks or legs are in contact with the cervix. There are three types of breech presentation: complete breech, in which the buttocks present and the thighs are well flexed on the abdomen; frank breech, in which the buttocks present and the thighs are extended across the abdomen and chest; and footling breech, in which there is no flexion and one foot or two feet are present. Breech presentations are more difficult to deliver vaginally. To decrease risks to the fetus, the majority of breech births are delivered surgically. These surgical deliveries, called *cesarean sections,* will be discussed later.

In about 1% of deliveries some other body part presents. These occur when the fetus has been in a transverse lie. The shoulder, hand, elbow, and iliac crest are possible presenting parts. In these cases a cesarean birth is also required.

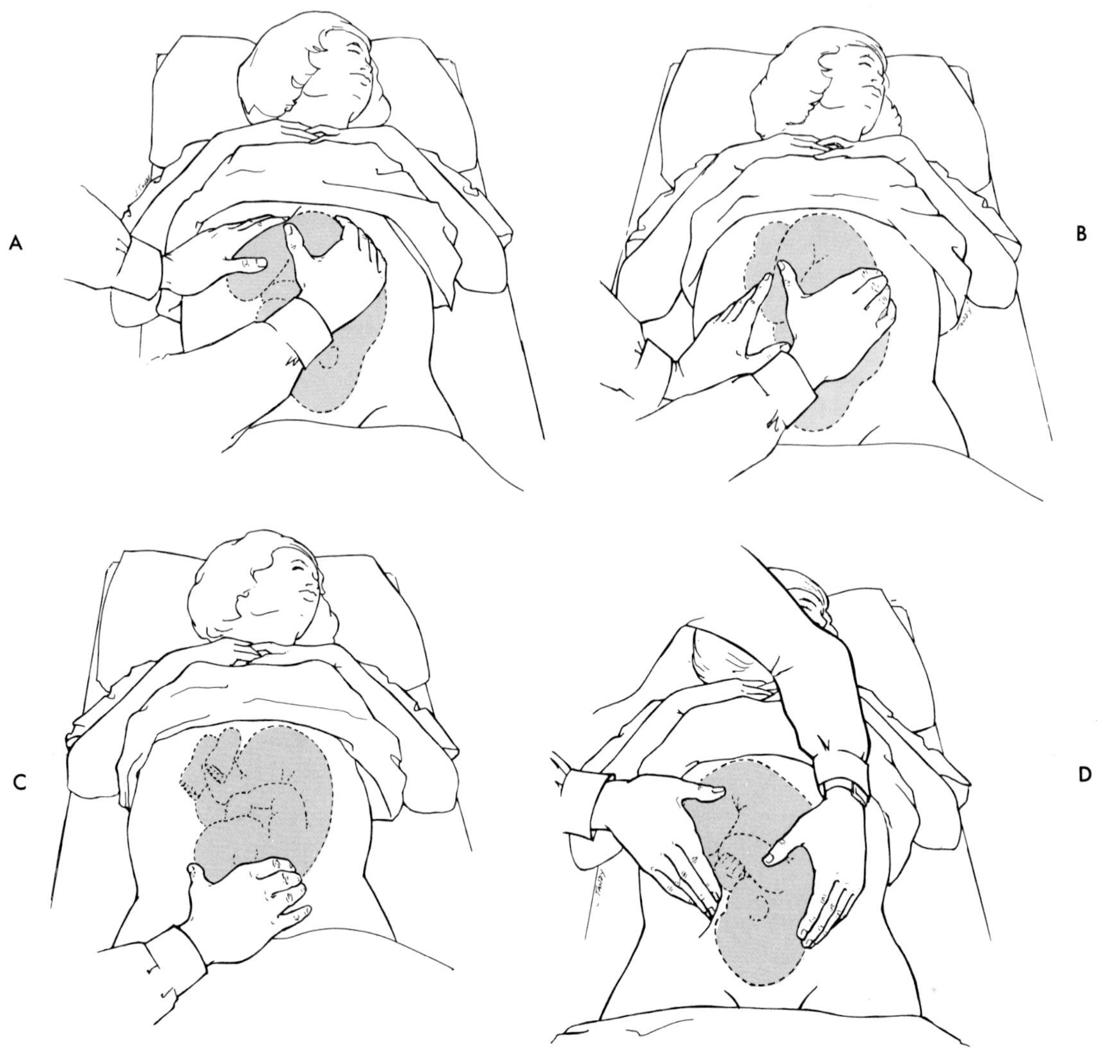

FIG. 43-4 Leopold's maneuvers.

Fetal position. Position is the relationship of the presenting fetal part to a quadrant of the maternal pelvis. Fetal position can be determined by abdominal inspection and palpation (Leopold's maneuvers, Fig. 43-4), vaginal or rectal examination, auscultation of fetal heart tones, or ultrasound or x-ray examination. Once the position is determined, it is expressed in abbreviated form. For example, the most common position for delivery is LOA, left occiput anterior, in which the occiput of the fetus points toward the left anterior segment of the maternal pelvis. ROA, right occiput anterior, is next most common. Many combinations are possible, as shown below and in Figs. 43-5 and 43-6.

MATERNAL PELVIS SIDE	PRESENTING PART	MATERNAL QUADRANT
R Right	O Occiput	A Anterior
L Left	B Brow	P Posterior
	M Mentum	T Transverse
	S Sacrum	
	SC Scapula	

Effect of fetal position on labor. A longitudinal lie, well-flexed attitude, with vertex presentation is the ideal. In this position the fetal skull bones are most able to mold to progress through the maternal pelvis. The fetal skull also provides a smooth, round surface, which is most effective in effacing and dilating the cervix. The smooth, regular shape also fills the cervix and prevents the umbilical cord from prolapsing, or coming before, the fetus. Cord prolapse is dangerous, because pressure on the vessels in the cord can restrict the blood flow to the fetus.

If a part other than the vertex presents, labor is generally longer, more tiring to the mother, and more likely to require surgical intervention.

Monitoring fetal status. The process of labor is stressful to the fetus, and it is important to monitor the fetus continuously during this time. Fetal heart rate (FHR) is a good indicator of the fetus's condition. The FHR is auscultated using a fetoscope or a Doppler instrument. This should be done every 15 to 30 minutes during the first stage of labor and every 5 minutes during the second

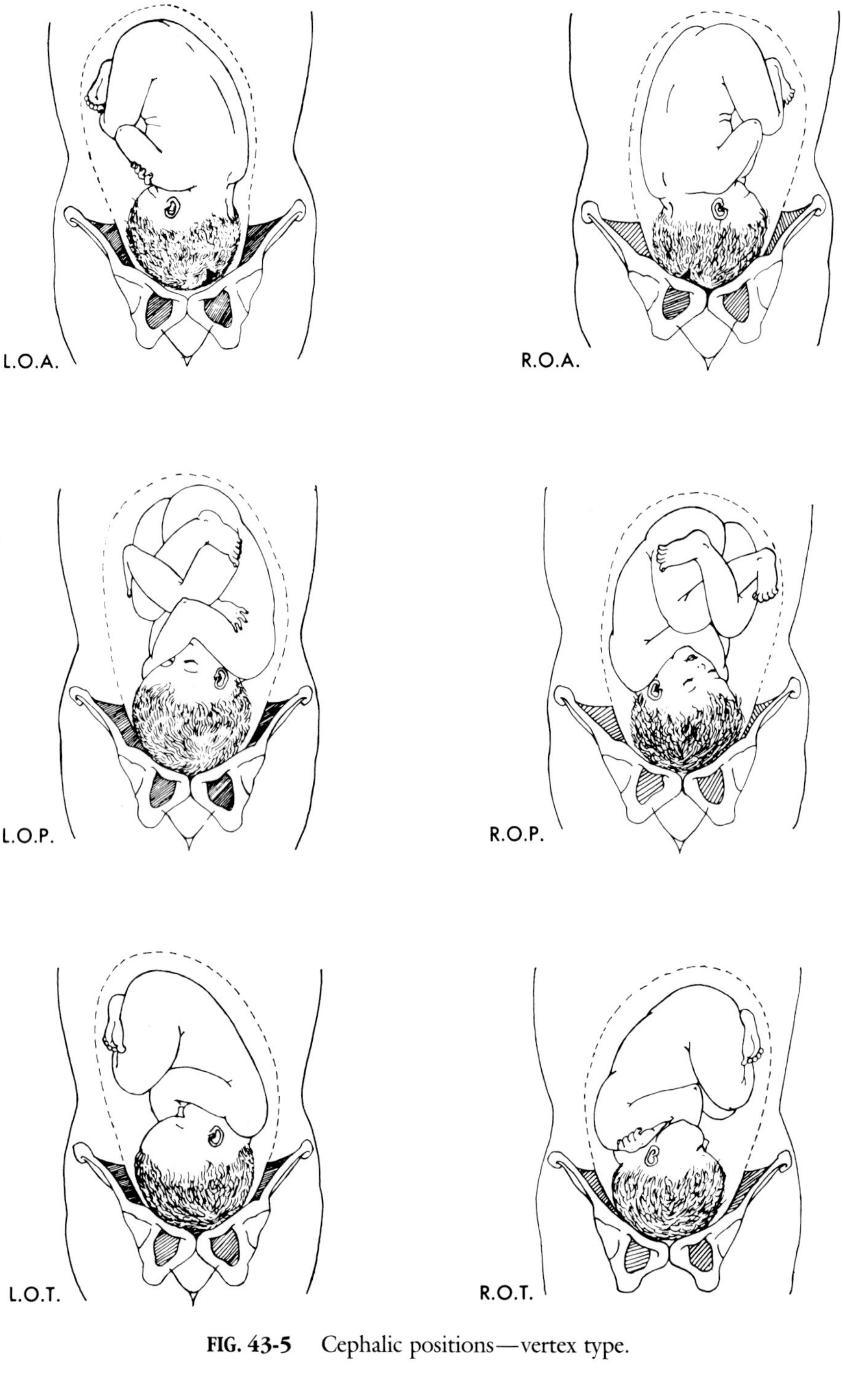

FIG. 43-5 Cephalic positions—vertex type.

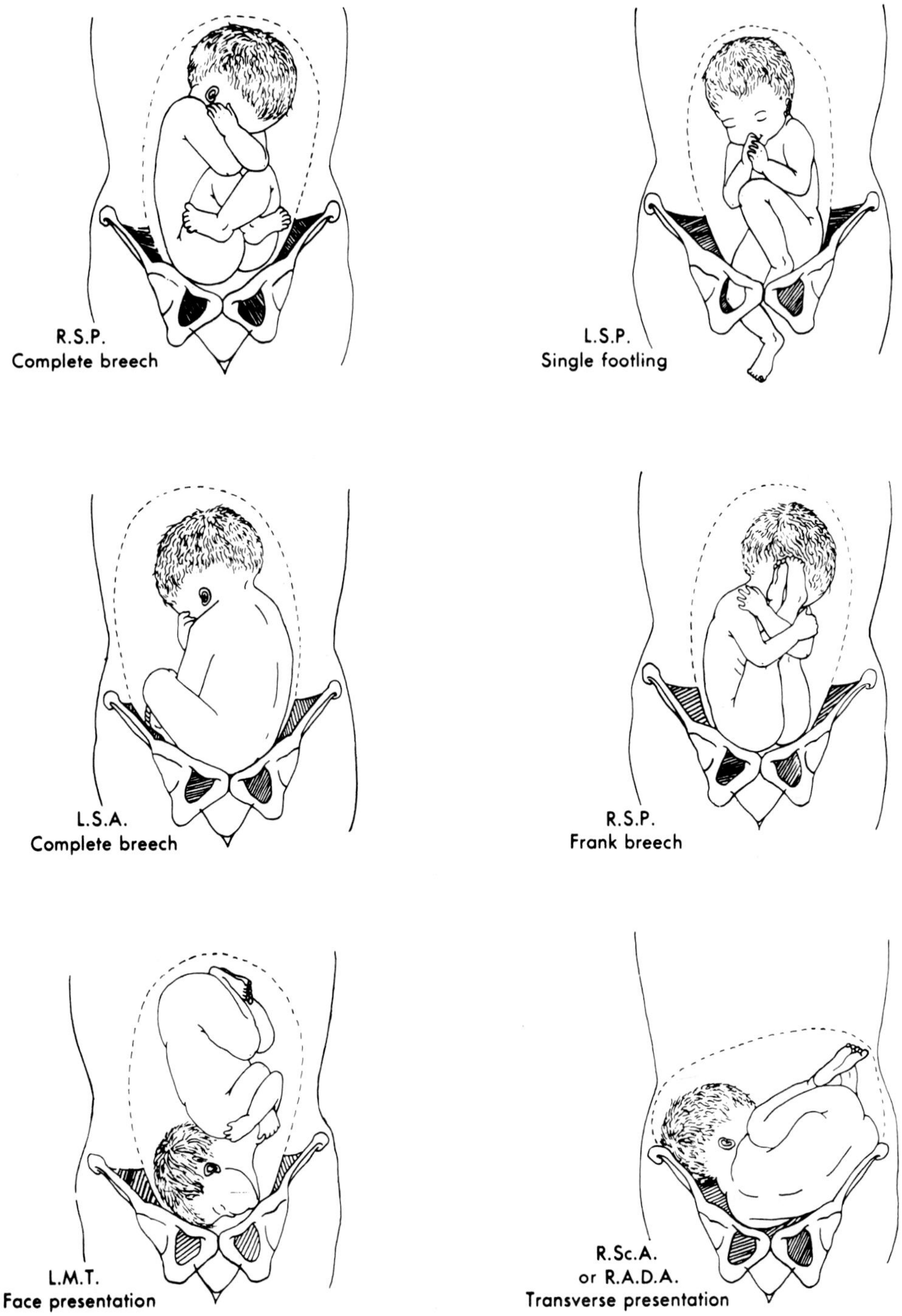

FIG. 43-6 Various presentations and positions.

stage. The FHR should also be taken immediately after rupture of the membranes, particularly if the head is not engaged (i.e., firmly settled into the pelvis). The normal FHR range is 120 to 160 beats per minute. An increase or decrease of 30 beats per minute indicates fetal distress and should be reported immediately.

Frequently electronic monitors, either internal or external, are applied. These monitors continuously track maternal contractions and the changes in fetal heart rate. Monitors are more accurate in detecting subtle changes of condition before they can be recognized by auscultation. Greenish discoloration of the amniotic fluid is significant: the color may result from stool, called **meconium,** being released from the fetal rectum in response to oxygen deprivation.

The Powers

The forces that move the passenger through the passage include involuntary uterine contraction and voluntary maternal pushing.

Uterine contractions. As already mentioned, during labor the muscles in the upper uterine segment, the fundus, thicken and contract at intervals. The intervals may be as much as 15 or 30 minutes apart in early labor and as frequent as every 2 or 3 minutes at the most active stage. Early contractions last 20 to 35 seconds; at the later stages they typically last 60 to 80 seconds. Each contraction has three parts: the increment, during which the muscles contract and the force increases in strength; the apex, during which the optimal force is exerted; and the decrement, during which the muscles relax.

These contractions are involuntary and originate at pacemaker points near the uterotubal junction. When a contraction occurs, the uterine cavity becomes smaller, and this forces the presenting fetal part or the bag of waters against the cervix. In addition, the thickening of the upper segment retracts, pulling the lower segment upward around the presenting part. In combination these actions efface and dilate the cervix. Before labor the nulliparous cervix is 2 to 3 cm long and 1 cm thick. The *os* (mouth or opening) is generally closed or open less than 1 cm. In a multiparous woman, the cervix may begin to efface and dilate before labor starts.

Labor progresses differently in nulliparas than in multiparas. In nulliparas, effacement usually precedes dilation. In multiparas, effacement and dilation usually progress simultaneously.

Effacement is described in percentages; total effacement is reached when no thickness of the cervix can be distinguished. Dilation is measured in centimeters; complete dilation is accomplished when a measurement of 10 cm is reached. This is the point at which the fetus is able to leave the uterus (Fig. 43-7).

Monitoring contractions. Contractions can be monitored by placing a hand on the fundus of the uterus and using palpation to detect the contraction. Contractions are timed from the beginning of one contraction to the beginning of the next. Electronic monitors measure and time contractions and correlate fetal heart rate to maternal contractions (Fig. 43-8).

Voluntary pushing. When the presenting part reaches the pelvic floor, the woman typically experiences an urge to bear down or push. Many women describe this as an urge to defecate. Pushing before the cervix is completely effaced and dilated will exhaust the woman and may actually slow the progress of labor. Once the cervix is fully effaced and dilated, the woman can assist in the progress of labor. To assist effectively, the woman must hold her breath and use her diaphragm and abdominal muscles to increase the intraabdominal pressure. Such pushing assists in forcing the fetus through the birth canal.

Positioning the woman in a manner that allows gravity to assist her efforts is helpful. Squatting or using a semiseated position is more effective than a supine position. Special birthing chairs, which provide support and facilitate voluntary pushing, are available in many birthing centers.

The Process

Mechanisms of labor. For the fetus to move through the maternal pelvis, several maneuvers are required. These turns and adjustments are called the *mechanisms of labor.* The mechanisms of labor in the vertex position are as follows:

Engagement
Descent
Flexion
Internal rotation
Extension
External rotation and restitution
Expulsion

Engagement occurs when the biparietal diameter of the fetal head crosses the inlet of the pelvis. When this occurs the head is said to be fixed or engaged in the pelvis. This tends to occur early in nulliparous women, often several days or weeks before labor begins. Multiparous women may not experience engagement until labor has started.

Descent. is the downward progress of the presenting part. The amount of progress is measured by comparing the lowest point of the presenting part to the ischial spines. This is measured in centimeters above or below the level of the spines and is referred to by *station.* For example, if the presenting part is even with the ischial spines, the station is 0; if the presenting part is 2 cm above the spines, the station is −2; if the presenting part is 2 cm below the presenting part, the station is +2 (Fig. 43-9).

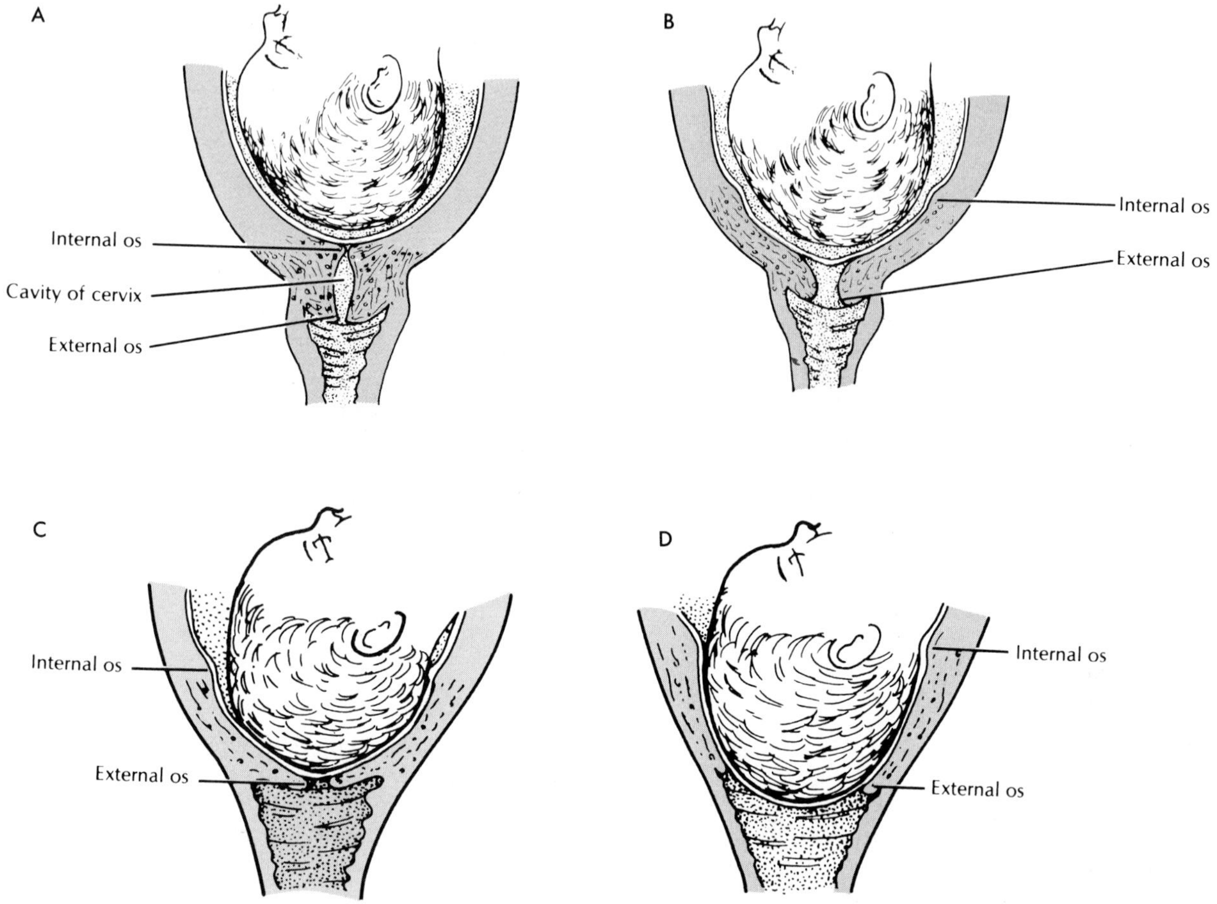

FIG. 43-7 Cervical effacement and dilation. Note how cervix is drawn up around presenting part (internal os). Membranes are intact, and head is not well applied to cervix. **A,** Before labor. **B,** Early effacement. **C,** Complete effacement (100%). Head is well applied to cervix. **D,** Complete dilation (10 cm). Some overlapping of cranial bones. Membranes still intact.

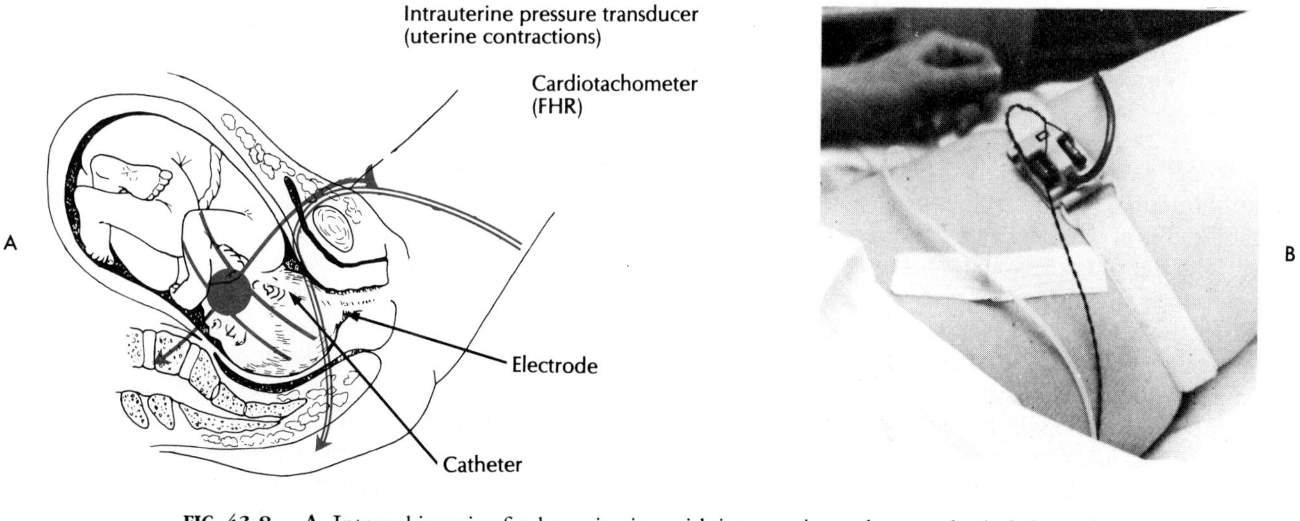

FIG. 43-8 **A,** Internal invasive fetal monitoring with intrauterine catheter and spiral electrode in place (membranes ruptured and cervix dilated). **B,** Device secured to woman's thigh.

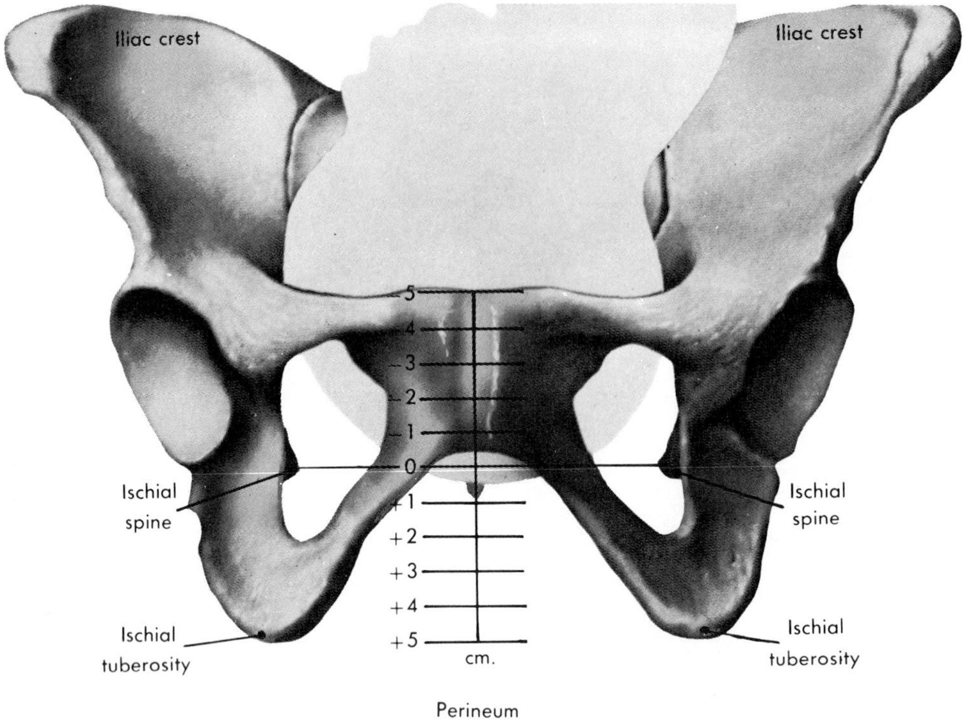

FIG. 43-9 Stations of presenting part, or degree of engagement. Location of the presenting part in relation to the level of ischial spines is designated *station* and indicates degree of advancement of the presenting part through pelvis. Stations are expressed in centimeters above (*minus*) and below (*plus*) the level of the ischial spines (*zero*). The head is usually engaged when it reaches the level of ischial spines. (From Phenomena of normal labor, Columbus, Ohio, 1964, Ross Laboratories.)

Flexion, which is the normal attitude, increases as a result of resistance from the cervix or pelvic floor.

Internal rotation enables the fetal head to progress through the maternal pelvis. The largest diameter of the fetal head aligns with the largest diameter of the pelvis.

Extension occurs when the occiput passes under the symphysis pubis. This bony structure acts as a stable point and provides leverage, enabling the head to leave the pelvis. The actual delivery of the head is done by extension. As soon as the head is delivered, it moves to realign with the body and shoulders. This is referred to as **restitution.**

External rotation occurs as the shoulders and body move through the birth canal, using the same maneuvers as the head. The shoulders are delivered similarly to the head, with the anterior shoulder pressing under the symphysis pubis, which again acts as a leverage point, and assists in delivery of the posterior shoulder. After the shoulders are delivered the delivery ends with **expulsion** in which the body of the infant leaves the pelvis. Delivery of the body occurs rapidly once the shoulders have been delivered (Fig. 43-10).

The first stage: dilation. The first stage begins with the onset of regular contractions and ends with complete dilation of the cervix. This is generally the longest stage of labor. In nulliparas this stage averages 10 to 12 hours; in multiparas the average is 6 to 8 hours. This stage is often divided into three substages:

1. Early labor: 0 to 4 cm dilation; contractions occur 5 to 8 minutes apart and last 20 to 35 seconds. During this stage the woman generally is alert, frequently is talkative, and tends to be receptive to coaching on breathing techniques. This coaching may be provided by the nurse or significant other and reviews techniques learned in the prenatal classes. Pain tends to be mild and easily controlled. Backache is a common complaint. Many women, particularly multiparas, prefer to remain home during this stage. If the bag of waters has not ruptured, many women walk during this stage. The nulliparous woman may express anxiety about her ability to cope with childbirth.
2. Midlabor: 4 to 8 cm dilation; contractions occur at 3- to 5-minute intervals and last 40 to 60 seconds. During this stage the woman becomes less talkative and focuses on breathing techniques. The intensity of the pain increases but still may be manageable without medication.
3. Transition: 8 to 10 cm dilation; contractions occur at 2- to 3-minute intervals and last up to 80 seconds.

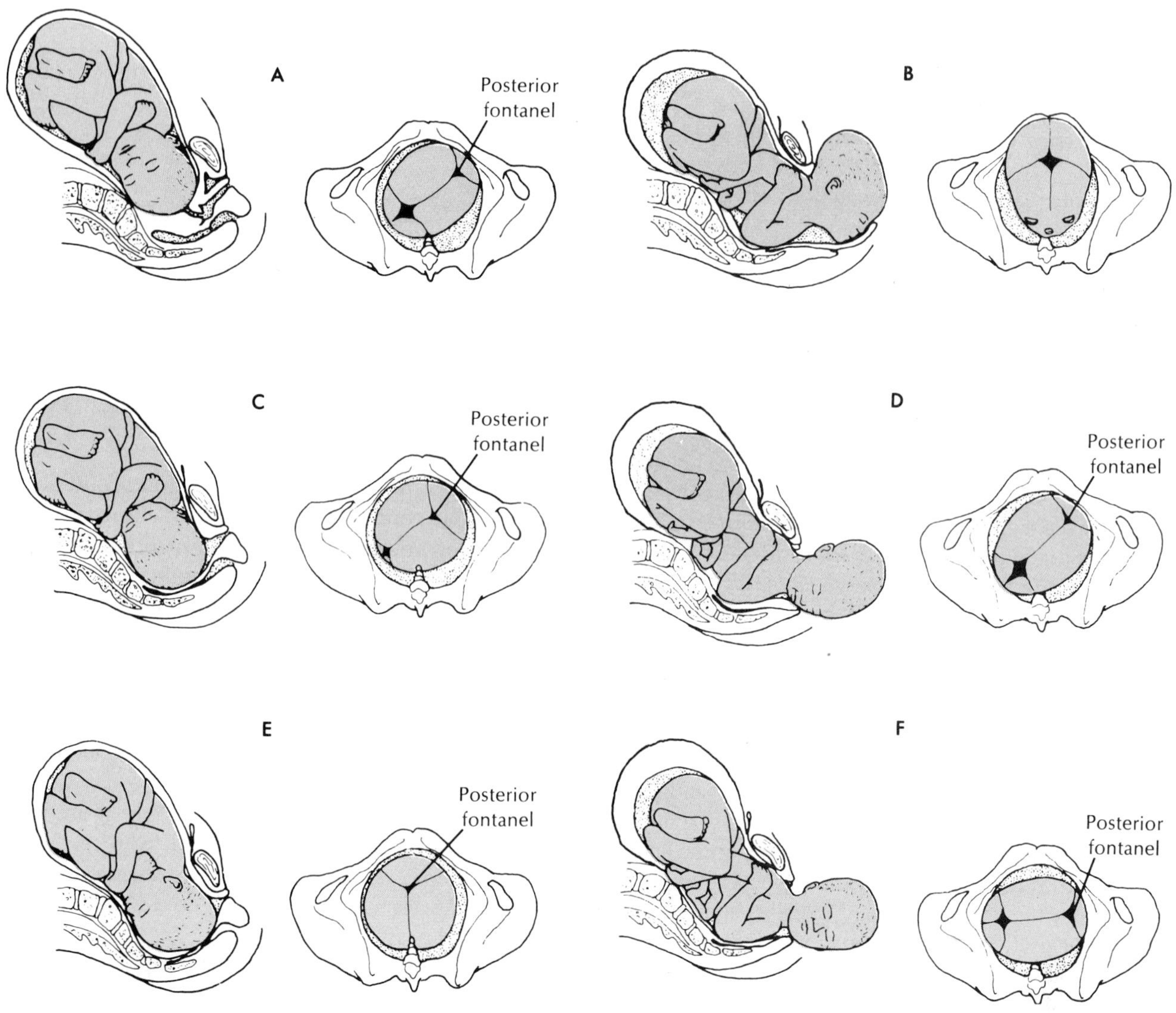

FIG. 43-10 Mechanism of labor in left occipitoanterior (LOA) presentation. **A,** Engagement and descent. **B,** Flexion. **C,** Internal rotation to OA. **D,** Extension. **E,** Restitution. **F,** External rotation.

This is a time of deep focus in which the woman may not wish to communicate with the nurse or significant other. If the woman has not requested pain medication earlier, she may desire it at this time. Many women experience nausea.

The second stage: delivery. The second stage begins with complete dilation at 10 cm and ends with the birth of the baby. The average length of this stage is 30 minutes to 2 hours in nulliparas and 20 minutes to 90 minutes in multiparas. Contractions continue to last 80 to 90 seconds but may be slightly less frequent.

Once the cervix is completely dilated, the woman is able to use the voluntary forces previously described. Generally, the woman feels the urge to push and is anxious to do so. Pushing is hard work, and the woman requires ongoing encouragement from the coach and nurse. Resting between contractions, if possible, is important to conserve energy.

During this stage the physician may provide anesthesia and perform an episiotomy. The episiotomy is a surgical incision of the perineum that allows easier delivery. The most common type of episiotomy is a midline incision in which the tissues of the perineum are separated at an anatomical junction. If the perineum is too small, the physician may perform a mediolateral incision in which muscle must be cut. This is generally more uncomfortable and is only done when necessary.

Immediately after delivery the baby's airway is established and the umbilical cord is clamped with two clamps and then severed between the clamps. If everything is normal, the baby is shown to the parents. The infant then either may be given to the mother to hold or may be positioned in a special warming unit that allows for close observation and care. If any problems occur with the infant, care is administered immediately. This emergency care may, of necessity, be performed in the delivery area.

The nurse should remain calm and supportive to the parents. The nurse should be aware that the parents may be alarmed and require support and explanations to allay their fears for the newborn.

The third stage: delivery of the placenta. The third stage begins with the delivery of the infant and ends with the delivery of the placenta. The average for both primiparas and multiparas is 5 to 20 minutes.

Generally speaking, the mother is less interested in the third stage. Focus and attention is usually directed to the newborn. Many women wish to inspect and possibly breast-feed the infant. When the placenta detaches from the uterine wall, a sudden outpouring of blood appears from the vagina. The cord protruding from the vagina lengthens, and the shape of the uterus becomes more rounded and firm. The woman may again experience contractions. The size and consistency of the placenta usually permit delivery with one or two pushes. Some women are curious to see the placenta; if so, it should be shown to them. During this time the physician repairs the episiotomy if one was performed. Total blood loss is normally from 200 to 300 ml; it is considered excessive if more than 500 ml of blood is lost during delivery. It is common for an **oxytocic** medication, such as Pitocin or Methergine, to be administered during this stage. These medications will cause the uterus to contract firmly. This causes compression of blood vessels inside the uterus and minimizes blood loss.

The fourth stage: stabilization. The time immediately after delivery is critical as the mother's body attempts to recover from the efforts of labor. Usually the mother is monitored closely for 2 to 4 hours after delivery in the birthing room or in a recovery room. Some women, particularly those who had a long or difficult labor and delivery, are exhausted and wish only to rest. Others appear to be euphoric and wish to talk about the experience or spend more time with the baby and their significant other.

It is important to monitor physiological changes closely during the fourth stage. Vital signs, uterine tone, vaginal drainage, and the perineal tissue are assessed. During the first hour assessments are done every 15 minutes. If observations are within normal limits, assessments are done every 30 minutes for the next hour. If all observations remain normal, the woman is transferred to a patient room for the remainder of her hospitalization.

Response of the newborn to birth. The process of delivery is stressful to the newborn. Rapid adaptation from the intrauterine climate to that of extrauterine life is essential if the newborn is to survive.

The physical condition of newborn infants is evaluated at birth. An evaluation guide called the Apgar score is used in most facilities (Table 43-3). This scoring is done at 1 and 5 minutes of age. The score can range from 0 to 10. The criteria used include heart rate, respiratory effort, muscle tone, reflex irritability, and skin color. A low score indicates serious problems that may require resuscitation. A high score indicates good condition, requiring only routine care.

Table 43-3 Apgar Scoring Chart

Sign	0	1	2
Heart rate	Absent	Slow—below 100	Above 100
Respiratory effort	Absent	Slow—irregular	Good crying
Muscle tone	Flaccid	Some flexion of extremities	Active motion
Reflex irritability	None	Grimace	Vigorous cry
Color	Pale blue	Body pink, extremities blue	Completely pink

Breathing must be established. In utero, the fetus's need for oxygen was met by the mother. Once the umbilical cord is severed, the newborn must breathe to obtain oxygen. Fetal lungs must be adequately mature so the alveoli can expand adequately. A substance called **surfactant** is produced that decreases surface tension within the alveoli and permits inflation. At the time of delivery a combination of chemical, thermal, tactile, and mechanical changes initiate the first breath.

The airway must be cleared of fluids that are present in the lungs. Some fluids are forced from the lungs as the thorax passes through the pelvis during delivery. A bulb syringe is used to remove excess fluid from the mouth and nasopharynx.

Warmth is necessary to prevent a rapid drop in body temperature. The environment in utero was approximately 99° F; the external environment in the delivery room is usually about 70° F. To prevent hypothermia the infant should be dried immediately to help reduce heat loss from evaporation. The baby then may be placed in contact with the mother's skin if she wishes to breast-feed, or the baby may be transferred to a radiant warming unit.

If there are no complications, the infant remains in view of the mother until her care is completed. Identification bracelets are placed on both mother and baby before they leave the delivery room. These will be used to verify infant identification and match it with that of the mother until discharge. Footprinting of the infant is another method of identification; this may be done in the delivery area or in the nursery.

NURSING ASSESSMENT AND INTERVENTIONS

Health Perception and Health Management

It is important to know how well prepared for childbirth the woman is; the woman who has attended classes and practiced breathing techniques will require a different level of explanation and support than one who has had no preparation.

If a hospital delivery is planned, admission is generally prearranged and much of the paperwork completed ahead of time to minimize delays. If home delivery is anticipated, the family should follow whatever directions the physician or midwife has given them.

When hospitalization is anticipated, it is a good idea for the prospective parents to prepare a suitcase with necessary items well in advance of the date of delivery. Making a "trial run" to the hospital also provides reassurance. This can reduce fears of not getting to the hospital on time. If there are children at home, plans should be made for their care. It is advisable that the parents-to-be anticipate as many problems as possible and make several alternative plans.

On admission an assessment begins. This typically includes the following:

1. Review of the prenatal record, including general medical history, past obstetrical history, and the history of this current pregnancy. This should include information about allergies and any current health problems, such as respiratory or other types of infection.
2. The mother is interviewed to gather information about signs and symptoms of the onset of labor, such as the nature and frequency of contractions; level of discomfort; and the presence of vaginal discharge such as bloody show or loss of amniotic fluid. If these data indicate that the woman is in labor, information regarding the type of preparation for childbirth, support person present, special cultural practices or expectations, type of anesthesia planned, method of infant feeding desired, and name of pediatrician are also obtained.
3. A physical examination is done, including a complete set of vital signs and fetal heart tones. These data will function as a baseline for further assessment. Heart and lung sounds are auscultated. The face, hands, legs, and sacrum are inspected for signs of edema. The abdomen is palpated to determine the fetal lie and presentation. The status of the membranes is assessed. If there is any question regarding ruptured membranes, a nitrazine test should be performed before the vaginal examination, since solutions used may make the test results unreliable. Contractions are timed to determine frequency, regularity, duration, and intensity. A vaginal examination is performed to determine the progress of labor, including position, dilation, effacement, and station.
4. Diagnostic tests include a urinalysis to check for the presence of glucose, protein, or ketones, which may indicate potential complications. If blood analyses were not performed during pregnancy, they should be done at this time. Information about hemoglobin and hematocrit levels, blood type and Rh factor, antibody titer, and screening for sexually transmitted diseases helps in assessment of actual or potential problems.

Nutritional and Metabolic Pattern

Gastrointestinal motility and absorption decrease during labor and delivery. Food eaten before labor may remain in the digestive tract and lead to complaints of nausea and vomiting. Once active labor begins, solid foods are generally withheld. It is important to know when food was last consumed in case administration of a general anesthetic becomes necessary. In addition, fluid intake should be assessed. Increased physical exertion and mouth breathing are common during labor. When these factors are combined with restricted oral intake, a fluid deficit may result. Some physicians allow small amounts of ice chips or clear beverages during labor. Orders for intravenous fluids, such as a 5% dextrose solution, to prevent fluid balance problems are common.

Elimination

Depending on the amount of fluid intake, urine output may be normal or decreased. Voiding every 2 hours is desirable. A full bladder can interfere with the progress of labor. When membranes are intact, use of the toilet is permitted. Once membranes are ruptured, use of the bedpan is preferred. If the presenting part is compressing the urethra, catheterization may be ordered.

Bowel elimination is assessed. Some women experience diarrhea with the onset of labor. Careful hygiene technique is important to reduce the possibility of contamination. Enemas were once routinely administered to empty the colon and maximize space in the pelvic cavity; today they are given only when specifically ordered. Large-volume enemas are sometimes used to stimulate or strengthen labor. Enemas *should not be given* if there is vaginal bleeding or premature labor, if the presenting part is not engaged, or if there is other than a vertex presentation. If membranes are ruptured, the enema should be expelled into a bedpan.

The urge to defecate during labor may indicate the start of the second stage of labor. Before allowing a woman to attempt to have a bowel movement, it is wise to inspect the perineum and assess dilation.

Activity/Exercise

Ambulation is generally encouraged so long as the membranes are not ruptured. Ambulation may also be permitted if the membranes have ruptured and the presenting part is fully engaged. Walking provides distraction and tends to strengthen the effectiveness of labor.

When ambulation becomes too uncomfortable, or if the mother has been given analgesics, she usually is encouraged to rest. Positioning becomes important; the woman should be encouraged to assume the position most comfortable for her. Sitting or semiseated positions are preferred by some women. Low back pain is common. A side-lying position is frequently more comfortable than supine. Changing position may help reduce discomfort. Side-lying positions reduce pressure on the vena cava. The left side is recommended if the fetal heart rate shows late deceleration or if the woman experiences hypotension. The Trendelenburg position is used if prolapse of the cord is suspected.

Sexuality/Reproductive

Assessment of vaginal drainage continues through labor. If not observed sooner, bloody show may be seen. Moderate amounts of discharge are common, and linens should be changed to provide comfort. Any bright red bleeding should be reported immediately.

Vaginal examination to assess the progress of labor continues through the first stage of labor. Contractions are monitored for frequency, duration, and intensity.

Coping/Stress Tolerance

Fears become apparent during labor and delivery, particularly in the primigravida. Many women have unrealistic expectations for themselves and feel that they should be able to be in control of labor. Controlled breathing techniques help, but the involuntary nature of labor troubles many women. Encouragement and support in breathing exercises, along with explanations regarding the progress of labor, are helpful. Fatigue and pain lower the woman's ability to cope. It is important to understand the cultural and religious background of each woman, since these factors may strongly influence her behavior.

The nurse should pay attention to the reaction of the support person. It is important to recognize that many times the woman's significant other will experience fears and anxieties. The father particularly may exhibit concerns about the process of labor and the pain the mother is experiencing. At times fathers will express guilt about their role, either in not being able to help enough or in being responsible for the pregnancy. It is important to tell the father that he is an important participant, not an unwanted guest in the process of childbirth. He should be encouraged to help make the woman comfortable and provide the companionship and caring needed.

Role/Relationship

Many women wish their spouse or a significant other to be with them during labor and delivery. Most childbirth education programs include this individual in the preparation. Often this person works as the "coach" to remind the woman of breathing techniques and provide encouragement.

In some situations this is not the case, and the woman faces labor and delivery alone. This may be at her request, or it may be a matter of circumstances. If she is alone, the nursing staff must provide extra support. Many other individuals, such as grandparents, siblings, and extended family, may be interested in the progress of labor. Depending on the situation, the nurse should try to pay attention to the needs of these family members.

Self-Perception

The prepared mother generally feels more able to deal with labor and delivery than the unprepared one. Multigravidas generally have more confidence, since they have previous experience to draw on. Women who have experienced problems during pregnancy or in past labors and deliveries may need reassurance that they can be successful. The nurse should continue to be supportive. Even an unprepared woman can participate in simple breathing exercises with coaching from the nurse.

Cognitive/Perceptual

Pain is a major concern during labor and delivery. Breathing exercises help reduce discomfort, but as the intensity of labor increases, most women require some form of analgesia and/or anesthesia. The physician will prescribe these medications with caution, because they pass through the placenta and affect the fetus. Timing is critical to prevent diminished or depressed respiratory effort at the time of birth. The condition of the mother and fetus must be carefully assessed before and after medication administration.

The most commonly used analgesics are meperidine HCl (Demerol) and butorphanol tartrate (Stadol), which may be given intramuscularly or intravenously. Antianxiety medications such as hydroxyzine HCl (Vistaril) and diazepam (Valium) may be administered to reduce apprehension and anxiety. These medications also potentiate the effects of narcotics. Occasionally, sedative/hypnotics such as pentobarbital (Nembutal) and secobarbital (Seconal) are given in early labor to promote relaxation and rest.

The form of anesthesia used will depend on the patient's wishes and physician's assessment of maternal and fetal need. Anesthetics are classified as general, regional, and local. Most vaginal deliveries today include some form of regional anesthetic (Fig. 43-11). Regional anesthetics include paracervical, epidural, spinal, and pudendal blocks (Table 43-4).

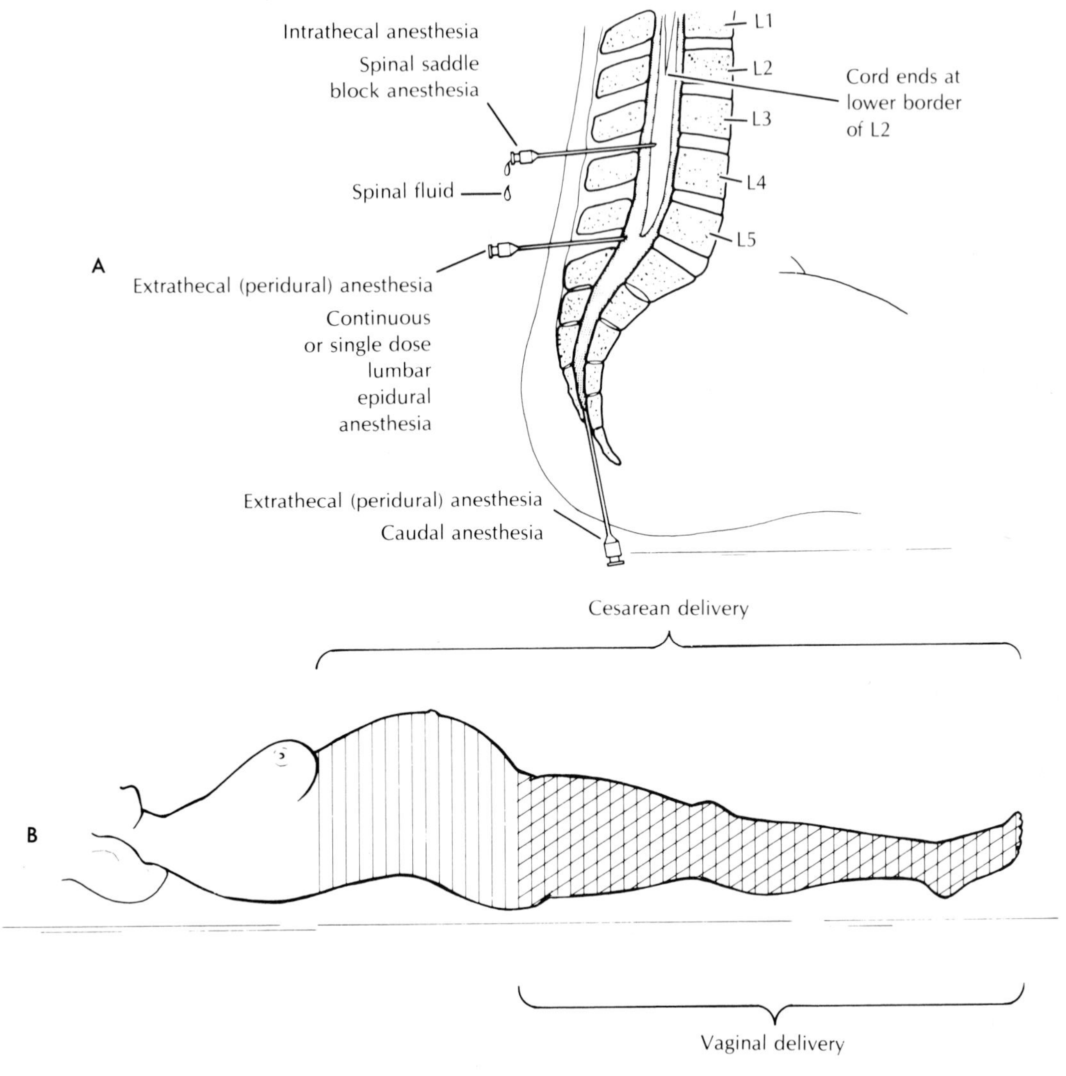

FIG. 43-11 **A,** Regional anesthesia in obstetrics. **B,** Level of anesthesia necessary for cesarean delivery and for vaginal delivery. (Courtesy Ross Laboratories, Columbus, Ohio.)

Table 43-4 Anesthesia for Labor and Delivery

Type of Anesthesia	Usual Dosage	Administration	Area Anesthetized or Effects	Possible Side Effects: Mother	Possible Side Effects: Fetus	Nursing Interventions After Administration
REGIONAL						
Paracervical block	5-10 ml of 1% solution of a "caine" drug	Injection, either side of cervix at 4 cm dilation	Cervix and uterus	Can slow labor	30% incidence of temporary slowing of fetal heart	Close monitoring of fetal heart tones and maternal vital signs and contractions
Pudendal block	5-10 ml of 1% solution of a "caine" drug	Injection into area of pudendal nerves for birth	Perineum	None unless allergic to drug	None	Reassurance and explanation; monitor fetal heart tones and maternal vital signs closely
Caudal and lumbar epidural	5-15 ml of 1%, 1.5%, or 2% solution of a "caine" drug	Caudal canal Epidural space at 4 cm dilation	Pelvic region	Hypotension; cannot "push" for delivery May slow labor if started too early	Slowing of fetal heart and fetal heart decelerates	Monitor fetal heart tones and maternal vital signs closely; use excellent aseptic techniques
Saddle block (low spinal)	1-1.5 ml of solution concentration depends on "caine" drug used	Injection under dura of spinal cord for birth	Pelvic region	Postspinal headache Hypotension	None	Intravenous and O_2 usually used
GENERAL INHALATION						
Nitrous oxide Ethylene Cyclopropane Ether Or other similar agents		Inhaled through mask	Complete body	Could aspirate if vomits	Respiratory depression; hypoxia	Be alert and prepared for vomiting (with aspiration of food) and excessive uterine bleeding owing to uterine relaxation
INHALANT ANALGESIA						
Methoxyflurane (Penthrane)	0.3% to 0.5% in first stage or at time of delivery	Volatile inhalant	Relieves pain	Hypotension; slow shallow respirations	Hypoxia and central nervous system depression	Inform woman of what she will experience. Allow her to administer as needed. Do not hold mask for her. Check vital signs frequently.
Trichloroethylene (Trilene)	0.5% in first stage or at time of delivery			Irregular pulse; rapid respiration		

Value/Belief

Cultural beliefs and practices have implications for labor and delivery, as they do in all aspects of life. The values and beliefs of women in labor should be respected. The nurse should seek information about specific cultural practices, values, and beliefs and incorporate these in the plan of care.

MEDICAL INTERVENTIONS

Although labor and delivery are essentially normal processes, sometimes complications arise. At times it becomes necessary for the physician to intervene to protect the mother or fetus.

Induction

As already discussed, the exact cause of labor is unknown. Induction is an attempt to start labor at a time other than when it begins spontaneously. This intervention may be necessary when membranes are ruptured more than 24 hours, in cases of severe pregnancy-induced hypertension, or in a postterm pregnancy. Occasionally an elective induction is performed when the woman has a history of precipitous (lasting under 3 hours) labors. This is done to prevent an emergency out-of-hospital delivery.

The physician assesses each woman carefully to determine that she is a good candidate for induction and that no harm will come to either mother or fetus.

The medically approved methods of inducing labor include the following:

1. Amniotomy: If the amniotic membranes have not ruptured, the physician may use a sterile hook to open the sac and allow drainage of the fluid; this procedure is called an **amniotomy.** Fetal heart rate is measured immediately before and after this procedure. The amount and color of amniotic fluid are assessed. If all criteria for induction were met, labor typically starts within 6 to 8 hours.
2. Prostaglandin (PGE) gel application: After assessment of the mother and fetus, the physician applies PGE gel intracervically using a plastic catheter. Contractions normally begin within an hour of instillation of the gel. Vital signs, fetal heart rate (FHR), and contractions are monitored carefully. It is common for an amniotomy to be performed in conjunction with the gel application. An internal fetal monitor is also routinely applied when PGE gel is used.
3. Oxytocin stimulation: Use of oxytocin is indicated to induce labor or to stimulate a labor that is not making adequate progress because of generalized inactivity, which is known as **uterine inertia.** A dilute form of the medication is administered intravenously. Pitocin is most commonly used, although Syntocinon, a synthetic form of oxytocin, is occasionally used. These medications are very powerful and are started by the physician or a specially trained nurse, if hospital policies permit. The RN may then monitor the progress of labor. Since the contractions that result from oxytocin can be very strong, it is essential to monitor the FHR and contractions really carefully and document care. The oxytocin infusion is stopped and the physician contacted if there are any signs of complications, such as changes in fetal heart rate, bradycardia, tachycardia, dysrhythmias, or excessive frequency, duration, or pressure of contractions.

Forceps Delivery

Forceps are a pair of spoonlike devices that fit around the fetal head to aid in expulsion of the fetus (Fig. 43-12). As with induction, there are certain criteria that must be met before the physician uses forceps. The nurse assisting in the delivery is responsible for providing the type of forceps requested by the physician. Close moni-

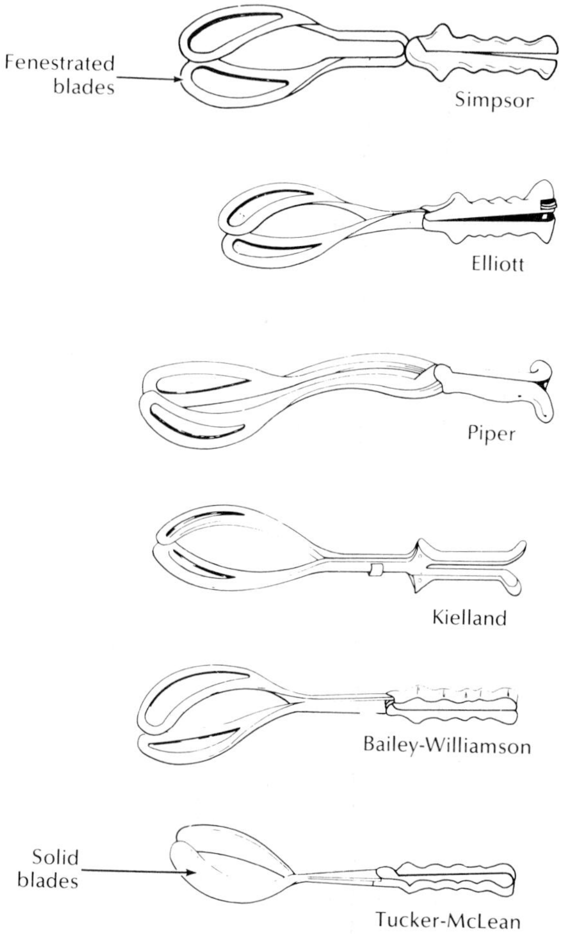

FIG. 43-12 Types of forceps.

Table 43-5 Nursing Process and the Patient in Labor

Pattern	Data Collection	Possible Nursing Diagnoses	Interventions
Health management	Does the woman appear prepared for labor and delivery? Has she taken prenatal classes? Has she received routine prenatal care? What if any unusual/untoward symptoms does she present? What is the status of fetal membranes?	Potential for injury Noncompliance Knowledge deficit	Assess level of knowledge and previous experiences. Provide emotional support. Provide explanations.
Nutritional/ metabolic	When was her last meal? What was consumed? Any nausea or vomiting? Any edema noted?	Altered nutrition: less than body requirement Fluid volume excess Fluid volume deficit	Initiate oral hygiene and comfort measures, ice chips if permitted. Monitor intravenous fluids if ordered.
Activity/ exercise	What is the status of fetal membranes? What is fetal heart rate? Fetal movement? Vital signs?	Potential for injury Activity intolerance	Encourage ambulation if fetal membranes intact. Use safety precautions if medicated for pain. Monitor FHR and vital signs.
Elimination	When was last bowel movement? Amount and consistency? What is pattern of urine elimination?	Constipation Altered patterns of urinary elimination Potential for infection	Administer enemas if ordered. Encourage voiding at regular intervals. Check frequency of voiding; check bladder for retention.
Rest/sleep	How long has she been in labor? How well has she slept recently?	Sleep pattern disturbance	Assist with positioning for optimal comfort. Encourage rest between contractions.
Cognitive/ perceptual	Is she knowledgeable of breathing techniques? What is level of pain? Duration? Location? How frequent are contractions?	Potential for injury Knowledge deficit	Review breathing techniques; explain and coach if untrained. Administer analgesics as ordered. Provide calm environment.
Role relationship	Who has accompanied to hospital? How interested/involved is this person?	Altered role performance Altered family processes	Listen; involve significant others in teaching. Possible social service contact if serious problems with dynamics observed.
Coping/stress	What fears or anxieties are verbalized?	Anxiety Fear Ineffective coping	Listen; provide explanations at patient's level of understanding. Provide written materials.
Value/belief	What is the patient's cultural background? What are her religious practices?	Spiritual distress	Incorporate cultural practices into care whenever possible. Consult minister, priest, rabbi for specific information if needed.

toring of the FHR before and during the forceps maneuvers is essential. It is also important to explain to the mother that these actions will not harm the baby.

Cesarean Delivery

Cesarean birth, also referred to as a *c-section,* is delivery through an abdominal and uterine incision. This type of delivery may be anticipated in advance or may be performed in cases of emergency. The number of cesarean deliveries has increased greatly during the last 20 years. Although there is concern in the medical community and the media about this trend, approximately 20% of deliveries continue to take place by the cesarean route.

Indications for cesarean birth can be maternal or fetal. The major maternal indications for cesarean delivery are (1) **fetopelvic disproportion,** in which the fetus is unable to pass through the maternal pelvis, (2) previous cesarean delivery, (3) breech presentation, (4) medical conditions that would endanger the mother's health, such as cardiac complications, (5) abnormal conditions of the placenta, such as placenta previa, (6) infections of the vaginal canal, and (7) pelvic abnormalities. The major fetal indicators are (1) fetal oxygen deprivation (hypoxia), (2) prolapse of the umbilical cord, (3) breech presentation, (4) malpresentations, such as transverse, and (5) other congenital anomalies. These conditions will be discussed in greater depth in Chapter 45.

Current medical practice is rethinking at least one of these criteria. The old rule was "once a cesarean, always a cesarean." Today many women who have previously delivered by c-section are candidates for vaginal birth after cesarean (VBAC). Depending on the woman's medical history, the nature of this pregnancy, and the reason for the earlier c-section, the physician may permit a trial labor. In these cases the woman must be very carefully monitored, and the facility must be prepared to perform an emergency cesarean if complications arise.

When a cesarean delivery is performed, incisions are made both in the abdominal wall and in the uterine wall. Depending on the technique used by the physician, different incisions may be employed.

Postpartum care of the woman experiencing cesarean delivery will be discussed in Chapter 44.

NURSING PROCESS SUMMARY

Table 43-5 offers guidelines for reviewing all health patterns to help the nurse focus observations when performing an assessment on a woman in labor. Significant observations or responses will indicate the need for further questioning. If the nurse is unsure of the significance of data it is important to consult with a more experienced nurse.

Table 43-5 also suggests possible diagnoses and interventions.

REFERENCES AND SUGGESTED READINGS

1. Bobak IM and Jensen MD: Essentials of maternity nursing, St Louis, 1991, The CV Mosby Co.
2. Burroughs A: Bleir's maternity nursing, ed 5, Philadelphia, 1986, WB Saunders Co.
3. Chute GE: Expectation and experience in alternative and conventional birth, JOGNN 14:61, 1985.
4. Doenges M and Moorhouse M: Nurse's pocket guide to nursing diagnosis with interventions, ed 2, Philadelphia, 1988, FA Davis Co.
5. Fischbach F: A manual of laboratory diagnostic tests, ed 3, Philadelphia, 1988, JB Lippincott Co.
6. Glazer G and Hulme A: Prostaglandin gel for cervical ripening, MCN 12:28, 1987.
7. Ingalls AJ and Salerno, MC: Maternal and child health nursing, ed 7, St Louis, 1990, The CV Mosby Co.
8. Jaffe MS and Melson KA: Maternal-infant health care plans, Springhouse, Pa, 1989, Springhouse Corp.
9. Ladewig PW, London ML and Olds SB: Essentials of maternal-newborn nursing, ed 2, Redwood City, Calif, 1990, Addison-Wesley.
10. Ladewig PW, London ML, and Olds SB: Maternal newborn nursing: a family-centered approach, ed 3, Menlo Park, Calif, 1988, Addison-Wesley.
11. Malestic SL: Don't these patients have a right to privacy, RN 53:3, 1989.
12. McKay S and Roberts J: Second stage of labor: what is normal? JOGNN 14:101, 1985.
13. OGN Nursing Practice Resource: The nurse's role in the induction/augmentation of labor, Washington DC, 1988, NAACOG.
14. Pillitteri A: Maternal-newborn nursing: care of the growing family, ed 3, Boston, 1985, Little, Brown & Co.
15. Pritchard JA, MacDonald PC, and Gant GF: Williams' obstetrics, ed 17, New York, 1985, Appleton-Century-Crofts.
16. Romond JL and Baker IT: Squatting in childbirth, JOGNN 14:406, 1985.

CHAPTER CHALLENGE

KEY POINTS

- Although various theories are proposed, the process that starts labor has not been determined.
- True labor and false labor can be confusing to the patient and health care personnel; even knowledgeable individuals can be mistaken.
- The birth process can occur in a variety of settings. The most important concern is protecting the welfare of both the mother and newborn.
- Vaginal delivery involves a complex interrelationship of the passageway, the passenger, and the powers.
- The first stage of labor is usually the longest stage. There are significant risks to both mother and fetus during this time; therefore both the mother and fetus must be carefully and continuously assessed.
- The fourth stage of labor, the time of stabilization, requires careful nursing assessment of the mother. Assessment of vital signs and fundal checks are essential to detect excessive blood loss.
- The process of delivery is stressful to the newborn. The Apgar scoring system is used 1 and 5 minutes after birth to assess the newborn's condition.
- Modification of functional health patterns occurs during labor and delivery. The nurse should assess all areas to detect problems quickly and report these promptly.
- In some cases the physician may have to intervene in the process of labor and delivery and use forceps or surgical means to deliver a healthy newborn.

STUDY QUESTIONS

1. The onset of labor is caused by:
   a. Excessive stretching of the uterus
   b. A decrease in progesterone
   c. An increase in estrogen
   d. Factors unknown at this time
2. A sign indicating that labor is near would be:
   a. Sudden, sharp pain in the lower abdomen
   b. Increased urination
   c. Increased discharge of pink-tinged mucus
   d. Production of colostrum
3. Regular contractions that increase in intensity and get stronger with ambulation indicate:
   a. True labor
   b. False labor
4. The best place for delivery is:
   a. The traditional hospital
   b. The home
   c. An alternative birthing center
   d. The one agreed on by the mother and physician
5. Complete dilation occurs when:
   a. The fetal head is visible on the perineal floor
   b. The presenting part is engaged in the pelvis
   c. The cervix is 10 cm
   d. The patient wishes to push
6. The patient has experienced a sudden change of behavior and tells everyone to leave her alone. She is probably in:
   a. Early stage one of labor
   b. Transition stage of labor
   c. Stage two of labor
   d. Stage three of labor
7. When membranes rupture before the onset of labor, the physician will observe the patient for:
   a. Signs of infection
   b. Possible prolapse of the cord
   c. Onset of active labor
   d. All of the above
8. The patient in labor is not fed during labor because:
   a. She may vomit and aspirate
   b. General/inhalation anesthetic cannot be given
   c. Digestion and peristalsis decrease when labor starts
   d. This will elevate the level of discomfort
9. An episiotomy may be performed:
   a. During stage one to hasten labor
   b. During stage one to prevent trauma to the fetus
   c. During stage two to prevent trauma to the perineum
   d. During stage three to facilitate delivery of the placenta
10. Apgar scoring is done to:
    a. Assess the condition of the newborn
    b. Assess the condition of the mother
    c. Assess the progress of labor
    d. Assess the position of the fetus

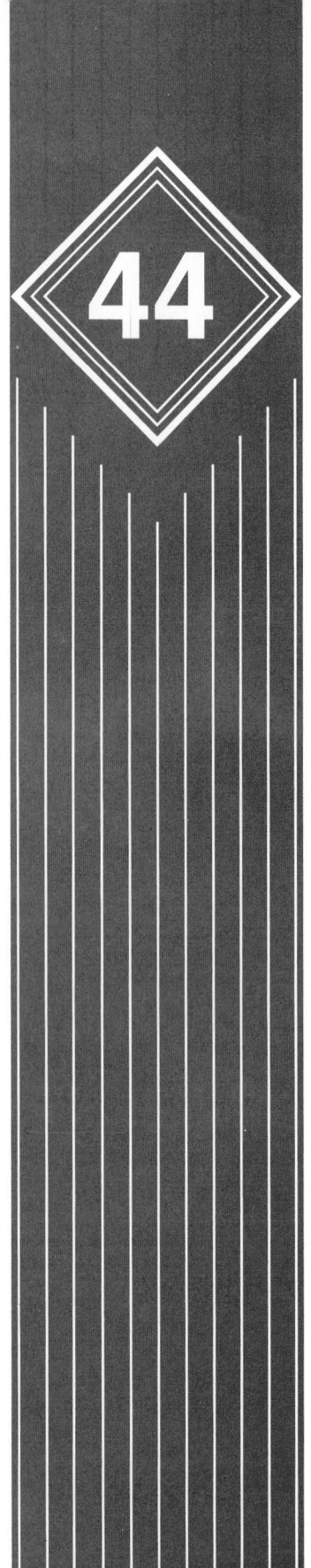

44

Care of the Mother and Newborn

GLORIA E. WOLD

LEARNING OBJECTIVES

After reading this chapter, the student should be able to do the following:

- Define the key terms.
- Describe postpartum assessment of the mother.
- Identify the physiological changes that occur in the postpartum period.
- Discuss the nursing responsibilities during the postpartum period.
- Explain the importance of teaching personal and infant care.
- Discuss the psychosocial adaptations that occur during the postpartum period.
- Describe the assessment of the normal newborn.
- Identify the physical characteristics of the normal newborn.
- Identify normal reflexes observed in the newborn.
- Describe common variations that may be observed in the newborn.
- Discuss nutritional needs and feeding of the newborn.

RELATED TOPICS OF INTEREST

- The family (Chapter 7)
- Diet therapy (Chapter 23)
- Care of the patient with a cardiovascular disorder (Chapter 32)
- Care of the patient with a urinary disorder (Chapter 33)

KEY TERMS

Define the following:

- acrocyanosis
- bonding
- colostrum
- engorgement
- harlequin sign
- lactation
- lochia
- meconium
- physiological jaundice
- puerperium
- vernix caseosa

The postpartum period, also called the **puerperium,** lasts from the time the woman delivers until the reproductive organs return to approximately the nonpregnant size and position. This consists of two stages. The immediate postpartum period, lasting up to 6 hours after delivery, is sometimes called the *fourth stage of labor* or the recovery stage. During this time the newly delivered mother requires special care and attention after the rigors of delivery. This is a time for close observation and assessment to ensure that no problems occur. The later postpartum stage follows the stage of recovery and lasts until about 6 weeks after delivery.

During the postpartum period the mother's body makes rapid physiological adaptations. The anatomical and physiological changes that took place over 9 months must reverse within just 6 weeks. Many psychological changes also occur as the woman and her family adjust to the new family member or members. (Fig. 44-1).

ANATOMICAL AND PHYSIOLOGICAL CHANGES

Uterus

After the birth of the baby and delivery of the placenta, the uterus contracts in response to oxytocin. This contraction compresses blood vessels at the site where the placenta separated from the uterine wall. This site, an area 8 to 10 cm (3 to 4 inches) in diameter, has open venous sinuses. If the uterus does not contract adequately, blood loss can be excessive. The placental site will heal by the process of exfoliation, in which necrotic tissue is sloughed from the uterine lining, leaving a fresh layer of endometrial tissue free from scars. This process is necessary if successive pregnancies are to occur.

Immediately after delivery the uterus can be felt at about the level of the umbilicus. It is the size of a small melon and weighs approximately 1000 g (2 pounds). Within a week it will be barely palpable at the level of the symphysis pubis and will have decreased in size to about 500 g (1 pound). Within 6 weeks the uterus will again be a pelvic organ approximately the nonpregnant size of 50 g (2 ounces). This decrease in size is called *involution.*

Involution is carried out by a process called *autolysis.* Autolysis is a result of sudden withdrawal of estrogen and progesterone. This sudden drop in hormone levels releases proteolytic enzymes into the endometrium; these enzymes cause the cells to lose protein materials and thereby shrink in size. The number of muscle cells remains the same, but the size of each cell changes dramatically.

The fluid waste discharged after delivery is called **lochia.** As the uterine lining is being shed, the necrotic tissue, blood, and mucus leave the body through the vagina. Lochia has a fleshy odor similar to menstrual discharge.

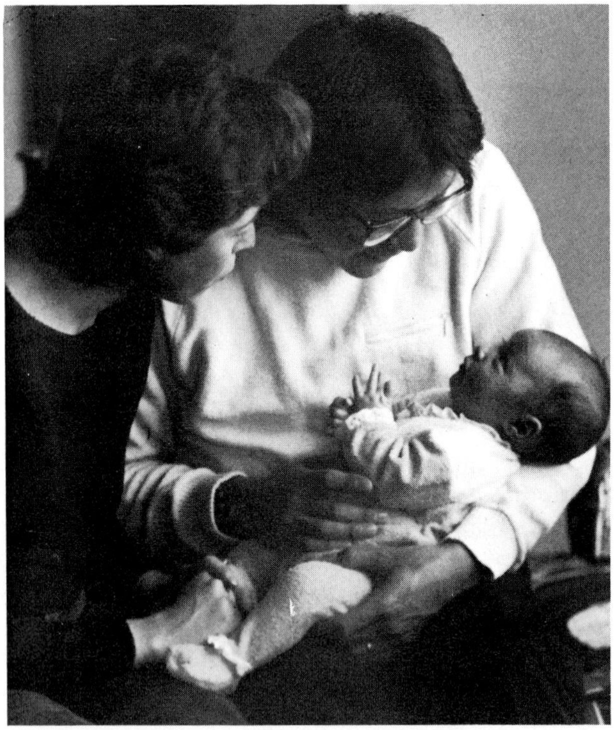

FIG. 44-1 Mother-father-baby interactions. (Courtesy Colleen Stainton.)

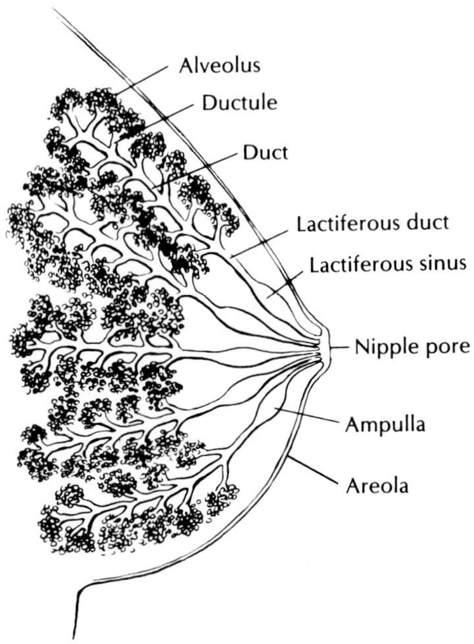

FIG. 44-2 Detailed structural features of human mammary gland.

Initially, the amount of blood content is greatest, resulting in a bright red drainage called *lochia rubra*. This is generally seen the first day or two after delivery. As healing of the placental site occurs, the discharge becomes a pink-to-brown color called lochia serosa. This generally occurs until the seventh day. After that the drainage is slightly yellow to white and is called *lochia alba*. This continues for another 10 days to 2 weeks. If fragments of the placenta remain in the uterus, the uterus will not be able to contract and seal blood vessels adequately. This can result in excessive blood loss and may require medical intervention. This will be discussed further in the area of complications.

Breasts

Breast changes begin to occur early in pregnancy. Increased amounts of estrogen stimulate enlargement of breast size as a result of increased adipose and fluid retention. Estrogen also stimulates the growth of the milk ducts to prepare for **lactation,** which is another term for the secretion of milk. Milk production is necessary if a woman plans to breast-feed her infant. This is a very basic yet complex process.

The first secretion produced by the breast is **colostrum.** This precursor to milk is thin, watery, and slightly yellow. It is rich in protein and low in sugar and fat. Colostrum may be produced as early as the last trimester of pregnancy, particularly in multigravidas. Its production continues for about 2 days after delivery, when true milk production begins.

Lactation is a combination of hormonal, neurological, and psychological responses. After delivery estrogen and progesterone levels drop rapidly. While the levels of estrogen and progesterone are diminishing, the level of prolactin is increasing. Prolactin, a hormone secreted by the anterior pituitary gland, is responsible for stimulating milk production in the mammary alveolar cells (Figs. 44-2 and 44-3, *A*). Stimulation of the nipples, particularly by the infant's sucking, causes the release of oxytocin from the posterior pituitary gland. Oxytocin stimulates contraction of the mammary ducts and causes the milk to be ejected from the breast. This cycle is called the *let-down reflex* (Fig. 44-3, *B*).

Embarrassment, fear of pain during breast-feeding, or lack of self-confidence in her ability to breast-feed may result in difficulty establishing the let-down reflex. In many women "let-down" also occurs during sexual orgasm. This may be troublesome if it is not expected.

Once lactation is established, the mother may feel a tingling or prickling sensation when feeding time approaches. If the mother nurses the baby at regular intervals and empties the breast, the supply of milk increases in response to the baby's demands. It is not uncommon for the breasts to become very full and uncomfortable when the milk supply initially comes in, since a combi-

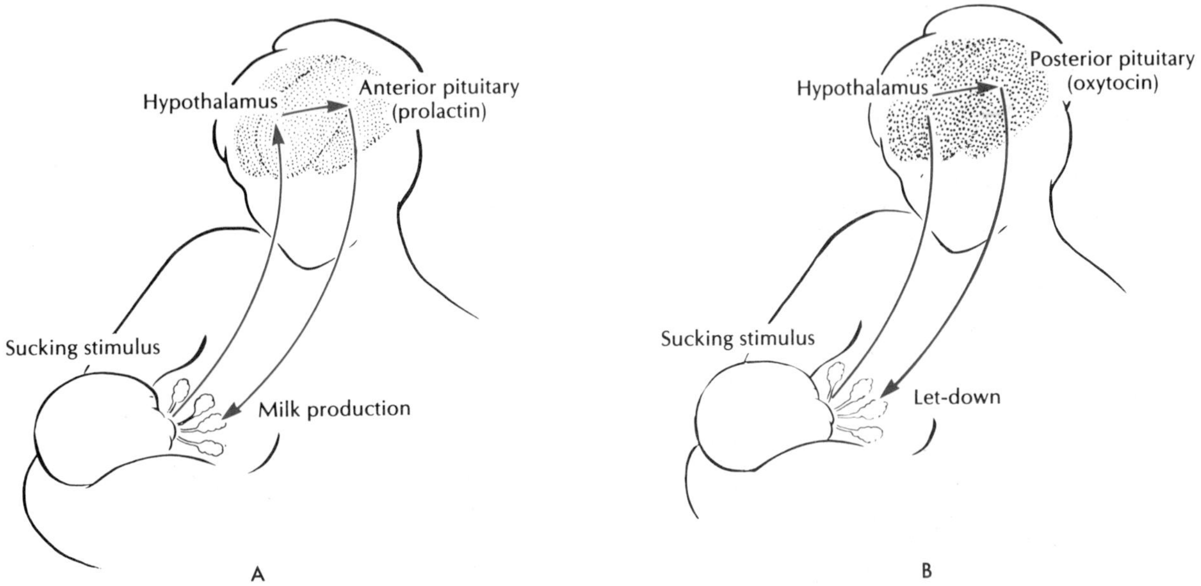

FIG. 44-3 Maternal breast-feeding reflexes. **A,** Milk production. **B,** Let-down.

nation of venous and lymphatic stasis also occurs during lactation. This fullness is called **engorgement.** Application of warm, moist washcloths to the breasts and nursing the baby more frequently usually resolve the problem. Once the supply is established, prolactin production decreases, and it is primarily oxytocin, released as the baby suckles, that maintains the supply of milk.

If the breast is not adequately stimulated, the lactation response may not be established. This can happen when the baby has a weak suck or is not put to breast often enough. If the breast is not emptied adequately, the pressure of the milk in the alveoli can also suppress milk production. Incorrect placement at breast may also lead to problems. If the baby's mouth grasps only the nipple and does not apply pressure on the lactiferous sinuses in the areola, milk will not be released and the needed stimulation will not occur. This also may lead to nipple trauma and soreness. The nurse should explain this to the new mother.

Two of the main causes for unsuccessful breast-feeding are lack of knowledge and poor self-confidence. Nurses can play an important role in supporting and encouraging the woman who wishes to breast-feed. To do this the nurse must be knowledgeable in correct techniques of breast-feeding. There are many good books available that can be useful when instructing a new mother; also many support groups such as LaLeche League provide information and encouragement (Figs. 44-4 and 44-5).

Breast-feeding has many benefits for the mother. One benefit is a more rapid involution of the uterus as a result of the release of oxytocin during breast-feeding, which stimulates contraction of the uterus. Another benefit is a lower incidence of breast cancer in women who have nursed for at least 3 months; several studies have validated this benefit. Also, many women who breast-feed report a special closeness to their infants, because they are providing a special and important nourishment.

Bottle-feeding is the choice of many other women. If the woman chooses not to breast-feed, lactation must be suppressed. This can be accomplished by use of medication or by mechanical means. The most commonly administered antilactogenic medication is bromocriptine mesylate (Parlodel), which suppresses prolactin secretion. This medication is started promptly after delivery and is taken twice daily for 14 to 21 days. If mechanical suppression is to be used, it must be started before milk production begins. This is accomplished by applying a supportive bra within 4 to 6 hours after delivery. Ice to the breasts will also decrease the discomfort that may result from engorgement. Any form of breast stimulation, such as pumping the breasts, should be avoided, and application of heat to the breasts should also be minimized, even when bathing. Maternal fluid intake should not be restricted.

NURSING ASSESSMENT AND INTERVENTIONS

Health Perception/Health Management

Women with uncomplicated deliveries remain in the hospital a short time after giving birth. It may be only a few hours or it may be 1 or 2 days after delivery when the woman and her baby are discharged. Even women who delivered by cesarean are rarely kept more than 5 to 7 days. This may be a result of financial concerns, type

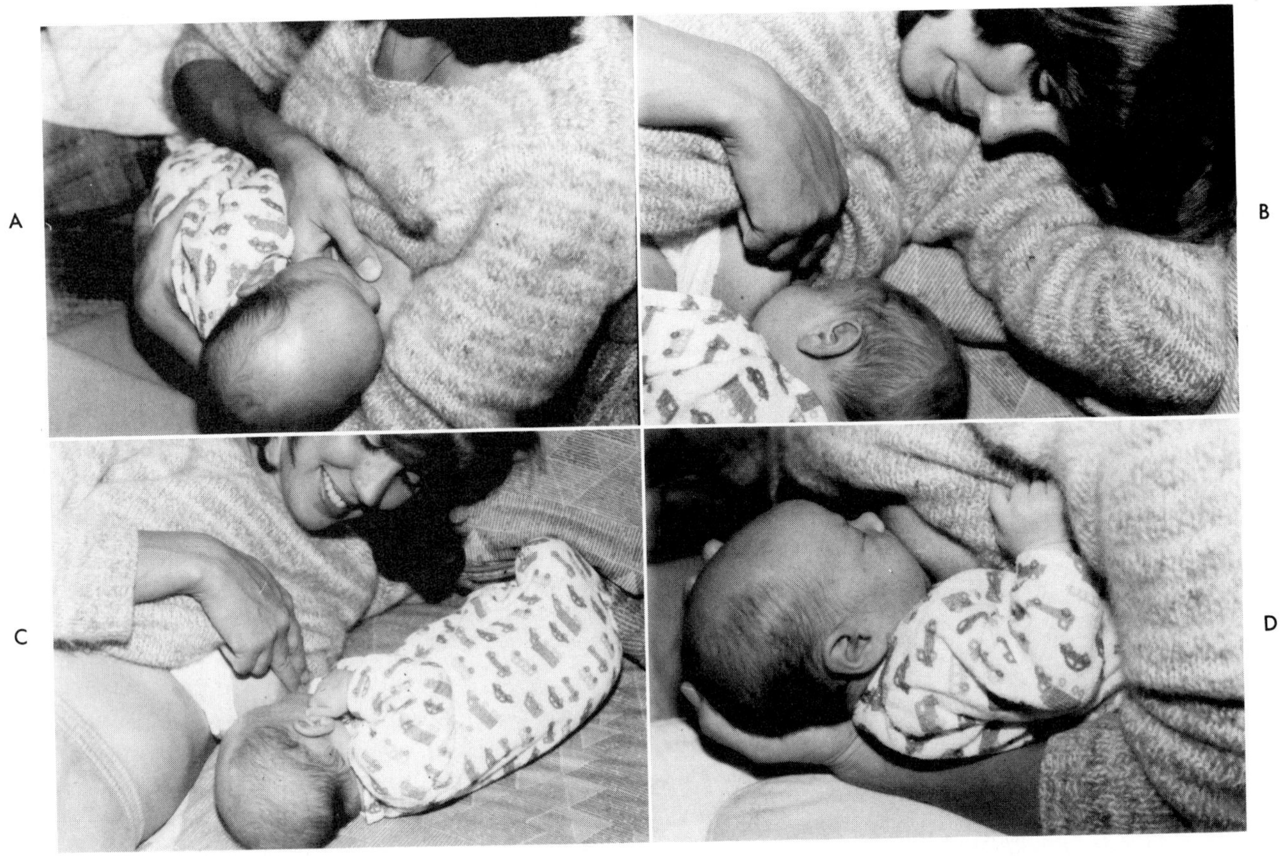

FIG. 44-4 Positioning the baby. **A,** Cradle hold. One arm and hand supports baby. Other hand supports breast (thumb above and fingers below). Breast is guided into baby's mouth. **B,** Side-lying position. Pillows support mother's head. Baby is turned toward mother. Mother depresses breast to facilitate baby's breathing. **C,** Variation on side-lying position. **D,** Football hold. Baby is held in one arm with hand supporting head. (Courtesy Marjorie Pyle, RNC, Lifecircle, Costa Mesa, Calif.)

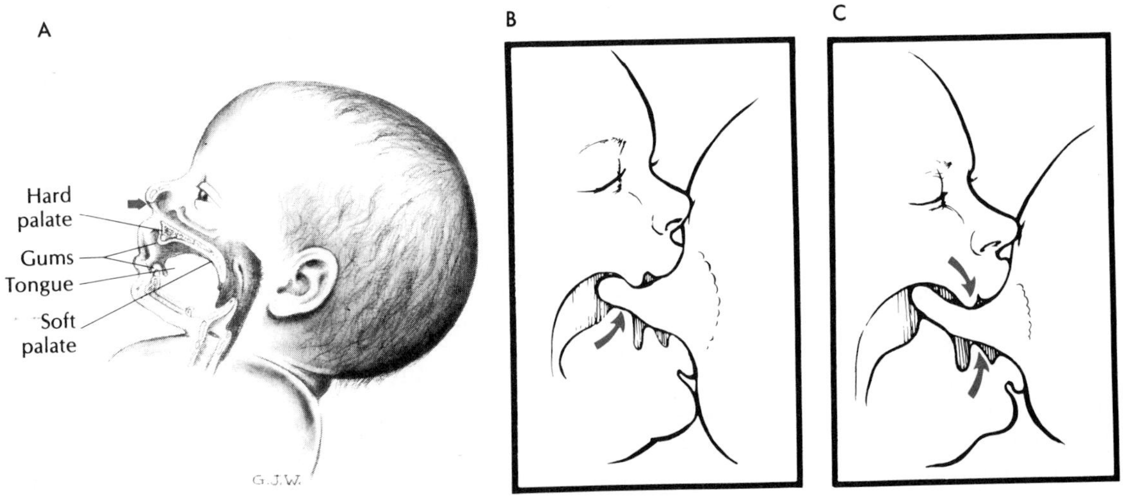

FIG. 44-5 Suckling process. **A,** Infant breathes through nose *(arrow)*. Tongue and palate meet closing esophagus. **B,** Tongue thrusts up and forward to grasp nipple. **C,** Gums compress areola and tongue moves backward, creating negative pressure for suction.

BOX 44-1 POSTPARTUM DANGER SIGNS

1. Fever with or without chills
2. Malodorous vaginal discharge
3. Excessive amount of vaginal discharge
4. Bright red vaginal bleeding after it has changed to pink or rust color
5. Edema, erythematous or painful area on the legs
6. Pain or burning sensation with urination or an inability to void
7. Breast changes such as localized pain, heat, edema, or malodorous drainage
8. Pain in the perineal or pelvic area

of insurance coverage, or personal preference. Since early discharge is increasingly common, it is important to assess the woman's ability to meet her own needs and those of her infant.

The home situation should be discussed. If any information obtained about the home situation appears unsafe or questionable, an appointment with a social worker is necessary before discharge. It is also important to review self-care concerns before discharge. This should include information about postpartum danger signs (see Box 44-1) and the importance of medical follow-up. It should also include review of infant and self-care activities and family planning information.

Nutritional/Metabolic

Recovery stage. The length of time spent in labor, and the physical exertion, often result in hunger. Most physicians allow a meal after delivery if the woman is alert and not nauseated. Fluids are very important during the recovery phase to replace the fluid and blood lost during delivery; a variety of fluids such as water and juices should be offered. If intravenous fluids are ordered by the physician, these should be administered promptly. When a general anesthetic has been used, such as during a cesarean delivery, the presence of bowel sounds should be verified before solid food is given.

If the woman has been using mouth-breathing techniques during labor, the mucous membranes and lips may be dry and cracked, and breath odor may be noticeable. Good oral hygiene will relieve these symptoms and reduce discomfort. A complete sponge bath enhances well-being and provides comfort by removing perspiration and other waste products from the skin.

Later postpartum stage. Diet remains an important concern during the postpartum stage. Many women are very aware of the weight gained during pregnancy, and wish to lose the excess as soon as possible. It is important that dieting not deprive the woman of necessary nutrition. If the woman has not gained excessive weight during pregnancy, the prepregnant weight is normally achieved in 6 to 8 weeks without dieting. Most physicians do not recommend any weight-loss diets until after this time. The nonlactating mother should continue to eat a well-balanced diet that includes the four basic food groups. Calorie intake should be the same as before pregnancy. Lactating mothers generally continue with the diet recommended during pregnancy; the extra calories, vitamins, and minerals are required by the body for lactation. A breast-feeding mother can consume more calories and lose weight at the same time. (See Diet Therapy, Chapter 23.)

Good personal hygiene continues to be important during the late postpartum stage. Excessive perspiration and a slight odor from drainage are common; regular bathing should be encouraged to minimize odors and promote comfort. After the first day, most women are permitted to be up ad lib and prefer to shower and shampoo by themselves. Vertigo may occur as a result of vascular shifts related to the heat of the shower. If this occurs while standing in the shower, the woman may experience syncope and injury may result. The first time the newly delivered woman takes a shower, the nurse should be particularly careful to provide for safety. This includes instruction on use of the emergency call signal and the length of time recommended and providing a chair in the shower room. The nurse should also check the patient frequently during her first shower to verify that safety is maintained. Tub baths are not recommended until after the postpartum examination at 6 weeks, so that no water that has been contaminated with body wastes enters the vaginal canal or uterus until healing is completed.

Sitz baths are sometimes ordered by the physician to reduce discomfort and to promote healing of the perineum. Vasodilation from the warm water helps reduce edema and speed tissue repair. If sitz baths are ordered, the patient should be instructed about water temperature and length of time. As with a shower, vascular changes may occur, and the nurse should check on the patient regularly to promote safety. It is important that proper cleaning of equipment take place between patients if community facilities are used. Today most facilities use a personal, portable sitz bath that the patient can take home at discharge.

If the woman has delivered by cesarean section, an abdominal incision is present, with sutures or staples that close the incision. This incision should be inspected in the same manner as any other surgical incision. It should remain intact with no abnormal erythema, and there should be very little drainage and no foul odor. The incision may be left open to the air or a surgical dressing may be applied, depending on the physician's orders. If no dressing is used to protect the wound, care should be used so clothing does not irritate the incision.

Elimination

Recovery stage. Diuresis and diaphoresis are common immediately after delivery. If, in addition, the woman received intravenous fluids, urinary output may be increased. The bladder should be supported above the symphysis pubis and palpated to check for fullness. Voiding is encouraged, because a full bladder may interfere with complete contraction of the uterus.

Many times the tissue edema from the delivery makes voiding difficult. The initial voiding should be within 4 to 6 hours after delivery. Measures to stimulate voiding should be tried. If these are unsuccessful, catheterization may be required. An indwelling catheter is routinely inserted before cesarean delivery and may remain in place for 1 or 2 days after delivery.

Later postpartum stage. Because most women are fatigued and the perineum is still painful, the nurse must encourage the woman to void at regular intervals of every 2 to 4 hours. If the woman is voiding frequently, and in small amounts (less than 100 ml), the nurse should suspect retention with overflow. The nurse should also question the patient about any symptoms of urgency, frequency, or dysuria. If any of these are noted they should be reported promptly. Incomplete emptying of the bladder will prevent the uterus from contracting normally; it also predisposes the patient to urinary tract infections.

It is particularly important to review proper cleansing technique after delivery. The woman should be instructed to gently cleanse and wipe from the anterior to posterior of the perineum. This method of cleaning prevents microorganisms from the rectal area being transported to the cleaner urinary or vaginal areas. Proper cleansing should be done after each urination or bowel movement.

Ideally, bowel elimination should occur before discharge from the hospital. Fear of discomfort because of an edematous, painful episiotomy or hemorrhoids may result in the woman's resisting the urge to defecate. Bowel peristalsis may continue to be slowed. When this fact is combined with decreased activity and loss of abdominal tone, constipation may result. To prevent this, many physicians order bulk enhancers or stool softeners. Occasionally, suppositories are administered to promote bowel evacuation. The nurse should inspect the perineum to be aware of problems and assure the patient that no harm will come from normal elimination. The importance of adequate bulk in the diet and adequate fluid intake should be stressed. Sitz baths after defecation provide cleansing and can soothe the perineum.

Cesarean section patients, particularly those who received general anesthesia, are likely to develop problems with bowel function. The combination of general anesthesia and lost abdominal tone increases the risk of ileus, so the nurse must pay close attention to bowel function and report any abnormal observations promptly.

Perineal pads, worn to absorb vaginal drainage, should be changed after each urination or defecation. It is essential to teach the woman about the importance of correct application and changing of the pad. Pads should be put in place from anterior to posterior and secured so as not to move about. If they are not correctly worn, contaminated areas could touch cleaner areas of the perineum and increase the risk of infection.

Activity/Exercise

Recovery stage. Vital signs should be monitored every 15 minutes during the recovery stage.

The woman's temperature may be slightly elevated if the woman is dehydrated. A temperature higher than 100.4° F (38° C) is significant and should be reported. Many women feel chilled after giving birth and appreciate an extra blanket or one that has been warmed.

Slight bradycardia, 50 to 70 beats per minute, is sometimes observed and is not considered abnormal if the other vital signs are within normal limits. Tachycardia may also occur as a response to increased blood loss or physical exertion.

Blood pressure may be slightly elevated from exertion, excitement, and possibly from the oxytocic medications. If the blood pressure is consistently elevated, or if the patient also complains of headache or visual disturbances, complications related to hypertensive disease of pregnancy could be occurring. These often persist even after delivery. The physician should be notified immediately. Decrease in blood pressure could be caused by altered intraabdominal pressure or hemorrhage. Changes should be watched closely and reported.

Little activity is observed during this stage. Most women wish to rest, hold the baby, or visit with their significant others.

Later postpartum stage. Vital signs normally stabilize within the first 2 hours after delivery; any abnormality persisting longer than this should be reported immediately. If vital signs have not stabilized within this time, the nurse should continue to monitor them and report significant changes.

A temperature of 100.4° F (38° C) or more on 2 successive days during the first 10 days after delivery, not including the first 24 hours after delivery, is considered indicative of puerperal infection. Any signs of infection occurring during the postpartum stage should be monitored closely. Good aseptic technique should be used when caring for the postpartum patient. Signs and symptoms of infection should be reviewed with the new mother before discharge. The nurse should stress the importance of contacting the physician promptly if any of these should occur.

Pulse and blood pressure are also assessed. Bradycardia may persist up to 10 days after delivery. Elevated blood pressure readings or a continued decrease in blood pressure may be significant and should be reported promptly.

Most women try to get as much rest as possible while in the hospital. This is important, but activity is also needed to prevent complications such as thrombophlebitis of the lower extremities. New mothers should be encouraged to be out of bed and move about in the room. If the baby is kept in a nursery away from the mother's room, this is a good target for ambulation. If the perineum is uncomfortable, the woman should be taught to stand using the muscles of the legs while squeezing the buttocks together. This technique also helps when she attempts to sit. If unsteadiness is observed, the woman should be accompanied when she ambulates. Ambulation is very important for women who delivered by cesarean section; they should be thought of as surgical patients and ambulated as soon as possible. It is important to remember that inactivity predisposes the woman to development of thrombophlebitis.

The flow of lochia may increase suddenly when the woman gets out of bed; secretions that pooled in the vagina drain out of the body when she stands. Once the lochia has changed to serosa or alba, excessive exercise or activity may result in the lochia's changing back to rubra. This is a good indicator to slow down and increase activity more slowly.

Many women wish to begin exercises to regain abdominal tone and their prepregnancy figure; however, most physicians do not recommend active exercises until after the 6-week examination. Nurses can teach isometric exercises that help toning without causing undue exertion.

Rest/Sleep

Rest and sleep are important through the postpartum period. After the difficulties most women encounter at the end of pregnancy, it is a pleasure to sleep in any position desired. Many women report that the night after delivery, they get the best sleep they have experienced in weeks.

Hospital noises interrupt the sleep of many new mothers; environmental noise should be kept to a minimum to promote rest and sleep. Sleep should not be disturbed unless it is necessary to protect the patient's well-being.

If she is breast-feeding, the new mother may choose to feed the infant at intervals through the night. This results in an interrupted night's sleep. This interrupted pattern may persist for weeks until the infant is capable of sleeping for 5 or 6 hours without a feeding. The nurse should instruct the patient on the importance of naps and rest periods during the day to compensate for lost sleep. If sleep deprivation becomes prolonged, it may actually interfere with milk production and the let-down reflex.

Sexuality/Reproductive

Recovery stage. The fundus and lochia are checked every 15 minutes for the first 1 or 2 hours after delivery. The fundus should remain contracted, firm, and midline. This is critical, since severe bleeding may result if the uterus does not tightly constrict the placental site. As discussed earlier, a full bladder can displace the uterus and prevent contraction of the uterus. The patient should be encouraged to empty her bladder before the nurse checks the fundus. The uterus is palpated by placing one hand over the lower segment of the uterus near the pubic bone. The side of the other hand is used to feel the location and consistency of the uterus (Fig. 44-6).

If the fundus is not firm, it will be difficult to locate. An atonic uterus, one which has lost muscle tone, feels soft or "boggy." The nurse may gently massage the fundus to increase contractility. Frequently small clots will be expressed during this maneuver, and the uterus will regain good contracted tone. If this does not result in contraction, the physician may order oxytocic medication. The most commonly ordered medications are pitocin, ergonovine maleate (Ergotrate), and methylergonovine maleate (Methergine). These are usually administered intravenously to obtain prompt response. Methergine may also be administered intramuscularly or orally. Vital signs must be monitored closely if these medications are being given, because they may cause alterations in blood pressure, bradycardia, nausea, headache, vertigo, and other side effects.

While the uterus is being palpated, the amount of lochia should be observed. If the uterus is contracting well, small to moderate amounts of drainage will be observed. If tone is poor the amount of lochia will be increased. It is important to learn what is considered scant, light, moderate, and heavy amounts. This is usually determined by number of absorptive pads saturated in a period of time, such as pads per hour (Fig. 44-7). The nurse should pay particular attention to the patient who has a small but steady trickle of lochia. Many times the blood loss in these patients is significantly greater than the loss in those who seem to bleed larger amounts. The nurse must also be sure to check under the buttocks of the patient who remains in the supine position; many times gravity causes drainage to miss the pad and pool under the patient.

Later postpartum stage. Daily checks are performed to assess breasts, fundus, lochia, perineum, rectum, and the vascular condition of the legs. These are often called the *postpartum checks.*

It is recommended that all new mothers wear a bra, even if the breasts are not overly large. The bra should be comfortable and fitted to provide support. Breast-feeding mothers should be encouraged to use bras large enough to accommodate the enlargement that occurs with lactation. Nonnursing mothers will need a bra that provides adequate compression to inhibit lactation without being uncomfortable.

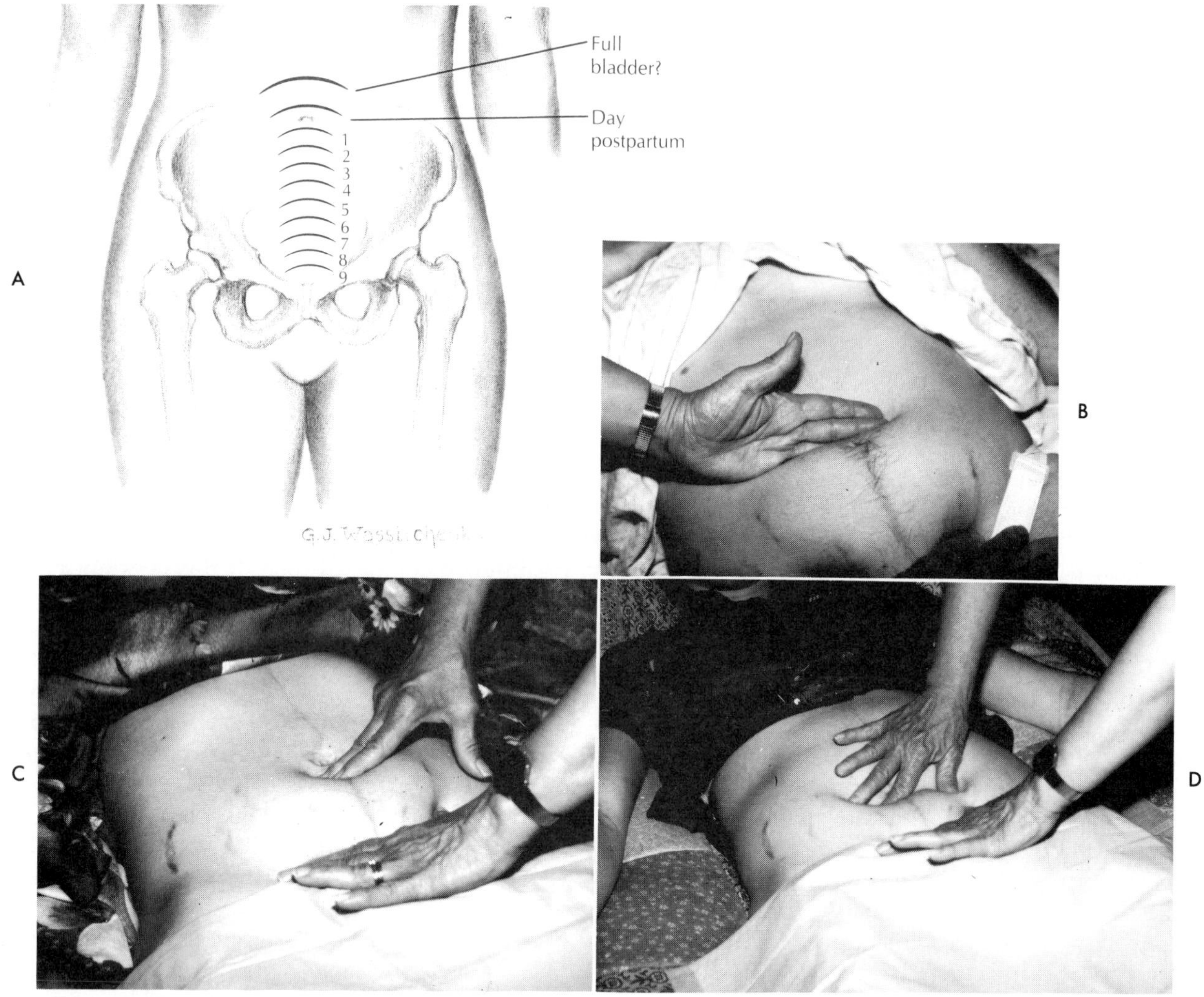

FIG. 44-6 Assessment of involution of uterus after delivery. **A,** Normal progress, days 1 through 9. **B,** Size and position of uterus 2 hours after delivery. **C,** 2 days after delivery. **D,** 4 days after delivery. (**B, C,** and **D** courtesy Marjorie Pyle, RNC, Lifecircle, Costa Mesa, Calif.)

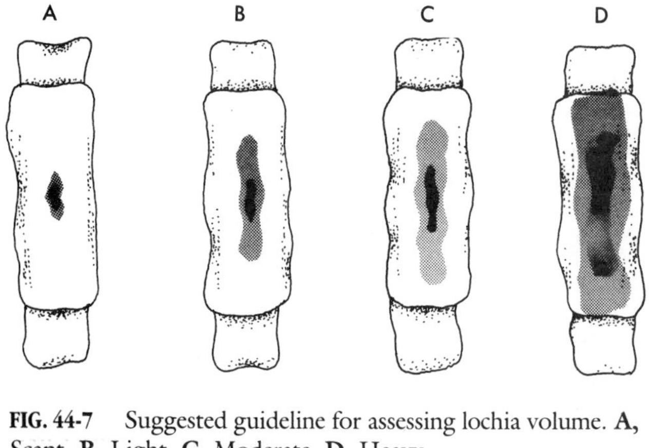

FIG. 44-7 Suggested guideline for assessing lochia volume. **A,** Scant. **B,** Light. **C,** Moderate. **D,** Heavy.

With the bra removed, the breasts should be inspected and palpated. The nurse should observe for erythema, heat, edema, and engorgement. Filling of the breast usually occurs first near the axillary region. Engorgement is usually not observed until the third postpartum day. Because most women have been discharged from the hospital before this occurs, it is important to teach methods of obtaining relief from engorgement before sending the mother home. If the woman is breast-feeding, interventions such as manual expression of milk and application of warm, moist heat are most useful. If the woman is not breast-feeding, compression of the breasts with a firm bra, wrapped ice packs, and analgesics are most often recommended.

The nipples should be inspected for inflammation, fissures, or soreness. The nipples generally do not cause any problems for nonlactating mothers; however, if the woman is breast-feeding, it is important to keep the nipples soft and supple. Most physicians recommend avoiding excessive use of soap or other chemicals on the nipple, because these dry the skin and may be ingested by the infant. Plain water and air drying may help prevent problems. Some physicians recommend allowing the nipples to dry after feeding without removal of the milk residue. If any additional moisturizer is needed, small amounts of unscented lanolin are used. If the woman is allergic to wool, lanolin should be avoided, because it is obtained from the wool of sheep. Modifications in the nursing schedule and positioning of the baby may be needed if sore or cracked nipples continue to be a problem. Many good references include more information on breast care.

The fundus is checked for the normal signs of involution. As in the recovery stage, the location and consistency of the uterine fundus are checked. It is normally located at the level of the umbilicus on the day of delivery. The first day postpartum it may be one fingerbreadth above or at the level of the umbilicus; after that it normally descends at the rate of one fingerbreadth per day. When assessing the fundus of a woman delivered by cesarean section, it is possible to carefully palpate on the sides of the incision to determine uterine tone and position.

As during the early recovery stage, the fundus should remain firmly contracted. Any atony should be handled as described. If massage does not result in adequate contraction, the physician should be notified. Lochia may begin to change within the first 2 days from the rubra to the serosa form. The amount of drainage is assessed. There is frequently less lochia observed after cesarean deliveries, because the uterine cavity is suctioned as part of the surgical procedure. The odor of the lochia should remain fleshy. If there is a fetid odor, infection may be present, and this should be reported promptly.

The perineum and rectum are inspected by having the woman assume a lateral position with the upper leg drawn toward the chest. The perineum should be intact. If an episiotomy was performed, the tissue may appear edematous and erythema is common. Ecchymosis is also common, particularly after a difficult delivery. Many physicians order some form of topical anesthetic, such as Tucks or Nupercaine ointment, to soothe the perineum. This should be applied to the perineum by means of a clean, lint-free tissue, not the fingers.

If localized edema, discoloration, and intense pain are observed in the perineal area, a hematoma may be present. This hematoma is caused by excessive bleeding into the tissue. A hematoma is most common after deliveries in which forceps were used. Hematomas may be obvious, or may be concealed in the vaginal canal. If the woman complains of persistent perineal pain or fullness in the vagina, the physician should be notified. This problem requires medical intervention.

Although the rectum and legs are not part of the reproductive system, these areas are typically included in postpartum checks.

Hemorrhoids (varicosities of the rectum) usually disappear quickly after delivery if there is no long-standing history of this problem. Topical anesthetics are used to relieve pain if ordered by the physician. Sitz baths also provide relief and should be offered if the physician has ordered them.

The legs should be examined by stretching and straightening the leg. The foot is then dorsiflexed. If pain occurs the patient is said to have a positive Homans' sign, which indicates inflammation of the blood vessels of the leg and possible thrombophlebitis. If Homans' sign is positive, the physician should be notified promptly.

Coping/Stress Tolerance

Many new mothers feel overwhelmed by the responsibility of motherhood. New mothers feel intimidated by the nurses' capability and skill with the newborn. They often feel inept and may not wish to ask questions that might be viewed as unintelligent. Establishing a rapport is essential; listening for fears and anxieties that are verbalized and anticipating those that are not verbalized are important nursing measures. False reassurances are not helpful; good teaching and encouragement are far more beneficial.

Often women experience a period of depression after delivery that is triggered by rapid hormonal shifts. This so-called postpartum depression may be mild or rather severe. It often appears between 2 and 7 days postpartum. Preparing the woman for the possibility of this and planning a course of action if it does occur are nursing responsibilities.

Occasionally the nurse may observe situations in which there are severe or long-standing coping problems. In these cases it is wise to consult with the physician, a nurse specialist, the social worker, or other professionals who can best help the woman cope with her problems.

Role/Relationship

Roles and relationships are affected by the addition of a new family member. These changes are most obvious when the first child is born, but adjustments take place any time an additional child joins a family. Time, money, and emotional resources must be divided to include the new member.

The mother faces the greatest number of changes. In our society the mother still fills the role of primary caregiver to the child. The total responsibility of this role 24 hours a day, seven days a week, is overwhelming to many women. Today, because many women are independent wage earners, the loss of freedom to come and go as they please is also a difficult adjustment. Even if the woman has made plans to return to work and has arranged for excellent child care, role conflict can lead to guilt and confusion. The nurse should be sensitive to the mother's concerns.

The responsibilities of fatherhood often become a reality when the father actually sees his child. The realization that a totally dependent individual needs him can be frightening to many men. The financial concerns of feeding, clothing, and sheltering his family take on new significance.

A two-income family may have only his wages, at least temporarily. Even if the mother returns to work, there are new expenses for child care. The wife is now also a mother, and many times the needs of the child will supersede the husband's needs or wishes. The freedom and spontaneity of a couple gives way to a life circumscribed by feeding schedules, diaper bags, and baby-sitters.

Because many men have little knowledge or experience in caring for infants, simple things, such as feeding, changing diapers, or even carrying a baby, may be intimidating. The nurse can help alleviate these fears by including the father in teaching whenever possible and by allowing him to verbalize his fears and concerns.

Additional role adjustments relate to friends and the extended family. Friendships and socialization may require adjustment. Parents now become grandparents and in-laws share grandchildren. These are all dynamic situations, and each family will make a variety of accommodations in the process of incorporating their new roles.

Self-Perception

It is common for the new mother to wish to discuss her perception of the labor and delivery. Time should be allowed for her to verbalize and work through her experiences. The reality may have differed greatly from her expectations, and explanations are needed to clarify things in her mind.

It is not uncommon for the new mother to be rather passive for the first day or two. This is what is often called the "taking in" stage. During this time the mother needs supportive care. Her primary focus may be on herself and on personal needs such as sleep, food, and attention. She may defer to the nurses and let others provide total care for the baby. This is followed by what is referred to as the "taking hold" stage. In this phase the woman is ready to assume greater authority and responsibility for herself and her baby.

Mood swings are common early in the postpartum period, related to recent stresses, fatigue, and rapid hormonal changes. This should be explained to the new mother so she does not become unduly concerned.

It is common for new mothers, particularly primiparas, to expect that they will regain their prepregnancy figure quickly after delivery. Many bring clothes that they hoped to wear home, only to be sadly disappointed. The nurse should be supportive and explain that time is required for the body to regain the prepregnancy tone and shape.

Cognitive/Perceptual

Control of discomforts during the postpartum period is important. If the woman is to resume a normal level of activity and get adequate rest, pain cannot be allowed to interfere.

The most common discomforts experienced are perineal pain from the episiotomy and the so-called afterbirth pains. Afterbirth pains are cramping sensations resulting from the contraction of the uterus. While any new mother may experience afterbirth pains, they are more common and may be more severe in multiparas.

Most physicians prescribe analgesics for these discomforts. Acetaminophen is commonly used, with or without codeine. Codeine is generally effective but is a controlled substance and also has side effects, such as constipation and vertigo, that may be undesirable in the postpartum patient. Salicylates, such as aspirin, are usually avoided, because they may interfere with clotting mechanisms. Recently ibuprofen (Motrin) has been popular. Ibuprofen is an analgesic, antiinflammatory, and prostaglandin inhibitor. It is often effective in reducing the severity of the cramping without altering the contraction of the uterine muscle. A cautionary note in using ibuprofen: ibuprofen is to be used with caution for persons with kidney or heart disease or those taking diuretics.

Another major challenge of the postpartum period involves learning. The new mother needs to know how to care for herself and how to care for the newborn. This can be overwhelming for the first-time mother. The nurse has limited time to teach all the necessary information. Most hospitals have teaching lists and printed handouts or booklets that include all of the key areas. To prevent the woman from becoming overwhelmed, teaching should be paced throughout the hospital stay, not left until discharge.

Value/Belief

Culture may prescribe activities or rituals for both mother and baby; these may include specific behaviors related to diet, hygiene, or activity. Each culture is unique as to what behaviors should occur or be avoided. Many books describe a variety of cultural practices related to childbearing. It is wise to have the patient verbalize her unique cultural practices; the nurse should listen nonjudgmentally. If any of the practices should be harmful to either mother or baby, it is important to explain the reasons the behavior should not be practiced. The ideal is finding a way to blend the cultural practice with safe health teaching.

THE NORMAL NEWBORN

Immediate Assessment of the Newborn

In addition to the Apgar scoring, which was done immediately after the delivery, the nurse performs other assessments to establish the gestational age of the newborn. Gestational age is the actual number of weeks since conception. This is important, because many problems observed in newborns are age related. Since many women are unsure of the exact date of conception, calendar-based gestational age is unreliable. Physical and neurological assessment based on established criteria are more reliable. Physical characteristics are evaluated within the first few hours of life. Neurological assessment is done 24 hours later, after the nervous system has had the opportunity to stabilize from the trauma of delivery.

Characteristics of the Normal Newborn

Body size and shape. The head of the newborn is disproportionately large for its body. The abdomen is prominent, with a smaller chest and narrow hips. The body is usually held in a moderately flexed position. There is a wide variation of size in normal newborns. The average newborn weighs 3400 g (7 pounds 8 ounces) and is approximately 50 cm (20 inches) in length. Height and weight charts are available for plotting these. The head circumference averages 33 to 35.5 cm (13 to 14 inches) and is generally about 2 cm (1 inch) larger than that of the chest, which averages 30 to 33 cm (12 to 13 inches).

Skin. The skin of the infant can exhibit a wide range of rashes and color changes. Most are not significant and disappear within a few days. However, parents may be concerned by these until the changes are explained.

Skin color. The skin color is normally pink to slightly reddish in appearance. The ruddiness results from normally elevated red blood cell concentration. The hands and feet may appear slightly blue; this is called **acrocyanosis** and is caused by poor peripheral circulation. It is most commonly observed when the infant becomes cold. Mottling, a lacy pattern with dilated vessels on pale skin, is also commonly seen. Another normal variation is called the *harlequin sign*; half of the newborn's body appears deep red and the other side of the body appears pale as a result of vasomotor disturbance, with some vessels constricting while others dilate. This may last for up to 20 minutes, and while disturbing to view, it is not harmful.

Jaundice, a yellow discoloration, is first detected over bony prominences on the face and on the mucous membranes. This is abnormal during the first 24 hours of life.

After 24 hours it is not necessarily abnormal. The hemoglobin and hematocrit levels of the newborn are frequently elevated; hemoglobin may range from 15 to 20 g/dl and hematocrit from 43% to 61%. After 24 hours **physiological jaundice** may appear, because the excessive levels of hemoglobin are no longer required for oxygen transport. When jaundice is observed, further assessment is required to determine the cause. The physician may order laboratory and diagnostic tests to determine the nature of the problem and begin treatment to prevent complications. Causes of jaundice will be discussed further in Chapter 45.

Skin appearance. At birth the skin is covered with a yellowish white cream cheese–like substance called **vernix caseosa**. This substance protects the infant's skin from amniotic fluid. When it is removed, the skin may appear dry and may crack, flake, and peel. A layer of soft hair called *lanugo* is commonly observed on the shoulders and back. Good turgor and tissue elasticity are normally observed.

A variety of observations may be made when assessing the skin. The most commonly observed are noted in Box 44-2.

BOX 44-2 — COMMON SKIN OBSERVATIONS IN THE NEWBORN

1. *Milia* are small white spots usually seen on the nose and chin. They are a result of occluded sebaceous glands and disappear spontaneously within a few weeks.
2. Newborn rash, technically called *erythema toxicum neonatorum,* is an elevated, hivelike rash that may result in small white vesicles. It is not contagious, and like milia disappears without treatment.
3. *Telangiectatic nevi,* "stork-bites," are flat, pink or red marks often seen on the eyelids, nose, or nape of the neck. These are dilated capillaries that become more vivid when the infant cries. They are not significant to the health of the infant and disappear at 1 to 2 years of age.
4. *Mongolian spots* are areas of increased pigmentation. The lumbar dorsal area is the most common location. The area may appear bluish-black. These are most often seen in darker-skinned races.
5. *Nevus flammeus,* "port-wine stain," is a reddish-purple discoloration often seen on the face. This is a capillary angioma below the epidermis. Unfortunately, these will not disappear spontaneously. Recently medical techniques have been developed that reduce or remove port-wine birthmarks.
6. "Strawberry birthmarks," *nevus vasculosus,* are capillary hemangiomas. These may continue to increase in size for several months. They normally then begin to shrink spontaneously and usually disappear early in childhood.

Head. The fontanels, which were discussed in Chapter 43, should be palpable. The anterior fontanel is normally large and diamond shaped and closes at approximately 18 months of age. The posterior fontanel is smaller and triangular in shape and normally closes at 2 months of age. The sagittal suture may be felt by running the fingers between the two fontanels.

The head of the newborn may also manifest many variations. Most of these are a result of the birth process and disappear without treatment shortly after delivery:

1. *Molding* is overlapping of the bones of the skull. The head may appear elongated and misshaped; this is a result of compression during delivery and normally disappears within a day or two.
2. *Caput succedaneum* is commonly seen with molding. It is the result of edema in the soft tissue of the scalp. The tissue feels spongy and may be felt over suture lines. This also disappears without treatment.
3. *Cephalhematoma* is caused by bleeding within the periosteum of a cranial bone. It is confined to a particular bone and does not cross suture lines. This is usually a result of difficult labor. Cephalhematomas may not be apparent immediately after delivery; they generally appear 1 to 2 days after birth. These normally absorb without treatment. Large hematomas may lead to anemia and jaundice, which require medical intervention.

Face. The newborn's chin is receding and the nose relatively flat. Fat pads make the cheeks appear full and round. Movements of the face should be symmetrical. The mouth should open freely, and the oral cavity should be intact with a closed palate. Small white nodules called *Epstein's pearls* may be observed on the hard palate. These are a result of epithelial cells and will disappear spontaneously within a few weeks. Occasionally an infant is born with teeth. This is rare but should be watched closely, because they may become loose and be aspirated. The oral cavity should be clean and free from lesions. A fungal infection may be acquired during passage through the birth canal if the mother is infected with *Candida albicans*. This results in thrush, a white, patchy coating of the mucous membranes that cannot be wiped off. Treatment with antifungal medications such as nystatin or gentian violet is required to treat this condition.

Eyes. The eyelids may appear edematous because of prophylactic antibiotic medication that was applied to the eyes after birth to prevent ophthalmia neonatorum, a gonococcal infection. The eyes appear wide-set. Strabismus (crossed eyes) and nystagmus (abnormal motion of the eyes) are commonly seen as a result of the newborn's immature nervous system. Most Caucasian infants have slate-gray to blue irises at birth; in darker-skinned races the irises may appear darker. The newborn does not produce tears, because the lacrimal structures have not fully matured. Vision has been found to be more acute than previously believed. Newborns are nearsighted and can see objects best at 8 to 10 inches; most prefer simple patterns in black and white and human faces. It is important that the parents know this, because eye contact with the baby is an important part of bonding.

Ears. The ears are normally positioned with the upper insertion of the pinna located even with the outer canthus of the eye. Low-set ears may indicate a chromosomal disorder. High-pitched sounds and the mother's voice generate the greatest attention. It is believed that the fetus becomes familiar with the mother's voice while still in utero.

Reflexes. A wide variety of reflexes are seen in the normal newborn. Some of these are protective reflexes, such as the rooting, sucking, gag, swallow, and sneeze reflex. Other reflexes such as the Babinski, Moro, tonic neck, startle, and stepping are related to the immature nature of the newborn's nervous system. Many of these reflexes are present for a limited time and then disappear. Table 44-1 identifies the nature and significance of the most commonly observed reflexes.

Genitals. The genitals in female newborns may be edematous. Discharge of blood-tinged mucus from the vagina, called *pseudomenstruation*, may occur in response to maternal hormones. The breasts may be enlarged in either sex. This is called *gynecomastia* and is also a result of maternal hormones. The labia majora cover the minora in term infants. The scrotum in the male may be enlarged

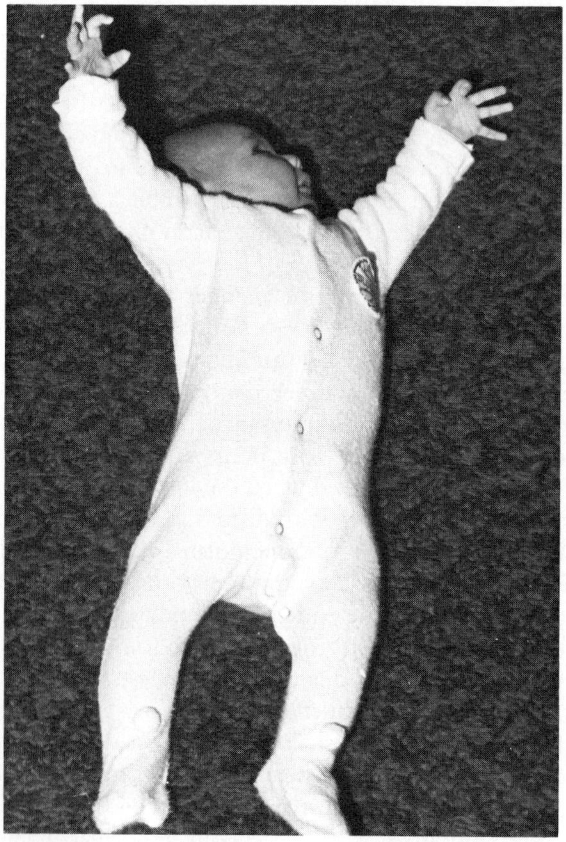

FIG. 44-8 Moro reflex.

Table 44-1 Assessment of Reflexes in the Normal Newborn

Reflex	Expected Behavioral Response	Comments
Moro	Sudden jarring or change in equilibrium causes extension and abduction of extremities and fanning of fingers, with index finger and thumb forming a C shape, followed by flexion and adduction of extremities; legs may weakly flex; infant may cry (Fig. 44-8).	Elicit by holding the infant above the examining table in a supine position with one hand beneath the sacrum and the other supporting the upper back and head; the infant's head is then suddenly allowed to fall about 30 degrees. Disappears after 3-4 months, usually strongest during first 2 months.
Startle	A sudden loud noise causes abduction of the arms with flexion of the elbows; the hands remain clenched.	Disappears by 4 months of age.
Tonic neck	When infant's head is quickly turned to one side, arm and leg will extend on that side, and opposite arm and leg will flex; posture resembles a fencing position (Fig. 44-9).	Disappears by 3-4 months of age, to be replaced by symmetrical positioning of both sides of body.
Dance or step	If infant is held so that sole of foot touches a hard surface, there will be a reciprocal flexion and extension of the leg, simulating walking (Fig. 44-10).	Disappears after 3-4 weeks, to be replaced by deliberate movement.
Crawling	When infant is placed on abdomen, he will make crawling movements with the arms and legs (Fig. 44-11).	Disappears at about 6 weeks of age.

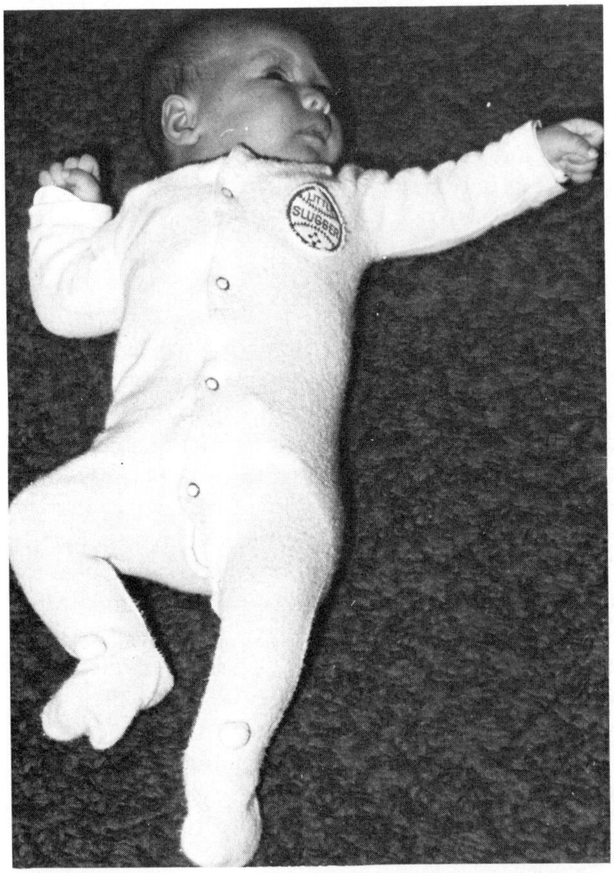

FIG. 44-9 Tonic neck reflex.

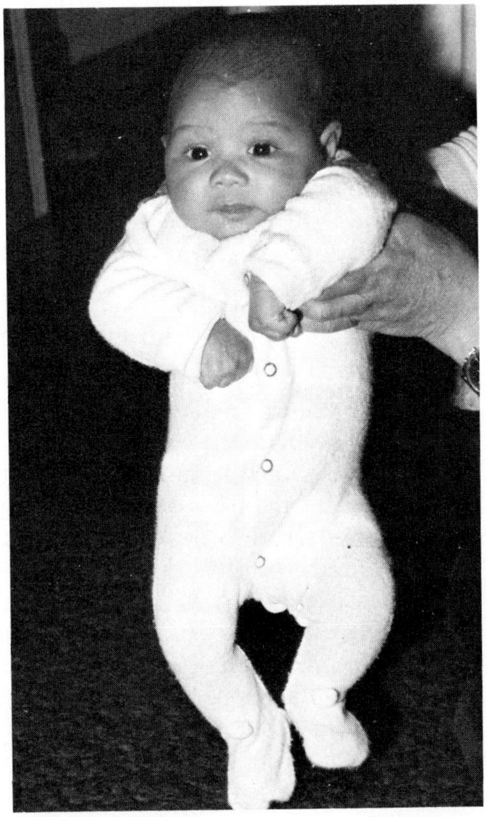

FIG. 44-10 Dance reflex.

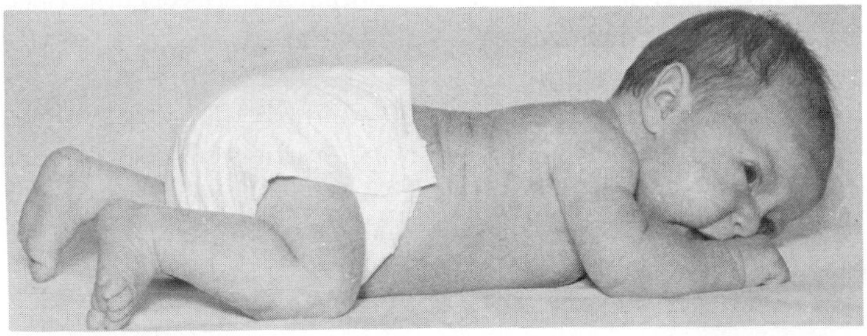

FIG. 44-11 Crawl reflex.

and edematous, indicating a hydrocele. The testicles are normally descended in term infants; in preterm infants they may not be descended (cryptorchidism). The penis should be inspected for position of the urethral meatus. Abnormal placement may result in problems with voiding. Circumcision is not normally done if there is any malplacement, since the foreskin may be used as part of the surgical correction.

Spine. The spine should be straight without curves. The normal cervical and lumbar curves will develop once the infant begins to stand. The spine should also be examined for dimples, tufts of hair, and masses that may indicate abnormalities of spinal column development.

Extremities. The arms and hands are generally flexed against the body. Both arms should move evenly. Trauma during delivery may result in fracture of the clavicle or in brachial palsy. Both hands should be free from webbing (syndactyly) or extra digits (polydactyly). A single crease in the palm of the hand, a simian line, may indicate chromosomal disorders. Nails often extend beyond the fingertips. Legs should be equal in length. If one leg appears longer or if the gluteal or popliteal folds are asymmetrical, a congenital hip dysplasia may be suspected. The hips should move freely. The feet may appear to be turned abnormally; this is often the result of the newborn's position in utero.

NURSING ASSESSMENT AND INTERVENTIONS

Health Management/Health Perception

Before giving the newborn to the mother, identification bracelets should be checked to prevent the possibility of giving the baby to the wrong mother.

The mother should be instructed about handwashing when caring for the baby to prevent the spread of microorganisms; this is particularly important when going from performing personal hygiene to caring for the infant.

The new mother should be instructed in safety practices to reduce the likelihood of injury to the infant. Positions that provide head support while carrying and burping should be demonstrated. The large size of the head requires care when handling the infant. The mother should also be taught never to leave the baby unattended in an unsafe location, such as a table or bed. The environment should be kept free of hazards, such as pins or other sharp objects. Bathing techniques and temperature taking should be demonstrated. The mother should be taught proper positioning of the infant. It is recommended that an infant be placed on its side after feeding to reduce the possibility of aspiration if the baby regurgitates. Bottles should never be propped for feeding, because this may lead to choking or aspiration. The use of infant car seats is now mandatory in most states.

State laws will require that certain diagnostic tests be performed on the newborn. The nurse must know the laws of the particular state. These tests are done to detect conditions that result in serious complications, such as neurological disorders and mental retardation. If any of these metabolic conditions are detected early in life and if proper treatment is started promptly, many of the complications may be eliminated or reduced. Most of the diseases tested for involve inborn errors of metabolism in which the newborn is unable to metabolize various nutrients. Some of the more common tests include those done to detect phenylketonuria (PKU), maple sugar urine disease (MSUD), galactosemia, and hypothyroidism. These tests involve either blood or urine samples. For most test results to be meaningful, the newborn must have consumed an adequate amount of either human milk or cow's milk formula. Because of early discharge of mothers and newborns this may not occur before the newborn goes home. If the tests are to be performed before the neonate is discharged from the hospital, completion of the necessary blood work should be verified and noted on the chart before the newborn is allowed to leave. If the tests are to be done later, usually at 2 to 5 days of age, the newborn will have to return to the hospital or physician's office. In these situations the nurse must be sure that the parents understand the importance of the tests and know specifically when the newborn is to be tested.

Nutritional/Metabolic

Newborns have low prothrombin levels at birth and are at risk for hemorrhage. Because newborns are not able to synthesize vitamin K in the colon until they have adequate intestinal flora, a vitamin K (Aquamephyton) injection is routinely administered to newborns. Injections are best administered in the vastus lateralis muscle.

Weight is monitored daily. It is considered normal for a newborn to lose up to 10% of its body weight in the first week of life, from a combination of factors. More weight is lost through the passing of meconium and urine than is taken in by the newborn. This is particularly true in breast-fed babies. Most newborns regain their birth weight within the first week.

Nutritional requirements. The normal newborn requires approximately 120 calories per kilogram of body weight each day. This includes proteins, carbohydrates, fats, vitamins, and minerals. Breast milk and prepared formulas are balanced to meet the needs of the newborn. Since newborns cannot concentrate urine efficiently, fluid intake needs are high; 140 to 160 ml/kg/day is necessary (1 kg = 2.2 lb).

With the improved formulas available today, the fluid and nutritional needs of infants can be met by either breast-feeding or bottle-feeding. The mother can choose which method she prefers. The nurse should provide support and teaching appropriate to the chosen method.

Breast milk is produced in three stages. Colostrum, the first substance produced, is creamy and yellow-white in appearance. It contains more protein, minerals, and fat-soluble vitamins than mature breast milk. It also contains high levels of immunoglobulins, which may transfer some immunity to the newborn. Production of colostrum begins in the last trimester of pregnancy and continues for 2 to 4 days after delivery. Transitional milk is produced for about 1 week. This may appear thinner and more watery. This milk is high in fats, lactose, and water-soluble vitamins and contains more calories than colostrum. Mature milk is generally established by 2 weeks after delivery. This may appear very thin and watery. It provides 20 kcal/oz and contains lactose, proteins, minerals, and vitamins. If the mother is eating properly, only vitamin D may need to be supplemented.

Formulas are prepared by modifying cow's milk to make it more similar to human milk. It appears thicker and more rich, but also contains 20 kcal/oz. Formulas are available in ready-to-feed and concentrated forms. The mother must be instructed in proper preparation and storage to prevent nutritional or digestive problems in her infant.

The first feeding is normally 15 to 30 ml of sterile water. This must be given with caution to verify that the infant is able to swallow normally and that no anomalies of the digestive tract are present. If this is taken without difficulty, either breast-feeding or bottle-feeding is begun. It is normal for infants to regurgitate mucus after the first few feedings. Food intake is necessary to prevent hypoglycemia, which is stressful to the newborn.

The frequency of feeding will depend on the type of feeding. Breast-fed babies tend to do best on an "on demand" schedule. Most breast-fed babies will nurse at 1- to 3-hour intervals. Bottle-fed babies tend to eat less frequently, usually every 2 to 4 hours, because formula is digested more slowly. Each baby will establish a pattern over a period of time. It is important not to overfeed, particularly with bottle-fed babies, since this can lead to regurgitation. Breast-fed infants may receive supplements of glucose water if this is ordered by the physician. However, this may interfere with the process of establishing lactation, since the neonate may not be adequately hungry when put to breast.

It is important to burp the baby at intervals. This should be done for both bottle- and breast-fed babies. While sucking the baby normally swallows air; if this air is not cleared from the stomach the infant may feel satisfied and stop eating. When the air clears the stomach, the infant may again appear hungry (Fig. 44-12).

Before starting, a feeding position that is comfortable for the mother should be chosen. The baby should be in a position that facilitates the flow of milk into the stomach. Many different positions are suitable for breast- or bottle-feeding.

Hypothermia. Maintenance of body temperature is a major concern when caring for the newborn. Prolonged exposure to a cold environment can result in increased oxygen consumption and depleted glycogen reserves. The newborn has a large surface area and a limited amount of protective adipose tissue. Heat is lost through radiation, evaporation, conduction, and convection. The nurse

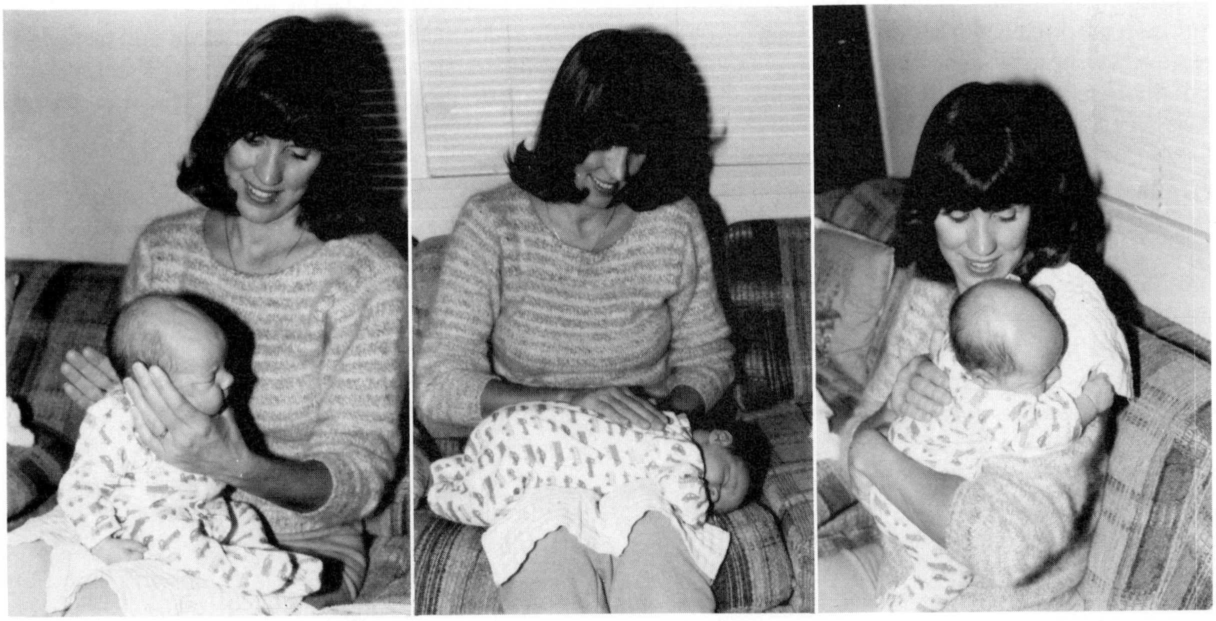

A B C

FIG. 44-12 Positions for burping an infant. **A,** Upright. **B,** Across the lap. **C,** Shoulder position. (Courtesy Marjorie Pyle, RNC, Lifecircle, Costa Mesa, Calif.)

Table 44-2 Precautions to Minimize Heat Loss in Infants

Heat Loss in Infants	Nursing Interventions to Prevent Heat Loss
Radiation: loss that occurs when heat transfers from the body to cooler surfaces and objects not in contact with the body	Keep body well wrapped to prevent radiant loss. Work quickly to avoid excessive time with skin exposed. Use radiant warmer to minimize loss.
Evaporation: loss when water is converted into a vapor	Dry infant thoroughly after delivery and dry promptly when bathing.
Conduction: loss of heat to a cooler surface by direct skin contact	Pad surfaces under infant, including tables and scales. Warm other equipment, such as stethoscopes, before use.
Convection: loss of heat to cooler air currents	Reduce drafts from open doors, windows, or air conditioning.

must be aware of ways heat is being lost and take precautions to minimize these when meeting the hygiene of the newborn (Table 44-2).

Temperature may be monitored with a skin sensor or thermometer. Before inserting a rectal thermometer it is important to verify that the anus is patent. Until stool is passed, most facilities use the axillary route. The normal axillary temperature is 97.7° to 98.6° F (36.6° to 37° C).

Skin care. Inspection and bathing of the neonate take place after the body temperature has stabilized. The first sponge bath is normally done using mild soap and water. The frequency and type of baths will depend on the policies of the facility. Any area of the body, particularly the perineal area, should be washed whenever soiled to prevent skin irritation.

The water should be approximately 100° F (38.7° C) to prevent chilling. The room should be warm, cold surfaces should be padded, a minimum amount of the body should be exposed, and the skin should be dried promptly. The order of the bath is essentially the same as for an adult, beginning with the eyes, face, and head, and ending with the anal region.

Special attention should be given to care of the umbilical area. At delivery the cord is moist. Over the next few days a drying process called *mummification* begins. It is important to avoid getting the cord wet during bathing. Most facilities have a routine to promote drying by use of alcohol or other substances that inhibit microbial growth. Odor or drainage from the cord is abnormal and should be reported promptly. Tub bathing is delayed until the fully dried cord drops off at about 10 days of age.

The mother should be given a demonstration of temperature-taking and bathing the newborn. If possible she should be encouraged to bathe the infant with a nurse observing. This will help her gain confidence and provides an opportunity to answer questions about care. It is also a good time to demonstrate safe methods of holding and positioning the infant (Fig. 44-13).

Circumcision, surgical removal of the foreskin, may be performed if the parents consent. There is little agreement among authorities about the necessity or desirability of circumcision. Because this is a surgical procedure, consent forms must be signed. If circumcision is performed, the site must be checked frequently for bleeding. Petroleum jelly is used to prevent the diapers from adhering to the site. Although the tip of the penis appears erythematous and painful, healing occurs quickly.

Elimination

The newborn should void within 24 hours of delivery. If this does not occur, the physician should be notified. The average newborn voids small amounts of poorly concentrated urine; it is normally clear and odorless. Occasionally a small pink or brownish discharge may be observed as a result of uric acid crystals that were formed in the bladder in utero. As the fluid intake increases and kidney function improves, urination becomes more frequent and assumes the normal color.

Bowel elimination should occur within 24 hours of birth. The initial stools of the newborn are odorless, black-green in color, and sticky in consistency. This is called **meconium** and is made up of vernix, lanugo, mucus, and other substances from the amniotic fluid. Occasionally the first stool is encased in mucus and called a *meconium plug*. If no stool is observed, the physician should be notified so tests can be done to determine the nature of the problem. Once the infant begins to take nourishment, the nature of the stool changes. Transitional stools, which occur on about the second day, tend to be greenish and loose. These are seen until about the fourth day, when the milk stool is seen. Breast-fed babies tend to pass stool frequently, sometimes with every feeding. The stool is pale yellow and sweet smelling. Small curds may be observed. Babies who are bottle-fed tend to have fewer stools, usually two or three per day. These are bright yellow in color and pasty in consistency; the odor may be slightly stronger than that of breast-fed babies. This type of stool will continue until solid food is introduced. Very watery stool, green stools (after the transition), or stools expelled with a great deal of force may indicate gastrointestinal irritation or infection and should be reported promptly. Newborns can lose a great deal of fluid rapidly and become dehydrated.

The skin of the perineum and buttocks can become irritated if waste products are left in contact for too long.

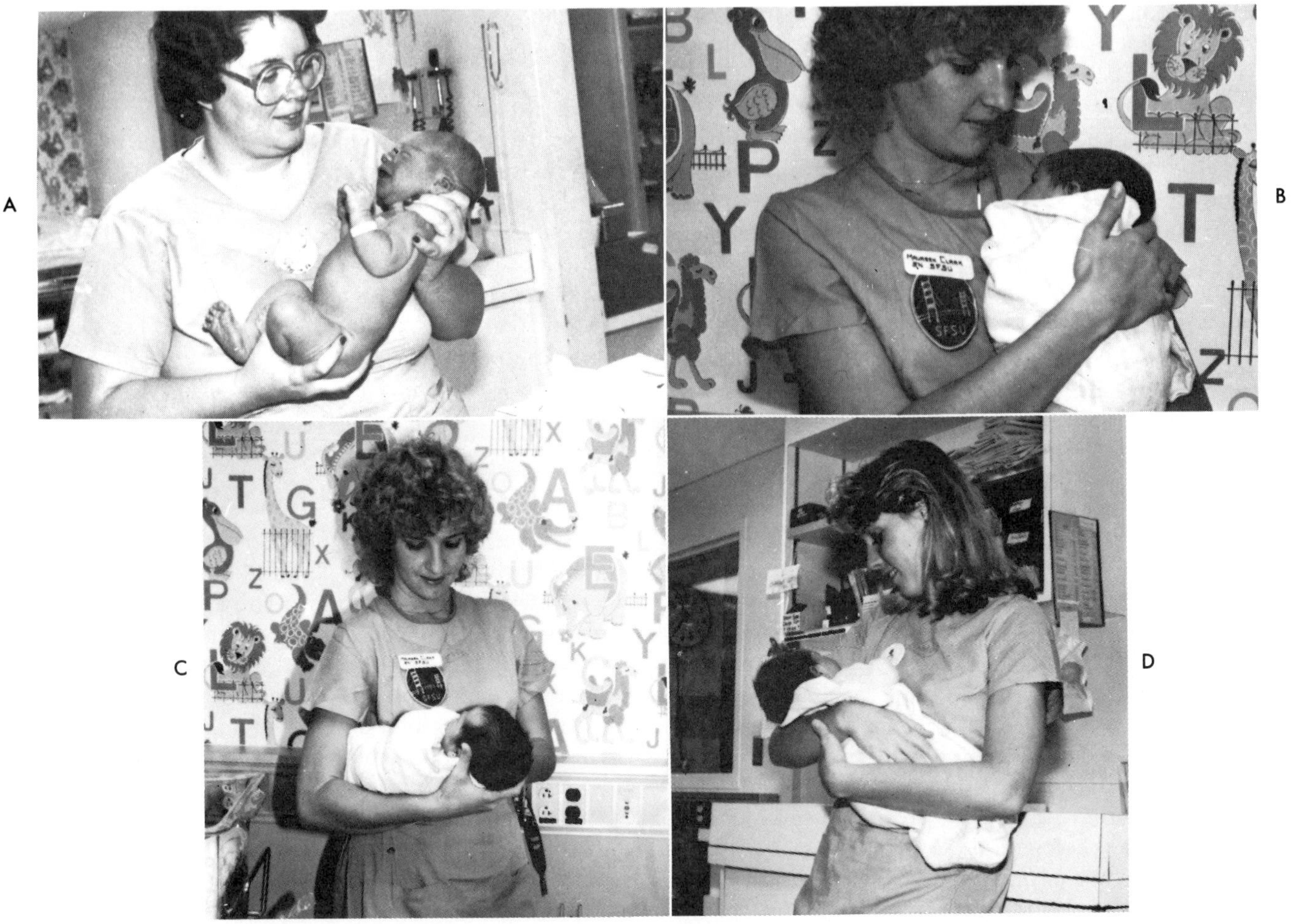

FIG. 44-13 Holding baby securely with support for head. **A,** Holding newborn while moving from one place to another. Baby is undressed to show posture. **B,** Holding newborn upright in "burping" position. **C,** "Football" hold. **D,** Cradle hold.

The mother should be taught to wash the skin, wiping from anterior to posterior, after each voiding or stool. Diapers should be changed promptly. Minimal use of powders and creams, which can irritate the skin, is recommended. Either disposable or cloth diapers may be chosen by the mother.

Rest/Sleep

Most newborns spend 16 to 20 hours per day sleeping. They may be observed to startle and make sucking motions during sleep. Breathing may be regular and even or irregular, depending on the sleep state. The time awake is spent crying, eating, or in quiet alertness. Each infant establishes a unique pattern. The pattern established by the newborn may be erratic and stabilizes over time as the nervous and digestive systems mature. Most infants do not exceed 5 continuous hours of sleep for some months, and this can be very disruptive to the mother's need for sleep.

Activity/Exercise

The newborn is able to do little independently. At birth, some infants are able to lift their heads and turn them from side to side. Most other activity is reflex in nature.

Maintenance of a clear airway is critical. Many infants require suctioning to remove mucus from the nose and mouth. Newborns are obligate nose breathers; they must be able to breathe through their nose while suckling. Therefore the nasal passageway must be kept open and free from mucus. A small bulb syringe is most commonly used. It must be decompressed before insertion and then gently released to suction secretions. Parents should have use of the bulb syringe explained before the first feeding. For the first few days a bulb syringe should always be kept with the newborn, particularly during feeding time.

Crying is the newborn's only means of communication. The cry can be used to indicate hunger, pain, or simply the need for attention. The cry of the newborn should be strong, vigorous, and of medium pitch. A high-pitched cry may indicate neurological problems.

The respiratory movements of a newborn are diaphragmatic and are best measured by counting the rise and fall of the abdomen. The normal respiratory rate is between 30 and 60 respirations per minute. Flaring of the nostrils, sternal retraction, or tachypnea could indicate distress and should be reported.

The normal range for the newborn heart rate is between 120 and 150 beats per minute. Rates as low as 100 beats per minute when sleeping, and as high as 180 beats per minute when crying, are not unusual. The heart beat should have a regular rate and rhythm. The apical beat can be auscultated between the fourth and fifth intercostal spaces. This is best done when the infant is asleep. Murmurs are rather common in the newborn. The physician will determine whether they are significant.

Blood pressure is approximately 80/40 in a healthy newborn. Electronic equipment with a specialized sensor is required to obtain accurate readings. Blood pressure readings are taken infrequently, unless complications occur.

Role/Relationship

The human infant is born quite defenseless. Without someone to meet his needs he could not survive. The parents, primarily the mother, are responsible for his physical and psychological development.

Parenting is not instinctive; a new parent must bond with the baby first. **Bonding** is defined as the initial phase in a relationship characterized by strong attraction and a desire to interact. (Fig. 44-14) Without bonding it would be difficult to keep up the effort and maintain the energy required to meet the needs of the newborn. The nurse cannot make bonding occur but can facilitate conditions that promote its development.

Early contact with the infant is important to establish bonding. A new mother normally wishes to touch and explore her baby. Holding the infant close and looking eye to eye help bonding to occur. It is normal for new mothers to talk in high-pitched tones to the new baby. The nurse should encourage early and frequent interaction between the newborn and the parents. Attachment should continue to increase when the infant begins to respond to its parents.

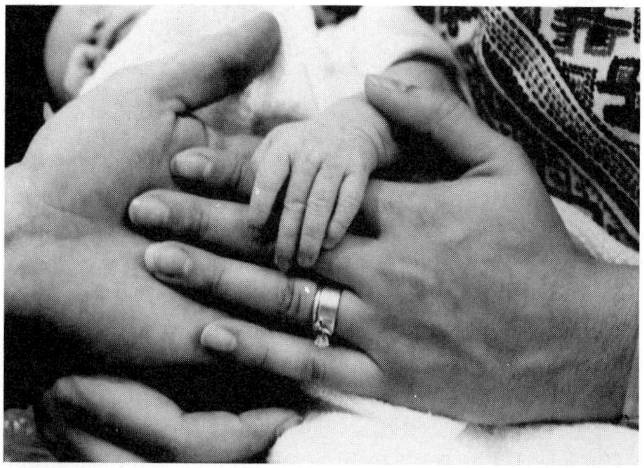

FIG. 44-14 Hands. (Courtesy St. Luke's Hospital, Kansas City, Mo.)

Periods of quiet alertness are best for interaction between the baby and parents. The nurse should explain the different levels of alertness to the parents so they can also recognize them. Care should be timed so that the mother is available to enjoy quiet moments with her newborn.

NURSING PROCESS SUMMARY

In performing an assessment on a postpartum patient or the newborn, Tables 44-3 and 44-4 will assist the nurse in reviewing all health patterns. This is simply a guideline to help focus observations; significant observations or responses will indicate the need for further questioning. If the nurse is unsure of the significance of data, it is important to consult with another nurse.

In addition, possible diagnoses and interventions are suggested.

REFERENCES AND SUGGESTED READINGS

1. Bobak IM and Jensen MD: Essentials of maternity nursing, St Louis, 1990, The CV Mosby Co.
2. Burroughs A: Bleir's maternity nursing, ed 5, Philadelphia, 1986, WB Saunders Co.
3. Doenges M and Moorhouse M: Nurse's pocket guide to nursing diagnosis with interventions, ed 2, Philadelphia, 1988, FA Davis Co.
4. Fischbach F: A manual of laboratory diagnostic tests, ed 3, Philadelphia, 1988, JB Lippincott Co.
5. Gay JT, Edgil AE, and Douglas AB: Reva Rubin revisited, Gynecol Neonatal Nurs 17:6, 1988.
6. Ingalls AJ and Salerno MC: Maternal and child health nursing, ed 7, St Louis, 1990, The CV Mosby Co.
7. Jaffe MS and Melson KA: Maternal-infant health care plans, Springhouse, Pa, 1989, Springhouse Corp.
8. Keefe MR: The impact of rooming in on maternal sleep at night, J Obstet Gynecol Neonatal Nurs 17:2, 1988.
9. Ladewig PW, London ML, and Olds SB: Essentials of maternal newborn nursing, ed 2, Redwood City, Calif, 1990, Addison-Wesley.
10. Ladewig PW, London ML, and Olds SB: Maternal-newborn nursing: a family-centered approach, ed 3, Menlo Park, Calif, 1988, Addison-Wesley.
11. Phillips CR: Rehumanizing maternal-child nursing, Mat Child Nurs 13:5, 1988.
12. Pillitteri A: Maternal-newborn nursing: care of the growing family, ed 3, Boston, 1985, Little, Brown & Co.
13. Pritchard JA, MacDonald PC, and Gant GF: Williams' obstetrics, ed 17, New York, 1985, Appleton-Century-Crofts.
14. Wilkerson NN et al: Synchronizing care with mother-baby rhythms, RN 13:4, 1988.

Table 44-3 Nursing Process and the Postpartum Patient

Pattern	Data Collection	Possible Nursing Diagnoses	Interventions
Health management	Is the patient interested in learning about personal care and that of the infant? Does she follow through on teaching? Did she follow through with prenatal care and does she have a physician to care for the baby? Has she made appointments for follow-up?	Altered health maintenance Noncompliance Knowledge deficit	Stress importance of medical care. Identify cause of noncompliance. Provide emotional support. Provide explanations. Teach and provide literature on postpartum care.
Nutritional/metabolic	Is diet adequate per recommended daily allowance? Is fluid intake adequate? How much weight has been gained/lost? Does she have an episiotomy? What is the condition of breasts and nipples? Is she breast-feeding?	Altered nutrition: less than body requirements; more than body requirements Fluid volume deficit Fluid volume excess Impaired skin integrity	Initiate dietary consultation. Review basic food groups and provide literature. Stress importance of diet if breast-feeding. Review perineal care and sitz bath.
Activity/exercise	What does she know about postpartum exercise? Who is available to help with care at home? How many other children are at home? Vital signs?	Potential for injury Activity intolerance Pain	Stress importance of pacing activities. Explore options for help at home.
Elimination	Has pattern of urine elimination changed? Has bowel elimination pattern changed? Is there any burning with urination? Pain with defecation? Constipation? Diarrhea?	Altered bowel elimination Altered patterns of urinary elimination Potential for infection	Discuss dietary interventions to prevent constipation. Teach Kegel's exercise. Review signs of urinary tract infection.
Rest/sleep	Has sleep pattern changed? Increased fatigue noticed? Does patient take naps or rest periods?	Sleep pattern disturbance	Discuss daily activities required and possibility of naps.
Cognitive/perceptual	Is there any pain? Nature? Duration? Location? Is she knowledgeable about newborn care? Growth and development and safety needs of newborns?	Potential for injury Knowledge deficit	Provide information regarding infant and child care. Provide materials on growth and development. Stress safety teaching.
Role/relationship	Does she feel confused about her changing role? Have interpersonal dynamics with husband, boyfriend, parents, friends changed?	Altered role performance Altered family processes	Listen; involve significant others in teaching. Possible social service contact if serious problems with dynamics observed.
Coping/stress	What fears or anxieties are verbalized? How has her self-image changed?	Anxiety Fear Ineffective coping	Listen; provide explanations at patient's level of understanding. Provide written materials.
Value/belief	What is the patient's cultural background? Religious practices?	Spiritual distress	Incorporate cultural practices into care whenever possible. Consult minister, priest, rabbi for specific information if needed.

Table 44-4 Nursing Process and the Newborn

Pattern	Data Collection	Possible Nursing Diagnoses	Interventions
Health management	Are the parents aware of the need for regular physical examination and the need for immunizations? Are the parents aware of normal growth and development during the first year of life?	Noncompliance Knowledge deficit	Identify cause of noncompliance. Provide emotional support. Provide explanations. Teach and provide literature regarding health needs of infant.
Nutritional/metabolic	What type of feeding is the infant receiving? Breast-fed? Formula? What type? How much consumed at each feeding? Any breaks in skin? How much weight has been lost? More than 10% of body weight? Body temperature?	Altered nutrition: less than body requirements Fluid volume deficit Altered body temperature: hypothermia Potential for infection	Monitor changes in weight. Provide support and information regarding breast/bottle feeding. Refer to support groups. Monitor temperature. Provide adequate warmth.
Activity/exercise	Is the airway clear of secretions? Can infant move freely? Symmetrically? Are gluteal folds equal? Can infant lift his head? Muscle tone?	Potential for injury Ineffective airway clearance	Stress importance of safety when handling infant. Teach proper positioning and holds. Keep bulb syringe available to remove mucus.
Elimination	How often does the infant void? What is the frequency, color, and consistency of stool? Are there any unusual observations about urine or stool?	Constipation Altered patterns of urinary elimination Potential for infection	Teach mother normal changes in bowel/bladder elimination. Teach proper cleansing of perineal area.
Rest/Sleep	What sleep pattern is observed? Does the infant wake readily for feeding? How many hours are spent asleep?	Sleep pattern disturbance	Discuss positioning after feeding. Explain normal variation of sleep patterns to parents.
Cognitive/perceptual	Does the infant respond to loud noises? Is eye-to-eye contact made? Does the infant appear to be in pain? Is crying continuous or intermittent?	Potential for injury	Discuss normal developmental/sensory changes.
Role/relationship	What is the parents' response to the infant? How does the mother handle the infant? Does the infant quiet with cuddling?	Altered role performance Altered family processes	Listen; involve significant others in teaching. Possible social service contact if serious problems with dynamics observed.
Coping/stress	What fears or anxieties are verbalized by the mother? What experience or knowledge regarding child care?	Anxiety Fear Ineffective coping	Listen; provide explanations at parents' level of understanding. Provide written materials.
Value/belief	What is the patient's cultural background? Family's religious practices?	Spiritual distress	Incorporate cultural practices into care whenever possible. Consult minister, priest, rabbi for specific information if needed.

CHAPTER CHALLENGE

KEY POINTS

- During the 6 weeks after delivery, the reproductive organs return to approximately the prepregnant size and location.
- The new mother should avoid dieting and excessive activity during the early postpartum period.
- Fatigue and depression are common as a result of hormonal and physiological changes.
- Complications can occur during the postpartum period. It is essential that the nurse assess each woman carefully.
- Before discharge the nurse should provide instruction concerning the danger signs of the postpartum period and verify that the woman knows when and how to contact her physician.
- Hormonal changes enable the woman to produce enough milk to meet the nutritional needs of the growing infant. Nutri-

KEY POINTS (cont'd)

tional needs of the lactating woman are similar to those during pregnancy.
- Motherhood is a learned skill. The new mother will require extensive teaching and encouragement about parenting skills.
- Early discharge requires that the nurse provide essential teaching in a brief period. The nurse should be careful to document teaching.
- The nurse should supplement teaching with written materials so the new mother has something to refer to when at home.
- There is a wide range of normal variation among newborns. The inexperienced nurse should verify any questionable observations with an experienced nurse or physician.
- Hypothermia and infection are two major areas of concern when providing care to the newborn.
- The nurse should provide demonstration and teaching to educate the mother about the hygiene needs of the newborn.

STUDY QUESTIONS

1. The postpartum period lasts until:
   a. Vital signs are stable 24 hours after delivery
   b. The woman is discharged from the hospital
   c. 1 week after discharge from the hospital
   d. The reproductive organs have returned to prepregnant size and position
2. Uterine contraction is necessary to prevent:
   a. Hemorrhage
   b. Thrombophlebitis
   c. Infection
   d. Afterbirth pains
3. When the nurse performs postpartum checks the fundus is displaced to the side. This is probably caused by:
   a. The woman's position in bed
   b. The trauma of labor and delivery
   c. An enlarged bladder
   d. Inadequate contraction of the uterus
4. On the first day postpartum the breasts are inspected. It is normal to observe:
   a. Soft breasts with colostrum production
   b. Engorged breasts producing milk
   c. Soft breasts and no secretions
   d. Breasts firm in the axillary region and producing milk
5. Nursing care in the postpartum stage focuses on:
   a. Assessment of vital signs and uterine contraction
   b. Assessment of urine and bowel elimination
   c. Assessment of activity and exercise tolerance
   d. All of the above assessments
6. Correct hygiene is very important to prevent:
   a. Urinary tract infections
   b. Contamination of the reproductive tract
   c. Transmission of microorganisms to the newborn
   d. All of the above
7. Assessment of the normal postpartum patient will typically reveal:
   a. Diaphoresis
   b. Malodorous vaginal drainage
   c. Temperature above 100.4° F (38° C)
   d. Swollen, painful breasts
8. Apprehension is common in the new mother. The nurse can reduce this by:
   a. Being efficient and competent
   b. Telling the mother what to do
   c. Listening to the mother's concerns
   d. Referring the mother for counseling
9. The newborn is given an injection of vitamin K to:
   a. Supplement breast-feeding
   b. Prevent hemorrhage
   c. Promote tissue development
   d. Help utilize calcium
10. The Apgar score includes assessment of:
    a. Respiratory effort
    b. Cartilage development of the ear
    c. Palmar creases
    d. Neurological maturity
11. Occluded sebaceous glands on the face and nose result in:
    a. Erythema toxicum neonatorum
    b. Strawberry birthmarks
    c. Milia
    d. Telangiectitic nevi
12. Edema observed on the head of the newborn that does not cross the midline of the skull is most likely:
    a. Cephalhematoma
    b. Caput succedaneum
    c. Cranial deviation
    d. Molding
13. A serious danger to newborns is risk of:
    a. Infection
    b. Hypothermia
    c. Aspiration
    d. All of the above

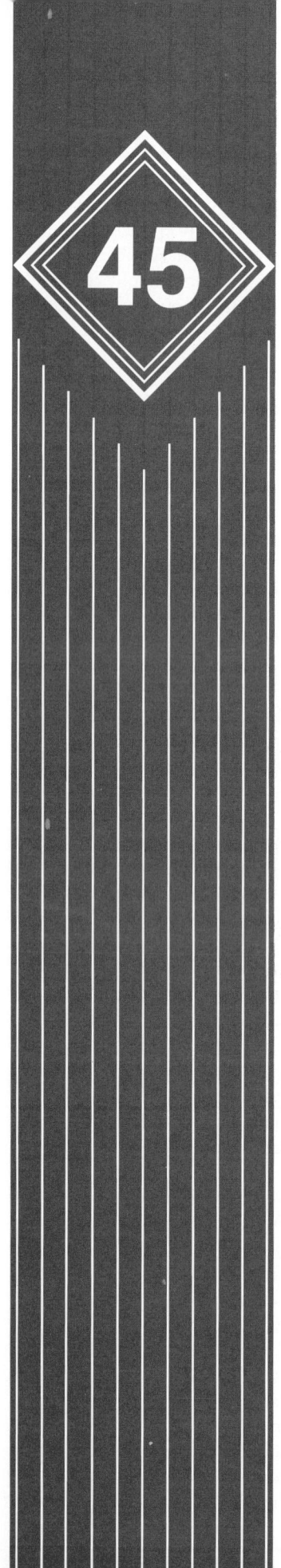

45

Care of the Mother and Newborn at Risk

GLORIA E. WOLD

LEARNING OBJECTIVES

After reading this chapter, the student should be able to do the following:

- Define the key terms.
- List those conditions that increase maternal and fetal risk.
- Discuss bleeding disorders that can occur during pregnancy.
- Identify diagnostic tests used to identify high-risk situations.
- Discuss the significance of maternal age to outcome of pregnancy.
- Discuss preexisting maternal health conditions that influence pregnancy.
- List the infectious diseases most likely to cause serious complications.
- Discuss the problems created by alcohol and drug abuse.
- Identify concerns related to preterm infants.
- Explain the hemolytic diseases of the newborn.
- Discuss nursing diagnoses related to high-risk conditions of the mother and newborn.

RELATED TOPICS OF INTEREST

- The adolescent (Chapter 10)
- Care of the patient with a cardiovascular disorder (Chapter 32)
- Care of the patient with an endocrine disorder (Chapter 35)
- Care of the patient with a reproductive disorder (Chapter 36)
- Care of the patient with AIDS (Chapter 40)
- The patient with an addictive personality (Chapter 50)

KEY TERMS

Define the following:

- anasarca
- atony
- chlamydia
- clonus(ic)
- dizygotic
- eclampsia
- gestational diabetes mellitus
- glycosylated hemoglobin
- hydramnios
- kernicterus
- monozygotic
- phototherapy
- pregnancy-induced hypertension (PIH)
- preeclampsia
- tonus(ic)
- TORCH infections

Although most pregnancies proceed normally, complications and high-risk situations can occur at any stage of the childbearing process, and the nurse must be aware of these so that appropriate, timely actions can be taken. Two lives are involved, and the nurse must provide care that protects the welfare of both.

HYPEREMESIS GRAVIDARUM

Etiology

Although mild morning sickness is common, hyperemesis gravidarum, also called *pernicious vomiting*, is a serious complication.

The exact cause of this condition is not known. Hormones, particularly human chorionic gonadotropin (HCG), are suspected: hyperemesis is more common with conditions in which there are high human chorionic gonadotropin levels, such as hydatidiform mole. Psychogenic factors may also be involved.

Clinical Manifestations

The mother experiences vomiting and retching that far exceeds that seen with normal morning sickness. Women with hyperemesis gravidarum may border on starvation and become severely dehydrated. Many serious complications that endanger both the mother and fetus can result. Acid-base imbalance related to the loss of excessive amounts of hydrochloric acid or intestinal juices may occur, resulting in alkalosis or acidosis. Potassium may become depleted, leading to cardiac dysrhythmias. Vitamin deficiencies can lead to jaundice and hemorrhage. If untreated, hyperemesis gravidarum can result in maternal and fetal death.

Assessment

The frequency, amount, and character of emesis should be assessed and reported. Fluid intake and output are measured carefully. Assessment of the fetal status is also important. The nurse must monitor fetal heart rate regularly and immediately report any significant changes.

Medical Management

Medical treatment is directed at meeting nutritional needs, thereby maintaining acid-base and electrolyte balance. Intravenous feeding must be monitored closely. Solid intake is restricted until vomiting stops and the woman feels capable of trying solid food. Bland solids, such as toast and crackers, or liquids are introduced slowly, and the woman's ability to tolerate these foods must be carefully assessed.

Nursing Interventions

Typically this patient is hospitalized and given parenteral fluids. Oral hygiene is essential, because the mouth may be irritated by the vomitus. Care is needed to reduce the mother's emotional distress; fear for herself and for her fetus are commonly observed. The nurse should provide emotional support and explanations.

NURSING DIAGNOSES	NURSING INTERVENTIONS
Altered nutrition: less than body requirements, related to pregnancy	Monitor food intake; Caloric record may be desirable. Offer dry crackers and bland food as tolerated. Provide a pleasant atmosphere at meal time.
Fluid volume deficit, related to decreased fluid intake and excessive fluid loss	Measure and record intake and output. Administer fluids as ordered. Assess skin turgor. Weigh daily at same time.
Potential for altered oral mucous membranes, related to dehydration and frequent emesis	Inspect oral cavity daily. Provide oral hygiene before meals and after each emesis, using soft bristle brush and oral swabs. Lubricate lips.
Fear, related to possibility of harm to fetus or self	Provide opportunities to verbalize fears. Provide continuity of care whenever possible.

MULTIPLE PREGNANCY

Etiology

Pregnancy involving twins occurs in approximately 1 of 90 births in the United States. Triplets occur in approximately 1 in 7600 births. Pregnancies involving more than three fetuses are even more rare. Pregnancies involving five or more embryos are often a result of fertility drugs.

Twins are classified as monozygotic or dizygotic. **Monozygotic** twins originate with one fertilized ovum, the embryonic disk divides, causing "identical twins." Because the genetic message is identical, the twins must be of the same sex and carry an identical genetic code. They share a placenta, but each has a separate umbilical cord. **Dizygotic** twins are the result of two separate ova being fertilized at the same time. These twins, while they share the uterus, have separate placentas. The sex and genetic makeup can vary; they are no more closely related than siblings born at different times (Fig. 45-1).

Pathophysiology

Maternal and fetal risks are increased during multiple pregnancy. Spontaneous abortions, maternal anemia, pregnancy-induced hypertension, hydramnios, and bleeding from placenta previa or abruptio placentae are more common in women with twins. Congenital anomalies, problems with entangled cords, and growth problems are common in the fetuses. An incomplete separation of the embryonic disk can result in conjoined ("Siamese") twins.

Labor may be complicated by loss of uterine tone resulting from overstretching of the musculature, abnormal presentations, and preterm labor. Many twin pregnancies and almost all pregnancies with more than two fetuses result in the need for cesarean delivery.

Clinical Manifestations

Multiple pregnancy is suspected when uterine enlargement exceeds the norm. Abdominal palpation using Leopold's maneuvers, auscultation of two distinct heart tones, and ultrasonography will reveal the presence of multiple fetuses.

BLEEDING DISORDERS

Vaginal bleeding during pregnancy is an indication that problems exist; women should be instructed to contact their physician if any bleeding occurs. Depending on the stage of pregnancy, several different conditions may cause the bleeding. Assessment, diagnostic tests, and nursing interventions for bleeding disorders will be addressed later in the Chapter.

ECTOPIC PREGNANCY

Etiology

In ectopic pregnancy implantation occurs somewhere other than within the uterus. The most common site of ectopic implantation is within the fallopian tube. Other possible sites include the abdominal cavity, ovary, ligaments, or cervix.

Ectopic pregnancy occurs when for some reason the progress of the fertilized ovum through the fallopian tube is slowed or obstructed. Pelvic inflammatory disease, resulting in tubal obstruction, is commonly a cause.

Pathophysiology

When the fertilized ovum implants and begins to develop in the fallopian tube, it soon grows to a size too large to be contained. This results in rupture of the tube and bleeding into the abdominal cavity.

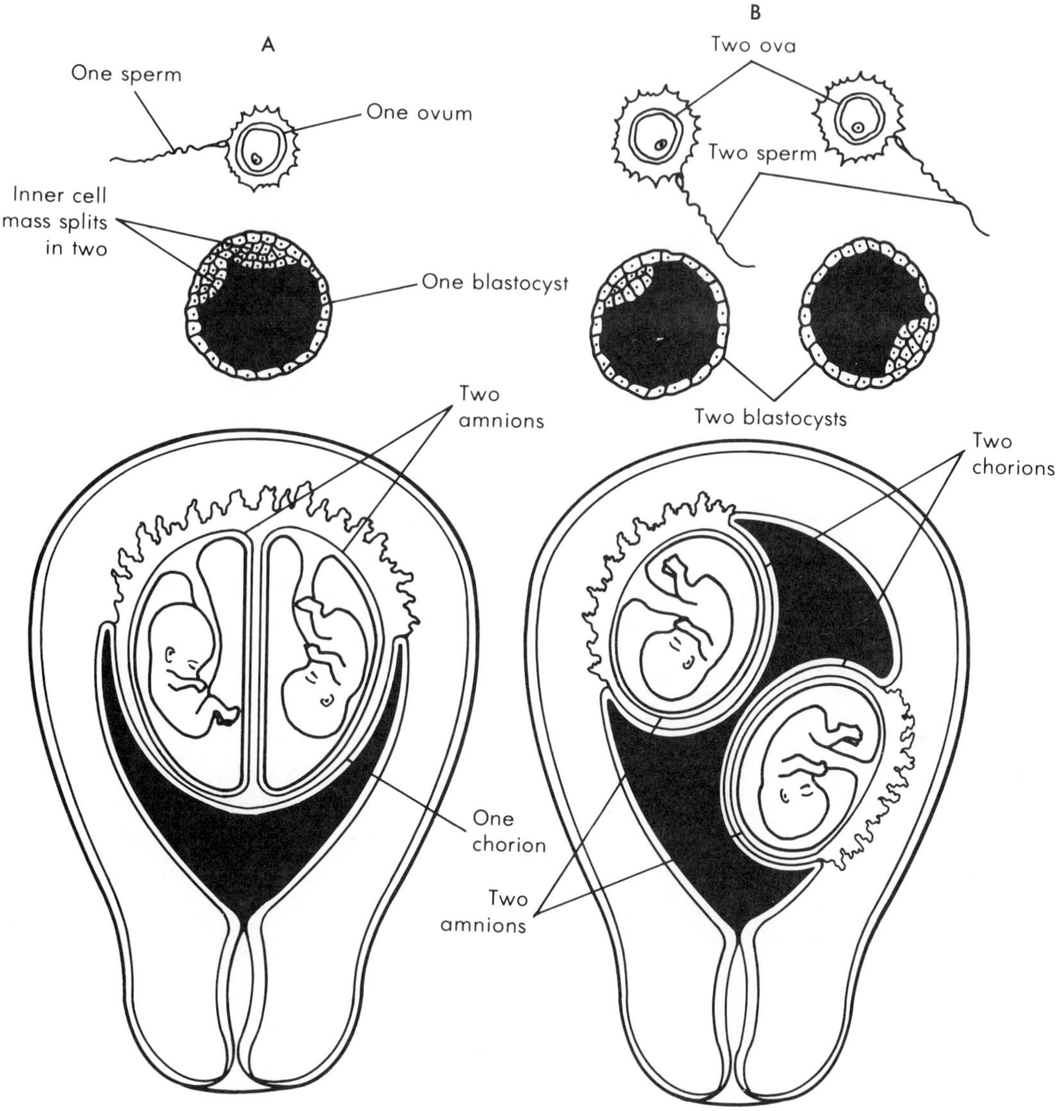

FIG. 45-1 Multiple pregnancies. **A,** Identical twins develop from one ovum and one sperm. **B,** Fraternal twins develop from two ova and two sperm.

Clinical Manifestations

Vaginal bleeding may be observed and hypovolemic shock may be present. Signs of peritoneal irritation include sharp, localized, one-sided pain or pain referred to the shoulder. The abdomen may become rigid and tender.

Medical Management

In the presence of ectopic pregnancy, rapid surgical treatment and blood loss replacement are generally indicated.

SPONTANEOUS ABORTION

Etiology

Abortion is the termination of pregnancy before the age of viability. Most abortions occur during the first trimester of pregnancy. It is estimated that as many as 20% of all pregnancies end in first-trimester spontaneous abortion. Many of these go unrecognized, with the woman merely thinking her menstrual period was delayed.

Spontaneous abortions may be caused by a number of factors. The most common cause is chromosomal abnormalities. Faulty implantation, teratogenic drugs, maternal infections, endocrine imbalances, and abnormalities of the reproductive tract are other common causes.

Pathophysiology

The pathophysiology depends on the specific cause.

Clinical Manifestations

The main presenting symptom is bleeding, which may or may not be accompanied by cramps or backache. Spontaneous abortions are classified as follows:

1. Threatened: Unexplained bleeding and cramping occurs. The fetus may or may not be alive. Membranes remain intact, and the cervical os remains closed.
2. Imminent: Bleeding increases and the cervical os begins to dilate. Membranes may rupture.
3. Complete: All products of conception are expelled from the uterus.
4. Incomplete: Some, but not all, of the products of conception are expelled.
5. Missed: The fetus dies and growth ceases, but the fetus remains in utero. Amenorrhea continues, but no uterine growth is measurable. In fact, the uterus may decrease in size.
6. Habitual: Three or more consecutive spontaneous abortions.

Medical Management

IV fluids may be administered, and blood loss may be replaced with transfusions when a spontaneous abortion occurs. A dilation and curettage (D&C) may be indicated to remove retained placental tissue.

PLACENTA PREVIA

Etiology

Placenta previa occurs when the placenta implants in the lower uterine segment. This may be covering the cervical os completely or marginally (Fig. 45-2, A).

The cause of placenta previa is unknown. It is more common in multiparas and seems to recur in the same woman.

Pathophysiology

In the last trimester of pregnancy, uterine size increases and the cervix begins to dilate. As the placenta separates from the uterus at the internal os of the cervix, sinuses at the site begin to bleed. The amount of bleeding depends on the amount of separation that occurs.

Clinical Manifestations

The main presenting symptom of placenta previa is painless vaginal bleeding occurring after 20 weeks' gestation.

Medical Management

Because of the relative safety of cesarean birth today, this is usually the treatment of choice for placenta previa. Some obstetricians may adopt a "wait and see" attitude and eventually deliver the baby vaginally.

ABRUPTIO PLACENTAE

Etiology

Abruptio placentae is premature separation of the placenta from the uterine wall. This generally occurs late in pregnancy, frequently during labor (Fig. 45-2, B).

The cause is unknown. Some predisposing factors include trauma, chronic hypertension, and pregnancy-induced hypertension.

Pathophysiology

When the placenta separates from the uterine wall, bleeding from uterine sinuses occurs, as in placenta previa. Three major forms of abruptio placentae have been identified:

1. Central: bleeding occurs in the center of the placenta; because the margins of the placenta remain

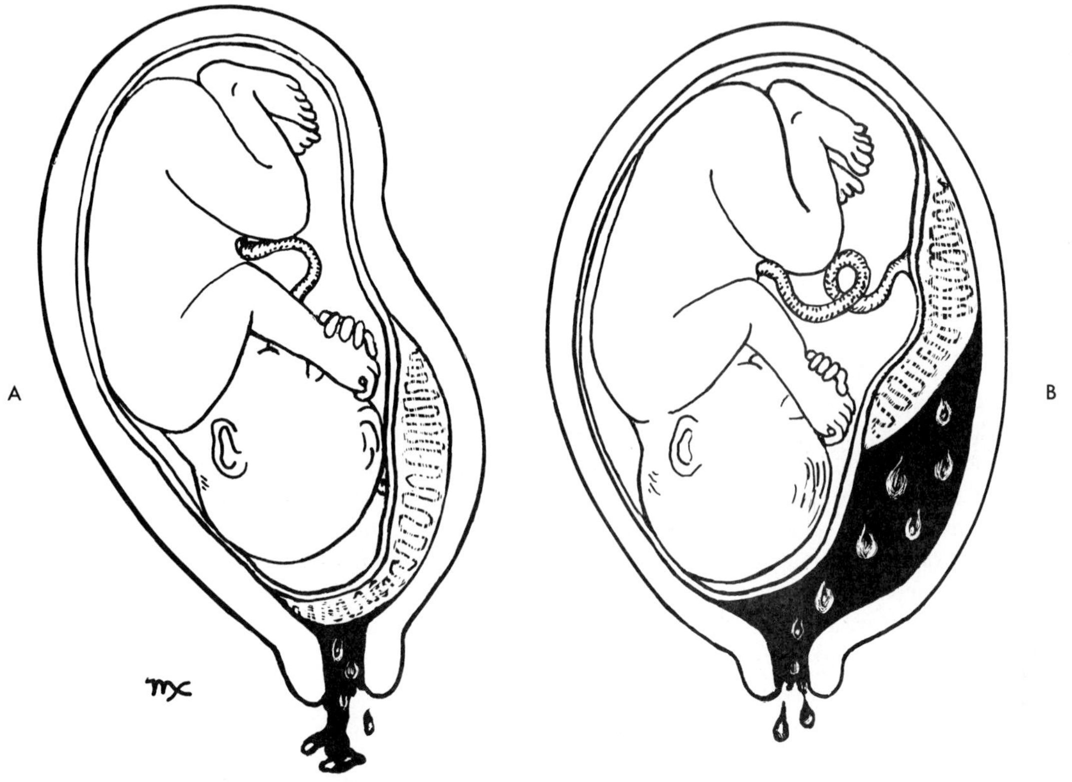

FIG. 45-2 **A,** A type of total placenta previa. **B,** Abruptio placentae, or separation of normally inserted placenta.

attached, the bleeding is not visible, resulting in a concealed hemorrhage.

2. Marginal: bleeding occurs when an edge of the placenta separates from the uterus; vaginal bleeding is apparent.
3. Complete: the entire placenta separates from the uterine wall; vaginal bleeding is profuse.

Clinical Manifestations

The major symptoms of abruptio placentae are sudden, severe pain accompanied by uterine rigidity. The uterus may also increase in size as a result of the hemorrhage. The first sign during labor may be very strong and constant contractions.

Assessment

When any vaginal bleeding occurs during pregnancy, the nurse should assess the following:

1. *The duration, amount, color, and characteristics of the bleeding.* This includes assessing (a) the time since the onset of bleeding, (b) what, if any, activity preceded the bleeding episode, (c) the number of pads saturated per hour, and (d) the color of the bleeding (bright red, dark red, or brown). If any clots or tissue is passed, it should be saved for examination by the physician.
2. *The vital signs.* Depending on the origin and severity of the bleeding, signs of shock may be present. In addition to pulse and blood pressure, it is important to observe for pallor, diaphoresis, cool, clammy skin, or dyspnea. These physical signs will seem out of proportion to the amount of bleeding if the hemorrhage is concealed, as in central abruptio placentae.
3. *Pain.* The nurse should note the location, nature, and duration of pain and whether bleeding is painless. This will help the physician determine the cause of the bleeding.
4. *Fetal heart rate.* Depending on the stage of pregnancy, this may be done with fetoscope or Doppler amplifier. If pregnancy is in the early stages, fetal heart sounds may not be heard. In labor when there is utero placental insufficiency, the fetus, in its struggle to obtain more oxygen, may be very restless and active. The fetal heart rate either greatly accelerates or slows.
5. *Emotional response.* The mother's fear for her own life and life of the fetus is common. Guilt that she

did something that caused the bleeding is also common.

Medical Management

Abruptio placentae in its more severe form is an obstetrical emergency. The treatment often, but not always, includes delivery by cesarean birth and blood replacement.

Diagnostic Tests

The most common laboratory tests include determination of hemoglobin and hematocrit levels. These tests determine the amount of blood loss. Blood typing and cross-matching of blood for transfusion are ordered in case blood replacement is necessary. Hormone studies may be ordered to determine fetal death. Ultrasound scans may be done to determine placental location. Vaginal and rectal examination are avoided, because they may cause increased bleeding.

Nursing Interventions

Nursing measures are structured to support and promote optimal physical and psychological functioning.

Oxygen should be available. If blood loss is significant, oxygen-carrying capability is decreased; therefore oxygen may be ordered to prevent maternal or fetal hypoxia.

Intravenous or blood replacement therapy may be required, and the nurse should be prepared for this.

Possible loss of the pregnancy is a crisis. It is important for the nurse to be supportive of the patient's and family's emotional needs. The nurse should remain with the woman as much as possible, listen to her concerns, give clear explanations about medical treatment, and prepare her for the possible loss.

NURSING DIAGNOSES	NURSING INTERVENTIONS
Fluid volume deficit, related to hemorrhage	Monitor and record vital signs every 15 minutes until stable, then every 1 hour as indicated. Measure and record intake and output. Weigh daily. Assess skin turgor and mucous membranes. Assist patient to ambulate.
Anticipatory grieving, related to possible loss of pregnancy	Allow time for patient to verbalize concerns about loss. Assist with grieving processes. Encourage contact with support system.
Fear, related to unknown outcome	Allow time to verbalize fears. Maintain continuity of care whenever possible.

DISSEMINATED INTRAVASCULAR COAGULATION

Etiology

Disseminated intravascular coagulation (DIC) is a potentially life-threatening disorder that results from alterations in the normal clotting mechanism. It may be seen with abruptio placentae, incomplete abortion, hypertensive disease, or infectious process.

Pathophysiology

As a result of stressing the coagulation processes in an attempt to prevent excessive blood loss, the body produces excessive amounts of thrombin, stimulating the conversion of fibrinogen to fibrin. Elevated fibrin levels result in multiple small clots forming in small blood vessels, which may lead to obstruction of vessels, ischemia, and damage to vital organs. This clot formation also traps platelets and can result in generalized hemorrhage.

Clinical Manifestations

The onset of symptoms is sudden. The patient may complain of chest pain or dyspnea and become extremely restless and cyanotic, occasionally expectorating frothy, blood-tinged mucus. Profound circulatory shock from hemorrhage may occur rapidly. Fetal and maternal death may occur.

Assessment

All women with complications that may result in DIC should be observed closely for signs of bleeding such as epistaxis (nosebleeds), bleeding gums, or petechiae. Maternal and fetal condition should continue to be monitored by assessment of vital signs, fetal heart rate, and intake and output and by good general observation.

Diagnostic Tests

Blood testing includes determination of hemoglobin and hematocrit. Clotting factor studies, such as fibrinogen levels, platelet counts, prothrombin time (PT) and partial thromboplastin time (PTT), are typically ordered. Laboratory tests may reveal various degrees of anemia and decreased fibrinogen and platelet counts. Prolonged prothrombin time (PT) and partial thromboplastin time (PTT) are also typical.

Medical Management

Emergency care for DIC includes IV administration of fibrinogen, blood, and other substances that will help restore normal clotting mechanisms, which pardoxically in DIC may include heparin and oxygen therapy. If the fetus is not yet born, deliverey should occur as soon as possible.

Nursing Interventions

Nursing interventions are directed at supporting medical treatment. Signs and symptoms must be reported promptly and completely. Caution should be used when providing care to minimize the risk of additional trauma to tissues, which may lead to further bleeding.

NURSING DIAGNOSIS	NURSING INTERVENTIONS
Potential impaired gas exchange, related to impaired oxygen-carrying capacity of the blood resulting from hemorrhage	Move patient slowly to prevent orthostatic hypotension. Avoid trauma during care. Check entire body for signs of bleeding. Monitor vital signs and laboratory values; report deviations from normal promptly.

POSTPARTUM HEMORRHAGE

Etiology

Postpartum hemorrhage is described in two stages: early postpartum hemorrhage is defined as blood loss greater than 500 ml in the first 24 hours after delivery; late postpartum hemorrhage occurs after the first 24 hours.

The most common causes of early hemorrhage are (1) uterine **atony**, often related to excessive distention of the uterus from multiple pregnancy, hydramnios (excessive amount of amniotic fluid), or a very large infant. Atony is also more common in grand multiparas or in cases in which labor has been prolonged or traumatic; (2) retained placenta or fragments of the placenta; and (3) lacerations of the perineum. The most common cause of late postpartum hemorrhage is retained fragments of the placenta.

Pathophysiology

The major action that prevents hemorrhage is contraction of the uterus, which seals off the uterine sinuses. Hemorrhage results when loss of tone or tissue remaining in the cavity prevents adequate contraction of the uterus.

Assessment

Nursing assessment of uterine contraction and lochia is part of routine postpartum assessment. If the uterus is found to be boggy or if the flow of lochia is heavy, hemorrhage should be suspected. Vital signs may also change if blood loss is substantial. Any alteration noted should be reported promptly.

Medical Management

The medical treatment for retained placental fragments is D&C, whereby the retained tissue is surgically removed. Blood transfusions are administered if hemorrhage is severe.

Nursing Interventions

Nursing interventions are directed at reducing blood loss. Initial care includes massage of the uterus; normally this increases the uterine tone and decreases bleeding. If the uterus remains atonic, the physician typically prescribes an oxytocin. Vital signs should be monitored carefully when oxytocin is administered. If bleeding continues, one may suspect that placental fragments have been retained. If a D&C is required, the nurse prepares the patient for surgery. Explanations of the necessity of surgery should be given to reduce apprehension. Consent forms must be signed and all other surgical preparations completed.

NURSING DIAGNOSES	NURSING INTERVENTIONS
Decreased cardiac output, related to postpartum blood loss	Monitor vital signs. Measure and record intake and output. Increase activity level slowly to avoid fatigue. Administer oxygen as needed.
Fear, related to possible surgical intervention	Allow opportunities to verbalize fears. Explain all treatments and procedures. Maintain continuity of care when possible. Include significant others.
Knowledge deficit, related to signs of hemorrhage	Select teaching strategies appropriate to patient's need. Demonstrate postpartum checks of fundus and lochia. Observe patient performing self-check. Review importance of contacting the physician if signs are abnormal or questionable.

Patient Education

Because today's patients leave the hospital in a relatively short time, it is important to teach the patient how to perform the postpartum checks of the fundus and lochia. They should be aware that it is important to call the physician if bleeding is excessive or persists longer than expected.

THROMBOPHLEBITIS

Etiology and Pathophysiology

Thrombophlebitis is clot formation in response to inflammation of the wall of the vein. Thrombophlebitis may involve either the deep or superficial veins. It is most often seen in the postpartum patient and is more common in women who deliver by cesarean section. Inactivity, venous stasis, and alteration in clotting factors resulting from pregnancy contribute to this problem.

Clinical Manifestations

The symptoms of thrombophlebitis include tenderness and warmth in a section of the vein. Erythema may be observed. Occasionally the patient will have a low-grade fever or elevated pulse. If the thrombus should break loose and travel through the circulatory system, pulmonary embolus—a life-threatening situation—may result.

Assessment

The nurse should assess for the presence of Homans' sign each day. Any complaints of pain in the lower extremities should be further examined. If thrombophlebitis is suspected, measurement of the calf circumference is desirable. Pedal pulses on the affected leg should be taken. It is also very important to observe for signs of pulmonary embolus.

Medical Management

Typically this includes bed rest, application of heat, use of elastic stockings, and possibly administration of anticoagulant medications. If pain is present, analgesics are administered.

Diagnostic Tests

If assessment indicates a problem, the physician may order venograms or other testing to confirm the diagnosis.

Nursing Interventions

Prevention of thrombophlebitis is an important nursing responsibility. Early ambulation, particularly of the c-section patient, is essential. If a thrombus develops, the nurse implements the medical treatment. Anticoagulants pose additional hazards for postpartum patients, because they increase blood loss through the vessels of the uterus. Assessment of lochia drainage must be done with great accuracy to detect signs of hemorrhage when anticoagulants are used.

NURSING DIAGNOSES	NURSING INTERVENTIONS
Altered tissue perfusion, related to reduced venous blood flow	Monitor vital signs every 4 hours. Observe and report any increase in TPR, dyspnea, cough, hemoptysis, or decrease in BP. Measure calves every 4 hours. Apply antiembolism stockings as ordered. Apply heat as ordered.
Altered tissue perfusion, related to reduced venous blood flow—cont'd	Elevate extremity, avoiding pressure in popliteal area. Instruct patient to avoid crossing legs. Have patient elevate legs while seated. Increase activity as ordered. Administer anticoagulants as ordered.
Potential for altered parenting, related to physical illness	Involve parents in infant care whenever possible. Explain all care and encourage parents to hold and touch infant. Increase contact time with infant when mother's physical condition permits.

Patient Education

It is important to explain to the patient all aspects of the treatment plan prescribed by the physician.

PREGNANCY-INDUCED HYPERTENSION

Etiology

Pregnancy-induced hypertension (PIH) is a serious complication of pregnancy and places both the mother and fetus at risk.

The cause of PIH is unknown. Many theories have been proposed, but to date none have been proven. This condition was formerly called *toxemia,* because it was thought that a toxin caused the symptoms. This term is no longer used. This condition is seen most often in primigravidas, particularly those under 20 or over 35 years of age. It is also more common in women from lower socioeconomic groups or individuals with poor nutritional status. A woman with a multiple pregnancy, diabetes mellitus, or family history of PIH is also at increased risk. PIH is a disease process unique to pregnancy. The only known "cure" is termination of the pregnancy.

Pathophysiology

Complex hormonal and vascular changes occur with PIH; these lead to increased blood pressure, decreased placental perfusion, decreased renal perfusion, altered glomerular filtration rate, and fluid and electrolyte imbalance.

Clinical Manifestations

The classic symptoms of PIH, in order of appearance, are (1) edema, (2) hypertension, and (3) proteinuria. These symptoms generally appear after the twentieth week of pregnancy. This is a progressive disease. Depending on the severity of the symptoms, PIH is classified as preeclampsia (which is further subdivided into mild or severe forms) and eclampsia.

Mild preeclampsia. There are few clinical symptoms in early **preeclampsia**. Change in the blood pressure readings—an increase of 30 mm Hg systolic and 15 mm Hg diastolic or a reading of 140/90 in a woman who has had normal blood pressure readings—indicates a problem. This is the reason it is important to establish baseline readings early in pregnancy. Generalized edema may be evident in the face, hands, and ankles. Weight may increase as much as 3 pounds (1.5 kg) per month in the second trimester and 1 pound (0.5 kg) per week in the third trimester. Urine testing frequently shows 1+ to 2+ albumin readings. The urine output is not less than 500 ml/24 hours.

Severe preeclampsia. The symptoms of severe preeclampsia may appear suddenly. Blood pressure readings increase, and readings of 160/110 or higher are common. Edema becomes increasingly obvious and may be observed in the face, hands, sacral area, abdomen, and throughout the lower extremities. Weight increases dramatically. As much as 2 pounds (1 kg) can be gained in a matter of a few days or a week. Urine testing for albumin shows 3+ to 4+ readings. The urine output is less than 500 ml/24 hours.

Eclampsia. Eclampsia is the most severe form of pregnancy-induced hypertension. The most dramatic characteristic is grand mal seizures, with **tonic** and **clonic** phases. This is generally followed by a coma that lasts from minutes to hours. If untreated, this sequence of seizure-coma may repeat.

Assessment

Blood pressure should be assessed routinely throughout pregnancy, labor, delivery, and the postpartum period. It is important to remember that PIH can occur anytime after the twentieth week and persist until 2 days after delivery. Weight should be recorded at each prenatal visit and compared to norms. Excessive or rapid weight gain, particularly when accompanied by edema, should be reported promptly. Assessment for edema should be done at each visit. Edema is typically described using a scale of 1+ to 4+:

1+ Minimal edema on pedal and pretibial areas
2+ Obvious edema of lower extremities
3+ Edema of face, hands, sacrum, and abdomen observed
4+ Indicates massive, generalized edema (**anasarca**)

Urine is typically tested for albumin using dipstick reagents. This should be done at each visit and on admission for labor. (If the bag of waters is ruptured, these dipstick readings may be inaccurate.) Questions about the occurrence of headaches, visual disturbance, or epigastric pain should be routinely asked, because these may also indicate problems with PIH.

If the patient is hospitalized for PIH, deep tendon reflexes and urinary output are monitored, as well as electronic monitoring of fetal heart rate.

Diagnostic Tests

Typical tests include hematocrit, BUN, and urine tests for specific gravity and protein. Often a 24-hour urine collection is obtained to determine protein loss. Electrolyte panels are commonly drawn. If symptoms indicate severe preeclampsia or eclampsia, liver function and platelet count evaluations are also done. If the physician determines that early induction of labor is required, tests for fetal maturity including estriol levels, amniocentesis, ultrasonography, and stress tests may be done.

Medical Management

The woman may or may not need to be hospitalized depending on the severity of symptoms. Very mild preeclampsia may be managed at home, but more severe symptoms require that the woman be hospitalized. Typically bed rest is ordered, preferably in the left lateral recumbent position, which will reduce pressure on the inferior vena cava and promote venous return. A well-balanced diet with adequate protein is important. Moderate sodium intake is allowed, but high-sodium foods should be avoided. Meals are allowed as long as the woman is alert and there are no signs of impending convulsions. Intravenous therapy may be initiated to keep a line open for emergency medications. Intravenous electrolytes may also be administered. In cases of severe preeclampsia or eclampsia, medications may be prescribed. Magnesium sulfate ($MgSO_4$) may be given to reduce the chance of convulsions. Sedatives and antihypertensives may also be ordered.

Nursing Interventions

The goal of nursing interventions is to be alert for signs and symptoms of preeclampsia, such as complaints of headache, edema, and blurred vision.

In mild cases routine intake and output is monitored; in severe cases it may be necessary to insert an indwelling catheter and record hourly urine output. Fetal condition must be monitored carefully. In mild cases routine auscultation of fetal heart rate is adequate; in severe cases fetal monitors will give more accurate information.

Daily weight is recorded to determine the amount of fluids eliminated from the body. Intake and output should be recorded. Blood pressure is monitored every 4 hours or more often if condition indicates. The nurse who is alert to encouraging compliance of treatment can be instrumental in preventing the patient from convulsing. Since stress may exacerbate this condition, it is important to keep the environment quiet and nonstressful.

Maintaining a stress-free environment is difficult, however, because enforced bed rest may last for several weeks. Enforced bed rest or hospitalization can be very disruptive for the patient and her family; there are financial implications, and the woman's condition can seriously affect family dynamics. Explanations of the necessity of treatment and clarification of care and treatment are essential.

NURSING DIAGNOSES	NURSING INTERVENTIONS
Altered family processes, related to protracted physical illness	Involve patient in family decision making whenever possible. Encourage family members to verbalize feelings about inability of wife/mother to participate in family activities.
Diversional activity deficit, related to environmental lack of stimulation	Elicit hobbies or interests that can be performed while at rest. Involve patient in conversation while performing care. Encourage family to visit and bring books or other recreational items. Provide change of scenery if possible.
Potential noncompliance, related to patient value system	Emphasize positive aspects of compliance. Expain importance of compliance to positive resolution of problem. Give positive reinforcement for compliant behavior. Determine values that lead to noncompliance.

Patient Education

All pregnant women must be taught the danger signs of pregnancy and the importance of regular medical supervision. Many of the symptoms of PIH, particularly the mild, early symptoms, will only be detected by maintaining regular physician contact. If PIH is diagnosed, it is important to explain the consequences of failure to comply.

High-quality protein, vitamin, and mineral intake should be encouraged. Salt restriction below normal dietary levels (4 to 6 g/24 hr) is usually not recommended.

It is important that the patient understand that bedrest is important because it slows metabolism of the body and relieves edema.

COMPLICATIONS RELATED TO INFECTIOUS PROCESSES

Infections

There are many microorganisms that can increase maternal and fetal risk. Many studies show an increase in mortality and morbidity when infection is present; thus it is important to prevent infection. If not prevented, infections should be recognized and treated promptly. The diseases of major concern are TORCH infections (Box 45-1) and AIDS (Box 45-2).

Etiology. The infectious diseases that may cause complications are numerous. While some are airborne or ingested, most are spread by direct contact, usually through sexual transmission. Others are contracted by use of contaminated needles or blood transfusions.

Nursing interventions. The presence of infection is not always evident. Because of the increased incidence of serious infectious diseases, the Centers for Disease Control (CDC) recommends that universal precautions be taken for *all* patients. These precautions are most important when dealing with blood and body fluids. When providing care to mothers and newborns the nurse is frequently exposed to blood and body fluids and must be particularly alert. Use of gloves, masks, gowns, and glasses is necessary when procedures that involve splashing of body fluids, such as amniotomy, are performed. Gloves should be used when cleaning or assessing the breasts or perineal area. Gloves should also be used when bathing the newborn. Handwashing, as always, is essential. Suctioning or resuscitation of the infant should be done using mechanical barriers or equipment such as mouth shields, suction devices, and ventilators. Care should be used when handling needles and syringes; these should be disposed of in special containers without breaking or recapping.

Psychological support is important to the patient with an infectious disease. Because many of these diseases are life threatening to the mother, fetus, or newborn, fear and anxiety are common. If the infection results in fetal mortality or defects, guilt may be expressed by the mother. The nurse must also cope with her own feelings about these serious infectious diseases. Caring for mothers and newborns with AIDS and other such diseases can create moral and ethical problems that must be resolved if the nurse is to function therapeutically.

NURSING DIAGNOSIS	NURSING INTERVENTIONS
Potential for infection, related to external factors	Practice good handwashing technique and correct use of protective gloving. Monitor vital signs, particularly temperature, every 4 hours. Observe for any drainage or discharge.

Patient education. Education on prevention of infection should start long before pregnancy. Infections acquired by a woman before she becomes pregnant can seriously affect the outcome of pregnancy. Immunization for rubella before childbearing years is essential, and the importance of having children routinely immunized should be stressed to all new mothers. Such hygiene practices as careful handwashing and proper storage and preparation of meats should be reviewed. Safe sex practices, including use of condoms, should be discussed with at-risk individuals, and the importance of regular medical care and treatment should be stressed.

BOX 45-1 TORCH INFECTIONS

T—Toxoplasmosis is caused by a protozoan, *Toxoplasma gondii,* which can be contracted by eating raw, contaminated meats or having contact with the feces of infected cats. The mother may be free of symptoms or may develop myalgia, enlarged posterior cervical lymph nodes, malaise, and rash that disappear in a matter of days. Diagnosis is confirmed by blood tests such as the IgM antibody test. The effects on the fetus can be profound: spontaneous abortion, stillbirth, neonatal death, blindness, retardation, and a wide range of congenital anomalies are associated with the disease. It is important to teach all pregnant women to avoid undercooked meats. If cats are present in the environment, the woman should wear gloves whenever chance of contact with feces exists.

O—Other; this includes the miscellaneous infections that may affect the mother and/or fetus. Urinary tract and vaginal infections can cause fever, chills, dysuria, pain, malaise, and changes in vaginal drainage. Any of these symptoms should be reported promptly to the physician. Culture and sensitivity tests will usually reveal the specific organism. The physician will base treatment on the causative organism and the severity of the problem. Treatment must be done cautiously because of the possibility of teratogenic effects from the antibiotics. Sexually transmitted diseases (STDs) are also a serious concern. Syphilis can cross the placental barrier and infect the fetus. **Chlamydia** may cause pneumonia or eye infections in the newborn. Gonorrhea can cause pelvic inflammatory disease (PID) in the mother and eye infections in the newborn.

R—Rubella, if contracted during the first trimester, can have profound effects on the fetus. A wide range of congenital defects, including congenital heart disease, mental retardation, and cataracts, may result. Diagnosis is made by serological tests for rubella titer. Immunization should ideally be given before a woman reaches childbearing age. If a pregnant woman does not have immunity, she should be cautioned to avoid risk of exposure to the disease. Because this immunization involves administration of an attenuated virus, it is given after delivery, frequently just before discharge. This is one time the physician can be certain that the woman is not pregnant. The woman should be further cautioned to avoid becoming pregnant for 2 to 3 months after vaccination, since the attenuated virus used for immunization may still be present in the mother.

C—Cytomegalovirus (CMV) is viral and belongs to the herpesvirus group. It is a very common infection that can be spread by close contact, breast-feeding, sexual relations, and kissing. More than half of all adults have antibodies to the virus. This virus is capable of crossing the placental barrier and causing serious damage to the fetus, including mental retardation, hearing problems, and congenital anomalies. It is unusual in that the mother may be totally asymptomatic and that it does not always cause fetal complications.

H—Herpes genitalis, also called herpesvirus type 2, causes painful lesions on the external genitals and can also involve the cervix. Intrauterine infection of the fetus can occur if the membranes rupture or vaginal delivery takes place when active lesions are present. If not treated the neonatal mortality rate is extremely high. Diagnosis is made on the basis of maternal symptoms and a culture of the lesions. Women with active herpes infection should be delivered by cesarean section.

BOX 45-2 AIDS

Acquired immunodeficiency syndrome is a major health concern today. It has had a significant impact on all areas of health care, including maternal nursing. The causative organism is the human immunodeficiency virus, HIV, which enters the body through blood, blood products, or sexual contact. It is capable of crossing the placental barrier and infecting the fetus in utero, causing congenital defects such as microcephaly (abnormal smallness of the head) and facial deformities. Because of the long incubation period, infants born to HIV seropositive mothers may show no indication at birth but develop signs of the infection later. These include failure to thrive, recurrent infection, interstitial pneumonia, neurological abnormalities, and others. Studies place the risk of perinatal transmission at 20% to 50%. Most children diagnosed with AIDS die within the first few years of life.

COMPLICATIONS RELATED TO EXISTING MEDICAL CONDITIONS

Diabetes Mellitus

Etiology. Diabetes mellitus is an endocrine disorder that affects metabolism and the utilization of glucose (see Chapter 35). This disease is not curable and is often difficult to control in the nonpregnant patient. In pregnancy, hormonal changes and stresses placed on all of the maternal body systems result in even more complex medical and nursing management. According to recent studies, diabetes is a risk factor in approximately 2% to 3% of pregnancies.

Pathophysiology. In diabetes the pancreas does not produce adequate amounts of insulin to metabolize glucose normally. Because glucose does not enter the cells without adequate insulin, blood glucose levels remain high. The cells release stored fat and protein for energy, leading to ketosis and a negative nitrogen balance.

Various forms of this disease have been classified. Type I, insulin-dependent diabetes mellitus (IDDM) requires regular administration of insulin for control. Type II, non-insulin-dependent diabetes mellitus (NIDDM), is most often controlled by diet or oral hypoglycemics. **Gestational diabetes mellitus** (GDM) is characterized by abnormal glucose metabolism, which is manifested only during pregnancy. A significant number of women who fall into this category will later manifest NIDDM.

Clinical manifestations. Alteration in blood glucose levels is the major manifestation of the disease. Blood glucose levels above 120 mg/dl significantly increase the risk of complications. When blood glucose levels are elevated, the classic symptoms of diabetes may be observed: polyuria, polydipsia, and polyphagia.

Effects on pregnancy. Improved control of this disease process has reduced the risk to both mother and fetus; however, the incidence of complications is still significant. Maternal complications include infections (urinary tract and vaginal), difficult labor related to increased fetal size (which frequently results in cesarean section), vascular complications (including retinopathy), azotemia, ketoacidosis, and increased incidence of hypertensive disorders. Fetal complications include spontaneous abortion, **hydramnios** (excessive amniotic fluid), large placenta, alteration in size for gestational age, congenital anomalies, increased incidence of respiratory distress syndrome, and fetal or neonatal death.

Assessment. Urine testing should be performed at all prenatal visits. If these indicate the presence of glucose, additional testing is required. For the known diabetic, assessment of diet, activity, and medication compliance is essential. The vascular system should be assessed regularly for possible complications, and the patient should be watched closely for signs of infection. The condition of the fetus is also assessed closely by serial ultrasonography and other medical measures.

Diagnostic tests. A 1-hour diabetes screening test or glucose tolerance tests may be ordered. If the woman is known to have diabetes, careful monitoring of blood glucose levels is important throughout pregnancy. **Glycosylated hemoglobin** tests are used to monitor glucose control during the preceding 1 to 3 months. Fingerstick blood testing is also useful.

Nursing interventions. Nursing care is directed at maintaining the patient in a euglycemic (normal blood glucose) status. The patient's insulin requirements will change significantly throughout pregnancy, labor, and delivery. The nurse must assess the patient carefully at each visit, complete all blood glucose level evaluations as ordered, and report any abnormalities to the physician promptly. Because of possible teratogenic effects, oral hypoglycemics are usually discontinued. Insulin may be required by both NIDDM and GDM patients to control blood glucose levels.

NURSING DIAGNOSIS	NURSING INTERVENTIONS
Potential noncompliance, related to prolonged and complicated medical regimen	Explain changes in diet, exercise, and insulin requirements related to changing needs of pregnancy. Emphasize benefits of compliance with plan of care. Identify patient values that affect compliance.

Patient education. The need for teaching will differ with the classification of the disease and the assessment of patient compliance. A woman who has been diagnosed before pregnancy will need reinforcement of diet, medication, and health practices. The nurse will also have to explain the effects pregnancy has on diabetes throughout the course of pregnancy, labor, delivery, and the postpartum period. For the gestational diabetic, teaching should stress the necessity of good control of the disease, including all of the teaching normally given to a new diabetic.

Cardiac Complications

Pregnancy increases the demands on the cardiovascular system. This is not a problem for the normal, healthy heart, which is able to adapt to the increased demands. However, women who have preexisting cardiac disease face increased risk when cardiac function is challenged by pregnancy.

Etiology. The most common cardiac problems of maternity patients result from rheumatic heart disease, congenital heart defects, or mitral valve prolapse. Occasionally a condition called *peripartum cardiomyopathy* is observed in patients who have no history of cardiac problems. This may be seen in the last month of pregnancy or during the postpartum period. The symptoms are similar to those of congestive heart failure.

Pathophysiology. During pregnancy increased blood volume, heart rate, and cardiac output are normal. In the woman with existing cardiac problems, the muscle, valves, or vessels are overly stressed by these changes and symptoms of the underlying pathological condition are exacerbated, resulting in cardiac decompensation, congestive failure, and other medical problems.

Clinical manifestations. The symptoms will depend on the underlying pathology. Edema, cyanosis, tachycardia, palpitations, dysrhythmias, chest pain, dyspnea, and fatigue may occur. Physical exertion may increase the symptoms.

Assessment. At each prenatal visit the patient's vital signs should be measured and her ability to participate in activity evaluated. Unusual fatigue with activity may reveal problems. Assessment should include checks for edema, weight gain, murmurs, cough, dyspnea, or abnormal lung sounds. It is important to compare these data with normal changes during pregnancy.

Diagnostic tests. Chest x-ray evaluation, electrocardiograms, echocardiograms, and auscultation are used to determine the type and severity of the cardiac problem. Blood gas analysis may be required if severe decompensation is observed.

Nursing interventions. Nursing care is directed at helping the woman to maintain normal physical and psychosocial function. During pregnancy the nurse should teach the importance of diet, medications, pacing activity, and adequate rest. This includes education about the specific disease and its management. Iron intake must be adequate to prevent anemia, which will further stress the heart. Sodium may be restricted to control the fluid volume and decrease cardiac stress. Stool softeners may be prescribed to decrease use of the Valsalva maneuver (holding the breath while bearing down) when defecating. The level of activity will be dictated by the severity of the cardiac problem. The nurse should be aware of the medical recommendations and help the woman incorporate these into her daily life. Patients with more severe cardiac problems will require the greatest adjustments, and the nurse must be highly sensitive to personal and family needs.

During labor, the semi-Fowler's or side-lying position with the head elevated will enhance respiratory effort and improve circulation. The efforts of labor may require oxygen administration, and the need for this should be explained. Administration of medications such as cardiotonics (digitalis), diuretics, prophylactic antibiotics, sedatives, and analgesics may be required as directed by the physician. The nurse should try to minimize unnecessary activity by the patient during labor and calmly explain everything to decrease anxiety. Fetal condition should be closely monitored for any signs of distress. A fetal monitor should be used for continuous assessment.

During delivery conservation of energy is important. Resting between contractions and using shorter, open-glottis pushing are recommended. The fetal status must be monitored very closely during this time.

Postpartum care will vary according to the severity of the cardiac problem. Methods of incorporating care of the infant into the mother's level of activity should be explored. To promote normal bonding, contact should be established as early as possible. Breast-feeding should be discussed with the physician, because the physical effort may be excessive to the mother and the transfer of medications in the breast milk may be harmful to the infant. As in all other areas of nursing, it is important to continue to assess the patient's status and give explanations for all care.

NURSING DIAGNOSIS	NURSING INTERVENTIONS
Activity intolerance, related to insufficient oxygenation resulting from decreased cardiac output	Plan nursing strategies to optimize rest. Teach methods that help conserve energy.
Activity intolerance—cont'd	Monitor vital signs and response to activity. Identify stressors. Discuss methods of stress reduction.

AGE-RELATED COMPLICATIONS

Adolescent Pregnancy

The number of adolescent pregnancies is increasing in most areas of the country. This trend is attributed to many sociological factors; breakdown of the traditional family and changes in social mores have resulted in earlier sexual activity. Teenagers account for an increasingly large percentage of births and abortions. Physiological immaturity, incomplete education, and unresolved developmental tasks are complicating factors. Most pregnant teenagers are unmarried. The psychological and economic support provided by a stable family is often missing. When combined with fear or denial of the pregnancy, the pregnant teenager often goes without medical attention until late in pregnancy. Lack of prenatal care increases the risk to the pregnant teenager and her infant. Teenagers under 15 years of age present the greatest risks. Older adolescents need not have increased risk if early prenatal care is obtained.

Assessment. Assessment of all health patterns for each adolescent is essential. While any and all nursing diagnoses are possible, most adolescents will experience the following.

NURSING DIAGNOSES	NURSING INTERVENTIONS
Ineffective individual coping, related to depression in response to identifiable stressors	Assess causative and contributing stressors. Demonstrate interest in the individual and willingness to help. Assist the patient to develop problem-solving strategies. Find methods of fostering feeling of achievement and self-esteem. Assist in developing or strengthening support systems.
Body image disturbance, related to pregnancy	Establish a trusting relationship. Promote social interaction. Provide education about discomforts of pregnancy.

Patient education. Education of the pregnant adolescent is essential. To work effectively with adolescents the nurse must be sensitive and nonjudgmental and knowledgeable about the stages of adolescence. Because no two adolescents are alike, a wide range of skills must be used to reach each individual.

Prenatal teaching is important. Nutrition is a major area of concern for the teenager. The young teen is often still growing herself, and her nutritional intake must meet her own needs and those of the fetus. Fad diets and food idiosyncracies are common in teenagers; this must be taken into account when teaching diet. Altered body image is a problem for even a mature woman. The teenager, particularly one who has not yet accepted the fact of pregnancy, may limit food intake to avoid gaining weight. This can be exceedingly dangerous to both mother and infant.

Preparation for labor and delivery is also essential. Many adolescents have little knowledge of human anatomy and have many fears and misconceptions about the process of childbirth. Many may have heard stories from friends that only increase their anxiety. The nurse should be factual without being harsh when describing the birth process.

Many adolescents plan to raise their infants; therefore instruction should also include child care and growth and development. Referral to community agencies that will provide ongoing support is important.

The adolescent father should not be ignored. It is important to consider the effect of pregnancy on him, particularly if he remains meaningfully involved with the teenage mother. Counseling is important for both, because the physical, financial, and emotional consequences of the pregnancy will affect both of them for the rest of their lives.

The Older Pregnant Woman

At the other end of the reproductive cycle are women who have their first child after they are 30 or more years of age. These women have a somewhat increased risk of maternal and fetal complications.

Changes in society, particularly the increased number of women with careers, have resulted in many women delaying pregnancy until later in life. Many women become aware of the "biological clock" as menopause approaches and wish to have a child while they are still able to do so. The potential for infertility increases with age. While most women who wait until later in life are well educated and have consciously decided to become pregnant, conception and pregnancy are not always easy. The likelihood of ectopic pregnancy and placenta previa and the incidence of various medical conditions, such as diabetes or hypertension, increase with age.

If the woman does become pregnant, studies show that each year after age 35 increases the risk of conceiving a child with Down's syndrome or other chromosomal anomalies. Amniocentesis is commonly done to detect genetic problems. Detection of genetic disorders can raise ethical dilemmas regarding abortion or raising a disabled child.

As women maintain better overall health and fitness, increased age appears to be less of an impediment to a normal pregnancy.

Psychosocial adjustment to parenthood at this time of life depends greatly on the individual and her particular situation. Changes in income, life-style, and work routines can present challenges that are stressful, even if the pregnancy is desired.

COMPLICATIONS RELATED TO THE NEWBORN

Newborns at Risk

Many maternal conditions can place the newborn in increased danger of illness or death. It is important to identify any maternal risk factors as soon as possible to decrease the risk to the fetus/newborn. Once these risks are identified, all medical and nursing measures possible should be undertaken to minimize the consequences to both the mother and newborn.

When risk factors are identified early, it is possible to be prepared to meet the needs of the newborn at risk. New equipment, such as fetal monitors and more sensitive diagnostic tests, has made recognition of problems occurring during labor and delivery easier. Despite all of our progress, however, many infants still are born in need of special attention.

At the time of delivery the newborn is assessed. The Apgar gives important information about the newborn's status at 1 and 5 minutes after delivery (see Chapter 43). This is followed by a more detailed assessment of size related to gestational age. It is important to distinguish between infants who are preterm and those who are small for gestational age. While both groups are at risk, the problems they present will be different.

Gestational age is significant with regard to neonatal mortality and morbidity (Figs. 45-3 and 45-4). Both preterm and postterm infants are at risk.

Gestational age is classified as follows:

Preterm	0 to 37 complete weeks of pregnancy
Term	38 to 41 complete weeks of pregnancy
Postterm	42 or more weeks of pregnancy

The preterm infant

Etiology. The exact causes of preterm labor are unknown. In some cases it is related to maternal or placental problems, but in other cases it cannot be determined whether preterm labor is related to any known problem. The end result is delivery of an infant 37 weeks or less in age.

Pathophysiology. The preterm infant is developmentally immature. The lungs are not producing sufficient amounts of surfactant to allow adequate oxygenation. Structures within the heart may not have adapted, as they normally do in a term infant, leading to oxygenation problems. Lack of subcutaneous fat, large surface area relative to body weight, and poor reserves of glucose and brown fat all contribute to problems with heat conservation. The digestive system is formed, but problems with absorption of nutrients are common. The renal system is

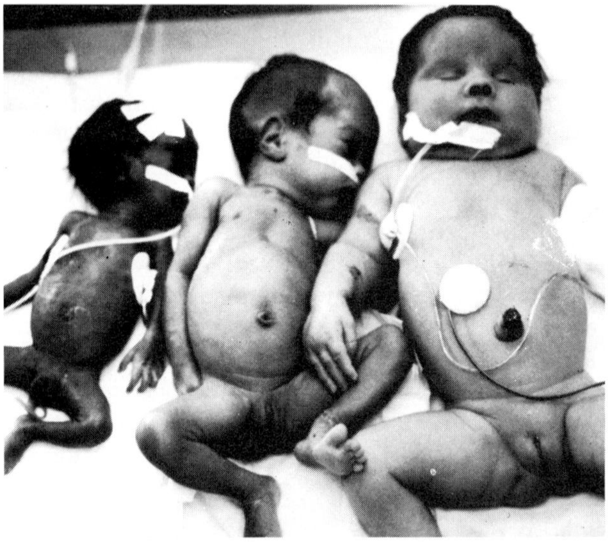

FIG. 45-3 Three babies of same gestational age, with weights of 600, 1400, and 2750 g, respectively, from left to right. Their weights are plotted in Fig. 45-4.

immature and ineffective. Fluid and acid-base imbalance is frequently observed. The infant in also neurologically immature; gag, suck, and swallow reflexes may be weak or absent, and other normal reflexes may be absent or atypical.

Clinical manifestations. The premature newborn's posture is froglike or flaccid. The color is usually ruddy, and cyanosis is common. The head appears very large in proportion to the body, and the bones of the skull are pliable with large, flat fontanelles. The skin is very thin and translucent with obvious blood vessels and little subcutaneous fat. There may be a layer of fine hair (lanugo) coating large areas of the body. Cartilage in the ears is pliable, and the ears can be easily folded. The genitals in males are small, and frequently the testes are undescended. In females the labia majora are small. The cry is weak, and reflexes are immature or absent.

Assessment. All systems of the premature newborn must be assessed carefully and continuously—changes occur rapidly and require continuous monitoring. Preterm infants are typically placed in an intensive care nurs-

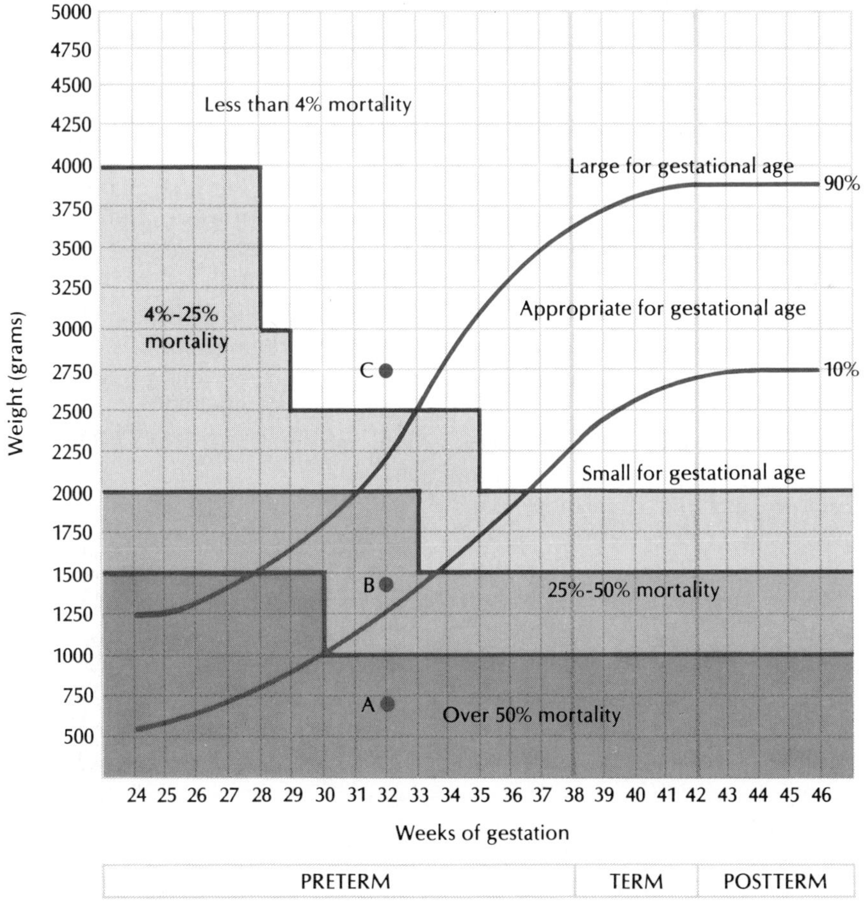

FIG. 45-4 Intrauterine growth status for gestational age and according to appropriateness of growth. Weights of infants shown in Fig. 45-3 are plotted at points *A, B,* and *C.* (Courtesy Mead Johnson & Co, Evansville, Ind. Modified from Battaglia FC and Lubchenco LO, J Pediatr 71: 59, 1967.)

ery and receive care from nurses specially trained to meet their needs.

Diagnostic tests. A wide range of diagnostic tests may be performed, based on the specific needs of the neonate.

Nursing interventions. The specifics of the care of the preterm newborn are too extensive for the scope of this text. The major goals include maintaining and stabilizing preterm neonates until they mature adequately. Respiratory regulation, thermal regulation, fluid and electrolyte balance, adequate nutrition, prevention of infection, sensory stimulation, and promotion of bonding with the parents are all major areas of concern for the nurse.

NURSING DIAGNOSIS	NURSING INTERVENTIONS
Hypothermia, related to exposure to cold	Monitor temperature every 4 hours or more often if necessary. Monitor heart rate and rhythm. Keep well covered and wrapped in blankets. Pad cold surfaces. Use radiant warmer if uncovered for extended periods of time. Keep skin dry. Avoid drafts.

Hemolytic diseases

Etiology. Hemolysis may result from basic incompatibility of blood groups, such as ABO incompatibility, or from a transfer of antibodies through the placenta.

Pathophysiology. Understanding Rh incompatibility requires an understanding of basic genetic laws. Rh incompatibility occurs only when the mother is Rh negative and the fetus is Rh positive. For this to occur the father of the fetus must be Rh positive (Fig. 45-5).

The term *Rh negative* indicates that the woman does not possess a specific blood antigen. If the woman is sensitized (i.e., exposed to the antigen), antibodies are produced. Exposure can occur through blood transfusion of incompatible blood or during pregnancy, when some fetal blood cells can enter the maternal circulation. This transfer of antigen may occur in cases of abortion or abruption, or at the time of delivery. Once Rh antibodies are developed by the mother, they remain in her blood, as do other antibodies.

When the woman becomes pregnant, antibodies may cross the placental barrier. If the fetal red blood cells contain the Rh antigen, the antibodies cause hemolysis (destruction). The higher the level of maternal antibodies, the greater the destruction of fetal RBCs.

Because sensitization most often occurs at delivery, the firstborn fetus generally has no signs of hemolysis; it is successive fetuses who are most likely to be affected. Today serious problems related to Rh incompatibility, such as erythroblastosis fetalis (profound hemolytic anemia in utero), are usually prevented by administration of a special gamma globulin.

ABO incompatibility is also an antigen-antibody process. Type O blood naturally contains anti-A and anti-B antibodies. These antibodies cross the placenta and cause hemolysis in the fetus if the fetus has blood types A or B. Incompatibility is also possible if the mother is A and the infant B or if the mother is B and the infant A. No sensitization is required, and it may affect the first and all successive pregnancies.

Clinical manifestations. The mother shows no clinical symptoms. Hemolysis may occur in utero, and detection must be made by diagnostic tests on amniotic fluid or suspected by changes in fetal condition or maternal diagnostic tests. Jaundice present at birth or observed during the first 24 hours of life is considered an indicator of a pathological condition. Severe jaundice, called **kernicterus**, may result in neurological damage. Anemia resulting from RBC destruction is also possible.

Assessment. The maternal blood type and Rh factor are determined during pregnancy. If the mother is Rh negative, it is necessary to know the blood type of the father. If he is also Rh negative, no Rh-based problems can occur. If he is Rh positive, the possibility of problems exists. It is also important to assess the woman's history for any occurrences that may have caused sensitization.

Diagnostic tests. Blood typing will reveal situations that require follow-up. Indirect Coombs' tests on maternal blood samples measure the number of maternal antibodies. Antibody titer tests determine the level of maternal antibodies. If the titer exceeds 1:16, amniocentesis may be performed to obtain fluid for further testing. Optical density studies, which measure bilirubin level, can be done on this fluid to assess fetal condition. (If the fetus is determined to be in grave danger, intrauterine transfusion may be necessary.) After delivery, direct Coombs' tests are done on infant blood to determine the presence of antibody-coated RBCs. Bilirubin levels of infant blood will measure the extent of RBC destruction.

Nursing interventions

Maternal. If the results of an Rh-negative mother's indirect Coombs' test are negative, the mother is given an intramuscular injection of anti-Rh gamma globulin (RhoGAM). This is currently recommended at 28 weeks of pregnancy and again within 72 hours of delivery. RhoGAM provides passive antibodies and prevents development of naturally occurring maternal antibodies. RhoGAM should also be given to an Rh-negative mother in cases of abortion, ectopic pregnancy, and amniocentesis.

Newborn. The newborn affected by a hemolytic process must be observed carefully; jaundice and anemia may become severe and lead to other complications. The nurse should monitor the bilirubin, hemoglobin, and hematocrit levels and notify the physician of any abnormal laboratory results. The infant suffering from severe jaundice

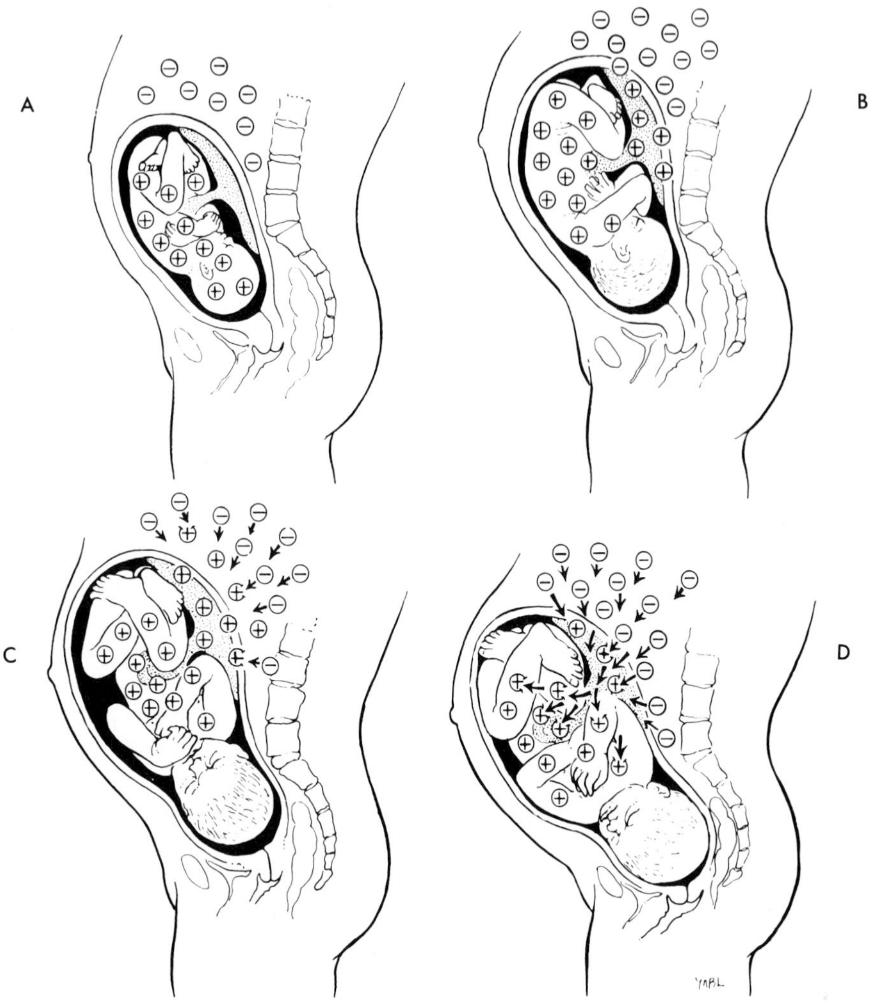

FIG. 45-5 Mechanism of erythroblastosis fetalis, which is caused by Rh incompatibility. **A,** Rh-positive fetus is carried by Rh-negative mother. **B,** Rh protein crosses placental barrier and invades mother's bloodstream. **C,** Mother's system manufactures antibodies to destroy foreign Rh protein. **D,** Antibodies cross back over placenta and destroy fetus's blood cells, which are intimately associated with Rh protein.

may be treated with phototherapy or may require transfusions. If the infant requires phototherapy, several precautions must be taken. **Phototherapy** involves exposing the skin to fluorescent lights, which converts the bilirubin to a water-soluble form that can be excreted in the urine. It is important to maintain body temperature and protect the infant's eyes during this treatment. Stools may be loose and the urine contains excessive waste products, so it is important to maintain skin integrity by careful cleansing and frequent diaper changes. Because fluid loss is increased, adequate fluids are important to maintain necessary hydration.

Patient education. Rh-negative women should be aware of the process involved in Rh sensitization. The nurse should answer all questions that the woman or her spouse or significant other may have.

Phototherapy is likely to be disturbing to the parents and can interfere with bonding of mother and newborn. The nurse must explain the reasons for treatment and provide opportunities for maternal-infant interaction. Today many newborns are sent home receiving this form of therapy. The nurse may be responsible for teaching the parents correct use of the equipment and the special care required by the infant.

Drug and Alcohol Syndromes

Etiology. The pregnant woman, who takes drugs or drinks alcohol not only places herself at risk but also endangers her fetus. Most drugs, including common substances such as alcohol and nicotine, are able to cross the placental barrier and affect the fetus. Depending on when in pregnancy a drug was taken, the amount taken, and the chemical properties of the drug, a wide range of fetal and maternal complications may occur.

Pathophysiology. The exact pathophysiology varies with the drug involved.

Clinical Manifestations and Assessment

Alcohol dependency. Use of alcohol may result in multiple anomalies called *fetal alcohol syndrome* (FAS). Characteristics of FAS are as follows:

1. Abnormalities of the central nervous system, including mental retardation, hyperactivity, and microcephaly. Withdrawal symptoms often occur within the first day of life. These include tremors, seizures, abnormal reflexes, inconsolable crying, sleeplessness, and inattention to stimuli.
2. Facial abnormalities, such as abnormal eyelid structure, and incomplete development of the facial bones, particularly underdevelopment of the jaw and upper lip.
3. Growth retardation and failure to thrive is commonly seen and may persist long after delivery. Most affected infants are small for gestational age at birth and exhibit feeding disorders and vomiting for months afterward.
4. Miscellaneous cardiac, renal, and skeletal abnormalities may occur.

Drug dependency also manifests a wide range of problems. The symptoms depend on the particular drug used but commonly include the following:

1. Congenital anomalies, particularly of the cardiac, genitourinary, and nervous systems
2. Abnormal behavior, with difficulty responding to the environment
3. Respiratory distress related to narcotic depression or aspiration of meconium
4. Growth retardation often related to poor nutritional status of the mother during pregnancy
5. Withdrawal symptoms, including disturbed CNS function such as exaggerated reflexes, hyperirritability, sneezing, yawning, sleeplessness, tremors, and seizures. Diarrhea, stuffy nose, perspiration, flushing, and other symptoms may occur.

Diagnostic Tests. Drug screening panels may be used to detect the presence of these substances in the mother's urine or blood. These tests may be unreliable, depending on the time interval since the mother last used the drug.

Nursing Interventions. Nursing care for the infant is directed at preventing further injury, particularly during the withdrawal phase. Observation of the newborn is essential to detect increasing instability. Infants of known drug and alcohol users are generally placed in a neonatal intensive care unit. Physical care includes careful temperature regulation and monitoring of vital signs. Small feedings are given, and the infant is observed for diarrhea, regurgitation, and vomiting. Positioning on the right side is helpful in preventing aspiration. Intravenous therapy may be required. Medications may be administered as ordered to prevent the most serious withdrawal symptoms. Stimuli that may aggravate seizures are minimized. The inconsolable behavior of these infants makes providing care to them exceedingly difficult and stressful.

The parents of the newborn should be included in care whenever possible. Depending on the severity of the problems encountered, the infant may remain in the hospital, be discharged to the parent, or placed in the custody of social services. It is a major challenge to establish a therapeutic relationship with the chemically dependent parent. Nurses should consult with social welfare or other departments that are best able to protect the newborn and also help the parent obtain the treatment needed to overcome the addiction.

NURSING DIAGNOSIS	NURSING INTERVENTIONS
Ineffective denial, related to acknowledgment of substance abuse/dependency	Use nonjudgmental approaches. Instill a sense of hope. Assist in developing improved self-esteem. Observe for medical signs of withdrawal; provide supportive care during detoxification. Assess potential for violent or suicidal behavior. Discuss coping strategies. Initiate referrals.

REFERENCES AND SUGGESTED READINGS

1. Aaronson LS and Macnee CL: Tobacco, alcohol and caffeine use in pregnancy, J Obstet Gynecol Neonatal Nurs 18:4, 1989.
2. Bobak IM and Jensen MD: Essentials of maternity nursing, St Louis, ed 3, 1990, The CV Mosby Co.
3. Burroughs A: Bleir's maternity nursing, ed 5, Philadelphia, 1986, WB Saunders Co.
4. Carpenito LJ: Nursing diagnosis, application to clinical practice, New York, 1989, JB Lippincott Co.
5. Cowen MJ et al: Maternal transmission of acquired immune deficiency syndrome, Pediatrics 73:382, 1984.
6. Doenges M and Moorhouse M: Nurse's pocket guide to nursing diagnosis with interventions, ed 2, Philadelphia, 1988, FA Davis Co.
7. Donner C and Cooper K: The critical difference: ectopic pregnancy, Am J Nurs 88:843, 1988.
8. Dunn PA et al: Care of the neonate with erythroblastosis fetalis, J Obstet Gynecol Neonatal Nurs 17:6, 1988.
9. Fischbach F: A manual of laboratory diagnostic tests, ed 3, Philadelphia, 1988, JB Lippincott Co.
10. Gabbe SG: Management of diabetes mellitus in pregnancy, Am J Obstet Gynecol 153:824, 1985.
11. Ingalls AJ and Salerno MC: Maternal and child health nursing, ed 7, St Louis, 1990, The CV Mosby Co.
12. Jaffe MS and Melson KA: Maternal infant health care plans, Springhouse, Pa, 1989, Springhouse Corp.
13. Klaus MH and Fanaroff AA: Care of the high risk neonate, Philadelphia, 1986, WB Saunders Co.
14. Klug RM: Children with AIDS, Am J Nurs 88:1127, 1986.
15. Ladewig PW, London ML, and Olds SB: Essentials of maternal-newborn nursing, ed 2, Redwood City, Calif, 1990, Addison-Wesley.
16. Ladewig PW, London ML, and Olds SB: Maternal newborn nursing: a family-centered approach, ed 3, Menlo Park, Calif, 1988, Addison-Wesley.
17. Minkoff HL: Managing AIDS in pregnant patients, Contemp OB-GYN 32(3):341, 1988.
18. Pillitteri A: Maternal-newborn nursing: care of the growing family, ed 3, Boston, 1985, Little, Brown & Co.
19. Prince NA et al: Perinatal nurses' knowledge and attitudes about AIDS, J Obstet Gynecol Neonatal Nurs 18:5, 1989.
20. Pritchard JA, MacDonald PC, and Gant NF: Williams' obstetrics, ed 17, New York, 1985, Appleton-Century-Crofts.
21. Taylor CM and Cress SS: Nursing diagnosis cards, Springhouse, Pa, 1988, Springhouse Corp.
22. Wiley K et al: Human immunodeficiency virus and precautions for obstetric, gynecologic and neonatal nurses, J Obstet Gynecol Neonatal Nurs 17:3, 1988.

CHAPTER CHALLENGE

KEY POINTS

- Complications can occur during any stage of the childbearing process.
- The nurse must continually assess pregnant women and newborns for any signs of complications.
- The nurse must educate all pregnant women and new mothers about the danger signs that indicate complications, stressing the importance of prompt medical attention.
- Hemorrhage is a danger sign both during pregnancy and after delivery.
- A wide range of infectious diseases present a threat to the mother and newborn.
- The Rh-negative mother may require special interventions to prevent sensitization, which may have an effect on future pregnancies.
- Preexisting health conditions, such as cardiac problems or diabetes mellitus, increase the risks of childbearing.
- The age of the mother is significant in childbearing. Both the very young and the older mother are at increased risk.
- Drug and alcohol use have a serious impact on the developing fetus.
- Newborns born to drug- or alcohol-abusing mothers may manifest a variety of anatomical and neurological defects.

STUDY QUESTIONS

1. A serious complication that may occur in hyperemesis gravidarum is:
   a. Abruptio placentae
   b. Acid-base imbalance
   c. Spontaneous abortion
   d. Jaundice
2. The implantation of two separate fertilized ova results in:
   a. Dizygotic twins
   b. Hydatidiform mole
   c. Ectopic pregnancy
   d. Monozygotic twins
3. In a ruptured ectopic pregnancy the nurse would observe:
   a. Bright red vaginal bleeding
   b. Dark red vaginal bleeding
   c. Signs of peritoneal irritation
   d. Elevated blood pressure readings
4. A spontaneous abortion in which all of the products of conception are delivered is called:
   a. Imminent
   b. Threatened
   c. Incomplete
   d. Complete
5. Painless vaginal bleeding after 20 weeks' gestation is most likely indicative of:
   a. Abruptio placentae
   b. Placenta previa
   c. Hydatidiform mole
   d. Ectopic pregnancy
6. Visual disturbances and weight gain in excess of 1 pound per week in the last trimester may indicate:
   a. Diabetes mellitus
   b. Hyperemesis gravidarum
   c. Pregnancy-induced hypertension
   d. Cardiac complications
7. Excess alcohol consumption may cause:
   a. Teratogenic effects
   b. Excessively large infants
   c. Hypoglycemia
   d. Jaundice
8. Rubella acquired during the first trimester often results in:
   a. Small for gestational age infants
   b. Teratogenic effects
   c. Fetal immunity to the disease
   d. Hemangiomas (strawberry birth marks)
9. Hemolytic disease of the newborn may occur when the:
   a. Mother is Rh positive and the father is Rh negative
   b. Mother is Rh positive and the father is Rh positive
   c. Mother is Rh negative and the father is Rh negative
   d. Mother is Rh negative and the father is Rh positive
10. Disseminated intravascular coagulation may be a result of which obstetrical complication(s):
    a. Placenta previa
    b. Abruptio placentae
    c. Retained placental fragments
    d. All of the above
11. Grand mal seizures may occur:
    a. Only during pregnancy
    b. During pregnancy or labor
    c. During pregnancy, labor, or delivery
    d. During pregnancy, labor, delivery, or the early postpartum period
12. The drug used to control the symptoms of severe eclampsia is:
    a. Magnesium sulfate
    b. RhoGAM
    c. Tegretol
    d. Meperidine hydrochloride

XI

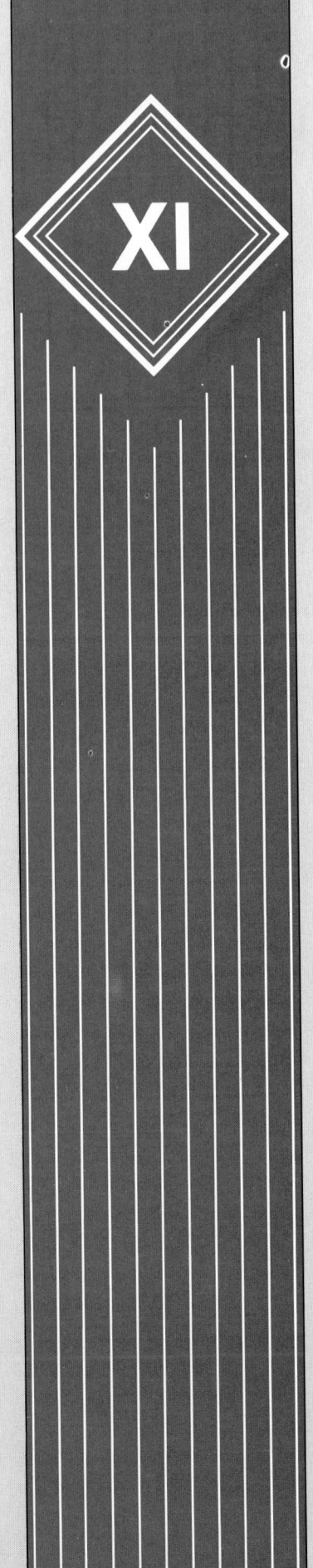

Pediatric Nursing

To me, nursing is more than a career; it is an art. It takes a special sort of person to take care of the ill. I try to keep in mind the sort of nurse I would want to take care of my family. I will love being an LPN. Every day at the hospital is a brand new experience. I find it fulfilling and very rewarding to see the patients I have worked with recover and eventually leave the hospital. I don't think one could possibly learn everything there is to know about nursing, and that is one aspect that is challenging. I feel the need to help others, and nursing is the choice I have made to help me fill that need.

JULIE KOTSCHWAR
Student Nurse

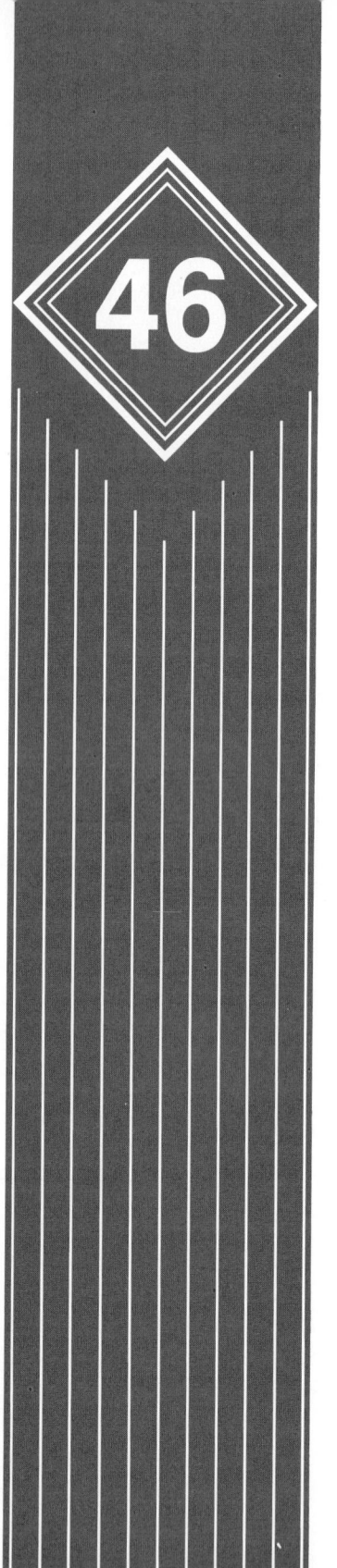

46

Basic Pediatric Nursing Care

GLADYS M. SCIPIEN

LEARNING OBJECTIVES

After reading this chapter, the student should be able to do the following:

- Identify three events that had a significant impact on the health care of children in the United States in the twentieth century.
- Describe the purposes and outcomes of the White House Conferences.
- Outline several methods in which the hospitalization of children car be positive experiences for them and their families.
- Explain the needs of parents in the course of their child's hospitalization.
- List ten methods of preventing injuries in 1- and 2-year-old children.
- Describe five methods in which growth and development principles are used by a pediatric nurse.
- List the two methods of computing drug doses and fluid needs for infants and children.
- Describe three alternative methods of feeding infants with health problems.
- Identify three methods of restraining infants and children for safety and/or procedures.
- Describe the differences in collecting urine and blood specimens from young children.

RELATED TOPICS OF INTEREST

- Communication (Chapter 4)
- Vital signs (Chapter 14)
- Admission, transfer, and discharge (Chapter 15)
- Safety (Chapter 17)
- Specimen collection (Chapter 21)
- Basic nutrition (Chapter 22)
- Mathematics review (Chapter 24)
- Principles and practice of medication administration (Chapter 25)
- The surgical patient (Chapter 26)
- Care of the mother and newborn (Chapter 44)

KEY TERMS

Define the following:

- anticipatory guidance
- birth defect (congenital anomaly)
- body surface area (BSA)
- bronchopulmonary dysplasia
- burping
- cleft lip
- cleft palate
- *en face*
- fontanel
- mortality
- morbidity
- trust
- weaning

HISTORY OF CHILD CARE IN AMERICA

For centuries children were considered miniature adults. In looking at medieval art, one observes the bodies of children were painted with the proportions and musculature of adults rather than the physical characteristics of infants and children. Childhood was considered an unimportant stage of life.

In colonial America children were expected to assume adult responsibilities as soon as they could. The value of a child was related directly to the work he could perform. Infant mortality was high. Epidemics were common, and there were no controls or treatment plans for diseases such as smallpox, diphtheria, measles, or dysentery. Farm accidents and burns from open fireplaces or from gun powder also contributed to high mortality.

With industrialization there was a population shift from rural to urban settings and families moved into cities, where they lived in overcrowded and unsanitary conditions. Young children worked in factories 12 to 14 hours a day. The economy was poor, and survival was a real issue as family life was sacrificed. Children had no legal rights, and there were no work laws.

These conditions continued until 1860 when Dr. Abraham Jacobi, a New York physician, first lectured to medical students on the special diseases and health problems of children. Until then no effort was made to provide health care to children and their needs were not considered to be different from those of adults.

Some physicians, nurses, and social workers became interested in working with children. Pioneering efforts in the investigation of childhood diseases resulted in the establishment of "milk stations." Until then milk was not refrigerated and contained hundreds of millions of bacteria, which contributed to the development of diarrhea and tuberculosis. At milk stations, infants were weighed and mothers were taught how to prepare milk before giving it to their babies. Mothers also had access to nurses who taught them the benefits of fresh air, clean water, adequate clothing, and the recreational needs of children. This crusade for pure milk resulted in improved sanitation, the pasteurization of milk, and increased interest in infant care.

In spite of the effort, as late as 1890 about 20% of the children died before their second birthday and about 50% did not live to the age of 21 years. Therefore families were large to compensate for these losses.

At the turn of the twentieth century deplorable social conditions continued. Children were being exploited in the work place. Many were homeless. Those in orphanages and foundling homes were subjected to cruel and inhumane treatment by caretakers. In 1909, with pressures to correct what was happening to children, President Theodore Roosevelt convened the first White House Conference on Children. It focused on such issues as child labor, dependent children, and infant care. In 1912 the U.S. Children's Bureau was established as a direct result of that conference. It was charged with investigating all aspects of child care, including infant mortality, child labor laws, conditions of social agencies, and the country's birthrate. This federal agency also published *Infant Care,* the most extensive collection of information on child care ever compiled.

With the end of World War I the second White House Conference was convened in 1919. It addressed the socioeconomic situation of mothers and children. The first federally supported health programs for mothers and children were established. The depression of 1929 paralyzed the United States and resulted in devastating social and economic conditions, which had their greatest effect on children. A White House Conference on Children was called in 1930 to study the economic effects on the health and well-being of children. Since then a conference has been held every 10 years, at the beginning of each decade.

These conferences have been responsible for many changes in child health and welfare, including funding for essential programs, legislation, and a shift from treating diseases to preventive health care. Those who attend are professionals who work with children, representatives of federal and state agencies and volunteer organizations, and members of various citizens' groups. Although these people cannot legislate, they raise the consciousness of public officials and private citizens regarding the status of children and families.

The United States did not recover from the 1929 depression for many years. In the interim the Children's Bureau was able to propose legislation that affected children. The most remarkable pieces of legislation were those authorized by the Social Security Act of 1937, which was signed by President Franklin D. Roosevelt. The health care needs of children were incorporated in Title V, and for the first time there was recognition of the needs of crippled children. The Women, Infants, and Children (WIC) program is one example of the benefits of this legislation.

Established in 1967, the Office of Child Development houses the Children's Bureau and the Bureau of Child Development Services, which operates such programs as Head Start. The Secretary of Health and Human Services is the cabinet officer responsible for all their activities.

An analysis of the progress made in child health and child care shows an increase in access to and a more equitable distribution of services in the 1960s. In the late 1970s and the 1980s the emphasis was on cost containment, which remains an important issue in the 1990s.

NURSING IMPLICATIONS OF GROWTH AND DEVELOPMENT

It is important for a nurse to know the basic principles of normal growth and development to understand what infants and children are like, what can be expected from them, what their needs are, and why they behave as they do. Although each child is unique, groups of children of the same age are more alike than they are different. For example, a number of general statements can be made about the babies in a newborn nursery and yet there are significant differences among them. In knowing their similarities, a nurse is better able to perform assessments, develop interventions, and, most important, identify problems.

The stages of growth and development are complex processes that occur as the body grows and the mind and personality unfold. As the newborn moves through infancy, toddlerhood, preschool age, school age, and adolescence, each stage consists of predictable, orderly events that are accomplished sequentially. When a nurse knows the normal milestones accomplished by a 6-year-old, for example, it is easier for her to identify a delay in the 6-year-old who has not mastered the developmental milestones expected. It is important to realize that there are differences in the rate at which a particular task is accomplished. One infant may sit up at 5 months of age and another at 7 months. However, *most* infants do so at 6 months of age. As one might expect, illness or a lack of stimulation interferes with normal development. Other variables that affect development include a baby's genetic makeup and a host of environmental factors, such as ethnic background, religion, family size, socioeconomic bracket, and education.

A student in pediatric nursing may ask why growth and development are important aspects of studying children. One of the primary responsibilities of a nurse is to identify an infant or child who is demonstrating a developmental delay in order to remedy the deficit as quickly as possible. For example, in performing a Denver Developmental Screening Test on a 14-month-old toddler, a nurse finds the toddler's language development consists of imitating speech sounds, rather than saying three words, including *mama* and *dada*. Nursing interventions should consist of encouraging parents and other adults to set aside time to speak to the child, to identify specific items in his environment, to name them, and to wait for the child's response. When adults make an early, conscientious effort to influence the toddler's language development, the toddler can overcome the delay and progress normally.

Understanding growth and development enables a nurse to select age-appropriate toys for the infant or young toddler and devise activities that appeal to the school-age child or adolescent who is hospitalized. Play is the work of an infant or toddler. It should be done in a safe environment, using toys that are safe. A child learns through every opportunity that is made available to him. One should observe a 2-year-old playing with a large, four-sided box to appreciate his curiosity or creativity. He can do more things with that box than any adult could ever imagine.

For a pediatric nurse a knowledge of growth and development also is the basis for anticipatory guidance with parents. **Anticipatory guidance** means to teach parents (and children when they are old enough to understand) what is likely to occur in the coming weeks and months so that the child's well-being will be protected and promoted at that time. For example, parents will know that their 9- or 10-month-old will begin to crawl from one place to another. It is normal, it is expected, and it should be allowed. However, parents must remove any harmful objects from the child's reach. Once a child becomes mobile, it is important to "child-proof" the environment, making it a safe one for the "curious crawler." Nurses play an intimate role in assisting parents to understand the physical and behavioral changes that occur rapidly in the developing infant or toddler. These principles also are useful in working with the school-age child, who will be exposed to many new experiences once he starts school, or the preadolescent, who should be prepared for the hormonal and growth changes he soon will be experiencing.

DIFFERENCES BETWEEN ADULTS AND CHILDREN

The differences between adults and children are significant, including rate of growth, level of understanding, and means of communicating. Each stage of childhood is unique, with its own set of characteristics. A nurse must use different skills with children of different age groups. The challenges that children present to a nurse are constant, exciting, and satisfying.

At birth, all body systems are not functioning at full capacity, affecting, for example, how newborns and young children respond to drugs: they are more susceptible than adults to the toxic effects of certain medications because of their limited ability to detoxify or eliminate drugs.

As the newborn grows, different systems of the body mature, teeth erupt, vision improves, nutritional patterns change, and speech develops. Gradually and through a series of complex processes, a totally dependent human being becomes a thinking, feeling, self-sufficient individual. Some of those processes are discussed here to explain the growth and development changes from childhood to adulthood.

Metabolism

The most obvious difference between an adult and an infant is size. The rate of metabolism is highest in the newborn infant because the ratio of total body surface area to body weight is much greater in the infant than it is in the adult. This proportion decreases as the child grows and matures. The basal metabolic rate (BMR) is a measure of metabolism when the body is at rest, and it changes dramatically as the body increases in size. When the nurse stops to consider that the newborn doubles his birth weight at 5 to 6 months and triples it at about 1 year of age, she better appreciates the rapid rate at which metabolism occurs in very young children.

Table 46-1 Caloric Needs of Infants, Children, and Adolescents

Age Group	Caloric Needs
Infants	
Birth-6 mo	115 kcal/kg
6-12 mo	105 kcal/kg
Children	
1-3 yr	100 kcal/kg
4-6 yr	85 kcal/kg
7-10 yr	86 kcal/kg
Adolescents	
Males	
11-14 yr	17 kcal/cm height
15-18 yr	16 kcal/cm height
Females	
11-14 yr	14 kcal/cm height
15-18 yr	13 kcal/cm height

Adapted from Food and Nutrition Board (1980).

The body uses energy provided by foods. Whereas the energy requirements for an infant are highest during the first 6 months of life, they are fairly constant from 4 to 10 years and vary in adolescence, depending on the teenager's physical development (Table 46-1).

Because metabolism is so high in infants and children, their ability to recover from surgery or a fractured bone is swift in comparison with that of an adult. With all bodily functions accelerated, healing occurs quickly. For example, a fractured femur at birth is united in 3 weeks, but an 8-year-old with the same type of fracture requires 8 weeks for union and a 20-year-old takes 20 weeks to heal.

Vital Signs

Body temperature, which also reflects metabolism, is fairly stable from infancy through adulthood. The one exception is the newborn infant, whose temperature can be affected by the environment. An air-conditioned delivery room may result in the newborn's temperature dropping to 97° F or lower, which accounts for the use of radiant warmers for newborns after delivery.

Despite the ability to regulate their temperatures, infants and toddlers are prone to wide variations, especially after crying for extended periods or after active play. Temperature elevations also occur rapidly in young children when infections are present.

Although a temperature is taken rectally initially in the

Table 46-2 Vital Signs (Averages)

Age	Heart Rate/Min	Respirations/Min	Blood Pressure
Newborn	120	35	70/50
1-11 months	120	30	90/60
2 years	110	25	96/68
4 years	100	23	100/70
6 years	100	21	105/70
10 years	90	19	108/70
12 years	88	19	110/70
16 years	77	17	120/78

newborn to assess a patent anus, axillary temperatures usually are done on infants and young children. Oral temperatures usually are taken on children 6 years and older.

There also are great variations in the heart rates of children. Although the apical beat of a newborn may be 152 per minute, very gradually the heart slows to 72 to 75 beats per minute by adolescence (Table 46-2). The presence of infection increases the heart rate, as does physical activity. During sleep a child's pulse is at its slowest rate. Any irregularities in volume, rate, and rhythm should be noted. Whereas an apical pulse is taken on infants and young children, a radial pulse is taken on older school-age children and adolescents. It should be counted for a full minute. The respiratory rate also slows as a child progresses from infancy to adolescence. A newborn is an obligatory nasal breather, which means he breathes only through his nose, and will not breathe through his mouth until he is 3 or 4 weeks old. A newborn's respiratory rate is extremely erratic, which requires counting it for 1 full minute to be accurate. The rate, depth, and quality of respirations should be assessed. The rate may be as rapid as 40 or 50 breaths a minute, gradually slowing to 32 to 35 a minute by 36 hours of age. In infants both abdominal and chest movements are observed when measuring respirations. The presence of a developing pulmonary disorder is suspected when the respiratory rate increases.

The blood pressure is low in a newborn. Gradually it rises, so that by the end of adolescence it is about 120/78. When doing a blood pressure reading, it is important to use the correct cuff size to ensure accuracy. The cuff should cover two-thirds the length of the upper arm or leg. The crying of an infant or toddler can result in a falsely elevated reading.

Urine Output

A nursing responsibility is the monitoring, measuring, and/or collection of urine. Output varies and depends on the size of the infant or child. Table 46-3 identifies average volumes excreted at given ages.

At birth the renal system, like many other systems of the body, is immature. Many tests done in adults are not done in young children because of this. For example, urea clearance is impaired in young children, so it is not measured in infants or toddlers younger than 2 years.

Table 46-3 Urine Output

Age	Volume
Preterm newborn	1-3 ml/kg/hr
Full-term newborn	3-4 ml/kg/hr
6 months	12 ml/hr
1 year	22 ml/hr
5 years	28 ml/hr
12 years	33-35 ml/hr

Measuring urine output in the infant or toddler who is not toilet trained can be a challenge. Most hospitals require routine weighing of diapers (before and after voiding) of all children who are not toilet trained. The weight of a dry disposable diaper is subtracted from the weight of a wet diaper. The difference in the weight in grams equals the milliliters voided; 1 g equals 1 ml of urine.

Teeth

The primary (deciduous, baby) teeth begin to descend between the sixth and ninth months of life. The central incisors are the first teeth to appear. By a child's third birthday, all 20 primary teeth are present. Permanent teeth begin to appear at about 6 years, and most are present by 12 years.

The eruption of teeth is distressing to the baby, whose gums are erythematous and edematous. The fussiness he demonstrates may result in refusal to eat. A cold teething ring provides some relief to painful gums.

Eating Patterns

Most infants are given solid foods at 5 or 6 months of age, when their teeth begin to erupt. Iron-fortified cereal is the first solid food given to a baby. Rice is easily digested and has low allergic potential, so it is commonly selected. However, oatmeal and barley are high-protein cereals that can be given also. After several months of breast milk or formula, the addition of solid foods to an infant's diet is a significant developmental step.

Although the order of introduction of foods other than cereal is arbitrary, the usual sequence is strained fruits, fruit juices, strained vegetables, and, finally, strained meats. As more teeth erupt, a finger-feeding food, such as zwieback, is offered. This helps the infant develop a hand-to-mouth cycle, which is basic to feeding himself.

It is important for each new food to be introduced at 4- or 5-day intervals, so that food allergies can be identified (the presence of an allergy may take several days to appear). Development of a rash, wheezing, or diarrhea may signify the baby's allergic response to a food.

By 9 months, several teeth have erupted and junior foods, which are of much coarser texture, can be offered. These fruits, vegetables, and meats taste different and encourage the infant to chew, as a result of the different texture. Finger foods given at this time include pieces of fruit (excluding grapes, which could choke the infant) and cooked vegetables.

The cost of baby foods is significant; therefore as the infant acquires more teeth and does not experience difficulty eating solids, parents are encouraged to prepare these foods at home. Cooking fresh or frozen foods and using a blender or food processor is encouraged. By 12 to 15 months toddlers should be eating table foods prepared for the family. Although using a spoon is messy, the typical toddler becomes angry and frustrated when he is "ready" to feed himself and a parent continues to feed him.

Weaning from the bottle or the breast is a major accomplishment in toddlerhood. That method of feeding has provided the child with a great deal of pleasure and satisfaction. However, solid foods also are pleasing to his taste buds, but when he feeds himself with a spoon, turning it upside down as he navigates the utensil toward his mouth, he loses much of the food; the same situation occurs with a cup. A plastic cup with a spout decreases the amount of milk or juice that is spilled. Most 9- or 10-month-old infants, who can sit in their high chairs, begin to demonstrate a readiness to wean. They are becoming much more active and squirm when they are held for feedings. In addition, they observe siblings and adults drinking from cups or glasses and desire to do the same. Gradually, bottle or breast feedings are replaced by the cup. Usually the bedtime feeding is the last one to be discontinued.

Vision

The eyes of a newborn undergo many changes before vision is comparable with that of an adult. At birth, visual acuity is 20/300, which makes it important for the adult holding a baby to assume an ***"en face"*** position (Fig. 46-1). Clear vision by the baby is achieved only at very close range. The baby should be held comfortably, so that

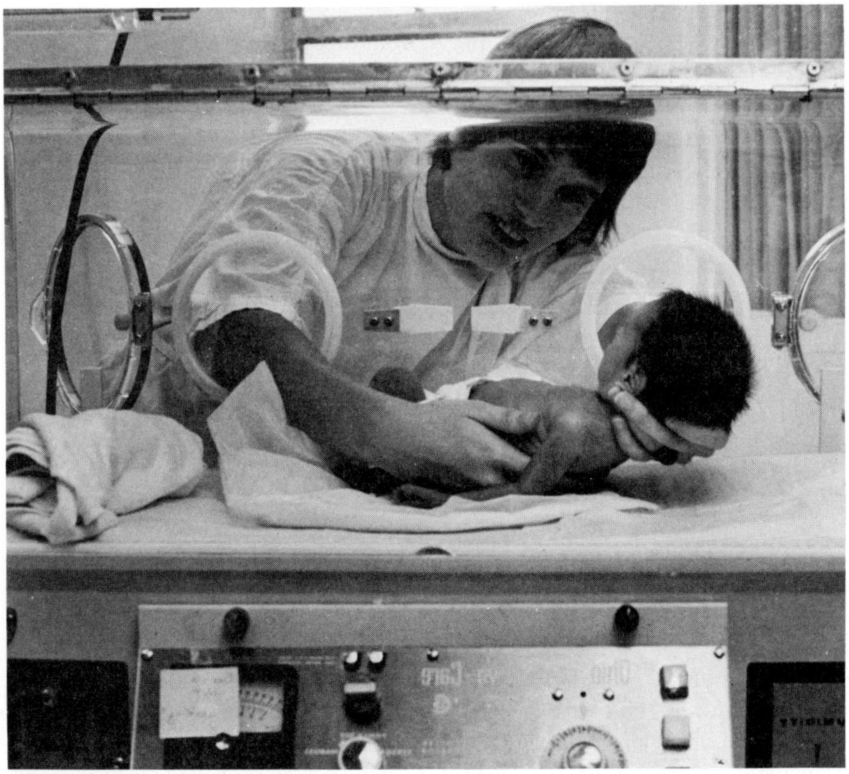

FIG. 46-1 Sometimes a mother must overcome a physical barrier to achieve the *en face* position.

eye contact can be made and the newborn can gaze on the face of the holder. Although tears are absent immediately after birth, by the second week of life, tear glands begin to function. Newborns can follow bright, colorful objects by the second or third week of life.

Although visual acuity is 20/200 by the fourth or fifth month, depth perception does not develop before the ninth or tenth month. One-year-olds, who enjoy playing with large objects (blocks, toys, and boxes), often bump into obstacles because their vision is only 20/100. By the fourth birthday, a child's vision is 20/20. When a child starts school, accommodation (changes in ciliary muscle and the lens in bringing light rays from various distances to focus on the retina) and refraction (the normal eye produces the proper image of the object on the retina) also are present. It takes almost 6 years of continual development for the parts of the eyes to function as they do in an adult.

Speech and Communication

Crying at birth is the earliest evidence of speech. The infant uses this method of communicating when he is hungry, in pain, or needs to be changed. Crying is gradually followed by other sounds, such as cooing, laughing, or babbling. By 9 months an infant practices and painstakingly repeats the noises he can make. While he begins to express himself, he also begins to imitate the vocal sounds of an adult. It is possible to have an actual conversation with the infant. Although no formal words are exchanged, it is a pleasant experience. The adult speaks, the infant responds, the adult answers, and so on. While each takes his turn at contributing to this verbal exchange, the "conversation" usually ends with laughter. As the infant begins to enjoy experimenting with these sounds, it is important to encourage these vocalizations; it is positive reinforcement for oral communication.

A 1-year-old has a three- or four-word vocabulary. It usually includes *mama, dada,* and *bottle.* In toddlerhood more words are understood than expressed. Children usually know 25 words by 18 months, but by 2 years, they may know more than 250 words. Speech develops rapidly at this stage, as children practice and learn new words and their meanings. Soon they can say a two- or three-word sentence. A preschooler has a fairly extensive vocabulary to convey his wants, needs, and desires.

An adult uses words confidently in speaking with others, but the same cannot be said for all children. That ability is determined by the child's stage of development, the amount of stimulation or encouragement he receives from adults, his health status, and many other factors. In addition, the development of language does not occur in isolation. It is related to the physiological, neurological, and psychosocial progress that occurs simultaneously.

A nurse should know what typifies speech at certain stages of childhood. That knowledge helps to identify a problem. For example, the lack of babbling or the inability of a 9-month-old to imitate sounds may indicate the presence of deafness. A deaf baby makes verbal sounds until 6 or 7 months of age, but without being able to hear, his verbalizations decrease and gesturing or some expression of body language (or nonverbal communication) increases.

A nurse uses verbal communication in a variety of ways. Talking softly to an infant while cuddling him is an important part of establishing a relationship with the baby. Although the toddler is leery of strangers, if the nurse talks with a parent first, the 2-year-old senses the trusting attitude of the adult and he begins to participate in the conversation. As a result of improving verbal skills, preschoolers and school-age children understand more and share their concerns more easily. Teaching 8- and 10-year-olds is particularly satisfying because they are eager to learn. On the other hand, adolescents who have refined their verbal abilities communicate a significant amount of information nonverbally through body language, gestures, or facial expressions.

One of the most important points a nurse should remember is to speak with a child at the child's stage of development. How a nurse talks with a 2-year-old differs greatly from her conversation with a 12-year-old. To be successful in establishing a relationship with a child and to be effective in teaching or sharing information, a nurse must communicate with him at the appropriate level.

HOSPITALIZATION OF A CHILD

Hospitalization is an anxiety-producing experience for a child and his family, primarily because of a basic fear of not knowing what will occur. It is an interruption in the child's normal development and routine, and it also separates him from his friends. Every member of the family is affected by the hospitalization because of its disruption in routines. Such an experience can be made less traumatic by anticipatory guidance, explanations, and preparation to help relieve fear and anxiety. However, infants and toddlers cannot understand. Therefore separation is especially painful for them. Preparation can be done for a scheduled admission; however, emergencies arise, and unplanned hospitalizations occur. In those instances, explanations should be given whenever possible and as soon as feasible to avoid traumatic situations.

Adequate preparation makes the transition from the security of a home to the unfamiliar atmosphere of a hospital less difficult. When preparation should begin and how much information should be given will vary. The age of the child influences his preparation. A physician provides a family with details about a treatment plan, length of stay, and expected results or outcomes. Parents can then reinforce the information by explanations to the child, using simple, age-appropriate terms. Usually there is time before the actual admission to provide opportunities for the child to talk about what is going to happen to him.

Preadmission Programs

Many hospitals have orientation programs for children who are to be admitted. The programs are based on the child's level of understanding and stage of development, with the purpose of familiarizing the child with hospital surroundings. These programs should dismiss the child's fantasies and correct his misconceptions. The programs include tours and audiovisual aids, such as movies, slides, and puppet shows. The child is given simple explanations of equipment used in the course of surgery and/or hospitalization.

It is helpful for children to handle some of the items they will see while hospitalized, such as masks and gowns, stethoscopes, and syringes. There should be time for questions. The nurse should encourage children to talk about what they have seen or heard. By doing so, problem areas or areas of concern can be identified. Some hospitals distribute coloring books or story books that focus on the information contained in the orientation program. This material reinforces information and also helps parents answer their children's questions. Brochures may be distributed at this time that describe hospital routines and list items children can bring with them to the hospital. Information is written simply, clearly, and at understandable levels.

Timing is important. Attendance at such a program should be enough in advance for the child to assimilate the information, but not so far in advance that the information is forgotten. Generally, the younger the child, the shorter the period between the time he is told that he is to be hospitalized and the actual admission date. A toddler usually is told only days before. However, an 8-year-old has a better understanding of time and the future; therefore he can be told that he is going to the hospital "in 2 weeks."

Every child should be allowed to prepare for this new experience in his own way. This preparation involves telling his friends and selecting pictures of family members, toys, or clothes he wishes to take, if they are permitted. Packing his bag with these items reinforces the eventuality.

Parents can benefit from such orientation programs too. They are provided with information that is helpful in answering a child's questions at home. Printed materials provide parents a reference guide for reviewing what the child has been told.

An emergency admission thrusts the child into an unknown environment surrounded by strange equipment, frightening sounds, and many unfamiliar adults. The incident that results in the hospitalization usually is sudden, serious, and possibly painful. The speed with which a health team responds to the emergency is critical, and there is little time for explanations. Whenever possible, a nurse must explain to the child and family what is happening. This can avoid an escalating crisis situation. When the child is stable and awake, a nurse can assess the child's perception of what happened, correct any misconceptions, and provide information not given initially.

Admission

In large hospitals children may be assigned to a nursing unit according to their age group. For example, a two-year-old will be admitted to the toddler unit and a teenager to the adolescent unit. Smaller, community hospitals attempt to assign children of similar ages in rooms large enough to accommodate two to four children.

Pediatric units are bright, colorful, and cheery areas with cartoon figures on the walls (or ceilings of treatment rooms), many pictures, and large photographs of sports figures and popular singers. The unit or room is decorated to reflect the age group admitted there. For example, an infant/toddler unit may have many age-appropriate toys, highchairs, play pens, and strollers. An adolescent area may have a lounge with a television, a stereo, records, tapes, and VCR, as well as a well-stocked refrigerator. The pediatric environment is different from adult units to decrease anxiety by including many items that are found in the home.

The child's first impression may influence his entire stay. Therefore when a child arrives on the unit, he should be greeted warmly and welcomed by name. After he is shown to his room and introduced to his roommate(s), he should be given a tour of the unit. Two important locations to be pointed out are the area in which snacks or liquid refreshments are available and the playroom where he will spend time when allowed out of bed. The play area is a safe, secure place for children. It contains an assortment of toys, games, and crafts for diversional activities. Newly admitted children also need explanations about when meals are served, how to operate their beds, and how to communicate with nurses by using a call bell or intercommunication system. Parents are usually allowed to visit 24 hours a day, but others may visit at designated times, such as 10 AM to 6 PM or 2 PM to 8 PM.

Hospital Policies

There are times when anxiety levels about the admission are high. Perhaps heart surgery is to occur or a brain tumor is suspected. In those instances, a nurse may elect to postpone a tour or an in-depth orientation. The development of a relationship with the family may be more important, because it can affect the entire course of a hospitalization. That is a nursing judgment.

Some hospitals have facilities that allow one parent to

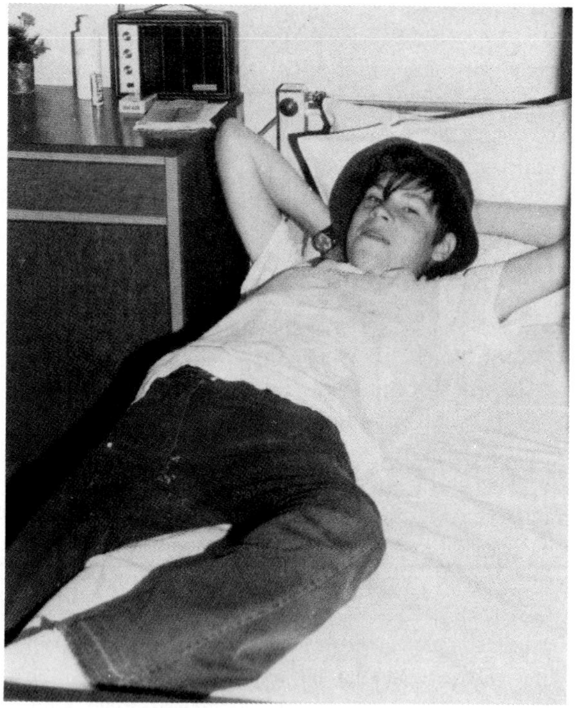

FIG. 46-2 When possible, an adolescent should wear his own clothes during a hospitalization.

"live-in" or "room-in," which means a parent can stay 24 hours a day. Beds, meals, and shower facilities are made available to them. Parents should be made aware that these accommodations are available. Hospitalization is especially traumatic to very young children, and having supportive parents stay increases their security.

Parents who are involved in care have a sense of contributing to the child's recovery, which is an important consideration. Having a parent present increases the teaching opportunities of a nurse. It also enables a nurse to assess a family's strengths, weaknesses, and potential problem areas. However, parents need time to relax and to get away from the child's bedside periodically. A room or other specified area on the nursing unit is set aside for live-in parents. There they can socialize, support each other, and share their thoughts. The presence of parents does not mean that nurses give up their responsibilities in caring for these infants and toddlers. Rooming-in can be an exhausting experience. Parents need breaks and relief to remain effective in supporting the child.

Certain hospitals allow children to wear their own clothes; this is important for a hospitalized adolescent (Fig. 46-2). However, if a child is scheduled for surgery or an intravenous line is started, hospital gowns are required because of the possibility of loss or damage.

After a child is admitted, a nursing history is obtained. An identification bracelet, usually worn on the wrist, is important to verify identity when medications are given or procedures are done. These bands may be placed on the ankles of infants and toddlers because they are curiosity items on their wrists. When the band is applied, the nurse should allow space for one finger to fit between the band and the skin. The band should not be constrictive, and the skin underneath should be checked for its integrity.

Vital signs, including blood pressure, are assessed. The height and weight also are measured and recorded. They are important baseline data. Height and weight may be used in calculating a child's body surface area, which is important information when treating a child with burns or in calculating fluid and electrolyte requirements. Most medical centers use body weight in kilograms to compute drug dosages. An important nursing responsibility is identifying the scale used to weigh a child, if more than one is available, so that the same scale is used for subsequent weighings.

All newly admitted infants and children have routine blood samples drawn by a laboratory technician. Urine specimens are collected. The laboratory values provide a physician with baseline information, and they may be diagnostic. Additional x-ray examinations or procedures will be ordered as appropriate to the child's specific health problem.

Parent Participation

It is essential to establish an effective, working relationship with parents as soon as possible. Parents are the most significant individuals to a child. Also, they know their child better than anyone else and may play an important role in assessing his responses. Therefore a nurse should project a positive attitude toward parents. It can be done by giving them a warm greeting, a smile, and establishing eye contact.

In obtaining a nursing history, it is important for the nurse to select a quiet place on the unit to listen to parents' responses and to provide them with opportunities to ask questions. The reason for hospitalization may be minor according to a physician, but a parent may perceive it as very serious. Parents may be fearful and anxious because of the seriousness of the illness, the procedures involved, or the pain a child will experience. Their apprehension then is transmitted to the child. Therefore it is important to convey interest and concern and try to decrease their anxieties.

Parents experience a series of reactions when a child is hospitalized. They too are in an unfamiliar environment, meeting different groups of people who ask many questions and give them much information. Perhaps the tests or procedures mentioned are unknown to them, and they may become frustrated because they do not understand much of what is being told to them. Parents often do not know hospital rules and regulations and what is expected of them. They lose control in this setting and feel powerless. To this point, they alone have cared for their son or daughter. Now a nurse assumes control over the child's care. If an accident is the cause for hospitalization, parents may blame themselves and feel guilty. When a nurse meets the emotional needs of a parent, that mother or father is better able to support the child.

On admission parents need specific information on routines, hospital policies that affect them, any limitations that exist, and what is expected of them. When parents are given information that they can apply immediately, their anxiety levels decrease and they feel more comfortable.

Later, diagnostic tests, medications, or procedures that are planned by the physician should be explained to the parents. It is not unusual for a parent to have selective hearing. Any change in plans generates anxiety and results in a parent being unable to process the information. Therefore the nurse should thoroughly explain the tests and treatments.

As the parents' comfort increases, they become more involved in meeting their child's physical needs. Mothers tend to spend more time with their hospitalized children and participate early in providing care. Fathers are often more reluctant, and they should be encouraged to become involved. If parents participate, they feel they are contributing to the child's recovery. Another strategy is for the nurse to ask for parents' assistance in establishing goals or revising a care plan.

The equipment that surrounds a child can be overwhelming, with the strange-sounding alarms or with electrodes placed on different parts of his body (Fig. 46-3). When a nurse explains the function of a monitor or some other device, it becomes less threatening. However, it is important to use terms a parent can understand.

Initially a parent may watch the nurse suction the child, perform chest physical therapy, or change a dressing. If a nurse uses these opportunities to describe what is done and why, parents become more interested. Eventually a nurse hears, "Do you think I can suction Billy today?" The information that has been exchanged between a parent and a nurse, the demonstrations that have occurred, and the teaching that has been done have motivated this parent to perform a procedure he or she has not done before. Parents can become skillful in performing a variety of technical skills if they are taught in a patient, nonthreatening manner and if questions are encouraged. Some activities in which parents become involved include gastrostomy tube feedings, tracheostomy suctioning, and intramuscular or subcutaneous injections.

Parents must be confident in their ability to perform given tasks in their child's care and should be encouraged to participate *only* in as many activities as they feel comfortable performing. Generally, the extent of parental involvement also is a good measure of a nurse's effectiveness as a teacher.

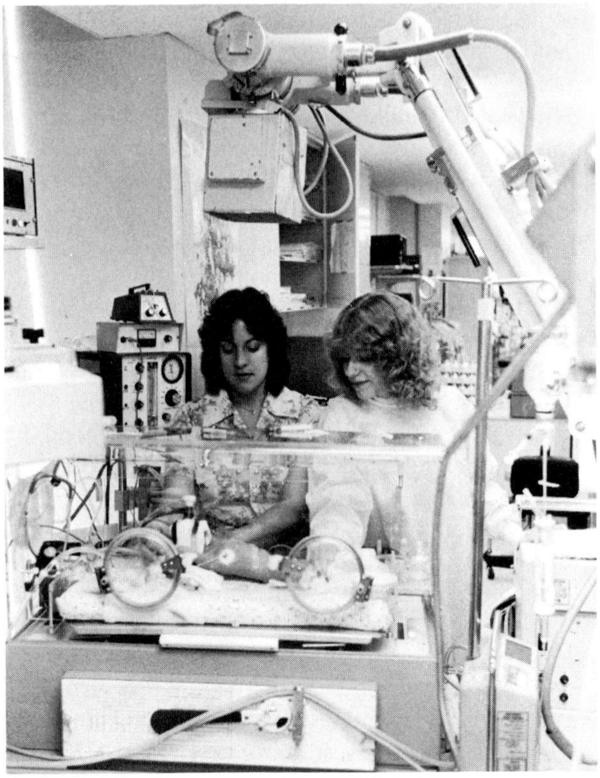

FIG. 46-3 A parent can be overwhelmed by the equipment that surrounds an infant.

The last phase of adaptation for parents of a hospitalized child relates to discharge. Teaching is an ongoing process throughout the hospitalization and should not be postponed until the time of discharge. Although there may be some activity restrictions for the child, any nursing intervention measures that are required can be done at home. After adequate instruction and supervision by a nurse, parents usually can provide care as competently as the nurse.

The pediatric nurse must gain the trust of the parents by (1) reviewing and interpreting information from the physician as needed, (2) asking the parents if they have any questions, (3) conveying concern for the parents' well-being, and (4) listening and being available. These activities are time-consuming, and yet for a nurse who works with families, they are some of the most satisfying.

Characteristics of a Pediatric Nurse

Pediatric nursing is different from other clinical specialties in nursing. First, the nurse must enjoy working with children of all ages. A great deal of time is spent with an individual child. Second, when a child has a health problem, it is the child, the disease, and the family that become a nursing concern; one cannot be separated from the other two. It is family-centered nursing in its truest sense.

The pediatric nurse must have keen observation skills, especially when caring for infants and toddlers or children who are critically ill. Some children have minimal communication abilities, and pain, thirst, or other discomfort must be interpreted. Also, the developmental ages of children can be assessed by watching them play or perform certain tasks. In addition, not all **birth defects (congenital anomalies)** are diagnosed in the newborn period and a nurse may identify a problem as a result of a physical assessment. When children are very ill, minor changes in their physical status can result in a variety of complications, and therefore any changes must be noted as early as possible. These examples typify the role observation plays in clinical practice.

Supporting a child through a difficult procedure or serious illness is an activity in which a pediatric nurse commonly becomes involved. Such an endeavor not only includes preparation for the event, it requires establishing a level of **trust,** which permits the child to express his fear, apprehension, and anxiety. To establish a trusting relationship, a nurse must convey respect to the child, talk with him at a level he can understand, and, most important, be honest with him.

Teaching is ongoing in pediatrics. It can range from explaining the effects of a medication to an 8-year-old to helping parents learn how to give an intramuscular injection to their infant. There also are innumerable opportunities to help children and parents adapt to a chronic illness or disorder, which requires a nurse's knowledge of community resources or volunteer agencies available for equipment or support.

A pediatric nurse also functions as a child and family advocate, whether those activities involve an ethical decision or the quality of care given. This may involve a nurse coordinating the activities of a health team and collaborating with members of different disciplines to provide a child with the expert care that is required.

Being able to communicate effectively with a child is essential. However, to enjoy and continue working in pediatrics, a nurse must recognize and appreciate the uniqueness that each child or adolescent brings to a nurse-patient relationship. It is that special quality—uniqueness—that should be understood, respected, and practiced by anyone who provides care for children.

SAFETY

Protecting a child from harm is a major issue in pediatrics. Anticipatory guidance for parents of infants and

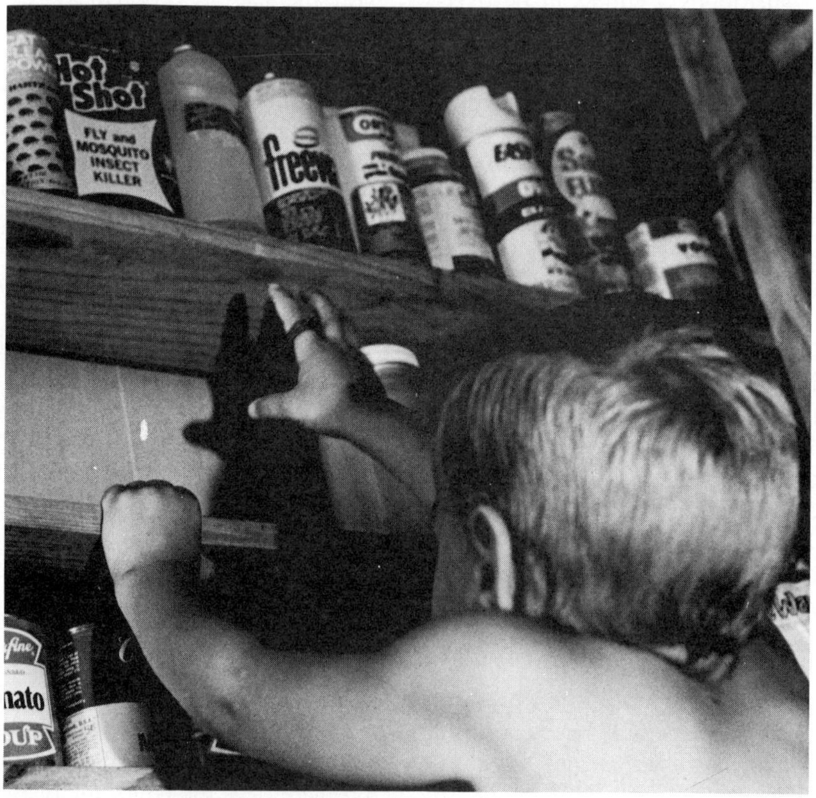

FIG. 46-4 Poisons and caustics must be placed where children cannot reach them.

toddlers and health teaching for school-age children and adolescents are two methods of preventing accidents. However, hazards and dangers are everywhere—in the home, at the playground, at school, and in the hospital.

The age of a child is an important consideration. The younger the child, the greater the dangers. For example, accidents are a leading cause of death in toddlers (Fig. 46-4). The risk-taking activities of adolescents also contribute to the **morbidity** and **mortality** of adolescence. Table 46-4 identifies common developmental characteristics, potential hazards, and preventive measures that can decrease the incidence of accidents and injuries.

Parents and children should talk and listen to each other to prevent many accidents. Maintaining open communication between and among all members of a family is one method of prevention. The adult who is a role-model, who thinks about safety, and who identifies potential dangers in the environment or a particular activity can influence a child immensely.

Table 46-4 Preventing Accidents

Age	Behavior	Accident/Hazard	Prevention
Newborn	Sleeping; poor head control; some body movement	Suffocation	Do not tuck blankets in. Do not use pillows. Do not use plastic bags in crib.
		Accidents	Use car seat. Check crib slats—they should be no more than 2⅜″ apart.
		Burns	Test bath water temperature. Never smoke or drink hot liquids while holding baby.
		Falls	Never leave baby alone. Always have one hand on baby. Carry newborn with two hands.
1-6 Months	Head control improving	Suffocation	Keep crib free of plastic bags. Do not use pillows.
	Placing objects in mouth	Foreign body aspiration Injury from toys: loose parts or sharp edges	Inspect all toys; remove button eyes or detach small wheels. Do not offer foods on which the baby can choke, such as grapes, nuts, potato chips, and raisins. Remove open safety pins, needles and nails from baby's reach.
	Moving body from one place to another	Falls	Do not leave baby unattended on bed, couch, or counter.
	Beginning to pull self to sitting position	Burns	Test bath water; hold infant securely. Keep hot liquids in cups away from child's grasp.
7-12 Months	Sitting up	Falls/drownings	Never leave infant unattended in highchair, on bed, or in tub.
	Crawling	Accidents	Use gates at bottom and top of stairs. Place guards around fireplaces; never leave infant alone near space heater.
		Suffocation	Do not leave plastic bags or balloons in crib or playpen.
	Feeding self	Aspiration/ingestion	Do not offer foods on which child can choke, such as popcorn, small, hard candies, or gum. Lock up all medications and poisonous household substances. Purchase medicines and household cleaners in childproof containers. Keep number of the local poison control center by telephone. Keep ipecac syrup on hand, and know how to give it. Childproof the entire house, including placement of poisonous houseplants out of reach.

Continued.

Table 46-4 Preventing Accidents—cont'd

Age	Behavior	Accident/Hazard	Prevention
1-2 Years	Holding on or walking	Falls, lacerations, and abrasions	Keep furniture with sharp edges and glass table tops out of child's way.
			Keep sharp kitchen utensils and garden equipment out of reach or locked up.
	Exploring environment		Always know where the toddler is playing.
			Supervise all outdoor play activities.
	Running		Do not allow child to run with objects in mouth.
			Begin teaching safety outdoors, including dangers of traffic, climbing, and walking in front of swings at playground.
		Motor vehicle accidents	Always use car seat.
			Keep toddler in fenced area.
			Install child-proof locks on car doors.
			Teach child to cross street holding an adult's hand.
			Keep car doors locked in garage or driveway.
			Do not allow play in driver's seat without adult present.
		Ingestion/inhalation	Keep insecticides, medications, and all harmful cleaners locked up.
		Suffocation	Supervise play with balloons.
			Do not allow plastic bags in play.
			Remove doors of refrigerators before discarding.
		Drowning	Keep bath water level low in tub.
			Never leave child alone in tub or wading pool; empty wading pool after use.
			Supervise child closely at beach.
			Never allow child near water without an adult.
			Fence in swimming pool.
			Enroll toddler in swimming class.
		Burns	Remove matches/lighters from reach.
			Teach fire safety.
			Keep handles of pots toward center of stove when cooking.
			Keep child away from stove while preparing meals.
			Keep child away from charcoal fires.
3-5 Years	Climbing; running	Falls, lacerations, and abrasions	Check yard, playground, and daycare center for potential hazards.
	Exploring environment outside the home		Begin teaching: safety in using playground equipment; dangers of pushing/shoving playmates; and avoiding strangers.
	Improving motor skills		Supervise child using scissors.
			Discourage approaching animals without an adult.
			Supervise action-related activities, such as tricycles and Big Wheels.
			Teach child his name, address, and telephone number.
		Motor vehicle accidents	Use care seat/safety belts in car.
			Review acceptable behavior in a moving car.
			Review crossing street at corner, watching lights and flow of traffic.
			Teach child to keep parent informed of whereabouts.
			Confine play to yard, not street.

Table 46-4 Preventing Accidents—cont'd

Age	Behavior	Accident/Hazard	Prevention
3-5 Years—cont'd		Burns	Practice fire drills in the home. Implement other practices similar to those for 1- to 2-year olds.
		Firearms	Never keep loaded guns/rifles in house or garage. Keep service guns locked. Instruct child never to touch gun or bullets.
6-11 years	Motor skills continuing to improve; enjoying large muscle activities; becoming increasingly independent; engaging in competitive sports; unsupervised activities	Motor vehicle accidents, injuries, and fractures	Review traffic safety. Use safety belts. Teach skate board safety—control speed and refrain from jumping. Teach bicycle safety—rules of the road, use of reflectors, and proper signaling. Review safety regarding use of lawn mowers, farm equipment, and tools. Teach child not to hide in or play near cars. Caution child about playing in vacant buildings, quarries, or sand pits. Teach proper use of protective gear in competitive sports. Teach child not to throw objects at people or moving vehicles. Teach child how to call fire department, police, and emergency medical assistance.
		Drownings	Review swimming and boating safety. Do not allow ice skating on pond unless its safety has been determined. Never allow the child to swim or skate alone.
		Inhalation/ingestions	Evaluate health education programs at school. Emphasize the hazards of glue sniffing and drug or alcohol use. Encourage family discussions about substance abuse.
12-18 Years	Rapid growth spurt; demonstrating risk-taking behaviors; demonstrating increased independence; engaging in extracurricular activities; reacting to peer group influence; driving a car	Motor vehicle, motorcycle, and bicycle injuries and fractures	Evaluate the high school's safety and health education programs. Review bicycle/motorcyle safety, including use of helmets. Enroll child in driver education classes. Establish limits regarding care, use, and consequences of drinking and driving. Encourage group participation in outdoor activities, such as running or jogging. Supervise competitive sports activities. Encourage enrolling in first aid classes. Maintain a physical conditioning program. Review water safety in seasonal activities.
		Drownings	Discourage risk-taking behaviors at pool or beach. Discuss dangers of swimming and skating alone. Keep guns empty and locked up. Teach proper care of firearms.
		Firearms	Supervise target practice in isolated areas.

COMMON PEDIATRIC PROCEDURES

Bathing

Bathing the child provides a nurse with the opportunity to do a complete skin assessment. When giving an infant a bath, the nurse should protect him from drafts and chilling. Bathing is usually done before a feeding to prevent regurgitating or vomiting. The water temperature is checked. If the umbilical cord is still attached, a sponge bath is given. The area around the cord and the cord itself should be cleaned with alcohol, which helps drying.

Water only is used to clean areas around the eyes. A mild soap is used on the rest of the body, which is bathed from the face and down the trunk. One section of the body should be exposed, washed, rinsed, and dried thoroughly before bathing another anatomical part. A baby's creases need special attention. Babies have very short necks, and if not cleaned and dried thoroughly, the skin may become impaired.

If a sponge bath is given at the bedside, the infant should be placed across the width of the bed so he faces the nurse. This practice allows greater control of any movement by the baby and decreases the likelihood of his rolling out of the crib. Cotton-tipped applicators are *never* used to clean the ear canal, because injuries can occur with any sudden movement. A wash cloth is adequate. Special care needs to be given to the genitalia. In females, the labia are separated and washed, from anterior to posterior. The penis and scrotum of a circumcised male are washed. In an uncircumcised male, the foreskin of the penis is retracted and cleansed. Daily retractions prevent the development of adhesions. Ointments and powders usually are not recommended.

Infants enjoy being placed in basins for baths. After washing the baby's face, the nurse lathers the trunk and extremities. She then dries her hands, which enables her to pick up the infant more securely and place him in the basin. The head needs the support of one hand; the other hand is used to rinse the infant, who should be allowed to play and splash the water, which encourages development. After the infant is removed from the basin, he is dried thoroughly.

When an infant's head is washed, he should be held football-style. In this position, an infant's hip rests on a nurse's hip. While one hand of the nurse supports the baby's head, the baby's back rests on the nurse's forearm. This position allows the infant to look at the nurse's face while the hair is washed. After the hair is lathered well, the head can be rinsed over the basin at the bedside. Some nurses prefer to wash an infant's hair at a sink under running water. Parents raise questions about the baby's soft spot (anterior **fontanel**). They should be assured the area cannot be injured by shampooing.

Most toddlers love to be placed in a tub for their baths. Toys should be provided. They are used in splashing, water play, and bathing. It is important to remember that water is fascinating to a toddler because it has no shape or form. Safety is an issue, and a child should *never* be left in a tub without supervision. Most young children should be allowed to enjoy themselves in a tub for 15 to 30 minutes.

Feedings

Formula. The position one assumes for feeding an infant should be comfortable for the adult and infant. The infant should be held securely in one's arms. A table or stand should be within arm's reach so the bottle can be set aside while the baby is burped.

Formula or juice should fill the nipple entirely to decrease the amount of air swallowed in the course of the feeding. It usually takes 15 to 20 minutes to complete a bottle feeding. Newborns should be burped after every ½ ounce, whereas older infants may burp after consuming 1 ounce of the feeding.

There are three common methods of **burping** an infant (see Chapter 44). The infant can be placed in a sitting position on one's lap. With one hand over his chin and chest supporting the body as he leans forward, the other hand gently pats or rubs the infant's back from the waist to the shoulders. The infant also can be placed flat across an adult's lap, using one hand to rub or pat his back and the other hand to secure the body. The third position is placing the baby upright, looking over a shoulder. One arm holds the baby and the other hand is free to rub his back from the waist to the shoulders. Once air has been released, the feeding can be resumed. This process is repeated until the desired amount has been consumed by the infant.

Solids. When solid foods are started, the infant should be fed in an infant seat. The safety strap should always be in place securely. When a baby is in an infant seat, his eyes can focus on the adult, while both hands of an adult are free to introduce solids to the infant. Once an infant achieves control, he can be held in the arms of an adult. Older infants (8 or 9 months old) can be placed in a high chair with a safety strap in place. It may be necessary to provide additional support. Baby blankets rolled up and placed on either side of the infant's trunk provide effective support.

Once a toddler has begun walking, placement in a high chair is a confinement he resists vigorously. In climbing out of a high chair, he may fall and sustain a significant injury, despite the fact that a safety strap was used. There are two points to remember when dealing with a toddler. First, his appetite decreases at this age and this is normal. Second, his resistance to the high chair is so intense that an injury can occur. It may be advantageous to try an alternative.

An unbreakable bowl containing small pieces of various foods placed on a chair or stool lets the toddler select what he wishes to consume as he strolls by. Such an intervention can avoid a difficult situation. While they take in less solid food, toddlers continue to drink liquids freely.

Special feeding needs: cleft lip/cleft palate. The baby born with a **cleft lip** or **cleft palate** cannot maintain closed suction around the nipple or use muscles to pull on it. There are several methods a nurse uses to provide nourishment until those defects are repaired. A soft, cross-cut nipple (cross cuts are made with a scalpel blade) is best. When placed in the mouth, the nipple *must not* be placed into the cleft.

Some infants do well using a Breck feeder, which is a small bulb syringe to which is attached a small piece (no more than 2 inches long) of rubber tubing. With the baby in her arms, the nurse inserts the tubing into the side of the baby's mouth and applies gentle pressure to the bulb of the syringe. Because sucking and swallowing are coordinated activities, initially this feeding method is slow. However, as the baby's coordination improves, the time required to feed him decreases.

These newborns should be fed in a sitting or semisitting position to prevent choking or aspiration. A feeding should not be interrupted unnecessarily. The infant with a cleft palate makes noises while he eats, and they differ greatly from a baby without this condition. However, by constantly interrupting his feeding, the infant becomes extremely frustrated, primarily because he *is* hungry but unable to eat. Once a successful feeding pattern is developed, it should be taught to parents.

Gavage. Some newborns and infants need gavage feedings. This involves passing a feeding tube through the nose or mouth, down the esophagus, and into the stomach. A number 8 or 10 tube is used. The length to insert the tube should be measured: the tip of the tube is placed at the tip of the baby's nose, extended to the tip of the ear, and down to the tip of the xiphoid process of the sternum.

Some restraint of infant activity may be necessary. For a newborn, the bottom of his shirt may be pulled up and over both arms. An older infant may need to be wrapped in a mummy restraint before proceeding. The mummy restraint is described in a later section.

While holding the baby's head, a nurse inserts the feeding tube quickly. If any cyanosis, choking, or resistance develops, the tube is withdrawn immediately. Once inserted, the tube is taped in place. If the tube was inserted through a naris, the tape should be applied with the tube flat against the skin under the nose. No tubing should be taped on the nose because it can cause skin impairment. Placement of the feeding tube in the stomach should be confirmed by pulling 1 to 2 ml of air into a syringe, placing a stethoscope on the area of the abdomen over the stomach, and listening for the rush of air as it is injected into the tube.

Although it is better to hold the infant during the gavage feeding, if a nurse is unable to do so, the infant should be placed on his right side with a blanket roll that maintains that position. A pacifier placed in his mouth encourages sucking during the feeding. The barrel of a 10 or 20 ml syringe is attached to the tubing and is lowered while formula is added to it. Then it is raised 6 to 8 inches above the baby so the formula can flow slowly by gravity. Infusing formula rapidly into the stomach can result in abdominal distention or vomiting. When the prescribed amount of formula has been given to the infant, the tubing is pinched and removed quickly. Pinching the tubing prevents dripping of formula into the pharynx, which causes gagging. It also prevents air from flowing into the stomach.

Infants need to be burped after a gavage feeding. They can be placed on their abdomens. However, if an infant is placed on his right side, it helps in emptying the stomach. At the conclusion of a feeding, a nurse records the type and amount of feeding given and the response of the infant to the feeding.

Gastrostomy. A gastrostomy tube is used to provide nourishment to an infant or child who cannot take feedings by mouth. A surgical procedure is done to place the tube into the stomach and to suture it to skin (Fig. 46-5). The tube remains in place for an indefinite period. To perform a gastrostomy feeding, the barrel of a 30- to 50-ml syringe is attached to the end of the gastrostomy tube and lowered while filled with formula. Then it is elevated 4 to 5 inches above the child, which allows the formula to flow in by gravity. The infant is given a pacifier to suck on during the feeding. It satisfies his sucking need and helps him realize that sucking satisfies hunger.

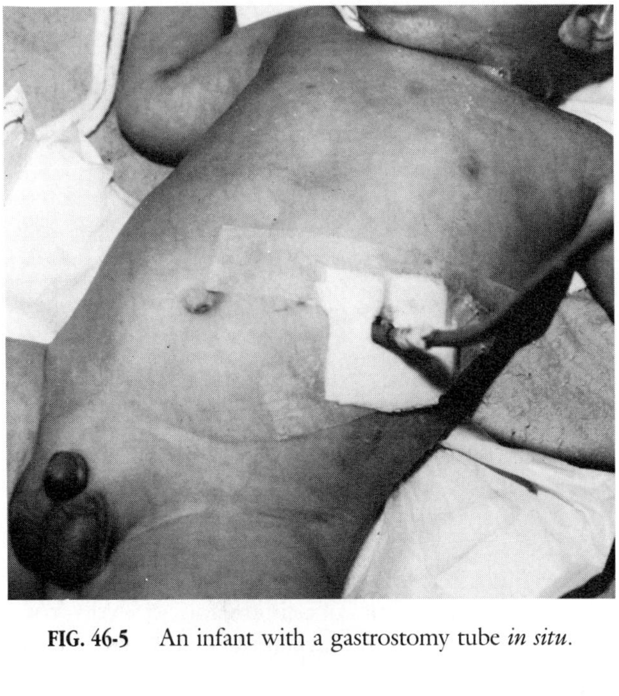

FIG. 46-5 An infant with a gastrostomy tube *in situ*.

At the end of a feeding, 5 to 10 ml of water is given through the gastrostomy tube to clear it. The barrel of the syringe is disconnected from the tube, and the tube is left unclamped to allow any air in the stomach to escape. Then the tube is clamped until the next feeding. It is necessary to record the amount and type of feeding, the child's response, and the condition of the gastrostomy site.

Restraints

There are times when, for a child's safety, he should be restrained after surgery or during a procedure or examination. Restraints are used only as a last resort. They should be applied correctly, and circulation and skin integrity are monitored closely. Any restraint should be removed every 3 to 4 hours so that the body area can be exercised. If extremities are restrained, they should be released one at a time so that the child cannot pull out an intravenous or a nasogastric tube. The ties of all restraints are attached to bedframes *only,* not to side rails.

Elbow restraint. Elbow restraints prevent flexion or bending of elbows. They allow an infant or toddler to move the upper extremities, but they protect the newly repaired cleft lip/palate or scalp vein infusion site. Clean tongue blades are slipped into the parallel pockets of a wraparound restraint (see Chapter 17). The shirt or pajama sleeve is pulled down to the wrist, and the elbow is placed in the center of this restraint. The restraint is wrapped around the arm and tied securely. The sleeve is cuffed over the bottom of the restraint to protect the skin. Both the axilla and the wrist should be checked for skin impairment.

Mummy restraint. A mummy restraint is used when the trunk and upper and lower extremities should be immobilized. A jugular venipuncture or the insertion of a nasogastric tube may require this type of restraint.

A square baby blanket is placed on a crib, and one corner is folded over. The infant is placed on his back on the blanket so the shoulders are at the level of the fold. The infant's arms are at his sides. One corner of the blanket is wrapped over the right arm and tucked under his left side. The opposite corner is placed over the left arm and placed securely under the right side of his body (Fig. 46-6).

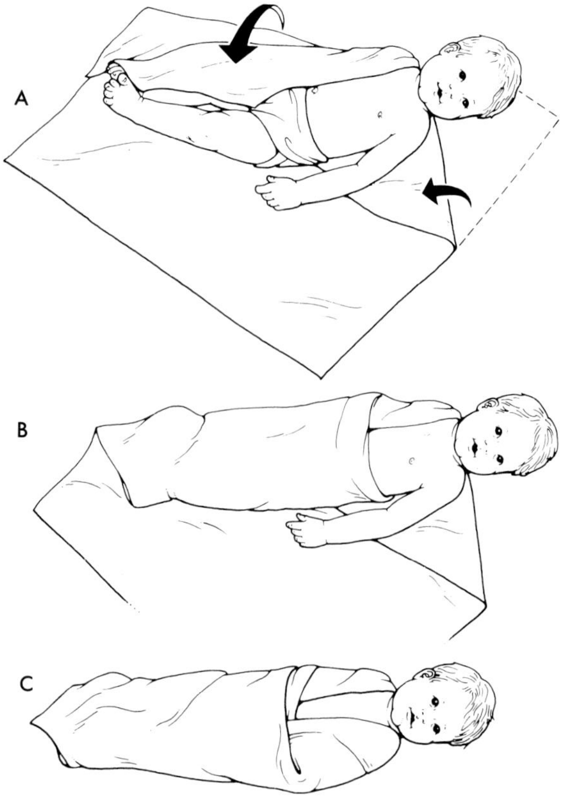

FIG. 46-6 Mummy restraint. **A** and **B,** Material is first folded over the right arm, and then corner is tucked under the left side. **C,** The opposite corner is then folded over the infant's left arm and tucked under the right side to secure.

A modified version may be necessary to expose the chest. While one corner of the blanket is placed around the right arm and tucked under the baby's body, the opposite corner encircles the left arm and it too is secured. The remaining corner beneath his feet is brought up to the abdomen and pinned, thereby leaving the chest exposed.

Clove-hitch restraint. This type of four-point restraint is used on all extremities of a child. Rolls of Kerlix, roller bandage, or strips of muslin can be used. The wrists and ankles are padded with gauze squares or other soft material. A clove hitch is *not* a square knot. A figure 8 is made with the material, slipped over the padded wrist or ankle, and tightened gently (see Chapter 17). Each restraint should be checked frequently so that circulation is not affected or there is no excessive pressure. A slip knot is used to tie the ends of these restraints to the bed frame.

Jacket restraint. A jacket restraint is sometimes used to keep an extremely active older infant or toddler safely in bed or in a high chair. It resembles a vest and has ties in the back. The child's arms are pulled through the jacket, and the jacket is tied in the back. The long ties are attached to a bed frame or under the seat of a highchair. While the child can move all body parts, he cannot climb out of the bed or high chair.

Urine Collection

Collecting a urine specimen can be a major problem in pediatrics when the child is not toilet trained. It is often a routine admission procedure that provides important information. In addition, kidney infections are common, and so urine should be collected and examined often.

A suprapubic bladder tap is done on newborns and infants (Fig. 46-7). Contamination is a minimal concern using this method. An infant is placed in a froglike position, similar to the position described below for femoral venipunctures. A physician prepares the skin above the bladder and inserts a 23-gauge, 1-inch needle into the bladder and removes several milliliters of urine. It is usually done 30 to 60 minutes after voiding.

Plastic urine collecting bags also are used. It is important to apply them correctly. Applying tincture of benzoin to the area increases the adhesiveness of these bags (Fig. 46-8). In girls special attention should be given to the narrow area between the vagina and the rectum. If the adhesive backing is not attached securely to this area, the anus is covered. As a result, a stool may contaminate the specimen.

When the bag is in place, a slit should be cut into the disposable diaper before it is placed on the child. By doing so the urine bag can be pulled through to the outside so it can be observed. As soon as the child voids, the bag is removed, decreasing the possibility of losing the urine specimen.

Catheterizations are done occasionally. The high possibility of contamination, especially in regard to introducing organisms into the urinary system, has resulted in avoiding this procedure as much as possible.

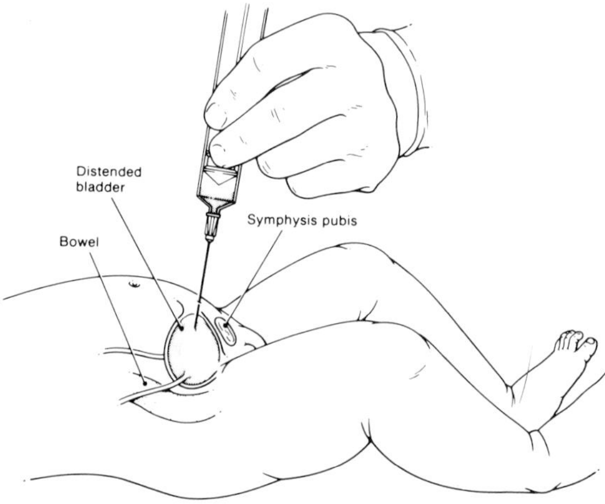

FIG. 46-7 Suprapubic bladder aspiration.

Venipunctures

In infants and toddlers, a jugular or femoral vein may be used to obtain a blood specimen. It is the nurse's responsibility to prepare the child and to position and restrain him. Holding the head or lower extremities absolutely immobile is critical.

When a jugular vein is used, the child is placed in a mummy restraint beforehand. The child's body is placed on the examining table so that his shoulders are at the edge of the table (Fig. 46-9). Turning the infant's head 45 degrees provides the best angle for successful entry.

For a femoral venipuncture, the infant is placed on his back with both legs in a froglike position (Fig. 46-10). It is necessary to apply gentle pressure to both knees to restrict movement. Once the needle has been removed from the vein, pressure should be applied to the site to prevent the formation of a hematoma.

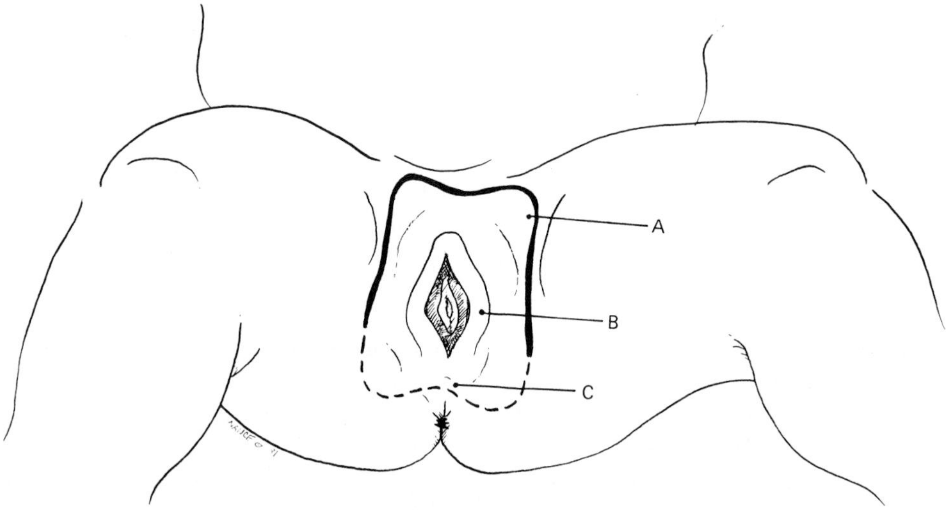

FIG. 46-8 Application of a pediatric urine bag for female infants. **A,** Pediatric urine bag. **B,** Labia majora. **C,** Pelvic floor (in female infants it is important to attach the bag securely at this point).

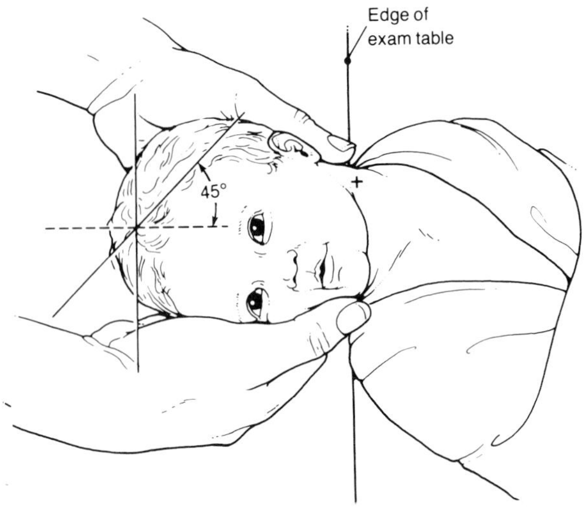

FIG. 46-9 Correct position for jugular venipuncture procedure. The puncture site is indicated by *x*. The mummy restraint is used.

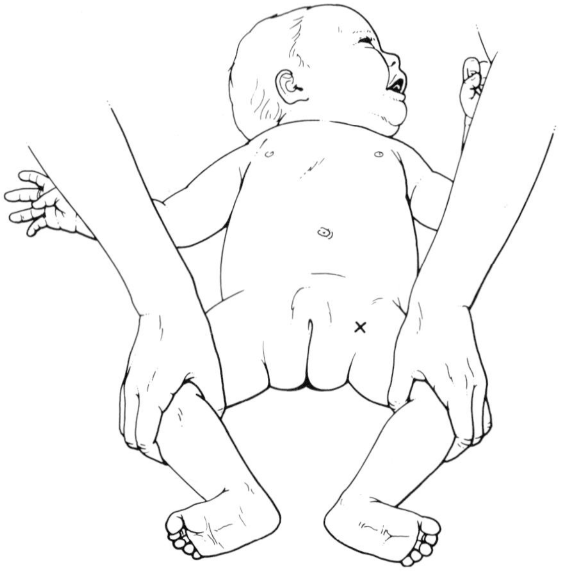

FIG. 46-10 Position for femoral venipuncture procedure. The *x* indicates the puncture site.

Lumbar Puncture

This procedure requires that an infant or child be positioned at the edge of the examining table or bed, on his side, facing the nurse who is holding him. The neck and legs are gently flexed, as demonstrated in Fig. 46-11. This angle increases the spinal curvature and helps the physician to gain entry into the subarachnoid space of the spinal canal. It is important to observe the child for any sign of difficulty. A toddler may need to have his legs wrapped in a blanket to decrease his activity. The child should be held securely in that position until the spinal tap has been completed.

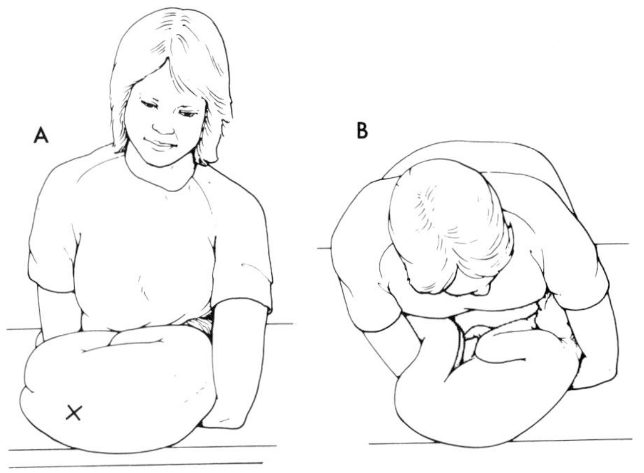

FIG. 46-11 **A,** Correct position for lumbar puncture procedure with infant at or over table edge; the *x* indicates the puncture site. **B,** View of lumbar puncture restraint from above.

Oxygen Therapy

Oxygen is used to improve a child's respiratory status. It is also used in children who have cardiac or neurological disorders. When a nurse administers oxygen to a newborn or infant, it is important to remember the harmful effects of oxygen on the developing pulmonary system. A variety of cellular changes occur and result in **bronchopulmonary dysplasia,** a serious lifelong problem. Oxygen is forced through sterile water to humidify it to counteract its drying effect.

Oxygen levels must be checked frequently (q2hr). An oxygen flow of 40% or less is considered safe. Levels higher than 40% should not be administered unless there is cyanosis or unless specifically ordered by a physician.

Infants and young children who are receiving oxygen are monitored on an oximeter, a flexible photoelectric device with an adhesive backing placed on the foot or hand of an infant or the finger of an adolescent. The monitoring screen gives an instant reading of the oxygen saturation of blood. There is a high correlation between this transcutaneous measurement and the child's actual arterial oxygenation.

Hood and incubator. Oxygen often is delivered to small infants through a plastic hood that fits over the baby's head (Fig. 46-12). It is an efficient method of providing oxygen at levels that can be controlled. More important, the body is accessible for starting an intravenous line or performing a procedure.

A less efficient method of delivering oxygen to an infant is with the use of a closed incubator. Imperfectly fitted lids, uncovered vents, and portholes that must be opened

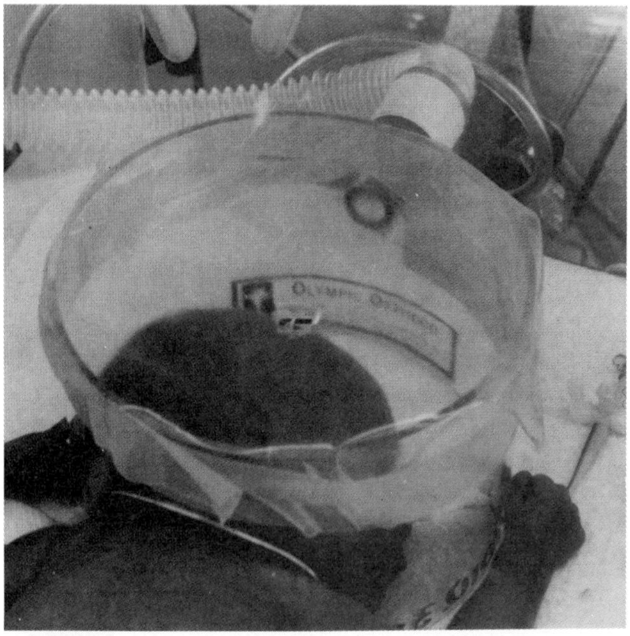

FIG. 46-12 A preterm neonate whose head is enclosed within a plastic circular hood that maintains a constant humidified and oxygenated environment.

often to perform an activity on the infant all contribute to fluctuations in oxygen levels. Maintaining a constant temperature within the incubator is a problem too. As the infant increases his metabolism in an effort to maintain his body temperature, he requires larger amounts of oxygen.

Mist tents. The purpose of using a mist tent is to improve a child's respiratory status by liquefying pulmonary secretions. It allows a nurse to observe a child easily through the plastic canopy. All of its working parts are outside of the tent, which is a distinct advantage when a toddler needs this form of therapy. Compressed air or oxygen runs through sterile water to form the therapeutic mist. A disadvantage is that the canopy must be opened for treatments and procedures, which lowers the concentration of the mist.

A nurse must organize all activities (to limit the number of times the tent is opened) so that the desired concentrations can be maintained and the child will have longer rest periods. The tent should be tucked under the mattress of a crib to maintain humidity levels. If the tent is functioning efficiently, dampness within it is significant and frequent (q3-4hr) linen and clothing changes may be necessary.

Nasal cannula. Delivering oxygen to newborns and all ages of children can be done using a nasal cannula. It is a mode of delivery commonly used with infants suffering from bronchopulmonary dysplasia. Maintaining the cannula's placement can be problematic in the infant, whose random head and hand movements disturb its position. Placing clear plastic tape around the oxygen tubing and over the nose/cheek prevents its disturbance. Adjusting the device at the back of an infant's head allows a nurse to fit the tubing to the child, and hooking it over the pinnae helps in stabilizing it. In older children the nasal cannula is held in place by adjustable elastic straps on the head.

Intake and Output

There are many health disorders that require the accurate monitoring of the amount of solids and liquids taken in and the amount excreted. For example, measuring and recording intake and output (I and O) is extremely important in infants with diarrhea, toddlers with burns, or adolescents with renal disorders. Infants who are hospitalized because they fail to thrive or to grow as expected are placed on "calorie counts," which requires the careful recording of all food ingested and liquids given. This intake is recorded at the bedside, and a nutritionist calculates the calories actually consumed by a child. It is helpful in determining whether the cause is organic or the result of an inadequate intake. These causes are ruled out before a maternal-infant problem is considered.

All fluids given to a child are documented on a record kept at the bedside. Adolescents assume this responsibility after an explanation. All urine voided is measured before discarding. The diapers of those who are not toilet trained are weighed. Older children may need to be reminded to save all urine. However, they are usually cooperative.

Weight

Fluid loss is reflected in a child's weight, especially that of infants and toddlers. The same scale should be used and the child should be weighed at the same time every day. Any error then becomes a constant one. What a child wears and what is attached to him is important and affects weight. For example, the weight of a naked infant with a nasogastric tube, electrodes, and an intravenous armboard differs significantly from that of the infant without these attachments. If this equipment has been removed, it should be noted on the graphic sheet.

Medication Administration

A critical responsibility of a pediatric nurse is the administration of medications. A nurse *must* know the drug's side effects and toxic signs and symptoms, as well as how to compute the dose correctly and administer it properly. Medication must be given to the right child at the appropriate time and by the correct route. Nurses also must observe and document a child's response to the drug.

There are no unit dosages in pediatrics because children are of various ages and weights. The two methods of calculating dosages for children are (1) body weight and (2) **body surface area (BSA).**

When weight is used, the recommended dose is given as milligrams/kilogram/dose, for example, 10 mg/kilogram/dose. A nurse calculates the appropriate dose a child requires from a standard dose. For example, an infant is to receive ampicillin 150 mg in liquid form and the standard dose on hand is 250 mg in 5 ml. To determine the dose required for a child, a nurse can use the "*desired* over *at hand*" rule.

$$\frac{\text{Desired amount}}{\text{Amount at hand}} = \frac{150 \text{ mg}}{250 \text{ mg}} = \frac{3}{5}$$

Another method is:

$$\frac{250 \text{ mg}}{5 \text{ ml}} = \frac{150 \text{ mg}}{x}$$

$$250x = 750 \text{ ml}$$

$$x = 3 \text{ ml}$$

When a child is burned or severely dehydrated, the body surface area is important. It can be determined by using a nomogram (see Fig. 24-1). A straight line is drawn connecting a child's height and weight on the nomogram. The point at which the line intersects the BSA column is the child's body surface area. If the child is of average size, it can be determined from weight alone (the enclosed area on the nomogram). A frequently used method of estimation is:

$$\text{BSA of child in m}^2 \times \text{dose per m}^2 = \text{estimated child's dose}$$

Intravenous medications. Medications are given through the infusion that is in progress. The intravenous sites in children differ from those of adults. A scalp vein is used in infants because their veins have no valves, so a needle can be inserted in either direction. In addition, the head can be moved from side to side without dislodging the needle.

A microdrip, in which there are 60 drops in each milliliter, is always used in young children. It makes computing the rate of flow less difficult. When 10 ml per hour is ordered, the intravenous flow rate is 10 drops/minute; if 37 ml per hour is required, the rate is 37 drops/minute. A calibrated volume control chamber that holds up to 150 ml prevents volume overload (Fig. 46-13). Only the desired amount of fluid is added to the chamber from the bottle or bag of solution. A 2-hour supply is the maximum amount added. For example, if a child receives 15 ml each hour, no more than 30 ml should be added to the control chamber. All infusions are monitored at least *hourly* and recorded on the flow sheet.

An intravenous medication is added to the control chamber after it has been prepared. Care should be taken to ensure that the medication is placed in the solution, not along the sides of the control chamber. The rate of flow should be adjusted so that the drug is received in the recommended time period for maximum effectiveness. The infusion site also should be monitored closely.

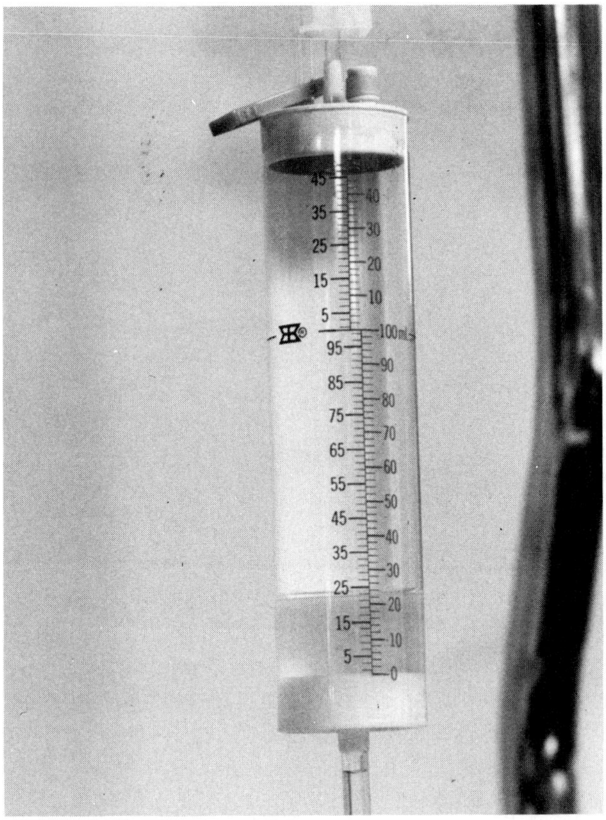

FIG. 46-13 A calibrated burette for use in administering intravenous fluids.

Converting an infusion line to a heparin lock is done when a child does not require additional intravenous fluids but a course of antibiotics may need to be completed. With a heparin lock, a child can move about more freely except for those brief periods when the drugs are infused. The extension tubing of the heparin lock should be irrigated regularly (q3-4hr) with 10 units of heparin so that the line remains open (see Chapter 26).

Intramuscular injections. The most common sites for intramuscular injections are (1) vastus lateralis and rectus femoris muscles, (2) the gluteal area for older children, and (3) the deltoid muscle. It should be remembered that infants have small muscle mass and a limited number of sites are available.

Needle size varies from 25-gauge, ⅝ inch long for use in infants to 22-gauge, 1 inch long for teenagers. All sites should be inspected for tenderness. Fig. 46-14 identifies the common injection sites.

Oral medication. Older children may know how to swallow pills, but attention should be given to infants and toddlers who are unable to do so. Liquid medication can

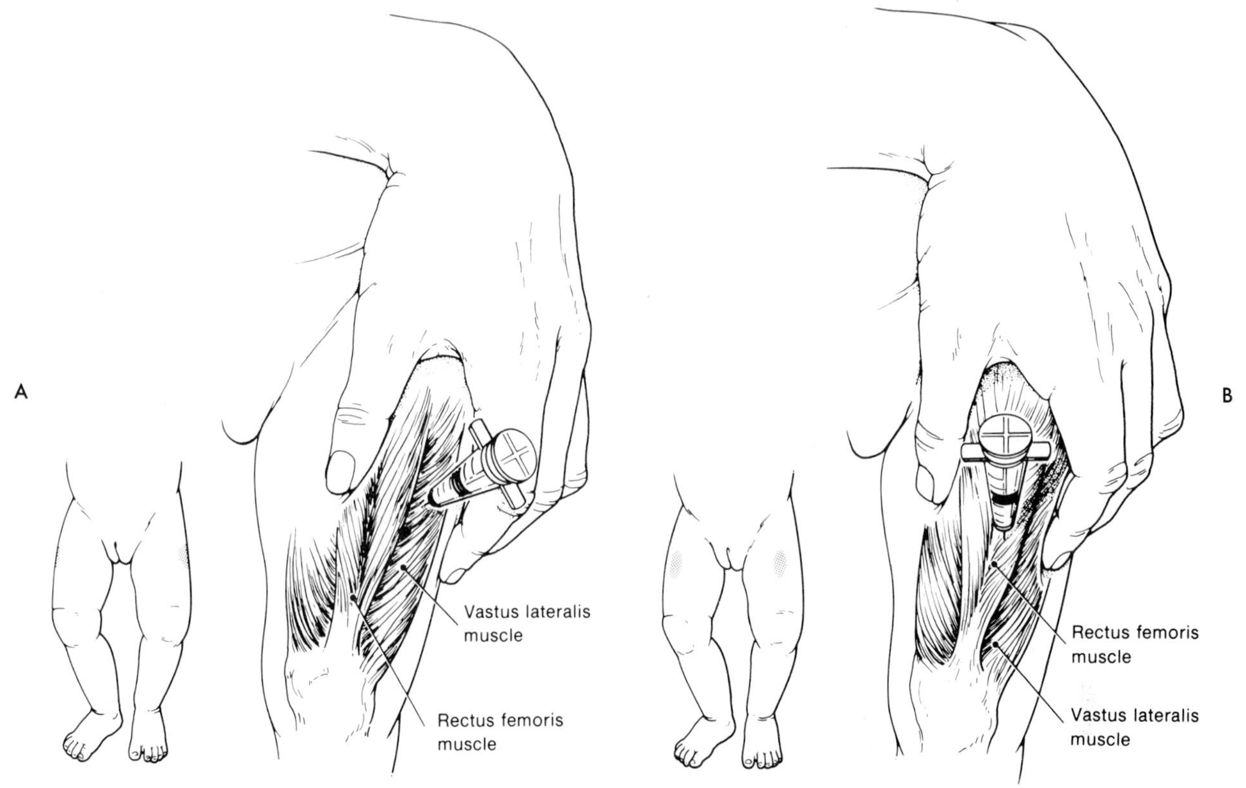

FIG. 46-14 **A,** The vastus lateralis muscle is the primary site for intramuscular injections in the thigh. The needle penetrates the midlateral thigh on a front-to-back course. **B,** An alternative site for intramuscular injections in the thigh is the anterolateral surface; the needle is directed into the rectus femoris muscle.

be given with a syringe (without the needle) or a medicine dropper. The drug should be given slowly and in small amounts, allowing an infant time to swallow. Liquids can be given by nipple too. A small plastic medication cup can be used for an older infant.

Medications in pill form may need to be crushed. After being pulverized, pills can be mixed in a very small amount of baby fruit or ice cream and administered.

Eye and ear drops. Administering eye and ear drops may require the assistance of a second nurse. Positioning is critical to administering them successfully. The child's head must be kept as immobile as possible and the eye should be opened for proper administration of eye drops. Likewise, after ear drops are given, the head should be kept still for the medication to run down the canal. For proper instillation of ear drops to children under 3 years, the pinna should be pulled *down and back.* For children older than 3 years, ear drops are given as to an adult—by pulling the pinna up and back.

REFERENCES AND SUGGESTED READINGS

1. Alexander D, White M, and Powell G: Anxiety of non-rooming-in parents of hospitalized children, Children and Health Care 15(1):14, 1986.
2. Bates TA and Broome M: Preparation of children for hospitalization and surgery: a review of the literature, J Pediatr Nurs 1(4):230, 1986.
3. Bausell RB and Soehen KL: Results of *Pediatric Nursing* survey on the importance of pediatric preventive behaviors, Pediatr Nurs 13(6):421, 1987.
4. Cyganski JM, Donahue JM, and Heaton JS: The case for the heparin flush, Am J Nurs 87(6):769, 1987.
5. Eland J: Pharmacologic management of acute and chronic pain, Issues Compr Pediatr Nurs 11(2-3):93, 1988.
6. Hughes D: *The health of America's children,* Washington, DC, Children's Defense Fund, 1987.
7. Killiam P and Smith K: Getting kids into car seats, MCN 13(2):124, 1988.
8. Klaus MH and Kennell JH: Bonding: the beginnings of parent-infant attachment, St Louis, 1983, The CV Mosby Co.
9. Lawrey GH: Growth and development of children, ed 8, Chicago, 1986, Year Book Medical Publishers, Inc.
10. Lee EJ, Jacobson JM, and Levanas V: Stressful life events and accidents at school, Pediatr Nurs 15(2):140, 1989.
11. McGovern K: Take the first step toward reducing medication errors, Nurs '87 17(12):49, 1987.
12. Papalia DE and Olds SW: A child's world, ed 4, New York, 1987, McGraw-Hill, Inc.
13. Parish L: Communicating with hospitalized children. Can Nurse 82(1):21, 1986.
14. Pass MD and Pass CM: Anticipatory guidance for parents of hospitalized children, J Pediatr Nurs 2(4):250, 1987.

15. Patterson KL and Ware LL: Coping skills for children undergoing painful medical procedures, Issues Compr Pediatr Nurs 11(2-3): 113, 1988.
16. Penatzer M: Common pediatric IV medications at a glance, Pediatr Nurs 14(1):56, 1988.
17. Pidgeon V: Children's concepts of illness: implications for health teaching, Matern Child Nurs 14(1):23, 25, 1985.
18. Ruddy-Wallace M: Temperament: assessing individual differences in hospitalized children, J Pediatr Nurs 2(1):30, 1987.
19. Scipien GM and others: Pediatric nursing care, St Louis, 1990, The CV Mosby Co.
20. Suri S: Simplifying urine collection from infants and children without losing accuracy, MCN 13(6):438, 1988.
21. Tichy AM: Stressors in pediatric intensive care units, Pediatr Nurs 14(1):40, 1988.
22. Trinkoff A and Baker S: Poisoning hospitalizations and deaths from solids and liquids among children and teenagers, Am J Public Health 76(6):657, 1986.
23. Vulcan B and Nikulich-Barrett M: The effect of selected information on mothers' anxiety levels during their children's hospitalizations, J Pediatr Nurs 3(2):97, 1988.
24. Weibley TT: Gavage tube insertion in the premature infant, MCN 12(1):24, 1987.
25. Whaley LF and Wong DL: Essentials of pediatric nursing, ed 3, St Louis, 1989, The CV Mosby Co.

CHAPTER CHALLENGE

KEY POINTS

- The medical and psychosocial needs of children were considered unimportant until the beginning of the twentieth century.
- The differences between adults and children are immense and demonstrate the challenges a pediatric nurse encounters daily in clinical practice.
- The traumatic effects of a child's hospitalization can be decreased by the child and his parents attending a preadmission orientation program.
- Rooming-in facilities allow a parent to become as involved as desired and provide the child with the security of an adult he knows, trusts, and loves.
- In understanding parental responses to the hospitalization of a child, the nurse is better able to address the parents' needs.
- When working with children, a nurse involves family members in the care given and considers the family as a unit.
- Accidents are a leading cause of death in children and adolescents, and potential hazards should be identified so they can be avoided.
- The preparation of medications for administration to infants and children requires precise computations of dosages.
- The urine of an infant can be obtained by using a plastic collecting bag or by the physician doing a suprapubic tap.
- Explanations that are provided to children always should be given at age-appropriate levels so they can be understood.

STUDY QUESTIONS

1. The president responsible for convening the first White House Conference was:
   a. F.D. Roosevelt
   b. R.B. Hayes
   c. G. Cleveland
   d. T. Roosevelt
2. The federal agency responsible for publishing *Infant Care*, the most extensive collection of information on child care, was:
   a. The Children's Bureau
   b. Child Development Office
   c. Social Security Office
   d. Library of Congress
3. With a sound knowledge of growth and development principles, a pediatric nurse can:
   a. Select appropriate diversional activities for a child
   b. Identify the child with a developmental delay
   c. Select the appropriate level for teaching a child
   d. Use the information in providing anticipatory guidance to parents
   e. All of the above
4. A new solid food is introduced to an infant at 4- or 5-day intervals to:
   a. Allow the infant time to develop a taste for the new food
   b. Permit proper digestion of the new food
   c. Identify the presence of an allergy to the new food
   d. Ensure a patent gastrointestinal tract
5. Accidents are a leading cause of death in:
   a. Infants
   b. Toddlers
   c. Preschoolers
   d. School-age children
6. Elbow restraints are commonly used in infants or toddlers hospitalized for:
   a. Fractured leg
   b. Arm laceration
   c. Cleft palate repair
   d. Hand surgery
7. The level of oxygen considered to be safe when administered to a newborn or infant is:
   a. 20%
   b. 30%
   c. 40%
   d. 50%
8. When a toddler is burned or severely dehydrated, his fluid requirements are calculated on the basis of:
   a. Height
   b. Weight
   c. Age
   d. Body surface area
9. An infant is to receive 12 mg of Gentamycin intramuscularly; the vial on hand contains 20 mg in each milliliter; the dose that should be withdrawn and given is:
   a. 0.5 ml
   b. 0.6 ml
   c. 0.7 ml
   d. 0.8 ml
10. When a physician orders the hourly rate of flow at 12 ml for an intravenous in a 3-month-old baby, the drops per minute using a microdrip are:
    a. 12
    b. 18
    c. 24
    d. 30
11. When a suprapubic bladder tap is done on an infant, it is important for a nurse to:
    a. Apply pressure to the site afterward
    b. Place the infant in a mummy restraint beforehand
    c. Notify a physician 15 minutes after the infant voids
    d. Hold the infant in a froglike position

47

Care of Children with Physical and Emotional Problems

GLADYS M. SCIPIEN

LEARNING OBJECTIVES

After reading this chapter, the student should be able to do the following:

- Define the key terms.
- Describe the major characteristics of three common communicable diseases of children.
- Develop a teaching plan for parents of an infant with a cleft palate.
- Identify the subjective and objective data to be obtained from a child and/or parents in the presence of a gastrointestinal problem.
- Describe the effects of cystic fibrosis on the respiratory and gastrointestinal systems.
- List four variables that influence the severity of a respiratory disorder in a young child.
- Develop a plan of care for a child with AIDS.
- List the signs and symptoms of a crisis in a child with sickle cell disease.
- Describe three acyanotic cardiac defects, their treatment, and management.
- Describe the nursing interventions of an adolescent with scoliosis.
- Identify methods of preventing urinary tract infections in children.
- List the clinical differences between hypoglycemia and hyperglycemia.
- Identify those drugs that have caused hearing impairments in children.

RELATED TOPICS OF INTEREST

- Communication (Chapter 4)
- The family (Chapter 7)
- The infant and young child (Chapter 8)
- The school-age child (Chapter 9)
- The adolescent (Chapter 10)
- Medical asepsis (Chapter 16)
- Basic nutrition (Chapter 22)
- Care of the patient with AIDS (Chapter 40)
- Basic pediatric nursing care (Chapter 46)

KEY TERMS

Define the following:

- anastomosis
- biopsy
- bolus
- bruit
- Colles' fracture
- collodion
- coxsackievirus
- cryptorchidism
- cushingoid
- cytomegalovirus (CMV)
- dander
- development delay
- Duchenne's muscular dystrophy
- exacerbation
- exocrine
- gluten
- hypertrophy
- hydrocephaly
- hydrostatic pressure
- hyphema
- immunosuppressed
- intrathecal
- Legg-Calvé-Perthes disease
- meningomyelocele
- metabolite
- narcotic abstinence syndrome
- nuchal rigidity
- Ortolani's test
- palliative
- pica
- sweat test
- tympanostomy tube
- Wilms' tumor

Many health problems of children differ from those of adults. Whereas some develop as a result of immature body systems, a significant number of disorders are related to the presence of a birth defect. Approximately 250,000 infants are born with birth defects each year. Although viruses, drugs (over-the-counter and prescription drugs and alcohol), and radiation have been implicated in the development of these anomalies in utero, the specific causes of most of them are unknown.

Some of these congenital malformations are evident at birth, such as cleft lip and palate. Many, however, are not apparent until later in infancy or in childhood, which necessitates thorough assessments to identify them as early as possible.

This chapter contains some of the common health problems of children. Although NANDA-approved nursing diagnoses are included, it should be remembered that each child is a unique, developing person, thus making it impossible to provide every appropriate nursing diagnosis. In addition, physicians order treatments and medications as appropriate for specific causes; therefore in some instances broad categories of medications, such as antibiotics or antihistamines, may be identified in the management of these disorders.

Many health problems occur more commonly at specific stages. Therefore, where possible, the content is organized developmentally. For example, health problems are categorized according to those seen at birth, later in infancy, and in toddlerhood.

Because it is beyond the scope of this chapter to address all disorders affecting children, readers are also referred to chapters within this text that address specific disorders within body systems, many of which provide specific pediatric focuses.

DISORDERS OF THE INTEGUMENTARY SYSTEM

Skin is the largest organ system of the body. Its major function is to protect the vital organs it envelops and to protect itself from trauma, radiation, fungi, and organisms. It also regulates body temperature and helps in secretion, excretion, and absorption. Any break in the skin's integrity results in an inflammatory response and a potential for infection. The epidermis is most commonly affected.

There are many causes of skin disorders, such as the following:

1. Viruses are responsible for such communicable diseases as measles and chickenpox (varicella).

2. The potential for severe, penetrating injuries always exists, especially in young children.
3. An allergic response to a food can be an external source of a skin reaction.
4. Diarrheal stools caused by food contamination can inflame skin in the perineal area of an infant or toddler.

Skin disorders usually are not life-threatening, but such complications as systemic infections can occur. Generally a disease runs its course, signs and symptoms are treated as they develop, and a child recovers. However, the condition may be a source of great discomfort to the child. Changes in the skin can influence how a child feels about himself: the adolescent with acne can be embarrassed by skin lesions, which influence his self-esteem and body image.

Nursing Assessment

Collection of *subjective data* must be comprehensive. It is important to collect all information to diagnose a child's skin disorder. Recent exposure to a known communicable disease, introduction of a new food, and acquisition of a pet are significant pieces of information. The nurse should obtain a description of associated symptoms, such as lacrimation, a cough, vertigo, or nausea. Pain, pruritus, fatigue, and erythema of a body part all develop with inflammation or infection.

Collection of subjective data includes noting the presenting problem (rash, fever, pustules), its onset (whether sudden or gradual), area in which the rash first appeared, any changes in the appearance of the lesions, and the pattern in which it spread to other parts of the body. Other clinical manifestations include pruritus, photophobia, the development of conjunctivitis, and increasingly oily skin. The nurse should ask if any medications were used, for how long, and their effect on the problem. Exposure to children with communicable diseases, immunization status, and family history of allergies and skin problems should be determined.

Collection of *objective data* includes inspecting the skin for color, dryness, erythema, irritation, and inflammation/infection. Also included is a thorough description of distribution and size of lesions, as well as skin turgor. Because many skin problems affect other organ systems, the nurse should examine the eyes for conjunctivitis and photosensitivity and should check the oral mucosa for lesions. She should examine the throat visually for exudate or irritation; tonsil size should be noted.

Table 47-1 Recommended Schedule for Active Immunization of Normal Infants and Children

Recommended Age	Immunization(s)	Comments
2 mo	DTP,* OPV*	Can be initiated as early as 2 wk of age in areas of high endemicity or during epidemics
4 mo	DTP, OPV	2-mo interval desired for OPV to avoid interference from previous dose
6 mo	DTP (OPV)	OPV is optional (may be given in areas with increased risk of poliovirus exposure)
15 mo	MMR*	MMR preferred to individual vaccines; tuberculin testing may be done
18 mo	DTP,†‡ OPV‡	
24 mo	HBPV*	
4-6 yr§	DTP, OPV	At or before school entry
14-16 yr	Td*	Repeat every 10 yr throughout life

From Committee on Infectious Diseases, American Academy of Pediatrics: Report of the Committee on Infectious Diseases, ed 20, American Academy of Pediatrics, Elk Grove Village, Ill, 1986, p 9.
*DTP = diphtheria and tetanus toxoids with pertussis vaccine; OPV = oral poliovirus vaccine containing poliovirus types 1, 2, and 3; MMR = live measles, mumps, and rubella viruses in a combined vaccine; HBPV = *Haemophilus* b polysaccharide vaccine; Td = adult tetanus toxoid (full dose) and diphtheria toxoid (reduced dose) in combination.
†Should be given 6 to 12 months after the third dose.
‡May be given simultaneously with MMR at 15 months of age.
§Up to the seventh birthday.
Note: For all products used, consult manufacturer's package insert for instructions for storage, handling, and administration. Biologics prepared by different manufacturers may vary, and those of the same manufacturer may change from time to time. Therefore, the physician should be aware of the contents of the package insert.
Author's Note: A conjugate vaccine (diphtheria toxoid-conjugate) to prevent *Haemophilis* b infection recently licensed for use in children 18 months or older is now recommended for all children at 18 months of age. (Recommendations of the ACIP, 1988.)

Communicable Diseases

The development of vaccines has decreased the prevalence of many communicable childhood diseases and eradicated others. Although most of these diseases are preventable today, outbreaks occur periodically because hundreds of thousands of children are either unimmunized or not immunized properly. The Academy of Pediatrics has developed a set of recommended immunization schedules, one of which starts in infancy and another designed for children who did not receive vaccines in the first year of life (see Tables 47-1 and 47-2). The goal is to immunize all children and prevent the complications that can occur if a communicable disease develops.

There also are some reasons for *not* immunizing certain children. For example, no immunizations are given to a child who is experiencing acute illness. None of the live

Table 47-2 Recommended Immunization Schedules for Children Not Immunized in First Year of Life

Recommended Time	Immunization(s)	Comments
LESS THAN 7 YEARS OLD		
First visit	DTP, OPV, MMR*	MMR if child ≥15 mo old; tuberculin testing may be done
Interval after first visit		
1 mo	HBPV*†	For children 24-60 mo
2 mo	DTP	OPV
4 mo	DTP (OPV)	OPV is optional (may be given in areas with increased risk of poliovirus exposure)
10-16 mo	DTP, OPV	OPV is not given if third dose was given earlier
Age 4-6 yr (at or before school entry)	DTP, OPV	DTP is not necessary if the fourth dose was given after the fourth birthday; OPV is not necessary if recommended OPV dose at 10-16 mo following first visit was given after fourth birthday
Age 14-16 yr	Td*	Repeat every 10 yr throughout life
7 YEARS OLD AND OLDER		
First visit	Td, OPV, MMR	
Interval after first visit		
2 mo	Td, OPV	
8-14 mo	Td, OPV	
Age 14-16 yr	Td	Repeat every 10 yr throughout life

From Committee on Infectious Diseases, American Academy of Pediatrics: Report of the Committee on Infectious Diseases, ed 20, Academy of Pediatrics, Elk Grove Village, Ill, 1986, p 11.

*DTP = diphtheria and tetanus toxoids with pertussis vaccine; OPV = oral poliovirus vaccine containing poliovirus types 1, 2, and 3; MMR = live measles, mumps, and rubella viruses in a combined vaccine; HBPV = *Haemophilus* b polysaccharide vaccine; Td = adult tetanus toxoid (full dose) and diphtheria toxoid (reduced dose) in combination.

†*Haemophilus* b polysaccharide vaccine can be given, if necessary, simultaneously with DTP (at separate sites). The initial three doses of DTP can be given at 1- to 2-month intervals; so, for the child in whom immunization is initiated at 24 months old or older, one visit could be eliminated by giving DTP, OPV, and MMR at the first visit; DTP and HBPV at the second visit (1 month later); and DTP and OPV at the third visit (2 months after the first visit). Subsequent DTP and OPV 10 to 16 months after the first visit are still indicated.

Table 47-3 Common Lesions in Communicable Diseases

Lesion	Description
Macules	Less than 1 cm in diameter; circumscribed alterations without elevations or depressions
Maculopapules	Macules that become slightly raised
Papules	Less than 1 cm in diameter; solid elevations with no visible fluid
Vesicles	Circumscribed elevations of the epidermis; less than 1 cm in diameter and contain a clear liquid; may develop from macules or papules

virus vaccines (mumps, measles, and rubella [MMR]) are given to children with leukemia or those receiving radiation therapy or steroids. The immune system is depressed in these children, and serious reactions can occur. In addition, MMR, especially the rubella component, threatens the developing fetus in the first trimester of pregnancy, so girls should receive this vaccination before puberty.

Normally newborns receive maternal antibodies, which provide them with immunity to some of these diseases for the first few months of life. One exception is whooping cough, or pertussis. Young infants, especially those younger than 3 or 4 months, are highly susceptible to this communicable disease, and they can become critically ill.

Communicable diseases continue to occur because children are exposed to a variety of potential sources, especially in day care centers and schools. Table 47-3 lists the different types of lesions in communicable diseases, and Table 47-4 identifies the common communicable diseases. Generally communicable diseases run their course, and children resume normal activities afterward. However, complications can occur. Parents should be advised that when signs and symptoms persist for an extended time, when they increase in severity, or when parents note a change in the child's overall behavior, such as increasing lethargy, a physician should be contacted.

Although prevention is the focus of pediatric health care, outbreaks occur. Some states have enacted legislation that requires up-to-date immunizations for eligibility for public school attendance. Until such action is a national effort and all children are immunized, communicable diseases will continue to plague children, parents, and school systems.

Isolation

A variety of conditions require isolation for children. Universal precautions are used when blood and body secretions are involved, and in pediatrics a number of

Table 47-4 Common Communicable Diseases

Disease	Causative Agent/ Transmission	Incubation Period	Clinical Signs and Symptoms	Nursing Interventions
Chickenpox (varicella)	Varicella zoster virus, direct contact, airborne droplets, and objects contaminated by infected person	10-21 days	Slight fever, anorexia, malaise. Rash starts as macule, progresses to papule, vesicle, ruptured vesicle, and finally crusted lesion. Lesions appear in crops, first on trunk, and then on scalp, face, and extremities. Vesicle appears as fragile "dewdrop" on erythematous base. Body part has lesions in all stages, which makes it easy to recognize. Vesicle begins to dry and form crust at site of dewdrop, in center of this lesion. Rash is extremely pruritic and causes significant discomfort until crusts form.	In hospital strict isolation is essential. Child should be kept at home until crusts form. Once vesicles begin to appear, pruritus may be intense. It must be controlled to decrease scar formation. Calamine lotion, starch baths, and oral antihistamines are helpful in relieving pruritus. Child also can be taught to apply pressure to area to decrease sensation. Finger nails are potential source of infection and should be clean and clipped short; "mittens" can be created by using socks. After bath, child's body should be patted dry to decrease possibility of breaking vesicles, which leads to scarring. Diversional activities occupy child. Aspirin has been implicated in development of Reye's syndrome when given to children who have signs and symptoms of chickenpox. Therefore Tylenol *only* should be given. Once crusts are formed, child can return to school. *Complications:* skin infections, cellulitis, pneumonia, and encephalitis.
German measles (rubella)	Rubella virus, direct contact, airborne droplets, and objects contaminated by infected person	14-21 days	Although some children have no symptoms before appearance of rash, others complain of headache, stiff neck, malaise, sore throat, and coryza. All symptoms disappear with eruption of pinkish-red macular, papular rash on face, which spreads down neck, arms, trunk, and legs. It disappears in 1-3 days. Skin does not peel afterward, and presence of rash does not cause discomfort.	Disease does not cause any discomfort to child. With exposure to rubella in first trimester of pregnancy, there are great dangers to the developing embryo; serious congenital anomalies can occur. Therefore these children should be isolated from contact with pregnant women. Some women may not yet know they are pregnant so children with rubella should not be taken to supermarkets or malls, where exposure can occur. *Complications:* extremely rare, except for developing fetus.
Regular measles (rubeola)	Rubeola virus; spread by cough or sneeze of infected person (airborne droplets), and objects contaminated by infected person	10-20 days	Child appears to have severe cold with high temperature (above 38° C), nasal congestion, cough, and conjunctivitis. About 24 hours after symptoms become more severe, Koplik spots appear on buccal mucosa of mouth; they are blue spots with white centers. One day later, macular, papular rash appears on face and spreads down body. Child most ill on second or third day of rash.	Child is sick and stays in bed. Eyes are light-sensitive; photophobia is common. Window shades down and dim lights help. Crusts that form on eyelids can be removed by warm water or saline compresses. Tylenol helps lower child's temperature. Nares can become excoriated as result of nasal discharge. Applying thin layer of petrolatum helps protect skin. Child should be dressed in light clothing. Encouraging large fluid intake when febrile is recommended. Pruritus is not problem, but if child complains of this discomfort, calamine lotion may relieve it. Parents may need to be assured that

Table 47-4 Common Communicable Diseases—cont'd

Disease	Causative Agent/ Transmission	Incubation Period	Clinical Signs and Symptoms	Nursing Interventions
			Elevated temperature (above 39° C), nasal discharge, harsh cough, and lacrimating, edematous, light-sensitive eyes are typical. Rash is pruritic and covers body. On fifth or sixth day of rash, there is sudden improvement, with normal temperature, improving coryza, and eyes no longer sensitive. Rash fades in same order that it appeared. Skin desquamates afterward and has brownish stain to it.	brown staining after warm bath is normal. They also should be advised that if child's temperature remains elevated, lethargy increases, or respiratory distress develops, child should be seen by physician. *Complications:* pneumonia, otitis media, encephalitis, and bronchiolitis.
Mumps (parotitis)	Virus, direct contact, airborne droplets, objects contaminated by secretions of oral cavity or respiratory tract of infected person	12-26 days	Low-grade fever, malaise, and edema, as well as pain in one or more salivary glands (usually bilateral; usually parotid). Swallowing is difficult and painful. Edema continues for 5-10 days.	Child should be isolated. Some discomfort can be relieved by Tylenol (liquid or suppository) and cool or warm compresses. Spicy or sour foods are avoided; bland foods only are offered. Adolescent males develop orchitis, which is painful and can result in sterility. Support to scrotum is important. Stretch bathing suit is most effective in relieving discomfort. *Complications:* sensorineural deafness, myocarditis, and arthritis.
Whooping cough (pertussis)	*Bordetella pertussis (Haemophilus pertussis),* airborne droplets, or direct contact	5-21 days	Signs and symptoms of respiratory tract infection that continue for 7-10 days. Cough gets progressively worse and ends in prolonged inspiration that is associated with high-pitched, crowing sound or "whoop." During these paroxysmal coughing episodes, face may become flushed, neck veins distend, eyes bulge, and tongue protrudes. Vomiting often occurs after infant expectorates thick mucus. From first symptoms to disappearance of cough may take as long as 6 weeks.	Infants are hospitalized and isolated. Sudden noises, such as lowering crib side, can precipitate coughing episode. Infant is kept elevated (in infant seat) and in humidified oxygen (mist tent). Suctioning may be required to keep airway patent. Small, frequent feedings are offered. Formula may need to be diluted with sterile water (1:1) to decrease thickness of oral secretions. If vomiting occurs, infant should be refed in 30 minutes. Exhaustion results from frequent, tiring coughing episodes. Environment should be quiet. At home, older child should be occupied—play activities distract him and decrease number of paroxysmal coughing episodes. Reduce factors that promote coughing, such as smoke, dust, temperature changes, and excitement. Have parents offer liquids frequently and in small amounts, especially apple juice, popsicles, ½ strength milk, ½ strength orange juice, jello, or any fluid that does *not* thicken secretions. *Complications:* hemorrhage (subarachnoid, retinal), dehydration, pneumonia, otitis media, convulsions, hernia, and prolapsed rectum.

Table 47-5 Types of Isolation

Condition	Specific Precautions	Special Considerations
STRICT ISOLATION		
Rubeola, varicella, herpes zoster, extensive infected burns (staphylococcus), vaccinia, pneumonitis, meningococcemia, neonatal vesicular disease (herpes simplex), congenital rubella	Private room with door closed; gowns, gloves, and masks are discarded in proper receptacles in child's room; wash hands on entering and leaving room; any articles leaving room must be double-bagged and properly identified before being sent to laundry, central supply, etc.	Rubella titers of all nurses assigned to children with congenital rubella must be reviewed; since baby sheds virus for many months, all women of childbearing age are endangered, including nurses, ancillary personnel, and visitors.
RESPIRATORY ISOLATION		
Bacterial meningitis, tuberculosis, pertussis, staphylococcal pneumonia, mumps	Private room with door closed; masks should be worn by susceptible individuals; all persons must wash hands on entering and leaving room; gowns and gloves are not necessary; articles contaminated by secretions must be treated separately and cleaned, as well as disinfected properly.	Children with bacterial meningitis are isolated until 24 hr after start of treatment.
PROTECTIVE ISOLATION		
Immunosuppression therapy, agranulocytosis, certain lymphomas and leukemias	Private room with door closed; gowns and masks worn; gloves used only by persons having direct contact with child.	No special handling of articles taken outside room.
ENTERIC PRECAUTIONS		
Shigellosis, salmonellosis, *Escherichia coli*, gastroenteritis, intestinal parasites, hepatitis	Single room; gowns used when having direct contact with child; gloves worn when handling diapers or bedpans; all persons must wash hands when entering or leaving room.	Children with hepatitis also are on needle and syringe precautions; gloves should be changed whenever contaminated by blood, excreta, or parasites.
DRAINAGE AND SECRETION PRECAUTIONS		
Impetigo, streptococcal skin infection, extensive burns not infected with staphylococcus or group A streptococcus, any extensive wound infection, staphylococcal skin and wound infections	Single room desirable but not necessary; gowns worn by those who have contact with patient; gloves must be worn by those who will have contact with affected areas; masks are worn only during dressing changes.	Care must be taken to dispose of all dressings properly; instruments used must be washed, dried, double-bagged, and labeled "contaminated" before sent to central supply room.

other precautions also are implemented. Table 47-5 identifies the different types of isolation used in pediatrics and the specific precautions that should be taken.

There are some sophisticated methods of isolation, especially at medical centers where children may be **immunosuppressed.** For example, a life island support system may be used, which consists of a bed within a plastic tent. All items that enter the tent are presterilized, the air is filtered, and contact with the child is accomplished through gloved sleeves, which are part of the tent. The system is expensive to construct and maintain, and the lack of human contact may be detrimental to the child. Another type of isolation environment is a positive-pressure laminar air flow room with a filtered air flow unit that constantly removes room air, preventing contamination. The advantage of this unit is that personnel and parents can enter the room to care for or visit with the child after donning sterile gowns, gloves, and masks.

In most hospitals, however, isolation consists of placing the infant or child in a single room and requiring everyone who enters to wear gown, gloves, and mask. The purpose is to prevent the transmission of pathogens from the child to others, although on occasion protective, or reverse, isolation is carried out to protect the child who is immunosuppressed.

The gowns used in an isolation room should be used

once and discarded. When a mask is worn, the nose and mouth *must* be covered. The mask should be changed every 30 minutes, because a moist mask is not effective. A mask should never be lowered to hang around the neck and should not be touched while it is worn in the room. When working with children, the nurse should show her face to them before donning a mask. Disposable, single-use gloves are used in isolation. They should be disposed of properly after use. Gloves that require sterilization and need special handling should not be used.

A second person outside the room should be available to assist with proper disposal of linens or other items removed from isolation. Contamination outside the child's room should be avoided by the following:

1. A linen bag is closed and tied in the isolation room.
2. A second person, outside, prepares another clean linen bag (some institutions use red exterior coverings to identify isolation contents more readily) into which the contaminated bag is placed.
3. The outer bag is tied and labeled before placed in the laundry chute.

This double-bagging procedure is used for all items removed from the child's room. A single break in technique causes contamination.

Thorough hand washing should be a routine practice after contact with any child, and it is imperative when caring for the child who has an infection. When a nurse or other person prepares to leave an isolation room after handwashing, paper barriers should be used to touch any equipment in the room or to open the door; the paper is then discarded.

Impetigo

Impetigo is an infectious disease of the superficial layers of the skin. There are two types: bullous impetigo and nonbullous impetigo. Bullous impetigo is seen in infants, and it is caused by staphylococci. Nonbullous impetigo is more common, and it affects children and young adults. It is caused by coagulase-positive streptococci and staphylococci. Skin cultures identify the organism.

In infants large, flaccid bullae develop on exposed areas. They fill with fluid, collapse, and become crusted. They are found frequently on exposed areas, such as the face, scalp, and extremities. The nonbullous lesions also begin on exposed areas of skin as macules that progress to pustules. They rupture and discharge a purulent fluid that forms straw-colored or brown crusts (Fig. 47-1).

Impetigo is a highly contagious disease that spreads rapidly, especially in warm, humid weather. Spread by direct contact with infected persons, it is seen among children who are victims of poor hygiene, malnutrition, and crowded living conditions. It may be a complication of any skin condition in which there are lesions, such as chickenpox or eczema. When impetigo is properly treated, healing occurs in 1 to 2 weeks.

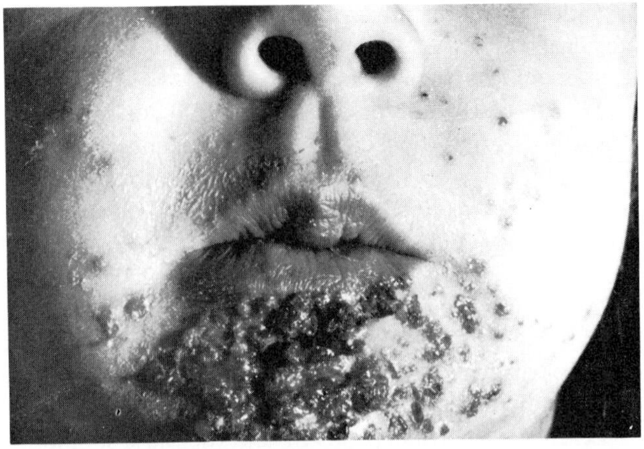

FIG. 47-1 Impetigo contagiosa.

Preventing the spread of impetigo is essential. Oral penicillin G is effective; however, it must be given three to four times a day. If compliance is unlikely, penicillin G benzathine (Bicillin) is given intramuscularly. Severe infections require hospitalization and the administration of intravenous antibiotics.

Skin lesions are cleansed thoroughly with hexachlorophene and Betadine. A physician may prescribe a topical antibacterial ointment. Soaks or compresses with normal saline or other solutions soften the thick crusts, which makes their removal less painful.

These lesions cause pruritus, and efforts should be directed toward decreasing the likelihood of scratching, which intensifies the problem. Nails must be cut short and kept clean. Benadryl may be given as ordered. Because impetigo is contagious, the items used by an infected child should be kept away from other children or family members.

Eczema

Eczema, or atopic dermatitis, is the earliest indication of an allergic response in an infant. It occurs more commonly in winter months and tends to run in families. There are three distinct stages to this skin disorder. In infancy, papules and vesicles form after erythema and pruritus occur. The cheeks are usually affected first and then the forehead, scalp, and flexor surfaces of the extremities. The entire body can be affected. Pruritus is intense, and as the infant scratches, vesicles rupture and a yellow, tenacious exudate covers the raw areas and then dries. When the acute process subsides, the crusts fall off and new epithelium forms. If secondary infections develop, scars can occur.

The childhood stage, which is less inflammatory, can occur during the ages of 3 to 5 years; however, it also can occur after the infantile stage. The childhood stage is characterized by pruritus, dryness, and papules that look like "goose bumps" at hair follicles. With scratching, irritation, and inflammation, there are pigment changes, especially on flexor surfaces, the wrists, knees, and elbows. Remission can occur at any time.

The third stage occurs in adulthood, with continued pigment changes, thickening of the skin, and dryness.

A careful history helps to identify the cause of this allergic response. In children younger than 2 years, foods, such as cow's milk, eggs, wheat cereals, and such fruits as oranges may be the cause. Dust, soaps, and harsh fabrics, such as wool, also may cause eczema. It is important to identify the aggravating factor that results in the scratch-itch-scratch cycle so that it can be avoided, because there is no cure for the problem.

Eczema is a chronic problem, and the cause should be identified as soon as possible. Pruritus must be controlled to avoid skin damage. Observing a child is important as is the administration of specific antipruritic or antihistamine drugs, which include trimeprazine (Temaril), cyproheptadine (Periactin), hydroxyzine hydrochloride (Atarax, Vistaril), and diphenhydramine (Benadryl). The most intense scratching occurs at night. Restraints, short, clean nails, and mitts over the hands can prevent injury to the skin.

Dry skin contributes to the pruritus, and bathing increases dryness. Warm baths followed immediately by the application of an occlusive lubricant or emollient, such as Eucerin, applied to the *wet* skin seals in the moisture. Sometimes wet wraps are applied to severely affected areas after an emollient has been applied to the body. The wraps are changed every 8 hours, and this treatment continues for 24 hours. The nurse should keep the dressings wet at *all* times. The solutions should be at room temperature, and the room itself should be warm to prevent chilling.

Topical steroids are used to control **exacerbation** and reduce inflammation. Systemic antibiotics are given for secondary infections that may develop. There are a variety of treatment protocols, and it is important to adhere to them.

Caring for the fussy, irritable, scratching child with eczema is time consuming for a nurse. The child's needs for love, attention, and methods of expressing his frustrations are greater than those of a normal child. A nurse should don a gown or apron to cuddle and hold the toddler as much as possible. Developmental needs must be met by providing smooth, washable, age-appropriate toys, as well as visual and auditory stimulation. Parents also need to express their feelings about this skin condition. Sometimes they are overwhelmed or discouraged by the required treatments. A nurse should explain the treatments and suggest methods that have been successful. She should write these instructions and give them to a parent. Reviewing what increases the pruritus (such as warm weather, overdressing, and exercise) can result in extended periods of remission.

Acne Vulgaris

Acne vulgaris is a chronic inflammatory disease of the sebaceous glands and hair follicles, which afflicts 80% to 90% of all adolescents in varying degrees. Even the most inconspicuous lesions are perceived by a teenager as noticeable, distressing, and embarrassing.

Acne begins with the hormonal changes at puberty. Androgen levels rise, and sebaceous glands, which have not been as active, secrete increased amounts of sebum and become occluded, resulting in the formation of a comedo, or blackhead. Skin bacteria form pustules. These eruptions last a short time and heal without damage. If the inflammation occurs in the dermis rather than the epidermis, a papule forms and it is more likely to develop into a cyst or abscesslike lesion with scars.

Treatment in females older than 16 years may include estrogens, which suppress sebaceous gland activity. Oral tetracycline also is prescribed. Corticosteroids, such as prednisone, reduce the inflammation. Ultraviolet light results in skin peeling, which provides relief. The role of diet is controversial. Most dermatologists consider cleanliness essential, so washing the face and using a mild astringent are important practices.

The nurse should promote a healthy self-image in the adolescent and provide information to prevent permanent damage to the skin. Teenagers should be cautioned about scrubbing the skin too vigorously, which may damage it. They are instructed not to use ointments, creams, or lotions, because these substances occlude follicles. Adolescents should be discouraged from picking at or squeezing the lesions, because these activities injure skin and cause scarring.

The nurse should reinforce that the teenager keep the face as clean as possible and then use astringents, such as alcohol. If topical ointments or steroids have been prescribed, the nurse should review the instructions with the teenager.

If tetracycline has been ordered, the teenager should be told to take it with water on an empty stomach; milk interferes with its absorption. Because phototoxicity and the inability to concentrate urine are side effects of tetracycline, this information should be shared with the adolescent. Isotretinoin (Accutane) also has been given orally, but it should not be ordered for sexually active females because it can cause birth defects. The nurse should also encourage adolescents to eat nourishing foods from all four food groups.

NURSING DIAGNOSES	NURSING INTERVENTIONS
Pain (pruritus), related to rash	Cut nails short, and keep hands clean. Put mittens (socks) on hands to prevent scratching. Teach older child to apply pressure to pruritic area to relieve sensation.

NURSING DIAGNOSES	NURSING INTERVENTIONS
Pain (pruritus), related to rash–cont'd	Apply topical antipruritics if ordered. Give oral antihistamines as ordered. Bathe child with mild soap and water; pat lesions dry. Use elbow restraints only when necessary. Notify physician of inflammation or infection.
Potential for infection, related to skin impairment	Isolate child from susceptible individuals. Review isolation techniques with parents and others. Identify high-risk children to whom disease may be fatal. Teach parents signs of immunization reactions. Notify school or day care of communicable disease. Review immunization records of all children. Participate in immunization programs.
Pain, related to the disease process	Assess level of discomfort. Devise support mechanism for scrotum if orchiditis is present. Apply petrolatum to excoriated areas around and under nose. Provide warm compresses to encrusted eyes. Use distraction strategies with child. Maintain bed rest. Give Tylenol for fever or discomfort, as ordered. Monitor temperature frequently. Provide bland liquids and solids. Keep lighting dim.
Body image disturbance, related to inflamed skin lesions	Explore adolescent's feelings about himself as a person. Assess his perception of how acne has affected such activities as his social interactions, dating, and school. Identify and encourage activities that enhance his strengths and feelings of self-confidence. Explore his understanding of acne, and review its possible causes and treatments. Listen to his expressed feelings, fears, and concerns. Provide reassurance and emotional support.

DISORDERS OF THE MUSCULOSKELETAL SYSTEM

Many disorders affect the musculoskeletal system. Some are congenital, and others are the result of infections or trauma. Almost all of these disorders affect mobility and skin integrity, and many require long-term treatment. Disorders that involve the skeleton and its associated structures also seem to occur more commonly at specific developmental stages. For example, Duchenne's muscular dystrophy becomes evident in preschoolers, Legg-Calvé-Perthes disease in school-age children, and scoliosis in adolescents.

Nursing Assessment

In assessing the musculoskeletal system, asking the right questions and using observational skills are critical to obtain the information that helps identify the disorder. Collection of *subjective data* includes learning the date the symptoms started and/or when alterations (gait change, for example) were noted, any traumatic incident that preceded those symptoms, and the type of first aid given at the scene. If signs and symptoms have been present for several days, especially joint pain, edema, or erythema, a chronological course of the presenting problem is helpful. Some illnesses, defects, or deformities, such as scoliosis, muscle weakness, and hip dysplasia, also affect family members, so obtaining family history may suggest the presence of one of these disorders in the child.

Although there are developmental differences that should be recognized, collecting *objective data* primarily involves inspection and palpation, as well as using a tape measure to assess symmetry and length of opposing parts. Vital signs should be measured, because, for example, an elevated temperature may confirm the presence of infection. In the course of a physical assessment, the nurse determines range of motion, measures leg lengths, observes a child's gait, and palpates the spinal column and extremities. The injured or affected part should be examined for edema, point of maximum tenderness, voluntary function, and range or limitation of movement.

Diagnostic Tests

A complete blood count, urinalysis, and erythrocyte sedimentation rate (ESR) in the presence of an acute infection are done. Serum enzymes are measured on children with muscle trauma and suspected muscle disease. For example, creatine phosphokinase (CPK) is elevated in the child with muscular dystrophy. X-ray studies are used widely in diagnosing musculoskeletal problems. Bilateral films are taken for comparison. In addition to diagnostic purposes, x-ray studies also enable monitoring the effectiveness of treatment and determining the extent of healing.

Clubfoot

Clubfoot is a condition in which there is a deviation from the normal shape or position of a foot. The cause

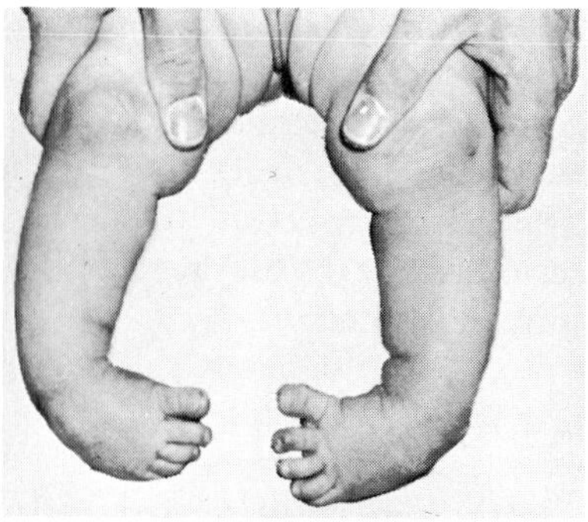

FIG. 47-2 Bilateral congenital talipes equinovarus (congenital clubfoot) in 2-month-old infant.

is unknown, but it is thought to be the result of arrested development during fetal life. When the insult occurs early in utero, *rigid clubfoot* develops. *Flexible clubfoot* is caused by malposition in the uterus and by intrauterine pressures. The flexible deformity occurs later in fetal development and involves joint tissues, not bone. With rigid clubfoot the bony deformity is in a major bone of the foot called the *talus*. The muscles, tendons, nerves, and vessels are not deformed. The most common type of clubfoot is pointed downward and inward. The degree of severity varies. Clubfoot may involve one foot (more common) or both feet (Fig. 47-2). It may occur by itself or in association with other diseases or defects.

Treatment for both rigid and flexible defects begins within the first week of life and involves gentle manipulation of the foot followed by the application of casts, elastic splints, or adhesive strapping. Because the infant grows rapidly, weekly manipulations and cast changes are necessary. Correction is usually achieved by 6 to 8 weeks of age. For the next 3 months the infant wears corrective shoes during the day and passive exercises are performed. At night bivalved casts are used to maintain the foot in a corrected position. If the foot is not corrected after 3 to 4 months, surgery is required to correct the deformity.

Nurses have an important role in detecting clubfoot so that early treatment can be started. Parents need to understand the treatment program for their child. Teaching cast care and skin care and reinforcing the physician's explanations are also nursing responsibilities. Parents may also require assistance in promoting normal development of the infant, who is restricted as a result of the therapy.

Congenital Hip Dysplasia

Congenital hip dysplasia is an abnormality of the hip joint at birth. One or both hips may be affected. The unstable hip can become subluxed or dislocated when manipulated. Subluxation is when the head of the femur rides on the edge of the acetabulum (socket). In dislocation of the hip, the head of the femur is totally outside the acetabulum. Congenital hip dysplasia may be caused by the action of maternal sex hormones, malposition in utero, or environmental factors after birth.

The most reliable test to detect the dislocated hip at birth is **Ortolani's test,** which is performed by a physician or nurse practitioner. A click heard or felt with this maneuver indicates a dislocated hip. The test is less useful after the first month of age. Other signs that indicate congenital hip dislocation include limited abduction of the hip, shortened leg on the affected side when the infant's hips and knees are flexed, and asymmetry of the skin folds of the buttocks, thighs, and knees. If the disorder is not detected early, when the child begins to walk he will have a ducklike waddle or "sailor's gait."

Treatment that starts when the child is younger than 2 months is most successful. The hip is gently manipulated to correct the dislocation. The proper position is maintained by using an abduction splint, such as a Frejka splint or other similar device. The splint is used continuously for approximately 2 to 3 months, followed by night splinting for another month. The hip will usually then develop normally.

If the child is older when the diagnosis of congenital hip dysplasia is made, traction (skin, skeletal, or both) is required. The hips are gradually moved into wide abduction after the head of the femur has been brought into the socket. After about 21 days a closed reduction is done. The hips are immobilized for 4 to 6 months in a hip spica cast or metal splint. Surgery may be required if the closed method of reduction is not successful. Hip development may not be normal if the child is older when treatment is started.

Nurses should be aware of the signs and tests used to detect congenital hip dysplasia. Although the nurse does not usually perform Ortolani's test, it is important for her to observe for other signs, such as asymmetrical creases and limited abduction. Older children should be observed for the ducklike waddle. The nurse should teach parents the purpose of the Frejka splint or any other splint that is used. The nurse should also demonstrate how to handle the child to keep the hips abducted. She should provide information to the parents about bathing, dressing, and diaper changes. It is common for an infant to be picked up by both feet to change a diaper. This should be discouraged for all babies, and must not be done with the infant with congenital hip dysplasia.

The older child with congenital hip dysplasia is in traction and spica casts for a long period. Parents should be informed of this before treatment is started so that they will be better prepared to meet the needs of their child while he is immobilized.

Osteomyelitis

Osteomyelitis is an inflammation of the bone, which usually involves long bones, such as the femur, tibia, humerus, or radius. In the majority of cases, *Staphylococcus aureus* is the cause. The bacteria enter through infections on the skin or through the mucous membranes after nose or throat infections. A fracture or other wound can also be the entry point. Once bacteria have entered, an injured area of bone seems to attract the bacteria. This injured area of bone provides a site for the development of osteomyelitis.

Bone is a rigid, closed space. The edema and inflammation cause pressure within the bone, which results in severe and constant pain. Pus forms and causes such intense pressure that necrosis (death) of the bone occurs. When infection spreads deeper into the bone, pain becomes even more severe. Without treatment, septicemia may occur. Septic arthritis may develop when bacteria invade the capsule surrounding the joint.

The child with osteomyelitis will first complain of pain in the involved area and refuse to move the extremity. Septicemia develops within 24 hours, and the child is febrile, anorexic, and weak. He may be irritable, lose function of the affected limb, and have edema and tenderness in the extremity. Clinical signs are used for early diagnoses. X-ray studies are useful only after bone destruction occurs, which takes several days.

The child must be hospitalized for treatment. Blood cultures are drawn, and intravenous antibiotic therapy is started. The child is made more comfortable with bed rest and analgesics. Splints or traction is used to rest the affected extremity, to decrease pain, to limit movement, which could spread infection, and to prevent contractures in soft tissues.

Surgery may be necessary if the child does not improve within 24 hours. Pus is removed for culture, and bone pressure is relieved. Chronic osteomyelitis may occur if treatment is inadequate.

Nursing management is similar to that for septic arthritis and is discussed under that section.

Septic Arthritis

Acute septic arthritis is an inflammation of a joint caused by pus-forming bacteria. This inflammation can occur in all age groups but most often affects children 1 to 2 years of age. The hip joint is most often affected, with the knee and elbow second. More than one joint can be involved. The source of the infection is usually from another site. Bacteria travel through the blood stream from a distant infection (such as otitis media) and invade the joint. *Staphylococcus* and *Streptococcus* bacteria are the organisms that most commonly cause septic arthritis.

The small child with septic arthritis protects the joint from movement. Tissue edema, warmth, and tenderness, fever, and an increase in white blood cell count are other clinical signs. In the infant, septic arthritis occurs most commonly in the hip.

Immediate treatment is necessary. A needle aspiration of the infected joint is done to obtain fluid for culture. Intravenous antibiotic therapy is started, and the antibiotic may also be instilled into the joint. Surgical treatment (arthrotomy) involves exploring the joint, removing pus, and irrigating the joint.

The nursing responsibilities in the care of the child with osteomyelitis or septic arthritis are similar. The child with osteomyelitis complains of fever and has an edematous and tender extremity. The child with septic arthritis also has an edematous and painful joint, limits movement of the joint, has fever, and is irritable.

The child is admitted to the hospital and placed on bed rest. The nurse may assist in obtaining blood and wound cultures and establishing intravenous access for antibiotic therapy. Analgesics may be given to relieve the child's pain and discomfort. The affected extremity is immobilized by the use of splints, casts, or skin traction. The nurse must assess the circulation of the extremity that is casted or in traction. The nurse monitors vital signs every 4 hours or more frequently if the child is febrile. A closed infusion and drainage system may be used for children with septic arthritis. It is the nurse's responsibility to monitor and record all fluids instilled and drainage output.

It is difficult for the small child to remain immobilized. The nurse should facilitate play and other diversional activities to meet the child's developmental and socialization needs. Parents should be encouraged to participate in the child's care also.

Fractures of the Forearm

Fractures of the forearm are common in childhood. They usually occur when the child attempts to break a fall by extending the palm of a hand or hands. The force of the fall is transmitted to the wrist and forearm, causing fractures in those parts. Fractures may be incomplete (greenstick) or complete (Fig. 47-3).

Greenstick, or incomplete, fractures involve only part of the thickness of a bone. A greenstick fracture in the distal or middle third of the forearm is reduced by closed manipulation, which involves restoring the bone to its normal position without surgery. The arm is then immobilized in a plaster of paris or fiberglass cast.

A **Colles' fracture** involves the distal end of the radius just above the wrist. The child's hand is displaced backward and outward. Fractures of any type are diagnosed by x-ray examination.

The nurse helps with the reduction and immobilization of fractures. The cast usually extends from the axilla to the midpalm. The arm is elevated for 24 to 48 hours. Ice bags may be applied to the forearm to reduce edema. Frequent circulation checks are essential. A sling can be used to support the hand, forearm, and elbow. Parents should be taught how to care for the cast, apply the sling,

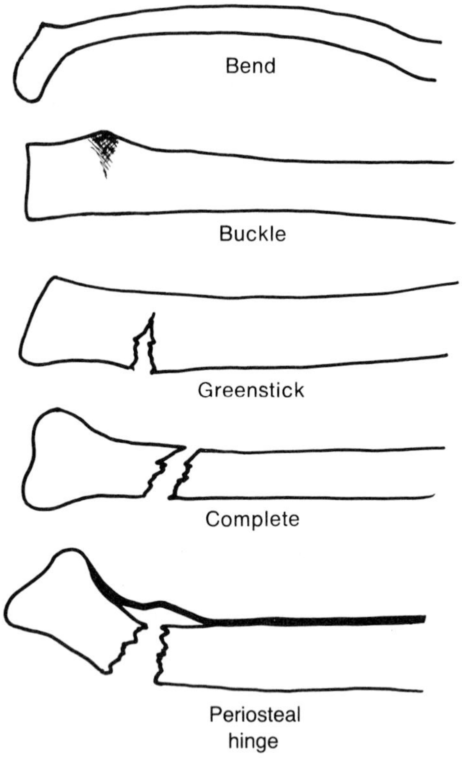

FIG. 47-3 Types of fractures in children.

and check circulation. X-ray studies are done periodically to check bone healing. The cast is removed after several weeks, and the child can then use his arm freely.

Duchenne's Muscular Dystrophy

Duchenne's muscular dystrophy is a genetic disease that results in progressive muscle wasting and weakness. The most common form is found in boys; it is a sex-linked recessive trait. The cause is not known, but a biochemical defect in muscle tissue is suspected.

The child with muscular dystrophy appears normal at birth and during infancy. Muscle weakness does not appear until 3 to 5 years of age. Stumbling, falls, and difficulty climbing stairs are usually the first symptoms noted. As the disease progresses, contractures and deformities develop. The child becomes confined to a wheelchair by 10 to 12 years of age. Scoliosis is extremely common, and vital organs become affected. As muscular dystrophy progresses, the cardiac and respiratory systems become impaired. Death is usually the result of respiratory and cardiac complications. Few boys survive beyond 20 years of age.

Various tests are used to diagnose muscular dystrophy. The CPK enzyme is elevated early in the disease. An electromyogram (EMG) may be done to determine whether abnormal nerves or muscles are the cause of muscle weakness. A muscle biopsy confirms the diagnosis. Treatment of the disease is supportive because there is no cure.

The diagnostic tests involved may be frightening and uncomfortable for the young child. The nurse is responsible for preparing the child and parents for these procedures. All explanations should be given at the child's developmental level. It is comforting to both the child and parents to have a nurse with the child during the tests.

The goal of treatment is to keep the child independent for as long as is possible. Activity is encouraged. Bed rest and inactivity are avoided because they contribute to muscle weakness. Braces may be used to support weak muscles and prevent abnormal postures. Electric wheel chairs are used when muscle weakness no longer allows the child to walk. Other activities of daily living, such as bathing, dressing, and toileting, must be modified according to the child's abilities. Parents require long-term support from nurses and other health care providers. An interdisciplinary approach aids both the child and family in dealing with the physical and psychosocial aspects of this disease. Genetic counseling may be of benefit to parents.

Juvenile Rheumatoid Arthritis

Juvenile rheumatoid arthritis (JRA) is an inflammatory disease of the joints. The cause is unknown but is thought to be caused by either an autoimmune process or a reaction to unknown infectious agents. The disease is characterized by inflammation and edema of the synovial membrane. Scar tissue develops as the disease progresses, and the joint may become contracted. Muscle tissues are affected by both inflammation and joint immobility, thereby contributing to joint contractures.

JRA has three subtypes. Approximately 45% of children with JRA have inflammation of only a few joints *(pauciarticular)*. About 35% have a symmetrical polyarthritis of the small joints of the hand and feet. Most of these children also have inflammation of the larger joints, such as the knees, ankles, and elbows *(polyarticular)*. When other body systems are involved, the disease is called *systemic JRA*.

Symptoms at the beginning of the disease vary. Some children become ill suddenly and others more gradually. Signs of JRA may be confined to the peripheral joints or may appear as a generalized body illness. Edema of a joint may be the first sign observed by a parent. Limited movement of the joint and warmth over the area are present. The child may walk with a limp. If the edema develops suddenly, the child also complains of pain and tenderness.

Systemic disease usually occurs suddenly. The signs and symptoms include fever, rash, discomfort, pallor, liver and spleen enlargement, enlarged lymph nodes, pericarditis, and arthritis in one or more joints. The rash is a salmon-pink, macular one, which appears intermittently on the chest, thighs, axilla, and upper arms.

JRA has a variable course, with children experiencing symptom-free periods and exacerbations. Children may not complain of joint pain but may refuse to move the affected limb or may walk with a limp. Morning stiffness is the child's inability to get out of bed in the morning or after a nap. Fever may occur periodically along with other symptoms. Diagnosis of JRA is made on the basis of the history and clinical signs and symptoms, as well as various laboratory findings. X-ray studies of joint areas and presence of immune complexes in both the blood serum and synovial fluid aid in diagnosis. Rheumatic factor (RF) is present in serum and joint fluid of most persons with rheumatoid arthritis. Antinuclear antibodies are also occasionally present.

JRA is an unpredictable disease and may continue for several years. The nurse should support both the child and parents. Nursing interventions are directed toward relieving the child's pain and discomfort and preventing joint contractures. Pillows are not placed under inflamed joints because they contribute to stiffness and contractures. Warm compresses and hydrotherapy help to improve joint movement. Passive motion of the affected extremities is necessary if the child cannot perform active movement. Splints are used to rest warm, swollen joints and prevent contractures. The nurse should stress to parents and the child that medications must be taken regularly, even when the child feels well. Regular medical follow-up is necessary. Eye examinations four times a year are necessary because loss of vision can occur with JRA.

Legg-Calvé-Perthes Disease

Legg-Calvé-Perthes disease is an aseptic (noninfectious) necrosis of the head of the femur. This disorder occurs in children between the ages of 3 to 11 years, with boys more often affected than girls. There are four stages of the disease. First, blood supply to the femoral epiphysis (growth plate) is interrupted (avascularity); bone stops growing and bone-forming cells die. Next, new blood vessels enter the dead bone and new bone is formed (revascularization); this new bone is not strong, and pathological fractures can occur. In the third phase (healing), new bone is formed and dead bone is removed. The fourth phase (residual deformity) occurs when healing is complete and the shape of the hip joint is fixed. The cause of the disease is unknown, and the disease may persist for years. It resolves itself eventually. The diagnosis is made by x-ray examination.

The child with Legg-Calvé-Perthes disease does not have symptoms until the second phase, when he complains of hip pain, has limited hip joint movement, and walks with a limp. However, damage to the femoral head has already occurred. Treatment consists of bed rest and traction to the affected leg. Then plaster casts are used to hold the leg in an abducted position. This position allows the head of the femur to sit deep in the hip socket. Abduction braces may be used instead of plaster casts. The child is allowed to bear weight in both the casts and braces. Treatment may last 2 to 4 years.

The child is admitted to the hospital for initial treatment. Analgesics may be necessary to relieve pain and discomfort. The nurse should explain to the child and parents the reasons for bed rest, traction, and abduction casts or braces. She should provide diversional activities for the child and assist the parents in developing plans for home care. Because treatment is long-term, nurses should give parents support and encouragement.

Crushing Injuries

Thousands of children sustain crushing injuries every year as a result of farm machinery or household appliances. These injuries cause extensive damage to soft tissues. The extent of the injury is determined by the force of the machinery, the area of the extremity in contact with the machinery, the length of time of exposure, and the force used to disengage the extremity from the machinery. After an injury, edema and bleeding develop. Large hematomas accumulate between the subcutaneous tissue and underlying muscle. The child may also suffer muscle damage and fractures.

Emergency treatment includes cleansing the wound, draining hematomas, suturing lacerations, and dressing the wound. Many children are hospitalized so that the extent of the damage, which may become more severe because of swelling, can be fully assessed. Antibiotics and tetanus antitoxin or toxoid booster are also given. Dressings are usually changed within 24 hours, and the injury is reevaluated. The child remains hospitalized if skin loss, paralysis, or severe swelling is present.

It is important for nurses in the emergency room to obtain a history of the injury, determining the age and type of machine involved, the area of the extremity crushed, the time of exposure, and the actions used to extricate the extremity.

Sterile technique is used to cleanse and dress the wound. Hematomas are drained before applying a pressure dressing, which aids in immobilizing the extremity. The extremity is elevated to decrease edema. The nurse assesses circulation in the extremity every 1 to 2 hours and administers analgesics before dressing changes as needed and to relieve pain and discomfort.

Discharge teaching includes medication instruction, the importance of elevating the extremity, and how to change the dressing. The nurse should stress to the parents the necessity of keeping clinic appointments after discharge. Any limitations on the child's activities should be explained to parents before discharge.

Sports Injuries

Although athletic activities provide exercise that contributes to health and fitness of children and adolescents, the repetitive trauma of training and exposure of growing bones and joints to impact and trauma in contact sports can cause injury to young athletes. Growth is a factor unique to the adolescent athlete, and this factor makes his musculoskeletal system vulnerable to injury, even though the high school or college athlete is more prone to injury than is the younger athlete.

The four types of musculoskeletal injuries sustained by children are (1) growth plate injuries; (2) injuries to the epiphysis (end of the bone); (3) avulsions (pulling away of tendons) at the site of insertion on the bone; and (4) stress fractures caused by excessive or rapid training techniques. The ankle and knee are most prone to develop subsequent problems after growth plate injuries. Limb length loss, angular deformity, or joint incongruity can result from these injuries.

The epiphysis forms part of the joint. Injury to this area can cause pieces to break off and limit joint function. Arthritis can also occur. The elbow, knee, hip, and ankle are most susceptible to this type of injury. Treatment consists of rest or casting the extremity to immobilize it. Surgery may be necessary to remove fragments in the joint.

Avulsion injuries occur in both upper and lower extremities. Overstretching causes the tendons to pull away from the bone insertion sites. Rest and immobilization are used for less severe injuries. Surgery to reattach the tendons may be necessary for severe injuries.

Stress fractures are usually caused by overzealous training activity over too short a period. There is a progressive loss of bony substance at a site. Running activities cause stress fractures of the tibia below the knee, and gymnastic activities can put pressure on the spine. Rest and immobilization are indicated for stress fractures to prevent complete fracture of the bone.

Injury prevention is the main goal of education regarding sports injuries. Children should compete on the basis of their maturational age and not just chronological age. Equipment should be appropriate to the activity the child is engaged in and must fit properly. Helmets and sufficient padding should be used for contact sports, such as football. Immediate attention should be given to any child's complaint of pain or dysfunction, to prevent serious and permanent damage.

Scoliosis

Scoliosis is a lateral curvature of the spine, and in approximately 70% of cases the cause is unknown (idiopathic). Although scoliosis can occur in any age group, adolescent girls are most frequently seen for treatment. The curve progresses as the child grows, and so treatment is started early to prevent its progression.

The Milwaukee brace is the most commonly used brace for the treatment of scoliosis. This device is individually fitted to the child and exerts longitudinal traction and lateral pressure. Time in the brace is gradually lengthened so that the child eventually wears it 23 hours a day. Exercises are done both in and out of the brace. It is adjusted at regular intervals. Once x-ray studies determine that bone has matured, the child is gradually weaned from the brace.

Severe curvatures of the spine may require the use of a Harrington rod or other device to mechanically correct the curvature. These devices are inserted surgically followed by spinal fusion. The child is required to wear a body cast for several months postoperatively.

Conservative treatment is more likely to be successful when scoliosis is detected early. Screening programs in the school-age years (10 to 13 years) have been beneficial in referring children for early diagnosis and treatment.

The child and parents require adjustment to any brace or cast used for treatment. Skin care is important in the cast. The skin should be examined for erythema and tenderness. The cast or brace can be adjusted if skin impairment develop. A smooth-fitting undershirt should be worn under the brace. Clothing over the brace should be loose. Adolescents are self-conscious, and body-image is a major concern. The importance of wearing the brace should be stressed; however, the empathetic nurse also should take the time to listen to the adolescent's concerns.

If surgery is performed, the nurse should do preoperative teaching and preparation with the adolescent. If a Stryker frame is to be used postoperatively, before the surgical procedure the child should be shown this piece of equipment and how it works. Postoperatively the adolescent is encouraged to cough and deep breathe. Incentive spirometry is used hourly. Log-rolling is used to change the child's position if he is in a regular hospital bed. The dressing is observed for any evidence of bleeding or drainage.

NURSING DIAGNOSES	NURSING INTERVENTIONS
Potential altered peripheral tissue perfusion, related to soft tissue swelling and/or constricting cast	Check color, temperature, sensation, and movement of fingers or toes q 30 min for first 8 hours; then q2hr; palpate pulses; check capillary refill.
	Observe for changes in sensory/motor function of affected extremity.
	Check for changes in sensation, tingling, prickling sensations, and muscle spasms.
	Elevate affected extremity after cast application and if edema develops.
	Encircle any drainage on cast, and record time marks are made.
	Observe for discomfort: facial grimaces, increasing irritability, and increased apical and respiratory rates.

NURSING DIAGNOSES	NURSING INTERVENTIONS
Potential altered peripheral tissue perfusion, related to soft tissue swelling and/or constricting cast—cont'd	Give analgesics as ordered, and evaluate child's response. Check cast for tightness by slipping finger under edge. Leave cast exposed to air to speed drying. If increasing discomfort, edema, and other complications occur, prepare child for bivalving/removing cast.
Potential for altered patterns of urinary elimination; potential for constipation, related to immobility	Monitor intake and output. Encourage voiding by providing privacy; use running water to enhance sensation of voiding. Ensure adequate intake by offering juices and other fluids often. Allow child choices in foods and fluids. Establish bowel program to maintain adequate function: ■ Provide foods high in fiber (raw fruits and vegetables). ■ Encourage activity as permitted by cast or traction. ■ Monitor frequency and consistency of stools. ■ Administer stool softener (Colace) if ordered. ■ Provide fracture pan to increase comfort during evacuation.

DISORDERS OF THE NEUROLOGICAL SYSTEM

Disorders that affect the nervous system are caused by birth defects, infections, and trauma, as well as many unknown factors. The residual neurological effects can in some instances impair function and profoundly influence a child's life. If a child's potentials are to be maximized, the presence of deficits must be identified early so that workable, realistic nursing interventions can be instituted.

Nursing Assessment

Although the presence of such birth defects as spina bifida and microcephaly are evident at birth, other disorders are more difficult to detect. For example, a child who is mildly retarded may not be identified as such until he starts school and "fails" kindergarten.

Collection of *subjective data* includes gathering such information as a history of loss of consciousness and seizures, increased irritability, a high fever, behavioral changes, delayed development, and poor school performance. A birth history is important, especially APGAR scores and any problems at delivery or immediately afterward. A family history may reveal seizure disorders, genetic problems, and substance abuse during the pregnancy.

Collection of *objective data* includes not only a complete physical assessment, but a neurological examination. What constitutes that assessment depends on the age of the child. Height, weight, and head circumference are obtained on infants, and their reflexes are tested. Children from 1 month through 6 years should have a Denver Developmental Screening Test. Generally a neurological assessment consists of six categories: cerebral function, cranial nerve intactness, cerebellar function, motor function, sensory integrity, and tendon reflexes.

Cerebral function testing includes asking the child to participate in various behavioral, intellectual, and emotional activities. Because the cerebellum is responsible for balance and coordination, performing activities of daily living assesses its function. Motor function is determined by observing, inspecting, and assessing muscle movement in response to verbal, tactile, and painful stimuli. Sensory integrity is measured by noting the child's response to various tactile stimuli, such as pain, pressure, temperature discrimination, and vibration sense. Deep tendon reflexes and cranial nerve testing complete the examination.

Diagnostic Tests

A complete blood count and urinalysis are ordered routinely, and a lumbar puncture is done, in which spinal fluid is collected for examination. Skull and/or spinal x-ray films are obtained, and a brain scan may be ordered. Because the senses may be affected, vision testing and audiometric studies are done. An electroencephalogram (EEG) provides valuable information to a neurologist, who also may request psychological testing. A ventriculogram and magnetic resonance imaging (MRI) usually complete the neurological workup done on these children.

Narcotic Abstinence Syndrome

A narcotic-addicted mother gives birth to a baby who suffers from **narcotic abstinence syndrome** (NAS). Because almost all narcotics cross the placenta, the newborn is an addict and demonstrates these signs within 24 hours. They include hyperreflexia, hypertonia, a high-pitched cry, tremors, sneezing, and yawning. These babies eat poorly, are mottled, have nasal congestion, and perspire profusely.

The infants receive such medications as tincture of opium, Paregoric, or phenobarbital as part of their withdrawal program. Swaddling also helps to decrease their irritability. An assessment tool, the Neonatal Abstinence Scoring Tool, is used to identify the progress the infant is making in being withdrawn. He is scored every 4 hours until he is free of symptoms and no longer on medication. The time required for some treatment may be as short as 2 weeks or as long as 3 to 4 months. The baby of a heavy user of intravenous drugs has a longer recovery. In addition, these babies are at risk of becoming HIV-positive as a result of the mother's drug use. Universal precautions are always instituted on delivery. The long-range implications are not known. However, research findings of NAS babies seem to indicate learning disorders and behavioral problems. AZT is given to those who are HIV-positive.

Hydrocephaly and Microcephaly

Hydrocephaly and microcephaly are apparent at birth. An abnormal increase in cerebrospinal fluid (CSF) volume within the intracranial cavity causes **hydrocephaly.** As the fluid accumulates, intracranial pressure increases, the scalp becomes thin and shiny, veins dilate, the cerebral cortex becomes thinner, and the cranial suture lines begin to separate (Fig. 47-4). The newborn may vomit and have a shrill, high-pitched cry, and his eyes may bulge in the classic "sunset" sign showing the upper scleras. A shunting procedure can be done to remove excessive cerebrospinal fluid (CSF) in the hydrocephalic newborn.

A head that is smaller than chest circumference is diagnosed as microcephaly. It occurs because (1) the brain is small or (2) the sutures close prematurely. With brain growth arrested, there is no treatment and these infants are profoundly delayed.

The nurse should measure the head circumference daily on these newborns. She should note the size and fullness of the anterior fontanel in the newborn suspected of having hydrocephaly. As the head circumference increases, positioning may be a problem and decubiti can develop. These infants should be turned often, and lamb's wool should be placed under their heads.

After a shunting procedure, the nurse should assess the incisions for signs of infection and should observe the anterior fontanel for fullness or tension. Irritability, vomiting, and a bulging fontanel are signs of increased intracranial pressure, which indicate the shunt is not functioning properly. Generally these infants do well; however, the shunt may need revision as the child grows.

Spina Bifida

Spina bifida is a congenital disorder in which there is a defective closure of the vertebral column. Normally the spinal cord and the cauda equina are protected by bone and the meninges, but on occasion the neural tube fails to fuse in the embryo and results in a variety of congenital defects. There are two types. Spina bifida occulta, which consists of a dimple, a tuft of hair, or a small, fatty mass over the defect, is found on a routine spinal x-ray examination. Spina bifida cystica is much more serious, with a protruding lesion along the vertebral column, which may or may not contain all the contents of the spinal column.

A meningocele is one form of cystica, which contains spinal fluid and meninges within the protruding mass. A much more serious defect is a **meningomyelocele,** because the contents of this mass include spinal fluid, meninges, spinal cord, and/or nerve roots. Both forms of cystica are covered by a thin, transparent layer of skin. Rupture, leakage, or infection of the skin covering the defect can jeopardize the newborn's life. Surgery is done almost immediately. Positioning and protecting the protrusion are critical before the defect is repaired.

A nurse plays an important role in determining whether a meningocele or a meningomyelocele is present. The dribble of urine, the absence of anal sphincter control, and extensive deformities of the feet signify a meningomyelocele. Paralysis, flaccidity, spasticity, or minimal lower extremity involvement may be present.

After surgery the newborn is kept on his abdomen, and the dressing on his back must remain dry and clean. Head circumference is measured daily, because hydrocephaly develops in 70% to 80% of these infants once the deficit has been closed. A bulging anterior fontanel, irritability, vomiting, and a high-pitched cry indicate increased intracranial pressure. Parents become involved in the infant's care as soon as they are emotionally ready to do so. These newborns have many long-term problems,

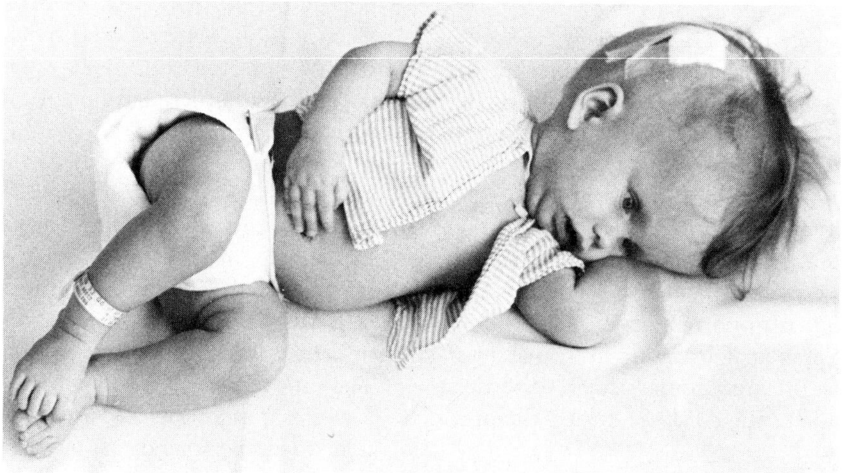

FIG. 47-4 Child with enlarged head caused by hydrocephalus.

BOX 47-1 CLINICAL MANIFESTATIONS IN DOWN'S SYNDROME

PHYSICAL CHARACTERISTICS (MOST FREQUENTLY OBSERVED)

Small rounded skull with a flat occiput

Inner epicanthal folds and oblique palpebral fissures (upward, outward slant of the eyes)

Small nose with a depressed bridge (saddle nose)

Protruding, sometimes fissured, tongue

Hypoplastic mandible (makes tongue appear large)

High-arched palate

Short, thick neck

Hypotonic musculature (protruding abdomen, umbilical hernia)

Hyperflexible and lax joints

Simian line (transverse crease on the palmar side of the hand)

Broad, short, and stubby hands and feet

INTELLIGENCE

Varies from severely retarded to low normal intelligence

Generally within mild to moderate range

SOCIAL DEVELOPMENT

May be 2 to 3 years beyond mental age, especially during early childhood

CONGENITAL ANOMALIES (INCREASED INCIDENCE)

Most common is congenital heart disease

Other defects include:
- Renal agenesis
- Duodenal atresia
- Hirschsprung's disease
- Tracheoesophageal fistula
- Hip subluxation
- Instability of the first and second cervical vertebrae (atlantoaxial instability)

SENSORY PROBLEMS (FREQUENTLY ASSOCIATED)

May include:
- Conductive hearing loss (very common)
- Strabismus
- Myopia
- Nystagmus
- Cataracts
- Conjunctivitis

GROWTH AND SEXUAL DEVELOPMENT

Growth in both height and weight reduced: obesity common

Sexual development delayed, incomplete, or both

Males infertile; females can be fertile

Premature aging common; lowered life expectancy

but an interdisciplinary team approach, access to community resources, and parental understanding of these long-range plans greatly influence and affect their early years.

Down's Syndrome

Down's syndrome, a chromosomal abnormality, has no known cause. However, the majority of cases can be traced to an extra chromosome 21 (group G). Maternal and paternal age increases the risk of this catastrophic condition. Other potential causes include translocation of chromosomes 15 and 21 or 22. Diagnosis of the disease is usually based on clinical manifestations (Box 47-1), but chromosomal studies are conclusive.

Physical problems associated with Down's syndrome include congenital heart malformations, respiratory infections, thyroid dysfunction, and leukemia.

Down's syndrome has no cure, but there are a number of interventions that can be employed, including corrective surgery for serious congenital anomalies, regular medical supervision, evaluation of sight and hearing, thyroid testing, and treatment of such symptoms as neck pain, weakness, and torticollis.

Care of the child with Down's syndrome presents a challenge to nurses. Ongoing support of the parents is critical, given the long-term nature of the disease. Families require extensive support at the time of diagnosis, and the nurse can assist with providing literature about the disease, support groups, home care, or even residential placement of the child.

The nurse should also assist parents in preventing physical problems, stressing good hygiene to prevent skin impairment. Because of poor muscle tone and inadequate drainage and pooling of mucus in the child's nose, parents should be instructed to clear the child's nose before feeding and to use a straight-handled spoon to push food toward the back and side of the mouth. Dietary intake needs special supervision to prevent obesity; calories should be calculated according to height and weight, not chronological age.

Cerebral Palsy (CP)

Cerebral palsy is a nonspecific term that refers to the presence of damaged motor centers of the brain. The damage occurs before, during, or after birth. Some causes include poor fetal growth, oxygen deprivation in utero, birth trauma, or infections after delivery. These children have a variety of neuromuscular disorders which can be moderate to severe and include the following:

- Involuntary movements, such as facial grimacing or mastication
- Spasticity with arching of the back and rigid extension of the extremities
- Seizures
- Abnormal reflexes
- Varying degrees of retardation
- Vision and hearing disorders

This disorder must be identified as early as possible and interventions instituted that can avoid complications. Initially parents need feeding instructions and assistance with methods of positioning and stimulating these infants to promote "normal" development. Later a variety of adaptive eating utensils encourages self-feeding. Braces, walkers, and carts are used for mobility (Fig. 47-5). Some children require orthopedic surgery to improve function. Medications do not help to relieve the spasticity or improve the uncontrollable movements. Such drugs as phenobarbital and phenytoin are effective in controlling seizures. Speech, hearing, and visual problems require attention. Dental care is important, especially when the child is receiving phenytoin. Physical therapy is a major component of treatment because it helps to maximize a child's functional abilities. The major goal is to nurture independence in the child and to foster a positive self-image, which helps him reach his highest level of functioning. Parents need much support and counseling, as well as direction toward community agencies and groups that help them with the long-term care these children require.

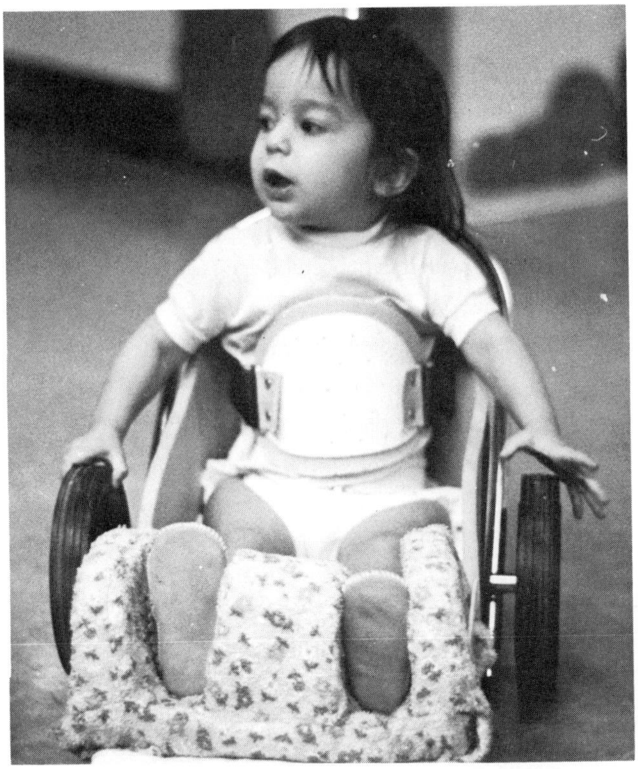

FIG. 47-5 Mobilizing device for a toddler.

Seizures

Any insult to the central nervous system can result in a seizure. The involuntary neuromuscular activity may affect a specific part or the entire body, with a loss of consciousness and loss of bowel and bladder control. The precise cause is unknown, but seizures are the sequelae of such conditions as high fevers (febrile seizures), metabolic disorders, alterations in fluids and electrolytes, brain damage, and infections of the nervous system. Anoxia during a seizure creates additional damage, so the seizure must be treated immediately. Medications help prevent and regulate seizure activity. If a brain tumor or hematoma is discovered, surgical intervention is necessary.

Nursing care is directed toward providing patient safety and documenting observations of seizure activity, as well as administering anticonvulsants, as ordered. Laboratory tests, x-ray studies, and an electroencephalogram confirm the diagnosis. Some drugs used include carbamazepine (Tegretol), phenytoin (Dilantin), and phenobarbital. A nurse should note a child's response to the medication, because the dose calculated, while within safe limits, may cause drowsiness. Although seizure activity should be controlled, the dose should allow the child to remain alert and active. However, as the child grows, the anticonvulsant dosage may not be adequate, and a seizure may occur. Long-term treatment is necessary, so follow-up clinic/physician visits are critical.

Meningitis

Meningitis is an inflammation of the meninges, which is caused by a number of bacterial and viral organisms. The bacterial causes include staphylococci, streptococci, meningococci, and *Haemophilus influenzae,* and the common viruses are coxsackie B, echovirus, mumps, rubella, and herpes. Symptoms of bacterial meningitis include a headache, abnormal reflexes, fever, vomiting, or **nuchal rigidity** (a stiff neck). The conditions of these children deterioriate rapidly. They may have seizures and have altered levels of consciousness. Meningococcal meningitis produces petechiae, and it is a serious infection with a higher mortality than other types of meningitis. The diagnosis is made on the basis of signs and symptoms, a lumbar puncture, and spinal fluid, nasopharyngeal, and blood cultures. Antibiotics are given intravenously, and although they are selected according to the causative organism, ampicillin, penicillin, chloramphenicol, or nafcillin is administered until laboratory results (cultures and sensitivity studies) are available. Fluid, antipyretics, and general comfort measures are instituted for the child, who is isolated for 24 hours after the start of antibiotics. Some children develop neurological sequelae despite aggressive treatment. The symptoms include seizures, hearing and vision impairments, and cognitive, language, perceptual, and behavioral problems.

The signs and symptoms of nonbacterial, or aseptic, meningitis are similar to those of bacterial meningitis except that there also can be nausea, vomiting, or abdominal pain. Many patients are treated with antibiotics until culture results are available. Antibiotics are discontinued then because they are not effective against viruses. This disease is benign, and it runs its course in 5 to 10 days without any residual effects.

Encephalitis

The term *encephalitis* refers to an inflammation of the central nervous system. Although it can be caused by mosquito bites or organisms such as bacteria, most cases are caused by viruses. Encephalitis may be primary, or it may develop after a viral infection, such as measles or varicella. A headache, fever, vomiting, stiff neck, seizures, lethargy, and unconsciousness are some of the clinical signs and symptoms. Signs and symptoms may be minimal or life-threatening. Obtaining a history is important, especially if recent exposure to mosquitos, ticks, or a communicable disease has occurred. A lumbar puncture and laboratory tests are done; however, some results may not be available for several weeks. Treatment is symptomatic, and recovery may be rapid or it may not occur for weeks or months. Permanent residual effects include seizures, neurological deficits, behavioral disorders, and mental retardation.

Vital signs and neurological signs should be monitored, and children with encephalitis should be observed for signs of increasing intracranial pressure. The nurse administers anticonvulsants, and notes responses. When the child regains consciousness, a developmental evaluation should be done. Observing the child during play activities often reveals the presence of neuromuscular dysfunction. Parents need support, counseling, and assistance. The child may have permanent disabilities, and parents must live with and accept the ultimate unknown outcomes, which are anxiety-producing.

Mental Retardation

Mental retardation refers to subnormal intellectual functioning, which is evident at some time during the developmental period. Generally mentally retarded children have intelligence quotients (IQ) below 70 or 75. Young infants and children can be evaluated using a Denver Developmental Screening Test (DDST), and others are assessed using a standardized intelligence test, such as the Stanford-Binet Test. There are four levels of mental delayedness (retardation), based on IQ (Box 47-2).

BOX 47-2 LEVELS OF DELAYEDNESS (RETARDATION)

Mild	IQ 50-70
Moderate	IQ 35-50
Severe	IQ 20-35
Profound	IQ 20 or below

There are many causes of delayedness. In newborns, chromosomal abnormalities such as Down's syndrome, the presence of microcephaly, anoxia, intracranial hemorrhage, or exposure to **cytomegalovirus (CMV)** or rubella in utero may result in delayedness. Social factors, such as maternal deprivation, and nutritional deficiencies also contribute to developmental delays. In children and adolescents, infections such as meningitis or encephalitis, brain tumors, and severe head injuries can result in neurological deficits. The child with a developmental delay, regardless of cause, concurrently has personal, social, and language limitations and impaired gross and fine motor skills, which affect his functioning in society.

Nurses play a major role in identifying children with intellectual impairments. The nurse should know growth and development principles to be able to recognize the cues given by an infant. Most child development experts believe that if an infant has not mastered a developmental milestone 3 months beyond the time expected, the infant should be assessed neurologically. For example, infants sit by 6 months of age. However, a baby who does not do so by 9 months deserves a thorough neurological workup. After a child has recovered from bacterial meningitis and parents state, for example, "He's not acting like himself" or "Those are baby things he's doing," a nurse should be concerned. His parents may be attempting to describe the neurological deficits they observe in their son.

Although a developmental screening test like the DDST is not diagnostic, it does compare the child's performance with that of an average child his chronological age. The 4-year-old child who is discovered to be functioning developmentally at a 2-year-old level is mentally retarded and should be treated at a 2-year-old level if any nursing interventions are to be successful. When a nurse does not acknowledge a child's developmental level and treats him according to his chronological age, the child becomes frustrated because those expectations may be unrealistic. A mentally retarded child desires to please and accommodate; however, requests made should be comparable with his abilities. He should never be set up to fail, which occurs when asked to do something beyond his capabilities.

The diagnosis of mental retardation, or the preferred term **developmental delay,** is devastating to parents who grieve for that "perfect" baby. Recognizing and admitting the presence of a problem may be a turning point in their lives as they develop new skills that enable them to cope and to care for that child. Community health and education services and programs, as well as parent groups, provide practical assistance to these parents and children.

Interventions are directed toward maximizing the potential of a child and the care-giving abilities of a family. Once the child's developmental level has been determined, programs focus on the acquisition of cognitive, language, and motor skills that enable him to function in society. Learning by a neurologically impaired child is in the same sequence as for any child, except that it is at a slower pace. The child should be stimulated frequently and at short intervals to acquire new skills. Goal-directed activities increase the child's self-worth, a positive self-concept, and ultimately independence.

In a hospital setting it is not unusual for a nurse to feel inadequate or insecure when assigned to a child who is delayed. These feelings may contribute to ignoring or isolating him further. If the nurse does an assessment of the child's competencies, selects age-appropriate activities (developmental age, *not* chronological age), and takes the time to understand the child, the hospital experience can be satisfying for both the child and the nurse.

NURSING DIAGNOSES	NURSING INTERVENTIONS
Potential for injury, related to involuntary neuromuscular activity and altered level of consciousness	Remove sharp, hard, potentially dangerous objects from child's immediate environment. Supervise closely when out of bed. Institute seizure precautions: ■ Place child in quiet room, near nurses' station. ■ Pad side rails of crib/bed. ■ Tape airway to head of bed. ■ Check oxygen and suction for readiness for use. ■ Keep emergency equipment at bedside. ■ Place seizure chart at bedside. ■ When seizure begins, note: time of onset; type of activity, length and pattern of seizure; incontinence; level of consciousness; time it ceases. ■ Note and record child's behavior before and after seizure. Monitor vital signs and neurological status q 30-60 min after seizure. Document child's response to medications given.
Grieving, related to the birth of a baby with spina bifida or cerebral palsy	Encourage parents to express feelings about baby. Provide information about treatment plans and long-term management.
Altered parenting, related to the loss of a "perfect" child	Anticipate variety of responses that typify grief: anger, hostility, aggression, and verbal outbursts. Explain normal responses to parents. Allow for time to listen as parents express feelings; be nonjudgmental. Offer support by sitting with them, speaking softly, or remaining silent. Accept their coping mechanisms, while assessing their grieving behaviors. Help parents identify available support systems. Assist parents in identifying routine aspects of caring for newborn. Offer constructive suggestions for holding and feeding baby when they express readiness to do so. Demonstrate behaviors of acceptance by holding baby, establishing eye contact with baby, and comforting him. Support parents when they need to make decisions. Seek out and refer parents to available community resources and parent support groups.

DISORDERS OF THE SENSORY SYSTEM

The sense of smell, or olfaction, is slight in a newborn and develops as the infant grows. Taste, or gustation, is present at birth. Problems with either sense are extremely rare. Therefore the discussion here focuses on the senses of sight and hearing, especially their impairment. Birth defects of the eyes and ears are rare and most of the problems that affect the eyes or ears usually result from trauma or infections. Intrauterine infections, such as rubella or cytomegalovirus, can affect vision and hearing. Hearing and vision impairments influence development and therefore have lifelong implications for the child and his family.

Nursing Assessment

Collection of ***subjective data*** includes an awareness that the presenting problem varies from patient to patient. In the course of a clinic visit a parent may state, "Her eye turns in"; "He's always rubbing his eyes"; or "He doesn't seem to hear me when I call him." Trauma to an eye or an ear is an emergency, and the type of trauma (blunt or sharp), a description of first aid received, and the time of the injury are important. A prenatal history may include exposure to viruses, such as rubella and cytomegalovirus, both of which can affect a developing embryo. A family history may reveal glaucoma or congenital cataracts. Pain, tenderness, and swelling also are common complaints in the presence of eye and ear problems. A history of eye or ear infections, vision and hearing problems, and use of ototoxic drugs to treat other health problems helps to identify a problem. A developmental history is valuable because, for example, communications skills are poor in a hearing-impaired infant. Visual problems can be detected by asking if the child tilts his head when examining a toy, holds objects close to the eyes, covers an eye while reading, or complains of headaches or being unable to see the blackboard at school.

Collection of *objective data* involves inspecting the eyes and noting any exudate. Pupillary reaction and convergence should be checked. Visual acuity should be tested using an age-appropriate chart. The ears should be inspected for placement, and a hearing evaluation should be done. Impedance audiometry and a series of audiometric tests should be completed. With sensory deficits, a Denver Developmental Screening Test should be administered to children younger than 6 years.

Diagnostic Tests

Urinalysis and a complete blood count are done routinely. Cultures of drainage from the eyes, ears, and nose identify the organism present in an infection. X-ray studies of the eye orbit, the sinuses, and the mastoid bone are ordered. A CT scan of the eye orbit also may be performed. When auditory and visual screening tests reveal deficits, the infants and children are referred immediately to audiologists, ophthalmologists, or other medical specialists to identify the specific problem and develop a treatment plan that allows the child to maximize his development.

Otitis Media

The most common ear problem in infants and children is otitis media, an infection of the middle ear. The eustachian tube connects the middle ear with the posterior nasopharynx, and in children under 2 years it is short and forms a relatively straight line. Therefore this age group is particularly prone to developing infections and effusion (a collection of fluid in the middle ear space). Infants with cleft palates and children with Down's syndrome also are more apt to develop otitis media. The disorder can affect one or both ears, and a variety of organisms, such as *Streptococcus pneumoniae, Haemophilus influenzae,* group A beta hemolytic streptococcus, and *Staphylococcus aureus* are common causes. Young children with otitis media have problems sleeping, may be irritable, may tug or rub their ears, and may have high fevers. Signs and symptoms in older children include rhinitis and cough, irritability, loss of hearing, or ear aches. These children receive antibiotics, such as ampicillin or amoxicillin, to eradicate the infectious process. Tylenol is used to relieve discomfort and/or high fevers. If fluid accumulates and remains in the middle ear space, surgery may be necessary. **Tympanostomy tubes,** sometimes called *pressure-equalizer (PE) tubes,* are inserted while the child is under general anesthesia, to drain the fluid. When a child receives antibiotics and his ear pain intensifies, it may be necessary to incise the tympanic membrane to allow the fluid to drain. The procedure is called a *myringotomy.* Children who are prone to several ear infections a year may be placed on an oral antibiotic during the cold months of the year.

A nurse who cares for the child with otitis media should inform parents to anticipate the development of otitis media when the child has a nasopharyngitis. She should emphasize the importance of giving antibiotics as prescribed to maintain blood levels and ensure an adequate course of treatment. Tylenol relieves ear pain, as does a heating pad or a hot water bottle covered by a towel. When a myringotomy has been done or tympanostomy tubes are in place, water should be prevented from entering the middle ear.

The major complication of recurrent otitis media is hearing impairment. Deafness is permanent; however, it can be prevented by effective teaching and adherence to the treatment protocol.

Periorbital Cellulitis

Periorbital cellulitis is a serious inflammatory problem because the infection can affect the eye or the central nervous system. Signs and symptoms include pain, tenderness, and extensive edema of the eyelids, as well as the distinctive magenta discoloration. Some organisms that cause this infection are *Haemophilus influenzae* type B, *Staphylococcus aureus,* and group A beta hemolytic streptococcus. Cultures of the eye and nose identify the specific organism. Intravenous antibiotics are instituted immediately and given aggressively.

The child is admitted as an emergency, with the affected eye closed and very painful. An intravenous line is established, and large doses of antibiotics, such as nafcillin, are started. Four-point restraints may be necessary if the child is young and parents are not present. Administering antibiotics as scheduled is critical. Warm packs to the eye provide relief as do analgesics. As the edema subsides and the eye opens, skin over the previously discolored area becomes dry and peels. A thin layer of petrolatum can be applied to the eyelid and surrounding area. The child usually recovers without complication.

Strabismus

Strabismus is when one or both eyes deviate rather than function as a unit. Eye movement is controlled by the extraocular muscles, and although strabismus is common in early infancy, convergence usually is established by the sixth month as the extraocular muscles strengthen. The affected eye may turn in (esotropia) or turn out (exotropia), or there may be vertical strabismus with the eye above the visual axis (hypertrophic) or below the visual axis (hypotrophic). Amblyopia, or the loss of vision, occurs in the affected eye, and if not corrected by 6 years of age, the visual deficit is permanent. Treatment is lengthy and may include one or more of the following options:

- Eyeglasses may be prescribed.
- The unaffected eye may be occluded with an elastic patch to force use of the deviating eye.
- The child may be taught a series of orthoptic exercises to assist in developing coordinated vision.
- Surgery may be performed, at which time the eye muscles are shortened or lengthened.

The eye care requires office or clinic visits every 4 to 6 months for several years. If glasses are prescribed, young children must be taught how to care for them. The occlusive, elastic bandages must be worn for 6 to 8 weeks and should be replaced if they become loose or are removed. A nurse teaches parents and the child about the specific treatment plan. Their cooperation is critical to preserving vision in the affected eye.

Eye Trauma

Blows to the eyeball by objects such as stones, baseballs, fists, and defective aluminum twist-off caps on soft drink bottles can cause trauma that ranges from pain to severe intraocular damage. A common result of the impact is hemorrhage into the anterior chamber, a condition called **hyphema.** An extensive hemorrhage requires hospitalization because 3 to 5 days after the initial episode, a second, more serious hemorrhage can occur. Long-term follow-up is essential because glaucoma and cataracts develop after such accidents.

Hyphema is painful, and the eyelid is very edematous. Children with this condition are on bed rest and receive ophthalmic topical steroids and dilating medications as frequently as every 2 hours. When the eye patch is removed, the eye should be evaluated in regard to edema and drainage, as well as its overall response to the medications. Patients should be in a quiet, restful environment. It is not unusual to sedate them initially to decrease the risk of a second hemorrhage. Children with this condition may be afraid of losing their vision, so they need support, reassurance, and a nurse's presence. A nurse should provide diversional activities that do not require vision and that are age appropriate. These activities could include word games, story-telling, visits with peers, or listening to the radio.

Ear Trauma

The ear can be damaged by a blow to the head (e.g., bat, ball, or punch), a sharp object placed in the ear, ototoxic drugs, certain viruses (rubella or cytomegalovirus), and sound pollution (e.g., excessive volumes of stereo tape players). Repeated episodes of otitis media also can impair a child's hearing. In *conductive* hearing loss, an obstruction (e.g., cerumen, eraser, or a pea) or a congenital malformation prevents the transmission of sound waves from the outer to the inner ear. Hearing aids are helpful to some children. *Sensorineural* hearing loss is more serious, because it is not treatable and it is permanent. In this disorder sound waves reach the inner ear, but they are not transmitted to the brain. Antibiotics that are known to be ototoxic include streptomycin, gentamicin, kanamycin, amikacin, and tobramycin; the diuretic *furosemide* (Lasix) is ototoxic also. Sound pollution has contributed to significant numbers of children and adolescents developing a hearing loss. Exposure to excessively loud music and noise from recreational activities such as model airplanes and snowmobiles may contribute to hearing loss.

Prevention of hearing loss is most important and children should be taught safety and supervised to avoid precipitating episodes. Dosage of any ototoxic drugs should be computed accurately and the drugs administered properly. A nurse should know whether other drugs taken by the adolescent potentiate the ototoxicity of a medication. Follow-up appointments for screening and audiometric testing are essential. Adolescents should be encouraged to use special muffs or plastic inserts when noise levels are excessive while snowmobiling or working with model airplanes. A hearing loss occurs very gradually and is not always apparent to the adolescent.

NURSING DIAGNOSES	NURSING INTERVENTIONS
Hyperthermia (temperature 39.5° C), related to increased metabolic rate or illness	Monitor temperature hourly when >38.5° C; notify physician. Administer antipyretics q 4 hr for temperature >38.5° C. Monitor and record effectiveness of antipyretic. Remove all clothes except diaper or underpants; open windows to cool environment. Remove all blankets. Give tepid sponge bath; avoid shivering. Provide large amount of fluids.
Sensory/perceptual alteration: visual impairment, related to bilateral eye patches	Inform child verbally when entering or leaving room. Identify self by name on entering room. Arrange to have sighted roommate. Explain all procedures. Allow child to handle any equipment to be used in examination. Maintain child's bed at lowest possible height from floor. Keep siderails up unless someone is with child. Provide opportunities for child to express his feelings. Administer ophthalmic medications as ordered.

NURSING DIAGNOSES	NURSING INTERVENTIONS
Sensory/perceptual alteration: visual impairment, related to bilateral eye patches—cont'd	Assess the edema and drainage from eyes and note response to ophthalmic medications. Refrain from using restraints (resistance can increase intraocular pressure).

DISORDERS OF THE GASTROINTESTINAL SYSTEM

One of the major function of the gastrointestinal (GI) system is to move food through the body. Any alteration in that process, whether it is congenital or mechanical, results in a variety of symptoms that the infant or child demonstrates. Certain problems can be identified on visual examination, such as the presence of a cleft palate or the absence of an anus. Other disorders, however, are internal, somewhere along the alimentary tract, which makes diagnosis more difficult. Other problems that can affect the GI system include parasites or infections, which result in gastroenteritis. Ingestion, digestion, absorption, and elimination occur through a series of complex processes. This section deals with an impairment of one or more of these mechanisms.

Nursing Assessment

Collection of *subjective data* from a child or family is important so that a baseline is established to determine the significance of the symptoms. A variety of systemic disorders can produce alterations in the GI tract.

A prenatal and birth history is especially important for infants. A formula intolerance should be noted, as should any food allergy that results in a GI disturbance. Introducing new solid foods also may result in symptoms. Noting any changes within the family unit (e.g., a newborn or a divorce) is useful because children often demonstrate GI symptoms in response to stress.

Collection of subjective data also includes a history of the present illness, including its onset and duration and any associated clinical manifestations. Significant symptoms may include nausea and vomiting, abdominal pain or cramping, rectal pruritus, anorexia, and weight loss.

Collection of *objective data* includes observation of signs of diarrhea, constipation, bloody stools, and changes in consistency and/or frequency of stools. Relevant objective data also include a child's general appearance, especially evidence of dehydration, such as the absence of tears when crying, sunken eyes, dry mucous membranes, a depressed anterior fontanel, and poor skin turgor. The nurse inspects the abdomen for symmetry, distention, and visible peristaltic waves. She auscultates for bowel sounds or bruits and palpates for tenderness, rigidity, guarding, organomegaly, and masses. Abdominal girth is measured.

Diagnostic Tests

A variety of diagnostic tests may be required for an infant or child who appears to have a GI disorder. The tests commonly include a complete blood count, electrolytes, urinalysis, urine culture, a sweat test, and a stool specimen for culture, blood, ova, and parasites. X-ray studies that the physician may order include flat and upright films of the abdomen, a barium enema, a barium upper GI series, bone age x-rays, and an intravenous pyelogram. The results of these tests may indicate the need for additional diagnostic procedures, such as an organ **biopsy** or an endoscopic examination.

Cleft Lip and/or Cleft Palate

A cleft lip and a cleft palate are deformities that may occur separately or together (Fig. 47-6). The cleft lip results from a failure of the maxillary and median nasal processes to fuse in the embryo, whereas the cleft palate is a failure of both sides of the palate to fuse during the same time. The cause is unknown.

A cleft lip may be a simple notch on one side of the upper lip, or it may be as extensive as total absence of the floor of the nose and upper gum (without tissue or structures below the nose). The cleft palate also may be unilateral or bilateral, and it may involve only the hard palate or the soft palate, or both. There are wide variations. Clefts of the palate result in an opening between the mouth and the nasal cavity, which causes feeding and respiratory problems. The clefts are identified visually at birth during a newborn assessment.

Whereas cleft lips are repaired by 2 or 3 months of age, palate surgery usually is started by 9 or 10 months of age, before speech begins. If a cleft palate is not repaired until later, undesirable speech patterns can develop. Although a cleft palate can be repaired by 12 months of age, revisions sometimes are necessary to correct nasal deformities and to reconstruct the nasopharynx to improve a child's speech. It is usually done at 4 or 5 years, especially in the case of a severe defect.

One or both of these defects creates a number of feeding or respiratory problems, frequent ear infections, impaired speech and tooth formation, and a potential problem in self-image. In the presence of a cleft lip or palate, the newborn cannot maintain a seal around the nipple to suck the formula. Devices that may be helpful are presented in Fig. 47-7.

Precautions against infections are required, because ear and respiratory infections are common, especially with a cleft palate. Feeding a baby in an upright position, not allowing him to lie on his back for extended periods, and placing him in an infant seat are successful methods of decreasing the frequency of ear and respiratory infections.

The infant who has just had a cleft lip repaired returns to the pediatric unit with a Logan's bar, or bow, in place. It is a protective device that is held in place by adhesive

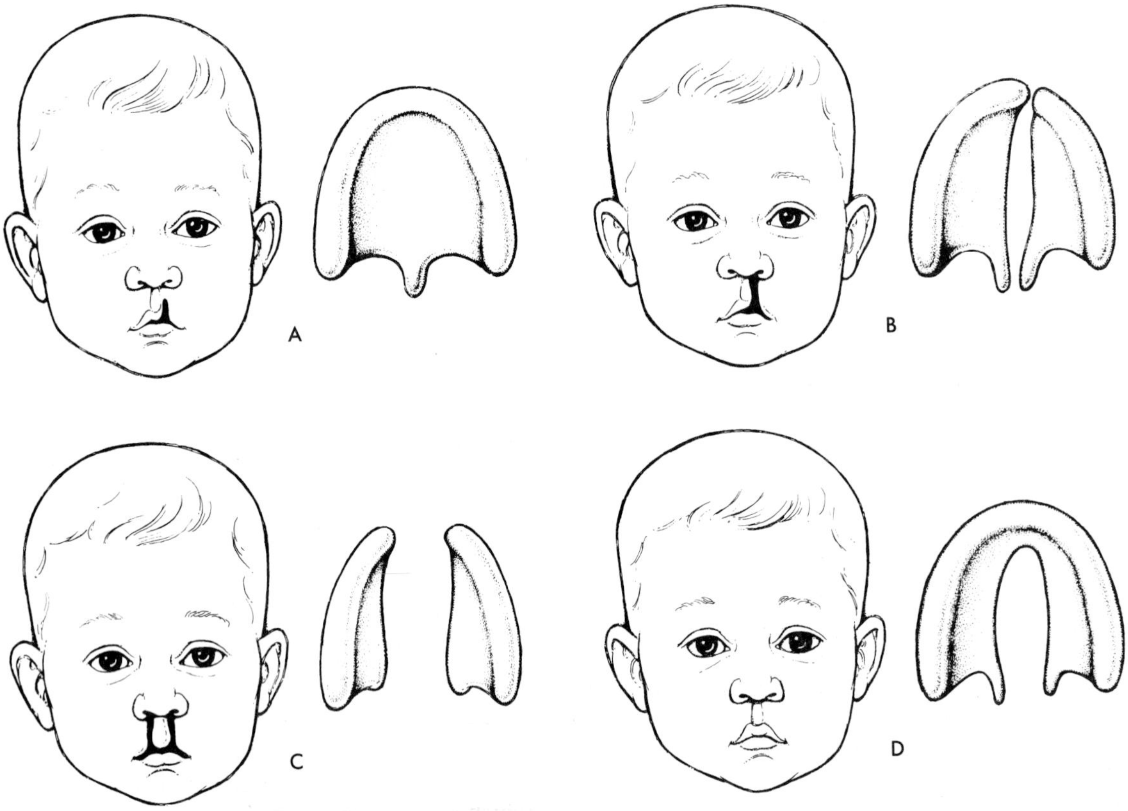

FIG. 47-6 Variations in clefts of the lip and palate at birth. **A,** Notch in vermilion border. **B,** Unilateral cleft lip and palate. **C,** Bilateral cleft lip and palate. **D,** Cleft palate.

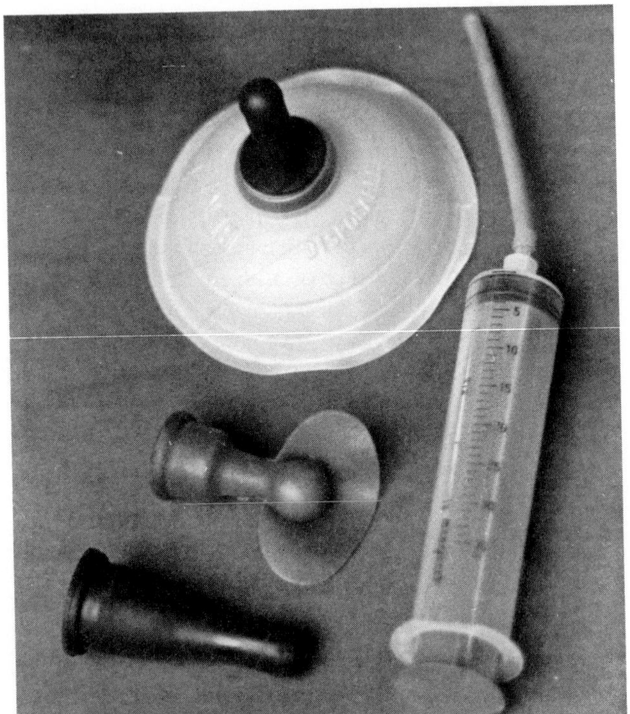

FIG. 47-7 Some devices used to feed an infant with a cleft palate. *Clockwise:* lamb's nipple, flanged nipple, special nurser, and syringe with rubber tubing (Breck feeder).

tape on either side of the repair. It looks like a miniature football face mask. Elbow restraints are applied in the recovery room. These infants are positioned in infant seats or on their sides. They are *never* allowed on their abdomens postoperatively because of the risk of damaging the plastic surgery. Also, these infants should be held if they are fussy; crying or fussing for any length should be prevented when possible to avoid strain on the suture line.

Postoperatively the infant with a cleft lip is fed carefully by dropper or plastic cup. The nurse keeps the suture line clean to prevent crusts from forming or infections from developing. Both events can result in separation of the suture line and damage the repair. Some plastic surgeons order fine mesh gauze to be placed over the suture line. It is kept moist with sterile saline until the sutures are removed. The gauze is removed for feedings and fresh sterile gauze is applied afterward.

The child who has had a cleft palate repaired is placed on his abdomen to facilitate removal of mucus and serosanguineous drainage. A mist tent liquifies secretions and prevents drying of the mucous membranes. The nurse should observe the child for any respiratory distress. Toddlers usually have elbow restraints applied in the recovery room. The nurse should administer analgesics as needed. The nurse uses paper cups to provide liquid nourishment, until sutures are removed. Straws or eating utensils are *never* given to these children because they may injure the suture line. Sterile water after feedings rinses the oral cavity of any debris.

Even after a palate repair, long-term care is essential. Malpositioned teeth require orthodontic follow-up. Speech may be affected and necessitate speech therapy. Frequent bouts of otitis media can affect hearing. A nurse provides information, counseling, and guidance to a family and serves as interdisciplinary team coordinator. Members of many disciplines are involved in working with children who have cleft palates but a nurse usually knows the child and family best as a result of daily contact. Hence it is commonly the nurse who coordinates the activities of the team of specialists who provide care to these infants and children.

Pyloric Stenosis

Pyloric stenosis is a condition in which the pyloric sphincter **hypertrophies.** It is seen most frequently in infants who are 2 to 6 weeks old and the first born. Initially the infant starts to vomit occasionally and then experiences severe, projectile vomiting within 20 to 30 minutes after every feeding. Infants with this disorder suck their fists vigorously. Peristaltic waves moving from left to right across the abdomen are evident. On palpation a surgeon feels the olive-shaped, enlarged pyloric sphincter.

These infants become dehydrated quickly. The anterior fontanel is depressed, the eyes are sunken, skin turgor is poor, and no tears are evident when the infant cries. The depletion of water and electrolytes needs correction, so intravenous therapy is started immediately. A barium swallow reveals the passage of barium through a very tight and narrow pylorus. Corrective surgery is called the *Fredet-Ramstedt* procedure, and it involves an incision into the muscle fibers of the pyloric sphincter, which releases the hypertrophy. Generally recovery is rapid.

Intravenous (IV) fluids should be administered and monitored closely. When feedings are given, a nurse observes the infant for peristaltic waves and projectile vomiting. It is important to note the time, type, character, and amount of the vomitus. Daily weights are done at the same time of day, on the same scale, and without clothes or a diaper. After surgery the nurse should frequently check the patency of the nasogastric tube and the rate of the IV. Once clear fluids are started, very small amounts of glucose water are given. For example, the infant is initially given 10 ml at hourly intervals for 4 hours. The amount is increased to 20 ml every 2 hours, and gradually the volume is increased to the limit ordered by the physician. Formula offered initially is one-fourth strength, then one-half strength, three-fourths strength, and full strength. When feedings are started, it is important to record the infant's response to them, including his weight each day.

Parents are anxious about feeding the baby, because of prior unfavorable feeding experiences. A nurse can be an effective role model by showing them how to feed the baby and by reassuring them that the surgery has been successful. The daily weight gain also verifies the positive outcome.

Hirschsprung's Disease

Hirschsprung's disease, also called *megacolon,* occurs as a result of the absence of parasympathetic nerve ganglion cells in the bowel. The affected part of the bowel cannot transmit coordinated peristaltic waves to pass fecal matter along its length. As a result the colon proximal to the affected part becomes greatly dilated from the fecal mass that accumulates (Fig. 47-8).

Infants with this disorder have bowel movements infrequently. The abdomen is protuberant, muscle wasting is apparent, and the mother describes the child's anorexia and lethargy. The infant's breath and stool have a foul odor. The fecal mass can be palpated.

Barium enemas and abdominal x-ray studies are done before treatment is started. However, a positive diagnosis can be made only with a biopsy. The affected part of the colon is removed, and a temporary colostomy is created, which allows the anastomosis to heal. The colostomy functions for 3 to 6 months.

The nurse should explain all of the procedures to parents. Before surgery the infant receives stool softeners and a clear liquid diet to decrease stool formation. The

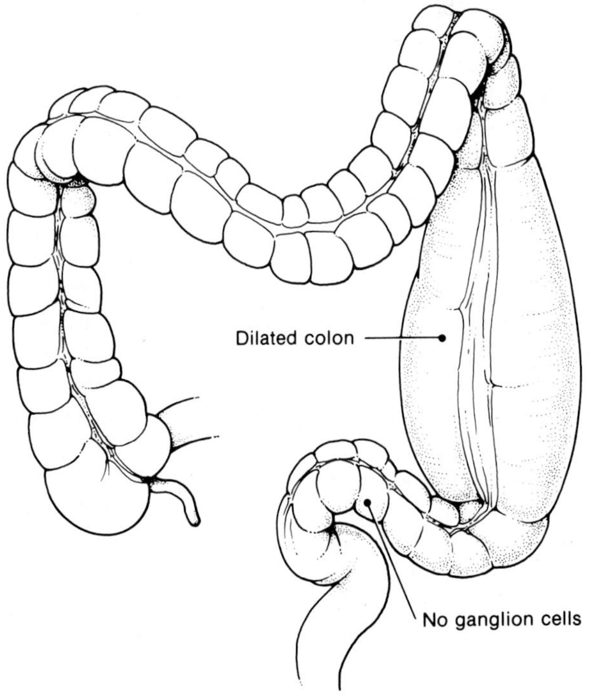

FIG. 47-8 The affected bowel in Hirschsprung's disease.

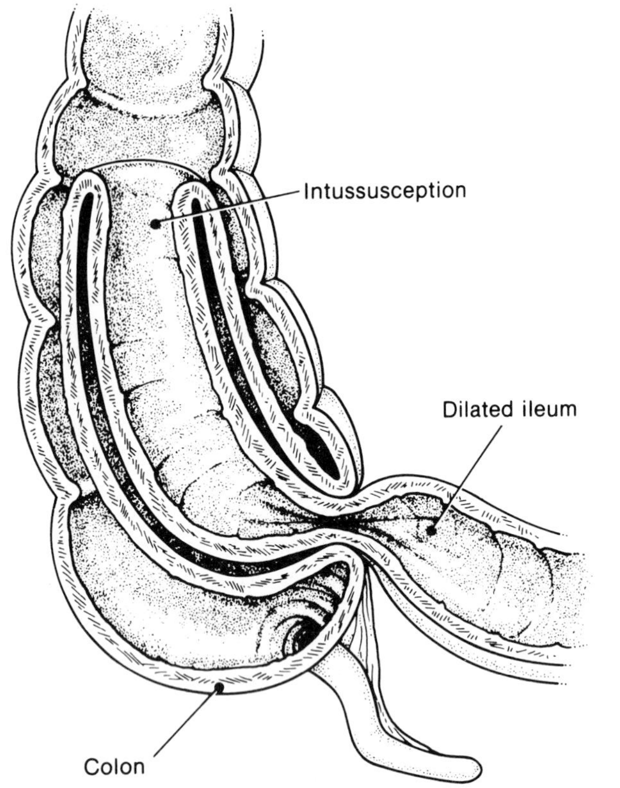

FIG. 47-9 Telescoping bowel in the presence of intussusception.

nurse may need to remove the fecal mass manually or by colonic irrigations. Specific medications ordered by the physician may be added to the irrigation to decrease the number of normal flora. The infant's bowel must be thoroughly cleaned before surgery is done. Postoperatively, colostomy care is similar to that provided to any patient (see Chapter 31). However, an infant's skin is sensitive, and the nurse should use care to preserve its integrity. Immediately after surgery an enterostomal therapist begins teaching parents to care for the colostomy. Intravenous fluids are given for several days after surgery, and a nasogastric tube remains in place until bowel sounds are present. Then clear fluids are started, and the diet is advanced gradually. Liquid stools resume 3 to 4 days after surgery, and as the infant's diet changes, stools assume a normal consistency. The nurse should describe the number, frequency, and character of all stools.

As progress continues and parents master colostomy care, the focus of care encompasses readmission. After several months the infant returns to the hospital for closure of the colostomy. Once the procedure is done, a regular diet is given. When stools are passed normally, the infant is discharged. Generally there are no long-term problems, and toilet training is accomplished without difficulty.

Intussusception

An intussusception occurs when a portion of the small intestine or colon telescopes into a more distal part (Fig. 47-9). It is seen most commonly in infants between 6 and 12 months. The infant suddenly starts to vomit, has a colicky abdominal pain, and passes stools that are like "currant jelly" (reddish-brown with mucus). The infant responds to the pain by crying, becoming pale, and pulling his legs up onto the abdomen. The cause is unknown.

An abdominal x-ray examination confirms the diagnosis. A barium enema may reduce the telescoped part of the bowel by **hydrostatic pressure.** If this procedure is successful, the infant resumes his regular diet and activity, but he should continue to be observed. If intussusception develops again, a surgeon may elect to reduce it manually.

Infants with this disorder should be monitored closely. If a barium enema has been given and the intussusception has been reduced, clear fluids are offered and the diet is gradually advanced as tolerated to a regular diet for age. Once normal stools are passed, the infant is discharged. If, however, the symptoms reappear, surgery may be necessary. The postoperative care is similar to that for any infant with an abdominal wound. The infant has a nasogastric tube for decompression and an intravenous line, which should be monitored at least hourly. The nurse should assess the incision and surrounding tissue. Once bowel sounds are present, clear fluids are started and the infant progresses to a regular diet for age as tolerated. Recovery is rapid, and there are no long-term problems.

Diarrhea and Gastroenteritis

Diarrhea is a disturbance in intestinal motility and absorption. It interferes with water and electrolyte absorption and increases the excretion of intestinal contents. The causes of acute diarrhea vary; however, most are considered infectious (Table 47-6). *Escherichia coli* is an example of a common causative organism. The severity of diarrhea is influenced by the infant's age, health status, and hygiene and the climate. Young children and those who are debilitated are more prone to diarrhea. Warm weather, which promotes bacterial growth, and improper food preparation increase the incidence. If organisms other than normal flora are growing in the intestinal tract, the diagnosis can be confirmed by stool culture. Usually the infant has been irritable and has had a low-grade fever, followed by vomiting, explosive, green, liquid stools, and abdominal distention.

With the sudden change in the frequency and character of stool, there is a rapid loss of fluid, which results in acid-base imbalance and dehydration. A depressed anterior fontanel, rapid, shallow breathing, hollow eyes, and a high fever are some of the signs of dehydration. Treatment is symptomatic and centers on the replacement of lost fluid and electrolytes. Control measures that are al-

Table 47-6 Causes of Diarrhea in Children

Acute Diarrhea	Chronic Diarrhea
OTHERWISE WELL CHILD	**OTHERWISE WELL CHILD**
Antibiotics	Carbohydrate intolerance
Contaminated foodstuffs	Dietary indiscretions
Dietary indiscretions	Irritable colon syndrome
Parasites	Milk protein allergy
Poisons	Parasites
	Polyposis
SICK CHILD	
Enteral	**SICK CHILD (NOT THRIVING)**
Appendicitis	Abetalipoproteinemia
Bacterial gastroenteritis	Acrodermatitis enteropathica
Carbohydrate intolerance	Carbohydrate intolerance
Hirschsprung's disease	Carcinoid tumors
Inflammatory bowel disease	Celiac disease
Milk protein allergy	Chronic pancreatitis
Nonspecific gastroenteritis (viral)	Cystic fibrosis
Necrotizing enterocolitis	Enterokinase deficiency
Pseudomembranous enterocolitis	Exocrine pancreatic hypoplasia
	Familial chloride diarrhea
	Ganglioneuroma
	Hyperthyroidism
	Immune deficiencies
	Inflammatory bowel disease
Parenteral	Lymphangiectasis
Upper respiratory tract infection (otitis media)	Maternal deprivation
Urinary tract infection	Polyposis
	Protein-calorie malnutrition
	Short bowel syndrome
	Stagnant loop syndrome
	Whipple's disease
	Zollinger-Ellison syndrome

ways instituted include isolation with special attention to hand washing. Such measures continue until three consecutive negative stool cultures are obtained.

Gastroenteritis can be viral or nonspecific in origin. Its onset is sudden and includes vomiting, a fever, and then diarrhea. Loose stools cause a distended abdomen, severe, crampy abdominal pain, and increased bowel sounds. The cause is presumed to be viral, and it is not usually identified by stool culture. Gastroenteritis also can be caused by bacteria, such as *Salmonella* or *Shigella* organisms. Food is the most common method of transmission, especially milk, eggs, meat, and shellfish. Contamination can occur also in the course of handling food. Signs and symptoms include nausea, vomiting, abdominal pain, fever, and watery diarrhea, which contains pus and mucus. Confirmation of the presence of *Salmonella* and *Shigella* requires reporting to the local health department. Household contacts should be identified, because carriers are without symptoms but excrete microorganisms for several weeks.

The infant with diarrhea, regardless of cause, requires observation. Fluids and electrolytes are replaced. The nurse should record the infant's responses to intravenous therapy. To rest the bowel, nothing is offered by mouth. Infants with diarrhea are weighed at least once a day and sometimes every 8 hours if the diarrhea is severe. The nurse should weigh the infant's diapers to measure additional water losses. All who enter the infant's room must follow appropriate isolation procedures. The nurse should teach family members how to enter and leave the room correctly. Rectal temperatures are *never* taken on infants who have diarrhea, because this procedure stimulates the anal sphincter to expel additional fluid.

Once the frequency of liquid stools has decreased or a firmer consistency is apparent, clear liquids are given by mouth. An oral electrolyte solution (Pedialyte) may be offered in satisfying amounts. If there is no increase in the number of stools and no return to watery stools, the infant can be advanced to half-strength formula or whole milk. With continued progress, full-strength formula is given. If the child is older, a physician may elect to resume solid foods and a BRAT diet is provided. The letters stand for *bananas* (fresh), *rice* cereal, *applesauce* (canned), and *toast*. These foods are nonirritating to the bowel.

Gradually the stools have firmer consistency and are less frequent. The infant's overall behavior changes dramatically as recovery occurs. He becomes more active, alert, and playful, and his appetite returns.

Failure to Thrive

Failure to thrive refers to an inadequate growth rate, one that is below the fifth percentile on the growth charts of the National Center for Health Statistics. The cause of this condition may be organic or nonorganic in origin. Infants and children who fail to thrive typically are very thin and malnourished, and they appear ill. They may be unclean and dehydrated and have open lesions, especially in the perineal area. Usually a nurse identifies developmental delays in motor activities, socialization, and language.

Organic failure to thrive is the result of the presence of a physical cause, such as cystic fibrosis, congenital heart disease, or malabsorption syndrome. Nonorganic failure to thrive usually has a psychosocial basis, such as an inadequate intake because of the parent's ignorance about nutrition, a disturbance in maternal-child attachment, or poor parenting skills. In essence, there is no physical reason for the infant's failure to gain weight. Nonorganic failure to thrive is seen more often in children from dysfunctional families.

When an infant whose height and weight are below normal standards is admitted for diagnostic workup, tests are done to determine a physical cause first. For example, a **sweat test** is given to rule out cystic fibrosis or a chest x-ray study is done to rule out cardiomegaly. When all physical causes for the problem have been eliminated, attention is directed toward a psychosocial reason for this deficiency.

A primary nurse should be the principal caregiver of a child who fails to thrive, because consistency is important in the development of trust. Daily weights are recorded, and inevitably these children usually gain a substantial amount of weight during the hospitalization.

The child's nutritional intake is monitored closely. The nurse carefully measures and records on a bedside calorie count sheet *all* food and fluid that the child consumes. The nurse should create an environment conducive to eating and should stay with the child and maintain eye contact. If the child has been only bottle fed, solids are started, which will require patience. The nurse should establish time limits for eating: 30 minutes is adequate.

When nonorganic failure to thrive is suspected, the nurse should observe and record interactions between the child and parent and should note how long parents stay, whether they seek out the primary nurse, and how the child responds to them or to other visitors. It may be difficult for the staff to establish a trusting relationship with these parents, but an effective nurse-parent relationship is critical to a successful outcome. The nurse should maintain a nonjudgmental attitude and help the parents feel comfortable and welcome. Also, she should *demonstrate* how to feed a baby, in addition to providing verbal instruction. The nurse can offer parents the opportunity to feed the baby, but only if the parents wish to do so. As parents become more involved, the nurse should praise them for their efforts.

Celiac Disease

Celiac disease is a genetic form of malabsorption syndrome and children with this disorder are usually between 9 and 18 months of age. They cannot tolerate a component of **gluten,** which results in changes in the intestinal mucosa. Ultimately they cannot absorb fats.

These children have diarrhea in the acute stage and often are admitted for failure to thrive. The abdomen is distended and the face is round, yet the extremities are very thin. Children with this disorder are anemic, listless, and anorexic and appear to be malnourished. Stools are bulky, greasy, large, and fetid.

X-ray studies confirm the mucosal changes, and laboratory examination of stools shows a high fat content. Hemoglobin, hematocrit, and serum iron levels are low. The diagnosis is confirmed with a biopsy of the small intestine. Wheat and rye products, which contain gluten, must be eliminated from the child's diet, and a gluten-free diet must be maintained for life.

Because these young children are severely malnourished and anorexic, they need small, frequent feedings. The nurse should observe and record their responses, especially their likes and dislikes. As new foods are introduced, the nurse should note new signs and symptoms that develop, such as abdominal distention or changes in stools. Daily weights reflect the child's progress in his ability to absorb nutrients.

Vitamins, especially vitamins A and D, as well as iron and folate, are administered to improve the child's overall physical status. Because celiac disease is chronic and removing gluten from the diet is imperative, a significant amount of teaching is done. Compliance with food limitations, initially under the supervision of the parents and later with the child assuming the responsibility, is necessary if the intestinal mucosa is to heal and gain its normal ability to absorb fats. Adhering to the dietary protocol and maintaining subsequent clinic or doctor's appointments are essential. The nurse and/or dietician should provide instructions on reading food labels, which is necessary to avoid wheat and rye products. Occasionally, an adolescent rebels against food restrictions and suffers an exacerbation. With the development of diarrhea and possibly other symptoms, the adolescent resumes his gluten-free diet.

Hernias: Inguinal and Umbilical (Fig. 47-10)

An inguinal hernia affects males primarily and occurs when a loop of intestine prolapses through the inguinal ring above the scrotal sac because of muscle weakness. It can be unilateral or bilateral. It is a common disorder in preterm infants. An inguinal hernia is usually evident before 5 years of age. A hydrocele or undescended testes may be present also. Inguinal hernias are usually asymptomatic and are found only in the course of a routine examination. However, a hernia can become strangulated or incarcerated, i.e., a portion of the intestines becomes tightly caught in the hernial sac, restricting blood supply. This condition is serious and usually requires that the child be sedated and placed in Trendelenburg's position and that ice be applied to the scrotum to decrease the edema. In most cases the hernia can be reduced by gently manipulating the trapped intestine. When surgery is done, an overnight hospital stay is usually not necessary.

The nurse should comfort and quiet the child with an incarcerated inguinal hernia so that the surgeon can reduce the incarceration. If surgery is planned, fluids are withheld and explanations are given. Postoperatively the wound is covered by a **collodion** dressing and kept dry. Diapers are left off, even if the child is not toilet-trained. Parents should be instructed not to give tub baths until healing is completed. Usually the collodion peels off at that time. Clear fluids are offered, and a regular diet is resumed when tolerated.

When there is a muscle wall weakness around the umbilicus, an umbilical hernia occurs as a small bulge or larger protrusion. There are no symptoms other than the protrusion, and this hernia rarely incarcerates. As a child uses his abdominal muscles in crawling, walking, and

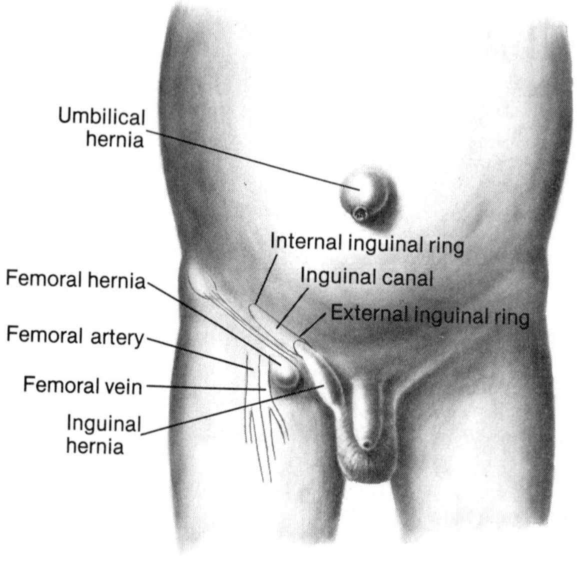

FIG. 47-10 Location of hernias.

running, the defect becomes smaller and eventually disappears. Elective surgery is performed only if the hernia is present beyond 5 years. Abdominal binders as a treatment should be discouraged.

Umbilical hernias that do not resolve are surgically corrected. The child is hospitalized and prepared for the experience. After surgery the child has a pressure dressing over the umbilical area, which should be kept dry and clean. Clear fluids are offered, and diet is progressively increased to regular diet as tolerated. Recovery is extremely rapid, and most children are discharged from the hospital within 48 hours.

Intestinal Parasites

Although a variety of parasites can be found in the intestines, the most common infestation among preschoolers and young schoolagers is pinworm infection. The pinworm, which is 2 to 12 mm long, attaches itself to the mucosa of the cecum or appendix. At night female pinworms crawl outside the body and deposit their eggs on the perianal and perineal skin. Anal pruritus, the most persistent symptom, results in the eggs being carried to the mouth, ingested, and hatched in the duodenum, where the cycle begins again. The original infection begins as a result of fecal contamination of food, soil, water, and hands. The diagnosis is made by placing clear cellulose tape over the anal opening for less than a minute at night or early in the morning and then putting the tape on a glass slide for examination. Pinworms are treated with pyrvinium pamoate, mebendazole, or piperazine citrate.

Parents are usually embarrassed by the presence of pinworms, and a nurse should be nonjudgmental. The nurse reviews with the parents instructions for administering the medication to the child. She should inform parents that if pyrvinium pamoate is given, the stool will be red.

Although the medication will destroy the parasites, other family members also may be infected and will need treatment. A parent can help the child refrain from scratching by washing the anal area frequently and using sprays to decrease pruritus. The nurse should educate the family about good personal hygiene, particularly washing hands before and after toileting and before preparing or eating food. She can also suggest that snug-fitting underpants will decrease contact of hands with the anal area.

Eating Disorders: Anorexia Nervosa and Bulimia

Anorexia nervosa and bulimia are two eating disorders of adolescence that involve self-image and self-control. They are related to stress, anxiety, and maladaptive coping skills of those affected. In anorexia teenage girls preoccupied with the concept of "thin is in" become obsessed about the size of their bodies. To avoid becoming fat they limit their food intake to such an extent that they lose 20% to 40% of body weight. Although thin, they consider themselves fat and refuse to maintain a normal body weight. Factors that play a role in this eating disorder are adolescent-related, including control issues with parents. Typically the anorexic is a high achiever, intelligent, a perfectionist, and a fierce competitor.

Bulimia is typified by eating enormous amounts of food in a relatively short time and then purging with laxatives or by vomiting. The reason for this cyclical binging and vomiting, or purging, is unknown. Individuals with bulimia are of normal weight or slightly heavier before bulemia. They tend to be unsuccessful in dieting and have very little control of eating, and many have been overweight children. Although their eating binges are pleasurable, they often are depressed afterward (Edmands, 1986).

These anorexic girls appear underweight and malnourished. They cannot explain the weight loss and deny any eating problems, which makes it difficult to obtain accurate information. Height and weight are measured. Urinalysis identifies a high ketone level, which is found in malnourished children. A low blood sugar, hemoglobin, hematocrit, and red cell count all indicate the teenager's poor nutritional state. The person with anorexia is bradycardic and hypotensive. The skin is dry.

Treatment for bulimia and/or anorexia focuses on improving dietary intake and providing psychotherapy for the affected adolescents and their families. Treatment usually requires hospitalization and long-term therapy.

In working with teenagers with eating disorders, a nurse must remember the psychological basis of the eating disorders, which results in feelings of inadequacy, ineffectiveness, and distorted body image. While being sensitive, and supportive, a nurse also should establish firm limits in managing the care of an adolescent with anorexia. Consistency is critical. A team approach is used because of the diverse needs of these individuals. The team determines and implements the therapeutic approach and communicates that plan to the adolescent so that expectations are understood. For example, the team may grant TV privileges if the individual gains a designated amount of weight each week.

If the teenager is severely malnourished, intravenous fluids and tube feedings may be started. Hyperalimentation is administered to those who refuse all oral intake. Otherwise, a well-balanced, sodium-limited 1000 to 1200 calorie diet may be ordered. A nurse must be firm at meal times to ensure some consumption of the diet. Observing the individual while she eats is essential; she should be observed also for at least 1 hour after feedings—she may regurgitate all that she has eaten. Calories are increased gradually, until the individual's weight increases by approximately 2 pounds each week. Rewards can be associated with compliance.

Monitoring daily weight is important. The adolescent should be asked to void before being weighed, because drinking large amounts of liquids can misrepresent a weight gain. As weight gain continues, the nurse should offer praise and other positive feedback.

As progress continues, the adolescent with an eating disorder becomes more and more involved in her care. She can begin to plan her own diet and take a more active part in selecting diversionary activities. By doing so, the teenager slowly begins to resume a sense of control.

Psychotherapy is long-term. Poor self-esteem, disturbances in body image, and impaired family interactions are not resolved easily. Once appropriate weight is attained, the person with an eating disorder should focus on identifying her strengths and developing coping skills that demonstrate her readiness for discharge.

Management of adolescents with bulimia is similar to the treatment plan of anorexic teenagers. The binge-vomit cycle serves to reduce the stress they experience. Improving their nutritional status and identifying the causes are critical to positive outcomes.

NURSING DIAGNOSES	NURSING INTERVENTIONS
Altered nutrition: less than body requirements, related to inadequate sucking	Demonstrate feeding techniques to parents. Supervise parent feeding infant. Position on side or place in infant seat (cleft lip). Position on abdomen (cleft palate). Feed in an upright position. Burp frequently. Offer feedings slowly. Rinse mouth with water after feeding. Encourage and praise parents for their efforts in feeding infant.
Fluid volume deficit, related to excessive losses through gastrointestinal tract	Monitor for increasing signs of dehydration. Monitor IV fluids q 1 hr; check site. Restrain if necessary to protect IV

NURSING DIAGNOSES	NURSING INTERVENTIONS
Fluid volume deficit, related to excessive losses through gastrointestinal tract—cont'd	Monitor intake and output; weigh diapers. Perform specific gravity on urine. Note character, amount, and time of vomiting or diarrhea. Assess skin turgor and mucous membranes. Identify presence of associated symptoms, abdominal cramping, and peristaltic waves. Perform daily weights. Assess overall behavior. Promote intestinal rest by food and fluid restrictions.
Knowledge deficit, related to lack of information regarding the cause, treatment, and management of the disorder	Provide parents with information about disease process. Attend conferences with physicians to be able to reiterate or clarify with parents present and future plans. Correct any parental misconceptions. Teach parents skills required in child's care. Provide written instructions for home care. Provide phone numbers to call for questions and lists of community resources for additional assistance.
Impaired skin integrity related to excretions on skin	Change diapers frequently. Wash and dry affected area after soiling. Expose skin to sunlight and/or air. Monitor and record characteristics, amount, and frequency of stools. Instruct parents in managing skin impairment. Assess infant for associated symptoms: abdominal distention and abdominal cramping.

DISORDERS OF THE RESPIRATORY SYSTEM

The main function of the respiratory system is to maintain adequate oxygen and carbon dioxide exchange between the body and the environment. The system is not fully developed at birth, and its structures are prone to malformation. The small lumens of the bronchi and bronchioles occlude easily with small amounts of mucus, which precipitates difficulties in breathing. A variety of microorganisms may be the causative agents in children with pneumonia. An inherited disorder, such as cystic fibrosis, or the response of the body to certain allergens also can result in a host of pulmonary problems.

Signs and symptoms of respiratory disturbances vary greatly in children of various ages. In addition, other problems may affect the lungs. For example, communicable diseases have pulmonary manifestations. Children with neurological impairments may demonstrate respiratory problems, as may children with allergies or other inherited disorders.

Nursing Assessment

The infant or child with a respiratory problem is acutely ill. The severity of the problem is related to several variables. The age of a child is significant, because younger children have less resistance and the size of their airways is much smaller. A child's overall physical status influences his response to a respiratory infection. For example, an anemic, malnourished child is much more susceptible than one who is in good health. The type of organism and the presence of other diseases, such as congenital heart disease or cystic fibrosis, also affect the severity of the respiratory disorder.

Collection of *subjective data* includes a description of the cough, respiratory difficulty, or congestion with its onset, frequency, duration, and progress. Associated signs and symptoms, such as flaring nares, cough, cyanosis, vomiting, decreased fluid intake, wheezes, hoarseness, sore throat, fever, and an increased respiratory rate, may be present. A history of frequent respiratory problems and hospitalization, a family history of allergies, or other cardiorespiratory disorders are all significant. A GI system history is pertinent also because some of the associated symptoms a child may have, such as frequent, bulky, fetid stools or the failure to gain weight may suggest a respiratory disease such as cystic fibrosis.

Collection of *objective data* includes the nurse assessing the child's general appearance and his respiratory status. The respiratory rate, depth, and rhythm, as well as the presence or absence of retractions (e.g., intercostal or substernal), reflect the severity of the disorder. The lungs are percussed for resonance and dullness, and auscultation may reveal abnormal breath sounds, such as rales, rhonchi, and wheezing, as well as prolonged inspiration or expiration.

Diagnostic Tests

A complete blood count is usually necessary, as is a chest x-ray examination. Throat cultures are also done to determine the source of any respiratory infection. If cystic fibrosis is suspected, a sweat test may be done and stools are examined for fat content.

A battery of pulmonary function tests are performed at a later date. These tests are important in evaluating changes in the lungs or determining the effectiveness of treatment protocols in the long-term follow-up of children with asthma or cystic fibrosis. They include functional residual capacity, tidal volume, vital capacity, and total lung capacity. Pulmonary function studies provide a physician with information about trapped air, airway obstruction, and ventilation.

Respiratory Distress Syndrome

Respiratory distress syndrome (RDS), found primarily in preterm infants, is caused by deficiency in *surfactant,* a protein complex that lines the alveoli. Normally when a baby takes its first breaths, high distending pressures allow the alveoli to snap open. Surfactant enables the alveoli to remain open because it acts like a detergent, reducing the surface tension of fluids that line the alveoli. Babies born prematurely with immature lungs do not have adequate amounts of surfactant. Therefore each subsequent breath is as difficult as the first because the alveoli continually collapse. RDS accounts for about 25,000 neonatal deaths each year.

Symptoms appear hours after birth. The respiratory rate exceeds 80 to 100 breaths per minute, and retractions, nasal flaring, grunty respirations, and cyanosis are present. Metabolic and respiratory acidosis develop as CO_2 accumulates. Treatment is supportive and consists of providing oxygen, correcting acidosis, and maintaining an appropriate ambient temperature to conserve the infant's use of oxygen.

Two new treatments are available in medical centers. The first is the administration of surfactant, which is obtained from amniotic fluid. The second is extracorporeal membrane oxygenation (ECMO), which shunts blood from the right atrium through a modified heart-lung machine and back into the infant's general circulation. In by-passing the lungs, blood continues to be oxygenated and the lungs can rest.

These newborns are critically ill. They are given humidified oxygen, and its levels must be monitored closely. If the infant cannot maintain acceptable oxygen saturation levels, he may need mechanical ventilation. Oral fluids are not offered. Intravenous fluids are initiated, and the infant's appropriate body temperature is maintained. The nurse must monitor the infant constantly.

The nurse does a pulmonary assessment hourly, and chest physical therapy, especially percussion, may be needed as often as every 2 hours. The nurse must keep the newborn's airway patent, suctioning him as often as his ever-changing status requires.

It is a stressful time for parents, who need support and explanations. They are frightened by the fragile status of their baby, especially when he is surrounded by complex equipment. The length of time for recovery varies. Whereas one baby may improve in a week, another may be ill for several weeks.

Bronchopulmonary dysplasia is a chronic respiratory problem that can follow RDS. If it is mild, the infant may be weaned from oxygen dependence in a few weeks. Those who have a severe form of this disorder may require oxygen at home for many months. Parents need support because of the chronic nature of the illness. The nurse should provide them specific instructions regarding nasal cannula care, monitors, chest physical therapy, and suctioning. Most infants are on diets appropriate for their age and require oxygen therapy at home. Parents should care for the infant in the hospital so that they can acquire the skills needed after discharge.

Sudden Infant Death Syndrome

Sudden infant death syndrome (SIDS), also known as *crib death,* is the most common cause of death in the first year of life. Its peak incidence is at 2 to 4 months, but it is rarely seen before 3 weeks or after 8 months of age. It is defined as "the sudden, unexpected and unexplained death of an apparently healthy infant" (Friedman, 1981).

An apparently healthy infant is put to bed and later is found dead. Its cause remains unknown; autopsy results reveal pulmonary edema and intrathoracic hemorrhages. There is no known way to prevent SIDS. Treatment lies in supporting parents and siblings who are grieving. Individuals who come in contact with the family after the infant's death—policemen, firemen, paramedics, physicians, and nurses—must show sensitivity and compassion. Someone knowledgeable about SIDS and skilled in helping families deal with grief should provide information, the autopsy findings, and counseling as soon as possible.

Bronchiolitis

Bronchiolitis develops after an infectious process affects the lungs. Widespread inflammation of the bronchiole mucosa with an increase in the production of exudate and mucus obstructs the infant's small airways. The respiratory syncytial virus (RSV) is the most common organism that causes the overdistention of lungs, dyspnea, cyanosis, and exhaustion. It is seen most commonly in the winter and spring, particularly in young infants.

Respirations exceed 60 to 80 per minute, and although they are labored, they are also very shallow. The infant has a hacking cough, eats and sleeps poorly, is irritable, and may be cyanotic. If RSV is identified, theophylline is given to prevent apnea.

If the cause is viral, antibiotics are not prescribed. The treatment is symptomatic. If the infant is cyanotic, a mist tent with humidity and oxygen liquifies secretions and decreases edema. These infants are kept in semi-Fowler's position to increase chest expansion. If tachypnea is present, intravenous fluids may be given. The acute phase lasts 3 to 5 days after a cough appears, and the infant begins to improve quickly.

Croup

Croup is a term applied to several pulmonary conditions characterized by a "barking," "brassy," inspiratory stridor, hoarseness, and various other signs of respiratory distress. In younger children the signs and symptoms are more severe. Edema of the glottis and larynx may spread to the trachea and bronchi as the infection moves downward.

A virus is the cause of croup in those from 3 months to 3 years of age, while a bacterial organism is usually the cause of croup in 3- to 7-year-olds. The older age group also seems more prone to the development of epiglottitis, an infectious form of croup caused by *Haemophilus influenzae* type B. It is a severe, rapidly progressive type: a 6-year-old may be asymptomatic and 3 to 5 hours later experience total airway obstruction.

Typically a child with croup may have a respiratory infection, which progresses to a sore throat, a cough, and croup. Hoarseness, inspiratory stridor, retractions, dyspnea, and restlessness occur. The body temperature may be normal, or it may reach 40° C. It lasts for several days, and then the infant or child improves.

However, the child with epiglottitis is acutely ill. Efforts are directed toward maintaining a patent airway. Often an endotracheal tube or a tracheotomy is necessary. Intravenous antibiotics also are ordered.

An infant or child with bronchiolitis or croup needs high humidity. He also needs oxygen if cyanosis is present or pulse oximeter levels are <95. Placed in mist tents, infants should be kept quiet with minimal disturbances, so nursing activities must be organized. Infants with severe respiratory distress may be given intravenous fluids and kept NPO. The nurse should assess their status for signs of improvement or deterioration.

The nurse should constantly observe the child with epiglottitis, because intubation may be necessary. Antibiotics are given intravenously. Sedatives are contraindicated because increasing restlessness is a criterion for a tracheotomy. Other signs and symptoms are treated as they appear. The nurse must record and report the degree of hoarseness, type and severity of retractions, the degree of respiratory difficulty, and the development of new signs and symptoms. If intubation is necessary, explanations must be provided to the child and the parents. Frequent reassurance by a nurse helps keep the child calm and quiet. This can be accomplished by her tone of voice, touch, and presence.

Asthma

Asthma is the most common cause of chronic disease in children younger than 17 years. Allergens responsible include inhalants, such as house dust, pollen, and mold spores, and the saliva and **dander** of dogs, cats, or other animals. Certain foods, such as egg whites, chocolate, and wheat, and strong odors, such as paint or smoke, can precipitate an asthmatic attack. A dramatic change in the seasons and vigorous exercise also cause bronchospasm.

An asthmatic attack, which may be of gradual or abrupt onset, consists of bronchospasm, mucosal edema, and increased secretions of tenacious mucus. The child experiences a tightness in his chest, uses accessory respiratory muscles, and may start paroxysmal coughing. Wheezing is audible, rales can be heard in the lung fields, and expirations become prolonged. As the spasm continues, dyspnea, retractions, cyanosis, and air hunger develop.

A medical diagnosis is made by chest x-ray examination, and examinations of peripheral blood (eosinophilia) and sputum, which contains bronchial casts and may contain bacteria and pus if a respiratory infection is present. Other diagnostic procedures include skin tests and pulmonary function tests.

Over time, if asthmatic episodes occur frequently, chronic emphysema, a "barrel chest," and decreasing pulmonary function occur. Treatment consists of avoiding allergens that trigger a bronchospasm, managing an acute attack, and long-term management.

In severe attacks, aminophylline is added to the IV solution to relax smooth muscle of the respiratory tract. Nebulizers with Isuprel, Bronkosol, or cromolyn sodium are given and followed by chest physical therapy. Oxygen is administered to maintain levels greater than 95%. An inhaler such as terbutaline sulfate may be used.

A nurse must observe these children closely. Their IV lines and their responses to medications or treatments must be monitored and pertinent data recorded. When aminophylline is infused, dysrhythmia may develop, so theophylline blood levels are evaluated frequently to ensure that therapeutic levels are maintained.

Positioning is an important intervention. High-Fowler's position maximizes pulmonary excursion. The nurse must auscultate breath sounds hourly to detect improvement or deterioration. These children are anxious, diaphoretic, and poorly oxygenated. The nurse must provide explanations, reassurance, and consolation.

When a child does not respond to therapy, he may be in *status asthmaticus,* which can be a life-threatening crisis in which respiratory failure can occur. All methods of treatment are intensified because these children are in great distress. The frequency of nebulizer treatments and chest physical therapy is increased to every 1 to 2 hours, aminophylline is given in an intravenous **bolus** added directly to the intravenous, and corticosteroids are prescribed. Assisted ventilation may be necessary.

The home should be assessed for a cause. Items such as curtains, wool rugs, or blankets may need to be replaced by synthetic fibers or plastic material. It may be necessary to find a new home for a pet, and foods that trigger a bronchospasm must be eliminated from the diet.

Initially the nurse provides a significant amount of information to the child and family about asthma and its treatment. Extensive explanations about the medications are required, and the nurse may need to review the information with the patient and family during subsequent hospitalizations. Breathing exercises should be taught to children with asthma when they can understand. As new products become available, more instruction is required. Compliance results in fewer visits to an emergency room, fewer hospitalizations, and less time lost from school. Asthma is a chronic problem that requires a child to assume more responsibility for his health, for adhering to medication protocols, and it is hoped for experiencing childhood and adolescence as normally as possible.

Cystic Fibrosis

Cystic fibrosis is a hereditary disease of the **exocrine** glands. It is one of the most common, serious childhood diseases in this country. Thick, tenacious excretions obstruct pancreatic ducts and bronchi. First the bronchioles are occluded and then the bronchi. Chronic lung disease develops, and it is followed by emphysema, which occurs from the obstructive overinflation.

Its signs and symptoms begin weeks, months, or years after birth. A dry, nonproductive cough develops. There are frequent respiratory infections, sometimes with severe respiratory distress. Alveoli are overaerated, and this results in a barrel-shaped chest. Eventually there is clubbing of fingers and toes.

More than 80% of children with cystic fibrosis have pancreatic involvement. It may be demonstrated early as a meconium ileus in the newborn. In spite of an excellent appetite, the child appears undernourished. His abdomen is distended, and stools are large, bulky, fetid, and have a high fat content. Trypsin is absent in about 80% of those affected.

A sweat test is done, and it confirms this diagnosis. A sweat chloride above 60 mEq/liter is diagnostic. The sweat sodium values are about 10 mEq/liter higher than the chloride results. X-ray studies reveal chronic lung disease and emphysema. Pulmonary function tests show increased airway resistance and residual lung volume and decreases in tidal volume and total lung capacity.

Intravenous antibiotics used to treat the infections are selected according to the organisms that are present, so cultures are done on sputum, as well as of the nasopharynx. Some drugs used are gentamicin, tobramycin, ticarcillin, and carbenicillin. Chest physical therapy is essential, and parents and others are taught its principles. When oxygen is necessary, levels should be monitored. A variety of nebulizer treatments also are required, in addition to expectorants and bronchodilators.

The pancreatic deficiencies must be treated also. These children require high-calorie, high-protein, and high-carbohydrate diets. Water-miscible vitamins are given in twice the usual doses. If there is liver involvement, vitamin K may be ordered. Pancreatic enzymes are given with *all* meals and snacks to produce more normal stools and increase the child's ability to absorb nutrients. In hot weather sweating is hazardous to these children, and they are encouraged to use table salt on their foods.

Preserving pulmonary function is critical, and so these children are taught to do breathing exercises, which usually follow chest physical therapy. Various exercise programs also can be effective in improving a child's pulmonary capacity. Children with cystic fibrosis are encouraged to participate in sports, especially swimming.

The life expectancy of a child with cystic fibrosis has improved dramatically with more aggressive treatment, the availability of new antibiotics, and an interdisciplinary approach to providing care. About 97% of males with cystic fibrosis are sterile, because of abnormal development of the vas deferens, epididymis, and seminal vesicles. Although fertility is decreased in females with cystic fibrosis, some have become pregnant and delivered full-term infants.

Cystic fibrosis remains a progressive, devastating disease, which results in death. While a nurse teaches the child and family about the disease, the medications, and the treatments required, she should emphasize the need for complying with follow-up visits: Pulmonary changes must be recognized early. Finally, because of the repeated hospitalizations and progressive deterioration, the nurse must be honest, supportive, and understanding.

NURSING DIAGNOSES	NURSING INTERVENTIONS
Ineffective airway clearance, related to excessive mucus secretions	Assess respiratory status for signs of adequate gas exchange. Note respiratory rate, quality, and depth. Administer bronchodilators and note child's response. Evaluate and document effectiveness of treatments in reducing respiratory distress. Assess breath sounds for quality, quantity, diminishing exchange, crackles, and expiratory wheezing. Determine degree of distress, tachypnea, dyspnea, nasal flaring, retractions, cyanosis, and changes in behavior. Monitor oxygen saturation levels with pulse oximeter; observe color of nail beds and mucous membranes. Administer antibiotics as ordered. Administer humidified oxygen. Obtain respiratory secretions for culture. Position in semi-Fowler's position. Perform chest physical therapy; auscultate breath sounds before and after. Ensure adequate hydration to liquify secretions. Administer nebulizer treatments as ordered. Promote lung expansion with deep breathing exercises and incentive spirometry.
Knowledge deficit, related to the disease, methods of treatment, and long-term management in the presence of a chronic disease	Provide explanations about respiratory tract and how disease affects its structures. Review dose, actions, side effects, and toxic signs and symptoms of medications given. Evaluate child's and family's understanding of what has been taught.

NURSING DIAGNOSES	NURSING INTERVENTIONS
Knowledge deficit, related to the disease, methods of treatment, and long-term management in the presence of a chronic disease—cont'd	Review environmental factors that cause an exacerbation, such as smoke and other allergens. Teach child signs of impending bronchospasm and what he should do immediately. Explore child's feelings about disease and care required. Allow parents time to verbalize concerns and fears. Instruct parents in technical skills, such as chest physical therapy and postural drainage. Provide instructions regarding maintenance of equipment that will be used at home. Arrange follow-up visits. Refer family to community resources, such as American Lung Association or Cystic Fibrosis Association, for participation in support groups. Furnish written instructions regarding medication schedule and treatment protocols. Make arrangements for genetic counseling. Assess child for disturbances in body image that result from progresssive illness and repeated hospitalizations. Provide emotional support to child and family through all aspects of care.

DISORDERS OF THE CARDIOVASCULAR SYSTEM

Most cardiac disorders in children are congenital, and their cause is unknown. Some conditions, such as carditis or valvular stenosis, occur when a child has rheumatic fever. These disorders are called *acquired cardiac disorders,* and they are the result of an infectious process. The presence of a child's heart problem and potential sequelae (e.g., impaired functioning) create anxiety in a family. However, many cardiac problems minimally restrict a child's activity.

Nursing Assessment

Collection of *subjective data* includes an awareness that although a newborn with severe congenital heart disease demonstrates a variety of signs and symptoms almost immediately, many disorders go unnoticed for a time. A family history may reveal the presence of heart disease, and a history of exposure to rubella, **coxsackievirus,** or **cytomegalovirus (CMV)** during pregnancy is significant, because of their association with congenital heart disease. Complaints of a poor weight gain, frequent respiratory infections, breathing difficulties during feeding, and exercise intolerance in an older child, as well as the presence of a "strep" throat, are typical concerns verbalized in an initial visit. Additional subjective data include reports of profuse perspiration, a congested cough, rapid respirations, and duskiness or cyanosis on exertion. Some associated symptoms include vertigo, syncope, and distended neck veins, and some parents describe the squatting behavior of their toddler.

Collection of *objective data* includes measuring vital signs, as well as height and weight, which are plotted on a growth chart. A blood pressure is measured on all four extremities. Assessing the child's skin is important too, especially to note the presence and degree of cyanosis. The mucous membranes of a dark-skinned child should be examined, because the membranes have a purple hue when cyanosis is present. The nurse should palpate bilaterally all pulses (radial, brachial, femoral, popliteal, and dorsal pedal) for rate, rhythm, and symmetry. She should also determine capillary refill, and fingertips and toes should be examined for any evidence of clubbing. To complete the collection of objective data, the abdomen is palpated for hepatomegaly, which is present in congestive heart failure. The heart is auscultated for rhythm and murmurs, and the lungs are evaluated for rales and wheezing. In the presence of cyanotic heart disease, a neurological assessment should be done.

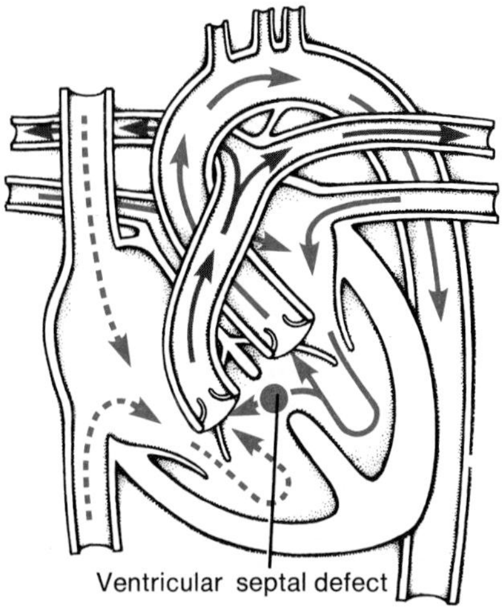

FIG. 47-11 Ventricular septal defect.

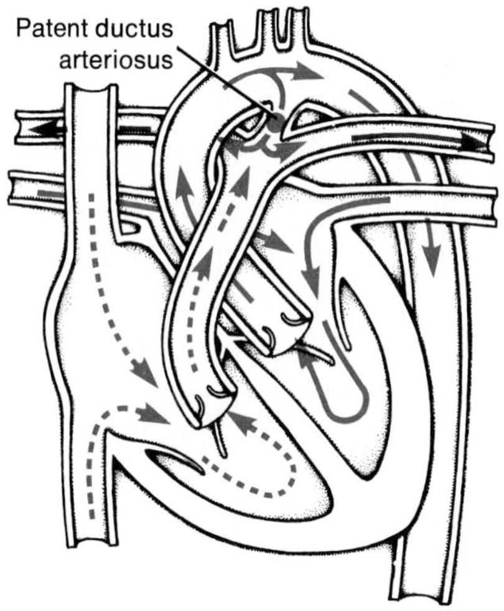

FIG. 47-12 Patent ductus arteriosus (PDA).

Diagnostic Tests

A complete blood count, blood chemistries, blood gases, urinalysis, urine culture, hemoglobin, and hematocrit are done routinely. Antistreptolysin-O titer is drawn if a streptococcal infection is suspected. However, none of these tests diagnose the disorder; they confirm the consequences of heart disease. The presence of a congenital heart is confirmed using an electrocardiogram, echocardiogram, and x-ray studies, as well as a cardiac catheterization. The results of all of these procedures must be available so that the cardiologist can make a diagnosis.

The child and family should be prepared for a cardiac catheterization, and all questions should be answered honestly. Often a nurse the child knows accompanies him to the cardiac catheterization. The child is sedated and placed in various positions during the procedure, as different specimens are obtained.

Afterward, vital signs are taken every 15 minutes for several hours. A nurse must assess the circulation of the catheterized extremity. Pulses, perfusion, color, and temperature are all significant. The pressure dressing that is in place must be examined at least every 15 minutes.

Congenital Defects

Acyanotic heart disease in infants and children often results in congestive heart failure (CHF), tachypnea, and poor growth patterns. These disorders may not demonstrate any clinical manifestations at birth.

A ventricular septal defect (Fig. 47-11) is an abnormal opening in the ventricular septum. It does not enlarge as the child grows, and 50% of these defects close spontaneously. Many children do not have any symptoms in the early years. An atrial septal defect is an opening in the atrial septum. Children with this defect also have a good prognosis. If CHF develops or if either opening is large, surgery can be done. The septal defect can be sutured closed, or a prosthetic patch may be inserted.

Patent ductus arteriosus (PDA) (Fig. 47-12) is the most common congenital cardiac anomaly seen in children. Often it is present in newborns exposed to rubella in utero and preterm infants who weigh less than 1200 g. A loud, machinelike murmur is a classic finding. Often

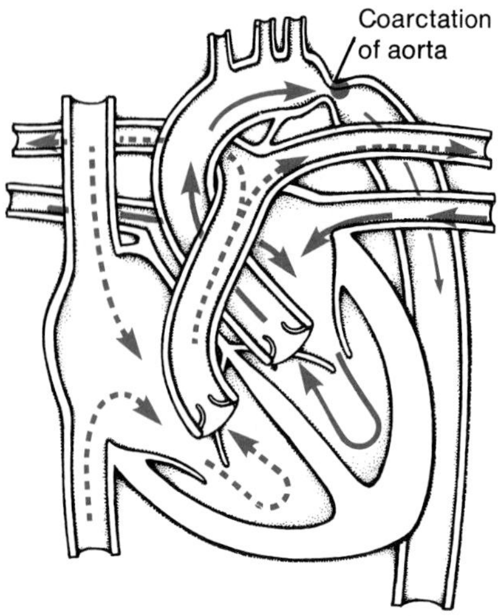

FIG. 47-13 Coarctation of the aorta.

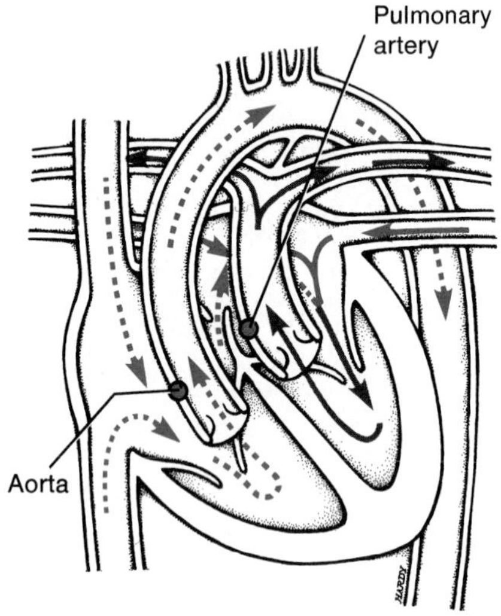

FIG. 47-14 Transposition of the great vessels.

it is present with other cardiac anomalies that may be life threatening, in which case the presence of patent ductus arteriosus is highly desirable, because it enables the mixing of oxygenated and unoxygenated blood. In many instances, this shunt can be closed by administering indomethacin. If this drug is given to an infant, the nurse must monitor his urine output, because indomethacin reduces renal blood flow. If treatment is unsuccessful, the PDA is ligated in a surgical procedure.

A coarctation of the aorta (Fig. 47-13) is a narrowing of the aorta, which results in differences in the blood pressures of the upper and lower extremities. The stenosis obstructs the flow of blood to the legs, although collateral circulation develops to carry blood around it. The blood pressures in both arms are higher than the readings in

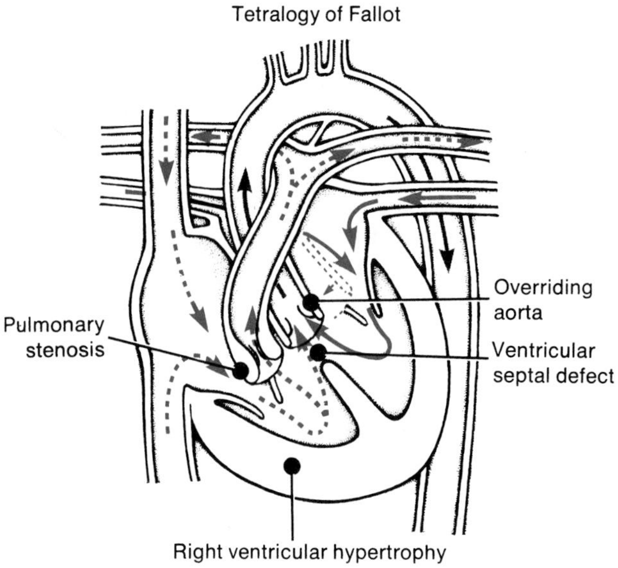

FIG. 47-15 Tetralogy of Fallot.

the legs. Unless there are other heart problems, upper extremity hypertension is the only sign. When detected, the stenosed area is resected in closed heart surgery and the prognosis is good.

Cyanotic heart disease is serious, and it is usually identified at birth, when the newborn becomes cyanotic after delivery. In transposition of the great vessels (Fig. 47-14), the aorta arises from the right ventricle and the pulmonary artery emerges from the left ventricle. As a result, unoxygenated blood from the body returns to the right side of the heart, which then pumps it back into general circulation. The pulmonary veins deliver oxygenated blood to the left heart, which then pumps it back to the lungs. Unless there are other heart anomalies such as PDA or a septal defect, the baby dies. (Their presence allows the mixing of oxygenated and venous blood.) During a cardiac catheterization a balloon-tipped catheter may be inserted through the septal defect and inflated. As it is pulled through the defect, the balloon tears the septum, allowing a better mix of oxygenated and unoxygenated blood. Severe hypoxemia can be avoided by this procedure. Congestive heart failure is a common complication. There are several types of corrective open heart procedures that should be done within the first year of life. In spite of a repair, these infants are at risk for bacterial endocarditis after surgery. Therefore they should receive antibiotics prophylactically before surgery and before extensive dental work.

Tetralogy of Fallot (Fig. 47-15) is the most common type of cyanotic congenital heart disease. This malformation consists of a ventricular septal defect, an aorta that overrides the septal defect, a hypertrophied right ventricle, and pulmonary stenosis. Infants experience "TET" spells, which are severe episodes of cyanosis and hypoxia. These anoxic episodes occur when oxygen requirements exceed the blood supply, as when the baby is crying. These infants should be comforted and placed in knee-chest position. In a very severe "TET" spell, intramuscular morphine sulfate may be required. Toddlers frequently assume a squatting position to relieve hypoxia. These children are very small for their age, have clubbed fingers and toes, and are usually cyanotic. Although "TET" spells do occur in older children, their chronic nature is reflected in the developmental delays that are seen in these children. Children with tetralogy of Fallot have high hemoglobin and hematocrit levels, which can cause polycythemia, emboli, and cerebrovascular accidents, as well as brain abscesses. **Palliative** procedures are done initially to increase oxygenation of blood. Corrective surgery is done later, after the child has gained weight and his anatomical structures have become larger, enabling a better repair.

Acquired Heart Disease

Acute rheumatic fever, an acquired heart disease, is an inflammatory disease that follows a group A beta hemolytic streptococcus infection. It is seen in children between 5 and 14 years of age, in the late winter and spring. A diagnosis is difficult to make because it is a disease that affects joints, the heart, subcutaneous tissue, and the nervous system. Anorexia, weight loss, and low-grade fever are general complaints. Hot, edematous joints, sudden, involuntary movements, an erythematous rash, and subcutaneous, nontender nodules over bony prominences, such as the knees and elbows, are specific to rheumatic fever. However, it is the rheumatic changes in the heart that are of great concern. Carditis, with an inflammation of the pericardium, myocardium, and valves, can cause permanent damage to all these structures.

Rapid treatment minimizes the inflammatory process and maximizes cardiac function by preventing damage to the heart valves. Penicillin destroys the streptococcus infection. Those who are allergic to penicillin receive erythromycin. The nurse should observe these children for signs and symptoms of congestive heart failure. Joint pain and fever are relieved by aspirin, and the nurse should position the child appropriately to minimize the pain of arthritis. Sometimes steroids are administered for the arthritis and the congestive heart failure. These children should be monitored for gastric ulcers when steroids are used and because of the stress they experience. If choreic movements occur, the child's lack of control of them is extremely frustrating for him. Bed rest is not mandated because these children curb their activity when they do not feel well. When pain is controlled, the child may become bored and present the nurse or family with the challenge to diversify activities to help pass the time. Absence from school is a concern, and once the acute phase is over, the child should be encouraged and assisted to keep up with his schoolwork. Teaching is an important responsibility of the nurse, and she must emphasize compliance with the antibiotics prescribed. The American Heart Association recommends that children who have had acute rheumatic fever receive prophylactic antibiotics indefinitely.

Bacterial endocarditis is an infection that can be acquired by children with congenital heart disease or those who have had rheumatic fever. It is caused by a variety of organisms. Hypertension and atherosclerosis also are problems that can develop in school-age adolescents. Those with a family history of hypertension and atherosclerosis are especially prone to acquiring these disorders.

NURSING DIAGNOSES	NURSING INTERVENTIONS
Altered nutrition; less than body requirements, related to fatigue, increased energy expenditure, and increased caloric needs	Encourage small frequent feedings q 2-3 hr, and limit them to 30 min to prevent fatigue. Use soft nipples, such as those used for premature infants, to decrease sucking effort. Provide rest periods between feedings. Assess infant's ability to tolerate feedings. Weigh daily, and monitor and record loss or gain. Identify child's feeding preferences: warmth of formula and favorite foods. Offer older children high-calorie, high-protein snacks between meals. Instruct parents to avoid adding medications such as Lanoxin and diuretics to bottle. Collaborate with nutritionist to develop diet high in calories and protein.
Activity intolerance, related to insufficient oxygenation	Monitor for signs of congestive heart failure. Assess for signs of decreased cardiac output: tachycardia, decreased peripheral perfusion, decreased peripheral pulses, and sluggish capillary refill. Assess chest expansion, respiratory rate, breath sounds, and quality of aeration. Monitor for frequency and severity of cyanotic episodes and syncope. Monitor oxygen saturation levels with pulse oximetry. Assist child in assuming knee-chest position. Assess all vital signs. Note degree of distress, exertion, or cyanosis with crying and increased activity. Administer oxygen properly. Determine infant's ability to be fed by mouth. Strictly monitor and record intake and output volumes.

DISORDERS OF THE HEMATOLOGICAL SYSTEM

Although trauma can result in significant blood losses, nutritional deficits, chronic systemic diseases, and inherited blood disorders account for the majority of the hematological disorders seen in infants and children. They can be short-term or long-term problems. Several disorders are fatal.

Nursing Assessment

Collection of *subjective data* begins when these infants are brought in for examination because they are pale, anorexic, edematous, irritable, and bruise easily. A nutrition history is important subjective information because the anemia may have developed as a result of a large milk intake to the exclusion of solid foods. A family history also can reveal the presence of inherited blood disorders, such as sickle cell anemia or hemophilia.

Collection of *objective data* reveals petechiae, purpura, bruises, jaundiced sclerae, poor capillary refill, and enlarged lymph nodes. There also is hepatosplenomegaly. Tachycardia, tachypnea, and edema may indicate the development of congestive heart failure because of the severe anemia.

Diagnostic Tests

A battery of tests should be done, including a complete blood count, hemoglobin, hematocrit, platelet count, and bleeding and clotting times. A reticulocyte count, peripheral blood smears, iron-binding capacity, and a stool for occult blood also are ordered. Abnormalities in the size, shape, and characteristics of cells must be identified. In addition, blood is now routinely screened for sickle cell disease in newborns. Bone marrow aspiration is performed to evaluate the production of blood cells by the bone marrow. This diagnostic procedure is always done on children suspected of having leukemia or other malignancies. In children the posterior iliac crest is the site from which the specimen is aspirated.

Iron-Deficiency Anemia

Iron-deficiency anemia occurs most commonly in infants and children younger than 2 years. It develops as a result of a dietary deficiency. For example, when solid foods are introduced, the infant offers resistance and demonstrates a preference for his bottle. Instead of continuing with these new foods, the parent provides a bottle of milk, which is a poor source of iron. Over time the oxygen-carrying capability of blood decreases and these infants and toddlers become markedly anemic, in spite of being overweight in some cases. They are extremely pale and listless and have poor muscle development; they are also prone to infections. Congestive heart failure may develop in those who are extremely anemic.

Treatment consists of administering ferrous sulfate preparations, such as Fer-in-Sol. The nurse should tell a parent that iron changes the color of bowel movements to tarry green. Iron-rich infant foods should be included in his diet. Because of the presence of baby fat, the infant appears well-nourished, and diet teaching may be a sensitive matter for a nurse to handle. The infant resists changing from an exclusively milk diet to one that includes new, unfamiliar foods, but his milk intake should be limited, and gradually the new foods satisfy his hunger. As red cell production increases, his activity improves rapidly.

Hemophilia

Hemophilia refers to a group of bleeding disorders in which there is a deficiency of one of the factors necessary for coagulation. The most common is *classic hemophilia*, in which the carrier-mother transmits the disease to an affected son. Factor VIII is deficient in this disease. The disorder is characterized by repeated bleeding episodes (e.g., after circumcision, eruption of a tooth, or sustaining the slightest break in the skin). When the toddler falls, he bleeds into soft tissue. The school-age child may bleed into a joint, which is called *hemarthrosis;* signs and symptoms include stiffness, warmth, tenderness, and limited movement. As the bleeding continues, the tissue around the joint becomes swollen, and over time, degenerative changes contribute to the development of contractures. Although there may be a family history of this disease, that is not always the case. For example, the first evidence of the disease may be when a newborn is circumcised and bleeds uncontrollably.

Protection from injury is critical. Cribs and playpens must be padded, and when the child begins to walk, a football helmet and elbow and knee pads should be worn. Aspirin and other drugs that affect platelet development should never be given. When bleeding episodes occur, ice bags and pressure should be applied immediately; ice bags must always be available in the home freezer unit. Joints should be elevated and supported in a slightly flexed position. Cryoprecipitate is always administered in a bleeding episode, and boys as young as 5 or 6 years learn to administer this replacement factor to themselves. These children and their families learn to recognize the earliest signs of bleeding, and they institute treatment immediately. Home management has resulted in earlier control of bleeding, fewer complications, and fewer interruptions in normal activities.

As a result of the development of home management programs, these children are admitted to the hospital only when there is an extensive blood loss. The child may be in pain and frightened by the episode, and the nurse should provide explanations and support. Although the constant threat of hemorrhage exists, these boys and their families lead active lives as a result of adjusting realistically to the presence of this disease with its limitations.

The Purpuras

A group of disorders known as the *purpuras* is characterized by bleeding into the skin. There also may be bleeding from mucous membranes and other organs. Platelet counts may be normal, as in Henoch-Schönlein syndrome, or they may be drastically reduced, as in idiopathic thrombocytopenic purpura (ITP), which is the most common form.

ITP occurs after a viral infection, with petechiae and ecchymotic lesions developing over all parts of the body. If tissue bleeding is extensive, blood transfusions may be necessary. Children with this disorder must be monitored for worsening or improvement. Corticosteroids reduce the bleeding, and precipitate remissions. Epistatic episodes upset the child, and nasal packing with Gelfoam may be necessary. While platelet counts are low, the child must be protected from injuries. This includes not participating in physical education classes and contact sports. Most children recover in about 6 weeks.

Leukemia

Leukemia is the most common form of childhood cancer. In this disease normal marrow elements are replaced by abnormal leukocytes. The leukemia is classified by the type of white blood cell that predominates in the marrow and peripheral blood. The majority of cases are acute lymphocytic or lymphoblastic leukemia; the remaining cases are classified as acute myelocytic or myeloblastic leukemia. Children with leukemia usually have a low-grade fever, malaise, hepatosplenomegaly, lymphadenopathy, and bruises. They also are anemic.

About 90% of those diagnosed go into a remission when treatment is started, and 50% remain in initial remission for at least 5 years. During that time they are free of the signs and symptoms of leukemia. The bone marrow is functioning adequately. At present, if they go into initial remission and remain free of symptoms for 3 years, drug therapy is discontinued.

A number of chemotherapeutic agents are given intravenously, **intrathecally,** and by mouth. They include prednisone, vincristine, Adriamycin, methotrexate, and cyclophosphamide. Unfortunately these drugs are very potent, and side effects, such as alopecia, immunosuppression, and ulcerations of the mouth, are common. The important issue in treating children with leukemia is that there are a limited number of drugs available, and although remissions occur, exacerbations occur also. There are many unknowns in this disease.

Infections are common, and the nurse should assess the patient several times a shift. Normal eating patterns are affected by fluctuations in appetite or mechanical difficulties in chewing when mouth ulcerations are present. When a toothbrush cannot be used, oral hygiene may consist of hydrogen peroxide and saline rinses or a mouth wash. Rectal ulcers may develop, so rectal temperatures should not be taken. Meticulous skin care with thorough rinsing and drying is essential in maintaining skin integrity.

The disease and the medications can result in physical changes in a child's appearance. The nurse should prepare the child and the family for the hair loss, the weight gain, or the **cushingoid signs.** She should provide opportunities to talk about these changes. Children can better cope with these feelings through role-playing or storytelling. When in remission, a child returns to his normal activities.

Exacerbations, however, result in irritability, pain, and renewed bleeding episodes. Positioning, the use of analgesics, and a quiet environment promote rest and comfort. Honest answers and accurate information are critical components in providing care to these children and their families. Nurses also should explore their own feelings of death in the presence of exacerbations. Although a variety of chemotherapeutic drugs are available and more effective supportive measures have made long-term survival a reality, the ultimate outcome is unknown.

Sickle Cell Anemia

Sickle cell anemia (a homozygous blood disorder) is inherited, and it occurs as a result of an abnormal type of hemoglobin in the red blood cell. With deoxygenation, the cell assumes an irregular, sickle shape. These abnormal cells increase the viscosity of the blood, which causes stasis and occludes small blood vessels. Sickling of erythrocytes is triggered by an infection, dehydration, or stress. There is a heterozygous form of this abnormality, which is called *sickle cell trait.* Its presence is usually discovered accidentally, and normally children with this condition have no problems.

The clinical signs and symptoms of sickle cell anemia include pallor, hepatosplenomegaly, jaundice, and growth retardation. However, the complications of this disease, the vasoocclusive crises, are responsible for the major problems these children experience. For example, the small blood vessels are occluded by the sickled cells during an infection, and there is soft tissue edema, pain, and infarction. The child is in "sickle cell crisis." These crises can involve any part of the body, such as the back, the abdomen, or a joint. The "hand-foot" syndrome is seen in children younger than 2 years. They experience soft tissue edema of their hands and feet, which is accompanied by severe pain. This disease is found primarily in the black population.

Children in crisis need intravenous and oral fluids, because dehydration causes decreased blood volume, sludging, increased blood viscosity, and further sickling. Pain is controlled by analgesics; however older children and adolescents may need morphine drips (continuous IV infusion with morphine as an additive) to control their severe pain. Applying local heat or massage and giving very warm baths for toddlers also are effective in controlling pain. The nurse should write the successful methods of controlling pain on a child's care plan so other nurses can use them.

Diagnosing sickle cell anemia is critical because then nurses can teach parents how to prevent infections and dehydration and thereby avoid a crisis episode. Older children are taught how to manage stress. Such interventions decrease the complications. Unfortunately, death usually occurs early in adulthood.

Children with sickle cell trait, which has little clinical significance, can expect to live a normal, uncomplicated life.

Acquired Immune Deficiency Syndrome (AIDS)

Pediatric AIDS is a tragic and usually fatal disease in children that affects the immune system. Although the majority of infants acquire the disorder from their infected mothers, other children, such as those with hemophilia, develop it from blood transfusions contaminated with the virus. The incubation period in children is about 6 months, whereas it may be several years in adults. If it is not suspected, the diagnosis may be delayed because its symptoms are vague and these symptoms could occur in any child. For example, children with AIDS fail to thrive and have repeated monilial infections, enlarged lymph nodes, and frequent episodes of otitis media and pneumonia. The majority of children acquire the virus from their mothers. The high-risk maternal group includes those women who are intravenous drug users and those with multiple sexual partners. It is not unusual for a mother to not realize she is infected until the infant is diagnosed with AIDS.

This disease has no cure, and the treatment for AIDS is symptomatic. The use of AZT in infants and toddlers has resulted in improving their neurological status (Pizzo, 1989). Nurses also report these children have better eating patterns and less frequent infections once they receive this medication. It is a most promising treatment on the basis of preliminary reports. However, opportunistic diseases continue to contribute to mortality, especially pneumocystosis (caused by *Pneumocystis carinii),* which requires the use of Pentam intravenously. Candidiasis is usually present and is treated with an antifungal drug, such as Nizoral. The management of children with AIDS also focuses on improving their nutritional status to increase their ability to resist infections. Although the children receive diets high in calories and protein, nurses must encourage them to eat. There are those who may require tube feedings or total parenteral nutrition because they do not tolerate oral foods.

Implementing universal precautions, including strict hand-washing techniques, is critical in preventing the spread of this virus. Although these infants and toddlers are not isolated on a pediatric unit, the nurse must protect them from developing infections. Because the patients are young, the nurse should provide activities that stimulate normal development. Both parents and community members are concerned about school attendance by children with AIDS. In some instances families are ostracized. Guidelines have been published by the Centers for Disease Control and the American Academy of Pediatrics, which state that these children and adolescents should be allowed to attend school unless they have open lesions or demonstrate such behaviors as biting. Unfortunately, the public has many unfounded misconceptions about the transmission of this virus, and much education is needed. From a nursing perspective, caring for children with AIDS is emotionally challenging: nurses must (1) help families cope with the multiple effects of this disease; (2) provide a loving environment in which the quality of an infant's life is maximized; and (3) accept the fact that, ultimately, an infectious process will shorten the child's life.

NURSING DIAGNOSES	NURSING INTERVENTIONS
Potential for injury, related to an alteration in coagulation	Inspect skin, nailbeds, and mucous membranes for any signs of bleeding. Examine urine and stool for evidence of bleeding, gross and occult, as ordered. Monitor vital signs, and assess for increase in apical pulse and respiratory rate and decrease in blood pressure. Observe for restlessness or apprehension. Use small-gauge needles for drawing blood, and apply pressure to site afterward. Assess capillary refill. Use soft toothbrush or nonirritating mouthwash for oral hygiene. Handle gently, and change position carefully. Do not administer aspirin-containing medications. Provide instructions on detecting and managing bleeding episodes.
Potential for impaired gas exchange, related to decreased hemoglobin levels	Maintain intravenous fluid rate as ordered. Monitor intravenous site and patency of IV. Assess child for signs of increasing respiratory distress. Administer oxygen to maintain oximeter levels above 95%. Elevate head of bed. Monitor and record intake and output.

NURSING DIAGNOSES	NURSING INTERVENTIONS
Potential for impaired gas exchange, related to decreased hemoglobin levels—cont'd	Offer large amounts of fluid by mouth. Provide quiet, restful environment. Minimize physical exertion by organizing and clustering activities.

DISORDERS OF THE GENITOURINARY SYSTEM

The major function of the kidneys is to maintain the equilibrium of body fluids. Although 5% to 10% of all infants are born with a malformation of the urinary tract, many of the malformations are clinically unimportant and others are surgically correctable. A majority of urinary tract anomalies are asymptomatic; however, some findings that are commonly associated with renal disease include low-set ears, widely spaced nipples, Wilms' tumor, and a family history of renal disease. The asymptomatic nature of many urinary problems presents a particular challenge to a nurse, because an early diagnosis is critical to prevent renal damage.

Nursing Assessment

The infant or child with a renal disorder may not be acutely ill, and the presence of the disorder may be detected only in the course of a routine examination. Young children often present with unrelated symptoms that do not focus on this body system.

Collection of *subjective data* includes noting that although hematuria, frequency, and urgency or incontinence may be verbalized complaints, such symptoms as chills or fever, lower abdominal pain, malaise, anorexia, or flank pain also are common. In collecting subjective information, a history of toilet-training efforts, the development of bedwetting, prior urinary tract infections, and a family history of renal disease are important data to explore with a parent. A child's current urinary habits, the number of voidings or wet diapers each day, a description of his stream, and the color and characteristics of urine all may be significant.

Collection of *objective data* includes the physical assessment, which begins with vital signs, a blood pressure reading, height and weight, as well as the child's overall physical status. The nurse palpates the abdomen for ascites and the presence of any masses or tenderness. She examines the area around the eyes, the external genitalia, and the extremities for any evidence of edema. It is advantageous to observe the child in the act of voiding for quality of stream, bloody urine, and pain as evident in his facial expressions.

Diagnostic Tests

Specimens are obtained for a complete blood count, urinalysis, midstream urine for culture, blood urea nitrogen, and serum creatinine levels. X-ray studies include a flat plate of the abdomen and intravenous pyelogram (IVP), which visualizes the upper urinary tract, a voiding cystourethrogram (VCUG), which studies the lower tract, computerized tomography (CT) scanning, and ultrasonography. These tests can be frightening to a young child, especially when they are done in rapid succession. A nurse should accompany the child to the radiology department to calm him and to solicit his cooperation.

Hypospadias and Epispadias

Hypospadias and epispadias are anomalies present at birth in which the urethral opening is not located at the tip of the penis. In hypospadias the urethra opens on the ventral surface of the shaft of the penis (Fig. 47-16), and in epispadias the urethral opening is on the dorsal surface. The urethral opening can be present anywhere along either surface of the penis. These disorders are usually repaired in one or two procedures before the age of 3 years. Circumcisions are never done on these infants because the foreskin is used to lengthen the urethra during surgery.

Postoperatively the nurse should monitor the child for wound infection and a urinary tract infection. Edema develops after surgery, so positioning is important to avoid wound separation. The nurse assesses the urethral and suprapubic catheters for drainage and documents the color and amount of urine. Pain is common and should be relieved. Bladder spasms develop also. Except in severe cases, recovery is uncomplicated and sexual function is normal.

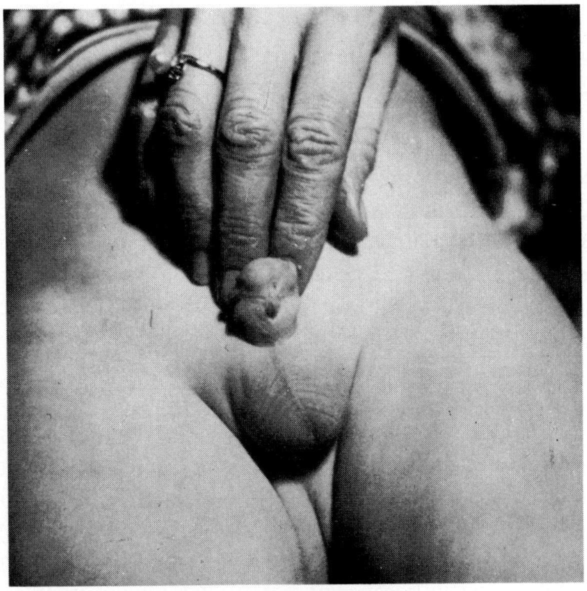

FIG. 47-16 Hypospadias.

Wilms' Tumor

Wilms' tumor, sometimes called a *nephroblastoma,* affects older infants and children younger than 3 years. Parents often first identify the firm, nontender mass as they bathe or dress the child. It is an embryonic tumor, which usually involves only one kidney. Signs and symptoms may include anorexia, malaise, and a fever. Undetected, its increased size causes abdominal pain, vomiting, and hematuria. On admission, abdominal palpations must be limited because they increase the danger of metastasis. A battery of diagnostic tests are done, and IVP and CT scan are particularly informative. Current treatment includes (1) surgery, when a nephrectomy is done; (2) chemotherapy using vincristine, Adriamycin, and actinomycin D, which eradicate any micrometastasis; and (3) radiation. Occasionally radiation may be used preoperatively to shrink the tumor mass.

Preoperatively a nurse collects urine specimens and explains the various procedures that are done. Surgery usually is done within 48 hours of admission, so there is limited time for preparation. Postoperatively the nursing care these children receive is similar to that provided to any child experiencing abdominal surgery. However, the nurse gives special attention to monitoring bowel sounds and noting any apparent distention. She assesses the patency of the nasogastric tube and carefully monitors the urinary output. Children with Wilms' tumors are at risk for intestinal obstruction once vincristine is started.

Diagnosis of Wilms' tumor is anxiety-provoking in parents, who feel guilty about not identifying the mass earlier, and the nurse should offer support and opportunities to discuss these feelings. The nurse should inform the parents about the side effects of both the chemotherapy and radiation. The length of treatment may be as long as 18 months, but the prognosis is excellent and survival rates have improved remarkably with aggressive treatment protocols.

Hydrocele

A hydrocele is an accumulation of fluid within the scrotal sac, and often it is present with an inguinal hernia. Generally the fluid is reabsorbed slowly over the first year of life. If not, surgery is necessary to remove the fluid and prevent the collection of additional fluid in the scrotal sac. Nursing interventions are identical to those provided to a child after an inguinal hernia repair.

Cryptorchidism

Cryptorchidism is when one or both testes fail to descend into the scrotum. It is found in 20% of preterm males, but most testes descend during the first year. The cause is unknown. If testes remain in the abdomen, sterility may result because normal body temperature is 2.2° C higher than scrotal temperature, and long-term exposure to the higher temperature is sufficient to cause damage. There is also an increased incidence of malignancy after adolescence. When the testes have not descended by the age of 6 to 8 years, chorionic gonadotrophin is given intramuscularly. If the testes do not descend after this treatment, surgery (orchiopexy) is done. During the procedure the testes are mechanically transplanted into the scrotum.

The surgery heightens a child's concerns about genital mutilation, and the procedure should be explained to the school-age child. Edema that develops can be relieved by ice packs around the scrotum. The suture line must be kept clean and dry. If the testes are secured in place with a suture to a rubber band taped to the thigh, its purpose should be explained to the child. The suture usually remains in place for several days, and the child recovers quickly and without complications.

Nephrosis

The cause of nephrosis is unknown. It affects toddlers and preschoolers and results in significant losses of plasma proteins, especially albumin, in the urine. Children develop a generalized edema. Initially the edema is periorbital, and then it is evident in dependent areas of the peritoneal cavity, legs, and external genitalia. As the disease progresses, skin over the abdomen becomes stretched and shiny, with prominent veins. The urine is foamy or frothy, and the blood pressure is normal. Nephrosis is a chronic disease. Most children respond to treatment and diurese after receiving steroids. However, a small number have exacerbations, fail to respond to steroids and other drugs, and die of progressive renal disease in 2 to 3 years.

Although the child cannot understand why he is "blown up," he does not feel ill but limits his activity because of the edema. Dietary restrictions are not necessary, although added salt in cooking or at the table is not allowed. A high-protein diet is desirable but is not tolerated well. A large amount of potassium is excreted and extra potassium is provided in juices, fruits (oranges, bananas, and grapes), and milk. Fluid restrictions are imposed rarely. Intake and output must be monitored carefully and the child should be weighed daily.

A challenge for the nurse is to maintain the child's skin integrity. Preventing skin impairment requires frequent positional and diaper changes, careful washing and drying of the skin and skinfolds, and liberal use of cornstarch or nonallergenic powder. If there is skin breakdown, use of ointments or powders should be discontinued because these materials trap organisms and contribute to infections. The nurse should practice meticulous handwashing.

Corticosteroids, the medical treatment, can decrease the amount of proteinuria, reverse the sequence of events, and promote the excretion of the edema fluid. The presence of edema and the use of steroids significantly contribute to the child's susceptibility to infection. Prednisone is commonly used. After several days of receiving this steroid, the child begins to void increasing amounts of urine. The output may be so great that it is necessary to weigh the child every 8 hours rather than once a day. Predisone is continued for about 2 weeks after diuresis occurs and the urine is protein free. This medication is then tapered over 2 months. These children develop cushingoid features, which include a moon face, fat pad over the base of the neck (Buffalo hump), abdominal striae, increased appetite, weight gain, and increased body hair. The nurse should reassure both the child and his parents that all of these features disappear 2 to 3 months after steroids are discontinued.

Urinary Tract Infections

Urinary tract infections (UTIs) are very common in children. Urine containing bacteria in excess of 100,000 bacteria per milliliter by culture indicates a UTI. Potentially these repeated infections can have long-term effects. These children may or may not be symptomatic. When a child has a positive urine culture, frequency, urgency, and dysuria, cystitis or an infection of the lower urinary tract is suspected. Those children with positive urine cultures, chills, fever, vomiting, and complaints of back pain have signs and symptoms suggesting an infection of the upper urinary tract, called *acute pyelonephritis*. Some bacteria responsible include *Escherichia coli* (the most common), *Proteus, Pseudomonas,* and various enterococci, which are normal fecal flora. Obstructions to urine flow and contaminated catheterizations contribute to UTI. Another cause of UTI is vesicoureteral reflux. The valve at the point where a ureter joins the bladder (vesicoureteral junction) does not close properly, which allows the urine to flow back up into the ureter. When voiding occurs, the urine refluxes into the ureter and returns to the bladder when voiding has stopped. The residual urine contributes to the infectious process. There is a high incidence of reflux in children younger than 2 years.

Clinical manifestations vary greatly, especially among different age groups. Neonates and infants have nonspecific symptoms, such as poor weight gain, poor appetite, and diarrhea. As a result they may have infections that seriously affect the urinary system. The 2- to 5-year-olds complain of abdominal pain, burning on urination, and urgency. Sometimes enuresis occurs in this age group. Females between 6 and 13 years tend to have recurrent, asymptomatic bouts of UTI. A female has an extremely short urethra, which can increase incidence of UTI. A nurse should consider a child's age when collecting a history.

The nurse must follow correct procedure when collecting a urine specimen for culture, since the diagnosis is made on those results. She must administer antibiotics as scheduled, so that therapeutic blood levels can be maintained, and she must carefully monitor and record the intake and output. Sometimes "forcing fluids" is prescribed to flush bladder contents. Follow-up urine cultures reflect a child's response to treatment. The nurse must do a significant amount of teaching if recurrent infections are to be avoided. Teaching includes the following recommendations:

1. Cleanse from anterior to posterior after voiding and defecating to avoid contamination.
2. Urinate frequently.
3. Maintain an adequate fluid intake to promote flushing the bladder.
4. Avoid using chemical irritants, such as bubble bath soap.
5. Take short tub baths or showers.
6. Avoid prolonged sitting in wading pools.
7. Avoid the use of feminine hygiene products that cause irritation.
8. Wear cotton underwear and pantyhose with a cotton crotch to avoid perineal irritation.

Enuresis

Enuresis is a problem that develops after a child has achieved bladder control. It is the repeated, involuntary urination that occurs in 4- or 5-year-olds. Nocturnal enuresis is more common, and it occurs more commonly in boys. Although urinary tract infections, a small bladder, or other disorders may cause nocturnal enuresis, its presence usually has a psychological basis, such as a family crisis, an impaired parent-child relationship, or a history of intense toilet-training. Enuresis is embarrassing to a child.

Anticholinergic drugs have been used with limited success. Restricting a child's fluids after the evening meal and waking the child so he can void before parents go to bed are other methods of dealing with this problem. Praising the child for periods of bladder control and not scolding or punishing him when he loses bladder control are effective too. Commercially available alarm systems have been used successfully in recent years. This conditioning method involves a urine-sensing device connected to an alarm, which is activated when the child voids. He learns to delay urination to avoid the alarm sounding and disturbing his sleep.

Acute Glomerulonephritis

Acute glomerulonephritis (AGN) is a serious disorder that usually follows one of the beta hemolytic streptococcus infections and affects school-age children, especially 6- and 7-year-olds. Its onset is abrupt with gross hematuria (urine is reddish-brown) and periorbital edema. Circulatory congestion is apparent with dyspnea and a cough, and the child is mildly or moderately hypertensive. He is pale, lethargic, and anorexic, with varying degrees of edema. An antistreptolysin O (ASO) titer confirms the presence of antibodies that reflect the recent streptococcal infection. Urinalysis during the acute phase characteristically shows hematuria, proteinuria, and increased specific gravity. Azotemia that results from impaired glomerular filtration is reflected in elevated blood urea nitrogen and creatinine levels in 50% of the cases. There is no specific treatment for AGN.

Vital signs, including a blood pressure, daily weights, and intake and output monitor the progress of this disease. Children usually confine themselves to bed rest. Dietary restrictions depend on the severity of the edema. No salt is added to foods. In moderately severe hypertension and edema, salt is restricted. Antibiotics may be ordered when there is evidence of a persistent streptococcal infection. Lasix and Apresoline are commonly used to control the hypertension. An increased urinary output and subtle decrease in weight are the first signs of improvement. As the diuresis continues, the hypertension resolves, the appetite improves, and the child recovers.

NURSING DIAGNOSES	NURSING INTERVENTIONS
Fluid volume excess, related to impaired kidney function resulting in edema	Accurately measure and record intake and output hourly. Perform urine dipsticks q 4 hr. Obtain weights daily or q 8 hr on same scale at same time. Assess pulses in all four extremities. Measure and record abdominal girths daily. Properly administer steroids. Check for pitting edema. Document diuretic response to steroid treatment (decrease in weight and proteinuria). Limit sodium or fluids as ordered. Auscultate lung fields, and observe for evidence of respiratory distress (dyspnea). Observe for signs of congestive heart failure. Monitor amount, color, and appearance of urine.
Urinary retention, related to hypospadias repair	Accurately measure and record intake and output volumes hourly. Maintain proper placement and patency of catheters. Assess patency of urinary drainage catheters hourly, and note presence of clots. Palpate bladder for distention. Measure abdominal girth q 4 hr. Assess child for signs of pain or discomfort. Prevent dislocation of urinary catheters by securing with tape to leg/abdomen. Assess catheter placement q 2 hr. Apply extremity restraints to ensure retention of catheters. Monitor frequency and duration of bladder spasms. Prevent pressure on catheters by using bed cradle.

DIABETES MELLITUS (DM)

Insulin-dependent diabetes mellitus (IDDM), or type I, is the most frequently seen endocrine disorder in children. There are three types of cells in the islands of Langerhans of the pancreas: alpha cells, which produce glucagon; beta cells, which produce insulin; and delta cells, which produce somatostatin. IDDM is a deficiency in the production of insulin. Individuals inherit a predisposition for the disease, and in the presence of certain environmental factors, they develop IDDM. An autoimmune process is involved also. Because of a defect in the immune system, a person is susceptible to viral infections that invade the beta cells and destroy them. No insulin is produced without beta cells. Insulin is needed to metabolize carbohydrates, fats, and proteins. With the lack of insulin, glucose is not available for cellular metabolism, and therefore glucose concentration rises in the blood, resulting in *hyperglycemia*. When the kidneys can no longer reabsorb the glucose, the glucose "spills" over into the urine, pulling water with it (polyuria). These increased urinary fluid losses cause dehydration and thirst, or *polydipsia,* which is characteristic of IDDM. Because glucose cannot enter the cells, protein is broken down and converted to glucose by the liver, increasing the hyperglycemia. Without carbohydrates for energy, fat and protein stores are depleted as the body tries to meet its energy needs. There is a weight loss and a comparable increase in appetite (polyphagia).

The onset of IDDM is sudden in school-age children. When hyperglycemia, vomiting, abdominal pain, a fruity odor to the breath, an altered level of consciousness, and possibly a coma occur, it is called *diabetic ketoacidosis,* a clinical manifestation of uncontrolled diabetes. As the body uses fat and proteins for energy, ketone bodies form, which are byproducts of fat metabolism. The number of ketone bodies increase and spill into the urine. The body also attempts to excrete the excess ketones through the lungs, which produces the acetone breath odor. Polyuria, polydipsia, polyphagia, and hyperglycemia are typical findings in IDDM.

When a child with ketoacidosis is initially admitted, glucose levels can be as high as 1000 mg/dl, and serum acetone levels are high, reflective of high ketone levels. Nursing activities involve maintaining intravenous lines and urinary catheters, strictly monitoring and recording intake and output, and administering insulin, as well as assisting in the collection of blood specimens. Treatment is aimed at establishing reasonably normal glucose levels and correcting fluid and electrolyte imbalances. These children are moderately to severely ill.

A great deal of teaching must be done during the course of a hospitalization, and the school-age child or adolescent is capable of assuming responsibility for urine and blood testing and administering insulin subcutaneously. There are three types of insulin: short-acting, intermediate, and long-acting. The dosage ordered depends on blood and urine results, food intake, and activity and exercise levels. Adjustments must be made during growth spurts, illness, infection, and surgery. Although they may be angry or fearful of injecting themselves, 5- and 6-year-olds can adjust to this lifelong health problem. Both the child and parents must learn what the signs and symptoms of hypoglycemia are (e.g., slurred speech, tremors) and how to reverse them, such as consuming orange juice or candy to raise the glucose level. These children should wear medical alert bracelets.

Properly instructed children can monitor their blood glucose levels and test their urine. They learn to maintain glucose levels of 80 to 120 mg/dl. Although it is costly and requires finger sticks, diabetic home management has resulted in better control of this disease. A nutritionist discusses foods and exchange plans with the family and the child. Food consumption must correspond with the time of administration and duration of action of the insulin. Meals and snacks are based on a balanced diet that includes all food groups, and sugar or readily available carbohydrates are restricted. Participating in exercise programs is encouraged, but an extra food intake is necessary to achieve the balance required between food and insulin when a child's activity increases. As the child learns to live with IDDM, he becomes skillful in managing all aspects of living with a chronic disease, making food substitutions, and participating in activities with peers.

As does any person with a chronic illness, the child with IDDM and his parents must make psychological adjustments and modifications in life-style. A nurse who supports the child and his parents and provides them with concrete suggestions about managing the disease can have a positive effect on their attitudes about and management of IDDM.

CHILD ABUSE

The term *child abuse* is used to describe physical and emotional abuse and neglect, as well as sexual abuse, of children. Abuse and neglect of children can result in a multitude of injuries, such as burns, lacerations, poisonings, head trauma, and fractures. In infants and small children, fractures of various types and severity are frequently seen as a result of child abuse.

Dislocations and fractures that are inconsistent with the history given by the parent should alert nurses to the possibility of abuse. The presence of new and old fractures in various stages of healing indicates that the fractures occurred at different times and is highly indicative of abuse. The twisting of small arms or legs can result in spiral fractures of these extremities. Abuse may also result in fractures of the skull, nose, or facial bones. An x-ray examination of the child's body (skeletal survey) is commonly done in situations of suspected child abuse.

The nurse caring for the abused child must have a nonjudgmental attitude toward the parents. If anger is directed toward parents, it seriously hampers the nurse's ability to intervene effectively. Most parents love their children even when they abuse them. They need assistance in developing appropriate measures to deal with the child's behaviors. The nurse must promote parenting skills and family functioning, and this can be done only if the nurse establishes a trusting relationship with the parents.

During the child's hospitalization the nurse can help parents recognize the difficulties involved with being a parent and help them develop self-esteem by providing support and positive reinforcement. The nurse should encourage the parents to be involved in their child's care. The nurse documents the interactions between the child and parents in an objective and factual manner. The serious nature of child abuse must not be overlooked. Parents should be informed that the abuse must be reported to proper authorities. They may become angry and upset; however, the situation must be handled honestly and in a straightforward manner. The goal is to protect the child.

The child needs consistent caregivers during hospitalization. His interactions and behaviors with nurses and other adults should be observed and documented to note the pattern of his relationships with others. Play activities can assist the child in expressing his feelings about the situation. Play therapy can help the child understand his feelings. Children protect their parents and often assume the responsibility for the abuse.

Discharge planning is of primary importance. Ideally the child would return to a secure and functional family; however, that is not always possible. If the child is to be placed in a foster home temporarily, both the parents and child must be prepared for this action. A nurse who has a good relationship with the family can be supportive to them. Community services are involved because the situation requires long-term intervention. Communication between all agencies involved with the family is mandatory. The community health nurse may be in the best position to coordinate these services to the child and his family.

REFERENCES AND SUGGESTED READINGS

APA: DSM-III-R: Diagnostic and statistical manual of mental disorders, ed 3, 1987.

Burns M: Pediatric urinary tract infection, Pediatr Clin North Am 34(4):1111, 1987.

Cohen FL: Neural tube defects: epidemiology, detection and prevention, J Obstet Gynecol Neonat Nurs 16(2):105, 1987.

Edmands MS: Overcoming eating disorders, J Psychosoc Nurs 24(8):19, 1986.

Eland J: Pharmacologic management of acute and chronic pediatric pain, Issues Compr Pediatr Nurs 11(2-3):93, 1988.

Friedman D: Taking the scare out of caring for seizure patients, Nurs '88 18(2):53, 1988.

Friedman SB et al: Statement on terminology from the National SIDS Foundation, Pediatrics 68(4):543, 1981.

Gates DM and McClure MJ: Forestalling the progress of heart disease, MCN 14(3):174, 1989.

Gawin FN and Ellingwood EH: Cocaine and other stimulants: actions, abuse, and treatment, N Engl J Med 318(18):1173, 1988.

Hartsell MB: Noninvasive oxygen monitoring, J Pediatr Nurs 2(1):64, 1987.

Hartsell MB: Chest physical therapy and mechanical vibration, J Pediatr Nurs 2(2):135, 1987.

Hayman LL: Reducing risk for heart disease in children, MCN (13):442, 1988.

Horner MM, Rawlins P, and Giles K: How parents of children with chronic conditions perceive their own needs, MCN 12:140, 1987.

Kaufman DH, Grothe G, and Brasser B: Early identification of ear infection and hearing loss in an early childhood population, School Nurse 3(1):18, 1987.

Lieber MT and Taub AS: Common foot deformities and what they mean to parents, MCN 13:47, 1988.

Linley JF: Screening children for common orthopedic problems, AJN 87(1):1312, 1987.

McKerrow K: Minimal hearing loss may not be benign, Am J Nurs 87(7):904, 1987.

Pizzo PA: Editorial response, N Engl J Med 320(12):806, 1989.

Smith JB: Ethical issues raised by new treatment options, MCN 14(3):183, 1989.

Stullenbarger B: Family adaptation to cystic fibrosis, Pediatr Nurs 13(1):29, 1987.

Tse AM: Seizures and societal attitudes: a teaching tool for children, siblings, classmates, parents, and classroom teachers, Issues Compr Pediatr Nurs 9(5):299, 1986.

Vulcan BM: Acute bacterial meningitis in infancy and childhood, Crit Care Nurs 7(5):53, 1987.

Webb C, Stergies D, and Rodgers B: Patient-controlled analgesia as postoperative pain management for children, J Pediatr Nurs 4(3):162, 1989.

CHAPTER CHALLENGE

KEY POINTS

- The postoperative care of a child who has had abdominal surgery includes intravenous fluids, hydration and electrolyte balance, nasogastric decompression, positioning, and relieving discomfort and pain.
- Adequate health protection measures for children include adhering to immunization schedules and controlling communicable diseases.
- Acute respiratory tract infections are a common cause of illness in infants and young children.
- When caring for an adolescent who has an eating disorder, nursing interventions should be directed toward enhancing the adolescent's self-image and self-control, thereby improving nutritional status.
- Interventions for a child with AIDS are directed toward preventing infections and providing a diet that ensures adequate nutrients to promote normal growth and development.
- Screening for scoliosis is an important component of the physical assessments of 10- to 14-year-old children.
- To effectively manage the care of a child who is developmentally delayed, the nurse must identify his developmental level.
- Decreased levels of secretion or the absence of insulin in a child results in the development of diabetes mellitus.

STUDY QUESTIONS

1. Important historical information to elicit when assessing a skin rash is:
   a. The pattern of spread
   b. The area in which the lesions first appeared
   c. The progression of the rash from its first appearance to the present status
   d. The presence of pruritus, scaling, and dryness
2. An adolescent who has acne tells the nurse that he has squeezed out several blackheads. The nurse explains that:
   a. Squeezing often causes rupture of the sebaceous follicle, inflammation, and scarring
   b. Squeezing causes keratinization of the sebaceous canal
   c. Squeezing causes oxidation of sebum
   d. It would be better to scrub or rub the skin vigorously
3. A nursing intervention that facilitates joint movement in the child with juvenile rheumatoid arthritis is:
   a. Placing pillows under the affected areas
   b. Massaging painful joints gently
   c. Applying warm compresses
   d. Raising the foot and head of the bed
4. With a diagnosis of Legg-Calvé-Perthes disease, the teaching and counseling done by a nurse must include its:
   a. Lengthy course
   b. Rapid resolution
   c. Extensive rehabilitation
   d. Debilitating sequelae
5. For children up to 6 years of age, the most effective standardized method of testing cerebral, motor, and cerebellar function is the:
   a. Boyd Developmental Progress Scale
   b. Developmental Attainment Form
   c. Denver Developmental Screening Test
   d. Guide to Normal Milestones of Development
6. In addition to preventing any strain on the suture line of a newly repaired cleft lip, a nurse implements measures that:
   a. Prevent speech defects
   b. Prevent crush formation
   c. Deter hemorrhage
   d. Discourage the use of straws or plastic cups
7. A BRAT diet for diarrhea consists of:
   a. Bananas (fresh), rice cereal, applesauce (canned), and tea (weak)
   b. Baked potatoes, rice cereal, applesauce (canned), and toast
   c. Bananas (fresh), rice cereal, applesauce (canned), and toast
   d. Bananas (fresh), rice cereal, applesauce (infant), and toast
8. When admitting a patient who is thought to have a coarctation of the aorta, a nurse identifies the characteristic:
   a. Excessive clubbing of the toes
   b. Lower blood pressure in the lower extremities
   c. Bounding femoral pulses
   d. Thready, poor-quality radial pulses
9. When working with the parents of children with cyanotic heart disease, it is important for nurses to stress the need for prophylactic antibiotics to decrease the likelihood of:
   a. Congestive heart failure
   b. Infections
   c. Pneumonia
   d. Bacterial endocarditis
10. The loss of consciousness or the "TET" spells demonstrated by an infant with tetralogy of Fallot can be relieved by:
    a. Placing the infant in the knee-chest position
    b. Keeping the baby prone
    c. Maintaining a high-Fowler's position
    d. Elevating the head of the crib 30 degrees
11. A urinary tract infection in a child often is closely associated with:
    a. Toilet training
    b. Difficulty in urination
    c. Vesicoureteral reflux
    d. Hydronephrosis
12. The parents of a child with nephrotic syndrome frequently relate that they have observed:
    a. Increased urination
    b. Frothy, foamy urine
    c. Increased appetite
    d. Listlessness

XII

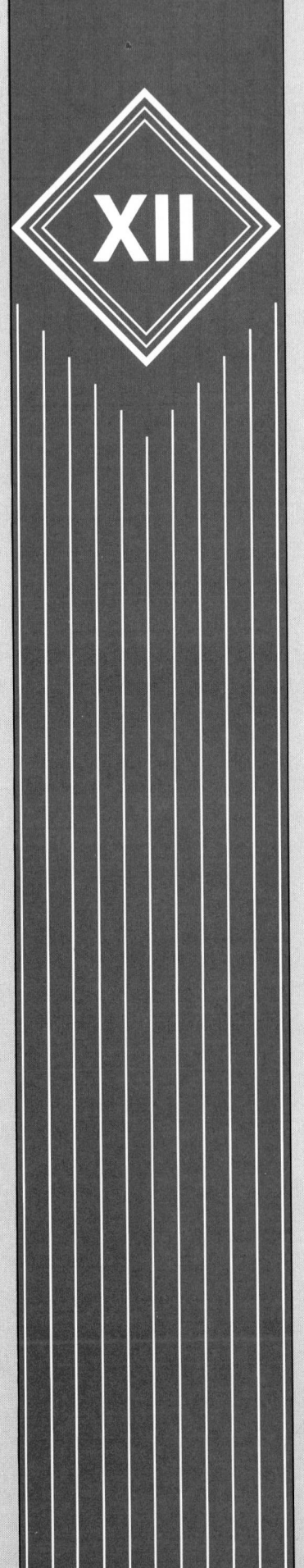

Geriatric Nursing

Nursing may be just a profession for some. I feel very sorry for these people. Nursing can be the most rewarding career of any field. There is no greater feeling in the world than when you have cared for a patient to the best of your knowledge and when you leave the room your patient says, “Thank you honey, you’ve really made my day.” Little do they know, but they have made my day also! It is a feeling you can’t describe with words. It is a total, all natural high. Only in the nursing profession can this be experienced. My only wish for fellow nursing students is that one day you feel “that” feeling.

TERESA SHARP
Student Nurse

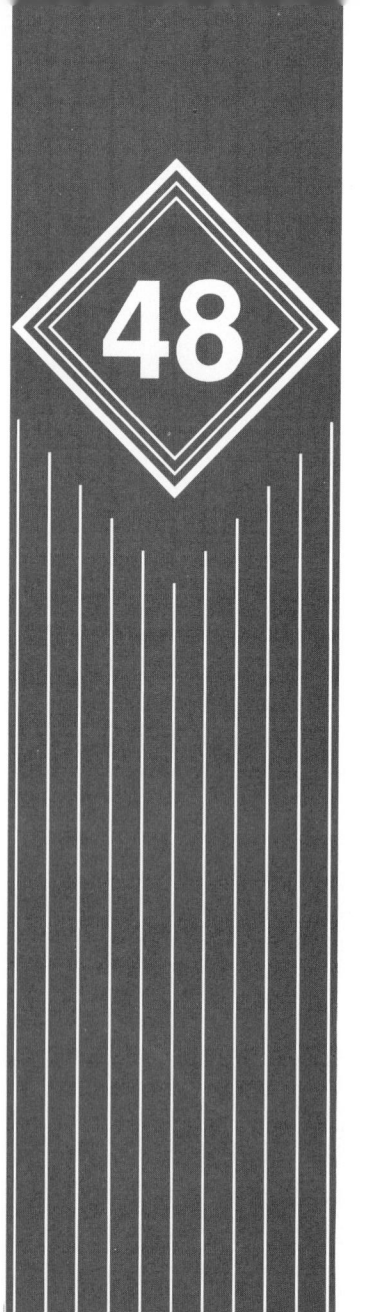

48

Care of the Aging

LINDA CUTCHEN-CLARK

LEARNING OBJECTIVES

After reading this chapter the student should be able to do the following:

- Define the key terms.
- Identify demographic information about the elderly population in the United States.
- Identify some of the common myths concerning the elderly.
- Describe biological and psychosocial theories of aging.
- Describe changes associated with aging for each of the body systems.
- Describe appropriate nursing interventions for common health concerns of the elderly.
- Describe how elders differ from younger individuals in their response to illness, medications, and hospitalization.
- Describe why finances and housing are major concerns for the elderly.
- Identify changes that occur with aging in intelligence, learning, and memory.
- Describe common psychosocial events that occur to the elderly.
- Describe ways to preserve dignity and to increase self-esteem of the elderly.

RELATED TOPICS OF INTEREST

- The family (Chapter 7)
- The adult (Chapter 11)
- Care of the patient with a cardiovascular or blood disorder (Chapter 32)
- Care of the patient with a respiratory disorder (Chapter 34)
- Care of the patient with an endocrine disorder (Chapter 35)
- Care of the patient with a neurological disorder (Chapter 38)
- Dying and death (Chapter 55)

KEY TERMS

Define the following:

- acuity
- aphasia
- ataxia
- atelectasis
- akinesia
- claudication
- chronological age
- collagen
- COPD
- dementia
- dysarthria
- dysphagia
- hemianopsia
- hemiplegia
- kyphosis
- lentigo
- matrix
- nocturia
- periodontal
- presbyopia
- presbycusis
- pruritus
- pyrosis
- senility
- shearing

OVERVIEW OF THE AGING ADULT

Description

Late adulthood is recognized as beginning between the ages of 55 and 65 and covering the remaining years until death. This could represent a span of 40 years or more. It may be more appropriate to think of late adulthood as several periods, including young elderly who are in their late fifties and sixties, elderly who are in their seventies, frail elderly who are over 80, and centenarians who are over 100 years of age.

Although late adulthood is tied to a chronological age, it is important to note that **chronological age** is a very poor indicator of old age. Some individuals are "old" in their fifties, and others in their nineties are physically and mentally active, involved contributors to society. Generally, people do not see themselves or others as being "old" if they are active and healthy.

Demographics

Currently there are approximately 30 million individuals over 65 years of age. This represents 12% of the United States population. Approximately 60% are women and 40% are men. The majority are Caucasian (90.5%). African-Americans and other races represent 9.5% of the elderly. It is projected that by the year 2020, 30% of the population will be over the age of 65.

Myths and Realities

The myths and stereotypes of aging and the elderly are numerous (Box 48-1). Most myths are generalizations that focus on the negative aspects of aging. In many cases research has proved such myths to be inaccurate.

Theories of Aging

Our current knowledge about aging and the aging process is very limited. In an attempt to explain aging and a person's response to aging, a number of theories have been proposed. Some of the biological and psychosocial theories of aging are listed in Box 48-2. Biological theories attempt to explain why the body ages; psychosocial theories try to give reasons for the responses and interactions the elderly have with society during late adulthood.

BODY SYSTEMS, AGING, AND RELATED NURSING INTERVENTIONS

All systems of the body experience age-related changes. The degree and rate at which changes occur vary among individuals, systems, and organs, as

BOX 48-1 COMMON MYTHS ASSOCIATED WITH AGING

Myth: All people become senile when they become old.
Reality: Studies and evidence indicate that decline is not inevitable. Creativity and intelligence do not appear to change. Memory and learning ability may show slight decline, since they are functions of the nervous system, which does experience some age-related changes. Serious decline in mental capabilities is generally a result of disease process—not age.

Myth: Old people are isolated and alone.
Reality: Studies have shown that the majority of elders have at least weekly contact with family. Many live within a half-hour's drive of at least one family member. Although it is assumed that the family is the main support and source of social activity, many older people have also developed a network of friends who provide support and relationships.

Myth: Most elderly are in nursing homes or care facilities.
Reality: Only 5% of elderly persons reside in hospitals or nursing homes. The majority of elderly own and live in their own homes.

Myth: Old people are poor.
Reality: While the poverty rate for people over 65 (12%) is above that of the rest of the population (10.5%), it is interesting to note that the median net worth of older households was over $60,000, compared with the U.S. average for other households of $32,000. The net worth for 16% of older households was below $5,000 and for 7% was above $250,000.

Myth: Old people are ill and disabled.
Reality: Most older people have at least one chronic condition, but these conditions generally do not limit their ability to manage their household and activities of daily living. In a study of noninstitutionalized elderly, approximately 7 of 10 individuals reported their health as "good" or "excellent" as compared with that of others their own age.

BOX 48-2 COMMON THEORIES OF AGING

BIOLOGICAL	
Programmed aging	Cells in the body can reproduce only 40 to 60 times. Aging takes place when more and more cells can no longer regenerate themselves.
Error	An error in protein synthesis causes successive errors in cells of the body, resulting in decline in biological functions.
Immunological	Through the immune system becoming less effective and/or less able to distinguish between foreign and host cells, aging occurs as a result of less protection from infection or disease and the immune system destroying body cells that it misreads as defective or foreign.
Free radical	In the metabolism of the body to produce energy, extra electrons are released that build up in the body and combine chemically, damaging cells and interfering with normal body function, resulting in aging.
Wear and tear	Cells of the body wear out from internal and external stress, which can include chemical damage, trauma, or dysfunction of body systems and buildup of waste products.
PSYCHOSOCIAL	
Erikson's developmental stages	In the last stage of life the task is acceptance of life and one's own life-style, which can result in ego integrity. Inability to achieve a level of acceptance results in anger and despair.
Disengagement theory	Aging is the process in which the elderly and society mutually withdraw from one another.
Exchange theory	Aging is reduced interaction between elders and society as a result of the decreasing value that interaction has for both.
Activity theory	Aging is a result of decreasing involvement of elders in the activities and events of the world.

does a person's ability to compensate. For each body system there are changes and conditions that are more commonly found in the elderly, and these changes produce needs and interventions that may be unique to the older individual. In this chapter the most common nursing diagnoses are identified and interventions given that focus on the older individual, but in all cases additional nursing diagnoses and interventions may be appropriate to meet the individual needs of the elder, or there may be interventions that would be appropriate regardless of age and that are discussed in other chapters.

Integumentary System

Age-related changes. The majority of age-related changes in the integumentary system are apparent to most people: the lack of pigment in the hair (graying); thinning hair and baldness; less **collagen** and elasticity in the skin, with less fat under the skin (wrinkles); age spots (**lentigo**); thinning of the epidermis and reduced numbers of oil and sweat glands (dry skin); and increased fragility of blood vessels (bruising).

Common concerns and nursing interventions

Pruritus. Elderly persons may complain of dryness and itching **(pruritus)** of the skin, especially in cold dry weather, because of reduced glandular secretions and moisture. The nursing diagnosis would be impaired skin integrity. Appropriate interventions would focus on the avoidance of activities and substances that would cause further drying of the tissues. Soap can be drying to the skin; this is true even of soaps designed for dry skin and of the residue left after incomplete rinsing. Older individuals should use soap sparingly. For sedentary elderly, bathing once or twice a week with partial baths at other times may be sufficient, because the normal body oils and perspiration are reduced. Water-based or light oil-based substances should replace alcohol rubs and alcohol-based substances for skin care. Application of water-based lotions to dry areas and after bathing can improve most individuals' comfort and avoid the oily feeling that some persons find uncomfortable.

Decubitus ulcers. Thin skin and lack of subcutaneous fat predispose elderly to decubitus ulcers when fragile skin is compressed between bony prominences of the body and other objects. The fragile skin of the elderly also bruises and tears easily. The major nursing diagnosis associated with decubitus ulcers is impaired skin integrity. Interventions include actions that will prevent pressure, friction, **shearing** forces, and moisture (most commonly associated with incontinence). Pressure points can best be prevented by frequent repositioning. There are many types of pads and aids available that are said to prevent pressure, but it is important to use aids that will minimize pressure without restricting circulation or creating pressure on surrounding areas.

The most common situation resulting in friction occurs when fragile skin rubs against the sheets of the bed. Besides the normal safety precautions taken to prevent injury to any patient, gentle handling during turning and transfers is required. It may be necessary to use additional assistance or equipment to adequately lift and move a patient rather than risk friction "burns" and tearing of the skin while trying to reposition a patient in bed. The use of tape on the skin of the elderly should be minimized, because the fragile skin can easily be torn in the process of removing tape. Urine, drainage, or fecal material left in contact with the skin even for a short period of time can cause it to break down. This can accelerate the formation of decubitus ulcers when it occurs at a pressure point such as the coccyx or hip. Urine, drainage, or fecal material should be removed and the skin washed, rinsed with clear water, and patted dry.

Prevention and healing of any decubiti depend on good nutritional status. A well-balanced diet with attention to protein, vitamins, and minerals is an important intervention for skin integrity in the elderly.

Gastrointestinal System

Age-related changes. Elderly persons experience a decreased secretion of saliva and enzymes in the intestinal tract, atrophy and decreased tone of the intestine, and decreased peristalsis. The normal changes of aging may be intensified by medications commonly prescribed for other conditions, lack of fluids, and lack of exercise. Elders also have a less active gag response, which increases the chances of choking and aspiration.

Common concerns and nursing interventions

Nutrition and obesity. Obesity is defined as weighing 20% over ideal body weight and is commonplace in the elderly. It would be prudent and perfectly normal for elders to consume less food than they did in their earlier, more physically active years. Expressed as the general nursing diagnosis altered nutrition, more than body requirements, the interventions would focus on reducing calories while providing the necessary nutrients in a diet acceptable to the elder. Adults 75 to 90 years of age need approximately 30 calories per kilogram of body weight (14 cal/lb), compared with 40 calories per kilogram (18 cal/lb) for persons 20 to 37 years of age. This normally represents a diet of 1800 to 2400 calories daily, depending on sex and ideal weight. With the reduction in calories, elders need to consume "quality foods" such as grains, vegetables, and fruits, which contain vitamins and minerals to meet their daily needs without large amounts of sugars and fats. Elders also need foods that provide protein and are good sources of calcium. In assisting an elder with a reduced-calorie diet, the nurse should keep in mind foods that may be poorly tolerated as a result of changes in the digestive tract, the elder's inability to eat certain foods because of dentures, difficulty in chewing and swallowing, and what the elder defines as acceptable to eat or individual food preferences.

Unless there is a medical condition requiring supplementation, a well-balanced diet precludes the need for daily vitamin supplements.

Weight loss. A very gradual weight loss over the later years is a normal response to loss of body mass associated with changes of body composition of fat, muscle, and fluid. A rapid weight loss may indicate illness and should be reported to the elder's physician.

Fluids/dehydration. Fluids are necessary for the body to function and remove waste products of metabolism. It is important for an elderly person to have a minimum of 1,500 ml of fluids daily. Frequently elderly individuals decrease fluid intake as a means of controlling incontinence when they have difficulty with mobility, which affects their ability to get to the bathroom, undress, and dress. Others have difficulty with hand grasp, so that pouring and drinking from a cup are difficult.

The general nursing diagnosis would be fluid volume deficit, and the interventions would depend on the cause of the deficit. If the deficit is caused by the elder trying to control occurrences of incontinence resulting from an inability to get to the bathroom in time, the most appropriate interventions would be to make arrangements to have fluids available *and* toilet facilities easily accessible. This can be done by arranging the room so that access to the bathroom is unobstructed; the elder is assisted to the bathroom on a scheduled basis, or a commode or urinal is kept where the elder can easily use it. Elders who have a fluid deficit because of difficulty picking up a cup or drinking may find one of the specially adapted cups with a double handle or a cutout for the nose to be a wonderful solution for a person who has difficulty bending his neck. Elders who are confused may need to be prompted to drink, and elders with severe impairments may need to be assisted to drink fluids on a scheduled basis.

Oral hygiene and dentures. Because many elderly people have dentures, people assume that it is normal to lose one's teeth during old age. However, it is not part of the normal aging process to lose teeth. Poor oral hygiene, untreated **periodontal** disease, and the fact that today's elder population matured before the introduction of many modern methods of dental prophylaxis are factors in the current elderly population having dentures. In the future, with good oral hygiene practices throughout life, many people will maintain their natural teeth for life.

The need for mouth care is generally related to the nursing diagnosis of self-care deficit or knowledge deficit. Recommended mouth care for the elderly consists of a thorough cleansing of all mouth structure with a soft-bristled toothbrush or foam-stick applicators in the early morning and at bedtime. Mouth care is also important when an elder has dentures. In addition to cleaning the dentures, the gums and tongue should be brushed and the mouth rinsed.

Loss of appetite. Elders may also experience or complain of a loss of appetite. Changes in taste resulting from decreased numbers of taste buds and saliva may make food taste different and less appealing. Missing teeth make chewing difficult and tiring. Loose-fitting dentures makes chewing difficult and can allow food under the denture resulting in lesions—both of which will decrease a person's desire to eat. The possible nursing diagnosis might be altered oral mucous membranes or altered nutrition, less than body requirements. Interventions begin with oral hygiene to eliminate debris that can interfere with taste or cause lesions. If dentures are in poor condition and fit poorly, interventions may include referral for dental services.

Interventions that may be appropriate when an elder is not eating adequately because of less taste or interest in food might include preparing the food using color and garnishes, using attractive dishes and table settings with good lighting and bright colors, and providing foods that have more seasoning if there are no restrictions. Homemade frozen dinners made from extra portions of an elder's favorite meal can be an easy and effective way to provide an interesting meal.

For individuals who have impaired mobility or activity intolerance that interferes with their ability to prepare food, community-based programs such as Meals-on-Wheels or home-delivered meals from a senior nutrition site can be a source of prepared meals. Also, a wide variety of fresh, canned, and frozen foods in small or single servings are available in stores.

For most individuals eating is also associated with a social setting, and food is less appealing when an individual eats alone. Older individuals may have lost their spouses, or they may be unable to leave their home. Common nursing diagnoses involve emotional reactions or altered relationships and might be expressed as hopelessness, grieving, or social isolation. Appropriate interventions would depend on the nursing diagnosis. For some individuals, listening to the radio or watching television at meal time or having a pet nearby to talk to during the meal can help to relieve some of the loneliness. Another option may be for the elder to participate in a congregate meal program in the community. This senior citizen program provides transportation, meals, and an opportunity for the elderly to socialize.

Pyrosis (heartburn) and food intolerance. It is not unusual for elders to complain of "heartburn," "sour stomach," and "gas." The nursing diagnosis may be pain after eating; this pain is frequently the result of a food intolerance or reflux of food into the esophagus. Reflux occurs when the sphincter at the proximal end of the stomach becomes less efficient, allowing food and digestive enzymes to flow back into the esophagus and cause irritation. Reflux can be controlled by eating small meals, avoiding eating before bedtime, and elevating the head of the bed by placing 4-inch blocks under the legs of the bed.

Lactose, which is the most common food substance to which individuals develop an intolerance, is primarily found in milk. Normally, the solution would be to avoid milk in the diet, but milk is a major source of calcium. A better answer would be to substitute other milk products, such as cheese and yogurt, that have been processed in such a way that they are better digested by lactose-intolerant individuals.

Dysphagia. Difficulty in swallowing (dysphagia) can be caused by neurological or vascular conditions that interfere with the coordination of swallowing. The major nursing intervention would be planning an appropriate diet, because it is usually more difficult for the elder to swallow fluids or foods such as soup, which contain firm foods in liquid, than semisolid or solid food.

A technique to assist swallowing involves sitting the individual up straight or slightly forward, chin down, and placing small amounts of moderately textured food in the mouth. This technique can help prevent aspiration and reduces swallowing difficulty.

Constipation. The elderly are prone to constipation as a result of the decreases in intestinal secretions and mobility, but fiber in the diet, fluids, and exercise are generally adequate measures for normal function. The general nursing diagnosis would be constipation. Nursing interventions would be to ensure adequate fluids, exercise, and a diet that contains fiber. If dietary fiber needs to be increased and the elder is unable to eat enough vegetables and fruits, a good source of fiber for the elderly is bran. Depending on the normal diet of the elder, up to 10 g of bran per day should be included in cereals, muffins, or breads or sprinkled over other foods. This can be achieved if the daily meals include 2 slices of whole-grain bread, 2 bran muffins or biscuits, and 2 spoonfuls of bran added to or sprinkled over other foods.

Urinary System

Age-related changes. Overall kidney function decreases with age. The number of functioning glomeruli is decreased approximately 50%. Even with this decrease the body has considerable reserve to support normal body functions unless kidney disease is present. Bladder capacity decreases approximately 50%, so that it may only hold 150 ml. The bladder and sphincters lose elasticity and are less responsive to the stimulus to urinate. Men commonly experience enlargement of the prostate gland.

Common concerns and nursing interventions

Nocturia. At least 50% of elderly men and 70% of elderly women have to get up two or more times during the night to empty their bladders (**nocturia**). This can be caused by age-related changes or medical conditions. The most significant age-related change is the decrease in bladder capacity. A decrease of bladder tone may also cause urine to remain in the bladder on emptying, causing a person to experience the sensation of a full bladder (frequency) within a brief period. Incomplete emptying of the bladder can also occur if a male has benign hypertrophy of the prostate gland, which causes the gland to enlarge, constricting the urethra and flow of urine. While nocturia does not jeopardize an individual's physical health, it is inconvenient, interferes with sleep, and can contribute to fatigue. Significant interruptions of sleep may generate the nursing diagnosis of sleep pattern disturbance. In such situations, nursing interventions would focus on decreasing or controlling nocturia by limiting fluids in the evening, taking diuretic medications in the morning, and minimizing the hazards for falls when an individual has to get up to urinate. A history of nocturia or an increase in the number of episodes would require medical evaluation, because it may indicate infection and the need for medical treatment.

Incontinence. Another related problem for many elderly individuals is incontinence. There are elders who will not leave their home for fear they will have an "accident" in public.

Having given birth, age-related changes in muscles and ligaments, and increased abdominal pressure can cause older women to experience incontinence when they laugh, cough, or sneeze. A common age-related problem is a decrease in the time between when an individual perceives the urge to urinate and the actual relaxation of the sphincters; therefore older men and women who have problems with mobility may experience incontinence when it takes them longer to get to the bathroom.

Nursing interventions for the nursing diagnosis of stress incontinence begins with an understanding that an elder is not trying to get attention by requesting to go to the bathroom frequently or is incontinent by choice. At no time should an elder be reprimanded or humiliated for having to urinate or having "accidents." It is more appropriate to make certain that an elder has frequent and easy access to a bathroom or a urinal or commode. Active, ambulatory elderly may feel comfortable going out in public if fitted with external collection devices, pants liners, or absorbent briefs.

Cardiovascular System

Age-related changes. The heart's muscle tissue loses fibers and strength with age. The valves of the heart become thick and more rigid. Nerve conduction and coordination is less efficient in the pacemaker of the heart. Cardiac output decreases approximately 1% each year after the age of 25 as heart contractions become weaker. It takes longer for the heart to contract and longer for the atria to fill. The heart is also less capable of de[illegible] with stress; typically it takes longer for the pulse t to normal after exercise. The vessels of the heart and body become less elastic and show calcification (arteriosclerosis) with advancing age. Systolic blood pressure generally rises to compensate for the increased resistance and loss of elasticity of vessels.

Common concerns and nursing interventions

Dysrhythmias. Changes in the structure of and blood supply to the heart and the pacemaker system may make the heart more susceptible to irregular heart rhythms (dysrhythmias). The dysrhythmias will cause the heart to be less effective in supplying blood to the body and can lead to heart failure. While the dysrhythmias and heart failure can be treated by the physician, the nursing diagnosis of decreased cardiac output will require nursing interventions such as observing the response to treatment by checking vital signs frequently, noting the characteristics of the pulse, accurately monitoring fluid intake and output, and observing and reporting the elder's response to medications. Other nursing interventions include minimizing stress on the heart by monitoring the elder's response to activity and providing appropriate rest periods before and after activity. (See Chapter 32 for more specific information regarding nursing interventions for cardiac conditions.)

Peripheral vascular disease. Vascular changes affect the arteries or veins of the elderly. Arterial conditions can be caused by spasms or atherosclerosis, which cause insufficient amounts of blood to tissues in the legs and feet. The elder may complain of cold feet, cramping (intermittent **claudication**), and numbness. Weakening of muscles and loss of elasticity in the veins are responsible for the most common venous condition in the elderly—varicose veins. The most common nursing diagnosis for peripheral vascular conditions would be altered peripheral tissue perfusion. Nursing interventions would include techniques to promote circulation, including walking to stimulate venous return, not standing in one place for long periods, and avoiding constriction of leg vessels, which occurs by crossing the legs or knotting stockings to hold them up. For varicose veins, elastic stockings are generally used to give veins needed support.

Other nursing diagnoses associated with peripheral vascular disease may be potential for infection and potential for impaired skin integrity. Nursing interventions would include cleanliness of the feet and legs; adequate shoes that will give protection, but not bind or rub; and teaching the elder to be aware of situations that may cause injury, because sensation for hot and cold is decreased.

Respiratory System

Age-related changes. The tissues of the lungs and bronchi become less elastic and more rigid with age. The chest wall is less able to expand because of changes in the skeletal system, such as **kyphosis** and calcification. Muscles associated with respiration are weakened, so that lung expansion and vital capacity are decreased. Overall, air exchange is reduced and secretions and residual air remain in the lungs.

Common concerns and nursing interventions

Chronic obstructive lung disease (COPD). A common respiratory condition of the elderly, **COPD,** is not a single disease but commonly a combination of chronic bronchitis, chronic asthma, and emphysema in varying degrees that result in progressive changes that are seen as individuals become older. By age 90 nearly everyone has some degree of emphysema; therefore the disease and the age-related changes cause most elders to experience some degree of COPD.

Nursing diagnoses would be ineffective airway clearance and impaired gas exchange and might also include ineffective breathing pattern. Nursing interventions for elders with mild to moderate COPD include measures to liquefy secretions through adequate intake of fluids and removal of secretions by teaching proper coughing technique to improve airway clearance. Interventions for impaired gas exchange would be the avoidance of smoking and areas of heavy air pollution, proper administration of prescribed medication, prevention of respiratory infections, and encouraging low-stress exercise such as walking for physical conditioning and breathing. Patient education in breathing techniques may help improve ineffective breathing patterns.

Since respiratory function affects many other systems and the functional ability of the individual, other nursing diagnoses and interventions may be appropriate for a patient with COPD; these are discussed in Chapter 34.

Pneumonia. Age-related changes and decreased resistance to respiratory infections cause more older individuals to contract pneumonia and die from pneumonia than persons of younger age groups. Even with modern antibiotics and sophisticated medical treatment, pneumonia can be life threatening for the elderly. This is especially true if an elder is hospitalized and has other chronic illnesses.

The nurse should recognize that elderly individuals do not always exhibit the usual signs and symptoms of pneumonia, such as high fever, cough, pain, and headache. Older individuals may show signs and symptoms only of lethargy, confusion, anorexia, and low or mild fever. Elders showing such signs and symptoms should be seen by a physician for appropriate treatment.

As with other respiratory conditions, nursing diagnoses would be ineffective airway clearance and impaired gas exchange. Interventions would be to liquefy secretions through adequate intake of fluids and prescribed medications, assisting removal of secretions by teaching proper coughing technique to improve airway clearance, and turning and deep breathing to improve gas exchange and prevent stasis of secretions.

Musculoskeletal System

Age-related changes. Some of the most obvious changes associated with aging occur in the musculoskeletal system. There is a reduction in the number and size of active muscle fibers with decreased muscle strength. The joints become less elastic and flexible with the loss and calcification of cartilage. There is demineralization and loss of supporting bone **matrix** in the skeleton. In the spine, changes in the bone structure and compression of intravertebral disks result in postural changes such as kyphosis.

Common concerns and nursing interventions

Arthritis. Two forms of arthritis may be found in the elderly. Rheumatoid arthritis, a systemic disease thought to be of immune factor origin, can affect persons of any age but is most common after the age of 60. Osteoarthritis, or degenerative joint disease, is a noninflammatory disorder in which the cartilage in the joints deteriorates and new bone forms on the surface. It is thought to be a normal response to aging. It is estimated that more than 90% of the population 40 years of age or older are affected, although a person may not experience symptoms for many years.

The primary nursing diagnoses will be impaired physical mobility and pain. Other nursing diagnoses may be (1) self-care deficits in bathing/hygiene, feeding, dressing/grooming; (2) impaired home maintenance management; (3) impaired social interaction; or (4) ineffective individual coping, since the chronic nature of arthritis affects the individual's functional ability and life-style. Interventions for elderly individuals with arthritis involve relieving stress on the affected joints through the use of rest and assistive devices such as splints, walkers, adapted utensils, and clothes with Velcro fasteners (Fig. 48-1). Range of motion and other forms of mild exercise are recommended to maintain muscle strength and joint motion. Heat and gentle massage can help to control pain and muscle spasms, and analgesic medications may be administered.

Osteoporosis. Generally considered a normal aging process because it is so common in the elderly, osteoporosis

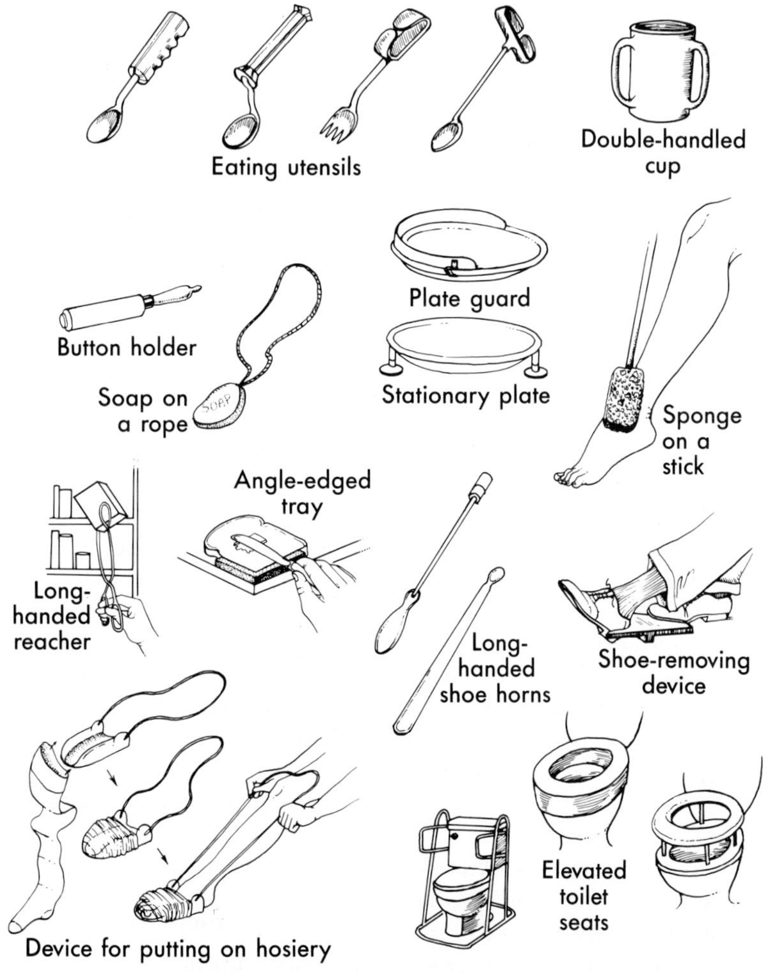

FIG. 48-1 Assistive devices for the elderly.

is a disease in which the bones become more porous and easily fractured. The cause is unknown, but it appears strongly related to estrogen deficiencies and low calcium levels in the blood. Most common symptoms are skeletal deformities from vertebral fractures and pain in the back or extremities from compression of nerves. Hip and wrist fractures are also common with falls.

Prevention in earlier years by eating a healthy diet, maintaining the recommended calcium intake, and engaging in weight-bearing activities is recognized as much more effective for retaining bone than any treatment later in life to replace bone once it has been lost.

A nursing diagnosis for an elder with osteoporosis might be health-seeking behaviors. The goal would be to improve the elder's health status. Interventions would include exercise in the form of walking or swimming to stimulate the formation of bone and avoidance of heavy lifting and bending to prevent vertebral fractures. Increasing the calcium intake to 1,200 to 1,500 mg per day would help to reduce bone loss.

Falls. Falls are the leading cause of accidental death in individuals over the age of 65. The consequences of falls are much more serious for the elderly than for younger people, because elders are more likely to be injured in the fall. Because of age-related changes in the musculoskeletal system, fractures are frequently the outcome of a fall.

Falls can result from disease processes and age-related changes with advanced age. Decreased circulation to the brain; diminished coordination, space, and position perception; decreased ability to balance; decreased muscle strength; changes in gait; and slowed nervous system response are some of the major factors contributing to falls in the elderly. Other factors include limited activity, side effects of medications, confusion, and environmental hazards such as low-light situations and objects obstructing the pathway.

Potential for injury is the related nursing diagnosis. Appropriate interventions are to provide an environment that is free of hazards, increased lighting for the decreased vision of the elderly, and assistive devices such as walkers and canes to aid balance. Other adaptations would be raised toilet seats, handrails on stairs, and grab bars in the bathroom to prevent falls (see Fig. 48-1). Elders should also be taught to sit on the side of the bed when they arise and to stand for several minutes before walking as a technique to cope with orthostatic hypotension that may be caused by poor vascular perfusion or medications.

Endocrine System

Age-related changes. The levels of hormones secreted and the response of body tissue to hormones change with age. A decrease in thyroid activity causes a lower basal metabolism rate. A reduction in pituitary hormone (ACTH) levels causes a decrease of adrenal gland function and reduced levels of steroids, progesterone, androgen, and estrogen. There is a gradual decrease in the release of testosterone, estrogen, and progesterone from the gonads. The beta cells in the pancreas produce a slow and insufficient release of insulin.

Common concerns and nursing intervention

Non-insulin-dependent diabetes mellitus. Two general types of diabetes are recognized: Type I or insulin-dependent diabetes mellitus (IDDM), in which the body fails to produce insulin, and Type II or non-insulin-dependent diabetes mellitus (NIDDM), considered to be the body's inability to produce and utilize insulin appropriately. Eighty-five percent to 90% of all adult diabetics have NIDDM, which often begins in middle age and does not always exhibit the usual symptoms of thirst, increased appetite, and large amounts of urine, as seen in IDDM. In the elderly, repeated infections, slow healing, and sensory and nervous system dysfunctions may be the more common signs.

The goal for interventions in NIDDM is to achieve and maintain a normal metabolic state through diet management, weight control, and exercise. Specific nursing diagnoses and interventions for diabetes are discussed in Chapter 35. In working with the elderly, the nurse should assist in adapting the diet, with as little change as possible to encourage compliance. Intake should be balanced, with recommended amounts of protein, carbohydrates, fats, vitamins, and minerals. Refined sugars should be avoided and a high-fiber diet is encouraged. The other aspects of care, especially important for the elderly, include preventing complications through blood testing to monitor glucose levels, good foot care, and instituting safety precautions to prevent injury and infections.

Reproductive System

Age-related changes. The major changes in the reproductive system related to aging are the diminished levels of male and female hormones—estrogen and progesterone in women and androgen and testosterone in men. The process of aging diminishes sexual function but does not preclude it. Although it takes longer for a man to be sexually aroused and achieve erection and ejaculation, men maintain the ability for sexual function into their eighties and nineties. For women, menopause is marked by a decrease in hormones, with tissue atrophy of the ovaries, fallopian tubes, cervix, and vulva. There is a decrease in the amount of vaginal secretions and the pH becomes more alkaline. Although age-related changes occur, they do not diminish the elderly woman's capacity to achieve orgasm and enjoy sexual relations.

Common concerns and nursing interventions

Sexual function. The misconceptions that elderly are impotent and asexual or that elderly are perverse if they are sexually active are probably the most common reasons for sexual dysfunction in the elderly. It has generally been found that if individuals continue to be sexually active on a regular basis, they retain the capability to respond sexually. In situations in which an elder indicates that sexual intercourse is difficult or uncomfortable because of vaginal dryness, the use of estrogen creams or water-soluble lubricants can relieve the discomfort.

Research and information from a variety of sources indicate that aging individuals have the potential to be sexual, continue to have interest in sex, and are indeed sexual beings. For many elderly, the lack of a sexual partner is the main factor for decreased sexual activity.

Sexuality also encompasses sexual identity as a man or woman, intimacy (emotional closeness to others), and touch. Regardless of age, it is important to feel good about oneself as a male or female and to have close relationships with other people.

The nurse must examine personal feelings about sexuality and the elderly and must become informed about age-related changes in sexual function to dispel misinformation. Sexuality of the elderly can also be supported by encouraging and helping them to look their best, complimenting them when they look nice, respecting and allowing them to have privacy, not ridiculing elders if they show affection for one another, and using touch to communicate acceptance. A pat on the arm or a hug can be a way of communicating concern and caring to almost anyone.

Special Senses

Age-related changes. Age-related changes in vision include **presbyopia,** or narrowing of the peripheral field of vision, decreased accommodation to near objects, and a decrease in visual **acuity** as the pupil becomes smaller and is less responsive to light. Depth perception is distorted and vision in dim light becomes difficult. There is some clouding of the lens of the eye. Yellowing of the lens and changes in color perception cause elders to have difficulty differentiating shades of the same color and colors such as green, blue, and violet. Although the age-related changes decrease visual capability, blindness is not a normal result of aging.

Age-related changes in hearing include **presbycusis,** which is the normal loss of hearing acuity, speech intelligibility, auditory threshold, and pitch associated with aging.

Hearing sensitivity decreases with age. The eardrum loses elasticity, the ossicles of the middle ear become more rigid, and there is atrophy of auditory nerve and end-organs in the inner ear. Because of exposure to a variety of loud noises throughout life and age-related changes, older individuals may have hearing losses of different tones, causing some sounds to be distorted and others to be absent.

Age-related changes affecting the sense of touch and position include a decrease in the number of receptor cells throughout the skin and joints. Elders have increasing difficulty sensing temperature and maintaining balance, which places them at risk for burns and falls.

The effects of aging on smell and taste are relatively minor. Olfactory receptors decline in number, which may reduce or alter a person's ability to smell. There is also a decrease in the number of taste buds, although it has not been proved to what degree taste is actually affected.

Common concerns and nursing interventions

Decreased vision. With increasing age comes decreasing visual capability as a result of the age-related changes previously described. The general nursing diagnosis for decreased vision would be sensory-perceptual alteration. A number of interventions can be used to compensate for age-related changes in vision; the nurse should make sure the patient's eyeglasses are clean and are used, increase the amount of light in the environment, reduce glare by use of shades on windows and lights, and use night lights to avoid abrupt light-to-dark changes. The use of low-vision aids such as large print, strongly contrasting colors (black on a white background), and magnifying glasses can compensate for the decrease in visual acuity.

Decreased hearing. The decreased ability to hear is frequently a frustration to both elders and individuals who are trying to talk to them. Hearing aids may help in situations in which amplification can improve hearing, but hearing aids cannot compensate for nerve damage or effectively screen out other distracting noises. To communicate with an individual with a hearing loss the nurse should speak at a normal or slightly slower pace without exaggerating or shouting, lower the tone of voice since hearing loss is frequently in the higher tones, and eliminate background noise whenever possible. Another effective communication technique is using nonverbal communication such as gestures, smiles, and nodding the head with the verbal message. The nurse should never project annoyance or impatience to the patient who has a hearing loss. Patience and acceptance of the patient are necessary in a therapeutic approach.

Nervous System

Age-related changes. With age there is a decline in the number of peripheral nerve cells and fibers, as well as brain cells. Physiologically, there is a slowing of nerve impulse transmission in the nervous system, resulting in a longer reaction time for the elderly. Autonomic nervous system changes include decreased efficiency in maintaining normal body temperature and in the pulse returning to normal after exercise or stress.

Common concerns and nursing interventions

Insomnia. It is not unusual for elders to state that they are not able to sleep. Studies of sleep patterns in various age-groups show that the sleep pattern changes with age. With aging there are fewer periods of deep sleep and frequent periods of wakefulness, giving the impression of sleeplessness even though the total sleep time is the same or only slightly reduced from that of young adulthood.

Many older people resort to sleeping pills in an attempt to treat their insomnia. Sleeping medications may help a person get to sleep, but they change the normal sleep patterns and may cause a person to wake up more during the night or feel drowsy and lethargic the next day.

Complaints of insomnia represent a nursing diagnosis of sleep pattern disturbance. Nursing interventions to help an elder sleep begin with encouraging a bedtime ritual. For most people this might include brushing the teeth, reading a book or the paper, using a favorite pillow, or listening to the radio. Exercise and activity during the day increase the likelihood of falling asleep at night. Research has also shown that the time it takes to fall asleep is related to the length of time from the last sleep period; therefore elders may find that they can fall asleep at night if they nap in the morning rather than taking an afternoon nap.

Confusion. *Confused* is a word frequently used to describe behavior in the elderly. To many people confusion is the same as **senility** or dementia—conditions that are not reversible. However, the majority of causes of confusion are reversible and should more properly be called *delirium.* Among the many causes of reversible confusion can be anemias, electrolyte imbalances, hypoxia, drugs, sensory deficits, pain, fatigue, crisis, and sensory overload.

If an elder suddenly becomes confused, it is important to look for a cause and have the elder seen by a physician for treatment. When an elder is experiencing delirium, the nursing diagnosis will be altered thought processes. Reality orientation is a useful intervention for delirium. Guidelines for reality orientation include the following:

- Call the patient by his correct name or as he wishes to be called
- Make eye contact
- Converse about familiar subjects
- Provide familiar objects in the elder's environment
- Explain events and procedures in concise, simple language
- Be honest
- Set a routine and be consistent
- Engage the elder in familiar and simple activities that have purpose, such as washing the face or brushing the teeth

A therapeutic dialogue involving reality orientation is provided on p. 1283.

Dementia/Alzheimer's disease. There are several causes of confusion that are irreversible and are considered to be true **dementia.** Almost all cases of dementia are either a result of arteriosclerosis combined with small CVAs or Alzheimer's disease.

Normally seen in individuals over 60 years of age, Alzheimer's disease is a progressive condition in which there is atrophy of the brain. There is loss of cortical neurons, the ventricles are enlarged, and senile plaques and neurofibrillary tangles are found in the cortex of the brain. The onset is gradual, usually beginning with memory failure and difficulty in focusing attention. Although the elder may become anxious about his inability to remember, it may be some time before family members become aware of the decline in mental function. As the disease progresses, memory becomes worse and the elder has difficulty with abstract reasoning and judgment. As mental capabilities decline, behavior deteriorates. The individual becomes less sociable and alert, has less tolerance for change, and may become agitated and untidy. In the late stage of the disease, the individual becomes disoriented as to time, place, and person. Deterioration in both mental and motor function results in incoherent speech and communication difficulties. Loss of motor function creates problems with eating, dressing, and toileting. In the terminal stage, the individual is unable to communicate. There is little or no response to surroundings or recognition of family members. Physically, the patient is unable to walk or control movement, becomes incontinent of urine and feces, and is susceptible to infections.

In dementia, regardless of the cause, the main nursing diagnosis is altered thought processes. Depending on the individual and the stage of the disease, other nursing diagnoses would include self-care deficit, potential for injury, impaired communication, and anxiety.

Interventions related to the nursing diagnoses attempt to maintain the ability of the individual to function. Activities of daily living such as dressing may need to be divided into small steps and explained as they are done in very specific and simple terms. The individual may need to be coached as to what to do when eating and given finger foods or only one item at a time. The environment should be calm, and distracting stimuli should be eliminated. Large groups or complex activities should be avoided, because they may cause the individual to become agitated or have a catastrophic reaction (angry and aggressive behavior, which is an overreaction to a situation with which he cannot cope).

When understanding and communication become impaired, nonverbal communication becomes more important. A calm, pleasant tone of voice, gestures that correspond to the verbal message, and maintaining contact through touch and listening skills should be used. Safety measures to prevent falls must be instituted.

Wandering is a behavior frequently associated with dementia. In some situations it may be an attempt to find the bathroom or familiar surroundings; it may be the individual's way of coping with anxiety. For an individual who is unable to locate the bathroom or his own room, easily read signs with universally accepted symbols and familiar objects can help a person find his way.

Restraining demented individuals can be detrimental and increase agitation. As long as there are safe areas, walking is a good activity for promoting sleep and reducing some of the anxiety and restlessness commonly found in dementia.

Care of an elder with dementia or Alzheimer's disease requires patience and calmness. Routine is very important, and changes should be introduced very slowly. It is important to remember that the individual no longer thinks logically or understands his surroundings.

Parkinson's disease.. Parkinson's disease is second only to cerebral vascular accident as the most common disorder affecting the nervous system in the elderly. It is a progressive, degenerative disease characterized by muscle rigidity, tremors, and **akinesia** (an abnormal state of motor and psychic hypoactivity). The individual has a masklike appearance, drooling, and shuffling gait and may experience emotional instability. In most cases, stress and frustration increase symptoms.

Drug therapy with levodopa, amantadine HCl (Symmetrel), and anticholinergic drugs such as benztropine mesylate (Cogentin) and trihexyphenidyl HCl (Artane) may help to slow the process of the disease or may temporarily improve a patient's condition, but side effects from the drugs can also cause confusion, blurred vision, delirium, and drowsiness.

Nursing diagnoses associated with Parkinson's disease include impaired physical mobility, potential for injury, and impaired verbal communication. Nursing interventions for an elder with Parkinson's disease include observing the response to drug therapy and maintaining mobility through exercise and activity. Range-of-motion exercises and massage help to relieve muscle spasms and maintain joint mobility. Interventions for a safe environment such as removing throw rugs and furniture from walkways, having hand rails or objects that will not tip over if the elder uses them to support himself, and good lighting are important, because the lack of balance and other characteristics of the disease can contribute to falls and injuries. The use of mobility aids such as canes and walkers as well as adaptive aids for activities of daily living can prolong the independence of an individual with Parkinson's disease.

The intellectual function of a person with Parkinson's disease is not impaired, but the tremors and akinesia cause difficulty in communication and much frustration for both the individual and others with whom he is trying to communicate. Giving the individual time to respond, encouraging efforts to communicate, and showing acceptance of the individual through actions and nonverbal communication can help to alleviate some of the feelings of frustration.

Transient ischemic attacks. The changes in the vascular system seen in the elderly include thickening of the vessel walls and the presence to some degree of atherosclerosis and arteriosclerosis. Specific medical diagnoses related to arterial conditions in the elderly are transient ischemic attack (TIA) and cerebrovascular accident (CVA or stroke).

TIAs are small spasms or occlusions in the vessels of the brain. Signs and symptoms of TIA vary, depending on the vessel's location in the brain. The most common signs and symptoms are changes in vision, headache, confusion, **ataxia,** and drop attacks (falling without losing consciousness). If the elder has not been seen by a physician for diagnosis of the symptoms, a referral to a physician for medical evaluation is appropriate.

The nursing diagnosis appropriate for an individual experiencing TIAs is potential for injury. Interventions for this condition would be providing a safe environment by removing hazards, use of safety devices and mobility aids to prevent falls and assist balance, and use of memory aids such as written instructions, schedules, and lists to assist the elder in coping with the confusion.

Cerebrovascular accident. CVAs are the third leading cause of death in the United States and increase in likelihood after 55 years of age. Symptoms of a CVA can include **hemiplegia, dysarthria, dysphasia,** sensory changes such as **hemianopsia, aphasia,** and intellectual and emotional changes. Nursing interventions immediately after the CVA involve support of life functions and are described in Chapter 38.

While some of the initial neurological involvement may disappear in 3 to 6 months, most individuals will have some residual dysfunction. The most common nursing diagnoses are impaired physical mobility, bathing/hygiene self-care deficit, and impaired verbal communication. Interventions will focus on the rehabilitation of the elder to maximize the elder's ability to accomplish activities of daily living and to be as independent as possible. Elders may need to learn to use the nondominant hand because of hemiplegia and may require adaptive and assistive devices for activities of daily living, such as adapted utensils, reaching devices, and pull-on or easily secured clothing (Fig. 48-1). Wheelchairs and canes may be necessary for the weakness, loss of balance, and loss of control of the legs. The nurse encourages or assists the individual to do exercises and activities prescribed by therapists as well as to follow the therapist's suggestions about actions that will be most beneficial for the elder's progress. Communication techniques for elders having aphasia include listening carefully, turning down or decreasing competing stimuli such as the radio or TV, and using pictures and appropriate gestures, speaking slowly, using direct short statements, and not interrupting. With all interventions, the nurse should make sure that the elder is not rushed and is given encouragement and praise for effort as well as success in performing tasks.

HEALTH CARE AND THE AGING ADULT

Symptoms and Illness

Normally we rely on a pattern of signs and symptoms to tell us when we are sick. When we assess a person we expect certain subjective and objective data to indicate illness. Elderly individuals do not always respond to illness in the same way as younger individuals. Elders frequently respond to illness and infections by exhibiting confusion or delirium, falling or postural instability, immobility, and incontinence. A change in behavior of an elder, especially involving the signs and symptoms listed, should be documented and reported. The change may indicate infection or illness long before any of the usual signs and symptoms appear.

Medications

There are some elders who do not take any medication, but others may be taking five or more medications per day (Box 48-3). Approximately 30% of the prescriptions for medication are given to 12% of the population (peo-

BOX 48-3 COMMON GROUPS OF DRUGS USED BY THE ELDERLY

DRUG GROUP	NURSING INTERVENTIONS
Antacids	Observe for signs and symptoms of diarrhea, constipation Teach elder to check sodium and sugar content on the label Encourage elder to take antacid 1 hour after meals and not with other medications Caution with history of cardiac or renal conditions
Antibiotics	Observe for confusion, changes in hearing Encourage fluid intake Monitor weight, intake and output, specific gravity of urine Observe for GI disturbances, diarrhea Observe for secondary yeast or fungal infections of mouth, vagina
Antidepressants/antipsychotics	Observe for tremor, spasms Teach techniques to use with vertigo when changing positions, and methods to counteract dry mouth Caution use with glaucoma, prostate, or cardiac conditions Observe for urinary retention
Antihistamines	Observe for changes in blood pressure Observe for anticholinergic effects—restlessness, delirium Caution use with glaucoma, prostate, or cardiac conditions
Antihypertensives	Observe for depression, anxiety, disorientation Monitor for bradycardia, angina, hypotension
Antiinflammatory agents	Teach importance of taking with food Avoid if there is a history of peptic ulcer Observe for nausea, vomiting, GI bleeding Observe for psychological disturbances
Cardiovascular agents	Explain importance of keeping appointments for laboratory examinations Observe for orthostatic hypotension Monitor heart rate and rhythm Observe for adverse reactions—confusion, depression, vertigo, lethargy
Diuretics	Observe for orthostatic hypotension, delirium, changes in mental function Should be taken in the morning
Narcotics	Observe for hypotension Observe for adverse or idiosyncratic reactions—hallucinations, agitation, confusion Monitor respiratory function
Oral anticoagulants	Monitor prothrombin times Observe for bleeding Explain importance of keeping appointments for laboratory examinations Avoid aspirin-containing products Institute safety measures to prevent injury
Oral hypoglycemic agents	Observe for signs of hypoglycemia—weakness, headache, malaise Monitor blood glucose levels
Tranquilizers/sedatives	Observe for signs of oversedation—lethargy, confusion, agitation Explain the need to avoid other depressants and alcohol Observe for adverse and idiosyncratic reactions—delirium, orthostatic hypotension, cardiac dysrhythmia

ple over 65). Elders also use a high percentage of the over-the-counter (OTC) drugs sold, such as antacids, laxatives, and analgesics; thus the elderly are at risk for adverse side effects and interactions of drugs.

Age-related changes in body function can also contribute to adverse reactions. Research indicates that the body's ability to absorb, transport, and eliminate drugs is decreased with age because of impaired circulation, changes in vessel walls, and a decrease in the number and efficiency of the glomeruli in the kidneys. Metabolism of drugs is also decreased as a result of decreased blood flow in the liver, fewer functioning liver cells, and a decrease in the liver enzymes that function to break down and transform drugs. As a result of all of the changes, many drugs remain in the body longer than in a younger person. Dosages may need to be reduced to prevent toxicity, since the normal adult dosage is for a 150-pound, 20-year-old individual. Many elders also have conditions such as congestive heart failure or kidney disease that further impair the body's ability to metabolize and excrete drugs.

Nursing interventions begin with assisting elders to take their medications properly. Most elders are interested in learning about the medications they are taking and appreciate techniques that will help them take the correct dose at the correct time, such as a chart or pill box with compartments labeled with the time and where the pills can be placed for each time they are to be taken. Nurses must also be alert to the possibility of drug interactions and symptoms of toxicities, which can easily be misinterpreted as "signs of old age." Confusion, fatigue, anorexia, falls, and vertigo are frequently indications of a drug reaction and should be reported to the physician for evaluation.

Hospitalization, Surgery, and Rehabilitation

Illness leading to hospitalization and surgical intervention requires knowledge of the aging process and the effects of anesthesia and immobility. Although responses are very individual, elders have less reserve to cope physically and emotionally with the effects of hospitalization and surgical intervention. They require longer postoperative recovery and convalescent periods, yet during these periods it is very important to minimize the normal effects of immobility on body systems, which can include stasis of secretions, orthostatic hypotension, and digestive and perceptual disorders. This is not to say that people in their eighties and nineties should not undergo surgery, but their rehabilitation should begin as soon as they are stabilized after surgical intervention. Especially important are measures to prevent complications of immobility and techniques to support coping skills and independence of the elder. Turning, deep breathing, coughing or other techniques for ventilation, and removal of respiratory secretions are important with the elderly because of the age-related changes in the respiratory tract that increase the risk of **atelectasis** and pneumonia. Depending on the type of surgery, older individuals should be ambulated within 8 to 24 hours to decrease the risks of stasis in the circulation, kidneys and bladder, and respiratory tract. Getting up, even to stand or take a few steps, can help to stimulate muscle activity, expand the lungs, and improve mental outlook. Older individuals should be encouraged to perform self-care activities but at their own level of tolerance and with rest periods. It is also important to remember that the hospitalization and surgical intervention may increase signs and symptoms of other chronic conditions, such as arthritis, which may be cause for complaints of discomfort or difficulty in doing activities of daily living.

SECURITY AND SAFETY CONCERNS FOR THE AGING ADULT

Finances

When asked what concerns them the most in their later years, elders will usually answer "health" and "finances." The two are frequently related. For the elderly, health care can become a major expense and devastate their financial security. Because of chronic health problems in addition to acute episodes, elders spend a greater percentage of their income on health care than younger individuals do. Many elderly have a fixed income from retirement pensions and only limited savings to pay for the rising costs of housing, food, and health care.

For individuals in lower socioeconomic groups, pensions may not be available, and low salaries and seasonal work prevent the accumulation of finances for later in life or can be insufficient to provide basic needs. A woman who remained at home as a homemaker and did not work outside the home may not have acquired any financial resources of her own and may become indigent when her husband dies.

Financial problems can arise when people have not planned carefully for retirement. Many people assume that adequate pensions will be available if they have to retire or if their spouses die and that Social Security pensions are available to everyone. Unfortunately, this is not true. Retirement planning, including financial planning, needs to begin early in life for both men and women. As people live longer, the retirement period could be as long as 40 years. Much of the planning involves education about the possible problems and options for retirement and financial security in the later years.

There are a number of agencies and senior programs in the community that can help elders who have limited resources. Such programs can include homemaking assistance, legal services, low-cost housing or housing improvement, multiservice senior programs, recreation programs, and information and referral services.

Housing

Housing represents a certain amount of a person's self-concept and status. It is also the largest expenditure in most persons' budgets; therefore it is a concern to many elders.

The majority of elders prefer to remain independent and have their own housing. Approximately 74% of the elderly own the home in which they live and 12% rent their house or apartment. Even when elders own their own home, the cost and difficulty of maintaining it frequently becomes a problem. Most elders are on a fixed income, which does not allow for rising costs of taxes and repairs, or mobility and medical problems make it difficult or impossible to keep a home in good condition.

If an elder chooses to have a smaller living space, it is frequently a mobile home or apartment. Other options for living arrangements might include retirement villages or senior housing apartments or single-family homes. Other innovative arrangements include group living and sharing a home.

PSYCHOSOCIAL CARE OF THE AGING ADULT

Intelligence, Learning, and Memory

Knowledge of the psychological aspects of aging begins with the understanding that aging has little influence on intelligence, ability to learn, and memory. "Intelligence" is very hard to define and measure. While many elders have had little formal education, they may be self-taught or know many things from experience. Research indicates that most older people retain their intelligence and are capable of learning throughout their lives, although it may require more time because of age-related changes in the senses and nervous system.

Loss, Grief, and Depression

Significant age-related changes experienced by the elderly in the psychosocial domain can include personal, social, and economic losses. There are changes in roles and retirement, and the loss of significant others—parents, siblings, children, spouses, and friends. Physical changes can result in losses of independence and space. For some elders their losses occur suddenly, concurrently, or within a short period. How well a person copes with grief related to loss and how long it takes for grief to be resolved depends on many factors. For some individuals, avoiding isolation and self-pity, helping others, joining groups, adopting a pet, setting goals, maintaining independence, and retaining a sense of humor are successful coping strategies for grief or isolation.

For others, the stress and grief related to real and perceived losses lead to either short- or long-term depression. Fatigue, sadness, insomnia, anorexia, helplessness, and hypochondria are frequent symptoms of depression in the elderly. These symptoms are commonly mistaken as changes that normally occur with aging. It is unfortunate that few elders receive treatment for depression, although it is more common in the elderly than any other age-group. Current research indicates that elders who receive psychotherapy for depression show improvement.

PROMOTING HEALTHY AGING

Successful aging requires self-esteem; it is the foundation of psychosocial health. Without self-esteem a person will lack the courage to interact or cope with new situations. Although it may not be possible to alter low self-esteem created and maintained throughout life, it may be possible to improve the self-esteem of an individual when it is related to the losses common to the elderly. Programs to increase self-esteem may include reality orientation, reminiscence, and pet therapy, all of which also encourage social interaction and positive reinforcement (Fig. 48-2).

Being valued by others and treated with respect build self-esteem. Addressing an elder as "Gramps" or "Grandma," unless the person is one's grandparent, is inappropriate. It is important to address an elder by name or what they choose to be called; it indicates respect for the individual. Giving an elder time to respond in a situation, respecting an elder's wishes or preferences, and listening to what an elder has to say are ways the nurse can communicate to the person that he is valued.

Supporting independence of an elder and providing ways for an elder to control his life contributes to self-esteem. Allowing elderly persons to make decisions that affect their care or to be a part of the decision-making process seems only natural but is frequently ignored. Another important nursing behavior is showing respect for an elder's privacy, space, and possessions in the home and in the hospital.

Besides the importance that independence has in maintaining self-esteem, the independence to live in their own way is necessary for many elders to exist; this independence needs to be preserved. Ebersole[6] speaks of the "least restrictive environment" for the frail elderly. Even if their ways of coping are not the most effective or acceptable to the nurse, intervention or change that is too aggressive can exceed an elder's ability to cope. The result may be mental deterioration, physical illness, and death.

■ ■ ■

To help the elderly, the nurse has a role as advocate to dispel the myths associated with aging and to educate people to the realities of aging and options that are available for the elderly. Excellent sources of information and resources for the elderly, their families, and care providers are the American Association of Retired Persons (AARP) and local Area Agency on Aging offices.

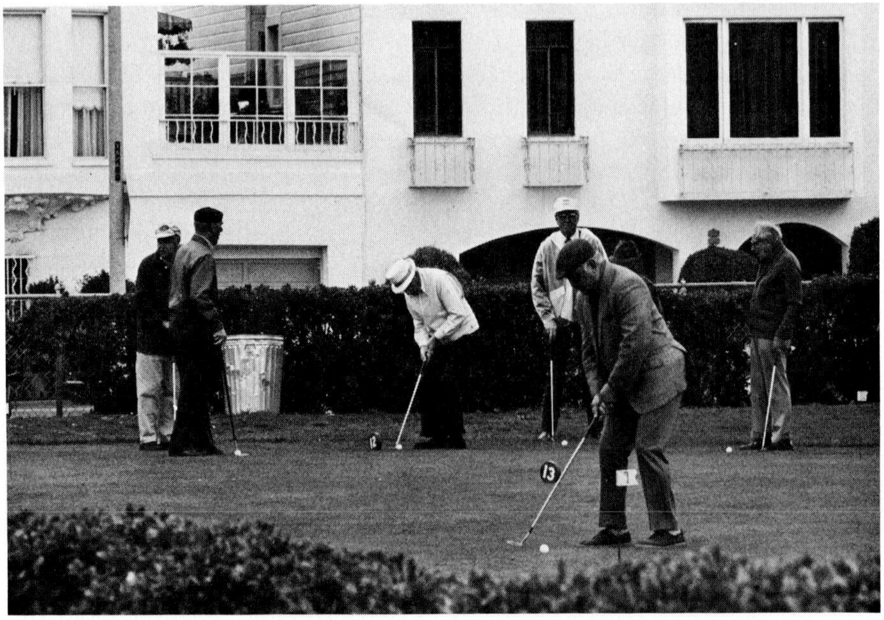

FIG. 48-2 Group activities and exercise promote health aging.

THERAPEUTIC DIALOGUE

NURSE: Good morning, Mrs. Brown. I am Nancy Smith. I am your nurse today.
PATIENT: Untie me, I can't get out of this mess.
NURSE: Mrs. Brown, what you see on your arm is a tube through which you are getting fluids and medication. Let me open up the drapes and put your glasses on so that you can see better.
PATIENT: Where are all of my things? Someone took them.
NURSE: Your clothes are here in this drawer. Let me show you. Your blue slippers and blue hair brush are also here.
PATIENT: Oh, my hair brush. My husband gave that to me for my seventy-fifth birthday. He is so thoughtful.
PATIENT: Where is he? He should be here any minute.
NURSE: Your husband will be in at 10:00. See the clock up on the wall? It is now 8:30 in the morning.
NURSE: While I get you a basin of water so that you can wash your face, would you like to brush your hair?
PATIENT: Oh yes, I must look a mess.

REFERENCES AND SUGGESTED READINGS

1. Aiken LR: Later life, ed 3, Hillsdale, NJ, 1989, Lawrence Erlbaum Associates, Inc.
2. Barker JC and Mitteness LS: Shedding light on nocturia, Geriatr Nurs 10(5):239, 1989.
3. Beck C and Heacock P: Nursing interventions for patients with Alzheimer's disease, Nurs Clin North Am 23(1):95, 1988.
4. Breitung JC: Caring for older adults, Philadelphia, 1987, WB Saunders Co.
5. Dimart J and Francis ME: Pressure sore prevention and management, J Gerontol Nurs 14(8):18, 1988.
6. Ebersole P and Hess P: Toward healthy aging, ed 3, St. Louis, 1990, The CV Mosby Co.
7. Eliopoulos C: Gerontological nursing, ed 2, Philadelphia, 1987, JB Lippincott Co.
8. Farrell J: Nursing care of the older person, Philadelphia, 1990, JB Lippincott Co.
9. Fox R: Atypical presentation of geriatric infections, Geriatrics 43(5):58, 1988.
10. Garrett JE: Multiple losses in older adults, J Gerontol Nurs 13(8):8, 1987.
11. Gioiella EC and Bevil CW: Nursing care of the aging client, Norwalk, Conn, 1985, Appleton-Century-Crofts.
12. Havis KA: Common dementia problems, Geriatr Nurs 11(2):76, 1990.
13. Hirst SP and Metcalf BJ: Promoting self-esteem, J Gerontol Nurs 10(2):72, 1984.
14. Kart CS: The realities of aging: an introduction to gerontology, ed 3, Boston, 1990, Allyn & Bacon.
15. Lewis C: Aging: the health care challenge, Philadelphia, 1985, FA Davis Co.
16. Louis M: Falls and their causes, J Gerontol Nurs 9(3):142, 1983.
17. Madson S: How to reduce the risk of postmenopausal osteoporosis, J Gerontol Nurs 15(9):20, 1989.
18. Matteson MA and McConnell ES: Gerontological nursing: concepts and practices, Philadelphia, 1988, WB Saunders Co.
19. Olson EV: The hazards of immobility, Am J Nurs 67(4):779, 1967.
20. Pettigrew D: Investing in mouth care, Geriatr Nurs 10(1):22, 1989.
21. A profile of older Americans. Prepared by AARP and AOA. Information researched and compiled by Fowlers DG, AOA Brochure no PF3049(1289)D996, 1989.
22. Santo-Novak D and Edwards RM: ℞: take caution with drugs for elders, Geriatr Nurs 10(2):72, 1989.
23. Steinke E and Bergen M: Sexuality and aging, J Gerontol Nurs 12(6):6, 1986.
24. Tideiksaar R: Home safe home, Geriatr Nurs 10(6):280, 1989.
25. Wolanin M: Confusion, prevention and care, St. Louis, 1981, The CV Mosby Co.

CHAPTER CHALLENGE

KEY POINTS

- Although the efficiency of body systems declines with age, the body has reserves and compensatory mechanisms that normally allow an individual to function well in late adulthood in the absence of disease.
- Regardless of age, individuals have the same basic needs for physiological function, safety, security, belonging, and self-esteem.
- While elders are experiencing age-related changes, the rate and response to such changes are individual and require individualized care.
- In the absence of disease that affects brain tissue or thought processes, individuals retain their intelligence, ability to learn, and memory throughout their life.
- The majority of elders have one or more chronic conditions that may have acute episodes or affect the care necessary when an elder is being treated for other, nonrelated medical-surgical events.
- With advancing age, more coordinated and active interventions are required to support the physiological and psychological equilibrium of the individual.
- Regardless of the normal age-related changes or disease processes that occur, supportive and restorative interventions are appropriate to maintain or improve the quality of life for an elder.

STUDY QUESTIONS

1. The percentage of people 65 years of age or older in the U.S. population is:
   a. 2%
   b. 5%
   c. 12%
   d. 25%
2. An accepted theory of aging would be:
   a. Immune—the immune system becomes less efficient and allows diseases to occur
   b. Socioeconomic—society withdraws economic support of the elderly
   c. Degeneration—a person deteriorates mentally and this causes him to deteriorate physically
   d. Incompetence—a person becomes incompetent to deal with the stresses of life
3. Insomnia is a complaint of many elders because:
   a. Patterns of sleep change with age
   b. Elders sleep less than younger individuals
   c. They become senile
   d. Medications they are taking cause insomnia
4. Finances are a major concern for most elderly because:
   a. The majority of elderly live in poverty
   b. The majority are not eligible for retirement benefits or pensions
   c. Most elderly have a fixed income
   d. Most families do not want to financially support elders
5. Improving self-esteem of the elderly in the hospital might best be accomplished by:
   a. Sending personal possessions home so they won't get lost
   b. Calling them "Grandma" and "Grandpa"
   c. Having the nursing staff plan daily recreational activities for each elder
   d. Being patient and listening to them when they talk
6. Nursing interventions to prevent decubitus ulcers in the elder would be:
   a. Padding of the bedrails and chair legs
   b. Increasing fluid intake during waking hours
   c. Lifting rather than pulling the person up in bed
   d. Raising the foot of the bed 4 inches
7. A technique to help communicate with an elder who has decreased hearing would be:
   a. Speaking in a higher tone of voice
   b. Speaking in a lower tone of voice
   c. Pausing after each word is spoken
   d. Standing to the side and speaking directly into the ear
8. When feeding an individual who has difficulty swallowing, it would be best to:
   a. Hold the chin up after each bite
   b. Put the solid foods in liquids
   c. Place the person in a semi-Fowler's position
   d. Sit the person slightly forward with the chin down
9. When working with an elder with dementia or Alzheimer's disease, it would be best to:
   a. Allow the elder to choose from a variety of recreational activities
   b. Include the elder in group activities whenever possible
   c. Have the elder do activities in small steps as you explain them
   d. Explain all steps of an activity to the elder before you begin
10. For individuals with lactose intolerance, it would be recommended to:
    a. Increase fiber in the diet
    b. Limit the amount of fat in the diet
    c. Substitute fresh milk for cream in the diet
    d. Substitute yogurt or cheese as a source of calcium

Identify the following statements as either T for True or F for False.

_____ 11. It takes longer for an elder to react than a younger individual.

_____ 12. Confusion can be a symptom of physical illness in the elderly.

_____ 13. Normal aging processes cause a decrease in intelligence as a person becomes elderly.

_____ 14. The majority of elderly people live in convalescent hospitals.

_____ 15. In addition to deaths of friends and family, losses experienced by the elderly can include independence and space.

XIII

Mental Health Nursing

Is it the excitement? You bet, and there is plenty of it. Or maybe it is the challenges and the changes of nursing that excited me. Nursing is certainly a challenging and ever-changing field. But then, there is also the reward that comes from that special feeling between a patient and a nurse, that unspoken communication that says, "I'm here for you, and I care." Life is such a precious thing. Every day, somewhere, someone is sick, maybe dying or in need of a helping hand. Let me be there to lend them my hand and contribute in some way to another's health and happiness, if only for a day. This is enough for me to say, "I love being a nurse."

BARBARA HUDSON
Student Nurse

49

Mental Health Concepts

MARY MILLER-WERLINGER

LEARNING OBJECTIVES

After reading this chapter, the student should be able to do the following:

- Define the key terms.
- Define mental health.
- Identify defining characteristics among people who are mentally healthy and those who are mentally ill.
- Describe the parts of the personality.
- Describe the factors that influence an individual's response to change.
- Identify barriers to healthy adaptation.
- Identify sources of stress.
- Describe factors that contribute to the development of emotional problems or mental illness.
- Identify the major components of a nursing assessment that focuses on mental status.
- Identify and describe the major mental disorders.
- Identify basic nursing interventions for patients experiencing various mental health problems.
- Describe the general care and treatment methods for patients experiencing mental health problems.
- Identify the key elements of effective (therapeutic) communication.

RELATED TOPICS OF INTEREST

- Communication (Chapter 4)
- The nursing process (Chapter 5)
- Cultural aspects of nursing care (Chapter 12)
- Diet therapy (Chapter 23)
- Care of the patient with a gastrointestinal or accessory organ disorder (Chapter 31)
- Care of the patient with a neurological disorder (Chapter 38)
- The patient with an addictive personality (Chapter 50)

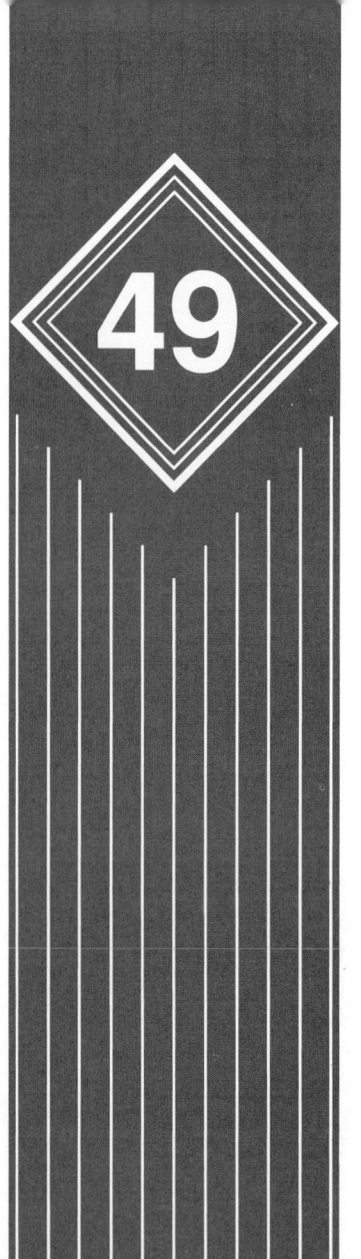

KEY TERMS

Define the following:

- adaptation
- affective disorders
- anxiety
- behavior
- catatonic state
- compulsion
- conflict
- coping responses
- defense mechanisms
- delusions
- depression
- feelings
- frustration
- illusion
- magical thinking
- mania
- mental health continuum
- mental illness
- mood
- motivation
- multiaxial system
- obsession
- personality
- phobia
- psychoactive
- psychosis
- somatization
- stress
- stressor

The LPN/LVN can expect to employ knowledge of mental health nursing principles in a variety of practice settings. Basic mental health concepts will be useful in understanding a patient's behavior as he responds to disease and dysfunction. Each person responds differently to change, such as the change created by illness and hospitalization. Response and **behavior** will vary in accordance with a person's basic personality and past experiences. All individuals have unique personalities and resources to deal with changing situations and the changing environment. An individual's mental health status may vary depending on the situation and the resources he has.

Mental health can be defined as one's ability to manage life's problems and to derive satisfaction from living throughout the various stages of life. No clear set of characteristics can be identified as specific to mental health. Mentally healthy individuals are characterized by (1) the development of mature patterns of problem solving, (2) an ability to cope with crisis beyond the assistance of family and friends, (3) a value system characterized by respect and trust for self and others, (4) having fulfilling interpersonal relationships, and (5) having satisfying work and work relationships.

Mental illness may be evidenced by behavior that is conspicuous, threatening, and disruptive of relationships or that deviates significantly from behavior that is considered socially acceptable.

Changes in society and in the economy have altered the status and situation of many individuals. It is estimated that one of every eight people in the United States is in need of mental health services. It is also estimated that one of every three people will develop a mental health problem at some point in his lifetime. In part these statistics may reflect our changing societal environment. Nurses may find themselves in daily contact with battered spouses, abused children, homeless, persons who are single parents, or substance abusers. Regardless of the practice setting, the nurse will frequently find a patient in need of emotional support.

Nurses are in a position to be a source of help to the patient. Nursing care is usually rendered in an interpersonal situation. Patients will express their feelings in a variety of ways. The nurse has the responsibility of assessing and intervening while maintaining a caring relationship of trust with the patient.

The emphasis of the mental health aspect of nursing is to assist the patient and family to achieve satisfying and productive ways of dealing with both the positive and negative aspects of daily living and to cope with situations that require a change in life-style.

This chapter is not intended to be a comprehensive course in psychiatric nursing. The focus of content will be on developing an awareness and understanding that regardless of the setting or the situation, the need for emotional well-being is a common thread among all patients.

HISTORICAL OVERVIEW OF MENTAL HEALTH

The history of mental health dates to primitive times. During early history, a mentally ill person was thought to be possessed by supernatural spirits or forces. The person was often ostracized, mistreated, and banished from the community. Historical records show that there was an interest in mental health and illness and its treatment during the Greco-Roman era. History has recorded the various directions that care and treatment of mental illness have taken (Box 49-1). The 1970s brought about treatment at the community level. A goal of community treatment is to return the individual to the home environment as soon as possible and to provide a support system within the community to facilitate treatment and return to as near normal functioning as possible.

Mental health concepts and principles are practiced in a variety of settings, including public health and home health care facilities and acute care hospitals. Psychiatric units and mental health centers are not the only settings in which mental health care is practiced; the patient in need of emotional support can be found in any health care setting. The community-based mental health movement and the holistic health movement brought about an awareness that all individuals, sick or well, have emotional needs.

BOX 49-1 HISTORICAL BACKGROUND

EIGHTEENTH CENTURY

In France, Phillippe Pinel freed the mentally ill from chains.

In the United States, Benjamin Rush founded Pennsylvania Hospital; he is regarded as the father of American psychiatry.

NINETEENTH CENTURY

Florence Nightingale founded modern nursing.

Dorothea Dix aroused public interest in the plight of the mentally ill and helped enact legislation to create mental hospitals.

Linda Richards became the first psychiatric nurse.

The first school for psychiatric nursing was established in Massachusetts.

Nursing care of the mentally ill was custodial in nature.

TWENTIETH CENTURY

Clifford Beers wrote *The Mind That Found Itself* and stirred public concern for mental illness.

Emil Kraepelin classified mental disorders.

Sigmund Freud developed psychoanalysis.

The National League for Nurses required psychiatric experiences in nursing education programs.

Johns Hopkins was the first school to incorporate psychiatry into the nursing school curriculum.

Psychotropic drugs were introduced.

The community-based mental health movement arose.

BASIC CONCEPTS RELATED TO MENTAL HEALTH

Nursing is a people-oriented profession. Every interaction that a nurse engages in with the patient affords an opportunity for assessment of the patient's emotional state. The nurse can create an environment that allows the patient to have as positive an experience as possible.

Mental Health Continuum

Mental health and mental illness can be viewed as being on opposite ends on a **mental health continuum**. On the illness end, the person is rarely in touch with reality. On the healthy side of the continuum, the person demonstrates high-level wellness. This form of wellness includes an assertive communication style, acceptance of strengths and weaknesses, and available energy to deal with life situations. The in-between point on the continuum can be regarded as normal mental health. Although some lack of insight may be evidenced, this level is characterized by adequate coping skills, satisfactory responses, and adjustments to life changes with some growth or possibly some mild regression.

Mental health	Mental illness
Adaptive (constructive)	Maladaptive (destructive)

The point at which a person is deemed to be mentally ill is determined by the behavior he exhibits as well as the context in which the behavior is observed. Mental illness results from an individual's inability to cope with a situation that he finds overwhelming. Often the maladaptive behavior is in response to acute anxiety.

Personality and Self-Concept

Personality refers to the relatively consistent set of attitudes and behaviors particular to an individual. Thoughts, feelings, values, and beliefs evolve into a consistent set of traits that characterize the person. Personality development is influenced by genetics and interactions with the environment. From infancy and throughout life a person has interactions that affect personal security, values, personal identity, and relationships with others.

Many theories exist about the growth process and the

development of the personality. All are attempts to explain why people behave as they do as well as how the individual evolves emotionally and physically.

Erickson provided a framework for understanding personality development in terms of task mastery. If a given task is not mastered, then a set of behaviors can be predicated. Freud described personality development as having three parts: id, ego, and superego (Box 49-2). A mature, well-adjusted personality is under the "leadership" of the ego.

Freud delineated the levels of awareness: conscious, preconscious, and unconscious. At the conscious level experiences are within the person's awareness; the person is aware of and can control thoughts. Preconsciousness refers to thoughts of which the person is not aware but that can be recalled to consciousness. The preconscious state helps to screen certain thoughts and repress unpleasant thoughts and desires. The unconscious level holds memories, **feelings,** and thoughts that are not available to the conscious mind.

Self is a complex concept that has four distinct parts that influence behavior. The four areas of self are (1) personal identity, (2) body image, (3) role, and (4) self-esteem. Personal identity is the organizing principle of the self; it is the "I." A person with a strong identity knows who he is and is not. Body image is the picture of and the feelings toward one's body. Body image includes feelings about the way one looks, the way one's body functions, sex, size, and whether one's body can help realize personal goals. Manifestations of body image include stance, posture, clothing, and jewelry. Role performance is the expected behavior of an individual in a social position. Roles are ascribed or assumed. An ascribed role involves no personal choice, such as being female or male. An assumed role is selected by the individual, such as occupation. In a lifetime an individual fills many overlapping roles and must combine these roles to achieve an integrated pattern of functioning. Self-esteem is the assessment one makes about personal worth. Self-esteem is the thoughts and feelings a person holds about himself. Self-concept is more than the total of the four parts—it is the frame of reference the individual uses for all he knows and experiences.

Through the process of growth and development, the individual accumulates and processes information that helps form a basic perception of who he is, how he looks, and how others react to him. How a person sees himself determines his behavior and interactions with others. Disturbances in self-concept are commonly seen in individuals with mental illness or emotional problems.

BOX 49-2 PARTS OF THE PERSONALITY

Id	The basic innate drive for survival and pleasure.
	Demands constant gratification.
	Composes the individual's entire personality at birth.
	The id is not changed by experience because it is not in contact with the external world. Its goals are to reduce tension, to increase pleasure, and to minimize discomfort.
Ego	The reality factor.
	Helps the individual perceive conditions accurately.
	Decides how to act and when to act.
	The ego is that portion of the psyche that is in contact with external reality—we might say the ego stands for reason and good sense, whereas the id stands for untamed passion (Freud, 1933).
Superego	The parental/societal value system.
	Strives for perfection and morality.
	The superego develops from the ego. It serves as a judge or censor over the thoughts and activities of the ego. Freud describes three functions of the superego: conscience, self-observation, and the formation of ideals.

Stress

Every individual is continually exposed to a variety of situations that produce stress. A person's mental health fluctuates according to his ability to adapt and deal with life situations. Any situation or event that requires change leads to stress. The situation or event may be either pleasant or unpleasant. **Stress** is the nonspecific response of the body to any demand made on it. By contrast, a **stressor** is a situation, activity, or event that produces stress. The meaning an individual gives to the stress determines whether the person feels distress. Mental health nursing concerns itself with behavior, particularly a person's response to stressors. Health factors affect this response. The stress of being ill greatly influences a person's emotional well-being. How stress is perceived by the person determines whether the stress produces anxiety in the individual. The nurse can be a resource in helping a patient develop adaptive patterns of behavior.

Anxiety

Anxiety is said to be a universal emotion and is a response to a stressful situation. It is a state of apprehension, a vague feeling whose source is often unknown. Anxiety is an internal process experienced when there is a real or perceived threat to the physical body or self-concept. *Anxiety is a major component of all mental health disturbances.* In mild forms, anxiety readies the body for action and reaction to danger. In severe forms, anxiety may be immobilizing and interferes with activities. Anxiety is usually described in terms of levels, and each level is associated with certain behaviors (Box 49-3). Signs of anxiety include vocal changes; rapid speech; increased pulse, respirations, and blood pressure; tremors; restlessness; increased perspiration; nausea; frequent urination; diarrhea; and occasionally vomiting.

Anxiety is created within the individual as the result of inner conflict, and subsequently behavior stems from the anxiety. Maladaptive behavior is often a defense against anxiety. A person learns a variety of ways to respond to anxiety as he moves through the various stages of growth and development. Behavior exhibited in response to stress and anxiety is the result of a combination of factors. The degree of anxiety experienced is influenced by the following:

How the person views the stressor (nature of the event)
The number of stressors (life situations) being handled at any one time
Previous experience with similar situations
The magnitude of change the event represents for the individual

Events that may precipitate feelings of anxiety include the following:

1. Threats to physical integrity—Decreased ability to perform activities of daily living
   Impending physiological disability: surgery, diagnosis of a life-threatening disorder
   Pain
   Infection
   Trauma
2. Threats to self-esteem and insults to the identity—
   Loss of spouse
   Difficulty at work
   Loss of job
   Change in jobs

Anxiety is relieved through various coping and mental mechanisms that will be discussed later in this chapter. These mechanisms are partly conscious and partly unconscious. They serve to protect the individual from situations perceived as dangerous. Anxiety is an inevitable part of life; part of the emotional growth process is to learn to deal with stress and anxiety in an adaptive or corrective manner.

Motivation

Motivation is the gathering of personal resources or the inner drive to perform a task or reach a goal. This inner drive may be generated by the perceived reward of having performed the task or from the perceived threat of punishment. Motivation is an important aspect in treating emotional problems.

BOX 49-3 LEVELS OF ANXIETY

An individual's response depends on the level of anxiety.

Mild	Slight increase in vital signs and an awareness of danger
	Able to think and make connections; heightened awareness
	Is ready for action
	Motivation is increased
Moderate	Feels tension
	Perception has decreased
	Remains alert but only to specific information
	May be prone to arguing, teasing, or complaining
	Physical symptoms may appear: headache, diarrhea, nausea, vomiting, low back pain
Severe	Experiences a feeling of impending danger
	Perceptual field significantly narrows and becomes distorted
	Communication may be distorted and difficult to understand
	Feels fatigued
	Changes in vital signs may be evident on assessment
Panic	Feeling of extreme terror
	Individual may become immobilized
	Reality is distorted
	Personality may disintegrate further
	Could cause harm to self and others

Frustration

Frustration refers to anything that interferes with goal achievement. Interference with goal-directed activity results in frustration. The concept is important in understanding the individual's response to frustration. Some people are more flexible and adaptable than others. When adaptive behavior fails, anxiety increases.

Conflict

Conflict refers to the presence of two drives. Some conflicts are easily resolved, whereas others are more complicated and lead to increased anxiety. If the conflict is of a serious nature, maladaptive patterns of resolving the situation may become evident. An example of conflict can be seen when a person is ill and needs to see a physican but does not because he feels he cannot afford to lose time from work.

Adaptation and Coping

Adaptation refers to an individual's abilty to adjust to changing life situations using various strategies. Any kind of change in routines or patterns of living causes varying degrees of stress. Illness, family problems, lack of money, or inadequate transportation may all be viewed as stressful to the individual. An inability to meet basic needs or role expectations can precipitate emotional upheaval. An emotionally healthy person finds ways of dealing with the stress and resolving it (problem solving); hence, adaptation occurs. Adaptation may be viewed as positive or negative, depending on the alternative that the individual selected. A person can grow or regress as the result of an experience.

Individuals may respond to anxiety through the use of coping responses. **Coping responses** are used to reduce anxiety brought on by stress. Common coping responses include overeating, drinking, smoking, withdrawal, seeking out someone to talk to, yelling, exercising, fighting, pacing, listening to music, and engaging in physical activity. Coping mechanisms are used consciously, and the individual chooses the behavior.

Defense Mechanisms

Another way of coping with anxiety is through defense mechanisms. **Defense mechanisms** are used to block conscious awareness of the threatening feelings. Usually these mechanisms operate at the unconscious level. Defense mechanisms are behavior patterns that protect the individual against a real or perceived threat. This type of coping behavior develops when an individual experiences (perceives) an unconscious conflict or a threat to personal integrity (physical or self-concept). This threat or conflict results in the creation of a state of anxiety within the individual, which is then relieved or diminished in some manner. Every individual uses defense mechanisms to maintain biological integrity and protect the self. If defense mechanisms are used inappropriately or are overused, this behavior is deemed to be a maladaptive pattern of coping. Table 49-1 shows commonly used defense mechanisms.

COMMON HUMAN RESPONSES ASSOCIATED WITH MENTAL ILLNESS

The LPN/LVN should have a basic understanding of the classifications (human responses) and treatment methods for mental illness. The patient on a medical unit may have a physiological disorder but may also have a history of emotional problems. A more common situation is the patient who is ill and is experiencing emotional disturbance as a result of the illness or the impact of the illness. It is important for nurses to be able to deal with both the physical and emotional aspects of patient care.

The *Diagnostic and Statistical Manual III Revised* (DSM-III-R), published by the American Psychiatric Association, is a **multiaxial system** that classifies mental disorders and is used by most hospitals and health care professionals in the United States. Various disorders and descriptive references are outlined. DSM-III-R, as it is commonly called, is the current tool used to facilitate medical diagnosis and is also used by nursing. This classification system is an excellent resource and a valuable tool for psychiatric nurses and physicians.

Mental disorders that will be discussed in this chapter include the following:

1. Organic mental disorders—delirium and dementia
2. Thought process disorders—schizophrenia
3. Affective disorders—depression
4. Anxiety disorders—phobias, general anxiety
5. Personality disorder
6. Psychophysiological disorder
7. Substance abuse and dependence
8. Eating disorders

A basic description of each of the major disorders (organic, thought process, affective, and anxiety) and a summary of treatment, prognosis, and related nursing diagnoses can be found in Table 49-2.

Organic Mental Disorders: Delirium and Dementia

Organic disorders differ from other mental health disorders in that there is an identifiable brain disease or dysfunction that is the basis for the behavior. Organic disorders may result from an underlying vascular disorder, brain infection, trauma, metabolic disturbance, or poisoning (see Table 49-2; see also Chapters 38 and 48 for a discussion of Alzheimer's disease). A predominant characteristic of this type of disorder is confusion and disorientation. Some individuals will interact appropriately during the day while environmental stimulation exists. When environmental cues are reduced during the late evening and night, some individuals will become disoriented. Teaching reality orientation techniques and providing a safe environment are two key aspects of nursing care.

Thought Process Disorders: Schizophrenia

Thought process disorders are characterized by bizarre, non-reality-based thinking. Persons with thought disorders represent the largest number of mentally ill patients. The personality in these patients is disorganized, disintegrates, and there is a distortion of reality (see Table 49-2). There are five subtypes of this category of illness:

1. Disorganized: Flat or inappropriate affect; incoherence
2. Paranoid: Delusions; auditory hallucinations
3. Catatonic: Features stupor, negativism, rigidity, excitement, posturing

Text continued on p. 1298.

Table 49-1 Commonly Used Defense Mechanisms

Mode	Description
Repression	The barring from conscious thought of painful, disagreeable thoughts, experiences, and/or impulses. Energy is expended so that the individual has less available energy. *Example:* A patient who was incontinent after surgery represses the embarrassment and totally suppresses the event.
Regression	Behavior, thought, or feelings used at an earlier stage of development are exhibited. *Example:* An 8-year-old who reverts to bed-wetting and thumb-sucking while hospitalized.
Identification	Individual incorporates a characteristic (thought or behavior) of another individual or group. The individual does not give up personal identity. *Example:* An employee who dresses similarly to the employer. *Example:* A teenager who dresses like his favorite rock singer.
Introjection	A quality or attribute of another is internalized and becomes part of the individual. *Example:* The child who follows his parents' instructions when the parents are not present (e.g., carefully crossing the street).
Reaction formation	The conscious behavior is completely opposite to the unconscious process. *Example:* A person who is excessively polite to an individual who is disliked.
Undoing	The individual engages in symbolic behavior that cancels out conscious thoughts that produce anxiety. The individual is aware of the behavior but not the purpose. *Example:* The husband who has an argument with his wife before work brings home a bouquet of flowers.
Isolation	The feelings associated with a thought or memory are not experienced with the thought or memory. *Example:* The person who has been in a car accident who recounts the experience but feels nothing while doing so.
Displacement	Emotions are expressed toward someone or something other than the source of the emotion. Unconsciously, the individual does not feel safe expressing the feelings directly. *Example:* The person has an argument with his employer and comes home and yells at the family.
Projection	Attributing to others characteristics that the person does not want to admit are his own. Blaming personal shortcomings on someone else. *Example:* A student who does poorly on an exam and states, "That test was unfair. The teacher did not present the material correctly."
Rationalization	A process of constructing plausible reasons to explain and justify one's behavior. The person denies his actual thoughts and justifies his actions by giving untrue, but seemingly more acceptable, reasons for his behavior. *Example:* The young boy who was instructed to make up his bed and clean his room before leaving for school chooses to play instead. In the afternoon, when he and his mother arrive home and she becomes angry at noticing his disregard of her instructions, states, "But Mom, Dad was in a hurry this morning and told me that if I wanted a ride to school, I'd better get in the car."
Denial	Reality is denied; it does not exist. *Example:* The person who has lost his job, yet buys a new car. *Example:* The patient who has suffered a severe myocardial infarction is told that he will have to severely restrict his physical activity. The evening nurse finds him on the floor of his room, doing sit-ups and push-ups.
Substitution	The individual replaces a highly valued, unacceptable object with a less valued, acceptable object. *Example:* The person who has a strong unconscious sexual attraction to a parent and marries someone who resembles that parent.
Sublimation	Sexual or aggressive energy/impulses are discharged in a socially acceptable way. *Example:* The teenager who engages in many competitive sports.
Conversion	Emotional conflicts are turned into a physical symptom, which provides the individual with some sort of benefit (secondary gain). *Example:* The individual who witnesses a murder, then experiences sudden blindness with no organic cause.
Suppression	An intentional exclusion of painful thoughts, experiences or impulses. (This is not considered a defense mechanism by some.) *Example:* A student who forgets to keep an appointment for academic counseling.
Compensation	An individual makes up for a "deficiency" in one area by excelling in or emphasizing another area. *Example:* A boy who is small in stature places his emphasis on academics rather than attempting sports.

Table 49-2 Human Responses Associated with Mental Illness

Characteristics	Treatment and Prognosis	Associated Nursing Diagnoses
ORGANIC MENTAL DISORDERS		
Dementia		
Slow and progressive worsening of symptoms: poor memory, impaired judgment, personality changes, decreased cognitive function	Determined by cause	Altered thought processes Potential for injury Anxiety Bathing/hygiene self-care deficit
Delirium		
Acute onset of symptoms: disorientation, incoherent thought content, impaired cognitive function, symptoms worsen at night, illusions, hallucinations	Determined by cause	Potential for injury Potential for violence: directed at others Altered thought processes Bathing/hygiene self-care deficit
Nursing interventions for patients with organic mental disorders Reality orientation techniques: Tell the patient who he is, who the nurse is, where he is, orient to day and time, and tell the patient what is expected of him at that point in time. Place large clock and calendar in strategic locations to serve as memory cues. Provide for safety: Bed in lowest position to the floor, side rails elevated, call light within reach, personal articles within reach on the bedside stand, sufficient night lighting from the bed to the bathroom. Provide for adequate nutrition. Assist with hygiene and toileting/grooming. Encourage and assist with mobility.		
THOUGHT PROCESS DISORDERS		
Schizophrenia		
Inappropriate emotional responses, incoherent, displays bizarre behavior, may exhibit hallucinations and delusions, has trouble relating to others	Antipsychotic medication therapy Long term-social support Prognosis is variable and depends on the extent of the symptoms and responses to treatment	Altered thought processes Sensory/perceptual alterations: visual, auditory, olfactory Anxiety Bathing/hygiene self-care deficits Impaired social interactions Altered role performance Altered family processes
Patient with paranoia may view the environment as threatening Symptoms present at least 6 months Affect is inappropriate or absent Ideas of reference, **magical thinking**	Paranoid type may be reluctant to seek treatment	
Nursing interventions for patients with thought process disorders Use simple statements in communication. Reality orientation. Be alert to the presence of hallucinations: do not argue with the patient or enter into the hallucination. Provide for nutrition. Approach the patient in an honest manner. Provide for safety. Encourage participation in self care; assist with self care as indicated.		
AFFECTIVE DISORDERS		
Bipolar affective disorder		
Mood swings with one or more manic episodes, alternating with or without episodes of depression	Antimanic medications (lithium) Family and individual support with education regarding symptoms and appropriate use of medication	Potential for injury Activity intolerance Potential for violence: directed at others Altered thought processes Violence, directed at others Impaired social interaction Altered nutrition: less than body requirements

Continued.

Table 49-2 Human Responses Associated with Mental Illness—cont'd

Characteristics	Treatment and Prognosis	Associated Nursing Diagnoses
AFFECTIVE DISORDERS—cont'd		
Bipolar affective disorder—cont'd		
Exhibits symptoms of mania: grand or self-confident mood, overresponse to stimuli, irritability, decreased need for and ability to sleep, increased physical activity, flight of ideas, rapid and pressured speech, "too busy" to eat or pay attention to self-care needs (hygiene and grooming), wears bright, garish clothes	Prognosis depends on response to medication and treatment	
Major depression		
Prolonged, intense unhappiness; symptoms include: lack of ambition, pessimism, multiple physical complaints, guilt feelings, isolation, anxiety, suicidal ideation, appetite disturbances, sleep disturbance, fatigue, constipation, limited attention span	Antidepressant medication therapy Electroconvulsive therapy (when medications are contraindicated or are ineffective) An estimated 50% of individuals have at least one additional episode of depression	Potential for violence: self-directed Hopelessness Ineffective individual coping Sleep pattern disturbance Powerlessness Altered nutrition: less than body requirements Impaired verbal communication Dressing/grooming self-care deficit

Nursing interventions for patients with affective disorders

Bipolar affective disorder

Planned activity (may have to remove patient from group activity).
Reduce environmental stimuli.
Use a kind but firm manner in addressing the patient.
Assist with grooming and hygiene.
Assist with selection of clothing.
Provide nutritional foods and snacks.
Provide for safety.
Be alert to changes in mood or behavior.
Administer prescribed medication.
Do not argue with patient.
Be consistent in assigning caregivers to the patient.
Assign patient to private (single) room.
Consider providing activities for the patient in his room.
Avoid placing the patient in competitive activities.
Weigh patient weekly.
Offer fluids frequently.
Monitor for dehydration.

Depression

Allow time for patient to respond to questions.
Present information to patient in simple terms.
Allow for rest periods.
Sit with patient and offer self (i.e., be there; be present in the patient's room; be available for interaction) if patient does not wish to initiate conversation.
Be alert for cues that indicate a potential for self-harm.
If potential for suicide gesture exists: check the environment for hazards, remove glass and sharp objects, check for clothing that might be used in a suicide attempt, move the patient closer to the nursing area, monitor patient frequently.

Table 49-2 Human Responses Associated with Mental Illness—cont'd

Characteristics	Treatment and Prognosis	Associated Nursing Diagnoses
ANXIETY DISORDERS		
Generalized anxiety		
Characterized by a steady, pervasive level of anxiety Can occur at any age; common around age 20-30 Lasts 6 months or longer Symptoms include apprehension, irritability, insomnia, poor concentration, fear of the unknown, conversation may be dominated by physical complaints, preoccupied or neglectful of hygiene/grooming	Occasionally, antianxiety medication therapy (therapy is effective in either diminishing anxiety or helping individual learn to cope with anxiety) Relaxation techniques	Anxiety Ineffective individual coping Fear
Panic disorders		
Severe anxiety Exhibits physical manifestations of anxiety Attacks occur suddenly and without apparent reason Attacks last minutes to hours and may recur several times a week Onset is frequently in the late twenties	Occasionally, antianxiety medication therapy Relaxation techniques	Anxiety Ineffective individual coping Fear
Nursing interventions for patients with anxiety disorders		
Encourage the patient to share thoughts and feelings. Be supportive. Provide appropriate assistance. Encourage the patient to participate in self-care. Encourage participation in simple decision making. Avoid reinforcing concerns over physical complaints. Explain all procedures and treatments. Be on time with treatments and medications.		
PERSONALITY DISORDERS		
May exhibit a range of behaviors, depending on the type of disorder present Common characteristics include poor impulse control (drinking, overeating, substance abuse, assaultive behavior), may perform self-destructive acts such as self-mutilation, may try to manipulate others or may demonstrate dependency on others, may have inappropriate behavior for the situation, may exhibit a disregard for rules and regulations	Medication therapy Support groups helpful (rehabilitative) Family counseling	Impaired social interaction Ineffective individual coping Altered family processes Potential for violence: self-directed or directed at others
Nursing interventions for patients with personality disorders		
Set limits on patient's behavior. Establish consequences for violating limits. Encourage ventilation of thoughts and feelings. Provide positive feedback when appropriate behavior or actions are exhibited. Encourage decision making. Encourage patient participation. Discuss incidents with patient. Approach in a calm, confident manner. Know where the patient is at all times.		

4. Undifferentiated: Delusions, hallucinations, incoherence, gross disorganization (does not fit criteria of other types)
5. Residual: Demonstrates the typical symptoms associated with schizophrenia without displaying evidence of gross disorganization, incoherence, delusions, and hallucinations

Affective Disorders: Bipolar Personality and Major Depression

Affective disorders (see Table 49-2) refer to disturbances in feeling or mood. **Mood**, as defined by DSM-III-R, is a prolonged emotion (depression or elation) that affects the psyche. Extremes in mood range from depression to mania. Research indicates that hereditary factors account for 60% to 80% of affective disorders.

Depression is a reaction to a real or perceived loss of a valued object. Depression may be prolonged and increasingly incapacitating. **Mania** (adj. *manic*) is characterized by overactivity and a euphoric state.

Anxiety Disorders: Generalized Anxiety and Panic Disorders

Anxiety disorders are characterized by a high degree of anxiety and/or avoidance behavior. Table 49-2 describes generalized anxiety disorders and panic disorders. Two other disorders classified as anxiety related include phobic disorders and obsessive-compulsive disorders.

A phobic disorder is characterized by a persistent dread or fear of an object or situation. A **phobia** transfers anxiety to some object in the environment. Common phobias include fear of heights, water, confined spaces, crowds, and snakes.

Obsessive-compulsive disorders frequently involve an undesirable but persistent thought about such things as violent behaviors, fear of contamination, or doubts about a situation (e.g., having turned off the burner of the stove). **Obsession** refers to the persistent thought or idea, while **compulsion** involves carrying out the obsession. Obsessive-compulsive disorders may be expressed in the form of constant handwashing, being obsessed with the cleanliness of one's house, checking the gas jets on the stove numerous times before leaving the house, or committing a violent act.

Several other responses associated with mental illness are noteworthy and will be briefly described.

Personality Disorders

Personality disorders are inflexible and maladaptive patterns of behavior or thinking that are associated with significant impairment of functioning. Box 49-4 outlines and describes the common disorders (see also Table 49-2). The disorder usually surfaces during adolescence or earlier and continues through adulthood. The associated behaviors are generally more troubling to others than to the individual. The disorders are characterized by impaired relationships, lack of insight, and difficulty handling change.

BOX 49-4 PERSONALITY DISORDERS

ABUSIVE PERSONALITY

Individual who uses violent or abusive behavior to cope with anxiety (tension conflict)

PARANOID PERSONALITY

Characterized by suspicion, secretiveness, distortion of reality, and oversensitivity; thinks that others are out "to get" him

BORDERLINE PERSONALITY

Has not established self-identity; fears being alone; experiences mood swings over a short period

ANTISOCIAL PERSONALITY

Has a history of difficulties with personal relationships; does not profit from experience or punishment; has no real loyalties to any person, group, or code; and has a tendency to rationalize behavior

Psychophysiological Disorders

Some physical disorders are thought to have a psychological basis. **Somatization** is the process whereby an individual's feelings, needs, and conflicts are manifested physiologically. Psychophysiological disorders are thought to have an emotional basis, manifested as a physical illness. Usually the individual has little or no awareness of the conflict underlying his illness and may even resent such an implication. Disorders thought to have emotional undertones include peptic ulcers, hypertension, asthma, certain skin disorders, arthritis, ulcerative colitis, coronary artery disease, and migraine headaches.

Substance Abuse and Dependence

Dependence on a substance may be defined as a disorder in which a person is psychologically or physically dependent, as on drugs or alcohol. Alcohol, the most abused drug in the United States, is a central nervous system depressant. Drugs that are abused usually alter the mood, giving the individual a euphoric feeling. Drugs that are abused include illicit drugs and certain prescription drugs such as diazepam (Valium) and chlordiazepoxide (Librium). (See Table 49-3).

Table 49-3 Frequently Abused Substances

Substance	Related Effects
Opiates Meperidine Morphine Codeine Methadone	Euphoria, relaxation, constricted pupils, slurred speech, impaired judgment
Barbiturates Amytal Nembutal Seconal	Euphoria, decreased inhibition, impaired judgment, slurred speech, incoordination
Amphetamines	Euphoria, hyperactivity, irritability, anorexia, weight loss, tachycardia, hypertension
Cocaine/crack	Euphoria, agitation, grandiose thinking, anorexia, weight loss, diaphoresis, insomnia
Hallucinogens	Perceptual distortion, heightened awareness, hallucinations, **illusions,** dilated pupils
Phencyclidine (PCP)	Euphoria, perceptual distortion, agitation, delusions, violence
Marijuana	Mild euphoria, loss of inhibition, relaxation, decreased motivation
Antianxiety drugs	Relaxation, feeling of confidence, relief of anxiety, drowsiness, hypotension

Alcoholism is the third leading cause of death in the United States. There are an estimated 10 million alcoholics over the age of 18. There are another 3.3 million teenagers under the age of 18 who are considered alcoholics. Alcohol abuse costs U.S. employers approximately $5 billion a year in absenteeism. Alcohol use has been referred to as a "defense mechanism" against anxiety. Alcohol abuse affects not only the person who is abusing it, but also other family members. Physiological effects of alcohol consumption involve the mouth, throat, stomach, intestines, liver, pancreas, nerves, brain, heart, lungs, and kidneys.

Immediate effects of alcohol are caused by its action on the brain and central nervous system. Judgment is impaired and sensations are dulled. Illnesses associated with alcoholism include delirium tremens, chronic gastritis, Laënnec's cirrhosis, peripheral neuropathy, nutritional deficiencies, and a predisposition to infection.

Delirium tremens (DTs) is an acute reaction to withdrawal from alcohol use. DTs occur several days to weeks after withdrawl from heavy alcohol consumption. Usual early symptoms of withdrawal include tremors of the hands, nausea, vomiting, tachycardia, diaphoresis, irritability, and anxiety. These symptoms may disappear in 5 to 7 days, unless DTs develop. Major symptoms of DTs include hypertension, **delusions,** hallucinations, agitated state, and seizures.

Nursing intervention focuses on vital sign assessment, maintenance of hydration and nutrition, providing for safety, giving prescribed medication, and providing a calm, quiet, nonstimulating environment.

Drug dependency continues to be a serious problem in the United States. Categories of drugs that are commonly abused include opiates, barbiturates, amphetamines, hallucinogens (not addictive), phencyclidine (PCP), and marijuana. Table 49-3 outlines the categories of abused drugs and the related effects of consumption.

Nursing intervention for patients with chemical dependency includes close monitoring, allaying anxiety and fear, particularly during the withdrawal period, providing for comfort, and providing a safe environment. The nurse must establish therapeutic communications with the patient (see Chapter 50).

EATING DISORDERS

Certain individuals develop nutritional problems known as eating disorders. Two common eating disorders are anorexia nervosa and bulimia.

Anorexia nervosa is a disorder characterized by extreme weight loss, fear of fat, and a distorted body image. Anorexia is usually seen in adolescent or young adult women. The individual is usually withdrawn and perceives herself as fat, regardless of her actual weight. Other characteristics include ritualistic and bizarre eating habits, hypotension, emaciation, depression, sleep disturbances, crying spells, amenorrhea, hypothermia, appearance of lanugo, and possible suicidal tendencies (see Chapters 23 and 31).

Bulimia refers to a cycle of binge eating followed by self-induced vomiting. Again, the population is usually prepubertal and pubertal females. The bulimic is usually an extrovert, a perfectionist, a high achiever, and is aware that her eating behaviors are abnormal, but may be secretive about the behavior. Other characteristics include laxative or diuretic abuse. Cardiac irregularities, electrolyte imbalance, gastric and esophageal irritation, tooth enamel erosion, broken nails, and scars on knuckles result from vomiting (see Chapters 23 and 31).

Nursing interventions for patients with eating disorders including keeping a calorie count (amount and type of food eaten), encouraging decision making, encouraging sharing of thoughts and feelings, monitoring physical activity, vomiting, and elimination, assessing weight daily, and gearing patient teaching to the importance of nutrition and its relationship to health. It is also important to help the patient explore the underlying emotional conflicts that may lead to the bulimic behavior and to identify appropriate means of dealing with stress.

Table 49-4 Therapeutic Techniques for Communication

Technique	Example	Rationale
Accepting	Yes. Nodding Go on.	Establishes relationship Implies you are listening
Offering self	I'll stay with you. I'll be here for a while.	Establishes relationship Offers assurance
Giving broad openings	Is there something you'd like to talk about? What are you thinking about?	Allows patient to go at own speed. Communicates respect
Making observations	You seem tense. I noticed you are pacing.	Verbalizes the implied and provides feedback about behavior
Using silence		Shows acceptance Places responsibility for communication on patient
Seeking clarification	I'm not sure I follow. What's the main point?	Allows you to check your perception
Voicing doubt	I find that hard to believe. Really? That seems quite unusual.	Helps the patient test reality This presents reality
Verbalizing the implied	PATIENT: It's just a waste of time to talk. NURSE: You feel like you're not solving your difficulties?	Helps the patient identify feelings
Restating	PATIENT: I'm exhausted. I'm always awake. NURSE: You're having trouble sleeping.	Emphasizes a point while clarifying content
Focusing	Let's talk about this some more. That point seems worth focusing on.	Allows you to help patient stay on meaningful topic
Reflecting	PATIENT: My #!*@ brother spends my whole check! NURSE: You are angry with your brother.	Allows you to focus on the feeling rather than the content; this allows the patient to identify his feelings
Summarizing	You've said that. We've talked about that, and now you are going to . . .	Provides a wrapping up for an episode in the conversation or for a complete interaction

Adapted from Hays JH and Larson KH: Interacting with patients, New York, 1965, Macmillan Publishing Co.

OVERVIEW OF TREATMENT METHODS

Communication and the Therapeutic Relationship

The nurse and patient become partners in a relationship built on trust. The relationship maximizes the patient's strengths, maintains self-esteem, and helps the patient cope. Communication skills are a key factor in establishing and maintaining this relationship. Communication and a trusting relationship are fundamental to all nursing practice; knowledge and skill in effective (therapeutic) communication are essential.

There are different types of relationships. Most relationships are social; that is, the participants are equally involved in exchanging information and meeting individual needs. In a therapeutic relationship both participants work toward goals that have been agreed on. The nurse assists the individual to learn new ways of interacting to function more effectively. The nurse attempts to establish a rapport with the patient and gain his trust to facilitate positive interactions that will lead to corrective behavior. In day-to-day interactions with a patient the nurse will find that the individual will be more responsive and amenable to instruction if he trusts the nurse and feels that the nurse is a competent professional.

Therapeutic communication is a dynamic process by which individuals share meaning. To be therapeutic, communication must assist with the corrective experiences that help the individual to meet predetermined goals. Therapeutic techniques for communication are included in Table 49-4. These techniques of communication can be used in every nursing situation. The therapeutic dialogues on the next page demonstrate therapeutic nurse-patient interactions.

Psychopharmacology

Psychotropic **(psychoactive)** medications are drugs used in conjunction with other therapies to help modify an individual's behavior. Medication is used to control symptoms. Monitoring for signs of effectiveness and evidence of side effects is an important nursing responsibility. It is clearly the role of the nurse administering these medications to understand their use. Commonly prescribed drugs are presented in Table 49-5.

Antidepressants. There are many antidepressant medications; four types that are currently in use include tricyclics, monoamine oxidase inhibitors (MAOI), and a newer group (similar to the tricylics) of which trazodone is a member. There is also another new antidepressant called Prozac (fluoxetine). The drugs work in different ways in the brain and assist with alleviating signs and symptoms of depression, such as decreased appetite or sleep, lack of alertness, and prolonged sadness. These medications do not take effect immediately; it is generally

2 to 4 weeks before improvement is noted. Antidepressants should be continued for several months to prevent recurrence of symptoms. The nurse should be familiar with each drug before administration.

Antimanics. The chief drug used to stabilize the mood and behavior of a patient with mania is lithium carbonate. A therapeutic blood level is required and may take 7 to 10 days to achieve. During the interim, antipsychotic medications are frequently used for control of behavior. Toxicity is a problem encountered with this drug, and the nurse should be aware of the signs. Patient education is an important factor in lithium administration.

Antipsychotics. Antipsychotic medications are for acute and chronic management of (1) schizophrenia, (2) organic mental disorders with **psychosis** (major disorder of organic or emotional origin, characterized by impairment of thought, communication, and memory and distortion of reality), and (3) the manic phase of a bipolar affective personality disorder. These drugs provide some symptomatic control, but are not a cure. There are a number of side effects associated with these drugs.

THERAPEUTIC DIALOGUE

EXAMPLE: Starting a conversation with a patient may include several approaches
What circumstances brought you to the hospital?
Tell me a little about what has been going on with you.
Mr. Jones, I am Nancy Smith. I'll be your nurse today.
Tell me how you are feeling today.

■ Mrs. Jung underwent a hysterectomy 2 days ago for severe fibroid tumors. She is 32 years old and has a 3-year-old child. She has been married 5 years. The nurse who admitted her after surgery enters the room and finds her crying.

NURSE: *(Walks over to Mrs. Jung and touches her arm and stands there quietly.)*
PATIENT: *(Continues to cry but looks up at the nurse and starts to quiet.)*
NURSE: You look upset; would you like to talk? *(Pulls up a chair and sits at eye level.)*
PATIENT: My whole life is ruined.
NURSE: Your life is ruined?
PATIENT: I wanted other children; we were going to have a large family.
NURSE: Tell me what a large family means to you.

Patients experiencing loss often need to cry. Crying begins to release emotion and should be accepted by the nurse. The close physical presence and touch communicate acceptance. Acknowledgement of feelings encourage further expression and then the patient's sense of loss can be explored.

■ Mr. Hill is a 65-year-old diagnosed with cancer of the lung. The day nurse is making initial patient rounds and enters the room. The nurse notices that Mr. Hill looks uncomfortable.

NURSE: *(Walks over to the bed.)* Good morning, Mr. Hill. You look uncomfortable.
PATIENT: I'm tired; I stayed awake all night.
NURSE: You had difficulty sleeping?
PATIENT: I have a lot on my mind. I couldn't sleep.
NURSE: *(Sits down next to the patient and pats his hand.)* Tell me what has been worrying you.

Patients should be encouraged to talk (ventilate). The nurse must be observant for nonverbal communication and for underlying meanings in the stated words. Talking brings emotions to the surface where they can be identified and dealt with.

It cannot be emphasized enough that the patient and the nurse bring their physiological, psychological, developmental, and spiritual components into the therapeutic relationship. Also brought into the relationship are previous life experiences, needs, aspirations, and frustrations. The nurse has an opportunity to help the patient explore a life event and the meaning that it has for him.

■ Mr. Ruiz is a 58-year-old Mexican-American with a diagnosis of diabetes mellitus and gangrene of the right foot. He is in his second postoperative day after an above-the-knee amputation. On arrival in Mr. Ruiz's room, the evening nurse notices he is holding the side rails and is grimacing.

NURSE: Mr. Ruiz, are you hurting? You seem to be uncomfortable.
PATIENT: *(In a tense voice)* I'm fine.

In checking the chart the nurse notices that Mr. Ruiz has not had any pain medication since early this morning.

NURSE: Mr. Ruiz, you haven't had anything for pain since early this morning according to this chart.
PATIENT: My leg hurts because of the way the nurses handled me today. They tossed me around like I was a bag of groceries!
NURSE: You believe that you were handled roughly?
PATIENT: *(Explains that a staff member from the physical therapy department was in to show him exercises and that the nurses got him up to a chair.)*
NURSE: *(Explains the reason behind the activity.)* I will be back with some medication for you, and I will help you get comfortable so that you can rest. Later this evening we will get you up to a chair again. I will be here to show you how to move into the chair so that you won't feel so strained.

Patients do not understand the reason for various hospital protocols and procedures. A nursing responsibility is assessing for nonverbal communication, and knowledge deficits (explaining treatments and procedures), demonstrating interest in the individual, and allaying anxiety. The vehicle for establishing trust and gaining understanding is communication.

Antianxiety agents. Antianxiety agents are used to help individuals who are experiencing moderate to severe anxiety. These agents reduce anxiety, but just enough so that tension is reduced and the patient remains motivated. Drugs in this category are commonly abused.

Other Forms of Treatment

Psychotherapy is a process in which feelings and thoughts are explored, new ways of perceiving the environment are taught, and interventions are reinforced. Psychotherapy includes psychoanalysis, family therapy, behavior modification, and group therapy.

Electroconvulsive therapy (ECT, shock treatments) involves the passing of an electrical current through electrodes to the brain, resulting in a seizure. ECT is used to treat severe depression and compulsive suicidal tendencies.

Adjunctive therapies include occupational therapy, recreational therapy, art therapy, and other similar therapies that allow the expression of feelings, help to increase the individual's self-esteem, and promote positive interactions.

THE NURSING PROCESS

There is a misconception that mental health principles are applicable only in a mental health facility or center. The goal of mental health nursing is to assist the individual to have a realistic and accepting view of self and to establish and maintain effective interpersonal relationships. The stress of being ill greatly influences an individual's mental state and level of functioning.

Ordinarily individuals feel "in control" of their lives. Illness reduces that control and may create instability and cause anxiety. When hospitalized, a person leaves behind the familiarity of home and work for the unfamiliar hospital setting. Activities may be limited, family visits may be restricted, possessions are locked up or returned home, and someone else is in control of the decision making. Most people do not expect to become ill or to have life-style alterations resulting from illness or accidents. Serious injury or illness may dramatically alter an individual's role performance (family, income, work), body image, life-style, and self-concept. Regardless of whether the situation is temporary or permanent, the individual's emotional state is disturbed.

Some patients will have difficulty with an illness or crisis. The "difficult" patient may cope by displaying denial, hostility, noncompliance, aggression, manipulation, apathy, or depression.

Behavior is learned, and patients bring their learned behavior patterns into the health care setting. All behavior has meaning; humans behave to meet needs and to communicate. The behavior the individual uses is based on past experiences and is the best available to the individual at the time. The interventions for nursing are to notice and respond therapeutically to all behavior. By understanding the relationship between stressors, anxiety, and behavior, the nurse can facilitate healthy adaptation.

Applying the Nursing Process

In every setting the nurse uses the nursing process to meet the many needs of the patient. The nursing process consists of five basic components: assessment, nursing diagnosis formulation, planning, intervention, and evaluation. The nursing process begins with the collection of data, which are then analyzed, and a nursing diagnosis is formulated. From the diagnosis, plans are outlined and then implemented. The nurse then evaluates these interventions to determine whether the goals have been achieved. The LPN/LVN participates in the nursing process by observing patient behavior and assisting in establishing the nursing diagnosis. Together with the RN, appropriate nursing interventions are outlined for the individual patient. The LPN/LVN and RN implement the plan and continue to observe and report behavior. It is from these observations that adjustments are made in the plans of care.

Box 49-5 outlines basic nursing assessments of emotional status. Other assessments include observation for potential for violence, level of anxiety, use of defense mechanisms, and use of coping methods.

The role of the LPN/LVN in the planning process is to offer suggestions for intervention believed to be helpful to the patient. RN and LPN/LVN work as a team to implement the plan of care.

Evaluation is ongoing. At intervals or when the patient's response dictates, the care plan is updated. Examination of the documentation and personal observations are all considerations when evaluating the plan of care (see nursing care plan, pp. 1304-1305).

All phases of the nursing process should be clearly documented. Most documentation is on an ongoing basis and should include the assessment criteria found in Table 49-5 on pp. 1306-1307. All facilities use various forms and methods in documentation. Information should be accurate and descriptive. Documentation of the patient's actual conservation is very valuable.

In summary, humans are complex in nature and possess both physical and psychological components. The individual is affected in various ways by any change that creates stress and anxiety. Nurses in any setting must consider the emotional aspect of the individual. The nurse can be a valuable resource in helping a patient develop adaptive patterns. To accomplish this, the nurse needs a basic knowledge of human behavior, basic mental health principles, and assessment.

BOX 49-5 ASSESSMENT OF EMOTIONAL STATUS

General appearance	Describe dress, makeup, and hygiene
General behavior	Describe general activity level, posture, gait, and response to examination
Speech pattern	Describe rate, tone, loudness, and quantity content of speech (descriptions include too detailed in response to questions, extreme distractibility, unable to complete an answer, uses rhyming)
Content of thought	Describe thinking being reality oriented, delusional, evidence of hallucinations, evidence of ideas of reference or other non-reality-based thinking
Mood/affect	Describe the general feeling state and affect
Sensorial function	Describe orientation, memory, attention, ability to think abstractly
Insight and judgment	Does the individual understand the present situation? What is the individual willing to do about it?
Potential for danger	Assess the individual's potential for violence or self-harm, degree of impulse control, previous history of violence or aggression toward others

REFERENCES AND SUGGESTED READINGS

1. Aguilera DC and Messick JM: Crisis intervention theory and methodology, ed 6, St Louis, 1990, The CV Mosby Co.
2. American Psychiatric Association: Diagnostic and statistical manual of mental disorders, ed 3, Washington, DC, 1987, The Association.
3. Antani-Otong: When your patient is depressed, Nurs 88, 18(9):70, 1988.
4. Bauer B and Hill S: Essentials of mental health care, Philadelphia, 1986, WB Saunders Co.
5. Burgess AW: Psychiatric nursing in the hospital and the community, ed 4, Englewood Cliffs, NJ, 1985, Prentice Hall, Inc.
6. Crawford A and Kilander V: Psychiatric mental health nursing, Philadelphia, 1986, FA Davis.
7. Grainger R: Dealing with feelings, Am J Nurs 90(2):14, 1990.
8. Johnson BS: Psychiatric mental health nursing adaptation and growth, Philadelphia, 1989, JB Lippincott Co.
9. Lewis S et al: Manual of psychosocial nursing interventions: promoting mental health in medical-surgical settings, Philadelphia, 1989, WB Saunders Co.
10. Lewis S, McDowell W, and Gregory R: Saving the suicidal patient from himself, RN 49(12):26, 1986.
11. Manderino M and Bzdek V: Mobilizing depressed clients, J Psychosocial Nurs, May 1986.
12. McClane A, editor: Classification of nursing diagnosis: proceedings of the seventh national conference, St Louis, 1987, The CV Mosby Co.
13. McConnell E: Do you really know what's troubling your patient? Nurs 90. 20(2):43, 1990.
14. Medried R: Strategies for handling angry patients and their families, Nurs 90 20(4):66, 1990.
15. Mereness D and Taylor C: Essentials of psychiatric nursing, ed 13, St Louis, 1990, The CV Mosby Co.
16. Pasquali E, Arnold H, and Debasio N: Mental health nursing, ed 3, St Louis, 1989, The CV Mosby Co.
17. Pelletier L and Kane J: Strategies for handling manipulative patients, Nurs 89 19(5):82, 1989.
18. Perko J and Kriegh H: Psychiatric and mental health nursing, East Norwalk, Conn, 1990, Appleton & Lange.
19. Powell A and Minick M: Alcohol withdrawal syndrome, Am J Nurs 88(3):312, 1988.
20. Sanders J and Buckingham S: Suicidal AIDS patients: when depression turns deadly, Nurs 88 18(7):59, 1988.
21. Schmitt D: Linda had lost her looks—and her will to live, Nurs 89 19(3):43, 1989.
22. Stuart G and Sundeen J: Principles and practice of psychiatric nursing, ed 4, St Louis, 1991, Mosby–Year Book, Inc.
23. Stuart G and Sundeen J: Pocket guide to psychiatric nursing, St Louis, 1988, The CV Mosby Co.
24. Taylor C: Mereness' essentials of psychiatric nursing, ed 13, St Louis, 1990, The CV Mosby Co.
25. Wilson H and Kneisel C: Psychiatric nursing, ed 3, Menlo Park, Calif, 1988, Addison Wesley.

NURSING CARE PLAN: THE PATIENT WITH DEPRESSION

PATIENT DATA: Mr. Cullin is a 68-year-old widower whose wife died 18 months ago. He was admitted to the open psychiatric unit for the diagnosis of major depression. Mr. Cullin has two grown children who live out of state. He has severe hypertension and beginning COPD.

On admission Mr. Cullin states, "I just can't go on all alone like this . . . . I have so little energy." Mr. Cullin has lost 20 pounds in 6 months; he weighs 180 pounds and is 5 feet 11 inches tall. Mr. Cullin rarely leaves home, although friends ask him out frequently. He complains of difficulty sleeping and reports 2 to 3 hours of sleep per night. When asked, he admits to thinking of killing himself; he states he attempted to do so with a mild overdose of his hypertension medication before this admission.

Possible nursing diagnoses for Mr. Cullin include potential for violence, self-directed; altered nutrition: less than body requirements; sleep pattern disturbance; dysfunctional grieving; and impaired social interaction.

GOAL: Patient will recognize and express feelings within 10 days.

Nursing diagnoses	Patient goals	Nursing interventions
Potential for violence: self-directed, related to suicidal thoughts, feelings of hopelessness and inability to cope as manifested by stating, "I can't go on alone," and overdose 2 days ago	Patient will not attempt suicide throughout hospitalization. Patient will express feelings when asked. Patient will verbalize one future-oriented goal not related to suicide.	Establish a relationship; keep staff assignment as consistent as possible. Provide a safe environment: no sharps, check to make certain patient swallowed medications. Use a kind, firm manner; tell patient that you can see that he is sad and that he still needs to do . . . At least two times per shift, while patient is awake, observe his suicide potential; ask "Are you thinking of hurting yourself now?" If yes, ask "How are you going to hurt yourself?" (Decide whether method is available.) "Can you agree not to hurt yourself for ______ *(specify time period)* without talking with me first?" If patient cannot commit to not acting, stay with him while appropriate alternative care is sought. Check on patient frequently q 30-45 min at varied intervals, such as 7:00, 7:25, 8:10, 8:35 . . . As patient begins to verbalize feelings, attempt to focus on anything that has gone right that he can feel good about. Ask what/how he can change to decrease feelings of loneliness. Assist patient to identify past meaningful activities (e.g., card game); attempt to have patient engage in these again. Have patient explore ways to cope: problem solving, physical activity, social activities, communication, etc.

NURSING CARE PLAN: THE PATIENT WITH DEPRESSION—cont'd

Nursing diagnoses	Patient goals	Nursing interventions
Impaired social interaction, related to fatigue and hopelessness, manifested by failure to interact with other patients and inability to make a decision, such as choosing clothing to wear	Patient will participate in unit activities when asked by day 3. Patient will remain out of bed and room by day 3. Patient will talk about one activity that he can do after discharge from hospital.	Encourage interaction with others (e.g., at mealtimes). Get patient out of bed and room. Have patient do short, focused activities (e.g., deliver flowers to a peer, call a family member). Plan for activities after discharge.
Altered nutrition; less than body requirements, related to grief, manifested by eating only about 40% of meals, weight loss of 20 lb in past 6 mo	Patient will eat 60% of all food offered. Patient will have adequate fluid intake. Patient will weigh 180 pounds.	Monitor eating. Encourage fluids. Try six small feedings. Present attractively prepared foods, foods patient likes.
Sleep pattern disturbance, related to lack of activity and feelings of hopelessness, manifested by sleeping only 2 to 3 hr/night	Patient will sleep 5-6 hr/night before discharge. Patient will verbalize ability to use relaxation techniques when awake at night.	Encourage planned naps only. Help patient to establish consistent sleep time. Teach progressive relaxation exercises. Plan a physical activity while patient is awake.

Mr. Cullin is treated with antidepressant medications (Pamelor [nortriptyline] and Desyrel [trazodone]), which he is tolerating well. He also has individual therapy with the unit psychologist. He is participating in the unit milieu and interacting with the nursing staff. Fourteen days after admission he has achieved the following:

1. No self-harm.
2. Discusses feelings one-to-one when asked; no spontaneous expressions as yet.
3. Verbalizes difficulty in thinking about returning home.
4. Two-pound weight gain; eating 70% of food and fluid offered.
5. Sleeping 5 hr/night with medication.
6. Has tried relaxation techniques but has not used them during the night.

Mr. Cullin is making progress; plans for activities, eating, coping, and socialization after discharge need additional interventions.

Table 49-5 Psychoactive Medications

Generic Name	Trade Name	Side Effects	Nursing Implications
ANTIDEPRESSANTS			
Tricyclics			
Amitriptyline Amoxapine Desipramine hydrochloride Imipramine hydrochloride Nortriptyline hydrochloride	Elavil Asendin Norpramin Tofranil Aventyl, Pamelor	Anticholinergic effects, including dry mouth, blurred vision, constipation, urinary retention, and tachycardia Other precautions: not used in patients with severe liver disease or immediately after a myocardial infarction; given with caution for persons with cardiac disease; abrupt withdrawal may cause sleep disturbance	Monitor B/P for hypotension Observe for urinary retention and constipation Suggest sugarless gum or candy for dry mouth Teaching: may experience increased appetite; caution patient against strenuous exercise and high temperature, because perspiration may be blocked by anticholinergic effects
Monoamine oxidase inhibitors			
Phenelzine sulfate Tranylcypromine sulfate	Nardil Parnate	Orthostatic hypotension, headache, abnormal heart rate and/or rhythm, blurred vision, dry mouth, fatigue, nausea and vomiting, constipation Other precautions: hypertensive crisis can result, especially if tyramine-containing foods are not restricted (e.g., red wine, beer, aged cheese, chocolate, licorice, yogurt, caffeine-rich foods, liver, and broad beans)	Monitor B/P, have patient stand up slowly and move legs before rising Teaching: foods high in tyramine must be restricted Consult physician before taking over-the-counter cough/cold products
Other			
Trazodone hydrochloride	Desyrel	See tricyclics	Teach patient to take with food to decrease vertigo
Fluoxetine	Prozac	Appetite loss, insomnia, anxiety, tremors, fatigue, weight loss, hyponatremia, diarrhea, frequent urination, painful menses	Teach patient to be alert for appetite loss Teach patient not to drink alcohol or take other antidepressant medications with Prozac
ANTIMANIC			
Lithium carbonate	Eskalith Lithobid	Possible toxicity at serum levels above 1.5 mEq/L Symptoms include nausea, vomiting, abdominal cramps, diarrhea, polyuria, polydipsia, coarse muscle tremor, ataxia, slurred speech, confusion, and seizures Long-term effects: possible kidney damage	Teach patient signs and symptoms of toxicity and to maintain high fluid intake and stable salt use Blood tests to assess level will be needed periodically
ANTIPSYCHOTICS			
Chlorpromazine Thioridazine hydrochloride Trifluoperazine hydrochloride Fluphenazine hydrochloride Perphenazine Thiothixene Haloperidol	Thorazine Mellaril-S Stelazine Prolixin Permitil Trilafon Navane Haldol	Anticholinergic side effects: dry mouth, blurred vision, constipation, urinary retention, postural hypotension, confusion Extrapyramidal side effects (EPS): akithesia (severe restlessness—"I can't stand still") Parkinsonian effects: rigidity, resting tremor, shuffling gait Dystonias: bizarre movements of the face and neck, torticollis, oculogyric crisis Other precautions: lowered seizure threshold, tardive dyskinesia (characterized by involuntary movements of lip, tongue, and jaw after medications are stopped or decreased) Rare side effects: neuroleptic malignant syndrome (hyperthermia, muscle rigidity, labile B/P, confusion, cardiovascular collapse)	Suggest sugarless candy or gum for dry mouth Teach patient the importance of taking medications and not stopping medications abruptly Patient should wear sunscreen product Baseline vital signs and blood counts Have patient move before rising Watch for EPS and use anticholinergic medications as ordered prn (Cogentin, Benadryl) Watch for neuroleptic malignant syndrome

Table 49-5 Psychoactive Medications—cont'd

Generic Name	Trade Name	Side Effects	Nursing Implications
ANTIANXIETY AGENTS			
Alprazolam Chlordiazepoxide hydrochloride Clorazepate dipotassium Lorazepam Oxazepam	Xanax Librium Tranxene Ativan Serax	Drowsiness, ataxia, muscle weakness, occasionally disinhibition Patient may complain of "morning hangover" and transient hypotension on arising Other precautions: must be used with caution in patients with depression, psychosis, or history of drug abuse	Watch for increased side effects in the elderly Explain to the patient the need to arise first to a sitting position, to equilibrate, before standing Teach patients not to operate machines while taking these medications, to avoid alcohol use, and not to stop medication abruptly

CHAPTER CHALLENGE

KEY POINTS

- Individuals have unique personalities.
- All behavior has meaning. An individual's behavior is the best that person is capable of, given the present environment.
- Corrective emotional experiences assist the individual to change. The nurse uses therapeutic communication to facilitate this.
- Personality refers to the relatively consistent set of attitudes and behaviors particular to an individual.
- Self is an important part of personality; self consists of identity, body image, role, and esteem.
- Anxiety is a universal response to a real or imagined threat to self.
- Defense mechanisms are automatic behaviors used to protect the individual from anxiety.
- Coping mechanisms are usually adaptive methods used by the individual to deal with feelings or stressors.
- Stress is the nonspecific response of the body to any demand made on it. Stressors are any factors causing stress.
- Mental health and illness can be viewed on a continuum.
- DSM III R is a multiaxial system used in the diagnosis of psychiatric disorders. This system consists of physical, psychiatric, and social factors affecting the individual.
- Psychiatric nursing is a science and an art. Each individual has unique value and potential for growth. The nurse in psychiatry uses self in the context of a therapeutic relationship; to accomplish this, the nurse must have self-knowledge.
- The nursing process is used in psychiatry and includes assessment, nursing diagnoses formulation planning, intervention, and evaluation. The care plan documents this process.
- Therapeutic communication is a dynamic method of interacting with patients for problem solving and growth.
- In psychiatry, medications are used to assist individuals with feelings and behaviors.
- Behavior is observed and then evaluated to determine a patient's progress and the effectiveness of the care plan.

STUDY QUESTIONS

1. Which of the following is an example of a personality trait:
   a. Body image
   b. Eye color
   c. Shyness
   d. All of the above
2. Which of the following is believed to be a source of anxiety:
   a. Fear
   b. Threat to self
   c. Another person
   d. Change
3. Which of the following is a common mechanism used to avoid the feeling of anxiety:
   a. Defense mechanism
   b. Coping mechanism
   c. Mood
   d. Stress
4. Which of the following is an example of the defense mechanism *identification*:
   a. An 8-year-old sucking his thumb
   b. Kicking the door when you are angry with another
   c. Developing blindness in reaction to witnessing a murder
   d. An employee dressing similarly to the employer
5. Which if any of the following characterizes a coping mechanism:
   a. It is a sign of mental illness
   b. It is used automatically
   c. It is used voluntarily
   d. None of the above
6. Which of the following is included as a fundamental goal of psychiatric nursing:
   a. Assisting patients in establishing and maintaining effective interpersonal relationships
   b. Ensuring patient medication compliance
   c. Looking for adaptation in patients
   d. The nurse learning about herself
7. The mental status examination assesses mental health functioning in the area of cognition, affect, and which, if any, of the following:
   a. Intelligence
   b. Behavior
   c. Relationships
   d. None of the above
8. Which of the following is included in the role of the LPN/LVN in the planning phase of the nursing process in psychiatry:
   a. Complete responsibility for formulation and documentation of the plan
   b. Setting patient goals
   c. Telling the physician the plan
   d. Offer suggestions for intervention and possibly share the plan with the patient
9. Which of the following is considered a therapeutic technique:
   a. Reassurance
   b. Self-disclosure
   c. Arguing
   d. Using silence
10. Which of the following is considered an anticholinergic side effect:
    a. Dry mouth
    b. Akinesia
    c. Bizarre face and neck movements
    d. Tremors
11. Which of the following interventions is for the suicidal patient with a nursing diagnosis of potential for violence: self-directed:
    a. Seclusion
    b. Providing a safe environment
    c. Checking every 4-5 minutes
    d. Telling the patient that he does not want to hurt himself

STUDY QUESTIONS (cont'd)

12. Which of the following nursing diagnoses is commonly associated with the manic phase of bipolar affective disorder:
    a. Impaired tissue perfusion
    b. Hopelessness
    c. Impaired social interaction
    d. Pain
13. True or false: individuals can usually identify the cause of their distress.
    a. T
    b. F
14. Five-year-old Johnny is admitted for treatment of pneumonia. Johnny clings to his mother and starts to suck his thumb. This is an example of the defense mechanism known as:
    a. Repression
    b. Suppression
    c. Regression
    d. Projection
15. Mr. Horvac is a 62-year-old businessman. He had a myocardial infarction 2 days ago. He has been allowed to perform self-grooming and hygiene and may be up to a chair for meals. The evening nurse finds him on the floor doing sit-ups. This is an example of the defense mechanism known as:
    a. Substitution
    b. Sublimation
    c. Identification
    d. Denial
16. What level of anxiety produces a disintegration of the personality along with a distortion of reality:
    a. Mild
    b. Moderate
    c. Severe
    d. Panic
17. True or false: stress always produces anxiety:
    a. T
    b. F
18. Freud described the personality as having three distinct parts. The ego:
    a. Seeks constant gratification
    b. Strives for perfection
    c. Composes the personality at birth
    d. Is referred to as the reality factor
19. Stress can be defined as:
    a. Anything that produces stress
    b. Any demand made on the body
    c. Two existing drives present at the same time
    d. A vague feeling of dread or impending doom
20. Dementia is classified as which of the following disorders:
    a. Thought process
    b. Affective
    c. Anxiety
    d. Organic
21. Mrs. Melmann has a history of mental disorder. She has been hospitalized for treatment of dehydration. The staff reports that Mrs. Melmann is making statements concerning the food being "poisoned." Mrs. Melmann may be experiencing which one of the following:
    a. Delusion
    b. Illusion
    c. Obsession
    d. Hallucination
22. The nurse enters the room to find Mr. Jablonski sitting in the chair, staring out the window. His lunch tray has hardly been touched. The nurse states, "Mr. Jablonski, I noticed that you did not eat much. Was there something wrong with the food?" The patient replies, "I can't eat this garbage. Oh, I hope I don't have cancer." The most appropriate response by the nurse would be:
    a. "Is there something else that you would rather eat?"
    b. "The dietary department worked very hard to prepare this meal."
    c. "Why don't you talk to your doctor about your laboratory reports?"
    d. "You think you have cancer."

50

The Patient with an Addictive Personality

ELIZABETH SCHENK

LEARNING OBJECTIVES

After reading this chapter, the student should be able to do the following:

- Define the key terms.
- Name three types of addictions, and explain each.
- Describe the terms *dependence* and *tolerance* as they relate to drug and alcohol use.
- Describe one educational effort and one legal effort that have been used to decrease the incidence of chemical dependency.
- Explain the concept of intervention as it relates to alcoholism.
- Describe what is meant by enabling behavior.
- Explain two reasons that have been proposed to explain the development of chemical dependency.
- Describe three disorders associated with alcoholism and two disorders/diseases associated with drug addiction.
- Describe what is meant by the term *drug addiction.*
- Identify the six types of drugs of abuse
- Discuss why nurses are at increased risk to develop chemical dependency.

RELATED TOPICS OF INTEREST

- Basic nutrition (Chapter 22)
- Diet therapy (Chapter 23)
- Care of the patient with a gastrointestinal or accessory organ disorder (Chapter 31)
- Mental health concepts (Chapter 49)

KEY TERMS

Define the following:

- abstinence
- abuse
- addiction
- Al-Anon
- Alcoholics Anonymous
- alcohol withdrawal syndrome
- alcoholism
- anorexia nervosa
- bulimia
- cannabis (marijuana)
- chemical dependence
- co-dependency
- delirium tremens (DTs)
- detoxification
- drug abuse
- drug addiction
- habituation
- hallucinogen
- physical dependence
- tolerance
- Wernicke's encephalopathy
- withdrawal symptoms

DEFINITIONS

The treatment of patients with addictive behaviors is an important concern for nurses. Treatment centers are in many areas, and more nurses are becoming involved in this specialty. Many patients in general hospitals also suffer from some type of addictive behavior. Persons may suffer from more than one **addiction** at the same time. An example of this is the alcoholic person who is also a drug addict and a compulsive gambler.

Alcoholism and drug addiction are commonly referred to as **chemical dependence.** Alcohol is a drug, and the person addicted to alcohol may be at greater risk for drug addiction. Other addictions include compulsive gambling, compulsive shopping, eating disorders, and sexual addictions. Co-dependency is also a problem requiring treatment. This chapter will deal mainly with alcoholism and drug addiction but will briefly cover co-dependency and eating disorders.

Most modern definitions of dependence concerning **drug addiction** and alcoholism consist of two parts—physical and psychological dependence. **Physical dependence** refers to a physiological state where the continuous and prolonged consumption of a drug or alcohol leads to the user adapting to its presence. **Tolerance** then develops. This is the ability to endure ordinarily injurious substances, such as drug or alcohol, without apparent physiological or psychological injury. If the use of alcohol or drugs stops, withdrawal symptoms occur. Psychological dependence refers to the craving for a drug or alcohol.

DUAL DIAGNOSIS

Chemical dependence is a primary illness; however, chemically dependent people often have other psychological effects, such as depression or anxiety. Many problems disappear when drinking and drug use cease; it is essential to diagnose and treat chemical dependence before other psychological problems are investigated.

Psychiatric and psychological symptoms may, however, make recognition of an addiction problem more difficult. Determining the correct diagnosis is a task for an expert in chemical dependence and in psychiatry or psychology. Persons with a dual diagnosis may be more difficult to treat and may require treatment with medication.

PREVENTION

Prevention of chemical dependence is a complex issue. Legal efforts have been made, by restricting the sale of alcohol to minors and by instituting heavier penalties for driving while intoxicated or drug trafficking. Unfortunately, many of these efforts have not been successful.

The key to prevention is, in part, education. This includes teaching fairly young children about the dangers of drug and alcohol use and **abuse.** Many elementary schools now start these programs as early as the first or second grades. In addition, work may be done with children to increase their self-esteem so that they may be better able to resist peer pressure to drink or use drugs as they become older.

Also, families and employers of alcoholics or drug abusers are being educated about these problems. They are taught that alcoholism is a disease that needs treatment. The alcoholic is usually surrounded by persons who enable his use and abuse. An example of this is the spouse who calls the employer on behalf of the drunk or hungover mate to report an illness, such as the flu. Without this enabling behavior, which includes making many excuses for the behavior of the alcoholic, the alcoholic might seek help sooner.

Prompt diagnosis and treatment can be important in assisting alcoholics to once again become productive members of society. It is often difficult to make the diagnosis of chemical dependence. Some indications of the problem include frequent illnesses or related illnesses, undue preoccupation with the use of chemicals, and mood swings. Other indications include violent or acting-out behavior, denial about the use of substances, and financial difficulties. The person tends to use the substance as an answer to all problems, loses control over the use, and loses the ability to express feelings. The use of defense mechanisms, especially denial, is common.

Prevention of complications must be considered. These complications occur not only because of effects of the substance, but also because of nutritional problems or infections. Complications for drug addicts often occur because of acquired disease from dirty needles or equipment and may prove fatal, such as with AIDS.

ALCOHOLISM

Etiology

Alcoholism is a common health problem and may add to the problems of persons with other health disorders. Excessive drinking of alcohol may lead to coma or death from acute alcohol poisoning or to numerous health problems if the drinking continues over a long period. The alcoholic begins to develop an increasing tolerance and physical dependence on alcohol. Blackouts from episodes of drinking may start to occur. Guilt, shame, and remorse are common; the alcoholic then drinks more to relieve these feelings. As the drinking increases, problems increase and relationships with others deteriorate. The person reaches a point where "he drinks to live and lives to drink."

Estimates are that about 90 million people use alcohol and at least 9 to 10 million persons are alcoholics or problem drinkers. In addition, alcoholism affects the functioning of another 30 million friends and relatives of alcohol abusers. Industries lose billions of dollars annually because of alcoholism. This includes medical expenses, lost wages, decreased production, motor vehicle accidents, and crime.[13]

The use of alcohol predates recorded history. Cultures from many parts of the world have developed alcoholic beverages that have been used to celebrate important events. Alcohol has been used as medicine, as a form of magic, and as a part of worship services. In the United States, legal positions on the use of alcohol have varied. In 1642 drunkenness was punishable by a fine. In 1790 a law was passed that gave every soldier a daily portion of liquor. Prohibition, which forbade the production and sale of alcoholic beverages, was passed in 1919 and repealed in 1933.

Theories of the Cause of Alcoholism

No one theory can explain the cause of alcoholism. Some believe that persons are more likely to develop alcoholism because of some physical reason, such as an inner urge controlled by the nervous system or a dysfunction of the endocrine system. It has been found that alcoholism is in part genetically determined. The incidence of alcoholism is high in families, and the risk of sons of alcoholic men developing alcoholism over their lifetime is 30% to 50%. Studies of twins have shown that the identical twin of an alcoholic will be an alcoholic in 60% of the cases, whereas only 30% of the fraternal twins of alcoholics will be alcoholics.

Other theories are based on the belief that some part of the personality leads to the development of alcoholism. Certain common personality traits have been identified in addicted persons. These include low stress tolerance, dependency, negative self-image, and feelings of insecurity and depression. It is not clear whether these traits are present before the development of alcoholism or are a result of it.[13]

A relationship has been found between various groups in society and alcohol use. For instance, Jews, Mormons, and Moslems have a very low rate of alcoholism, whereas the French have a high rate.

Some people still believe that alcoholism develops as a result of either a moral fault or a sin of the alcoholic. Much of the early treatment of alcoholics was based on this theory. Today, alcoholism is generally accepted as a disease that is treatable.

Pathophysiology

Alcohol is a central nervous system depressant. The so-called stimulating effect of alcohol occurs because the first areas affected are the higher centers of the brain that govern self-control and judgment. As alcohol continues to be ingested, other areas of the brain are affected. Unconsciousness may set in, respirations may be affected, and death may occur.

Alcohol does not require digestion and is absorbed in both the stomach and the intestine. An empty stomach increases absorption. After ingestion, small amounts of alcohol are lost through breathing and in the urine, but 90% of alcohol is broken down by the liver. The active ingredient in alcoholic beverages is ethyl alcohol, or ethanol. Twelve ounces of beer, 4 ounces of wine, and 1½ ounces of "hard" liquor contain a similar amount of alcohol.

Alcohol has a diuretic effect. Increased amounts of electrolytes, especially potassium, magnesium, and zinc, may be excreted in the urine of a heavy drinker. Prolonged use of alcohol has a toxic effect on the intestinal mucosa that results in decreased absorption of thiamine, folic acid, and vitamin B_{12}.

Alcohol is not converted to glycogen and provides the body with calories but no minerals or vitamins. One ounce of alcohol provides 200 kcal, but these are "empty calories" (calories with no nutritional value). Blood alcohol levels depend on the amount of alcohol ingested and the size of the individual. Most states designate blood alcohol serum levels of 100 mg/dl (0.10%) as the legal limit for driving a motor vehicle. Increasing blood alcohol levels have increasingly more serious side effects (Box 50-1).

BOX 50-1 BLOOD ALCOHOL LEVELS AND RELATED SIDE EFFECTS

LEVEL	SIDE EFFECTS
50-75 mg/dl (0.05%-.075%)	Pleasant, relaxed state, mild sedation, loosening of inhibitions
100-200 mg/dl (0.1%-0.2%)	Overt signs of intoxication: loosening of tongue, clumsiness, beginning emotional changes
200-400 mg/dl (0.2%-0.4%)	Severe intoxication: difficulty speaking, stumbling, emotional lability
400-500 mg/dl (0.4%-0.5%)	Stupor, coma
Over 500 mg/dl (0.5%)	Usually fatal

Assessment

It is important to collect both subjective and objective data about the patient suffering from substance abuse. Subjective data include the person's normal using or drinking pattern, as well as the date and time of the last drink or use of drugs. The specific drink or drug used and the quantity used are important. See Box 50-2 for an example of a chemical use history that may be helpful in determining the drinking or using pattern. (See therapeutic dialogue and see latter part of chapter for specific information of drugs mentioned.)

Any history of tremors, hallucinations, delusions, or DTs should be assessed. Past periods of abstinence, normal diet patterns, the presence of problems (legal, occupational, family), and any family history of chemical dependency are assessed. It is important to remember that the defense mechanism of denial will usually be present in untreated chemical dependence. The information

THERAPEUTIC DIALOGUE

NURSE: Welcome to our unit, Mr. Smith. My name is Sue Jones and I am the nurse on duty tonight. Can you tell me why you are here?

PATIENT: They made me come.

NURSE: Can you tell me more about what you mean?

PATIENT: My family ganged up on me and had this meeting. They called it an intervention. They set it up for me to come here.

NURSE: That must be hard for you. Why did they have the meeting?

PATIENT: I only drink on the weekends, and then not that much.

NURSE: How much is not much?

PATIENT: About 10 beers, more or less.

NURSE: What is the most you've ever had on the weekend?

PATIENT: About a case and a half. But that's unusual.

NURSE: Mr. Smith, I know that it is sometimes hard to get really honest about drinking. But I want to assure you that information you share with me will be shared only with the treatment team. Also, we're not here to judge you. It's important for you to tell me as honestly as you can what and how much you've been drinking, as well as the time of your last drink. This is important so that we can help prevent withdrawal symptoms and complications that could happen. I'm not sure you've told me the whole story.

PATIENT: You don't think I'm terrible?

NURSE: No, I don't. I think that you're sick and need help, but I don't think you're terrible.

PATIENT: I guess I drink about a case a day, every day. I also use cocaine several times a week.

(Interview continues.)

BOX 50-2 CHEMICAL USE HISTORY

CHEMICAL CLASS	DRUG NAME	DATE LAST USED	AMOUNT	FREQUENCY	LENGTH OF USE	USUAL AMOUNT	METHOD OF USE
Barbiturates							
Tranquilizers							
Alcohol							
Marijuana							
Opium							
Heroin							
Narcotics							
Cocaine							
Stimulants							
Hallucinogens							
Inhalants							
PCP (dust)							
Amphetamines							
Caffeine							
Hash/hash oil							
Analgesics							
Others							

gained from the person may not always be accurate, and it is helpful to validate it with families or significant others.

Objective data that can be important include abnormal responses to preoperative medication, anesthetics, or sedatives. The presence of tremor, morning nausea, or skin conditions should be assessed, as well as mental functioning, general behavior, and the relationship of weight to height. The presence of tachycardia, hypertension, neuropathies, and petechiae are significant. The presence of ascites and a blood or urine specimen positive for alcohol or drugs should alert the nurse to take further history.

Diagnostic Tests

Routine blood tests will often reveal abnormalities that are directly related to alcoholism. These include liver enzymes, hypoglycemia, and abnormal blood protein levels. Magnesium levels may be decreased. It is not uncommon to find anemia and other evidence of poor nutrition in alcoholic patients.

Disorders Associated with Alcoholism

Fetal alcohol syndrome. Fetal alcohol problems occur frequently in newborns whose mothers drank frequently during pregnancy. These women have a higher incidence of delivering infants with birth defects, such as mental retardation, growth disorders, and malformed body parts, as well as a high incidence of spontaneous abortions, stillbirths, and infant deaths. Even moderate drinking can result in infants with birth defects.

Alcohol withdrawal. When alcohol is not available to a person who has developed a physiological dependence, withdrawal symptoms occur. These symptoms range from mild tremors to severe agitation and hallucinations. The type and seriousness of the symptoms depend on several factors. Alcoholics at high risk include older persons, persons who have had a previous history of delirium tremens, persons with nutritional problems, and persons with other illnesses. Symptoms of alcohol withdrawal **(alcohol withdrawal syndrome)** include diaphoresis, tachycardia, elevated blood pressure, tremors, nausea and/or vomiting, anorexia, restlessness, hallucinations, and convulsions.[30]

The tremors associated with alcohol withdrawal usually are seen 6 to 48 hours after the last drink. They may persist from 3 to 5 days. The hands are involved first, but the tremors may become generalized with involvement of the feet, tongue, and trunk. Seizures may occur from 12 to 24 hours after the last drink. Usually these are grand mal seizures and are not preceded by an aura.

Delirium tremens, or DTs, is an acute complication of alcohol withdrawal that interferes with brain metabolism. The rate of death can be as high as 15%, even with treatment. Signs that indicate DTs may occur include tremors, increased activity, confusion and disorientation, fear, and an elevated temperature. DTs often occurs suddenly, 3 to 4 days after the last drink. The condition lasts from 2 days to a week, but at times can last as long as 4 weeks.

Other disorders that occur with alcoholism include those found in Box 50-3.

NURSING DIAGNOSES	PATIENT GOALS
Potential activity intolerance	Patient will maintain optimal activity.
Anxiety	Patient will verbalize less anxiety.
Potential altered body temperature	Patient's body temperature will be maintained in normal range.
Ineffective individual and family coping	Patient and family will learn to cope in healthier fashion.
Ineffective denial	Patient will admit use of mood-altering substances and effect on life.
Fear	Patient will verbalize fewer fears.
Fluid volume excess or deficit	Patient will maintain normal fluid volume.
Altered health maintenance	Patient will demonstrate appropriate health maintenance activities.
Impaired home maintenance management	Patient will be able to manage at home.
Hypothermia	Patient will maintain normal body temperature.
Incontinence	Patient will demonstrate continence.
Potential for infection	Patient will remain free of infection.
Potential for injury	Patient will remain free of injury.
Knowledge deficit	Patient will verbalize knowledge of disease concept and medical aspect. Patient will verbalize need for continued abstinence. Patient will verbalize importance of expressing feelings to stay sober. Patient will verbalize knowledge of drugs to avoid and the importance of being honest with physician and dentist. Patient will verbalize knowledge of defense mechanisms and signs and symptoms of impending relapse. Patient will verbalize knowledge of aftercare, including AA and Narcotics Anonymous (NA).
Impaired physical mobility	Mobility will be maintained at optimal level.
Noncompliance	Patient will comply with treatment regime.
Altered nutrition: less than body requirements	Patient will maintain adequate nutrition.
Powerlessness	Patient will verbalize powerlessness over alcohol.
Bathing/hygiene, dressing/grooming self-care deficit	Patient will be able to handle self-care.
Self-esteem disturbance	Patient will verbalize positive self-esteem.
Sensory/perceptural alteration	Patient will compensate effectively for sensory/perceptual alterations.
Sleep pattern disturbance	Patient will sleep at least 6 hours nightly.
Impaired social interaction	Patient will maintain positive social interactions with others.
Spiritual distress	Patient will verbalize sense of spirituality.
Altered thought processes	Patient will maintain ability to think clearly.
Potential for violence	Patient will control behavior.

BOX 50-3 DISORDERS THAT MAY OCCUR WITH ALCOHOLISM

SYSTEM	DISORDERS
Hepatic	Hepatitis, cirrhosis, fatty liver (see Chapter 31)
Gastrointestinal	Cancer of the mouth and esophagus, irritation of the stomach or pancreas, difficulty in absorbing food (see Chapter 31)
Neurological	Organic brain disease with confusion, Wernicke's encephalopathy (pathological condition of brain caused by thiamine deficiency), disorders of peripheral nerves (neuropathies) (see Chapter 38)
Cardiovascular	Enlarged heart, high blood pressure, increased cholesterol levels, low blood sugar, anemia, coronary artery disease, congestive heart failure (see Chapter 32)
Musculoskeletal	Disorders of muscles (myopathies) (see Chapter 30)
Immunological	Increased susceptibility to infection (see Chapter 39)

Nursing Interventions

Care for the alcoholic patient in the acute phase usually involves **detoxification** efforts to prevent acute withdrawal. Detoxification is undertaken in a controlled setting where the patient can be closely watched and treated for complications as needed.

Nursing diagnoses. Nursing diagnoses that may apply to the alcoholic patient are presented below. The actual diagnoses will depend on the condition and nursing assessment of the patient.

Medications

Medications used in the initial period of detoxification include chlordiazepoxide (Librium) or a similar drug. The drug is used in decreasing doses for its sedating and anticonvulsant effect during detoxification. The dosage can be as great as 50 mg every 3 hours during the first 24 hours. Anticonvulsant therapy may include phenytoin (Dilantin) and magnesium sulfate. The anticonvulsant may be continued for a longer period if the person has a history of seizures. Because nutritional problems are common with alcoholism, multivitamin supplements including thiamine and vitamin B_{12} are usually prescribed.

Specific medications may differ from setting to setting. In some, alcohol or paraldehyde will be used in the detoxification process. Whatever the medication used, it is important to realize that alcoholics may require large doses of medication to safely withdraw from alcohol. If medication does not control the withdrawal, restraints may be needed for safety of both the patient and the staff.

Another medication that may be used is disulfiram (Antabuse), which blocks the enzymatic action needed to metabolize alcohol. If the person drinks, the drug will cause nausea, vomiting, palpitations, and general ill feelings. Antabuse is used voluntarily by the patient to help maintain sobriety. It is important for him to know what effects will occur if he drinks while taking this drug. It is usually continued for some time after treatment.

Nutrition Therapy

Many alcoholics enter treatment in a poor nutritional state. They may have received most of their calories from alcohol or had no appetite for food. As the condition of the alcoholic improves, the appetite usually improves also. The emphasis is on three well-balanced meals a day, with free access to snacks. Many patients crave sugar in this period. If the alcoholic has developed cirrhosis of the liver, dietary modifications may be needed. In cases of DTs, intravenous feedings or feedings through a nasogastric tube may be necessary.

Patient Education

Educating the alcoholic about the disease is important. This should include information about the disease concept and medical aspects of the disease, including complications, the need for continued **abstinence,** and signs and symptoms of relapse. The importance of aftercare, including Alcoholics Anonymous (AA), the importance of being honest with a physician, and the importance of expressing feelings are also stressed. The patient should be advised about what drugs to avoid and about products that contain alcohol, such as mouthwash and after-shave.

Education of the alcoholic should also include the family and significant other. These persons need understanding and education to help themselves and the alcoholic to recover. **Al-Anon** may be helpful.[6] Al-Anon is a group of persons closely related to alcoholic persons who meet for support and self-help.

Rehabilitation

The object for treatment for alcoholism is to assist patients to completely stop drinking alcohol. They need to understand that they can never take one drink or mood-altering drug without the danger of relapse. Alcoholics who are not currently drinking are not considered cured—only recovering.

Group therapy is often used. The goal of this is to enable the person to see the relationship between alcohol and the negative consequences that have been suffered. Positive reinforcement, caring, emotional support, and encouragement are also important. The group can point out negative behaviors and defense mechanisms and offer possible solutions to its members.

Many recovering alcoholics attend **Alcoholics Anonymous** (AA). This is a group of self-acknowledged alcoholics whose goal is to stay sober and to help other alcoholics gain sobriety. AA groups meet regularly in most communities. Local AA groups are sometimes listed in the telephone book or in a local directory of meetings. A phone call to AA will bring help in the form of a telephone call or a visit by an AA member to the alcoholic desiring help.

The foundation of AA is a 12-step program that assists the alcoholic in admitting his or her powerlessness over alcohol and other drugs. The success of AA has led to the formation of other groups that share the same 12-step approach. These groups include Al-Anon, Families Anonymous, and Overeaters Anonymous. See Box 50-4 for a listing of the 12 steps.

Planned Confrontations

Some still believe that it is only when the alcoholic desires and seeks help that treatment can be effective.

BOX 50-4 **TWELVE STEPS OF ALCOHOLICS ANONYMOUS**

1. We admitted we were powerless over alcohol—that our lives had become unmanageable.
2. Came to believe that a power greater than ourselves could restore us to sanity.
3. Made a decision to turn our will and our lives over to the care of God as we understood him.
4. Made a searching and fearless moral inventory of ourselves.
5. Admitted to God, to ourselves, and to another human being the exact nature of our wrongs.
6. Were entirely ready to have God remove all these defects of character.
7. Humbly asked him to remove our shortcomings.
8. Made a list of all persons we had harmed, and became willing to make amends to them all.
9. Made direct amends to such people whenever possible, except when to do so would injure them or others.
10. Continued to take personal inventory and when we were wrong promptly admitted it.
11. Sought through prayer and meditation to improve our conscious contact with God as we understood Him, praying only for knowledge of His will for us and the power to carry it out.
12. Having had a spiritual awakening as a result of these steps, we tried to carry this message to alcoholics, and to practice these principles in all our affairs.

From Alcoholics Anonymous, New York, 1976, Alcoholics World Service, Inc.

Unfortunately, often by the time an alcoholic realizes the need for help, much has been lost. Recently a process called *intervention* has been used to assist the alcoholic in asking for help. Interventions are planned confrontations by individuals who care about the person. They present facts or data about specific and descriptive events. The tone of the intervention should be nonjudgmental. The goal of the intervention is to have the alcoholic see and accept reality so that the need for help is realized. It is best to have immediate help ready.[22] See nursing care plan on p. 1318.

DRUG ABUSE

Because alcohol is in itself a drug, alcoholism and **drug abuse** are considered part of the disease of chemical dependence. Persons who abuse substances often use drugs and alcohol. Much of the information covered in the section on alcoholism also pertains to the use of drugs.

The history of nonmedical drug use is thousands of years old. As early as 5000 BC, the Sumerians referred to a "joy plant" (thought to be the opium poppy plant). Since then, drugs have played a significant role in almost every culture. In recent years the incidence of drug abuse has risen. Drugs are often readily available.

The terms *habituation* and *addiction* have been used to define the nature and extent of drug use. Drug **habituation** includes repeated use of a drug to a point where there is psychological dependence. Drug **addiction** includes craving, psychological dependence, and physical dependence. *Drug dependence* or *chemical dependence* are other terms that may be used.

The drug types discussed in this chapter will include stimulants, depressants, hallucinogens, narcotics, cannabis, and deliriants.[13]

Stimulants

Stimulants are natural or synthetic drugs that have a strong stimulating effect on the central nervous system that is accompanied by a feeling of alertness and self-confidence. Other results include dilation of the pupils, increase in pulse and blood pressure, reduction of fatigue, reduction of appetite, and an increase in concentration. However, when the feeling of alertness wears off, the person experiences fatigue and depression. Drugs included in this category are amphetamines, cocaine, caffeine, and nicotine.

Stimulants have the potential to produce tolerance, but usually not physical withdrawal. Psychological dependence is common. Side effects of stimulant use include restlessness, dizziness, insomnia, headaches, diarrhea, constipation, and lack of appetite. Persons who ingest a large amount of stimulants over a period of time may experience extreme agitation and anxiety. Death may occur as a result of a cerebral hemorrhage or myocardial infarction. Persons can collapse from exhaustion while using stimulants. Withdrawal can lead to profound depression and may lead to suicide.

Amphetamines. Amphetamines are synthetic psychoactive drugs that are available in capsule or tablet form. Medical uses of amphetamines include the treatment of narcolepsy, obesity, fatigue, and depression. Ritalin, an amphetamine-like drug, is used to treat children who are hyperactive. Common amphetamines include dextroamphetamine (Dexedrine), methamphetamine (Methedrine), and amphetamine (Benzedrine). Street names include pep pills, dexies, bennies, ups, speed, crystal, meth, and whites.

Cocaine. Cocaine is a psychoactive drug that comes from the leaves of the South American coca bush. It was first used by early South American tribes. Its use was encouraged by the Spaniards, who found that the natives worked longer and harder and needed less food when they used cocaine.

At one time cocaine was used as an ingredient in many products, including syrups, nasal sprays, cigarettes, li-

NURSING CARE PLAN: THE PATIENT WITH ALCOHOLISM

Mr. Smith is a 54-year-old certified public accountant who is admitted to a treatment facility. He gives a history of drinking as much as a fifth of whiskey a day. Presently, he is slightly intoxicated and his blood alcohol level is 0.12%. His admission liver function studies are abnormal, and his urine drug screen is negative for any other drugs. He is separated from his wife of 30 years. However, she drove him to the facility and admitted that she still cared for him, but that his drinking was the cause for her leaving him. Mr. Smith has never been treated for alcoholism before. Except for hypertension, his health is good. He has been drinking heavily, according to his wife, for about 5 years, since their son was killed in an automobile accident. On admission, he has a slight tremor and is cooperative, but tearful.

Nursing diagnoses	Patient goals	Nursing interventions
Ineffective individual coping	Patient will learn to cope in healthier fashion.	Teach patient alternative ways to relax, such as biofeedback and relaxation techniques. Reinforce positive actions of patient. Encourage patient to share with other patients.
Ineffective denial	Patient will recognize effects of alcohol on life.	Assist patient to complete drug and alcohol history. Encourage patient to participate in group. Confront inconsistencies in drug history or story. Share abnormal laboratory values and implications with patient.
Potential for injury	Patient will remain free of injury.	Observe closely for signs of alcohol withdrawal. Medicate as ordered.
Knowledge deficit	Patient will verbalize knowledge of: disease concept, medical aspects, need for abstinence, importance of expressing feelings, drugs to avoid, importance of honesty to physician, defense mechanisms, aftercare, and AA.	Teach patient after withdrawal and when ready to listen.
Powerlessness, as a result of alcoholism	Patient will verbalize knowledge of powerlessness.	Assist patient to learn about and taking first step of AA.
Self-esteem disturbance	Patient will verbalize positive self-concept.	Give patient positive reinforcement of work. Demonstrate to patient that he is not unique. Help patient to process past events.

quors, and Coca-Cola. It was also recommended as a treatment for alcoholism. In 1914 the nonmedical use of cocaine was prohibited. Medical uses now include (1) an anesthetic of choice for some procedures of the nose and throat and (2) as an ingredient of Brompton's cocktail, used for pain control in patients with cancer.

Cocaine is used by sniffing, smoking, or injecting. Cocaine may also be free-based (a process of heating the drug to separate it from impurities). When free-base cocaine is injected, it produces a "high" that is more intense and short-lived than when cocaine is smoked.

A newer form of cocaine that is increasingly available is called *crack*. It is less expensive than other forms and highly addicting. Other street names for cocaine include blow, coke, dust, flake, nose candy, rock, snow, superblow, toot, and white.

Chronic sniffing of cocaine can destroy the nasal tissues. Smoking it can cause lesions in the lungs. Tolerance and psychological dependence can develop, and an overdose can cause convulsions, respiratory paralysis, and death. A cocaine psychosis has been reported, which is characterized by a loss of pleasure and orientation, hallucinations, and insomnia. Abrupt withdrawal from cocaine does not lead to physical withdrawal.[15]

Caffeine. Caffeine is the most accepted and used psychoactive substance in the United States. Many beverages, medications, and other products contain caffeine. It has been used as an additive in carbonated beverages since the early 1900s. Because of its availability and widespread use, most persons do not view caffeine as a drug.

In its pure state, caffeine is a white powder or white needle-shaped crystals. It stimulates the central nervous system (CNS) and digestive system and the kidneys. Body metabolism is increased, and blood pressure is raised. Large doses of caffeine cause tachycardia, headaches, nervousness, insomnia, and stomach distress. Physical dependence occurs with a regular intake of 350 mg for an adult (a cup of brewed coffee contains 75 to 155 mg). Withdrawal symptoms include severe headache, irritability, and fatigue.

Nicotine. It is far easier to become addicted to cigarettes than to alcohol or other drugs. Smoking is also physically damaging. It has been linked to heart and blood vessel disease, chronic bronchitis, emphysema, and cancer.

The tobacco plant belongs to the genus *Nicotiana,* a member of the nightshade family. There is evidence that tobacco was used as long ago as A.D. 200 Tobacco is chewed or inhaled. The nicotine in tobacco stimulates the CNS and suppresses the appetite. Withdrawal symptoms include decreased heart rate, weight gain, impaired psychomotor performance, nervousness and anxiety, headaches, fatigue, and insomnia.

Depressants

Depressants are synthetic drugs that have a depressant action on the CNS. Drugs included in this category are barbiturates and tranquilizers. Methaqualone is a nonbarbiturate sedative-hypnotic that is also a depressant. Commonly called Quaalude, the drug is no longer available as a legal prescription drug, but is available on the streets. Other specific examples of depressants include Valium, Seconal, Librium, and Ativan. These will be discussed further later in the chapter.

Barbiturates. Barbiturates are synthetic drugs that are classified as *sedative-hypnotics.* They arise from barbituric acid and are used medically to treat high blood pressure, epilepsy, and insomnia, and to sedate patients before and during surgery.

Barbiturates are swallowed (capsule or elixir), used as a suppository, or injected. The drugs were first synthesized in the early 1900s. Street names of barbiturates include yellow jacket (pentobarbital), red devil (secobarbital), phennie (phenobarbital), blue heaven or blue devil (amobarbital), barbs, downs or downers, rainbows, blues, or goof balls.

Barbiturates cause depression of the CNS, including slowing of physical and mental reflexes. Continued use of these drugs can cause physical and psychological dependence, as well as tolerance. Barbiturates produce a feeling of well-being and relief from anxiety. Side effects include difficulty in breathing, lethargy, nausea, and dizziness. Alcohol and other CNS depressants potentiate the effects of barbiturates. **Withdrawal symptoms** include irritability, restlessness, anxiety, and sleep disturbances. In severe forms, withdrawal causes convulsions and delirium.

Tranquilizers. Minor tranquilizers are psychoactive drugs that are taken to reduce anxiety. First developed in 1950, they are commonly prescribed and are available in capsules, tablets, and liquid. Common types of tranquilizers are those found in the benzodiazepine family and include chlordiazepoxide (Librium), diazepam (Valium), oxazepam (Serax), lorazepam (Ativan), and clorazepate (Tranxene).

Minor tranquilizers slow the activities of the CNS. They also have anticonvulsant and muscle-relaxant properties and produce a sense of well-being. When the effects of the drug wear off, users frequently feel increased anxiety. Tranquilizers can cause physical and psychological dependence, and tolerance to them can develop.

Other CNS-depressing drugs potentiate the action of tranquilizers. Signs of an overdose include sleepiness, confusion, loss of consciousness, and decreased reflexes. Withdrawal symptoms include anxiety, diaphoresis, insomnia, vomiting, tremors, delirium, and seizures. Because of the dangers of seizures, detoxification should be medically supervised.

Hallucinogens

Hallucinogens are natural and synthetic drugs that affect the mind and produce changes in perception and thinking. Included in this category are phencyclidine (PCP), lysergic acid diethylamide (LSD), mescaline, psilocybin, and 3,4-methylenedioxyamphetamine (MDA). They are found in the streets in a wide range of forms, including powder, peyote buttons, mushrooms, capsules, and tablets. LSD may be found on blotter paper, chips, and sheets of paper containing tattoos or stamplike pictures of cartoon figures. Hallucinogens are usually taken orally, although MDA can be sniffed and injected. They may be put on sugar cubes or mixed in other food. PCP may be sprinkled on tobacco or marijuana and smoked. When it is combined with marijuana, it is called

BOX 50-5 **COMMON STREET NAMES OF HALLUCINOGENS**

LSD	Acid, barrels, blotter, domes, microdots, purple haze, windowpane
Mescaline	Buttons, cactus, mesc, mescal buttons
MDA	Love drug, mellow drug of America
Psilocybin	Magic mushroom, shroom
PCP	Angel dust, animal tranquilizer, crystal, dust, hog, embalming fluid, KJ killer, peace pill, synthetic marijuana

sheba. PCP may be injected or snorted. Common street names include those found in Box 50-5.

Most of the effects of hallucinogens are psychological, although nausea and vomiting are not uncommon reactions. These drugs act as stimulants at first and produce depressed appetite, dilated pupils, and increases in body temperature, heart rate, and respirations. Hallucinogens have a profound psychological effect on people, often described as a process of amplification, with the drug acting as a catalyst. This effect is called a *trip*. A person's attempts to resist the effects of the drug seem to increase the chances of a negative experience, or a bad trip, which is characterized by tremendous confusion, unpleasant sensory images, and extreme panic. With large doses of PCP, there may be respiratory or cardiac arrest. Flashbacks may occur with the use of hallucinogens: the user reexperiences the effects of a drug without having taken it again.

Narcotics

Narcotics are drugs that are derived from the opium poppy or are produced synthetically. In general, narcotics lower the perception of pain. Narcotics include heroin, morphine, opium, codeine, meperidine, and methadone. Narcotics are injected, sniffed, smoked, or taken by mouth. Street names for heroin include H, horse, junk, hard stuff, smack, or scag.

Effects of narcotics include (1) shallow breathing, (2) reduced hunger, thirst, and sexual drive, and (3) drowsiness. The person may experience euphoria, lethargy, heaviness of limbs, and apathy. Overdoses of narcotics can cause coma, convulsions, respiratory arrest, and death. If narcotics are injected, there is risk of hepatitis B, AIDS, or other infections, such as septicemia. With narcotics, tolerance and physical and psychological addiction develop. Withdrawal may be painful and should be medically supervised. Clonidine (Catapres) is often used for detoxification. Symptoms of withdrawal include nausea, cramps, chills, sweating, restlessness, and increased nasal secretions.

Cannabis

Cannabis, or **marijuana,** comes from the Indian hemp plant. It can grow wild or is fairly easily cultivated. It is usually smoked as a cigarette (joint or reefer) or in a pipe or bong. Slang terms for marijuana include dope, grass, herb, joint, pot, reefer, roach, smoke, snuff, and weed. Marijuana has been used for medical and nonmedical purposes for more than 3000 years. Its popularity as a street drug began in the nineteenth century. It is commonly abused today. Hashish, or hash, is more concentrated than marijuana and produces more intense symptoms.

Marijuana's role in reducing eye pressure in glaucoma and in controlling side effects of chemotherapy is being evaluated. Physical effects of marijuana include drying of the eyes and mouth, increase in appetite, reddening of the eyes, and impairment of short-term memory. It raises the heart rate and blood pressure while lowering the body temperature and producing loss of coordination and possible confusion. Research shows that marijuana may affect chromosome division and cause birth defects. Marijuana is fat soluble and may be stored in the body for as long as several months.

Psychological effects of marijuana include an altering of perception of the senses. The user has a sense of well-being and intoxication, although depression and panic may ocur. Psychological addiction occurs, and anxiety reactions may occur.

Deliriants

Deliriants are any chemicals that produce fumes or vapors that, when inhaled, cause symptoms similar to intoxication. They may be called inhalants. The fumes or vapors from inhalants are sniffed through the nose, or the vapors are put into a bag or captured in a balloon to increase the concentration of the inhaled fumes.

The use of inhalants is traced back to ancient Greece. Sniffing of commercial products and solvents was first documented in the 1950s. The deliriants or inhalants have a psychoactive or mood-altering effect when the vapors are inhaled or sniffed. Most fall into one of three categories: solvents, aerosol sprays, or anesthetics. Solvents include commercial products such as glue, gasoline, kerosene, lighter fluid, Wite-Out (correction fluid), and nail polish remover. Products such as hair sprays, deodorant, insecticides, and cookware sprays are examples of aerosols. Anesthetics that are used recreationally include ether, chloroform, and nitrous oxide. Amyl nitrate and butyl nitrate, drugs used for cardiac disease, are also abused. These may be called *whippets*.

Almost all inhalants are CNS depressants that slow the user's heart rate, brain activity, and breathing. Other effects include slurred speech, blurred vision, inflamed mucous membranes, light-headedness, ringing in the ears, watering eyes, loss of coordination, and excessive nasal secretions. With high doses, the user may lose consciousness or have seizures. The effects are immediate and usually last 20 to 45 minutes.

The prolonged use of inhalants may lead to liver, kidney, blood, and bone marrow damage. The sniffing of toluene, found in gasoline and commercial cleaners, has been linked to irreversible brain damage. This can be manifested as forgetfulness, inability to think clearly, depression, irritability, hostility, and paranoia. Use of large amounts of aerosols or solvents can cause death as a result of cardiac arrest after dysrhythmias. Death from inhalants is usually caused by suffocation because of the displacement of oxygen in the lungs. Sniffing inhalants from a bag or balloon increases the risk of suffocation.

Some inhalants cause tolerance or dependence. Symptoms of withdrawal include chills, hallucinations, headaches, stomach pains, cramps, and delirium tremens. The psychological effects of deliriants include a feeling of stimulation and energy. At higher doses, the user may feel intoxicated.

Assessment

Subjective factors to assess include those found in the section on alcoholism. See Box 50-2 for a drug history format that can be used. The objective factors found in the discussion of alcoholism also are pertinent, with the addition of the presence of "track marks"—if the person has been mainlining (injecting the drug directly into a vein), needle marks, scars, or small scabs can be seen on the hands, forearms, or insteps. However, many other veins are used as points of entry to conceal addiction, including the dorsal vein of the penis or the conjunctival artery of the eyelid.

Diagnostic tests. Diagnostic testing for drug abuse can be done on urine or blood samples. The amount of time after use that drugs can be detected in the urine varies from a very short time for alcohol and cocaine to a long time for benzodiazepines and cannabis. It is possible to have a minimally positive drug test for cannabis because of a long period of "passive inhalation" (close contact with someone smoking and exhaling marijuana fumes). Urine testing is not commonly done to detect alcohol because alcohol is metabolized very rapidly; alcohol blood levels are much more accurate. A breath test is used by law enforcement agencies to determine alcohol levels in the blood.

Nursing Diagnosis and Expected Patient Outcomes

The reader is referred to p. 1315 in the section on alcoholism.

Nursing Interventions

Rehabilitation of the drug-dependent person follows the guidelines discussed for the treatment of the alcoholic. One difference between drug and alcohol abuse is that, in most cases, the possession and use of drugs is illegal. In the United States, the illicit use of narcotics has been a crime since the 1914 Harrison Narcotic Act was passed.

Methadone Maintenance

One approach to the treatment of narcotic addiction is the methadone maintenance program. Methadone is a synthetic drug, and the average daily dose costs much less than heroin or morphine. The drug is given legally as a part of a rehabilitation program. Methadone itself is addictive. Because methadone is easily available through legal channels, some experts believe that it is essentially the same as taking maintenance doses of other drugs, such as insulin. Other persons disagree, however, because they believe that the use of methadone encourages addiction and replaces one drug with another.

Cocaine Withdrawal

Although cocaine does not produce physical tolerance, the psychological tolerance is very strong. Research has shown that long-term cocaine use has yielded symptoms similar to those of Parkinson's disease. It depletes dopamine in the brain. Because of this, bromocriptine (Parlodel) has been used to assist in controlling the symptoms of withdrawal from cocaine and to prevent relapse.

Risk of Disease

Addicts who inject drugs are at risk for diseases such as hepatitis and AIDS. Often addicts share needles and equipment or reuse them without sterilization between use. Addicts may also demonstrate resistance to more responsible use because of blackouts or the character traits that accompany the disease. Many intravenous drug users test positive for the AIDS virus. Although supplying clean needles to drug users has been advocated by some, this is controversial. Those who oppose this recommendation feel that it would encourage IV drug use.

Patient Education

The reader is referred to the discussion of this topic in the section on alcoholism (p. 1316).

CO-DEPENDENCY

Co-dependency has been defined as the set of maladaptive and/or immature responses, behaviors, and feelings experienced by someone closely associated with an actively chemically dependent person. Commonly reported symptoms of co-dependency include the following[35]:

1. Self-esteem that relies heavily on feeling needed by others
2. Need to control others even when it is unrealistic to do so
3. Tendency to develop complicated relationships with chemically dependent people

Co-dependency becomes significant because persons in recovery often find that they need to address their co-dependency to gain complete peace of mind. Without this they are at increased risk of relapse and problems with relationships. Also, research has found that nursing as a profession tends to attract those who are from alcoholic homes and those who are co-dependent in nature. These nurses may have increased risk of "burnout" from nursing. Al-Anon or Adult Children of Alcoholics groups may provide treatment for the person who is troubled because of co-dependency.

EATING DISORDERS

An eating disorder has been described as an obsession with weight and an addiction to food. It is also, however, a way of coping with feelings and an attempt for the persons to feel better about themselves. It is an addiction, and much of the discussion concerning alcoholism and drug addiction applies here.

Anorexia nervosa and bulimia are two common eating disorders.[14] **Anorexia nervosa** results in weight loss, to 15% less than the expected norm, based on age and height. There are also (1) an intense fear of becoming obese and (2) a distortion of body image. The person feels "fat" even when emaciated. Menstrual periods may cease with this disorder. **Bulimia** is defined as episodes of binge eating, during which there is a feeling of lack of control. Regular, self-induced vomiting or the use of laxatives to purge is common. Other symptoms may include restrictive dieting, fasting, or vigorous exercise to prevent weight gain. There is also an excessive concern with body shape and weight.

Eating disorders are a way to "anesthetize" intense negative feelings and to cope with stress and relieve tension. Most of the time activities relative to eating and exercise become a part of a ritual. Most persons with eating disorders fear losing control.

Both anorexia nervosa and bulimia are common in young women. Treatment for these is important — without treatment, these conditions can be fatal. Treatment includes helping the person learn to trust others and to exercise his or her rights in a relationship. Patients are assisted in expressing their feelings, and individual patient education and nutritional counseling are crucial. While this treatment is carried out, the patient may require nutrition intravenously or by nasogastric tube to sustain life.

IMPAIRED NURSES

Over the past several years, many states have developed programs to assist nurses who are impaired by either alcohol or drugs. Part of the reason for this is that the rate of chemical dependence among nurses and other health providers is greater than that of the general public.[16] Before the start of peer assistance programs, through either state boards or state nursing associations, often nurses would be fired or be free to move to other facilities, where the abuse could continue.

In 1980 two states, Maryland and Ohio, had peer assistance programs in place. By the fall of 1983, 25 states either had programs in place or were planning to start them. At present only a few states do not have programs. These programs work closely with state boards of nursing.

Peer assistance programs have several goals: (1) to assist the nurse who is impaired to receive treatment, (2) to protect the public from the untreated nurse, (3) to help the recovering nurse reenter nursing in a systematic, planned, and safe way, and (4) to assist in monitoring the continued recovery of the nurse for a period of time.

The reentry of the nurse may include a restriction on access to narcotics for a period of time.

The basis of these programs is one nurse helping another nurse. Most volunteers in these programs are recovering nurses or nurses who work in the area of chemical dependence or psychiatric nursing.

If a colleague is suspected, it is important to notify the supervisor, who will often notify the state nursing association or state board of nursing. The best way to help a colleague who is abusing drugs or alcohol is to not cover up the use and to report it to persons who can help arrange for appropriate help.

REFERENCES AND SUGGESTED READINGS

1. Adams F: Drug dependency in hospital patients, Am J Nurs 88 (4):477, 1988.
2. Alcoholics Anonymous, New York, 1976, Alcoholics World Services, Inc.
3. Am J Nurs: Which nurse is likely to become chemically dependent? 88(6):791, 1988.
4. American Nurses Association: Addiction and psychological dysfunction in nursing: the profession's response to the problem, Kansas City, Missouri, 1984, ANA.
5. Beattie M: Co-dependent no more, Minneapolis, 1987, Hazelden Foundation
6. Captain C: Family recovery from alcoholism: mediating family factors, Nurs Clin North Am 24(1):55, 1989.
7. Caroselli-Karinja M: Drug abuse and the elderly, J Psychosoc Nurs Ment Health Serv 23:25, 1985.
8. Cermak T: Diagnosing and treating co-dependence, Minneapolis, 1986, Johnson Institute.
9. DaDalt R: Changing patterns of drug diversion, Am J Nurs 86: 792, 1986.
10. DiCicco-Bloom B et al: The homebound alcoholic, Am J Nurs 86 (2):167, 1986.
11. Edens K et al: How to use intervention in your profession, Minneapolis, 1987, Johnson Institute.
12. Estes N and Heineman M: Alcoholism: development, consequence, and interventions, ed 3, St Louis, 1986, The CV Mosby Co.
13. FitzGerald K: Alcoholism: the genetic inheritance, New York, 1988, Doubleday & Co.
14. Flood M: Addictive eating disorders, Nurs Clin North Am 24 (1): 45, 1989.
15. Gay G: Clinical management of acute and chronic cocaine poisoning, Ann Emerg Med 11:77, 1982.
16. Green P: The chemically dependent nurse, Nurs Clin North Am 24(1):81, 1989.
17. Haack M and Hughes T: Impairment in nursing: clinical perspectives and program development, New York, 1988, Springer-Verlag New York, Inc.
18. Huffman A: Body and behavioral experiences in recovery from alcoholism, Rehabil Nurs 12(4):188, 1987.
19. Hughes T: Models and perspectives of addiction: implications for treatment, Nurs Clin North Am 24(1):1, 1989.
20. Hutchinson S: Chemically dependent nurses: the trajectory toward self-annihilation, Nurs Res 35:196, 1986.
21. Jack L: Use of milieu as a problem-solving strategy in addiction treatment, Nurs Clin North Am 24(1):69, 1989.
22. Johnson V: Intervention, Minneapolis, 1987, Johnson Institute.
23. Johnson V: I'll quit tomorrow, New York, 1973, Harper & Row Publishers, Inc (classic).
24. Kelley R: The path to addiction and recovery, Am J Nurs 87(2): 176, 1987.
25. Kirk E and Bradford L: Effects of alcohol on the CNS: implications for the neuroscience nurse, J Neurosci Nurs 19(6):316, 1987.
26. Long B and Phipps W: Medical-surgical nursing, St. Louis, 1988, The CV Mosby Co.
27. M, Alice. Two reports, one disease, Am J Nurs 88(5):660, 1988.
28. Matteson M and McConnell E: Gerontological nursing: concepts and practice, Philadelphia, 1988, W B Saunders Co.
29. Mosby's medical and surgical nursing dictionary, ed 2, St Louis, 1986, The CV Mosby Co.
30. Nuckols C and Greeson J: Cocaine addiction: assessment and intervention, Nurs Clin North Am 24(1):33, 1989.
31. Powell A and Minick M: Alcohol withdrawal syndrome, Am J Nurs 88:312, 1988.
32. Sullivan E, Bissell L, and Williams E: Chemical dependency in nursing: the deadly diversion, Menlo Park, Calif, 1988, Addison-Wesley Publishing Co, Inc.
33. Tweed S: Identifying the alcoholic client, Nurs Clin North Am 24 (1):13, 1989.
34. Vandegaer F: Cocaine — the deadliest addiction, Nurs '89, 19 (2):72, 1989.
35. Williams E: Strategies for intervention, Nurs Clin North Am 24 (1):95, 1989.
36. Zerwekh J and Michaels B: Co-dependency: assessment and recovery, Nurs Clin North Am 24(1):109, 1989.

CHAPTER CHALLENGE

KEY POINTS

- Examples of compulsive addictions include alcoholism, drug addiction, compulsive overeating, and compulsive gambling.
- Alcoholism and drug addiction are commonly referred to as chemical dependence.
- Dependence may be psychological and physical and is defined as the need to continue the use of drugs and/or alcohol to prevent withdrawal.
- Persons with chemical dependence may also suffer from a psychiatric diagnosis (called dual diagnosis)
- There is a genetic component to the development of chemical dependence
- Alcohol provides the body with "empty calories," and heavy drinking can cause damage to many body systems, especially the liver.
- Denial and delusion are commonly found in persons with untreated chemical dependence.
- Alcoholics may require large doses of medication to safely withdraw from alcohol.
- Many of the problems found with alcoholism may be the result of nutritional problems.
- Alcoholics Anonymous or a related 12-step group has been effective in treating the addicted person, because it helps the person accept the powerlessness over drugs or alcohol.
- The basic types of drugs that are abused are stimulants, depressants, hallucinogens, narcotics, cannabis, and deliriants.
- Drug addiction includes craving, psychological dependence, and physical dependence.
- Drug addicts who inject drugs are at increased risk for the development of chemical dependence.
- Nurses are at increased risk of the development of alcoholism and chemical dependence.

STUDY QUESTIONS

1. What is a true statement about a person who is alcoholic:
   a. The person has a moral problem
   b. The person is at increased risk to develop drug addition
   c. The person will be cared for only in a treatment center
   d. The person will never be able to stay sober
2. What blood alcohol usually indicates that a person is legally intoxicated:
   a. 0.05%
   b. 0.001%
   c. 0.075%
   d. 0.10%
3. Which common defense mechanism is usually present in the untreated chemically dependent person:
   a. Denial
   b. Sadness
   c. Laughter
   d. Sarcasm
4. Alcohol is classified as which type of drug:
   a. Depressant
   b. Stimulant
   c. Deliriant
   d. Hallucinogen
5. What is the most common psychoactive drug used today:
   a. Cocaine
   b. Nicotine
   c. Alcohol
   d. Caffeine
6. Antabuse causes a reaction when which substance is ingested:
   a. Alcohol
   b. Nicotine
   c. Heroin
   d. Amphetamine
7. What is not a goal of peer assistance programs for nurses:
   a. To ensure that nurses receive the treatment they need
   b. To protect the public from the untreated nurse
   c. To ensure that the nurse never works again as a nurse
   d. To assist in monitoring the recovering nurse
8. The wife who calls the place of employment of her intoxicated husband and says he is sick is exhibiting what kind of behavior:
   a. Enabling
   b. Caring
   c. Disabling
   d. Realistic

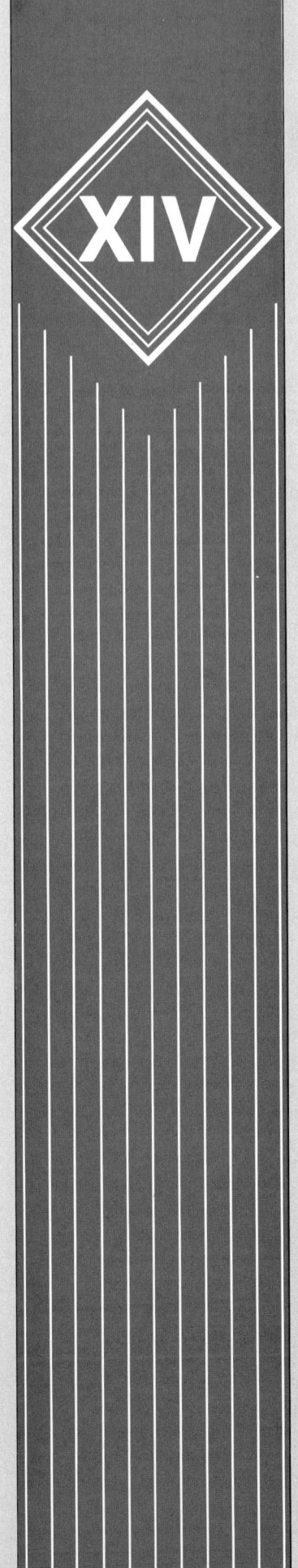

XIV

Community Health Nursing

I love many things about nursing. First of all, it's not routine; there is a new experience every day. Secondly, it is a joy to know that I can help people when they need it most. The patients rely on me, so I do my best. Thirdly, I love to help people and know that they appreciate my help. Lastly, I love to learn new things and apply them to my patients to the best of my ability. Nursing is a job that will never be boring or routine. It is very fulfilling.

JOHNNA DAVIS
Student Nurse

51

Home Health Nursing

SANDRA KLOCKE

LEARNING OBJECTIVES

After reading this chapter, the student should be able to do the following:

- Define the key terms.
- Describe how home health care differs from community and public health care services.
- List at least three types of home health agencies.
- List at least four services that may be provided by home health care.
- Describe two major ways home care differs from hospital care.
- Define skilled nursing services.
- Describe the role of the LPN/LVN in the delivery of skilled nursing care.
- Identify one function the LPN/LVN does not practice in home health care.
- Relate the nursing process to home health care practice.
- List two sources of reimbursement for home care services.

RELATED TOPICS OF INTEREST

- The evolution of nursing (Chapter 1)
- Legal aspects of nursing (Chapter 2)
- Ethical aspects of nursing (Chapter 3)
- The nursing process (Chapter 5)
- Documentation (Chapter 6)
- The family (Chapter 7)
- Admission, transfer, and discharge (Chapter 15)
- Hospice care (Chapter 56)

KEY TERMS

Define the following:

- accreditation
- certification
- DRG
- home health care
- Medicaid
- Medicare

Home health care services enable individuals of all ages to remain in the comfort and security of their homes while receiving health care. Family support, familiar surroundings, and participation in the care process contribute to feelings of worth and dignity. Services may include skilled nursing, physical therapy, speech language pathology, occupational therapy, medical social services, homemaker–home health aide (also referred to as home health aide), nutritional support, respiratory therapy, acquisition of medical supplies and equipment, and homemaker and companion care. The approach to patient care is one of teamwork and blending of disciplines. Historically and currently professional nurses are the backbone of home health care and the discipline primarily involved in the administration and management of agencies. Although home care has traditionally been a part of public and community health services, the focus is much narrower.

DEFINITIONS

Home health care preserves individual independence and integrity and keeps families together.

The following are definitions of home health care as viewed from four different perspectives:

OFFICIAL: A component of comprehensive health care in which services are provided to individuals and their families in their place of residence for the purpose of promoting, maintaining, or restoring health, or of minimizing the effects of illness and disability.

PATIENT: Skilled and compassionate care provided on a one-to-one basis in the comforting and familiar surroundings of the home. It is based on individual needs and personalized schedules and is provided over a period of time so that adjustment, change, and learning can most effectively take place.

FAMILY: A means to keep the family together as a functioning, integrated unit. The goals are learning to adapt to change, preventing dysfunctional patterns, and attaining family wellness within the confines of an individual member's illness or disability. It provides needed emotional support and linkage with the larger community support systems.

PROVIDER: Challenges all disciplines involved to provide excellent care in often less than excellent conditions and surroundings. Independence, creativity, communication, and excellent clinical skills are integral parts of daily practice. It is an opportunity for nurses to demonstrate the best of their profession and themselves in cooperation with the health care team to patients and families with physical and psychological needs.

Home care was formerly simply defined as providing physical care to the sick in their homes, but the scope and complexity of the concept and practice have grown.

HISTORICAL OVERVIEW

Roots of the concept can be traced to the New Testament, when visiting the sick was a form of charity. Sixth century monks practiced home care as an important aspect of their work in the community. One of the earliest organized systems for home care was developed in 1617 by St. Vincent de Paul, who organized the Sisterhood of the Dames de Charite to meet social welfare and visiting nursing needs.

In the 1700s families were primary caregivers. The poor were hospitalized, whereas those with financial means were cared for in their homes by the visiting physician.

The first home care program in the United States was organized in 1796 as the Boston Dispensary. In 1859 William Rathbone of Liverpool, England, established the Metropolitan Nursing Association, the first organized district nursing service, because of the outstanding home care his dying wife received. He believed that many people with long-term illnesses could be better cared for in their own homes than in a hospital—a belief central to home care today.

The first visiting nurse service in the United States was formed in Philadelphia in 1886. It was directed by nurses who provided care to all ages of persons with both acute and chronic care needs.

Lillian Wald and Mary Brewster developed a visiting nurse service for the poor in New York City in 1893 at the Nurses' Settlement House on Henry Street. In the late 1800s and early 1900s visiting nurse associations were formalized and public health departments became widespread.

Metropolitan Life Insurance had a major impact on the growth and nature of home services when in 1909 it began offering nursing services to its millions of industrial policy holders. This initiated third-party payment for services. Payment until then had been provided primarily on a charitable or patient-paid basis.

The Social Security Act of 1935 first provided governmental rather than local charitable funding for selected services, such as maternal health, communicable disease, and the training of public health professionals. It subsidized assistance for the poor and aged. Amendments to the Act in 1950 further defined services and opened the door to direct payment for providers.

A revolution, however, occurred in 1965 when Title XVIII (known as Medicare) and Title XIX (known as Medicaid) amendments to the Social Security Act were enacted. **Medicare** provided direct federal monies for the health care of all citizens 65 and older (or disabled), regardless of socioeconomic status. The companion **Medicaid** bill covered the care needs of the poor and indigent of all ages. When Medicare became effective in 1966, it revolutionized home care by (1) changing it to a medical rather than nursing model of practice, (2) defining and limiting services it would reimburse, and (3) changing the payment source and even changing the reason home care was provided.

The next major influence on home care came in 1983. Congress enacted the prospective payment system as a part of the Tax Equity and Fiscal Responsibility Act for hospitals receiving Medicare reimbursement. This system, based on major diagnostic categories and diagnosis related groups (**DRG**s) paid a set rate (according to diagnosis) for the hospitalized patient's care rather than the "cost" or charges traditionally billed by institutions. The net effect of the change was a major shift of patients out of the hospital into their homes, extended-care facilities, or skilled nursing facilities. Such patients were discharged earlier in their convalescence and thus required more nursing care. This created a challenge to home care in terms of volume of patients seen, necessity of more skilled nursing care over intensive times, and the evolution of highly technical procedures in the home. Existing agencies expanded, and new ones developed to meet the demand.

TYPES OF AGENCIES

In the broadest terms home care services can be delivered by any individual, service group, organization, or agency with the desire to provide services to the elderly, disabled, or ill of any age. The type and qualifications of personnel used, quality of services delivered, and standards of care can vary widely and often depend on funding sources.

The agency may have to comply with federal, state, and local laws and regulations via the following:

LICENSURE by the state: This gives legal permission to operate within that state only. Regulations vary widely. Not all states have such laws.

CERTIFICATION by state certifying body designated by the federal government: Rules governing certification are federally mandated. Only certified agencies may receive Medicare payment. Many states piggyback Medicaid reimbursement to certification as do some insurers.

CERTIFICATE OF NEED granted by some states according to rules and formulas devised by state regulators: Cost of starting and running the agency, availability of personnel, and need for their services are generally considered in this process.

ACCREDITATION by an outside agency who evaluates and judges how well the agency meets certain standards set by the accrediting organization: This accreditation may be granted by the National League for Nursing Community Health Accreditation Program, the Joint Commission for Accreditation of Healthcare Organizations, or the National Homecaring Council. Other groups may accredit special programs or specialized agencies.

It is still possible for some agencies to operate under no specific rules or regulations.

Before Medicare, home health care was provided primarily by visiting nurse associations, nursing divisions of state or local health departments, and hospitals. Now agencies are classified according to (1) tax status—for profit or not for profit; (2) location—freestanding or institution based; and (3) governance—private or public. Table 51-1 summarizes and describes the six generally accepted types of home health agencies. The structure of some of these agencies is subject to change and variation. For example, some visiting nurse associations have reorganized and placed their home health agencies into private, nonprofit structures to ensure reimbursement that will cover the cost of providing services. Similarly, it is possible to have an official or voluntary hospital-based agency.

Growth in number of agencies has mirrored the growth of home care. In 1966 there were approximately 2000 agencies. In 1989 the number had grown to more than 8000 agencies operating nationwide. Medicare-certified agencies numbered 2864 in 1980, 6007 in 1986, and 5787 in 1988. The recent decrease in number can be linked with a decline in official, voluntary, and combined agencies, who find it difficult to compete with the resources of private agencies in metropolitan areas. Agencies in rural areas are having difficulty with increasingly stringent Medicare paperwork and documentation requirements, as well as with recruiting sufficient qualified staff.

SERVICE COMPONENTS

Most home health agencies follow the basic Medicare model of services offered. Functions and scopes of practice are dictated by state licensing boards and professional organizations. Primary services include the following:

- Skilled nursing
- Physical therapy
- Speech-language pathology
- Occupational therapy
- Medical social services
- Home health aide

Other therapy services, such as respiratory, or professional services such as nutritional counseling, pharmacy, podiatry, dentistry, and psychiatric or mental health, may be offered. Support services, such as homemaker, companion, and respite, may be provided but are not directly reimbursed by Medicare. The service mix depends on patient diagnosis, patient/family needs, and availability of resources. Medicare and Medicaid home care services are based on the medical model of treatment and depend on the physician for entry into the formalized system. Medicare requires a plan of treatment signed by the physician, outlining all disciplines, treatment, frequency, and duration. These orders must be recertified every 62 days. Third-party payers may or may not have similar requirements. Only the primary services will be explained in this chapter.

Skilled Nursing

Skilled nursing services are provided and directed by currently licensed registered nurses. Some agencies require that nurses have a bachelor's degrees in nursing, whereas others hire graduates of all types of RN programs and teach them agency policies and specific procedures. Not all nurses can be effective home health nurses. Limited skilled nursing services may be provided by the LPN/LVN under the supervision of the RN.

Service goals

Skilled nursing services revolve around the following four major goals:

RESTORATIVE: The return to a previous level of functioning as appropriate and realistic

IMPROVEMENT: Achieving better health and a higher level of functioning than previous

MAINTENANCE: Preservation of functional capacities and independence by maintaining current level of health

PROMOTION: Teaching health life-styles that minimize the effect of illness or disability and prevent the recurrence of illness

Provider attributes. Nurses practicing in the home setting are caregivers, teachers, counselors, case managers, and advocates. They must be technically proficient, self-motivated, innovative, and independent decision makers. Common sense, flexibility, compassion, empathy, patience, honesty, and dependability are essential. Nurses who depend on the security of the institutional setting, immediate medical direction, and frequent peer support find the independence of home care practice difficult.

Home health nursing requires that nurses and other providers adapt to the patient, family, and home environment. Staff are visitors in the patient's home. Strong communication skills are essential for teaching, counseling, interviewing, and listening. High energy level, cheerfulness, and a positive attitude are valuable attributes as nurses often work with patients and families who are under stress. Respect of the patient's dignity, privacy, and needs of autonomy is an integral part of providing effective nursing services.

Services are generally provided in the patient's home;

Table 51-1 Home Health Agencies

Type of Agency	Status	Governed By	Supported By	Services Offered	Staffed By	Time of Service	Example
Voluntary	Public; nonprofit; freestanding	Community-based board of directors	Tax deductible contributions; grants; fees from all sources	Community health; public health; home health	RN; LPN/LVN; aide; homemaker; social worker; therapists	Generally ½-8 hr	Visiting nurse association
Official	Public; nonprofit; freestanding	State, county, city, or other local unit of government and volunteer board representatives of the area	State, local, or county revenues; grants; fees from limited sources; charitable contributions	Community health; public health; home health	RN; LPN/LVN; aide; homemaker; may have social workers; therapists	Generally ½-4 hr	State health departments; county health departments; city health departments
Combination	Public; nonprofit; freestanding	Jointly operated by the two types of agencies above under a combined board of directors	State, local, or county revenues; grants; fees from limited sources; charitable contributions	Community health; public health; home health	RN; LPN/LVN; aide; homemaker; may have social workers; therapists	Generally ½-4 hr	County-based visiting nurse association
Hospital	Private; nonprofit or for profit; institution-based; hospital	Hospital board of directors	Fees from all sources	Home health; community health (limited)	RN; LPN/LVN; aide; social worker; therapists	Generally ½-4 hr	XYZ hospital home health agency
Proprietary	Private; for profit; freestanding	Governed and owned by individual corporation, or other organization; many paid boards of directors appointed by owner	Fees from most sources; may or may not participate in Medicare/Medicaid	May have limited home health; private duty; homemaker	RN; LPN/LVN; aides	1-24 hr	Home health care of XYZ
Private not for profit	Private; nonprofit; freestanding	Governed and owned by individual, corporation, or other organizational structure; board appointed by owner	Fees from most sources; may or may not participate in Medicare/Medicaid	May have limited home health services; private duty; homemaker	RN; LPN/LVN; aides	½-24 hr	ABC home health agency
Other	Private; for profit or nonprofit; institution based	Based within formalized institution; governed by that board or designated board	Fees from all sources	Home health services; limited homemaker	RN; LPN/LVN; aide; therapists; may have homemaker; social worker	½-4-8 hr	ABC nursing home—home health agency; ABC rehabilitation facility home care

hence nurses must feel comfortable with the unknown, as well as accept differences in ethnic cultures, mores, and value systems. Commitment to professional standards of practice, ongoing continuing education, and skills updates are important.

Nursing process. Home health nursing uses the basic nursing process to assess the needs, establish a patient-centered plan of care, implement nursing actions, evaluate the effectiveness of actions, and plan for modification or resolution of identified problems. Interventions may range from wound care to intravenous chemotherapy. Teaching could involve diabetes instruction or the management of complex support equipment in the home. Teaching is always patient centered with the primary goals of self-care and independent functioning within the confines of the illness or disability (Fig. 51-1). In the counseling role a nurse may provide emotional support to the dying patient and his family or provide skilled psychiatric interventions (if properly qualified). Case management may include only supervision of the home health aide or involve the coordination of complex care plans with services, supplies, and equipment provided by many different disciplines.

RNs have been the primary providers of skilled service by both tradition and regulation. Skilled service has become, however, a growing field of practice for the LPN/LVN as agencies cope with increased staffing needs, nursing shortages, and recognition of the contributions the LPN/LVN can make to home care.

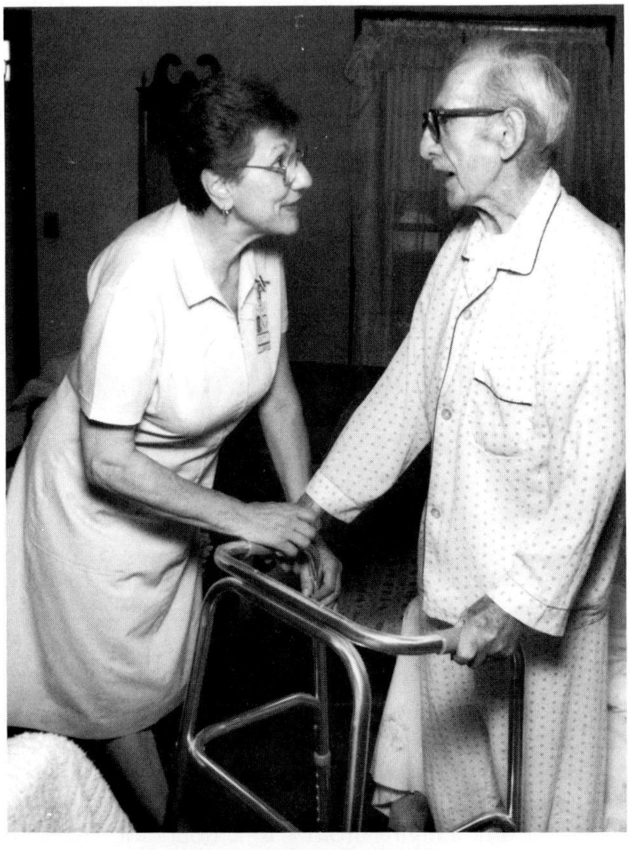

FIG. 51-1 The nurse assists an elderly patient to ambulate. (Photo by Marilu Halamandaris, *CARING* Magazine.)

Licensed Practical/Vocational Nurse Role

LPNs/LVNs must be supervised by the RN. Although LPNs/LVNs cannot make detailed patient assessments or clinical judgments, their observations, reporting, documentation, teaching, and technical care capabilities are important to home care.

Provider attributes. Personal and professional attributes described for RNs also apply to the LPN/LVN. Independent practice is not allowed, but self-direction, motivation, creativity, clinical proficiency, flexibility, compassion, empathy, and patience are all essential attributes. Good communication skills, both written and verbal, are necessary. The ability to work alone, follow directions, recognize important changes in condition, and assist in patient teaching is needed. Evaluation of care interventions and recommendations for alteration of the plan of care are a part of the role. The concept of teamwork must be understood and practiced.

Functions. Depending on the agency, agency policies, and state practice acts, the LPN/LVN may provide the following services in the home as directed and supervised by the RN:

1. Catheter care and teaching
2. Ostomy care and teaching
3. Wound care and sterile dressing changes
4. Obtaining specimens for cultures
5. Injection administration
6. Prefilling of insulin syringes
7. Fingersticks for blood sugar readings
8. Monitoring of physical status (such as lung sounds, bowel sounds, pulses, edema, and weights)
9. Teaching, monitoring, or setting up medications
10. Enteral feedings
11. Specimen collection
12. Therapeutic diet teaching or reinforcement
13. Tracheostomy care including suctioning
14. Enemas for special conditions
15. Emotional support
16. Preventive health measures
17. Patient and family teaching

Assistance with highly technical procedures, such as intravenous therapies, home dialysis, and respirator management, may be allowed in some states.

Home health care offers a new and challenging area of practice for the LPN/LVN who enjoys practicing nursing in a less restrictive environment. The need for this level of nursing practice will continue to grow. Commitment to quality of care is a common thread through skilled nursing services: hence the LPN/LVN must also pursue frequent inservice updates and continuing education to ensure current practice.

PHYSICAL THERAPY SERVICES

Services must be provided by a qualified and licensed physical therapist. A physical therapy assistant under the supervision of the licensed therapist may deliver limited services. The goals of treatment must be restorative for Medicare reimbursement but may be maintenance or preventive for other payer sources. The therapist completes a detailed assessment of the patient and then determines treatment, education, and assistive devices needed for rehabilitation. These are included as a part of the physician-approved plan of treatment. Treatments range from muscle strengthening to transcutaneous nerve stimulation and ultrasound treatments. The therapist actively teaches the patient and family the rehabilitation plan to promote self-care and independence. Communication with the physician and RN promotes continuity of care.

SPEECH LANGUAGE PATHOLOGY SERVICES

To be Medicare reimbursed, speech services must be provided by a master's-prepared clinician who has been certified by the American Speech and Hearing Association. Other insurers may accept a practitioner prepared at the bachelor's level. Therapy goals include minimizing communication disorders and their physical, emotional, and social impact. Independent functioning and maximum rehabilitation of speech and language abilities are primary treatment goals. Services may be provided after stroke or after surgery. Therapies may range from language relearning to working with eating or swallowing disorders or teaching lipreading to those with hearing disorders. Pathologists work closely with the patient and family for rehabilitation or adjustment to a new disability.

OCCUPATIONAL THERAPY

Occupational therapy services deal with life's practical tasks. Therapists are prepared at the bachelor's level and may earn the occupational therapist registered (OTR) designation if they meet the registration requirements of the National Occupational Therapy Association. Some services may be provided by the certified occupational therapy assistant under the supervision of the OTR. Based on a complete evaluation of functional level, the therapist will choose and teach therapeutic activities designed to restore functional levels. Services include (1) techniques to increase independence, (2) design, fabrication, and fitting of orthotic or self-help devices, and (3) assessment for vocational training. Patient-centered education is an integral part of attaining independence in self-care.

MEDICAL SOCIAL SERVICES

Medical social services are provided by social workers prepared at the master's level. Bachelor's-prepared workers may provide services under mastered social worker (MSW) supervision. Their focus is on the emotional and social aspects of illness. The patient, family, or other support systems are evaluated for social, emotional, and environmental factors. The care plan includes education, counseling, payment source identification, and referrals. Coping with stress and crisis intervention are also part of social worker services. Social services in home health are generally short term.

HOMEMAKER–HOME HEALTH AIDE SERVICES

Medicare refers to the homemaker–home health aide (HM-HHA) as a home health aide (HHA). These workers are an integral part of the home health care team. They provide the basic support services that can enable an elderly individual, disabled adult, or dependent child to remain at home. Medicare requires a primary skilled or therapy service (speech or physical) be necessary before HHA services can be provided. Medicaid and some insurers have less stringent requirements. Many insurers do not reimburse this care. Family members and individuals are often willing to pay privately to prevent institutionalization.

Most aide services fall into one of three categories: (1) personal care: assistance with bathing, oral hygiene, eating, dressing, or toileting; (2) physical assistance: with transfers, medications, ambulation; or (3) household chores: cooking, light housekeeping, shopping, laundry. Medicare will not cover visits made solely for the third reason.

Although "training" of aides has long been required by Medicare, rules governing type, length, and content of preparation have been nonexistent; hence, skills and standards were not uniform. As a part of the Omnibus Reconciliation Act of 1987, new standards for training and competency evaluation have been formulated and are now effective.

Medicare requires 2 weeks of on-site supervision of the aide, principally by an RN. A licensed physical therapist may provide the supervision if skilled nursing is not involved. Private payers, however, often do not have such requirements. Aide services are sometimes provided in blocks of time ranging from 1 to 2 hours for Medicare to 8 to 24 hours for private or other payment sources.

THE TYPICAL HOME HEALTH PROCESS

Referral

The entry point to the home health care system is by referral. This can come from the patient, family, social service agency, hospital, physician, or another agency. Agencies have a variety of methods of intake for referrals ranging from a formalized hospital discharge planning process with a central agency intake coordinator to a direct call from the physician to the agency staff.

Admission

The initial evaluation and admission visit are made by an RN within 24 to 48 hours of the referral. This may be completed by an RN in a formal role as admission nurse or by a staff nurse who will serve as the primary nurse on the case. The physician often is contacted for general orders before this visit, but agencies may make an evaluation visit without orders if allowed to do so by agency policy. The evaluation and admission process generally includes as a minimum:

1. Complete patient evaluation including physical and psychosocial factors
2. Environmental assessment relating specifically to safety and ability to provide services effectively in the home
3. Identification of primary functional impairments
4. Identification of the impact of the disease or disability on the patient and family
5. Assessment of the family or significant other support system
6. Determination of knowledge and adherence to treatments and medications
7. Determination of the desire for care and services
8. Involvement of the patient and family in the development of the plan of care and goals
9. Notification to the patient of his rights as a patient, along with information on costs, payment sources, and billing practices
10. Provision of initial nursing interventions

The admission process typically takes a minimum of 1 hour. It will take longer if the patient is confused or in need of nursing care. In some hospital-based agencies an abbreviated evaluation visit may be made while the patient is still in the hospital.

Care Plan

If the patient is to be admitted, the physician must be contacted for specific orders before delivery of care. A treatment plan is drafted cooperatively with the physician. This plan describes the current physical status of the patient, medications, treatments, the disciplines needed to provide care, the frequency and duration of services, and the goals and the time frame for implementation. A plan of treatment must be signed by the physician and serves as the traditional physician orders. Although the treatment plan can be altered at any time, based on patient needs, through additional written, signed orders, it *must* be reviewed and renewed on a regular schedule for Medicare and Medicaid patients. Separate care plans may be written that are discipline specific, such as nursing and physical therapy. A separate detailed home health aide care plan is always required.

Visits

Visits for interventions by ordered disciplines are made to meet the patient-centered goals. Skilled nursing visits typically take 30 to 45 minutes but could increase to several hours for complex procedures. Therapy visits range from 30 minutes to 1 hour. Aide visits average 1 to 2 hours but could be longer, depending on needs and payment source. Revisions to the plan of care and referrals to other agencies occur during this period. Patients may be visited as infrequently as one time a month for diabetic monitoring to several times a day over a short period to provide complex care. Several visits per week are typical. Patients may receive only skilled nursing services or may be visited by all disciplines. They may remain on the caseload a week or years, but 60 to 90 days is common.

Documentation

Throughout the care process concise and complete documentation is essential. This documentation may be handwritten, dictated, or entered into a computer. A number of agencies use the problem-oriented record system—many in combination with the nursing diagnosis system.

Documentation that follows the nursing process model provides an accurate picture of care. It reflects the effectiveness of the plan of care and progress toward goals or it reflects the nature and reasons for lack of progress or deterioration and includes alternative interventions. Communications with the home care team and referral sources must also be documented.

Documentation is influenced by other factors. Staff must recognize the record as a legal document subject to close scrutiny at any time. Professional standards and quality of care are closely linked to legal implications, as well as to internal evaluation purposes.

Reimbursement sources have a major influence on documentation requirements by setting forth specific forms and formats that must be followed. Medicare requires extensive paperwork. Private insurer requirements are generally less cumbersome.

Discharge Planning

Discharge planning for home care, as in hospitals, begins with admission. When patient goals or other specific criteria are met, the discharge occurs. Patient and family participation in discharge planning is encouraged. The physician is consulted regarding the discharge and issues the final order. Many agencies follow up on a postdischarge basis to track patient progress and elicit patient satisfaction information.

QUALITY ASSURANCE

Quality assurance programs provide documentation for outside organizations and for internal measures for improvements and refinements of policies and procedures. Assessing quality involves evaluating all aspects of agency operation. Three major elements are included:

1. *Structural criteria:* The agency's overall organization, philosophy, policies, procedures, bylaws, personnel practices, supervision, orientation, contracts, and physical facilities.
2. *Process criteria:* evaluation of care delivery. The activities of the health professionals and paraprofessionals and support in the management of patient care, documentation, and patient care conferences are scrutinized.
3. *Outcome criteria:* measurement of change in patient behavior, the results of patient care in terms of changes, health indicators, and satisfaction. Care standards and expected outcomes are an integral part of this area.

Specific criteria and measures are developed in each area and evaluated for compliance and effectiveness. Evaluation may be accomplished in some areas by management, by a multidisciplinary committee, or by groups of outside professionals and consumers.

In the past, measures of quality of the agency, care delivered, and staff were subjective with little standardization and agreement. Quality assurance plans now reflect standards, objectives, and measurable outcomes and include plans for remediation or improvement as an integral part of the process.

REIMBURSEMENT SOURCES

Reimbursement for home health services comes from a variety of sources, and covered services and disciplines vary. Medicare and Medicaid are major sources of income for the majority of agencies, but reliance on these sources for reimbursement has decreased in recent years.

Medicare

Medicare is a federal program that requires agencies to be certified as meeting the federal conditions of participation, which set forth specific requirements for organization, staffing, training, types of services covered, and agency evaluation. Regulations further mandate eligibility requirements. Beneficiaries of services must be 65 or older, disabled, or have end-stage renal disease. In addition, they must be (1) under the care of a licensed physician, (2) homebound, and (3) in need of skilled nursing or therapy services on an intermittent basis.

Types of services covered and length of coverage are further delineated in guidelines developed by the Health Care Financing Administration (HCFA). Ten regional fiscal intermediaries, who act on behalf of HCFA, receive claims for payment, process reimbursement, and determine coverage.

Medicaid

The Medicaid program pays for home care services to indigent and low-income persons of all ages. It is administered by the state but is both state and federally subsidized. Many states require Medicare certification for participation in the Medicaid program. Services covered vary from state to state, but most include the basic services covered by Medicare plus expansion of aide and personal care services. This program has recently been allowed, through a waiver process, to pay for around-the-clock services to children who require high-technology care and equipment. Children who have lived in an institution can go home and be a part of the family unit (Fig. 51-2).

Third Party

Third-party insurers pay for limited home care services. Coverage, requirements, and payment rates vary. Reim-

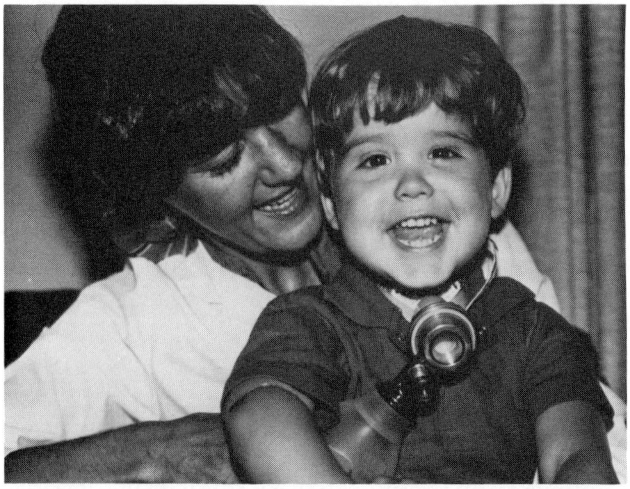

FIG. 51-2 Child with Ondine's disease, chronic obstructive pulmonary disease, and collapsible airway syndrome. With the services of home health care he has been able to recover at home. (Photo by Marilu Halamandaris, *CARING* Magazine.)

bursement often is tied to posthospitalization recoveries. A few progressive companies are paying for nursing and aide services for new mothers who return home within 24 hours of delivery.

Private Pay

Individuals may also pay directly for home health services. Charges may be the standard full charge or may be scaled down based on the ability of the patient to pay.

Other Sources

Health maintenance organizations (HMOs) and preferred provider organizations (PPOs) have negotiated contracts with home health agencies to provide services to their patients. Both organizations are prepaid health plans operated independently or through employer groups. Again, requirements and coverage differ.

Current trends support the growth of home care as an economical, humane, preferred health delivery system for certain types of care. Advances in medical knowledge coupled with high-technology health care have increased the number of individuals surviving birth traumas, prematurity, infectious diseases, acute illnesses, accidents, and other maladies that formerly were fatal. Many illnesses are medically managed and controlled rather than cured. This has increased the number of potentially debilitating chronic illnesses. Dependency and disability are more prevalent in all age groups. One in seven persons now needs help with basic activities of daily living. Home care provides needed assessment and evaluation of chronic illnesses to prevent acute episodes. Aides and homemakers can provide necessary support in activities of daily living to enable the patient to remain in the home.

The birth rate has declined, resulting in an aging population. In the 1900s only 2% of the population was 65 or older. That figure was 12.3% in 1989 and is projected to reach 20% by the 2030. It is estimated that 80% of this group has at least one chronic disability. The age group older than 85 years is the fastest growing group today. It is estimated that by the year 2000 there will be a tenfold increase in persons older than 100 years. About 40% of those 85 and older need help with physical activities. Assistance in daily living is essential to this group. Skilled nursing and therapy offer rehabilitation and prevention of deterioration, as well as methods to cope with physical changes.

Federal and private insurers are trying to cap the rapidly rising cost of health care by shortening hospital stays and controlling admissions. Home care agencies are filling the gap for patients who are released early but who still require complex care or rehabilitation. In many cases, home care services can prevent hospitalization by offering enteral, parenteral, intravenous, and blood transfusion services.

The movement toward deinstitutionalization of technology-dependent children and adults is now possible as Medicaid and third-party payers change reimbursement criteria. Home care support makes "family life" a reality for people who once thought of hospital personnel as parents.

An emphasis on healthy living and illness prevention is supported by home health providers as part of the plan of care. This one-on-one education teaches specific techniques to avoid recurrences of illness or deterioration of condition.

Finally, individuals want to be at home as long as possible. Care provided by home health agencies and support from social service agencies and others are now making this possible throughout the life span.

REFERENCES AND SUGGESTED READINGS

1. Aitken MJ: Matching models to environments: a planning guide to the solution of pediatric home care models, Home Healthc Nurse 7(2):13, 1989.
2. Department of Health and Human Services: Code of Federal Regulations (Title 42), Washington, DC, 1989.
3. Harper MS: Providing mental health services in the homes of the elderly, Caring 8(6):5, 1989.
4. Harris MD: Home health administration, Owings Mills, MD, 1988, National Health Publishing.
5. Health Care Financing Administration: HCFA statistics, Bureau of Data Management and Strategy, Pub No 03229, Washington, DC, 1986, US Government Printing Office.
6. Home care services: past, present, and future, Caring 7(12):4, 1988.
7. Home health and hospice manual: Regulations and guidelines, Subscriber Digest, Bulletin No 17, Owings Mills, MD, 1989, National Health Publishing.
8. Maurano L: Pediatric home care: past, present, and future, Home Health Care Pract 1(2):1, 1989.
9. Mesenheimer CG: Quality assurance for homecare, Rockville, MD, 1989, Aspen Publishers, Inc.
10. Newacheck PW, Fox, HB, and McManus MA: Home care needs of chronically ill children, Caring 7(6):4, 1988.
11. Shaughnessy P, Bauman M, and Kraner A: Measuring the quality of home health care: some important considerations, Caring 9(2): 4, 1990.
12. Stanhope M and Lancaster J: Community health nursing process and practice for promoting health, ed 2, St Louis, 1988, The CV Mosby Co.
13. Stewart R: Manual of community and home health nursing, Boston, 1987, Little, Brown & Co, Inc.
14. Stuart-Siddal S: Home health care nursing: administrative and clinical perspectives, Rockville, MD, 1986, Aspen Publishers, Inc.

CHAPTER CHALLENGE

KEY POINTS

- Home health care allows individuals to maintain personal control and to participate in the direction of their own care.
- Families are an important part of the success of home care services as health care workers provide care, supervision, assistance, and support in attaining the care plan goals.
- Home health care is not a new concept; however, legislative, regulatory, and current health care trends have changed the way it is provided.
- A number of different professional and paraprofessional disciplines provide home care services based on a coordinated plan of care approved by a physician. Teamwork is an essential component of the concept.
- Home health agencies are organized groups that employ or contract with professionals and paraprofessionals to provide services. Different types of agencies may be subject to varying federal, state, and local laws and regulations.
- Skilled nursing care is the most frequently provided serivce. RNs and LPNs/LVNs under the supervision of RNs provide direct care of different levels of complexity.
- Providers of care in the home must possess special qualities to effectively practice in this nontraditional environment.
- Home health care agencies strive to provide the highest quality of services in an economical manner. Success is evaluated through quality assurance plans.
- Home health services are reimbursed by federal, state, local, group, and private sources.

STUDY QUESTIONS

1. Home health care includes all of the following except:
   a. Enables individuals of all ages to remain in their homes while receiving health care
   b. Can assist patients and families in achieving better health and a higher level of functioning than previous
   c. Is completely regulated by federal and state laws
   d. Teaches healthy life-styles that minimize the effects of illness or disability and can prevent the recurrence of illness
2. Home health services can be provided by:
   a. Only certified home health agencies
   b. Only licensed home health agencies
   c. Only accredited home health agencies
   d. Any individual, group, organization, or agency
3. Organized agencies are classified according to:
   a. Tax status
   b. Location
   c. Governance
   d. All of the above
4. Which of the following services is not generally provided by a home health agency:
   a. Skilled nursing
   b. Nutritional support
   c. Home health aide
   d. Physical therapy
   e. Recreational therapy
   f. Medical social services
5. Which of the following statements is NOT true:
   a. Home care providers are guests in patients' homes
   b. Nurses providing services must be goal oriented and develop rigid schedules for meeting goals
   c. Patient teaching is an important aspect of nursing services
   d. Quality assurance includes evaluating outcomes
6. LPNs/LVNs may do all of the following except:
   a. Observe and report changes in a patient's condition
   b. Independently change the plan of treatment
   c. Provide sterile dressing changes
   d. Participate in patient and family teaching
7. Sources of payment for home care might include which of the following:
   a. Medicare/Medicaid
   b. Blue Cross/Blue Shield
   c. Health maintenance organization
   d. Individuals
   e. All of the above
8. Home health care is a growing part of the health care delivery system because of all of the following except:
   a. A nursing shortage has forced hospitals to reduce the number of beds
   b. High-technology health care has improved survival rates of serious illnesses and traumas
   c. The aging population is creating increasing numbers of people with chronic illnesses
   d. Early hospital discharges create a need for further care after hospitalization

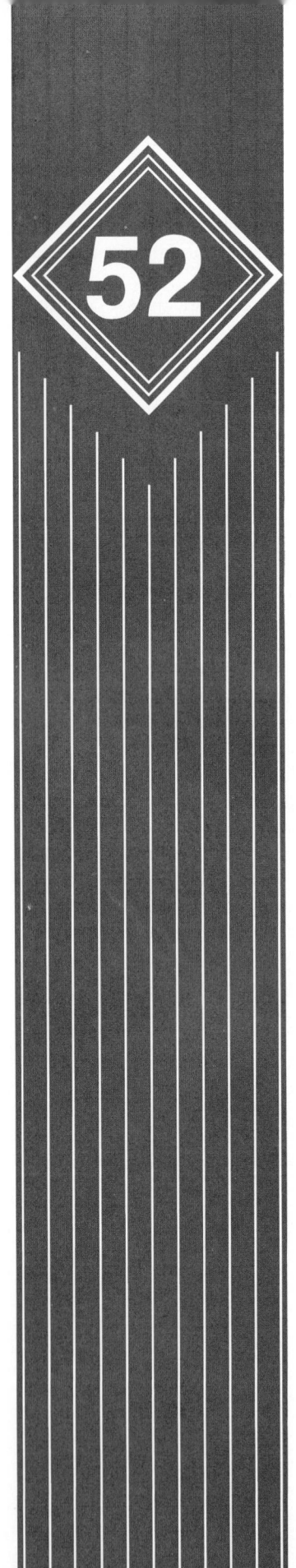

52

Rehabilitation Nursing

SALLY L. PERSONS BECK

LEARNING OBJECTIVES

After reading this chapter, the student should be able to do the following:

- Define the key terms.
- Define the philosophy of rehabilitation nursing.
- Describe the rehabilitation team concept and functions of each member.
- Discuss the stages of disability adjustment.
- Discuss three major disabling conditions.
- Provide the nursing diagnosis, goals, and interventions for three major disabling conditions.

RELATED TOPICS OF INTEREST

- Care of the patient with a musculoskeletal disorder (Chapter 30)
- Care of the patient with a neurological disorder (Chapter 38)
- Home health nursing (Chapter 51)

KEY TERMS

Define the following:

- cervical cord injury
- comprehensive rehabilitation plan
- evaluation conference
- flaccid
- functional assessment
- holistic approach
- intervention
- lumbar cord injury
- physiatrist
- rehabilitation
- spastic
- spondylolisthesis
- thoracic cord injury
- traumatic brain injury

Rehabilitation is the process of maximizing an individual's abilities and resources to promote optimum growth and function by focusing on the individual's decision-making ability. This begins with preventive care in the initial stage of the accident or disease, it continues through the restorative phase, and it involves adaptation to a new life.

Rehabilitation is reaching maximum achievable independence. It is restoration to the fullest physical, mental, social, vocational, and economic capacity possible for a given individual. When individuals no longer regard themselves as disabled, they become more responsive and participative members of their families and communities.

The focus in rehabilitation should be on *ability,* not *disability.* This usually requires training, education, and strengthening. Comprehensive rehabilitation helps each person as an individual see that he or she has more reasons to pursue successes than to give up. For those who have the courage to try, the reward is newfound achievement and independence.

Rehabilitation nursing is an "attitude" along with knowledge and skills that must be basic to all phases of patient care. The concept of rehabilitation should be infused into general care, and the maintenance and preventive aspects should be ongoing throughout the individual's life. *Rehabilitation nursing is a vital part of health care, not just a phase of it.*

REHABILITATION PROFESSIONALS: THE REHABILITATION TEAM

Rehabilitation is a creative process. It requires a team to work together and contribute specialized services for a common goal (Box 52-1). The team members represent a variety of disciplines. A multidisciplinary team concept is used at a rehabilitation center. Professional staff members use their knowledge and skills to develop and implement a care plan—a plan designed to help the patient reach a maximum level of independence. This requires a **holistic approach.**

REHABILITATION NURSING

Disease and injuries can occur slowly or suddenly and result in devastating disabilities. Life-styles are dramatically altered, and families may be torn apart. Rehabilitation can make a difference. It can turn tragedy to triumph.

The rehabilitation nurse focuses on creative problem-solving techniques. The goal is to provide a supportive environment that encourages independence while helping the patient to adapt to a different life-style. The major emphasis is on "how to" and "why" and involves active patient participation. Quality rehabilitation must be consistent.

BOX 52-1 THE REHABILITATION TEAM

MEMBER	ROLE	GOAL
Patient	Key member	Participates in goal setting; takes control of own life
Physiatrist	Rehabilitation physician	Team leader; coordinator of program
Rehabilitation nurse	Care provider; educator	Provides support; promotes independence
Physical therapist	Designs exercise program	Provides therapy; assesses needs; provides training
Occupational therapist	Assesses independent living needs	Recommends equipment modifications; adapts equipment
Speech pathologist	Designs rehabilitation communication program	Assists in regaining communication skills; educator
Therapeutic recreation therapist	Recreation planner	Activates leisure time; promotes interest in activities
Clinical psychologist	Emotional evaluator	Assists patient in developing realistic positive attitudes
Chaplain	Consultant	Provides support and guidance
Vocational rehabilitation counselor	Vocational planner	Helps obtain training and employment

A rehabiliation nurse must focus on means to enable the patient to move from a totally dependent state to a level of independence. Each patient should receive individual treatment by specific nurses and therapists so bonds of trust and friendship can develop through a difficult rehabilitation process. Extensive family and patient education, modern adaptive equipment, numerous community integration activities, specialized programs, and professional effective team therapies combine to help patients learn to maximize their lives.

Basic rehabilitation can be used whether the patient has arthritis, multiple sclerosis, mental illness, cerebral vascular accident (CVA, or stroke), spinal cord injury, burn, or traumatic brain injury (TBI). It is the nurse's responsibility to apply appropriate concepts and techniques.

Basic nursing measures, such as position changes, are essential to maintain body alignment. This prevents skeletal and muscular deformities (contractures) and decubitus ulcers (pressure sores).

Rehabilitation nursing is a challenge that requires knowledge, teamwork, coordination, planning, and patience. Rehabilitation professionals must learn to care for disabled persons and must stay informed regarding current knowledge and techniques.

A COMPREHENSIVE REHABILITATION PLAN

The more comprehensive the rehabilitation program, the better the chance for achieving substantial results. All major services that are needed to treat a patient's disability should be provided. The goal of rehabilitation specialists should be to help individuals return to home, work, or school.

There is a newly developed problem-oriented format used for medical evaluations that lists patient problems rather than a single diagnosis. The list includes the disease or injury, significant consequences and complications, physical function limitations that reflect the extent of the physical disability, and psychological, social, and vocational data. With this new approach, specific therapeutic techniques and **interventions** can be directed toward each of the limitations.

Initially, medical services are primary and vocational services are minimal. Gradually, medical services decrease and vocational services increase. Part of the medical **comprehensive rehabilitation plan** involves team consultations, which include functional assessment, evaluation conference, and family conference. **Functional assessment** is completed on patient admission (at least within 24 hours of admission) and examines the patient's functional abilities. This assessment should include the patient's (1) level of response, (2) attitude, cooperation, and motivation, (3) bladder program, (4) bowel program, (5) skin condition, (6) sleep/activity tolerance, (7) diet and nutrition, and (8) activities of daily living (ADLs), such as bed/car transfer, toilet transfer, light hygiene, bath, and positioning. At the **evaluation conference,** the patient is thoroughly evaluated. A complete medical team reviews the available data and sets realistic goals. At a family conference the patient's functional status, goals, and future plans are discussed. This conference is usually arranged by the rehabilitation social worker.

In today's society employment fulfills many basic human needs. It provides a sense of identity and independence, a feeling of accomplishment and status, and an opportunity to use skills to be responsible. It is a source of earnings and security. When introduced, individuals usually share information about occupation immediately after exchanging names. And with jobs tied to personal identity, any loss of identity can create considerable anxiety, depression, or various emotional concerns. Jobs provide not only personal satisfaction and socialization benefits, but a reason to get out of bed in the morning. The workplace is where an individual is expected to be, a place to come home from, and a reason to be tired.

Disability Adjustments

After acute medical treatment, often the first barrier identified is the person's change in social status. Disabled persons are classified as some type of minority, and at times people tend to attribute negative characteristics to them. Others may see them as less attractive, less desirable, or less capable. As a result of their disability, these persons may lose their social status and serious economic consequences may result. The disability may be so great that the cost of medical care depletes the family's resources. The tendency to stereotype and discriminate against the "disabled and handicapped" can be reversed if employers and other members of society will consider them to be what they are—people with physical and/or mental limitations.

Stages of Adjustment

Numerous experts have proposed various stages of adjustment. Generally it is felt that each phase is accompanied by a characteristic emotional experience, and a predominant emotional reaction changes as the person progresses through the phases of adjustment. A synopsis of the various stages is provided (Box 52-2). The duration and individual reactions vary in time, intensity, and order. A person may skip a phase altogether.

BOX 52-2 STAGES OF ADJUSTMENT

STAGE	DEFINITION	CHARACTERISTICS
Reaction stage	Shock	Withdrawal; anxiety; blunted emotions; depression; anger
Adjustment stage	Defensive retreat	Persistent or reoccurring denial; refusal to accept limitations
Understanding stage	Acknowledgment	Realistic attitude; depression; goal setting
Acceptance stage	Adaptation	Utilizes assets; independence; development of self-image

AN OVERVIEW OF MAJOR DISABLING CONDITIONS

Rehabilitation is a bridge for the patient, spanning the gap between uselessness and usefulness, between hopelessness and hopefulness, between despair and happiness. A few of the major conditions follow for which dedicated rehabilitative efforts are required.

Decubitus Ulcer

A decubitus ulcer is a bedsore or pressure sore. It is the most common severe skin problem faced in the health care setting. Decubitus is Latin for "a lying down." *Ulcer* refers to the cavity created by the sloughing away of dead tissue. Pressure sores result from continued pressure, which decreases blood supply to a given area. They can occur with patients who are sitting, lying, or standing. Constrictive clothing, improperly fitted shoes, or maligned bracing equipment can result in decubitus ulcers.

Normally, our bodies are aware of pressure. When one of the transmitting systems is impaired, the risk of skin breakdown increases. The brain is constantly receiving information, processing it, and sending messages in response to the sensation of pressure. For example, a patient with a spinal cord injury, paralyzed from the waist down and sitting in a chair, does not feel pressure below the level of the cord injury. When pressure occludes the flow of blood to an area, messages of pain are sent but not received.

Decubitus ulcers can be prevented. Both the family and patient must practice a total prevention program. Rehabilitation nurses can facilitate and encourage prevention through education. Nursing assessment involves observation of skin color, turgor, temperature, and condition. Assessment must include the patient's movement and sensation.

NURSING DIAGNOSIS: Impairment of skin integrity, actual or potential

GOAL: Patient's skin integrity maintained, clean, dry, and intact

INTERVENTIONS:
- Bathe daily using warm water and mild soap
- Massage the skin with mild lanolin-based lotions to increase circulation and maintain integrity
- Dry skin thoroughly
- Assess perineal and perianal areas to observe for excoriation, vaginal discharge, and pain
- Apply lotions or cornstarch to area as needed
- Assess feet and hands to observe for signs of rash, dryness, or skin breaks

INTERVENTIONS: Cleanse and trim nails when necessary
Assess condition of hair
Assess patient for shaving needs
Maintain physical comfort
Change bed linen daily, and keep linen clean, dry, and wrinkle free
Provide adequate warmth
Change position every 1-2 hours
Maintain adequate nutrition

Multiple Sclerosis

Multiple sclerosis (MS) is one of the most common neurological diseases. The cause is unknown. It is defined as a chronic, progressive disease characterized by scattering of demyelinating lesions in the central nervous system (CNS), which affects the white matter of the brain and spinal cord. Assessment involves observations/findings, such as fatigue, sensory impairment (numbness and tingling), dizziness, weakness of extremities, visual disturbance, speech impairment, difficulty in chewing and swallowing, staggering gait, bladder or bowel dysfunction, mood swings, depression, irritability, apathy, inattention, lack of judgment, and weeping. Nursing diagnoses/goals/interventions for multiple sclerosis follow.

NURSING DIAGNOSIS: Hygiene, feeding, and/or toileting self-care deficit, related to limitations in physical mobility imposed by disease process

GOAL: Patient's self-care needs will be met

INTERVENTIONS: Maintain quiet and relaxing environment
Encourage self-care
Avoid use of heating pads (heat diminishes muscle strength and increases potential for burns)
Plan all activities to avoid fatigue
Plan bladder and bowel dysfunction program, if appropriate
Encourage fluids

NURSING DIAGNOSIS: Potential for body image and self-esteem disturbance, related to altered perception of self

GOAL: Patient will accept changes in body image and self-esteem

INTERVENTIONS: Establish means of communication
Acknowledge concerns about body image
Be supportive of emotional changes, and encourage verbalization of feelings

NURSING DIAGNOSIS: Potential for ineffective airway clearance, related to motor weakness and/or immobility

GOAL: Patient will maintain a patent airway

INTERVENTIONS: Suction as needed
Assist and teach patient to cough and deep breathe
Maintain patent airway

NURSING DIAGNOSIS: Knowledge deficit regarding disease process

GOAL: Patient and/or significant other will demonstrate understanding of home care and follow-up instructions through interactive discussion and actual return demonstration

INTERVENTIONS: Explain nature of disease
Explain that warm weather and hot baths may increase weakness
Explain importance of avoiding fatigue
Explain importance of regular exercise and rest
Discuss symptoms of disease progression
Discuss symptoms of cold and influenza and report to physician
Encourage socialization and independence

Cerebral Vascular Accident

A cerebral vascular accident (CVA) can be defined as a sudden onset of neurological symptoms as a result of an abnormal condition of the blood vessels of the brain, characterized by occlusion by an embolus or cerebrovascular hemorrhage, resulting in ischemia of the brain tissues normally perfused by the damaged vessels. CVA is often accompanied by other medical problems associated with the diseases of the blood vessels, such as hypertension, heart disease, or peripheral vascular disease. Nursing concerns include depression, contractures, bowel and bladder dysfunction, urinary tract infections, pneumonia, or seizures. Rehabilitation potential is directly related to the duration and depth of coma. The earlier the return of extremity function, the better the prognosis. In addition to the nurse, other rehabilitation professionals usually involved are the speech pathologist, occupational therapist, physical therapist, clinical psychologist, and vocational rehabilitation counselor if appropriate. (See Chapter 38 for nursing interventions for CVA.)

Low Back Pain

Back disorders constitute a substantial percentage of all disabilities. Usually the pain is in the lower lumbosacral region. Various back disorders are diagnosed as acute sprain, chronic strain, degenerative disk disease, and **spondylolisthesis.** The range of medical intervention may include total bed rest, medications to ensure relaxation and to relieve inflammation and pain, or home exercise programs. Surgery is sometimes required. Vocation implications include careful analysis of sitting, standing, moving, lifting, pulling, pushing, and climbing requirements of the job. It is also important to identify potential sources of stress in the job. The individual with chronic back pain poses a definite challenge to achieve vocational success.

Low back pain is defined as pain in the lower back that may be caused by a variety of diseases that affect bone, but is generally the result of (1) stress on the vertebral process or (2) herniated disk. Assessment and observations include back pain (low and intense), radiating leg pain, muscle spasm, muscular weakness, obesity, and faulty posture. Nursing diagnoses/goals/interventions follow.

NURSING DIAGNOSIS: Pain, related to the disease process

GOAL: Patient will express minimal discomfort or absence of pain

INTERVENTIONS: Maintain bed rest with firm mattress
Administer medications as ordered: analgesics, muscle relaxants, antiinflammatory agents
Application of hot or cold compresses as ordered
Physical therapy as ordered
Increase activity as allowed

NURSING DIAGNOSIS: Knowledge deficit regarding home care management

GOAL: Patient and/or significant other will demonstrate understanding of home care and follow-up instructions through interactive discussion and actual return demonstration

INTERVENTIONS: Stress importance of prescribed rehabilitation plan
Demonstrate use of transcutaneous electrical nerve stimulation (TENS)
Provide diet instructions
Discuss medication: name, schedule, purpose, dosage, and possible side effects
Promote follow-up visits with physician

Emotional Disabilities

A disability may cause behavioral, emotional, role, body image, and self-concept changes and alterations in family dynamics. Emotional disabilities are generally grouped into diagnostic categories defined by the American Psychiatric Association, such as organic, mental, and personality disorders. The more seriously disabled individuals are usually socially isolated and vocationally inadequate and possess strong dependency needs. Additionally, they lack self-confidence and social skills necessary to effectively communicate with others. It should be emphasized that even severely disabled psychiatric patients can be helped to improve their lives through work. Work is therapeutic. Emotional disability requires close vocational counselor involvement and support.

Spinal Cord Injuries

Spinal cord injuries have increased mainly because of an increase in motor vehicle accidents. The majority of individuals paralyzed are young. Because of improved medical care, they now survive the injury, and because of their youth, they have vocational potential. Functional disabilities are related to injury level. After acute nursing intervention, other concerns involve bowel and bladder functional impairment, ambulation functions, dressing, personal hygiene, exercise, and communication (speech and writing). Rehabilitation potential is directly related to nursing concerns. It is important for the rehabilitation professional to carefully consider education, interests, aptitudes, and physical requirements when assessing rehabilitation potential.

A spinal cord injury is any injury in which the spinal cord is compressed by fracture or displaced vertebrae, bleeding, or edema. Spinal cord injuries can be divided into the following:

1. **Cervical cord injury:** Level of injury is at cervical spine C2 to C6 and involves paralysis of all extremities and trunk, respiratory failure, bladder and bowel disturbance, bradycardia, perspiring, elevated temperature, and headache.
2. **Thoracic cord injury:** Level of injury is at thoracic spine T1 to T12 and involves paralysis of lower extremities. Initially muscles are **flaccid** and later become **spastic.** Paralysis of bladder, bowel, and sphincters; pain in chest or back; abdominal distention; and loss of sexual function are other potential symptoms.
3. **Lumbar cord injury:** Level of injury is at lumbar spine L1 to L2 with paralysis of lower extremities, bladder, and rectum, and loss of sexual function.

NURSING DIAGNOSIS: Ineffective breathing pattern, related to neurogenic or traumatic injury

GOAL: Patient will have a patent airway

INTERVENTIONS: Maintain patent airway
Administer assisted ventilation
Closely monitor for signs of respiratory failure, and be prepared to assist with tracheotomy if needed.
Monitor vital signs and consciousness every 1 to 2 hours
Assess motor/sensory function to ensure adequate rhythm and pattern of respiration

NURSING DIAGNOSIS: Hygiene, feeding, and toileting self-care deficit, related to neurophysiological impairment

GOAL: Patient's self-care needs will be met

INTERVENTIONS: Maintain IV fluids as ordered
Maintain NPO until chewing, swallowing, and gastrointestinal (GI) function is established
Provide nutritional support as ordered
Connect indwelling catheter to closed gravity drainage
Teach self-catheterization to thoracic- and lumbar-injured patients
Administer catheter care

INTERVENTIONS: Administer oral hygiene every 2 to 4 hours
Administer skin care every 2 to 4 hours
Explain importance of skin care
Teach muscle-building exercises

NURSING DIAGNOSIS: Knowledge deficit regarding diagnosis and potential home management

GOAL: Patient and significant other will demonstrate understanding of home care and follow-up instructions

INTERVENTIONS: Ensure patient and significant other are informed about disease prognosis
Prepare for chronicity and duration of rehabilitation process
Discuss medications: name, dosage, routine, possible side effects, and purpose

Traumatic Brain Injury

Although there are numerous disabilities, each with its own nursing and vocational implications, few present the challenges of the patient with **traumatic brain injury** (TBI). In spite of mandatory seat belt laws and drinking/driving reforms, the number of head injuries resulting from motor vehicle accidents continues to rise. Again, as a result of medical advances, there are an increasing number of survivors.

Head injuries can be classified as either penetrating or closed head injuries. In penetrating injuries, an object lacerates the scalp, fractures the skull, and injures the soft tissue in its path, thus destroying nerve cells. In a closed head injury, the brain collides with an inner surface of the skull. This results in widespread damage called *shearing* (when the brain mass is rotated in the cranial vault). Thus there is violent twisting action, which causes the upper section of the brain to rotate with the lower end anchored securely in a stationary position.

There appears to be direct correlation between the amount of disability resulting from a traumatic brain injury and the degree of expertise and aggressiveness of those providing medical care during the acute period. Successful vocational outcome correlates with duration and depth of coma, duration of posttraumatic amnesia, preinjury level of functioning (positive achievement), rate of improvement in the 1-year postinjury stage, age of onset (the younger the age of the patient with a head injury, usually the better the prognosis), and the presence of realistic vocational goals.

Head injuries can be classified as mild, moderate, severe, or catastrophic. Mild head injury is characterized by brief or no loss of consciousness, which constitutes the majority of head injuries. Neurological examinations are often normal. Postconcussive syndrome can persist for months, years, or indefinitely. Signs and symptoms include fatigue, headache, dizziness, lethargy, irritability, personality changes, cognitive deficits, decreased information-processing speed, and memory, understanding, learning, and perceptual difficulties. These symptoms lead to feelings of incompetence, guilt, and frustration. Family members may become impatient and frustrated.

In the moderate head injury there is a characteristic period of unconsciousness from 1 to 24 hours. There are usually cognitive impairments, which include planning, sequencing, judgment, reasoning, and computation skills. Generally there are some psychosocial problems, which include self-centeredness, denial, mood swings, agitation, depression, lethargy, sexual dysfunction, emotional lability, low frustration tolerance, poor judgment, or behavioral outbursts.

Patients with severe head injuries experience unconsciousness or posttrauma amnesia in excess of 8 days. There are cognitive, psychosocial, and behavioral disabilities.

Catastrophic head injury is characterized by a coma lasting several months or longer. These individuals may appear to be awake. However, they generally never regain significant meaningful communication with their environment.

In rehabilitative assessing of the patient with TBI, inconsistent performance, anger, and frustration should be expected, and ineffective behavior will be changeable (unless it is neurogenic in origin). Cognitive barriers to rehabilitative recovery include problems in thinking and reasoning (impaired memory), impaired concentration and attention, and impaired informational processing speed. Psychosocially, there appears to be a lack of initiative. However, this is a normal consequence of a head injury. Egocentric (self-centered) behavior is 100% normal in a head-injured individual, as is depression. Generally, the more the memory improves, the more the patient becomes depressed. Abstinence from alcohol should be considered primary with any patient with a head injury. Alcohol increases the chance of impulse and seizure activity.

IF ANYONE ELSE MAKES AN ERROR, IT'S RECORDED AS AN ERROR
...IF A TBI PATIENT DOES IT, IT'S RECORDED AS BRAIN DAMAGE!!!

Continuous and honest involvement of the family, as both a vicitim of the injury and an equal participant in the rehabilitation process, is critical to the successful rehabilitation of the head-injured patient. It should be remembered that the entire family is a victim of the traumatic brain injury. Often the head-injured person's awareness and acceptance of the disability is determined by the flexibility of the family system itself.

The rehabilitation professionals must be available and be honest in reporting to families, including "I don't know," when appropriate. Equal communication with all family members is important, as is encouraging the family to become involved in counseling and education. The family should be encouraged to be aware of each others' needs and interests, they should be assisted in becoming involved in a support group, and technical terminology should be avoided. It is important the family understand that rehabilitation is not a birthright.

Nursing assessments involve observing altered levels of consciousness, including headaches, dizziness, mental changes (irritability, restlessness, confusion, stupor, coma), pupillary response (size, equality, response to light), airway patency, seizure activity, projectile vomiting, drainage from ears and nose, elevated temperature, and elevated or decreased blood pressure.

NURSING DIAGNOSIS: Ineffective airway clearance, related to impaired neurological function

GOAL: Patent airway will be maintained

INTERVENTIONS:
- Maintain patent airway, endotracheal tube, or tracheostomy, as ordered, with suctioning prn
- Administer oxygen, humidification, or mechanical ventilation as ordered
- Assist patient in coughing and deep breathing
- Check blood pressure, pulse, and respiration every 15 to 30 minutes; report any pupillary or mental changes immediately, since changes signal respiratory embarrassment

NURSING DIAGNOSIS: Bathing, feeding, and toileting self-care deficit related to neurological impairment

GOAL: Patient's self-care needs will be met

INTERVENTIONS:
- Administer oral hygiene every 2 to 4 hours
- Administer skin care every 2 hours prn
- Provide for all hygiene needs as indicated
- Provide for patient's elimination needs
- Initiate voiding measures as indicated
- Encourage early ambulation as ordered
- Perform active or passive range-of-motion (ROM) exercises to all extremities

NURSING DIAGNOSIS: Potential for alteration in body image disturbance, related to actual/perceived changes in physical and personal self-image

GOAL: Patient will accept changes in body image and self-esteem

INTERVENTIONS:
- Provide emotional support
- Encourage verbalization of feelings about body image
- Provide for alternative communication methods if vocalization is impaired, such as Magic Slate or pencil and paper

NURSING DIAGNOSIS: Knowledge deficit regarding disease process and home management

GOAL: Patient and/or significant other will demonstrate understanding of home care and follow-up instructions through interactive discussion and actual return demonstration

INTERVENTIONS:
- Discuss nature of disorder, treatment, and procedures
- Explain to family the need to encourage verbalization about body image change or limitation
- Explain need for ambulation and planned rest periods
- Discuss possible residual effects, such as dizziness, headache, and memory loss, which may persist for 3 or 4 months after trauma
- Discuss medications
- Explain need to avoid taking over-the-counter medications
- Discuss symptoms of progression of condition to report to physician
- Explain importance of ongoing outpatient care

Begin as soon as possible with vocational planning. As soon as the patient can participate, include him or her. Early intervention is necessary.

Use calm, controlled, and consistent manner
Use short-term, goal-directed techniques
Accentuate the positive
Coordinate vocational and psychosocial adjustment
EXPECT THE UNEXPECTED
Use group methods and videotaping
Use positive reinforcement
BE REDUNDANT
Assume nothing: *review, review, review*

Specific considerations for return-to-work evaluations include the following:

1. Initiate evaluation early.
2. Evaluate all areas of work repertoire (obtain detailed preinjury work information).
3. Identify compensatory mechanisms.
4. Seek a broad range of input from family, team, and other patients.
5. Above all, determine whether the patient's work and jobs were the central life focus.

Regardless of personality types, any disability, particularly a TBI, is a crisis that threatens many aspects of the patient's and family's life: job income, pleasures, family, community ties, health, and life itself. The fears are very real.

■ ■ ■

Rehabilitation nurses must take their responsibility seriously as professionals who can significantly affect the future of those with disabilities. Nurses must facilitate changing restraint to openness, turning inertia into action. Focus must be on the assets and successes of people who have disabilities.

Emerson summed it up succinctly when he wrote:

> It is one of the most beautiful compensations of this life that no man can sincerely try to help another without helping himself.

REFERENCES AND SUGGESTED READINGS

1. Casselt B: Treating pressure sores stage by stage, RN, Jan 1986.
2. Fraser RT, McMahon BT, and Vogenthaler D: Contemporary challenges to the rehabilitation counseling profession, Baltimore, 1988, Paul H Brookes Publishing Co.
3. Hood GH and Dincher JR: Total patient care, ed 7, St Louis, 1988, The CV Mosby Co.
4. Long, Jo; RN.,C.R.R.N. Rehabilitation Clinician; Immanuel Rehabilitation Center, Omaha, NE, Personal clinical notes, 1989.
5. Minchow, Mary; BA, Vocational Rehabilitation Counselor III; Clinical Documentation of Spinal Cord Injuries and Their Vocational Implications, Personal workshop notes, Sept, 1988.
6. Mosby's medical, nursing, and allied health dictionary, ed 3, St Louis, 1990, The CV Mosby Co.
7. National Institute on Disability and Rehabilitation Research: Stroke, Rehab Brief, XI (11), Washington, DC, Office of Special Education and Rehabilitation Services, 1989, The Institute.
8. Nebraska, The State of; Department of Education, Division of Rehabilitation Services, Data from 1989.
9. Passerella P and Gee Z: Starting right after stroke, Am J Nurs 87 (6):802, 1987.
10. Potter P and Perry A: Basic nursing: theory and practice, St Louis, ed 2, 1990, The CV Mosby Co.
11. Reich N and Otten P: What to wear: a challenge for disabled elders, Am J Nurs 87(2): Feb 1987.
12. Stolov WC and Clowers MR: Handbook of severe disability, 1981, US Department of Education Rehabilitation Services Administration.
13. Tucker SM and others: Patient care standards: nursing process, diagnosis, and outcome, ed 4, St Louis, 1988, The CV Mosby Co.

CHAPTER CHALLENGE

KEY POINTS

- Rehabilitation is the process of maximizing the use of an individual's capabilities or resources to foster optimal growth and functioning.
- The patient is the most important team member and must be involved in planning the programs and learning in detail about the disabilities, the ways of accomplishing the goals, and the options available.
- Rehabilitation nursing is directed toward the prevention of complications of disease or trauma and the maintenance and/or restoration of function.
- Basic rehabilitation can be used regardless of disability. It is the nurse's responsibility to apply appropriate concepts and techniques.
- A disability can have a number of effects on both the patient and the family, including behavioral and emotional changes and changes in roles, body image, self-concept, and family dynamics.
- A nurse must consider all the effects of an illness on a patient and the family to plan and implement holistic nursing care that assists both the patient and family in attaining a state of maximal functioning and well-being.
- A comprehensive rehabilitation plan is multifaceted and may involve a functional assessment, evaluation conference, and family conference.
- Stages of adjustment include shock, denial or defensive retreat, acknowledgment or constructive response, and adaptation. Individual reactions vary in time, intensity, and order.
- Decubitus ulcers are the most common severe skin problem faced in the health care setting.
- The number of spinal cord injuries and traumatic brain injuries has increased because of an increase in motor vehicle accidents. Medical advancements result in an increasing number of survivors.

STUDY QUESTIONS

1. Another name for decubitus ulcer is:
   a. Adaptation
   b. Bed sore or pressure sore
   c. Contracture
   d. Skin turgor
2. Rehabilitation is:
   a. Maximizing an individual's abilities and resources to promote optimum growth and function
   b. Becoming functionally independent
   c. A creative process
   d. All of the above
3. The number of spinal cord injuries has increased mainly because of:
   a. Better coma care
   b. Mandatory seat belt laws
   c. Increased vehicle accidents
   d. Rehabilitation centers
4. The rehabilitation team may consist of:
   a. Therapeutic recreation therapist
   b. Rehabilitation nurses
   c. Medical social worker
   d. All of the above
5. A physiatrist:
   a. Prevents disability
   b. Maintains functional ability of patient
   c. Treats communication disorders
   d. Is a medical specialist in rehabilitation
6. A rehabilitation nurse requires:
   a. Special knowledge, skills, and attitudes
   b. Skills to assist patients in becoming independent
   c. Being goal directed
   d. All of the above
7. Rehabilitation:
   a. Assists individuals with disabilities
   b. Identifies patients' health care needs
   c. Is designed to help prevent harm
   d. Is a process of gathering, verifying, and communicating data about a patient
8. A comprehensive rehabilitation plan:
   a. Organizes orderly procedures
   b. Assists patients in reaching their maximum potential
   c. May involve functional assessment, evaluation, and conferences
   d. All of the above
9. Nursing assessment of the TBI patient includes:
   a. Monitoring altered states of consciousness
   b. Observing for seizure activity
   c. Monitoring vital signs
   d. All of the above
10. With a TBI patient, the nurse should:
    a. Be redundant
    b. Use long-term, goal-directed techniques
    c. Avoid group methods and videotaping
    d. Use calm and inconsistent manner

XV

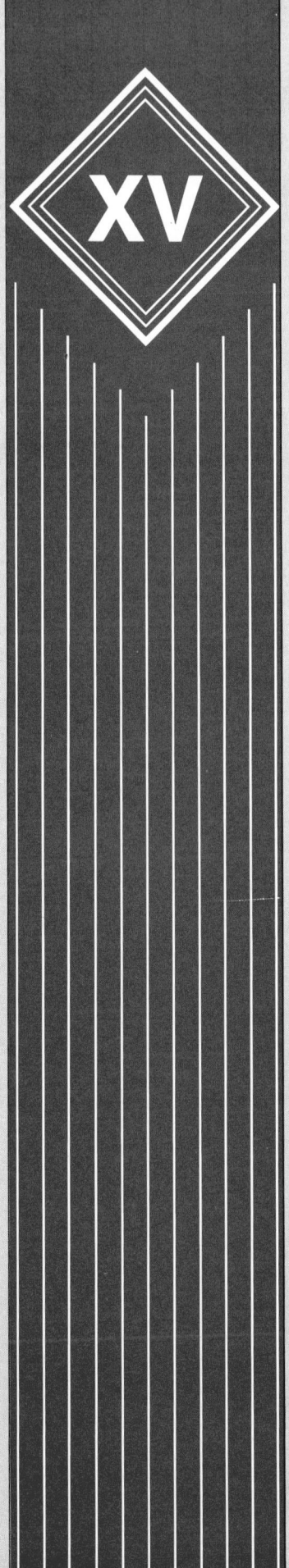

Emergency Nursing

I love nursing, because the special smiles tug at our hearts—the special smiles from a patient who had been labeled by others as grumpy, hard to get along with, a real bear, etc.; that special smile that lets you know that you have made a difference that day or minute—that your being there, caring, and being kind was appreciated. I have been a sickly person all my life. If not for the special nurses who cared, I would not be here today. I feel that I am helping and caring for others who need that special care and smiles as much as I needed them in the past. Nursing can be a very rewarding and caring profession.

CAROL RUNGE
Student Nurse

53

Cardiopulmonary Resuscitation

GLORIA DePOLE COSCHIGANO

LEARNING OBJECTIVES

After reading this chapter, the student should be able to do the following:

- Define the key terms.
- List the reasons CPR should be performed.
- Discuss the legal implications of CPR.
- Name six causes of sudden death.
- List the steps in performing one-rescuer CPR on the adult victim.
- Name the steps in performing two-rescuer CPR on the adult victim.
- List the steps in performing CPR on the pediatric victim.
- Recognize the causes of airway obstruction.
- Name the steps in performing the Heimlich maneuver on the conscious choking victim.
- Describe the steps in performing the Heimlich maneuver on the unconscious victim.
- Discuss management of airway obstruction in the pediatric individual.

RELATED TOPICS OF INTEREST

- Legal aspects of nursing (Chapter 2)
- Ethical aspects of nursing (Chapter 3)
- First aid (Chapter 54)

KEY TERMS

Define the following:

- ABC
- anaphylaxis
- biological death
- BLS
- brain death
- cardiac arrest
- carotid pulse
- clinical death
- external cardiac compressions
- CPR
- EMS
- stridor
- ventilator
- xiphoid process

Cardiovascular disease remains the number one killer in the United States. However, communities with large numbers of people trained in cardiopulmonary resuscitation **(CPR)** and a rapid response emergency medical services **(EMS)** system can successfully resuscitate victims of "sudden death," especially those "deaths" caused by cardiovascular disorders. It is important for the licensed practical/vocational nurse to be able to perform CPR, both as a responsible member of the community and as a member of the health care team.

LEGAL IMPLICATIONS

The Good Samaritan Acts protect the CPR rescuer just as they protect the provider of first aid (see Chapter 2). However, it is important that the rescuer be thoroughly familiar with the CPR technique. Certification in basic life support **(BLS)** may be obtained through local chapters of the American Heart Association or the local American Red Cross Association. The rescuer must perform CPR according to the standards designated by the certifying agency.

ETHICAL IMPLICATIONS

Reasons why individuals choose not to become involved in performing CPR include (1) lack of motivation, (2) fear of doing harm, (3) lack of knowledge, and (4) fear of contracting communicable diseases. However, once CPR is started, it may not be discontinued except for the following reasons:

- The victim recovers.
- The rescuer is exhausted and cannot continue CPR.
- Trained medical personnel arrive on the scene and take over CPR.
- A licensed physician arrives on the scene, pronounces the victim dead, and orders CPR to be discontinued.

EVENTS REQUIRING CPR

There are many situations that require resuscitation efforts (Box 53-1). CPR is indicated in any syndrome where respiration or respiration and circulation are absent. The two purposes of CPR are:

- To keep the lungs supplied with oxygen when breathing has stopped
- To keep the blood circulating and carrying oxygen to the brain, heart, and other parts of the body

BOX 53-1 **EVENTS REQUIRING CPR**

Cardiac arrest The most common cause of cardiac arrest is myocardial infarction (MI). In addition, shock from hemorrhage, trauma to the heart, respiratory arrest, and drugs may precipitate a cardiac arrest.

Drowning Children are common victims of drowning and boating accidents. Persons using alcohol and/or drugs near bodies of water are often victims of drowning. It is important to note that near-drowning victims may recover completely after long periods of submersion. The low water temperature that produces hypothermia reduces the metabolic rate and decreases oxygen demands. Because of this, CPR must be initiated even after 4 to 6 minutes are known to have elapsed.

Electrical shock Persons exposed to high-voltage electricity may be subject to accidental electrocution. Electrical shock may paralyze the breathing muscles and cause cardiac arrest by interfering with the normal rhythm of the heart. The rescuer who is initiating CPR must be careful not to be exposed inadvertently to the electrical current himself. The rescuer must ensure that the current is deenergized before beginning CPR.

Anaphylactic reaction Exposure to a known allergen (food, poisons, drugs) or an insect bite may produce a severe allergic reaction known as **anaphylaxis.** This reaction may cause spasms or edema of the upper airway and could progress to cardiovascular collapse. CPR must be initiated immediately, as with any other emergency situation.

Asphyxiation Asphyxiation or suffocation may be caused by inhaling a gas other than oxygen, resulting from fires, chemical spills, or gas leaks. In addition, children and adults may suffer respiratory arrest and ultimately cardiac arrest from choking on food or small objects that are placed in the mouth. The Heimlich maneuver and CPR are performed in this instance.

Drug overdose Intentional or accidental abuse of alcohol and drugs may cause respiratory and cardiac arrest. Besides treating this as a poisoning emergency, CPR should be performed as necessary.

Clinical death means that heartbeat and respiration have ceased. **Biological death** results from permanent cellular damage caused by lack of oxygen. The brain is the first organ to suffer from this lack of oxygen. In many cases CPR can reverse clinical death if initiated before 4 minutes of cardiopulmonary arrest. After 10 minutes without CPR, **brain death** is certain. Therefore it is extremely important that CPR is begun as quickly as possible.

ADULT ONE-RESCUER CPR

To remember the steps of one-rescuer or two-rescuer CPR, remember the **ABC**s:

A Airway

The initial assessment in determining the need for CPR is to determine responsiveness. This is done by gently shaking the victim and shouting, "Are you OK?" This precaution will prevent the rescuer from injuring a person who is alert, but sleeping. OK is a word that is understandable in any language.

B Breathing

Mouth-to-mouth ventilation is the quickest method of supplying oxygen to the victim's lungs. The rescuer's exhaled air has enough oxygen to supply the victim's needs until life support systems take over. The head-tilt/chin-lift position and an airtight seal must be maintained throughout rescue breathing.

To preserve the open airway, the rescuer should be at the victim's shoulders and the thumb and index finger of the hand that is maintaining the head-tilt should be used to gently pinch the nostrils closed. The rescuer should then take a deep breath, seal the lips around the outside of the victim's mouth (creating an airtight seal), and give *two* full breaths lasting 1 to 1½ seconds each (Fig. 53-1). It is important that the amount of exhaled air be enough to cause the victim's chest to rise. The victim will exhale spontaneously, and the rescuer will see the chest fall. Gastric distention (air in the stomach instead of the lungs) can result from excessive air volume and rapid breathing.

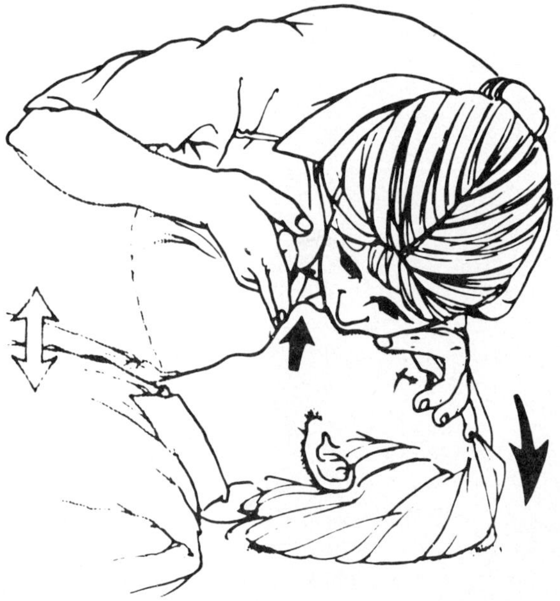

FIG. 53-1 (American Heart Association CPR Manual.)

If the initial attempt to ventilate the victim is unsuccessful, the rescuer should reposition the head and attempt to ventilate again. Improper chin and head position is the most common reason for difficulty with ventilation. If the second attempt at ventilation is also unsuccessful, the rescuer should proceed with foreign body airway obstruction management procedures.

C Circulation

Once the ventilations have been performed, it is important to assess for the presence of the pulse. Pulselessness (cardiac arrest) indicates the need for external cardiac compressions. Respiratory arrest may occur without cardiac arrest. Performing external cardiac compressions on a victim with a pulse may result in severe physical damage. Rescue breathing should be initiated at one breath every 5 seconds, or 12 times per minute. Cardiac arrest will follow if respiratory arrest continues.

The carotid pulse is the most reliable and accessible for the CPR rescuer. While the head-tilt is maintained with one hand on the forehead, the rescuer should locate the victim's thyroid cartilage (Adam's apple) with two or three fingers of the other hand. The rescuer should then gently slide these fingers into the groove between the trachea and the muscles on the side of the neck until the **carotid pulse** is felt. The pulse must be palpated gently on one side to avoid obliteration of the artery.

If there is no pulse, the diagnosis of **cardiac arrest** is confirmed. At this point it is important to activate the EMS system (if not already done). If another person is present, he or she should call the local emergency phone number. If the rescuer is alone and help can be summoned, CPR should be performed for 1 minute and then the EMS system is activated. If the rescuer is alone and not able to activate the EMS system, the only option is to continue CPR.

Performing **external cardiac compressions** will circulate blood to the heart, lungs, brain, and the rest of the body. If external cardiac compressions are performed properly, 20% to 50% of the normal output of the heart can be maintained. This will bring enough oxygen to the body to sustain life. Proper hand position will enable as much blood to be circulated as possible. Hands should be positioned as follows:

1. With the middle and index fingers of the hand that is nearest the victim's legs, the rescuer palpates the lower edge of the victim's rib cage on the side next to the rescuer.
2. The fingers are then run up the rib cage to the substernal notch (where the ribs meet the sternum on the lower part of the chest).
3. Keeping the middle finger on this notch, the rescuer places the index finger next to the middle finger on the lower end of the sternum.

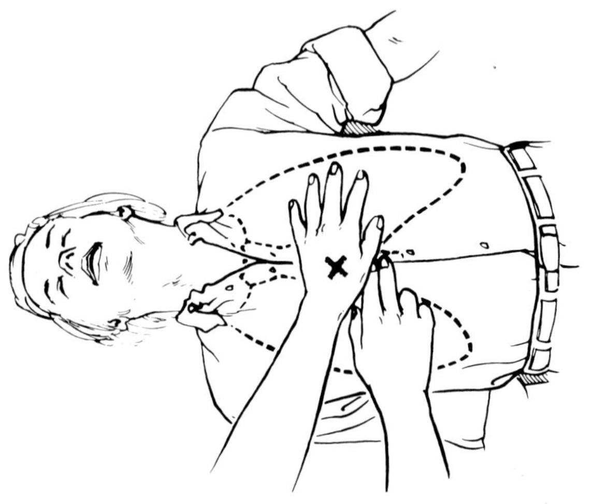

FIG. 53-2 (American Heart Association CPR Manual.)

4. The heel of the hand nearest the victim's head is placed on the lower half of the sternum, as close as possible to the index and middle fingers (Fig. 53-2).
5. The fingers may be extended or interlaced, but must be kept off the chest.

Proper compression techniques are important to deliver the appropriate amount of force to simulate the pumping action of the heart. Compression techniques are as follows:

1. The elbows are locked in place, with the arms straight and the shoulders positioned over the hands so that the thrusts of external cardiac compressions are in a downward motion. Some of the force of the compressions will be lost if there is a rolling or rocking motion.
2. The rescuer leans forward, creating pressure to depress the sternum 1½ to 2 inches in the adult. The motion is smooth, never rolling or jerking (Fig. 53-3).

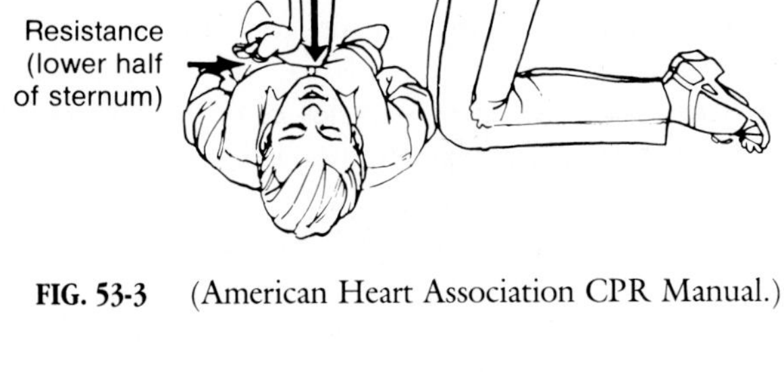

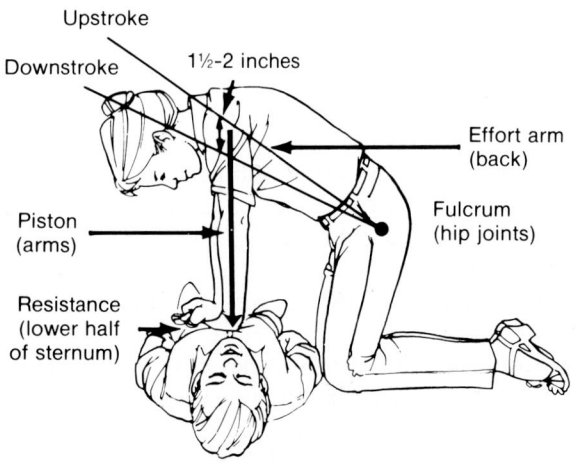

FIG. 53-3 (American Heart Association CPR Manual.)

3. External chest compression pressure is released completely to allow the chest to return to position. This allows blood to flow into the heart. The time allowed for release should equal the time required for compression. There should not be a pause between compressions.
4. Hand positions must be maintained at all times—the hands should not be lifted or moved in any way. Hands should stay in contact with the chest at all times.
5. Complications of external chest compressions as a result of improper technique or poor hand placement include lacerated liver, fractured ribs, and ineffective resuscitation.

The sequencing of breathing to external compressions in one-rescuer and two-rescuer CPR will be discussed in the following paragraphs:

Steps to Adult One-Rescuer CPR

A Airway

- Determine unresponsiveness.
- Call for help.
- Position the victim (and rescuer).
- Open the airway.

B Breathing

- Determine breathlessness.
- If victim is not breathing, give 2 breaths.
- If unable to give 2 breaths, reposition the head and reattempt to venitlate.
- If still unable, proceed with foreign body airway obstruction management procedures.

C Circulation

- Determine pulselessness.
- If pulse is present, continue rescue breathing at 12 times per minute, or one breath every 5 seconds. Activate the EMS system.
- If pulse is not present, activate the EMS system (if not done previously). Perform 15 chest compressions at a rate of 80 to 100 per minute. Count "1 and, 2 and, 3 and, 4 and, 5 and, 6 and, 7 and, 8 and, 9 and, 10 and, 11 and, 12 and, 13 and, 14 and, 15."
- Continue with 2 breaths and 15 compressions for 4 cycles.
- Reassessment: After 4 cycles of 2 breaths and 15 compressions, reevaluate the victim for:
  1. Return of the pulse
     If absent, continue CPR with 2 ventilations followed by compressions.
  2. Return of breathing
     If present, monitor breathing and pulse closely.

TWO-RESCUER CPR

Because artificial ventilation must be combined with external cardiac compressions, it is less fatiguing to perform CPR with two rescuers. The Red Cross now teaches two-rescuer CPR only to professionals and paraprofessionals.

When One-Rescuer CPR is in Progress

If CPR has been started with one rescuer, the most logical time for entrance of the second rescuer is after a completed cycle of 15 compressions and 2 breaths.

The second rescuer identifies himself by saying, "I know CPR," moves to the head, opens the airway, and checks the carotid pulse. The other rescuer positions himself or herself at the chest and finds proper hand placement for chest compressions. This should take no longer than 5 seconds.

The next step is to call for help—even if no one is in sight, someone may be within hearing distance and can activate the EMS system.

Next, the victim should be properly positioned. For maximum effectiveness of CPR, the victim must be placed horizontally on a firm, flat surface. (The floor is usually the best place. In the clinical setting, a cardiac board is placed under the victim's back.) Caution must be taken if a suspected neck or back injury is present (see Chapter 54 for discussion on rolling a victim). The victim's arms are placed alongside the body and the legs straight. The rescuer should kneel beside the victim at the level between shoulder and the waist.

The most important action in the successful resuscitation of the victim is the immediate opening of the airway. The tongue is the most common obstruction to the airway. Sometimes opening the airway may be all that is needed to relieve obstruction and allow the victim to breathe spontaneously.

The head-tilt/chin-lift is the recommended technique to open the airway. It is accomplished by the rescuer placing one hand on the victim's forehead and applying firm pressure with the palm of the hand to tilt the head back. To complete the technique, the rescuer places the fingers (not the thumb) of the other hand under the lower, bony portion of the jaw near the chin, and lifts the chin forward (Fig. 53-4). If the soft tissue of the chin instead of the bony area is pressed, the airway may become occluded by the fingers. Dentures should remain in the mouth if they can be maintained in place without difficulty. They will give support to the mouth and cheeks during mouth-to-mouth breathing.

If the victim has a suspected neck injury and extending

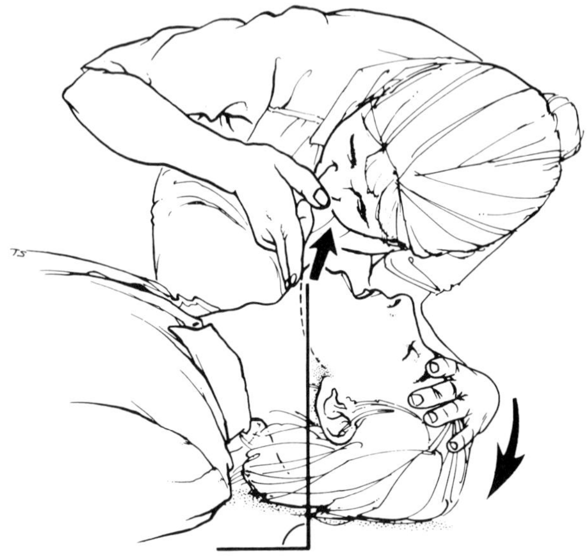

FIG. 53-4 (American Heart Association CPR Manual.)

the neck is contraindicated, the jaw-thrust technique may be used. In this technique the rescuer grasps the angles of the victim's lower jaw and lifts with both hands, displacing the mandible forward, thus tilting the head backward without extending the neck. The rescuer's elbows must remain on the surface on which the victim is lying.

Once the airway is open, it is important to assess the victim for spontaneous breathing. The rescuer places his ear over the victim's mouth and nose while maintaining the open airway position. The rescuer then:

- Looks to see the chest rise and fall
- Listens to hear breath sounds
- Feels for the flow of air against the cheek

This step should take 3 to 5 seconds. If it is determined that the victim is not breathing, rescue breathing should be initiated.

If there is no pulse, the ventilator gives 1 breath and the compressor gives 5 compressions, counting "1 and, 2 and, 3 and, 4 and, 5." The rate of compressions is 80 to 100 per minute. At the end of the fifth compression, a pause should be allowed for ventilation (1 to 1½ seconds per breath).

When No CPR is in Progress

If both rescuers arrive at the scene at the same time, it is important to establish priorities. One rescuer should activate the EMS system while the other initiates one-rescuer CPR. If the EMS system can be activated by another person, the two rescuers should proceed as follows:

One rescuer goes to the victim's head and does the following:

1. Determines unresponsiveness
2. Positions the victim
3. Opens the airway
4. Checks for breathing
5. If breathing is absent, says "no breathing" and gives 2 ventilations
6. Checks for pulse; if pulse is absent, says "no pulse"

The second rescuer, at the same time, does the following:

1. Finds the location for external cardiac compressions
2. Assumes proper hand position
3. Begins external cardiac compressions after the "no pulse" statement is made by the first rescuer; the sequencing remains 5 compressions for every 1 breath

It is the responsibility of the **ventilator** (rescuer at the head of the victim) to evaluate the effectiveness of chest compressions by checking the carotid pulse and monitoring for the spontaneous return of circulation and breathing.

Switching Procedures

Switching the positions of the ventilator and the compressor prevents fatigue of either rescuer and allows time for the ventilator to evaluate the effectiveness of CPR. The switch is initiated by the rescuer performing chest compressions at the end of the 5 : 1 sequence. After giving a breath, the ventilator moves to the chest and gets into position to give compressions. The compressor moves to the victim's head and checks the pulse for 5 seconds. If no pulse is felt, he or she gives a breath and states the command to "resume CPR."

PEDIATRIC CPR—CHILD/INFANT

The basic steps of CPR and foreign body airway obstruction management are the same whether the victim is an infant, child, or adult. For the purpose of BLS, an infant may be defined as anyone younger than 1 year. A child may be defined as anyone between the ages of 1 and 8 years.

A Airway

Unresponsiveness should be determined. The child should be gently shaken. The heels of the feet of an infant may be tapped.

Help should be called for. The victim should be positioned on a firm, flat surface for effectiveness of CPR. Performing CPR while carrying an infant may be advantageous if help could be obtained more quickly. However, this technique is not as effective.

The head-tilt/chin-life technique is used to open the airway. However, care must be taken not to hyperextend the neck in infants. The shorter trachea may become occluded by this maneuver. The head should not be tilted in the case of a head injury: the jaw thrust may be used instead.

B Breathing

After the airway is open, the rescuer looks for movement of the chest, listens for breath sounds, and feels for exhaled airflow. If there is no breathing, the rescuer inhales and seals the mouth and nose of the infant. He or she pinches the nostrils closed and seals the mouth of the child.

Two breaths (1 to 1½ seconds per breath) are given with a pause between breaths. The volume of air in an infant's lungs is smaller than an adult's, thus the rescuer's breaths should be adjusted to allow for appropriate rise and fall of the chest. Gastric distention is very common in infants and children during CPR as a result of overinflation of the lungs.

C Circulation

Assessment of the pulse should be made on the carotid artery of the child and the brachial artery of the infant. If there is a pulse, rescue breathing should be continued. It there is no pulse, external cardiac compressions must be performed also.

When performing external cardiac compressions in the infant, the rescuer must do the following:

1. Visualize an imaginary line between the nipples.
2. Place the index finger of the hand farthest from the infant's head under this line as it intersects the sternum (breastbone).
3. Using the middle and ring fingers, compress the breastbone on this area (one finger's width below the line between the nipples). Because of the variations in sizes of infants, this measurement should be used only as a guide.
4. The breastbone is compressed to a depth of ½ to 1 inch at a rate of at least 100 times per minute. Count aloud very quickly "one, two, three, four, five." Compression and release action should be done smoothly.
5. At the end of each compression, pressure is released and the sternum is allowed to return to normal position without removal of the fingers from their placement. The movements should be smooth, not jerky.
6. The sequence of compressions to ventilation is 5:1 (5 compressions to 1 breath).

When performing cardiac compressions in the child, the following must be done:

1. The lower margin of the child's rib cage is palpated with the middle and index fingers, while the head tilt is maintained by the other hand.
2. The substernal notch (where the ribs and breastbone meet) is located.
3. With the middle finger on this notch, the index finger is placed next to the middle finger.
4. Looking at the landmark, place the heel of the hand next to where the index finger was.
5. The chest is compressed with the heel of one hand at a rate of 80 to 100 times per minute. The fingers should not touch the ribs.
6. The compressions should be smooth, allowing the chest to return to the natural position after each compression.
7. The sequence is 5 compressions to 1 breath.
8. If the child is older or large, the adult method of CPR should be used.

FOREIGN BODY AIRWAY OBSTRUCTION MANAGEMENT

Food, particularly meat, is the most common cause of choking or airway obstruction in the adult. Factors that contribute to this are large or poorly chewed pieces of food, the ingestion of alcohol, and loose-fitting dentures. Foreign objects (for example, marbles, beads, or food) are the most common cause of airway obstruction in children. The Heimlich maneuver is the most effective method of removing foreign body airway obstructions.

If the victim has a good air exchange, he is able to cough forcibly, although there may be wheezing between coughs. *DO NOT INTERFERE* with the victim at this point. However, he should be monitored closely, because he may regress to a state of poor air exchange.

If the victim is experiencing poor air exchange, he may have a weak, ineffective cough, make a high-pitched, "crowing" noise while inhaling, have increased respiratory difficulty, and develop cyanosis. With complete airway obstruction, the victim cannot speak, breathe, or cough, and may clutch his neck (Fig. 53-5). This sign is the universal distress signal. To assess the inability to speak ask the victim, "Are you choking?" Complete airway obstruction will prevent oxygen from entering the lungs and being circulated to the brain and vital organs. Unless prompt action is initiated, the victim will become unconscious and death will result.

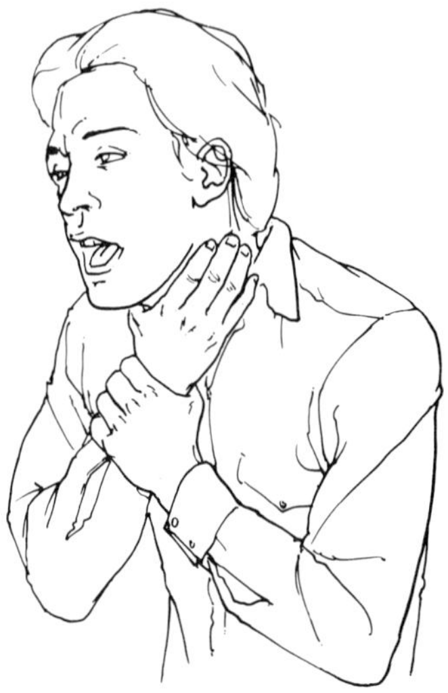

FIG. 53-5 (American Heart Association CPR Manual.)

Management of Foreign Body Airway Obstruction in the Conscious Victim

Abdominal thrusts given below the diaphragm (the Heimlich maneuver) are recommended for relieving foreign body airway obstruction. These thrusts put pressure on the diaphragm, forcing air from the lungs to move and expel the foreign object. The victim may be in a sitting position. Standing behind the victim, the rescuer wraps his arms around the victim's waist. He should then make a fist with one hand and place the thumb of the fist against the middle of the victim's abdomen slightly above the navel and well below the tip of the xiphoid process. He then presses the fist into the victim's abdomen with a quick upward thrust (Fig. 53-6). The rescuer repeats each thrust until the foreign body is expelled or the victim becomes unconscious. If the victim is pregnant or markedly obese, chest thrusts may be used instead of abdominal thrusts.

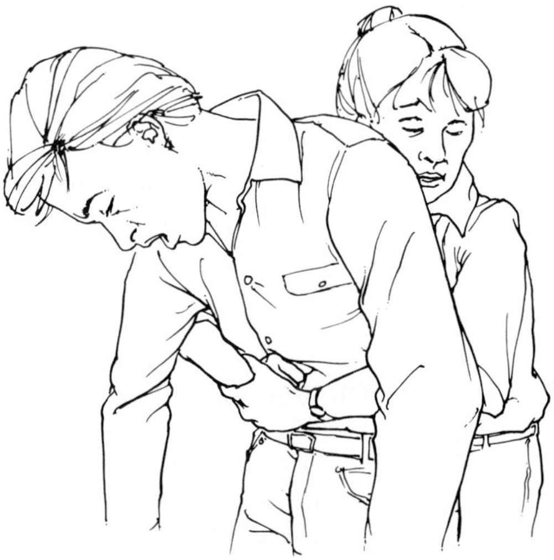

FIG. 53-6 (American Heart Association CPR Manual.)

Management of Foreign Body Airway Obstruction in the Unconscious Victim

If the conscious victim becomes unconscious, he should be placed in a supine position with the face up. Because regurgitation is a common occurrence in an unconscious victim, a finger sweep should be performed. In performing the finger sweep, the rescuer opens the victim's mouth by grasping both the tongue and the lower jaw between his thumb and fingers and lifting upward. This draws the tongue from the back of the throat and away from the foreign body. The index finger of the rescuer's available hand is inserted along the side of the cheek and deeply into the throat to the base of the tongue. A hooking motion is used to dislodge the object and bring it into the mouth, where it can be grasped and removed. Care should be taken not to push the foreign body farther down into the throat with this maneuver.

The rescuer should then open the airway and attempt to ventilate (if the foreign body has been dislodged, the victim will need artificial respirations and possibly external cardiac compressions). If ventilation is unsuccessful, 6 to 10 abdominal thrusts should be performed. To perform abdominal thrusts on an unconscious victim, the rescuer should kneel astride the victim's thighs and place the heel of one hand against the victim's abdomen, in the midline slightly above the navel but well below the tip of the **xiphoid process.** The rescuer should press into the abdomen with a quick, upward thrust. The mouth should be opened again and a finger sweep performed. All the above steps should be repeated until the foreign body is dislodged and spontaneous breathing is restored.

Foreign Body Airway Management in the Infant

Of all deaths from foreign body aspiration, 65% are in the infant age group. Aspirated materials include food, such as candies and nuts, and small objects. Infants and children experience acute respiratory distress with coughing, gagging, and **stridor.** The victim may become unconscious.

The child is treated as the adult with performance of the Heimlich maneuver. However, there is a potential for injury in using this maneuver in the child less than 1 year old. Infants should have a combination of back blows and chest thrusts, as follows:

- The infant is straddled over the rescuer's arm with head lower than the trunk and supported firmly at the jaw.

- With this arm resting on the rescuer's thigh, the other arm delivers four back blows between the infant's shoulder with the heel of the hand (Fig. 53-7).
- The rescuer places his free hand on the infant's back so that the victim is sandwiched between the two hands, one supporting the neck, jaw, and chest, while the other supports the back.
- While continuing to support the head and neck, the rescuer turns the infant and places him on the thigh with the head lower than the trunk.
- Four chest thrusts are performed with the hands in the same position as when performing external cardiac compressions (Fig. 53-8).
- The finger sweep technique is never used, because the foreign body would most likely become lodged farther because of the shortened trachea of the infant. However, if the object is visualized when the mouth is open, it may be removed.

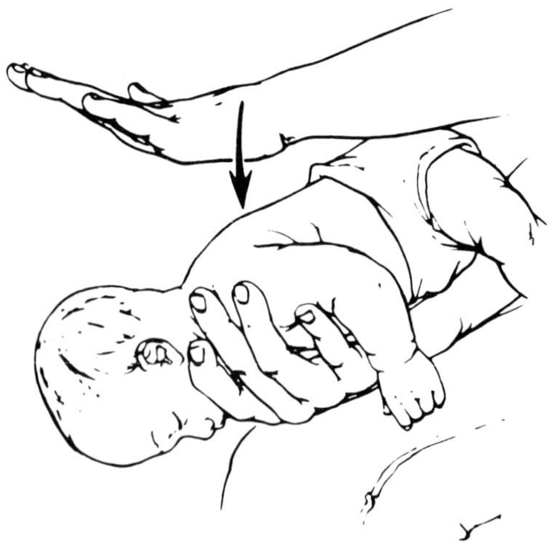

FIG. 53-7 (American Heart Association CPR Manual.)

CHAPTER CHALLENGE

KEY POINTS

- Personnel trained in CPR and a rapid response EMS system can be successful in resuscitation of victims of cardiac arrest or apparent sudden death.
- The rescuer must perform CPR according to the standards designated by the American Heart Association or the American Red Cross.
- There is a moral obligation to continue CPR once it has been initiated.
- The best recovery from cardiopulmonary arrest occurs when CPR is begun within 4 minutes from cardiopulmonary arrest. After 10 minutes without CPR, brain death is certain.
- **A**irway, **B**reathing, and **C**irculation are the three steps to remember in one- or two-rescuer CPR.
- Rescue breathing can supply enough oxygen to meet the victim's needs until the EMS takes over.
- A tight seal of the nose and mouth during rescue breathing will help prevent gastric distention.
- If external cardiac compressions are performed accurately, enough oxygen can be supplied to the heart, lungs, brain, and the rest of the body to sustain life.
- The chest must be compressed to a depth of 1½ to 2 inches in the average-sized adult.
- The sequencing for adult one-rescuer CPR is 2 breaths for every 15 compressions.
- CPR should not be interrupted for more than 5 seconds, except for special circumstances.
- The sequencing for two-rescuer CPR is 1 breath for every 5 compressions.
- The responsibility of the ventilator in two-rescuer CPR is to evaluate the effectiveness of CPR by monitoring the carotid pulse and observing for the spontaneous return of circulation and breathing.
- According to basic child life support standards, an infant is defined as anyone younger than one year of age. A child is defined as anyone between the ages of 1 and 8 years.
- Two fingers are used during chest compressions in the infant.
- The heel of one hand is used during chest compressions of the child.
- If a victim is choking but has good air exchange (is coughing forcibly), do not interfere.
- The Heimlich maneuver is the most effective method of removing foreign body airway obstruction.
- The finger sweep technique must be avoided when managing foreign body airway obstruction in the infant.

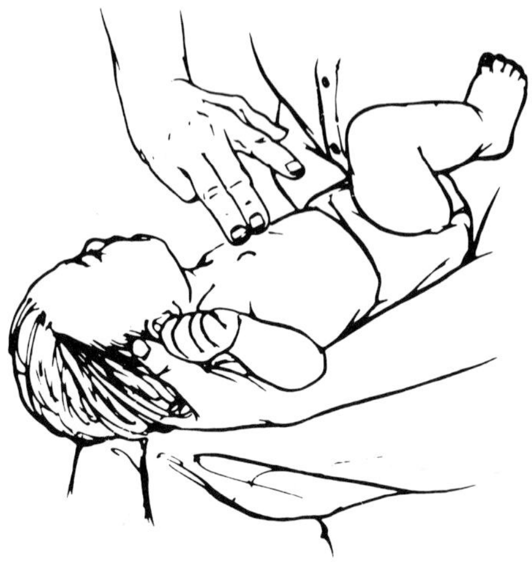

FIG. 53-8 (American Heart Association CPR Manual.)

REFERENCES AND SUGGESTED READINGS

1. American Heart Association: Instructor's manual for basic life support, American Heart Association, 1987.
2. American Red Cross: Instructor's manual for community CPR, American National Red Cross, 1988.
3. American Red Cross: American Red Cross CPR: basic life support for the professional rescuer, Instructor's Manual, American National Red Cross, 1988.
4. Curley M and others: Assessment and resuscitation of the pediatric patient, Crit Care Nurs 7(3):26, 39, 1987.
5. Gatch G and others: Foreign body aspiration in children, AORN J (46)5:850, 1987.
6. Standards and guidelines for cardio-pulmonary resuscitation (CPR) and emergency cardiac care (ECC), JAMA 255:2905, 1986.
7. Willens JS and others: Performing CPR on adults, Nurs '89 19(1):34, 1989.

STUDY QUESTIONS

1. In performing CPR on an adult with one rescuer, give the ratio of compressions to breaths:
   a. 12 compressions, then 15 breaths
   b. 8 compressions, then 1 breath
   c. 15 compressions, then 2 breaths
   d. 5 compressions, then 1 breath
2. You may stop CPR for all of the following reasons except:
   a. When a licensed physician arrives
   b. When the heart begins beating again
   c. When another rescuer trained in CPR takes over for you
   d. When you determine efforts are useless
3. When one is doing a primary assessment to check the condition of the body's two most important systems, this is called:
   a. Circulatory and respiratory assessment
   b. ABCs assessment
   c. Neurological examination and respiratory assessment
   d. Circulatory and neurological assessment
4. When giving abdominal thrusts to an unconscious child, the correct position to place the child is:
   a. Lying on his abdomen
   b. Lying on his side
   c. Lying on his back
   d. Sitting position
5. When you give CPR to a child, the ratio of compressions to breaths is:
   a. 5 compressions to 1 breath
   b. 5 compressions to 5 breaths
   c. 10 compressions to 2 breaths
   d. 15 compressions to 2 breaths
6. The universal distress signal for choking is:
   a. Low-pitched wheezing
   b. Clutching at the throat
   c. Coughing with great force
   d. Color changes
7. How far should you compress the chest of an adult during CPR:
   a. 1 to 1½ inches
   b. 1 to 2 inches
   c. 2 to 3 inches
   d. ½ to 1 inch
8. When you start CPR, your arms should be:
   a. Bent
   b. Straight
   c. Crossed
   d. Flexed inward
9. If a choking victim is greatly overweight or in the late stages of pregnancy, you should give:
   a. Chest thrusts
   b. Abdominal thrusts
   c. Xiphoid process pressure
   d. No pressure
10. In performing CPR to an adult with a two-rescuer team, give the following ratio of compressions to breaths:
    a. 12 compressions to 1 breath
    b. 10 compressions to 2 breaths
    c. 5 compressions to 1 breath
    d. 15 compressions to 2 breaths

54

First Aid

GLORIA DePOLE COSCHIGANO

LEARNING OBJECTIVES

After reading this chapter, the student should be able to do the following:

- Define the key terms.
- List priorities of assessment to be performed when arriving at a situation requiring first aid.
- Discuss moral, legal, and physical interventions of performing first aid.
- List five causes of shock.
- State four symptoms of shock.
- List nursing interventions to treat shock.
- Discuss three methods of controlling hemorrhage.
- Define four types of wounds.
- Discuss types of treatment including bandaging of wounds.
- Discuss methods of treating three types of common poisonings.
- State the characteristics of assessment of bone, joint, and muscle injuries.
- Discuss emergency care for suspected injuries.
- Define three types of burns.
- List four nursing interventions in the first aid treatment of burns.
- Describe the nursing interventions of heat and cold emergencies.

RELATED TOPICS OF INTEREST

- Signs, symptoms, and physical assessment (Chapter 13)
- Care of the patient with an integumentary disorder (Chapter 29)
- Care of the patient with a musculoskeletal disorder (Chapter 30)
- Cardiopulmonary resuscitation (Chapter 53)

KEY TERMS

Define the following:

- anaphylaxis
- crepitus
- cyanosis
- embolism
- emergency medical system (EMS)
- epistaxis
- Good Samaritan laws
- hematemesis
- hematuria
- hemoptysis
- melena
- oliguria
- pleural space
- shock
- tachycardia
- tetanus toxoid
- vesicle

First aid is the immediate, *temporary* assistance given to a person who is injured or has become ill. First aid includes assessing the victim for life-threatening conditions, performing appropriate interventions to sustain life, and keeping the person in the best possible physical and mental condition until he can enter the **emergency medical system (EMS).** It is important to remember that first aid *does not replace* medical care but is used to preserve life until medical help is obtained. Because minutes are precious in preventing permanent disability and injury, the nurse must be prepared to handle emergency conditions and administer first aid.

OBTAINING MEDICAL EMERGENCY AID

The nurse's ability to recognize the need for medical assistance and knowledge of how to obtain medical emergency aid can mean the difference between life and death to an injured or ill person. It is important to know the right phone number to call (both in the community and in the institutional setting). In most communities the emergency medical number is 911; however, the fire department, police department, or local hospital may be the correct number to call for assistance in some localities. Box 54-1 provides important information to convey when calling in a medical emergency from the community.

MORAL AND LEGAL RESPONSIBILITIES OF THE NURSE

Good Samaritan laws have been enacted in most states to protect health professionals from legal liability when providing emergency first aid. If the nurse follows a reasonable and prudent course of action, the chances of legal problems are very small. Before the nurse administers first aid, she must have verbal permission from the victim; the victim also has the right to refuse first aid. The law assumes that an unconscious person would give consent if he were able. Once the nurse has initiated first aid, she has a moral and legal obligation to continue until the victim can be cared for by someone with comparable or better training; for example, an EMT or a physician can arrive at the scene and assume first aid care of the victim.

ASSESSMENT OF THE EMERGENCY SITUATION

Assessment of life-threatening problems is the first priority in an emergency situation. Assistance may be required to care for victims of some injuries or illnesses or to call EMS. In these cases the nurse may need to shout several times to get someone's attention. While seeking help the nurse should continue the primary survey by checking for (1) an open airway, (2) breathing,

BOX 54-1 INFORMATION TO CONVEY IN A MEDICAL EMERGENCY

1. Location of the emergency
2. What has happened (either by direct observation or by gathering data from others)
3. The numbers of people that need assistance
4. Obvious injuries and the victim's apparent condition
5. First aid measures that have been administered
6. Presence of Medic-Alert bracelet or any known history of medical problems
7. The victim's names
8. Name of person making the phone call
9. The physical characteristics of the rescue (stairs, elevators)
10. Always hang up last

and (3) circulation (pulse and severe bleeding). This is known as checking the ABCs. An immediate life-threatening situation of highest priority is arrested or abnormal breathing. To assess whether the victim is breathing properly, the airway must be opened with a chin lift–head tilt maneuver. The nurse determines whether the chest is rising, listens for breath sounds, and places the cheek near the victim's mouth to feel the passage of air from the victim's breathing (Chapter 53). Rhythm, depth, and rate of respirations should be assessed. The following are signs that the victim is having problems breathing: cyanosis, wheezing, stridor, and snoring.

An arrested or abnormal pulse is also a life-threatening situation. The rate, rhythm, and strength of the carotid pulse are assessed. It is important to observe for signs of external bleeding and internal bleeding, which may result in shock. Skin color, temperature, pupil reaction, pulse, and respiration must be monitored. Poisonings are also life threatening. The nurse should observe for burns or stains in and around the person's mouth or hands. Depressed respirations and circulatory collapse may also result from poisonings.

After the initial assessment for life-threatening problems, the victim must be observed for indications of skull injury and brain or spinal cord damage, which require attention as soon as possible. Decreasing level of consciousness, abnormal pupil reaction, and lack of movement in the arms or legs may indicate injury to the head or spinal cord. Fractures, dislocations, and superficial ecchymosis or wounds require attention after the more serious conditions are treated.

SHOCK

Shock results from the failure of the cardiovascular system to provide sufficient blood circulation (oxygen) to all parts of the body. To maintain circulatory homeostasis, the following mechanisms must be present: a functioning heart to circulate blood and a sufficient amount of blood volume. The capability of the vascular system, accommodating blood flow to the capillaries and returning it to the right side of the heart, is also necessary to maintain adequate circulation. Inability of the body to compensate for failure of one or more of these mechanisms results in shock.

BOX 54-2 TYPES OF SHOCK

Hypovolemic shock: also known as hemorrhagic shock; this is caused by a decrease in fluid volume from bleeding, prolonged vomiting or diarrhea, or loss of fluid from surgery or trauma.

Cardiogenic shock: results from poor heart function caused by various cardiovascular abnormalities. The heart is unable to maintain sufficient blood pressure to all body parts.

Neurogenic shock: caused by failure of the nervous system to maintain the normal contraction of the blood vessels. Common causes are spinal anesthesia and quadriplegia in which the blood pressure is lower because there is not enough blood to fill the dilated blood vessels.

Septic shock: results from severe infection. Toxins from the microorganisms cause loss of fluid through the blood vessel walls.

Psychogenic shock syncope: caused by the nervous system's reaction to an emotional stimulus. The blood vessels dilate temporarily, decreasing blood flow to the brain, which results in unconsciousness or syncope.

Anaphylactic shock: **anaphylaxis** results from a sudden, severe, allergic body reaction to a foreign substance. The allergen or foreign protein causes the sudden release of histamine, which decreases the amount of blood for circulation because of the release of plasma through the capillary walls as a result of capillary hyperpermeability.

Classification of Shock

Shock is classified according to the cause. The most common causes of shock are severe loss of blood, intense pain, extensive trauma, burns, poisons, emotional stress or intense emotions, extremes of heat and cold, electrical shock, allergic reactions, and a sudden or severe illness. Box 54-2 provides examples of types of shock.

Assessment

The signs and symptoms of shock can be disguised by other signs of injury; some may appear in only the late stages of shock. The nurse must be aware of the following when assessing the victim for shock:

Level of consciousness. The victim may experience changes in behavior, restlessness, anxiety, confusion, syncope, and agitation. As the condition worsens, the victim becomes more lethargic. Coma and death can result.

Skin changes. The skin becomes cool, pale, and ashen-looking. As shock progresses, **cyanosis** (especially of the lips and nail beds) develops.

Cardiovascular blood pressure. Initially the blood pressure may be normal, but as shock progresses, there is steady decrease in blood pressure.

Pulse. The pulse rate usually increases (**tachycardia**) in all types of shock. It also becomes weak and thready in character.

Respirations. The respiratory rate increases. Respirations may also be shallow, rapid, labored, or irregular as a result of vasoconstriction in the lungs, causing fluid to accumulate.

Urinary output. With decreased circulation of fluid volume, the amount of urinary output is decreased (**oliguria**).

Neuromuscular changes. Decreased oxygen to the tissues results in weakness and/or tremors of the arms and legs. Eyelids close and the pupils dilate.

Gastrointestinal. Because of loss of fluids and fluid shifts, the victim will complain of thirst. Nausea, vomiting, and dry mucous membranes may also be present.

Nursing Interventions for the First Aid Treatment of Shock

The nurse must *immediately treat* the cause of shock. Priority interventions are to establish an airway (Chapter 53), control bleeding, and reduce pain. Appropriate positioning of the victim in shock is determined by the type and extent of injuries; the following general guidelines are recommended. The victim should lie flat with the head slightly lower than the rest of the body, unless the victim has sustained head and/or chest injuries (Fig. 54-1). If the victim is unconscious or is vomiting or bleeding around the nose and mouth, he should be positioned on the side to allow the airway to clear and to encourage drainage. The head and shoulders should be elevated if the victim is having problems breathing. If neck or spinal injuries are suspected, the victim must not be moved unless it is necessary to prevent further injury.

The nurse must maintain the shock victim's body temperature, keeping him warm and dry by placing blankets or other coverings under the victim to prevent heat loss in surfaces beneath him. The victim should be covered with any available material, such as a blanket or clothing; however, overheating should be avoided. The victim should never be given anything to eat or drink because internal injuries may be present, surgery may be needed immediately, and the patient may aspirate the fluid. A moistened cloth will relieve dry mouth or mucous membranes. In a clinical setting, fluids will be replaced by IV therapy.

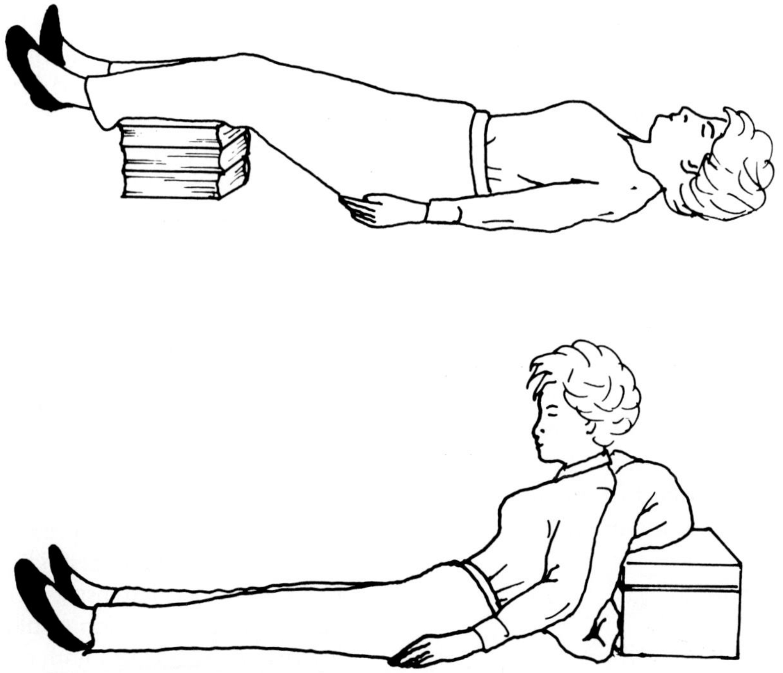

FIG. 54-1 Body positioning for shock.

The nurse must take measures to relieve pain in the shock victim. Nursing interventions include supporting the injury, avoiding rough handling, and adjusting tight or uncomfortable clothing or bandages. It is important not to give analgesics or drugs unless directed by a physician. Because the victim may be very frightened, it is essential to give him emotional support and reassurance.

BLEEDING/HEMORRHAGE

An average adult male has approximately 12 pints of blood circulating in his bloodstream. Blood is necessary to transport oxygen and nutrients to all parts of the body.

The Effects of Blood Loss

The loss of blood (hemorrhage) from internal or external bleeding causes a decrease in oxygen supply to the body. Decreased blood volume also causes the blood pressure to fall; thus the heart must pump faster to compensate for the decrease in blood volume and blood pressure. The body will attempt to clot the blood to halt bleeding. Clotting usually requires 6 to 7 minutes. If uncontrolled, bleeding can result in shock and death.

Types of Bleeding

Depending on the depth of the wound, bleeding may come from one or all of three sources—capillaries, veins, and arteries. Capillary bleeding, the most common type of external hemorrhage, results from damaged or broken capillaries and is characterized by the oozing of minor cuts, scratches, and abrasions.

Venous bleeding occurs when a vein is severed or punctured. The result is a slow, even flow of dark red blood. Besides shock from blood volume loss, a danger of venous bleeding is the entrance of air into the severed vein, which could result in **embolisms** traveling to the vital organs—heart, lung, and brain.

Arterial bleeding is the least common type of injury, because arteries are located deep in the body and are usually protected by bones, fat, and other structures. When an artery is severed or punctured, the bleeding is characterized by the heavy spurting of bright red blood in the rhythm of the heart beat. The most common arteries that can be affected are:

- Femorals (in the upper thigh and groin)
- Radials (in the lateral aspect of the lower arms)
- Brachials (in the medial aspect of the upper arm)
- Carotids (on either side of the neck)

Nursing Interventions for the First Aid Treatment of Bleeding

Direct pressure. The best general treatment of bleeding is to apply direct pressure over the bleeding site. This can be accomplished by placing a dressing or the cleanest material possible over the wound and applying firm pressure with the hand (Fig. 54-2). Then a bandage should be applied with the knot tied snugly over the wound to exert direct pressure. If bleeding continues after the bandage is applied, pressure should be resumed with the hand as well as the bandage. Bleeding should be controlled in 10 to 30 minutes. The bandage supplying direct pressure should not be removed except by a physician, even if it becomes saturated with blood. Another layer of dressing may be placed on top and firm pressure continued.

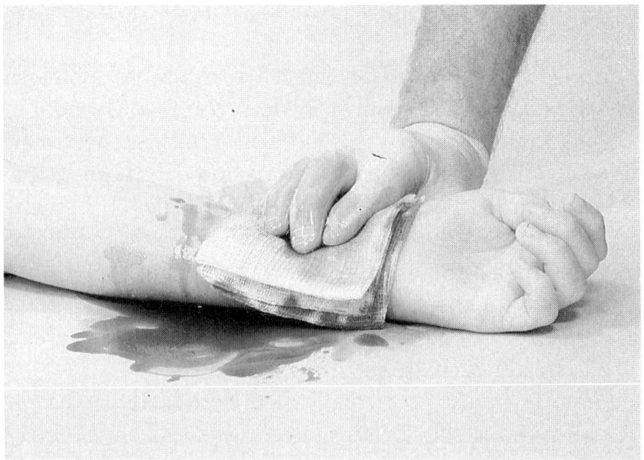

FIG. 54-2 Applying pressure to wound site.

Raising the bleeding part of the body above the level of the heart will decrease the amount of blood flow and increase the body's ability to clot at this site. This technique should be used with direct pressure *only* if there are no suspected or known fractures or conditions that may be exacerbated by this maneuver. A splinted fracture, however, may be elevated if no other contraindications are present.

Indirect pressure. If direct pressure and elevation do not control bleeding, indirect pressure may be applied to any of the 26 pressure points situated along main arteries. To apply indirect pressure the fingers or the heel of the hand is used to compress the artery against the underlying bone located between the heart and the wound. This can be done only if there are no suspected fractures beneath the area where pressure must be applied. The most common pressure points are over carotid, subclavian, brachial, and femoral arteries.

Application of a tourniquet. Bleeding can almost always be controlled by the three-step measure of direct pressure, elevation, and indirect pressure. A tourniquet must be used *only* when these methods have failed and the victim's life is in danger. Extensive damage to the part may occur because of the cessation of blood flow to the area; there is a risk of sacrificing a limb to save a life. An improperly, loosely applied tourniquet will not stop arterial flow but will hinder venous flow. Thus bleeding may be increased

SKILL 54-1

APPLYING A TOURNIQUET

1. Use a strong piece of cloth (e.g., towel, necktie, belt). Never use rope or wire, which could cut the skin.
2. Place pressure on the nearest pressure point to control bleeding while applying the tourniquet.
3. Apply a pad (piece of cloth, handkerchief, dressing) over the artery to be compressed to prevent damage to the skin.
4. Place the tourniquet between the wound and the heart, allowing uninjured skin to be present between the wound and the tourniquet. Wrap the material around the limb twice and tie a half-knot on the upper surface of the limb.
5. Place a stick or rod (approximately 6 inches long) over the knot and secure it in place.
6. Twist the stick enough times to stop the bleeding.
7. Secure the stick firmly wth the free ends of the tourniquet. Do not cover the tourniquet.
8. Write "T" or "TK" (meaning tourniquet) on the victim's forehead and the time it was applied. Attach a note to the victim's clothing describing the time and location of the tourniquet.
9. Treat for shock and transport to the nearest medical facility.
10. Never loosen a tourniquet once it has been applied. *Always* seek medical attention once a tourniquet has been applied.

STEP 7

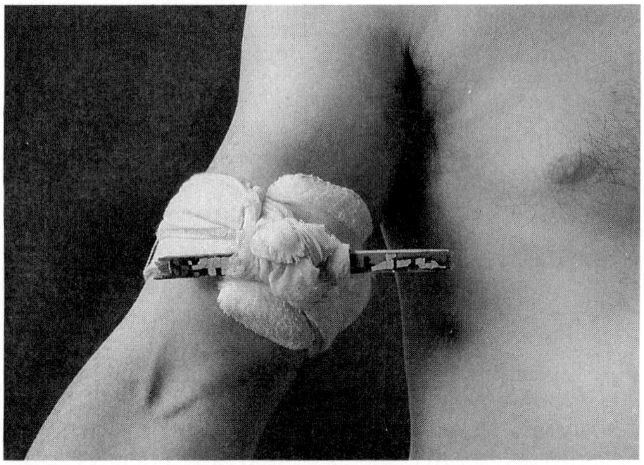

instead of controlled. Skill 54-1 provides techniques that should be followed when applying a tourniquet.

Epistaxis

Epistaxis is very common but is seldom a serious emergency. However, profuse bleeding from the nose can lead to shock. There are several causes of epistaxis. Trauma (especially a direct blow to the nose), infections, including the common cold, high blood pressure, and strenuous activity may precipitate epistaxis.

Nursing interventions for epistaxis. The person with epistaxis must be kept quiet in a sitting position, leaning forward. If the victim is unable to sit up, he should remain supine with the head and shoulders raised (if this position is not contraindicated by other injuries). Pressure is applied by pinching the nostrils and placing cold compresses on the nose and face. Pressure should be applied beneath the nostril above the upper lip. If bleeding continues, and if it is severe, medical assistance should be sought. The patient may be nauseated or vomiting.

Internal Bleeding

Internal bleeding is a potentially life-threatening situation. It is difficult to diagnose and can progress rapidly. Common causes of internal bleeding include fractures, knife or bullet wounds, crushing injuries, organ injuries, and medical conditions such as ruptured aneurysms.

Assessment. All the signs and symptoms of shock may

prevail, as discussed on p. 1365. Initially the victim may experience only vertigo or dizziness. The victim may also expectorate blood (**hemoptysis**) or vomit blood (**hematemesis**). Dark, tarry stool (**melena**) or blood in urine (**hematuria**) may also be present. Pain, tenderness, or a dislocation where injury is suspected could indicate internal bleeding, as would obvious bleeding from the mouth, rectum, or any other body opening.

Nursing interventions to control internal bleeding. Internal bleeding is a priority medical emergency, and every effort should be made to obtain medical care immediately. The victim should be placed on a flat surface with legs slightly elevated if this is not contraindicated by other injuries. An airway is established, and treatment for shock is instituted. A cold compress or ice is positioned on the area of the suspected injury. Body temperature is maintained with blankets and vital signs are measured (assessed) every 5 minutes. The victim should not be given anything to eat or drink. Oxygen may be administered if it is available. The nurse decreases the victim's fear and anxiety by giving support and reassurance.

WOUNDS AND TRAUMA

A wound is an injury to the internal or external soft tissues of the body. The basic rules for the first aid treatment of all wounds include these:

1. Stop bleeding.
2. Treat for shock.
3. Prevent infection.

Closed Wounds

Closed wounds involve the underlying tissues of the body; the top layer of skin is not broken. Examples of closed wounds are ecchymoses, contusions, strains, and sprains. They most commonly occur during injury from falls, automobile accidents, or contact sports.

The following signs and symptoms are most likely to occur with a closed wound: (1) *edema* may appear within 24 to 48 hours; (2) *discoloration* is likely to occur caused by the formation of a hematoma or blood clot—initially the discoloration is blackish-blue and then turns to green or yellow within a few days; (3) *deformity* of the limbs is caused by fractures and dislocations; (4) *shock* may follow from the force of the trauma; (5) there may be *pain and tenderness* at the site; and (6) signs of *internal bleeding* may be present.

Nursing interventions for the first aid treatment of closed wounds. If the wound is small, ice packs may be applied, and padding and a soft roller bandage may be used for pressure. If the wound is large, the patient should be treated for shock; cold compresses and a pressure bandage are applied. Medical assistance should be obtained immediately. (See p. 1375 for nursing interventions in the treatment of dislocations and fractures.)

Open Wounds

Open wounds are openings or breaks in the mucous membrane or skin. Regardless of the type, there is always danger of bleeding or infection. Infection is more common in wounds that do not bleed freely, because active bleeding tends to flush bacteria from the wound. Following are five general types of open wounds—abrasions, incisions, lacerations, punctures, avulsions—and their nursing interventions.

Abrasions. Abrasions are caused by a rubbing or scraping of the outer layers of the skin. Bleeding is limited to oozing of blood: there is danger of infection from contamination with dirt and bacteria. Examples of abrasions include rope and road burns, scratches, and abrasions of the knees and elbows.

Nursing interventions in the first aid treatment of abrasions. The wound should be washed with soap and water, from the inside to the outside. All dirt should be removed if possible. Strong antiseptics should not be used, because they may irritate the skin. The abrasion is covered with a sterile dressing. If the abrasion is deep or a **tetanus toxoid** injection is needed, a physician should be consulted. Assessment of whether tetanus toxoid injection is needed should be made on all wounds that have been made by a soiled object or are themselves dirty.

Incisions. Incisions are smoothly divided wounds made by sharp instruments. Infection is not as likely to occur, because blood flows freely from the wound. However, bleeding may be extensive and muscles, tendons, and nerves may be damaged. Common examples of incisional wounds include cuts from knives, broken glass, razors, or edges of paper.

Nursing interventions in the first aid treatment of incisions. The incision is carefully cleaned with soap and water and covered with a sterile dressing; an antiseptic is used only at a physician's recommendation. A "butterfly" bandage or Steri-Strips may be used to hold together the edges of the wound. Bleeding is controlled by applying pressure. Medical attention should be sought if the incision is deep and/or bleeding is profuse.

Lacerations. Lacerations are wounds that are torn with jagged, irregular edges. Bleeding may be profuse, and tissue destruction and infection may occur. Auto accidents, blunt objects, and heavy machinery accidents are common causes of lacerations.

Nursing interventions in the first aid treatment of lacerations. The laceration should be carefully cleaned with soap and water. Bleeding is controlled by applying pressure (See Fig. 54-2). Adhesive strips, Steri-Strips, or a "butterfly" bandage are used to close the edges of the laceration. The wound should be covered with a sterile dressing, and the victim should be taken to a physician for treatment.

Puncture wounds. Puncture wounds are caused by the penetration of sharp objects into body tissues. The surface opening may be small; however, the object may penetrate deeply, causing severe damage to tissues and organs. Infection is common, since bleeding is minimal. Tetanus bacteria, in particular, may multiply rapidly after a puncture wound. Nails, needles, bullets, knives, animal bites, and insect stings are common causes of puncture wounds.

Nursing interventions in the first aid treatment of puncture wounds. If the wound is deep the object should not be removed (it may have to be cut from the tissues). The wound site should be immobilized and the patient taken to the physician immediately.

Avulsions. An avulsion is the forcible tearing of tissue from the body. The force of industrial or automobile accidents may amputate fingers, toes, or whole limbs of the body. Bleeding is usually extensive, and shock usually results. In some cases, a detached part may be reattached by a surgeon if it is sent to the hospital with the victim.

Nursing interventions in the first aid treatment of avulsions. The *ABC*s of emergency care should be followed (See Chapter 53), with airway being the first priority. Hemorrhage must be controlled; a tourniquet should be used as a last resort (see Skill 54-1). Because of this trauma and subsequent loss of blood, the nurse must monitor and treat for shock. If the severed part is found, it should be separated from as much dirt and debris as possible with gloved hands and covered with sterile gauze, a towel, or clean cloth. It should be put in a plastic bag, sealed shut, and the bag placed in ice or cold water. The part is transported with the victim. The severed part *must not* be frozen, immersed in a solution or water, treated with antiseptic, or thrown away.

Special Types of Wounds

Eye injuries. Foreign bodies such as dirt, sand, cinders, or pieces of metal are the most common causes of eye injury. They not only cause discomfort, but if not removed, may cause inflammation or infection. The natural flow of tears when a foreign body is present very often leads to the flushing out of a foreign object. The victim should not rub the eye, since this can scratch the tissues of the eye and further embed the object.

Assessment. The victim should be observed for: edema or lacerated eyelids and/or erythema on the surface of the eye. Sometimes the nurse may see a visible scratch on the surface of the eye. Excessive tearing of the eye may also be noted, and the victim may complain of discomfort. Changes in vision or visual acuity may occur.

Nursing interventions to remove a foreign body from the eye. Initially the eyelids should be flushed with clean water, if available, holding the eyelids open and flushing from the inner canthus to the outer canthus of the eye. If the foreign object is under the upper eyelid, it may be removed by bringing the upper lid over the lower lid. As the upper lid returns to its normal position, the undersurface will be wiped by the action of the eyelashes. A foreign body of the upper lid may also be removed by grasping the eyelashes of the upper lid and averting it over a cotton swab or similar object. The foreign object may then be removed with the corners of a piece of sterile gauze.

Particles under the lower lid may be removed by pulling down the lower lid, exposing the inner surface. The corner of a piece of sterile gauze can be used to remove the foreign body. If the foreign body cannot be removed by these measures, if the eye is scratched, or if the object is embedded in the eye, no attempt should be made to disturb it, because this could cause further damage. A cup or cone can be positioned over the area of injury, and then a bandage can be loosely applied to both eyes. The head is stabilized with sandbags or pillows and the victim is transported in a supine position to the physician as quickly as possible.

Chest injuries. Chest wounds are extremely dangerous and need immediate medical attention. In most wounds of the chest, air escapes into the chest (**pleural space**). Normally this space is a vacuum; therefore air entering this space may cause an increase in pressure, which will result in a pneumothorax (collapse of the lung).

Assessment. The nurse should assess the following:

Sharp pain at the site of the injury
Pain associated with breathing
Difficult and labored breathing
Failure of one or both sides of the chest to expand normally with inspiration
Expectorating bright red or frothy blood (hemoptysis)
Symptoms of shock: rapid, weak, thready pulse, vertigo, and hypotension
Cyanosis of the skin and mucous membranes
There may be a sucking or hissing sound as air flows in and out of the chest
Distention or edema of the neck and arm veins

Nursing interventions for the first aid treatment of penetrating chest wounds. If the chest wall has been penetrated by a sharp object, the object should not be removed; this could result in further bleeding and the entrance of air into the chest wound. The object is immobilized with dressings and tape. The *ABC*s of treatment should be employed (See Chapter 53). The victim should be treated for shock; however, the victim's head may need to be elevated slightly to facilitate breathing.

If there is a sucking chest wound (without the penetrating object in place), an airtight dressing must be applied. Any material available may be used—gauze, plastic wrap, clothing, or even the nurse's hand if that is the only thing available. This dressing must be large enough so that it is not sucked into the hole in the chest, and it should be as airtight as possible. Liquids should be withheld, since aspiration could result.

Nursing interventions for the first aid treatment of crushing chest wounds. The most common injury to the chest is fractured ribs. Simple fractures (one or two ribs) may not need to be bound, strapped, or taped. If the injury to the chest is extensive, the fractured ribs should be immobilized with gauze or clothing. Dressings should be applied carefully to open wounds to avoid pressure on the chest. The victim's head and shoulders should be elevated slightly to facilitate breathing.

Dressings and Bandages

General principles of bandaging. Bleeding should be controlled before applying the bandage. The dressing is opened carefully, using sterile materials if possible. If sterile equipment is not available, the cleanest material possible should be used. The dressing should cover the entire wound. Wounds should be bandaged firmly but not too tightly; tight bandages can interfere with circulation to the tissue. Loose ends may be caught on objects. The part should always be bandaged in the alignment that is desired; a joint should never be bent after it is bandaged. The tips of the fingers and toes should remain exposed if possible, to check for circulation. The nurse should assess for edema and circulation frequently. Knots should be tied over the top of open wounds to control bleeding unless this is contraindicated.

Application of common types of bandages

The bandage compress. The bandage compress is the most common type of dressing. It consists of several thicknesses of gauze, covered with tape or gauze.

The triangular bandage. The triangular bandage is made of a piece of cloth that is folded diagonally and cut along the fold. This is used most commonly as a sling to support injured bones. Skill 54-2 describes the application of an arm splint using a triangular bandage.

The roller bandage. The roller bandage is used to support an injured part, apply pressure to a dressing for control of bleeding, or secure a splint to immobilize a part (Fig. 54-3). Roller bandages should be applied uniformly to ensure even pressure. The skin should be covered completely; it is safer to use a greater number of evenly spaced overlapping turns than fewer, tighter turns of the bandage. The roller bandage is started at the point of dressing or at the part of the limb with the smallest circumference (e.g., the wrist or ankle). The roller bandage is fastened either with tape or a square knot. Circular or spiral roller bandages are used to cover a cylindrical part. A figure-eight may also be used, especially if splints must be used.

SKILL 54-2

APPLYING AN ARM SPLINT USING A TRIANGULAR BANDAGE

1. Place one end of the base of the open triangle over the uninjured shoulder.
2. Place the apex of the triangle behind the elbow of the injured arm.
3. Bend the arm at the elbow with the hand elevated slightly (4 to 5 inches).
4. Bring the forearm across the chest and over the bandage.
5. Take the lower end of the triangle and bring it over the shoulder of the injured side. Tie the bandage on the neck at the uninjured side, so that the knot is on the side of the neck.
6. Twist the remaining end of the bandage and tuck it in at the elbow.
7. Remember to keep fingertips exposed to assess circulation.

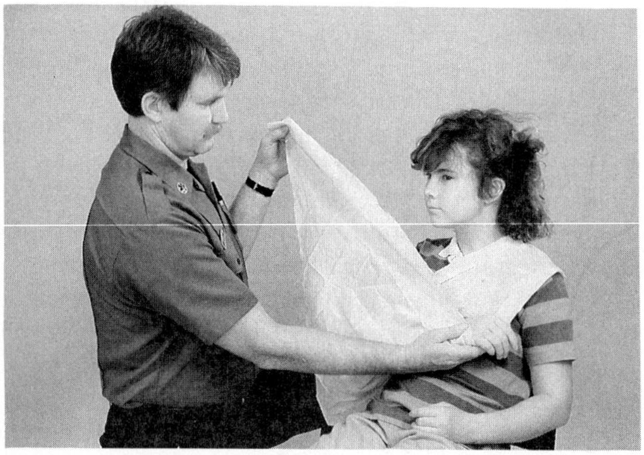

STEP 1

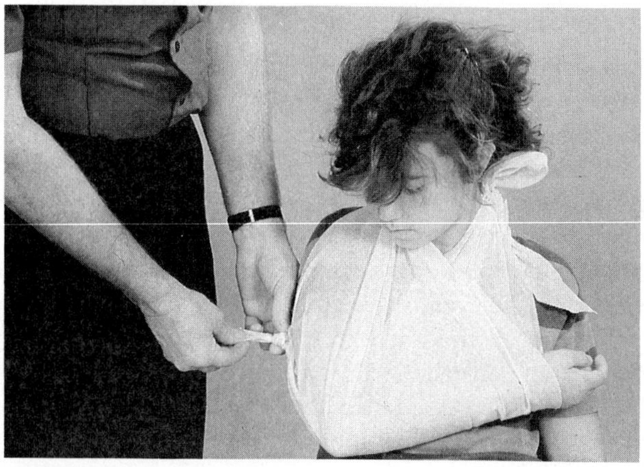

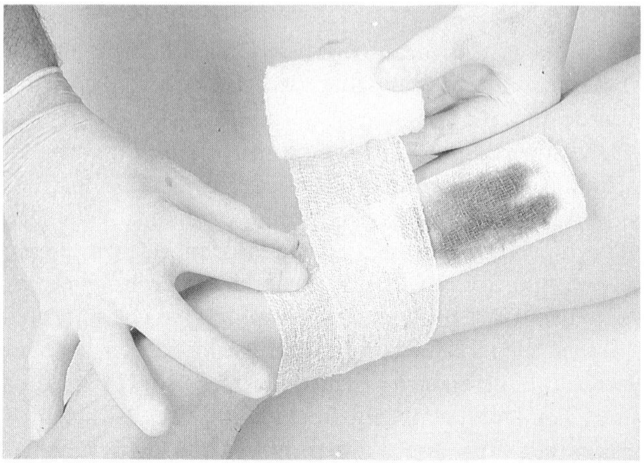

FIG. 54-3 Use of roller bandage.

POISONS

Each year thousands of people die from self-inflicted or accidental poisonings. Of these people, the majority are children. A poison is any substance (solid, liquid, or gas) that even in small amounts causes damage to the body or interferes with the function of its system. There are poison control centers throughout the country that are equipped to give information about poisons and methods of treatment on a 24-hour-a-day, 7-day-a-week basis. Most poisons act rapidly and require immediate first aid.

General Assessment of Poisonings

Acute signs and symptoms of poisonings may be delayed for hours. The following may be indications of poisonings: severe nausea, vomiting, or diarrhea; seizures, twitching, or paralysis; decreased level of consciousness or unconsciousness; restlessness, delirium, agitation, or panic; color changes: pale flushed or cyanotic skin; signs of burns, edema around the mouth or other areas of the body; pain on swallowing, tenderness, cramps; characteristic odor on the breath; unusual urine color (red, green, bright yellow, black, bronze); slow, labored breathing or wheezing; abnormal constriction or dilation of the pupils; skin irritation, erythema, and/or edema; and shock or cardiac arrest.

Ingested Poisons

Poisoning by mouth is the most common, especially in children. Common substances include household cleaning products, garden and garage supplies (e.g., insecticides, gasoline), drugs, medications, food, and plants.

Nursing interventions in the first aid treatment of ingested poisons. The nurse should waste no time in calling the poison control center to describe the poison ingested and receive instructions. An airway must be maintained. If the victim is an adult and is conscious, the poison is diluted by giving 1 to 2 glasses (8 to 16 ounces) of water (for a child, 1 glass [8 ounces]), unless drugs are the cause of the poison, because water would increase the rate of absorption. If the victim is conscious and the poison is *not* a corrosive, and only when the nurse is directed to do so by the poison control center or other medical facility, vomiting should be induced. The following methods may be used.

One tablespoon of syrup of ipecac with 6 to 8 ounces of water should be given to a child, and 2 tablespoons of ipecac with 1 to 2 glasses (8 to 16 ounces) of water to an adult. Milk or carbonated beverages should never be given with syrup of ipecac. If vomiting does not occur within 20 to 30 minutes, the dose is repeated once only. If syrup of ipecac is not available, vomiting may be induced by carefully tickling the back of the throat with a spoon or tongue blade.

Vomiting should not be induced if the victim is having a seizure, is semiconscious or unconscious, or if the nurse suspects the victim has swallowed any caustic or corrosive substance, such as a strong acid, lye, gasoline, or rat poison. The nurse should not induce vomiting if the victim has a serious heart condition or is in the later stages of pregnancy. If the poison is corrosive, it should be diluted with water and medical help sought immediately. The nurse should treat for shock and administer CPR if needed. The substance's container and any vomitus should be brought to the medical facility to help identify and treat the poison. An antidote should never be given until the poison control center has been consulted.

Inhaled Poisons

Because inhaled poisons can be present without warning and are absorbed very rapidly, prompt first aid measures are important. Common sources of inhaled poisons include carbon monoxide (from autos, fires, heating systems, propane engines, and paint remover), carbon dioxide (from sewers or industry), and refrigeration gases. Chlorine (used in cleaning and industry) and fumes from sprays and other liquid chemicals may also give off poisonous fumes.

Nursing interventions in the first aid treatment of inhaled poisons. The nurse must first assess the danger. The victim should be removed from the dangerous area only if there is no danger to the rescuer. Clothing should be loosened from the victim's throat and chest. An airway must be maintained, and CPR may have to be started. The victim should remain quiet and inactive while being transported to the nearest medical facility.

Absorbed Poisons

Poisons, caustic chemicals, and poisonous plants that come in contact with the skin can be rapidly absorbed, causing burning, skin irritation, allergic responses, or severe systemic reactions. Poison ivy, poison oak, and poison sumac are the most common plants that can elicit a poison response.

Nursing interventions in the first aid treatment of poisoning by absorption. The first action must be to quickly remove the source of the irritation and then to wash the contacted area with soap and water. Skin preparations that are effective in the treatment of contact poisonings include baking soda, Burow's solution, or oatmeal to dry **vesicles.** Calamine lotion and hydrocortisone cream (5%) are effective to relieve pruritus.

Injected Poisons

Injections of drugs to which an individual is allergic and the venom from insects, reptiles, and animals can cause allergic reactions that can range from mild to severe. Emergency care involves minimizing the travel of the poison to the heart. The reaction to an insect bite may be mild or severe.

Minor reactions to insect bites. If the individual has been stung by a bee, the stinger should be removed with the *side* of a tweezer or knife in a scraping motion. If the nurse attempts to grasp the barbed stinger with tweezers, venom may be forced further into the skin. Nursing interventions include washing the bite with soap and water and applying cold packs to relieve pain and slow the absorption of the poison.

Severe reactions to insect bites. Within as little as 60 minutes or up to several hours, a victim of a bite or sting may experience a severe allergic reaction. Uticaria, wheezing, edema of the lips and tongue, generalized pruritus, and respiratory arrest are the most common symptoms of anaphylactic shock (severe allergic reaction). (See Chapter 39.)

Nursing interventions in the first aid treatment of major reactions to insect bites. The victim should lie down and the nurse should immobilize the area of the bite. A constricting band is then applied above the edematous area. The band should only stop venous blood flow, not arterial; therefore, a pulse should be present below the constriction. The affected part should be kept in a dependent position, below the level of the heart. The victim should be transported to the hospital immediately, and if possible the type of animal or insect that caused the bite should be identified. Some people who know that they are allergic wear Medic-Alert tags and carry medication (antihistamines) to take after a bite. This can be self-administered. The nurse should give this medication only if directed to do so by the physician.

DRUG AND ALCOHOL EMERGENCIES

Drugs (including alcohol) are chemical substances that can affect body functioning and can be subject to abuse and overdose.

Alcohol

Alcohol is the most commonly abused drug in the world. It is a depressant that can cause many symptoms, even death.

Assessment. Signs and symptoms of *mild* intoxication include nausea, vomiting, diarrhea, lack of coordination, and poor muscle control. Flushing, erythema of the face and eyes, visual disturbances, and rapid mood swings may be present. Slurred or inappropriate speech, inappropriate behavior, and lethargy (sleepiness) may also occur.

Serious alcohol intoxication is usually caused by consuming a large quantity of alcohol over a short period of time. Signs and symptoms include drowsiness that progresses to coma; rapid, weak pulse; and depressed, labored breathing or respiratory arrest. Loss of control of urinary and bowel functions and confusion, restlessness, and hallucinations may occur. Tremors that may progress to grand mal seizures, nausea, vomiting, expectorating blood from the respiratory tract, and diarrhea may be present. This person may also experience loss of memory, visual disturbances, lack of muscle coordination, and depressed reflexes.

Drugs

Abuse of drugs is a major problem in the world today. Not only are illegal drugs abused, but also prescription and over-the-counter medications. In assessing the drug abuser the nurse observes for signs and symptoms of loss of reality orientation, hallucinations, and varying degrees of consciousness; coma could be a result. Slurred speech, extremes in mood swings, inappropriate behavior, and anxiety may also be present. The victim may have a fever, flushed skin, and be experiencing diaphoresis (sweating). Lack of coordination and impaired judgment may make safety a real problem. Depending on the drug, the pulse and blood pressure may increase or decrease, the pupils may constrict or dilate, and the appetite may increase or decrease. Obvious hypodermic needle marks on the arms, legs, and neck may be present. The victim may complain of diarrhea or pain in the abdomen, legs, or joints. He may also experience tremors or seizures.

Nursing interventions in the first aid treatment for drug and alcohol emergencies. Because an accurate nursing history is important, the nurse must obtain as much information as possible about the substance ingested and keep the containers if possible. The life-threatening situations are handled first and an airway is established. If the victim is unconscious, his head should be turned to the side. Clothing is loosened to assist ventilation. If the victim is having muscle twitching and is drowsy, the nurse should not attempt to arouse him, because this may precipitate a seizure. If a fever is present, it can be reduced by applying cool, wet compresses. The nurse should protect the victim from hurting himself during a seizure or hallucination by removing harmful objects. The nurse should not attempt to restrain a patient during seizure activity.

The nurse may induce vomiting, particularly if the drug was taken within 30 minutes. Vomiting should never be induced if the victim is stuporous because of the danger of aspiration. The nurse must be calm, supportive, and nonjudgmental, especially if the patient is very agitated or excited. The intoxicated person should never be left alone. Careful assessment of mental status and vital signs must be performed frequently. A substance abuse victim can go into respiratory arrest very quickly. The victim must be transported to a medical facility promptly.

THERMAL AND COLD EMERGENCIES

Heat Injuries

Excessive heat affects the body in several ways. In a hot environment, heat builds up in the body. The body automatically attempts to get rid of the excessive heat by increasing the amount of perspiration produced and slowing down muscular activity. If this mechanism fails for an external (environmental) or internal reason, heatstroke or heat exhaustion could result. Heatstroke and heat exhaustion represent a different reaction to excessive heat; for this reason signs, symptoms, and treatment are also different.

Heat Exhaustion

Heat exhaustion is the most common type of heat injury and is the result of prolonged perspiration and the loss of large quantities of salt and water. It occurs most often in hot humid weather, when adequate fluids are not replaced (common in the elderly who have a diminished thirst mechanism despite dehydration).

Nursing assessment of the victim of heat exhaustion would include observing for signs and symptoms such as headache, dizziness, nausea, weakness, and diaphoresis.

Mental confusion and brief loss of consciousness may occur. The victim has a normal body temperature with pale, cold, clammy skin. The victim may complain of abdominal cramps and loss of appetite. Breathing may be rapid and shallow and the pulse may be weak and rapid.

Nursing interventions in the first aid treatment of the victim with heat exhaustion. The victim must be cooled off as quickly as possible by moving him to a cool area, but avoiding chilling. As much clothing as possible should be removed and constrictive clothing loosened to allow the circulation of air to cool the body. The victim should lie down with feet 8 to 12 inches higher than the head. The victim may be cooled with cold, wet compresses, and a fan or air conditioner should be used if available.

If the victim is completely conscious and alert, fluids may be replaced with a solution of 1 teaspoon salt in a glass of water. This should be administered every 15 minutes over an hour. If the victim is drowsy or vomiting, fluids should not be given by mouth. In the clinical setting IV fluids are given. The victim should be transported to a medical facility as soon as possible.

Heatstroke

Heatstroke is the most serious heat injury; death can result if heatstroke is untreated. The most common cause of heatstroke is vigorous physical activity in a hot, humid environment. The body becomes overheated, but the cooling mechanism of perspiration does not operate. Deprived of this mechanism, the body stores excessive heat. (Body temperature may rise to 106° F.) Brain and central nervous system damage can result.

Assessment. The signs and symptoms of the heatstroke include rapidly rising body temperature, hot, dry, red skin, and no visible perspiration. The pulse is rapid initially, then slows and weakens as the blood pressure falls. Breathing becomes deep and rapid. The victim complains of headache and dry mouth, and he may experience vertigo, decreased level of consciousness, and may collapse. Muscle twitching and convulsions may occur.

Nursing interventions in the first aid treatment of the victim of heatstroke. It is important to cool the victim as quickly as possible, moving him to a cool area. Establishing and maintaining an airway is a priority nursing intervention. The victim should be undressed (retaining undergarments only). The victim's bare skin should be cooled as quickly as possible with cold water or ice compresses. Cold packs can be placed around the victim's neck, under the arms, and around the ankles to cool the blood in the main arteries. A fan or air conditioner should be used if available. Treatment continues until the victim's temperature falls below 100° F. The victim should be monitored for chilling as the body temperature falls, and the temperature should be checked every 10 to 15 minutes to ensure that it does not rise again. Cooling efforts are continued until the victim is able to obtain medical assistance.

Exposure to Excessive Cold

When the body is exposed to severe cold, blood vessels constrict, body heat is lost, and destruction of tissue may result. Cold, moist air, fatigue, smoking, drugs, alcohol, dehydration, and age accelerate the potential for injury.

Frostbite. Frostbite is the most common and dangerous local cold injury involving freezing and damaging of body cells. Ice crystals actually form in the body fluid and underlying tissues. These crystals draw water from the cells, causing destruction of tissue integrity. Common areas affected by frostbite are the ears, nose, fingers, and toes.

Assessment. Initially the frostbitten skin takes on a red flush, and the victim may complain of numbness, tingling, and/or pain. Progressively the part becomes hard and loses all sensation. The color of the part changes to a grayish white color as circulation diminishes further. If thawing occurs, the color may change to blue-purple or black, indicating severe damage or death of tissues. Vesicles and edema may occur. If frostbite is very severe, complete loss of function of the part may result from the damage.

Nursing interventions in the first aid treatment of frostbite. If there is a possibility that the part will become refrozen after it has been thawed, it is better to leave it frozen until the victim arrives at a medical facility. Severe tissue damage can result from thawing and refreezing a frozen part. The victim should be treated for shock and an airway established and maintained. Any constricting clothing should be removed to encourage circulation.

If there is no risk of the part being refrozen, it should be warmed in this manner. The frozen part is immersed in warm water (preferably a bathtub) at 102° to 105° F for 20 to 45 minutes. Water temperature should be checked frequently, not allowing it to cool. If a tub is not available, a hot, moist towel may be used. The nurse must be very careful *not to rub the part;* underlying tissue may become bruised and damaged by friction. If water is not available, the part may be warmed by placing it against a warm part of the body—the armpit, abdomen, or between the legs. The frozen part should never be placed near an open flame or oven. Gentle warming must be performed to avoid burns and damage.

Once the part is warmed, the victim is encouraged to gently move the part. If the legs or feet are involved, however, the victim should not be allowed to walk. The thawed part is wrapped in clean towels or dressings and elevated. The entire body should be kept warm, and warm fluids should be offered to drink. Alcohol should never be given, and the victim should not smoke, because this will cause further vasoconstriction. All frostbite injuries, no matter how minor, should be seen by a physician.

Hypothermia. Hypothermia is the lowering of the body temperature below the normal level (95° F or below). The brain, heart, lungs, and other vital organs are affected by this drop in temperature. Hypothermia occurs most frequently when the air is windy, cold, and moist, or precipitation is present. The victim may be exhausted or intoxicated; elderly persons or those living in a poorly heated environment are subject to hypothermia.

Assessment. Initially, the victim may shiver uncontrollably; shivering ceases when the body temperature is below 90° F. Speech becomes slow, slurred, and incoherent, and the victim demonstrates memory lapses, disorientation, and poor judgment. Safety is a problem, because the gait becomes uncoordinated and muscle activity may decrease or cease. The skin appears mottled and edematous, and the patient complains of generalized numbness. A weak, irregular pulse develops, with a depressed respiratory rate. The victim becomes lethargic, with decreasing levels of consciousness. Finally, there is a loss of all reflexes and the victim appears to be dead.

Nursing interventions in the first aid treatment of hypothermia. Although a person in the final stages of hypothermia may appear to be dead because of the effects of the lowered metabolic rate, many such victims can be revived. First aid is always instituted in an attempt to treat hypothermia. CPR should always be initiated if necessary, even though the victim may appear dead. The victim should be placed in a supine position with the head lower than the feet. The victim is rewarmed slowly; rapid exposure to warmth can precipitate shock. The victim is moved to a warm area, and all wet clothing is removed and replaced with dry ones. The nurse should cover the victim with warm blankets.

If the victim is completely conscious, warm fluids can be given to drink. Alcohol should never be given because of its vasodilatory effect on the peripheral vessels, which causes the central temperature core to drop further. Medical help must be obtained as soon as possible.

BONE, JOINT, AND MUSCLE INJURIES

The four major types of injuries that occur to bones, tendons, ligaments, and muscles are fractures, dislocations, sprains, and strains.

Fractures

A fracture is a break in the continuity of a bone. Fractured bones seldom are an immediate threat to life. In administering first aid to an injured victim, establishing an airway and treating hemorrhage are considered priority situations. There are several types of common fractures:

- Open or compound fractures: an open wound exists over the fracture site. Very often the affected bone may be seen protruding through the skin.
- Closed fractures: the skin overlying the injury is intact.
- Comminuted fractures: the bone is shattered into two or more fragments or pieces.
- Greenstick fractures: an incomplete break occurring most commonly in children because their bones are pliable.

Assessment. The physician, using x-ray diagnostic procedures, can determine whether a bone is definitely fractured. Fracture is suspected if there are pain and tenderness in the area of the fracture; pain also develops during movement, and the victim complains of an inability to move the affected part. A deformity of the limb may be obvious with edema and discoloration (cyanosis, erythema) of the area. Fragments of bone may be protruding

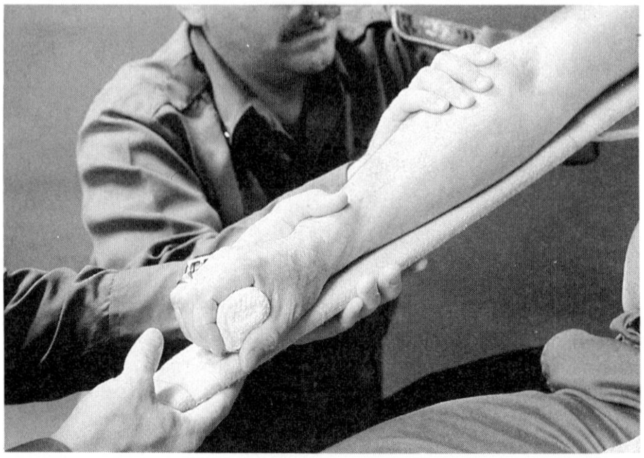

FIG. 54-4 Immobilization of fractured arm.

through the skin. If the affected part is moved, a grating sound is heard. This is called **crepitus** and is caused by the broken bones scraping against each other. The victim may state that he heard or felt the bone snap.

Nursing interventions in the first aid treatment of fractures. The victim should not be moved unless he is in danger. The *ABCs* of first aid take priority. Next the nurse must control bleeding in open fractures by cutting away the clothing around the wound and covering with a large sterile pressure dressing. The nurse should not attempt to reduce the fracture; this could cause further damage to the bone and tissue. The victim is treated for shock.

The fracture should be immobilized, but no attempt to realign the bone should be made. The rule is: "Splint the part where it lies." A fracture can change from a simple break to comminuted or splintered by moving it improperly. The splint should be lightweight but rigid. It must be long enough to extend past the joints above and beyond the fracture. It should be wider than the thickest part of the injury. The splint must be padded on the inner surface to avoid contact with the skin. The fracture is supported while gently sliding the splint under the limb. A roller bandage or similar material is used to secure the limb in place (Fig. 54-4). Circulation in the limb is monitored by assessing color, temperature, pulses below the injury, complaints of numbness and tingling, and evidence of edema.

Dislocations

Dislocations occur in joints. They usually result from a blow or fall. Common areas are the jaw, shoulder, elbow, wrist, finger, hip, and ankle.

General assessment of the victim with dislocations. The victim may complain of pain and edema in the area of the dislocation. A deformity of the part may be observed. The part may be rigid and the victim is unable to move it. A common observation in the dislocated joint of an extremity is shortening of the affected part.

General nursing interventions for the victim of a dislocation of the joint. The nurse should never attempt to reduce a dislocation or push the joint back into place; this will further damage delicate ligaments, tendons, and the bone. The joint must be splinted in the same manner as a fracture. The nurse should be sure the splint is large enough to support the limb in the line of the deformity. The limb is bound to the body or supported in a sling. This is useful in dislocations of the shoulder and elbow.

Strains and Sprains

Strains are injuries to muscle tissue that result from stretching and tearing from overexertion. Sprains are injuries to joints resulting from stretched and/or torn ligaments. This may be caused by twisting it beyond the normal range of motion. The most commonly affected joints are the knee and ankle. Permanent damage can occur to the tissue and joint if sprains are left untreated.

Assessment of the victim with strains or sprains. Injuries to muscle or ligaments result in the following signs and symptoms:

Strains: spasms, or "knotting" of the muscles, acute pain, stiffness, and weakness on movement; back pain radiating down the leg; discoloration

Sprains: pain and/or tenderness around a joint; immobility of the joint; rapid and marked edema; discoloration around the joint

Nursing interventions in the first aid treatment of strains and sprains. A suspected musculoskeletal injury should be treated as a fracture, until fracture is definitely ruled out. In the treatment of sprains and strains, the nurse should remember the word *RICE,* which stands for:

R Rest the affected extremity.

I Ice applications to the part until the edema and pain subside (24 to 72 hours is most common). This may be followed by warm compresses to encourage healing by increasing blood flow. The skin is assessed frequently for evidence of burns.

C Compression: an Ace bandage or compression bandage should be used to support the injured part.

E Elevation: the part is elevated above the level of the heart to promote venous flow and therefore reduce edema.

Spinal Cord Injuries

Assessment of spinal cord injuries. To assess for paralysis, the nurse asks the victim if he can move his hands and/or feet and asks the victim if he feels pain or sensation. The nurse may test for sensation by touching or pinching the skin. Abrasions and ecchymosis, especially

SKILL 54-3

MOVING THE VICTIM WITH A SUSPECTED SPINAL CORD INJURY

1. Carefully roll the victim, supporting the entire length of the body, just enough to slip a solid board underneath the victim for support. This board must extend beyond the victim's head and feet.
2. While another person steadies the victim's head, place a towel or padding in the space underneath the victim's neck (never put the head on a pillow).
3. Place additional padding (rolled up blankets, towels, sandbags, etc.) around the head and neck to hold the head in place, keeping the neck in line with the body.
4. Secure the victim to the backboard with bandages or improvise these so that the entire body is immobilized. Tape the head in place.
5. In the event of an emergency situation in which the victim is wearing a helmet, the nurse should immobilize the victim with the helmet left in place.

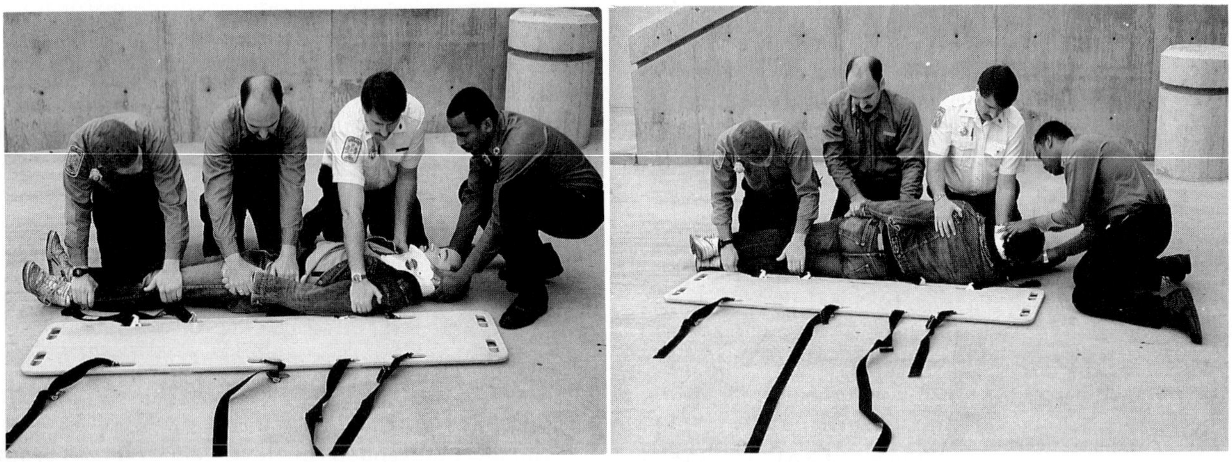

STEP 1

on the shoulders, back, and abdomen, may indicate injury to the spinal cord.

Nursing interventions in the emergency care for suspected spinal injury. Spinal cord precautions are taken in all cases of head trauma and multiple traumas. An airway is established, keeping the head in a neutral position (never hyperextending the neck). If the victim vomits, he should be moved (by several people as one unit) on the side to allow drainage.

CPR is administered if necessary. Hemorrhage and shock must be treated. The head and neck must be kept in line with the body when moving the victim. Even a slight movement of the head can cause spinal damage. The nurse should not attempt to move the victim without at least three assistants. (See Skill 54-3).

BURN INJURIES

Burns are a leading cause of accidental injuries, especially among children. Burns may be caused by heat from fire or steam, electricity from faulty wiring, chemicals such as lye, strong cleaning products, and acids, and solar radiation and radioactive materials.

Burns may be classified according to the depth or the extent of the body surface area burned. The principal complications of all burns are shock from loss of fluids and electrolytes and trauma and infection because of the loss of skin as a barrier.

Shallow Partial-Thickness Burns

Shallow partial-thickness burns (previously classified as first-degree burns) are the least serious of all burns, involving only the outer layer of the skin. The most common first-degree burns are simple sunburn or contact with hot objects. Healing is usually spontaneous and uncomplicated. Signs and symptoms include erythema of the skin and pain.

Nursing interventions for the first aid treatment of shallow partial-thickness burns. The burn should be cooled immediately by soaking in cold (not ice) water or applying cold compresses to the area for as long as it takes to decrease pain (up to 30 minutes). The nurse should never put grease, butter, salt water, or topical burn ointments or sprays on the burn. A sterile dressing should be placed over the burn site to ease pain.

Deep Partial-Thickness Burns

Deep partial-thickness burns (previously classified as second-degree burns) involve the entire first layer of skin (epidermis) as well as some of the underlying tissue; scarring from vesicles and infection may occur. Common causes of second-degree burns are severe sunburn, scalding liquids, direct flame, and chemical substances.

Assessment. Signs and symptoms include the following. Deep erythema of the skin, or mottled skin with vesicular formation, may be seen. Considerable edema may result, lasting over several days. There may be a weeping of fluid through the skin surface (loss of plasma), and the person complains of intense pain.

Full-Thickness Burns

Full-thickness burns (previously classified as third-degree burns) involve destruction of the skin and underlying tissue, including fat, muscle, and bone. The area is usually charred and healing is difficult. The skin may be thick and leathery, with black or dark brown, cherry red, or dry and milky white colors. The victim may not complain of pain, since nerve endings may be severed by the burn. There is a hyperpermeability of capillaries, with plasma seeping into the interstitial spaces—thus fluid loss; the wounds weep a great deal of fluid and blood. Thus a fluid and electrolyte imbalance occurs. Hypovolemic shock and infection are common complications. Medical attention is urgent. Common causes of full-thickness burns are direct flame (ignited clothing), explosions, and gasoline or oil fires.

Nursing interventions in the first aid treatment of moderate to severe burns (deep partial-thickness and full-thickness). An airway must be established before edema occurs. Respiratory and cardiac function is assessed. The nurse should remove all of the victim's clothing, shoes, and jewelry, which may be constricting and even smoldering. Leaving clothing on can cause more severe burns. CPR is administered if necessary. The victim is treated for shock. The victim should be kept warm, with the burned area elevated. The nurse should inspect for burns around the mouth and nose, which could affect respiratory status.

If medical help will be arriving within 15 to 30 minutes, the nurse should withhold oral fluids. If medical help is delayed, ½ glass of water mixed with ½ teaspoon of salt plus ½ teaspoon baking soda may be given to replace electrolytes. If vomiting occurs, fluids should not be given.

The burn should be cooled immediately, using cool compresses. This should be used only for partial-thickness burns. Cool compresses could cause hypothermia in more extensive burns. Clothing is removed from the burned area. The victim's shoes should always be removed; often heavy boots may be smoldering and can cause a more severe burn. Vesicles should not be broken, and the nurse should not touch a burn with anything except sterile dressings. Antiseptics, ointments, sprays, or creams should not be applied on a burn; this could interfere with medical treatment and cause further complications. Loose sterile dressings should be applied over the burn. The victim should be checked frequently to be sure that edema has not caused further constriction of the area near the burn.

REFERENCES AND SUGGESTED READINGS

1. American Red Cross: Multimedia standard first aid, New York, 1987, American Red Cross.
2. American Red Cross: Standard first aid, New York, 1988, American Red Cross.
3. Flight MR: Law, liability and ethics for medical personnel, Albany, NY, 1988, Delmar Publishing.
4. Hafen BQ: First aid for health emergencies, ed 4, New York, 1988, West Publishing Co.

4a. Hood G and Dincher J: Total patient care: foundations and practice, St. Louis, 1988, The CV Mosby Co.

5. Mosby's medical, allied health, and nursing dictionary, St. Louis, 1989, The CV Mosby Co.
6. Nurses' Service Organization: Nurses' guide to avoiding malpractice lawsuits, Springhouse, PA, 1986, Springhouse Corp.
7. Phipps W, Long B, and Woods N: Medical-surgical nursing: concepts and clinical practice, St. Louis, 1991, The CV Mosby Co.
8. Rosenberg SN: The Johnson & Johnson first aid book, New York, 1985, Warner Books, Inc.

CHAPTER CHALLENGE

KEY POINTS

- First aid is used to preserve life until medical help arrives, not to replace medical care.
- Airway problems, circulatory problems, profuse bleeding, and poisonings are life-threatening situations that require priority emergency care.
- Shock should be suspected in all traumatic injuries, diseases, and physical and emotional stress situations.
- Shock can be prevented and kept from worsening by administering prompt, effective treatment.
- Steps for controlling bleeding include direct pressure, elevation, and indirect pressure. A tourniquet is seldom used, and only as a last resort.
- The chief responsibilities of the nurse caring for an open wound are to stop bleeding and prevent infection.
- The major concerns in a chest wound are to control bleeding and maintain breathing and oxygenation.
- When bandaging a part it is important to assess frequently for evidence of impaired circulation: edema, pain, change of color, coolness.
- Any substance, if abused or misused, may be considered a poison and needs medical assistance immediately.
- The nurse should never induce vomiting in a poisoned victim unless directed to by the poison control center or medical facility.
- Reactions to a poisonous bite may take a few minutes to several hours to appear. First aid measures should be taken immediately.
- The main objectives in administering first aid to a victim with a fracture are to immobilize the area, treat for shock, and prevent further injury.
- The nurse should always splint a fractured part in the position it is in and should never attempt to realign a fracture.
- A splint must extend past the joint above and below the fracture.
- First aid treatment must always be given for a musculoskeletal injury as if it is a fracture.
- The spinal cord can be damaged by edema, resulting from internal hemorrhage or external pressure from fractured vertebra. Every precaution must be taken to immobilize the victim to prevent a spinal injury from resulting in cord damage.
- The dangers from burn injuries are shock, loss of fluids, and infection.
- In heat emergencies, it is important to cool the victim as soon as possible.
- The greatest danger in the treatment of frostbite is that the part becomes thawed and then refrozen. Severe tissue damage may result.
- Although a victim of hypothermia may appear dead because of low metabolic levels, many victims have been revived.

STUDY QUESTIONS

1. A rapid, weak pulse is an indication of:
   a. Fright
   b. Shock
   c. High blood pressure
   d. A normal finding
2. A tourniquet should be applied:
   a. In any case where there is severe bleeding from an artery
   b. In any case where there is severe bleeding from a vein
   c. As a second step to control bleeding
   d. Only as a last resort, when all other methods have failed to stop bleeding
3. If a finger is amputated, it should be:
   a. Discarded, since it is of no value
   b. Placed in a container of water and sent to the hospital with the victim
   c. Repositioned at the victim's injury site
   d. Wrapped in sterile dressings, covered with a plastic bag filled with ice, and sent to the hospital with the victim
4. In caring for an injured victim, your first consideration should be to:
   a. Care for the burns
   b. Treat for shock
   c. Care for possible fractures
   d. Establish an airway
5. To help prevent shock you should:
   a. Maintain normal body temperature
   b. Keep the victim as warm as possible
   c. Keep the victim as cool as possible
   d. Not worry about body temperature
6. You must stop profuse bleeding from a leg wound. The first procedure would be to:
   a. Apply a tourniquet to the leg above the wound
   b. Apply direct pressure to the wound with a compress
   c. Flush the wound with water
   d. Apply a tourniquet to the leg below the wound
7. You find an unconscious woman in a car that is on fire. She is breathing. Her arm is fractured. She has several lacerations that are bleeding profusely. What do you do first:
   a. Splint the fractured arm
   b. Get her out of the car
   c. Give mouth-to-mouth resuscitation
   d. Stop the bleeding
8. In the situation described above, what do you do next:
   a. Splint the arm
   b. Get her out of the car
   c. Give mouth-to-mouth resuscitation
   d. Stop the bleeding
9. A man fell from a tree. It is uncertain what types of injuries he has sustained. The safest position to treat shock would be:
   a. On his back, with head and shoulders elevated
   b. Lying flat in the position in which he fell
   c. On his back with his head lower than his feet
   d. In a sitting position
10. You find a child with an open bottle of aspirin. What do you do:
    a. Wait for signs and symptoms
    b. Search the label
    c. Call the poison control center
    d. Give large quantities of milk to drink
11. You suspect a fracture in a victim's lower leg. What parts would you keep from moving:
    a. Hip, ankle, fractured bone ends
    b. Ankle, knee, fractured bone ends
    c. Hip, ankle, knee
    d. Spine, hip, ankle
12. Bleeding from most wounds is controlled best and most easily by:
    a. Pressure points
    b. A tourniquet
    c. Direct pressure
    d. A gauze bandage

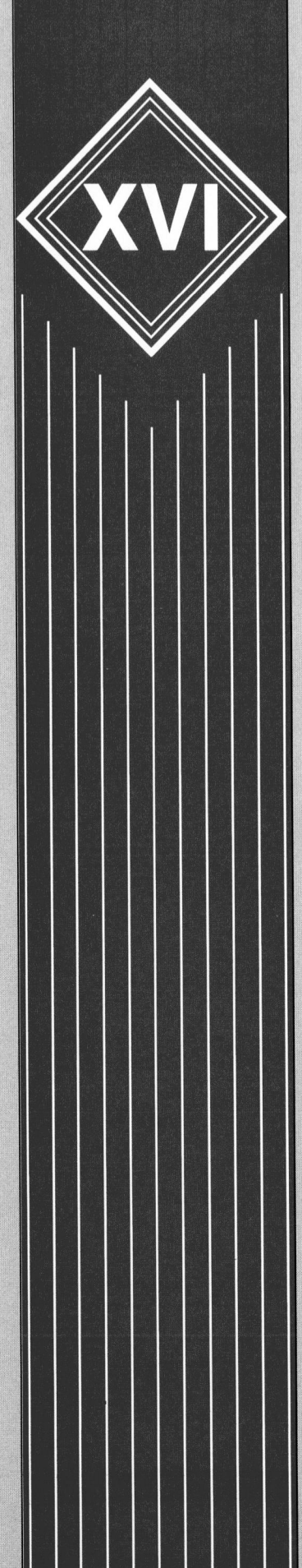

XVI

Dying and Death

I walk into my patient's room and see a person with physical needs. I reach out with all the knowledge my teachers imparted to me and diminish another's pain. I look up into my patient's eyes and see anxiety, fear, inner turmoil. I slow my step to hold a hand, give a smile, offer reassurance, or keep silent and just listen. This to me is the art of nursing. I never know when I step onto the floor what opportunities I will receive each day to lighten someone's burden. I give to my patients, and they give back to me, enriching my life by their presence. In nursing you always receive abundantly more than you give.

LUETTA MCKELVEY
Student Nurse

55

Dying and Death

LINDA RICKEL

LEARNING OBJECTIVES

After reading this chapter, the student should be able to do the following:

- Define the key terms.
- Identify how the changes in the health care system affect nursing care of the dying patient.
- Define grief, loss, and death.
- Explain how the concept of loss impacts on the grief reaction.
- Describe the stages of dying and death.
- Identify needs of the grieving patient and family.
- Recognize the five aspects of human functioning and how each interacts with the others during the grieving/dying process.
- Describe nursing interventions that may facilitate deaths in special circumstances (perinatal, pediatric, geriatric, and suicide).
- Describe techniques in assisting the dying patient to say "goodbyes."
- Identify unique physical symptoms of the near-death patient.
- Discuss nursing interventions that may be helpful to the dying patient.
- Describe nursing responsibilities in care of the body after death.
- Describe approaches in assisting grieving families to expand their social network.
- Explain concepts of euthanasia, DNR, organ donations, fraudulent methods of treatment, and the Dying Person's Bill of Rights.

RELATED TOPICS OF INTEREST

- Legal aspects of nursing (Chapter 2)
- Ethical aspects of nursing (Chapter 3)
- Cultural aspects of nursing care (Chapter 12)
- Home health nursing (Chapter 51)
- Hospice care (Chapter 56)

KEY TERMS

Define the following:

- bereavement
- death
- DNR
- grief
- grief therapy
- grief work
- hospice
- living will
- loss
- mourning
- perinatal death
- postmortem care
- social network
- suicide

Care of dying patients and their families can be one of the most challenging aspects of nursing care. Because dying is the final stage of human growth and development, it is essential that nurses be as knowledgeable about the process of dying as they are about the process of birth. Because health care usually emphasizes the cure of disease and the promotion of health, the death of a patient may represent a form of failure to health care providers. Research in the United States has shown that health care personnel caring for dying patients often withdraw from the patients socially while providing adequate physical care.[5]

When nurses deal with grieving families and dying patients, they are confronted with their own mortality and other discomforting issues that accompany loss. Such factors can influence quality of care. All losses have the possibility of triggering the grief process. The severity of the loss may vary, but the stages of grief that accompany the loss are still present. Understanding loss, the grief process, and the task of dying can assist the nurse in delivering quality care to those patients and families experiencing death.

CHANGES IN HEALTH CARE RELATED TO DYING AND DEATH

Before the 1950s it was common for patients to die at home in their own beds with assistance only from their family. From the 1950s to the 1980s the health care system became very mechanized and dying occurred mostly in institutions and often with very sophisticated machinery attached to the dying individual to prolong life. As recently as 1983 when diagnosis related groups (DRGs) came into play, this trend again changed. Generally, only those persons considered medically at risk for complications or who need immediate hospital recovery time after surgery or special procedures are placed in hospital beds. Currently, the recuperating or terminally ill patient is often discharged to home, convalescent center, or nursing home. Nurses practicing in home health care settings have felt this impact as they provide care to the terminally ill patient. At home these patients are now receiving IV infusions, including blood products, and other technical and mechanical assistance. Nurses in health care facilities and homes are the health care providers most often available to the grieving family during the crisis of death. These nurses are often licensed practical/vocational nurses.

HISTORICAL OVERVIEW

Opportunities to learn the dynamics surrounding grief, **dying,** and death are relatively new. It was in the 1960s that pioneers in death and dying theory, such as Kübler-Ross[11] and Glasser and Strauss[9] produced in this field works that stimulated the health care industry. Dying and death became topics of research and seminars. In the 1970s **hospices** in the United States became recognized as health care delivery systems (see Chapter 56). **Grief therapy** was introduced in the 1980s when Benoliel and Martocchio[5] added new insights into the needs and caring of the dying patient. Care providers are assisting patients and families to become involved in determining treatment options and to choose the setting, circumstances, and management of the dying process.

The future will offer opportunities for individuals to exercise more control over their care as living wills are upheld in courts of law as legal documents and terminal health care shifts away from hospital settings. This shift will continue to provide a primary role for nurses in the care of the dying person at home and the family experiencing loss.

LOSS

When any aspect of one's self is no longer available to a person, that person suffers a **loss.** Not all losses are obvious or immediate. Obvious losses are such events as the death of a loved one, divorce, or breakup of a relationship. Not so obvious are the losses precipitated by illness, aging, and changing schools, jobs, or neighborhoods.

Individuals experience many losses throughout life, and these losses often are related to age. They can occur as one experiences the loss of childhood dreams, the loss as an adolescent when a romance fails, and the loss felt when leaving the family home for college or marriage and establishing a home of one's own. Later as one ages, the individual experiences menopause, retirement, and loss of hair, teeth, hearing, sight, and "youth." All of these losses give the individual experience with loss and promote emotional growth and the activation of coping skills. These skills can later be used to cope with even more significant losses. Early experiences with loss can prepare individuals to deal with loss throughout the life cycle (Table 55-1).

Table 55-1 Losses

Types	Example
Physiological	Loss of body function, body structure, valued physical attribute Loss of body image through loss of extremity or breast
Psychological	Loss of self-esteem, self-concept, self-identity Loss of a job
Sociocultural	Loss of social identity, social role, or family constellation or cultural heritage Loss through divorce Loss of a loved one or significant other caused by death
Material	Loss of possessions, such as money, home, pet, car Loss of home by fire Loss of belongings through theft

TYPES OF LOSS

When death occurs after a long illness, each family member is affected psychologically, socioculturally, and materially. The person experiencing the death is affected in all of these areas, as well as physiologically.

Each person experiences loss as it individually affects him or her. Each loss is followed by a time of grief and grieving.

GRIEVING AND GRIEF

Grief is the subjective response of emotional pain to actual or anticipated loss. Grief is a natural part of human experience. ***Bereavement*** is defined as the experience of having lost something or someone by death. **Mourning** refers to culturally defined patterns for expressions of grief. Mourning patterns include funerals, wakes, memorials, black dress, and defined time of social withdrawal.

Stages of Grief/Dying

The purpose of knowing about the stages of grief and dying is to recognize what emotions and behavior can occur and to plan interventions accordingly as they appear. Kübler-Ross' *Stages of Dying*[11] and Martocchio's *Manifestations of Grief*[14] are essential for the nurses' understanding of the human reactions to the dying process (Table 55-2). The grief theory models seem to demonstrate that in the normal grief process, there is an onset, active grief work, and a resolution or reorganization of the survivors' lives after the loss.

Supportive Care During the Dying/Grieving Process

To give compassionate nursing care and support to the family and patient during both the grieving and dying process, the nurse should consider the five aspects of human functioning. By using the nursing process, the nurse does an assessment in each aspect: physical, emotional, intellectual, sociocultural, and spiritual, to fully understand and adequately provide interventions in these areas.

Physical. While interviewing and observing the patient, the nurse should assess such areas as sleeping patterns, body image, activities of daily living (ADLs), mobility,

Table 55-2 Reactions to the Dying Process

	Stage	Reaction	Description
PATIENT			
Kübler-Ross*:			
Stages of grieving/dying	Denial and isolation	"No—not me." "There must be a mistake."	Serves as a buffer to the patient to shield oneself until the individual is able to mobilize alternate defenses.
	Anger	"Why me?"	Hostility may be directed toward caregivers or loved ones.
	Bargaining	"Yes, but"	Bargaining is often made with God. It is an attempt to postpone death and is a positive way to maintain hope.
	Depression	"Yes, me"	Sadness and grief. Time of introspection. Usually request only significant others to be with them. The patient struggles with painful realities of life and preparing for death.
	Acceptance	"I am ready."	Resolved to the fact that death is imminent. Peaceful acceptance and positive feelings are often present.
SURVIVORS			
Martocchio†:			
Manifestations of grief and bereavement	Shock and disbelief	"Maybe this is not happening." "This is just a dream/nightmare."	Survivors feel a sense of unreality. Often reject offers of comfort and support. Disbelief may remain even though death is comprehended intellectually.
	Yearning and protest	"Why do I feel this way?"	Survivors may express anger toward the deceased for leaving them.
	Anguish, disorganization, and despair	"Living is a chore." "All the joy is gone out of life."	Reality and permanency of the loss is recognized.
	Identification in bereavement	"I am just like him (dying or dead person)." "I will carry on her (dying person) goals."	Bereaved may adopt behavior, ideals, mannerisms, or goals of the deceased.
	Reorganization and restitution	"Life goes on." "The sun has risen on a new day."	Life stabilizes but some of the pain of loss may last for a lifetime.

*From Beck CK, Rawlings R, and Williams S: Mental health–psychiatric nursing: a holistic life-cycle approach, ed 2, St Louis, 1988, The CV Mosby Co.
†From Martocchio B: Grief and bereavement healing through hurt, Nurs Clin North Am 20(2):327, 1985.

general health, medications, and pain. The nurse also should address the basic needs of nutrition, elimination, oxygenation, activity, rest, sleep, and safety.

Goals for interventions should be (1) energy conservation, (2) pain reduction techniques, (3) comfort measures, (4) promotion of sleep and rest, and (5) increasing self-esteem through body image acceptance.

Emotional. Preparing for one's death is a personal endeavor filled with anxiety and fear.[16] Assessing the patient and family's anxiety level, guilt, anger, level of acceptance, and identification is important. Major fears of the dying patient include fears of abandonment, loss of control, pain and discomfort, and the fear of the unknown.

The nurses can intervene appropriately when they are able to accept the patient and family's individual feelings, offer encouragement and support, and give the patient "permission to die" by assisting the patient in saying "good-bye."

Intellectual. Intellectual assessment includes an evaluation of the patient and family's educational level, their knowledge and abilities, and expectations they have in regard to how and when death will occur. Some aspects of the intellectual dimension can be altered during the dying process because of physiological changes, medications, the patient's emotional state, or the disease process. Being alert to these changes will avert problems if the patient's memory or sensations are decreased.

Intervention is directed toward patient/family education and support. Keeping all informed of procedures, changes in condition of the patient, and hospital policies contributes to well-informed decisions being made when necessary.

Social. Assessing the patient and family's support systems is valuable. Ascertaining if family members desire to assist in the patient's daily care will not only lessen the family's sense of loss of control but also will clarify what tasks the family will do and what will be done by nursing staff. Not making these needs and desires clear can result in distrust and hostility between family and nursing staff. Each family and each individual member in that family are unique in what they wish to do. The nurse should never assume that families *want* to deliver daily care. Many do, but others do not, and they need the opportunity to make that choice.

During the social assessment, it is necessary to learn whom the patient considers significant others. Although families are considered important, it is crucial to learn whom the patient considers the most supportive person in his or her life. It may be a friend, coworker, or church member. This person should become a part of the patient's supportive network and be included in planning the patient's care. The nurse encourages these social support persons to become involved and at the same time

NURSING CARE PLAN: PERSON FACING DEATH

Mrs. Hannah is 64 years old and has been admitted to the hospital for weakness and debilitation caused by widespread metastatic cancer of the colon. She is anxious to return home, and both she and her family are aware of her terminal state.

The nursing history identified that (1) she is unable to care for herself because of severe weakness, (2) she appears anxious and wants to be home with her family, and (3) she is grieving the loss of her health and expresses fears regarding her death.

GOAL: Prevent injury, assure safety, and provide for activities of daily living, including adequate nutrition, hydration, and elimination.

Nursing diagnoses	Patient goals	Nursing interventions
Bathing/hygiene, dressing, toileting self-care deficit, related to advanced disease	Patient will carry out ADLs at highest ability.	Provide assistance with basic ADLs but allow patient/family to assist when able. Provide sufficient time for ADLs.
Severe anxiety, related to impending death	Patient will verbalize statements that reflect anxiety.	Allow patient to verbalize feeling and concerns. Explore how patient sees the dying event. Teach family members how to offer support effectively.
Social isolation, related to hospitalization	Patient will be reunited with family.	Allow family to visit as much as possible. Involve patient in group activities.
Grieving, related to deteriorating health	Patient will be able to verbalize feelings of loss.	Allow patient to express feelings, including anger. Assist patient in identifying positive aspects of her life that can be used now.

maintains and promotes the patient's independence whenever possible.

Spiritual. The nurse assesses the spiritual dimension by gaining insight into the patient's philosophy of life, his religious resources, and how the rituals of his faith group have significance in dealing with his death.

Interventions in this area can come from clergy, friends, family, health care providers, and significant others. Supporting the patient and family's belief system and values is important (Chapter 12). By completing the nursing process of assessment, diagnosis, planning, implementation, and evaluation, the nurse can develop a nursing care plan as shown on p. 1386.

Special supportive care. Often death occurs outside the realm of serious illness, injury, or aging. Perinatal, pediatric, suicidal, and geriatric deaths are some examples that warrant special consideration.

Perinatal death. The death of a child is often viewed as one of the most devastating losses that can occur in a family. If the death of the child occurs before, during, or shortly after birth, it is called **perinatal death.**

Special considerations by health care providers should be addressed so that the parents and family can grieve adequately. Because there are no or few memories that loved ones can share about the child, "acting as though it never happened" places parents in jeopardy of living with unresolved grief. When possible, the parents should see, touch, and hold the infant, so that the reality of the situation can be faced and resolution of the grief can occur. Listening attentively and allowing the parents to express their feelings over their loss is beneficial. Referring to the baby as "your baby," "your son," or "your daughter," or using the given name can reinforce that the baby was indeed a unique individual who was loved and will be missed. The usual cultural rituals after death should take place for the baby, such as a funeral or memorial service.

Pediatric death. Children faced with death present a need for special nursing skills. Nurses should be aware of how children view or understand death, both for themselves and for others[3] (Box 55-1).

BOX 55-1 CHILDREN'S BELIEFS ABOUT DEATH

AGE (Years)	BELIEF SYSTEM
3	See death as a separation. Unable to comprehend permanency.
3 to 5	Fear death but see it as reversible. View death as a loss of an object.
6 to 10	Generally see death as permanent. Often have morbid feelings about death. Fear pain and mutilation.
11 to 18	Recognize death as permanent and irreversible. Attitudes and beliefs greatly influenced by parents. Often act as if they are invincible.

Children facing death are usually aware that they are going to die. They often try to protect their parents. They need to be told the truth in language they can understand and be allowed to share their fears, feelings, and opinions.

Parents and loved ones have much difficulty in accepting the reality of a child's impending death. Death of a child is an "out of sequence" death and therefore is often more difficult to accept. Parents often harbor extreme guilt. They may express hostility and anger toward health care providers, God, or the world in general. When a grandchild is dying, the grandparents suffer a double grief—for themselves and for their son or daughter. Siblings also are extremely affected and need much support at this time. Supportive group therapy is often beneficial for the survivors after a child's death, as well as during the dying process.

Suicide. Survivors of **suicide** suffer all the emotions of grief, in addition to profound guilt or shame. Because of this, they are at high risk for suicide themselves, and a grief counselor may be very helpful. Because suicide is usually not considered acceptable, many families of suicide victims are not given the same support from the church, community, or workplace as those whose loved ones have died from other causes. Because of the family's anger, fear, and shame, others do not reach out to help them.[8]

Geriatric death. It is often assumed that the elderly will display some understanding and acceptance toward the death process. This is not always true. The elderly patient must be treated as an individual, and the nurse should assess the patient's needs in the same way as for any patient facing a terminal illness. It is important to include the elderly person in his or her own care and in decisions to undergo or refuse extensive therapeutic or resuscitative measures. Even when aggressive technological options are rejected, patients still need to have intensive nursing care and pain control. Families who suffer the loss of an elderly person may accept the death but nonetheless must experience the grieving process.

Other considerations in caring for dying patients include such issues as euthanasia, DNR, organ donations, fraudulent treatment methods, and the Dying Person's Bill of Rights.

ISSUES RELATED TO DYING AND DEATH

Euthanasia

Euthanasia (*Gk,* easy death) is the relatively painless killing or permitting of death of a terminally ill person for reasons of mercy, sometimes referred to as *mercy killing*. Nurses face legal or ethical issues when dealing with the terminally ill patient in regards to prolonging life by artificial means.

Euthanasia is sometimes considered when death is inevitable and there is no chance of returning to a functioning life situation. Active euthanasia is considered a crime and is illegal in the United States.

Do Not Resuscitate

Patients and families should control any decisions relative to any conditions that withhold or withdraw treatment. Death with dignity remains a concern for all. A do not resuscitate (**DNR**) decision should be a joint decision of the patient, family, and health care providers. All facts regarding the patient's condition should be explained to the patient and family, as well as all treatment options. DNR means *only* not to resuscitate. It does not mean to withhold any other care, such as hygiene, nutrition, fluids, or medications.[4] All DNR orders and the discussion with the patient and family should be thoroughly documented in the patient's chart (Box 55-2).

Some patients request or have a **living will**, which describes their wishes regarding their medical care. This document can assist the family and health care providers in carrying out an individual's wishes. In some states the living will is legally binding. Courts in some states where living wills are not recognized as legal documents have upheld treatment decisions that a competent, rational adult has made for himself.

Organ Donations

Patients and families also have the right to give permission before the patient's death for organ donations upon death. Nurses often are present when such requests are given. Organs cannot be bought or sold, and all donations must be voluntary. These donations can include the following:

BODY ORGANS	BODY TISSUE
kidney	cornea
heart	bone
lung	skin
heart-lung	heart valve
liver	
pancreas	

BOX 55-2 **LEGAL ISSUES**

Characteristics of Acceptable Do Not Resuscitate (DNR) Orders

A medical order **not** to resuscitate a patient is an acceptable order when:

- The order is documented in the written medical record
- The order specifies the exact nature of the treatment to be withheld
- Patients, when they are able, and families participate in the decision
- The decision not to resuscitate is discussed with caregivers, including the nurses
- The order is periodically reviewed
- Staff realize the order is not equivalent to medical or psychological abandonment of patients

Do not resuscitate (DNR) orders are commonly understood to mean the withholding of CPR, which is used to treat cardiac arrest. It involves external chest compression and some form of artificial respiration. Because of potential misunderstanding of what the DNR order specifically means, it is advisable that the DNR order be written identifying the exact condition not to be treated and the specific intervention to be withheld. The practice of not writing the DNR order is unacceptable. In fact, the medical record, read as a whole, should reveal the clear responsibility for the DNR order, the rationale for it, and the process used in its formulation. Some hospitals and nursing homes may have more specific requirements in their policies that the medical/surgical nurse should follow.

Every competent adult has the right to refuse treatment, even life-sustaining procedures, such as CPR. The patient's informed consent should be obtained by the physician who will write the order, and should be documented in the medical record. Or, if unable to consent, the patient's family participation should be sought and documented. The patient's incapacity to participate must also be documented to reflect the rationale for involving the family. In some states the law may be that when it is two physicians' opinion that a patient lacks capacity to consent, a surrogate is sought from a list provided in the law. That surrogate must consent to the DNR order.

DNR orders must be reviewed periodically, because the patient's status may change or new knowledge may come to light about the patient's condition. Continual review of the DNR order helps reassure staff that they are not abandoning the patient; it will also ensure that the "hopeless" patient is still cared for.

Fraudulent Methods of Treatment

Often patient and family seek unconventional methods of treatment to prolong the patient's life. Such treatments may include special diets, enemas, unproven drugs, and machines or devices. Nurses may assist patients and families in sorting out which treatments are real and which are fraudulent. Fraudulent treatments are those that are misrepresented, whether by concealment or nondisclosure of facts, for the purpose of inducing another to use the product. Any treatment that does not offer the patient informed consent with information regarding options, results, and approvals from federal agencies should be suspect.

BOX 55-3 THE DYING PERSON'S BILL OF RIGHTS

I have the right to be treated as a living human being until I die.

I have the right to maintain a sense of hopefulness however changing its focus may be.

I have the right to be cared for by those who can maintain a sense of hopefulness, however changing this might be.

I have the right to express my feelings and emotions about my approaching death in my own way.

I have the right to participate in decisions concerning my care.

I have the right to expect continuing medical and nursing attention even though "cure" goals must be changed to "comfort" goals.

I have the right not to die alone.

I have the right to be free from pain.

I have the right to have my questions answered honestly.

I have the right not to be deceived.

I have the right to have help from and for my family in accepting my death.

I have the right to die in peace and dignity.

I have the right to retain my individuality and not be judged for my decisions which may be contrary to beliefs of others.

I have the right to discuss and enlarge my religious and/or spiritual experiences, whatever these may mean to others.

I have the right to expect that the sanctity of the human body will be respected after death.

I have the right to be cared for by caring, sensitive, knowledgeable people who will attempt to understand my needs and will be able to gain some satisfaction in helping me face my death.

From Barbus A: The dying patient's bill of rights, Am J Nurs, p. 99. Jan. 1975.

Rights of Dying Patients

Death with dignity is the goal in caring for the dying patient. Box 55-3 shows the Dying Person's Bill of Rights.

THE DYING PATIENT

Assisting the Patient in Saying Good-bye

Many terminally ill patients are fully aware that they are dying. One of their most difficult tasks is in the "saying of good-byes" to their loved ones. Saying good-bye acknowledges leaving and may be expressed in verbal, nonverbal, concrete, and symbolic ways. By working through these tasks, the family members are moving toward the completion of unfinished business with the patient. Unfinished business will compound the transition through the grieving process. This is an area where nurses can assist the dying person and the family. (See therapeutic dialogue.)

First, the nurse can provide a private, comfortable environment. The patient may request that the nurse or another health care provider be present or very nearby to be of assistance if emotional expression becomes overwhelming. Patients can be assisted in saying their good-byes through role playing, letter writing, or audio or video recording. Helping patients focus on what they want to say can be facilitated by asking them to talk to their loved ones as if they were going to be separated for

THERAPEUTIC DIALOGUE

■ Family Support

FAMILY MEMBER: I can't go back in that room. He just lies there and stares. I don't know what to do or say.

NURSE: Being near someone who is dying can be uncomfortable.

FAMILY MEMBER: It makes me so sad to see him like that. Do you think he knows I'm there?

NURSE: It's very possible that he does. Would you like me to go in with you?

FAMILY MEMBER: Yes, please. I wonder if he can hear me?

NURSE: It must be very difficult for you not to be certain that he is hearing you. If there is something you want to say to him, get close, take his hand, and speak directly to him. Most people in his condition can hear but are very weak and may not have the strength to respond.

FAMILY MEMBER: I just feel like I am not able to do anything for him anymore.

NURSE: Just being there is letting him know that you care. That's something very important to any person.

FAMILY MEMBER: I suppose you're right. I guess I'm ready to go in now. You will stay close, won't you?

NURSE: Yes, I'll be right here next to you.

a long time. They should be encouraged to express those feelings and thoughts they would most want their loved ones to know in their absence. Asking a dying person what he would want to say to his 6-year-old when the child is 12 can help the patient formulate appropriate letters or tape recordings. Often dying patients become depressed because they do not have a purpose in life. Working on tasks, such as poems, letters, and recordings, affords patients feelings of control and productivity in their last days.

Physical Care

The nurse has an important responsibility in assisting patients to meet their physical needs. Providing adequate nutrition and maintaining elimination patterns are priorities in providing for the dying patient's physical needs (see Chapter 56). Keeping the patient clean, dry, well groomed, odor free, and comfortable decreases the chances of skin breakdown and also provides the patient with feelings of self-esteem and self-worth.

Adjusting the environment to increase comfort and safety is paramount. Siderails should be used for both safety and assisting weak patients to adjust their own positions when possible.

Assessments and Interventions for the Dying Patient

Care of the dying patient has many facets. The core of nursing interventions in the care of the dying focuses on communication, relief of symptoms and pain, knowledge of available resources, facilitation of problem solving, and fostering involvement in and control of decisions affecting the patient's care.

The patient near death continues to need meticulous nursing interventions. Because of the increased weakness and deterioration of the body, the patient's physical needs are important. Although patients may appear comatose, unconscious, or unresponsive, this appearance is often a result of extreme fatigue, and the nurse will find that patients are aware of those activities occurring around them. Table 55-3 shows signs of approaching death as expressed in physical needs and the appropriate interventions.

Changes in vital signs include (1) slow, weak, and thready pulse, (2) lowered blood pressure, and (3) rapid, shallow, irregular, or abnormally slow respirations. Mouth breathing occurs, which leads to dry oral mucous membranes. The patient often has a detached look in the eyes. There is a diminished sensory and motor function in the lower extremities, progressing to the upper extremities. There is diminished touch sensation; pressure and pain sensations remain intact. As death becomes imminent, the pupils will become dilated and fixed, Cheyne-Stokes respirations will occur, the pulse will become increasingly weaker and more rapid, and the blood pressure will continue to fall. There is diminished peripheral circulation. The skin is cool and clammy; profuse diaphoresis may occur. If collection of mucus occurs in the throat, noisy respirations will be heard. This noise is referred to as the *death rattle*. A period of peace may immediately precede the moment of death. The clinical signs of death are the following:

1. Unreceptivity and unresponsibility
2. No movement or breathing
3. No reflexes
4. Flat encephalogram
5. Absence of apical pulse
6. Cessation of respirations

Table 55-3 Nursing Interventions for the Patient Near Death

Physical Needs	Nursing Interventions
1. Decreased sensations and reflexes	1. Good skin care and range-of-motion exercises
2. Decreased circulation	2. Frequent positioning
3. Decreased sphincter control (urinary and bowel incontinence)	3. Meticulous hygiene and skin care
4. Decreased hearing and sight	4. Clear and slow verbal communication; stand within patient's vision
5. Decreased need for pain medication	5. Evaluate and differentiate between pain and anxiety
6. Increased need for touch	6. Touch gently
7. Usually conscious	7. Involve patient in care; explain all actions

Postmortem Care

When the patient has been pronounced dead by a physician or professional nurse, the nurse assumes the responsibility of caring for the body **(postmortem care)**. During this phase of care, the nurse cleans, identifies, and positions the body by following the facility's procedure (Skill 55-1). At the time of death, the nurse must also make notation of any valuables, such as watch, rings, or money, and secure these articles so that they may be delivered to the family according to facility policy.

Documentation

Documentation of the care given to the dying patient must be objective, complete, legible, and accurate. As death approaches, documentation should be frequent and include the signs of impending death as they occur. Re-

SKILL 55-1 CARE OF THE BODY AFTER DEATH

1. Gather equipment to organize procedure.
2. Wash hands to reduce number of organisms.
3. Don clean gloves to protect nurse from contamination.
4. Close patient's eyes and mouth if needed to provide a more normal appearance.
5. Remove all tubings and other devices from patient's body to make patient look more peaceful.
6. Place patient in supine position for access for procedures.
7. Replace soiled dressings with clean ones to avoid odor.
8. Bathe patient as necessary to reduce odor.
9. Brush or comb hair for more normal appearance.
10. Apply clean gown for appearance.
11. Care for valuables and personal belongings for legal considerations.
12. Allow family to view body and remain in room to provide emotional support.
13. After the family has left the room, attach special label if patient had a contagious disease to protect those who handle the body.
14. Close door to room to prevent exposure to patients and visitors.
15. Await arrival of ambulance or transfer to morgue out of respect for patient.
16. Document procedure and disposition of patient's body for legal documentation.

cording who was present at the time of the patient's death is important. The nurse should continue to chart until the last entry states where and to whom the body was transferred.

SUPPORT OF THE GRIEVING FAMILY

The grieving family and significant others' needs should be met by a caring, compassionate health care provider. If an individual is alone at the time of the loved one's death, it is essential that all attempts be made to contact someone—family, clergy, or friends—to be with the grieving individual. Words that convey sympathy should be expressed, and if appropriate, a spontaneous touch, such as a hand on the arm or embrace, can be used as a comforting gesture. Any questions should be answered, and the family should be encouraged to view, touch, and talk to the dead family member. Be nonjudgmental as the individual expresses anger, guilt, or unfairness. Assist in notifying the mortician and any individuals involved in the procurement of donated organs.

Informing others can be a major emotional step for family members. Being present and offering assistance in this area can be very supportive. Directing family members to support groups and other referral agencies (churches, therapists, social workers) will facilitate the expansion of the family's **social network,** as well as foster relatedness and decrease isolation.

Grief work as described by Martocchio is as follows[14]:

1. Emancipation of the bereaved from bondage to the deceased
2. Readjustment to an altered environment
3. Development of new or renewed relationships
4. Learning to live in a comfortable fashion with memories of hurt, happiness, suffering, and joys associated with the deceased

EVALUATION CRITERIA FOR THE GRIEVING FAMILY

Resolution of grief has begun when, after the loss, the grieving person and/or family can complete the following tasks[15]:

1. Have positive interactions with others
2. Participate in support groups with others similarly bereaved to share expressions of loss and offer companionship
3. Establish goals, and work to achieve them
4. Discuss the meaning of the loss and its effect on the person's life

Dealing with the grief that comes with the loss of a loved one requires support and understanding. Six months to 2 years may elapse before an individual can complete his or her grief work and begin the full process of resolution.

REFERENCES AND SUGGESTED READINGS

1. Barbus A: The dying person's bill of rights, Am J Nurs, p. 99, Jan 1975.
2. Beare P and Myers J: Principles and practice of adult health nursing, St. Louis, 1990, The CV Mosby Co.
3. Beck CK, Rawlins R, and Williams S: Mental health—psychiatric nursing: a holistic life-cycle approach, ed 2, St. Louis, 1988, The CV Mosby Co.
4. Bedell SE and others: Do not resuscitate orders for critically ill patients in the hospital: how are they used and what is their impact? JAMA 256(2):233, 1986.

5. Benoliel JQ: Loss and terminal illness, Nurs Clin North Am 20(2):439, 1985.
6. Conboy-Hill S: Psychosocial aspects of terminal care: a preliminary study of nurses' attitudes and behavior in a general hospital, Int Nurs Rev 33(1):19, 1986.
7. Crispell K and Gomez C: Proper care for the dying: a critical public issue, J Med Ethics 13(2):74, 1987.
8. Glasser BG and Strauss AL: Awareness of dying, Chicago, 1965, Aldine Publishing Co.
9. Johnson R: Documenting patients' end-of-life decisions, Nurse Pract 13(6):41, 45, 52, 1988.
10. Kübler-Ross E: On death and dying, New York, 1969, Macmillan Publishing Co.
11. Kübler-Ross E: To live until we say good-bye, Englewood Cliffs, NJ, 1978, Prentice Hall Press.
12. Martocchio B: Authenticity, belonging, emotional closeness, and self-representation, Oncol Nurs Forum 14(4):23, 1987.
13. Martocchio B: Grief and bereavement healing through hurt, Nurs Clin North Am 20(2):327, 1985.
14. McIntosh JL and others: Suicide and its aftermath: understanding and counseling the survivors, New York, 1987, WW Norton & Co., Inc.
15. Rawlins R and Heacock P: Clinical manual of psychiatric nursing, St. Louis, 1988, The CV Mosby Co.
16. Rickel L and others: Therapy with dying clients. In Beck C, Rawlins R, and Williams S, editors: Mental health-psychiatric nursing, ed 2, St. Louis, 1988, The CV Mosby Co.
17. Ross-Aloalmolki K: Supportive care for families of dying children, Nurs Clin North Am 20(2):457, 1985.
18. Rouse F: Legal and ethical guidelines for physicians in geriatric terminal care, Geriatrics 43(8):69, 1988.

CHAPTER CHALLENGE

KEY POINTS

- Care of the dying patient has moved from the home to hospitals and back again over the past 50 years.
- In 1969 Kübler-Ross was instrumental in identifying the five stages of death and dying: denial, anger, bargaining, depression, and acceptance.
- Losses occur thoughout the life cycle and provide the individual experience with loss and promote emotional growth and development of coping skills.
- The effect a loss will have on a person is individualized and may be determined by duration, abruptness, extent, time required for treatment or replacement, or financial impact of the loss.
- The major concerns of the dying patient are (1) fears of abandonment, (2) fears of loss of control, (3) fears of pain and discomfort, and (4) fears of the unknown.
- Special considerations by health care providers should be extended to those families suffering perinatal, pediatric, geriatric, or suicidal deaths.
- Euthanasia is an ethical and legal issue faced by nurses. Active euthanasia is illegal in the United States.
- A do not resuscitate (DNR) order means only that. It does not mean to withhold hygiene, hydration, nutrition, or medications.
- The Dying Person's Bill of Rights speaks to the elements that may characterize dying with dignity.
- Assisting a patient in saying his "good-byes" is an intervention nurses can initiate.
- The physical care requirements of the dying patient are primarily nursing responsibilities. Providing adequate nutrition, elimination, hygiene, safety, and comfort are nursing priorities.
- Continuing to speak to and include the patient in his or her care is essential, since as death approaches, the dying patient becomes weaker. Patients may appear comatose and yet be aware of activities around them.
- Signs of impending death are (1) slow, thready and weaker pulse, (2) lowered blood pressure, (3) rapid shallow, irregular, or abnormally slow respirations, and (4) mottling of lower extremities.
- Postmortem care is the care administered to the body after death. Skill procedures should be followed. The skills include cleansing, positioning, and labeling the body.
- When caring for the dying patient, the nurses' responsibility frequently includes the family. Once death has occurred, the nurse can assist the grieving family in informing others, seeking counseling or support groups, and expanding their social network.

STUDY QUESTIONS

1. Dying is considered:
   a. Undesirable at any time
   b. A failure for the nurse
   c. Impossible with modern medical devices
   d. The final stage of human growth and development
2. Grief work is completed:
   a. When the family returns to work, school, and other social activities
   b. After the funeral, wake, or memorial service
   c. As soon as the bereaved can talk freely
   d. On an individualized schedule
3. All the following statements are true about loss except:
   a. Losses occur throughout the life cycle
   b. Experiencing losses is an opportunity for growth
   c. All losses are obvious
   d. Loss is followed by grief
4. Which of the following defines *living wills*:
   a. The will to live
   b. A nationally recognized legal document
   c. A document written by a person describing his or her wishes regarding medical care
   d. A family's request to prolong the life of a dying person
5. Kübler-Ross' stages of death and dying are:
   a. Grief, loss, fear, and pain
   b. Denial, anger, bargaining, depression, and acceptance
   c. Denial, grief, loss, isolation, and acceptance
   d. Denial, isolation, bargaining, and resolution
6. Perinatal death refers to:
   a. The death of an infant before, during, or shortly after birth
   b. The death of a child
   c. The death of a family member
   d. The death of anyone who has donated organs
7. Euthanasia is a term that can be defined as:
   a. Prolonging life by artificial means
   b. An easy death
   c. Suffering from an incurable condition
   d. Presence of flat electroencephalogram
8. Postmortem care is:
   a. Death occurring at home
   b. Care of the body after death
   c. Care given to family members
   d. Physician pronouncing the patient dead
9. The following statement is true in supporting family members after the death of a patient:
   a. Do not touch the family in any way
   b. Express words of sympathy, and offer other assistance
   c. Reassure them that the patient "is at peace"
   d. Refer all questions to the physician

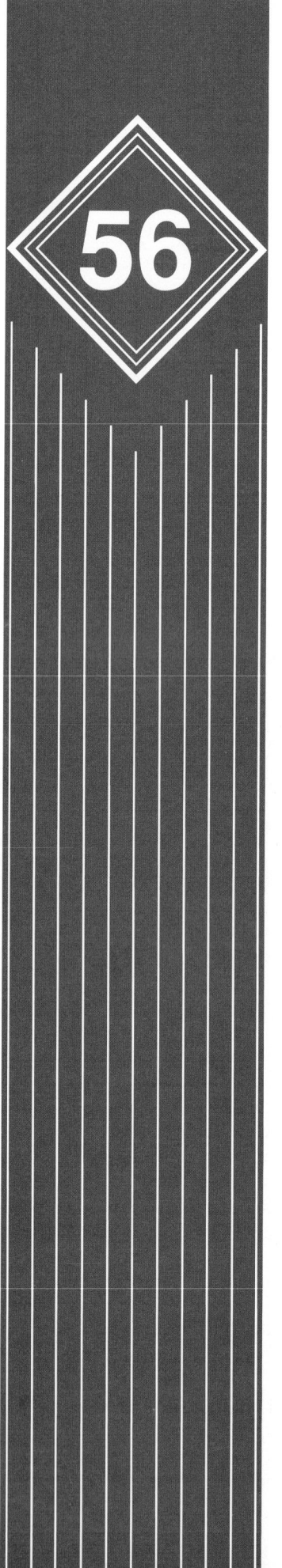

56

Hospice Care

JOSEPHINE M. ESTRADA

LEARNING OBJECTIVES

After reading this chapter, the student should be able to do the following:

- Define the key terms.
- Differentiate between curative and palliative care.
- Define the term *hospice*.
- Define the philosophy of hospice care.
- List three requirements for hospice admission.
- List the roles of the interdisciplinary team.
- List three common symptoms related to the terminally ill.
- Develop a care plan with nursing goals related to these symptoms.
- Discuss two ethical issues in hospice care.
- List three common hospice settings.
- Identify the role of hospice in the family's bereavement period.

RELATED TOPICS OF INTEREST

- Ethical aspects of nursing (Chapter 3)
- Care of the patient with cancer (Chapter 41)
- Home health nursing (Chapter 51)
- Dying and death (Chapter 55)

KEY TERMS

Define the following:

- bereavement
- curative
- holistic care
- hospice
- interdisciplinary hospice team
- pain
- palliative
- primary caregiver
- psychosocial
- respite
- spiritual
- stomatitis
- TENS

HOSPICE MOVEMENT

Hospice is a philosophy of care that has been revived during the past decade. The concept originated in Europe and now has spread throughout the world. **Hospice** is from the Latin word *hospitium,* meaning hospitality, lodging. It is defined as a resting place for travelers on a difficult journey.

In the middle ages, hospices were places of refuge for the poor and the sick and for travelers on religious journeys. Hospices emerged because the religious orders of monks and nuns believed that service to one's neighbor was a sign of love and dedication to God. A typical medieval hospice was a combination guest house and infirmary, providing food, shelter, and illness care to the guests until they were refreshed and renewed for their journey or until they died. One of the earliest hospices was founded around AD 450 in Syria. Many hospices were established across Europe and to the Mediterranean region. In the late nineteenth and early twentieth centuries, religious groups started hospices in Dublin and London to care for the poor. As centuries passed, these hospices grew into hospitals as the religious concept gradually became dissociated from medical care.

The concept was renewed in the 1960s in London by Cicely Saunders, a nurse who later became a physician. Because of her interest in persons who were terminally ill with cancer, she became intensely involved in improving methods of pain control. She began her work at St. Joseph's Hospice, operated by the Irish Sisters of Charity. In 1968 she opened St. Christopher's Hospice of London, which has become a model for modern hospice care. This hospice offers in-patient care, home care, and bereavement services. It also serves as a national and international education, training, and research center for professionals involved in the hospice approach to terminal care.

Hospice migrated to the United States in the early 1970s. Since then, physicians, nurses, clergy, social workers, and many other nonprofessional volunteers have worked together to develop more than 800 hospice programs in the United States. There are five identifiable kinds of hospices:

1. Free-standing: this type is not connected to a hospital but offers inpatient care, as well as home care.
2. Inpatient: this is also known as *hospital-associated* and is a separate section within the hospital.
3. Home health agency hospice: care is provided in the home with a close family member or significant other as a primary caregiver. Visiting nurses make home visits to coordinate care.
4. The roving hospice team: the roving hospice team works with dying patients wherever they are located. They do not have any designated beds.
5. Hospital-based and medical school affiliation: this type of hospice program is located within a hospital and is associated with a medical school.

ISSUES AND RESPONSES OF THE TERMINALLY ILL

When a patient with a life-threatening illness has exhausted all treatment and the disease has not been arrested or cured, he must decide whether continued active therapy is feasible or beneficial. By this time, he may have already experienced many debilitating physical and emotional symptoms caused by the treatments or the progressive disease itself. Not all terminally ill patients experience all symptoms, but all have experienced at least some symptoms at one time or another.

At this point, when decisions for the appropriate type of care must be made, it is important to establish an honest and open communication among the patient, family, and physician. The patient's total physical, psychosocial, and spiritual needs are evaluated and openly discussed by those involved in the care. Dying and death are now realities affecting family roles, life-style patterns, and future goals. This total situation leads to deciding between palliative care and further **curative** measures. **Palliative** care is alleviating or controlling those symptoms that create physical, psychosocial, or spiritual distress. It stresses quality of life and is directed toward living life to the fullest until death occurs naturally.

HOSPICE APPROACH

Hospice care becomes appropriate when active treatment is no longer effective and supportive measures are needed to assist the terminally ill patient through the dying process. It offers the dying person a safe passage from life to death in a way that preserves dignity and important relationships. Not every terminally ill patient is suited to this type of care, because there are families and patients who choose to fight for life until the end. Hospice is appropriate mainly for those individuals who feel that the quality of life is more important and vital than the length of life.

To provide effective hospice care, an understanding of the philosophy and its relationship with the patient's responses and points of view is needed. The basic goals of hospice address the following:

1. Controlling or alleviating symptoms
2. Allowing the patient and family to be involved in decision making to maintain dignity
3. Encouraging both the patient and family to live life as fully as possible
4. Providing continuous support to maintain confidence and reassurance to achieve those goals

This approach is defined as **holistic care,** because it focuses on physical, psychosocial, and spiritual issues, using an interdisciplinary team to provide this care. Specific standards of practice have been adopted by the National Hospice Organization as official guidelines in hospice care (Box 56-1).

BOX 56-1 NATIONAL HOSPICE ORGANIZATION STANDARDS

1. Appropriate therapy is the goal of Hospice care.
2. Palliative care is the most appropriate form of care when cure is no longer possible.
3. The goal of palliative care is the prevention of distress from chronic signs and symptoms.
4. Admission to a Hospice program of care is dependent on patient and family needs and their expressed request for care.
5. Hospice care consist of a blending of professional and non-professional services.
6. Hospice care considers all aspects of the lives of patients and their families as valid areas of therapeutic concern.
7. Hospice care is respectful of all patient and family belief systems, and will employ resources to meet the personal philosophic, moral, and religious needs of patients and their families.
8. Hospice care provides continuity of care.
9. A Hospice care program considers the patient and the family together as the unit of care.
10. The patient's family is considered to be a central part of the Hospice care team.
11. Hospice care programs seek to identify, coordinate and supervise persons who can give care to patients who do not have a family member available to take on the responsibility of giving care.
12. Hospice care for the family continues into the bereavement period.
13. Hospice care is available 24 hours a day, 7 days a week.
14. Hospice care is provided by an interdisciplinary team.
15. Hospice programs will have structured and informal means of providing support to staff.
16. Hospice programs will be in compliance with the standards of the NHO and the applicable laws and regulations governing the organization and delivery of care to patients and families.
17. The services of the Hospice program are coordinated under a central administration.
18. The optimal control of distressful symptoms is an essential part of a Hospice care program requiring medical, nursing and other services of the interdisciplinary team.
19. The Hospice care team will have:
    a. a medical director on staff
    b. physicians on staff
    c. a working relationship with the patient's physician
20. Based on patient's needs and preferences as determining factors in the setting and location for care, a Hospice program provides in-patient care and care in the home-setting.
21. Education, training and evaluation of Hospice services is an ongoing activity of Hospice care programs.
22. Accurate and current records are kept on all patients.

To assist the dying patient, the team considers not only the patient but also his family regarding decisions affecting care. Hospice considers the patient and family as a unit, because families experience the stresses of dying as much as the patient. Stress extends into the **bereavement** period after the patient dies. To be admitted into the program for care, established criteria are considered:

1. There must be medical direction, and the physician of the patient must approve and willingly participate in the plan of care. The physician must also certify that the patient's disease is life threatening and that curative measures are no longer feasible.
2. The patient and family must agree to participate in this type of service.
3. The patient and family must understand and agree that care will be planned according to comfort and that life support measures may not necessarily be performed.

Also important is the availability of a **primary caregiver.** This person is usually a member of the immediate family or can be a significant other. This person becomes vital when the patient can no longer care for himself safely. A primary caregiver is essential if hospice services are provided in the patient's home, but if the services are provided in a free-standing or inpatient facility, the primary caregivers are the staff working in the facility. Once these criteria for admission are considered and agreed upon, the interdisciplinary team focuses on the appropriate plan of care.

Most hospice programs use a core of professionals who are responsible for coordinating the overall program and are referred to as the **interdisciplinary hospice team** (Table 56-1). These professionals may have various educational backgrounds. The team usually consists of a medical director who is a licensed physician, a hospice coordinator who is usually a registered nurse, a social worker, a chaplain, and a volunteer coordinator. Each of these professionals has a responsibility to establish the care that will be delivered. The medical director is a liaison between the hospice team and primary physician and provides consultation relating to the medical aspects of care. The hospice coordinator coordinates the program by explaining the services to potential patients, admitting them into the program, assigning the primary team, and facilitating the team meetings. The social worker evaluates the psychosocial needs of the patient and family, is a resource for potential community services if financial matters are a concern, counsels when communication dif-

Table 56-1 Interdisciplinary Hospice Team

Team Member	Background	Function/Responsibility
Medical director	Licensed physician	Is a liaison between the hospice team and primary physician Provides consultation relative to medical aspect of care
Hospice coordinator	Licensed registered nurse	Coordinates the hospice program Explains the service, admits the patients, and then assigns the primary team Facilitates team meetings
Social worker	Certified as a social worker with a bachelor's or master's degree	Evaluate the psychosocial needs Is a resource for potential community services Assists with obtaining equipment and supplies Counsels when there are communication difficulties
Chaplain coordinator	Seminary degree; Clinical Pastoral Education (CPE) experience	Is a liaison between hospice team and pastoral community Coordinates pastoral support for the patient/family
Volunteer coordinator	Experience in volunteer work	Recruits and trains the volunteer Coordinates assignment of the volunteers
Bereavement coordinator	Background in bereavement counseling	Assesses the bereaved family after the death of the patient Coordinates and facilitates bereavement support group Provides bereavement counseling
Pharmacist	Licensed registered pharmacist	Provides drug consultation
Dietician	Licensed dietician	Provides diet counseling
Physical therapist	Registered physical therapist	Recommends appropriate safety devices Performs and instructs patient and family in passive exercises and transfer training

HOSPICE WEEKLY UPDATE

PATIENT NAME: Edgar DATE: 5-30-89

PRIMARY NURSE: Kay PRIMARY PHYSICIAN: Cooper

PRIMARY CAREGIVER: Dodie PASTOR: Miles

SOCIAL WORKER: Mary CHURCH: Episcopal

VOLUNTEER: Phyllis DIAGNOSIS: Ca prostate c̄ met.

MEDS AND FREQUENCY: Phenergan 50 mg. Ⓡ q̄ 6 hr
Morphine rectal supp. 20 mg. q̄ 6 hr.
Hydrochlorothiazide 25 mg. q̄ day
O_2 at 2L
*Other meds but hasn't taken
* reg. this wk. because of N & V*
Roxanol 20 mg. q̄ 4-6 hr. prn
Hydrocortisone 20 mg. ii daily
Tagamet q̄ HS
Bentyl 10 mg. bid
Sudafed prn.

ALLERGIES: NKA

NURSING/MEDICAL UPDATE:

WEIGHT: 140 DATE: 5-30-89

VITAL SIGNS: 104/54 - 112 - 16

MENTAL ACUITY: more forgetful ? recall more diff.

NEURO: OK

CARDIAC:

RESPIRATORY: c/o pain Rt chest deep inspiration; tender in this area when palpated

BOWELS: sluggish

INTAKE/OUTPUT: 1 qt. in / out good

APPETITE: none

ACTIVITY LEVEL: fair, but very weak

SKIN INTEGRITY: good

PAIN SITES:	INTENSITY	CONTROL
		good

PROGRESS NOTES: Pt. over the weekend became very nauseated & vomited until nothing left in stomach, then has "dry heaves," which is triggered spontaneously.
Afraid that his oral meds are causing this & afraid to take them -- informed pt. that I doubted it was the medication specifically. c/o Rt ear plugged & sore throat starting last Fri. -- throat sl. red -- ear exam normal. Had diff. breathing over weekend, O_2 was ordered & pt. obtains notable relief, did not have O_2 on during my visit.
Frustrated because his memory recall poorer lately.

PLAN: Could increase Phenergan supp to every 3-4 hr. if needed.
Social worker will call wife next week to check on spouse concerns.

Hospice Team Signatures: J. Doe
B. Smith
W. Browne
M. Carson
T. Thompson

☐ Check - Reported to Primary Nurse

FIG. 56-1 Hospice weekly update.

ficulties are present, and obtains any necessary equipment and/or supplies needed for the safety and comfort of the patient. The chaplain coordinator contacts the patient's own pastor in the community to be part of the team for spiritual support. The pastor's role is vital to assist the patient and family to cope with fears and uncertainty. Support can include dealing with unfinished business and regrets and providing opportunities for reconciliation, prayer, and spiritual healing. Funeral planning and performing the burial services are included in this role also, along with continued support for the family throughout the bereavement period.

The patient's primary physician provides medical support, focusing on symptom control. His involvement is essential to the success of the team care plan. The nurse becomes a liaison between the patient, family, physician, and interdisciplinary team regarding information about the status of the patient and effectiveness of symptom control. The nurse (1) evaluates the patient's response to treatment, (2) instructs the patient and family in management and effects of medications, illness, and basic nursing care, and (3) provides emotional support as possible.

The volunteer coordinator is responsible for training and assigning volunteers who will provide added support. When families are responsible for the total care of the patient in the home, "burnout" of the caregiver becomes a concern. This is when the services of volunteers become vital. They provide companionship, family relief through **respite** care, and emotional support. With use of the volunteer, family can grocery shop, run errands, and participate in other activities, knowing their loved one is not alone. Volunteers become dependable friends, whose services the family can request and accept without guilt or feeling that they are imposing.

Other team members include: a pharmacist, for drug consultation; a dietician, for diet counseling and meal planning; a physical therapist, to provide safety devices, passive exercises, or transfer training; an occupational therapist, to assist in activities of daily living; and a music therapist, to provide diversional therapy to assist with pain management.

Each hospice patient and family is assigned a specific primary team who will be responsible for delivering the care (Table 56-2). A team care plan is developed by the total interdisciplinary team. Weekly team conferences are held to discuss effectiveness of care (Fig. 56-1). Observations by all members are reported and evaluated, and changes regarding care are made accordingly. The team must function as a cohesive unit to use all expertise and resources to provide quality patient care.

SYMPTOM CONTROL AND NURSING CARE

Pain

Of all the symptoms a dying patient experiences, pain is the most dreaded. To the healthy person, pain is usually temporary, but to the dying it can be constant and terrifying. **Pain** takes on many forms, such as physical, **psychosocial,** and spiritual, and becomes a major factor that

Table 56-2 Primary Hospice Team

Team member	Background	Function/Responsibility
Primary physician	Licensed physician	Responsible for the medical aspect of symptom control for patient
Primary nurse	Licensed registered nurse	Is an advocate between patient, family, physician, and interdisciplinary team Evaluates patient's response to treatment Instructs the patient and family in management and effects of medication, illness, basic nursing, etc.
Secondary nurse	Licensed practical/vocational nurse	Works under supervision of physician and registered nurse to provide bedside nursing interventions appropriate to the terminally-ill patient Assists in the physical, emotional, and spiritual support of the patient and family
Primary pastor	As required by church affiliation	Supports patient and family to cope with fears and uncertainty Provides opportunities for reconciliation, prayer, and **spiritual** healing. Responsible for funeral planning and performing burial services Continues to support the family during bereavement period
Hospice volunteer	Completion of volunteer training of at least 24 hrs	Provides companionship for patient/family Available for family relief for respite care and emotional support Continues to be supportive throughout the bereavement period
Nurse's aide	Certified as a nurse's aide	Administers personal care and assistance with activities of daily living (ADLs).

should be addressed and alleviated. According to Munley,[19] although 50% of those dying with a malignancy usually do not have physical pain, and 10% may have mild pain, 40% suffer severe pain. The stress related to suffering and trying to control or alleviate it causes anxiety, anger, depression, restlessness, and isolation. The family caring for persons in this situation become frustrated and helpless as they try to control the pain, creating further feelings of guilt and inadequacy. Another issue that contributes to pain and emotional stress is the financial burden of high medical bills, inadequate funds, and unemployment. Spiritual pain may also surface, especially if there has not been any form of religious support or practices within the family unit. The patient and the family may develop a sense of hopelessness regarding the patient's impending fate, and fears related to the dying process, such as lingering, suffering, and isolation, may come into focus.

Initially, the physician may order diagnostic tests to determine if the cause of pain is related to tumor invasion or other pathological factors. Removing the cause may be impossible; therefore controlling the pain becomes vital in successful management of the person who is terminally ill. Many studies have been done regarding effective pain control, and the consensus is that a pain assessment must be done to effectively control pain. Many programs use a pain assessment form to determine what mode of therapy will be effective. Questions used for evaluation are directed to the patient:

1. Where is your pain? (The use of a body chart can be helpful for the patient to identify the location.)
2. What kind of pain do you have? (Is it sharp, dull, continuous; a pain scale [where 0 is no pain, and 10 is severe] is useful.)
3. How long have you had pain?
4. When does your pain occur, and how often?
5. How long does your pain last?
6. What other problems add to your pain?
7. What relieves your pain? (Position of comfort, medications used, and environment can be addressed here.)

Answers to these questions are important in determining appropriate therapy. Even if the cause of pain is not apparent, the need for control is imperative.

Oral administration of medications is preferred, so that patients and families can independently manage the schedule and administration. Mild to moderate pain is controlled effectively in many cases with nonsteroidal antiinflammatory drugs. These drugs are also beneficial to use with narcotic analgesics, decreasing the required dose of narcotic. Narcotic analgesics, such as the opiates, are commonly used when severe pain cannot be controlled with nonsteroidal antiinflammatory drugs. When oral administration is not feasible because of nausea or vomiting, many of these drugs can be given rectally and parenterally. Morphine has become the drug of choice in hospice care, because it can be administered orally, sublingually, rectally, and parenterally.

Ineffective pain management is usually associated with undermedication or overmedication. Some causes of undermedication are (1) fear that the patient will become addicted; (2) fear that the patient will become dependent too soon and a stronger drug will be needed; (3) not taking the medication until the pain is intense, making it difficult to control; and (4) attempting to relieve pain with ineffective medication, holding in reserve for later the stronger ones, such as morphine. Overmedication may occur when several different narcotic analgesics are taken at the same time or close together because relief is not obtained soon enough. The goal is to prescribe a sufficient dose of an effective drug to alleviate pain and at the same time allow the patient to remain alert enough to participate in activities of daily living. Medication should be administered on a regular basis so that the pain does not return.

Another effective method of pain control is the use of heat or cold packs at the site of discomfort. Acupuncture and transcutaneous electrical nerve stimulation **(TENS)** units have been used also. Some behavior techniques that can be beneficial are relaxation, hypnosis, and biofeedback.

Nursing interventions. The nurse's role focuses on teaching the patient and family the effects and schedule of the medications so they can control the patient's pain. The patient and family should understand that pain can be controlled and that using large doses of narcotics is common and necessary to achieve that control. The nurse can assist the family in setting a schedule for administering the medications and then can monitor the patient's response to and compliance with the established treatment. Patient education regarding other techniques, such as massage, positioning for comfort, and heat or cold packs, is also the nurse's responsibility. It is important to give positive feedback to the patient and family when management of the pain is successful.

Nausea and Vomiting

Nausea is usually worse than vomiting because often it is obvious only to the patient, and so it tends to be ignored. Sometimes the drugs used for pain control cause nausea, and therefore it is recommended to give antiemetics with the narcotic analgesic. Anxiety has also been known to cause nausea, which then leads to vomiting. Patients who vomit are anxious about why they are vomiting, and this worsens the symptom. Constipation also can cause nausea. If nausea and vomiting occur because of obstruction from tumor invasion, it will be necessary to seek medical intervention. Evaluating the cause may not be easy, but once corrected it can often be prevented.

Nursing interventions. Educating the patient and family regarding the problems that could cause or prevent nausea and vomiting is necessary. The patient should be encouraged to take the ordered antiemetics 30 minutes before meals and at bedtime on a regular basis. If vomiting occurs, eating should be discouraged for a period to allow the bowel to "rest." Relaxation and rest periods should be encouraged to avoid unusual stimulation. When the nausea and vomiting have subsided, the patient should begin drinking liquids or eating soft, bland foods. Small light meals should be served initially, with the diet as bland as possible, avoiding sweet, greasy, spicy, or strong-smelling foods. Fluids are important to prevent dehydration. The patient should eat slowly and in a pleasant atmosphere. If anxiety is causing nausea and vomiting, the patient should be encouraged to verbalize his fears.

Constipation

Constipation is one of the most common problems for the terminally ill patient. Sometimes this problem causes more anxiety and discomfort than pain itself. Because constipation can cause other symptoms, such as abdominal pain, nausea, or vomiting, prevention of the problem is important. Factors that contribute to constipation are poor dietary intake, the use of narcotics for pain control, and inactivity. When a patient begins to take medication for pain control, the use of a stool softener and stimulant laxative is necessary. Suppositories and enemas may be needed if oral laxatives produce no results. A rectal examination performed by the nurse may be necessary to check for an impaction. If an impaction is present, manual removal is necessary for relief.

Nursing interventions. The following points are important for the nurse to educate the patient and family in prevention of constipation:

1. Narcotics may cause constipation, so laxatives must be given with the narcotic.
2. Patients who are not eating continue to produce waste in the bowel and can get impacted with feces.
3. High fluid intake should be maintained.
4. The patient should have a bowel movement at least every 3 days.
5. If possible, eating foods high in fiber is helpful.

Anorexia/Malnutrition

Anorexia may be caused by nausea, vomiting, constipation, dysphagia, **stomatitis**, and infections. These complications lead to difficulty in eating, which in turn causes loss of appetite. Odors of food cooking, inability to tolerate sweet foods, or a bitter taste in the mouth also contributes to the problem. This makes food less enjoyable, so the patient does not eat. Poor intake lowers the body's metabolism, which decreases the need for nourishment. Thus hunger is not realized. This cycle leads to malnutrition, resulting in muscle weakness and weight loss.

Nursing interventions. If anorexia is related to stomatitis or infections, good oral hygiene is important. A technique to alleviate discomfort is using swabs soaked in flavored mouthwash to cleanse the mouth. Small, frequent drinks or crushed ice can be useful to relieve dry mouth. If odor of food causes anorexia, the patient should not be in the kitchen during meal preparation. The meals should be as attractive as possible, using foods chosen by the patient. High-protein supplements are helpful when eating is impossible. Weighing the patient should be avoided because he or she may be depressed and discouraged by attention to weight loss.

Other Common Symptoms

Weight loss and dehydration can lead to a decrease of soft tissue, especially on the bony areas of knees, hips, elbows, and buttocks. Increased weakness is also noted in the last stages of a terminal illness. With increased weakness, activity decreases and the patient spends most of the time reclining. This leads to potential skin breakdown and the formation of decubiti.

Nursing interventions. It is important at this time to teach the patient and family the basics of good skin care. Cleanliness promoted by bathing can be refreshing, as well as therapeutic, in promoting comfort and the feeling of self-worth. The skin should be inspected frequently and kept as dry and clean as possible. Avoiding harsh soaps, strong detergents, or irritations from buttons, snaps, or food crumbs should be stressed. An Eggcrate mattress, sheepskin, or air-flotation mattress and heel and elbow protectors can cushion the bony areas. If decubiti occur, cleaning with hydrogen peroxide, drying well, and applying a skin protector are effective measures.

BEREAVEMENT PERIOD

The family, especially the caregiver, continues to need support during the bereavement period when the patient dies. Even though the family feel they have prepared for the death, facing the future without the person who died is difficult. Hospice care does not conclude once the patient dies, but continues for at least 1 year. Depending on the size of the program, special bereavement teams with counselors are available for the family. The team may facilitate a bereavement support group, which meets on a regular basis, providing these families the opportunity to communicate and share their feelings. Volunteers and pastors keep in touch by phone calls, cards, and remembering the bereaved person on holidays and anniversaries.

ETHICAL ISSUES IN HOSPICE

Some ethical issues when dealing with hospice patients include withholding or withdrawing nutritional support, right to refuse treatment, or "do not resuscitate" (DNR). Families find it difficult to discontinue nourishment, even when death is clearly approaching. If the patient is unconscious, decisions regarding these issues may fall upon one family member. This may create guilt if other family members disagree. There are no simple answers to any of these concerns. It is hoped that the patient's wishes are made known in advance, such as in a living will, or that a power of attorney has been appointed.

Death is a lonely experience, and can be done only alone, but the period leading to that point should not be lonely. It is important for the hospice team to be sensitive to the patient and family's needs and maintain honesty at all times. The patient and the family should be included in all aspects of care and decision-making. Opportunities for expression of concerns and fears should be provided, because this will make the process less fearful and threatening. Allowing the patient and family to live fully and comfortably until death occurs naturally is the main goal of hospice care.

REFERENCES AND SUGGESTED READINGS

1. Archer DN and Smith AC: Sorrow has many faces: helping families cope with grief, Nurs '88 18(5):43, 1988.
2. Billings JM: Outpatient management of advanced cancer, Philadelphia, 1985, JB Lippincott Co.
3. Breslin R: Food: the essence of life—in sickness and in health, Caring 5(10):76, 1986.
4. Carusso DM: Sexuality and the terminal patient, Caring 5(10):68, 1986.
5. Chase D: Dying at home with hospice, St Louis, 1986, The CV Mosby Co.
6. Colburn L: Pressure ulcer prevention for the hospice patient, Am J Hospice Care 4(2):22, 1987.
7. Dixon C, Emery AW, and Hurley R: Nutrition and patient with limited life expectancy, Am J Hospice Care 2(3):27, 1985.
8. Enck R: Constipation: etiologies and management, Am J Hospice Care 5(5):17, 1988.
9. Hill CS: Narcotics and cancer pain control, CA 38(6):322, 1988.
10. Kerr D: Mouth care for the dying, Am J Hospice Care 6(1):23, 1989.
11. Lannie VJ: The positive aspects of anguish: a hospice philosophy, Am J Hospice Care 1(4):33, 1984.
12. MacFarlane B: Pain management using TENS, Continuing Care 7(11):21, 1988.
13. McCaffery M and Beebe A: Pain: clinical manual for nursing practice, St Louis, 1989, The CV Mosby Co.
14. Mishkin B: Courts entangled in feeding tube controversies, Nutr Clin Prac 1(4):209, 1986.
15. Mishkin B: Withholding and withdrawing nutritional support, Nutr Clin Prac 1(1):50, 1986.
16. Munley A: The hospice alternative: a new concept for death and dying, New York, 1983, Basic Books, Inc, Publishers.
17. O'Connor P: The role of spiritual care in hospice, Am J Hospice Care 5(4):31, 1988.
18. Olsson G and Parker G: A model approach to pain assessment; Nurs '87 17(5):52, 1987.
19. Paradis LL: Hospice handbook: a guide for managers and planners, Rockville, Md, 1985, Aspen Publishers, Inc.
20. Siegler M and Shiedermayer D: Should fluid and nutritional support be withheld from terminally ill patients, Am J Hospice Care 4(2):32, 1987.
21. Ufema JK: How to talk to dying patients, Nurs '87 17(8):43, 1987.
22. Wormer K: Guilt feelings in the spouse of the terminally ill, Home Healthc Nurse 3(5):21, 1985.

CHAPTER CHALLENGE

KEY POINTS

- Palliative care is appropriate when cure is not possible but care is still needed. This becomes the goal of hospice care.
- The goal of palliative care is to control pain and other symptoms for the prevention of distress.
- Admission to a hospice program is the decision of a patient and family, because not all persons need or desire hospice care.
- Hospice care consists of a blending of professionals and nonprofessionals to meet the total needs of the patient and family.
- Hospice care is delivered by an interdisciplinary team, because no individual or profession can meet all the needs of terminally ill patients and families all the time.
- Hospice care considers all aspects of the lives of patients and their families. Stresses and concerns may arise in many ways when families are faced with a terminal illness.
- A hospice care program considers the patient and family together as the unit of care, because families experience much stress and pain during the terminal illness of one of their members.
- Family participation in care giving is an important part of palliative care.
- Hospice care is available 24 hours a day, 7 days a week, because needs may arise at any time.
- Hospice care is respectful of all patient and family belief systems, seeking resources to meet the physical, psychosocial, and spiritual needs of the total family unit.
- Hospice care for the family continues into the bereavement period. Needs of the family continue after the patient dies.

STUDY QUESTIONS

1. Palliative care is defined as:
   a. Aggressive therapy
   b. Custodial care
   c. Care related to symptom control
   d. None of the above
2. The basic goals of hospice care are:
   a. Control symptoms
   b. Allow patient and family decision making
   c. Provide continuous support
   d. All of the above
3. The interdisciplinary team consists of a:
   a. Nurse, physician, social worker, pastor, volunteer
   b. Physician, pastor, volunteer, nurse
   c. Social worker, volunteer, pastor, dietician
   d. Physician, social worker, volunteer, physical therapist
4. Common symptoms related to the terminally ill are:
   a. Pain
   b. Nausea and vomiting
   c. Constipation
   d. None of the above
   e. All of the above
5. One of the most common drugs used in pain control in hospice is:
   a. Demeral
   b. Codeine
   c. Methadone
   d. Morphine
6. What measures can alleviate or reduce the symptoms of nausea and vomiting:
   a. Taking pain medication on a regular basis
   b. Taking antiemetic medication on a regular basis
   c. Greasy, spicy diet
   d. Active exercise
7. What symptoms are associated with anorexia:
   a. Stomatitis
   b. Weight loss
   c. Nausea and vomiting
   d. a and b only
   e. All of the above
8. Effective measures in contolling pain are:
   a. Giving the pain medication PRN only
   b. Regular administration of pain medication
   c. Relaxing and massaging techniques
   d. c only
   e. b and c only
9. What is one of the most common side effects of taking narcotic analgesics:
   a. Nausea
   b. Vomiting
   c. Constipation
   d. Muscle weakness
   e. Anorexia
10. The bereavement follow-up period after the death of the patient is:
    a. 2 years
    b. 1 year
    c. 6 months
    d. 1 month

XVII

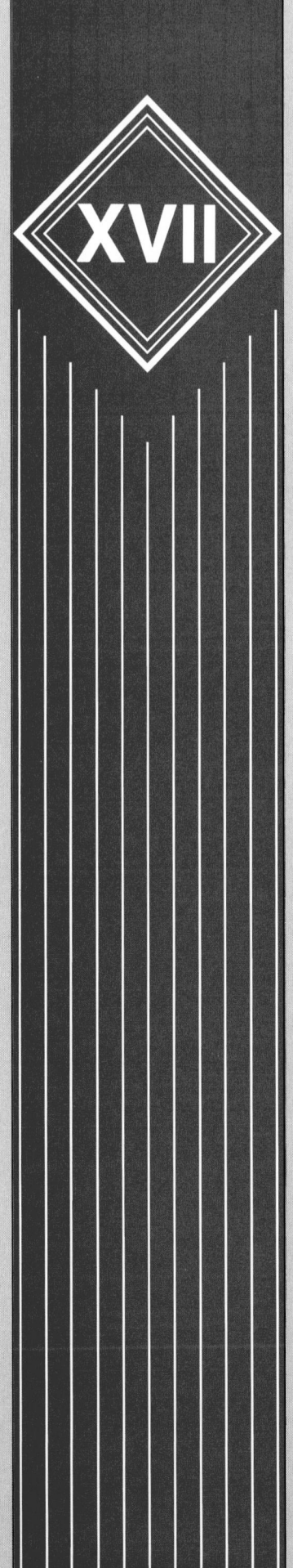

The World of the Graduate

I have always had a longing deep down inside of me to be needed and helpful to people in need. Nursing helps to fulfill this lifelong desire. Caring for a patient in some way during the day, whether by giving a bath, a medication, or just a pat on the arm, helps to fill the need I have to help. Nursing is especially rewarding when a patient gives you a special look, a little smile, or any small gesture that says, "Thank you, you helped." When I've done the best I can and feel that I have helped in some way, there is a sense of satisfaction that cannot be achieved in any other way.

MARLA WEBER
Student Nurse

57

The World of the Graduate

CAROLYN DEAN

LEARNING OBJECTIVES

After reading this chapter, the student should be able to do the following:

- Define the key terms.
- Describe the three methods to apply for a job.
- Describe what could be expected from an orientation to a new job.
- List two advantages of membership in professional organizations.
- Define confidentiality.
- Explain the difference in the three leadership styles discussed in this chapter.
- List five guidelines for being an effective leader.
- Identify two reasons why an evaluation is important.
- Identify the three types of physicians' orders and legal aspects of each.
- List three ways you can ensure accuracy when transcribing physicians' orders.
- Describe the Nurse Practice Act.
- List four reasons the state board of nursing could revoke a nursing license.
- Identify three important functions of the state board of nursing.
- List the pertinent data necessary to compile an effective shift report.

RELATED TOPICS OF INTEREST

- Legal aspects of nursing (Chapter 2)
- Ethical aspects of nursing (Chapter 3)
- Communication (Chapter 4)
- Principles and practice of medication administration (Chapter 25)
- Home health nursing (Chapter 51)
- Rehabilitation nursing (Chapter 52)
- Hospice care (Chapter 56)

KEY TERMS

Define the following:

- assessment
- confidentiality
- endorsement
- evaluation
- leadership
- malpractice
- management
- negligence
- nurse practice act
- responsibility
- resumé
- role
- transcribing

FUNCTIONING AS A GRADUATE

The **role** of a graduate nurse will be both exciting and challenging. The LPN/LVN is a valuable member of the health care team and functions in various settings. This chapter will provide some guidelines on being a conscientious nurse while assuming a new role. There are many nursing opportunities from which to choose.

Methods to obtain a job after graduation are (1) letter of application, (2) resumé, and (3) interview.

Letter of Application

The letter of application should always be brief, neatly typed, and with correct spelling. A sample letter of application is found in Box 57-1. The letter should state the exact position for which you are applying and any information about yourself and your qualifications. Box 57-2 provides guidelines for writing the letter of application.

The Resumé

The resumé is a one- or two-page written document that has certain information about you. It is a brief outline of personal and professional life. It also describes your skills and interests. Future employers will be impressed with a well-prepared resumé; therefore take the preparation of your resumé seriously. It should be well organized, neat, and accurate. Prepare one that is basic, properly arranged, and contains the most recent information. Use a variety of action words and self-descriptive words, as listed in Box 57-3. There are several types of resumés— keep yours brief and informative. The employer is seeking the employee with the most potential for the job. The resumé may be the first means by which the employer gains an impression of you. A sample resumé is presented in Box 57-4.

The Personal Interview

The interview is important, and every effort should be made to make it a success. First impressions are sometimes incorrect, and whether they are positive or negative, they have a lasting effect. Prepare carefully for the interview, and make a good impression. Box 57-5 provides steps to a successful interview.

It is beneficial to understand the types of questions that an employer might ask. Practice answering the questions in Box 57-6 in a sincere, honest manner.

The employer is not the only person who should ask questions during

BOX 57-1 **SAMPLE LETTER OF APPLICATION**

(return address) 1314 East 17th Street
Sedalia, MO 65301
(date) Sept. 3, 1990

Mr. Greg Derk *(inside address)*
Personnel Manager
North Central Hospital
615 South Tryon Street
Kansas City, MO 64156

Dear Mr. Derk: *(salutation)*

I am interested in the position of LPN on a surgical unit for which you advertised an opening in the Kansas City Star on Sunday, Sept. 2.

I will graduate on Sept. 23 from North Central Missouri College and will take the LPN licensure examination in October. Throughout my education, I have maintained a keen interest in medical/surgical nursing. In addition, I worked part-time as a nurse assistant on a surgical floor at St. Francis Hospital in Marceline for a year while I was in nursing school. My resumé is enclosed for further information about my background and experience.

I am a highly motivated individual and perform well in stressful situations. I am energetic, systematic, organized, efficient, and provide quality nursing care to patients. I am enthusiastic about my career in nursing and look forward to reviewing my qualifications with you.

I will be in Kansas City on Friday, Sept. 7, and if it is convenient for you, I would like to talk with you then about this position. You can reach me by phone at (816) 827-1032. I look forward to hearing from you.

(complimentary close) Sincerely yours,

(provide signature)
Sue Renfro

Enclosure

BOX 57-2 **GUIDELINES FOR WRITING LETTER OF APPLICATION**

1. Include your full address above the date of your letter.
2. Address the letter appropriately. If you are responding to a classified advertisement that provides a return box only, use the address given and the salutation *Ladies and Gentlemen.* If you have learned about a position through your school office or through a friend, you should have the name of the person in charge of employment. In this case, include the name in the inside address as follows:

   Mr. Thomas L. Leeper
   Personnel Manager
   The Azzaro Corporation
   3689 Wilson Street
   Atlanta, GA 30315

   The proper salutation is *Dear Mr. Leeper:*.
3. In the first paragraph, state your interest:

   The nursing position that you advertised in the *Atlanta Times* on Monday, June 2, is of interest to me.

   or

   Miss Cathie Royer, the placement counselor at Greenville College, has suggested that I apply for the nursing position that is available in your facility.
4. In the second paragraph refer to your **resumé**, which you will enclose. This paragraph should highlight the main points of your education and experience.
5. In the final paragraph of your application, indicate your interest in a personal interview and the times you are available.
6. The complimentary close may be a simple *Sincerely yours.* Include your signature above your typewritten name, and indicate the enclosure.

BOX 57-3 **KEY WORDS FOR RESUMÉ AND COVER LETTER PREPARATION**

ACTION WORDS

accelerated	generate	provide
actively	implemented	recommend
adapted	improve	reduced
administer	increased	reinforced
analyze	influence	reorganized
approve	interpret	responsibilities
coordinate	launched	responsible
completed	lead	revamped
conceived	lecture	revise
conduct	maintain	review
control	manage	schedule
created	motivated	significantly
delegate	organize	simplicity
demonstrate	originate	set up
develop	participated	solve
direct	perform	strategy
effect	plan	structure
eliminated	pinpointed	streamline
established	proficient	successfully
evaluate	program	supervise
expanded	proposed	support
expedite	proved	teach
founded		

SELF-DESCRIPTIVE WORDS

active	economical	pleasant
adaptable	efficient	positive
aggressive	energetic	practical
alert	enterprising	productive
ambitious	enthusiastic	realistic
analytical	extroverted	reliable
attentive	fair	resourceful
broad-minded	forceful	respective
conscientious	imaginative	self-reliant
consistent	independent	sense of humor
constructive	logical	sincere
creative	loyal	sophisticated
dependable	mature	systematic
determined	methodical	tactful
diplomatic	objective	talented
disciplined	optimistic	will travel
discreet	perceptive	will relocate

BOX 57-4 **SAMPLE RESUMÉ**

LINDA PATTERSON
2777 EAST EIGHTH
TRENTON, MO 64683

PHONE: (816) 359-8888

JOB OBJECTIVES: Staff LPN leading toward inservice or home health care.

EDUCATION: North Central Missouri College, Trenton, MO 64683
Licensed Practical Nurse: Graduation, Sept. 1990; License, 1990

Kirksville Health Center, Kirksville, MO 63501
Advanced Cardiac Life Support, 1990
Advanced Fluid and Electrolyte Course, 1990

EXPERIENCE: St. Francis Hospital, Marceline, MO 64668, August 1989 to July 1990, Nurse Assistant

Brookfield Nursing Center, Brookfield, MO 64628, January 1989 to July 1989, Nurse Assistant

Grim-Smith Hospital, Kirksville, MO 63501, June 1988 to December 1988, Nursing Assistant

HONORS AND ACTIVITIES: North Central Community College: Dean's Honor Roll; Class Secretary; Intramural sports.

High School: Member, National Honor Society; Class President; Who's Who Among American High School Students; Girls' State delegate; Member, concert and marching band; Softball; Basketball.

Community: Girl Scout; Community Betterment; Youth Leadership Award from the governor–1989; Extension Club president.

REFERENCES:

Mrs. Lynn Myers
Health Occupations Division
Trenton Junior College
Trenton, MO 64683
(816) 359-3948

Mrs. Carol Jacobs
Director of Nursing
St. Francis Hospital
Marceline, MO 64668
(816) 359-3939

Ms. Cherie Urton
Instructor
Trenton Junior College
1301 Main Street
Trenton, MO 64683
(816) 359-4562

BOX 57-5 STEPS TO A SUCCESSFUL INTERVIEW

1. Be well groomed.
2. Arrive at the interview a few minutes earlier than the appointment; if there is a receptionist or secretary, tell him or her who you are, and give the name of the person you are to see.
3. Be cheerful and polite.
4. Know something about the position for which you are applying.
5. Be patient while waiting for an interview.
6. Smile, and give name distinctly when greeting the interviewer.
7. Use a firm handshake.
8. Address interviewer by name, using Mr., Mrs., or Ms.
9. Use appropriate body language.
10. Look directly at the interviewer.
11. Let the interviewer take the initiative.
12. Answer questions concisely. Try to make the interview interesting and informative. Use the time effectively.
13. Articulate.
14. Be factual when answering questions.
15. Avoid being critical.
16. Convey genuine interest and enthusiasm.
17. Avoid discussing personal problems, unless applicable to job.
18. Be prepared to relate qualifications and experiences.
19. Ask about job description, work schedule, and fringe benefits.
20. If asked, state salary desired; if salary offered is unacceptable, do not mislead the interviewer.
21. Inquire about starting salary, pay increases, and maximum salary allowed.
22. If asked, indicate preference of position desired.
23. Look for clues when the interview is over. Usually an employer will ask, "Do you have any more questions?" This is probably a good time to say, "No thank you, but I enjoyed our interview and hope that you will consider me for the position with your company."
24. Express appreciation for the interview.
25. Suggest when and where you might be contacted, if necessary.
26. Send additional information promptly, upon request.

an interview. The applicant, too, has the right to certain information. A list of questions appropriate for an applicant to ask a prospective employer in an interview are found in Box 57-7.

For a good working relationship, your skills and nursing care values should be in harmony with the objectives of the job description.

BOX 57-6 QUESTIONS FREQUENTLY ASKED IN AN INTERVIEW

1. Tell me about yourself . . . about your family?
2. Where did you go to school?
3. What are your future plans?
4. In what position are you most interested?
5. Why do you think you might like to work for our facility?
6. What jobs have you held? Why did you leave?
7. Why do you think you would like this particular type of position?
8. What interests you about our nursing services?
9. What hours can you work?
10. What jobs have you enjoyed the most? The least? Why?
11. What type of nursing interests you?
12. In what professional organizations have you participated?

BOX 57-7 QUESTIONS TO ASK THE EMPLOYER IN AN INTERVIEW

1. How does one advance?
2. If I were required to relocate, how much of the expense would the facility pay?
3. Is any overtime required for this position? How much? How is overtime compensated?
4. If I wish to go back to further my education, would the facility pay any expenses?
5. How permanent is this position?
6. Is there an incentive program for continuing education?
7. What is your policy on pregnancy leaves?
8. Do I have a choice about where I would be assigned?
9. Will the facility compensate me for use of my own vehicle? Telephone?
10. Is a degree essential to advancement?
11. When will you be making a decision on this position?
12. May I provide any further information?

Terminating Employment

Resigning from a position properly is another skill that you should have. Employers will sometimes question a resumé that reflects frequent job changes; therefore it is in your best interest to remain at the first place of employment at least 1 year. If this is impossible, the proper resignation procedure should be followed. A verbal statement and a letter of resignation, if given, may be beneficial in obtaining your next position. If the facility has a formal

BOX 57-8 **SAMPLE LETTER OF RESIGNATION**

406 Martin Lane
Edinburg, MO 64683
May 6, 1990

Ms. Nel Pitts, R.N.
Director of Nurses
Memorial Hospital
Edinburg, MO 64683

Dear Ms. Pitts:

Because of unforeseen circumstances, I must resign my position as staff L.P.N. on 1-E. My husband has been transferred to another city, and I must seek employment there.

I would like my resignation to be effective as of May 29, 1990.

I would appreciate it if I could have my accrued benefits added to my terminal salary check.

I thank you for all the courtesies extended to me during my employment. The staff has been helpful, and I have enjoyed my 4 years of employment at Memorial Hospital. I hope that in the future I can seek employment again at this facility.

Sincerely yours,

(provide signature)
(Mrs.) Jenny Dean, L.P.N.

resignation form, it should be completed neatly and legibly. If a letter of resignation is expected, it should be brief and courteous. In concise terms, state your reason for leaving. Address the letter to your immediate supervisor or employer. It is delivered in a sealed envelope. A sample letter of resignation is found in Box 57-8.

THE GAP BETWEEN STUDENT AND GRADUATE

Know Who You Are

Sometimes it is difficult to clearly understand the exact responsibilities of each health team member. Job descriptions to fit some of the new roles have not been written. The LPN/LVN is responsible to an RN or to the physician. The role of the LPN/LVN, like the roles of others associated with health care, is constantly changing. As the services of health care facilities are extended to meet the increasing demand of the population, the role of the LPN/LVN cannot remain static. Many technical and scientific changes in the health care system have resulted in a multiplicity and complexity of functions placed on nurses. As a result, those who work with patients must be extremely careful not to lose sight of their principal concern, the human being. Patients quickly recognize nurses who have a genuine concern for their individual needs. Your enthusiasm and zest for nursing are clearly evident in the personalized quality of care given.

Confidentiality

Consider as confidential all information the patient gives. The information may be exchanged with other members of the health care team only in the performance of your duties. Release of information to anyone other than the health care team without the consent of the patient is a violation of his or her right to privacy. Important reminders concerning **confidentiality** are listed in Box 57-9.

Expectations of an LPN/LVN in the Community

The LPN/LVN participates in activities that promote the community's attitude towards positive health care.

BOX 57-9 CONFIDENTIALITY REMINDERS

1. Discuss patient information only in conferences or reports.
2. Keep confidential all information gathered from medical records, reports, or conferences.
3. Be nonjudgmental in observations of patients, hospital staff, family members, or other personnel.
4. Do not store patient statistics on any retrievable or permanent computer system unless authorized.
5. Do not keep or copy any patient information except when necessary for required report. All notes should be destroyed after submitting required report.
6. Never copy any original medical records for any reason unless ordered by a physician.
7. Do not leave patient chart where unauthorized persons can access it.
8. It is generally not the nurse's responsibility to release patient information to the police, media, relatives, or visitors.
9. Familiarize yourself with how patient information is to be handled within the facility.
10. You are ethically obligated to treat information about your patient as confidential.

The nurse uses community resources to promote a better understanding of the health services available to the general public and promotes and participates in community health projects and other health-oriented activities.

Professional Organizations

If you want a voice in your vocation, it will be a benefit to join that vocation's organizations. No organization can be any more active or effective than its members.

Two national organizations are designed to support and meet the needs of the LPN/LVN: the National Association for Practical Nurse Education and Service (NAPNES) and the National Federation of Licensed Practical Nurses (NFLPN).

NAPNES was founded in 1941 to promote an understanding of practical nursing schools and continuing education for the LPN. The organization also developed a position on the education of the practical nurse and defines ethical conduct and publishes standards of practical/vocational nursing practice. The *Journal of Practical Nursing* is the official publication, and *NAPNES Forum* is the newsletter that informs members of activities. Membership is open to students, graduates, faculty, and others who are interested in the practical/vocational nurse. For more information, write to: NAPNES, 1400 Spring Street, Suite 310, Silver Spring, MD 20910.

NFLPN was founded in 1949 to promote the licensed practical nurse. The membership is limited to practical/vocational nursing students and graduates. It informs members of the most current issues of interest and makes available to its members malpractice, personal liability, health, and accident insurance. The NFLPN also lobbies on both the state and national levels for issues that are of interest and concern to its members. The *Licensed Practical Nurse* is the official publication. For further information write to: NFLPN, 214 South Drive, PO Box 11038, Durham, NC 27703.

Members who constitute these two organizations all share the common goals of the LPN/LVN.

The National League for Nursing (NLN) was founded in 1952 and is involved with all types and levels of nursing. The NLN is a large organization that has divisions called *councils*. The Councils of Practical Nursing Program (CPNP) is the division of the NLN that accredits educational programs and provides continuing education for faculty. The official publication is *Nursing and Health Care*. Professional testing services, studies, and surveys on nursing education are provided by the NLN organization. Membership is open to all nurses and others interested in health care.

Updating and Continuing Education

The health care system is changing daily as a result of rapidly developing technology, and it is critical to keep current on nursing trends and issues. More excellent opportunities to learn new nursing skills are available to the nurse today than ever. Facilities are offering employees continuing education through seminars or workshops by current videos, journals, and textbooks.

To renew nursing licenses, some states require a given number of hours per year in continuing education units (CEUs). This is to improve the quality of patient care by educating nurses on the most recent trends in nursing interventions.

LPNs/LVNs who wish to pursue further education may receive credit for education. Progressive LPN/LVN to RN programs have been developed throughout the nation, making it possible for an LPN/LVN to become an RN in a shorter period of study. There are various names for these programs, such as *career ladder, upper mobility, level I and level II, 1 + 1,* and *accelerated/associate degree nursing program.*

CAREER OPPORTUNITIES

Never before has nursing been so exciting; today the new graduate has a variety of job opportunities available. The options will require considerable thought to make the correct decision. The job opportunities for the LPN/

LVN are expanding and extend beyond those in the nursing home and hospital.

Hospital Nursing

In hospital nursing, the responsibilities of the LPN/LVN will depend on the policies and philosophy of the facilities. Hospital schedules usually are of three shifts: 7AM to 3PM; 3PM to 11PM; and 11PM to 7AM. Some may schedule two 12-hour shifts: 7AM to 7PM and 7PM to 7AM. Most offer different options to meet the personal needs of the employee. In the hospital, the LPN/LVN is usually the bedside nurse, and the RN is usually the charge nurse. In many hospitals total patient care is given. Total patient care can best be described as follows: the nurse assigned to the patient gives the bath, makes the bed, gives the medications, performs various procedures necessary, and charts; each caregiver has fewer patients but gives total care to those patients for the entire shift.

In some hospitals other work experiences may be available for the LPN/LVN. Such areas are intensive care units, renal dialysis, pediatrics, surgery, and emergency room. These areas usually require specialized education beyond the LPN/LVN education. Many hospitals offer further education to the LPN/LVN who is interested in one of these specialties.

Also, same day surgery units within the hospital setting are more common, to keep the expense of health care at a minimum. In this type of unit, patients are admitted, have surgery, and are discharged in the same day. The LPN/LVN must be skilled in preoperative, postoperative, and recovery care.

Private Duty Nursing

The private duty nurse gives total care to one patient. The setting for the private duty nurse may change from patient to patient, but basically the job description is the same. This type of nursing is totally independent nursing care service. Private duty nursing may take place in the hospital, home, or other facility. The nurse is paid directly by the patient or responsible person. When the setting for private duty nursing is in a health care facility, the nurse is expected to follow the policies and procedures of that facility.

Home Health Nursing

Home health care is expanding rapidly. The hours of employment with this type of nursing may fit into your life-style. Some facilities prefer you to have some experience in hospital nursing first, for you to function with a broader knowledge base. An established health care program that is funded and operated by local, state, or federal government agencies provides the nursing care. The LPN/LVN will work under the supervision of an RN or physician. The nursing care may be given in the home or in a community health center. The nurse may have an opportunity to do patient teaching in public or community health. This may range from prenatal classes to teaching patients to give their insulin injections. The nurse is allowed to be flexible and works autonomously. Therefore skillful time management and an interest in working independently are helpful in this area.

Armed Services Nursing

There are various branches of services that offer educational benefits to nurses. The United States Army offers the LPN/LVN financial assistance with education; however, basic training is required. This area offers a wide range of experience, including traveling and working in Veterans Administration hospitals. If you are interested in armed services, such as army, navy, or air force, it is advisable to contact the recruiter in your area.

Industrial Nursing

The focus in industrial nursing is on promoting wellness and preventing accidents. Safety is emphasized, and usually the nurse is first-aid oriented. The industrial nurse may do physical assessment, health surveys, insurance forms preparation, and health education, as well as nursing intervention for patients injured in industrial accidents. The LPN/LVN will work under the supervision of a registered nurse or physician. Depending on the size of the industrial site, this type of nursing may offer shifts and benefits different from those of other career opportunities.

Office Nursing

The LPN/LVN may work in a physician's office, clinic, or other health practice. In these settings, the nurse may be responsible for various duties other than nursing skills, such as receptionist, bookkeeper, and laboratory assistant, and may be responsible for ordering supplies. The LPN/LVN who makes this choice must be flexible and be able to adjust easily to various roles.

Nursing Home and Extended-Care Facilities

The job opportunities in the field of geriatrics are increasing daily. In the nursing home or extended-care facilities, a large number of LPN/LVNs are needed, and in many instances they function as charge nurses. The amount of responsibility for the LPN/LVN depends on the facility and the level of care given. Working at this type of setting requires many special qualities, such as patience, interest in working with the same people over a long period, good communications, and leadership skills.

Hospice Nursing

Hospice nursing offers care to terminally ill patients in either an institution or home setting, usually under the auspices of home health nursing. The qualifications for a hospice nurse are to have a clear understanding of his or her own feelings concerning death and to understand the philosophy of the hospice setting. The nurse closely supports the patient and family without interfering with family interpersonal relationships.

THE GRADUATE AS A TEAM LEADER OR CHARGE NURSE

Structure and Role of the Charge Nurse

In nursing homes or extended care facilities, LPNs/LVNs may be assigned as charge nurses. They work under the supervision of registered nurses or physicians. There may be times when the registered nurse or physician is on call but not physically present in the facility. Therefore it is necessary for the LPN/LVN to be well oriented to the position, thus ensuring more efficiency and less apprehension.

As a team leader or charge nurse, you will have **responsibility** that requires special skills, such as time management, assessment, and evaluation. There will be workshops and seminars offered specifically for each of these areas. The employer should provide opportunities for the LPN/LVN to develop these skills before he or she is assigned to be charge nurse.

The word *leader* is defined as a person who holds a position of authority and who guides others to perform in a particular manner. The ability to influence the behavior of those one works with requires certain traits and skills. The leader must be motivated and have the ability to successfully guide team members toward a mutual goal of providing excellent nursing care to all patients.

It is of value to the team leader or charge nurse to do a self-study to evaluate the types of leadership styles most appropriate.

There are various styles of **leadership.** An effective charge nurse realizes the highest quality of patient care can be achieved through motivation and cooperation of other members of the nursing team.

Types of leadership are authoritative, participative or democratic, and the laissez-faire process.

Authoritative (autocratic) **management** is a directive style of supervision characterized by designated persons or groups with the right to rule and command others in whatever way they see appropriate. Common characteristics found in the groups with authoritative management are (1) low degree of participation in making decisions, (2) obedience to the leader, (3) lack of trust, and (4) feelings of tension. A decrease in self-worth, apathy, and uncooperativeness could appear in a strong authoritarian system. However, there are advantages to this type of leadership— it often gets the job done.

Democratic management allows groups to participate in decision making and creates mutual acceptance and trust. There is development of self-interests and freedom to change or expand. The group senses that their feelings and thoughts are important. Personal satisfaction is achieved, and each individual is helped to become a fully functioning person.

Laissez-faire management is best described as open and permissive, with a minimum of group functioning. No leader is invested with responsibility, and no one assumes the role. There are few rules, guidelines, or regulations, because they are seen as infringement on the rights and dignity of the person.

As you practice the different leadership styles, you will see a combination of the three will be most effective. It is beneficial to have a knowledge of the different styles and characteristics of each. The authoritative charge nurse demonstrates more power, relies on rules and conformity, and is less flexible. Less responsibility is delegated to the staff, and more of the decision making is performed by the authoritative charge nurse. This leadership could produce anxiety in staff if frustration develops from a feeling of powerlessness. The authoritative nurse usually has a very organized staff. The charge nurse who is a democratic or participative leader usually has a more content staff. This charge nurse keeps the team members informed and asks for suggestions for feedback, which often results in more harmonious staff members. The laissez-faire charge nurse is one who is nonjudgmental of others but also often lacks direction and control. This nurse accepts people as they are and expects reciprocal relationships. This leader is usually friendly, warm, and helpful.

When you are the charge nurse in a nursing home or extended-care facility, it will be you from whom others will be seeking advice and guidance. You are expected to make the correct decisions effectively for the shift. Every nurse needs a basic set of guidelines to assist in functioning efficiently as a charge nurse. Box 57-10 provides guidelines to assist in more effective leadership.

Time Management

Using time to good advantage will be of great value. Learn good time management skills, and practice them frequently until they become fully developed. These skills will help you manage not only at work but also in daily living. See Box 57-11 for 10 steps to effective time management.

Manage your time so you can accomplish both what you must do and what you *want* to do.

Assessment

Assessment may be defined as observing, gathering, verifying, and communicating pertinent data. Acuity of observation develops rapidly in the effective leader. The

BOX 57-10 GUIDELINES FOR EFFECTIVE LEADERSHIP

1. Orient the team you will be working with. They deserve to hear what is expected of them by you. Each one should be aware of his or her job description. The workplace will be less stressful if everyone is familiar with any uniqueness you or others may have concerning the nursing care given.
2. Keep notepad and pencil with you (document on notepad pertinent information that may be needed later). Also have available a pocket calculations guide on drug doses and IV drop rate.
3. Develop your own system of abbreviations for your information—use only standard abbreviations on legal documents.
4. Make patient rounds as soon as report is over. If you are to be responsible for the direct care of a certain number of patients, make certain you can document accurate information concerning their conditions. Note on your "pocket notes" date and time, and briefly state what you observe or hear. This is helpful if the patient's condition changes during the shift.
5. Check all equipment and supplies that you will be responsible for during your shift. You may assign these duties to another responsible person if available. These checks can become part of the routine and will certainly assist in the proficiency of the staff.
6. Everyone performs his or her best when the team works together and each receives recognition for his or her performance.
7. Keep informed of the events within the facility.
   a. Attend necessary meetings.
   b. Become familiar with rules and regulations of the facility in which you are employed.
   c. Learn what surveys or inspections will be conducted.
   d. Learn where the policy and procedure documents are kept; also ensure that they are updated and located in a central area.

BOX 57-11 10 STEPS TO EFFECTIVE TIME MANAGEMENT

1. Set goals, plan, and evaluate feedback relative to your goals.
2. Set priorities—know what you want, how you want it, and when you want it.
3. Use "do" lists daily, weekly, monthly. Mark off tasks as completed.
4. Do not procrastinate. Identify and confront underlying problems that lead to procrastination, and resolve them.
5. Be organized. Avoid time wasters and learn to delegate.
6. Have self-discipline—it generates pride and satisfaction.
7. Do one of four things with paperwork: complete it, act on it, save it (if valid reason), or destroy it (if it is of no value).
8. Keep motivated—think in a positive manner.
9. Learn to use computers efficiently—thoroughly learn a computer program.
10. Learn your peak time when energy and attention levels are optimal; match your energy level with complexity of task to be completed.

nursing assessment must be systematic, accurate, and comprehensive. Increase your perception by systematically looking for details for which you should be alert. Assess the patient in an organized manner. Document your assessments. Also, be alert to the safety of the patient's environment. As your assessment skills develop, you will be better able to identify patient needs.

Evaluation

As charge nurse or team leader you will be expected to evaluate yourself and other nursing staff. The plan for **evaluation** should be consistent and fully explained to each person evaluated. The evaluation should not be viewed as a negative procedure. Adequate guidelines are necessary for the evaluation process to be of value. Evaluations are important in nursing for nurses to give the best care possible. The evaluation process should be continuous. Present an atmosphere of support and acceptance for those being evaluated. The evaluation process in nursing is an assessment of a series of actions. There are three persons involved in the evaluating process: (1) the evaluator, (2) the person being evaluated, and (3) the person receiving the report. For the evaluation procedure to be a success, everyone involved must respond positively to the evaluation. The leader's success depends on promoting a positive morale of the team members. There should always be a follow-up on the evaluation, when the person being evaluated and the evaluator discuss the progress and achievements that have occurred. There must be open communication for the evaluation to be a success. The evaluator should follow the same guidelines for all evaluations. Evaluations are of benefit to the employee and employer. The ultimate beneficiary of a successful evaluation program is the patient: with continued improvement in individual performance, the nursing interventions are much more successful.

Computers in Nursing

Computers have been in health care for 20 to 30 years. First they were used for financial records; however, now they are used to assist with documentation, care plans, staff scheduling, and patient monitoring. The routine clerical tasks can be performed by the computer, but the competent bedside nurse is still needed to do the skilled nursing care. Nurses do not need to know the complexities of the computer but should be computer literate. It would be helpful to understand the basics of operating the computer and to be familiar with computer terminology. The use of computers in nursing is a reality. If properly developed, automation will allow the nurse to have more time for direct patient care as the computer assumes more routine clerical functions.

Transcribing Physicians' Orders

Physicians' orders are written, telephoned, or verbal. The written orders are recorded on the chart by physicians. Some facilities employ ward clerks or ward secretaries to transcribe the physicians' orders. But in long-term care facilities, there usually are no ward clerks. In facilities that do employ ward clerks, the clerks usually do not work at night. Therefore in many facilities, the nurse is expected to transcribe the order from the chart. There will be times when the order will be difficult to read—*NEVER GUESS*. If in doubt, get a second opinion. Also if the written order does not read like a "routine order" or if it is a little different from usual, check with the physician or other responsible person. It is imperative to check on the written order before carrying out the order. If in doubt about physician's order, always recheck for clarity.

The policy for verbal or telephone orders varies in different facilities. Be certain to check the policy of the facility for the LPN/LVN regarding accepting verbal or telephone orders. The order given by telephone or verbal communication is more subject to error. If you are responsible for accepting this type of order, be certain of the accuracy. Clarify the order by repeating it to the person giving it. This gives both people a chance to hear the order. Always write a telephone or verbal order immediately. If it is given too rapidly, ask that it be repeated more slowly. When the correct spelling of a medication is questionable, refer to a list of commonly ordered medications or to the *Physicians' Desk Reference* (PDR). Be cautious when medications look alike when written, have similar spelling, or sound alike. There are several drugs that sound alike but have very different actions.

When **transcribing** from physicians' orders, the precautions in Box 57-12 will assist in avoiding errors.

When there is an order for a medication to be discontinued or changed, the steps in Box 57-13 should be followed (again, this procedure will vary in different facilities):

Orders to be transcribed are diet, preoperative and postoperative, all medical treatments, activity, procedures, medications, x-ray and other diagnostic studies, and laboratory tests. When a patient undergoes surgery, all preoperative orders are automatically canceled. The physician must rewrite the orders postoperatively if the orders are to be continued. Many physicians have routine postoperative orders, which have been prepared beforehand. This sheet is placed in the patient's chart, and the orders are transcribed as discussed. There will be a procedure for each order according to policy of the facility. When transcribing any order, follow completely through

BOX 57-12 **PRECAUTIONS FOR TRANSCRIBING ORDERS**

The information that follows applies to all physicians' orders.

1. Check that orders are written on the correct chart.
2. If there is more than one order, read through *all* orders before beginning.
3. Process stat orders first. (A stat order signifies that a single dose of medication is to be given immediately and only once.)
4. If there is some confusion during a telephone order, have another nurse listen in on the line for clarification.

The items below are basic guidelines and may vary from one facility to another. Check the agency's policy.

5. The medication needed should be ordered from the pharmacy: include the date, patient's name, room number, time, medication, route of administration, dosage, and frequency.
6. Record the orders in the required areas, such as Kardex, Medex, or medication card. Be certain to include the date.
7. A stat medication may need to be written on a card of a different color. Write STAT on the card, and also write the room number, patient's name, drug dose, route, and time. Pay special attention to STAT orders—the card should be destroyed after the order is given and recorded. STAT orders are to be carried out *immediately,* not at the next routine time for medication administration or procedure performance.
8. Check and recheck to see if all orders have been carried out and recorded in the proper record. (Have a second nurse verify for accuracy until you gain experience.)
9. Each order should be checked off on the physicians' order sheet and signed with your name or initials.
10. Those nurses responsible for administering medications are notified of any new order.
11. Most facilities use a sign that indicates a new order. A red flag may be placed on each chart, or perhaps the physician places the chart in a specific place, such as on the ward clerk's desk.
12. Preferably the charge nurse may be assigned to examine all patients' charts for new orders. This may happen during each shift.

BOX 57-13 PROCEDURE FOR DISCONTINUING OR CHANGING A MEDICATION

1. Mark old medication order off the Kardex or Medex by crossing through with a highlighter marking pen. If it is an order change, write new order.
2. Notify the nurse responsible for carrying out new orders about discontinued and newly ordered medications.
3. See that the old medication card is destroyed, if medication card is used.
4. Check off on physicians' order sheet.

BOX 57-14 SAMPLE OF A SHIFT REPORT

348,A Mabel Lauritsen, age 86, patient of Dr. Hartman, in with congestive heart failure and stasis ulcer of the right leg. She is alert and cheerful, has had a comfortable day. She has a slight increase of the edema in her lower extremities. Received an additional 40 mg of Lasix orally at 10 AM; weight is 165 lb, down 10 lb since admission 2 days ago. Vital signs unremarkable except BP 168/100. Has an IV of D_5W with 20 mEq of KCl infusing at 60 ml per hr with a credit of 600 ml. IV site is without edema or erythema. Has been up about 1 hour today. Appetite has been good. Received Bancap tablets two at 2 PM for pain in right leg. Intake 480 ml IV, 350 ml oral; voided 650 ml of clear, amber urine. Lung sounds clear except for fine rales in base of right lung. She is expectorating a small amount of mucus. No dyspnea noted. Bowel sounds present; abdomen soft. Had moderate amount soft brown stool. Pedal pulses are present bilaterally. Has a 2 by 3 cm stasis ulcer of right leg treated with whirlpool and Betadine dressing. The dressings to be changed qid; TED hose are on. There is an order for Hematest of stools × 3, clean catch urine for C&S, and a chest x-ray. She is to be NPO after midnight for surgery at 9 AM for débridement of the ulcer of her right leg. A preoperative consent form is needed. Social services will be seeing the patient and her daughter Ann Zahrt for discharge planning a few days after surgery.

all steps one order at a time, and then check it off on the order sheet. The nurse transcribing orders should record the time and sign full name on each order. When appropriate, complete the proper requisition slip. As a charge nurse, report any new orders or changes to other staff members so that optimum care will be provided to the patient.

End-of-Shift Report

As an LPN/LVN, you are often responsible for giving an end-of-shift report. See Box 57-14 for an example. The following material will assist you in organization of data for a more efficient and accurate report.

The purpose of the shift report is to provide the next shift with pertinent information about the patient. The quality of nursing care the patient receives is contingent on how well each shift communicates with the other.

Before beginning the report, plan your communication. Be cognizant of what you want to express. Consider your choice of words. Be precise. Use accepted medical/nursing terminology. Practice pronouncing difficult vocabulary to enhance pronunciation.

Before starting the report, write down all necessary information, such as vital signs, type of intravenous fluids, rate of infusion, and credit left in intravenous bottles and continuous bladder irrigations. Report the condition of the IV site. Record the patient's appetite, intakes, and output for feces, urine, and gastric secretion. Report output from drain tubes, such as Davols, Hemovacs, T-tubes, Malecot drains, Solcotrans, and closed chest tubes. Report color of all body excretions. Have information of analgesics given, the time administered, and effect. Record the amount of patient-controlled analgesia used. Write down narcotic credits from the patient-controlled analgesia. Write down the assessment results of your patient's lung sounds, bowel sounds, abdomen (soft or distended), and condition of the skin—report abnormal color and turgor for dehydration or edema. Note circulatory checks if pertinent, as well as presence or absence of pedal pulses. If the patient has a bruit, report it. Note dressing changes, amount and color of exudate, and the condition of the incision. Note any abnormal symptoms, such as dyspnea, tachycardia, or abnormal mental status or level of consciousness. Note neurological deficits, such as flaccid extremity, drooping side of face, hemianopia, or difficulty swallowing (dysphagia).

Once all of the above data are compiled, use Kardex and begin the report. Be systematic and report the following:

1. State patient's room and bed number, name, age, physician, all diagnoses, date of surgery if patient is postoperative.
2. Summarize patient's day/evening/night.
3. Report all pertinent nursing care.
4. Describe change in patient's condition. Usually most facilities report only abnormal vital signs except first postoperative day, and then last set of vital signs are given.
5. Report special medications, intravenous solutions, infusion rate, IV credits. State time, method, and dosage of analgesics given and the effect.
6. Report all intakes and outputs.

7. Report status of lungs and bowel sounds.
8. Report mental status and level of consciousness.
9. Report circulatory checks, pedal pulses, and skin abnormalities in turgor or color.
10. State diagnostic procedures, such as CT scans, x-rays studies, MRI, endoscopy, proctoscopy, thoracentesis, and surgery. Report diet changes, special permits, preoperative procedures, daily weights, activity status, Accuchecks, Hematest for stools, clean catch urine for analysis and/or C&S, sputum specimen for C&S, respiratory therapy, and physical therapy orders. Report all nursing interventions, such as dressings, packs, ostomy care, and oxygen.
11. Discuss patient and family education.
12. Note other services, such as social services, pastoral care, and discharge planning.
13. State any pertinent information helpful in patient care.
14. Report "no code" status.
15. Present the report in an unbiased, nonjudgmental manner.

LEGAL ASPECTS

LPNs/LVNs are legally liable for their actions. The LPN/LVN should understand the legal framework within which he or she practices nursing. A knowledge of the laws that govern the activities, rights, and responsibilities of the LPN/LVN is needed. Each state has a Nurse Practice Act, and this is the most important law governing nursing practice. Familiarize yourself with this vital information.

The LPN/LVN is held liable for any harm a patient suffers as a result of his or her actions. It is recommended that nurses carry **malpractice** insurance. You should buy professional liability insurance to cover the substantial expense of defending a law suit. It can be purchased through a private insurance company or one of your practical/vocational nursing organizations. The facility you work in often provides malpractice insurance. However, it is still good practice to have your own policy. The nurse should read any policy carefully before purchasing it to ascertain if it covers all aspects of professional work. Some policies exclude such types of lawsuits as defamation. Other policies exclude coverage for liability arising from performing certain procedures, such as x-ray therapy. If a lawsuit is filed against a nurse who has such insurance protection, the nurse should notify the insurance company immediately and cooperate with the insurance representative during the course of the lawsuit. This will prevent jeopardizing the nurse's coverage under the terms of the policy. It is important that you practice at the level for which you were educated.

THE LICENSURE EXAMINATION

The graduate practical/vocational nurse's first responsibility after completion of an approved course of study is to successfully pass the National Council Licensure Examination for Practical Nurses (NCLEX-PN). The NCLEX-PN covers all areas of the practical/vocational nursing curriculum and has been designed to test your nursing knowledge, including your ability to apply the principles of that knowledge to given clinical situations in a safe and effective manner.

It is recommended that all new graduates prepare themselves for the NCLEX-PN by systematically reviewing their practical/vocational nursing curriculum. There are excellent comprehensive review books available to assist the student in this endeavor.

On successful completion of the examination, you can practice as a LPN/LVN. An application to take the NCLEX-PN must be completed and sent to the board of nursing in the state in which you reside. Your school of nursing will send a transcript of your records along with your money order or certified check for the required fee for licensing. Application questions and fees may vary for different states. Therefore if you plan to apply in another state, you must contact that state for requirements and fee. The examination is a national licensure examination. Endorsement can be obtained from one state to another. The scores are on a pass/fail basis. At the present, if the test is failed, it may be taken as many times as necessary to pass. The state board of nursing has the authority to refuse any graduate the right to take the examination. Sometimes graduates do not understand that completing the required hours of theory and clinical practice does not automatically make them eligible to take the examination. If there is a question as to the moral character of the applicant, an individual state board hearing may occur. A recommendation as to the applicant's moral character may be written by a person who is knowledgeable about the applicant. Often a nurse educator will be asked to submit such a letter to the state board of nursing. The state board has the authority to accept or reject an applicant to sit for the national licensure. The director of the school of nursing must recommend the graduate to sit for the national licensure. After receiving the license, the LPN/LVN is responsible for renewing it and keeping the state board informed of any changes of address, name, and employment (i.e., active or inactive) status. The nurse cannot legally practice nursing without a license.

The NCLEX-PN makes it possible to practice nursing in other states if one has successfully passed the examination and if the nurse's education fulfills the issuing state's requirements. When the nurse moves to another state, he or she must apply for a license or temporary practice permit before practicing nursing. This licensure from one state to another is called **endorsement.** If the nurse travels with a patient from one state to the other or to Canada, the license the nurse has in her possession is valid for the length of the stay in the other state or Canada.

THE NURSE PRACTICE ACT

The **Nurse Practice Act** is a statute enacted by the legislature of any of the states or by appropriate officers of the districts or possessions.

The Nurse Practice Act is the licensing law. It defines the title and regulations governing the practice of nursing. The act delineates the legal scope of the practice of nursing within the geographical boundaries. Its provisions assist the nurse in staying within the legal scope of nursing practice in each state. Some states have separate governing boards for professional and practical/vocational nursing. The Nurse Practice Act defines the regulations for practical nursing and includes requirements for an approved school of nursing. It also states the requirements for licensure and conditions for which a license may be revoked or suspended (see Chapter 2).

THE STATE BOARD OF NURSING

The state board of nursing consists of members who represent the different levels of nursing and who are appointed by the governor. The purpose of the board is to protect the public by administering the Nurse Practice Act. The board is responsible for approving schools of nursing, administering the licensing examinations, and renewing and issuing licenses. The board has the authority to suspend or revoke a license. Some of the conditions in which a nursing license may be suspended or revoked because of inability to perform competently are drug addiction, alcohol abuse, and lack of mental or physical well-being. A nursing license can be revoked also for **negligence** in patient care, endangering a patient's life, or failing to comply to the standard and requirements of the Nurse Practice Act of the state in which the nurse is practicing.

REFERENCES AND SUGGESTED READINGS

1. Becker BG and Fenderler DT: Vocational and personal adjustments in practical nursing, ed 6, St Louis, 1990, The CV Mosby Co.
2. Behrens E: Charting your success with an effective resumé, LPN, Spring: 14-18, 1986.
3. Hill SS and Howlett HA: Success in practical nursing, Philadelphia, 1988, WB Saunders Co.
4. Hollowell JW and Eldrid JW: The nursing shortage: the increasing risk of legal liability and how to avoid it, J Pract Nurs 39(2):28, 1989.
5. Kurzen CR: Contemporary practical vocational nursing, Philadelphia, 1989, JB Lippincott Co.
6. Mosby's medical, nursing, and allied health dictionary, ed 3, St Louis, 1990, The CV Mosby Co.
7. O'Leary J: What employers will expect from tomorrow's nurses, Nurs Health Care 7(4):207, 1986.
8. Potter PA and Perry AG: Basic nursing: theory and practice, St Louis, 1987, The CV Mosby Co.
9. Practices-nurse's reference library, Springhouse, Penn, 1984, Springhouse Corp.
10. Ringsven MK and Jorenbt BM: Basic community and home care nursing, New York, 1988, Delmar Publishers, Inc.

CHAPTER CHALLENGE

KEY POINTS

- A well-prepared resumé broadens interview opportunities.
- Notice of resignation should be given at least 2 weeks and preferably 1 month in advance.
- Charting notes may be used in court.
- The release of information to anyone other than the health care team is a violation of the patient's right to privacy.
- The LPN/LVN is liable for her own actions.
- The nurse may be found guilty of invasion of privacy, slander, or libel if the patient's health care information is not kept confidential.
- Nurses are responsible for their own actions.
- The nurse should follow the correct procedure while transcribing physicians' orders.
- Nurses must understand legal obligations and responsibilities to patients.
- The purpose of the shift report is to accurately communicate pertinent patient information from one shift to another.
- Learning does not stop at graduation.
- Endorsement enables a nurse to practice in another state without retaking the NCLEX-PN.
- The main function of the state board is to assure safety to the consumer of nursing services.

STUDY QUESTIONS

1. Which of the following is not one of the three types of leadership:
   a. Authoritative   c. Feudal
   b. Democratic   d. Laissez-faire
2. The function of the state board of nursing is to:
   a. Establish certain nursing procedures in the hospital
   b. Legislate and execute laws pertaining to nursing
   c. Separate schools of nursing in the state
   d. Establish in-service programs in the hospital
3. Which of the following organizations are totally committed to practical/vocational nursing and its continuing education:
   a. NAPNES and NLN
   b. NAPNES and NFLPN
   c. NLN and ANA
   d. ANA and NFLPN
4. Of the following, which is the National Organization for Licensed Practical Nurses:
   a. NAPNES   c. ANA
   b. NLN   d. NRN
5. The physician's order that is the least subject to error is:
   a. Written   b. Telephone   c. Verbal
6. In private duty nursing:
   a. You must always work fixed hours and days
   b. You care for three or four patients
   c. The pay is the same as for a registered nurse
   d. You are directly responsible to the individual employer for salary and schedule
7. Which physician's order is always carried out first:
   a. PRN order
   b. One-time-only order
   c. STAT order
   d. Routine order
8. A statute enacted by the legislature of any of the states to delineate the legal scope of the practice of nursing within the geographical boundaries of the jurisdiction is called the:
   a. NLN act
   b. Nurse Practice Act
   c. Joint Commission on Accreditation of Hospitals
9. All of the following would be helpful in giving a quality change-of-shift report except:
   a. Patient's room, bed number, name, diagnosis, physician's name
   b. Summary of patient's day, evening, night
   c. Diagnostic procedures, pertinent nursing care
   d. Nurse's perception of patient's uncooperative manner
10. All of the following characteristics are useful for effective leadership except:
    a. Organizational skills
    b. Nonjudgmental attitude
    c. Standardization of abbreviations
    d. Projection of confidence, knowledge, and integrity

CREDITS

We thank Mosby–Year Book for the use of its extensive art library during the preparation of this text. We also acknowledge the following Mosby–Year Book authors and their books from whom we have borrowed select illustrations and display material.

Beare PG and Myers JL: Principles and practice of adult health nursing, 1990.
Bobak I, Jensen M, and Zalar M: Maternity and gynecologic care: the nurse and the family, ed 4, 1989.
Clayton BD and Stock YN: Basic pharmacology for nurses, ed 9, 1989.
Dison N: Simplified drugs and solutions for nurses including mathematics, ed 9, 1988.
doCarmo PB: Basic EMT skills and equipment: techniques and pitfalls, 1988.
Ebersole P and Hess P: Toward health aging: human needs and nursing, ed 3, 1990.
Glanze WD, Anderson KN, and Anderson L: Mosby's medical, nursing, and allied health dictionary, ed 3, 1989.
Haas A and Haas K: Understanding sexuality, ed 2, 1990.
Hamilton PM: Basic maternity nursing, ed 6, 1989.
Havener WH: Synopsis of ophthalmology, ed 5, 1979.
Harkness-Hood G and Dincher JR: Total patient care: foundations and practice, ed 7, 1988.
Ingalls AJ and Salerno MC: Maternal and child health nursing, ed 7, 1991.
Kaye D and Rose LF: Fundamentals of internal medicine, 1983.
Korones SB: High-risk newborn infants: the basis for intensive nursing care, ed 4, 1986.
LaRocca J and Otto S: Pocket guide to intravenous therapy, 1988.
Long BC and Phipps WJ: Medical-surgical nursing: a nursing process approach, ed 2, 1989.
Malasanos L et al: Health assessment, ed 4, 1990.
McCance KL and Huether SE: Pathophysiology: adults and children, 1990.
Meeker MH and Rothrock J: Alexander's care of the patient in surgery, ed 9, 1991.
Nolte J: The human brain: an introduction to its functional anatomy, ed 2, 1988.
Perry AG and Potter PA: Clinical nursing skills and techniques, ed 2, 1990.
Perry AG and Potter PA: Pocket guide to basic skills and procedures, ed 2, 1990.
Phillips C: Family-centered maternity/newborn care, ed 2, 1987.
Phipps WJ et al: Medical-surgical nursing: concepts and clinical practice, ed 4, 1991.
Potter PA and Perry AG: Basic nursing: theory and practice, ed 2, 1991.
Potter PA and Perry AG: Fundamentals of nursing: concepts, process, and practice, ed 2, 1989.
Prior JA, Silberstein JS, and Stand JM: Physical diagnosis: the history and examination of the patient, ed 6, 1981.
Saunders WH et al: Nursing care in eye, ear, nose, and throat disorders, ed 5, 1979.
Schneeburg NG: Essentials of clinical endocrinology, 1979.
Schottelius BA and Schottelius DD: Textbook of physiology, ed 18, 1978.
Scipien GM et al: Pediatric nursing care, 1990.
Seeley RR, Stephens TD, and Tate P: Anatomy and physiology, 1989.
Seidel HM et al: Mosby's guide to physical examination, ed 2, 1991.
Sorentino SA: Mosby's textbook for nursing assistants, ed 3, 1991.
Thibodeau G: Anthony's textbook of anatomy and physiology, ed 13, 1990.
Thibodeau G: Structure and function of the body, ed 8, 1988.
Thompson JM et al: Mosby's manual of clinical nursing, ed 2, 1989.
Tucker SM: Fetal monitoring and fetal assessment in high-risk pregnancy, 1978.
Whaley LF: Understanding inherited disorders, 1974.
Whaley LF and Wong DL: Essentials of pediatric nursing, ed 3, 1989.
Whaley LF and Wong DL: Nursing care of infants and children, ed 4, 1991.
Williams SR: Essentials of nutrition and diet therapy, ed 5, 1990.
Wilson JR et al: Obstetrics and gynecology, ed 8, 1987.
Worthington-Roberts B and Williams SR: Nutrition in pregnancy and lactation, ed 4, 1989.
Zschoche D: Mosby's comprehensive review of critical care, ed 3, 1985.

ANSWER KEY

Chapter 1

1. d
2. a
3. c
4. a
5. b
6. d
7. b

Chapter 2

1. c
2. d
3. d
4. e
5. b

Chapter 3

1. d
2. b
3. b
4. d
5. c

Chapter 4

1. c
2. b
3. a
4. c
5. e
6. a
7. b
8. d

Chapter 5

1. b
2. c
3. a
4. True
5. True
6. False
7. False

Chapter 6

1. c
2. e
3. b
4. e
5. a
6. b
7. d
8. d
9. e
10. b
11. d
12. c

Chapter 7

1. c
2. a
3. a
4. b
5. a
6. b
7. a
8. c
9. a
10. c
11. a

Chapter 8

1. b
2. a
3. c
4. d
5. b
6. a
7. c
8. a
9. d
10. b
11. c
12. c
13. a
14. a
15. a
16. b
17. b
18. b

Chapter 9

1. a
2. c
3. b
4. a
5. b
6. a
7. b
8. c
9. b
10. c

Chapter 10

1. a
2. c
3. b
4. b
5. a
6. d
7. a
8. b
9. c
10. c
11. b
12. a
13. c
14. a
15. a

Chapter 11

1. b
2. c
3. a
4. b
5. c
6. a
7. b
8. c
9. a
10. c
11. b
12. a
13. c

Chapter 13

1. d
2. a
3. a
4. d
5. c
6. d
7. a
8. b
9. b
10. b
11. a
12. a
13. c

Chapter 14

1. a
2. a
3. b
4. c
5. d
6. b
7. d
8. a
9. b
10. c

Chapter 15

1. a
2. b
3. c
4. a
5. b
6. b
7. d
8. a
9. d

Chapter 16

1. a
2. c
3. a
4. b
5. a
6. d
7. b
8. a
9. b
10. d
11. c
12. b
13. a
14. c
15. d
16. a
17. c

Chapter 17

1. c
2. d
3. a
4. d
5. a
6. a
7. d
8. c
9. d
10. b

Chapter 18

1. d
2. c
3. b
4. a
5. d
6. b
7. b

Chapter 19

1. a
2. b
3. c
4. a
5. c
6. d
7. d
8. a
9. a
10. d
11. c
12. b
13. a
14. d
15. b
16. d

Chapter 20

1. d
2. c
3. b
4. d
5. c
6. b
7. a
8. d
9. c
10. d
11. b
12. d
13. a
14. a
15. d
16. c
17. c
18. d
19. c
20. b

Chapter 21

1. d
2. a
3. c
4. b
5. a
6. d
7. d
8. a
9. c
10. d
11. b
12. c

Chapter 22

1. a
2. c
3. b
4. a
5. a
6. d
7. c
8. c
9. c
10. j
11. i
12. f
13. c
14. h
15. b
16. a
17. e
18. d
19. g

Chapter 23

1. c
2. a
3. b
4. c
5. d
6. d
7. c
8. b
9. a
10. a. R; b. A; c. A; d. R; e. R; f. R; g. R; h. A; i. A; j. R
11. a. R; b. R; c. A; d. A; e. A; f. R; g. R; h. A; i. A; j. R

Chapter 24

Section I

1. a
2. b
3. b
4. c

Section II

1. b
2. b
3. a

Section III

1. c
2. d
3. c
4. a
5. b

Section IV

1. c
2. c
3. d
4. a

Chapter 25

1. a
2. d
3. c
4. b
5. a
6. d
7. a
8. d
9. a
10. d
11. b
12. b
13. a
14. b

Chapter 26

1. d
2. d
3. c
4. a
5. c
6. b
7. c
8. a
9. d
10. b
11. a
12. c
13. c
14. d
15. e
16. a
17. f

Chapter 27

1. c
2. b
3. c
4. b
5. d
6. a
7. d
8. c
9. d
10. a

Chapter 28

1. b
2. a
3. d
4. a
5. b
6. d
7. a
8. c
9. b
10. c
11. a
12. Fluid compartments:
    Intracellular
    Extracellular
    Interstitial
    Intravascular
13. A high percentage of an infant's body weight is fluid, and as aging occurs, the amount of body fluid decreases. A geriatric patient has less fluid to lose before an imbalance will develop.
14. Active transport requires the use of energy.
15. Glucose is carried into the cells using insulin as the transporter.
16. Hypertonic solutions pull fluid from the cells, causing the cells to shrink; hypotonic solutions move into the cells, causing them to enlarge or expand; isotonic solutions cause no abnormal fluid shift.
17. pH.
18. Acidosis — the hydrogen ion concentration increases; alkalosis — the hydrogen ion concentration decreases.
19. The buffers are the first line of defense. When they are exhausted, the lungs come to their aid as the second line of defense. The kidneys are available as the last line of defense.
20. Bananas, oranges, melons, tomato juice, and raisins.
21. Teach the patient to relax, breathe slowly, and breathe into a paper bag to rebreathe carbon dioxide.

Chapter 29

1. b
2. a
3. d
4. b
5. b
6. c
7. d
8. c
9. c
10. d
11. d
12. c
13. c
14. c
15. a
16. c
17. b
18. a
19. e

Chapter 30

1. c
2. b
3. d
4. a
5. a
6. b
7. a
8. b
9. d
10. b
11. c
12. a
13. b
14. c
15. d
16. a
17. b
18. c
19. d
20. b
21. d
22. b
23. c
24. d

Chapter 31

1. b
2. c
3. c
4. d
5. b
6. a
7. b
8. a
9. c
10. a
11. b
12. d
13. a
14. c
15. d
16. c
17. d
18. a
19. b
20. a

Chapter 32

1. c
2. c
3. a
4. c
5. b
6. b
7. b
8. b
9. b
10. a
11. b
12. b
13. a
14. d
15. b
16. b
17. c
18. b
19. a
20. a
21. c
22. d
23. d
24. b
25. d
26. c
27. d
28. b
29. d
30. b

Chapter 33

1. c
2. a
3. a
4. d
5. c
6. a
7. c
8. d
9. c
10. a
11. d
12. c

Chapter 34

1. a
2. c
3. c
4. b
5. a
6. b
7. d
8. a
9. c
10. c
11. c
12. d
13. c
14. d
15. d
16. d
17. c
18. a
19. d

Chapter 35

1. c
2. a
3. d
4. a
5. b
6. b
7. a
8. b
9. d
10. c
11. d
12. b

Chapter 36

1. b
2. d
3. a
4. b
5. c
6. a and d
7. d
8. b
9. c
10. a
11. d
12. a
13. b
14. c
15. a
16. d
17. c
18. a
19. b
20. d

Chapter 37

1. b
2. b
3. c
4. b
5. a
6. b
7. b
8. d
9. c
10. a
11. b
12. a
13. a
14. c
15. d
16. b
17. c
18. b
19. a
20. c
21. b
22. d
23. c

Chapter 38

1. a
2. c
3. b
4. a
5. c
6. b
7. a
8. c
9. b
10. b
11. b
12. d
13. c
14. a
15. c
16. d
17. d
18. a
19. c
20. c
21. a
22. b
23. d
24. a
25. c
26. b
27. a
28. b
29. c

Chapter 39

1. a
2. b
3. a
4. c
5. d
6. a
7. d
8. d
9. c
10. b
11. b
12. a

Chapter 40

1. d
2. b
3. e
4. c
5. a
6. c
7. d
8. a
9. b

Chapter 41

1. b
2. d
3. a
4. a
5. b
6. a
7. d
8. a
9. c
10. a
11. c
12. c
13. b
14. c
15. d

Chapter 42

1. a
2. b
3. c
4. b
5. a
6. b
7. a
8. b
9. b
10. c

Chapter 43

1. d
2. a
3. a
4. d
5. c
6. b
7. d
8. c
9. c
10. a

Chapter 44

1. d
2. a
3. c
4. c
5. d
6. d
7. a
8. c
9. b
10. a
11. c
12. a
13. d

Chapter 45

1. b
2. a
3. c
4. d
5. b
6. c
7. a
8. b
9. d
10. d
11. d
12. a

Chapter 46

1. d
2. a
3. e
4. c
5. b
6. c
7. c
8. d
9. b
10. a
11. d

Chapter 47

1. b
2. a
3. b
4. c
5. c
6. b
7. c
8. b
9. d
10. a
11. c
12. b

Chapter 48

1. c
2. a
3. a
4. c
5. d
6. c
7. b
8. d
9. c
10. d
11. T
12. T
13. F
14. F
15. T

Chapter 49

1. c
2. b
3. a
4. d
5. c
6. a
7. b
8. d
9. d
10. a
11. b
12. c
13. a
14. c
15. d
16. d
17. b
18. d
19. b
20. d
21. a
22. d

Chapter 50

1. b
2. d
3. a
4. a
5. b
6. a
7. c
8. a

Chapter 51

1. c
2. d
3. d
4. e
5. b
6. b
7. e
8. a

Chapter 52

1. b
2. d
3. c
4. d
5. d
6. d
7. a
8. d
9. d
10. a

Chapter 53

1. c
2. d
3. b
4. c
5. a
6. b
7. a
8. b
9. a
10. c

Chapter 54

1. b
2. d
3. d
4. d
5. b
6. b
7. b
8. d
9. b
10. c
11. b
12. c

Chapter 55

1. d
2. d
3. c
4. c
5. b
6. a
7. b
8. b
9. b

Chapter 56

1. c
2. d
3. a
4. e
5. d
6. b
7. e
8. e
9. c
10. b

Chapter 57

1. c
2. b
3. b
4. a
5. a
6. d
7. c
8. b
9. d
10. c

Glossary

ABC Airway; Breathing; Circulation.

abduction Movement of a limb away from the body.

abrasion Scraping or rubbing away of a surface, such as the skin, by friction.

accommodation Adjustment of the eye to variations in distance.

accountability Responsible attitude regarding moral and legal requirements of proper patient care.

accreditation Process whereby a professional association or nongovernmental agency grants recognition to a school or institution for demonstrating ability in a special area of practice or education.

acetabulum Large, cup-shaped cavity at the juncture of the ilium, the ischium, and the pubis; contains the ball-shaped head of the femur.

acetone Colorless, aromatic ketone found in small amounts in normal urine and in larger quantities in the urine of patients with diabetes mellitus.

acetylcholine Neurotransmitter substance widely distributed in body tissues, with a primary function of mediating synaptic activity of the nervous system.

achalasia Inability of a muscle to relax, particularly the cardiac sphincter of the stomach.

Achilles tendon Common tendon of the soleus and gastrocnemius muscles; the thickest and strongest tendon in the body.

achlorhydria Abnormal condition characterized by the absence of hydrochloric acid in the gastric juice.

ACLS (advanced cardiac life support) Includes providing basic life support plus using adjunctive equipment for establishing an intravenous line, administering fluid and drugs, monitoring the heart, performing defibrillation, controlling dysrhythmias, and providing postresuscitation care.

acrocyanosis Condition characterized by cyanotic discoloration, coldness, and sweating of the extremities.

acromion Lateral extension of the spine of the scapula, forming the highest point of the shoulder and connecting with the clavicle at a small, oval surface in the middle of the spine; also called the *acromion process*.

active transport Movement of materials across the membrane of a cell; chemical activity allows the cell to admit larger molecules than could otherwise enter.

acuity Sharpness or acuteness of hearing or sight.

acute pain Intense pain of short duration, lasting less than 6 months; a warning of actual or potential tissue damage.

adaptation Ability to adjust to change.

adaptive immunity Immunity that is acquired, not innate or natural.

adduction Movement of a limb toward the axis (center) of the body.

adenosine triphosphate (ATP) Compound that stores energy in muscles; the energy is released when it is hydrolyzed to adenosine diphosphate.

adhesion Band of scar tissue that binds together two anatomical surfaces that are normally separate.

adipose tissue Collection of cells containing stored fat (depot fat).

adjunct Additive substance or treatment to increase the effectiveness of a primary procedure or to facilitate its performance.

ADL Activities of daily living.

admission Entry of a patient into a health care facility.

adolescence Period that begins with puberty and extends for 8 years or longer, until the person is physically and psychologically mature and ready for adult responsibilities.

adrenal gland Either of two secretory endocrine organs located on the superior surface of the kidneys.

adrenalin Adrenal hormone and synthetic adrenergic vasoconstrictor.

adrenocorticotropic hormone (ACTH) Hormone of the anterior pituitary gland that stimulates growth of the adrenal gland cortex and the secretion of corticosteroids.

adverse drug effect Harmful, unintended reaction to a drug administered at a normal dosage.

afebrile Without fever.

affect Outward evidence of a person's feelings or emotions.

afferent Proceeding toward a center, as applied to arteries, veins, lymphatics, and nerves.

against-medical-advice (AMA) Patient leaves a health care facility without a physician's order for discharge.

ageism Attitudes, actions, or institutional structures that discriminate against individuals on the basis of age.

agility Ability to move with quick, easy grace.

aging Process of growing old, which begins at conception and ends at death.

agnosia Brain damage resulting in total or partial inability to recognize familiar objects or persons.

agonist Drug having a specific cellular affinity that produces a predictable response.

AIDS Acquired immune deficiency syndrome.

akinesia Loss or reduction of the capacity to initiate, maintain, and perform voluntary motor activities.

Al-Anon International organization that offers guidance and counseling for the relatives, friends, and associates of alcoholics.

albuminuria Condition of excess serum proteins in the urine; also called *proteinuria*.

alcohol sponge Sponge bath using alcohol and water to reduce body temperature.

alcohol withdrawal syndrome Clinical signs and symptoms associated with stopping alcohol consumption, including tremor, hallucinations, autonomic nervous system dysfunction, and seizures.

Alcoholics Anonymous International nonprofit organization founded in 1935, consisting of abstinent alcoholics whose purpose is to help other alcoholics stop drinking and maintain sobriety.

alcoholism Extreme dependence on excessive amounts of alcohol, associated with a cumulative pattern of deviant behaviors.

alignment Maintaining of body structures in their appropriate anatomical positions.

alimentary canal Musculomembranous tube, about 9 meters (30 feet) long, extending from the mouth to the anus and lined with mucous membrane.

allergen Substance that can produce a hypersensitive reaction in the body but is not necessarily harmful.

alopecia Partial or complete baldness resulting from aging, endocrine disorder, drug reaction, anticancer medication, or skin disease.

alveoli Small, saclike structures through which gas exchange takes place in the lungs.

amenorrhea Absence of menstruation.

amino acids Building blocks of protein; 22 amino acids have been identified as vital for human life. The body can synthesize 13 of these, termed *nonessential*, whereas the remaining 9 must be obtained from dietary sources and are called *essential*.

amniotomy Rupture of the amniotic sac.

ANA Standards of Nursing Practice Evaluation that serves as a basis for comparison of similar occurrences, set forth by the American Nurses' Association.

anabolism Constructive metabolism characterized by conversion of simple substances into the more complex compounds of living matter.

analysis Separation of substances into their constituent parts.

anaphylaxis Severe and sometimes fatal hypersensitivity reaction to a sensitizing substance (allergen).

anaplasia Change in the structure of cells; a loss of differentiation, characteristic of a malignancy.

anasarca Generalized massive edema.

anastomosis Surgical joining of two ducts or blood vessels to allow flow from one to the other.

anatomy Study of the structure of the human body.

androgen Any steroid hormone that produces male physical characteristics.

anemia Decrease in hemoglobin in the blood to levels below the normal range.

anesthesia Absence of normal sensation, especially sensitivity to pain, induced by an anesthetic substance for surgical purposes.

animism Ascribing of human characteristics to nonhuman or inanimate objects.

anion Negatively charged ion, atom, or molecule.

ankylosis Fixation of a joint, often seen in an abnormal position.

anomaly Deviation from what is considered normal.

anorexia Lack or loss of appetite, resulting in the inability to eat.

anorexia nervosa Psychoneurotic disorder characterized by a prolonged refusal to eat; self-imposed starvation.

anoxia Abnormal lack of oxygen.

answer Response of a defendant to the complaint of a plaintiff.

antagonist Drug that exerts an opposite action to that of another drug.

anterior Front of a structure.

anterior fontanel Diamond-shaped area at the superior, anterior area of the head.

antibody Protein molecule essential to the immune system, produced by lymphoid tissue in response to bacteria, viruses, or other antigenic substances; an antibody is specific to an antigen.

anticipatory guidance Psychological preparation of a patient for an event expected to be stressful, as in the preparation of a child for surgery by explaining what will happen and what it will feel like. It is also used to prepare parents for normal growth and development of their children.

antigen Substance, usually a protein, that causes the formation of an antibody and reacts specifically with that antibody; helps form immunity in humans.

antidiuretic hormone (ADH) Hormone that decreases production of urine by increasing reabsorption of water by the renal tubules.

antioxidant Chemical or other agent that delays or prevents the breakdown of a substance by oxygen.

anuria Cessation of urine production, or a urinary output of less than 100 to 250 ml per 24 hours.

anxiety Vague sense of impending doom characterized by uneasiness and physiological changes; usually results from a real or perceived threat to the self.

aorta Main trunk of the systemic arterial circulation.

apex Pertaining to the top, the end, or the tip of a structure—as the apex of the heart.

aphasia Defective or absent language function caused by injury to certain areas of the cerebral cortex.

apnea Absence of spontaneous respiration.

appeal Request for review and/or retrial of legal issues.

approved Status of a nursing program that meets minimum standards set by the state.

apraxia Impairment in the ability to perform purposeful acts or to manipulate objects.

aqueous humor Clear, watery fluid circulating in the anterior and posterior chambers of the eye.

arachnoid membrane Thin, delicate membrane enclosing the brain and the spinal cord, interposed between the pia mater and the dura mater. The subarachnoid space lies between the arachnoid membrane and the pia; the subdural space lies between the arachnoid membrane and the dura.

ARC AIDS-related complex.

areolar gland One of the large sebaceous glands in the areolae encircling the nipples on women's breasts.

arrhythmia See *dysrhythmia*.

arteriole Blood vessel in the smallest branch of arterial circulation. Blood flowing from the heart is pumped through the arteries to the arterioles.

arteriosclerosis Degenerative thickening, calcification, and decreased elasticity of arterial walls.

artery One of the large vessels carrying blood away from the heart.

arthrocentesis Puncture of a joint with a needle to withdraw fluid.

arthrodesis Surgically induced fixation of a joint to relieve pain or to provide support.

arthroplasty Surgical reconstruction or replacement of a painful, degenerated joint.

arthroscopy Examination of the interior of a joint performed by inserting a specially designed endoscope through a small incision.

articulation Gliding, rotation, and angular movement of a joint.

ascites Abnormal intraperitoneal accumulation of fluid.

asepsis Absence of germs. Surgical asepsis protects against infection before, during or after surgery by the use of sterile techniques.

asphyxia Severe lack of oxygen to the blood, leading to hypercapnia, loss of consciousness, and, if not corrected, death.

assessment Evaluation or appraisal of a patient.

asthma Respiratory disorder characterized by recurring episodes of labored breathing, wheezing on expiration, coughing, and viscous, mucoid bronchial secretions.

astigmatism Eye condition in which light rays cannot focus clearly on a point in the retina.

asymptomatic Without indication of disease; without subjective or objective signs and symptoms.

ataxia Impaired ability to coordinate movement; a staggering gait.

atelectasis Collapse of lung tissue, preventing respiratory exchange of carbon dioxide and oxygen.

atheroma Abnormal mass of fat or lipids deposited on the arterial wall.

atherosclerosis Arterial disorder characterized by yellowish plaques of cholesterol, lipids, and cellular debris in the walls of the arteries.

atrioventricular valve Value in the heart through which blood flows from the atria to the ventricles.

atrium Chamber or cavity, such as the right and left atria of the heart.

atrophy Decrease in size or physiological activity of a part of the body because of disease or lack of use.

attachment Close, mutual relationship between two people that involves contact and proximity and endures through time.

attitude Fetal position in the uterus.

audiometry Testing of hearing acuity.

auditor Person appointed to examine patients' charts and health records to assess the quality of care.

auditory hallucination Perception of sound without an external stimulus.

auscultation Act of listening for sounds within the body to evaluate the condition of various organs.

autistic behavior Self-absorbed, isolated, repetitive behavior and lack of communication with others.

autograft Surgical transplantation of any tissue from one part of the body to another in the same individual.

autoimmunity Abnormal characteristic or condition in which the body reacts against constituents of its own tissues.

autonomy Ability or tendency to function independently.

axilla Pyramid-shaped space forming the underside of the shoulder between the upper part of the arm and the side of the chest; also called *armpit*.

axis Line that passes through the center of the body or through a part of the body.

axon Cylindrical extension of a nerve cell that conducts impulses away from the neuron cell body. Axons may be bare or sheathed in myelin.

azotemia (uremia) Excessive nitrogenous compounds in the blood.

B cell Type of lymphocyte that responds to stimulation of antigens entering the body, causing an immunological response.

babbling Incoherent sounds made by an infant while vocally playing with sounds.

back rub (massage) Manipulation of the soft tissue by rubbing and kneading to increase circulation, improve muscle tone, and promote relaxation in the patient.

basal metabolic rate (BMR) Amount of energy used by the body at rest to maintain vital functions such as respiration, circulation, temperature, peristalsis, and muscle tone.

base of support Stance with the feet slightly apart to provide better stability for work.

bath basin Small plastic pan used to hold water for bathing a patient.

bath mitt Wash cloth folded over the hand to form a mitt; prevents wet ends of cloth from touching the patient.

battered woman syndrome Repeated episodes of physical assault on a woman by a man with whom she has a close relationship.

bedpan Shallow pan for use as a toilet by a person confined to bed.

bedside commode Chair with a hole in the seat containing a vessel for urination and defecation.

behavior Actions that occur intentionally or spontaneously and are observable and measurable.

beneficence Bringing about of good.

benign neoplasm Localized tumor that has a fibrous capsule, limited potential for growth, and cells that are well differentiated.

beriberi Disease of the peripheral nerves caused by deficiency of or inability to assimilate the vitamin *thiamin*.

bereavement Common depressed reaction to the loss of a loved one.

bicarbonate (HCO_3) Salt of carbonic acid; a base or alkaline.

biological age Person's present position with respect to potential life span, which may be younger or older than chronological age and encompasses measures of vital organ functions.

biological death Total absence of activity in the brain and central nervous system, the cardiovascular system, and the respiratory system as observed and declared by a physician.

biopsy Removal of a small piece of living tissue for microscopic examination to confirm or establish a diagnosis.

birth defect (congenital anomaly) Abnormality, particularly a structural one, present at birth, which may be inherited genetically, acquired during gestation, or inflicted during parturition.

blanching Causing to become pale by applying digital pressure.

blastocyst Undifferentiated embryonic cell before germ layer formation.

BLS (basic life support) Phase of emergency cardiac care that prevents circulatory or respiratory arrest (or insufficiency) by prompt recognition and intervention.

body mechanics Field of physiology that studies muscular actions and the function of muscles in maintaining the posture of the body.

body surface area (BSA) Total area exposed to the outside environment.

bolus Round mass, specifically a masticated lump of food ready to be swallowed.

bonding Parent's feeling and attachment behavior toward infant after delivery.

bony prominence Area of the body where bones can be easily palpated. Bony areas have greater potential for impaired skin integrity than other areas of the body.

Bowman's capsule Cup-shaped end of a renal tubule containing a glomerulus.

bradycardia Heart rate of less than 60 beats per minute.

bradykinesia Abnormal condition characterized by slowness of all voluntary movement and speech, as caused by Parkinsonism and certain tranquilizers.

bradypnea Abnormally slow respiratory rate of less than 12 breaths per minute.

brain death Irreversible form of unconsciousness characterized by a complete loss of brain function while the heart continues to beat.

brainstem Portion of the brain comprising the medulla oblongata, the pons, and the mesencephalon. It performs motor, sensory, and reflex functions. The 12 pairs of cranial nerves are attached to the base of the brain.

Braxton Hicks contractions Irregular tightening of the pregnant uterus that begins in the first trimester and increases in frequency, duration, and intensity as pregnancy progresses. Contractility of uterine muscle increases in pregnancy. Near term, strong Braxton Hicks contractions are often difficult to distinguish from the contractions of true labor; also called *false labor*.

bronchiole Small airway of the respiratory system extending from the bronchi into the lobes of the lung.

bronchitis Acute or chronic inflammation of mucous membranes of the tracheobronchial tree.

bronchopulmonary Of or pertaining to the bronchi and the lungs of the respiratory system.

bronchopulmonary dysplasia Abnormal development of the bronchi and lungs.

bronchoscopy Visual examination of the tracheobronchial tree, using the standard metal bronchoscope of the narrower, flexible fiberoptic bronchoscope.

bronchus Large passage into the lungs through which pass inspired air and exhaled waste gases.

bruit Abnormal sound or murmur heard while auscultating an organ, gland, or vessel, as the liver or an artery.

buffer Substance or group of substances that can absorb or release hydrogen ions to correct an acid-base imbalance.

bulimia Eating disorder involving an insatiable craving for food, often resulting in episodes of continuous eating followed by periods of depression, self-deprivation, and/or purging.

burnout Mental or physical energy loss related to a job, accompanied by feelings of hopelessness or loss of creativity.

burping Belching or eructation.

bursa Fibrous sac between certain tendons and the bones beneath them. Lined with a synovial membrane that secretes synovial fluid, the bursa acts as a small cushion that allows the tendon, as it contracts and relaxes, to move over the bone.

cachexia Ill health, malnutrition, and wasting as a result of chronic disease.

calcitonin Hormone produced in the thyroid that participates in regulating the blood level of calcium.

calcium (Ca^{++}) White, alkaline earth metal element occurring mainly in the bones of the body.

callus Bony deposit formed between and around the broken ends of a fractured bone during healing.

calyx Cup-shaped part or organ; e.g., renal calyx.

candidiasis Any infection caused by a species of *Candida*, usually *Candida albicans*.

cannabis or marijuana Psychoactive drug derived from hemp plants.

canthus Angle at the medial (inner) and lateral (outer) margins of the eyelids.

capillary One of the tiny blood vessels joining arterioles and venules. Through its walls blood and tissue cells exchange various substances.

carbohydrate Any of a group of organized compounds. The most important are sugar, starch, cellulose, and gum.

carcinoembryonic antigen (CEA) Antigen present in very small quantities in adult tissue. A greater than normal amount is suggestive of cancer.

carcinogen Substance or agent that produces cancer.

carcinoma Malignant epithelial neoplasm that tends to invade surrounding tissue and to spread to distant regions of the body.

carcinoma in situ Premalignant neoplasm that has not invaded surrounding membranes or tissue, but has characteristics of invasive cancer; frequently seen on the uterine cervix.

cardiac arrest Sudden cessation of cardiac output and effective circulation. Immediate initiation of cardiopulmonary resuscitation is required to prevent heart, lung, kidney, and brain damage.

cardiac output Volume of blood expelled by the ventricles of the heart.

cardiovascular Of or pertaining to the heart and blood vessels.

caregiver role Function of giving care to elderly parents, other elderly family members, or spouse.

carotid pulse Pulse of the carotid artery, felt by gently pressing a finger into the groove between the larynx and the sternocleidomastoid muscle in the neck.

carrier Person or animal who harbors and spreads a microorganism causing disease in others, but who does not become ill.

catabolism Complex, metabolic process in which energy is liberated for use in work, energy storage, or heat production by the destruction of complex substances to form simple compounds.

cataract Abnormal progressive condition of the lens of the eye, characterized by loss of transparency.

catatonic state Extreme immobility and muscular rigidity, usually associated with panic or schizophrenia.

cation Positively charged ion, atom, or molecule.

CDC *See Centers for Disease Control.*

cell Fundamental unit of all living tissue.

cellular immunity Acquired immunity characterized by the dominant role of small T cell lymphocytes.

Centers for Disease Control (CDC) Division of the U.S. Public Health Service, in Atlanta, Georgia; investigates diseases, especially those with epidemic potential.

center of gravity Midpoint or center of weight of a body or object. In the standing adult human the center of gravity is in the midpelvic cavity, between the symphysis pubis and the umbilicus.

centrifuge Equipment that spins test tubes at high speeds.

centriole Intracellular organelle, associated with cell division.

cerebellum Part of the brain located in the posterior cranial fossa behind the brainstem. It consists of two lateral cerebellar hemispheres, or lobes, and a middle section called the *vermis*. Its functions are concerned with coordinating voluntary muscular activity.

cerebral dominance Specialization of each of the two cerebral hemispheres in the integration and control of different functions.

cerebrospinal fluid Fluid that flows through and protects the four ventricles of the brain, the subarachnoid space, and the spinal canal.

cerebrovascular accident Occlusion of a blood vessel in the brain by a thrombus, an embolus, or cerebrovascular hemorrhage, resulting in decreased blood supply.

cerebrum Largest and uppermost section of the brain, divided by a central sulcus into the left and the right cerebral hemispheres.

certification Process in which an individual, an institution, or an educational program is evaluated and recognized as meeting certain predetermined standards.

cerumen Earwax; a yellow or brown waxy secretion in the external ear canal.

ceruminous gland One of a number of tiny structures in the external ear canal, believed to be a modified sweat gland. It secretes a waxy cerumen instead of water sweat.

cervical cord injury Spinal injury that may affect upper extremities, trunk, lower extremities, and bladder and bowel function.

chancre Skin lesion, usually of primary syphilis, that begins at the site of infection as a papule and develops into a red, bloodless, painless ulcer with a scooped-out appearance.

chart or health care record Patient record that includes all the forms used to document care.

charting by exception Process of recording only new data or changes in patient status or care; charting the exceptions to the previously recorded data.

charting, documenting, or recording Process of noting data in a patient record, usually at prescribed intervals.

chemical dependence Total psychophysical state of one addicted to drugs or alcohol who must receive an increasing amount of the substance to prevent abstinence signs and symptoms.

Cheyne-Stokes respiration Abnormal respiratory pattern characterized by periods of apnea alternating with deep, rapid respirations.

child abuse Attack on a child by an adult caretaker that results in physical, emotional, and/or sexual injury or trauma.

chlamydia Microorganism that lives in the epithelium of the urethra and cervix. It is one of the most common sexually transmitted diseases and a frequent cause of sterility.

chloride (Cl^-) Salt compound in which the negative element is chloride.

cholecystokinin Hormone produced by the mucosa of the upper intestine; stimulates contraction of the gallbladder and secretion of pancreatic enzymes.

cholesterol (dietary) Fat-soluble sterol found in animal fats and oils, organ meats, and egg yolk.

cholesterol (serum) Fat-soluble sterol found in the blood stream and continuously synthesized in the body, primarily in the liver.

choroid Thin, highly vascular membrane covering the posterior five sixths of the eye between the retina and sclera.

chromatin Material within the cell nucleus from which the chromosomes are formed. It consists of fine, threadlike strands.

chronic obstructive pulmonary disease (COPD) Progressive and irreversible condition characterized by diminished inspiratory and expiratory capacity of the lungs.

chronic pain Pain lasting longer than 6 months; may be continuous or intermittent and as intense as acute pain.

chronological age Age of an individual expressed as the time that has elapsed since birth.

chum Close friend, often of same gender and age.

chux Waterproof disposable pad.

Chvostek's sign Facial spasm occurring when the facial nerve is tapped above the mandibular angle, next to the earlobe in patients who are hypocalcemic (positive sign).

cilia Small, hairlike processes on the outer surfaces of some cells, aiding metabolism by producing motion, eddies, or current in a fluid; most often associated with the respiratory passageway.

circumcision Surgical removal of the foreskin of the penis.

classification Sorting of objects into groups according to certain attributes, such as color, size, or shape.

claudication Weakness of the legs with cramplike pains in the calves, caused by poor circulation of blood to the leg muscles.

cleft lip Congenital anomaly consisting of one or more clefts in the upper lip, resulting from failure of the maxillary and median nasal processes to close.

cleft palate Congenital defect characterized by a fissure in the midline of the palate, resulting from failure of the two sides to fuse during embryonic development.

climacteric Cessation of menses; commonly refers to *menopause*.

clinical death Total absence of activity in the brain and central nervous system, the cardiovascular system, and the respiratory system as observed and declared by a physician.

clonus(ic) Abnormal pattern of neuromuscular activity, characterized by rapidly alternating involuntary contraction and relaxation of skeletal muscle.

closed bed Hospital bed made with all linens pulled toward the head of the bed.

CMV (cytomegalovirus) Member of a group of large, species-specific, herpes-type viruses with a wide variety of disease effects.

co-dependency Situation in which a person is overly affected by and concerned with controlling other people's behaviors.

code Discreet signal used to summon a special team.

cognitive behavior Mental processes characterized by knowing, thinking, learning, and judging.

cognitive learning Learning concerned with problem-solving abilities, intelligence, and conscious thought.

cohabitation Two people living together in a sexual relationship without marriage.

coitus Sexual union of two people of the opposite sex.

collagen Tiny protein fibrils that form inelastic fibers of the tendons, ligaments, and fascia.

Colles' fracture Fracture of the radius at the epiphysis within 1 inch of the joint of the wrist, easily recognized by the resulting dorsal and lateral position of the hand.

collodion Clear or slightly opaque, highly inflammable liquid composed of pyroxylin, ether, and alcohol. It dries to a strong, transparent film that is used as a surgical dressing.

color blindness Inability to distinguish colors of the spectrum.

colostrum Fluid secreted by the breast during pregnancy and during the first days of postpartum before lactation begins.

colporrhaphy Surgical procedure in which the vagina is sutured, as for the purpose of narrowing or repairing the vagina.

command hallucination Imaginary voice commanding the individual to do something.

communication Any process in which information is transferred and received.

community health nursing Blend of nursing and public health, promoting prevention, education, and maintenance.

compartment syndrome Pathological condition caused by progressive development of arterial compression and reduced blood supply.

compatibility State in which two or more drugs can be given at the same time without producing undesired side effects or without canceling or changing the therapeutic effects of the other.

complaint Pleading by a plaintiff made under oath to initiate a law suit.

comprehensive rehabilitation plan Planned, orderly sequence of services for a handicapped individual, designed to help him realize his maximum potential.

compressor Individual in two-rescuer cardiopulmonary resuscitation (CPR) who performs external cardiac compressions.

compulsion Act carried out, to some degree against a person's conscious will, to avoid anxiety.

computed tomography Painless x-ray technique that films a cross section of tissue (CT scan); also called *computerized axial tomography*.

computer terminal Machine at a nursing work station used to access the larger mainframe computer for data processing.

concrete stage Stage of cognitive development that involves reasoning about tangible or familiar situations.

condyle Rounded projection at the end of a bone that anchors muscle ligaments and articulates with adjacent bones.

confidentiality Process of keeping information and records private or secret.

conflict Two incompatible goals occurring at the same time.

confront To challenge.

congruent In agreement or harmony.

conjunctiva Mucous membrane lining the inner surfaces of the eyelids and the anterior part of the sclera.

conjunctivitis Inflammation of the conjunctiva.

connective tissue Tissue that supports and binds other body structures. The types are *bone*, *cartilage*, and *fibrous tissue*.

conservation Mental process of understanding the sameness of a situation or object in spite of a change in some aspect, e.g., that the mass or quantity of an object is the same even if it changes shape or position.

consumer One who uses goods or services.

contact lens Small, curved glass or plastic lens shaped to fit the eye and to correct refraction or inability of the lens of the eye to focus accurately.

contamination Soiling or infection with something undesirable, as bacteria in a wound; also known as *sepsis*.

context Meaning of language within a particular setting.

continuity-of-care Continuing of care in from one setting to another.

contracture Abnormal, usually permanent condition of a joint, characterized by flexion (bending) and fixation caused by atrophy and shortening of muscle fibers.

convalescence Period of recovery after an illness, injury, or surgery.

conversion Unconscious defense mechanism in which repressed emotions are transformed into physical signs and symptoms; also called *conversion hysteria* or *conversion reaction*.

cooing Hum of contentment made by an infant.

coping Voluntary pattern of behavior used to relieve stress or anxiety.

cordotomy Operation in which an incision is made high in the thoracic area and two laminae are removed; then the pain pathways in the spinothalamic tract (anterior and lateral aspect of the cord) on the side opposite the pain are severed.

corium Layer of skin just below the epidermis, containing blood and lymphatic vessels, nerves and nerve endings, glands, and hair follicles.

cornea Convex, transparent, anterior part of the eye, comprising one sixth of the outermost tunic of the eye bulb.

coronary (in anatomy) Of or pertaining to encircling structures, as the coronary arteries of the heart.

corpuscle Any cell of the body; a red or white blood cell.

cortex Outer layer of a body organ or structure, as distinguished from the internal substance.

corticosteroid Antiinflammatory drug for relief of inflammation and pruritus (itching).

cortisol Steroid hormone occurring naturally in the body.

countertraction Force that counteracts the pull of traction.

Couvade syndrome Man's physical and emotional reaction to his partner's pregnancy.

coxsackievirus Any of 30 serologically different enteroviruses associated with a variety of signs and symptoms and primarily affecting children during warm weather.

craniotomy Any surgical opening into the skull, performed to relieve pressure, to control bleeding, or to remove a tumor.

creatinine Substance formed from the metabolism of creatine, commonly found in blood, urine, and muscle tissue.

crepitus Crackling sound heard as a result of bone fragments rubbing together or air in the subcutaneous tissue.

crisis Time of change or turning point in life when patterns of living must be modified to prevent disorganization of the person or family.

cryosurgery Use of subfreezing temperatures to destroy tissue.

cryptorchidism Failure of one or both of the testicles to descend into the scrotum; also called *undescended testis.*

cue Word, phrase, or symptom that indicates the nature of something perceived. Cues are grouped to assist the nurse in interpretations of data.

culdoscopy Diagnostic procedure to visualize the pelvic organs.

cultural healing beliefs Beliefs that reflect a specific culture's orientation to health and illness.

culture (1) System of symbols shared by a group of humans and transmitted by them to upcoming generations; also group design for living, i.e., goals, attitudes, roles, and values.

culture (2) Living cells in a special medium that can support growth of microorganisms.

cumulative action Increased activity demonstrated by a drug when repeated doses accumulate in the body.

curative Method of combating or preventing; a treatment designed to cure.

curettage Scraping of material from the wall of a cavity or other surface with an instrument called a *curet.*

cushingoid Having the habitus and facies characteristic of Cushing's disease: fat pads on the upper back and face, striae on the limbs and trunk, and excess hair on the face.

custom Habitual practice; the usual way of acting under given circumstances.

cyanosis Blue discoloration of the skin and mucous membrane caused by inadequate oxygen in the blood.

cytology Study of cells: their formation, origin, structure, biochemical activities, and pathology.

cytomegalovirus (CMV) Member of a group of large, species-specific, herpes-type viruses with a wide variety of disease effects.

damages Money awarded to a plaintiff by a court as compensation for any loss, detriment, or injury to the plaintiff's person, property, or rights caused by the wrongdoing or negligence of the defendent.

dander Dry scales shed from the skin or hair of animals or feathers of birds that may cause an allergic reaction in some individuals.

data base Large store of information.

death Cessation of life.

débridement Removal of dirt, foreign objects, damaged tissue, and cellular debris from a wound or burn to prevent infection and to promote healing.

decentering Coordination mentally of two or more ideas or characteristics, such as space and length.

decorticate rigidity Abnormal postural reflex characterized by flexion of the arms, wrists, and fingers. The legs may also be flexed.

decubitus ulcer Inflammation or sore in the skin over a bony prominence. It results from ischemic hypoxia of the tissue because of prolonged pressure on the part.

defendant Party named in a plaintiff's complaint and against whom the accusations are made.

defense mechanism Involuntary behavior used to protect the individual from feeling anxiety.

dehiscence Separation of a surgical incision or the rupture of a wound closure.

delirium tremens (DTs) Acute and sometimes fatal psychotic and physical reaction caused by withdrawal of alcohol after excessive intake of alcoholic beverages over a long period; characterized by agitation, tremors, excitement, disorientation, mental confusion, vivid hallucinations, and other signs and symptoms.

delusion False belief, held as true in spite of evidence to the contrary.

dementia Progressive, organic mental disorder characterized by confusion and impaired intellectual function, memory, and judgment.

demographics Statistical study of human populations, especially with reference to size and density, distribution and vital statistics, and typical characteristics.

dendrite Branching process that extends from the cell body of a neuron. Each neuron usually possesses several dendrites, which receive impulses conducted to the cell body.

denial Unconscious defense mechanism in which emotional conflict and anxiety are avoided by refusing to acknowledge those thoughts, feelings, desires, impulses, or external facts that are consciously intolerable.

dentin Chief material of teeth, surrounding the pulp and situated inside the enamel and cementum.

denture Artificial tooth or set of teeth not permanently fixed or implanted.

deposition Sworn pretrial testimony given by a witness in response to oral or written questions and cross examination.

despair Second response to separation from attachment figure, involving quiet hopelessness, sadness, and mourning.

detoxification Treatment to diminish or remove from a patient's body the toxic effects of chemical substances, such as alcohol or drugs, usually as an initial step in treating a chemically dependent person.

developmental delay Preferred term for mental retardation.

diabetic retinopathy Disorder of the retinal blood vessels caused by diabetes mellitus.

diagnosis related group (DRG) Designation in a system that classifies patients by age, diagnosis, and surgical procedure, producing 300 categories used in predicting use of hospital resources. Cost reimbursement systems by government health plans (Medicare and Medicaid) are based on a patient's DRG.

diaphragm Domelike muscular partition between the thoracic and abdominal cavities.

diaphysis Shaft of a long bone, consisting of a tube of compact bone enclosing the medullary cavity.

diarthrosis Freely movable joint in which contiguous bony surfaces are covered by articular cartilage and connected by ligaments lined with synovial membrane.

diastole Time between contractions of the atria or the ventricles during which blood enters the relaxed chambers from systemic circulation and the lungs.

diencephalon Division of the brain between the telencephalon and the mesencephalon. It consists of the hypothalamus, thalamus, metathalamus, and the epithalamus and includes most of the third ventricle.

diet therapy Treatment of disease or medical/surgical conditions by diet.

dietary fiber Generic term for nondigestible chemical substances in plants.

differentiation Process of cellular development in which unspecialized cells or tissues are modified to achieve specific and characteristic physical forms, physiological functions, and chemical properties.

diffusion Process in which solid, particulate matter in a fluid moves from an area of higher concentration to lower concentration, resulting in even distribution of the particles in the fluid.

digestion Conversion of food in the gastrointestinal tract into absorbable substances.

dilemma Situation requiring a choice between two equally desirable or undesirable alternatives.

diplopia Double vision caused by defective function of the extraocular muscles or by a disorder of the nerves that innervate the muscles.

disaster-preparedness plan Formal plan of action, usually prepared in written form, for coordinating the response of the hospital staff in the event of a disaster within the hospital or the surrounding community.

discharge Release of a patient from a health care facility.

discovery Pretrial procedure allowing one party to examine vital witnesses and/or documents held exclusively by the adverse party.

disengagement stage Time in family life when a child or children leave home, leaving the couple or single parent to live alone.

disinfection Destruction of disease-causing microorganisms.

disorientation Mental confusion characterized by inadequate or incorrect perceptions of place, time, or identity.

diuresis Increased formation and secretion of urine.

diverticulitis Inflammation of one or more diverticula (pouchlike herniations through the colon).

diverticulosis Presence of pouchlike herniations through the muscular layer of the colon.

dizygotic Pertaining to twins from two fertilized ova.

DNR Do not resuscitate.

documentation Written material associated with a computer or a computer program.

dominant group Social group that controls the value system and the rewards in a society.

dorsal (supine) Pertaining to the back or posterior; the back.

drainage Removal of fluids from a body cavity or a wound.

dramatic play Play that acts out adult roles.

drawsheet Sheet smaller than a bed sheet, usually placed across the middle of the bottom sheet to keep the mattress and bottom linens dry; can also help turn or move a patient in bed.

DRG See *diagnosis related groups*.

drip factor Number of drops an IV tubing set delivers per milliliter; factor needed for determining the drip rate of an IV.

drug abuse Use of a drug for nontherapeutic effect, especially one for which it was not prescribed or intended.

drug addiction Condition characterized by an overwhelming desire to continue taking a drug in which one has been habituated through repeated consumption. The drug produces a particular effect that is usually an alternation of mental activity, attitude, or outlook.

dumping syndrome Profuse perspiring, nausea, vertigo, and weakness in some patients who have had a subtotal gastrectomy.

dura mater Outermost and most fibrous of the three membranes surrounding the brain and spinal cord.

Duchenne's muscular dystrophy Abnormal congenital condition characterized by progressive symmetric wasting of the leg and pelvic muscles. It is an X-linked recessive disease that appears insidiously between 3 and 5 years of age and spreads from the leg and pelvic muscles to the involuntary muscles. It usually results in death within 10 to 15 years of the onset of symptoms; also called *pseudohypertrophic muscular dystrophy*.

dysarthria Difficult, poorly articulated speech, usually the result of a damaged central or peripheral motor nerve.

dysmenorrhea Painful menstruation.

dysphagia Difficulty in swallowing.

dysplasia Abnormal development of tissue.

dyspnea Shortness of breath or difficulty breathing.

dysrhythmia Any disturbance or abnormality in normal rhythmic pattern, especially heart or brain waves.

dysuria Painful urination.

eclampsia Gravest form of toxemia of pregnancy, characterized by grand mal convulsion, coma, hypertension, proteinuria, and edema.

ectoderm Outermost of the three primary cell layers of an embryo; gives rise to the nervous system; the organs of the special senses, as the eyes and ears; the epidermis and epidermal tissue, as fingernails, hair, and skin glands; and the mucous membrane of the mouth and anus.

ectopic (of an object or organ) Situated in an unusual place, away from its normal location.

edema Abnormal accumulation of fluid in the tissue.

effacement Shortening of the vaginal portion of the cervix and the thinning of its walls as it is stretched and dilated by the fetus during labor.

efferent nerve Nerve that transmits impulses away or outward from a nerve center, such as the brain or spine.

ego integrity Feeling of acceptance of life for what it has been, with no wish to relive it.

egocentric Self-centered; unable to consider another's viewpoint.

electrolyte Element or compound that, when melted or dissolved in water or other solvent, dissociates into ions and can conduct electric current.

electromyogram (EMG) Record of the intrinsic electric activity in a skeletal muscle.

embolism Abnormal circulatory condition in which an embolus travels through the blood stream and lodges in a blood vessel.

embolus Foreign object, tissue, tumor, or piece of thrombus that circulates in the blood stream.

emesis basin Small, kidney-shaped basin used to collect vomitus.

empathy Ability to recognize and to some extent share the emotions and states of mind of another and to understand the meaning and significance of that person's behavior.

emphysema Overinflation and other destructive changes of alveolar walls, resulting in loss of lung elasticity and decreased gas exchange.

EMS (emergency medical system) Network of advanced cardiac life support, usually consisting of a signaling center that receives calls, an ambulance team, and a medical facility.

en face Position in which the mother's face and the infant's face are approximately 8 inches apart and on the same plane, as when the mother holds the infant up in front of her face or when she nurses the child.

enamel Hard, white substance that covers the dentin of the tooth crown.

endocrine gland Ductless gland that delivers hormones to specific groups in the body.

endocrinologist Physician specializing in the study of the endocrine system and treatment of endocrine disorders.

endoderm Innermost of the cell layers that develops from the embryonic disk of the inner cell mass of the blastocyst. From the endoderm arises the epithelium of the trachea, bronchi, lungs, GI tract, liver, pancreas, urinary bladder and canal, pharynx, thyroid, tympanic cavity, tonsils, and parathyroid glands.

endogenous infection Infection caused by nonpathogenic bacteria.

endometriosis Gynecological condition characterized by abnormal growth and function of endometrial (uterine) tissue.

endorphin Substance produced by the brain that mimics the effects of opiates, such as morphine.

endorsement Statement of recognition of the license of a health practitioner in one state by another state.

engagement Fixation of the presenting part of the fetus in the maternal pelvis. The lowest part of the presenting part is at or below the level of the ischial spines.

engorgement Swelling of breast tissue caused by an increased flow of blood and lymph preceding true lactation.

engrossment Father's initial response to newborn.

enteral Pertaining to the intestines.

enteral nutrition Administration of nutrients into the GI tract; usually refers to tube feeding.

enteric Pertaining to the intestines.

enucleation Removal of the eyeball.

environment All of the factors that influence the life and survival of a person.

enzyme Protein produced by living cells that catalyzes chemical reactions without being changed in the process.

epidermis Superficial layers of the skin, made up of an outer, dead portion and a deeper, living, cellular portion.

epididymitis Acute or chronic inflammation of the epididymis (sperm duct).

epiphysis Head of a long bone, which is separated from the shaft of the bone by the epiphyseal plate until the bone stops growing, the plate is obliterated, and the shaft and the head become united.

epistaxis Bleeding from the nose.

epithelium Covering of the external and internal organs of the body, including the lining of the vessels.

erythema Redness or inflammation of the skin or mucous membranes.

eschar Scab or dry crust resulting from a burn, infection, or skin disease.

essential nutrients Carbohydrates, proteins, fats, minerals, vitamins, and water necessary for growth, normal function, and body maintenance. These substances must be supplied by food—they are not synthesized by the body in the quantities required for normal health.

estrogens Hormones that produce female physical characteristics.

ethics Science or study of moral values or principles, including ideals of self-determination, kindness, and justice.

ethnic stereotype Fixed concept or expectation about how members of an ethnic or cultural group act or think.

ethnicity Group's sense of belonging associated with its common social and cultural heritage.

ethnocentrism Tendency to view members from one cultural or ethnic group in terms of the standards of behavior, values, and customs of a person's own group.

etiology Study of all factors involved in the development of a disease.

eustachian tube Tube that joins the nasopharynx and the tympanic membrane.

euthanasia Deliberate bringing about of death in a person who has an incurable disease or condition, either actively by administering a lethal drug or passively by withholding treatment and allowing the person to die.

evaluation Judgment of patient and nursing behavior regarding the extent to which the established goals of care have been met.

evaluation conference Thorough evaluation of a patient by a medical, nursing, sociological, psychological and spiritual team to establish rehabilitation goals.

√**evisceration** Protrusion of an internal organ through a wound or surgical incision, especially in the abdominal wall.

exacerbation Increase in the seriousness of a disease or disorder, as marked by greater intensity in the signs and symptoms of the patient.

excoriation Injury to the surface layer of skin caused by scratching or abrasion.

exocrine Of or pertaining to the process of secreting outwardly through a duct to the surface of an organ or tissue or into a vessel, as a gland that secretes through a duct.

exocrine gland Gland that secretes through a series of ducts.

exogenous infection Infection caused by microorganisms not present in the human body.

exophthalmos Marked protrusion of the eyeball.

expectant stage Time in family life when the woman is pregnant, necessitating some changes in life-style.

extended family Nuclear family plus other relatives who live together.

extracellular Occurring outside a cell or cell tissue or in cavities or spaces between cell layers.

extravasation Passage or escape into the tissues, usually of blood, serum, or lymph.

exudate Fluid, cells, or other substances that have been slowly exuded, or discharged, from cells or blood vessels through small pores or breaks in cell membranes. Perspiration, pus, blood, and serum are sometimes identified as exudates.

family Two or more persons who are related by blood, marriage, or adoption, and who live together over a period of time.

family conference Consultation between the rehabilitation team and the family to discuss the patient's functional status, goals, and future.

family interaction Total of all roles and behaviors shown in a family at a given time.

fanfold Folded like a fan lengthwise, such as the top linen on a hospital bed.

fasciculation Localized, uncoordinated, uncontrollable twitching of a single motor muscle group innervated by a single motor nerve.

fat Substance composed of lipids or fatty acids, ranging from oil to tallow.

fatigue State of exhaustion or a loss of strength or endurance.

√ **febrile** Having an elevated body temperature above 99.6° F or 37.5° C.

feces Waste from the intestine; BM (bowel movement).

feedback Cyclic part of the process of communication that regulates and modifies the content of messages.

feelings All emotional and physical responses and sensations. Feelings are indicators of well-being.

fibrin Stringy, insoluble protein; a product of the action of thrombin on fibrinogen in the clotting process.

fibroblast Flat, elongated, undifferentiated cell in connective tissue that forms fibrous, binding, and supporting tissue.

fibromyositis Any one of a large number of disorders in which the common element is stiffness and joint or muscle pain.

filtration Process in which liquid passes through a membrane or partial barrier but the solid particles are too large to pass.

flaccid Weak, soft, and flabby; lacking normal muscle tone.

flagella Hairlike projections that extend from some unicellular organisms and aid in their movement.

flatus Air or gas in the intestine that is passed through the rectum.

flossing Mechanical cleansing of tooth surfaces with stringlike waxed or unwaxed dental floss.

fluid Body fluid, either intracellular or extracellular, that is involved in the transport of electrolytes and other vital chemicals to, through, and from tissue cells.

fluoroscopy Technique in radiology for visually examining a part of the body or the function of an organ using a fluoroscope.

focus charting Expansion of the *data* and *need* columns in nurses' notes to include topics concerning the whole patient, such as behavior or treatment and response. The charting format is DAR (data, action, response).

follicle-stimulating hormone (FSH) Gonadotropin, secreted by the anterior pituitary gland, that stimulates the growth and maturation of graafian follicles in the ovary.

fomite Nonliving material, such as bed linens, that may convey pathogenic microorganisms.

fontanel Space covered by tough membranes between the bones of an infant's cranium. The anterior fontanel, roughly diamond-shaped, remains palpable until about 2 years of age. The posterior fontanel, triangular in shape, closes about 2 months after birth.

footboard Board placed at the foot of the patient's bed so the feet rest firmly against the board at right angles to prevent footdrop.

foramen Opening or aperture in a membranous structure or bone, such as the apical dental foramen and the carotid foramen.

foramen magnum Passage in the occipital bone through which the spinal cord enters the spinal column.

fossa Hollow or depression, especially on the end of a bone, such as the olecranon fossa or the coronoid fossa.

fracture pan Small bedpan often used for patients with fractures to help prevent pain by reducing the amount of movement required for its placement.

frustration Feeling experienced when there is interference with goal-directed activity.

functional assessment Admission examination of the patient's functional abilities.

gait Manner or style of walking.

gang Group whose membership is formed on the basis of skilled performance of some activity; a group of persons having informal and unusually close social relations.

ganglion One of the nerve cells, chiefly collected in groups outside the central nervous system.

Gate control theory Theory proposing that pain impulses transmitted from nerve receptors through the spinal cord to the brain can be altered or blocked in the spinal cord or brain.

gauge Measurement that designates space within a needle (lumen).

generation gap Conflict between parents and offspring.

generativity Concern about providing for others that is equal to the concern of providing for the self.

geriatrics Medical and nursing specialty concerned with the physiological and pathological changes of later maturity, including study and treatment of health problems.

gerontology Study of the individual in later maturity and the aging process from physiological, pathological, psychological, sociological, and economic points of view.

gingiva Gum of the mouth; a mucous membrane with supporting fibrous tissue that overlies the crowns of unerupted teeth and encircles the necks of teeth that have erupted.

Glasgow coma scale Standardized system for assessing the degree of conscious impairment in the neurologically impaired patient.

glaucoma Elevated pressures within the eye caused by obstruction of the outflow of aqueous humor.

glioma Malignant tumor of the brain.

global cognitive dysfunction Loss of thinking and reasoning powers caused by severe brain damage.

glucagon Hormone produced by the alpha cells in the islets of Langerhans in the pancreas that stimulates the conversion of glycogen to glucose in the liver.

gluten Insoluble protein constituent of wheat and other grains.

glycogen Polysaccharide that is the major carbohydrate stored in animal cells.

glycosylated hemoglobin test Diagnostic test that measures the glucose bound to hemoglobin; used as an index of blood sugar control.

goal Purpose toward which an endeavor is directed, as the outcome of diagnostic, therapeutic, and educational management of a patient's health problem.

Golgi apparatus One of many small membranous structures found in most cells, composed of various elements associated with formation of carbohydrate and protein compounds.

Good Samaritan Law Law that has been enacted in almost every state and province that provides immunity to volunteers at the scene of an accident, provided they are not grossly negligent, do not injure the victim, and are acting in good faith.

Graafian follicle Mature ovarian vesicle that ruptures during ovulation to release the ovum.

graduated Container marked with lines that indicate measurement, such as number of milliliters; used to measure urine output, for example.

gravid- Combining form meaning *pertaining to pregnancy* or *pregnant*.

gravida Combining form meaning *pregnant woman with* (specified) *quantity of pregnancies*.

gray matter Gray tissue that makes up the inner core of the spinal column, arranged in two large lateral masses connected across the midline by a narrow commissure; also, gray tissue on the surface of the cerebral hemisphere comprising the cerebral cortex.

grief Nearly universal pattern of physical and emotional responses to bereavement, separation, or loss.

grief therapy Mental treatment aimed at helping a patient deal with the pain of loss.

grief work Adaptation process of mourning a loss.

growth hormone Hormone released by the anterior pituitary gland that produces normal growth of the body.

gyrus One of the tortuous convolutions of the surface of the brain caused by infolding of the cortex.

habituation Psychological and emotional dependence on a drug, tobacco, or alcohol, resulting from the repeated use of the substance but without the addictive, physiological need to increase dosage.

hallucinogen Substance that causes excitation of the central nervous system, characterized by hallucination, mood change, anxiety, sensory distortion, delusion, depersonalization, increased pulse, temperature, and blood pressure, and dilation of the pupils.

handroll Device, usually a washcloth rolled and placed in the patient's hand, to support the hand while squeezing.

Hazard Communication Act Act that requires hospitals to inform employees about harmful exposures, thus reducing the risk of injury or illness to employees.

head injury Any traumatic damage to the head resulting from penetration of the skull or from too rapid acceleration or deceleration of the brain within the skull.

health Physical, mental, and social well-being, and the absence of disease or other abnormal condition.

health care facility Agency or institution that provides health care, e.g., hospital, nursing home, clinic, or home health agency.

health care system Complete network of agencies, facilities, and all providers of health care in a specified geographical area.

health history Collection of information obtained from a patient and from other sources. The history provides a data base on which a plan for diagnosis, treatment, care, and follow-up of the patient may be made.

hematemesis Vomiting of bright red blood.

hematocrit Measure of the packed cell volume of red cells, expressed as a percentage of total blood volume.

hematoma Escaped blood trapped in tissues of the skin or in an organ as a result of trauma.

√ **hematuria** Blood in the urine.

hemianopsia Blindness in one half of the visual field.

hemiplegia Paralysis of one side of the body.

hemoccult Test for blood in stool.

hemoglobin Complex, protein-iron compound in the blood that carries oxygen to the cells from the lungs and carbon dioxide away from the cells to the lungs.

hemophiliac Person with an inherited disorder characterized by excessive bleeding caused by a clotting defect.

hemopoiesis Formation and development of the various types of blood cells.

hemoptysis Expectorating of blood from the respiratory tract.

Heparin Lock Device used with an Angiocath or Butterfly needle allowing maintenance of an IV route without continuous administration of IV fluid.

heterograft (xenograft) Tissue from another species used as a temporary graft, as in treating severe burns with pig skin grafts, when sufficient tissue from the patient is not available.

heterozygous Having two different genes for a particular characteristic; an inherited gene from one parent and the alternative gene from the other parent.

hilum (hilus) Depression or pit at that part of an organ where vessels and nerves enter.

hilus Depression or pit at the part of an organ where vessels and nerves enter.

hirsutism Excessive body hair.

HIV Human immunodeficiency virus.

holistic health care System of comprehensive or total patient care that considers the physical, emotional, social, economic, and spiritual needs of the person, the response to the illness, and the impact of the illness on the person's ability to meet self-care needs; also called *comprehensive care*.

home health care Nursing care provided in the patient's home.

homeostasis Relative constancy in the internal environment of the body, naturally maintained by adaptive responses that promote healthy survival.

homograft (allograft) Transfer of tissue between two genetically dissimilar individuals of the same species.

homozygous Having two identical genes for a particular characteristic, inherited from each parent. An individual homozygous for a genetic disease caused by recessive genes manifests the disorder.

hormone Complex chemical substance produced in one part or organ of the body that initiates or regulates the activity of an organ or a group of cells in another part of the body.

hospice System of family-centered care provided outside the hospital, designed to assist the dying patient to maintain a satisfactory lifestyle through the terminal phases of dying.

host Organism on which a parasite lives and receives nourishment.

humoral immunity One of the two forms of immunity that respond to antigens such as bacteria and foreign tissue. It is mediated by the B cells.

hydrocephaly Pathological condition characterized by an abnormal accumulation of cerebrospinal fluid, usually under increased pressure, within the cranial vault and subsequent dilation of the ventricles. In infants the head grows at an abnormal rate with separation of the structures, bulging fontanels, and dilated scalp veins. Typical behavior includes irritability with lethargy and vomiting.

hydronephrosis Distention of the renal pelvis and calyces of the kidney.

hydrostatic pressure Pressure exerted by a liquid.

hygiene Practice of cleanliness that is conducive to health.

hypercalcemia Abnormally high level of calcium in the blood.

hypercapnia Excessive amounts of carbon dioxide in the blood.

hyperglycemia Abnormally high level of glucose in the blood.

hyperkalemia Abnormally high level of potassium in the blood.

hyperlipidemia Excess of lipids in the blood.

hypermenorrhea Abnormally heavy or long menstrual periods.

hyperplasia Increase in the number of cells of a body part.

hyperreflexia Neurological condition characterized by increased reflex reactions.

hypersensitivity Excessive reaction to a particular stimulus.

hypertension Elevated blood pressure; blood pressure readings consistently elevated above 140/90.

hyperthermic Much higher than normal body temperature.

hypertonic Having a greater concentration of solute than another solution, hence exerting more osmotic pressure than that solution, as a hypertonic saline solution that contains more salt than is found in intracellular and extracellular fluid.

hypertrophy Increase in the size of an organ caused by an increase in the size of the cells rather than the number of cells.

hyperventilation Breathing rate that is greater than metabolically necessary for the exchange of respiratory gases.

hyphema Hemorrhage into the anterior chamber of the eye, usually caused by a blunt or percusive injury; also called *hyphemia*.

hypocalcemia Abnormally low level of calcium in the blood.

hypoglycemia Abnormally low level of glucose in the blood.

hypokalemia Abnormally low level of potassium in the blood.

hypotension Abnormal condition in which the blood pressure is not adequate for tissue perfusion and oxygenation.

hypothermia Abnormal condition in which the body temperature is below 95° F (35° C).

hypotonic Having a smaller concentration of solute than another solution, hence exerting less osmotic pressure than that solution. Example is a hypotonic saline solution that contains less salt than is found in intracellular or extracellular fluid.

hypoventilation Abnormal condition characterized by cyanosis, clubbing of the fingers, Cheyne-Stokes breathing, and generally decreased respiratory function.

hypoxia Inadequate amount of oxygen available at the cellular level, characterized by cyanosis, tachycardia, hypertension, peripheral vasoconstriction, vertigo, and mental confusion.

hysterosalpingo-oophorectomy Surgical removal of one or both ovaries and oviduct(s) along with the uterus.

icterus Yellow color of the skin, mucous membranes, and sclera of the eyes (jaundice).

ideas of reference Obsessive delusion that statements or actions of others refer to oneself, seen in paranoid disorders.

identity Sense of uniqueness as a person; of internal stability, sameness, and continuity, which resist extreme change.

idiopathic Without a known cause.

idiosyncratic Unique hypersensitivity to a particular drug.

ileal conduit Method of urinary diversion in which the ureters are joined to a segment of ileum.

illness Abnormal process in which aspects of the social, physical, emotional, or intellectual condition and function of a person are diminished or impaired, compared with that person's previous condition.

illusion False perception or experience occurring in response to an environmental stimulus.

immune response Reaction of the body to foreign substances.

immune serum Serum of an animal or human containing antibodies against a specific disease; used to confer passive immunity to that disease.

immunity Quality of being insusceptible to or unaffected by a particular disease condition.

immunization Injection of diluted and/or weakened organisms or products produced by organisms to promote resistance to disease.

immunocompetent Ability of the immune system to function appropriately.

immunodeficiency Abnormal condition of the immune system in which cellular or humoral immunity is inadequate and resistance to infection is increased.

immunogen Any agent or substance capable of provoking an immune response or producing immunity.

immunoglobulins Proteins capable of acting as antibodies; present in serum, body fluid, and body secretions.

immunosuppressed Administration of agents that significantly interfere with the ability of the immune system to respond to antigenic stimulation by inhibiting cellular and humoral immunity.

immunosuppressive Substance or procedure that lessens or prevents an immune response.

immunotherapy Special treatment of allergic responses: administering increasingly large doses of the offending allergens to gradually develop immunity.

immunotropic Tendency to have an influence on or be influenced by the immune system.

implantation Process involving the attachment, penetration, and embedding of the blastocyst in the lining of the uterine wall during the early stages of prenatal development.

incision Cut produced surgically by a sharp instrument to create an opening into an organ or space in the body.

incus One of the three ossicles in the middle ear; resembling an anvil.

induration Hardening of a tissue, particularly the skin, because of edema, inflammation, or infiltration by neoplasm.

industry Interest in doing work of the world, formation of responsible work habits and attitudes, and mastery of age-appropriate tasks.

infant First 12 to 24 months of life.

infant mortality Statistic rate of infant death during the first year after live birth, expressed as the number of such births per 1000 live births in a specific geographical area or institution in a given period.

infarct Localized area of necrosis in tissue, a vessel, or an organ resulting from tissue anoxia; caused by an interruption in the blood supply to an area.

Infection process cycle Five-point cycle that enables microorganisms to move from place to place and cause infection. If the cycle is broken, the microorganisms cannot grow, spread, or cause disease.

inferiority Feeling inadequate, defeated, lazy, unable to learn or do tasks, and unable to compete, compromise, or cooperate, regardless of actual competence.

inflammation Protective response of body tissues to irritation or injury, such as pain, swelling, redness, heat, and lack of function.

inflammatory bowel disease Refers to both Crohn's disease and ulcerative colitis, involving inflammation and tissue changes in intestinal walls.

inhibit To restrain the action or function of an organ or cell as to reduce a physiological activity by an antagonistic stimulation.

initial/establishment stage Period when a couple establishes a home.

innate immunity Natural and permanent form of immunity to a specific disease.

inner canthus of the eye Inner angle at the medial and lateral margins of the eyelid.

innominate Without a name. The term is traditionally applied to certain anatomical structures, often identified by their descriptive names, such as hipbone, brachiocephalic artery, and brachiocephalic vein.

insertion Place of attachment, such as of a muscle to the bone it moves.

institutionalize To place a person in an institution for psychological or physical treatment or for the protection of the person or society.

insulin Naturally occurring hormone, secreted by the beta cells of the islets of Langerhans in the pancreas as a response to increased levels of glucose in the blood.

insulin reaction Adverse effects caused by excessive levels of circulating insulin.

integument Covering or skin.

intelligence Ability to learn from experience, to acquire and retain knowledge, to solve problems, and to respond to a new situation.

interagency Between two health care facilities.

interdisciplinary team Multiprofessional health team, such as doctors, nurses, social workers, and pastors, working together in caring for the terminally ill patient.

intermittent claudication Weakness of the legs with cramping pains, occurring usually after an extended period of walking or exercise and normally relieved by rest.

interrogatories Series of written questions submitted to a witness or other persons having information of interest to the court.

interstitial Of or pertaining to the space between the tissues, as interstitial fluid.

intervention Action performed to prevent harm from occurring to a patient or to improve the mental, emotional, physical, or social function of a patient.

intimacy Reaching out and using the self to form a commitment to and an intense, lasting relationship with another person, or even a cause, an institution, or a creative effort.

intraagency Within a health care facility.

intracellular Located within the cell.

intraoperative Occurring during surgery.

intrathecal Of or pertaining to a structure, process, or substance within a sheath, as the cerebrospinal fluid within the theca of the spinal canal.

intravascular Located within the vessel.

intussusception Prolapse of one segment of bowel into the lumen of another segment.

involuntary Occurring without conscious control or direction.

iridectomy Surgical removal of part of the iris.

iris Circular, contractile disc suspended in aqueous humor between the cornea and the crystalline lens of the eye and perforated by a circular pupil.

iron-deficiency anemia Decrease of hemoglobin in the blood caused by inadequate supplies of iron, characterized by pallor, fatigue, and weakness.

irradiation Exposure to x-rays.

ischemia Deficiency of blood supply caused by circulatory obstruction.

ischium One of the three parts of the hip bone, joining the ilium and the pubis to form the acetabulum.

isolation and self-absorption Inability to be intimate, spontaneous, or close with another.

isolation Separation of a seriously ill patient from others.

isotonic Having the same concentration of solute as another solution, hence exerting the same amount of osmotic pressure as that solution.

joint Any of the connections between bones. Each is classified according to structure and movability, as fibrous, cartilaginous, or synovial.

judgment Final decision of the court regarding a case before it.

jurisdiction Power and authority of a constitution of the state and/or local system to pronounce the sentence of the law.

JVD Jugular vein distention, which reflects increased right arterial pressure.

Kaposi's sarcoma (KS) Malignant tumor, seen more commonly in men.

Kardex or nursing Rand Card filing system, usually kept at the nursing station, that allows quick reference to the particular needs of each patient for nursing care.

Kegel's exercises Also called *pubococcygeus exercises*, a regimen of isometric exercises in which a woman executes a series of voluntary contractions of the muscles of her pelvic diaphragm and perineum;

may increase the contractility of her vaginal muscles or improve the retention of urine.

keratoplasty Surgery to excise an opaque portion of the cornea.

kernicterus Abnormal toxic accumulation of bilirubin in central nervous system tissues caused by hyperbilirubinemia.

ketoacidosis Abnormal accumulation of ketones in the body, resulting from faulty carbohydrate metabolism, occurring primarily as a complication of diabetes mellitus.

ketones Acetone bodies found in diabetes mellitus; breakdown of fatty acids causing increased levels of ketone bodies in the blood, called *ketosis*.

kilocalorie Unit that denotes the heat expenditure of an organism and the fuel or energy value of food, often abbreviated kcalorie or kcal.

Korotkoff sounds Sounds heard when taking a blood pressure using a sphygmomanometer and stethoscope. As air is released from the cuff, pressure on the brachial artery is reduced and blood is heard pulsing through the vessels.

KS See *Kaposi's sarcoma.*

kwashiorkor Malnutrition disease primarily of children, caused by severe protein deficiency and usually occurring when the child is weaned.

kyphosis Abnormal, convex curvature of the thoracic spine.

labia majora Two large folds of skin, one on each side of the vaginal orifice outside the labia minora.

labia minora Two small folds of skin between the labia majora, extending from the clitoris backward on both sides of the vaginal orifice, ending between it and the labia majora.

labile Unstable; characterized by a tendency to change or to be altered.

labyrinthitis Inflammation of the inner ear canal resulting in vertigo.

lactation Synthesis and secretion of milk from the breasts for the nourishment of an infant or child.

lalling Infant's movement of tongue with crying and vocalization.

laminectomy Surgical chipping away of the bony arches of one or more vertebrae.

language Combination of sounds into a meaningful whole to communicate thoughts and feelings.

lanugo Soft, downy hair covering a normal fetus. It begins to shed in the fifth month of life and is almost entirely shed by the ninth month.

lanula Half-moon structure, such as the crescent-shaped, pale area at the base of the nail of a finger or toe.

laparoscopy Any surgical incision into the peritoneal cavity, often performed on an exploratory basis.

larynx Organ of voice that is part of the air passage connecting the pharynx with the trachea.

law Rule, principle, or regulation established and promulgated by a government to protect or to restrict the people affected.

Legg-Calvé-Perthes disease Aseptic (noninfectious) necrosis of the head of the femur, characterized initially by epiphyseal necrosis or degeneration and followed by regeneration or recalcification.

leisure Freedom from obligations and formal duties of paid work, and opportunity to pursue, at one's own pace, mental nourishment, enlivenment, pleasure, and relief from fatigue of work.

lens Crystalline lens of the eye; a curved transparent disc that is capable of refracting light.

lentigo senilis Irregular areas of dark pigmentation of the skin in the elderly.

leukemia Malignant neoplasm of blood-forming organs.

leukocyte White blood cell; one of the formed elements of the circulating blood system.

leukopenia Abnormal decrease in the number of white blood cells to fewer than 5000 cells per cubic millimeter.

leukoplakia Precancerous change in a mucous membrane characterized by thickened, white, firmly attached patches.

leukorrhea Normal white vaginal discharge.

liability Something one is obligated to do or an obligation required by law, usually financial in nature.

licensure Granting of permission by a competent authority to an organization or individual to engage in a practice or activity that would otherwise be illegal.

lie Relationship between the long axis of the fetus and the long axis of the mother.

ligament One of many predominantly white, shiny, flexible bands of fibrous tissue binding joints together and connecting various bones and cartilages.

lightening Subjective sensation reported by many women late in pregnancy as the fetus settles lower in the pelvis, leaving more space in the upper abdomen.

lipoprotein Protein and lipid molecule, which facilitates transport of lipids in the blood stream. They are classified according to their composition and density.

litigate To carry out a lawsuit or to contest one.

living will Instrument by which a dying person makes his wishes known to those who will survive him.

lochia Discharge that flows from the vagina after childbirth.

lordosis Increased curve in the lumbar region of the spine.

loss Any aspect of one's self that is no longer available to that person.

lumbar cord injury Spinal injury involving paralysis of the lower extremities.

lumen Space within a tube, such as a needle; also, a cavity or channel within an organ, specifically the blood vessels of the cardiovascular system.

luteinizing hormone Produced by the anterior pituitary gland, it stimulates the secretion of sex hormones by the ovary and the testes and is involved in the maturation of sperm and ova.

lymphadenopathy Disease of the lymph nodes, including hypertrophy and proliferation of lymphoid tissue.

lymphocyte Lymph cell or white blood cell; develops in the bone marrow.

lymphokine Chemical factor released by the T cell that attracts macrophages to the site.

lysosome Cytoplasmic, membrane-bound particle containing hydrolytic enzymes that function in intracellular digestive processes.

macrophage Cell that "eats" pathogenic microorganisms.

macule Small, flat blemish or discoloration that is flush with the skin surface.

magical thinking Belief that merely thinking about an event in the external world can cause it to occur.

magnesium Silver-white mineral that is found in combination with other elements in the body.

magnetic resonance imaging (MRI) Medical imaging that uses nuclear magnetic resonance as its source of energy.

malignant neoplasm Tumor that progressively spreads to other areas of the body.

malleolus Rounded, bony process on each side of the ankle.

malpractice Professional negligence that is the most likely cause of injury or harm to a patient, resulting from a lack of professional knowledge, experience, or skill, or from negligence.

mammography Radiography of the soft tissues of the breast to identify neoplastic processes.

management Act, art, or manner of managing or handling, controlling, or directing: careful, tactful treatment.

mandatory Required by a command, order, or law.

manubrium One of the three bones of the sternum, presenting a broad, quadrangular shape that narrows where it unites with the superior end of the sternum.

marasmus Extreme malnutrition and emaciation, occurring chiefly in young children, with wasting of subcutaneous tissue and muscle; results from lack of calories and proteins.

mastoiditis Infection of one of the mastoid bones.

matrifocal/matriarchal family Family in which a woman has the main authority and power.

matrix Basic substance from which a specific type of tissue develops.

mattress pad (cover) Material that fits over a mattress to protect it from soiling.

meconium Newborn's first fecal material after birth.

mediastinum Portion of the thoracic cavity in the middle of the thorax, between the pleural sacs containing the two lungs.

Medicaid Health insurance program for the indigent and poor passed in 1965 as the Title XIX Amendment to the Social Security Act. It provides payment for certain home care services.

medical asepsis Removal or destruction of disease organisms or infected material.

medical diagnosis Traditional approach to diagnosis as practiced by physicians focusing on the defect or dysfunction within the patient. Medical diagnosis is focused on the physical and biological aspects of specific diseases and conditions.

Medicare Health insurance program for the aged and disabled passed in 1965 as the Title XVII Amendment to the Social Security Act. It dramatically changed the delivery of home health services.

medicated tub bath Therapeutic bath in which medication is dispersed in water, usually in treating dermatological disorders.

medicine Art and science of diagnosis, treatment, and prevention of disease and the maintenance of good health.

medulla Most internal part of a structure or organ.

medulla oblongata Most vital part of the brain; continuing as the bulbous portion of the spinal cord just above the foramen magnum and separated from the pons by a horizontal groove.

melanin Black or dark brown pigment that occurs naturally in the hair and skin and in the iris and choroid of the eye.

melanoma Malignant neoplasm, primarily of the skin.

membrane Thin layer of tissue that covers a surface, lines a cavity, or divides a space, such as the membrane that lines the abdominal wall.

menarche First menstrual period; physiological marker of puberty in female.

meninges Any of the three membranes that enclose the brain and spinal cord, comprising the dura mater, the pia mater, and the arachnoid.

meningomyelocele Developmental defect of the central nervous system in which a hernial sac containing a portion of the spinal cord, its meninges, and cerebrospinal fluid protrudes through a congenital cleft in the vertebral column; also called *myelomeningocele*.

meniscus Curved upper surface of a liquid in a container.

menopause Permanent ceasing of ovulation and menstruation, which causes loss of reproductive ability.

menorrhagia Abnormally heavy or long menstrual periods.

menstruation Periodical discharge through the vagina of a bloody secretion from the shedding of the endometrium.

mental health continuum Mental health and mental illness can be viewed as opposite ends on a continuum. The point at which the person is deemed mentally ill is determined by behavior, as well as by the circumstances in which the behavior is seen.

mental illness Pattern of behavior disturbing to the individual or to the community in which he lives.

mesentery Broad, fan-shaped fold of peritoneum connecting the jejunum and ileum with the dorsal wall of the abdomen.

mesoderm Middle of three cell layers of the developing embryo, lying between the ectoderm and the endoderm. Bone, connective tissue, muscle, blood, vascular and lymphatic tissue, and the membranes of the pericardium and peritoneum are derived from the mesoderm.

metabolism Combination of all chemical processes that take place in living organisms, resulting in growth, generation of energy, elimination of wastes, and other body functions as they relate to the distribution of nutrients in the blood after digestion.

metabolite Substance produced by metabolic action or necessary for a metabolic process.

metastasis Process by which tumor cells spread to distant parts of the body.

microorganism Tiny living plant or animal that can be seen only via a microscope; may be pathogenic.

micturition Urination.

middle age Period of life from mid-40s to mid-60s or 70.

midlife crisis Major turning point in one's life related to identity crisis and self-absorption; involves changes in commitments to career and/or spouse and children, as well as emotional turmoil for the individual and others.

milliequivalent (mEq) Number of grams of solute dissolved in 1 ml of a normal solution.

mineral Inorganic substance ingested as a compound (such as sodium chloride) rather than as a free element. Minerals help regulate many body functions.

minority group Group of people who, because of their physical or cultural characteristics, receive unequal and different treatment from others in the society. Minority group members view themselves as victims of collective discrimination.

miotic Causing constriction of the pupil of the eye.

miter Fold and tuck made on the corner of a sheet; gives hospital bed a finished appearance.

mitochondria Powerhouses of the cell. They are bean shaped and convert food to an energy form (ATP) for the cell.

monocyte Large, mononuclear leukocyte.

monozygotic Pertaining to twins who develop from a single ova; identical twins.

mood Particular state of mind or feeling, such as humor or temper.

morals Generally accepted customs of conduct and right living in a society.

morbidity (1) Illness or abnormal condition or quality; (2) in statistics, the rate at which an illness or abnormality occurs, calculated by dividing the entire number of people in a group by the number in that group who are affected with the illness or the abnormality; (3) the rate at which an illness occurs in a particular area or population.

mores Folkways of central importance, accepted without question and embodying the fundamental moral views of a group.

morphology Study of physical shape and size.

morula Solid, round mass of cells resulting from the cleavage of the fertilized ovum in the early stages of embryonic development.

motivation Inner drive that leads an individual to complete a task or meet a goal.

motor Pertaining to motion, the body apparatus involved in movement, or the brain functions that direct purposeful activities.

motor neuron One of various efferent nerve cells that transmit nerve impulses from the brain or from the spinal cord to muscular or glandular tissue.

mourning Reaction activated by a person to assist in overcoming a great personal loss.

multiaxial system System used for organizing information in a psychiatric diagnosis.

multigravida Woman who has been pregnant more than once.

multipara Woman who has been delivered of more than one viable infant.

multiple myeloma Malignant neoplasm of the bone marrow.

muscle tone Muscle strength; the normal state of balanced tension in muscles.

myalgia Diffuse muscle pain, usually accompanied by malaise, occurring in many infectious diseases.

mydriatic Causing dilation of the pupil of the eye.

myelin Fatty sheath covering neurons.

myelogram X-ray film taken after injection of a radiopaque medium into the subarachnoid space; demonstrates any distortions of the spinal cord, spinal nerve roots, and subarachnoid space.

myelosuppression Inhibition of the production of blood cells and platelets in the bone marrow.

myocardial infarction (MI) Occlusion of a coronary artery caused by atherosclerosis or an embolus; heart attack.

myocardium Thick, contractile, middle layer of uniquely constructed and arranged muscle cells that form the bulk of the heart wall.

myositis Inflammation of muscle tissue.

myringotomy Surgical incision of the eardrum.

NANDA North American Nursing Diagnosis Association.

narcotic abstinence syndrome (NAS) Affects babies born to narcotic-addicted mothers whose addiction is passed on to the child. The baby will demonstrate signs of hyperreflexia, hypertonia, a high-pitched cry, tremors, sneezing, and yawning.

narrative charting Traditional style of charting in which the nurse documents in story form all pertinent patient observations, care, and responses in the *nurse's notes* section.

negative feedback In physiology, a decrease in function in response to a stimulus.

neglect Failure of caregivers to provide a child with basic necessities of life.

negligence Commission of an act that a prudent person would not have done or the omission of a duty that a prudent person would have fulfilled, resulting in injury or harm to another person.

neonate Infant during first 4 weeks of life.

neoplasia New and abnormal growth of cells, which may be benign or malignant.

neoplasm Any abnormal growth of new tissue, which may be benign or malignant.

nephron Structural and functional unit of the kidney, resembling a microscopic funnel with a long stem and two convoluted sections.

nephrotoxin Substance destructive to the kidney.

neurilemma Layer of cells composed of one or more Schwann cells, which enclose the segmented myelin sheaths of peripheral nerve fibers. The nerve fibers of the brain and the spinal cord are not enclosed by neurilemma.

neuromuscular junction Area of contact between the ends of a large myelinated nerve fiber and a skeletal muscle fiber.

neuropathy Any abnormal condition characterized by inflammation and degeneration of the peripheral nerves.

neurotransmitter Any one of numerous chemicals that modify or result in the transmission of nerve impulses between synapses.

neurotropic Having a tendency to influence or be influenced by the nervous system.

nocturnal emissions Ejaculation of semen during sleep; physiological marker of puberty in male.

nodule Small, nodelike structure.

nonrapid eye movement (NREM) One of two major stages of sleep; consists of four distinct phases of sleep in which very little movement can be observed.

nonspecific immunity Passive immunity; acquired immunity transmitted naturally through the placenta to a fetus or through the colostrum to an infant, or artificially by injection.

normotensive Having normal blood pressure.

nosocomial infection Infection acquired during hospitalization.

noxious Harmful, injurious, or detrimental to health.

nuchal rigidity Pain and stiffness of the neck.

nuclear family Mother, father, and child(ren) in the family unit.

nullipara Woman who has not been delivered of a viable infant.

Nurse Practice Act Outlines the legal scope of nursing within the geographical boundaries of the jurisdiction.

nurse's notes Nurse's written documentation of patient observations, care, and responses.

nursing Practice in which a nurse assists the individual, sick or well, in the performance of those activities contributing to health or its recovery (or to a peaceful death) that he would perform unaided if he had the necessary strength, will, or knowledge.

nursing assessment Identification by a nurse of the basis, preferences, and abilities of a patient. Assessment provides the scientific basis for a complete nursing care plan.

nursing care plan Plan of care based on a nursing assessment and a nursing diagnosis; lists nursing actions necessary to meet a patient's needs.

nursing diagnosis Statement of a health problem or a potential problem in the patient's health status that a nurse is licensed and competent to treat.

nursing process Process that serves as an organizational framework for the practice of nursing; assists in a systematic approach to nursing assessment of the patient.

nutrient density Nutrients relative to calories. Food providing a high quantity of one or more nutrients in a small number of calories is nutrient dense.

nutrition All the processes involved in taking in nutrients and in their assimilation and use for proper body functioning and maintenance of health.

nystagmus Involuntary, rhythmic movement of the eyes. Oscillations may be horizontal, vertical, rotary, or mixed.

obesity Abnormal increase in the proportion of fat cells, mainly in the viscera and subcutaneous tissues of the body; overfatness.

objective data Data that are both observable and measurable. Vital signs and laboratory reports are examples of objective data.

objective data collection Process in which data relating to the patient's problems are obtained through direct physical examination, laboratory analysis, and radiological studies.

obsession Thought recognized by the individual as irrational and recurring despite the wish to avoid it.

occiput Back of the head; of or pertaining to the occipital region.

occult Hidden or difficult to observe.

occupied bed Hospital bed that must be made up while it is occupied by a patient.

olecranon Projection of the ulna that forms the point of the elbow and fits into the olecranon fossa of the humerus when the forearm is extended.

oligohydramnios Abnormally small amount or absence of amniotic fluid.

oliguria Diminished capacity to form and pass urine, less than 240 ml in 8 hours.

oncology Study of tumors.

open bed Fanfolded top linens on a hospital bed, for easy access for patient.

ophthalmoscope Device used to examine the interior of the eye.

opportunistic infection Infection in a person whose resistance to disease has been decreased by other disorders, such as diabetes mellitus, cancer, or AIDS, or by a procedure, such as surgery or catheterization.

oral hygiene Maintenance of tissues and structure of the mouth; includes brushing teeth, dental flossing, and cleaning of dentures.

oral swabs Swabs impregnated or soaked with various solutions for oral hygiene, such as glycerin and lemon juice.

orientation Awareness of one's physical environment with regard to time, place, and the identity of other persons; the ability to adapt to such an existing or new environment.

orifice Entrance to or outlet of any cavity in the body.

orthopedic bed Bed designed to accommodate a patient with fractures.

orthopnea Abnormal condition in which a person must sit or stand to breathe.

Ortolani's test Procedure used to evaluate the stability of the hip joints in newborns and infants. A click or a popping sensation (Ortolani's sign) may be felt if the joint is unstable, because the head of the femur moves out of the acetabulum under pressure from the examiner's hands during rotation and abduction.

OSHA Occupational Safety and Health Administration.

osmosis Movement of a pure solvent, as water, through a semipermeable membrane from a solution with lower solute concentration to one with higher solute concentration.

osseous Pertaining to bone.

ossicle Small bone, as the malleus, the incus, or stapes of the middle ear.

osteoclasia Destruction and absorption of bony tissue by osteoclasts, such as during growth or the healing of fractures.

osteoclast Large type of multinucleated bone cell that functions in periods of growth or repair, such as the breakdown and resorption of osseous tissue.

otitis Inflammation or infection of the ear.

outer canthus of the eye Outer angle at the medial and lateral margins of the eyelid.

ovulation Release of a mature ovum (egg) from the ovary.

oxidation Process in which the oxygen content of a compound is increased.

oxytocic Any one of the numerous drugs that stimulate the smooth muscle of the uterus to contract.

pain Unpleasant sensation caused by noxious stimulation of the sensory nerve endings.

palliation Therapy to relieve or reduce uncomfortable symptoms but not to cure.

palliative To sooth or relieve intensity of uncomfortable symptoms but not to produce a cure.

palpation Technique where the examiner feels texture, size, consistency, and location of body parts.

Papanicolaou test Method of examining stained cells obtained from lesions, sputum, urine, and other material by aspiration, scraping, a smear, or washings of the tissue. The "pap" test is a vital part of the female pelvic examination to detect cancer of the cervix.

papule Small, solid, raised skin lesion, less than 1 cm in diameter.

-para Combining form meaning *woman who has given birth to children in a number of pregnancies*.

parallel play Playing alongside a peer or same-aged child.

paralysis Abnormal condition characterized by loss of muscle function or loss of sensation.

paranoia Transitory mental state characterized by illogical thought processes and generalized suspicion and distrust.

parasympathetic Of or pertaining to the craniosacral division of the autonomic nervous system, consisting of the oculomotor, facial, glossopharyngeal, vagus, and pelvic nerves. The parasympathetic slows heart rate, increases intestinal peristalsis and gland activity, and relaxes sphincters.

parathyroid gland One of several small structures, usually four, attached to the thyroid gland.

parathyroid hormone Secreted by the parathyroid glands; maintains a constant concentration of calcium in the blood.

parenchyma Tissue of an organ, as distinguished from supporting or connective tissue.

parenteral Not in or through the digestive system; generally refers to needle routes.

parenteral nutrition Administration of nutrients by a route other than the alimentary canal, such as intravenously.

parenthood stage Stage of family life at birth of a child.

partial bath Patient's incomplete bath. A nurse usually must bathe the back, legs, and feet.

passive transport Movement of small molecules across the membrane of a cell by diffusion.

patella Flat, triangular bone at the front of the knee joint, which attaches to the ligamentum patellae also called *kneecap*.

patent Condition of being open and unblocked, such as a patent airway.

pathogen Any microorganism capable of producing disease.

patient Recipient of a health care service.

patients' rights Legal and regulatory rights to participate in the planning of care, be informed of services, know by whom and how payment will be made, have privacy and grievance procedures, and be shown respect for personal possessions.

patient-controlled analgesis (PCA) Method by which a patient can control intravenous analgesia by pressing a button.

patrifocal/patriarchal family Family in which a man has the main authority and power.

PCP Pneumocystic carinii pneumonia.

pediculosis Infestation of lice; may be of the head, facial hair, skin, and pubic region.

peer Person deemed an equal for the purpose at hand. A peer is usually about the same age and mental level.

peer review Appraisal by professional coworkers of equal status of the way an individual nurse or other health professional conducts practice, education, or research; uses accepted standards as measures against which performance is weighed.

pellagra Disease resulting from deficiency of the vitamin *niacin*.

pepsin Enzyme secreted in the stomach that catalyzes hydrolysis of protein.

peptic ulcer Loss of the mucous membrane of the stomach, duodenum, or any part of the GI system exposed to gastric juices.

perception Understanding based on impressions and feelings.

percussion Technique used to evaluate size, border, and consistency of some organs and to discover the presence and evaluate the amount of fluid in a body cavity.

perennial Present at all seasons of the year; permanent, consistent.

perinatal death Death of an infant before, during, or shortly after birth.

perineal care Care given the genitalia.

periodontal disease Disease of the tissues around the teeth.

perioperative period Entire surgical inpatient period, from admission to date of discharge.

periorbital edema Swelling around the eyes, which may indicate a pathological condition of the kidney.

periosteum Fibrous, vascular membrane covering the bones, except at their extremities; consists of an outer layer of collagenous tissues containing a few fat cells and an inner layer of fine, elastic fibers.

peripheral nervous system Motor and sensory nerves and ganglia outside the brain and spinal cord.

peripheral parenteral nutrition (PPN) Administration of a nutritionally adequate solution into a peripheral vein.

pernicious anemia Progressive decrease in blood hemoglobin, affecting mainly older people and resulting from lack of the factor essential for absorbing vitamin B_{12}.

personality Unique pattern of the mental, emotional, and behavioral traits of an individual.

PGL Persistent generalized lymphedema.

phagocytosis Process by which certain cells engulf and dispose of microorganisms and cell debris.

phalanges Any one of 14 tapering bones composing the finger of each hand and the toes of each foot.

pharynx Throat; a tubular structure about 13 cm long that extends from the base of the skull to the esophagus.

phimosis Narrowing of the prepuce opening so that the foreskin of the penis cannot be retracted.

phlebothrombosis Abnormal condition in which a clot forms within a vein.

phobia Irrational, exaggerated fear of an object, activity, or situation.

phosphate (HPO_4) Salt element of phosphoric acid.

physiatrist Physician who specializes in the field of rehabilitation.

physician's orders Specific orders by a physician for a patient's medical care.

physiology Study of functions of the various organs and tissues of the body.

pia mater Innermost of the three meninges covering the brain and the spinal cord. It is closely applied to both structures and carries a rich supply of blood vessels, which nourish the nervous tissue.

pica Craving to eat substances that are not foods, as dirt, clay, chalk, glue, ice, starch, or hair.

PIH Pregnancy-induced hypertension.

pinocytosis Process by which extracellular fluid is taken into a cell. The cell membrane develops a saccular indentation filled with extracellular fluid and then closes around it, forming a vesicle or a vacuole of fluid within the cell.

pituitary gland Small gland attached to the hypothalamus and couched in the sphenoid bone, supplying numerous hormones that govern many vital processes.

placebo Inactive substance, such as saline, distilled water, or sugar, prescribed as if it were a needed medication.

plaintiff Person who files a lawsuit initiating a legal action.

pleural effusion Accumulation of nonpurulent fluid in the space between the visceral and parietal pleura.

pleural space Potential space between the visceral and parietal layers of the pleurae.

pleurisy Inflammation of the parietal pleura of the lungs, characterized by dyspnea and stabbing pain, leading to restriction of ordinary breathing with spasm of the chest on the affected side.

pluralistic society Society in which numerous distinct ethnic, religious, or cultural groups coexist within one nation.

pneumonia Acute inflammation of the lungs, often caused by inhaled pneumococci.

poisoning Condition or physical state produced by the ingestion, injection, or inhalation of or exposure to a poisonous substance.

polydipsia Excessive thirst.

polyphagia Excessive hunger.

√ **polyuria** Excretion of abnormally large amounts of urine.

pons Prominence on the ventral surface of the brainstem, between the medulla oblongata and the cerebral peduncles of the midbrain. The pons consists of white matter and a few nuclei and is divided into a ventral portion and a dorsal portion.

portal of entry Route by which microorganisms enter the human body.

position Relationship of a fetal reference point with respect to its location in the maternal pelvis.

postmortem care Care of the body after death.

posterior Back part of a structure; toward the back.

posterior fontanel Triangular-shaped area at center back of head.

postictal period Time immediately after a convulsion (usually a grand mal seizure).

postprandial After a meal.

posture Position of the body with respect to the surrounding space; the sense of balance.

potassium ($K+$) Alkali metal element that is necessary to the life of all plants and animals; the chief intracellular electrolyte.

potentiation Synergistic action in which the effect of two drugs given at the same time is greater than the effect of the drugs given separately.

PQRST Method used when gathering information during a patient interview: P—provocative, palliative; Q—quality, quantity; R—region, radiation; S—severity scale; T—timing.

preadolescence (prepubescence) Period from about age 9 or 10 until the onset of puberty, characterized by an increase in hormone production.

preeclampsia Abnormal condition of pregnancy characterized by the onset of acute hypertension after the twenty-fourth week of gestation.

premenstrual syndrome Group of signs and symptoms occurring about a week before menstruation, associated with fluid retention.

presbycusis Normal loss of hearing, speech, and pitch associated with aging.

presbyopia Decreasing elasticity of the lens and decreasing power of accommodation, so that vision of near objects is blurred or indistinct.

preschooler Ages 3 to 5½ years.

presentation Part of the fetus that first appears in the pelvis.

primary caregiver First or responsible person in decision making or providing care to an ill person.

primipara Woman who has given birth to one viable infant.

prn *(pro re nata)* When required.

problem list for POMR Prioritized master list of the patient's active, inactive, temporary, and potential medical and other problems; serves as an index to the rest of the record.

problem-oriented medical record (POMR) Method of recording data about the health status of a patient in a problem-solving system. Parts included are the data base, problem list, initial plan, and progress notes.

procidentia Downward displacement of an organ; usually applied to a prolapsed uterus.

progesterones Female hormones that prepare the uterus to accept a fetus and maintain the pregnancy.

progress notes Notes made by a nurse, physician, or other team member that describe the patient's condition and the treatments given and planned.

proliferate To produce or multiply.

prone Lying face down.

proprioception Awareness of the position of one's body; pertaining to stimuli originating from within the body regarding spatial position.

proprioceptor Any sensory nerve ending, such as those located in muscles, tendons, and joints, that responds to stimuli originating from within the body regarding movement and spatial position.

prosthesis Artificial replacement for a missing body part.

protein (dietary) Any large group of naturally occurring, complex, organic nitrogenous compounds necessary for proper growth, development, and maintenance of health.

protest Initial grief response in separation from attachment figure.

pruritus Itching.

PSRO (Professionsl Standards Review Organization) Physicians review the services provided under Medicare, Medicaid, and Maternal-Child Health programs to ensure standards are being met and to ascertain the need for the program.

psychoactive material Substance that affects mental activity.

psychological age Behavioral capacity of the person to adapt to changing environmental demands; includes capacities of memory, learning, intelligence, skills, feelings, and motivations for exercising behavioral control or self-regulation.

psychosocial Intellectual, emotional, and social components of the individual.

psychotic State characterized by gross distortion of reality and impaired social functioning.

ptosis Drooping of the eyelids.

pubarche Beginning development of certain secondary sex characteristics preceding physiological puberty.

puberty State of physical development when sexual reproduction first becomes possible, with menstruation and spermatogenesis (10 to 14 years for females; 12 to 16 years for males).

public health nursing Nursing assessment, identification of high-risk groups, intervention directed at disease prevention, and health education and promotion for all ages, groups, and individuals.

puerperium Time after childbirth, approximately 6 weeks, during which anatomical and physiological changes brought about by pregnancy resolve.

pulmonary edema Accumulation of extravascular fluid in lung tissues and alveoli, caused most commonly by congestive heart failure.

pulmonary embolus (PE) Occlusion of a pulmonary artery by foreign matter, such as fat, air, tumor tissue, or a thrombus, that usually arises from a peripheral vein.

pulse deficit Condition that exists when the radial pulse rate is less than the ventricular rate.

pulse pressure Difference between systolic and diastolic pressure, usually 30 to 40 mm Hg.

pulverized Crushed into a powdered form.

punctum Tiny opening in the margin of each eyelid that opens into the tear duct.

pupillary reflex Adjustment of the eyes for near vision, consisting of pupillary constriction.

purulent Producing or containing pus.

pustule Small elevation of the skin containing fluid that is usually purulent.

PWA Person with AIDS.

pyrexic fever Having a body temperature above 98.6° F (37° C).

pyrosis Heartburn; painful burning centered in the esophagus just below the sternum, often caused by reflux of gastric contents into the esophagus or by gastric hyperacidity.

quadratectomy Removal of a quadrant of the breast along with overlying skin.

quality assurance Evaluation of services provided and results achieved as compared with accepted standards.

RACE Rescue patients; sound the Alarm; Confine the fire; and Extinguish or evacuate.

racism Any ethnocentric activity—cultural, individual, or institutional, deliberate or not—that is based on a belief in the superiority of one racial group over other racial groups, thus maintaining the oppression and control of these groups.

radial pulse Pulse of the radial artery, felt at the wrist over the radium.

Range-of-motion exercise Any body action involving the muscles, the joints, and natural directional movement.

rapid eye movement (REM) sleep Period of sleep when dreams occur, characterized by rapid movement of the closed eyes.

reagent Substance producing a chemical reaction.

receptor Sensory nerve ending that responds to various kinds of stimulation.

reconstituted/blended family Divorced or widowed adult and a new spouse, with each adult's own child(ren) plus the child(ren) of the new partnership, if any, who live together.

recumbent Lying down; reclining.

referred pain Pain felt at a site other than its origin.

reflection Therapist's repetition of statements made by the patient; helps to clarify information.

reflex Reflected action, particularly an involuntary action or movement.

rehabilitation Process of assisting an individual after a disabling event has occurred.

remission Partial or complete disappearance of the clinical and subjective characteristics of a chronic or malignant disease.

residual urine Urine left in the bladder after the patient has voided.

residue Bulk in the colon that includes undigested food, fiber, bacteria, body secretions, and cells.

respite Period of relief from responsibilities for the care of a patient.

responsibility Moral, legal, or mental accountability.

restraint Any one of numerous devices used in aiding the immobilization of patients.

resume Summary of one's career and qualifications, prepared typically by an applicant for a position; a brief biography.

retention Inability to urinate.

retraction Visible sinking in of soft tissue of the chest between and around the firmer tissue of the ribs as occurs with increased respiratory effort.

retrovirus Member of a family of viruses that alter genetic structure of the host cell by changing RNA to DNA, reversing the usual flow of genetic information.

reversibility Performance of opposite mental actions with the same problem or situation, such as addition and subtraction, multiplication and division.

review of systems (ROS) System-by-system review of the body functions. ROS is begun during the initial interview.

rhizotomy Resection of a posterior nerve root just before it enters the spinal cord, usually performed to control severe pain in the upper trunk or to relieve severe spasms.

ribosome Cytoplasmic organelle composed of ribonucleic acid and protein that functions in the synthesis of protein.

role Character assigned or assumed; a socially expected behavior pattern usually determined by an individual's status in a particular society.

ROM Range of motion.

rubor Redness, especially when aconnmpanying inflammation.

Rule of nines Formula for estimating the amount of body surface covered by burns. In the adult 9% is assigned to head and each arm, 18% to each leg, 18% to the anterior and posterior trunk, and 1% to the perineum.

SOAPE charting Charting format used in POMR. Components include subjective data (S) reported by the patient; objective data (O) acquired by inspection, percussion, auscultation, and palpation and by tests, usually measurable findings; assessment (A) of the problem; plan (P) of care; and evaluation (E) of patient's response to the treatment plan.

SOAPIER charting Same as SOAPE charting except that intervention (I) and revision (R) are added. Interventions are specific actions carried out, and revisions are the changes to be made to the original plan.

sanguineous Pertaining to blood. dark

sarcoma Malignant neoplasm of connective tissues arising in fibrous, fatty, muscular, synovial, vascular, or neural tissue.

satiety Feeling of fullness and satisfaction from food.

scale Small, thin flake of keratinized (dried-out) epithelium.

scar Connective tissue that is avascular, pale, contracted, and firm after the earlier phase of healing.

school age Period from about 6 to sixteen years of age.

sclera Tough, inelastic, opaque membrane covering the posterior five sixths of the eyeball. It maintains the size and form of the eye and attaches to muscles that move it.

scoliosis Lateral or S curvature of the spine.

scurvy Condition resulting from lack of ascorbic acid (vitamin C) in the diet.

sebaceous gland One of the many small organs in the dermis (skin); secretes oil.

sebum Oily secretion from the sebaceous glands.

secondary gain Material, emotional, or social advantage acquired as a result of a symptom or an illness.

self-bath Bath done by the patient in bed or at the bedside.

self-despair Feeling that life has not been satisfactory and having a desire to relive it.

semicircular canals Any of three bony, fluid-filled loops in the osseous labyrinth of the internal ear, associated with the sense of balance.

semilunar valve Valve with half-moon–shaped cusps, as the aortic valve and the pulmonary valve.

senescence Mental and physical decline associated with aging.

sensitivity Susceptibility to a substance, such as a drug or an antigen.

separation anxiety Fear and apprehension caused by separation from familiar surroundings and significant persons.

septum Partition, as the interauricular septum that separates the atria of the heart.

sequela Any abnormal condition that occurs after a disease, treatment, or injury.

seriation Mental ordering of objects according to height, weight or strength.

seroconversion Point at which a pathogenic organism can be identified in the blood.

serosanguineous Composed of serum and blood.

sex education Factual teaching about anatomy and physiology related to the sex act and reproduction.

sex hormones Biochemical agents that influence structure and function of sex organs and appearance of sexual characteristics.

sexuality education Learning about self as a sexual being.

shearing Force causing two contacting parts to slide upon one another.

sibling Brother or sister.

sign Objective finding of an examiner, such as a fever, or a rash.

Sims Position in which the patient lies on the side with the superior knee flexed and the thigh drawn upward toward the chest. The chest and abdomen are allowed to fall forward.

single parent One parent who lives with the child(ren).

Sitz bath Bath in which only the hips and buttocks are immersed in water or saline solution; the time allotted is 20 to 30 minutes.

skin graft Portion of skin implanted to cover areas where skin has been lost by burns or injury.

skin impairment Irritated skin that breaks open and becomes a decubitus ulcer which can penetrate to the bone.

smear Material placed on a microscopic slide or culture medium.

Snellen test Chart test used to determine visual acuity.

social age Roles and habits of a person with respect to other members of society, resulting from the person's life course through various social institutions.

social network Interconnected group of cooperating significant others, related or not, with whom a person interacts.

sodium Soft, gray, alkaline metal that is the chief electrolyte in interstitial fluid.

somatization Physical manifestation of an individual's feelings, emotional needs, or conflicts.

souffle cup Small, white, pleated paper cup used to contain nonliquid oral medications.

spastic Of or pertaining to spasms or other uncontrolled contractions of the skeletal muscles.

specific immunity (or active acquired immunity) Form of acquired immunity that results from production of antibodies in the cells.

specimen Small sample, such as of blood or urine.

speech Uttering of vocal sounds that form words and express thoughts.

spermatogenesis Production of spermatozoa.

sphygmomanometer Device for measuring arterial blood pressure.

spiritual life That aspect of life involving religious beliefs or value systems.

spondylolisthesis Partial forward dislocation of a vertebra over the one below it, most commonly the fifth lumbar vertebra over the first sacral vertebra.

stagnation or self-absorption Regression into adolescent or younger behavior, characterized by physical and psychological invalidism.

stapedectomy Removal of the stapes of the middle ear and insertion of a graft to restore hearing.

stapes One of three tiny ossicles in the middle ear, resembling a stirrup.

stasis Disorder in which the normal flow of a fluid through a vessel of the body is slowed or halted.

statute Legislative act declaring, commanding, or prohibiting something.

sterile Free of germs.

sterilization Destruction of microorganisms using heat, water, chemicals, or gases.

stethoscope Device for listening to heart, vascular, lung, and bowel sounds.

stomatitis Any inflammatory condition of the mouth; may result from drugs used for cancer.

strabismus Cross-eye.

stress Specific response by the body to a stimulus that disturbs normal functioning.

stressor Any factor that causes stress. Common ones include change and loss.

stridor Abnormal, high-pitched, musical respiratory sound caused by an obstruction in the trachea or larynx.

subculture Large group of people who, although members of a still larger cultural group, has shared characteristics exclusive to its subgroup.

subjective data Patient's perceptions and feelings about himself and what is happening to him. Only the patient can give subjective data.

subjective data collection Process in which data relating to the patient's problems are elicited from the patient.

sublingual Beneath the tongue.

subluxation Partial dislocation.

sudoriferous gland One of about 3 million tiny structures within the dermis that produce sweat.

suicide Self-inflicted death.

sulfate (SO_4) Salt of sulfuric acid, which is plentiful in the body.

summons Document issued by a clerk of the court on the filing of a complaint.

supine Position in which the patient lies horizontally on the back.

suppression Cessation of urine production (anuria).

suppuration Production of purulent (puscontaining) matter.

surface tension Tendency of the surface of a liquid to contract; causes liquids to rise in a capillary tube, affects the exchange of gases in the pulmonary alveoli, and alters the ability of various liquids to wet another surface.

surfactant Certain lipoproteins that reduce the surface tension of pulmonary fluids, allowing the exchange of gases in the lungs and contributing to the elasticity of pulmonary tissues

surgery Branch of medicine concerned with diseases and trauma requiring operative procedures.

surgical asepsis Protection against infection by destruction of all microorganisms and their spores or reproductive cells.

suture Surgical stitch taken to repair a tear, incision, or wound.

sweat test Method for evaluating sodium and chloride excretion from the sweat glands; often the first test performed in the diagnosis of cystic fibrosis.

sympathetic nervous system Part of the nervous system that accelerates heart rate, constricts blood vessels, and raises blood pressure.

symptom Subjective indication of a disease or a change in condition as perceived by the patient.

synarthrosis Any one of many immovable joints, such as those of the skull segments, in which a fibrous tissue or a hyaline cartilage connects the bones.

syncope Brief lapse of consciousness; fainting.

syndrome Complex of signs and symptoms.

synovectomy Excision of a synovial membrane of a joint.

syntaxic (consensual) communication Communication in which two people can understand the meaning of their dialogue together, explore and agree on meanings of words used, and speak in cause-effect relationships.

systole Contractions of the heart, driving blood into the aorta and pulmonary arteries; the first heart sound heard on auscultation during the blood pressure procedure.

T-cell A small, circulating lymphocyte that participates in cellular immune responses, such as graft rejection and delayed hypersensitivity.

tachycardia Abnormally rapid heart rate of more than 100 beats per minute.

tachypnea Abnormal rate of breathing, greater than 26 breaths per minute.

tactile fremitus Tremulous vibrations of the chest wall felt on palpation.

TBI Traumatic brain injury.

tendon One of many white, glistening, fibrous bands of tissue that attach muscle to bone.

tenesmus Persistent, ineffectual spasms of the rectum or bladder, accompanied by the desire to empty the bowel or bladder.

TENS See *transcutaneous electrical nerve stimulation.*

tepid Moderately warm to the touch.

teratogenic Any substance, agent, or product that interferes with normal prenatal development, causing the formation of one or more developmental abnormalities in the fetus.

testosterone Male hormone that contributes to development of male characteristics.

tetanus toxoid Active agent prepared from detoxified tetanus toxin that produces an antigenic response in the body, conferring permanent immunity to tetanus infection.

tetany Condition characterized by cramps, muscle twitching, and possibli convulsions.

therapeutic Beneficial, such as a dose of medication that produces a helpful effect.

therapeutic communication Process in which a nurse helps the patient to a better understanding through verbal or nonverbal communication.

third-party-payers Entities other than the giver or receiver of the service responsible for payment, e.g., Medicare or insurance companies.

thoracic cord injury Spinal injury that usually involves partial trunk and lower extremity paralysis.

thrill Fine vibration felt by the examiner, indicating an organic murmur.

thrombocytes (platelets) Smallest cells in the blood. They are disk-shaped, contain no hemoglobin, and are essential for clotting of the blood.

thrombophlebitis Inflammation of a vein that often accompanies formation of a clot.

thrombus Accumulation of platelets, fibrin, clotting factors, and the cellular elements of blood, attached to the interior wall of a vein or artery and sometimes occluding the lumen.

thymus gland Located in the mediastinum, the primary gland of the lymphatic system.

thyroid gland Highly vascular organ at the front of the neck; secretes thryoxin.

tibia Second longest bone in the skeleton, located at the medial side of the leg. It articulates with the fibula laterally, the talus distally, and the femur proximally, forming part of the knee joint.

tinnitus Tingling or ringing in one or both ears.

tissue Collection of similar cells that act together in the performance of a particular function.

TMJ Temporomandibular joint.

toddler Ages 1 to 3 years.

tolerance Ability to consume ordinarily injurious quantities of such substances as drugs or alcohol without apparent physiological or psychological injury.

tongue depressor Wooden blade used to facilitate examination of the throat.

tonus(ic) Normal state of balanced tension in the tissues of the body, especially the muscles.

tophus Abnormal stone, containing sodium urate deposits, that develops in periarticular fibrous tissue, typically in patients with gout.

tort Civil wrong, other than a breach of contract.

total parenteral nutrition (TPN) Administration of a nutritionally complete solution through a central vein.

toxicity Degree to which something is poisonous.

tracheotomy Incision made into the trachea through the neck below the larynx, performed to gain access to the airway below blockage with a foreign body, tumor, or edema of the glottis.

tract In neurology, the neuronal axons grouped together to form a pathway.

traction Having a limb, bone, or group of muscles under tension with weights and pulleys; aligns or immobilizes the part and relieves pressure on it.

traditional or block chart Conventional patient chart broken down into sections or blocks; included are admission data, physicians' orders, history and physical, nursing care plan, nurses' notes and graphics, progress notes, and test data.

transcribing Making a copy of, in longhand or on a typewriter.

transcutaneous electrical neural stimulation (TENS) Alteration of pain sensations by stimulating peripheral nerves; uses application of electric current to the skin.

transfer Moving a patient from one unit to another within an institution or moving a patient from one health care facility to another.

transformation Shift from one state to another, such as water to ice to vapor.

transient ischemic attack (TIA) Episode of cerebrovascular insufficiency, usually owing to partial occlusion of an artery by an atherosclerotic plaque or embolism.

trauma Physical injury caused by violent/disruptive action.

trichomoniasis Vaginal infection caused by the protozoan *Trichomonas vaginalis.*

trophic Having to do with nutritional status.

Trousseau's sign Test for latent tetany, in which carpal spasm is induced with a sphygmomanometer cuff on the upper arm.

trust Risk-taking process whereby an individual's situation depends on the future behavior of another person.

tube feeding Administration of nutritionally balanced, liquified foods or formula into the stomach, duodenum, or jejunum by way of a nasoenteric tube or a feeding ostomy.

turgor Normal resiliency of the skin caused by outward pressure of cells and interstitial fluid. Decreased turgor indicates dehydration; increased turgor indicates edema.

tylectomy Partial mastectomy/lympectomy; the removal of involved breast tissue (about one fourth or one third of the breast), preserving contour and muscle function.

tympanic membrane Thin, semitransparent membrane in the middle ear that transmits sound vibrations.

tympanoplasty Surgical procedure performed on the eardrum to restore or improve hearing in patients with conductive deafness.

tympanostomy tube Tubes inserted under general anesthesia to drain accumulated fluid from the middle ear space; also called *pressure equalizer (PE) tubes.*

Type I diabetes mellitus insulin-dependent diabetes mellitus.

Type II diabetes mellitus non-insulin-dependent diabetes mellitus.

umbilical cord Bluish-white, gelatinous structure that transports maternal blood from the placenta to fetus.

umbilicus Point on the abdomen at which the umbilical cord joined the fetus. In most adults it is marked by a depression.

universal donor Person with type O, Rh factor–negative blood. Such blood may be used for emergency transfusion with minimal risk of incompatibility.

Universal Precautions CDC-recommended "universal blood and body fluid precautions" (prevent injury from needles and sharps; wear protective devices during resuscitation; avoid patient and equipment contact if draining lesion exists in health care worker).

urate Any salt of uric acid, as sodium urate.

ureter One of a pair of tubes that carry urine from the kidney to the bladder.

urinal Metal or plastic receptacle for urine—may be designed for male or female patients.

urolithiasis Calculus (stone) formed in any part of the urinary tract.

urticaria Itching skin eruption characterized by welts of varying sizes with well-defined, inflamed margins and pale centers (also called *hives*).

value system Accepted mode of conduct and set of norms, goals, and values binding any social group.

values Personal beliefs about the worth of an idea or behavior.

valve Combining form meaning *a thing that regulates the flow of.*

vegan Vegetarian whose diet excludes all foods of animal origin.

vehicle Fluid or structure in the body that passively conveys a stimulus.

vein One of many vessels that convey blood from the capillaries to the heart as part of the pulmonary system.

vena cava One of the two large veins returning blood from peripheral circulation to the right atrium of the heart.

ventilator Person in two-rescuer CPR who performs rescue breathing technique.

ventricle Small cavity, such as the one filled with cerebrospinal fluid in the brain, or the right and left ventricles of the heart.

venule Any one of the small blood vessels that gather blood from the capillary plexuses and anastomose to form the veins.

vertigo Dizziness; a sensation of faintness or an inability to maintain normal balance in a standing or seated position.

vesicle Small, thin-walled, raised skin lesion containing clear fluid; a blister.

viable Capable of developing, growing, and otherwise sustaining life.

virulence Power of a microorganism to produce disease.

viscus Internal organs within a body cavity, primarily the abdominal organs.

visual analog scale Rating scale using a line to represent a continuum. The ends are marked for two extremes of pain.

vital signs Measurements of temperature, pulse, respiration, and blood pressure.

vitamin Organic compound essential in small quantities for normal physiological and metabolic functioning of the body.

vitreous humor Transparent, semigelatinous substance filling the cavity behind the crystalline lens of the eye.

vomer Bone forming the posterior and inferior part of the nasal septum, having two surfaces and four borders.

weaning (1) Gradually eliminating breast or bottle feeding, replaced by cup and table feeding. (2) Withdrawing a person from something on which he is dependent.

wellness Dynamic state of health in which an individual progresses toward a higher level of functioning, achieving an optimum balance between internal and external environments.

Wernicke's encephalopathy Inflammatory, hemorrhagic, degenerative condition of the brain caused by thiamine deficiency, seen in association with chronic alcoholism.

wheal Elevated lesion; an individual lesion of urticaria.

whirlpool bath Immersion of the body or part of the body in a tank of hot water agitated by a jet of equally hot water and air.

white matter Tissue surrounding the gray matter of the spinal cord, consisting mainly of myelinated nerve fibers but with some unmyelinated nerve fibers, embedded in a spongy network of neuroglia.

widow(er)hood Status of the surviving spouse after the death of husband or wife.

Wilms' tumor Malignant neoplasm of the kidney, occuring in young children. The tumor, an embryonal adenomyosarcoma, is well encapsulated in the early stage, but may later extend into the lymph nodes and the renal vein or vena cava and metastasize to the lungs or other sites.

withdrawal symptoms Unpleasant, sometimes life-threatening, physiological changes that occur when certain drugs are withdrawn after prolonged, regular use.

wound Any physical injury involving a break in the skin; caused by an act or accident rather than by a disease.

xerostomia Dryness of the mouth caused by cessation of normal salivation.

xiphoid process Small, fragile bone located at the distal end of the sternum.

young adulthood Chronologically a period of life from the mid-20s to the mid-40s.

Index

D

J

Q

R

S

COMMON ABBREVIATIONS

° C	degrees Centigrade
° F	degrees Fahrenheit
ʒ	dram
@	at
♀	female
♂	male
>	greater than
<	less than
↑	increase
↓	decrease
1°	primary
2°	secondary
△	change
aa	of each
ABG	arterial blood gas
ac	before meals
ad lib	freely as desired
ADL	activities of daily living
a.m.a.	against medical advice
BE	barium enema
bid	two times a day
BP	blood pressure
BRP	bathroom privileges
BUN	blood urea nitrogen
c̄	with
c/o	complains of
cap	capsule
CBC	complete blood count
cc	cubic centimeter
CDC	Centers for Disease Control
cm	centimeter
CO	carbon monoxide
CO_2	carbon dioxide
CPR	cardiopulmonary resuscitation
CT	computed tomography
D_5W	5% dextrose in water

dl	deciliter
DNR	do not resuscitate
dx, Dx	diagnosis
ECG, EKG	electrocardiogram
EEG	electroencephalogram
elix	elixer
ER	emergency room
ESR	erythrocyte sedimentation rate
ETOH	ethyl alcohol
f℥	fluid ounce
FUO	fever of unknown origin
Fx, fx	fracture, fractional urine test
g, gm, Gm	gram
GI	gastrointestinal
gr	grain
gt, gtt	drop, drops
GTT	glucose tolerance test
h	hour
H&P	history and physical examination
Hct, HCT	hematocrit
Hgb	hemoglobin
HIV	human immunodeficiency virus (AIDS)
hs	at bedtime
I&O	intake and output
IDDM	insulin-dependent diabetes mellitus
IM	intramuscular
IV	intravenous
IVP	intravenous push; intravenous pyelogram
IVU	intravenous urogram
K	potassium
kg	kilogram
KUB	kidney, ureters, and bladder (radiograph)
KVO	keep vein open
L	liter
m	meter
m, min, ♏	minum

mcg	microgram
mg	milligram
ml	milliliter
mm	millimeter
mm Hg	millimeters of mercury
MRI	magnetic resonance imaging
O_2	oxygen
OD	right eye; optical density; overdose
OS	left eye
OZ, ℥	ounce
pc	after meals
PERRLA	pupils equal, round, and reactive to light and accommodation
pH	hydrogen ion concentration (acidity and alkalinity)
PO, po	orally
p.r.n.	when required, as often as necessary
q	every
qd	every day
qh	every hour
qid	four times a day
qod	every other day
ROM	range of motion
Rx	take; treatment
s̄	without
sos	if necessary
SQ, subq, SC	subcutaneous
ss	half
SSE	soapsuds enema
stat	immediately
tid	three times a day
TLC	tender loving care
TKO	to keep open
TPR	temperature, pulse, and respirations
WBC	white blood cell, white blood count

NURSING CARE PLANS